Practical Pediatric Imaging

Diagnostic Radiology of Infants and Children

Third Edition

Practical Pediatric Imaging
Diagnostic Radiology of Infants and Children
Third Edition

EDITOR

DONALD R. KIRKS, M.D.

Chairman, Department of Radiology
Radiologist-in-Chief, Children's Hospital
John A. Kirkpatrick Professor of Radiology
Harvard Medical School
Boston, Massachusetts

ASSOCIATE EDITOR

N. THORNE GRISCOM, M.D.

Department of Radiology
Children's Hospital
Professor of Radiology
Harvard Medical School
Boston, Massachusetts

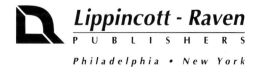
Lippincott - Raven
PUBLISHERS
Philadelphia • New York

Acquisitions Editor: James D. Ryan
Developmental Editor: Brian Brown
Manufacturing Manager: Dennis Teston
Production Manager: Jodi Borgenicht
Production Editor: Raeann Touhey
Cover Designer: Patricia Gast
Indexer: Kathy Pitcoff
Compositor: Maryland Composition
Printer: Quebecor Kingsport

Printed in the United States of America

9 8 7 6 5 4 3 2 1

Library of Congress Cataloging-in-Publication Data
Practical pediatric imaging : diagnostic radiology of infants and
   children / editor, Donald R. Kirks ; associate editor, N. Thorne
Griscom.—3rd ed.
      p.   cm.
   Includes bibliographical references and index.
   ISBN 0-316-49473-9
   1. Diagnosis, radiologic.   2. Children—Diseases—Diagnosis.
3. Pediatric radiology.   4. Pediatric diagnostic imaging.
I. Kirks, Donald R.   II. Griscom, N. Thorne
   [DNLM: 1. Diagnostic Imaging—in infancy & childhood.   WN 240
P8945   1997]
RJ51.R3P725   1998
618.92′00754—DC21
DNLM/DLC
for Library of Congress

To the memory of my parents, Cornelia and Raymond Kirks.
They opened the doors.

To the inspiration of my mentor, role model, and closest personal friend, Derek Harwood-Nash.
His spirit of giving, love of teaching, and commitment to
excellence will always be remembered.

To my wonderful and devoted wife, Jan, with love.
You provide advice, support, and encouragement.

To our children, John and Julie, and their spouses, Kathleen and Derek.
Your father loves you.

Contents

Contributing Authors

William S. Ball, Jr., M.D.   *Chief, Section of Neuroradiology, Department of Radiology, Children's Hospital Medical Center; Professor of Radiology and Pediatrics, University of Cincinnati College of Medicine, Cincinnati, Ohio.*

Patrick D. Barnes, M.D.   *Chief, Division of Neuroradiology, Department of Radiology, Children's Hospital; Associate Professor of Radiology, Harvard Medical School, Boston, Massachusetts.*

Carol E. Barnewolt, M.D.   *Department of Radiology, Children's Hospital; Instructor in Radiology, Harvard Medical School, Boston, Massachusetts.*

George S. Bisset III, M.D.   *Vice-Chairman, Department of Radiology, Duke University Medical Center; Professor of Radiology and Pediatrics, Duke University School of Medicine, Durham, North Carolina.*

Carlo Buonomo, M.D.   *Department of Radiology, Children's Hospital; Assistant Professor of Clinical Radiology, Harvard Medical School, Boston, Massachusetts.*

Patricia E. Burrows, M.D.   *Chief, Division of Cardiovascular/Interventional Radiology, Department of Radiology, Children's Hospital; Professor of Radiology, Harvard Medical School, Boston, Massachusetts.*

Taylor Chung, M.D.   *Department of Radiology, Children's Hospital; Instructor in Radiology, Harvard Medical School, Boston, Massachusetts.*

Robert H. Cleveland, M.D.   *Department of Radiology, Children's Hospital; Associate Professor of Radiology, Harvard Medical School, Boston, Massachusetts.*

Leonard P. Connolly, M.D.   *Division of Nuclear Medicine, Department of Radiology, Children's Hospital; Assistant Professor of Clinical Radiology, Harvard Medical School, Boston, Massachusetts.*

N. Thorne Griscom, M.D.   *Department of Radiology, Children's Hospital; Professor of Radiology, Harvard Medical School, Boston, Massachusetts.*

Gary L. Hedlund, D.O.   *Department of Pediatric Imaging, The Children's Hospital; Clinical Associate Professor of Radiology, University of Alabama at Birmingham, Birmingham, Alabama.*

Fredric A. Hoffer, M.D.   *Director, Body MRI, Department of Diagnostic Imaging, St. Jude Children's Research Hospital; Associate Professor of Radiology, University of Tennessee at Memphis, Memphis, Tennessee.*

Diego Jaramillo, M.D.   *Chief, Section of Body CT/MRI, Department of Radiology, Children's Hospital; Associate Professor of Radiology, Harvard Medical School, Boston, Massachusetts.*

Francine M. Kim, M.D.   *Department of Radiology, LeBonheur Children's Medical Center; Assistant Professor of Radiology, University of Tennessee at Memphis, Memphis, Tennessee.*

Donald R. Kirks, M.D.   *Chairman, Department of Radiology, Radiologist-in-Chief, Children's Hospital; John A. Kirkpatrick Professor of Radiology, Harvard Medical School, Boston, Massachusetts.*

Tal Laor, M.D. *Department of Radiology, Children's Hospital; Assistant Professor of Radiology, Harvard Medical School, Boston, Massachusetts.*

Robert L. Lebowitz, M.D. *Chief, Division of Diagnostic Radiology, Department of Radiology, Children's Hospital; Professor of Radiology, Harvard Medical School, Boston, Massachusetts.*

Alan E. Oestreich, M.D. *Department of Radiology, Children's Hospital Medical Center; Professor of Radiology and Pediatrics, University of Cincinnati College of Medicine, Cincinnati, Ohio.*

Harriet J. Paltiel, M.D. *Department of Radiology, Children's Hospital; Assistant Professor of Radiology, Harvard Medical School, Boston, Massachusetts.*

Tina Young Poussaint, M.D. *Division of Neuroradiology, Department of Radiology, Children's Hospital; Instructor in Radiology, Harvard Medical School, Boston, Massachusetts.*

Richard L. Robertson, M.D. *Division of Neuroradiology, Department of Radiology, Children's Hospital; Instructor in Radiology, Harvard Medical School, Boston, Massachusetts.*

Caroline D. Robson, M.B., Ch.B. *Division of Neuroradiology, Department of Radiology, Children's Hospital; Instructor in Radiology, Harvard Medical School, Boston, Massachusetts.*

Jane C. Share, M.D. *Chief, Section of Ultrasonography, Department of Radiology, Children's Hospital; Assistant Professor of Radiology, Harvard Medical School, Boston, Massachusetts.*

Janet L. Strife, M.D. *Radiologist-in-Chief, Children's Hospital Medical Center; Professor of Radiology and Pediatrics, University of Cincinnati College of Medicine, Cincinnati, Ohio.*

George A. Taylor, M.D. *Chief, Division of Body Imaging, Department of Radiology, Children's Hospital; Professor of Radiology and Pediatrics, Harvard Medical School, Boston, Massachusetts.*

S. Ted Treves, M.D. *Chief, Division of Nuclear Medicine, Department of Radiology, Children's Hospital; Professor of Radiology, Harvard Medical School, Boston, Massachusetts.*

Introduction to the Foreword

"There is a tide in the affairs of men,
Which, taken at the flood, leads on to fortune;"

William Shakespeare
Julius Caesar

This was one of Derek Harwood-Nash's favorite quotations. With his unexpected death, the world of radiology lost one of its most charismatic, influential, dynamic, and effective leaders. Because of his professional success and academic productivity, radiology, pediatric radiology, and neuroradiology are forever positively changed! His "flood of fortune" touched the minds and hearts of many students, colleagues, and friends around the world. Derek was a clinician, a scientist, a teacher, a mentor, a role model, an academic leader, and my closest personal friend. He was one of the most sensitive and caring people that I have ever known; Derek was one of those rare individuals who would much rather give than receive. In dedicating this textbook to him, I remember and celebrate the tide that was the life of Derek Harwood-Nash and the flood of fortune that came to him. This flood of fortune was shared with all of radiology; we are better for having known him!

Derek had agreed to write the foreword to the revised edition of this textbook. We had discussed the significant changes and increased content of the new edition. I have included the foreword that he wrote for the Second Edition of *Practical Pediatric Imaging: Diagnostic Radiology of Infants and Children*.

The medical care of infants and children throughout the world has been improved and enriched by Derek's many contributions. His remarkable life and career have influenced and enhanced the lives of his students, professional colleagues, and many radiology friends. Our challenge is to continue the flood tide of Derek Harwood-Nash. Never forget his pursuit of excellence and his love of teaching. Emulate his spirit of giving as we care for our patients, enjoy our friends, and love our families.

Derek, no one did it better! There is a tide. . .

Donald R. Kirks, M.D.

Foreword to the Second Edition

Success is but a journey, not a destination. The Second Edition of *Practical Pediatric Imaging: Diagnostic Radiology of Infants and Children* is yet another milestone, another crossroad, another panorama stretching out to the horizon of today. Today, diagnostic imaging of the infant and child is a mature, innovative, and, above all, quintessential component of the care of the sick child. Pediatric diagnostic imaging has successfully embraced its burgeoning new procedures together with both dramatic and subtle improvements and refinements in its classic techniques. Pediatric imaging is now a recognized specialty and for many a lifelong odyssey. The Society for Pediatric Radiology in North America is the oldest specialty organization within radiology.

What lies over the horizon is not certain. What is certain is that we have a suitable passport for the next stage of the journey, with a major road map and traveler's guide for pediatric imaging, all contained in this most significant new edition by Dr. Donald R. Kirks and his associates at Children's Hospital Medical Center in Cincinnati.

One definition of a split second could be the interval between the completion of one edition of a textbook and the immediate requests, perchance demands, for the next. This is only matched in passion by the dismay felt by one's spouse, family, and secretary.

This second edition is both timely and expert. The great distinction of and personal pride in contributing a foreword to a book such as this is matched by the opportunity for an extensive preview of its contents. The quality of the contributors to *Practical Pediatric Imaging,* prominent pediatric radiologists all, is of the highest order and will be evident to any reader. Single authorship of general textbooks is surely now beyond the skills and energy of even the most talented. The success, style, and significance of Dr. Kirks's first edition, of which he was the sole author, has provided both stimulus and template for the second.

Our own residents and fellows at the Hospital for Sick Children in Toronto considered the first edition a premier general textbook on pediatric imaging, appropriate for day-to-day use. Our faculty considered it a useful reminder in each's organ system interests and an essential source of additional information for other systems and for facts long forgotten or not yet appreciated. The second edition will surely continue in tune with the first. Of particular attraction to me in the new edition are the original and adapted techniques of clinical penmanship: the imaging triage; the comprehensive lists but with perspective; the heading of each illustration's legend; the presentation of both the general and the particular; and the practical, subdivided reference lists at the end of each chapter. This edition was not intended to be an encyclopedic reference book, but rather a constant and readily available practical source of knowledge and diagnostic direction for trainees, for general radiologists whose prime persuasion is not pediatric imaging, and in particular for those who have no immediate access to a pediatric radiologist. There are now not enough fully trained pediatric radiologists to serve all demands everywhere. *Practical Pediatric Imaging,* Second Edition, will in large part serve as a counterbalance.

Plato, in *The Republic,* stated that those who have torches will pass them on to others. Dr. Kirks, a leader, a teacher, and a clinician with remarkable expertise and energy, together with his colleagues from a premier department, has done just that. The journey continues, as does the success.

And now another split second, and hopefully then . . .

Derek C. Harwood-Nash

xiii

Preface

"If we want things to stay as they are, things will have to change."

Giuseppe di Lampedusa
The Leopard

It has been said that one must know the past and understand the present in order to predict the future. The first clinical x-ray obtained in America was of Eddie McCarthy, a 14-year-old boy from Hanover, who fell and injured his left wrist while skating on the Connecticut River (1). Two weeks later on Monday, February, 3, 1896, and just over two months after Roentgen's momentous discovery, Professor Edwin B. Frost at Dartmouth College performed an x-ray of the boy's injured left wrist. The image, made with a 20-minute exposure, was felt to show an ulnar fracture. Motion artifact significantly degrades the gelatin-plate image (1). We know that there had to be an associated radial fracture (2).

Pediatric radiology is the oldest of the diagnostic radiology subspecialties (3). It started in the early 1900s, when departments of radiology were organized in children's hospitals (4). The Society for Pediatric Radiology (SPR), the oldest subspecialty organization in diagnostic radiology, was founded in 1958; it has continued to grow during the subsequent 40 years. However, the oldest of the radiologic subspecialties had "growing pains" (5). Pediatric radiology primarily consisted of conventional radiography and fluoroscopy into the 1980s, with most pediatric imaging and vascular/interventional procedures being performed by adult radiologists. The pediatric radiologist of the late 1990s is trained to perform and interpret all imaging procedures for the diagnosis and treatment of diseases of infants and children. Because of the increasing centralization of pediatric health care and the development of effective sedation and monitoring programs, pediatric radiology is now a microcosm of adult radiology; it includes conventional radiology, fluoroscopy, ultrasonography (US), computed tomography (CT), magnetic resonance imaging (MRI), nuclear medicine (NM), and vascular/interventional (V/I) procedures. During this decade, pediatric radiology has become pediatric imaging; the oldest subspecialty of diagnostic radiology has finally "come of age" (6).

Children's Hospital, Boston is the largest pediatric medical center in the United States; there are over 325,000 ambulatory and emergency visits, 19,000 hospital admissions, 17,000 surgical procedures, and 119,000 radiologic examinations per year. The increased centralization of pediatric health care has led to a modest increase in the volume of conventional pediatric radiologic examinations but a dramatic growth in the number of time-intensive and physician-intensive pediatric imaging studies and interventional procedures. Current annual volumes in our department are as follows: conventional radiology, 88,000; US, 10,500; NM, 4,000; CT, 8,800; MRI, 6,700; V/I procedures, 1,800.

Pediatric radiology is much more than an age-related, service-oriented subspecialty that involves only patient care (6). In order for the subspecialty to continue to mature as an academic discipline, we must continue to advance the science of pediatric radiology through clinical, translational (experimental to clinical practice), and health services (technology assessment, utilization management, appropriateness criteria, practice guidelines, patient access, cost-effectiveness, outcomes) research. Training of future pediatric radiologists must be in an academic environment that emphasizes critical thinking, careful analysis, and scientific inquiry. It is imperative that we collaborate with clinical and basic researchers to train a cadre of pediatric radiology investigators both skilled in and familiar with investigative techniques. We must study not only clinical applications of pediatric imaging but also fundamental mechanisms of disease and innovative methods of preventive medicine.

There have been many changes in the Third Edition of *Practical Pediatric Imaging: Diagnostic Radiology of Infants and Children.* Several contributors to the Second Edition with whom I had worked at Children's Hospital Medical Center, Cincinnati agreed to participate in this revision. The authorship has been significantly expanded to include faculty of the Department of Radiology, Children's Hospital, Boston. The contributing authors used the Second Edition as a framework for extensive revisions, additions, and deletions. The discussion and illustrations have been expanded and modified to reflect more accurately the current practice of pediatric imaging. Although conventional radiography and fluoroscopy remain the cornerstones of pediatric radiology, there are increasing applications of US, NM, CT, MRI, and V/I techniques for the diagnosis and treatment of pediatric disease. The reference list of each chapter has been significantly updated. A separate chapter on head and neck imaging was added because of its increased clinical importance. Finally, in an effort to retain continuity of style. Thorne Griscom and I have edited the revised manuscript in its entirety.

Despite extensive changes in text, tables, illustrations, and references, the purpose of this edition is the same as the First and Second Editions—to provide an overview of pediatric radiology for trainees in diagnostic radiology and pediatric radiology, general diagnostic radiologists, medical students, pediatric residents, and pediatric physicians in medical as well as surgical subspecialties. Although all aspects of pediatric radiology are not covered in this text, imaging of more common pediatric diseases is discussed and illustrated. It is our hope that the reader, regardless of the level of training or knowledge, will be stimulated to learn more about pediatric diseases and pediatric imaging. If this textbook helps the reader to better understand pediatric radiology and thus, improves the quality of health care of infants and children, we will have accomplished our goal.

> *"When I look upon a child,*
> *I am filled with admiration for that child,*
> *not so much for what it is today,*
> *as for what it might become."*
>
> Louis Pasteur

Donald R. Kirks, M.D.

REFERENCES

1. Spiegel PK. The first clinical x-ray made in America—100 years. *AJR* 1995;164:241–243.
2. Stansberry SD, Swischuk LE, Swischuk JL, Midgett TA. Significance of ulnar styloid fractures in childhood. *Ped Emerg Care* 1990;6:99–103.
3. Kirks DR. The Society for Pediatric Radiology: 30 years later. *AJR* 1988;151:151–152.
4. Griscom NT. Pediatric radiology in North America. In: Gagliardi R, Krabbenhoft K, McClennan B, eds. *A history of the radiologic sciences: diagnosis.* Reston, VA: Radiology Centennial, Inc. 1996, 345–368.
5. Kirks DR. Academic pediatric radiology: best of times; worst of times. *Invest Radiology* 1988;23:540.
6. Kirks DR. Pediatric radiology: flexibility, viability, credibility, and opportunity. *Radiology* 1993;187:311–312.

Preface To the Second Edition

"All is flux, nothing stays still.
Nothing endures but change."

Heraclitus
c. 540–480 B.C.

What changes have been made in the Second Edition of *Practical Pediatric Imaging: Diagnostic Radiology of Infants and Children?* First, the authorship has been expanded to include faculty of the Department of Radiology, Children's Hospital Medical Center, Cincinnati (CHMC). The contributors used the first edition of the text as a framework for extensive revisions. Second, both text and illustrations have been expanded and modified to reflect the current practice of pediatric imaging. To retain continuity of style, I have edited the revised manuscript in its entirety.

Conventional radiography and fluoroscopy remain the cornerstones of pediatric radiology; however, the transition from pediatric radiology to pediatric imaging is reflected in the greater use of ultrasonography, nuclear medicine, computed tomography, magnetic resonance imaging, and vascular/interventional techniques for the diagnosis and treatment of pediatric disease.

The first edition of this textbook was written in the early 1980s. Pediatric radiology was just advancing beyond plain films and contrast studies. Although subspecialization in diagnostic radiology began with age-related pediatric radiology in children's hospitals in the early 1900s, pediatric radiology did not make its transition to pediatric imaging until the late 1980s.

The change from pediatric radiology to pediatric imaging was brought about by greater centralization of pediatric health care; there has been regionalization and consolidation of pediatric beds in children's, university, and community hospitals. As a result, the severity of illness of hospitalized pediatric patients has increased dramatically. This tertiary care of infants and children requires sophisticated diagnostic and therapeutic procedures as well as radiologic consultation with pediatric physicians in various subspecialty disciplines. Moreover, safe pediatric sedation programs have been developed that require meticulous physiologic monitoring and excellent radiology nursing care. The pediatric radiologist is now able to evaluate complex disease processes, apply the newest technologies, develop integrated evaluations, and perform aggressive therapeutic intervention. At the beginning of the 1990s, pediatric radiology has become a microcosm of adult diagnostic radiology. Pediatric radiology has finally come of age!

CHMC is the largest pediatric institution in the United States, with 355 patient beds; there are more than 275,000 ambulatory and emergency visits, 18,000 hospital admissions, 16,000 surgical procedures, and 105,000 radiographic examinations per year. An analysis of the types and volume of examinations performed in the Department of Radiology emphasizes the increased complexity of pediatric imaging: conventional radiology, 87,000; ultrasonography, 7,500; nuclear medicine, 3,500; computed tomography, 3,800; magnetic resonance imaging, 2,400; vascular/interventional procedures, 1,000.

The purpose of this textbook is to provide an overview of pediatric imaging. The material is directed primarily to trainees in diagnostic radiology, but also to general diagnostic radiologists, medical students, pediatric residents, and pediatric physicians in medical as well as surgical subspecialties. Although the entire subspeciality of pediatric radiology is not covered in this text, imaging of more common pediatric diseases is discussed and illustrated. It is hoped that the reader, regardless of level of training or knowledge, will be stimulated to ask questions and to learn more about pediatric disease and pediatric imaging. If the information in this book answers some of these questions and somehow improves the quality of pediatric health care, our goal will have been accomplished.

> *"If you ask me a question that I don't know, I won't answer."*

Yogi (Lawrence Peter) Berra
Attributed

Donald R. Kirks, M.D.

Preface to the First Edition

"Many men are stored full of unused knowledge. Like loaded guns that are never fired off, or military magazines in times of peace, they are stuffed with useless ammunition."

Henry Ward Beecher
Proverbs from Plymouth Pulpit
1887

Why write another textbook of pediatric radiology? Although there are numerous textbooks of radiology, organ imaging, and modality applications in infants and children, a practical overview of pediatric diagnostic imaging, including newer modalities, is not currently available. I hope that this textbook will fill a void in pediatric radiology.

This text grew out of a series of introductory lectures given to residents in both radiology and pediatrics at the three institutions where I have worked. Several residents noted that this practical information was not readily available for review and suggested that the material be expanded and organized into textbook format.

Pediatric radiology includes the application of all modalities (conventional radiography, ultrasonography, nuclear medicine, computed tomography, angiography, interventional techniques, nuclear magnetic resonance) to the diagnosis of diseases of infants and children. I have divided this text into eight chapters: one on techniques, since these are unique in children; the other seven by traditional organ systems. The role and application of newer imaging modalities are discussed and illustrated throughout the book.

Each chapter is divided into general abnormalities with differential diagnoses and common specific disease entities with important radiologic features. I have made liberal use of tables, line drawings, and figures in order to discuss and illustrate differential diagnostic considerations as well as the radiology of common pediatric diseases. Algorithms and personal imaging approaches are included when appropriate. References at the end of each chapter are grouped by general category or specific abnormality. Appendices for preparation, technique, and radiation exposure are included at the end of the book.

The material in this textbook is directed to four potential audiences. First, trainees in diagnostic radiology should be able to read through the entire text during the three or four months of pediatric radiology in their residency. Second, radiologists may find some information helpful when evaluating children in their daily practices. It should be stressed that at least 90 percent of all pediatric imaging is superbly performed by general radiologists. Third, pediatricians, pediatric residents, and medical students should find the tables of differential diagnoses and discussions of common radiologic abnormalities helpful in broadening their understanding of pediatric diseases. Finally, pediatric physicians in various medical and surgical subspecialties may need a practical radiologic approach, including newer imaging modalities, to common abnormalities of infants and children. I hope that the reader, regardless of individual interest, will be stimulated to question and to learn more about pediatric disease in general and pediatric imaging in particular.

"The greater our knowledge increases, the greater our ignorance unfolds."

John F. Kennedy
Address, Rice University
Houston, Texas
September 12, 1962

Acknowledgments

"I want to thank everyone who made this Yogi Berra Day necessary."

Yogi (Lawrence Peter) Berra
Yogi Berra Appreciation Day
Yankee Stadium, Bronx, New York
September 1963

This textbook could not have been written without the teaching, stimulation, encouragement, and help of many mentors, colleagues, fellows, residents, and radiologic technologists.

I trained in diagnostic radiology at the University of California, San Francisco Medical Center. Clinical radiology, teaching, and research were stressed in that excellent academic department under the chairmanship of Alexander R. Margulis. Mentors who particularly influenced me during my more malleable years of radiology training were Hideyo Minagi, Richard Greenspan, and John Amberg. Hideyo remains a confidante, role model, and close personal and family friend.

I have trained and worked with three of the finest pediatric radiologists in the world. Hooshang Taybi showed me how much there is to learn in the subspecialty of pediatric radiology. Guido Currarino is a brilliant clinical radiologist and academician; his clinical acumen, depth and breadth of knowledge, professional dedication, and academic determination are unparalleled. This textbook is dedicated to Derek Harwood-Nash who stressed excellence in patient care, teaching, writing, and research. He was a mentor and constant source of inspiration and encouragement.

The residents in both radiology and pediatrics at Brooke Army Medical Center; Children's Hospital Medical Center in Oakland; Children's Medical Center in Dallas; Duke University Medical Center; Children's Hospital Medical Center (CHMC), Cincinnati; and Children's Hospital, Boston (CH,B), have always shared interesting cases, sought my opinions, expressed their thanks for my teaching efforts, and stimulated me to learn more about pediatric disease and pediatric imaging.

I am indebted to many clinical colleagues at CH,B. Numerous pediatric physicians—Michael Scott, Peter Black, Joe Volpe, Gerry Healy, Jim Kasser, John Emans, Jim Lock, John Mayer, Richard Jonas, Mary Ellen Wohl, Alan Leichtner, Alan Retik, Bill Harmon, Gary Fleisher, Hardy Hendren, Holcombe Grier, Phil Pizzo, Fred Lovejoy, and Paul Hickey—have supported my efforts to build a strong clinical and academic pediatric radiology department. Many of them have also sought my radiologic opinions and challenged my traditional thinking about pediatric imaging.

I am fortunate to work in one of the greatest pediatric institutions in the world. CH,B has a long tradition of excellence in pediatric patient care, education, and research. There has been a strong institutional commitment to and support of the Department of Radiology under the leadership of Ed Neuhauser, John Kirkpatrick, and myself. The Board of Trustees and the President of CH,B, David S. Weiner, maintain a positive atmosphere that is conducive to excellence of clinical care and academic pursuits.

The Department of Radiology at CH,B has an outstanding faculty of pediatric radiologists. Several authors from the Second Edition also contributed to this textbook. Contributors expanded and completely revised the Second Edition; the result is an overview of pediatric radiology in the late 1990s. My special thanks to Thorne Griscom for his excellent editorial assistance. His thoughtful comments and insistence on clarity of style and succinctness of presentation are greatly appreciated.

I acknowledge the many excellent fellows who trained in pediatric radiology during my six years at CHMC and six years at CH,B. In chronological order from 1986, these fellows are Alan Brody, Ed Burton, Beth Ey, Dick Patterson, Phil Stalker, Sam Auringer, Kathy Garrett, Gary Hedlund, Paula Shultz, Jane Matsumoto, Bill Shiels, Jeff Foster, Beth Hingsbergen, Connie Maves, Marcie Piccolello, Keith White,

Antonio Souza, Eli Vazquez, Bill Beckett, Dave Frankel, Don Frush, Jodie Cressman, Jeff Jacobson, Beth Kline, Bernadette Koch, Ron Pobiel, Janice Allison, Brad Betz, Vesna Kriss, Susan Connolly, Vickie Gylys-Morin, Connie Kaminsky, Tal Laor, Carol Barnewolt, Greg Bates, Heather Bray, Taylor Chung, Lynn Fordham, Yves Patenaude, Kimberly Applegate, Mike D'Alessandro, Lisa Martin, David Wilkes, Tim Bonsack, Jerry Dwek, Ed Lebowitz, Terri Vaccaro, David Bloom, Kirsten Ecklund, Janice Gallant, Francine Kim, Callie Robson, Santiago Medina, Cynthia Christoph, Carol Hankins, Brent Adler, Kathleen Buckley, John Januario, Ariane Neish, Steve O'Connor, Jim Carrico, Caroline Carrico, Kee Chung, Molly Dempsey, Laura Fenton, Janet Reid, Liat Ben-Sira, Sunny Chung, Evan Evans, Steve Kraus, Claudia Reynders, Laura Varich, and José Vazquez. The superb patient care, careful research, and exemplary teaching by all these fellows is greatly appreciated; their probing questions, open discussions, irreverent arguments, constructive criticisms, stimulating ideas, and innovative research have all been important in the writing of this textbook.

Pediatric radiologic technologists are a hard-working and conscientious group with a positive impact on pediatric health care. Dedicated pediatric technologists at all six institutions where I have worked contributed radiographs and images used for illustrations. My special thanks to Linda Poznauskis who helped Taylor Chung and me to update Appendices 1, 2, and 4. Ginny Grove, Elaine Ward, Paulette Fontaine, Eileen Walsh, Jane Choura, and Laura Freeman typed and modified manuscripts of the contributing authors; they worked from diskettes of the Second Edition, numerous drafts, handwritten revisions, and dictation to produce the final manuscript. I could never have completed this revision without the dedication, help, and support of my executive assistants, Jane Choura and Laura Freeman. They spent many late evenings and numerous weekends typing and correcting the final manuscript. Their enthusiasm, hard work, efficiency, coaxing, humor, and cajolery got us all through this "labor of love."

The medical division of Lippincott–Raven has been extremely helpful and cooperative throughout the revision of the Third Edition. The advice and encouragement of Raeann Touhey, Production Editor, and Jim Ryan, Editor-in-Chief, are appreciated.

Most important, I acknowledge the help of my family. My wife, Jan, and our children, John and Julie, supported and encouraged me throughout the initial writing and subsequent first revision of the textbook. On many occasions, family activities were changed, postponed, or cancelled so that I could work on "the book." My particular thanks to Jan, who helped me to edit and proofread the entire manuscript and page proofs of the First Edition. She tolerated many nights, during the revision of this Third Edition, of my sitting at the dining room table, scribbling on draft manuscript pages, cluttering up the house with reprints and drafts, and mumbling into a dictaphone.

Practical Pediatric Imaging

Diagnostic Radiology of Infants and Children

Third Edition

Practical Pediatric Imaging: Diagnostic Radiology of Infants and Children, Third Edition.
D. R. Kirks, editor and N. T. Griscom, associate editor.
Lippincott–Raven Publishers, Philadelphia © 1998.

CHAPTER 1

Techniques

Taylor Chung and Donald R. Kirks

The child is not a small adult. This oft-quoted aphorism is appropriate for any discussion of pediatric radiology. It is particularly pertinent to techniques. Most general diagnostic radiologists and radiologic technologists are uncomfortable when examining infants and young children. Unfortunately, this uncertainty is usually transmitted to the child and frequently to the parents. The result is often an inadequate examination that is either confusing or uninterpretable (1). Pediatric imaging is no better than its techniques and technologists (2).

Imaging has assumed an increasingly important role in the evaluation, diagnosis, understanding, and follow-up of pediatric diseases and abnormalities (3–5). Because of the explosive technical advances of the last two decades, a variety of imaging modalities is available for diagnostic evaluation of children. The radiologist must be involved in the selection and sequencing of diagnostic evaluations. The prospective benefits of each examination must be carefully balanced against the costs and particularly against any potential risks.

This introductory chapter points out some of the unique technical aspects of pediatric radiology. Guidelines for conventional radiologic examinations are discussed and illustrated. The techniques and applications of modern imaging modalities (nuclear scintigraphy, ultrasonography, computed tomography [CT], magnetic resonance imaging [MRI], digital radiography, angiography, interventional techniques) in children are also discussed. Appendices 1 through 10 provide tabular information on pediatric imaging techniques, radiation dosage, and contrast media.

DEVELOPMENT OF PEDIATRIC RADIOLOGY

Pediatric radiology is the application of diagnostic radiology to aid in the understanding, diagnosis, therapy, and follow-up of diseases of infants and children. Its history includes the emergence of pediatrics and radiology as medical specialties, the growth of these two parent specialties, their fusion into pediatric radiology (3), and the explosive growth of pediatric radiology as a subspecialty of diagnostic imaging (6–19).

X-rays were discovered by Wilhelm Konrad Roentgen on November 8, 1895. Roentgen's brilliance and scientific

T. Chung and D. R. Kirks: Department of Radiology, Children's Hospital, Harvard Medical School, Boston, Massachusetts 02115.

1

inquisitiveness permitted him to characterize all of the basic properties of these rays by December 28, 1895. For this work he received the first Nobel Prize for physics in 1901. On February 3, 1896, at Dartmouth College in New Hampshire, the first clinical radiograph on this continent was made of a 14-year-old boy who injured his wrist while skating on the Connecticut River (6). A radiology department specifically for children was established in Graz, Austria in 1897. Pediatric radiologic activities on this continent began at the Hospital for Sick Children in Toronto in 1896 and at Children's Hospital, Boston, in 1899. However, after an initial burst of activity and enthusiasm, pediatric radiology lagged significantly behind the growth of both radiology and pediatrics, until the late 1940s (7).

The first textbook of pediatric radiology in any language, *Living Anatomy and Pathology: The Diagnosis of Diseases in Early Life by the Roentgen Method*, was published in 1910 by Thomas Morgan Rotch, professor of pediatrics at Harvard Medical School. This book seems to have had little impact (18,19). It was not until 1945 that the second American text, *Pediatric X-Ray Diagnosis*, was published by John Caffey, also a pediatrician. Caffey had become the radiologist at Babies Hospital in New York City in 1929. His textbook began to define and systematize the knowledge base of pediatric radiology. This textbook is currently in its ninth edition (3).

The Society for Pediatric Radiology was founded in 1958 by 33 radiologists to study problems peculiar to the practice of pediatric radiology and to aid in the education of members and others interested in those problems (7–14,16,17). Caffey was made an honorary counselor; Edward B. D. Neuhauser was elected the first president of the organization, and Frederic N. Silverman, Caffey's first trainee, was named the president-elect. Membership in the Society is limited to those whose principal interest is the practice of pediatric radiology; over 1000 radiologists around the world are currently members of the organization. In 1994, *Pediatric Radiology* became the official journal of the Society for Pediatric Radiology (SPR) and the European Society of Paediatric Radiology (ESPR). The growth of the SPR has confirmed and strengthened pediatric radiology as an important and dynamic subspecialty within diagnostic radiology (16).

The first 60 years (1896–1956) of pediatric radiology in the United States was beautifully chronicled by Caffey (7). The initial growth of pediatric radiology was at least as dependent on pediatrics and pediatric surgery as on radiology. Many of the pediatric radiologists of the 1940s and 1950s had their primary training in pediatrics and little or no training in radiology. However, the 1960s to the early 1990s were times of continual technologic explosion in diagnostic radiology. The development and refinement of angiography, angiocardiography, nuclear scintigraphy, ultrasonography, CT, digital radiography, teleradiology, MRI and MR spectroscopy, and vascular/interventional techniques have completely changed pediatric radiology. In fact, diagnostic pediatric radiology is now pediatric imaging. The dramatic expansion of imaging modalities available to evaluate pediatric disease has solidified the position of pediatric radiology as an important, viable subspecialty within diagnostic imaging (15–19). Currently, more than 60 pediatric radiology fellowship training positions are available to physicians with sufficient training in diagnostic radiology to qualify for the American Board of Radiology examination. The most recent milestone was in 1995, when the first examinations for the Certificate of Added Qualification (CAQ) in Pediatric Radiology were given by the American Board of Radiology.

PROBLEM-ORIENTED PEDIATRIC RADIOLOGY

For many years radiologists have simply attempted to improve the accuracy of various imaging techniques. They have been interested in the ability of a diagnostic modality to detect patients with disease (sensitivity) and to exclude patients without disease (specificity). As new techniques have developed, they have been quickly applied to pediatric radiology. The availability of many imaging modalities requires problem-oriented decisions to determine which techniques should be used or omitted in any given clinical situation (5,20,21). The radiologist must be willing to state that certain studies are *definitive* rather than hiding behind the term *complementary*. Moreover, the radiologist must know what examinations are obsolete or less frequently needed (5,18,20–23). Radiation exposure, delay in both diagnosis and therapy, and cost must be minimized. One must be aware of what is done *to* the pediatric patient (risk) as well as what is done *for* the child (benefit).

RISKS OF PEDIATRIC RADIOLOGY

The risks and nonmonetary costs of pediatric imaging include radiation exposure, physical trauma, psychological trauma, alteration of environment, oversedation, and adverse reactions to contrast media. The radiologist is also increasingly aware of cost. Because of the rising costs of medical care, examinations with a low diagnostic yield or that simply duplicate information must be omitted (23).

Radiation risks of diagnostic radiology in the pediatric patient are either deterministic or stochastic in nature. Deterministic radiation injuries (tissue injury, cataract production) occur when a number of cells are involved; a threshold dose is required (24). Above the threshold, the severity of the injury is proportional to the dose. There is no evidence that deterministic injuries occur as a result of low-dose diagnostic procedures. However, diligent attention to the cumulative radiation exposure and fluoroscopy time is required during difficult interventional procedures to ensure that threshold doses for skin erythema and epilation are not exceeded.

Stochastic radiation injuries (genetic effects and carcinogenesis) are believed to be caused by injury to a single cell (24). Typically, a threshold dose is not required. The probability of the injury is proportional to the dose, but the severity of the injury is independent of the dose. If one assumes a linear relation without a threshold for genetic effects, "any radiation is bad!" Irradiating the gonads of another's child is like irradiating the gonads of one's own child, as the cumulative effect is on the gene pool. Dose may be decreased by performing only examinations that are clinically indicated, tailoring the examination, decreasing exposure with fast film-screen combinations, using correct exposure techniques, shielding the patient's gonads or breasts when possible, preventing repeat exposures due to motion with proper immobilization, continuing education of technologists and physicians, updating quality improvement programs, and using low-dose digital radiography or nonionizing radiation (ultrasonography, MRI) techniques whenever feasible (1,2,25–27).

There are also physical risks to infants caused by immobilization or injury during radiologic examinations. These physical risks (falls, abrasions) are avoidable if proper techniques are used by trained technologists. Electrical or mechanical hazards may occur if imaging and accessory equipment is not properly grounded and mechanically maintained through planned, comprehensive, periodic equipment maintenance programs. Changes in environment and body temperature, which are problems primarily of the neonate, can be prevented with adequate care and warming devices (28).

The risks of oversedation cannot be adequately stressed (29). Registered nurses (RNs) are integral members of a radiology department. Although radiologists have the ultimate responsibility, RNs greatly facilitate the entire sedation process including presedation evaluation, monitoring during sedation, and postsedation recovery. This allows the radiologist to concentrate on the imaging procedure and also streamlines the work flow.

Contrast media may harm the patient by damaging tissues during injection, entering undesired sites, altering cardiovascular hemodynamics, or causing a systemic reaction (1). Contrast reactions are less frequent and less severe in children than in adults, particularly when low-osmolality contrast media are used (30,31). In addition, many radiology information systems (RIS) have a warning system. For patients who have had an adverse reaction to contrast media or latex, a warning label is automatically generated for any radiologic examination.

THE PROBLEM-ORIENTED APPROACH

To minimize risks and maximize benefits from any imaging examination, the procedure must be tailored to the specific clinical problem (1,3,5). This approach is especially important in pediatric radiology because of radiation considerations. Ideally, every examination should be approved and supervised by the radiologist after a discussion of the history, physical examination, laboratory data, diagnostic considerations, and expected yield of various imaging techniques with the referring physician. However, the physical and temporal constraints of busy clinical practices and radiology depart-

ments preclude this ideal approach, at least for the simpler examinations. Appendices 1 and 2 list pediatric radiology techniques and tabulate the preparation of children for those procedures and the radiographic projections used. The suggested projections (Appendix 2) are used for conventional examinations with relatively low radiation doses. The examination and clinical history are reviewed by a radiologist and additional films are obtained if necessary. Special procedures, imaging examinations, and fluoroscopic studies require precise tailoring to the clinical problem. Verbal consultation or review of the patient's chart is critical before supplementary imaging procedures.

The newer diagnostic imaging techniques have increased our ability to identify abnormalities, stage disease, and monitor therapy. However, these improvements increase the responsibility of both referring physicians and radiologists to choose the most appropriate examination from among the the many possibilities. The radiologist must also decide how many films or sections are needed. As one increases the number of films or images in an examination or the number of examinations during a diagnostic evaluation, one increases the probability of making the correct diagnosis but by decreasing amounts (1). Diagnostic certainty can never reach 100%. Imaging, especially in children, is a compromise. The best compromise depends on the specific clinical problem, the method of evaluation being used, the radiologic abnormality being searched for, and the experience of the radiologist (5,20,21,23). Therefore, diagnostic approaches vary from one radiologist to another and from one institution to another. Throughout this book, the authors point out an approach to problem-oriented pediatric radiology. Suggested guidelines for conventional examinations are listed in Appendices 1 and 2. Other diagnostic evaluations are suggested as tables or algorithms in other chapters.

ROLE OF THE RADIOLOGIST

The radiologist plays the central role in the diagnostic imaging process (Fig. 1-1). In the era of cost containment, capitation, and clinical practice guidelines, the radiologist must act as "gatekeeper" and be actively involved in developing the optimal sequence of diagnostic evaluation. One must be thoroughly familiar with the history, physical examination, and initial laboratory studies in order to determine what, if any, imaging modalities are indicated for diagnostic evaluation, subsequent therapy, and follow-up. Diagnostic radiologists must use whatever is in their armamentarium to make a correct diagnosis, as long as the expected benefit is greater than the expected risks and costs. Because of their familiarity with radiologic methods, inherent risks, and expected diagnostic yields, radiologists must assume responsibility for the proper selection of examinations. They must determine if the requested examinations are indicated, what examinations should be performed, what views should be

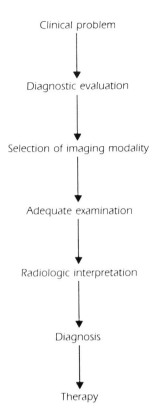

Clinical problem

↓

Diagnostic evaluation

↓

Selection of imaging modality

↓

Adequate examination

↓

Radiologic interpretation

↓

Diagnosis

↓

Therapy

FIG. 1-1. Diagnostic imaging process.

obtained, what the sequence of examinations should be, and whether contrast studies or other supplementary imaging examinations are required. These decisions require open communication between the radiologist and the referring physician; such cooperation greatly improves the quality of patient care.

Each radiologic consultation must follow an ordered, detailed, meticulous sequence (Fig. 1-2). The patient should arrive in the radiology department with a request form stating the pertinent clinical information and the anatomic part for radiologic evaluation. The patient's chart must accompany the inpatient scheduled for special examinations such as ultrasonography, nuclear scintigraphy, CT, magnetic resonance, angiography, vascular/interventional procedures, gastrointestinal and other flouroscopic examinations, and radiologic examination of the urinary tract. Pertinent patient data are entered into the radiology information system at registration (Fig. 1-3A). The request form (with the chart, if available) is combined with the patient's x-ray folder by clerical personnel, and both are given to the pediatric radiologic technologist. In many departments, outpatients and inpatients have separate waiting areas (Fig. 1-3B) and radiographic rooms. This keeps inpatients in hospital gowns from waiting with fully clothed outpatients. Also, the throughput for outpatients is higher, since examinations of inpatients tend to be more time-consuming. Critically ill patients and patients on stretchers wait in the staging area while the request and film jacket are reviewed by the technologist. If

the requisition is for a conventional radiologic examination that has not been recently performed on the child, he or she is brought directly into the appropriate radiographic room and the examination is performed. The radiologist is immediately available if the examination is not a conventional study, if a similar examination has been recently performed, or if the technologist has any questions regarding the request form.

The question of whether to allow a parent in the radiographic room with a child is difficult to answer (2,32). In our experience, the presence of a parent or other adult family member is helpful, not disruptive, especially when the child is frightened. A parent can be a great help in immobilization, not only for conventional radiologic examinations but also for gastrointestinal and urologic fluoroscopic examinations, ultrasonography, CT, magnetic resonance, and nuclear medicine studies. Before the examination, the radiologist or the technologist explains the procedure to the parents and the child. The parents are encouraged to stay and participate. Protective shielding is provided for parents. Occasionally, when their presence causes uncooperative behavior by the child, the radiologist will need to ask the parents to wait outside.

The patient is returned to the staging area (Fig. 1-4) while the films are processed, checked by the technologist, combined with the x-ray jacket and request form, and checked by the radiologist. Meticulous attention to detail by the technologist and radiologist is essential for accurate diagnosis.

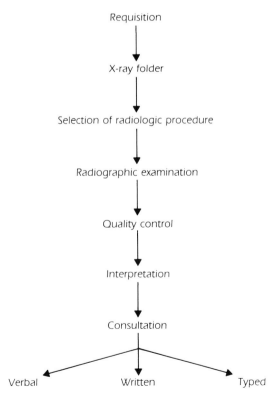

Requisition

↓

X-ray folder

↓

Selection of radiologic procedure

↓

Radiographic examination

↓

Quality control

↓

Interpretation

↓

Consultation

↙   ↓   ↘

Verbal   Written   Typed

FIG. 1-2. Sequence of radiologic evaluation.

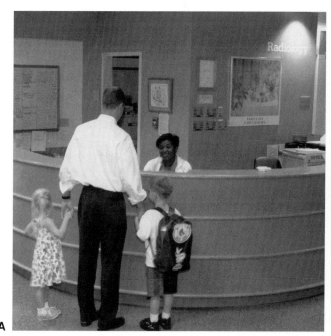
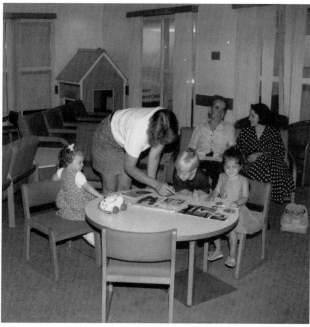

A   B

FIG. 1-3. Reception area. A: Patient is registered in the radiology department. **B:** Spacious waiting area for conventional outpatient radiology. Toys and books are readily available.

Views or examinations should be repeated only if they are needed for better evaluation of the clinical problem. However, assuming that radiologic examination was warranted in the first place, the patient may have to be exposed again

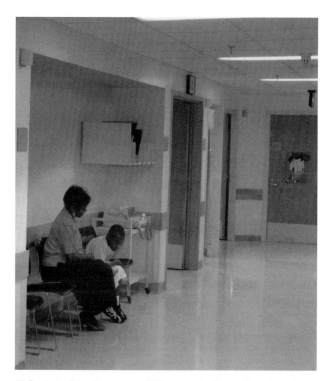

FIG. 1-4. Staging area. This area is immediately adjacent to the radiographic rooms and serves as a temporary holding area for the child and parent to wait while films are processed. The area is large enough for stretchers and wheelchairs.

if the initial films are inadequate. After this initial review of the images, the radiologist may need to examine the patient, obtain further history from the parents, or discuss the preliminary findings with the referring physician. Supplementary information and physical examination are helpful adjuncts to the radiologic examination and resolve many diagnostic problems. After completion and review of the radiologic examination, the patient is either sent home or returned to his or her hospital room.

The radiologist who first reviews the films acts as a triage point in the main reading room (Fig. 1-5A). All examinations from the emergency department, operating rooms, and outpatient clinics requiring a preliminary report are reviewed by a resident or fellow supervised by a faculty member, and a final interpretation is rendered immediately. More routine inpatient examinations are quickly reviewed for any findings that may require immediate medical attention; the films are then matched by the file room personnel with previous studies and hung on a multiviewer for interpretation by another team of radiologists (resident, fellow, and faculty) assigned to read inpatient studies. Each inpatient's films occupy one panel of the multiviewer assigned to his hospital location (Fig. 1-5B). After the radiologic impression is reached, a report is dictated, typed, approved, and filed in the patient's chart. A brief report is handwritten on the front of the x-ray folder. The latter is valuable for radiologic colleagues and clinicians discussing an examination without benefit of the primary interpretation. A verbal report is always given over the telephone when the request form specifies a preliminary report or when there is a significant positive finding. The large main reading room also serves as the location for scheduled work rounds conducted daily by radiologists for

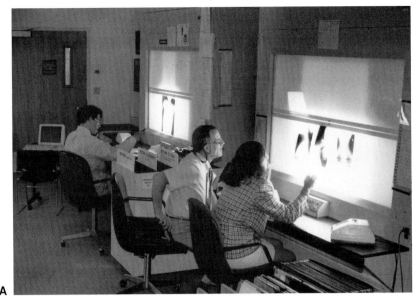

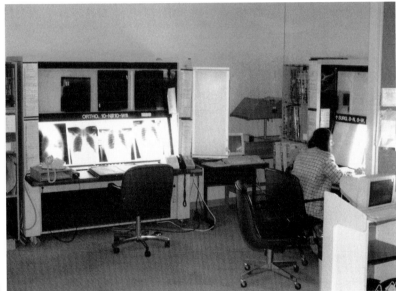

FIG. 1-5. Main reading room. A: A staff radiologist (*middle*) in charge at the point of triage in the reading room, overseeing the resident on the left for emergency examinations and interpreting an outpatient case on the right with a fellow. **B:** Inpatient films are placed on multiviewers for final interpretation. A panel is used for each patient so current studies are readily available for review.

clinical teams (Fig. 1-6A) and for unscheduled individual consultation (Fig. 1-6B).

PEDIATRIC RADIOLOGIC TECHNIQUES

Personnel and Surroundings

Diagnostic radiology is no better than its radiologic technologists; this is particularly true of pediatric radiology. However, not all technologists enjoy working with children; many become frustrated by their lack of cooperation. Consequently, pediatric technologists must be selected with care. They must be conscientious, dedicated individuals who enjoy working with children and have sufficient patience

and firmness to develop rapport with and handle ill children and their anxious parents (2).

A common mistake in general hospitals is to expect all technologists to be able to radiograph children. This lackadaisical attitude toward pediatric radiologic technology has developed despite widespread acceptance of specialization by technologists in nuclear medicine, ultrasonography, CT, MRI, angiography, and vascular/interventional procedures. It is critical that some technologists develop special skills in pediatric radiology, even when infants and children represent only a small part of the patient population. This practice allows the pediatric technologists to develop their skills and to gain confidence as well as expertise (1). Emergency coverage by pediatric radiologic technologists and radiologists should be provided for special pediatric procedures.

During the 1980s the importance of nursing support for

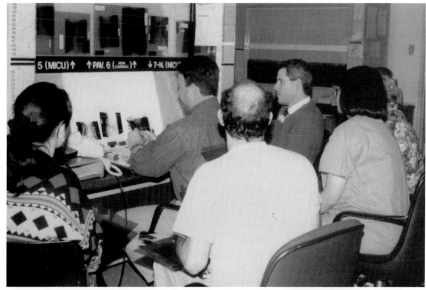

A

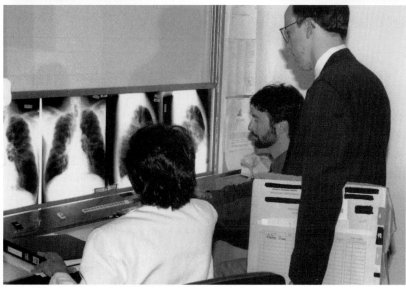

B

FIG. 1-6. Interaction with other physicians. A: Intensive care unit team reviewing films with radiologists. B: Individual consultation.

radiology became increasingly apparent. Nurses are valuable in all aspects of pediatric radiology but particularly for CT, MRI, and vascular/interventional examinations. They provide presedation evaluation, monitoring, intravenous access, and observation after sedation.

A warm, sympathetic attitude on the part of technologists, radiologists, clerks, nurses, and other personnel in the radiology department fosters the development of rapport with the child and parents. Colorful uniforms and lead aprons enhance the environment and help the child feel more secure. Decorations such as brightly colored animals and figures on the walls create a pleasant atmosphere for the child (Fig. 1-7). Stuffed animals and toys are kept in the radiography rooms, staging areas, and waiting rooms. Toys and decorations tend to distract young children and help them to adjust to the strange, threatening environment of a radiology department (see Fig. 1-3B).

Radiologic Equipment

Generators

Rooms used for pediatric radiology require generators capable of a kilovoltage (kVp) range of 60–150. The technique for all exams should be determined by the required radiographic contrast balanced against the increased dose that occurs at lower kVp. The contrast improvement by a reduction from 60 to 50 kVp is insignificant, but the patient dose is increased by at least a factor of 2! Optimal kVp settings for iodine range from 65 to 75, and for barium from 90 to 110 depending on the size of the patient. High kVp (130–140) is frequently required for examinations of the airway and mediastinum and, in large adolescents, the lungs.

The generator must provide reproducible exposures with a duration of 5–30 milliseconds regardless of the patient

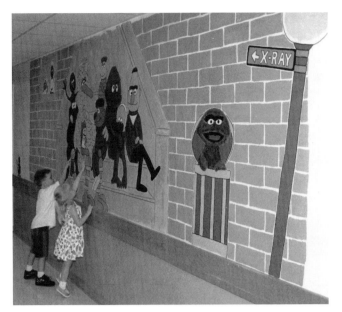

FIG. 1-7. The radiology department is a friendly place for children.

size. Exposure durations of less than 5 milliseconds are not reproducible because of limitations in automatic exposure control devices. Therefore, minimum tube current settings down to 100 mA must be available for examination of small patients and extremities. Some falling-load generators designed for adult imaging provide no tube currents below 300–400 mA and therefore require drastic reduction in kVp. This improper technique adjustment does not compromise image quality but can increase the radiation dose to the patient by a factor of 3.

Exposure durations greater than 30 milliseconds are not capable of preventing motion in any patient, let alone an uncooperative infant or young child. Since the kVp should not be changed, higher tube currents are used to reduce exposure times for large patients. Maximum tube currents of 500 mA are more than adequate for large patients, although this depends partly on the speed of the image receptors.

Even today, most fluoroscopy is performed with an x-ray beam which is continuously on when the exposure switch is depressed. Some generators are now capable of pulsing the x-ray beam during fluoroscopy; this improves the sharpness in the image by freezing motion. Some of these generators are capable of reducing the frequency of the pulses during fluoroscopy, which allows reduction in patient and personnel dose without significant loss of image quality (33). Variable rate, pulsed fluoroscopy is an important method of minimizing patient doses, especially in special procedure labs used for diagnostic and interventional studies.

Specific recommendations for generators for general pediatric radiography and fluoroscopy are as follows: maximum kVp of 150; operator selectable tube currents from 100 to 400 mA (50-kW rating at 100 kVp); minimum switchable exposure times of 1 millisecond; either three-phase 6- or 12-pulse or frequency invertor.

X-ray Tube and Collimator

Currently, fast image receptors (400 speed and higher) and 50-kW rated generators provide excellent image quality when equipped with an x-ray tube with a small focal spot to decrease geometric unsharpness (34). The 10-kW and 30-kW load factors have been used successfully for the small and large focal spots in routine pediatric radiographic and fluoroscopic rooms. This allows a focal spot combination of 0.3/0.6 mm or possibly 0.4/0.8 mm depending on the angle of the anode. A larger focal spot, ideally 0.9 mm with a load factor of 50 to 70 kW, is necessary in the special procedures lab, especially if digital subtraction imaging is to be performed. The 0.3-mm focal spot is also appropriate for pulsed fluoroscopy.

Since automatic collimation is no longer mandated by federal regulations and since the technologist typically reduces the size of the x-ray beam below that of the image receptor, a good-quality, multitiered, manual collimator is recommended. Added filtration in the collimator or x-ray tube port selectively removes low-energy x-rays from the beam and significantly reduces patient entrance exposure, although with some loss of radiographic contrast. While others have shown that numerous materials can be successfully used for adults (35–38), these published filter thicknesses must be decreased for pediatric imaging to avoid significant loss in radiographic contrast. Shaped filters can effectively reduce specific organ doses during frequently repeated exams, as in films of the spine for scoliosis (39–41) (Fig. 1-8).

Grids

Grids are designed to pass primary radiation and absorb scatter radiation. They are composed of alternating strips of lead and interspace material of low x-ray attenuation, such as aluminum, wood, and carbon. The grid ratio is the ratio of the height of the lead strips to the distance between them. In general, the higher the ratio, the more scatter, but also the more primary radiation the grid absorbs; more radiation must enter the patient to penetrate both the patient and the grid to reach the film. Radiographic contrast is improved by high grid ratios but at the expense of increased patient dose.

Since small patients are imaged with x-ray beams of small area, scatter levels are usually low. The radiation dose to small patients can be significantly reduced by omitting the grid with little loss of radiographic contrast due to scatter (42,43). However, a grid is generally required for examinations of the abdomen, pelvis, spine, and skull in children 5 years of age or older. Grids with 8:1 ratios are adequate for general pediatric radiology. If kilovoltages over 100 are commonly used, a 10:1 linear grid is recommended. Image intensifiers with maximum fields of view of 9 in. or less should be equipped with a removable 6:1 or 8:1 grid.

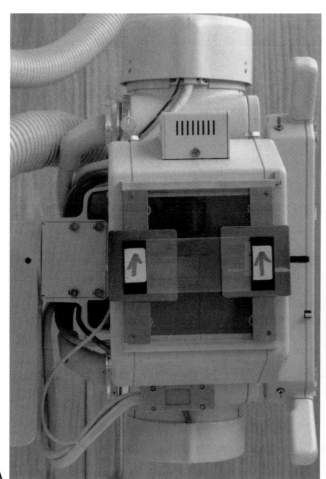
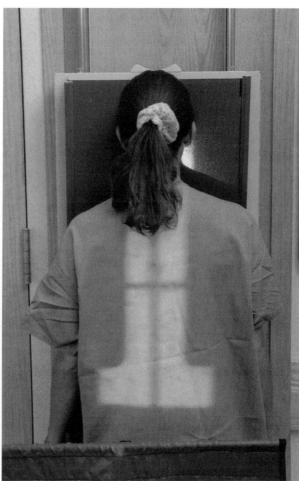

A   **B**

FIG. 1-8. Breast shielding in spine film for scoliosis. A: Magnetically mounted breast shields and wedge compensation filter on collimator of x-ray tube. **B:** Collimator light on patient's back indicates the area of the primary x-ray beam. Note that the breasts are shielded. Also, note the placement of the shield between the x-ray tube and the patient's gonads. The PA projection further decreases the dose to the breasts.

Cassettes

Cassettes provide good film-screen contact. Poor contact allows light from the screen to spread; the image is consequently blurred. Cassettes should have a curved back to ensure proper film-screen contact. Plastic cassettes tend to be more rugged than metal ones, resist damage when dropped, and are warmer to the touch. Color-coded cassettes allow identification of multiple film-screen combinations within the department. Because pediatric patients range in age and size from the newborn to the young adult, the entire spectrum of cassette sizes must be available: 8 × 10 in., 24 × 30 cm, 30 × 35 cm, 35 × 43 cm, 24 × 24 cm, 35 × 35 cm, 14 × 17 in., and 14 × 36 in. The patient identification marker and time may be flashed directly on the film outside the darkroom with a special identification camera (Fig. 1-9).

The front of the cassette, like the tabletop, the exposure detector wafer, and the grid, cause unwanted attenuation of the x-ray beam. The patient's dose must therefore be increased. The amount of tabletop and cassette front attenua-

tion varies with composition and thickness (44–46). Most manufacturers offer specifically designed pediatric cassettes using carbon fiber–reinforced plastic in the front cover. Similarly, tabletops constructed of carbon fiber–reinforced plastic material allow reductions in exposure of as much as 30% (44). The use of carbon fiber–reinforced plastic covers and interspaces (44,47) in grids also reduces attenuation of primary radiation without significant loss of image quality.

Film-Screen Combinations

The choice of a film-screen combination should consider image quality, patient dosage, and cost. Calcium tungstate phosphor intensifying screens, developed by Thomas Edison in 1896, were used for several decades. In the 1970s developments in rare-earth phosphors resulted in a breakthrough in screen technology. The first rare-earth screens used lanthanum and other rare-earth elements that increased the speed of the screens without an unsharpness-producing in-

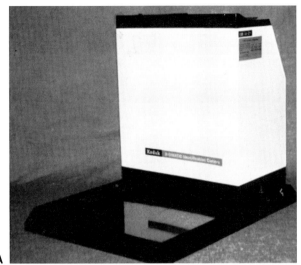

A

B

FIG. 1-9. Film identification. **A:** Identification camera may be kept in the radiography room or in the work area. **B:** Identification mark on the film of an 18-year-old male. The name, radiology (medical record) number, date of examination, birth date, and time of examination are included.

crease in thickness. These screens increase x-ray absorption efficiency and x-ray-to-light conversion efficiency. This speed increase is accompanied by an increase in quantum mottle, since the number of x-ray quanta (radiation exposure) used to produce the image is decreased. Quantum mottle is due to the statistical distribution of x-ray photons across the surface of the screen. It is directly proportional to the speed of the system and inversely proportional to the number of x-ray photons used to form the image. Clinical studies have led to the establishment of a number of functional, low-dose, pediatric film-screen radiographic systems (25,26,46,48).

The higher cost of the rare-earth screens is justified by the markedly reduced radiation dosage (20% to 50% of the radiation dosage of a par-speed system). The exposure of the patient to primary radiation and of radiology personnel to secondary radiation is reduced. The increased speed of the rare-earth system allows shorter exposure times and reduces retakes required because of motion. Since the relative speed of rare-earth image receptors is dependent on the effective energy of the x-ray beam reaching the receptor, technique charts that vary the kVp as opposed to the mA cannot be established by linear extrapolation. For example, a common pediatric rare-earth system, Lanex/TML, is approximately 3 times faster than a par-speed system at 60 kVp, 4 times faster at 80 kVp, and approximately $3\frac{1}{2}$ times faster at 100 kVp (49). The relative speed of this system is 400; par-speed film has a relative speed of 100. Problems in setting up these technique charts can be avoided by using relative speed diagrams (50).

Standard 400-speed rare-earth image receptors do not provide images sharp enough for bone radiology. Unfortunately, sharper image receptors that produce better bone detail also increase the quantum mottle. This results in an image that is perceived to be more noisy. Therefore, the faster image receptor must be made slower to obtain images with acceptable levels of perceived quantum mottle. This problem is overcome by the use of a 400-speed rare-earth image receptor for general work and a 100-speed rare-earth image receptor for extremities. The use of image receptors of two different speeds provides low-dose radiography for the entire spectrum of pediatric radiology.

A number of rare-earth film-screen systems for the adult chest and a specific system tailored to the unique needs of pediatric imaging have recently become available. One system uses a film with an added dye which prevents light from the front screen from reaching the rear emulsion of the film and vice versa. This improves the sharpness of the image (51) but reduces the speed of the system. The loss of speed is partly compensated for by using cassettes with carbon fiber fronts to reduce x-ray attenuation and screens with increased x-ray-to-light conversion efficiency. The result is an image with reduced quantum mottle and increased sharpness. One example of this type of film-screen combination designed for general pediatric work has a relative speed of 320 to 350; the system designed for pediatric extremity exams has a speed of approximately 200. Therefore, in comparison to standard rare-earth film-screen combinations operating at speeds of 400 and 100, respectively, for general and extremity pediatric imaging, extremity doses are significantly reduced, but doses to other areas of the patient's body are increased by 15 to 20%.

Radiologic Examination

Identification

Departmental personnel and technologists must check carefully to ensure that the right patient is radiographed and the appropriate examination performed. This verification is particularly necessary during conventional examinations on inpatient infants, as the patients may not communicate, the parents seldom are present, and the chart may not be available. In this situation, patient identification tags must be checked against the radiographic request form.

There are several systems for film identification. We prefer to use an identification camera (Fig. 1-9A); with it, each film can immediately be identified through the closed cassette outside the darkroom or even in the radiography room. This device records on the film not only the identification card information but also the time.

On the identification card we place the child's name, medical record (radiology) number, birth date, and date of examination (Fig. 1-9B). The age of the patient (obtained from the birth date) is extremely important when interpreting pediatric radiologic examinations, particularly when assessing skeletal maturation.

Side markers (left or right) are always important, particularly to prevent overlooking anomalies of situs. Markers with a bubble of mercury may be used to indicate whether the beam was horizontal or vertical.

Immobilization

Inadequate immobilization is one of the most important causes of poor-quality pediatric radiographs (1,2,32). Proper immobilization techniques improve image quality, decrease the length of the examination, and decrease the need for repeat studies. Parents, technologists, nurses, and aid personnel, all properly protected by lead aprons, can provide highly effective immobilization for conventional radiography. Proper immobilization is less traumatic to the patient than manual restraint. Infants frequently fall asleep with adequate mechanical immobilization, especially when they are swaddled with warmed blankets. Although restraints may not be necessary for the cooperative child (over 4 years old), immobilization is almost universally needed for younger patients to achieve proper positioning.

A combination of commercially available and custom-designed immobilization devices may be used. An immobilization board is one device suited for use on a horizontal radiographic table. The Tame-Em immobilizer (Tayman Industries, Severna Park, MD) consists of a Lucite immobilization board and plastic adjustable straps with Velcro fasteners

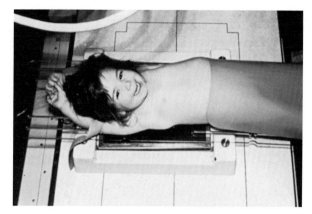

FIG. 1-10. Immobilization of young child. A 3-year-old girl is immobilized for a chest radiograph on the Tame-Em immobilizer. Velcro bands are placed around the arms and legs; a vinyl sheet of lead covers the lower abdomen and gonads. Note the expression of happiness.

at each end (Fig. 1-10). After proper immobilization, supine radiographs may be obtained by a vertical x-ray beam. This immobilizer board also fits onto a plastic base that holds cassettes for vertical beam or horizontal beam radiography, which permits supine anteroposterior (AP) and lateral radiographs of the chest in the infant after a single immobilization. The Vezina Octostop System (Entreprises Octostop Inc., St-Laurent, Quebec, Canada) has a padded wooden board with a plastic octagon at each end so that the immobilized patient can be placed in eight different positions (52) (Fig. 1-11). The importance of upright radiography of the infant has been overemphasized. When upright radiography is necessary, one may use the Pigg-O-Stat device (Modern Way Immobilizers, Memphis, TN). It consists of a saddle with a plastic holder that keeps the infant in the erect position (Fig. 1-12). The device is on wheels, so it can be brought to and from an upright cassette holder. It is mounted on a rotating and sliding platform to permit adjustment for lateral and oblique radiographs. This device is not ideal, as the plastic holder produces artifacts, and small infants tend to slump into a lordotic position. Moreover, the Pigg-O-Stat device permits the child to rotate during exposure, and the plastic sleeve restricts the depth of inspiration.

We have found several custom-designed devices to be useful for immobilization for conventional radiographs (53). The chest and torso box is used for infants and young children for vertical AP and horizontal lateral projections (Fig. 1-13). The chest stand is used for children who are old enough to sit at the end of the x-ray table (Fig. 1-14). If necessary, a parent can hold the child at the elbows keeping the arms up and can also hold the head to eliminate rotation. A box is used for standing radiographs of the feet (Fig. 1-15). A wooden bench with a back support and a slot for a film cassette can be used for decubitus radiographs (Fig. 1-16). The back support gives both the technologist and the child a greater sense of security than an unsupported cassette alone.

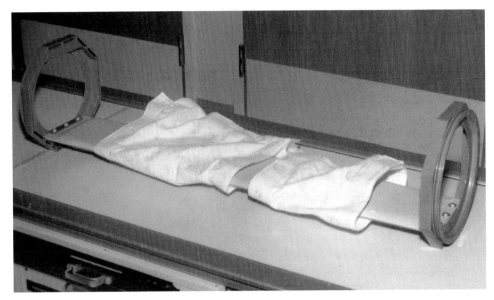

FIG. 1-11. An octagon board for immobilization.

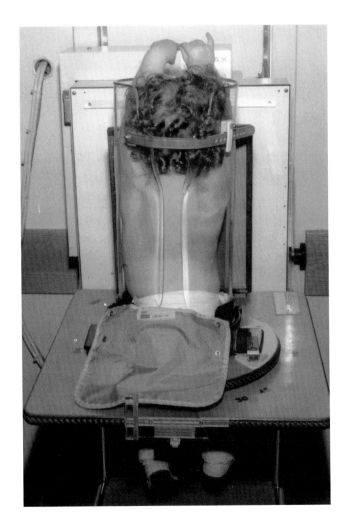

FIG. 1-12. Infant immobilized for upright chest film. Infant immobilized and supported by the Pigg-O-Stat device. The device can be rotated 90° for a lateral projection. Note the presence of shielding for the pelvis.

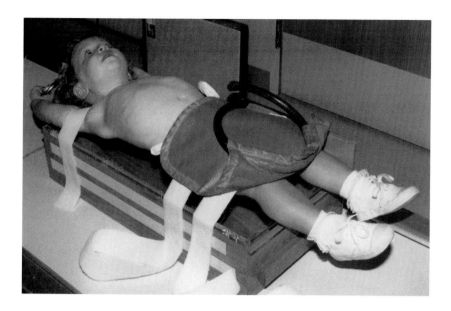

FIG. 1-13. The chest and torso box. The chest and torso box used for a cross-table lateral chest radiograph on a young child. The child is immobilized with Velcro straps at the shoulders and the legs, which eliminates rotation. An AP radiograph can easily be obtained by placing the x-ray cassette in the box underneath the patient.

Proper immobilization may also require the use of adhesive tape, Velcro straps, foam rubber blocks and wedges, towels, diapers, sandbags, Ace bandages, stockinettes, clear plastic or acetate sheets, and balsa wood blocks (Fig. 1-17). The hands and feet of children can be radiographed while

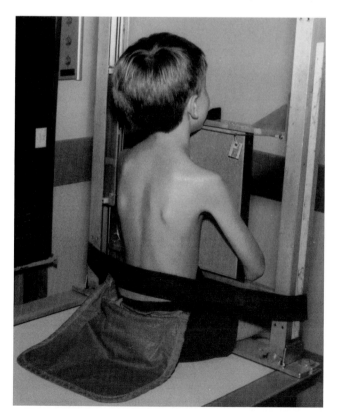

FIG. 1-14. Chest stand at the end of the x-ray table. A cooperative young child can be easily immobilized for an upright (sitting) PA chest radiograph with the support of a Velcro strap on the lower back. Note that the gonads are shielded.

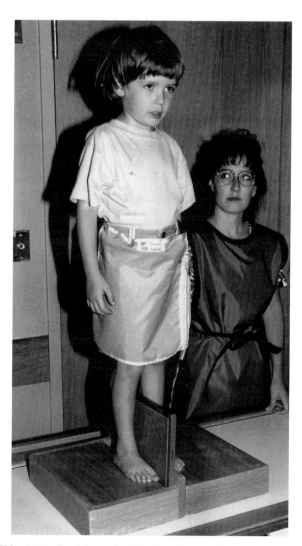

FIG. 1-15. Foot box. A child standing on the foot box for a lateral radiograph of the foot. Note that a parent wearing a lead apron is nearby for safety reasons and that the child has a gonadal shield in place.

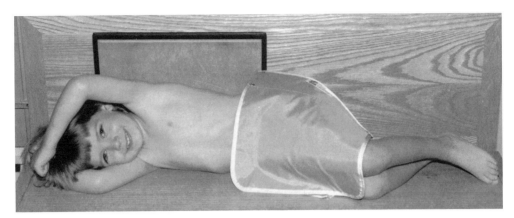

FIG. 1-16. Wooden bench. A cooperative older child can be easily and safely positioned for a decubitus projection on a wooden bench with a back support. There is a slot for stabilizing the cassette.

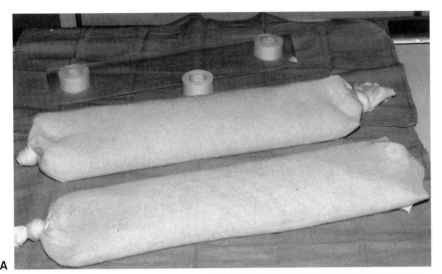

A

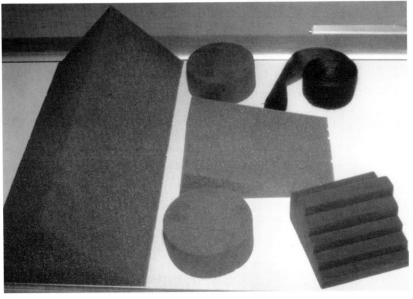

B

FIG. 1-17. Items frequently used for immobilization. A: Sandbags, tape, clear Plexiglas strip. B: Sponges of various shapes and sizes, Velcro strap.

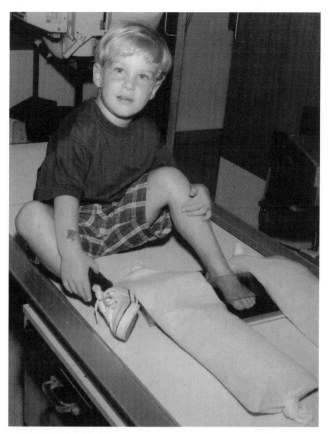

FIG. 1-18. Immobilization for AP view of foot. This child's left foot is immobilized using a combination of Plexiglas and sandbags.

cally (gonads) and somatically (eye, thyroid, bone marrow). Dose reduction can be accomplished for the site examined as well as other body regions (Table 1-1) (1,25).

The gonads must be shielded whenever they are within 5 cm of the primary beam (1). The testes can be shielded during nearly every examination of the abdomen and pelvis (Fig. 1-21). Because of the location of the ovaries and their variable position, they obviously cannot be fully shielded during examinations of the abdomen and pelvis. However, if two views that include the ovaries (pelvis to include hips) are requested in a female, one view (pelvis with the hips in neutral position) should be obtained without gonadal shielding and the other view (pelvis with the hips in frog-leg lateral position) with shielding. Positioning can be used in some cases to reduce the radiation dose to critical organs. An example is the performance of scoliosis exams posteroanterior (PA) instead of AP. This significantly reduces the dose to breast tissue because entrance doses are up to 50 times as great as exit doses (see Fig. 1-8).

Contact gonadal shields are easy to make from readily available material. With a template (Fig. 1-22) for sex and age, they are cut into a variety of sizes and shapes from 1.0 mm lead vinyl sheeting (Fig. 1-23). Gonadal exposure in an AP or PA film that includes the gonads can be reduced by 95% in boys and up to 50% in girls with proper contact shielding (54). In male patients, proper positioning of the shield avoids obscuring any bony detail of the pelvis (see Fig. 1-21). In female patients, the position of the ovaries in the pelvis varies tremendously depending on bladder disten-

compressing them with a piece of plastic (Fig. 1-18). Extremity radiographs can be obtained by immobilizing the child on a board or on the table and then taping the extremity in place over the film. Older children can be immobilized with sheets (Fig. 1-19).

Fluoroscopy and fluoroscopic procedures are performed on a conventional radiographic and fluoroscopic table. A digital spot-film camera permits last-image hold, storage of data, significant dose reduction, and image manipulation. Judicious use of last-image hold during fluoroscopy in place of separate exposures for digital spot films can significantly decrease patient dose. Proper immobilization for patient positioning and table movement during pediatric fluoroscopy is critical. A custom-made seat is used to keep children secure for upright fluoroscopy in modified barium swallow studies (Fig. 1-20).

Reduction of Radiation Exposure

Any radiation is considered harmful to the child. All efforts must be made to reduce radiation exposure without decreasing diagnostic information. Reduction of radiation exposure should be focused on sites that are sensitive geneti-

TABLE 1-1. *Methods of reducing radiation exposure*

Dose reduction to area examined:
  Select imaging modality that minimizes radiation
    Ultrasonography
    Magnetic resonance imaging
    Nuclear scintigraphy
    Low-dose techniques
  Avoid repeat examinations
  Tailor examinations
  Reduce number of exposures
  Choose appropriate film–screen combination
  Use digital fluoroscopy
  Use appropriate projection
  Use adequate filtration
  Use good geometry
  Process films adequately
Dose reduction to unexamined areas:
  Select imaging modality that minimizes radiation
    Ultrasonography
    Magnetic resonance imaging
    Nuclear scintigraphy
    Low-dose techniques
  Use tight collimation
  Shield breasts and gonads
  Immobilize patient
  Use proper positioning

Modified from Poznanski (1).

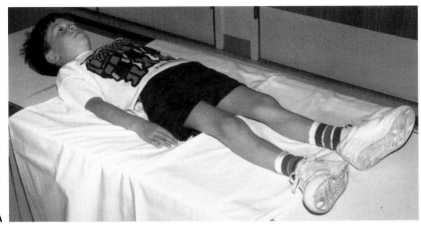

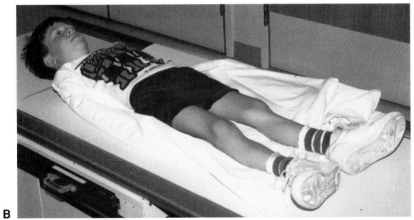

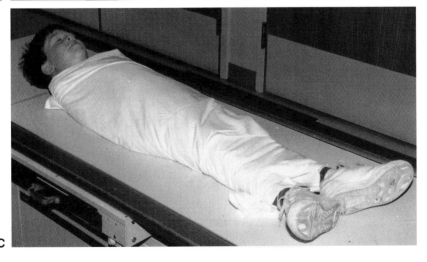

FIG. 1-19. Immobilization with a body wrap. A large folded sheet immobilizes this child's body and extremities. **A:** The child is positioned on the sheet. **B:** One side of the sheet is wrapped over the right arm and under the body. **C:** The other side of the sheet is wrapped around the child.

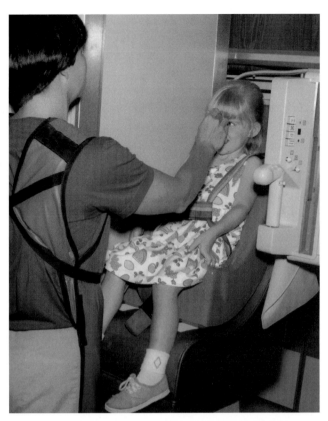

FIG. 1-20. Chair for modified barium swallow. This seat is mounted on the elevated footrest on a conventional fluoroscopic table (positioned upright). The child is secured to the seat by safety belts and immobilized.

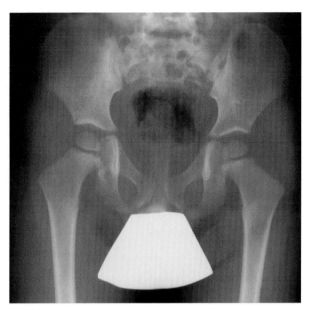

FIG. 1-21. Male gonadal shielding. The gonads of a 3-year-old male are adequately shielded without obscuring any bony anatomy.

tion. After selecting the contact shield according to the age of the patient, the lower margin of the shield is placed at the level of the pubis. The upper margin of the shield should be just below the iliac crests (Fig. 1-24) (55).

Radiation Dosage in Children

Estimations of the the skin dose and gonadal dose for any given radiologic examination are available. Appendix 3 lists,

according to patient age, the entrance skin doses, midline doses, and gonadal doses per radiograph for many examinations. All of these doses in mrads were calculated from measured free-in-air exposures (when available) using the radiographic technique factors listed in the other columns of the appendix. The midline dose is included because it is a better indicator of radiobiological risk than skin entrance doses (56). The gonadal doses assume that no shielding is used—this of course is often not true—and that the x-ray field is collimated to the size of the body part examined rather than the size of the image receptor system. These figures are based on 100-, 400-, and 1100-speed image receptors, respectively, for extremity, general, and scoliosis examinations.

The doses listed in Appendix 3 are significantly affected by the choice of kVp. For example, assume a change of + 10 kVp for an AP abdomen exam of a 1- to 3-year-old as shown below:

AP Abdomen (400 speed)

Pat. age	SID (cm)	PID (cm)	Grd Rat	kVp	mAs	Pat Thk (cm)	Free A expos. (mR) ±10%	Skin ±15%	Midline ±30%	M/F Gonads ±30%
								Doses (mrad)		
1–3 yr	107	8	8	60	5.8	13	30	28	11	3.2/11
1–3 yr	107	8	8	70	3.0	13	21	20	8.6	2.2/7.8
1–3 yr	107	8	8	80	1.8	13	16	16	7.3	1.7/6.4

The entrance (free-in-air) exposure is increased 43% at 60 kVp and decreased 24% at 80 kVp from the exposure at 70 kVp. The midline dose increases 28% and decreases 14% with the same kVp changes. As the kVp increases, however,

the gonadal dose decreases significantly. Clearly, the changes in radiation exposure due to the choice of radiographic technique are significant.

The values in Appendix 3 should be used only to compare

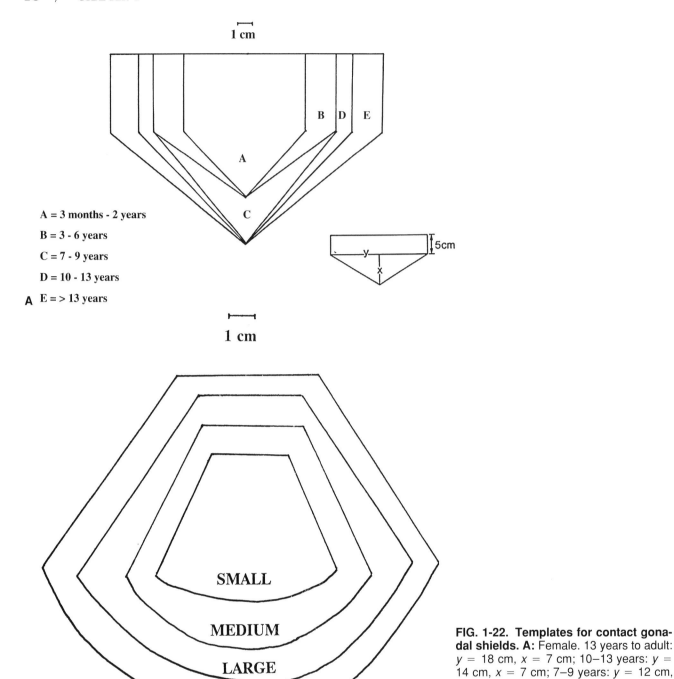

1 cm

B D E

A

A = 3 months - 2 years

B = 3 - 6 years

C = 7 - 9 years

D = 10 - 13 years

E = > 13 years

A

C

y

x

5cm

1 cm

SMALL

MEDIUM

LARGE

ADULT

B

FIG. 1-22. Templates for contact gonadal shields. A: Female. 13 years to adult: $y = 18$ cm, $x = 7$ cm; 10–13 years: $y = 14$ cm, $x = 7$ cm; 7–9 years: $y = 12$ cm, $x = 7$ cm; 3–6 years: $y = 12$ cm, $x = 4$ cm; 3 months–2 years: $y = 8$ cm, $x = 4$ cm. Modified from Godderidge (55). **B:** Male.

doses relative to differences in patient size or in the type of exam. The actual exposure and dose to a specific patient is dependent on the radiographic technique used, the patient's unique anatomy and disease state, and the unique performance and setup of the specific x-ray equipment. Use of nonoptimal radiographic techniques or equipment can more than double the doses listed in the appendix. The specifications of the x-ray equipment that affect these calculated patient doses are listed at the end of Appendix 3.

A few generalizations can be made from Appendix 3. The maximum gonadal dose occurs when the gonads are unshielded and in the primary x-ray beam. This gonadal dose for females is similar to the midline dose. For males, the gonadal dose is greater, if the gonads lie in front of the midline of the patient, less if the reverse.

The gonadal dose decreases rapidly with distance from the primary x-ray beam. When the gonads are 10 cm from the edge of the primary beam, the gonadal dose is approxi-

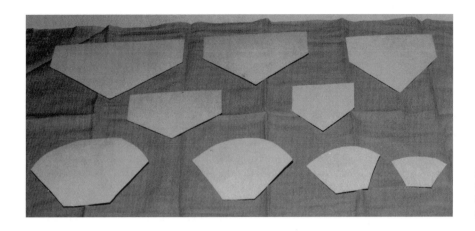

FIG. 1-23. Contact gonadal shields.
Contact gonadal shields are cut from sheets of lead vinyl using the templates shown in Fig. 1-22.

mately 1% to 2% of the entrance skin dose (57). Gonadal doses less than 0.25 mrad are less than the daily gonadal dose from background radiation (58). Examinations of the head, neck, chest, and extremities do not cause any significant gonadal doses.

The dose values in the table can be significantly reduced by appropriate shielding when the gonads are in the primary beam. Contact shielding of the male gonads can reduce doses up to 90% (57). The reduction factor for females is not as large because the shield is often not accurately placed. The reduction by shielding is much smaller when the gonads are outside the primary beam. This is because external shielding cannot attenuate internally scattered x-rays, the major source of dose when the gonads are outside the primary beam.

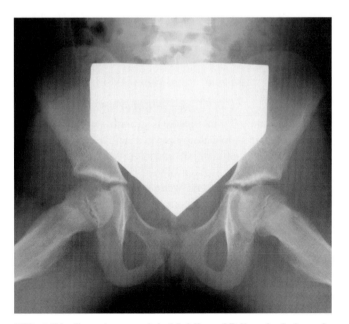

FIG. 1-24. Female gonadal shielding. AP (frog-leg) view of the pelvis in a 7-year-old female. The lower margin of the contact gonadal shield is placed just at the pubis. The upper margin of the shield extends to just below the iliac crests.

ROUTINE RADIOLOGIC EXAMINATIONS

In the ideal practice of pediatric radiology, there would be no routine radiologic examinations—only problem-oriented evaluations. In reality, there must be general guidelines for patient preparation and radiologic projections. These technique guidelines for preparation (Appendix 1) and projections (Appendix 2) have evolved over the past 25 years. The methods listed in Appendix 1 and Appendix 2 work at Children's Hospital, Boston, and can work for you!

The clinician should provide pertinent clinical information and diagnostic questions with all written or verbal radiography requisitions. The patient's hospital chart should accompany inpatients for fluoroscopy, gastrointestinal radiography, radiologic examination of the urinary tract, ultrasonography, nuclear scintigraphy, magnetic resonance, and vascular/interventional procedures. The clinician should be encouraged to consult the radiologist (a clinical colleague who happens to use imaging methods for diagnosis) regarding indications, techniques, complications, radiation dosage, and the expected diagnostic yield of any particular imaging study.

The normal sequence of diagnostic radiologic examinations is as follows: plain films, cross-sectional and other imaging studies, excretory urography, and barium studies. Barium may interfere with nuclear scintigraphy, body CT, body MRI, and ultrasonography. All special imaging procedures in children (nuclear medicine, ultrasound, CT, MRI, angiography, and vascular/interventional procedures) should be scheduled and orchestrated by a radiologist with a special interest in pediatric imaging. Gastrointestinal tract and urinary tract x-ray examinations, unless urgent, should be scheduled at least a day in advance.

Preparation for Radiologic Examinations

If both genitourinary and gastrointestinal radiographic examinations are to be performed, the genitourinary studies should be performed first. Discussion between the clinician and the radiologist is mandatory before excretory urography in patients with impaired renal function, hypertension, or dehydration. Patients should not have solid food, milk, or apple juice for 4 hours prior to excretory urograms. No preparation is needed for voiding cystourethrograms (Appendix 1).

The correct preparation of infants (2 years of age and younger) for gastrointestinal contrast studies must be thoroughly understood by radiologic and nursing personnel. Infants should never be kept without oral feedings longer than 4 hours prior to any examination (Appendix 1). No colon preparation is indicated for patients with acute abdominal conditions or suspected Hirschsprung disease.

A pneumocolon (air contrast barium enema) is a time-consuming, detailed examination requiring vigorous preparation (Appendix 1). The indications (suspected polyp or inflammatory bowel disease) for this infrequent examination must be thoroughly understood by both clinician and radiologist.

Radiographic Projections

The projections in Appendix 2 are guidelines for conventional radiographic examinations in children. If the views have not been specified on the requisition, the technologist should obtain films according to this list. In any questionable case the technologist should check with the radiologist. Comparison views are done only after the approval of the radiologist. Some generalizations regarding radiographic projections for specific anatomic areas are discussed below.

Head

A skull series includes AP, Towne, and lateral views. These are usually taken supine to make immobilization and positioning easier (Fig. 1-25). Cross-table lateral positioning is used if the child is unable to assume the position for a tabletop lateral view and in cases of trauma to the head and neck. The cross-table lateral view allows better visualization of the sutures and sella turcica. A supplementary submento-vertex (basal) view may be useful for demonstrating the foramen magnum, petrous ridges, basilar foramina, and coronal sutures.

Mastoid films, rarely performed after the advent of CT, in children require patience, careful technique, and expertise on the part of a dedicated technologist. Towne, lateral, and Stenvers views are particularly helpful for comparing the development, aeration, and density of the two mastoids.

The paranasal sinuses, facial bones, and orbits are well demonstrated by Waters, Caldwell, and lateral (to include from the nose to the thoracic inlet) projections. These radiographs are performed upright when the child is old enough to sit alone. The tripod oblique view of the orbit visualizes only the orbital end of the optic canal. Complete visualiza-

tion of the orbital end, bony canal, and cranial end of the optic canal requires CT or MRI.

Neck and Upper Airway

A lateral film is adequate for evaluating most upper airway abnormalities and the size of the adenoids. Detailed evaluation of the upper airway sometimes requires AP and lateral radiographs during inspiration and expiration. Problems regarding adequacy of inspiration, the effect of adenoidal enlargement on the nasopharyngeal air column, and retropharyngeal soft tissue swelling are clarified by fluoroscopy. Lateral airway films should be taken during inspiration with the neck extended. A physician must accompany any patient with moderate or severe respiratory stridor if radiographs are obtained in the radiology department. Patients with stridor should not be forced into a supine, flexed, or hyperextended position; patients with upper airway obstruction should be radiographed in whatever position the compromised child finds most comfortable.

Spine

Because of the high radiation dose and limited yield, oblique views of the spine are not routine in children except in the examination of the bony fusion mass after spinal fusion surgery and in the demonstration of pars defects in the lumbar spine of the older patient. Erect views of the thoracolumbar spine from the external auditory meatus to the iliac crest are usually adequate for the assessment of scoliosis. Breast shielding is critical in female patients (see Fig. 1-8). Bending films are obtained in scoliosis patients only if specifically requested.

Extremities

Comparison views, except in hip examinations, are recommended only if joint disease is strongly suspected. Radiographs of a hip should almost always include the entire pelvis including the contralateral hip, in AP and frog-leg lateral projections. Skeletal maturation is assessed from a single view of the left hand and wrist in children over 1 year of age. If the chronologic or bone age is less than 1 year, radiographs of the left hemiskeleton should be obtained for a more accurate assessment of skeletal maturation (see Chapter 5) (59). A skeletal survey for suspected child abuse and a metastatic series are similar (Appendix 2), whereas a long-bone series includes only AP views of the upper and lower extremities.

Chest

Chest films are obtained in the supine position (AP and cross-table lateral projections) in uncooperative children and

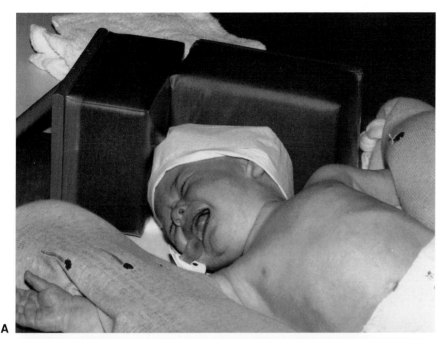

A

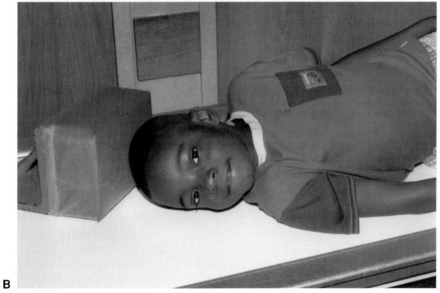

B

FIG. 1-25. Positioning for supine lateral projection of the skull. A: A small sheet is used to make a head wrap for this infant. The head is positioned for a lateral projection with the wrap sheet under the cushioned immobilization devices. Sandbags are used as restraints for the extremities. **B:** A cooperative child can easily assume the position for the lateral skull radiograph. The head cushion is used as a gentle reminder for the child to hold his head still.

in young infants. Most children older than 1 year of age can sit upright with support. In addition to evaluation for pleural fluid, lateral decubitus views of the chest are occasionally performed for the suspicion of a foreign body in the bronchus. A ''cardiac series'' (two or four views with barium in the esophagus) is performed only very rarely in children.

Abdomen

The second view of the abdominal series in a young infant is frequently a supine or prone cross-table lateral view rather than an upright AP view. Three views (supine, prone, horizontal beam film) are often obtained to evaluate the acute abdomen.

Radiographic Techniques

The techniques listed in Appendix 4 are those used in the Department of Radiology at Children's Hospital, Boston. They are based on 90-second film processing, three-phase generators, and rare-earth film-screen combinations. These techniques serve only as guidelines; variations will depend on individual equipment, screens, film, and developing factors. For the abdomen and extremities, only AP techniques are listed. The amount of increase in technique from an AP film to a lateral of the abdomen depends on the size of the patient. In general, the kilovoltage should be increased by 3 or 4 kV to go from an AP to a lateral extremity view.

The child between 6 months and 4 years of age, large enough to resist immobilization and not always willing or able to cooperate, is the most challenging to radiograph. Techniques with the shortest exposure times are recommended for these difficult infants and young children. Motion remains the most common cause of technical failure. Increased kilovoltage and milliamperage permit use of faster times. Generators should permit exposures as short as 5 milliseconds.

Contrast Media

The contrast media listed in Appendix 5 are those commonly used in pediatric radiology. Generic name, percentage of contrast media in the solution, trade name, iodine content, osmolality, manufacturer, and uses are shown. Contrast agents for urinary tract and intravascular use and for selected gastrointestinal tract examinations are also listed. Barium compounds for routine gastrointestinal studies are not given in Appendix 5 but are discussed in Chapter 8. Osmolalities, concentrations, and iodine content were obtained from the figures supplied by the manufacturers (60).

Types of Contrast Media

Contrast agents for intravascular use and for direct injection into the genitourinary system contain iodine. These commercially available contrast media are ionic or nonionic, and include high-osmolality and low-osmolality compounds.

Osmolality is determined by the amount of dissolved solute per unit of solvent. A monomer ionic contrast medium in solution has two dissolved ions per molecule: the cation and the large organic iodine-containing anion. This medium is designated as a ''ratio 1.5'' contrast medium, a number derived by dividing the number of iodine atoms per molecule (3) by the number of ions per molecule in solution (2) (60). A nonionic, monomeric contrast medium is designated as a ratio 3 contrast medium (3:1), as is the monoacidic dimer (6:2).

Conventional intravascular contrast media have high osmolalities and can have a profound effect on serum osmolality and the hemodynamic status of infants and children. Most hemodynamic disturbances caused by contrast media when used for angiography or angiocardiography are related to an abrupt increase in serum osmolality; thus, it is advantageous to use the lowest possible osmolality contrast agent in children (31,61).

Intravascular contrast media formulations, including those that have a significantly reduced osmolality, are listed in Appendix 5. Ioxaglate is an ionic dimeric compound; iohexol, iopamidol, and ioversol are nonionic contrast agents.

Indications for Low-Osmolality Contrast Media

The low-osmolality contrast agents are safer than the high-osmolality agents. Decreased morbidity and mortality have been documented in animals, in healthy volunteers, and in

patient trials (62–65). Recent reviews indicate a decrease in reactions (vomiting, movement, local pain at injection site) from nonionic low-osmolar contrast agents compared to ionic high-osmolar contrast agents, especially in children (31,61).

The availability of low-osmolality contrast agents that are much safer but also much more expensive poses a dilemma for both the general radiologist (62,63,66) and the pediatric radiologist (61). The incremental cost cannot readily be transferred to the patient under current billing limitations, and much of the increased expense must be absorbed by hospitals, clinics, and radiologists. Nevertheless, our department switched to using nonionic, low-osmolality contrast media in all examinations and procedures requiring intravascular administration in 1990. Children now rarely become nauseated or feel discomfort at the site of injection of contrast media. As a result, the imaging examinations proceed with fewer delays; image degradation due to motion occurs less often; and, most importantly, the children are not as fearful of repeat examinations.

SPECIAL RADIOLOGIC TECHNIQUES

Neonatal Radiography

The radiology and radiography of the neonatal period (first month of life) are unique. The causes and radiologic appearances of diseases differ from those in older infants and children (67–69). Moreover, techniques must be modified for radiologic examination of the neonate (1). Some of these modifications are discussed and illustrated in this section; neonatal diagnostic radiology is presented by organ system in the following chapters.

The problems of radiologic examination are related to the fragile clinical condition and thermal lability of the neonate. It is hazardous to move the extremely ill neonate or his incubator to the radiology department, and therefore radiology must usually come to the baby (mobile examination). If the neonate is stable enough to be transported to the radiology department for a contrast examination or special imaging, particular attention must be paid to monitoring vital signs and keeping the child warm.

Mobile Radiographic Equipment

Because of the necessity, nearly absolute, to keep the neonate in the incubator and the incubator in the nursery, most departments use mobile (mobile: capable of being moved; portable: capable of being carried) equipment. Many problems previously associated with mobile equipment can be overcome by separating the x-ray unit from its power supply during exposure, through use of a capacitor-discharge or battery-powered generator.

One may use a capacitor-discharge mobile unit that plugs into a wall outlet or a battery-operated frequency inverter mobile unit. The unit should provide an operator-selectable

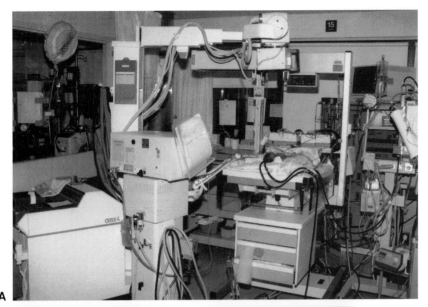

A

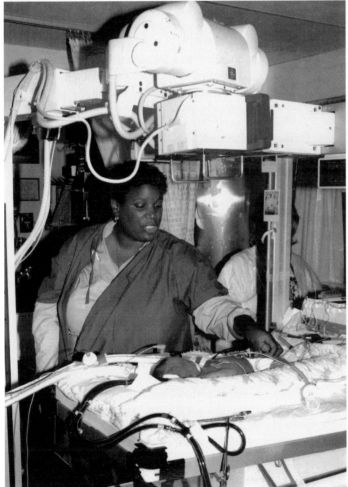

B

FIG. 1-26. Mobile neonatal radiography. A: This neonate is critically ill and requires extracorporeal membrane oxygenation (ECMO). The mobile unit needs to be small and maneuverable to fit into an instrument-packed unit. **B:** The technologist is placing a contact gonadal shield on the diaper of the neonate. The mobile unit is positioned for an AP chest film.

kilovoltage range from 55 to 120. These units have a fixed tube current that cannot be changed by the operator. In the case of the battery-powered unit, the tube current should be at least 100 mA to allow the short exposure times necessary to freeze patient motion. These units allow the operator to select the product of tube current and exposure time, mAs. The minimum mAs setting must be 0.5 or less. The mobile unit must be heavy duty and yet small enough to fit over the incubator or underneath the heating panel in the open nursing unit (Fig. 1-26). It must be capable of providing reproducible, consistent exposures at its minimum kVp and mAs settings. Ideally, one mobile unit should be permanently stationed in the neonatal nursery.

Film-Screen Combinations

Grids should not be used for neonatal radiography because scatter is minimal. Plastic film cassettes are ideal because they are heavy duty, color-coded, and not cold to touch. The problem of quantum mottle caused by rare-earth systems in the neonate has been discussed previously. We currently use a rare-earth system specifically tailored to pediatric radiography, as was discussed in the section on film-screen combinations.

Techniques

Films in the neonatal intensive care unit should be obtained by an experienced pediatric technologist who is aware of the tenuous condition of these infants; therapeutic tubes, catheters, and monitoring wires should be disturbed as little as is consistent with appropriate diagnostic quality (Fig. 1-27). The technologist should have a good rapport with the nursing staff and must immediately notify them of any change in the condition of the child or in the position of the tubes and monitors. The technologist must wash and gown when entering the intensive care unit. Cleanliness is maintained by wrapping the cassette in a disposable plastic bag or sterile sheet (1).

The techniques must allow short exposure times. Standard mobile technique for a neonatal chest film is a 40-in. distance

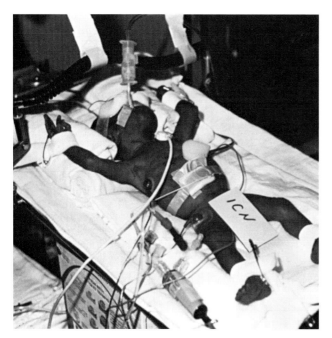

FIG. 1-27. Sick newborn. The radiologic technologist must be careful with the tubes, catheters, and monitoring lines of ill newborns, who are very fragile.

using average factors of 60 kVp at 0.7–1.2 mA with a 400-speed film-screen combination. Supine films of the chest or abdomen may be obtained by placing the cassette directly under either the child or his bedding. An unwrapped cassette should never be in contact with the patient. However, placing the wrapped cassette directly beneath the baby produces less magnification, increases detail, and prevents mattress artifacts.

Although sick neonates are usually not active, positioning and immobilization are still usually necessary to avoid projecting an extremity or one of many tubes and lines on the chest or abdomen. Artifacts such as mattress material, incubator holes, skin folds, and extraneous opacities on the neonate should be avoided if possible.

Radiation Exposure

Although good collimation is an excellent method of gonadal protection for chest radiographs, we still shield the gonads if possible even when they are not in the primary beam. Several contact gonadal shields should be kept in the neonatal nursery. Wrapped in a plastic bag or sterile cloth, they are placed over the gonads before the exposure.

There is a common misunderstanding about radiation exposure from mobile neonatal radiography to nursing personnel. Frequently, as soon as the technologist enters the unit or nursery, someone yells "x-ray" and the nurses vacate the premises. Poznanski (1) showed that 1 foot is the magic distance for vertical beam films with mobile equipment (Fig. 1-28A); that is, personnel in the neonatal nursery need not wear lead aprons or leave their patients so long as they are at least 1 foot outside the primary x-ray beam. There is some danger from horizontal beam films (supine cross-table views), however, and in that case the technologist must be certain that other neonates and unprotected personnel are not in the path of the primary x-ray beam (Fig. 1-28B).

Fluoroscopy

It is almost always necessary to bring the neonate to the radiology department for fluoroscopy and contrast studies. This can be done safely if there is proper communication among the neonatologist, radiologist, intensive care nurse, radiology nurse, and radiologic technologist. The technologist must prepare the fluoroscopy room so that equipment for maintaining body temperature (28), suction, and resuscitation is readily available. An attendant from the nursery (preferably both a nurse and a physician) should accompany the neonate.

Supplementary Conventional Radiography

Horizontal Beam Radiography

The horizontal beam technique (x-ray beam parallel to the floor) is valuable in pediatric radiology (Table 1-2) (70–73).

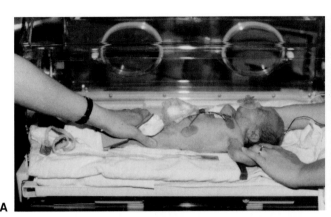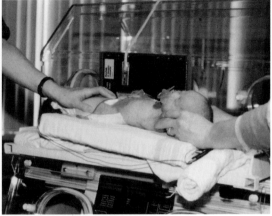

A   B

FIG. 1-28. Techniques for newborn abdomen radiography. A: AP supine view of the abdomen in the isolette. Exposure is no more than background if one stays at least 1 foot from the primary (vertical) beam. **B:** However, the adjacent isolette is exposed to the primary beam when the horizontal beam technique is used for a lateral view of the abdomen.

A cross-table, horizontal beam lateral view may be used as one of the three views of a skull series (Appendix 2). It is always used during cerebral angiography. If supine chest radiography is performed in the newborn nursery or for infants and uncooperative young children, the lateral view is obtained by the horizontal beam technique (see Fig. 1-13). In the decubitus position, the dependent lung is normally underaerated, whereas the elevated lung is normally hyperaerated. Thus, the horizontal beam AP view of the chest

TABLE 1-2. *Potential uses of horizontal beam radiography*

Skull
  Horizontal lateral view
    Sella turcica
    Sutures
  Paranasal sinuses
    Fluid level
  Cerebral angiography
Spine
  Myelography
  Fracture
Skeleton
  Hip dislocation
  Fracture
Chest
  Routine lateral view
    Neonate
    Infant
  Airway evaluation unless contraindicated
  Pneumonia
  Foreign body in airway
  Pneumothorax
  Pneumomediastinum
  Pleural effusion
Abdomen
  Obstruction
  Pneumoperitoneum
  Ascites
  Necrotizing enterocolitis

in the decubitus position may be used for the diagnosis of pneumonia in the nondependent lung (72) and airway foreign body (70) as well as pleural effusion in the dependent lung. A cross-table, supine lateral view of the abdomen is the most sensitive radiologic examination for pneumoperitoneum in the neonate (73). In infants with necrotizing enterocolitis, the cross-table lateral view detects air in the portal venous system (71) as well as pneumoperitoneum (73). The cross-table, prone lateral view is excellent when low colonic obstruction is suspected in the neonate (Fig. 1-29). Other examples of the value of horizontal beam radiography are illustrated in later chapters.

Mobile Radiography

As previously discussed, a mobile radiographic unit is preferable for neonatal radiology. Such units are small, easily maneuvered, and battery-operated or readily charged from standard 110- or 220-volt lines. Capacitor-discharge units are adequate for mobile (bedside) radiographs of the chest, abdomen, and extremities in infants and children. Because the actual kilovoltage of a capacitor-discharge unit falls 1 kV for every 1 mA required for the exposure, these units are not good choices for radiographs of the spine or abdomen in large teenagers. For example, if 10 mA is required, the kVp at the beginning of the exposure will be 10 kVp higher than the at exposure termination. Battery-operated mobile units that produce constant kilovoltage waveforms (55–120 kVp) and tube currents (100–150 mA) during exposures are better suited for procedures that require more than a few mAs of total exposure.

Fluoroscopy

Image intensification is mandatory for fluoroscopy of children. A number of techniques significantly reduce expo-

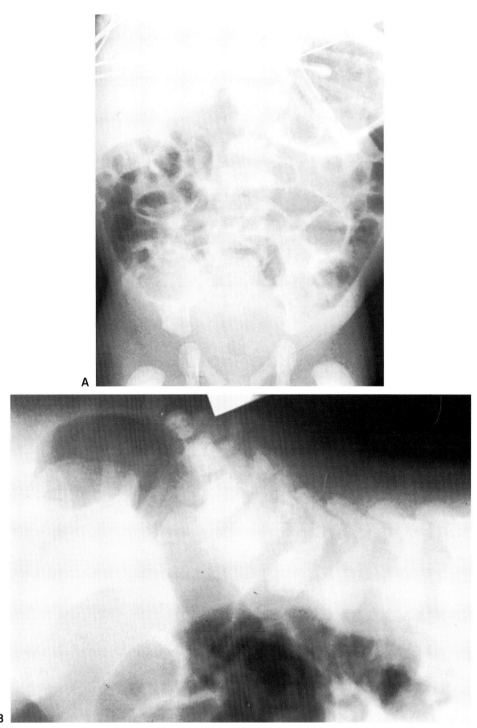

FIG. 1-29. Value of prone cross-table lateral film. A: AP supine film of the abdomen. This neonate has abdominal distention. Gas is seen within what appears to be small and large bowel, but no air is seen in the rectum. The possibility of low colonic obstruction cannot be excluded. **B:** Prone cross-table lateral film shows air in the rectum and excludes low colonic obstruction. Bowel distention is paralytic ileus due to sepsis.

sures during fluoroscopy of children with acceptably small losses in image quality. Opening the adjustable iris in front of the TV camera reduces exposure during those parts of an exam when increased quantum mottle is acceptable

(33,43,74). This range of exposures can be increased if necessary by adding adjustable video camera gain (27).

The power curve (kVp plotted against mA) of the automatic brightness system (ABS) illustrates the change of kilovoltage and tube current in response to the change in thickness of patient anatomy in the x-ray beam. This power curve is usually designed by the manufacturer for adults and can result in fluoroscopic techniques with as little as 45 kVp and 1 mA when infants are imaged. This technique increases the patient dose rate to levels three to four times higher than with the appropriate technique of 65 kVp and 0.2 mA. To achieve these substantial dose savings with minimal loss of image quality, the ABS should be modified by the manufacturer to deliver the appropriate kV despite the wide range of pediatric patient sizes.

If the room is equipped with variable–rate pulsed fluoroscopy, the ABS must control the pulse width (ideally 3–4 milliseconds) and tube current during the pulse to provide the proper kV regardless of patient size. Unfortunately, most manufacturers can only provide variable–rate pulsed fluoroscopy with one fixed-pulse width and one fixed-tube current. This results in the ABS seeking the optimum kVp for only one size of patient; this is clearly unsatisfactory for pediatric fluoroscopy. Investigators have shown that a reduction of the pulse rate from 30 frames per second to 7.5 frames per second can be accompanied by a reduction of patient entrance exposure by a factor of 2 with no difference in the noise perceived in the image (75). The loss of temporal information caused by a reduction from 30 to 7.5 frames per second is acceptable for examinations that do not involve rapid motion of the patient's anatomy (75, 76).

During the 1980s, spot films were usually obtained by photographing the output phosphor of the image intensifier on 100- or 105-mm film. This type of optically coupled spot-film camera decreased the radiation dose by at least 75% from that of a conventional spot-film device, which used a cassette film-screen combination.

In the 1990s, digital spot-film cameras have virtually replaced 100- or 105-mm film. These digital imaging devices decrease radiation dose an additional 50% when compared to 100-mm cameras; image quality is similar or better, and the digital camera allows more efficient management of the images. Digital spot-film cameras allow image retention (last-image hold), image manipulation, digital data storage, and information transfer to remote sites (27,77). The image manipulation features allow the enhancement of the most critical image. Most digital systems allow frame averaging to smooth the quantum mottle, although at the cost of sharpness. This loss of sharpness can then be recovered by digital edge enhancement, which improves sharpness along with the undesirable enhancement of quantum mottle. If these two image manipulations are balanced properly, digital systems can produce nonsubtracted images with enhanced edges with no net increase in noise level.

Some digital spot-film cameras can also produce digitally subtracted images using a mask and a temporally separated contrast image. This technique enhances small changes in contrast in the image; the required gain applied to the image also enhances the quantum mottle. This noise enhancement in the subtracted image requires a 10-fold increase in dose

compared to nonsubtracted digital images for acceptable noise levels of the image. It is imperative that the manufacturer of digital spot-film cameras with both capabilities allows the dose level to the patient to be changed appropriately depending on the mode of imaging.

The faster exposure times used with a 105-mm or digital camera are particularly valuable for the uncooperative child (48). Videotape should be used to record motion, and spot films should be used to document anatomy. One minute of fluoroscopy is equivalent to 25 conventional spot films produced with a 400-speed cassette film-screen combination, 45 105-mm camera images, 55 digital spot-film images, or 5 digitally subtracted spot-film images.

Conventional Tomography

In theory, the resolution of tomography in children is greater than in tomograms of the same area in adults, as less tissue is radiographed (1). In practice, however, tomography is much less frequently performed in children than in the adult. Tomography is difficult to perform in infants because of respiration and motion. Sedation is often needed for younger patients, and it is difficult even for a very cooperative child to remain completely motionless. With the availability of multiplanar two-dimensional and three-dimensional reformations of CT images, conventional tomography is now mainly used in selected cases of developmental abnormalities of the spine (block vertebra, hemivertebra) (Fig. 1-30) and complex fractures of the spine and extremities.

Nuclear Medicine

Nuclear medicine imaging relies on the external detection of radiopharmaceuticals within the human body. Nuclear medicine imaging methods are relatively noninvasive, safe, and sensitive and are therefore well suited for the evaluation of pediatric patients. The functional information that scintigraphy provides often complements the anatomic information from other imaging modalities. Sometimes nuclear medicine provides the only imaging evidence of pathology. Following their administration by any of a variety of routes, radiotracers and radiopharmaceuticals are imaged as they pass through, are taken up by, or localize in normal and abnormal structures and tissues. These agents are taken up or localized in organs, systems, or lesions by several mechanisms (Table 1-3). The images obtained depict both normal and pathologic processes. Radiopharmaceuticals are given in very small amounts and are physiologically innocuous, i.e., they do not produce significant pharmacologic, hemodynamic, osmotic, or toxic effects. Radiation exposures from their use in diagnostic imaging usually fall in the lower range of radiation exposures from common radiologic examinations. For a complete review of radiation doses in pediatric nuclear medicine, the reader is referred to the work of Stabin (78).

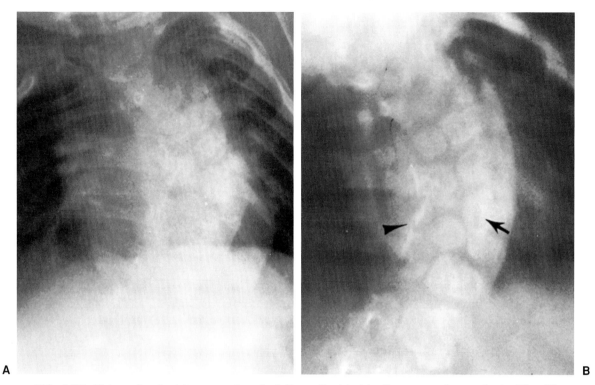

FIG. 1-30. Value of spinal tomography. A: A 7-month-old girl with progressive scoliosis. The AP radiograph shows angular thoracic scoliosis. **B:** AP tomogram confirms a hemivertebra *(arrow)*, a laminar bar *(arrowhead)*, and rib fusions.

The basic principles of nuclear medicine will not be reviewed here. In order to optimize the scintigraphic evaluation of children, however, radiopharmaceutical dosages, imaging techniques, instrumentation, and personnel training will be considered (79).

TABLE 1-3. *Radiopharmaceuticals: mechanisms of uptake and localization*

Regional perfusion or blood flow: 99mTc-MIBI, 99mTc-ECD, 99mTc-HMPAO, 201Tl
Blood pool, first-pass studies: 99mTc-pertechnetate, 99mTc-RBCs
Phagocytosis: 99mTc-Sulfur colloid
Cellular transport: 99mTc-MAG3, 99mTc-DISIDA, 123I-orthoiodohippurate
Glomerular filtration: 99mTc-DTPA
Specific cellular localization: 99mTc-DMSA, 123I-iodine, 123I-MIBG
Capillary blockade: 99mTc-MAA
Dilution, diffusion, or direct infusion: 99mTc-DTPA, 111In-DTPA, 99mTc-pertechnetate, 99mTc-Sulfur colloid
Ventilation: 133Xe, 81mKr
Ciliary motion: 99mTc-Sulfur colloid
Fluid transport in lung: 99mTc-DTPA
Lymphatic flow: 99mTc-Sulfur colloid
Adsorption: 99mTc-MDP
Infection: 67Ga, 99mTc-WBCs, 111In-WBCs
Gastrointestinal content flow: 99mTc-Sulfur colloid
Splenic sequestration: 99mTc-denatured RBCs

Radiopharmaceutical Dosages

In estimating the dose to be administered for pediatric scintigraphy, the goal is to keep the child's absorbed radiation to a minimum possible while obtaining a study of diagnostic quality. Lower and higher administered doses result in futile or unnecessary radiation exposure. Administered doses are generally calculated by adjusting the usual adult doses for body weight or body surface area; calculations based on body weight are simpler. Special consideration must be given to neonates and infants, for whom the concept of minimal total dose must be applied. The minimal total dose is the radiopharmaceutical dose below which the study will be inadequate regardless of the body weight or surface area. The minimal total dose depends on the type of examination, the duration of the examination, and the available instrumentation. In some cases, dynamic studies require a higher photon flux and thus higher doses than static studies. Table 1-4 lists the usual radiopharmaceutical dose schedule at Children's Hospital, Boston (80). These are given only as a guide; other institutions and physicians will vary in their practices and preferences.

Imaging Techniques

Imaging techniques include dynamic and static planar scintigraphy, single photon emission computed tomography

TABLE 1-4. *Pediatric nuclear medicine procedures and usual radiopharmaceutical doses[a]*

Procedure	Radiopharmaceutical	Route of administration	Dose/kg		Minimal total dose		Dose/70 kg		Comments
			mCi	MBq	mCi	MBq	mCi	MBq	
Radionuclide angiocardiography	99mTc-Petechnetate	Intravenous	0.2	7.4	2.0	74	10–20	370–740	
Thyroid scintigraphy	99mTc-Petechnetate	Intravenous	0.03	1.11	0.2	7.4	2.0	74	
Detection of ectopic gastric mucosa	99mTc-Petechnetate	Intravenous	0.1	3.7	0.2	7.5	10	370	
Scrotal scintigraphy	99mTc-Petechnetate	Intravenous	0.1	3.7	2.0	74	15	555	
Pulmonary perfusion scintigraphy	99mTc-MAA	Intravenous	0.05	1.85	0.2	7.4	3	111	
Right-to-left shunts	99mTc-MAA	Intravenous	0.02	0.74	0.1	3.7	1	37	<10,000 particles
Pulmonary perfusion scintigraphy	133Xe on saline	Intravenous	0.3	11.1	5	185	30	1110	
Regional cerebral perfusion	99mTc-HMPAO	Intravenous	0.2–0.3	7.4–11.1	1.0	37	10–20	370–740	
Regional cerebral perfusion	99mTc-ECD	Intravenous	0.2–0.3	7.4–11.1	1.0	37	10–30	370–1110	
Myocardial perfusion scintigraphy	99mTc-MIBI	Intravenous	0.4	14.8	2	74	10–30	370–1110	
Detection of tumor activity	99mTc-MIBI	Intravenous	0.4	14.8	2	74	10–30	370–1110	
Hepatobiliary scintigraphy	99mTc-Disofenin	Intravenous	0.05	1.85	0.5	18.5	2.5	92.5	
Hepatic and splenic scintigraphy	99mTc-Sulfur colloid	Intravenous	0.05	1.85	0.1	3.7	3.0	111	
Detection of bleeding	99mTc-Sulfur colloid	Intravenous	0.05	1.85	0.1	3.7	3.0	111	
Gated and non-gated blood imaging, detection of bleeding	99mTc-RBCs	Intravenous	0.2	7.4	1.0	37	20	740	
Splenic scintigraphy	99mTc-Heat-treated RBCs	Intravenous	0.05	1.85	0.5	18.5	3.0	111	
Skeletal scintigraphy	99mTc-Methylene diphosphonate (MDP)	Intravenous	0.2	7.4	1.0	37	20	740	Radionuclide angiography[b]
Renal cortical scintigraphy	99mTc-Dimercapto-succinic acid (DMSA)	Intravenous	0.05	1.85	0.2	7.4	3.0	111	
Dynamic renal scintigraphy, indirect radionuclide cystography	99mTc-MAG3	Intravenous	0.2	7.4	1	37	10	370	Radionuclide angiography[b]
Dynamic renal scintigraphy, indirect radionuclide cystography	99mTc-DTPA	Intravenous	0.1	3.7	0.3	11.1	8	296	Radionuclide angiography[b]
Dynamic renal scintigraphy, indirect radionuclide cystography	99mTc-Gluco-heptonate	Intravenous	0.2	7.4	1	37	10	370	Radionuclide angiography[b]
Localization of inflammation, infection	99mTc-WBCs	Intravenous	0.2	7.4	0.5	11.5	20	740	
Localization of inflammation, infection, tumor activity detection	67Ga-citrate	Intravenous	0.04	1.48	0.25	9.25	3	111	SPECT dose: maximum 5 mCi (185 MBq)
Myocardial perfusion scintigraphy	201Tl as thallous chloride	Intravenous	0.03	1.11	0.15	5.55	2.0	74	
Detection of tumor activity, brain	201Tl as thallous chloride	Intravenous	0.03–0.05	1.11–1.85	0.5	18.5	2.0	74	
Detection of neuroblastoma, pheochromocytoma	123I-MIBG	Intravenous	0.2	7.4	1.0	37	10	370	

(continued)

TABLE 1-4. *Continued*

Procedure	Radiopharmaceutical	Route of administration	Dose/kg		Minimal total dose		Dose/70 kg		Comments
			mCi	MBq	mCi	MBq	mCi	MBq	
Detection of neuroblastoma, pheochromocytoma	^{131}I-MIBG	Intravenous	0.014	.52	0.1	3.7	1.0	37	
Gastroesophageal reflux, gastric emptying, aspiration	^{99m}Tc-Sulfur colloid	Oral	0.015	.55	0.2	7.4	1.0	37	
Thyroid scintigraphy	^{123}I NaI	Oral	0.005	0.185	0.025	0.93	0.3	11.1	
Localization of inflammation, infection	^{111}In-WBCs	Intravenous	0.005	0.185	0.05	1.85	0.3	11.1	

Procedure	Radiopharmaceutical	Route of administration	Dose
Radionuclide cystography	^{99m}Tc-Petechnetate	Intravesical	Total dose: 1–2 mCi [37–74 MBq]
CSF shunt	^{99m}Tc-Petechnetate	Shunt	Total dose: 0.5 mCi [9.25 MBq] 0.05–0.1 ml
Esophageal motility	^{99m}Tc-Sulfur colloid	Oral	Concentration 0.005 mCi [0.2 MBq]/ml, Total dose: 0.2–1.0 mCi [7.4–3.7 MBq] in 30 ml
Ventilation	^{133}Xe Gas	Inhalation	Total dose: 8–30 mCi [296–1110 MBq]
Ventilation, membrane transport, and vascular washout	^{99m}Tc-DTPA aerosol	Inhalation	Total dose: 30 mCi [1110 MBq] in 3 ml in aerosolizer
Ventilation and cilliary motion	^{99m}Tc-Sulfur colloid	Inhalation	Total dose: 30–40 mCi [1110–1480 MBq] in 2–3 ml in aerosolizer
Cisternography, CSF shunt assessment, rhinorrhea	^{111}In-DTPA	Intrathecal	Total dose: 0.05–0.5 mCi [1.87–18.5 MBq]
Cisternography, CSF shunt assessment, rhinorrhea	^{99m}Tc-DTPA	Intrathecal	Total dose: 1.0–3.0 mCi [37–111 MBq]
Lymphoscintigraphy	^{99m}Tc-Sulfur colloid, ^{99m}Tc-Antimony sulfide	Intradermal	Each dose: 1 mCi [37 MBq]/0.1 ml
Dacryoscintigraphy	^{99m}Tc-Petechnetate	Conjunctival	Total dose: 0.1–0.2 mCi [3.7–7.4 MBq] in 100 μl
Salivagram	^{99m}Tc-Sulfur colloid	Sublingual	Total dose: 0.3 mCi [11.1 MBq] in 100 μl
Metastatic survey	^{131}I NaI	Intravenous/oral	Total dose: 1–2 mCi [37–74 MBq]

[a] Usual doses at Children's Hospital, Boston; from Treves (79).
[b] Radionuclide angiography doses are: 0.2 mCi [7.4 MBq], minimum 2–3 mCi [74–111 MBq], maximum 10–20 mCi [370–740 MBq].
WBC, white blood cell.

(SPECT), and positron emission tomography (PET) (81–84).

Dynamic scintigraphy provides information about rapid time-dependent phenomena, such as blood flow or cell transport, by continuous sequential image recording. The duration of the study and the rate at which images are obtained and displayed depend on the process being studied. For example, radionuclide angiocardiographic determination of ventricular ejection fraction requires a minimum recording rate of 25 frames per second for 25 seconds, whereas hepatobiliary scintigraphy for suspected cholecystitis is recorded with serial 30-second frames for 60 minutes. Static scintigraphy can be obtained in either a whole-body or "multispot" format. Whole-body imaging requires continuous recording as the gamma camera moves along the body. The global evaluation that this provides is especially useful in skeletal scintigraphy, where specific patterns of abnormal tracer distribution can be identified in certain disease states, such as child abuse and metastatic disease. Whole-body scintigraphy requires that the patient remain still longer than is needed for spot images. Multispot scintigraphy results in images of better spatial resolution than is provided by the whole-body technique. Planar scintigraphy with modern systems achieves spatial resolution on the order of 6–9 mm.

Magnification scintigraphy is an essential part of pediatric nuclear medicine. It is frequently required in evaluating osteomyelitis, avascular necrosis of bone, and renal scarring or pyelonephritis. Optical magnification using a pinhole collimator with a 2- to 3-mm aperture provides the highest spatial resolution (1.5–2.0 mm) attainable in nuclear medicine.

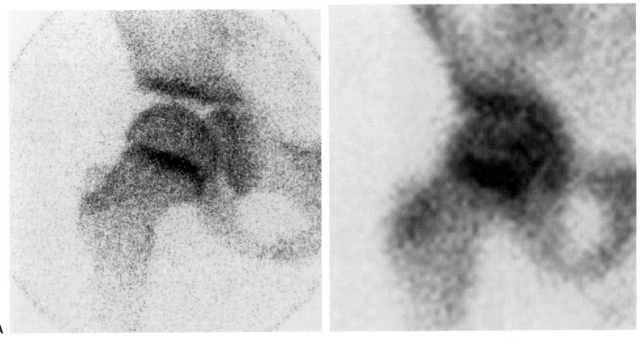

A   B

FIG. 1-31. Magnification skeletal scintigraphy. Magnification skeletal scintigraphy (^{99m}Tc-MDP) of the right hip of a 5-year-old patient. Note the markedly superior spatial resolution of pinhole collimation **(A)** over electronic magnification **(B)**.

Electronic magnification (zoom) increases the image size but does not improve resolution and is not a reasonable alternative to pinhole collimation (Fig. 1-31) (82,85).

SPECT shows radionuclide distribution accurately and in three dimensions. Pediatric applications of this technology include renal, skeletal, myocardial, and brain imaging. Resolution on the order of 6–9 mm can be achieved with current technology if high- or preferably ultrahigh-resolution collimation is used and strict attention is paid to optimal patient positioning and quality control of the imaging unit (84).

PET assesses regional tissue physiology with positron-emitting isotopes of biologically important elements such as oxygen (^{15}O, $T_{1/2}$ = 2.1 minutes), nitrogen (^{13}N, $T_{1/2}$ = 10 minutes), and carbon (^{11}C, $T_{1/2}$ = 20.1 minutes). Additionally, fluorine-18 (^{18}F, $T_{1/2}$ = 110 minutes) can replace hydrogen in many biomolecules. Demonstration of altered metabolic activity in viable tumor, ischemic myocardium, and epileptogenic zones indicates the useful clinical applications of PET.

Instrumentation

The gamma camera is the principal detection instrument for nuclear medicine. Gamma cameras can be classified according to the number of detectors which they possess. The most common system, a single-detector system, has one crystal, a collimator, and photomultiplier tubes. Dual- and triple-detector systems are also widely used. Single- and dual-detector systems designed for planar scintigraphy alone or both planar scintigraphy and SPECT are available. Some are able to acquire images in the whole-body format. Triple-detector systems are specially designed and optimized for SPECT but are also capable of planar imaging.

Single-detector systems are the most versatile and the most commonly used. Dynamic scintigraphy, whole-body and multispot static planar scintigraphy, pinhole magnification scintigraphy, and SPECT can be performed with a single-detector gamma camera. The configuration of single- and some dual-detector systems allows easy access to the patient. This can be critical for an acutely ill child and also allows a reassuring parent or technologist to calm an anxious child during image acquisition.

The primary advantage of multiple-detector systems over single-detector systems is the shorter examination time. This limits the need for sedation in all children and allows rapid completion of studies in acutely ill children. Dual-detector systems enable the simultaneous acquisition of opposing planar projections, whereas triple-detector systems allow the simultaneous acquisition of planar images in various obliquities (Figs. 1-32, 1-33, 1-34). Compared to SPECT on a single-detector system, SPECT images of an equal count density can be obtained in half the time with a dual-detector and one third the time with a triple-detector system. While multiple-detector systems shorten imaging time, the required configuration limits physical access to the patient. Pinhole collimation is impossible with some dual- and all currently available triple-detector systems.

Whether performing planar imaging or SPECT, collimator choice is critically important. Because of the small size of the structures imaged in children, a high-resolution or, better, an ultrahigh-resolution collimator should be used whenever the photon flux and the energy of the gamma rays permit this.

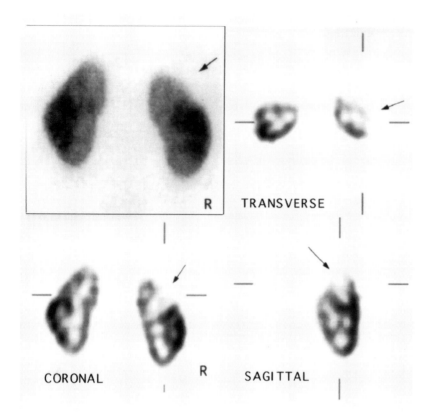

FIG. 1-32. Renal ^{99m}Tc-DMSA scintigraphy in acute pyelonephritis. Planar image *(arrow, top left)* suggests reduced tracer uptake in the upper pole of the right kidney. Single photon emission computed tomography (SPECT) verifies the cortical defect of pyelonephritis in three planes *(arrows)*.

A relevant consideration for all SPECT systems is that manufacturers seldom address peculiarities of pediatric imaging. Special modifications in table size, restraining devices, and autocontouring may therefore be desirable or even necessary.

PET systems are designed exclusively for coincidence detection of the 511-keV gamma rays emitted during positron annihilation. Because of the expense of PET systems and the on-site cyclotron necessitated by the short physical half-lives of many PET radiopharmaceuticals, PET is not widely available. Imaging 511-keV photons is, however, possible with single- and dual-detector SPECT devices fitted with high-energy collimators. Methods of coincidence detection on a dual-detector SPECT system are also being developed. These new techniques for imaging positron emitters with a conventional gamma camera and the fact that ^{18}F has a physical half-life long enough for remote production suggest that PET will soon be used more widely.

No single instrument can perform all nuclear medicine examinations optimally, especially in pediatrics. Compromises between versatility and performance are necessary.

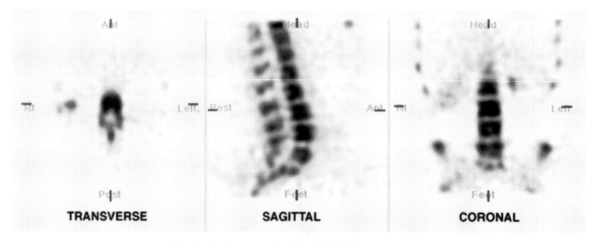

FIG. 1-33. Normal skeletal SPECT of the spine.

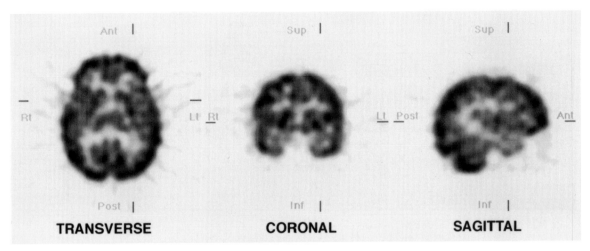

Ant | Sup | Sup |

Rt   Lt   Rt   Lt   Post   Ant

Post | Inf | Inf |

TRANSVERSE   **CORONAL**   **SAGITTAL**

FIG. 1-34. Normal perfusion brain SPECT.

Personnel

Pediatric nuclear medicine technologists and physicians must be able to handle children and parents during examination. They must be patient, understanding, and compassionate. An ability to allay the child's natural fears and a willingness to help distract the child during the examination will minimize the need for sedation. In fact, sedation should rarely be required for pediatric scintigraphy, as most examinations can be performed with simple restraining techniques after the child's trust is gained (Fig. 1-35). A small video monitor playing a program of interest to the child, placed for easy viewing, is helpful in distracting and relaxing many patients during the examination (Figs. 1-35 and 1-36). How-

ever, neurologically impaired patients undergoing brain SPECT usually need sedation.

Training in pediatric nuclear medicine is a prerequisite for all practitioners; this cannot be overemphasized. Pediatric nuclear medicine practitioners must know the fundamental principles of their science. In adult practice, imaging protocols can be applied to most patients. In pediatric nuclear medicine it is often necessary to tailor an examination according to the information required and the ability of the child to cooperate. Understanding the strengths and limitations of various imaging techniques allows the examination to be adapted to the child rather than forcing the child to adapt to the examination. Technologists and physicians must have a detailed knowledge of equipment capabilities and

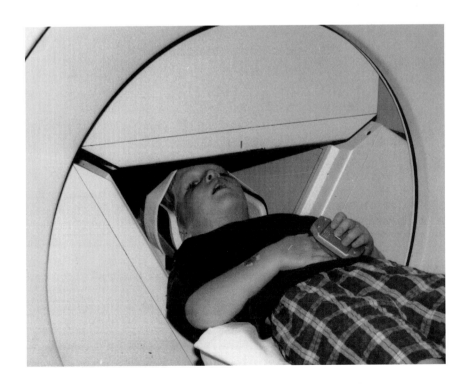

FIG. 1-35. Cooperative young child undergoing a brain SPECT.

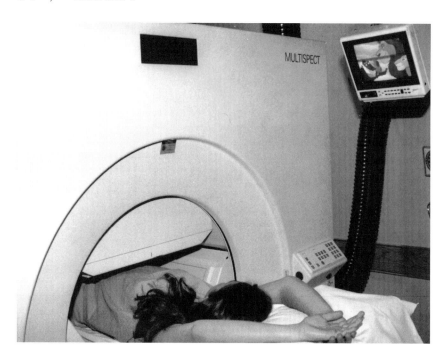

FIG. 1-36. Use of video during nuclear scintigraphy.

of such considerations as pinhole magnification, electronic zoom, collimators, and the use of SPECT reconstruction filters. Since the most frequent route of radiopharmaceutical administration is intravenous, technologists must be expert at placing and securing intravenous lines.

Ultrasonography

Ultrasonography is ideal for imaging children for a number of reasons: (a) It uses no ionizing radiation; (b) there is no evidence that the energy levels used in diagnostic ultrasound harm humans (86); (c) sedation is almost never required; (d) all examinations can be performed at the bedside if necessary, which eliminates the need to transport a sick child to the radiology department; (e) the paucity of fat in the pediatric abdomen and the smaller size of the patient allow detailed visualization of abdominal anatomy; (f) the sonographer has direct access to the child and can assess his or her overall status and specific symptoms.

Equipment

State-of-the-art pediatric ultrasonography is performed using real-time ultrasound equipment. Real-time ultrasonography permits both dynamic and static anatomic evaluation of the pediatric patient. A wide range of transducer frequencies (2–10 MHz) is used in children because of their large variation in size. Nearly every type of examination performed in adults is performed in children as well.

Doppler ultrasonography can be used to evaluate blood flow (87–95). Structures and processes evaluated by Doppler in children include the following:

1. Intracranial arterial and venous structures in the premature infant, the asphyxiated infant, or the infant being treated with extracorporeal membrane oxygenation (ECMO)
2. Hepatic vascularity in suspected portal hypertension and before and after liver transplantation
3. Renovascular disease
4. Renal transplantation
5. The painful scrotum
6. Peripheral venous structures, for patency prior to placement of vascular catheters, and, occasionally, during placement of catheters
7. Deep venous thrombosis
8. Vascular anomalies of the soft tissues

Pulsed Doppler and color flow Doppler ultrasonography, the most commonly used Doppler modalities in pediatrics, demonstrate the direction and velocity of blood flow. Power Doppler shows the amplitude of blood flow better than standard color Doppler techniques. However, power Doppler does not reveal the direction of blood flow and is very motion-sensitive; the image is significantly degraded by patient motion (96). The role of power Doppler in pediatric ultrasonography continues to be clarified (97).

In general, whenever a mass is identified during ultrasonography, its vascularity should be evaluated with Doppler sonography. The inferior vena cava should be evaluated to look for tumor thrombus, and the aorta and the vessels of the organ of origin should be interrogated to show the vascular supply of the lesion. Whenever a cyst or cyst-like lesion is discovered, Doppler evaluation is used to show whether the lesion is a vascular structure.

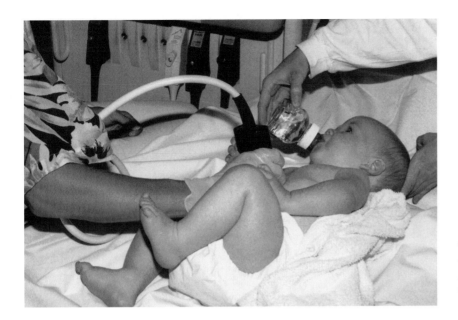

FIG. 1-37. Glucose water as pacifier. This technique can be particularly useful when Doppler studies are being performed and the child must be kept very still. Bottles of glucose water and nipples should be readily available in the ultrasound suite.

Scanning Techniques

Sedation is almost never needed for ultrasonography. A pacifier or the finger of a parent in the mouth will often keep a restless infant still. If the stomach need not be empty, feeding the baby may induce sleep. Glucose water can be substituted for the baby's formula (Fig. 1-37). If a baby or small child is extremely restless, the technologist may need help in holding the child still. It is often best if a familiar person such as a parent does this (Fig. 1-38). Immobilization with sandbags or other devices is rarely necessary.

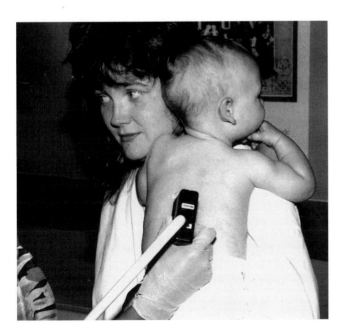

FIG. 1-38. One possible position for ultrasonagraphy. The baby's mother holds her son against her chest while his kidneys are scanned in the sagittal plane.

Babies must be kept warm during the examination. Warm gel is used for acoustic coupling. The gel, which cools rapidly, should be removed from the skin immediately after the examination. Warming lights angled toward the baby and away from the ultrasound machine help maintain body temperature, as does covering the baby's head. In the intensive care unit, the study must often be done through side ports in the incubator after carefully washing transducers and hands.

The general approach to the older child is similar to that for adults. Parents are encouraged to stay in the examining room, unless the patient is an adolescent who prefers privacy.

Commonly Performed Examinations

Ultrasonography is best done by a thorough, orderly approach, followed fairly rigidly. After routine images, additional images of an area of interest are often needed. Suggested imaging sequences for common ultrasonographic examinations and suggestions for transducer selection are provided next.

Pediatric Abdomen

A screening abdominal ultrasound examination should be standardized. After beginning with transverse views of the liver and its vessels, transverse views of the pancreas, gallbladder, and right kidney follow. The relationship of the superior mesenteric artery and vein is evaluated; abnormal orientation of these vessels suggests malrotation. Then longitudinal views are obtained of the liver, pancreas, gallbladder, aorta, inferior vena cava, and right kidney. The left upper quadrant is saved for next-to-last because children are most ticklish there. Longitudinal and transverse views of the spleen and left kidney are obtained. Views of the urinary bladder and the space behind it show the presence or absence of ascites. The child is then placed prone for additional images of the kidneys, unless the likelihood of renal pathology is low.

A transducer of the highest frequency which allows adequate penetration should be used for abdominal ultrasound. In the infant, a 5-MHz linear array or sector transducer is used. A 7.5-MHz linear array transducer can be used in prematures. In toddlers and small school-aged children, a 5-MHz transducer is appropriate. For older or chubby children, transducers appropriate for adults are used.

Pediatric Urinary System

In ultrasonographic screening of the urinary system, the bladder should be imaged before the kidneys and ureters; the child who is not toilet-trained may urinate as the transducer is moved over his abdomen. The kidneys should be imaged in the longitudinal and transverse planes beginning with the patient supine. If the kidneys are not seen in their expected locations, an ectopic kidney should be searched for in the lower abdomen and pelvis. A dilated ureter, if present, will be seen in the coronal plane and will connect with the renal pelvis.

The child is then placed prone for additional images of the kidneys in the longitudinal and transverse planes. The most reproducible renal lengths (important in the child being followed for vesicoureteral reflux) are obtained in the sagittal plane with the child prone (Fig. 1-39).

If hematuria or hypertension is present, views of the aorta, inferior vena cava, and adrenal beds should be added to

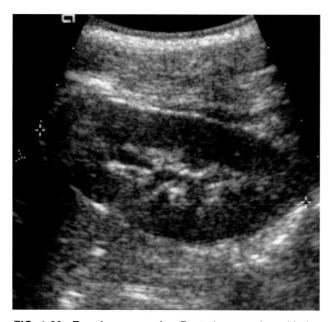

FIG. 1-39. Renal sonography. Posterior scanning with the child in the prone position or held in a parent's arms (as in Fig. 1-38) is routinely performed to measure the renal length.

this routine. Doppler interrogation of the kidneys, if this technology is available, should also be done.

Pediatric Pelvis

A distended urinary bladder is needed to see the uterus and ovaries. If the bladder is empty, the patient is encouraged to take fluids by mouth and is rescanned at short intervals until bladder distention is adequate. If the oral intake is contraindicated and prompt examination is needed, filling the bladder by intravenous fluids or urethral catheter should be considered. In the sexually active female, transvaginal ultrasonography is performed when appropriate.

The normal uterus is visible at all ages. The ovaries may not be visible in the young child, as they are small and can be obscured by bowel gas.

Brain and Hip

The reader is referred to Chapter 2 for techniques of cranial ultrasonography and to Chapter 5 for ultrasound of the hip.

Common Indications

Ultrasonography is pivotal in pediatric imaging and is frequently the first imaging study performed. Table 1-5 lists abnormalities that are commonly imaged by ultrasonography; their sonographic findings are discussed in later chapters (98–129).

Computed Tomography

CT, conceptualized by Oldendorf in 1961 and developed as an imaging modality by Hounsfield in 1973, has had a tremendous impact on diagnostic radiology in general and pediatric radiology in particular (130–175). The basic advantage of CT is that it demonstrates tissue anatomy with precision and clarity. The spatial resolution and anatomic detail of CT are superior to that of any other cross-sectional imaging modality except MRI, and occasionally they are superior to MRI. It permits two-dimensional visualization of entire anatomic sections of tissue, which helps determine the extent of disease. The technique is not operator-dependent and permits accurate measurement of tissue attenuation. Contrast enhancement shows blood flow to an organ or a lesion. Bolus contrast injection permits excellent visualization of vascular structures, such as the inferior vena cava, renal veins, aorta, brachiocephalic vessels, and circle of Willis. Anatomic and physiologic information can be obtained even in severely compromised organs. Structures can be visualized despite overlying gas and bone.

CT is less invasive rather than noninvasive (136,142), as it uses radiation and requires alteration of the patient's envi-

TABLE 1-5. *Pediatric indications for and abnormalities evaluated by ultrasonography*

Central Nervous System
  Brain
    Intracranial hemorrhage
    Periventricular leukomalacia
    Stroke
    Asphyxia
    Hemorrhage before or during ECMO therapy
    Ventricular dilatation
    Vascular abnormality (Doppler)
    Structural abnormality in the newborn
    Meningitis
    Congenital infection
    Craniomegaly
    Intraoperative: shunt, tumor
  Spine
    Spinal dysraphism
    Intraoperative: tumor; syrinx
Face and Neck
  Adenopathy
  Abscess
  Branchial cleft cyst
  Fibromatosis colli
  Lymphatic malformation
  Vascular anomaly
  Thyroglossal duct cyst
  Thyroid mass
Chest
  Congenital heart disease
  Pleural effusion
  Diaphragm motion
  Intrathoracic mass
  Chest wall mass
  Pericardial effusion
Extremities
  Developmental dysplasia of hip
  Joint effusion
  Soft tissue mass
  Foreign body
  Infection
  Deep venous thrombosis
  Vascular shunts

Genitourinary System
  Kidney
    Urinary tract infection
    Hydronephrosis
    Multicystic dysplastic kidney
    Other cystic disease
    Urolithiasis
    Renal vein thrombosis
    Aortic or renal artery thrombosis
    Hypertension
    Renal transplantation
    Neoplasm
  Adrenal Gland
    Hemorrhage
    Neuroblastoma, other tumors
  Scrotum
    Cryptorchidism
    Torsion of testis
    Epididymitis or orchitis
    Torsion of appendix, testis, or epididymitis
    Hernia
    Trauma
    Tumor
    Precocious puberty
  Uterus and ovaries
    Pregnancy
    Precocious puberty
    Amenorrhea, primary and secondary
    Ambiguous genitalia
    Ovarian torsion
    Pelvic mass
Gastrointestinal Tract
  Pyloric stenosis
  Appendicitis
  Intestinal duplication
  Ascites
  Choledochal cyst
  Cholelithiasis
  Hepatosplenomegaly
  Liver transplant evaluation
  Pancreatitis
  Abscess
  Tumor of solid organ or bowel
  Mass

ECMO, extracorporeal membrane oxygenation.

ronment. Sedation and contrast enhancement are frequently required. The paucity of fat in children makes delineation of the anatomy of the mediastinum and retroperitoneum difficult without contrast enhancement.

Basic Physical Principles

Conventional radiography is based on the variable attenuation of an x-ray beam as it passes through tissue. Because only the sum total of this attenuation is recorded on radiographic film, conventional radiographs record differences in attenuation of approximately 10%; this prevents detailed characterization of soft tissue densities. The densities that can be visualized on conventional diagnostic radiographs are air, fat, soft tissue, bone, and heavy metal; distinction between two soft tissues is difficult and often impossible.

CT passes many highly collimated x-ray beams through one cross-sectional slice of tissue from different angles. This multitude of data permits a computer to determine and record the x-ray absorption in a specific volume element (voxel) as small as $0.2 \times 0.2 \times 1.0$ to 10.0 mm. This detection system is much more sensitive than conventional radiography, distinguishing differences in attenuation coefficient as small as 0.1%. It permits identification of various components (subarachnoid space, white matter, gray matter, and ventricles) of soft tissue (brain). The technique is based on the ability of a computer to determine the attenuation coefficient (density) of each tissue voxel within a section.

Equipment

There have been many advances since the first clinical applications of CT were reported by Ambrose in 1973. *First-generation CT systems* consisted of a pencil beam x-ray source and a single detector. A frame was moved linearly so that the beam scanned through the tissue section and the detector moved concomitantly to record numerous attenuation coefficients. After this first linear scan (''translation'') had been completed, the entire frame was rotated on a gantry through a small angle (''rotation''), and another dataset was recorded. *Second-generation CT systems* used a similar translation-rotation movement but had a fan beam source of x-rays and multiple detectors. *Third-generation CT systems* use a fan beam source of x-rays linked with multiple detectors so that the rotational motion of the gantry (without translation) permits increased scan speed and enhanced resolution. *Fourth-generation CT systems* have fixed detectors within the circular gantry so that only the fan beam x-ray source rotates about the patient. *Ultrafast* or *cine CT systems* have fixed detectors within a circular gantry with electronic focusing and movement of the x-ray beam about the patient. *Helical (spiral) CT* utilizes slip-ring technology in the gantry such that the source-detector assembly can rotate continuously (175). With this design, the patient on the table is advanced through the gantry at a constant speed while being exposed continuously to x-rays.

State-of-the-art CT scanners (helical CT systems) produce images of 1.0- to 10.0-mm-thick anatomic sections with a reconstruction time of 4.5 seconds. When operating in the helical mode, one such system provides a continuous 30-second scan at a maximum mA of 330 or a 60-second scan at 240 mA. When operating in the conventional incremental mode, these systems have a scan time of 1 second, a half-scan time of 0.6 second, and an interscan delay of 1 second for a maximum of 33 images at 400 mA or 92 images at 240 mA. With this increase in speed, especially in the helical mode, cooperative adolescents can be scanned during a single breath hold, thus almost eliminating motion artifacts and misregistration. Scans on children too young to hold their breaths nevertheless yield adequate images (167). The need for sedation decreases with increasing familiarity with helical CT scanning (168). Helical CT also allows high-quality multiplanar and 3-D reformations. As the scan data represent a volume rather than a group of planes, one can retrospectively reconstruct data into highly overlapping transaxial images. These can then be used to generate multiplanar and 3-D reformations with smoother margins (175).

CT is a system with great sensitivity but variable specificity; it is still not a radiologic microscope (136). However, it does provide remarkable precision, as it detects density changes within tissue pixels as small as 0.2 mm in diameter.

Techniques

The problems of CT in young children are several: rapid respiratory rate, uncontrolled voluntary movement, little in-

trinsic contrast because of a paucity of fat, and small size of structures of interest. Radiation doses, which are not small, must be taken into account in every case.

Patient Preparation

Food and liquids should be withheld from all infants and children who will be sedated or receive IV contrast medium. This helps accomplish two goals: it makes the child thirsty enough to drink oral contrast, and it diminishes nausea during bolus IV contrast injection. In general, our protocol requires patients to have no solid food for 4 hours and no liquid for 3 hours before receiving IV contrast or sedation. For the newborn this usually translates to withholding the last feeding. Psychological preparation is also very important in obtaining cooperation from frightened children.

Sedation and Monitoring

Sedation is almost always required under age 5, especially when IV contrast is to be used. IV pentobarbital at a dose of 2–6 mg/kg has been used quite safely and successfully in children (176–181). The advantages of IV sedation are its rapid onset and predictable effect (176). It is titratable to the desired effect, and administration of the optimal dose is usually possible. Children under 12 months of age can also be sedated well with oral chloral hydrate at a dose of 50–100 mg/kg. Appendix 6 is the sedation formulary used in the Department of Radiology, Children's Hospital, Boston, in July 1997. As with any potent barbiturate or narcotic, pentobarbital can cause respiratory depression and arrest. The smallest effective dose should always be used.

All sedated children should be monitored both visually, by medical and nursing personnel, and by mechanical means. Pulse oximetry with respiratory monitoring and electrocardiography (ECG) are the safest monitoring tools (29,182).

Patient Positioning and Immobilization

Care should be taken in aligning the patient on the table in the gantry. Seemingly insignificant errors in positioning may lead to serious image distortion, especially in infants and younger children. For scanning the chest or abdomen, the upper extremities are placed above the head and immobilized by use of tape, or hook and loop straps. A strap is placed over the abdomen and another over the thighs and knees. All tubes, catheters, and lines should be removed from the field of view if possible. Artifacts caused by hardware can cause significant degradation of the study (Fig. 1-40).

For routine brain CT examination, the patient is supine and the head is positioned in a foam head holder. The chin is tilted down 15°, which usually allows a scan plane parallel to the skull base and avoids irradiation of the lens. This desired angle can also be achieved by tilting the gantry by

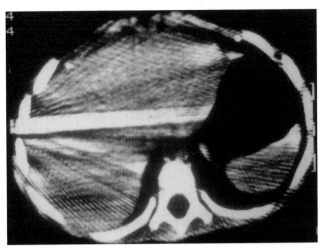

FIG. 1-40. CT artifact. Spray artifacts caused by overlying monitoring wire.

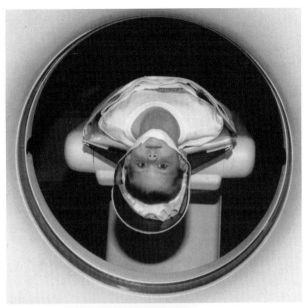

A

an amount determined from a lateral scout projection (Fig. 1-41). For direct coronal imaging of sinuses, orbits, facial bones, and temporal bones, the patient is placed in the coronal head holder (Fig. 1-42) with a 15° sponge under the shoulders to assist hyperextension of the neck. Abnormalities of the cervical spine, neck, and airway preclude direct coronal imaging. Velcro straps are placed around the torso to secure the patient and act as a gentle reminder to remain still (Fig. 1-42A).

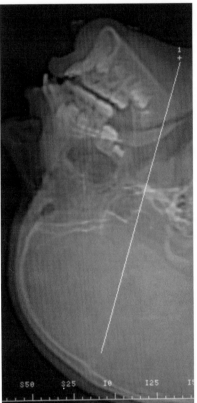

B

FIG. 1-42. Direct coronal CT scan of the head. A: A cooperative 5-year-old boy positioned on the CT table for a direct coronal study. The child's head is supported by the head holder, which is padded with foam and sheets. A Velcro chin strap and Velcro body straps are placed to stabilize his position and to remind him not to move. B: Example of a lateral scout projection of a 10-year-old child for a direct coronal examination of the sinuses. The scan plane (cursor line), perpendicular to the hard palate, is achieved by head positioning and angulation of the gantry.

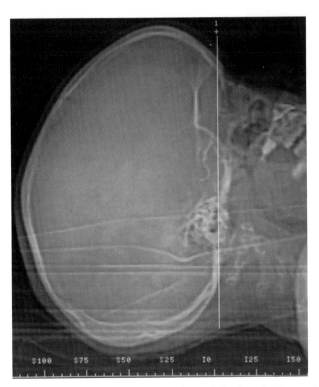

FIG. 1-41. Lateral scout projection of the head. Plane of axial sections (cursor line) is parallel to the skull base to avoid irradiation of the lens.

Intravenous Contrast for Body Imaging

Extensive noncontrast scanning in children is usually not necessary. Noncontrast scans are useful when the detection of calcification or hemorrhage is important, as in the initial evaluation of abdominal masses or when looking for urinary calculi. Noncontrast scans are routine when looking for metastatic disease of the lungs.

Intravenous contrast, used in most other circumstances, can be quite helpful in separating normal from abnormal structures in young children. Contrast should be administered as a rapid intravenous bolus. Drip contrast infusion results in poor tissue and especially vascular opacification and should be avoided. We currently perform rapid hand injections in all patients. The wider use of helical CT in children may lead to greater use of power injectors (169,170,171). When performing incremental (nonhelical)

CT, nonionic intravenous contrast (300–320 mg of iodine per ml) at a dose of 1.5–2 ml/kg (maximum 120 ml) is given. When a combined scan of the chest and abdomen is requested, we suggest delivering half of the total dose at the top of the mediastinum and the remainder, by a second bolus, at the level of the diaphragm. When an abnormality is suspected in the pelvis, one third of the contrast dose can be reserved and given as a bolus at the level of the pelvic inlet.

IV contrast enhancement for spiral CT differs from that for conventional (nonhelical) CT in two important ways: volume required and method of administration (173). Because of the very short scanning time, the volume of contrast can be reduced. In adults, the volume may be reduced by 25% to 50% without sacrificing vascular and tissue opacification (162). Similar reductions can be achieved in children. Excellent opacification can be routinely obtained using nonionic intravenous contrast (300–320 mg of iodine per ml),

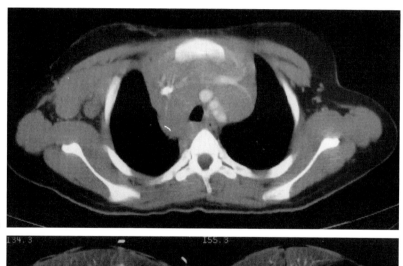

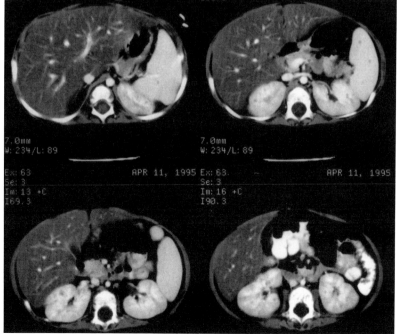

FIG. 1-43. Vascular opacification. Excellent opacification with 1.5 ml/kg of 320 mg of iodine/ml nonionic contrast. **A:** Spiral CT of the mediastinum in a 15-year-old with Hodgkin lymphoma. **B:** Spiral CT of the upper abdomen in a 16-month-old baby with leukemia and disseminated candidiasis of the spleen and kidneys.

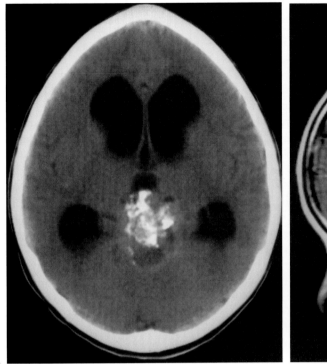
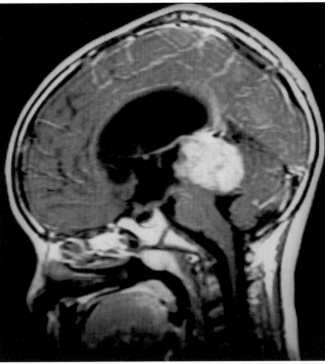

A   B

FIG. 1-44. Pineal mass. A 5-year-old boy with developmental delay and the recent onset of mutism. A: A screening CT examination of the brain without intravenous contrast demonstrates hydrocephalus and a large, partially calcified pineal region mass. B: Conventional spin-echo T1-weighted sagittal midline MRI section with intravenous administration of gadolinium shows a large enhancing pineal tumor with distortion of the adjacent cerebellum, brainstem, and aqueduct of Sylvius.

at a dose of 1.0–1.5 ml/kg by rapid bolus injection (Fig. 1-43). This is especially helpful when the amount of contrast is limited by diminished cardiac or renal function or tenuous venous access. For a combined chest and abdomen spiral CT, a single rapid bolus of contrast at a dose of 2 ml/kg can be administered at the beginning of the scan, rather than separate injections at the top of the mediastinum and at the diaphragm.

Intravenous Contrast for Neuroimaging

Most brain CT examinations are performed without contrast administration. This is because of the common indications: trauma—rule out hemorrhage; suspected shunt malfunction—rule out hydrocephalus. MRI is preferred to a contrast-enhanced CT examination for other indications such as vascular anomalies and newly diagnosed intracranial

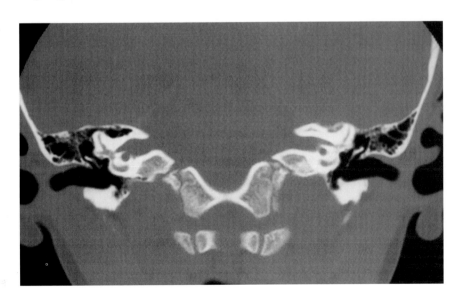

FIG. 1-45. Direct coronal CT of the temporal bones. Note the exquisite demonstration of the normal ossicles, middle ear, and mastoids.

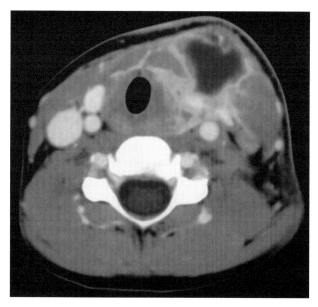

FIG. 1-46. Neck abscess. There is excellent vascular opacification. The left jugular vein is distorted by a low-density left anterior neck abscess.

tumors (Fig. 1-44). When intravenous contrast is needed, a dose of 2 ml/kg (maximum 100 ml) is given as a bolus, and the scan is begun at the end of the bolus. Intravenous contrast is rarely needed for CT study of the sinuses, orbits, facial bones, or temporal bones (Fig. 1-45). CT of the neck, however, is usually performed with intravenous contrast (2 ml/kg, maximum of 100 ml) so that vascular structures of the neck can be distinguished from abnormalities (Fig. 1-46).

Gastrointestinal Contrast

Oral contrast is given for most examinations of the abdomen for tumor, adenopathy, and infection. It is crucial in the evaluation of patients with possible inflammatory bowel disease, abdominal abscess, lymphoma, or metastatic disease because without GI contrast fluid-filled bowel loops may be impossible to distinguish from interloop abscesses, intraperitoneal fluid collections, and abdominal lymph nodes (Fig. 1-47). Oral contrast may be omitted when evaluating parenchymal lesions in the liver, when evaluating a child after blunt abdominal trauma, and when the child is nauseated and likely to vomit during injection of intravenous contrast. If the child cannot or will not take the contrast orally, a nasogastric tube (no. 8 French) may be inserted into the stomach. Contraindications to the use of oral contrast include the absence of a gag or cough reflex, intubation with an uncuffed endotracheal tube, unresponsiveness, and coma. Recommended schedules and volumes of oral contrast are given by patient age in Appendix 7.

Occasionally it is useful to opacify the distal colon and rectum. In those situations, a 1.5% solution of Hypaque can be slowly administered to the child through a small catheter in the rectum. Recommended volumes are 30–50 ml for infants, 50–100 ml for young children, and 100–150 ml for older children.

Scanning Protocols for Body Imaging

When incremental CT techniques are used, dynamic scanning, short slice acquisition times, and thin collimation are the keys to high-quality examinations. Slice acquisition times of less than 2 seconds are necessary to stop normal

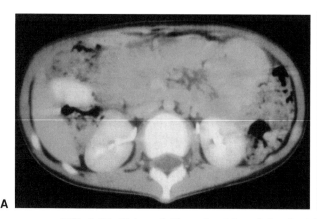
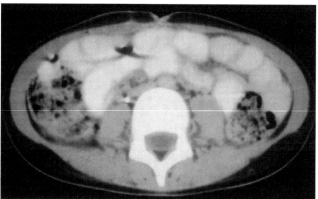

A

B

FIG. 1-47. Value of GI contrast for abdominal CT. A: Scan obtained after inadequate oral contrast administration shows paucity of peritoneal fat and difficulty in distinguishing adenopathy from fluid-filled bowel loops. **B:** Repeat CT after additional oral contrast shows contrast-filled bowel and no evidence of adenopathy.

respiratory motion in children. Scans of 1 second or less are preferable in younger children and can be achieved using partial rotation scans. Suggested slice collimation varies with age. In general, 5-mm collimation should be used in children less than 2 years of age and 7- to 10-mm collimation in older children.

Helical (spiral) CT is now commonly used for children. This technique allows significant decrease in scanning time and may reduce the amount of intravenous contrast required. It also improves lesion conspicuity, permits better multiplanar reconstructions, and reduces radiation dose. Its main disadvantages are decreased spatial resolution along the z axis, increased sensitivity to large-amplitude motion, and increased data processing and storage requirements (172,183,184). Spiral scans can usually be performed in children less than 12 years of age without suspended respiration with few or no misregistration artifacts. Suspended respiration is usually reserved for cooperative adolescent patients. For each spiral CT scan the radiologist must specify several scanning and reconstruction parameters, including the collimation, table speed, total scan time, and images for reconstruction, always keeping in mind the goals of the particular study and the radiation dose to the child. Imaging parameters recommended for chest and abdomen/pelvis CT in children are listed in Appendix 8. The choice of reconstruction intervals is based on the particular clinical problem being addressed. The optimal overlap for reconstructed images is approximately 50% of the original slice thickness. For example, if the original slice thickness is 10 mm, little will be gained by reconstruction from slices with more than 5 mm overlap.

Scanning Protocols for Neuroimaging

For routine neuro-CT examinations, in which motion is seldom a problem, incremental rather than helical scanning is used. Ten-millimeter contiguous axial sections are performed from the skull base to the vertex. Five-millimeter axial sections are used in the neonate, and occasionally through the posterior fossa at other ages. Direct coronal sections, 3–5 mm thick, are preferred to axial sections with coronal reformatting for evaluation of the sinuses and orbits. Evaluation of temporal bone pathology is performed with 1- to 3-mm axial and direct coronal sections. Neck CT is usually performed with 5-mm contiguous sections using helical CT techniques.

With the advent of MRI, CT cisternoventriculography and CT myelography are rarely performed. The former is helpful in evaluating the communication between cystic spaces within the cisterns and ventricles. The latter is useful when metallic instrumentation precludes MR imaging.

Contiguous 1-mm incremental axial imaging, or helical imaging, with multiplanar and 3-D reformations is often helpful in the preoperative evaluation of craniofacial malformations, craniocervical anomalies, and congenital scoliosis. Other specific imaging parameters are listed in Appendix 8.

Indications

Radiologists are becoming increasingly concerned with defining strict indications for the wide variety of available imaging modalities. This is particularly true of CT, as the value of diagnostic information likely to be obtained must be weighed against the risk to the child and other costs. The radiation dosage, risks of sedation, complications of intravenous contrast material, and environmental change caused by pediatric CT must not be overlooked (155).

Broad indications for CT in infants and children have been derived through clinical experience (136,141,150,155). Examples of pediatric abnormalities that may be evaluated by CT are listed in Table 1-6. Technical and clinical advances in CT have increased the number of patients who, after CT,

TABLE 1-6. *Pediatric indications for and abnormalities evaluated by CT*

Central nervous system and craniofacial structures
  Hydrocephalus
  Intracranial hemorrhage
  Infarction or infection
  Abnormal head size
  Gross congenital malformation
  Craniosynostosis (3-D reformation)
  Head trauma
  Facial trauma
  Orbital trauma
  Sinusitis
  Choanal atresia
  Temporal bone (trauma, infections, mass, maldevelopment)
  Spinal column abnormality
Chest
  Mediastinal tumor involvement
  Metastatic disease
  Opaque hemithorax
  Diffuse lung disease (bronchiectasis, interstitial disease)
  Complications of pulmonary infections
  Primary chest tumor
Abdomen
  Blunt trauma
  Neoplasms of liver, adrenal, kidney, retroperitoneum
  Adenopathy
  Abscess
  Infection in immunocompromised host
  Complex fluid collections
  Extent and complications of inflammatory bowel disease
Musculoskeletal
  Soft tissue tumor
  Osteoid osteoma
  Developmental hip dysplasia
  Femoral anteversion
  Leg length discrepancy
  Tarsal coalition

need no further diagnostic procedures. However, the availability of CT is no excuse for technically sloppy conventional radiography, nuclear scintigraphy, ultrasonography, angiography, or myelography.

Magnetic Resonance Imaging

Since the advent of clinical MRI in the early 1980s, its applications to pediatric disease have grown steadily (185–216). The lack of ionizing radiation, superb soft tissue contrast, multiplanar capabilities, and the ability to image blood vessels (magnetic resonance angiography, or MRA) without the use of intravenous contrast agents are important advantages of MRI over other imaging modalities. In addition to illustrating normal and pathologic anatomy, assessments of tissue perfusion and chemical composition with specialized MR methods are becoming available; this allows physiologic evaluation in the clinical setting.

Basic Physical Principles

A detailed presentation of the physics of MRI (217) is beyond the scope of this text, though a brief description is merited. The basis of MRI lies in the behavior of the nuclei of certain elements (^{1}H, ^{13}C, ^{19}F, ^{23}Na, ^{31}P, ^{39}K) in very strong magnetic fields. Clinical MRI utilizes the hydrogen nucleus, abundant in the human body. A typical imaging field strength to which these protons are subjected is 1.5 Tesla (T), approximately 30,000 times greater than the earth's magnetic field. The protons, acting like small bar magnets in this strong external magnetic field, tend to align themselves either parallel (low-energy state) or antiparallel (high-energy state). This polarization results in the formation of a net magnetization vector **M**, which is made up of contributions from each individual proton. Because more protons align themselves parallel than antiparallel to the field, **M** points in the same direction as the external field, by convention the z axis.

When the magnetization vector **M** is tipped from its equilibrium position along the z axis into the x–y plane, it precesses at the Larmor frequency. The magnitude of this frequency is given by the product of the proton's gyromagnetic ratio (4258 Hz/Gauss) and the strength of the external field. These frequencies are in the radiofrequency (RF) range at typical imaging field strengths. For instance, at 1.5 T, the Larmor frequency is approximately 64 MHz. The precession of **M** results in the emanation of RF waves from the sample at the Larmor frequency, the so-called signal. The tipping of **M** from its equilibrium position, necessary to generate a signal, is performed using an RF pulse applied at the Larmor frequency. A 90° pulse causes a complete tip from the equilibrium z axis to the x–y plane and results in maximal signal.

When the RF pulse is removed, **M** will gradually return to its original alignment. The time it takes for **M** to return (relax) to its original direction along the z axis (longitudinal relaxation) is the T1 relaxation time. The time it takes for the protons to become completely out of phase or incoherent within the transverse (x–y) plane (transverse relaxation) is the T2 relaxation time. It is while **M** is tipped away from the z axis that the sample emits RF signals due to the precession of **M**. Collecting multiple RF signals following repeated tippings or "excitations" of **M** forms the raw data from which images are made. Both the tipping of **M** and the "listening" to **M** are performed with radiofrequency coils tuned to the Larmor frequency. These act like antennae tuned to a radio broadcasting station.

The final element in the formation of an MR image is the application of small, position-dependent, magnetic fields within the bore of the magnet. These magnetic field gradients are superimposed on the large external field and cause the Larmor precession frequency to become a function of position. For full three-dimensional localization capabilities, three mutually orthogonal gradient coils represent integral components of MR scanners. How and when these gradients are applied during both tipping and listening to **M** with the RF coils determines slice selection as well as the phase and frequency in-plane imaging dimensions.

The MR Image

In very simplistic terms, the MR image reflects the distribution of protons (proton density) in the section of the body represented by the image. The difference in contrast of various tissues seen in the image depends on the characteristics of the tissue. These characteristics or parameters include proton density and T1 and T2 relaxation times, which by now have been fairly well documented for different tissues at different field strengths (209). Additional contrast factors include susceptibility effects at air-tissue and bone-tissue interfaces, chemical shift considerations, and whether the protons are stationary or in motion, as is true of flowing blood and pulsating cerebrospinal fluid (CSF). There are also many extrinsic parameters that contribute to tissue contrast. These include (a) the strength of the external magnetic field; (b) the specific pulse sequence and parameters used to acquire the MR signals, specified as the TR (repetition time between spin excitations), the TE (echo time or time elapsed between excitation and signal acquisition), the TI (the time elapsed between an inversion or 180° flip of all spins and the excitation pulse), and the precise flip angle(s) used for excitation.

Tissue appearance on an MR image depends on all of the above intrinsic and extrinsic parameters. In general, the whiter or brighter the tissue is, the stronger the signal. TR is the time between two consecutive 90° RF pulses. TE is the time the MR unit waits after the 90° RF pulse to receive the RF signal, the echo from the relaxing protons. The selection of TR and TE determines the relative T1 and T2 weighting of the image.

T1-weighted images have short TR (<800 milliseconds)

and short TE (<30 milliseconds). The short TR allows signals from tissues to be differentiated according to T1 relaxation. The short TE makes the image insensitive to T2 decay or relaxation. Fat, for example, has a shorter T1 relaxation time than water. Therefore, within the relatively short TE, the protons in fat recover more longitudinal magnetization than those of water and thus exhibit a stronger signal. Fat is therefore brighter than water on a T1-weighted image.

T2-weighted images have long TR (<2000 milliseconds) and long TE (<60 milliseconds). The long TR makes the image insensitive to differences in T1 relaxation, so that signals from tissues are differentiated by T2 relaxation. Tissues with short T2 will not have much signal left if the MR unit waits for a relatively long time (long TE) before ''listening.'' Fat has a shorter T2 relaxation time than water; thus the transverse magnetization of the protons in fat decays faster. Therefore, when the MR unit listens to the signal after a long TE, the signal from the protons of water will have a stronger signal than those from fat. Water is therefore brighter than fat on a T2-weighted image.

Many other pulse sequences (gradient echo, inversion-recovery, fast spin-echo, echo-planar) have been designed to achieve different contrast effects on different tissues and to shorten the time to acquire the least amount of data needed to produce an optimal image (202). In-depth discussion of MR pulse sequences and methods of fast acquisition can be found in reviews dedicated to the subject (218–220).

Image Quality

The goal of MRI in pediatrics is to maximize image quality while covering the region of interest in the shortest possible time. Speed is especially important when a sedated child or an unsedated but anxious child is in the scanner. Signal-to-noise ratio (SNR), contrast-to-noise ratio, spatial and temporal resolution, and scanning parameters (TR, TE) determine the image quality. Unfortunately, changes made to enhance image quality often increase scan times. To illustrate, the acquisition time of a sequence is determined by multiplying the number of phase-encoding steps (the number of spatial resolution steps along the y axis), the TR of the pulse sequence, and the number of signal averages. If the matrix size is increased to achieve better spatial resolution, the number of phase-encoding steps and the acquisition time increase. In addition, as the voxel becomes smaller to achieve better resolution, the SNR will decrease. The number of signal averages can be increased to improve the SNR; again, this increases acquisition time.

In general, the longer the TR, the greater the signal and the more slices available from a single scan, but again, the longer the acquisition time. If fat suppression is used to enhance the contrast-to-noise ratio, there is a decrease in the number of slices available. To cover the region of interest adequately and to have improved conspicuity with fat suppression, a longer TR or even a second pulse sequence may be required.

MR images are highly sensitive to motion. For reduction of gross patient motion of infants and young children, sedation and restraints are necessary. Enough time must be spent to ensure the patient's comfort. Foam sponges, pillows, Velcro straps, and tape are all used to immobilize the child without sacrificing comfort. Sedated infants can be swaddled in prewarmed blankets.

Many software techniques have been developed to combat intrinsic motion (excursion of the diaphragm; pulsations of the heart, blood vessels, and CSF; peristalsis of the gastrointestinal tract; and ocular motion). These include signal averaging with multiple acquisitions, respiratory-ordered phase encoding (221), spatial presaturation (222), rephasing gradients (223), and gradient moment nulling (224). Combinations of these techniques are routinely used, especially in long TR/long TE sequences, to suppress motion artifacts in the MR image along the phase-encoding direction.

Techniques

Preparation, Sedation, and Monitoring

Patients and parents are informed about the MR unit and its intolerance of motion. They are warned of the loud knocking sounds created by the rapid switching of the gradient coils. Ear plugs or earphones are offered to older children. An adult companion is allowed to stay in the scan room if it makes the patient more comfortable. A radiology nurse meticulously screens the patient and parent before they enter the scan room. The screening checklist includes questions about recent surgery, metallic implants, surgical clips, pacemakers, and metallic foreign bodies. All metallic accessories such as chains, earrings, and watches are removed. Radiographs are needed if the patient is unsure about metallic material in the body.

Sedation is needed for most patients under 6 years of age and occasionally for older children who cannot hold still for the entire examination (225,226). Chloral hydrate in a dose of 50–100 mg/kg administered orally is usually used in children less than 12 months of age. If intravenous contrast administration is needed for the examination, an intravenous line is placed before sedation. Pentobarbital sodium (Nembutal) in a dose of 2–3 mg/kg administered intravenously is the usual sedative for children more than 12 months old. A second dose may be administered in 30–60 seconds if needed. The total dose should not exceed 6 mg/kg (see Appendix 6).

A radiology nurse monitors the patient during the sedation. Pulse oximetry and respiratory and EKG monitoring are always used (225,226). Shielded telemetry and oximetry systems are now widely available. It is helpful to have sedation and recovery rooms adjacent to the scan room; this allows better communication and coordination between MRI technologists and nurses. An extra detachable MR scanning table allows a child to be sedated and positioned while the

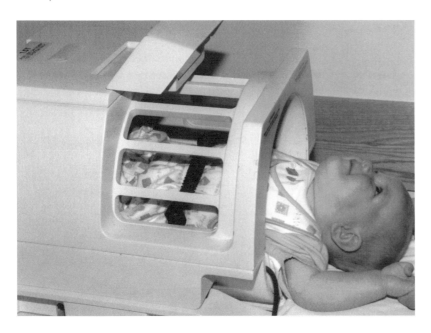

FIG. 1-48. Infant in adult head coil for MR examination of abdomen. Note that the head coil readily provides coverage of the infant's abdomen and pelvis or chest and abdomen.

preceding examination is continuing; the table and the child are then transferred into the scan room. All monitor and support devices such as intravenous poles must be MR-compatible.

General anesthesia is required in patients who have a serious underlying cardiorespiratory condition or who have failed intravenous sedation. The anesthesiology team must be aware of the hazards of the powerful magnetic field. Shielded monitoring wires and extended ventilatory hoses are needed because most anesthesia machines are not MR-compatible and therefore must be kept outside the scan room.

Scanning Techniques

Proper positioning of the patient is vital. In general, the body part of interest is positioned, as much as possible, within the central bore of the magnet where the magnetic field is the most homogeneous. In pediatric imaging, the body part is often small. Therefore, placing surface coils immediately adjacent to the region of interest greatly enhances the SNR and allows the use of thin slices (1–3 mm) and high-resolution matrices (256 or 512). Most commercially available surface coils are designed for adults, and pediatric radiologists need to adapt them for pediatric applications. The following is a brief description of the coils and techniques used at our institution on a 1.5-T Signa System (General Electric Medical Systems, Milwaukee, WI).

MRI of the infant brain may be performed with an adult extremity coil. In older children and adolescents, the adult head coil is adequate. A field of view (FOV) of 24 cm is standard for brain imaging in all three planes. For total spine or craniospinal imaging, a surface coil of appropriate size or a flat surface coil in a movable coil holder/multiple array coil is placed underneath the supine patient. The entire neuroaxis can thus be imaged without moving the patient, who may be sedated. A 32-cm FOV is used in a sagittal localizer followed by an FOV of 21–24 cm in the sagittal and coronal plane and an FOV of 12–18 cm in the axial plane.

MRI of an infant's chest, abdomen, or pelvis can be performed using the adult head coil (Fig. 1-48) with a 24- to 28-cm FOV. For a toddler, our experience has been good with the 5 × 11 in. flat surface coil or "license plate" to cover the chest or abdomen and pelvis. However, there will always be some loss of signal anteriorly, away from the surface coil. Most recently, the torso phase-array coil has provided excellent images with much more homogeneous signal intensity throughout the FOV with improved signal-to-noise ratio (SNR). For older children and adolescents, the adult body coil is used. Specific FOV will depend on the region of interest. Frequently, one can start with a large FOV for the localizer images and then decrease the FOV to the region of interest.

Musculoskeletal imaging requires high resolution and a smaller FOV. The use of different surface coils can maximize SNR. For example, imaging of both ankles can be performed with both feet either in the extremity coil or in the head coil (Fig. 1-49) depending on the size of the patient. A unilateral hip study can be performed with an adult shoulder coil taped over the patient's hip (Fig. 1-50). If both hips need to be assessed, a flat surface coil with the patient prone or a torso phase-array coil can be used.

Scanning Protocols

Each MR examination must be tailored to the clinical situation. Unlike in adults, there are no routine or automatic protocol MR examinations in children. The radiologist needs to be present, supervising the examination and adapting the

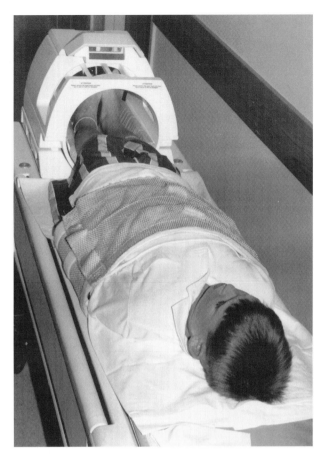

FIG. 1-49. **Head coil to image both ankles.** An 8-year-old boy.

protocols to the particular case. General guidelines are listed in Appendices 9 and 10.

For general screening of the brain, at least two imaging planes and three sequences are obtained. They usually consist of a conventional spin-echo (CSE) T1-weighted sagittal localizer sequence followed by fast spin-echo (FSE) proton density and T2-weighted axial sequences (202).

For general screening of the spine and spinal neuroaxis, a CSE T1-weighted sagittal localizer sequence with a large FOV to cover the entire spine is obtained. Then, FSE proton density and T2-weighted sagittal sequences are usually performed, followed by a CSE T1-weighted axial sequence through the levels of interest.

Intravenous administration of gadolinium (0.2 ml/kg with a maximum single dose of up to 10 ml) is used with CSE T1-weighted imaging for the initial evaluation and follow-up of CNS neoplasms. T1-weighted imaging is usually performed in more than one plane. More detailed protocols and applications of MRI for the central nervous system are discussed in subsequent chapters.

For most MRI of the abdomen and pelvis, a sagittal large FOV localizer is first performed using either a fast gradient recalled echo (GRE) sequence or a fast multiplanar inversion-recovery (FMPIR) sequence. This is usually followed by a CSE T1-weighted coronal sequence. In patients with

paraspinal masses, it is important to have one coronal section through the vertebral canal. Then, a FSE T2-weighted axial sequence with fat suppression is performed. When necessary, after administration of gadolinium, a CSE T1-weighted coronal or axial sequence is acquired. Contrast enhancement is used primarily for imaging neoplastic and infectious processes. Additional fat suppression sequences are optional.

For most MRI of the musculoskeletal system, a combination of a CSE T1-weighted sequence, GRE sequence, CSE proton density and T2-weighted sequences with or without fat suppression, and an FMPIR sequence is utilized. Abnormality of the bone marrow is detected on the T1-weighted, FSE T2-weighted (with fat suppression), and FMPIR images. The cartilaginous structures including the physeal cartilage are seen with high conspicuity on the GRE and CSE proton density with fat suppression sequences. The ability to image cartilage and to detect changes in the bone marrow are major advantages of MRI over other modalities (210).

Indications

Table 1-7 lists examples of pediatric abnormalities that are evaluated by MRI (186,188,195,199,211).

Potentials for the Future

With continued improvements and innovations in software and hardware design, MR units with faster scanning

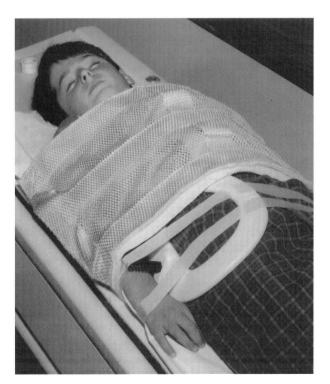

FIG. 1-50. **Shoulder coil to image right hip.** A 9-year-old boy.

TABLE 1-7. *Pediatric indications for and abnormalities evaluated by MRI*

Brain
  Developmental abnormalities (migrational anomalies)
  Myelination disorders
  Neoplasms (surgical anatomy, staging, radiotherapy planning, follow-up after treatment)
  Inflammation, infection
  Infarction, hemorrhage
  Vascular malformations
  Phacomatoses
  Unexplained seizure
  Unexplained hydrocephalus
  Unexplained neuroendocrine disorder
Orbit (tumor, infection, inflammation)
Spine
  Developmental malformations
  Neoplasm
  Infection
  Trauma
  Atypical scoliosis
Chest
  Airway evaluation
  Vascular rings and slings
  Coarctation of the aorta
  Venous thromboses, access evaluation
  Mediastinal masses
  Congenital heart disease (before and after surgery)
  Chest wall pathology (neoplasm, infection)
  Foregut malformations (sequestration)
  Diaphragmatic hernia
Abdomen and pelvis
  Developmental anomalies before and after surgery (anorectal malformations)
  Congenital anomalies of the genitourinary tract
  Neoplasms arising from abdomen and retroperitoneum (neuroblastoma, Wilms tumor, hepatoblastoma, etc.)
  Infection (abscess)
  Liver transplant evaluation
  Vascular abnormalities
  Venous thromboses, access evaluation
  Budd-Chiari syndrome
  Hemosiderosis
  Pelvic neoplasms (ovarian origin, rhabdomyosarcoma, sacrococcygeal teratoma)
Musculoskeletal
  Trauma to joints (damage to ligaments and cartilage, physeal injuries)
  Infection
  Neoplasms
  Osteonecrosis

capabilities like echo-planar imaging (EPI) are becoming available. With the faster image acquisition times (50–100 milliseconds), artifacts from physiologic motion are reduced. Preliminary work has shown that EPI is useful in imaging the coronary arteries and in determining myocardial perfusion in adults (227). Cine-MRI techniques have been used to assess ventricular function (228) and estimate peak velocities across stenoses (229). These techniques have been adapted to image congenital heart disease (204,216).

Similarly, utilization of MRI to assess physiologic func-

tion of the CNS of children has been reported. Both perfusion studies (214,230) and spectroscopy (212,213) of the brain are feasible. MR spectroscopy has also been used in other parts of the body including developing bone marrow (215). Combined anatomic and functional MR examinations of various organ systems will probably soon be routine.

Digital Imaging

Digital imaging is the generation or conversion, processing, display, and storage of images in digital format. The images are composed of a two-dimensional array of *pixels* (picture elements), each of which is digitally encoded. The smallest unit of digital information is the *bit* (binary digit), which computers commonly handle in groups of eight, *a byte*.

The advantage of digital imaging is the ability to present precisely a large amount of information for measurement and display. Once the raw dataset is in digital form, it is theoretically nondegradable, easily transportable, and reproducible. Upon reproduction, various schemes of digital signal processing can be applied to enhance particular portions of the spectrum of the images; an example is edge enhancement (high-pass filtering). Digital imaging is particularly appealing for pediatric imaging (231–235).

Principles

With projection imaging, a three-dimensional distribution of an object property (absorption of x-rays) produces a two-dimensional image on a receptor. This image may be displayed in analog form on film. However, using a scanning process, the two-dimensional distribution on the receptor may be sent to a computer and stored as a one-dimensional set of data. The computer again converts the one-dimensional dataset to a two-dimensional image, which may be displayed on a cathode ray tube monitor (soft copy) or printed on film (hard copy).

All digital imaging has a projection source, detectors, and digital technology components. The system consists of a source of imaging energy, a detection device that converts the transmitted energy to digital data, and a digital method of constructing the image. The source, detector, and digital technology are different for CT, ultrasonography, MRI, nuclear medicine, digital angiography, digital fluoroscopy, and computed radiography.

Applications

Computed Tomography

Computed tomographic imaging employs a two-dimensional fan beam from an x-ray tube as the source of imaging energy. This beam scans the body from many angles. Thousands of precise absorption measurements in digital form are taken by specially designed electronic (xenon or solid state) detectors. These digital measurements (attenuation, position) are the basis for all CT image construction (preprocessing, postprocessing) and storage.

Ultrasonography

Sonography uses high-frequency sound waves that are reflected by various organ surfaces and internal architectural structures. A piezoelectric crystal is both the source and the detector of these high-frequency vibrations. The time between emission of the ultrasound wave and arrival of the reflected wave is a measure of the skin-to-interface (skin-to-organ) distance. This time interval and the spectrum of the reflected sound energy can be digitized. Plotting the many thousands of such measurements generates an ultrasound cross-sectional image.

Magnetic Resonance Imaging

MRI uses a strong magnetic field and radiofrequency energy to generate a synchronized precessional motion of receptive elements in body tissues. The image is formed from different proton densities in tissues and different rates of spin energy decay. The relaxation parameters are related to binding forces with the biochemical environment and the abundance of receptive atoms. Digital technology permits signal processing, image reconstruction, and image storage.

Nuclear Medicine

The imaging energy source for scintigraphy is the isotope attached to a radiopharmaceutical injected into the body. The detection system, a gamma camera, uses a collimator and photomultiplier tubes that direct the gamma rays emitted from the body to a scintillation crystal. The raw data from the scintillation crystal eventually yields an image after computer reconstruction and signal processing. This image can be stored in computer memory.

Digital Subtraction Angiography

Digital subtraction angiography (DSA) uses x-rays as the source and an image intensifier as the detector. Digital technology includes both analog-to-digital conversion of beam attenuation and image storage. DSA stores an image before contrast injection and then stores several more images as the contrast medium passes through the vessels. The digitally subtracted image (the difference between the preinjection image and the post-injection images) provides a highly detailed delineation of vascular anatomy.

Digital Fluoroscopy

The essential elements of digital fluoroscopy are short x-ray exposure time, phototimed by the x-ray generator; digitization of the video signal received from a television camera, which is connected to an image intensifier; storage of the digital image in a computer; and production of hard copies by a laser imager.

The fluoroscopic images are transformed into digital format by dividing the image into pixels in a matrix. Maximum spatial resolution of images depends on the size of the matrix and the input field to be digitized. A matrix size of $1024 \times 1024 \times 8$ bits deep has proved clinically acceptable with fields up to 10 in. If each pixel is represented by 8 bits (1 byte), such systems are able to resolve 256 shades of gray. The advantages of digital fluoroscopy (or any digital system) are reduction of quantum mottle via frame averaging to improve low-contrast resolution, edge enhancement to improve high-contrast resolution, contrast (window) and brightness (level) control by the operator, potential for reduced radiation dose, immediate image display, last-image hold, and correction of exposure prior to hard-copy film.

Computed Radiography

Computed radiography uses x-rays as a source and either a two-dimensional or a one-dimensional imaging plate as a detector. Digital technology permits measurement of attenuation values and digital image processing as previously described.

Computed radiography utilizes a photo-stimulable phosphor as the image receptor. Standard conventional imaging equipment is used to expose the image receptor plate, which is coated with europium-activated barium fluorohalide compounds in crystal form held in an organic binder. These crystals trap energy when exposed to ionizing radiation. The energy released by each picture element on the plate represents the subject contrast originally contained in the x-ray pattern in space. The image plates are reusable.

The luminescence stimulated by the scanning laser is collected through a light guide into a photomultiplier tube that produces an analog electrical signal. These signals are digitized to form an image in a 2048×2048 image matrix. Computed radiographs generated by the image processor may be viewed as soft copy on a high-resolution video monitor or as hard copy on a single-emulsion film printed by a laser camera.

Picture Archiving and Communication Systems

Picture archiving and communication systems (PACSs) are computer-driven systems designed for electronic storage and retrieval (archiving) and transmission (communicating) of digital images. The implementation of PACSs in radiology departments ranges from modules that address specific needs, such as availability of radiographs on monitors in intensive care units, to a totally digital radiology department (236). The integration of PACSs into a modern radiology department with multiple modalities is much easier with the development of a standard for network interfaces known as DICOM (Digital Imaging and Communications in Medicine) by the ACR-NEMA (American College of Radiology and National Electrical Manufacturers' Association) (237). Ideally, if all vendors of medical imaging equipment and medical information systems support DICOM, problems arising from networking and interfacing among various imaging units and computer systems can be greatly reduced. Total integration of PACSs, radiology information systems, and hospital information systems is now possible.

Teleradiology

Teleradiology is the electronic transmission of digital radiographic images over a telecommunication linkage for interpretation at remote sites. From the transmission of video signals of a radiograph via cable closed-circuit television in the early 1970s, teleradiology systems have evolved to transmission of diagnostic quality images over high-speed telecommunication lines (238). In 1995, the American College of Radiology passed a resolution on guidelines of equipment specifications for teleradiology systems used for official authenticated written interpretation without hard copy films. The digitization system needs to have a resolution of $2048 \times 2048 \times 12$ bits (approximately 7 megabytes of data for a 14×17 in. radiograph); and the display system needs to have a resolution of $2048 \times 2048 \times 8$ bits (239). An uncompressed 7-megabyte image can be transmitted through a T1 data communication link capable of 1.544 megabits/second data transmission rate in approximately 36 seconds (235). Modern teleradiology can eliminate geographic restrictions on final interpretation of diagnostic images. Small rural medical facilities and outpatient clinics unable to support a full-time radiologist can have immediate access to larger medical centers for timely interpretation of imaging studies.

Nonvascular Interventional Procedures

A steady increase in number and types of pediatric nonvascular interventional procedures has occurred in the last decade (240–261) (Table 1-8). This increase stems mainly from the growing recognition that many pediatric nonvascular interventional procedures, like their counterparts in the adult world, can achieve the same results as surgery without being as invasive and usually with less morbidity and a more rapid recovery.

Preprocedure imaging is vital to the success of interventional procedures. Frequently, a combination of ultrasound, CT, and MRI can determine the most direct and safest ap-

TABLE 1-8. *Pediatric interventional procedures*

Vascular
  Embolization
  Sclerotherapy
  Angioplasty
  Fibrinolytic therapy
  CVL and PICC insertion
  Foreign body removal
  Transjugular liver biopsy
  TIPS
Nonvascular
  Aspiration: abscess, pleural effusion, fluid collection
  Drainage: abscess, pleural effusion, fluid collection
  Biopsy
  Gastrointestinal procedure
    Balloon extraction (coin)
    Balloon dilatation (esophagus, biliary duct)
    Percutaneous gastrostomy/gastrojejunostomy
  Genitourinary procedures
    Percutaneous nephrostomy
    Balloon dilatation (ureter)
    Percutaneous pyeloplasty
    Stone removal

CVL, Central venous line; PICC, peripherally-inserted central catheter; TIPS, transjugular intrahepatic portosystemic shunt.

proach to the abnormality, avoiding important adjacent vascular and visceral structures (Fig. 1-51). Viable tissue is distinguished from necrotic tissue, for biopsy (Fig. 1-52). In general, procedures are performed with ultrasound guidance alone (aspiration, biopsy) or with a combination of ultrasound and fluoroscopy (abscess drainage, nephrostomy). Ultrasound allows real-time, continuous imaging and guidance for the needle placement, rapid needle positioning, and imaging-guided redirection if needed. With the exceptions of bony and nonperipheral lung parenchymal lesions for which CT is necessary, we favor the use of ultrasound guidance.

Adequate sedation preventing significant discomfort can often be achieved by intravenous administration of sedatives and narcotics (see Appendix 6). This applies to short-duration procedures such as aspirations, biopsies, and simple drainages. For children under 7 years of age, we usually use IV pentobarbital (2–6 mg/kg), and for older children, we use IV midazolam (0.05 mg/kg). These sedatives are combined with occasional use of IV fentanyl citrate (1–3 μg/kg). Preprocedure placement of anesthetic cream (lidocaine 2.5% and prilocaine 2.5%) to the site of entry (262) helps, as does the addition of sodium bicarbonate to the local anesthetic injection (0.5–1.0 cm^3 of 1 mEq/cm^3 of sodium bicarbonate solution mixed with 1% xylocaine solution to a total volume of 10 cm^3). If a long, complicated procedure is anticipated or if the procedure is likely to cause significant discomfort, general anesthesia is required. Even a cooperative older child or adolescent cannot be expected to remain still when frightened and in pain. A moving target undoubtedly increases the risk and failure rate of the procedure.

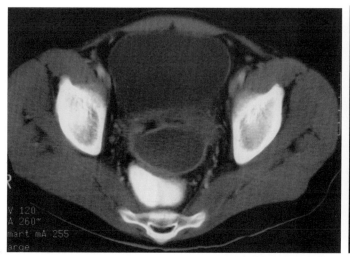 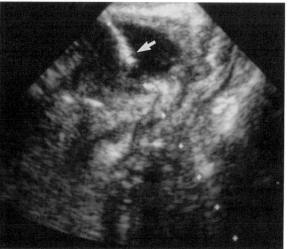

A   B

FIG. 1-51. Transrectal abscess drainage. A: CT shows a pelvic abscess in a 15-year-old boy with a perforated appendix. An anterior approach is blocked by the urinary bladder and a transgluteal approach is complicated by the presence of small vessels just deep to the internal obturator muscles. **B:** Transrectal sonography. A needle *(arrow)* is guided from a transrectal approach into the abscess cavity.

Aspiration and Drainage

Indications

Indications for imaging-guided aspiration and drainage are similar to those in adults. The pathology in question is usually infectious, and percutaneous drainage of an abscess can often facilitate recovery. Cytologic examination of ascites or pleural fluid occasionally yields the diagnosis of Bur-

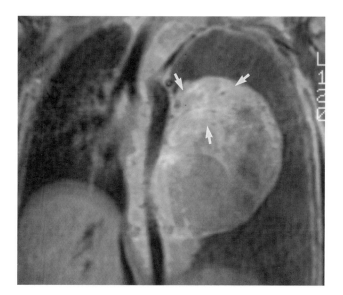

FIG. 1-52. Viable area within tumor. T1-weighted coronal MR image of a child with a thoracic neuroblastoma. Area of viable tissue *(arrows)* for biopsy is indicated by presence of contrast enhancement in the upper portion of the tumor; compare the appearance of enhancing viable tumor to the nonenhancing necrotic lower portion.

kitt lymphoma (252). The most common indications for ultrasound-guided aspiration are hip aspiration for possible septic arthritis (258) (Fig. 1-53), thoracentesis, and paracentesis. Less common indications include aspiration of lung abscess (263), peritoneal inclusion cyst (264), and ovarian cyst. The most common indications for drainage are intraabdominal and intrapelvic abscess, obstructive hydronephrosis, lung abscess (265,266), and empyema (267). Less common indications include drainage and treatment of lymphocele (268), infected bilomas (247), and urinoma (251).

Technique

Whenever possible, ultrasonography is used for guidance in all aspirations and drainage procedures. In aspirations, the needle tip can be monitored continuously while the surrounding structures (lung parenchyma adjacent to pleural effusion) progressively collapse around the needle. Spinal needles (18–22 gauge) or Chiba needles are used depending on the expected viscosity of the fluid.

In drainage procedures, a 21-gauge Chiba needle is often used initially. With a modified Seldinger technique, over a 0.018-in. wire, a 4-Fr coaxial dilating system that accepts a 0.038-in. wire is placed. After sequential dilation, 8- to 14-Fr self-retaining catheters are placed. Fluoroscopy is used to monitor the dilatations and the placement of the catheters. Small collections may require tight pigtail loops of 1-cm diameter (Fig. 1-54). When the collection is large and peripheral, a one-step trocar technique can sometimes be used. For deep pelvic collections, as in adults, transrectal drainage either with transabdominal sonographic guidance (253) or transrectal sonographic guidance (261) has been shown to be effective.

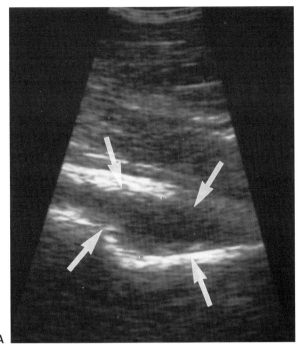

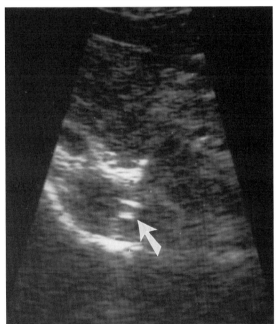

FIG. 1-53. Hip aspiration with sonographic guidance. A: Preaspiration sonography shows a hip effusion *(arrows)* of moderate size. **B:** The tip of a 20-gauge spinal needle *(arrow)* is clearly seen within the joint effusion.

Biopsy

Indications

Indications for percutaneous biopsy include the need for tissue to determine the microscopic pathology of medical diseases (glomerulonephritis, metabolic liver disease), tumors, and infectious processes. Percutaneous biopsy of solid organs (liver, kidney) for the pathologic diagnosis of chronic

diseases and for diagnosis of rejection has gradually replaced incisional biopsy.

However, percutaneous biopsy of nonresectable neoplastic lesions in infants and children is not yet a routine procedure, even in many pediatric centers. In adults, cytology from fine needle aspiration is often adequate to diagnose carcinoma. More tissue is needed in children because neoplasms are often sarcomas, lymphomas, and other small round cell tumors. Core biopsies are therefore often required. In addition, many common pediatric neoplasms have cytogenetic findings that aid in diagnosis and prognosis. The most common example is neuroblastoma; in this tumor, the number of N-myc oncogenes and the DNA index (ploidy), together with the patient's age, can indicate prognosis and dictate treatment (269). Percutaneous biopsy establishes a pathologic diagnosis without surgery and allows preoperative chemotherapy to reduce the burden of tumor. Thus, a nonresectable lesion is sometimes converted to a resectable one (270), and sometimes more of the organ of origin can be saved (271).

Occasionally, an infectious organism can be identfied only by biopsy. The percutaneous route may be the least invasive way of obtaining tissue for culture.

Technique

Most percutaneous biopsies of lesions of solid organs (liver, kidney) or of the retroperitoneum are performed with sonographic guidance. Large peripheral lesions in the lung can be biopsied under fluoroscopic guidance; others require CT guidance. Biopsy of vertebral lesions can be guided by CT; sometimes, CT will reveal a more accessible soft tissue component so that biopsy of the vertebra itself can be

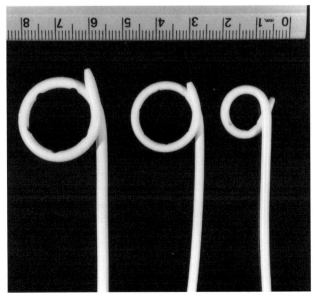

FIG. 1-54. Self-retaining or "pigtail" drainage catheters. Note the sizes of the loops of the "pigtails." From left to right: 10-Fr adult size loop, 8.5-Fr smaller loop; 8.5-Fr with 1-cm-diameter loop.

avoided. Prebiopsy imaging of large neoplastic lesions by CT or MRI can be extremely helpful in distinguishing viable from necrotic tissue (Fig. 1-52).

For tumor biopsies, we prefer to use 15- or 16-gauge automated spring-loaded core biopsy needles. Multiple passes are made to obtain enough tissue for both histopathologic and cytogenetic analyses. For biopsy of the liver or kidney, 18-gauge spring-loaded needles can yield adequate samples (272,273). Coaxial biopsy systems allow multiple passes through a single puncture of the pleura in lung biopsies and the liver capsule in liver biopsies. In the lung, we prefer a 19-gauge sheath with a 20-gauge needle, and in the liver, a 17-gauge sheath with an 18-gauge needle. In patients with coagulopathy, the coaxial system allows the biopsy track in the liver to be embolized at the completion of the biopsy with Gelfoam (Upjohn Co., Kalamazoo, MI) or Avitene (Medchem Products Inc., Woburn, MA) (274). Vertebral biopsy is performed with a 14-gauge Terkel trephine needle set. In all biopsies, it is best to discuss the case with the referring surgeon. The pathologist should be alerted so that an immediate touch preparation can determine whether the samples are diagnostic. The pathologist can also determine whether the volume of tissue is adequate.

Other Procedures

Percutaneous placement of gastrostomy tubes and gastrojejunostomy tubes by interventional radiologists with sedation has replaced surgical gastrostomy and percutaneous endoscopic gastrostomy (PEG) in some pediatric centers. Both the antegrade (244,250) and retrograde techniques (254,256) are safe and effective. Jejunal feeding tubes can also be placed through a PEG site or a surgical gastrostomy site under fluoroscopy (255,275).

Balloon dilatation of esophageal strictures after repair of esophageal atresia or caused by reflux esophagitis may be therapeutic (245). Removal of blunt foreign bodies (coins) from the esophagus with balloon catheters has also been successful (276–278).

Percutaneous nephrostomy and the Whitaker test (260,279) can be performed easily with sonographic guidance. The initial puncture is through a posterior calyx. Placement of the drainage tube and nephrostography are done with fluoroscopic guidance. Intravenous injection of contrast material is not needed. Ureteral dilation, stone removal, and pyeloplasty (280) can also be performed from an antegrade percutaneous approach.

Angiography and Vascular Interventional Procedures

Indications

The availability of Doppler ultrasound, MRI, MRA, and CT has decreased the need for conventional angiography, a more invasive procedure (Table 1-9). Most pediatric angiography is now performed in conjunction with endovascular intervention. Current indications for cerebral angiography

TABLE 1-9. *Indications for pediatric angiography*

CNS
  Hemorrhage
  Ischemia
  Trauma
  Vascular anomalies
  Myelopathy
Viscera
  Systemic hypertension
  Portal hypertension
  Ischemia after organ transplantation
  Gastrointestinal bleeding
  Vascular anomalies
  Complication of or placement of indwelling catheter
Extremities
  Vascular anomalies
  Presurgical evaluation of congenital anomalies of hands and feet
  Penetrating injuries
  Ischemic vasculopathies
  Thrombosis
Thorax
  Congenital cardiovascular disease
  Hemoptysis
  Pulmonary arteriovenous fistula
  Pulmonary embolism
  Complication of or placement of indwelling catheter

CNS, central nervous system.

include subarachnoid hemorrhage, unexplained cerebral ischemia, a vascular complication of trauma, and vascular anomaly (281). The most common indications for visceral angiography include hypertension, ischemia after organ transplantation, gastrointestinal bleeding, and vascular anomaly (232,257,282–286). Extremity angiography is required before reconstruction of complex anomalies of the hands and feet, following penetrating injury, and to diagnose ischemic vasculopathies. Thoracic angiography is performed for congenital heart disease, hemoptysis, cyanosis suggesting pulmonary arteriovenous fistula, and pulmonary thromboembolism. Complications of indwelling catheters are the main indications for venography. The diagnosis and treatment of thromboembolic disease, often due to an underlying coagulopathy, is occasionally required in pediatric practice. Imaging-guided placement of central venous catheters has become a common procedure in some pediatric radiology departments. In each institution, the indications will depend on the risk/benefit ratio, which is partly based on the skills and experience of the local interventional radiologists and other physicians.

Techniques

Pediatric vascular procedures require a number of technical modifications of standard adult practice (257,281,282). The femoral arteries of young children are small, easily traumatized, and prone to spasm and thrombosis (287). Sedation with physiologic monitoring or general anesthesia is usually required. The advantages of general anesthesia include the absence of patient movement, monitoring of physiologic pa-

TABLE 1-10. *Suggested contrast dosages for pediatric angiography*

Vessel	Contrast dosage in ml or ml/kg by child's weight[a]				
	<10 kg	10–20 kg	20–40 kg	>50 kg	Maximum
Cerebral					
Vertebral artery (ml)	2–3	3–5	4–6	7–9	10
Internal carotid artery (ml)	3–4	5–7	7–9	8–12	12
External carotid artery (ml)	2	3–4	4–5	5–6	6
Common carotid artery (ml)	4–5	6–7	8–9	10–12	12
Extracerebral					
Aorta (ml/kg)	1.5	1.2–1.5	1.0–1.5	0.8–0.9	60
Inferior vena cava (ml/kg)	1	1	0.8	0.8	40
Celiac (ml/kg)	1.0–1.2	0.9–1.0	0.8–0.9	0.8	60
Hepatic or splenic artery (ml/kg)	0.7–0.8	0.7	0.6	0.5	35
Superior mesenteric artery (ml/kg)	0.8–1.0	0.8–0.9	0.7–0.8	0.7	50
Inferior mesenteric artery (ml/kg)	0.5–0.7	0.5	0.4–0.6	0.4	25
Renal artery (ml)	1–2	3–5	5–7	7–10	10
Adrenal artery (ml)	0.5–1.0	1.0–1.5	1.5–2.0	2	2

[a] Nonionic, low-osmolality contrast: 300–320 mg iodine/ml for conventional film angiography; 180, 240, or 300 mg iodine/ml for digital subtraction angiography.

Modified from Harwood-Nash and Fitz (288), Kirks (286), and Kirks et al. (285).

rameters, correction of fluid and blood pressure alterations, and ability to affect vascular tone and blood flow. Small children lose heat rapidly under general anesthesia; devices such as electrical warming blankets, warm air infusers, and wrapping the head and trunk in plastic maintain body temperature quite effectively. Use of special padding, such as egg carton foam, to prevent pressure injury to the skin and peripheral nerves is recommended for long procedures. Careful monitoring of the volumes of fluid and contrast medium administered is also important. Pressurized systems for injecting flush solutions into arterial sheaths and catheters should be restricted by a flow-limiting valve or infusion pump. Urinary catheters are mandatory for long procedures to prevent overdistention of the bladder and to monitor urine output accurately.

Contrast Media

Low-osmolality, nonionic contrast media are recommended. If full-strength contrast (320 mg iodine/ml) is used,

the total volume should be restricted to 4–6 ml/kg at one session, although larger quantities are usually well tolerated over a long procedure if renal function is normal. Hand injections of contrast material for localization should be kept to a minimum. The use of dilute contrast medium (140–240 mg iodine/ml), especially for DSA, and the aspiration of contrast medium from catheters before flushing reduce the volume of contrast medium used. The contrast volumes recommended for individual vessels are based on weight and are relatively greater for infants than for older children (Table 1-10) (281–288).

Arterial Access

Arterial access, especially in the chubby infant, is often the most difficult part of the vascular procedure. Percutaneous cannulation of the femoral artery, using the modified Seldinger technique, is the most common approach (282). In the newborn, the umbilical artery or even the femoral venous approach may be tried. High runoff vascular lesions

TABLE 1-11. *Systems for pediatric angiography*

System	Device of choice, by child's weight		
	<10 kg	10–20 kg	>20 kg
Needles (disposable)	22-gauge Angiocath[a] 21-gauge × 1 in. TW[c]	20-gauge Potts[b]	19-gauge thin wall[d] or 20-gauge Potts[b]
Wires	0.018 in.	0.025 in.	0.025–0.035 in.
Catheters	3–4.0 Fr	4–4.1 Fr	4–5.0 Fr
Sheaths	4.0 Fr	4.0 Fr	4–5.0 Fr

[a] Deseret Pharmaceutical Co., Sandy, UT.
[b] Becton-Dickinson, Rutherford, NJ.
[c] Argon Medical Corp., Garland, TX.
[d] Cook Inc., Bloomington, IN.

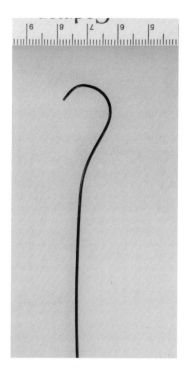

FIG. 1-55. Preshaped catheter for aortography and selective angiography. This 3-Fr catheter has two small side holes near the tip permitting a maximum flow rate of 7 ml/sec. The preformed cobra shape permits selective catheterization of renal and other arteries in infants less than 12 kg and obviates the trauma of catheter exchange (Cook Incorporated, Bloomington, IN).

such as hepatic hemangioendotheliomas and anomalous systemic arteries to the lungs may have a small abdominal aorta; an axillary or brachial artery approach may make catheterization of the feeding vessels easier.

A general guideline for needles and catheters (Table 1-11) is to use the smallest and least traumatic system which is feasible. We prefer the double-wall arterial puncture technique, usually entering the skin 1 cm below the inguinal crease and directing the needle nearly horizontally to enter the common femoral artery just below the inguinal ligament. A bolster may be placed under the pelvis to make the arterial pulse easier to palpate and to make the femoral artery more horizontal; it should be removed after cannulation to avoid pressure injury. A bolus of 100 U of heparin per kilogram of body weight is given as soon as the catheter has been inserted into the artery and repeated after 2 hours, if necessary. If small catheters are used, heparinization usually does not need to be reversed at the end of the procedure.

Repeated catheter exchanges should be avoided in infants and small children. A multiple-sidehole catheter with a preshaped curve can be used for both aortography and selective angiography, providing the sideholes are distal (Fig. 1-55). Most pediatric vascular procedures can be performed with 3- and 4-Fr catheters. The shape of the distal curve must be proportional to the diameter of the pediatric aorta (Fig. 1-56) (282,285). Commercially available 4-Fr catheters have curves that are much wider than a child's aorta and require

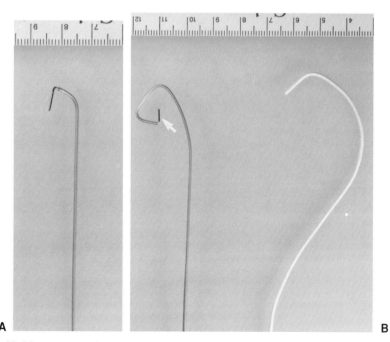

FIG. 1-56. Multipurpose selective catheter. A: This 4-Fr polyethylene catheter is preshaped with a short distal curve, ideal for cerebral angiography. It can be steam-shaped for selective catheterization of other vessels (Cook Incorporated, Bloomington, IN). **B:** The same multipurpose catheter *(left)* has been shaped over a mandrel *(arrow)*. Steaming will set the new curve. A commercially available 4-Fr Cobra catheter *(right)* is shown for comparison.

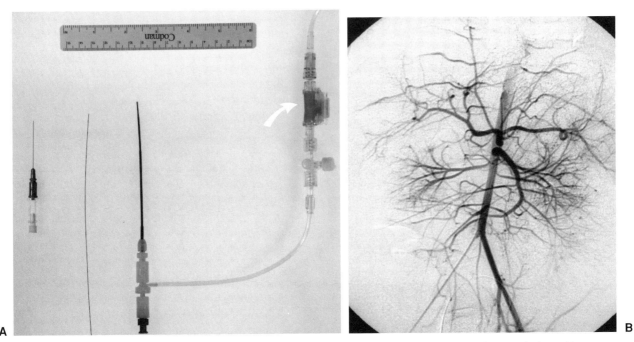

FIG. 1-57. Arterial sheath for infant. A: The dilator is tapered to 0.018 in. to permit cannulation with a 22-gauge Teflon-coated needle. A flow-limiting valve *(arrow)* limits flush solution to 3 ml/hour. **B:** Abdominal aortogram in a 3-week-old infant demonstrates arterial spasm of the iliac artery around a 4-Fr introducer sheath.

large access needles; polyethylene catheters that can be custom-shaped are preferable.

Arterial sheaths, with introducers tapered to 0.018 or 0.025 in., are used to protect the femoral artery and ensure continuous access during procedures that require more than minimal manipulation (Fig. 1-57). They are perfused with heparinized flush solution, using a check-flow valve to limit flow to 3 ml/hour.

At the end of the procedure, the pedal pulses should be checked before the catheter is removed. If pulses are not present, contrast material may be injected into the iliac artery under fluoroscopy. If the femoral artery is completely occluded because of spasm, 1–3 μg per kilogram of dilute nitroglycerin may be injected through the catheter during withdrawal. Other methods of dealing with arterial spasm include infiltration of the tissue around the artery with lidocaine, and simple removal of the catheter and observation. The patient and especially the lower extremities must be kept warm in order to maintain good perfusion of the lower extremities. If pedal pulses are not palpable 4 hours after catheter removal, the patient should be heparinized, providing there are no contraindications. If pulses have not returned after 24 hours of heparinization, consideration should be given to intravenous thrombolytic infusion.

In the first week of life, the umbilical artery can be catheterized directly or by exchanging an umbilical artery line over a guidewire. Appropriate catheters include 3- to 5-Fr diagnostic catheters, 4-Fr sheath, or 4- or 5-Fr infusion or flexible delivery catheters (Fig. 1-58) (for coaxial use with a microcatheter). Although selective catheterization is more difficult through the umbilical artery than through a femoral artery sheath, the former approach causes many fewer femoral artery thromboses and facilitates staging of procedures.

Applications

Modern angiography systems have variable fluoroscopic and film acquisition radiation dose rates. In general, dose and image quality are directly proportional. Intensifier field size, collimation, filming rate, and gonadal shielding should be monitored carefully to minimize radiation exposure.

Vascular Interventional Techniques

Endovascular therapeutic techniques currently used in pediatrics are listed in Table 1-8.

Embolization

Pediatric embolization techniques are similar in general to those used in adults, but the indications are often different. The best results will be achieved if the operator understands the natural history of the lesions involved, is experienced in pediatric vascular interventional techniques, and uses catheters and/or delivery systems modified for smaller vessels. Neonatal lungs tolerate only a limited amount of embolic

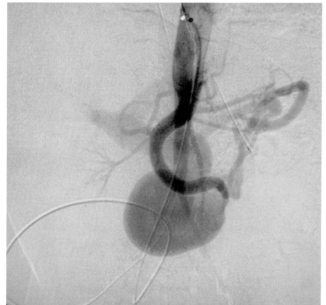
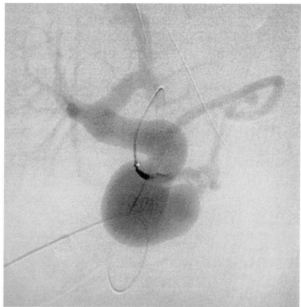
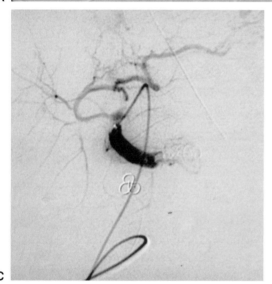

FIG. 1-58. Embolization of abdominal arteriovenous fistula via umbilical artery. A: Abdominal aortogram using a 4-Fr infusion catheter (Tracker 38 special, Target Therapeutics, Fremont, CA). **B:** Selective angiogram prior to placement of coils in the arteriovenous fistula between the gastroepiploic artery and the superior mesenteric vein. **C:** Angiogram immediately after coil placement demonstrates complete occlusion of the fistula.

material before the development of fatal pulmonary hypertension. Right-to-left shunting readily occurs across a patent foramen ovale.

Indications. In children's hospitals, most embolizations are performed for the treatment of vascular malformations (289–294). Other indications include the presurgical or primary treatment of hypervascular tumors (295,296), treatment of acute or chronic bleeding from a variety of causes and at a variety of sites, and ablation of splenic or renal tissue in the treatment of hypersplenism or hypertension (297,298). Embolization techniques are also useful in occluding anomalous or hypertrophied systemic arteries to the lungs, coronary fistulae, and surgical systemic-to-pulmonary shunts.

Technique. Embolization requires supraselective catheterization of supplying arteries (289). Small arterial sheaths and catheters, especially microcatheters of variable stiffness, should be used (290). Common embolization materials in-

clude Gelfoam and Avitene for temporary occlusion as well as polyvinyl alcohol foam particles, platinum coils, and wire coils for permanent occlusion. Tissue adhesive and detachable balloons are useful devices but are not currently approved by the Food and Drug Administration. Sclerosants such as sodium tetradecyl and 100% ethanol are used for direct injection into venous and sometimes lymphatic malformations (291,294).

Angioplasty

Indications. Pediatric indications for balloon dilatation angioplasty include (a) arterial obstructions, such as renal artery stenosis; (b) venous obstructions, such as catheter-related stenosis, inferior vena cava (IVC) stenosis, and hepatic vein stenosis (Budd-Chiari syndrome) (299); and (c) vascular obstructions following organ transplantation (300,301).

Technique. Arterial angioplasty in small children can be performed by using small balloon catheters designed for adult coronary or distal extremity arterial stenoses. Hemodynamic monitoring, anticoagulation and vasodilation medication are necessary.

Pediatric Thrombolysis

Indications. The vast majority of pediatric vascular occlusions are caused by catheterization (287,302). Thrombolytic therapy is effective in restoring lower extremity circulation in 70% to 84% of patients with femoral artery thrombosis after cardiac catheterization (302). Other indications include central venous thrombosis, neonatal aortic thrombosis, renal vein and dural venous sinus thrombosis, pulmonary artery thrombosis, and thrombosed Blalock-Taussig shunts or other vascular anastomoses (303–305).

Technique. Techniques of administration include systemic (intravenous) high-dose infusion of streptokinase, urokinase, or tissue plasminogen activator and selective, direct infusion of clot. The loading dose for systemic urokinase is 4000 U/kg given over 30 minutes, followed by 4000 U/kg/hour; there is no maximum dose. Tissue plasminogen activator is given as an infusion of 0.1–0.5 mg/kg/hour. Infusions are carried out in the intensive care unit, with close observation and frequent monitoring of clotting parameters (prothrombin time [PT], partial thromboplastic time [PTT], fibrinogen) and hemoglobin levels. Low-dose direct clot infusion is used in the presence of contraindications to high-dose intravenous thrombolytic therapy, after failure of intravenous treatment, and when frequent angiographic monitoring of the thrombus is necessary. Bleeding remote from the arteriotomy site is rare in children undergoing thrombolytic infusion. Intracranial hemorrhage has been reported in neonates (304). Some neonates have low plasminogen levels and this may contribute to failure of thrombolytic therapy (303).

New Applications

Transjugular liver biopsy is indicated in the presence of undiagnosed severe liver disease complicated by coagulopathy (306). Transjugular intrahepatic portosystemic shunt (TIPS) has been performed in children as young as 5 years of age prior to liver transplantation (307). The current indication for TIPS is GI bleeding from esophageal varices, not controlled by endoscopic sclerotherapy. The applicability of this technique in children with portal hypertension is limited by the high incidence of portal vein occlusion and hypoplasia.

Radiologic manipulation and insertion of central venous catheters is becoming more common. These procedures involve the use of sonographic or venographic guidance of venous cannulation and subsequent fluoroscopic guidance of catheter placement (308).

REFERENCES

General Information

1. Poznanski AK. *Practical approaches to pediatric radiology.* Chicago: Year Book, 1976.
2. Godderidge C. *Pediatric imaging.* Philadelphia: WB Saunders, 1995.
3. Silverman FN, Kuhn JP. *Caffey's pediatric x-ray diagnosis: an integrated imaging approach.* 9th ed. St. Louis: Mosby, 1993.
4. Sty JR, Hernandez RJ, Starshak RJ. *Body imaging in pediatrics.* New York: Grune and Stratton, 1984.
5. Hilton SV, Edwards DK. *Practical pediatric radiology.* 2nd ed. Philadelphia: WB Saunders, 1995.

Development of Pediatric Radiology

6. Spiegel PK. The first clinical x-ray made in America—100 years. *AJR* 1995;164:241–243.
7. Caffey J. The first sixty years of pediatric roentgenology in the United States. *AJR* 1956;76:437–454.
8. Hope JW. Pediatric radiology. *AJR* 1962;88:589–591.
9. Singleton EB. Society for pediatric radiology. *AJR* 1964;91:706–709.
10. Baker DH. Pediatric radiology: the first decade—the second decade. *AJR* 1968;103:224–225.
11. Gwinn JL. Pediatric radiology. *AJR* 1974;120:470–471.
12. Griscom NT. Parts and wholes: The Society for Pediatric Radiology and the general radiologic community. *AJR* 1978;130:799.
13. Kirks DR. The Society for Pediatric Radiology: 30 years later. *AJR* 1988;151:151–152.
14. Kirks DR. International pediatric radiology '87: inaugural conjoint meeting of The Society for Pediatric Radiology and the European Society of Pediatric Radiology. *AJR* 1987;149:1300.
15. Forman HP, Leonidas JC, Kirks DR. Clinical activities of pediatric radiologists in the United States and Canada: 10-year follow-up. *Radiology* 1990;175:127–129.
16. Kirks DR. Pediatric radiology: flexibility, viability, credibility, and opportunity. *Radiology* 1993;187:311–312.
17. Griscom NT. The foundation and early meetings of The Society for Pediatric Radiology. *Pediatr Radiol* 1995;25:657–660.
18. Griscom NT. History of pediatric radiology in the United States and Canada: images and trends. *RadioGraphics* 1995;15:1399–1422.
19. Griscom NT. Pediatric radiology in North America. In: Gagliardi R, Krabbenhoft K, McClennan B, eds. *A history of the radiologic sciences: diagnosis.* Reston, VA: Radiology Centennial, Inc., 1996, 345–368.

Problem-Oriented Pediatric Radiology

20. Sauvegrain J. Problem-oriented pediatric radiology. *Ann Radiol* 1978; 21:89–90.
21. Rigler LG. Is this radiograph really necessary? *Radiology* 1976;120: 449–450.
22. Griscom NT. Examinations that are sometimes overused or that are now obsolescent or obsolete. *Curr Opin Pediatr* 1991;3:1–3.
23. Seibert JJ, Bryant E, Lowe BA, et al. Low efficacy radiography of children. *AJR* 1980;134:1219–1223.
24. Wagner LK, Eifel PJ, Geise RA. Potential biological effects following high x-ray dose interventional procedures. *J Vasc Intervent Radiol* 1994;5:71–84.
25. Wesenberg RL, Rossi RP, Hendee WR. Radiation exposure in radiographic examinations of the newborn. *Radiology* 1977;122:499–504.
26. Wesenberg RL, Rossi RP, Hilton SV, et al. Low-dose radiography in pediatric radiology. *AJR* 1977;128:1066–1067.
27. Wesenberg RL, Amundson GM. Fluoroscopy in children: low exposure technology. *Radiology* 1984;153:243–247.
28. Barbier JY, Shackelford GD, McAlister WH. A radiant-heating device for control of body temperature of infants during radiography. *Radiology* 1973;108:215–216.
29. Fisher DM. Sedation of pediatric patients: an anesthesiologist's perspective. *Radiology* 1990;175:613–615.
30. Gooding CA, Berdon WE, Brodeur AE, Rowen M. Adverse reactions to intravenous pyelography in children. *AJR* 1975;123:802–804.
31. Cohen MD, Herman E, Herron D, et al. Comparison of intravenous

contrast agents for CT studies in children. *Acta Radiol* 1992;33: 592–595.

32. Shiels WE II. Handling of the acutely ill or injured child. In: Kirks DR, ed. *Emergency pediatric radiology. A problem-oriented approach.* Reston, VA: American Roentgen Ray Society, 1995, 1–5.

Radiologic Equipment

33. Bednarek DR, Rudin S, Wong R, Andres ML. Reduction of fluoroscopic exposure for the air-contrast barium enema. *Br J Radiol* 1983; 56:823–828.
34. Sprawls P Jr. *Physical principles of medical imaging.* Rockville, MD: Aspen Publishers, 1987.
35. Koedooder K, Venema HW. Filter materials for dose reduction in screen-film radiography. *Phys Med Biol* 1986;31:585–600.
36. Kohn ML, Gooch AW Jr, Keller WS. Filters for radiation reduction: a comparison. *Radiology* 1988;167:255–257.
37. Jangland L, Axelsson B. Niobium filters for dose reduction in pediatric radiology. *Acta Radiol* 1990;31:540–541.
38. Thierens H, Kunnen M, Van der Plaetsen A, Segaert O. Evaluation of the use of a niobium filter for patient dose reduction in chest radiography. *Br J Radiol* 1991;64:334–340.
39. Becker J. Adjustable compensating filters for pediatric 72-inch spine radiography. *Radiol Technol* 1979;51:11–16.
40. Gray JE, Stears JG, Frank ED. Shaped, lead-loaded acrylic filters for patient exposure reduction and image-quality improvement. *Radiology* 1983;146:825–828.
41. Butler PF, Thomas AW, Thompson WE, et al. Simple methods to reduce patient exposure during scoliosis radiography. *Radiol Technol* 1986;57:411–417.
42. Drury P, Robinson A. Fluoroscopy without the grid: a method of reducing the radiation dose. *Br J Radiol* 1980;53:93–99.
43. Rudin S, Bednarek DR, Miller JA. Dose reduction during fluoroscopic placement of feeding tubes. *Radiology* 1991;178:647–651.
44. Hufton AP, Russell JGB. The use of carbon fibre material in table tops, cassette fronts and grid covers: magnitude of possible dose reduction. *Br J Radiol* 1986;59:157–163.
45. Herman MW, Mak HK, Lachman RS. Radiation exposure reduction by use of Kevlar cassettes in the neonatal nursery. *AJR* 1987;148: 969–972.
46. Burton EM, Kirks DR, Strife JL, et al. Evaluation of a low-dose neonatal chest radiographic system. *AJR* 1988;151:999–1002.
47. McDaniel DL. Relative dose efficiencies of antiscatter grids and air gaps in pediatric radiography. *Med Phys* 1984;11:508–512.
48. Skucas J, Gorski JW. Comparison of the image quality of 105 mm film with conventional film. *Radiology* 1976;118:433–437.
49. Skucas J, Gorski JW. Application of modern intensifying screens in diagnostic radiology. *Med Radiogr Photogr* 1980;56:25–36.
50. Rossi RP, Hendee WR, Ahrens CR. An evaluation of rare earth screen/film combinations. *Radiology* 1976;121:465–471.
51. Bunch PC. Performance characteristics of high-MTF screen–film systems. *Proc SPIE* 1994;2163:14–35.

Immobilization

52. Vezina JA. Octagon board for pediatric immobilization. *J Can Assoc Radiol* 1970;21:290–294.
53. Poznauskis L. Immobilization. In: Godderidge C, ed. *Pediatric imaging.* Philadelphia: WB Saunders, 1995;145–158.
54. United States Department of Health, Education and Welfare. *Gonad shielding in diagnostic radiology.* DHEW, 1975.
55. Godderidge C. Female gonadal shielding. *Appl Radiol* 1979;8:65–67.

Radiation Dosage in Children

56. Hall EJ. *Radiobiology for the radiologist.* Hagerstown, PA: Harper and Row, 1978.
57. Kereiakes JG, Rosenstein M. *Handbook of radiation doses in nuclear medicine and diagnostic x-ray.* Boca Raton: CRC Press, 1980.
58. Hall EJ. *Radiation and life.* New York: Pergamon Press, 1976.
59. Elgenmark O. Normal development of ossific centres during infancy and childhood. A clinical, roentgenologic, and statistical study. *Acta Paediatr Suppl* 1946;33:1–79.

Contrast Media

60. Fischer HW. Catalog of intravascular contrast media. *Radiology* 1986; 159:561–563.
61. Cohen MD. A review of the toxicity of nonionic contrast agents in children. *Invest Radiol* 1993;28:S87–S93.
62. Wolf GL. Safer, more expensive iodinated contrast agents: how do we decide? *Radiology* 1986;159:557–558.
63. McClennan BL. Low-osmolality contrast media: premises and promises. *Radiology* 1987;162:1–8.
64. Siegle RL. Rates of idiosyncratic reactions. Ionic versus nonionic contrast media. *Invest Radiol* 1993;28:S95–S98.
65. Thomsen HS, Dorph S. High-osmolar and low-osmolar contrast media. An update on frequency of adverse drug reactions. *Acta Radiol* 1993;34:205–209.
66. White RI Jr, Halden WJ Jr. Liquid gold: low-osmolality contrast media. *Radiology* 1986;159:559–560.

Neonatal Radiology

67. Swischuk LE. *Imaging of the newborn, infant, and young child.* 4th ed. Baltimore: Williams and Wilkins, 1997.
68. Wesenberg RL. *The newborn chest.* Hagerstown, PA: Harper and Row, 1973.
69. Poznanski AK, Kanellitsas C, Roloff DW, Borer RC. Radiation exposure to personnel in a neonatal nursery. *Pediatrics* 1974;54:139–141.

Horizontal Beam Radiography

70. Capitanio MA, Kirkpatrick JA. The lateral decubitus film. An aid in determining air-trapping in children. *Radiology* 1972;103:460–462.
71. Kirks DR, O'Byrne SA. The value of the lateral abdominal roentgenogram in the diagnosis of neonatal hepatic portal venous gas (HPVG). *AJR* 1974;122:153–158.
72. Kaufman AS, Kuhn LR. The lateral decubitus view: an aid in evaluating poorly defined pulmonary densities in children. *AJR* 1977;129: 885–888.
73. Seibert JJ, Parvey LS. The telltale triangle: use of the supine cross table lateral radiograph of the abdomen in early detection of pneumoperitoneum. *Pediatr Radiol* 1977;5:209–210.

Fluoroscopy

74. Leibovic SJ, Caldicott WJH. Gastrointestinal fluoroscopy: patient dose and methods for its reduction. *Br J Radiol* 1983;56:715–719.
75. Aufrichtig R, Xue P, Thomas CW, et al. Perceptual comparison of pulsed and continuous fluoroscopy. *Med Phys* 1994;21:245–256.
76. Hernandez RJ, Goodsitt MM. Reduction of radiation dose in pediatric patients using pulsed fluoroscopy. *AJR* 1996;167:1247–1253.
77. Ablow RC, Jaffe CC, Orphanoudakis SC, et al. Fluoroscopic dose reduction using a digital television noise-reduction device. *Radiology* 1983;148:313–315.

Nuclear Medicine

78. Stabin MG. Internal dosimetry in pediatric nuclear medicine. In: Treves ST, ed. *Pediatric nuclear medicine.* 2nd ed. New York: Springer-Verlag, 1995, 556–582.
79. Treves ST. *Pediatric nuclear medicine.* 2nd ed. New York: Springer-Verlag, 1995.
80. Treves ST. Introduction. In: Treves ST, ed. *Pediatric nuclear medicine.* 2nd ed. New York: Springer-Verlag, 1995, 1–11.
81. Phelps ME, Mazziotta JC, Schelbert HR. *Positron emission tomography and autoradiography: principles and applications for the brain and heart.* New York: Raven Press, 1986.
82. Sorenson JA, Phelps ME. *Physics in nuclear medicine.* 2nd ed. Philadelphia: WB Saunders, 1987.
83. Drane WE, Abbott FD, Nicole MW, et al. Technology for FDG SPECT with a relatively inexpensive gamma camera. Work in progress. *Radiology* 1994;191:461–465.
84. Groch MW, Erwin WD, Bieszk JA. Single photon emission computed

tomography. In: Treves ST, ed. *Pediatric nuclear medicine*. 2nd ed. New York: Springer-Verlag, 1995, 33–87.

85. Davis RT, Zimmerman RE, Treves ST. Magnification in pediatric nuclear medicine. In: Treves ST, ed. *Pediatric nuclear medicine*. 2nd ed. New York: Springer-Verlag, 1995, 24–32.

Ultrasonography

86. AIUM. Bioeffects considerations for the safety of diagnostic ultrasound. *J Ultrasound Med* 1988;7:S1–S38.

87. Grant EG, White EM, Schellinger D. Cranial duplex sonography of the infant. *Radiology* 1987;163:177–185.

88. Mitchell DG, Merton D, Needleman L, et al. Neonatal brain: color Doppler imaging. Part I. Technique and vascular anatomy. *Radiology* 1988;167:303–306.

89. Dean LM, Taylor GA. The intracranial venous system in infants: normal and abnormal findings on duplex and color Doppler sonography. *AJR* 1995;164:151–156.

90. Taylor GA, Walker LK. Intracranial venous system in newborns treated with extracorporeal membrane oxygenation: Doppler US evaluation after ligation of the right jugular vein. *Radiology* 1992;183:453–456.

91. Hernanz-Schulman M. Applications of Doppler sonography to diagnosis extracranial pediatric disease. *Radiology* 1993;189:1–14.

92. Patriquin H. Doppler examination of the kidney in infants and children. *Urol Radiol* 1991;12:220–227.

93. Ingram S, Hollman AS. Colour Doppler sonography of the normal paediatric testis. *Clin Radiol* 1994;49:266–267.

94. Jequier S, Patriquin H, Filiatrault D, et al. Duplex Doppler sonographic examinations of the testis in prepubertal boys. *J Ultrasound Med* 1993;12:317–322.

95. Yazbeck S, Patriquin HB. Accuracy of Doppler sonography in the evaluation of acute conditions of the scrotum in children. *J Pediatr Surg* 1994;29:1270–1272.

96. Rubin JM, Bude RO, Carson PL, et al. Power Doppler US: a potentially useful alternative to mean frequency-based color Doppler US. *Radiology* 1994;190:853–856.

97. Babcock DS, Patriquin H, LaFortune M, Dauzat M. Power Doppler sonography: basic principles and clinical applications in children. *Pediatr Radiol* 1996;26:109–115.

98. Babcock DS, Mack LA, Han BK. Congenital anomalies and other abnormalities of the brain. *Semin Ultrasound CT MR* 1982;3:191–199.

99. Mack LA, Alvord EC. Neonatal cranial ultrasound: normal appearances. *Semin Ultrasound CT MR* 1982;3:216–230.

100. Grant EG. Sonography of the premature brain: intracranial hemorrhage and periventricular leukomalacia. *Neuroradiology* 1986;28:476–490.

101. Han BK, Babcock DS, McAdams L. Bacterial meningitis in infants: sonographic findings. *Radiology* 1985;154:645–650.

102. Taylor GA, Fitz CR, Miller MK, et al. Intracranial abnormalities in infants treated with extracorporeal membrane oxygenation: imaging with US and CT. *Radiology* 1987;165:675–678.

103. Cohen HL, Haller JO. Advances in perinatal neurosonography. *AJR* 1994;163:801–810.

104. DiPietro MA. The conus medullaris: normal US findings throughout childhood. *Radiology* 1993;188:149–153.

105. Naidich TP. Sonography of the caudal spine and back: congenital anomalies in children. *AJR* 1984;142:1229–1242.

106. Korsvik HE. Ultrasound assessment of congenital spinal anomalies presenting in infancy. *Semin Ultrasound CT MR* 1994;15:264–274.

107. Kraus R, Han BK, Babcock DS, Oestreich AE. Sonography of neck masses in children. *AJR* 1986;146:609–613.

108. Friedman AP, Haller JO, Goodman JD, Nagar H. Sonographic evaluation of noninflammatory neck masses in children. *Radiology* 1983;147:693–697.

109. Glasier CM, Seibert JJ, Williamson SL, et al. High resolution ultrasound characterization of soft tissue masses in children. *Pediatr Radiol* 1987;17:233–237.

110. Haller JO, Schneider M, Kassner EG, et al. Sonographic evaluation of the chest in infants and children. *AJR* 1980;134:1019–1027.

111. Glasier CM, Leithiser RE Jr, Williamson SL, Seibert JJ. Extracardiac chest ultrasonography in infants and children: radiographic and clinical implications. *J Pediatr* 1989;114:540–544.

112. Yousefzadeh DK, Ramilo JL. Normal hip in children: correlation of

113. Harcke HT, Grissom LE. Performing dynamic sonography of the infant hip. *AJR* 1990;155:837–844.

114. Miralles M, Gonzalez G, Pulpeiro JR et al. Sonography of the painful hip in children: 500 consecutive cases. *AJR* 1989;152:579–582.

115. Stark JE, Weinberger E. Ultrasonography of the neonatal genitourinary tract. *Appl Radiol* 1993:50–53.

116. Strife JL, Souza AS, Kirks DR, et al. Multicystic dysplastic kidney in children: US follow-up. *Radiology* 1993;186:785–788.

117. Dinkel E, Orth S, Dittrich M, Schulte-Wissermann H. Renal sonography in the differentiation of upper from lower urinary tract infection. *AJR* 1986;146:775–780.

118. Kangarloo H, Gold RH, Fine RN, et al. Urinary tract infection in infants and children evaluated by ultrasound. *Radiology* 1985;154:367–373.

119. Hayden CK Jr, Santa-Cruz FR, Amparo EG, et al. Ultrasonographic evaluation of the renal parenchyma in infancy and childhood. *Radiology* 1984;152:413–417.

120. Brenbridge AN, Chevalier RL, Kaiser DL. Increased renal cortical echogenicity in pediatric renal disease: histopathologic correlations. *J Clin Ultrasound* 1986;14:595–600.

121. Finkelstein MS, Rosenberg HK, Snyder HM III, Duckett JW. Ultrasound evaluation of scrotum in pediatrics. *Urology* 1986;27:1–9.

122. Luker GD, Siegel MJ. Pediatric testicular tumors: evaluation with gray-scale and color Doppler US. *Radiology* 1994;191:561–564.

123. Teele RL, Share JC. Ultrasonography of the female pelvis in childhood and adolescence. *Radiol Clin North Am* 1992;30:743–758.

124. Stark JE, Siegel MJ. Ovarian torsion in prepubertal and pubertal girls: sonographic findings. *AJR* 1994;163:1479–1482.

125. Barr LL. Sonography in the infant with acute abdominal symptoms. *Semin Ultrasound CT MR* 1994;15:275–289.

126. Sivit CJ. Diagnosis of acute appendicitis in children: spectrum of sonographic findings. *AJR* 1993;161:147–152.

127. Paltiel HJ. Imaging of neonatal cholestasis. *Semin Ultrasound CT MR* 1994;15:290–305.

128. Haller JO. Sonography of the biliary tract in infants and children. *AJR* 1991;157:1051–1058.

129. Teele RL, Share JC. *Ultrasonography of infants and children*. Philadelphia: WB Saunders, 1991, 214–316.

Computed Tomography

130. Harwood-Nash DC, Breckbill DL. Computed tomography in children: a new diagnostic technique. *J Pediatr* 1976;89:343–357.

131. Naidich TP, Epstein F, Lin JP, et al. Evaluation of pediatric hydrocephalus by computed tomography. *Radiology* 1976;119:337–345.

132. Brasch RC, Korobkin M, Gooding CA. Computed body tomography in children: evaluation of 45 patients. *AJR* 1978;131:21–25.

133. Maravilla KR, Kirks DR, Maravilla AM. Computer reconstructed sagittal and coronal CT scans. Applications in neurological disorders of infants and children. *Pediatr Radiol* 1978;7:65–69.

134. Burstein J, Papile LA, Burstein R. Intraventricular hemorrhage and hydrocephalus in premature newborns: a prospective study with CT. *AJR* 1979;132:631–635.

135. Berger PE, Munschauer RW, Kuhn JP. Computed tomography and ultrasound of renal and perirenal diseases in infants and children: relationship to excretory urography in renal cystic disease, trauma, and neoplasm. *Pediatr Radiol* 1980;9:91–99.

136. Kirks DR, Harwood-Nash DC. Computed tomography in pediatric radiology. *Pediatr Ann* 1980;9:66–76.

137. Kirks DR, Korobkin M. Chest computed tomography in infants and children: an analysis of 50 patients. *Pediatr Radiol* 1980;10:75–82.

138. Kirks DR, Merten DF, Grossman H, Bowie JD. Diagnostic imaging of pediatric abdominal masses: an overview. *Radiol Clin North Am* 1981;19:527–545.

139. Riddlesberger MM Jr, Kuhn JP. The role of computed tomography in diseases of the musculoskeletal system. *J Comput Tomogr* 1983;7:85–99.

140. Yamada H. *Pediatric cranial computed tomography*. Tokyo: Igaku-Shoin, 1983.

141. Kirks DR. Computed tomography of pediatric urinary tract disease. *Urol Radiol* 1983;5:199–208.

142. Kirks DR. Practical techniques for pediatric computed tomography. *Pediatr Radiol* 1983;13:148–155.

143. Kirks DR, Fram EK, Vock P, Effmann EL. Tracheal compression by mediastinal masses in children: CT evaluation. *AJR* 1983;141: 647–651.

144. Kaufman RA. Liver-spleen computed tomography. A method tailored for infants and children. *J Comput Tomogr* 1983;7:45–57.

145. Siegel MJ. Computed tomography of the pediatric pelvis. *J Comput Tomogr* 1983;7:77–83.

146. Lallemand DP, Brasch RC, Char DH, Norman D. Orbital tumors in children: characterization by computed tomography. *Radiology* 1984; 151:85–88.

147. Sarwar M. *CT of congenital brain malformations.* Boston: Martinus Nihoff, 1985.

148. Miller JH, Greenspan BS. Integrated imaging of hepatic tumors in childhood. Part I. Malignant lesions (primary and metastatic). *Radiology* 1985;154:83–90.

149. Terrier F, Weber W, Ruefenacht D, Porcellini B. Anatomy of the ethmoid: CT, endoscopic, and macroscopic. *AJR* 1985;144:493–500.

150. Daneman A. *Pediatric body CT.* New York: Springer-Verlag, 1987.

151. Taylor GA, Fallat ME, Eichelberger MR. Hypovolemic shock in children: abdominal CT manifestations. *Radiology* 1987;164:479–481.

152. Feldman F, Singson RD, Rosenberg ZS, et al. Distal tibial triplane fractures: diagnosis with CT. *Radiology* 1987;164:429–435.

153. Brick SH, Taylor GA, Potter BM, Eichelberger MR. Hepatic and splenic injury in children: role of CT in the decision for laparotomy. *Radiology* 1987;165:643–646.

154. Kaufman RA. Technical aspects of abdominal CT in infants and children. *AJR* 1989;153:549–554.

155. Siegel MJ. *Pediatric body CT.* New York: Churchill Livingstone, 1988.

156. Wells RG. CT of the orbit in pediatrics. *Appl Radiol* 1988;15 and 23.

157. Fredericks BJ, Boldt DW, Tress BM, Cattapan E. Diseases of the spinal canal in children: diagnosis with noncontrast CT scans. *AJNR* 1989;10:1233–1238.

158. Taylor GA, Guion CJ, Potter BM, Eichelberger MR. CT of blunt abdominal trauma in children. *AJR* 1989;153:555–559.

159. Kleinman PK, Spevak MR. Advanced pediatric joint imaging. *Radiol Clin North Am* 1990;28:1073–1109.

160. Strand R, Humphrey C, Barnes PD. Imaging of petrous temporal bone abnormalities in infancy and childhood. In: Healy G, ed. *Common problems in pediatric otolaryngology.* Chicago: Mosby–Year Book, 1990, 121–130.

161. Griscom NT. CT measurement of the tracheal lumen in children and adolescents. *AJR* 1991;156:371–372.

162. Costello P, Dupuy DE, Ecker CP, Tello R. Spiral CT of the thorax with reduced volume of contrast material: a comparative study. *Radiology* 1992;183:663–666.

163. Jabra AA, Fishman EK, Taylor GA. CT findings in inflammatory bowel disease in children. *AJR* 1994;162:975–979.

164. Medina LS, Siegel MJ. CT of complications in pediatric lung transplantation. *RadioGraphics* 1994;14:1341–1349.

165. Eggli KD, King SH, Boal DKB, Quiogue T. Low-dose CT of developmental dysplasia of the hip after reduction: diagnostic accuracy and dosimetry. *AJR* 1994;163:1441–1443.

166. Vannier MW, Pilgram TK, Marsh JL, et al. Craniosynostosis: diagnostic imaging with three-dimensional CT presentation. *AJNR* 1994;15: 1861–1869.

167. Cox TD, White KS, Weinberger E, Effmann EL. Comparison of helical and conventional chest CT in the uncooperative pediatric patient. *Pediatr Radiol* 1995;25:347–349.

168. White KS. Reduced need for sedation in patients undergoing helical CT of the chest and abdomen. *Pediatr Radiol* 1995;25:344–346.

169. White KS. Pediatric CT scanning techniques. In: Kirks DR, ed. *Emergency pediatric imaging. A problem oriented approach.* Reston, VA: American Roentgen Ray Society, 1995, 95–98.

170. Siegel MJ, Luker GD. Pediatric applications of helical (spiral) CT. *Radiol Clin North Am* 1995;33:997–1022.

171. Kaste SC, Young CW. Safe use of power injections with central and peripheral venous access devices for pediatric CT. *Pediatr Radiol* 1996;26:499–501.

172. Dean LM, Taylor GA. Pediatric application of spiral CT. In: Fishman EK, Jeffries RB Jr, eds. *Spiral CT: principles, techniques and clinical applications.* New York: Raven Press, 1995, 159–166.

173. Berland LL. Slip-ring and conventional dynamic hepatic CT: contrast material and timing considerations. *Radiology* 1995;195:1–8.

174. Ambrosino MM, Genieser NB, Roche KJ, et al. Feasibility of high-resolution, low-dose chest CT in evaluating the pediatric chest. *Pediatr Radiol* 1994;24:6–10.

175. Brink JA, Davros WJ. Helical/spiral CT: technical principles. In: Zeman R, ed. *Helical/spiral CT: a practical approach.* New York: McGraw-Hill, 1995, 1–26.

176. Strain JD, Harvey LA, Foley LC, Campbell JB. Intravenously administered pentobarbital sodium for sedation in pediatric CT. *Radiology* 1986;161:105–108.

177. Thompson JR, Schneider S, Ashwal S, et al. The choice of sedation for computed tomography in children: a prospective evaluation. *Radiology* 1982;143:475–479.

178. Strain JD, Campbell JB, Harvey LA, Foley LC. IV Nembutal: Safe sedation for children undergoing CT. *AJR* 1988;151:975–979.

179. Hubbard AM, Markowitz RI, Kimmel B, et al. Sedation for pediatric patients undergoing CT and MRI. *J Comput Assist Tomogr* 1992;16: 3–6.

180. Nelson MD Jr. Guidelines for the monitoring and care of children during and after sedation for imaging studies. *AJR* 1993;160:581–582.

181. Pereira JK, Burrows PE, Richards HM, et al. Comparison of sedation regimens for pediatric outpatient CT. *Pediatr Radiol* 1993;23: 341–344.

182. American Academy of Pediatrics Committee on Drugs. Guidelines for monitoring and management of pediatric patients during and after sedation for diagnostic and therapeutic procedures. *Pediatrics* 1992; 89:1110–1115.

183. Katakura T, Kimura K, Midorikawa S, et al. Improvement of resolution along patient axis in helical-volume CT. *Radiology* 1990;177(P): 108.

184. Heiken JP, Brink JA, Vannier MW. Spiral (helical) CT. *Radiology* 1993;189:647–656.

Magnetic Resonance Imaging

185. Johnson MA, Pennock JM, Bydder GM, et al. Clinical NMR imaging of the brain in children: normal and neurologic disease. *AJR* 1983; 141:1005–1018.

186. Zimmerman RA, Bilaniuk LT. Applications of magnetic resonance imaging in diseases of the pediatric central nervous system. *Magn Reson Imaging* 1986;4:11–24.

187. Holland BA, Haas DK, Norman D, et al. MRI of normal brain maturation. *AJNR* 1986;7:201–208.

188. Cohen MD. *Pediatric magnetic resonance imaging.* Philadelphia: WB Saunders, 1986.

189. Dietrich RB, Kangarloo H. Kidneys in infants and children: evaluation with MR. *Radiology* 1986;159:215–221.

190. Bisset GS III, Strife JL, Kirks DR, Bailey WW. Vascular rings: MR imaging. *AJR* 1987;149:251–256.

191. Barnes PD, Lester PD, Yamanashi WS, et al. Magnetic resonance imaging in childhood intracranial masses. *Magn Reson Imaging* 1986; 4:41–49.

192. Barkovich AJ, Kjos BO, Jackson DE Jr, Norman D. Normal maturation of the neonatal and infant brain: MR imaging at 1.5T. *Radiology* 1988;166:173–180.

193. Dietrich RB, Kangarloo H, Lenarsky C, Feig SA. Neuroblastoma: the role of MR imaging. *AJR* 1987;148:937–942.

194. Boechat MI, Kangarloo H. MR imaging of the abdomen in children. *AJR* 1989;152:1245–1250.

195. Barnes PD. Magnetic resonance in pediatric and adolescent neuroimaging. *Neurol Clin* 1990;8:741–757.

196. Auringer ST, Bisset GS III, Myer CM III. Magnetic resonance imaging of the pediatric airway. Compared with findings and surgery and/or endoscopy. *Pediatr Radiol* 1991;21:329–332.

197. Meyer JS, Hoffer FA, Barnes PD, Mulliken JB. Biological classification of soft-tissue vascular anomalies: MR correlation. *AJR* 1991;157: 559–564.

198. Surratt JT, Siegel MJ. Imaging of pediatric ovarian masses. *RadioGraphics* 1991;11:533–548.

199. Wolpert SM, Barnes PD. *MRI in pediatric neuroradiology.* St. Louis: Mosby–Year Book, 1992.

200. Dangman BC, Hoffer FA, Rand FF, O'Rourke EJ. Osteomyelitis in children: gadolinium-enhanced MR imaging. *Radiology* 1992;182: 743–747.

201. Jaramillo D, Hoffer FA. Cartilaginous epiphysis and growth plate: normal and abnormal MR imaging findings. *AJR* 1992;158: 1105–1110.

202. Ahn SS, Mantello MT, Jones KM, et al. Rapid MR imaging of the pediatric brain using the fast spin-echo technique. *AJNR* 1992;13: 1169–1177.

203. Barkovich AJ, Kjos BO. Gray matter heterotopias: MR characteristics and correlation with developmental and neurological manifestations. *Radiology* 1992;182:483–499.

204. Fellows KE, Weinberg PM, Baffa JM, Hoffman EA. Evaluation of congenital heart disease with MR imaging: current and coming attractions. *AJR* 1992;159:925–931.

205. Quencer RM. Intracranial CSF flow in pediatric hydrocephalus: evaluation with cine-MR imaging. *AJNR* 1992;13:601–608.

206. Burrows PE, MacDonald CE. Magnetic resonance imaging of the pediatric thoracic aorta. *Semin Ultrasound CT MR* 1993;14:129–144.

207. Gylys-Morin V, Hoffer FA, Kozakewich H, Shamberger RC. Wilms tumor and nephroblastomatosis: imaging characteristics at gadolinium-enhanced MR imaging. *Radiology* 1993;188:517–521.

208. Shady KL, Siegel MJ, Brown JJ. Preoperative evaluation of intraabdominal tumors in children: gradient-recalled echo vs. spin-echo MR imaging. *AJR* 1993;161:843–847.

209. Jaramillo D, Laor T, Mulkern RV. Comparison between fast spin-echo and conventional spin-echo images of normal and abnormal musculoskeletal structures in children and young adults. *Invest Radiol* 1994;29:803–811.

210. Laor T, Chung T, Hoffer FA, Jaramillo D. Musculoskeletal magnetic resonance imaging: how we do it. *Pediatr Radiol* 1996;26:695–700.

211. Siegel MJ. MR imaging of the pediatric abdomen. *Magn Reson Clin North Am* 1995;3:161–182.

212. Tzika AA, Vigneron DB, Ball WS Jr, et al. Localized proton MR spectroscopy of the brain in children. *J Magn Reson Imaging* 1993; 3:719–729.

213. Wang Z. Zimmerman RA, Saeuter R. Proton MR spectroscopy of the brain: clinically useful information obtained in assessing CNS diseases in children. *AJR* 1996;167:191–199.

214. Tzika AA, Massoth RJ, Ball WS Jr, et al. Cerebral perfusion in children: detection with dynamic contrast-enhanced T2*-weighted images. *Radiology* 1993;187:449–458.

215. Mulkern RV, Meng J, Oshio K, et al. Spectroscopic imaging of the knee with line scan CPMG sequences. *J Comput Assist Tomogr* 1995; 19:247–255.

216. Higgins CB. *MRI in congenital heart disease: morphology, function and flow.* In: *American College of Radiology Syllabus for the categorical course on cardiovascular imaging.* Reston, VA: American College of Radiology, 1995, 87–89.

217. Horowitz AL. *MRI physics for radiologists.* New York: Springer-Verlag, 1995.

218. Cohen MS, Weisskoff RM. Ultra-fast imaging. *Magn Reson Imaging* 1991;9:1–37.

219. Haacke EM, Tkach JA. Fast MR imaging: techniques and applications. *AJR* 1990;155:951–964.

220. Mulkern RV. Technical developments in abdominal magnetic resonance fast imaging. In: Beltran J, ed. *Current review of magnetic resonance imaging.* Philadelphia: Current Medicine, 1995, 1–18.

221. Bailes DR, Gilerdale DJ, Bydder GM, et al. Respiratory ordered phase encoding (ROPE): a method for reducing respiratory motion artifacts in MR imaging. *J Comput Assist Tomogr* 1985;9:835–838.

222. Felmlee JP, Ehman RL. Spatial presaturation: a method for suppressing flow artifacts and improving depiction of vascular anatomy in MR imaging. *Radiology* 1987;164:559–564.

223. Haacke EM, Lenz GW. Improving MR image quality in the presence of motion by using rephasing gradients. *AJR* 1987;148:1251–1258.

224. Mitchell DG, Vinitski S, Burk DL Jr, et al. Motion artifact reduction in MR imaging of the abdomen: gradient moment nulling versus respiratory-sorted phase encoding. *Radiology* 1988;169:155–160.

225. Bisset GS III, Ball WS Jr. Preparation, sedation, and monitoring of the pediatric patient in the magnetic resonance suite. *Semin Ultrasound CT MR* 1991;12:376–378.

226. Bisset GS III. Pediatric sedation and monitoring in the emergency setting. In: Kirks DR, ed. *Emergency pediatric radiology. A problem-oriented approach.* Reston, VA: American Roentgen Ray Society, 1995, 61–63.

227. Edelman RR, Li W. Contrast-enhanced echo-planar MR imaging of myocardial perfusion: preliminary study in humans. *Radiology* 1994; 190:771–777.

228. Doherty NE III, Fujita N, Caputo GR, Higgins CB. Measurement of right ventricular mass in normal and dilated cardiomyopathic ventri-

229. Martinez JE, Mohiaddin RH, Kilner PJ, et al. Obstruction in extracardiac ventriculopulmonary conduits: value of nuclear magnetic resonance imaging with velocity mapping and Doppler echocardiography. *J Am Coll Cardiol* 1992;20:338–344.

230. Hossmann KA, Hoehn-Berlage M. Diffusion and perfusion MR imaging of cerebral ischemia. *Cerebrovasc Brain Metab Rev* 1995;7: 187–217.

Digital Imaging

231. Wagner ML, Singleton EB, Egan ME. Digital subtraction angiography in children. *AJR* 1983;140:127–133.

232. Tonkin IL, Stapleton FB, Roy S III. Digital subtraction angiography in the evaluation of renal vascular hypertension in children. *Pediatrics* 1988;81:150–158.

233. Broderick NJ, Long B, Dreesen RG, et al. Phosphor plate computed radiography: response to variation in mAs at fixed kVp in an animal model. Potential role in neonatal imaging. *Clin Radiol* 1993;47:39–45.

234. Franken EA Jr, Berbaum KS, Marley SM, et al. Evaluation of a digital workstation for interpreting neonatal examinations. A receiver operating characteristic study. *Invest Radiol* 1992;27:732–737.

235. Goldberg MA, Rosenthal DI, Chew FS, et al. New high-resolution teleradiology system: prospective study of diagnostic accuracy in 685 transmitted clinical cases. *Radiology* 1993;186:429–434.

236. Huang HK, Kangarloo H, Cho PS, et al. Planning a totally digital radiology department. *AJR* 1990;154:635–639.

237. Ackerman LV. DICOM: the answer for establishing a digital radiology department. *RadioGraphics* 1994;14:151–152.

238. Batnitzky S, Rosenthal SJ, Siegel EL, et al. Teleradiology: an assessment. *Radiology* 1990;177:11–17.

239. *ACR standards for teleradiology.* American College of Radiology Standards 1995:57–60.

Nonvascular Interventional Procedures

240. Stanley P, Bear JW, Reid BS. Percutaneous nephrostomy in infants and children. *AJR* 1983;141:473–477.

241. Stanley P, Atkinson JB, Reid BS, Gilsanz V. Percutaneous drainage of abdominal fluid collections in children. *AJR* 1984;142:813–816.

242. Ball WS Jr, Towbin R, Strife JL, Spencer R. Interventional genitourinary radiology in children: a review of 61 procedures. *AJR* 1986;147: 791–796.

243. Towbin RB, Strife JL. Percutaneous aspiration, drainage and biopsies in children. *Radiology* 1985;157:81–85.

244. Keller MS, Lai S, Wagner DK. Percutaneous gastrostomy in a child. *Radiology* 1986;160:261–262.

245. Hoffer FA, Winter HS, Fellows KE, Folkman J. The treatment of post-operative and peptic esophageal strictures after esophageal atresia repair: a program including dilatation with balloon catheters. *Pediatr Radiol* 1987;17:454–458.

246. vanSonnenberg E, Wittich GR, Edward DK, et al. Percutaneous diagnostic and therapeutic interventional radiologic procedures in children: experience in 100 patients. *Radiology* 1987;162:601–605.

247. Hoffer FA, Teele RL, Lillehei CW, Vacanti JP. Infected bilomas and hepatic artery thrombosis in infant recipients of liver transplants. Interventional radiology and medical therapy as an alternative to retransplantation. *Radiology* 1988;169:435–438.

248. Towbin RB, Ball WS Jr, Bisset GS III. Percutaneous gastrostomy and percutaneous gastrojejunostomy in children: antegrade approach. *Radiology* 1988;168:473–476.

249. Towbin RB, Ball WS Jr. Pediatric interventional radiology. *Radiol Clin North Am* 1988;26:419–440.

250. Towbin RB. Pediatric interventional procedures in the 1980s: a period of development, growth, and acceptance. *Radiology* 1989;170: 1081–1090.

251. Hoffer FA, Winters WD, Retik AB, Ringer SA. Urinoma drainage for neonatal respiratory insufficiency. *Pediatr Radiol* 1990;20:270–271.

252. Hoffer FA. Imaging guided aspiration and biopsy in children. *Semin Intervent Radiol* 1991;8:188–194.

253. Pereira JK, Chait PG, King SJ, et al. Transrectal drainage of deep pelvic abscesses in children (abstract). *Radiology* 1992;185(P): 231–232.

254. Malden ES, Hicks ME, Picus D, et al. Fluoroscopically guided percutaneous gastrostomy in children. *J Vasc Intervent Radiol* 1992;3: 673–677.

255. Hoffer F, Sandler RH, Kaplan LC, et al. Fluoroscopic placement of jejunal feeding tubes. *Pediatr Radiol* 1992;22:287–289.

256. Chait PG, Weinberg J, Connolly BL, et al. Retrograde percutaneous gastrostomy and gastrojejunostomy in 505 children: a 4 1/2 year experience. *Radiology* 1996;201:691–695.

257. Hubbard AM, Fellows KE. Pediatric interventional radiology: current practice and innovations. *Cardiovasc Intervent Radiol* 1993;16: 267–274.

258. Zawin JK, Hoffer FA, Rand FF, Teele RL. Joint effusion in children with an irritable hip: US diagnosis and aspiration. *Radiology* 1993; 187:459–463.

259. Towbin RB, Kaye R, Bron K. Intervention in the critically ill patient. *Crit Care Clin* 1994;10:437–454.

260. Fung LC, Khoury AE, McLorie GA, et al. Evaluation of pediatric hydronephrosis using individualized pressure flow criteria. *J Urol* 1995;154:671–676.

261. Chung T, Hoffer FA, Lund DP. Transrectal drainage of deep pelvic abscesses in children using a combined transrectal sonographic and fluoroscopic guidance. *Pediatr Radiol* 1996;26:874–878.

262. Ogborn MR. The use of a eutectic mixture of local anesthetic in pediatric renal biopsy. *Pediatr Nephrol* 1992;6:276–277.

263. Lorenzo RL, Bradford BF, Black J, Smith CD. Lung abscesses in children: diagnostic and therapeutic needle aspiration. *Radiology* 1985;157:79–80.

264. Hoffer FA, Kozakewich H, Colodny A, Goldstein DP. Peritoneal inclusion cysts: ovarian fluid in peritoneal adhesions. *Radiology* 1988; 169:189–191.

265. vanSonnenberg E, D'Agostino HB, Casola G, et al. Lung abscess: CT-guided drainage. *Radiology* 1991;178:347–351.

266. Yellin A, Yellin EO, Lieberman Y. Percutaneous tube drainage: the treatment of choice for refractory lung abscess. *Ann Thorac Surg* 1985;39:266–270.

267. Lee KS, Im JG, Kim YH, et al. Treatment of thoracic multiloculated empyemas with intracavitary urokinase: a prospective study. *Radiology* 1991;179:771–775.

268. Gilliland JD, Spies JB, Brown SB, et al. Lymphoceles: percutaneous treatment with povidone-iodine sclerosis. *Radiology* 1989;171: 227–229.

269. Look AT, Hayes FA, Shuster JJ, et al. Clinical relevance of tumor cell ploidy and N-myc gene amplification in childhood neuroblastoma: a Pediatric Oncology Group study. *J Clin Oncol* 1993;9:581–591.

270. Pierro A, Langevin AM, Filler RM, et al. Preoperative chemotherapy in ''unresectable'' hepatoblastoma. *J Pediatr Surg* 1989;24:24–29.

271. McLorie GA, McKenna PH, Greenberg M, et al. Reduction in tumor burden allowing partial nephrectomy following preoperative chemotherapy in biopsy proven Wilms tumor. *J Urol* 1991;146:509–513.

272. Cozens NJA, Murchison JT, Allan PL, Winney RJ. Conventional 15 G needle technique for renal biopsy compared with ultrasound-guided spring–loaded 18G needle biopsy. *Br J Radiol* 1992;65:594–597.

273. Webb NJ, Pereira JK, Chait PG, Geary DF. Renal biopsy in children: comparison of two techniques. *Pediatr Nephrol* 1994;8:486–488.

274. Sawyerr AM, McCormick PA, Tennyson GS, et al. A comparison of transjugular and plugged-percutaneous liver biopsy in patients with impaired coagulation. *J Hepatol* 1993;17:81–85.

275. Lu DSK, Mueller PR, Lee MJ, et al. Gastrostomy conversion to transgastric jejunostomy: technical problems, causes of failure, and proposed solutions in 63 patients. *Radiology* 1993;187:679–683.

276. Campbell JB, Davis WS. Catheter technique for extraction of blunt esophageal foreign bodies. *Radiology* 1973;108:438–440.

277. Campbell JB, Condon VR. Catheter removal of blunt esophageal foreign bodies in children. Survey of The Society for Pediatric Radiology. *Pediatr Radiol* 1989;19:361–365.

278. Kirks DR. Fluoroscopic catheter removal of blunt esophageal foreign bodies: a pediatric radiologist's perspective. *Pediatr Radiol* 1992;22: 64–65.

279. Newhouse JH, Pfister RC, Hendren WH, Yoder IC. Whitaker test after pyeloplasty: establishment of normal ureteral perfusion pressures. *AJR* 1981;137:223–226.

280. Faerber GJ, Ritchey ML, Bloom DA. Percutaneous endopyelotomy in infants and young children after failed open pyeloplasty. *J Urol* 1995;154:1495–1497.

Angiography and Vascular Interventional Procedures

281. Burrows PE, Robertson RL, Barnes PD. Angiography and the evaluation of cerebrovascular disease in childhood. *Neuroimaging Clin N Am* 1996;6:561–588.

282. Stanley P. Angiographic procedure. In: Stanley P, ed. *Pediatric angiography*. Baltimore: Williams and Wilkins, 1982, 1–34.

283. Moore AV, Kirks DR, Mills SR, Heaston DK. Pediatric abdominal angiography: panacea or passe? *AJR* 1982;138:433–443.

284. Clayman AS, Bookstein JJ. The role of renal arteriography in pediatric hypertension. *Radiology* 1973;108:107–110.

285. Kirks DR, Fitz CR, Harwood-Nash DC. Pediatric abdominal angiography: practical guide to catheter selection, flow rates, and contrast dosage. *Pediatr Radiol* 1976;5:19–23.

286. Kirks DR. Pediatric renal angiography. *Appl Radiol* 1978;11:83–91.

287. Burrows PE, Benson LN, Williams WG, et al. Iliofemoral arterial complications of balloon angioplasty for systemic obstructions in infants and children. *Circulation* 1990;82:1697–1704.

288. Harwood-Nash DC, Fitz CR. Neuroradiological techniques and indications in infancy and childhood. In: Kaufman HF, ed. *Progress in pediatric radiology*, vol 5. Basel: Karger, 1976, 2–85.

289. Lasjaunias P, Berenstein A. Endovascular treatment of craniofacial lesions. *Surgical neuroangiography*. Vol. 2. Berlin: Springer-Verlag, 1987.

290. Burrows PE, Lasjaunias PL, Ter Brugge KG, Flodmark O. Urgent and emergent embolization of lesions of the head and neck in children: indications and results. *Pediatrics* 1987;80:386–394.

291. Dubois JM, Sebag GH, De Prost Y, et al. Soft-tissue venous malformations in children: percutaneous sclerotherapy with Ethibloc. *Radiology* 1991;180:195–198.

292. McHugh K, Burrows PE. Infantile hepatic hemangioendotheliomas: significance of portal venous and systemic collateral arterial supply. *J Vasc Intervent Radiol* 1992;3:337–344.

293. Friedman DM, Verma R, Madrid M, et al. Recent improvement in outcome using transcatheter embolization techniques for neonatal aneurysmal malformations of the vein of Galen. *Pediatrics* 1993;91: 583–586.

294. Burrows PE, Fellows KE. Techniques for management of pediatric vascular anomalies. In: Cope C, ed. *Current techniques in interventional radiology*. Philadelphia: Current Medicine, 1995, 12–27.

295. Davis KR. Embolization of epistaxis and juvenile nasopharyngeal angiofibromas. *AJR* 1987;148:209–218.

296. De Cristofaro R, Biagini R, Boriani S, et al. Selective arterial embolization in the treatment of aneurysmal bone cyst and angioma of bone. *Skeletal Radiol* 1992;21:523–527.

297. Kumpe DA, Rumack CM, Pretorius DH, et al. Partial splenic embolization in children with hypersplenism. *Radiology* 1985;155:357–362.

298. Stanley P, Shen TC. Partial embolization of the spleen in patients with thalassemia. *J Vasc Intervent Radiol* 1995;6:137–142.

299. Lois JF, Hartzman S, McGlade CT, et al. Budd-Chiari syndrome: treatment with percutaneous transhepatic recanalization and dilation. *Radiology* 1989;170:791–793.

300. Barth MO, Gagnadoux MF, Mareschal JL, et al. Angioplasty of renal transplant artery stenosis in children. *Pediatr Radiol* 1989;19: 383–387.

301. Aliabadi H, McLorie GA, Churchill BM, McMullin N. Percutaneous transluminal angioplasty for transplant renal artery stenosis in children. *J Urol* 1990;143:569–573.

302. Wessel DL, Keane JF, Fellows KE et al. Fibrinolytic therapy for femoral arterial thrombosis after cardiac catheterization in infants and children. *Am J Cardiol* 1986;58:347–351.

303. Corrigan JJ Jr, Jeter M, Allen HD, Malone JM. Aortic thrombosis in a neonate: failure of urokinase thrombolytic therapy. *Am J Pediatr Hematol Oncol* 1982;4:243–247.

304. Strife JL, Ball WS Jr, Towbin R, et al. Arterial occlusions in neonates: use of fibrinolytic therapy. *Radiology* 1988;166:395–400.

305. Vogelzang RL, Moel DI, Cohn RA, et al. Acute renal vein thrombosis: successful treatment with intraarterial urokinase. *Radiology* 1988;169: 681–682.

306. Furuya KN, Burrows PE, Phillips MJ, Roberts EA. Transjugular liver biopsy in children. *Hepatology* 1992;15:1036–1042.

307. LaBerge JM, Ring EJ, Gordon RL, et al. Creation of transjugular intrahepatic portosystemic shunts with the wallstent endoprosthesis: results in 100 patients. *Radiology* 1993;187:413–420.

308. Chait PG, Ingram J, Phillips-Gordon C, et al. Peripherally inserted central catheters in children. *Radiology* 1995;197:775–778.

Practical Pediatric Imaging: Diagnostic Radiology of Infants and Children, Third Edition.
D. R. Kirks, editor and N. T. Griscom, associate editor.
Lippincott–Raven Publishers, Philadelphia © 1998.

CHAPTER 2

Skull and Brain

Richard L. Robertson, William S. Ball, Jr., and Patrick D. Barnes

Pediatric neuroradiology, a subspecialty of both pediatric radiology and neuroradiology, applies imaging techniques to the diagnosis of pediatric central nervous system (CNS) disease (1). This component of pediatric radiology is often difficult because of the complexities of normal anatomy, the frequency of normal variants, the variety of congenital abnormalities, and the unique effects of neurologic disease on the developing skull, brain, spine, and spinal cord (1–4). Furthermore, the need for high-resolution imaging requires an immobilized child, and this may require sedation or anesthesia. The three-volume textbook published in 1976 by Harwood-Nash and Fitz, *Neuroradiology in Infants and Children* (5), documented that the development of pediatric neuroradiology had developed into a unique subspecialty. Recent textbooks have further expanded on the basic principles of the subspecialty (6,7).

TECHNIQUES

A variety of imaging modalities may be used to evaluate pediatric CNS disease (Fig. 2-1). Imaging of the skull and brain currently includes plain radiography, ultrasonography (US), computed tomography (CT), magnetic resonance imaging (MRI), cerebral angiography, and nuclear medicine. Pediatric neuroradiologic evaluation must be flexible enough to fit the individual diagnostic requirements of the child, the clinical problem, and the neurologic disease (1,4–7).

US, CT, and MRI have become the focal points of neuroradiologic investigation. A normal cross-sectional imaging examination may make further invasive studies needless. The appearance is often so characteristic (hematoma, ger-

R. L. Robertson and P. D. Barnes: Division of Neuroradiology, Department of Radiology, Children's Hospital, Harvard Medical School, Boston, Massachusetts 02115.

W. S. Ball, Jr.: Section of Neuroradiology, Department of Radiology, Children's Hospital Medical Center, University of Cincinnati College of Medicine, Cincinnati, Ohio 45229.

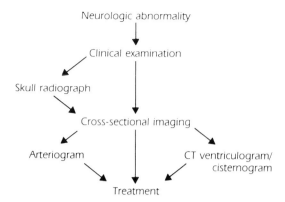

FIG. 2-1. Imaging protocol for pediatric neurologic disease. Cross-sectional imaging has become the focus of the neuroradiologic evaluation. Modified from Kirks and Harwood-Nash (3).

minal matrix hemorrhage, hydrocephalus) that treatment can be instituted solely on the basis of the imaging examination (3,4).

Conventional Radiography

Radiography of the skull should ordinarily include three projections (Appendix 2): anteroposterior (AP) or posteroanterior (PA) view, Towne view, and lateral view (vertical beam) or cross-table lateral view (horizontal beam). Basal (submentovertex) and oblique projections, as well as fluoroscopy, may occasionally be necessary. Skull radiography is most frequently used for demonstrating fractures and evaluating craniosynostosis. It may also clarify skull findings suggested by CT or MRI.

Ultrasonography

Rapid, noninvasive evaluation of the neonatal and young infant brain is performed with real-time US with the anterior fontanel as an imaging window (3,4,6–12). Supplemental windows include the posterior and posterolateral fontanels (mastoid view) and the temporal squamosa. Intracranial structures including the ventricles, parenchyma, and vessels are readily visualized in both coronal and sagittal planes (Fig. 2-2). Ventricular size, parenchymal and intraventricular hemorrhage, extracerebral fluid collections, cystic lesions, and solid parenchymal masses may be evaluated. Intracranial blood flow may be interrogated with Doppler techniques.

Examinations should be performed using a 5.0-MHz or 7.5-MHz sector transducer with aqueous gel as the coupling agent. Examinations are recorded on static images and can be videotaped in the nursery for later dynamic viewing and interpretation. Sedation is rarely necessary. The examinations are usually performed in the nursery without removing the infant from the isolette.

The transducer is placed on the anterior fontanel and the

sonographic beam is initially oriented in the coronal plane. Structures are usually visualized in each of five coronal planes (see Fig. 2-2A) as follows: plane 1 (frontal horns of the lateral ventricles); plane 2 (cingulate sulcus, corpus callosum, cavum septi pellucidi, caudothalamic groove, caudate nucleus, foramen of Monro, anterior third ventricle, thalamus, middle cerebral arteries); plane 3 (lateral ventricles, posterior third ventricle, quadrigeminal plate cistern, hippocampal sulci, tentorium, fourth ventricle, and cerebellum); plane 4 (trigone, choroid plexus); plane 5 (occipital horns). The sonographic beam is then shifted 90° to delineate structures in five sagittal and parasagittal planes (Fig. 2-2B) as follows: planes 1 and 5 (choroid plexuses, trigones, occipital horns, temporal horns); planes 2 and 4 (bodies of lateral ventricles, heads of caudate nuclei, caudothalamic grooves); plane 3 (anterior cerebral arteries, cingulate sulcus, corpus callosum, cavum septi pellucidi, third ventricle, massa intermedia, aqueduct of Sylvius, fourth ventricle, pons, cerebellum). These standard views are often supplemented by additional views. Views steeply angled through the anterior fontanel can delineate superficial lesions. More posteriorly angled views are important for delineating the deep cerebral white matter and cortex posteriorly and superiorly. Laterally angled parasagittal views are useful for assessing the frontal, parietal, and temporal lobes and convexities. Images obtained with a linear array transducer are used to show abnormalities such as extraaxial fluid and sagittal sinus thrombosis. Views through the posterior fontanel are useful for confirming small amounts of intraventricular hemorrhage not visible on routine anterior fontanel views. Views through the posterolateral fontanel (mastoid view) may also be used to detect small amounts of subarachnoid hemorrhage in the posterior fossa and basal cisterus (13). Pulsed Doppler and color flow Doppler US can be used to assess relative velocity (magnitude and direction) of intracranial blood flow as well as the resistive index. Power Doppler is a newer technology that improves the detection of blood flow, although does not provide flow magnitude or direction and is highly susceptible to motion artifact.

Cranial US is most frequently used in premature infants

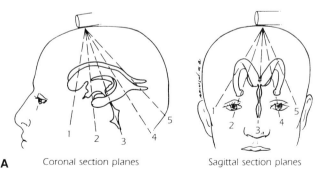

A   Coronal section planes   Sagittal section planes   B

FIG. 2-2. Infant cranial sonography. Transfontanel real-time ultrasonographic examination includes imaging in a minimum of five coronal **(A)** and five sagittal-parasagittal **(B)** planes.

to detect and follow intracranial hemorrhage and periventricular leukomalacia. Other uses include screening for the sequelae of hypoxia-ischemia in term infants and detecting hemorrhage or infarction in infants undergoing extracorporeal membrane oxygenation (ECMO). Doppler US is often used to evaluate intracranial vascular abnormalities. Many lesions (particularly cystic ones) identified by US should be evaluated by Doppler to assess their vascularity. Although intracerebral mass lesions (cystic or solid) may be detected by real-time US, CT or MRI is usually required to characterize them.

Computed Tomography

CT techniques for evaluating the pediatric CNS include noncontrast imaging; contrast-enhanced imaging; axial and coronal imaging of the brain, sinuses, orbits, and temporal bones; sagittal, coronal, and oblique reformatting; 3-D reconstruction; helical imaging; and stereotactic CT for neurosurgical biopsy or excision, for radiosurgery, or for radiation therapy using image fusion techniques (CT plus MRI). Cerebrospinal fluid (CSF)–enhanced CT studies are done using water-soluble, low-osmolar, nonionic contrast media specifically approved for evaluation of the ventricular system (via ventriculostomy or ventricular shunt catheter) or for evaluation of the subarachnoid spaces (cisternography) (6,7).

Most CT examinations of the brain are done without contrast enhancement using 7- to 10-mm contiguous axial sections from the skull base to the vertex (6,14). Occasionally, 5-mm sections are obtained through the posterior fossa or the supratentorial region, especially in the neonate and young infant. The most common indications for emergency CT are trauma, unexplained seizure, hydrocephalus with suspected shunt malfunction, and acute neurologic deficit possibly due to hemorrhage (15–19). The decision for intravenous contrast enhancement is made after viewing the noncontrast study and depends on the clinical indication. CT angiography (CTA) utilizes a spiral acquisition performed during the administration of an intravenous contrast bolus to image the cerebral vasculature. CTA may be extremely useful in evaluating cerebrovascular disease. MRI is often preferred to contrast-enhanced CT if the situation (often the presence of a mass) allows the additional time for an MRI to be performed. In general, for imaging of the sinuses, orbits, facial bones, and temporal bones, direct coronal imaging is preferable to thin axial sections with reformatting. However, significant abnormalities of the cervical spine, neck, and airway must be excluded before direct coronal imaging. All studies are planned using the appropriate lateral or frontal scout images.

Magnetic Resonance Imaging

MR techniques useful for imaging of the pediatric CNS include MRI with conventional spin-echo (CSE), fast spin-echo (FSE), gradient echo (GE), and fat suppression techniques (20). Other techniques currently available or undergoing development include MR angiography (MRA), perfusion MRI, spectroscopy, image fusion (CT/MRI, SPECT/MRI), 3-D display, echo-planar imaging, diffusion MRI, CSF flow imaging, and magnetization-transfer enhancement, STIR, and FLAIR imaging (6,7,14,21–23). Sagittal T1 CSE images are often followed by axial proton density FSE or FLAIR images and axial T2 FSE images. Angled coronal T2 FSE or STIR images are often obtained, particularly in the evaluation of seizure disorders. Gadolinium-enhanced T1 CSE images are often used in one or more planes, particularly for the initial and follow-up evaluation of CNS tumors and especially for recurrence or CSF seeding. A 5-mm section thickness is routinely used for brain imaging, usually with a 2.5-mm interslice gap, occasionally with a 1-mm interslice gap. Often, 3-mm T1 sections in the sagittal and coronal planes are used to evaluate the perisellar region. Axial 3-mm T1 sections may be used with enhancement to evaluate the internal auditory canals and cerebellopontine angles. Similarly, thin sections with fat suppression (STIR) are often employed to image the orbits (24).

Follow-up brain MRI studies, particularly for possible tumor recurrence, should often duplicate the technique of previous studies to facilitate comparison. Vascular flow-enhanced studies may be done using multiple single-slice (SPGR) or multislice (FMPSPGR) GE techniques. GE techniques are used to enhance vascular flow, CSF, or magnetic susceptibility effects due to iron, calcium, or hemorrhage. A number of 2-D and 3-D time-of-flight (TOF) and phase contrast (PC) techniques are available for MRA (25). The 3-D TOF technique is more often used than the 2-D or 3-D PC technique for rapid MRA of the carotid-basilar structures, circle of Willis, and cerebral arterial territories. The 2-D technique is preferred for imaging of the dural venous sinuses and jugular veins; either 2-D or 3-D TOF MRA technique is used for evaluating the carotid and vertebral arteries in the neck.

Cerebral Angiography

Cross-sectional imaging by US, CT, and MRI has greatly decreased the number of cerebral angiograms performed in children (6,7). Modern microsurgical and interventional techniques, however, have also increased the importance of visualizing the vascular anatomy in certain conditions. Cerebral angiography should be considered in evaluating children with intracranial hemorrhage, vascular malformation, aneurysm, trauma, and cerebrovascular occlusive disease. The percutaneous femoral artery approach is usually employed. Selective injections of the internal carotid arteries and vertebral arteries are typically performed. Catheter size and contrast dosage are determined by the age and weight of the patient (see pages 53–56).

Nuclear Medicine

With recent improvements in radiopharmaceuticals and instrumentation, nuclear medicine now offers a variety of techniques used for functional neuroimaging. Radiopharmaceuticals such as ^{99m}Tc-hexamethylpropylene amine oxime (HMPAO) and ^{99m}Tc-bicisate (ECD) are taken up by brain tissue in proportion to regional perfusion (26,27). Because abnormalities of perfusion are frequently associated with local changes in cerebral physiology and blood flow, single photon emission computed tomography (SPECT) of the distribution of such agents may demonstrate important functional abnormalities despite normal anatomy on CT or MRI. Perfusion brain SPECT is used to localize epileptogenic foci in patients with refractory epilepsy who are being considered for excisional surgery. Ictal perfusion SPECT is more sensitive than interictal SPECT and appears to be at least as effective as interictal positron emission tomography (PET) (14). Ictal SPECT is best obtained using intravenous ECD during a seizure (27). SPECT may also be used to show the distribution of agents, such as thallium-201 or 2-methoxyisobutylisonitrite (MIBI) ^{99m}Tc-MIBI, that depict abnormalities of the blood-brain barrier and cellular metabolism (14,27). These agents sometimes can differentiate tumor recurrence from treatment-related necrosis or gliosis. Another indication for SPECT is evaluation of cerebrovascular disease, as seen in sickle cell disease and moyamoya. Image registration techniques, e.g., MRI/SPECT fusion, are useful for precise anatomic localization by MRI of a functional abnormality detected by SPECT. ^{111}In-diethylenetriamine pentacetic acid (DTPA) cisternography may be used to assess CSF kinetics and CSF shunt patency (14,27).

Sedation, Anesthesia, and Monitoring

Sedation may be required for CT, MRI, nuclear medicine, or other procedures. As described in Chapter 1, we prefer oral chloral hydrate for young infants and intravenous pentobarbital for children over 1 year of age. If sedation is contraindicated or difficult, intravenous or inhalation anesthesia is provided by an anesthesiologist (7,14). Vital signs and oxygen saturation are monitored by system-compatible equipment. It is critical to develop a detailed protocol (see Chapter 1) for the sedation and monitoring of pediatric patients. The program includes training and support of qualified personnel as well as continuous quality improvement.

IMAGING GUIDELINES

General Guidelines

Structural Imaging

MRI has in many instances replaced more invasive diagnostic procedures such as angiography, pneumoencephalog-

raphy, ventriculography, and cisternography. Although US remains the procedure of choice for evaluating fetal and infant CNS abnormalities and CT continues to be preferred for trauma and acute neurologic deficits, MRI is now considered the definitive modality for evaluation of the pediatric CNS in most clinical circumstances. Neoplasia, certain vascular and hemorrhagic lesions, and inflammatory processes of the brain are best evaluated with MRI (6,7,14,28). Furthermore, MRI is more sensitive and specific than CT or US for the evaluation of myelination, neurodegenerative disorders, and developmental malformations of brain. Moreover, MRI has become the definitive modality for imaging the patient with intractable or unexplained focal seizures, unexplained hydrocephalus, or neuroendocrine dysfunction (6,7).

Functional Imaging

SPECT, PET, MR spectroscopy (MRS), and MR perfusion imaging (pMRI) are currently used for functional assessment of the developing CNS (14). PET uses specific metabolic tracers to assess oxygen utilization and glucose metabolism, but SPECT is widely available, is relatively simple, and is undergoing rapid technical advancements. Clinical and investigative applications of PET and SPECT include focus localization in refractory childhood epilepsy (29), assessment of progression or recurrence versus treatment effects in CNS neoplasia, the evaluation of moyamoya for surgical revascularization, and cortical activation techniques in the elucidation of childhood behavior disorders.

MRS and pMRI are applications of the same nuclear magnetic resonance (NMR) phenomena as conventional MRI (21–23,30). MRS offers a noninvasive in vivo approach to biochemical analysis. Furthermore, MRS provides quantitative information regarding cellular metabolites, since signal intensity is linearly related to steady-state metabolite concentration. If MRS can detect cellular biochemical changes before morphologic changes are evident by any imaging technique, further insight into assessment and prognosis will be available. With recent advances in instrumentation and methodology, single-voxel and multivoxel proton MRS can now be performed with relatively short acquisition times to determine concentrations of metabolites in healthy and diseased tissues. Currently, proton MRS is used for assessment of the developing brain, perinatal brain injury, childhood CNS neoplasia, and neurodegenerative disorders (21,30).

pMRI is currently being used to evaluate cerebral hemodynamics by the application of a dynamic, contrast-enhanced, T2*-weighted MRI technique (22). This new technique is undergoing further development to demonstrate and quantify normal and abnormal cerebrovascular dynamics by analyzing hemodynamic parameters including relative cerebral blood volume, relative cerebral blood flow, and mean transit time; all are complementary to the findings of conventional MRI. Current applications include evaluation of cerebrovascular disease and differentiation of tumor progression or regression from treatment effects.

Other emerging applications of MRI that may further enhance sensitivity and specificity are echo-planar imaging (EPI), diffusion-weighted MRI, CSF flow imaging, and magnetization transfer contrast enhancement (6,14). Further advances in computer display technology include image fusion (MRI/SPECT, CT/MRI), 2-D reformatting, and 3-D volumetrics/reconstructions to assist in the planning of stereotactic radiotherapy and radiosurgery, craniofacial reconstructive surgery, and other neurosurgical procedures.

Imaging Approaches

Developmental Malformations

Disorders of dorsal neural tube closure include anencephaly, the Chiari malformations, and cephaloceles (6,7,31,32). US or CT usually suffices for screening. MRI is useful when the US or CT fails to satisfy the clinical investigation or if specific treatment more specific than shunting for hydrocephalus is planned. MRI may also provide a more complete delineation, useful for prognosis and genetic counseling of complex CNS anomalies

Disorders that arise at the time of ventral neural tube closure include the holoprosencephalies, septooptic dysplasia, cerebral and cerebellar hypoplasias, and the Dandy-Walker spectrum (33,34). US or CT may be adequate for diagnosis. MRI is reserved for more definitive evaluation, particularly when surgical intervention is anticipated; one example is the Dandy-Walker spectrum, when the decision for cyst shunting versus shunting of both the cyst and the ventricles is based on the presence or absence of a widely patent aqueduct of Sylvius. Patients with craniosynostosis are initially evaluated with plain films. Those with involvement of more than one suture, especially when associated with a craniofacial syndrome, often require evaluation by three-dimensional CT and occasionally by MRI.

Disorders of neuronal proliferation, differentiation, and histogenesis include micrencephaly, megalencephaly, aqueductal anomalies, cystic cerebral anomalies (porencephaly), the neurocutaneous syndromes, vascular malformations, and developmental tumors. MRI is now the preferred modality for both screening and definitive evaluation of the dysplastic, neoplastic, and vascular manifestations of the neurocutaneous syndromes (35–39). After initial screening with US or CT, MRI is the modality of choice for treatment planning and follow-up of vascular malformations and developmental tumors. MRI is often required to delineate the more subtle disorders of neuronal migration and cortical organization including schizencephaly, heterotopia, pachygyria, polymicrogyria, cortical dysplasia, and callosal dysgenesis (40,41). The perfusion characteristics of structural and functional cortical dysplasias in children with refractory partial epilepsy are best investigated with SPECT (29). For added precision, SPECT data may be fused with MRI data to provide a high-resolution display of the functional information. Myelination and disorders of myelination are assessed only by MRI (6,7,42). Encephaloclastic processes are destructive lesions of the formed brain that result from a variety of insults including hypoxia-ischemia and infection (6,28,43). They include hydranencephaly, porencephaly, multicystic encephalomalacia, hydrocephalus, leukomalacia, dystrophic calcification, hemorrhage, infarction, demyelination, and atrophy. MRI may demonstrate subtle abnormalities, as in periventricular leukomalacia, not revealed by US or CT. Although arachnoid cysts are often readily delineated by US or CT, MRI may be necessary to exclude solid tumor and for surgical planning. When conventional MRI is equivocal, diffusion MRI may distinguish an arachnoid cyst from an epidermoid.

Infection

US or CT with contrast enhancement adequately evaluates meningitis and its complications, including subdural effusion, cerebral infarction, ventriculitis, hydrocephalus, abscess, and empyema (28,43). Recurrent infectious or noninfectious meningitis may require investigation for a parameningeal focus (sinus or mastoid infection, dermal sinus, primitive neurenteric connection, CSF leak, dermoidepidermoid). Infectious or postinfectious encephalitis is usually viral or postviral in origin. The latter category includes acute disseminated encephalomyelitis (ADEM). MRI is more sensitive than CT in demonstrating encephalitis and ADEM. The congenital TORCHS (toxoplasmosis, rubella, cytomegalovirus, herpes, syphilis) infections and their calcifications are adequately evaluated with US or CT. In the absence of calcification, MRI provides more diagnostic information. Brain abscess or empyema may be associated with a sinus infection, trauma, surgery, sepsis, immune deficiency, or uncorrected cyanotic congenital heart disease; contrast-enhanced CT is critical for diagnosis and follow-up.

Neoplastic Diseases

Intracranial tumors in childhood may be classified as follows: posterior fossa tumors, tumors about the third ventricle, and cerebral hemispheric tumors (6,7,44,45). Common posterior fossa tumors of childhood include medulloblastoma, cerebellar astrocytoma, brainstem glioma, and ependymoma. Tumors about the third ventricle (suprasellar and pineal regions) frequently encountered in childhood include optic glioma, craniopharyngioma, and germ cell tumors (germinoma, teratoma). Hemispheric cerebral tumors of childhood include astrocytoma (fibrillary or pilocytic), choroid plexus papilloma, ganglioglioma, other glial tumors, and embryonic tumors (primitive neuroectodermal tumor, glioblastoma). Rare intracranial tumors include sarcomas, meningeal tumors, and metastases. Although US or CT will detect the vast majority of intracranial masses of childhood, MRI is best for definitive evaluation, treatment planning, and following tumor response and treatment effects. Furthermore, the superior sensitivity of MRI allows it to detect tumors occult to CT and US. MRI is particularly helpful in the explanation of focal or partial seizure disorders, hydrocephalus, neuroendocrine disorders, cervicomedullary junction tumors, and leptomeningeal neoplastic processes. MRI is an important adjunct to CT in the evaluation of parameningeal or extradural tumors, such as sarcomas and neuroblastomas, that encroach on or invade the CNS. Craniospinal MRI with gadolinium enhancement shows CSF tumor seeding well, especially in medulloblastoma, germ cell tumors, and malignant glial tumors. MRI is sensitive to treatment effects such as ischemic or hemorrhagic radiation vasculopathy. Functional or metabolic imaging (SPECT, PET, MRI, MRS) may differentiate radiation necrosis from tumor progression (21,23,46).

Trauma

CT remains the procedure of choice for cranial imaging in acute trauma (15,16,47). US is primary for perinatal trauma, particularly in the premature infant. CT remains superior to US, however, for delineating extracerebral hemorrhage and posterior fossa hemorrhage, more frequent in the term neonate. CT is sensitive and specific for acute hemorrhage and for the sequelae of fractures. MRI is used when neurologic deficits persist and CT is negative or nonspecific; examples are nonhemorrhagic lesions such as brainstem infarction, white matter shear injury, cortical contusion, gliosis, and multicystic encephalomalacia. MRI is often more specific than CT for hemorrhage after the acute and subacute stages; MRI may distinguish dilated subarachnoid spaces (communicating hydrocephalus, atrophy) from chronic subdural hematomas due to child abuse or other trauma when US or CT only show nonspecific extracerebral fluid collections. Furthermore, the demonstration of hemosiderin by MRI is pathognomonic of previous hemorrhage. In children with hemorrhage out of proportion to the reported trauma, MRI may detect an underlying vascular malformation, demonstrate a hemorrhagic neoplasm, or suggest child abuse (6,7,48).

Vascular Diseases and Hemorrhage

Occlusive or hemorrhagic cerebrovascular disease characteristically causes an acute neurologic deficit (19,49). Occasionally, the deficits may be episodic or migrainous. A fixed deficit (static encephalopathy) may indicate a prenatal or perinatal injury. CT is the primary imaging choice in acute situations; it readily shows intracranial hemorrhage. Intracranial vascular malformations in childhood include arteriovenous fistulas, arteriovenous malformations, cavernous malformations, venous anomalies, and telangiectasias (capillary malformations). Aneurysms are very rare in childhood but may be congenital, associated with a syndrome, or due to trauma or infection. A Galenic malformation is a classic type of vascular malformation occurring in infancy; it causes congestive heart failure, hydrocephalus, or both. Neoplastic or inflammatory neovascularity causes acute hemorrhage on rare occasions. Hemorrhage due to coagulopathy occurs in hemophilia, leukemia, immune thrombocytopenic purpura (ITP), and disseminated intravascular coagulopathy (DIC). Hypertensive hemorrhage is rare in childhood but must always be considered in a child with hypertension and encephalopathy.

Whereas US is reliable for the diagnosis of hemorrhagic complications of prematurity (germinal matrix hemorrhage, intraventricular hemorrhage), CT better shows subarachnoid, subdural, and posterior fossa hemorrhages more reliably. MRI is often reserved for more definitive evaluation and to decide on the need for angiography. MRI usually distinguishes hemorrhagic infarction from hematoma and often characterizes the specific type of vascular malformation. MRA also helps to delineate vascular malformations. When CT demonstrates a focal high density that may be either calcification or hemorrhage, MRI may provide further specificity, e.g., by distinguishing vascular malformation from a neoplasm.

Prenatal or perinatal hypoxia-ischemia may result in imaging findings of periventricular leukomalacia, cortical and subcortical border zone cerebral injury, or extensive injury including involvement of the brainstem and basal ganglia. Imaging demonstrates edema, necrosis, or hemorrhagic infarction. The long-term result is static encephalopathy (cerebral palsy); imaging may demonstrate porencephaly, hydranencephaly, atrophy, leukomalacia, or encephalomalacia. There may or may not be calcifications. MRI is occasionally indicated to clarify negative or nonspecific US or CT findings. Further developments in diffusion imaging and MRS will make the diagnosis and prognosis more precise in hypoxic-ischemic injury.

Neurovascular occlusive disease, arterial or venous, may be caused by stenosis, thrombosis, or embolization (49). The result is ischemic edema, ischemic infarction, or hemorrhagic infarction. Arterial occlusive disease occurs with meningitis, cyanotic congenital heart disease, sickle cell disease, metabolic disease (mitochondrial cytopathies), moyamoya syndrome, dissection, vasculitis, and migraine. Conditions commonly associated with cerebral venous or dural venous sinus occlusive disease include infection, dehydration, perinatal encephalopathy, cyanotic congenital heart disease, L-asparaginase therapy for leukemia, polycythemia in the newborn, DIC, and oral contraceptives. MRI is more sensitive and specific than US or CT for multiple infarctions, hemorrhagic infarction, and venous thrombosis. MRA and CTA aids in the diagnosis of arterial or venous occlusion, but cerebral angiography may be required to confirm the diagnosis and plan therapy. pMRI is capable of quantitating cerebral blood flow and blood volume in such cases (22).

Neurodegenerative Diseases

The neurodegenerative diseases are rare disorders producing progressive neurologic impairment in the absence of any other identifiable cause such as tumor or infection (6,7,50). The diagnosis is made by clinical presentation, metabolic testing, or biopsy. MRI is superior to CT in evaluating disease extent and distribution. Occasionally, MRI may demonstrate characteristic imaging findings, e.g., iron accumulation in Hallervorden-Spatz disease. MRS contributes to the metabolic characterization of these disorders.

Hydrocephalus

Hydrocephalus, or "water in the head," is not a disease entity but a pathologic condition in which there are enlarged cerebral ventricles unrelated to cerebral atrophy or dysgenesis. Hydrocephalus is dynamic; there is an active, progressive increase in ventricular volume associated with increased intraventricular pressure due to obstruction of the CSF flow or a mechanical imbalance between CSF production and absorption (5). When there is obstruction in the ventricles, the term noncommunicating hydrocephalus is applied (Table 2-1). Extraventricular obstruction is termed communicating or external hydrocephalus (see Table 2-1). Rarely, hydrocephalus is caused by CSF overproduction by a choroid plexus papilloma or villous hypertrophy.

Hydrocephalus may be due to developmental or acquired causes. Developmental causes include Chiari II malformation (particularly after myelomeningocele repair), aqueduct stenosis, encephalocele, cyst, universal craniosynostosis, stenosis of one or more skull foramina (jugular foramen stenosis in achondroplasia), immaturity of arachnoid villi, and Galenic malformation. Hydrocephalus may follow intraventricular hemorrhage or infection and may be due to the mass effect of a tumor (18,51).

Tumors occurring in the lateral ventricles, at the foramina of Monro, next to the cerebral aqueduct, or within or compressing the fourth ventricle are likely to produce noncommunicating hydrocephalus. Most tumors causing ventricular obstruction can be demonstrated by CT, although MRI may improve delineation of the extent and characterization of the lesion. Tectal glioma, which causes lateral and third ventricular obstruction, may be difficult to identify on CT but is readily shown by MRI (see Fig. 2-89).

Communicating (external) hydrocephalus is usually associated with enlargement of the entire ventricular system, although the fourth ventricle may not be as distended as the lateral and third ventricles. The extracerebral CSF spaces are often enlarged as well. Benign macrocrania is a self-limited type of communicating hydrocephalus that seen in some infants. The condition typically presents as macrocephaly without neurologic symptoms or signs. There is frequently a familial tendency to large head size. The wide spaces are believed to be due to immaturity of the arachnoid villi and impaired CSF absorption. The subarachnoid and ventricular dilatation typically resolves or stabilizes by 2 years of age (52,53).

Imaging, usually in the clinical setting of a large or increasing head circumference, is obtained to determine whether hydrocephalus is present, its severity, and, when possible, its cause (18,54). Ventricular enlargement may be accompanied by periventricular edema if the hydrocephalus is acute or severe. Splaying of the sutures or bulging of the fontanels may be evident. CSF flow dynamics in hydrocephalus may be studied with cine-MRI (55).

Imaging is also commonly performed to determine ventricular size after shunting of hydrocephalus, to assess complications of ventricular shunting, and to evaluate for shunt malfunction and increasing ventricular size if new neurologic symptoms develop (Table 2-2) (6,56,57). Nonenhanced CT is the procedure of choice in this setting because it is widely available, is compatible with life support devices, rapid, and often requires no patient sedation.

TABLE 2-1. *Classification of obstructive hydrocephalus*

Intraventricular obstructive hydrocephalus ("noncommunicating hydrocephalus")
  Lateral ventricle
    Trigone: coarctation, neoplasm, ventriculitis
    Body: coarctation, neoplasm, ventriculitis
  Foramina of Monro: coarctation, neoplasm[a], ventriculitis, hemorrhage, tuber, shunt complication
  Third ventricle
    Anterior: craniopharyngioma[a], glioma, sellar mass, aneurysm
    Posterior: pineal neoplasm, quadrigeminal cyst, galenic AVM, arachnoid cyst
  Aqueduct: ventriculitis, hemorrhage[a], aqueduct stenosis[a], Arnold-Chiari malformation[a], neoplasm[a], infection[a]
  Fourth ventricle: ventriculitis, hemorrhage[a], Dandy-Walker cyst, neoplasm, Arnold-Chiari malformation[a]
Extraventricular obstructive hydrocephalus ("communicating hydrocephalus")
  Cerebellar subarachnoid space: hemorrhage[a], infection[a]
  Basal cisterns: hemorrhage[a], infection[a], neoplastic seeding
  Tentorial hiatus: Arnold-Chiari malformation[a], achondroplasia
  Cerebral subarachnoid space: hemorrhage[a], infection[a], increased CSF protein, subdural hematoma, meningeal infiltration
  Arachnoid granulations: congenital absence, trauma, hemorrhage[a], infection[a], subdural hematoma

---

AVM, arteriovenous malformation; CSF, cerebrospinal fluid.
[a] More common.
Modified from Harwood-Nash and Fitz (5).

NORMAL SKULL RADIOLOGY

Many radiologists are uncomfortable when interpreting the skull radiograph of an infant or child. The skull of the newborn, infant, and young child is a dynamic structure that

TABLE 2-2. *Complications of shunts for hydrocephalus*

Ventricular end
  Blockage: ependymal impaction, choroid plexus plugging, perforation, hemorrhage, ventriculitis, disconnection,[a] debris,[a] malposition, thrombosis
  Migration[a]: cerebral perforation, distraction
  Hemorrhage[a]
  Infection[a]
  Hematoma: epidural, subdural, intracerebral
  CSF hygroma
  Isolated or "trapped" fourth ventricle[a]
  Upward brainstem herniation
  Secondary craniosynostosis[a]
  Calvarial thickening[a]
  Inappropriate ADH secretion
  Shunt-dependent ventricles[a]
Distal end
  Blockage: malposition, disconnection[a], debris, thrombosis, adhesions
Atrial end
  Thrombosis[a]: calcification, pulmonary emboli, cor pulmonale, SVC obstruction
  Migration: transmyocardial, pericardial effusion, pulmonary artery
  Infection[a]: septicemia, pneumonia, septic emboli, endocarditis
Peritoneal end
  Perforation: stomach, rectum, intestine, bladder
  Infection[a]: peritonitis, adhesions
  CSF[a]: "pseudotumor," encystment
  Bowel obstruction
  Entrapment in inguinal hernia or hydrocele
Miscellaneous: congestive heart failure, shunt glomerulonephritis, metastatic seeding

ADH, antidiuretic hormone; CSF, cerebrospinal fluid; SVC, superior vena cava.
[a] More common.

reflects underlying brain growth and associated somatic growth (58–61). In addition to growth changes, the skull may also show changes due to chromosomal abnormality, bone dysplasia, infection, intracranial mass, increased or decreased intracranial pressure, metabolic disease, and hematologic disease. It is sometimes more difficult to identify normal anatomy, normal variants, and artifacts than to recog-nize pathologic abnormalities. One must be familiar with the normal in order to interpret the abnormal (5). The radiology of the pediatric skull is simplified by understanding the basics of embryology and development, using an ordered approach to the skull radiograph, and systematically analyzing the facial bones, bony calvaria, and skull base. These principles are also readily applied to the interpretation of skull findings on CT, including the scout projection images, and on MRI. Furthermore, the skull radiograph often clarifies unusual or confusing skull findings on CT or MRI. For example, a skull fracture may be questionable or invisible on CT and yet obvious of plain films.

Embryology and Development

The skull base (mendosal suture to anterior portion of the ethmoid bone) is formed by endochondral ossification and becomes the floor for the brainstem, cerebellum, and cerebral hemispheres. Chondrocranial growth parallels skeletal growth and is independent of brain growth. The bony calvaria (frontal, parietal, greater wings of sphenoid, squamous temporal bones, and squamous occipital bones) is formed by membranous ossification. The mendosal sutures (Fig. 2-3), which disappear during the first year of life, mark the junction of the cartilaginous and membranous portions of the occipital bone. The inner table of the bony calvaria grows solely in response to the growth of the intracranial contents and has no known inherent growth potential (61).

The cerebral hemispheres, derived from the forebrain, determine the shape of the cranial vault. The brain weight of a newborn is 25% that of the adult brain. There is rapid infantile brain growth, so the brain reaches 50% of its adult weight by 8 months, 75% by 2½ years, 90% by 6–7 years, and nearly 100% by 12 years of age (61).

The distance from the sella turcica to the sphenoethmoidal synchondrosis reaches adult dimensions by 10 years of age. The sphenoccipital synchondrosis remains open until 14–20 years of age and is a site of endochondral growth to elongate the skull base. This synchondrosis may be widened and demineralized in patients with rickets due to abnormal endo-

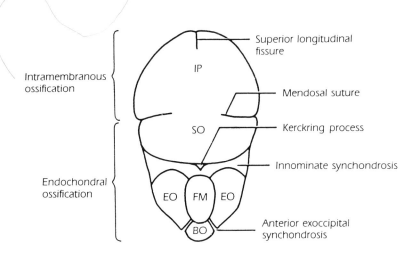

FIG. 2-3. Formation of the occipital bone. The occipital bone contains the foramen magnum *(FM)* and forms from interparietal *(IP)*, supraoccipital *(SO)*, exoccipital *(EO)*, and basioccipital *(BO)* ossification centers. Note that the mendosal sutures are the junction of intramembranous ossification and endochondral ossification.

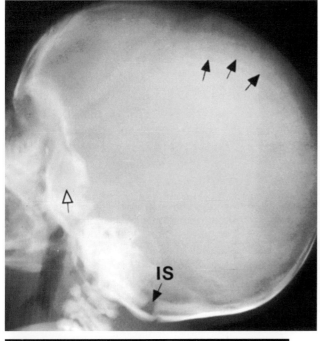

A

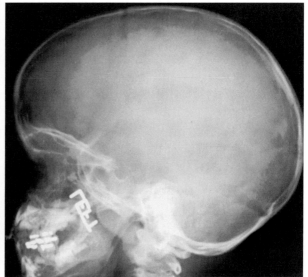

B

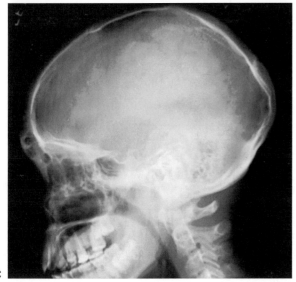

C

FIG. 2-4. Normal craniofacial relationships. The craniofacial relationship is estimated by comparing the area of the face with that of the cranium. **A:** Full-term newborn. The skull/face area ratio is about 4:1. Note also the crescentic scalp folds *(closed arrows)*, innominate synchondrosis *(IS)*, and intersphenoid synchondrosis *(open arrow).* **B:** Three-year-old male. Skull/face area ratio of 2.5:1. **C:** Sixteen-year-old male. Normal adult skull/face ration of 1.5:1.

chondral ossification (5). The sella turcica reaches adult size by 7–10 years of age. Because the growth of the skull base is dependent on normal endochondral bone formation, the foramen magnum and chondrocranium are small and shortened in achondroplasia. Poor growth of the cranial base and facial structures is also present with trisomy 21, rickets, progeria, and hypothyroidism.

At birth the cranial vault dwarfs the facial bones not only because of rapid brain growth in utero but also because the maxilla, mandible, and paranasal sinuses grow and develop relatively late. The craniofacial proportions may be estimated by comparing the area of the face with that of the skull (vault and base) on the lateral radiograph (Fig. 2-4). The normal skull/face area ratio decreases with age approximately as follows: premature newborn 5:1; term newborn 4:1; 2 years 3:1; 3 years 2.5:1; 12 years 2:1; adult 1.5:1.0.

Bony Calvaria

Sutures

Sutures consist of connective tissue between the edges of the calvarial bones. As remnants of the original membranous cerebral capsule, sutures permit progressive ossification by direct osteoblastic transformation during expansile brain growth (5). The calvaria is then reshaped by the standard osteoclastic-osteoblastic sequence. The bony edges of sutures are tapered and have no interdigitations in the neonate (Fig. 2-4A). However, the sutures of older children have interdigitations at the outer table surface (Fig. 2-4B; see Fig. 2-6) but a relatively straight margin on the inner table. The primary sutures, major or minor, join at fontanels (Figs. 2-5 and 2-6). Major primary sutures include the sagittal,

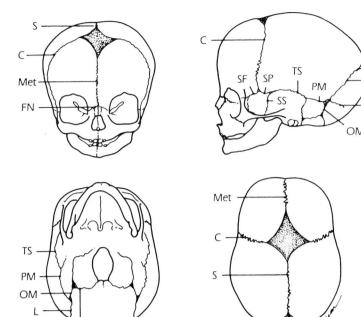

FIG. 2-5. Normal neonatal sutures and synchondroses. Anterior, lateral, basal, and vertex views of the normal neonatal skull. Sagittal suture *(S)*; coronal sutures *(C)*; metopic suture *(Met)*; frontonasal suture *(FN)*; sphenofrontal suture *(SF)*; sphenoparietal suture *(SP)*; sphenosquamosal suture *(SS)*; temporosquamosal suture *(TS)*; parietomastoid suture *(PM)*; occipitomastoid suture *(OM)*; lambdoid suture *(L)*; mendosal suture *(Men)*; innominate synchondrosis *(IS)*.

metopic, coronal, lambdoid, and squamosal (temporosquamosal) (Fig. 2-5). Minor primary sutures include frontoethmoidal, frontonasal, zygomatic (zygomaticotemporal, zygomaticofrontal, sphenozygomatic), parasphenoid (sphenofrontal, sphenoethmoidal, sphenoparietal, sphenosquamosal, sphenozygomatic), parietomastoid, occipitomastoid, and mendosal.

Fontanels

Fontanels are broad areas of connective tissue (residual membranous cerebral capsule) at the junctions of the major sutures (Fig. 2-5). The anterior fontanel is a diamond-shaped unossified area between the two frontal and two parietal bones. It usually disappears by 2 years of age, although it may close as early as 4 months of age (5). A fontanel may feel closed even when radiographs show that it is still unossified. The smaller posterior fontanel may or may not be detectable at birth. If present, it usually closes by 3–6 months of age. The anterolateral fontanel (pterion) closes at about 3 months of age, whereas the posterolateral fontanel (asterion) often persists until 2 years of age.

Skull Base

Sella Turcica

The sella turcica includes, from anterior to posterior, the limbus sphenoidale, chiasmatic sulcus, tuberculum sellae, sellar floor within the pituitary fossa, and dorsum sellae. The optic struts, anterior clinoids, optic foramina, carotid canals, and posterior clinoids are located lateral to the sella turcica. The growth of the pituitary fossa may be affected not only by disturbances of normal endochondral growth and pituitary gland development but also by lesions in adjacent (para-, retro-, supra-, ante-, perisellar) areas.

Synchondroses

Synchondroses are cartilaginous tissues between the endochondral bones of the skull base. The frontosphenoidal synchondrosis separates the body of the sphenoid from the frontal bone and disappears at approximately 2 years of age. The intersphenoid synchondrosis separates the presphenoid from postsphenoid portions of the body of the sphenoid bone and should disappear by 1 year of age. This synchondrosis is located just below the tuberculum sellae and is commonly seen in neonates (Fig. 2-4A). It should not be confused with the rare basipharyngeal canal (remnant of Rathke pouch), which extends almost vertically from the middle of the sellar floor and is therefore inferoposterior to the more common intersphenoidal synchondrosis (58–60). The sphenooccipital synchondrosis separates the body of the sphenoid from the basiocciput. It usually closes at 14 years of age but can persist until early adulthood (5). The small anterior exoccipital synchondroses between the basiocciput and the exoccipitals (see Fig. 2-3) and the larger posterior exoccipital synchondroses (innominate synchondroses) (see Fig. 2-5) disappear by 2–4 years of age (62).

Common Normal Variants

The radiologist should be aware that the pediatric skull is a dynamic structure (60). The general skull size and shape should always be evaluated before progressing to detailed

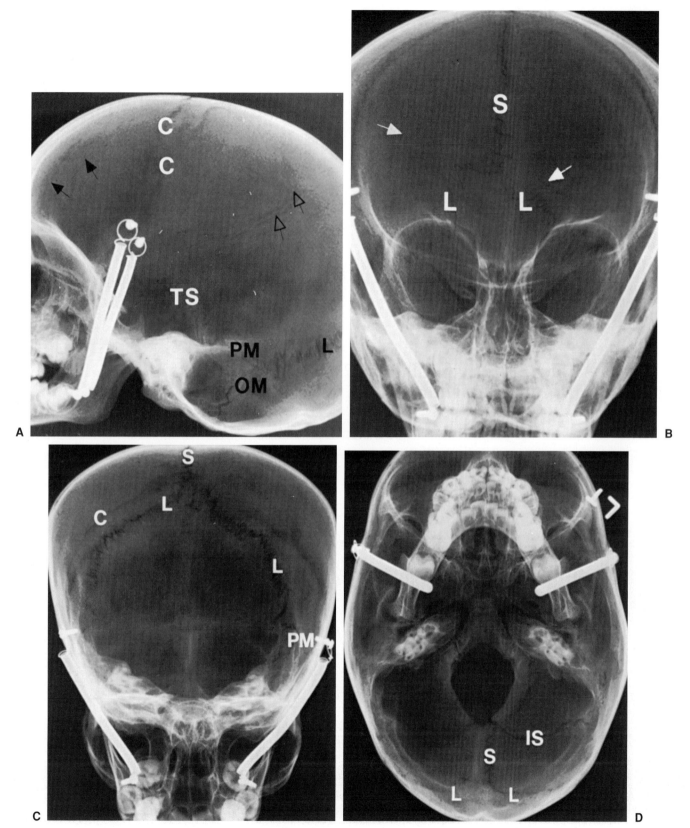

FIG. 2-6. Normal pediatric skull. Lateral **(A)**, posteroanterior **(B)**, Towne **(C)**, and basal or submentovertex **(D)** views of skull specimen of a 3-year-old child. Letter labels are the same as those used in Fig. 2-5. Note the prominent frontal *(closed arrows)* and parietal *(open arrows)* vascular grooves.

TABLE 2-3. *Common normal variants of the pediatric skull*

Shape
  Molding
  Bathrocephaly
Density
  Demineralization of premature neonate
  Hyperostosis of newborn
Soft tissue artifacts
  Folded ear
  Skin folds[a]
  Hair braids
  Radiopaque densities: EEG paste, dirt, hair
Bony calvaria
  Vascular markings[a]
  Sutures
    Transient sutural diastasis of newborn
    Pseudowidening
    Pseudofracture[a]
    Accessory sutures[a]
    Wormian bones
Posterior parietal variants (see Table 2-5)
  Parietal underossification and irregularity
  Parietal foramina
  Diploic veins[a]
  Convolutional markings[a]
Fontanels
  Accessory fontanels
  Fontanel bones
Skull base
  Synchondroses
  Sella turcica—infantile
  Bathrocephaly
  Occipital ossicles
  Kerckring process

EEG, electroencephalography.
[a] More common.

analysis. One must first know the normal pediatric skull anatomy and its normal variations before interpreting a finding as an abnormality (63). The first question is always: "Could this be a normal variant?" There are myriad pseudo-abnormalities of the skull (particularly in the neonate and young infant) that may trap the unwary (Table 2-3).

Vault Molding

There may be considerable molding of the cranial vault during delivery. Frequently, both parietal bones are displaced posteriorly and superiorly, with concomitant rotation of the occipital and temporal bones as well as suture overlap (Fig. 2-7). This molding usually disappears within 2–3 days. The sutures may also transiently widen, perhaps because of postpartum cerebral swelling.

Cranial Vault in the Premature Infant

The premature infant has a relatively unossified cranial vault with a rounded shape as seen on lateral skull radiographs. The normal craniofacial ratio in premature infants may be as high as 5:1 or even 6:1.

Soft Tissue Artifacts

The hair and scalp often cause confusing shadows on skull radiographs. Skin folds produce crescentic soft tissue densities (see Fig. 2-4A). Hair braids, matted hair, dirt, or elec-

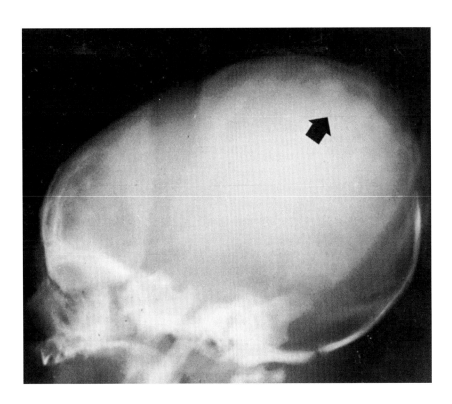

FIG. 2-7. Skull molding. Male newborn with abnormal skull shape. Lateral skull radiograph shows that both parietal bones are displaced posteriorly and superiorly *(arrow)*, and there is widening of the coronal and lambdoid sutures.

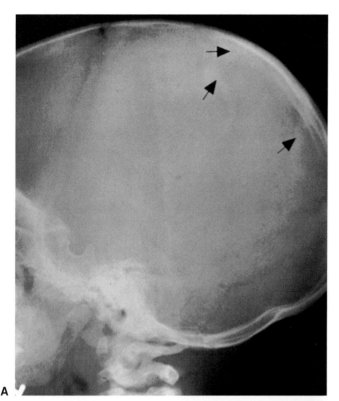

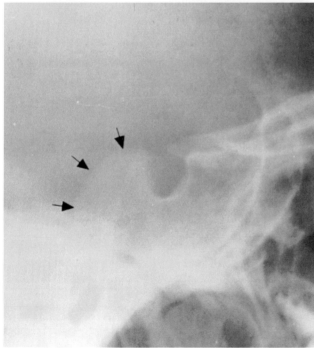

FIG. 2-8. Artifacts. A: This 15-month-old girl had her hair in braids. Several densities *(arrows)* are seen that mimic intracranial calcifications. **B:** Folded ear. The dependent ear of this 4½-year-old male was folded forward during tabletop lateral skull radiography. The folded ear *(arrows)* mimics a dense clival mass.

troencephalography paste may mimic intracranial calcifications (Fig. 2-8A). A folded earlobe may simulate a calcified clival or parasellar mass (Fig. 2-8B).

Vascular Markings

Vascular markings occur in varying degrees of prominence in several areas of the cranial vault. These markings are due to dural venous sinuses, diploic or emissary veins, and meningeal vessels (Table 2-4). Vascular markings are usually not present in the newborn skull (see Fig. 2-4A). Occasionally, frontal diploic venous markings are noted in the neonate and may be confused with a fracture (59). Vascular markings become more apparent as the bony calvaria develops into an inner table, diploic space, and outer table. Dural venous sinus grooves may be initially identified at about 3 years of age. The right transverse sinus is larger than the left in 60% of patients, equal to it in 20%, and smaller in 20%. Diploic venous markings may be present in the frontal bone in the neonate. Parietal diploic venous markings are frequently stellate (see Fig. 2-6A). Emissary vein foramina connect dural sinuses to extracranial venous pathways. Although these foramina may enlarge with increased intracranial pressure, they may also be large in normal patients. Meningeal vascular grooves are usually not evident until 12 years of age.

Sutural Pseudodiastasis

Because at birth membranous ossification is incomplete at sutural margins, sutures may be prominent in the normal neonate (see Fig. 2-4A). This pseudospread of sutures is further accentuated in conditions with physiologic (prematurity) or pathologic (osteogenesis imperfecta, hypophosphatasia, rickets, hypothyroidism, pyknodysostosis, cleidocranial dysplasia) underossification of the skull.

During periods of rapid brain growth (at 2–3 years and 5–7 years), one may see physiologic sutural diastasis (58).

TABLE 2-4. *Vascular markings of the pediatric skull*

Dural venous sinus grooves
  Sagittal sinus
  Transverse sinus
  Sigmoid sinus
  Occipital sinus
Diploic venous markings
  Frontal diploic veins
  Parietal diploic veins
Emissary vein foramina
  Postmastoid region
  Occipital (inio-endineal)
  Emissary veins of Santorini (parietal foramina)
  Midline frontal
Meningeal vascular grooves
  Meningeal artery
  Meningeal veins

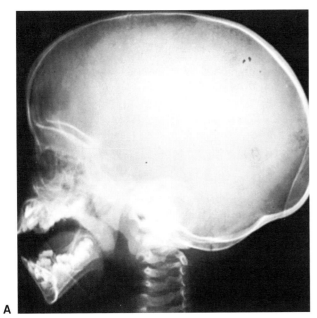

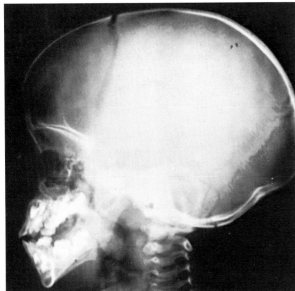

FIG. 2-9. "Physiologic" sutural diastasis. A: Normal admission skull radiograph of 2-year-old male with known child abuse and deprivation. **B:** Definite coronal and lambdoidal sutural diastasis after 2 weeks of hospitalization and treatment of deprivation. Note the accentuated interdigitations of the spread sutures.

Slight widening of the upper portions of the coronal sutures is present, but there is no accentuation of sutural interdigitations. Moreover, the sagittal suture and sella turcica remain normal in appearance.

Exaggerated physiologic sutural diastasis may occur after treatment of prematurity, chronic illness, deprivational dwarfism (64) (Fig. 2-9), and hypothyroidism. Brain volume increases with a concomitant decrease in the size of sulci and the ventricles, the increased brain volume presumably representing catch-up growth.

Wormian Bones

Wormian bones are intrasutural ossicles that occur most frequently in the lambdoid, posterior sagittal, and squamosal sutures. They are usually a normal variant. However, if their formation is marked (Fig. 2-10), one should suspect osteogenesis imperfecta, cleidocranial dysplasia, hypothyroidism, hypophosphatasia, pyknodysostosis, pachydermoperiostosis, certain trisomies, healing rickets, or chronic hydrocephalus (5).

Posterior Parietal Variants

The parietal bones begin to ossify during the seventh or eighth week of fetal life as islands of bone in the membranous cerebral capsule. With development, ossification radiates in a uniform fashion except for a small region along the sagittal suture just in front of the lambda (65). This parietal notch normally disappears by the fifth fetal month, but vestiges may be observed postnatally as bony defects in the region of the obelion (65). These bony defects (Fig. 2-11) include parietal incisura, parietal irregularity, parietal fissuring, small and large parietal fontanels, obeliac bones, Wormian bones, persistent midline parietal foramen, and small or large parietal foramina (Table 2-5).

Convolutional Markings

Convolutional markings are due to pressure on the inner table of the skull by the surface of the growing brain. Although grooves on the floor of the anterior and middle fossae are related to cerebral convolutions, the digital

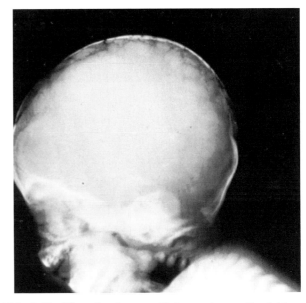

FIG. 2-10. Wormian bones. Male newborn with cleidocranial dysplasia.

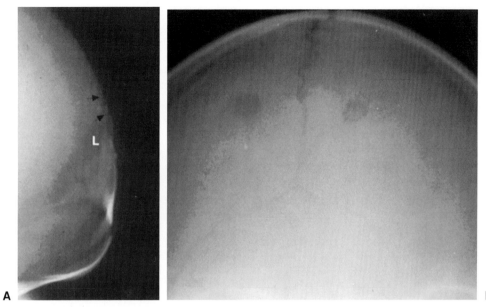

FIG. 2-11. Posterior parietal normal variants. A: Coned-down lateral view of a normal male newborn. Parietal fissuring and irregularity *(arrows)* are noted above the lambdoid suture *(L).* **B:** Small parietal foramina. PA view of the skull shows bilateral rounded lucencies. These emissary vein foramina are in the region of the obelion.

impressions of the rest of the cranial vault are probably due to pulsations of CSF within sulci (5). Brain growth is 60% complete by 12 months of age, 80% complete by 3 years, and 95% complete by 8 years. There are periods of exuberant brain growth (at 2–3 years and 5–7 years) that produce a "relative" increase in intracranial pressure with physiologic coronal sutural diastasis and accentuation of normal convolutional brain markings. These convolutional markings are a reflection of normal brain growth and should not be confused with the "hammer-beaten silver" appearance of increased intracranial pressure, uni-

TABLE 2-5. *Normal variants of the posterior parietal region*

Parietal underossification[a]
Parietal thinning
Parietal incisura
Parietal irregularity and fissuring[a]
Small parietal fontanel
Large parietal fontanel
Obeliac bones
Wormian bones
Persistent midline parietal foramen
Small parietal foramina (foramen of emissary veins of Santorini)[a]
Enlarged parietal foramina (Catlin mark)
Parietal diploic veins[a]
Convolutional markings[a]
Accessory fontanels
Fontanel bones

[a] More common.
Modified from Currarino (65).

versal craniosynostosis, or developmental lacunar skull (see "Lacunar Skull," page 91).

Bathrocephaly

Bathrocephaly ("step in the head") is an unusual normal variant of the neonatal skull. It is a posterior bulging of the interparietal portion of the occipital bone (Fig. 2-12). There is frequently an associated interparietal (inca) bone and an upward convexity of the supraoccipital portion of the occipital bone. Bathrocephaly is probably a developmental variant of the mendosal sutures (5). It disappears by remodeling after a few months and has no clinical significance.

Occipital Ossicles

Occipital ossicles are small, round bones located in the innominate synchondrosis just above the foramen magnum (Fig. 2-13). Single or multiple, they simply represent accessory centers of ossification that have no clinical significance. They may be associated with a Kerckring process, a midline bony process just above the foramen magnum (63).

Systematic Approach to the Pediatric Skull

A systematic approach to the skull radiograph allows complete analysis of normal structures and detection of abnormalities. As with all radiologic examinations, the observer should start at the periphery and work toward the critical

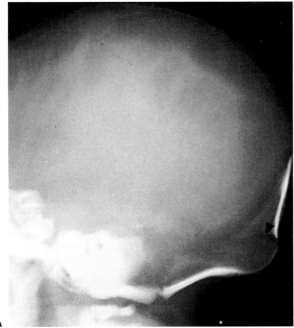

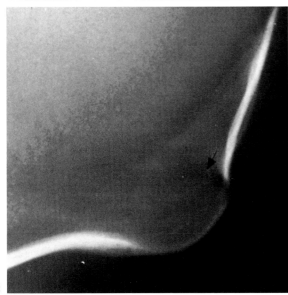

FIG. 2-12. Bathrocephaly. A: Lateral skull view of normal newborn. Note bulge behind mendosal suture *(arrow)*. **B:** Coned-down view of the occiput. There is rounded bulging of the interparietal portion of the occipital bone, which is just below the mendosal suture *(arrow)*.

organ (brain). Table 2-6 lists an analytic approach to skull radiographs.

GENERAL ABNORMALITIES

Abnormalities of Skull Shape

An estimation of shape requires at least two and preferably three radiographic views of the skull. There is considerable variation in skull shape. Long, broad, and tall heads may

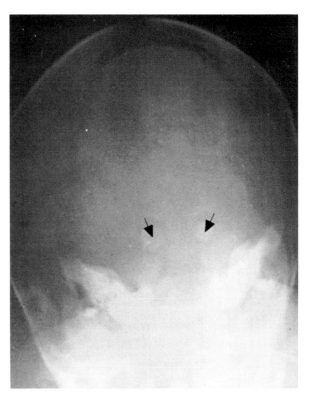

FIG. 2-13. Occipital ossicles. Two rounded ossicles *(arrows)* are noted just above the foramen magnum.

occur without skull abnormality in certain families or races. However, the skull is generally spheroid. Abnormalities of skull size (see following) may have associated abnormalities of skull shape. In general, abnormalities of skull shape may be due to abnormal brain growth, an intracranial mass, a vault abnormality, and abnormal suture or synchondrosis fusion (Table 2-7).

TABLE 2-6. *Approach to pediatric skull radiography*

Cervical spine and foramen magnum
Craniofacial relationship
   Skull configuration: shape, volume
   Skull/face area ratio
Soft tissues: use "bright light"
Facial bones: orbits, maxilla, nasal bones, mandible
Calvaria
   Bony skull vault: outer table, diploic space, inner table
   Sutures
   Fontanels
   Vascular markings
   Convolutional markings
Skull base
   Occipitocervical junction
   Foramen magnum
   Mastoids and petrous ridges
   Synchondroses
   Sella turcica
Intracranial calcifications
   Physiologic
   Pathologic

TABLE 2-7. *Abnormalities of skull shape*

Abnormal brain growth
  Decrease: atrophy[a], dysgenesis, encephalocele, microcephaly[a]
  Increase: hamartomatous, unilateral megalencephaly, neurofibromatosis, macrocephaly[a]
Intracranial mass
  Cerebrospinal fluid: encysted temporal horn, Dandy-Walker cyst[a]
  Brain: superficial neoplasm, porencephalic cyst
  Arachnoid: arachnoid cyst[a]
  Subdural: chronic subdural hematoma or hygroma[a]
Vault abnormalities
  Dysmorphic syndromes
    Frontal bossing: achondroplasia, severe anemia, otopalatodigital syndrome, progeria, Hallermann-Streiff-François syndrome
    Low nasal bridge: achondroplasia, Down syndrome, cleidocranial dysplasia
  Neoplasms: teratoma, progonoma, meningioma, dermoid
  Fibrous dysplasia
  Hyperphosphatasia
  Trauma: cephalohematoma[a], molding, depressed fracture, surgery[a]
  Paranasal sinus abnormalities: mucocele, neoplasm
  Hypertelorism
    Primary: morphogenetic, Grieg syndrome
    Secondary: cleidocranial dysplasia, encephalocele, Cooley anemia, median cleft face, Crouzon disease, Apert syndrome, hypothyroidism, fibrous dysplasia, trisomy 13, hypercalcemia, Hurler syndrome
  Extrinsic: molding, positional flattening, scoliosis capitis
  Abnormal bone formation: achondroplasia, osteogenesis imperfecta, hypophosphatasia, rickets
Abnormal fusion of sutures and synchondroses
  Craniosynostosis
  Primary isolated[a]
  Primary associated with syndromes
  Secondary
  Premature fusion of synchondroses

[a] More common.
Modified from Harwood-Nash and Fitz (5); and Swischuk (60,68).

Abnormalities of Skull Size

Abnormal skull size is due to increased intracranial volume, decreased intracranial volume, or increased cranial vault thickness without change in size of intracranial contents (5). Cranial size almost always reflects the size of the brain. Head size is best evaluated with serial tape measurements of the occipitofrontal circumference using a standard head circumference chart; there is good correlation between skull size as measured on radiographs and clinical measurement (66).

The skull size may be abnormally increased (macrocrania) or decreased (microcrania). Macrocrania is caused by increased brain volume, extraaxial CSF collections, hydrocephalus, intracranial mass, or calvarial thickening (Table 2-8). Microcrania is almost always due to a decrease in the size of the underlying brain (micrencephaly). A decrease in the size of the brain and skull may be seen with genetic or chromosomal abnormalities, intrauterine insults, or neonatally acquired disorders (see Table 2-8). When skull size is more than 2 standard deviations below normal for chronologic age, neurologic or mental impairment is usually present.

Abnormal Skull Density

The cranial vault consists of an inner table, diploic space, and an outer table. It usually has a uniform bony density that is best assessed on the lateral skull radiograph. The skull may have increased (Table 2-9) or decreased (Table 2-10) density. These density abnormalities may be localized to a portion of the skull or involve the entire cranial vault (Fig. 2-14).

Skull Defects

Skull radiography in a child may show a single bony defect or multiple lucencies throughout the cranial vault. One must decide if a radiolucent defect is a normal anatomic structure, a normal variant, or a pathologic entity. The location of the defect, the presence or absence of a soft tissue mass, the skull table(s) involved, and the nature of the borders of the defect provide important clues in the differential diagnosis of such lesions (Table 2-11). Disease entities that produce multiple skull defects frequently have an unfavorable prognosis (Fig. 2-15). Normal anatomy and normal variants are more likely to cause a single skull defect or paired defects rather than multiple scattered defects (5).

Increased Intracranial Pressure

Plain radiography of the skull formerly was commonly used to detect an increase in intracranial pressure, the signs of which are still occasionally useful. Increased intracranial pressure (Table 2-12) may be due to increased cerebrospinal fluid volume and pressure (hydrocephalus), brain swelling (edema, cerebritis), mass within the parenchyma (abscess, neoplasm), subdural mass (hematoma, hygroma), failure of sutures to permit normal skull expansion (universal craniosynostosis), or idiopathic (pseudotumor cerebri) (5,18). The skull, particularly in infancy, is able to adapt to gradual increases in intracranial volume so that chronic hydrocephalus may simply produce calvarial enlargement when compared with the face. Rapid increases in intracranial pressure may produce sutural diastasis, especially in infancy. More chronic pressure results in sellar changes and increased convolutional markings, particularly in later childhood and adolescence.

The skull changes of increased intracranial pressure depend on the ability of the sutures to spread (67). In neonates and infants, the sutures are open and easily separated by increased intracranial pressure. In older children and adults with closed sutures, increased intracranial pressure is mani-

TABLE 2-8. *Abnormalities of skull size*

Macrocrania
  Increased brain volume
    Normal large brain: benign, familial
    Megalencephaly
      Anatomic: achondroplasia, neurofibromatosis, tuberous sclerosis, cerebral gigantism, Russell-Silver dwarf, Beckwith-Wiedemann syndrome
      Metabolic: mucopolysaccharidosis, gangliosidosis, Tay-Sachs disease, Canavan disease, Alexander disease
    Brain edema: trauma, intoxication, inflammation, ischemia
  Increased ventricular volume and pressure: hydrocephalus[a], hydranencephaly
  Intracranial mass
    Subdural: subdural hygroma, subdural hematoma, benign macrocrania[a]
    Brain: neoplasm, porencephalic cyst, arteriovenous malformation
    Dura: sarcoma
    Cerebrospinal fluid: hydrocephalus[a]
    Arachnoid: arachnoid cyst[a]
  Calvarial thickening: anemia[a], fibrous dysplasia, hyperostosis syndromes, hyperphosphatasia
  Chondrodystrophies
  Craniosynostosis

Microcrania
  Syndromes: Cornelia de Lange, Cockayne, Seckel; Rubenstein-Taybi, Riley-Day, Smith-Lemli-Opitz
  Chromosomal: trisomy 21[a], trisomy 13, trisomy 18
  Intrauterine insult[a]: radiation, infection, aminopterin, ischemia, idiopathic
  Neonatal abnormality: ischemia[a], encephalitis, encephalomalacia, hypoxia[a]
  Brain atrophy[a]
  Large encephalocele
  Universal craniosynostosis
  Idiopathic microencephaly
  Congenital: holoprosencephaly, anencephaly, cerebral hypoplasia, tuberous sclerosis
  Metabolic: homocystinuria, phenylketonuria, Fanconi syndrome, Fahr disease

[a] More common.

TABLE 2-9. *Increased skull density*

Localized
  Congenital: tuberous sclerosis, hemiatrophy
  Infection: chronic osteomyelitis
  Tumor: fibrous dysplasia, osteoma, hemangioma, meningioma, chordoma, sarcoma, primary bone tumor, metastases
  Trauma: depressed fracture, cephalohematoma
Generalized
  Congenital: tuberous sclerosis, Van Buchem syndrome, Kenny-Caffey syndrome, pyknodysostosis, osteopetrosis, craniotubular dysplasia, otopalatodigital syndrome, mucopolysaccharidoses, hyperphosphatasia, acrodysostosis, Cockayne syndrome, Pyle disease
  Trauma
    Treated hydrocephalus
    Irradiation
  Endocrine
    Hypervitaminosis D
    Hypoparathyroidism
    Hypercalcemia
    Pseudohypoparathyroidism
    Hyperparathyroidism
Miscellaneous
  Chronic anemia[a]
  Dilantin therapy[a]
  Idiopathic
  Healing rickets
  Cerebral atrophy
  Congenital heart disease
  Myelosclerosis
  Fluorosis
  Microcephaly
  Metastatic disease
  Leukemia, lymphoma

[a] More common.

fested by increased inner table markings and sellar changes. With increasing age, the frequency of sutural diastasis decreases whereas that of sellar change increases. Sutural diastasis is a common sign of increased intracranial pressure

TABLE 2-10. *Decreased skull density*

Localized
  Parietal thinning[a]
  Neoplasm or cyst
    Cyst: encysted ventricle, porencephalic cyst, arachnoid cyst[a]
    Intracranial tumor
    Chronic subdural hematoma or hygroma[a]
    Leptomeningeal cyst
  Neurofibromatosis
Generalized
  Congenital
    Lacunar skull[a]
    Hydrocephalus
    Osteogenesis imperfecta
    Cleidocranial dysplasia
    Hypophosphatasia
    Melnick-Needles syndrome
    Progeria
  Endocrine
    Rickets[a]
    Hyperparathyroidism
    Hypothyroidism
Miscellaneous
  Prematurity[a]
  Hydrocephalus
  Amino protein poisoning
  Increased intracranial pressure[a]

[a] More common.

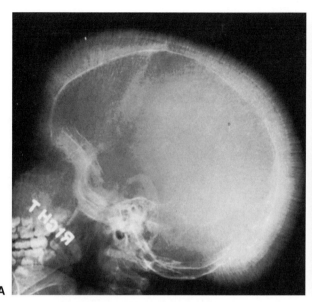
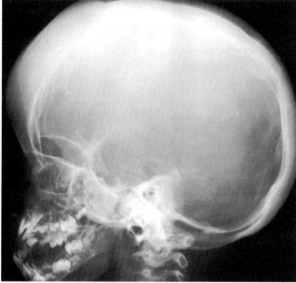

FIG. 2-14. Increased skull density. A: Six-year-old female with untreated thalassemia major. The diploic space of the cranial vault formed by intramembranous ossification is markedly thickened and sclerotic, with vertical densities producing a "hair-on-end" appearance. Note the extramedullary hematopoiesis in the maxillary antra. **B:** An 8-year-old child with severe iron deficiency anemia. There is thickening and increased density of the cranial vault.

TABLE 2-11. *Lytic skull defects*

Congenital
   Lacunar skull[a]
   Convolutional markings[a]
   Meningoencephalocele
   Dermal sinus, dermoid[a]
   Epidermoid[a]
   Cranium bifidum
   Neurofibromatosis (lambdoid defect)
   Anomalous apertures
     Parietal foramina[a]
     Emissary vein foramina
   Wormian bones
   Encephalocele
Infection
   Osteomyelitis[a]: bacterial, fungal
   Syphilis
Neoplasm
   Dermoid, epidermoid[a]
   Hemangioma
   Metastasis[a]
   Sarcoma
   Superficial intracranial mass
   Leukemia, lymphoma
   Primary bone tumor
Trauma
   Surgical defect[a]
   Fracture[a]
   Healed cephalohematoma
   Leptomeningeal cyst
   Radiation necrosis
Miscellaneous
   Aneurysmal bone cyst
   Fibrous dysplasia
   Hemophiliac pseudotumor
   Histiocytosis[a]
   Caffey disease
   Hyperparathyroidism

[a] More common.

until about 12 years of age (60,67). However, young patients with increased intracranial pressure may demonstrate both sutural diastasis and sellar demineralization. Children under 10 years of age with prominent convolutional markings solely because of normal brain growth have no sutural diastasis or sellar changes.

The coronal suture is usually the first suture to demonstrate diastasis (67). In the neonate, it is manifested as an exaggerated V-shaped configuration (Fig. 2-16) (5,59,60). The anterior fontanel may also bulge. In older children,

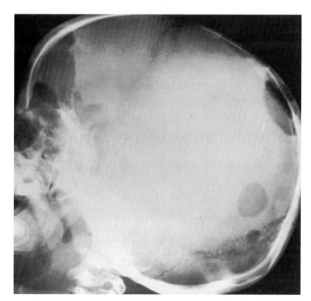

FIG. 2-15. Multiple skull defects. Two-year-old girl with Letterer-Siwe type of histiocytosis.

TABLE 2-12. *Causes of increased intracranial pressure*

Congenital
  Hydrocephalus[a]
  Arnold-Chiari malformation
  Dandy-Walker syndrome
  Cloverleaf skull: severe universal craniosynostosis
  Congenital neoplasm
Infection
  Meningitis,[a] meningoencephalitis
  Cerebritis
  Subdural empyema
  Ventriculitis
  Abscess
  Parasitic disease
Neoplasm
  Primary brain tumor[a]
  Metastatic disease: neuroblastoma, leukemia/lymphoma
Trauma
  Subdural hematoma or hygroma[a]
  Cerebral edema[a]
  Cerebral contusion
  Cerebral hemorrhage
Miscellaneous
  Hydrocephalus[a]
  Cerebral infection[a]
  Lead encephalopathy
  Drug therapy
  Hyperthyroidism
  Hypervitaminosis A, hypovitaminosis A
  Hypoparathyroidism
  Leukemia, lymphoma
  Pseudotumor cerebri
  Craniosynostosis (universal)

[a] More common.

there is stretching of the coronal sutural interdigitations with diastasis. After the coronal suture, the usual sequence of diastasis is sagittal, lambdoid, and finally squamosal. The submentovertex view is excellent for confirming or excluding coronal sutural spread. If one remains uncertain about the presence of coronal diastasis, the sagittal suture should be examined in both AP and Towne projections, as there is less difficulty distinguishing a normal from an abnormal sagittal suture (68). The uppermost portion of the coronal suture should not measure more than 3 mm after 3 months of age (68). Although intricate measurements of sutures are available (67), they are difficult to apply in day-to-day radiologic practice. In general, if one feels that the sutures may be diastatic, they probably are separated. CT, US, or MRI should be performed to detect any intracranial abnormality.

In older children, increased intracranial pressure causes bony demineralization of the sella turcica and accentuation of the convolutional markings (Fig. 2-17). The earliest demineralization involves the posteroinferior floor of the sella at the base of the dorsum sellae. If there is third ventricular enlargement, there may be associated sellar enlargement, erosion of the posterior clinoids, shortening of the anterior clinoids, and enlargement of the chiasmatic sulcus.

Abnormal Sella Turcica

The sella turcica reflects changes of chronically increased intracranial pressure, changes in sellar or pituitary volume, and bony dysplasia (69–72). Increased intracranial pressure

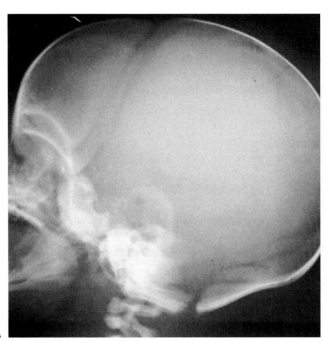

A

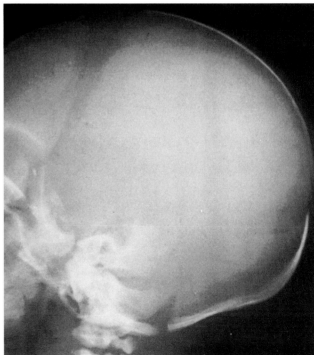

B

FIG. 2-16. Acute increased intracranial pressure in the neonate. A: Lateral skull radiograph at 1 day of age is normal. **B:** The patient had a spontaneous subarachnoid hemorrhage with associated increase in intracranial pressure at 8 days of age. Note the exaggerated V-shaped configuration of the coronal suture. This particularly involves the upper part of the suture.

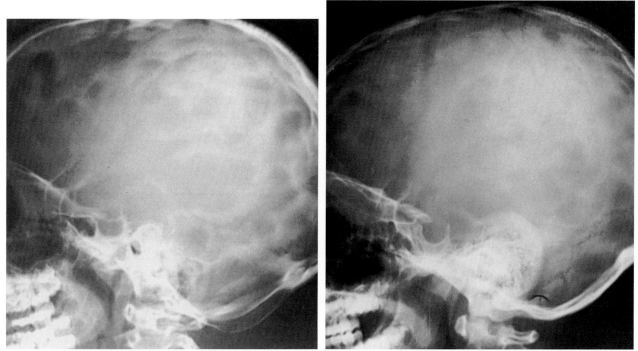

A   B

FIG. 2-17. Chronic increased intracranial pressure in the older child. A: Eight-year-old girl with increased intracranial pressure due to meningeal sarcoma. There is marked accentuation of the convolutional markings with enlargement and demineralization of the sella turcica. **B:** Five-year-old boy with increased intracranial pressure due to central nervous system leukemia. There is accentuation of convolutional markings, sutural diastasis with pronounced interdigitations, and demineralization of the posterior part of the floor of the sellar fossa.

changes are discussed above. Enlargement of the pituitary fossa occurs with an intrasellar mass, rebound hypertrophy of the pituitary gland (hypothyroidism, Nelson syndrome), the empty sella syndrome, long-standing increased intracranial pressure, and contiguous bone destruction (5,71) (Fig.

2-18A). A small pituitary fossa may be seen as a normal variant. It may also be present with hypopituitarism (Fig. 2-18B), septooptic dysplasia, and primary growth hormone deficiency (presumably because of pituitary gland hypoplasia or aplasia). A small pituitary fossa may also be due to

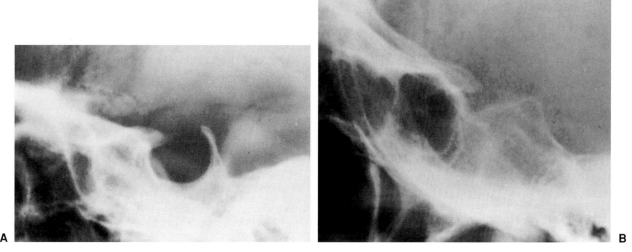

A   B

FIG. 2-18. Abnormalities of sellar size. A: Hypothyroidism. There is enlargement of the pituitary fossa due to hypertrophy of the pituitary gland. **B:** Hypopituitarism. There is a small pituitary fossa presumably because of hypoplasia of the pituitary gland.

previous surgery, local irradiation, or a primary bone dysplasia.

Intracranial Calcification

Intracranial calcifications in infants and children can occur in the dura, arachnoid, brain, cerebral vasculature, or mass lesions (73–77). Lourie has devised the mnemonic PINEAL, the pineal also being the most common site of physiologic calcification (74). Causes of pediatric intracranial calcifications are listed using this mnemonic, which is spelled with two E's and two A's for completeness: PINEEAAL (Table 2-13) (74). If the radiologic appearance and location are considered in conjunction with clinical data, the cause of many of these calcifications is readily diagnosed. CT is

TABLE 2-13. *Intracranial calcification in infants and children—"PINEAL"*

*P*hysiologic factors
  Pineal[a]
  Choroid plexus
  Habenular commissure
  Ligaments: petroclinoid, interclinoid
  Dura: falx, tentorium
*I*nfection
  TORCHS complex: toxoplasmosis[a], rubella, CMV, herpes, syphilis
  Abscess
  Tuberculoma
  Fungal and other granuloatous disease
*N*eoplasms
  Craniopharyngioma[a]
  Oligodendroglioma
  Choroid plexus papilloma
  Pineal tumor
  Lipoma of corpus callosum
  Ependymoma
  After radiation therapy
*E*ndocrine
  Hyperparathyroidism
  Hypervitaminosis D
  Hypoparathyroidism, pseudohypoparathyroidism
*E*mbryologic factors
  Neurocutaneous syndromes: tuberous sclerosis[a], Sturge-Weber syndrome[a], neurofibromatosis, Hippel-Lindau disease, ataxia-telangiectasia
  Fahr disease
  Cockayne syndrome
  Basal cell nevus syndrome
*A*rteriovenous disease
  Infarction
  Aneurysm
  Hematoma, hemorrhage
  Arteriovenous malformation
  Hemangioma
  Irradiation[a]
*A*rtifacts[a]: contrast media, braids, EEG paste, dirt
*L*eftover *L*'s: lipoma, lipoid proteinosis, lissencephaly

CMV, cytomegalovirus; EEG, electroencephalogram.
  [a] More common.
Modified from Lourie (74).

much more sensitive and specific than plain radiographs and MRI for the diagnosis of intracranial calcifications. Calcifications may be demonstrated by US as increased echogenicities with characteristic acoustic shadowing.

Physiologic calcifications may occur in membranes or cerebral organs. Some common physiologic calcification sites include the interclinoid ligament (over 1 year of age), falx (over 3 years old), petroclinoid ligament (over 5 years old), pineal and habenula (over 10 years old), and glomus of the choroid plexus (over 3 years old) (5). Physiologic calcification of the pineal gland in young children is so rare that calcification in this region in a child less than 10 years of age, especially if the calcification is more than 1 cm in diameter, suggests a pineal neoplasm. Asymmetric, extensive, or precocious calcification (less than 10 years of age) of the choroid plexus suggests neurofibromatosis, tuberous sclerosis, or choroid plexus papilloma.

SPECIFIC ABNORMALITIES

Congenital and Developmental Abnormalities

Congenital and developmental abnormalities of the CNS have been classified by van der Knaap and Valk according to time of onset during gestation (78). This approach focuses on the timing rather than the etiology of an insult as the major determinant of the type of malformation. Using this classification scheme (Table 2-14) (78), the common, important congenital malformations and deformities of the CNS are discussed below.

Craniosynostosis

Craniosynostosis, or craniostenosis, is the premature closure of a calvarial suture or sutures. It may be primary, or it may be secondary to metabolic disease, bone dysplasia, hematologic disorder, prematurity, external compression of the calvarium, failure of brain growth, or decreased intracranial pressure (Table 2-15) (6,79,80). The distinction between secondary and primary craniosynostosis has genetic, prognostic, and therapeutic implications (61,80).

The etiology of primary craniosynostosis is unknown. It may be related to an anomaly of the skull base and thus considered a disorder of ventral induction. Faulty dural development, dysplasia, metabolic alteration, and local sutural injury have also been postulated (7,60,79,80). When a suture prematurely closes, normal bone growth along its edges is impaired, whereas growth in other directions at other sutures is excessive. This combination of delayed growth perpendicular to the fused suture with compensatory accelerated growth in other directions leads to the specific calvarial deformities of each type of craniosynostosis.

Most significant synostoses have developed in utero and are detectable at or shortly after birth. To be deforming, closure must occur during fetal life or early infancy, as bony

TABLE 2-14. *Classification of congenital CNS defects*

1. Abnormalities of dorsal induction
   a. Primary neurulation (3–4 weeks gestation)
      1) Anencephaly
      2) Cephalocele
      3) Myelomeningocele
      4) Chiari malformation
      5) Hydromyelia
   b. Secondary neurulation (4 weeks–7 months gestation)
      1) Lipomyelomeningocele
      2) Dermal sinus
      3) Tethered cord/tight filum
      4) Myelocystocele
      5) Meningocele
      6) Diastematomyelia
      7) Neurenteric cysts
      8) Split notochord syndrome
      9) Caudal dysplasia syndrome
      10) Developmental tumors
          a) Lipoma
          b) Dermoid/epidermoid
          c) Teratoma
2. Abnormalities of ventral induction (5–10 weeks gestation)
   a. Holoprosencephaly
   b. Septooptic dysplasia
   c. Agenesis of the septum pellucidum
   d. Cerebral hemihypoplasia
   e. Hypoplasia of the cerebellar hemispheres or vermis
   f. Dandy-Walker spectrum
   g. Craniosynostosis
   h. Diencephalic cyst
   i. Joubert syndrome
3. Abnormalities of neuronal proliferation, differentiation, and histogenesis (2–5 months gestation)
   a. Micrencephaly
   b. Megalencephaly (unilateral or bilateral)
   c. Congenital vascular malformations
   d. Congenital CNS tumors
   e. Aqueductal anomalies/stenosis
   f. Colpocephaly
   g. Porencephaly
   h. Hydranencephaly
   i. Multicystic encephalopathy
   j. Neurocutaneous syndromes
4. Disorders of migration and cortical organization (2–5 weeks gestation)
   a. Schizencephaly
   b. Neuronal heterotopias
   c. Pachygyria
   d. Lissencephaly
   e. Polymicrogyria
   f. Hypoplasia or aplasia of the corpus callosum
5. Disorders of myelination (7 months gestation–2 years of age)
   a. Hypomyelination/dysmyelination
6. Secondarily acquired defects of formed structures (encephaloclastic) (>5 months)
   a. Colpocephaly
   b. Hydrocephalus
   c. Porencephaly
   d. Hydranencephaly
   e. Multicystic encephalopathy
   f. Leukomalacia
   g. Hemiatrophy
7. Unclassified
   a. Arachnoid cysts

Classification of these disorders is based primarily on the timing of the insult necessary to produce the radiologic finding. Whether the disorders are related to neuronal proliferation and histogenesis or other factors is controversial.

Adapted and modified from van der Knaap and Valk (78).

remodeling is able to maintain normal skull shape after 1 year of age if only one suture is closed. There is a 3:1 male predominance, with some instances of isolated coronal or sagittal synostosis being familial. The order of frequency of involvement for various synostoses is as follows: sagittal 56%, multiple 14%, unilateral coronal 11%, bilateral coronal 11%, metopic 7%, and lambdoid 1% (5). Frequent combinations include coronal and lambdoid, sagittal and metopic, sagittal and lambdoid, and universal craniosynostosis.

Analysis of skull shape clinically or by plain skull radiographs is usually the best clue to the presence of craniosynostosis (60,80). Closure of various sutures leads to predictable responses in other sutures and particular alterations in growth, so the diagnosis of synostosis can be made from skull shape alone if it is clear that external molding has not occurred. However, characteristic changes also occur along the involved suture (80). These changes include sutural narrowing, parasutural sclerosis, sharpening of suture edges, and bony bridging across the suture. Perisutural sclerosis in isolation, however, is not evidence of impending synostosis (81). Sutures may be either partially or totally fused. Even with partial anatomic fusion, the skull shape is characteristically altered, indicating that there is complete functional closure. Inner table convolutional markings may also be in-

TABLE 2-15. *Classification of craniosynostosis*

Primary (idiopathic)
  Dolichocephaly (sagittal)[a]
  Brachycephaly (bilateral coronal[a] or lambdoid)
  Plagiocephaly (unilateral coronal[a] or lambdoid)
  Trigonocephaly (metopic)
  Oxycephaly (universal)
Secondary
  Part of syndrome
    Crouzon disease
    Apert syndrome
    Carpenter syndrome
    Treacher-Collins syndrome
    Craniotelencephalic dysplasia
    Arrhinencephaly
    Cloverleaf skull (Kleeblattschädel syndrome)
Associations
  Metabolic diseases
    Rickets
    Hypercalcemia
    Hyperthyroidism
    Hypervitaminosis D
    Bone dysplasias
      Hypophosphatasia
      Achondroplasia
      Metaphyseal dysplasia
      Rubinstein-Taybi syndrome
    Down syndrome
    Skull hyperostoses
    Hurler disease
  Shunt for hydrocephalus[a]
  Microcephaly[a]: dysgenesis, atrophy
  Hematologic: sickle cell, thalassemia

[a] More common.

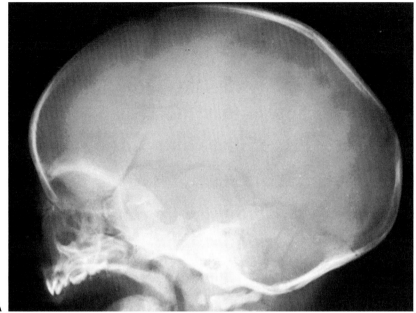

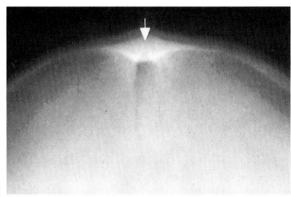

FIG. 2-19. Sagittal craniosynostosis. A: The skull of this 2-month-old female is dolichocephalic. **B:** Coned-down frontal skull film shows bony bridging of the sagittal suture *(arrow)* and parasutural sclerosis.

creased due to decreased compliance of the expanding skull, particularly with multiple or universal synostoses. Equivocal craniosynostosis may be confirmed by fluoroscopy, nuclear scintigraphy, CT, or three-dimensional CT (82). Three-dimensional CT is generally more helpful than plain skull radiographs or axial CT for assessing cosmetic improvement and detecting premature resynostosis following surgical correction. CT is also frequently performed to assess the underlying brain in patients with complex or multiple craniosynostoses.

There is no brain growth impairment with single craniosynostosis, so craniectomy is performed in these isolated fusions for purely cosmetic purposes. Multisutural or universal craniosynostosis may lead to chronic increased intracranial pressure with papilledema, cranial nerve palsy, and impaired brain growth, so early surgical correction is mandatory.

Sagittal Craniosynostosis

Premature closure of the sagittal suture produces a long, narrow skull that is termed dolichocephaly or scaphceph-

aly. This characteristic shape is readily apparent clinically and radiologically (Fig. 2-19). Usually, fusion begins in the midportion of the suture and progresses in both anterior and posterior directions. There may be narrowing, sclerosis, ridging, and bridging of the sagittal suture (see Fig. 2-19). Diastasis of the coronal and lambdoid sutures occasionally occurs in response to sagittal craniosynostosis.

Coronal Craniosynostosis

The coronal suture is the second most common suture to be involved in craniosynostosis. Craniosynostosis of the coronal suture may be unilateral (Fig. 2-20) or bilateral (Fig. 2-21). The skull is short in its AP diameter and wide (brachycephaly). The entire coronal suture may be fused, with extension into the sphenofrontal suture and sphenoethmoidal synchondrosis. There is flattening of the ipsilateral frontal area and foreshortening of the anterior fossa (see Figs. 2-20 and 2-21). The shallow orbits have oval, oblique margins that together with the elevated lesser wing of the sphenoid and expanded greater wing produce a "harlequin eye" appear-

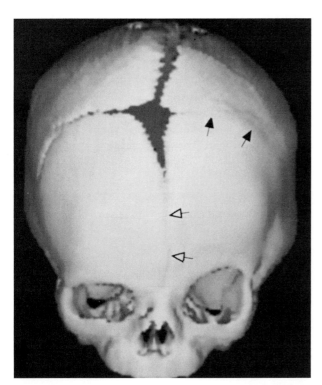

FIG. 2-20. Three-dimensional CT of unilateral coronal craniosynostosis. There is a harlequin eye appearance of the left orbit, bridging and obliteration of the left coronal suture *(closed arrows)*, and deviation of the metopic suture *(open arrows)*.

ance (see Fig. 2-21). Hypertelorism may be present. As best seen on the AP skull radiograph, there is tilting of the crista galli, ethmoid complex, and nasal septum to the side of a unilateral coronal fusion.

Metopic Craniosynostosis

Premature fusion of the metopic suture produces trigonocephaly (triangle-shaped head as seen from the top) and hypotelorism (Fig. 2-22). The forehead has a pointed shape that is best demonstrated by a tangential view (between a basal view and a steep Waters projection), axial CT, or three-dimensional CT. The lateral skull radiograph shows a shallow anterior cranial fossa and parasutural sclerosis of the metopic suture. The orbits are angled upward and medial to produce the "quizzical eye" appearance, and there is hypotelorism (Fig. 2-22A) (83). Most of the milder, later-diagnosed cases of metopic synostosis reshape themselves spontaneously.

Lambdoid Craniosynostosis

Lambdoid craniosynostosis is the rarest of the isolated craniosynostoses. With unilateral lambdoid synostosis, there is severe flattening of the ipsilateral occipital region, producing plagiocephaly. The sclerotic, thin, sharp-edged lambdoid

suture is identified. With bilateral lambdoid synostoses, the entire occipital area is flattened and inner table convolutional markings are prominent above the site of the synostosis. In young infants that sleep supine, considerable posterior flattening occurs in many normals, sometimes even with perisutural sclerosis. However, this positional plagiocephaly is not lamboid synostosis and will reshape itself without surgery.

Cloverleaf Skull

The cloverleaf skull *(Kleeblattschädel)* is a grotesque malformation due to fusion of coronal, lambdoid, and sagittal

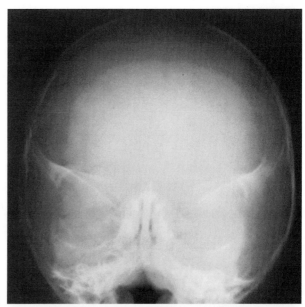

A

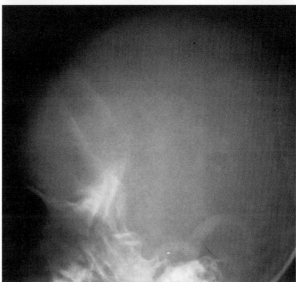

B

FIG. 2-21. Bilateral coronal craniosynostosis. A: Anteroposterior view shows bilateral harlequin eye appearance. **B:** Skull is brachycephalic with flattening of the frontal bone and foreshortening of the anterior fossa. Both coronal sutures are sclerotic.

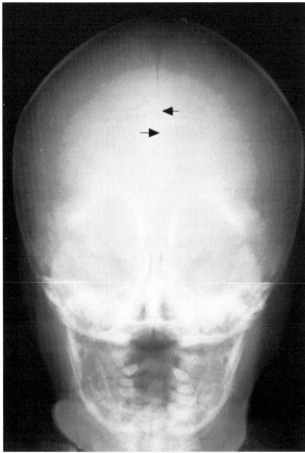

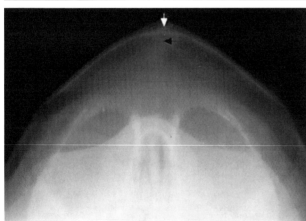

FIG. 2-22. Trigonocephaly. A: Anteroposterior view of the skull shows parasutural sclerosis of the metopic suture *(arrows)*, medial and upper angulation of the orbits producing a "quizzical" appearance, and hypotelorism. **B:** Tangential view confirms the pointed forehead and parasutural sclerosis along the metopic suture *(arrows)*. (Courtesy of Guido Currarino, M.D., Dallas, Texas.)

sutures. Bulging occurs at the bregma and squamosal areas (Fig. 2-23), producing a cloverleaf configuration to the calvarium. A lacunar skull is frequently associated, and exophthalmos is severe. CT or MRI usually demonstrates underly-

ing hydrocephalus and brain dysgenesis. Approximately one third of patients with cloverleaf skull have bony changes of thanatophoric dwarfism.

Craniosynostosis Secondary to Brain Atrophy

It is important to distinguish craniosynostosis secondary to brain atrophy from primary universal craniosynostosis be-

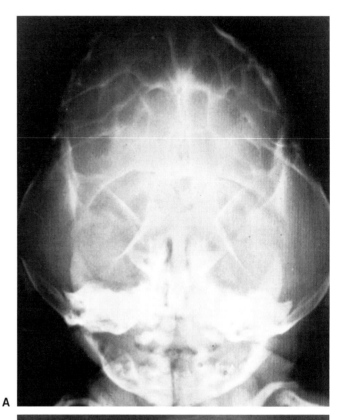

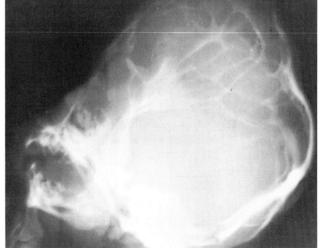

FIG. 2-23. Universal craniosynostosis with cloverleaf skull. Frontal **(A)** and lateral **(B)** skull films in a 2-day-old boy. Note marked bulging of the bregma and temporal regions. There is a lacunar skull and fusion of all major sutures.

cause surgical intervention is not indicated in the former but is mandatory in the latter (79). If there is lack of brain growth (micrencephaly leading to microcephaly), the stimulus for sutural patency is absent. The skull is small, with postural flattening of the occiput, thick cranial vault, lack of convolutional markings, small fontanels, and narrow sutures without sclerosis, bridging, or ridging. The cranial vault appears smooth and bland rather than active and dynamic, as there is little or no underlying brain growth (Fig. 2-24) (79). Sinus and mastoid overpneumatization is characteristic.

Lacunar Skull

Lacunar skull (craniolacunia, *Lückenschädel*) is a mesenchymal dysplasia associated with myelomeningocele, myelocele, and encephalocele (84,85). Patients may have severe lacunar skull and underlying brain dysgenesis without spinal dysraphism or cranioschisis, but this situation is the rare exception rather than the rule. Mild irregularities of both inner and outer tables of the cranial vault may be demonstrated by CT in normal infants but should not be confused with a true lacunar skull. Essentially all patients under 3 months of age with meningomyelocele or encephalocele have some radiologic evidence of lacunar skull; and, conversely, a lacunar skull almost always indicates the presence of a myelomeningocele or encephalocele.

Lacunar skull is a defect in ossification of the calvaria unrelated to increased intracranial pressure. Intraventricular pressure is normal in some patients with lacunar skull. Moreover, the calvarial defects (lacunae) disappear by 6 months of age, whether or not a shunt has been placed (85).

The radiologic appearance of lacunar skull is characteristic. There are multiple oval lucencies due to thinning of the inner table and diploic space, with interspersed linear bony ridges (Fig. 2-25). These lacunae are most prominent in the parietal and upper occipital bones; the frontal bones are less frequently involved. A frontal cranium bifidum, defective ossification of the frontal bone along with the upper metopic suture, is frequently present as well.

Lacunar skull should not be confused with prominent convolutional markings in normal children or the hammer-beaten silver appearance of increased intracranial pressure (see Fig. 2-17). Normal convolutional markings are present at a time of maximal brain growth (3–7 years); the sutures and sella turcica are normal. Lacunar skull is present in the neonate with encephalocele or myelomeningocele but disappears by 6 months of age. Chronic increased intracranial pressure in older children may produce marked accentuation of the convolutional markings, but there is also associated sutural diastasis or sellar demineralization (see Fig. 2-17).

Disorders of Dorsal Induction

Dorsal induction is the process whereby the notochord induces thickening of the adjacent ectoderm to form the neural plate. Neural folds develop from each side of the plate to form the primitive neural tube, a process referred to as

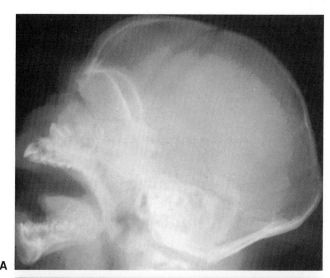

A

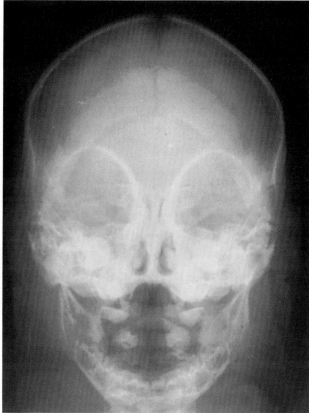

B

FIG. 2-24. Microcephaly. Lateral **(A)** and anteroposterior **(B)** views of the skull in this 4-month-old girl with marked craniofacial disproportion. There is slight occipital flattening, no convolutional markings, a small anterior fontanel, and early closure of sutures. This type of microcephaly, due to underlying brain atrophy or dysgenesis, should not be confused with primary universal craniosynostosis.

primary neurulation. Malformations due to disorders of dorsal induction originate during the first month of gestation. The intracranial manifestations of abnormal dorsal induction include anencephaly, cephaloceles, and the Chiari malformations.

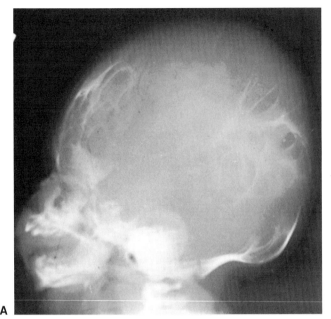

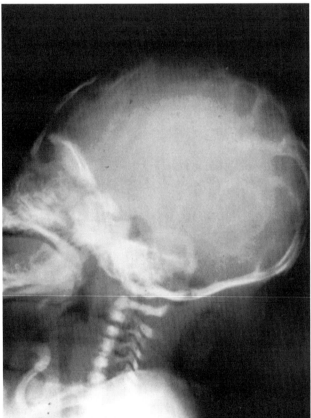

FIG. 2-25. Lacunar skull of a newborn. A: Known myelo-meningocele. **B:** Occipital encephalocele.

Anencephaly

Anencephaly occurs when normal closure of the cranial end of the neural tube fails at 24 days gestation, resulting in complete absence of the cranium and brain above the

brainstem (5,6). The malformation is fatal in utero or within a few days of birth. Elevation of α-fetoprotein is present in maternal serum and amniotic fluid. The diagnosis can be made with prenatal US.

Cephaloceles

Cephaloceles are extensions of one or more intracranial structures through a skull defect. Depending on the elements present, cephaloceles may be classified as meningoceles (meninges only), encephaloceles or encephalomeningoceles (meninges and brain tissue), and encephalocystomeningoceles (meninges, brain, and ventricles) (6,7). Cephaloceles are also categorized by location and may extend through either the calvaria or the skull base. Cephaloceles result from failure of primary neural tube closure, faulty induction of bone growth, pressure erosion from an intracranial mass, or failure of fusion of the ossification centers at the skull base (31,86).

Occipital cephaloceles comprise up to 71% of cephaloceles seen in North America (31,87). Occipital cephaloceles may be present in conjunction with the Dandy-Walker spectrum or as a part of the Meckel-Gruber syndrome. Cervico-occipital cephalocele is a component of the Chiari III malformation. Most occipital cephaloceles contain brain tissue (occipital lobes or cerebellum). The brain tissue within the cephalocele is usually dysplastic. Anomalies of the venous sinuses are also frequently present, and one of the sinuses may extend through the calvarial defect. Documentation of the aberrant course of the venous sinus is important when surgery is contemplated. MRI is useful in occipital cephaloceles to demonstrate the contents of the cephalocele, the position of the dural venous sinuses (with MR venography), any associated CNS anomalies, and hydrocephalus (Fig. 2-26) (6,7).

Frontoethmoid cephaloceles are uncommon in North America and Europe but are the most common type in Southeast Asia (31,86). Frontoethmoidal cephaloceles may be subdivided, according to the osseous defect, as nasoethmoidal (between the nasal bones and nasal cartilage), nasofrontal (between the frontal and nasal bones) (Fig. 2-27), nasoorbital (between the frontal process of the maxilla anteriorly and the lacrimal bone and lamina papyracea of the ethmoid bone posteriorly), and interfrontal (through the metopic suture). Frontoethmoidal encephaloceles may present with hypertelorism or as a glabellar mass. Associated anomalies include agenesis of the corpus callosum, holoprosencephaly, migrational defects, and hydrocephalus.

Nasal dermoids and nasal gliomas are embryologically related to nasofrontal cephaloceles (6,88). The foramen cecum at the anterior border of the crista galli is normally patent early in gestation but then closes. Dura normally projects through the foramen early in fetal life. Incomplete regression of the dural projection may result in a nasofrontal cephalocele, dermoid-epidermoid, or nasal glioma. Nasal

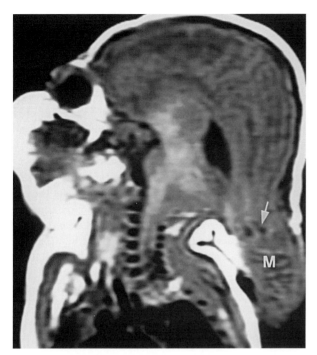

FIG. 2-26. Occipital encephalocele. Newborn infant. Sagittal T1 MRI demonstrates a large occipital scalp mass *(M)* containing CSF *(arrow)* and cerebral tissue. There is associated microcephaly.

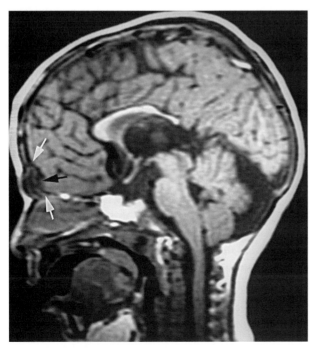

FIG. 2-27. Frontal meningocele. A 6-year-old boy with sagittal T1 MRI showing a midline frontal bone defect *(white arrows)* and a cerebrospinal fluid intensity fluid-filled mass *(black arrow)*. There is also callosal dysgenesis and a Dandy-Walker spectrum anomaly.

gliomas are ectopic, dysplastic brain tissue found in the nasal cavity or subcutaneous tissues; they probably arise from herniation of brain tissue through a patent foramen cecum. With closure of the foramen, the neural tissue becomes isolated from the intracranial contents.

Sphenoidal cephaloceles are rare (31,87). The osseous defect occurs through the floor of the sella turcica and sphenoid body with potential herniation of the infundibulum and third ventricle through the defect. The masses may be sphenoidal (Fig. 2-28), sphenoethmoidal, or, rarely, sphenopharyngeal. Agenesis of the corpus callosum, hypertelorism, and midline facial clefts may coexist. Sphenoid wing cephaloceles are usually associated with neurofibromatosis.

Parietal cephaloceles are uncommon and are often atretic. Associated anomalies include Dandy-Walker spectrum malformations, callosal agenesis, holoprosencephaly, Chiari II malformations, and venous sinus abnormalities (6,31). The superior sagittal sinus may extend through the bony defect. The straight sinus is often absent, and an anomalous falcine sinus may extend into the defect (Fig. 2-29).

Chiari Malformations

The Chiari type I malformation is defined as downward displacement of the cerebellar tonsils below the foramen magnum but without displacement of the medulla and fourth ventricle. Tonsillar herniation of less than 5 mm below the foramen magnum is unlikely to be clinically significant (89,90). In children between the ages of 5 and 15 years, tonsillar ectopia of up to 6 mm may not produce symptoms (90). Chiari I malformations are associated with hydrocepha-

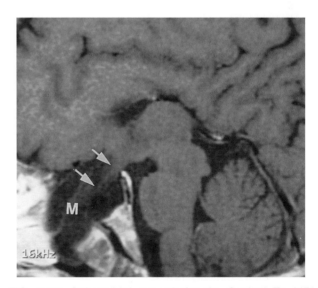

FIG. 2-28. Sphenoidal encephalocele. Sagittal T1 MRI demonstrates a cerebrospinal fluid–containing mass *(M)* extending through the defective sphenoid body and sella turcica into the nasal cavity and nasopharynx. The cyst-like mass also contains a portion of the optic nerves and chiasm *(arrows)*.

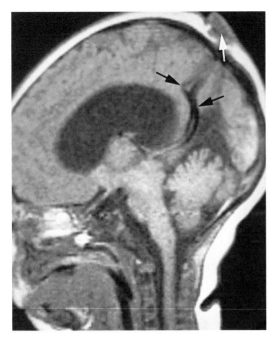

FIG. 2-29. **Parietal cephalocele**. A 4-month-old infant. Sagittal T1 MRI demonstrates a parietal cerebrospinal fluid intensity scalp mass *(white arrow)*. Deep anomalous veins are seen in the midline *(black arrows)* beneath the cephalocele.

lus, bony anomalies of the craniocervical junction, basilar invagination, scoliosis, and hydrosyringomyelia. As many as 25% of Chiari I patients will have hydrosyringomyelia (Fig. 2-30) (91). Chiari I malformations may be acquired

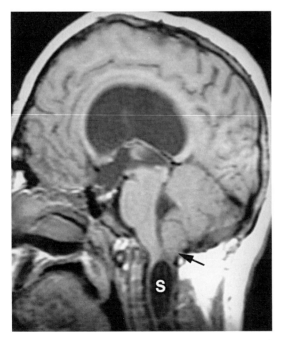

FIG. 2-30. **Chiari I malformation**. A 12-year-old boy. Sagittal T1 MRI demonstrates the cerebellar tonsils *(arrow)* and cervicomedullary junction located below the foramen magnum. Syringohydromyelia *(S)* and hydrocephalus are present.

after placement of a lumboperitoneal shunt or may develop in the absence of any predisposing factor. Supratentorial anomalies other than hydrocephalus are rarely present (6).

Chiari type II malformations are complex congenital anomalies affecting the brain, spinal cord, skull, and vertebral column (6,7,92–96). The malformation is characterized by a small posterior fossa with caudal displacement of the inferior cerebellum and tonsils, pons, medulla, and fourth ventricle into the upper cervical canal (Fig. 2-31). The anomaly is almost always accompanied by a myelomeningocele. The presence of a leaking myelomeningocele results in inadequate enlargement of the cerebral ventricles, and this produces a small posterior fossa. With continued cerebellar growth, there is progressive herniation of hindbrain elements into the upper cervical canal (95). The medulla becomes elongated and descends behind the upper cervical spinal cord, which is fixed in position by the dentate ligaments. This relationship produces the typical cervicomedullary "kink" of a Chiari II malformation (97). Hydrocephalus, if not present at birth, almost always develops after repair of the myelomeningocele (6).

The many supratentorial anomalies which occur with Chiari II malformations are demonstrated by US, CT, and MRI (6,7,92–96,98). Callosal dysgenesis or agenesis is frequent. Colpocephaly (prominence of the posterior body and trigone of the lateral ventricles) is common and is probably due to the callosal abnormality. Stenogyria (small, pointed gyri) may be seen in the medial portions of the occipital lobes (94). The falx may be fenestrated; this allows interdigitation of gyri across the midline. Enlargement of the massa intermedia is often present. The quadrigeminal plate exhibits an unusual pointed appearance referred to as tectal beaking. The cerebral aqueduct may be stenosed, dilated, or shortened. Subependymal heterotopias may also occur.

The skull is abnormal in Chiari II malformation (93). Marked thinning of the parietal and occipital bones is responsible for the Lückenschädel (lacunar) appearance of the skull. This appearance is unrelated to hydrocephalus and usually resolves after the first 6 months of life with or without ventricular shunting (84,85,93). Scalloping of the temporal bones may be due to pressure effects from the development of the cerebellum within a small posterior fossa.

After surgical repair of a myelomeningocele, the neurologic deficit should be static. The onset of new neurologic symptoms in postoperative patients should initiate prompt radiologic investigation of the brain and spinal cord. Hydrocephalus due to shunt malfunction is common in this setting. Special attention should be paid to the size of the fourth ventricle, which should be small or slit-like. Even a fourth ventricle which seems to have a normal size may be encysted or entrapped (Fig. 2-32) (99). Other possible causes of neurologic deterioration in patients with Chiari II malformations include syrinx formation, stenosis at the craniocervical junction, and retethering of the spinal cord.

A Chiari type III malformation is a rare disorder in which there is a posterior cervicooccipital cephalocele containing

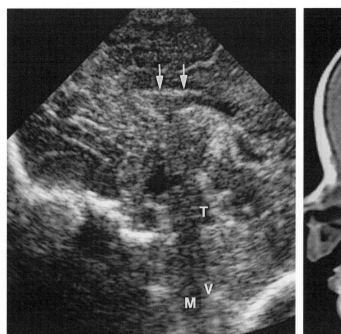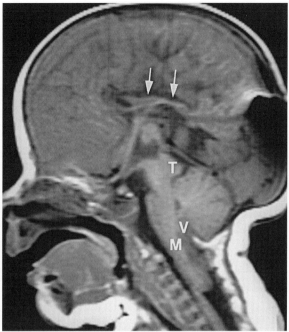

FIG. 2-31. Chiari II malformation. Newborn girl with meningomyelocele. US **(A)** and sagittal T1 MRI **(B)** show caudal placement of the medulla *(M)* and cerebellar vermis *(V)*. The cerebellum is featureless. No fourth ventricle is identifiable by sonography. Note the beaked tectum *(T)* and hypogenesis of the corpus callosum *(arrows)*, demonstrated by both ultrasound and MRI.

dysplastic cerebellum, fourth ventricle, and sometimes brainstem (Fig. 2-33) (6,7).

The Chiari type IV malformation consists of hypoplasia of the cerebellar vermis, cerebellar hemispheres, and brainstem with no inferior displacement of posterior fossa structures; it was not described by Chiari. It is considered a form of vermian cerebellar hypoplasia (6,7).

Disorders of Ventral Induction

Ventral induction is the process whereby the cranial end of the neural tube expands to form the brain, and mesoderm induces the overlying ectoderm to form the facial structures. With expansion and diverticulation of the neural tube, three subdivisions of the brain are formed: the prosencephalon (forebrain), the mesencephalon (midbrain), and the rhombencephalon (hindbrain). The prosencephalon subsequently divides into the telencephalon (cerebral hemispheres, caudate nuclei, and putamina) and the diencephalon (thalami, hypothalami, and globi pallidi) (6). Disruption of normal development during ventral induction (weeks 5–10 of gestation) may produce holoprosencephaly, septooptic dysplasia, posterior fossa cystic malformations, agenesis of the septum pellucidum, and perhaps craniosynostosis (7).

Holoprosencephaly

Holoprosencephaly is a spectrum of disorders resulting from lack of normal cleavage of the telencephalon into two cerebral hemispheres and lack of separation of the telencephalon from the diencephalon (5,6,100). Associated facial anomalies include cyclopia (single orbit with a proboscis but

FIG. 2-32. Entrapped fourth ventricle. Axial CT shows a markedly dilated fourth ventricle *(4V)* in an infant with Chiari II malformation and shunted hydrocephalus after repair of a myelomeningocele.

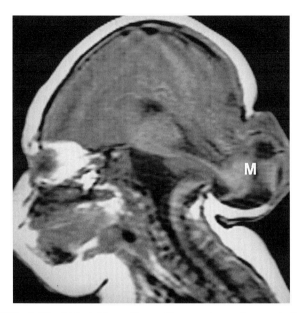

FIG. 2-33. Chiari III malformation and cervicooccipital meningocele. Newborn with large occipital mass. Sagittal T1 MRI demonstrates a large occipital scalp mass *(M)* containing cerebrospinal fluid as well as cerebral and cerebellar tissue. There is posterior kinking of the malformed brainstem, absence of the corpus callosum, and severe microcephaly.

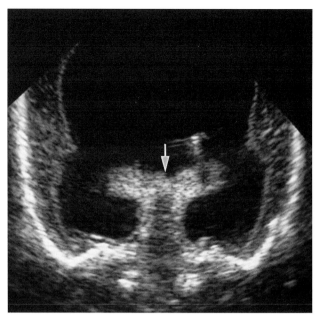

FIG. 2-34. Holoprosencephaly. Neonate. Coronal US shows a large monoventricular chamber and fusion of the basal ganglia and thalami across the midline *(arrow).*

no nose), ethmocephaly (severe hypotelorism with median proboscis), cebocephaly (hypotelorism with rudimentary nose), and hypotelorism alone. The more severe facial anomalies are associated with the more severe intracranial abnormalities (83,100,101).

Alobar holoprosencephaly is the most severe form of holoprosencephaly (6,7,101). Affected individuals are usually microcephalic. A monoventricle is present with failure of separation of the thalami and no attempt at hemispheric cleavage (Fig. 2-34). A mantle of cortical tissue is present anteriorly but no falx cerebri, corpus callosum, or olfactory nerves. The membranous roof of the third ventricle may dilate to form a large dorsal cyst (Fig. 2-35). A single (azygous) anterior cerebral artery is present but the superior sagittal sinus, straight sinus, and internal cerebral veins are absent. Affected infants are stillborn or die soon after birth.

Semilobar holoprosencephaly is an intermediate form. As in the alobar form, affected individuals are microcephalic. The cerebral hemispheres are partially cleaved from each other posteriorly. The splenium of the corpus callosum may be present even when the development of the more anterior portions of the corpus callosum are undeveloped (6,12, 102,103). There is partial separation of the thalami, and the temporal horns may be partially formed (Fig. 2-36). The falx and interhemispheric fissure may be present posteriorly. Facial anomalies are less severe and are a less constant feature than in the alobar type.

Lobar holoprosencephaly is the mildest form of holoprosencephaly. Facial anomalies are usually not present; the brain is almost always normal in size (7,101). The occipital

and temporal horns of the lateral ventricles are well formed. However, there is failure of cleavage of the two cerebral hemispheres frontally. As in all forms of holoprosencephaly, the septum pellucidum is absent. The corpus callosum may be incomplete or dysplastic as well.

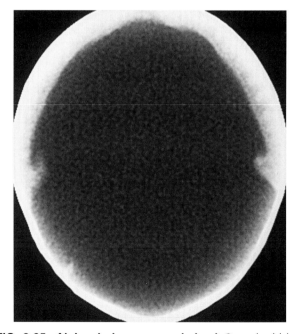

FIG. 2-35. Alobar holoprosencephaly. A 2-week-old boy with macrocephaly. Axial CT demonstrates a large monoventricular chamber anteriorly and a huge dorsal cyst posteriorly. There is no interhemispheric fissure or falx.

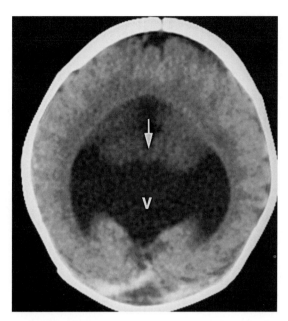

FIG. 2-36. Semilobar holoprosencephaly. Axial CT in a newborn demonstrates partial fusion of the thalami in the midline *(arrow)* and a monoventricular chamber *(V)* extending across the midline.

Septooptic Dysplasia

Septooptic dysplasia (de Morsier syndrome) is an abnormality of ventral induction characterized by complete or partial absence of the septum pellucidum and hypoplasia of the optic nerves (Fig. 2-37) (104). Schizencephaly or heterotopia is present in at least 50% of cases (Fig. 2-38) (87). Hypothalamic and pituitary dysfunction is seen in up to two thirds of patients. The most frequent pituitary abnormalities are deficiencies of growth hormone and thyroid-stimulating hormone. Ectopia of the posterior pituitary bright spot may also occur. By MRI, two groups of patients are identified: (a) those with partial absence of the septum pellucidum, hypothalamic dysfunction, and schizencephaly or neuronal heterotopia and (b) those with complete absence of the septum pellucidum and hypoplasia of the cerebral white matter without other anomalies (104,105). The frontal horns of the lateral ventricles have a squared-off appearance with inferior pointing on coronal MRI; hypoplasia of the optic nerves may be evident in severe cases (6).

Other causes of absence of the interventricular septum include Chiari II malformation, holoprosencephaly, callosal agenesis, and severe hydrocephalus (6).

Posterior Fossa Cystic Malformations

The posterior fossa cystic malformations have traditionally been divided into Dandy-Walker malformation, Dandy-Walker variant, mega cisterna magna, and Blake pouch or arachnoid cyst (5,7). More recent categorization of these lesions emphasizes that posterior fossa cysts comprise a continuum of malformations (106–108). The pathogenesis of these lesions is uncertain; however, one possibility is that maldevelopment of the anterior and posterior membranous

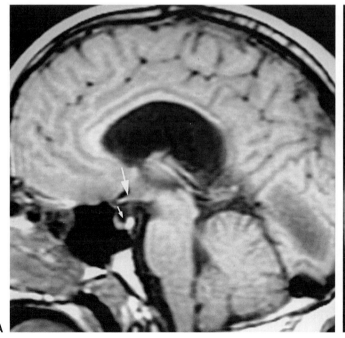

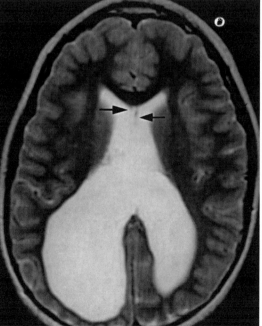

FIG. 2-37. Septooptic dysplasia. A 12-year-old boy with endocrine dysfunction. Sagittal T1 MRI **(A)** shows a hypoplastic optic chiasm *(large arrow)* and a partially empty sella *(small arrow)*. Axial T2 MRI **(B)** demonstrates asymmetric ventriculomegaly with only a few septal leaflet remnants *(arrows)*.

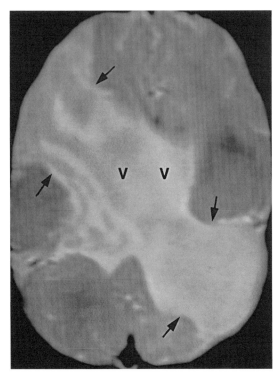

FIG. 2-38. Absence of the septum pellucidum and schizencephaly. Axial T2-weighted MRI demonstrates bilateral cerebral clefts *(arrows)* communicating with the dilated lateral ventricles *(V)*. There is absence of the septal leaflets in this child with septooptic dysplasia.

areas of the fourth ventricle during the fifth week of gestation causes the cystic malformation (6,107,108).

The classic Dandy-Walker malformation has complete or partial vermian agenesis, a retrocerebellar cyst communicating with the fourth ventricle, an enlarged posterior fossa, torcular elevation above the lambda, and absence of the falx cerebelli (Figs. 2-39 and 2-40) (106). Supratentorial anomalies (hypogenesis or agenesis of the corpus callosum, polymicrogyria, cortical heterotopias, occipital encephalocele, holoprosencephaly) may coexist. Macrocephaly and hydrocephalus are common. The developmental delay that may occur is probably due to associated supratentorial anomalies or hydrocephalus. MRI evaluation of the cerebral aqueduct for patency is extremely important in these patients prior to shunting the ventricles or the posterior fossa cyst (7). If the aqueduct is occluded, shunting of one compartment may lead to herniation of the other (106).

Lesions lacking some of the features of a Dandy-Walker malformation are considered to be part of the Dandy-Walker spectrum. In the Dandy-Walker variant, the cerebellar vermis is hypogenetic; the posterior fossa is usually normal in size, but there is a posterior fossa cyst (Fig. 2-41). If the cerebellar vermis is completely formed and an enlarged retrocerebellar CSF space is present without significant mass effect, the term mega cisterna magna is used (Fig. 2-42). If the retrocerebellar CSF collection has a mass effect on a completely formed cerebellum, the diagnosis of an arachnoid or Blake pouch cyst is made (Fig. 2-43) (106).

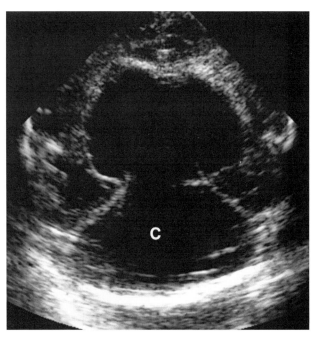

FIG. 2-39. Dandy-Walker malformation. Coronal plane US in a neonate shows a large anechoic posterior fossa cyst *(C)* with supratentorial extension and marked ventriculomegaly.

Disorders of Neuronal Proliferation and Differentiation

Megalencephaly

Megalencephaly (large brain) may be bilateral or unilateral (109). Bilateral megalencephaly may be present in cere-

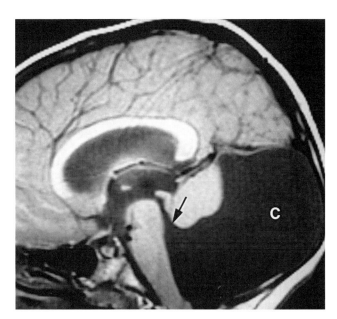

FIG. 2-40. Dandy-Walker malformation. An 8-year-old girl with sagittal T1 MRI demonstrates absence of the inferior cerebellar vermis, a large retrocerebellar cerebrospinal fluid intensity cyst *(C)* continuous with the fourth ventricle *(arrow)*, and hydrocephalus. From Strand et al. (106).

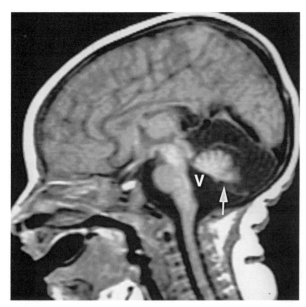

FIG. 2-41. Dandy-Walker variant. A 1-month-old boy. Sagittal T1 MRI demonstrates partial absence of the cerebellar vermis inferiorly *(arrow)*, a moderate-sized posterior fossa cerebrospinal fluid intensity space continuous with a partially formed fourth ventricle *(V)*, and no hydrocephalus. From Strand et al. (106).

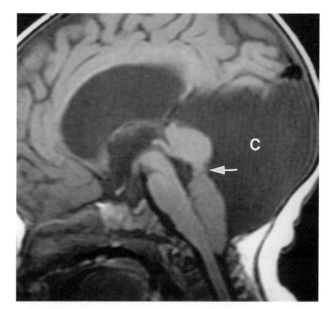

FIG. 2-43. Blake pouch cyst. A 6-month-old. Sagittal T1 MRI demonstrates a large retrocerebellar cerebrospinal fluid intensity cyst *(C)* compressing the deformed cerebellar vermis *(arrow)* and producing massive hydrocephalus.

bral gigantism (Soto syndrome), the phakomatoses, and Beckwith-Wiedemann syndrome. Familial megalencephaly may also occur but is usually mild and asymptomatic (6,7).

Unilateral megaloencephaly is a hamartomatous over-growth of the cerebral hemisphere and may occur as an isolated finding or in association with hemihypertrophy, linear sebaceous nevus syndrome, neurofibromatosis type 1, and unilateral hypomelanosis of Ito (109–113). These patients have intractable seizures, developmental delay, and hemiparesis. Imaging of unilateral megalencephaly demonstrates

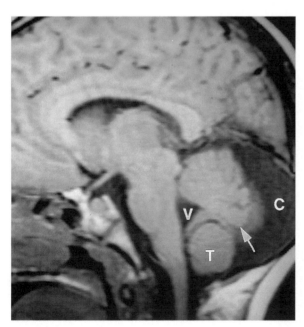

FIG. 2-42. Mega cisterna magna. A 7-year-old boy. Sagittal T1 MRI demonstrates a completely formed cerebellar vermis *(arrow)*, cerebellar tonsil *(T)*, and fourth ventricle *(V)* with a moderate-sized retrocerebellar cerebrospinal fluid intensity fluid space *(C)*. From Strand et al. (106).

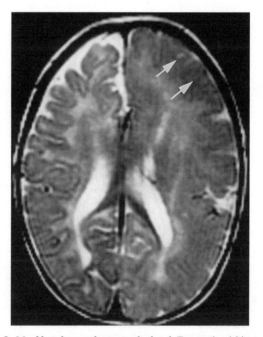

FIG. 2-44. Hemimegaloencephaly. A 7-month-old boy with intractable seizures. Axial T2 MRI demonstrates gyral thickening *(arrows)*, loss of gyral-sulcal detail, and decreased gray-white matter differentiation throughout the larger left cerebral hemisphere.

thickening of the cortex and enlargement of the ipsilateral lateral ventricle (Fig. 2-44). Polymicrogyria, pachygyria, or agyria may be present. The white matter of the involved hemisphere is often hypointense on T1-weighted and hyperintense on T2-weighted MRI.

Aqueductal Abnormalities

Narrowing of the aqueduct of Sylvius may be congenital or acquired. Congenital narrowing of the aqueduct may be due to stenosis, gliosis, forking, or membrane formation (6). With the exception of membrane formation, which affects the distal end of the aqueduct, narrowing usually occurs at the level of the superior colliculi or at the intercollicular level (114). Forking of the aqueduct (separation into anterior and posterior channels) may accompany spinal dysraphism (92,94). Infections and tumors may lead to acquired aqueductal stenosis.

MRI of aqueductal stenosis demonstrates enlargement of the lateral and third ventricles but a normal-sized fourth ventricle (Fig. 2-45). There may be associated dysplasia of the tectum with nodular thickening or beaking. The aqueduct may not be visible at all or may be ballooned proximally. An aqueductal web is shown as a thin band at the distal end of a dilated aqueduct. Tectal gliomas may also produce

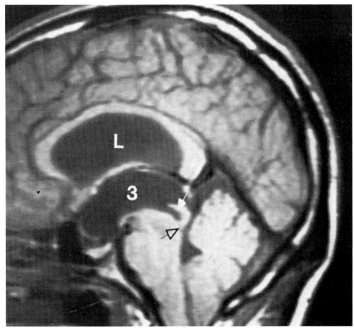

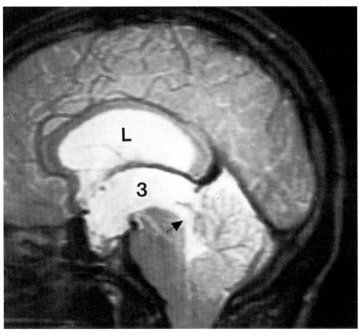

FIG. 2-45. Aqueductal stenosis. A: There is marked dilatation of the lateral *(L)* and third *(3)* ventricles as well as disproportionate dilatation of the proximal aqueduct *(solid arrow)*. The distal aqueduct *(open arrow)* and fourth ventricle are normal in size. **B:** Increased T2-weighted signal intensity secondary to gliosis within the midbrain *(solid arrow)* obscures the transition between the dilated proximal and stenotic distal aqueduct.

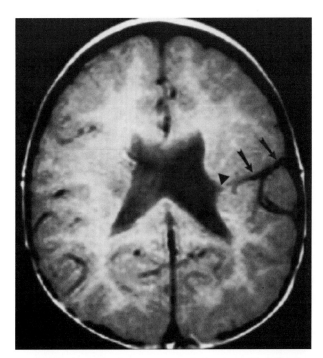

FIG. 2-46. Closed-lip schizencephaly. Axial T1 MRI demonstrates a narrow low-intensity cerebral cleft *(arrows)* extending from a dimple of the lateral ventricle *(arrowhead)* to the cortical surface. The cleft is lined by gray matter.

aqueductal obstruction (see Fig. 2-89); these small mass lesions of the tectum are best imaged by MRI. They have increased signal on both proton density and T2-weighted images.

Disorders of Neuronal Migration and Cortical Organization

In gestational order these include schizencephaly, heterotopia, agyria (lissencephaly), pachygyria, and polymicrogyria (diffuse and focal cortical dysplasias) (115–117). Agenesis of the corpus callosum is also included in this spectrum of disorders. Characteristic clinical manifestations of focal defects include congenital hemiparesis and focal seizures, especially refractory epilepsy; the latter may be amenable to excisional surgery. More diffuse defects are associated with developmental delay.

Schizencephaly

Schizencephaly literally means a split in the brain. Schizencephaly includes a spectrum of migrational cortical anomalies that manifest as gray matter–lined clefts within the hemispheres. The clefts may be unilateral or bilateral, symmetric or asymmetric, and they may occur anywhere in the cerebral hemispheres. The cleft characteristically extends from the lateral ventricle to the peripheral subarachnoid space and is lined by a pial-ependymal seam. Yakovlev and

Wadsworth subgrouped schizencephaly into those with fused lips and those in which the lips are separated and the cleft open (118,119). Rarely, an incomplete cleft that does not extend entirely across the hemisphere is encountered. Absence of the septum pellucidum is found in 75% to 100% of cases of schizencephaly (120). Schizencephalic clefts are found in at least half of patients with septooptic dysplasia (104). Polymicrogyria often lines the cortical margins of the clefts.

A schizencephalic cleft is best seen on T1-weighted MRI (Fig. 2-46, see Fig. 2-38). Heterotopic gray matter or polymicrogyria lines the entire length of the cleft (120). On proton density and T2-weighted images, the lining of the cleft remains isointense to gray matter. Differentiation of schizencephaly from a porencephalic cyst by MRI is based on demonstration of gray matter along the entire length of the cleft in schizencephaly, whereas with porencephaly the cleft extends through both gray and white matter so that there will also be white matter abutting the CSF cyst. The exact etiology of schizencephaly is not known, although it is thought to be the result of migrational arrest due to early gestational injury (frequently ischemic) to the periependymal germinal matrix.

Neuronal Heterotopias

Neuronal heterotopias result from of an arrest in axial migration of neurons from the subependymal zone to the cortical region. They are commonly found in association with other migrational disorders (lissencephaly, polymicrogyria, schizencephaly), although they may occur as an isolated abnormality. Isolated heterotopias typically present with seizures, often refractory to medical therapy. They are best identified with MRI, appearing as nodular or laminar masses within the subcortical or subependymal white matter regions (Figs. 2-47 and 2-48) (121). They are usually isointense to gray matter on T1-, intermediate-, and T2-weighted sequences, although they are occasionally hyperintense to gray matter on intermediate-weighted images. When periventricular, they often give a lumpy appearance to the ventricular wall. Heterotopia rarely divides the white matter region into laminated zones.

Lissencephaly

Lissencephaly (agyria) is a rare congenital malformation of the CNS resulting from an arrest in normal neuronal migration. It includes a spectrum of malformations from total failure to develop cerebral sulci and gyri (agyria) to the development of coarse, broad, flat gyri with shallow intervening sulci (pachygyria) (120,122–124). Three clinical types of lissencephaly have been described (6,7). Type 1 lissencephaly is associated with microcephaly. Included in this group are the Miller-Dieker, Norman-Roberts, and Neau-

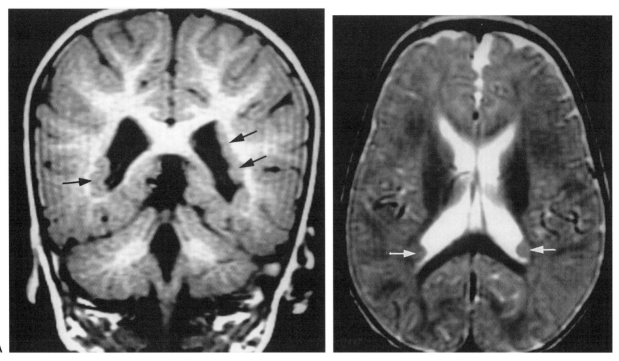

FIG. 2-47. Familial neuronal heterotopias. A 4-year-old girl with coronal T1 **(A)** and axial T2 **(B)** MRI showing bilateral subependymal nodules *(arrows)* of gray matter.

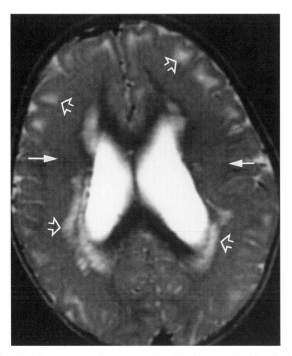

FIG. 2-48. Laminar heterotopias. An 18-month-old girl with severe developmental delay. Axial T2 MRI demonstrates gray matter bands *(closed arrows)* replacing most of the subcortical and periventricular cerebral white matter bilaterally. High intensity dysplastic cortical and periventricular white matter abnormalities *(open arrows)* are also noted.

Laxova syndromes. Deletion of the short arm of chromosome 17 has been identified in Miller-Dieker syndrome. Affected individuals are severely retarded. Patients with type 2 lissencephaly have macrocephaly. Disorders in this category include the Walker-Warburg and cerebrooculomuscular syndromes. The Walker-Warburg syndrome is characterized by lissencephaly, hydrocephalus, retinal dysplasia, and vermian hypoplasia with or without a Dandy-Walker malformation (Fig. 2-49). An encephalocele may be present. When these features are associated with congenital muscular dystrophy, the disorder is termed the cerebrooculomuscular syndrome. Type 3 is isolated lissencephaly.

Agyria is rarely the sole manifestation of a migrational defect; there is frequently a mixed pattern with intervening areas of pachygyria (Fig. 2-50). The surface features of the brain, abnormalities in cortical thickness and distribution, and the presence or absence of periventricular heterotopias are best demonstrated by MRI. MRI is also sensitive to the abnormalities of myelination that accompany these disorders. With agyria, the cortical surface remains smooth and does not develop normal cerebral sulci and gyri. The gray matter mantle is typically broad and contains thickened bands of disorganized neuronal architecture interspersed with zones of cortical necrosis. The interface between the white and gray matter is smooth and lacks the normal pattern of interdigitation. The cranial vault is usually small. A small midline anterior calcification, best seen by CT, may be noted in the roof of the cavum septi pellucidi (122). Lissencephaly may be found in association with congenital infection by cytomegalovirus (CMV).

Nonobstructive dilatation of the ventricular system is often present and is most marked posteriorly (colpocephaly) (5). The Sylvian fissures are often shallow and vertically oriented and extend to the vertex. This abnormal appearance is due to lack of normal frontal, parietal, and temporal lobe opercularization that is necessary for the formation of a horizontally oriented Sylvian fissure (see Fig. 2-50).

Pachygyria

With pachygyria the maturational arrest occurs later than with agyria and produces a cortex that is less disorganized but still immature. The gyri are decreased in number, broad, and flat; intervening sulci are shallow. Involvement of the entire brain is rare. Areas of pachygyria are mixed with areas devoid of gyral architecture (agyria) (see Fig. 2-50) or with normal brain. Colpocephaly may be present (Fig. 2-51). MRI best demonstrates the thickened layer of cortex and additional heterotopias within the white matter (see Fig. 2-51). The centrum semiovale appears decreased in volume as a result of increased cortical thickness. Myelination is typically delayed, producing persistent T2 prolongation (hyperintensity) beyond 2 years of age. On CT the presence of periventricular calcifications suggests CMV infection,

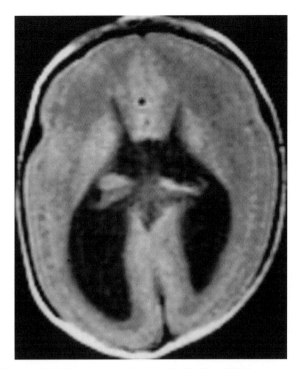

FIG. 2-49. Lissencephaly and Walker-Warburg syndrome. Newborn with abnormal neurologic exam and a large head. Axial proton density MR demonstrates an agyric cerebral cortical pattern, hypoplastic white matter, and hydrocephalus.

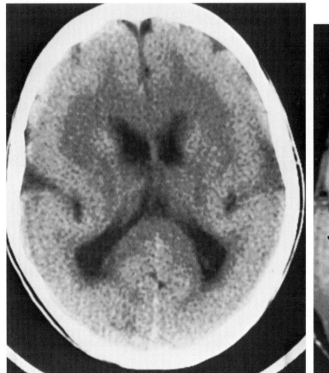

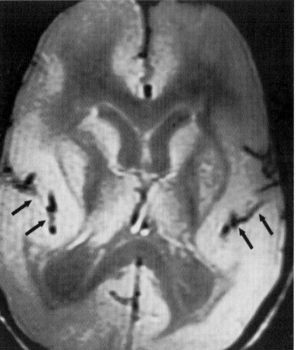

A

B

FIG. 2-50. Lissencephaly and pachygyria. Axial CT **(A)** and T2 MRI **(B)** demonstrate areas of pachygyria and agyria, lack of cortical gray-white matter differentiation, plus ventricular and Sylvian dysmorphia. The shallowness and vertical orientaion of the Sylvian fissures *(arrows)* are due to lack of opercularization.

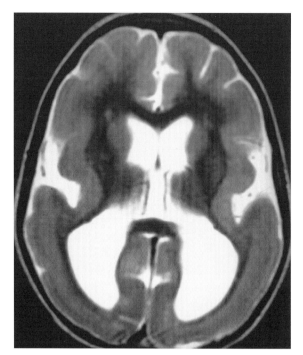

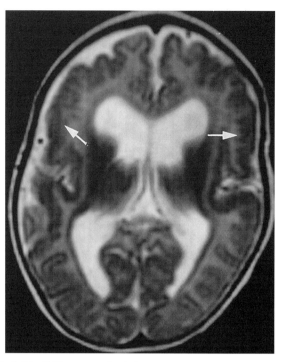

FIG. 2-51. Pachygyria and colpocephaly. A 15-year-old girl. Axial T2 MRI demonstrates marked gyral thickening with fewer than normal sulci, wide Sylvian fissures, hypoplastic cortical and subcortical white matter, and dilatation of the posterior horns of the lateral ventricles (colpocephaly).

FIG. 2-52. Diffuse cortical dysplasia and polymicrogyria. A 3-month-old girl with previous cytomegaloviral infection. Axial T2 MRI demonstrates bilateral serrated cortical hypointensities *(arrows)* in the peri-Sylvian frontal and temporal regions, ventricular dilatation, and widening of the Sylvian fissures and extracerebral spaces.

which presumably caused the migrational arrest and disorganization.

Polymicrogyria

Polymicrogyria (microgyria) was first described by Heschl and literally means many small gyri (125). It is the major component of the cortical dysplasias, diffuse or focal. Bresler later refined Heschl's original classification and coined the term polymicrogyria to indicate a late migrational or postmigrational anomaly in which the surface of the brain takes on a "cobblestone" appearance (126). This anomaly may be diffuse or focal and is often found in association with other manifestations of migrational arrest or abnormalities of neuronal differentiation and proliferation including agyria, pachygyria, cortical heterotopias, megalencephaly, and hemimegalencephaly. The identification of the abnormal gyri may be difficult on MRI even with cortical surface renderings. The cortex is serrated or thickened and isointense to gray matter on both T1- and T2-weighted sequences (Figs. 2-52 and 2-53).

Polymicrogyria often lines the complete cleft of a schizencephalic defect and the partial cleft of focal cortical dysplasia. Hyperintense T2 signal may persist within the white matter and represents a delay in myelination. As in pachygyria, the volume of white matter is decreased and lacks the normal number of interdigitations with the overly-

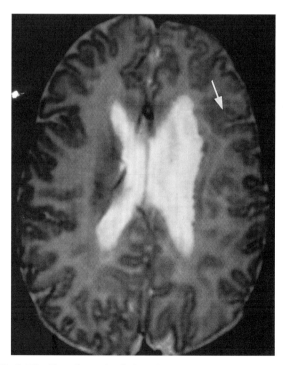

FIG. 2-53. Focal cortical dysplasia and polymicrogyria. A 3-month-old girl with focal seizures. Axial T2 MRI demonstrates left frontal cortical partial cleft *(arrow)* with serrated cortical thickening and dimpling of the underlying enlarged lateral ventricle. Multiple small hypointense heterotopias are seen along the margin of the left lateral ventricle.

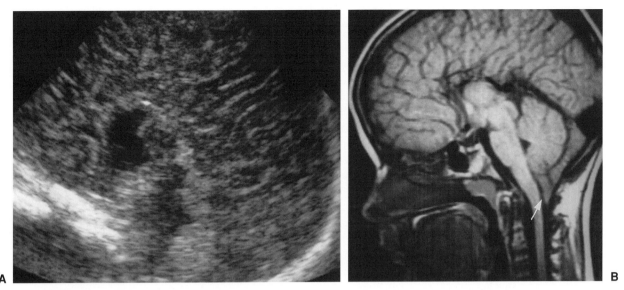

FIG. 2-54. Agenesis of the corpus callosum. Sagittal US **(A)** and sagittal T1 MRI **(B)** show total absence of the corpus callosum with a characteristic radiating gyral pattern. MRI also demonstrates a Chiari I malformation; the cerebellar tonsils *(arrow)* are well below the foramen magnum.

ing cortex. Differentiation of pachygyria from polymicrogyria is often not possible even with MRI. Occasionally there are anomalous veins or arachnoidal cysts associated with the polymicrogyria-lined clefts.

Dysgenesis of Corpus Callosum

Dysgenesis of the corpus callosum includes complete or partial absence of the interhemispheric callosal commissural fibers that bridge the two hemispheres. This abnormality may be isolated or be associated with other midline developmental anomalies, such as the Chiari malformations, Dandy-Walker spectrum, holoprosencephaly, septooptic dysplasia, median cleft face syndromes, sphenoethmoidal encephaloceles, and Aicardi syndrome (6,7,12,127). Aicardi syndrome occurs only in females; it includes agenesis of the corpus callosum with interhemispheric cysts (frequently neuroepithelial), lacunar chorioretinopathy, mental retardation, and infantile spasms (128,129).

The corpus callosum develops as a bud from the lamina terminalis between the 8th and 20th weeks of gestation (127,130). During the 7th week of gestation, the rostral end of the neural tube, the lamina terminalis, undergoes thickening to form the commissural plate (130). The groove in the superior surface of this plate fills with cells that help to guide axons across the midline. The corpus callosum normally grows cephalad and then posteriorly to end in the splenium. When the corpus callosum is dysgenetic, it is the posterior body, splenium, and rostrum that are absent. The presence of these posterior components without more anterior portions of the corpus callosum suggests destruction of the previously formed anterior elements. An exception to this general rule is holoprosencephaly in which only the splenium

and posterior portion of the body of the corpus callosum may be present (103). Although US (Fig. 2-54A) and CT may demonstrate findings of callosal dysgenesis (131), MRI is preferred for evaluating the extent of the callosal anomaly and any associated malformations (Figs. 2-54 and 2-55). With absence of the corpus callosum, the cingulate gyri remain everted and the cingulate sulcus does not form. As a re-

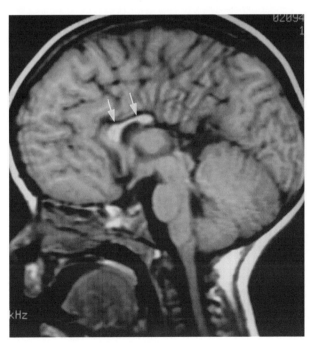

FIG. 2-55. Partial agenesis of the corpus callosum. A 5-year-old boy. Sagittal T1 MRI demonstrates remnants of the corpus callosum anteriorly *(arrows)*. This includes the genu and a portion of the anterior body.

sult, gyri on the medial surface of the brain radiate to the roof of the third ventricle (131). Furthermore, the axons which normally cross through the corpus callosum are diverted and run along the medial surface of the lateral ventricles. These white matter tracts, the bundles of Probst, are well delineated on coronal images. The lateral ventricles are separated and the third ventricle extends dorsally between the two lateral ventricles; the frontal horns of the lateral ventricles have a "steer head" configuration on coronal images because of the eversion of the cingulate gyri. The third ventricle, in addition to being abnormally elevated, is usually dilated. The bodies of the lateral ventricles typically have a parallel configuration on axial images, and colpocephaly is commonly present (see Fig. 2-51). Interhemispheric clefts or arachnoid cysts may be demonstrated by MRI as masses in the interhemispheric fissure (Fig. 2-56); there may be communication of these CSF intensity masses with the third ventricle. There is frequently associated hydrocephalus. Associated heterotopic gray matter may produce nodules that project into the walls of the lateral ventricles. Sagittal T1-weighted MRI sections best demonstrate dysgenesis of the corpus callosum, whereas T2-weighted images best identify the abnormal Probst bundles and associated heterotopic gray matter (127).

Lipoma of the Corpus Callosum

A lipoma of the corpus callosum is a benign, midline cranial tumor associated with dysgenesis of the corpus callo-

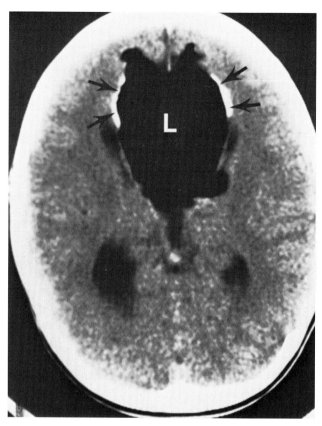

FIG. 2-57. Agenesis of the corpus callosum with lipoma. Large midline lipoma *(L)* associated with agenesis of the corpus callosum. Note the dystrophic calcification in the wall of the lipoma *(arrows).*

sum in at least half of cases. It is a congenital malformation presumably due to entrapment of multipotential cells (102).

The fat-containing tumor is commonly located within or replaces the genu of the corpus callosum but may be found anywhere in the midline. In older children, the wall of the mass frequently contains a rim of calcification. CT demonstrates the fat and calcium within the mass (Fig. 2-57); however, MRI better demonstrates the extent of the lipoma, its relationship to surrounding vascular and neural structures, and the associated dysgenesis of the corpus callosum (Fig. 2-58).

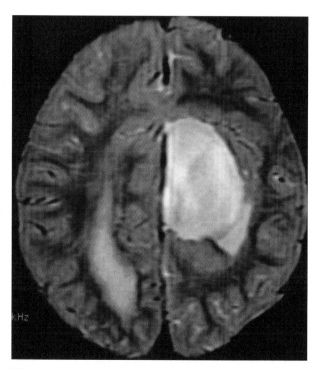

FIG. 2-56. Agenesis of the corpus callosum with an interhemispheric cyst. A 2-year-old boy. Axial T2 MRI demonstrates a large left paramedian cerebrospinal fluid intensity cyst. Note the parallelism of the right lateral ventricle. Sagittal images verified agenesis of the corpus callosum.

Myelination

Normal Myelination

Neuronal and glial proliferation of the gray matter and axonal myelination of the white matter occur in a predictable pattern in the developing brain. The process of maturation is primarily the result of complex genetically predisposed determinants and, to a lesser extent, environmental factors. Myelination begins during the fifth month of fetal life and continues into adulthood. However, at no other time during childhood is the process of myelination so readily apparent and so rapidly changing as during the first 24 months of life.

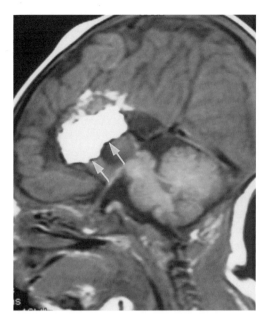

FIG. 2-58. Agenesis of the corpus callosum with lipoma.
A 3-month-old boy. Sagittal T1 MRI demonstrates a high-intensity, midline lipoma and absence of the corpus callosum. Hypointensities *(arrows)* along the margins of the lipoma represent calcification and chemical shift artifact.

The ability to assess myelination using US and CT is poor at best. The T1- and T2-weighted relaxation characteristics of white matter show the degree of myelination, however (Figs. 2-59 through 2-61). White matter is relatively hydrophilic (infantile pattern) or hydrophobic (adult pattern), depending on the amount and distribution of axonal myelin. In the immature neonate, white matter, lacking myelin, appears hypointense on T1-weighted and hyperintense on T2-weighted MRI (see Fig. 2-59). The progress of myelination gradually causes white matter to become hyperintense on T1-weighted and hypointense on T2-weighted images. This reversal in MRI appearance and development of an adult pattern is complete after 18–24 months of age.

The diagnosis of delay in maturation depends on knowledge of the normal pattern for the age. Studies by Barkovich et al. (132), Bird et al. (133), and Dietrich et al. (134) provide standards of normal myelination on MRI (Table 2-16). In general, normal myelination proceeds in a caudal-cranial direction, as does neurologic development. CNS myelination first begins in the spinal cord and dorsal brainstem and progresses rapidly into the cerebellar white matter tracts, the long tracts of the midbrain, the posterior thalami, the posterior limb of the internal capsule, and the deep white matter tracts of the corona radiata and centrum semiovale leading to the paracentral cortex. This process is first noted on MRI at 40–44 weeks gestational age and progresses rapidly during the first 3 months of life (Fig. 2-60). Myelination of the corpus callosum first begins within the splenium at 2–3 months and progresses anteriorly to the genu and rostrum by 6–8 months. In keeping with the importance of visual

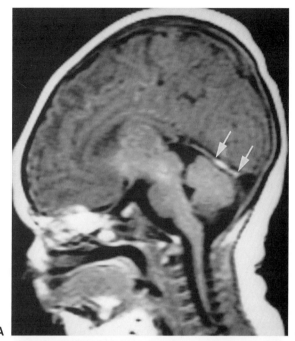

A

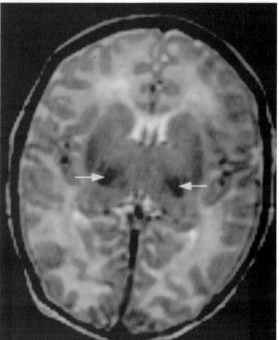

B

FIG. 2-59. Normal newborn brain MRI. Sagittal T1 MRI **(A)** shows the normal hyperintense myelinated appearance of most of the brainstem and cerebellum. There is the normal isointense-to-hypointense premyelinated appearance of the corpus callosum and cerebrum. Linear hyperintensity along the tentorium *(arrows)* probably represents a small amount of hemorrhage, a common finding in newborns. Axial T2 MRI **(B)** demonstrates the normal watery hyperintensities of the premyelinated white matter throughout most of the cerebrum and a normal hypointense cortical ribbon bilaterally. Normal hypointense myelination is demonstrated in the posterior limbs of the internal capsule *(arrows)* bilaterally.

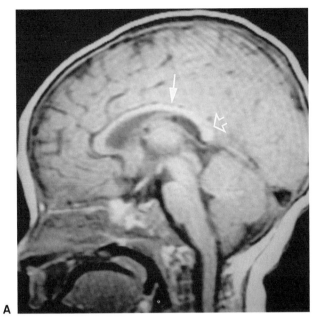

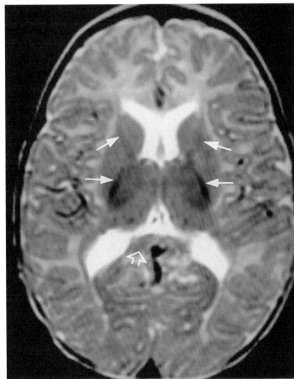

FIG. 2-60. Normal brain MRI at 5 months of age. Sagittal T1 MRI **(A)** shows relative hyperintensity of the myelinating corpus callosum, particularly of the splenium *(open arrow)* and body *(closed arrow)*. Axial T2 MRI **(B)** demonstrates hypointense myelination of the anterior and posterior limbs of the internal capsule *(closed arrows)* bilaterally and of the splenium of the corpus callosum *(open arrow)*.

Myelination of the centrum semiovale extends from a central focus first posteriorly and then anteriorly to the frontal cortex. By 10–12 months, T1-weighted images are less helpful in showing the further progress of myelination (132). According to Barkovich et al., T2-weighted images are more helpful for determining the adequacy of myelination between 12 and 24 months of age (Fig. 2-61) (132).

Abnormal Myelination

A variety of factors cause delay in myelination or hypomyelination, including hypoxia-ischemia, infection, malformative syndromes, trauma, and metabolic disease.

Differentiation among the numerous etiologies of delayed myelination is not always possible. The history may suggest the cause. Distinguishing demyelination (destruction after normal formation) from dysmyelination (abnormal formation) is often difficult, particularly in early infancy. Involvement of cortex, diffuse loss of brain substance, and undermyelination in the distribution seen with periventricular leukomalacia suggests a hypoxemic-ischemic insult. With many leukodystrophies, on the other hand, although myelination is delayed, the overlying cortex and the volume of white matter remain normal, particularly early. When there is doubt, a repeat examination may show whether areas of increased signal within the white matter are indeed abnormal and whether they are static or progressive.

Acquired Injury of Formed Structures

Besides affecting future development, an in utero insult may destroy previously formed CNS structures. The expres-

TABLE 2-16. *Normal myelination of brain*

Anatomic region	Age when changes of myelination appear (months)	
	T1-weighted images	T2-weighted images
Middle cerebellar peduncle	Birth	Birth to 2
Cerebellar white matter	Birth to 4	3–5
Posterior limb of internal capsule		
Anterior portion	Birth	4–7
Posterior portion	Birth	Birth to 2
Anterior limb of internal capsule	2–3	7–11
Genu of corpus callosum	4–6	5–8
Splenium of corpus callosum	3–4	4–6
Occipital white matter		
Central	3–5	9–14
Peripheral	4–7	11–15
Frontal white matter		
Central	3–6	11–16
Peripheral	7–11	14–18
Centrum semiovale	2–4	7–11

Note: T1-weighted sequence of 600/20 ms (TR/TE). T2-weighted sequence of 2500/70 ms.

From Barkovich et al. (6, 132).

response in normal development, the optic tracts and radiations begin to myelinate early; myelination usually appears anteriorly during the first 2 or 3 months and extends to involve the calcarine cortex by 4–6 months (see Fig. 2-60).

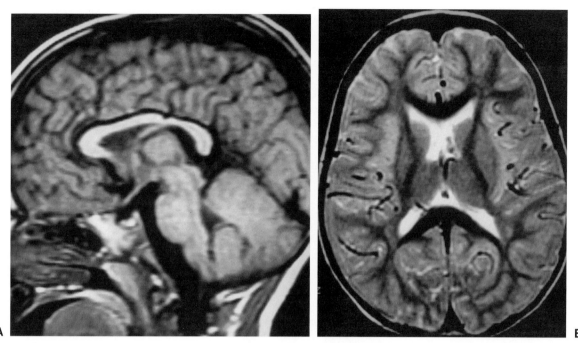

A B

FIG. 2-61. Normal brain MRI at 2 years of age. Sagittal T1 MRI **(A)** demonstrates normal hyperintensity of the normally formed and normally myelinated corpus callosum. Axial T2 MRI **(B)** demonstrates the normal hypointensity of myelination in the cortical and subcortical white matter, periventricular white matter, and capsular white matter and in the genu and splenium of the corpus callosum. The small hyperintensities in the temporoparietal periventricular white matter bilaterally represent normal myelination variants.

sion of the insult will depend on both its severity and the timing, since the response of the developing brain to injury changes during gestation. First and early second trimester insults are not accompanied by a glial response and so only tissue destruction may be evident. Later injuries incite an astroglial response. Hydranencephaly, porencephaly, and encephalomalacia are manifestations of in utero injuries.

Hydranencephaly

Hydranencephaly is an encephaloclastic disorder in which much of the supratentorial brain is replaced by thin-walled sacs (Fig. 2-62) (135). Hydranencephaly has been produced experimentally by bilateral occlusion of the supraclinoid segments of the internal carotid arteries (ICAs) (6). Relative preservation, due to intact vertebrobasilar arterial supply, of the occipital lobes, inferior temporal lobes, thalami, brainstem, and cerebellum supports the theory of ICA occlusion as the etiology. In utero infection with toxoplasmosis or cytomegalovirus has also been implicated. Because hydranencephaly occurs after brain structures have been formed, the falx is usually present and the thalami have separated; this distinguishes hydranencephaly from alobar holoprosencephaly (7). Patients with hydranencephaly may be microcephalic, normocephalic, or macrocephalic depending on CSF dynamics (6). In the macrocephalic infant, differentiation of hydranencephaly from very severe hydrocephalus

may be difficult. CSF shunting may be worthwhile in both cases, to preserve brain tissue and function in severe hydrocephalus and to prevent massive head enlargement in hydranencephaly.

Porencephaly

The response of the brain to focal, multifocal, or diffuse injury changes during gestation. Prior to the end of the second trimester, parenchymal injury fails to incite a glial reaction (6,7,135). The result is therefore a porencephalic cyst. Porencephalic cysts are thin-walled and of CSF intensity; they have no internal septations (Fig. 2-63).

Encephalomalacia

After damage to the brain during the second or early third trimester, a glial reaction does occur. This glial response is manifested as prolonged T1 and T2 intensity around the region of injury; moreover, there are septations within the region of destroyed brain (Fig. 2-64).

Arachnoid Cysts

Intracranial arachnoid cysts are extraaxial and may be primary or secondary. Primary arachnoid cysts are congenital

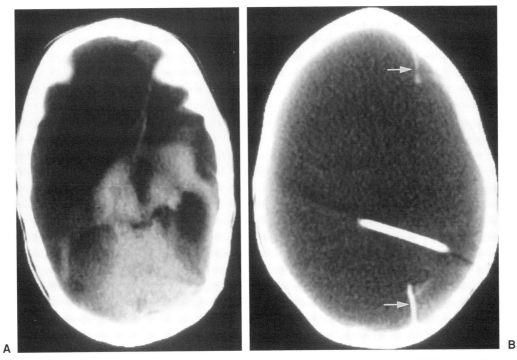

FIG. 2-62. Hydranencephaly. Axial CT **(A, B)** demonstrates extensive supratentorial low densities and a partially intact falx *(arrows)*. Cerebellar, brainstem, and diencephalic tissue densities are present. A ventricular catheter is identified.

lesions; these CSF-filled cavities arise within the arachnoid membrane, are lined by arachnoid tissue, and do not freely communicate with surrounding subarachnoid spaces (136). Secondary or acquired arachnoid cysts are loculations of CSF produced by arachnoidal scarring due to inflammation, infection, or trauma; these also do not communicate with the subarachnoid CSF. Arachnoid cysts slowly increase in size and displace surrounding cranial structures.

Arachnoid cysts are located, in declining order of frequency, in the middle cranial fossa and Sylvian fissure, sellar

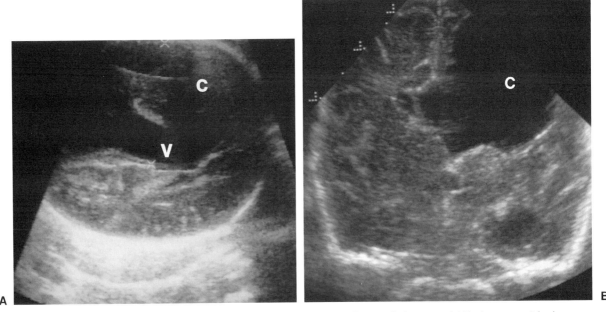

FIG. 2-63. Porencephaly and congenital hydrocephalus. Prenatal ultrasound **(A)** shows ventriculomegaly *(V)* and adjacent cyst-like sonolucency *(C)*. Postnatal coronal plane US **(B)** shows asymmetric ventriculomegaly and a communicating left frontal sonolucent porencephalic cyst *(C)*.

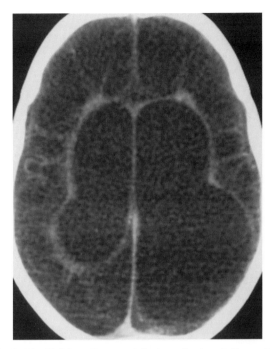

FIG. 2-64. Multicystic encephalomalacia. A 5-month-old boy. Axial CT demonstrates extensive cerebral low density with septations throughout. There is marked asymmetric ventricular dilatation.

and suprasellar region, quadrigeminal plate cistern, posterior fossa, interhemispheric fissure, adjacent to the clivus, and over the frontal convexities (7,137). The adjacent brain may be hypoplastic or dysplastic. Arachnoid cysts may occur within and expand the cleft of schizencephaly or focal cortical dysplasia.

On imaging, arachnoid cysts have the density and intensity characteristics of CSF (Fig. 2-65) (6,7,136). The wall of the cyst is usually not perceptible. Mural calcification and enhancement should not be present. Vessels typically pass around but not through the lesion. Often there is thinning of the overlying calvaria. Hydrocephalus is present in up to 60% of cases and is particularly frequent with midline cysts. The hydrocephalus may be either communicating or non-communicating (138). Hemorrhage into the cyst and superimposed infection occasionally occur.

Infection

Congenital Infections

The most common congenital infections affecting the CNS are those due to bacteria, cytomegalovirus, toxoplasmosis, human immunodeficiency virus (HIV), rubella, herpes simplex type 2, and syphilis (139). With the exception of bacterial infections and herpes, these diseases are transmitted to the fetus through the placenta. Bacterial infections often ascend through the vagina and cervix. Herpes is typically acquired during parturition. Congenital infections

differ from those of later life in that they occur while the nervous system is developing and thus can disrupt organogenesis. The manifestations of congenital infections, therefore, depend more on the timing than on the nature of the insult (6). Infections in the first trimester and early second trimester commonly result in brain malformations. Later infections are associated with encephaloclastic lesions, obstructive hydrocephalus, and variable degrees of gliosis.

Cytomegalovirus

Cytomegalovirus (CMV) infection is the most common of the TORCHS (toxoplasmosis, rubella, CMV, HIV, herpes, syphilis) infections; it occurs in approximately 1% of all live births. Up to 55% of infected infants have neurologic signs attributable to the virus. The manifestations include microcephaly, impaired hearing, seizures, chorioretinitis, and developmental delay. Affected children may also have hepatosplenomegaly and petechiae.

The mechanism by which CMV affects the developing brain is unknown. It is postulated that there is an affinity of the virus for the germinal matrix or vessels. Depending on the timing of the infection, the result is varying degrees of cortical dysplasia, ventricular enlargement, gliosis, delayed myelination, parenchymal calcification, and cerebellar hypoplasia. The severity of the cortical dysplasia is related to the timing of the insult. Early second-trimester infections produce lissencephaly, late second-trimester infections cause polymicrogyria, and third-trimester infections result in little or no cortical abnormality (140).

Cranial CT is preferred for the detection of the intracranial calcifications, which are typically periventricular in location (Fig. 2-66). CT will also depict the more severe cortical abnormalities and cerebellar hypoplasia. MRI is useful in evaluating subtle dysmorphic features of the brain, delayed myelination, and gliosis. Both imaging modalities will demonstrate the broad, smooth gyri of lissencephaly. MRI shows the nodular appearance of polymicrogyria to better advantage than CT (see Fig. 2-52).

Toxoplasmosis

Toxoplasmosis is produced by the intracellular protozoan *Toxoplasma gondii* (28,141,142). Maternal infection usually occurs through the ingestion of oocytes from undercooked pork or beef. Fetal infection is hematogenous and transplacental. Toxoplasmosis is the second most common of the TORCHS infections and has an incidence of 1 in 1000–3500 live births (143). Seizures, mental retardation, hydrocephalus, and chorioretinitis are common. As with other congenital infections, the degree of neurologic impairment is related to the timing of the insult; earlier fetal infections cause more devastating sequelae. Early infection may produce hydranencephaly, whereas late third-trimester

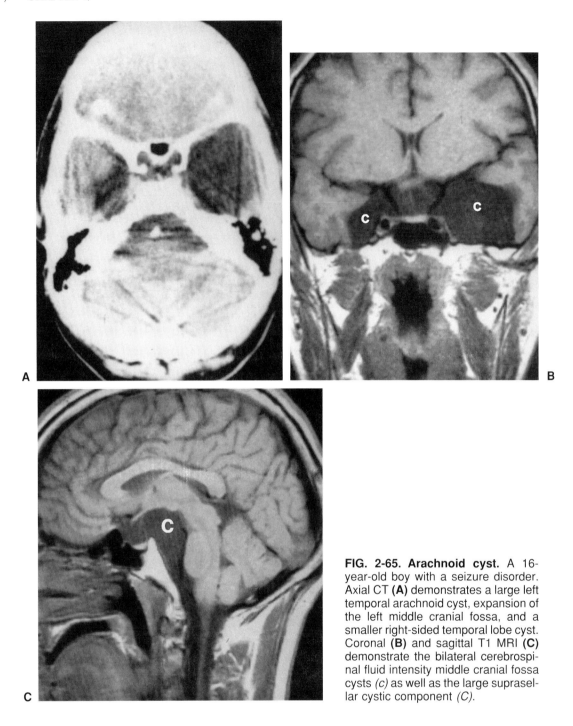

FIG. 2-65. Arachnoid cyst. A 16-year-old boy with a seizure disorder. Axial CT **(A)** demonstrates a large left temporal arachnoid cyst, expansion of the left middle cranial fossa, and a smaller right-sided temporal lobe cyst. Coronal **(B)** and sagittal T1 MRI **(C)** demonstrate the bilateral cerebrospinal fluid intensity middle cranial fossa cysts *(c)* as well as the large suprasellar cystic component *(C)*.

infection may produce only parenchymal calcifications. Cortical dysplasia is infrequent in congenital toxoplasmosis, in contrast to CMV. Parenchymal calcifications in toxoplasmosis are more random than with CMV infection; they may be periventricular, cortical, or in the basal ganglia (Fig. 2-67). Toxoplasmosis produces a granulomatous meningeal reaction which can lead to aqueductal obstruction and hydrocephalus. Affected infants may be either macrocephalic or microcephalic depending on whether hydrocephalus or parenchymal destruction dominates. The intra-

cranial abnormalities of toxoplasmosis are readily demonstrated by either CT or MRI.

Rubella

Congenital rubella has decreased markedly in incidence because of screening programs for pregnant women and the availability of immunization. Rubella is a nonarthropod-borne virus. Maternal infection is acquired by the respiratory

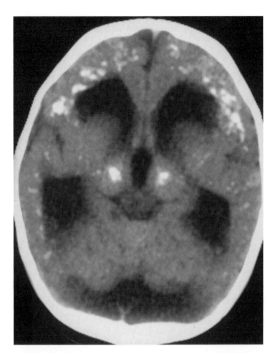

FIG. 2-66. Cytomegaloviral infection in newborn. Axial CT demonstrates extensive bilateral periventricular and basal ganglia calcifications with uneven lateral ventriculomegaly, cerebral and cerebellar hypoplasia, and microcephaly.

route; the virus is transmitted to the fetus through the placenta (6,144). Infections occurring early in gestation are more likely to produce CNS abnormalities than those occurring in the second and third trimesters. Manifestations of the

infection include microcephaly, cerebral infarctions, chorioretinitis, cataracts, glaucoma, sensorineural hearing loss, metaphyseal abnormalities (see Chapter 5), and cardiovascular disease (28). The neuroimaging features of rubella include calcifications in the basal ganglia and cortex, infarctions, and delayed myelination.

Herpes Simplex Type 2

Neonatal herpes infection is usually the result of maternal to fetal transmission of the deoxyribonucleic acid (DNA) virus, herpes simplex type 2, during parturition (145). Nonneurologic signs of infection include cutaneous, ocular, and mucous membrane lesions, jaundice, fever, and respiratory distress (141). CNS involvement results in seizures or lethargy.

Neuroimaging reveals a diffuse encephalitic process in contrast to the more focal involvement, typically of the temporal lobe, seen in HSV-1 infections in older children and adults (see page 118). There are diffuse or multifocal areas of edema (Fig. 2-68). Meningeal enhancement may be present. Regions of gliosis, delayed myelination, and multicystic encephalomalacia may be evident late in the course of disease (28).

Syphilis

Fetal infection with the spirochete *Treponema pallidum* occurs most commonly during the maternal phase of secondary syphilis (28). The signs of congenital infection include condylomata, lymphadenopathy, meningitis, bone destruction, and periostitis (see Chapter 5). The usual neurologic

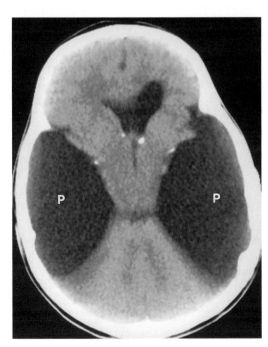

FIG. 2-67. Toxoplasmosis. Axial CT shows bilateral porencephaly *(P)*, hydrocephalus, and scattered, punctate calcifications.

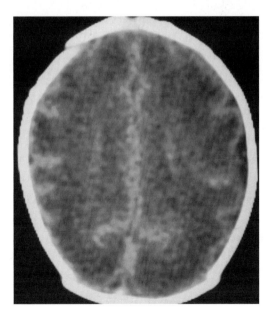

FIG. 2-68. Herpes simplex type 2 encephalitis. Newborn with seizures. Axial CT demonstrates extensive bilateral cerebral low density due to edema.

manifestation of the infection is a basal meningitis (146). The meningitis may extend along perivascular spaces, but parenchymal lesions are uncommon. Hydrocephalus may be present in chronic meningovascular syphilis. Aneurysm formation and intracranial hemorrhage are rare complications.

Human Immunodeficiency Virus

Childhood infection by HIV type 1, a ribonucleic acid (RNA) retrovirus, is usually acquired in utero. Transmission of the virus may also occur with transfusions of infected blood products, though new cases of this are now very rare. The virus is both lymphotropic and neurotropic (28). The severity of symptoms is variable, and symptoms are typically delayed at least for some months. In its most severe form, HIV infection results in the full-blown acquired immunodeficiency syndrome (AIDS). Fifty to 90% of infected children will develop neurologic symptoms. CNS manifestations may result either directly from infection by the virus itself (the major effect) or from opportunistic infections (toxoplasmosis, CMV, *Mycobacterium avium intracellulare,* papovavirus) or neoplasia, usually lymphoma. Opportunistic infections and neoplasia are less common in childhood HIV infection than in infected adults. CNS lymphoma develops in only 5% of pediatric patients (147). Vascular thrombosis, distal embolization, or hemorrhage is caused by a dilational vasculopathy affecting the circle of Willis. Progressive encephalopathy is the most common CNS manifestation of the disease. Affected children may also develop movement disorders, ataxia, developmental delay, and microcephaly.

Neuroimaging of children with HIV infection most commonly shows atrophy. Calcification commonly occurs in the basal ganglia and is most easily appreciated on CT (Fig. 2-69). Calcifications may also be present in the frontal lobe white matter and cerebellum (6,148). MRI may demonstrate delayed myelination. Mass lesions are occasionally present, from superimposed infection or tumor. Toxoplasmosis often produces ring-enhancing lesions in the basal ganglia. Lymphoma is commonly hypointense or mildly hyperintense on T2-weighted MRI images, usually enhances markedly, and has less mass effect than the size that the lesion suggests. Regions of demyelination in the white matter, particularly in the parietal lobes, suggest progressive multifocal leukoencephalopathy due to papovavirus infection. When present, arterial dilatation may be appreciated on both spin-echo and MRA images. Ischemic infarctions may be evident. Occasionally, hemorrhage secondary to thrombocytopenia occurs (6,149).

Postnatal Infections

Osteomyelitis of the Skull

Skull infections are unusual at any age but are even rarer in children (5). Osteomyelitis of the skull may be primary

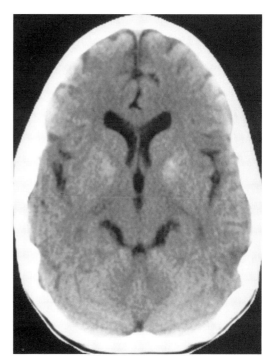

FIG. 2-69. HIV encephalopathy. An 8-year-old boy with known human immunodeficiency virus infection. Axial CT demonstrates bilateral basal ganglia calcifications and poor gray-white matter differentiation.

(tuberculosis, syphilis, coccidioidomycosis, actinomycosis, blastomycosis) or secondary (after sinusitis, mastoiditis, trauma, craniotomy, skin infection, or sepsis). Skull radiographs show a moth-eaten lucency of the diploic space and destruction of one or both tables of the skull (Fig. 2-70). There may be soft tissue swelling if infection extends through the outer table. CT or MRI may be indicated to exclude an abscess or venous sinus thrombosis. Sclerotic densities may coexist with destruction if the infection is chronic. Bone scintigraphy, as elsewhere in the skeleton, may identify osteomyelitis before it is apparent on plain radiographs. Gallium imaging is helpful, in selected cases, for assessing the response of cranial osteomyelitis to therapy.

Meningitis

Meningitis may be either viral or bacterial. Meningitis producing significant neurologic sequelae is almost always bacterial. Meningeal infection is often followed by infection of the brain (meningoencephalitis). In the newborn period, meningitis is most often due to group B *Streptococcus, Escherichia coli,* or *Listeria monocytogenes* (28). Other bacteria encountered with some frequency in newborns are *Staphylococcus, Proteus,* and *Pseudomonas.* Meningitis in children at ages 3 months to 2 years is commonly the result of *Hemophilus influenzae* type B infection. In older children, meningitis due to *Streptococcus pneumoniae* and *Neisseria menin-*

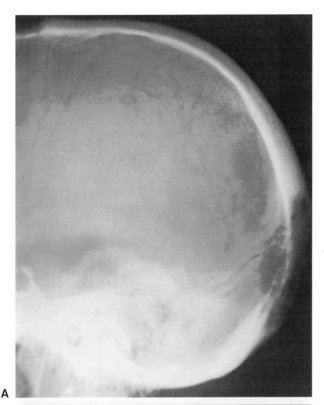

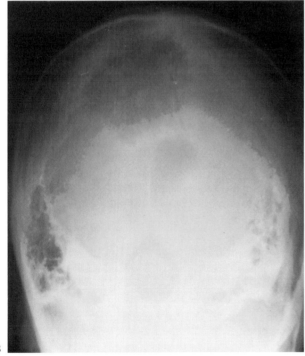

FIG. 2-70. Skull osteomyelitis. A 10-year-old girl with disseminated coccidioidomycosis. Lateral **(A)** and Towne **(B)** views of the skull show lytic destruction involving the outer table of the frontal and occipital bones.

gitidis is more frequent (150). Infections by *S. aureus* or *S. epidermidis* may be associated with ventricular shunt malfunction or dermal sinus tract infection.

Causes of meningitis in the newborn include maternal urinary tract or genital infection, premature rupture of the membranes, and nosocomial factors, e.g., the intensive care unit environment (28). Because of the immaturity of the neonatal immune system, infections at this age are often particularly severe. Infection usually occurs hematogenously and leads to ventriculitis and arachnoiditis. Venous or arterial occlusions may develop and produce hemorrhagic or ischemic infarctions. Hydrocephalus resulting from meningeal inflammation is common. Abscess formation is relatively rare; gram-negative bacteria such as *Citrobacter* are the usual offenders (28).

Imaging of acute neonatal meningitis reveals edema with or without ischemic or hemorrhagic infarction (151). CT or MRI may show enhancement of the ependyma or leptomeninges (28). Rim-enhancing abscesses are occasionally identified (Fig. 2-71). By US, ventriculitis appears as increased intraventricular echoes, ventricular wall thickening, and hyperechoic periventricular regions (43,151). Encephalomalacia, hydrocephalus, ventricular encystment, atrophy, and calcifications may develop later.

Meningitis in older children may be produced by hematogenous dissemination of infection to the CNS starting in the choroid plexus, contiguous spread from adjacent mastoiditis or sinusitis, CSF leaks, congenital or acquired fistulae, trauma, or surgery (28). Fever, meningismus, headache, seizures, and photophobia are common symptoms. As in the neonate, meningitis in the older infant and child may produce arterial, venous, or dural sinus occlusions and parenchymal infarction. Subdural effusions are often small and bilateral but may be asymmetric or unilateral (Fig. 2-72). Surgery for subdural effusions is usually not necessary unless the collections are large or purulent. Recurrent meningitis suggests a parameningeal focus such as mastoiditis or an abnormal communication between the CNS and adjacent structures. Traumatic fistulae, dermal sinus tracts, encephaloceles, inner ear anomalies, and primitive neurenteric communications may lead to recurrent CNS infection (28).

Imaging of meningitis after infancy is often negative in the acute stage. Subdural effusion, dilated subarachnoid spaces, and ventricular enlargement may be present. Ependymal or leptomeningeal enhancement may be evident (152). Single or multiple low-density foci from arterial infarction are occasionally demonstrated. Atrophy, encephalomalacia, and hydrocephalus may develop later (28).

Cerebritis and Abscess

Bacterial infection of the brain initially produces cerebritis (purulent inflammation of the brain) and, if not successfully treated, abscess. Infection of the brain may be divided into four stages: early cerebritis, late cerebritis, early capsule for-

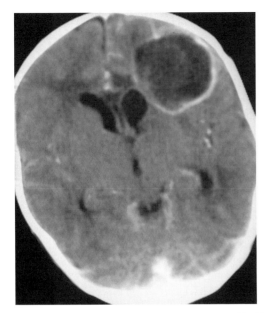

FIG. 2-71. Gram-negative abscess. Newborn with *Enterobacter* meningitis. Axial enhanced CT shows a large left frontal low-density abnormality with peripheral ring enhancement.

mation, and late capsule formation (abscess) (153,154). In early cerebritis, inflammation and tissue necrosis occur without capsule formation. In late cerebritis, the region of necrosis becomes better defined, surrounded by edema. Early capsule formation occurs as reticulin and collagen are laid down at the periphery of the lesion and the surrounding edema subsides. In the late capsule stage, the collagen perimeter is thicker and more distinct. The capsule is often thicker on the cortical side because of the greater vascularity there, which allows for more collagen deposition. The progression from cerebritis to abscess takes 1–2 weeks (153,154).

Infection of the brain may arise hematogenously from systemic infection or from a distant site, by direct inoculation due to penetrating trauma, by extension from a contiguous infection (sinusitis), or after septic thrombophlebitis of the bridging veins. Children with uncorrected or palliated cyanotic heart disease and pulmonary arteriovenous malformations are at increased risk of cerebritis because of right-to-left shunting bypassing the pulmonary capillary filtration mechanism.

Cerebritis is treated medically with antibiotics. Surgery is not indicated at this stage. If the infection evolves into a well-encapsulated abscess, antibiotic therapy alone may be ineffective and surgical drainage or excision is warranted.

The neuroimaging of cerebral suppuration depends on the stage of infection (6). The edema associated with early cerebritis exhibits T1 and T2 prolongation, causing respectively hypointensity and hyperintensity, on MRI (Fig. 2-73) and hypodensity on CT (Fig. 2-74). Patchy enhancement may be present. As the infection progresses to abscess formation, there is central heterogeneity in the region of necrosis. In

the later phases, the center of the abscess becomes more homogeneous. Brain abscesses are typically low in attenuation on CT with rim enhancement (see Fig. 2-74). The abscess rim is often mildly hyperintense on unenhanced T1-weighted MRI sequences in the subacute phase. The abscess rim becomes thicker and displays more intense enhancement as the lesion evolves to a more chronic stage (see Fig. 2-73). The rim of a chronic abscess is typically isointense on T1-weighted imaging and hypointense on T2-weighted

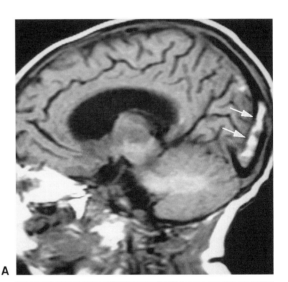

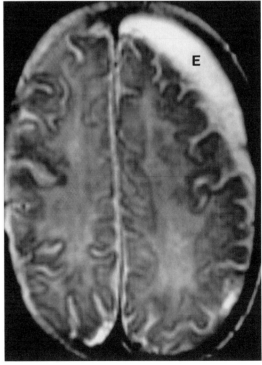

FIG. 2-72. Subdural effusion and dural venous sinus thrombosis. A 4-month-old girl with pneumococcal meningitis. Sagittal T1 MRI **(A)** shows abnormal hyperintensity *(arrows)* along the superior sagittal sinus. Axial T2 MRI **(B)** demonstrates a large left frontal subdural effusion *(E).*

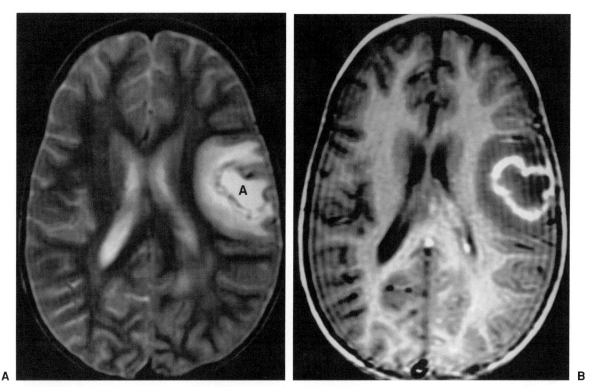

FIG. 2-73. Cerebral abscess. A 2-year-old girl with hemolytic uremic syndrome. Axial T2 MRI. **A:** Left frontotemporal intracerebral high-intensity collection *(A)* with surrounding edema and mass effect. **B:** Axial gadolinium-enhanced T1 MRI shows a thickened and markedly enhancing abscess rim.

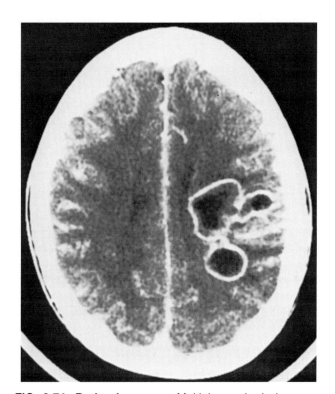

FIG. 2-74. Brain abscesses. Multiple cerebral abscesses appear on CT as well-defined, low-attenuation fluid collections surrounded by thin enhancing rims.

scans. The T2 shortening that occurs may be the result of the low water content of the collagen in combination with a small amount of blood products or free radicals (155).

Empyema

Subdural and epidural empyemas occur more commonly in adolescents than in younger children and usually follow sinusitis. Subdural collections are more frequent and may be unilateral or bilateral. There may be mass effect on the underlying brain. Parenchymal edema, cerebritis, and abscess may accompany the empyema (28). Imaging reveals crescentic or lens-shaped extracerebral collections with peripheral enhancement (Fig. 2-75).

Encephalitis

Encephalitis is a nonsuppurative inflammation of the brain sometimes accompanied by meningeal inflammation. Encephalitis may be the result of a viral infection; it may also be an immunologic response to a recent infection or vaccination (acute disseminated encephalomyelitis) (28; see page 119). Viral infections of the brain may be sporadic (herpes simplex virus type 1, or HSV-1) or occur in epidemics (arboviruses). The inflammation may predominantly affect the meninges

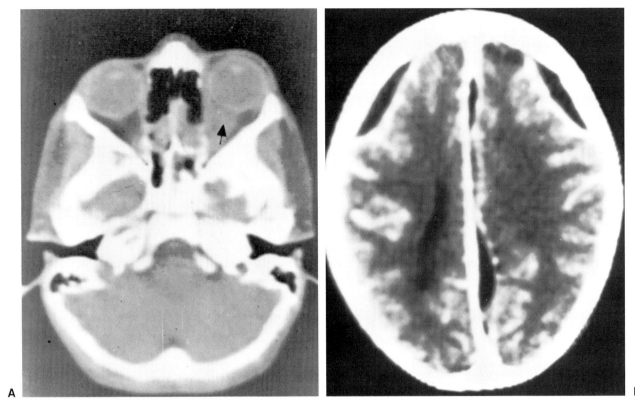

A   B

FIG. 2-75. Sinusitis with orbital abscess and subdural empyema. An 8-year-old comatose boy with pansinusitis and left orbital proptosis. **A:** Orbital CT shows pus within the ethmoid sinuses and a left orbital abscess *(arrow)* displacing the globe anteriorly. **B:** Extracerebral fluid collections are present over the frontal convexities and within the interhemispheric fissure. Note contrast enhancement at the brain-subdural interfaces.

(mumps and coxsackievirus), cortex (HSV-1, arboviruses, and rabies), or white matter (eastern and western equine encephalitis virus, progressive multifocal leukoencephalopathy, and subacute sclerosing panencephalitis) (6,156). The radiologic and clinical manifestations of encephalitis are not specific for the causative agent. However, sometimes certain viruses produce typical imaging findings.

Herpes Simplex Type 1 Infection

Infection by HSV-1 is probably the most common cause of sporadic meningitis and encephalitis in childhood (28,157). It is usually associated with orofacial herpetic lesions (6). Involvement of the CNS usually results from reactivation of a latent and distant infection rather than primary CNS infection. Retrograde transport of the virus to the Gasserian ganglion occurs via the branches of the trigeminal nerve. The viral infection may then spread along meningeal branches of the Vth cranial nerve to the middle cranial fossa, leading to meningitis or necrotic meningoencephalitis of one or both temporal lobes. The infection typically spreads to the subfrontal region and insula and spares the basal ganglia.

MRI is more sensitive than CT for HSV-1 infection, although both exams may be negative early in the course of the illness (158,159). The characteristic appearance of HSV-1 infection is low density on CT with T1 and T2 prolongation on MRI in one or both temporal cortices. The cortex is frequently thickened and enhancement is often present (Fig. 2-76). Petechial hemorrhages are common.

Progressive Multifocal Leukoencephalopathy

Progressive multifocal leukoencephalopathy (PML) is an opportunistic leukoencephalitis produced by a papovavirus. PML occurs primarily in individuals with conditions resulting in compromised cell-mediated immunity such as AIDS, with congenital immunodeficiency syndromes, or receiving immunosuppressive therapy for malignancies (6). The disease is less common in children than in adults. The primary imaging manifestation is regional demyelination, most common in the parietal and frontal lobes. The lesion may extend across the corpus callosum.

CT may show regions of low attenuation. MRI is more sensitive and demonstrates areas of T1 and T2 prolongation in the white matter. Mass effect and enhancement are uncommon (160).

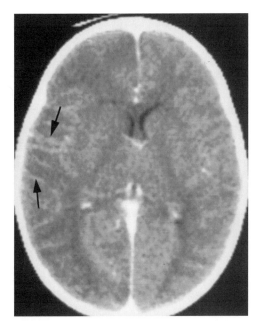

FIG. 2-76. Herpes simplex 1 encephalitis. A 4-year-old boy with encephalitis. Axial contrast-enhanced CT shows right frontotemporal cerebral low-density and moderate leptomeningeal enhancement *(arrows)*.

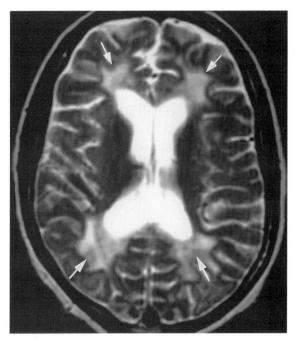

FIG. 2-77. Subacute sclerosing panencephalitis. Axial T2 MRI. Frontal and temporoparietal periventricular white matter hyperintensities *(arrows)* are consistent with encephalitis. The dilated ventricles and enlarged cortical sulci are due to cerebral atrophy.

Subacute Sclerosing Panencephalitis

Subacute sclerosing panencephalitis (SSPE), predominantly a disease of childhood, is probably the result of reactivation of a latent measles infection. As many as half of the patients with SSPE have had a documented measles infection prior to 2 years of age (28). These children develop changes in mental status and behavior, seizures, and irritability (6,28).

Imaging is nonspecific and reveals atrophy and patchy regions of increased water in the white matter on both MRI and CT (Fig. 2-77). Enhancement and mass effect are not present.

Rasmussen Encephalitis

Rasmussen encephalitis is a chronic focal encephalitis. Although a number of viruses have been found in involved regions of the brain, a single infectious agent has not been identified (6,28,161). Affected individuals present with intractable focal seizures. The diagnosis of Rasmussen encephalitis can be confirmed only by brain biopsy or autopsy. Imaging demonstrates focal cortical edema followed by progressive regional or hemispheric atrophy (Fig. 2-78).

Acute Disseminated Encephalomyelitis

Acute disseminated encephalomyelitis (ADEM) is a postinfectious or parainfectious inflammatory condition of the brain and spinal cord. The onset of symptoms (seizures, leth-

argy, focal neurologic deficits) usually occurs several days after a viral infection or immunization. The most commonly associated illnesses are measles, mumps, chicken pox, rubella, and pertussis (6). ADEM is probably due to an immu-

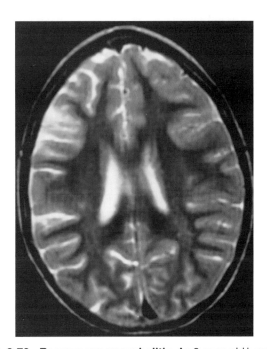

FIG. 2-78. Rasmussen encephalitis. An 8-year-old boy with refractory epilepsy. Axial T2 MRI. There is mild right cerebral atrophy with dilatation of cortical sulci and slight enlargement of the right lateral ventricle.

nologic response to a viral infection that results in the formation of antibodies to a CNS antigen. Most affected children make a complete recovery from the illness; however, occasionally fixed neurologic deficits and movement disorders remain. Treatment with corticosteroids may be beneficial.

In ADEM, regions of demyelination appear on CT as areas of low attenuation and on MRI as foci of T2 prolongation (high intensity) in the subcortical white matter, brainstem, and cerebellum (Fig. 2-79). The basal ganglia may also be abnormal (162). Enhancement of the lesions is variable (163).

Tuberculosis

Although now uncommon in the United States, tuberculous meningitis remains a frequent cause of death in children worldwide (164). Infection of the CNS is usually the result of miliary spread of *Mycobacterium tuberculosis* (6,28,150). A severe granulomatous meningitis of the basal cisterns develops which, if untreated, may cause death in a few weeks. The meningeal involvement probably results from rupture of cortical tuberculomas into the subarachnoid space. The extensive basal meningitis causes hydrocephalus in most patients (164,165). The basal inflammatory changes may also induce a vasculitis of the lenticulostriate and thalamoperforator vessels leading to infarction of the basal ganglia and thalami.

Imaging reveals parenchymal tuberculomas as nodular or ring-enhancing lesions, often at the gray-white matter junction or in a periventricular location. The lesions occasionally calcify. Focal density or intensity abnormalities may be present in the basal ganglia and thalami due to infarction. Hydrocephalus and marked enhancement of the basal leptomeninges are typical (Fig. 2-80) (28,164,166).

Fungal Infections

Fungal diseases of the CNS may result from infection by pathogenic fungi in immunocompetent patients or from infection with either pathogenic or saprophytic fungi in immunocompromised individuals (6,28). Common pathogenic fungi are *Blastomyces, Histoplasma, Coccidioides,* and *Nocardia.* Common saprophytes are *Cryptococcus, Actinomyces, Aspergillus, Candida,* and the fungus causing mucormycosis. Fungal infections of the CNS are less common in children than in adults. They typically produce a granulomatous basal meningitis similar to that seen in tuberculosis. Parenchymal abscesses and granulomas may also be present (146). Aspergillosis or mucormycosis may cause a vasculitis with parenchymal infarction or hemorrhage.

Sarcoidosis

Sarcoidosis, a disease of unknown etiology, produces noncaseating granulomas in many organ systems (6,28,167).

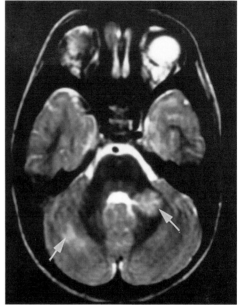

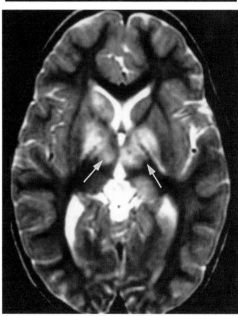

FIG. 2-79. Acute disseminated encephalomyelitis. A, B: Axial T2 MRI. There are nodular and patchy hyperintensities *(arrows)* in the right cerebellum, left middle cerebellar peduncle, basal ganglia and thalamus bilaterally, and within the subcortical as well as periventricular cerebral white matter.

CNS sarcoid is uncommon in children. Presenting complaints include cranial neuropathies, hydrocephalus, hypothalamic dysfunction, and focal neurologic deficits. The most frequent imaging manifestation of sarcoid is a basal granulomatous meningitis with hypothalamic involvement. Contrast enhancement of the meningeal process is usually intense. Parenchymal masses (granulomas) may also be present. The masses are isointense on T1-weighted MRI, mildly hyperintense on T2-weighted images, and usually enhance (168,169).

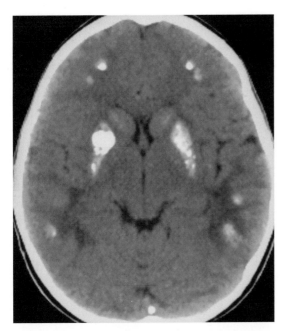

FIG. 2-82. Radiation effects. A 12-year-old girl treated for ependymoma 8 years earlier. Bilateral basal ganglia and cerebral white matter calcifications as well as bilateral white matter low densities (demyelination) are present.

cerebellar signs (ataxia), brainstem signs (cranial nerve palsies), or meningeal signs (head tilt). Common pediatric infratentorial neoplasms include embryonal tumors (medulloblastoma), cerebellar astrocytomas, brainstem gliomas, and ependymomas (Table 2-18). Less frequent tumors include dermoid-epidermoid, teratoma, ganglioglioma, gangliocytoma of Lhermitte-Duclos, choroid plexus papilloma or carcinoma, sarcoma, acoustic neuroma, meningioma, and hemangioblastoma. Nonneoplastic lesions included in the differential diagnosis of posterior fossa masses are the Dandy-Walker spectrum of retrocerebellar cysts, arachnoid cyst, cavernous malformation, cholesterol granuloma, abscess, and hemorrhage. Skull base or petrous-temporal tumors that may invade the posterior fossa include carcinomas, metastases, sarcomas, histiocytoses, neuroblastomas, primitive neuroectodermal tumors (PNETs), paragangliomas, and chordomas.

Cerebellar Astrocytoma

Cerebellar astrocytoma and medulloblastoma are the two most common posterior fossa neoplasms of childhood (5–7,194). The pilocytic subtype of cerebellar astrocytoma is by far the most common, followed by the fibrillary, mixed, and the infrequent anaplastic forms (195). The majority of astrocytomas are slow growing, sharply demarcated, and well differentiated. These are usually noninvasive, do not metastasize, and have the best prognosis of any CNS neoplasm of childhood, usually requiring only surgical excision. Cerebellar astrocytomas usually arise within the vermis or hemisphere. They infrequently arise in the cerebellopontine

angle or middle cerebellar peduncle. There is a broad spectrum from noncystic solid tumors to microcystic but solid-appearing tumors to macrocysts containing tumor nodules or laminar wall tumor. Most of these tumors cause hydrocephalus by compression or displacement of the fourth ventricle or aqueduct. Cerebellar astrocytomas are derived from astrocytic neuroglial cells.

Skull radiographs frequently demonstrate sutural diastasis. By CT, the cystic or microcystic component is commonly of low density, whereas a more solid tumor is isodense to brain. With the more common cystic cerebellar astrocytoma, CT shows a well-defined area of uniform decreased density or fluid representing the cystic component of the tumor; mural nodules are isodense to normal surrounding cerebellum (Fig. 2-84) (194). The cyst is variable in size and is surrounded by a rim of tissue that usually enhances after contrast administration. The mural nodules are frequently medial or anterior, may be multiple, and may enhance markedly after contrast administration (Fig. 2-84B). The cyst contents on both T1- and T2-weighted MRI are frequently more intense than CSF because of increased protein content. The mural nodule is seen to better advantage on MRI, where it appears iso- or hyperintense on T2-weighted sequences. The mural nodule and rim of the cyst usually enhance intensely following gadolinium administration (Fig. 2-85).

Contrast enhancement of the nodular component is characteristic (6,7). Occasionally, the tumor is a large mass of uniform low density without abnormal enhancement; this may be difficult to distinguish from a developmental cystic malformation, although its attenuation values are higher than those of CSF. Infrequently, the tumor appears as a uniform isodense or a mixed-density mass with either homogeneous or inhomogeneous enhancement. When a cerebellar astrocytoma occurs in the midline, differentiation from medulloblastoma and ependymoma may be difficult; cerebellar astrocytomas, however, rarely demonstrate tumor hyperdensity, hemorrhage, or calcification. The pattern of contrast enhancement of these tumors is quite variable; the pattern may be diffuse or focal, nodular or rim-like, and homogeneous or irregular. By MRI the macrocystic component usually displays intensity patterns characteristic of proteinaceous fluid rather than CSF (195). The microcystic component is

TABLE 2-18. *Posterior fossa tumors of childhood*

Cerebellar astrocytoma[a]	Choroid plexus tumors
Medulloblastoma[a]	Mixed glioma
Medulloepithelioma	Lhermitte-Duclos gangliocytoma
Brainstem tumors:	Schwannoma
Glioma[a]	Neurofibroma
Tectal	Lymphoma
Pontine/diffuse	Germ cell tumors
Cervicomedullary	Dermoid/epidermoid
Ependymoma[a]	Hemangioblastoma
Tetroma	Acoustic neuroma
Ganglioglioma	Meningioma

[a] More common.

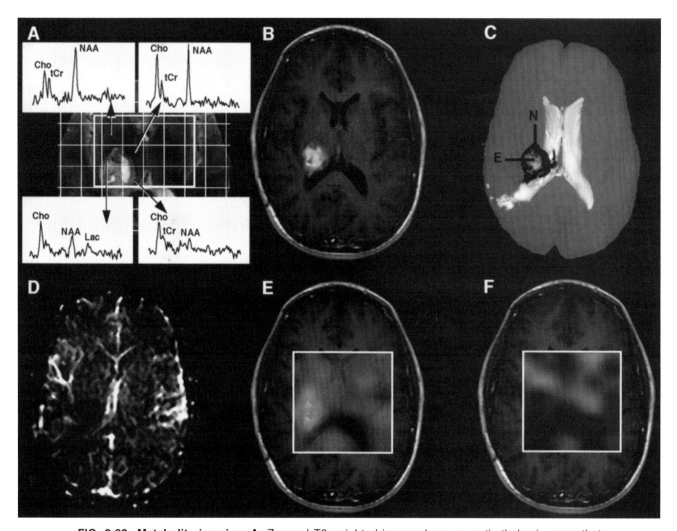

FIG. 2-83. Metabolite imaging. A: Zoomed T2-weighted image shows a cystic thalamic mass that enhances with gadolinium. This is a biopsy-proven fibrillary astrocytoma, recurrent after resection 5 years earlier. The white box shows the four regions selected for magnetic resonance spectroscopy *(MRS)* analysis. The upper spectra exhibit prominent *N*-acetyl aspartate *(NAA)*, total creatine pool *(tCr)*, and choline-containing compounds *(Cho)* peaks that correspond to normal tissue *(left)* and normal tissue plus tumor tissue *(right)*; tumor contains a relatively high Cho peak. The lower spectra contain primarily tumor tissue and show a stronger Cho signal suggesting a higher level of Cho due to tumor and a discernible lactic acid *(Lac)* peak, possibly due to metabolic acidosis. **B:** Postgadolinium axial MRI image following stereotactic radiation treatment shows a decrease in the size of the cyst within the tumor. **C:** Segmentation shows the contrast-enhancing *(E)* and nonenhancing *(N)* portions of the tumor; the volume of the cyst has been reduced from 20.6 to 2.4 cm³, although E (4.5 cm³) and N (6.8 cm³) have remained essentially unaltered. **D:** Calculated MR map of relative cerebral blood volume *(rCBV)*. The rCBV is reduced (95%) in the region of the tumor compared to the contralateral side. Metabolite distribution maps illustrating increased Cho in the tumor region **(E)** and depicting absence of NAA in the tumor and ventricles **(F)**. This case demonstrates the potential value of volume MRI/MRS in providing morphologic, hemodynamic, and metabolic assessment in the follow-up of pediatric brain tumors. (Courtesy of A. Aria Tzika, Ph.D., Boston, MA.)

usually of low intensity on T1 MRI and isointense to hyperintense on proton density and T2 MRI images. The nodular or laminar solid component is usually T1-isointense; it is isointense to hyperintense on proton density and T2 images, although tumor nodule hypointensity has also been observed. Gadolinium enhancement is quite variable and is similar to that described for contrast enhancement with CT (see Fig. 2-85).

Medulloblastoma

Medulloblastoma, a malignant, invasive tumor that arises in the primitive cerebellum from the granular layer of the medullary velum, is considered a primitive neuroectodermal tumor (PNET). These neoplasms occur predominantly in children and arise from the neuronal series rather than from the glial series. The usual site of origin is the vermis in the

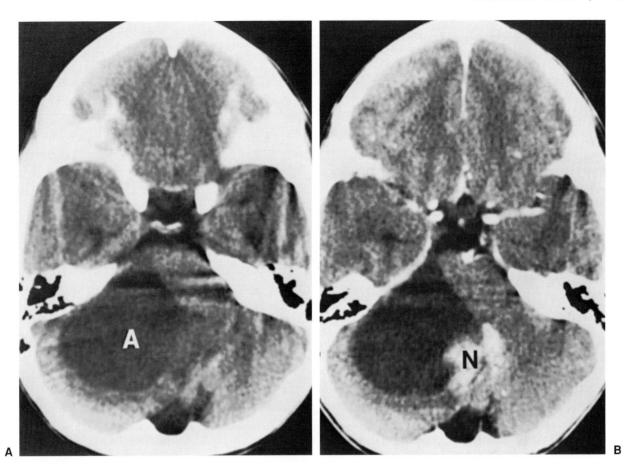

FIG. 2-84. **Cerebellar astrocytoma. A:** Large cyst *(A)* occupies the right posterior fossa. **B:** There is contrast enhancement of the mural nodule *(N)*.

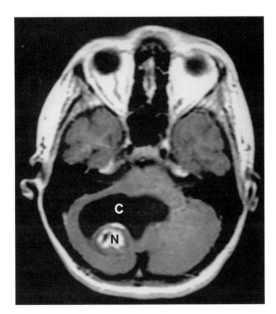

FIG. 2-85. **Cerebellar astrocytoma.** A 9-year-old girl with ataxia. Gadolinium-enhanced axial T1 MRI demonstrates a right cerebellar hemispheric cystic mass *(C)* with enhancing nodular component *(N)*.

region of the inferior medullary velum. The most malignant infratentorial neoplasms in children, they are second in incidence to cerebellar astrocytoma. Medulloblastoma usually presents with hydrocephalus and increased intracranial pressure due to ventricular obstruction. These neoplasms tend to invade the fourth ventricle. There is a propensity for metastasis along CSF pathways, with tumor seeding to the spinal cord, over the cerebral hemispheric convexities, and in the suprasellar subarachnoid space (196–199). Medulloblastoma is the most common childhood tumor producing intracranial and intraspinal seeding; these CSF metastases may be present at initial diagnosis.

The most frequent abnormality on skull radiography is sutural diastasis. Calcification on skull radiographs is unusual but may be demonstrated by CT in as many as 25% of tumors. CT demonstrates a midline, frequently ill-defined mass in the posterior fossa that may be hyperdense, isodense, or even hypodense (6,199,200). The more typical appearance is that of a homogeneous, hyperdense mass on unenhanced scans with marked but uniform contrast enhancement (Fig. 2-86). The CT appearance may be indistinguishable from that of an ependymoma or vermian astrocytoma.

On MRI, probably because of their uniform cellularity, the tumors are more homogeneous than either astrocytomas or ependymomas; they are hypointense or isointense on T1-

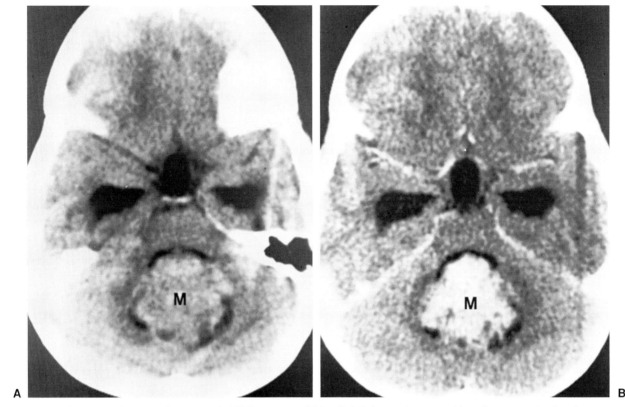

FIG. 2-86. Medulloblastoma. A: Midline mass *(M)* is slightly hyperdense and is adjacent to the fourth ventricle. **B:** Marked homogeneous contrast enhancement of medulloblastoma *(M)*. Note the associated obstructive hydrocephalus.

weighted and hypointense to mildly hyperintense on T2-weighted sequences (Fig. 2-87) (198). As seen best on sagittal projections, the tumor originates from the region of the inferior medullary velum. There is shift of the fourth ventricle anteriorly or superiorly, or in both directions. There is usually marked contrast enhancement of the midline mass on both CT and MRI (see Figs. 2-86 and 2-87). Necrotic portions of the tumor do not enhance. The CT hyperdensity and the occasional T2 hypointensity frequently correlate with tumor hypercellularity. MRI is the modality of choice for accurate determination of tumor location and extent and identification of secondary CSF metastases (see Fig. 2-87) (198,201).

Brainstem Tumors

Brainstem tumors in children are predominantly gliomas; most are astrocytomas of varying subtypes and histologic variation (202–205). Histologically there are pilocytic, anaplastic, and glioblastomatous forms; there are occasionally mixed gliomas or neuronal tumors. These brainstem tumors are commonly referred to collectively as brainstem gliomas.

Most brainstem tumors occur in children. They account for 10% of all pediatric intracranial neoplasms (5). Patients typically present with cranial nerve abnormalities, pyramidal tract signs, or cerebellar dysfunction. Rarely do these tumors present with obstructive hydrocephalus. Brainstem gliomas most commonly arise in the pons, followed in frequency by the midbrain, medulla, cerebral peduncles, and cervical cord; a brainstem glioma may involve several areas. From the pons, these tumors tend to infiltrate the medulla caudally and the midbrain rostrally (Fig. 2-88). There may be symmetric growth with circumferential expansion or asymmetric growth with exophytic extension in any direction. Occasionally, the tumor appears confined to the pons, midbrain, or medulla.

An anatomic classification of brainstem tumors based on combined clinical and imaging findings has been developed to guide therapy and predict outcome (6,7). The categories include diffuse, focal, and cystic types. Focal midbrain, thalamic, and cervicomedullary tumors are usually of lower grade and have a better prognosis than pontine or diffuse brainstem gliomas. Cystic or necrotic tumors of the pons or entire brainstem are frequently high-grade malignancies (glioblastoma). Tectal tumors may be relatively benign in behavior, occurring as low-grade gliomas, hamartomas, or occasionally only gliosis; these often produce obstructive hydrocephalus and are more readily detected by MRI than CT (Fig. 2-89) (206,207).

Skull radiographs are usually normal. CT may demonstrate enlargement, distortion, or abnormal density of the brainstem; there is frequently compression of the prepontine

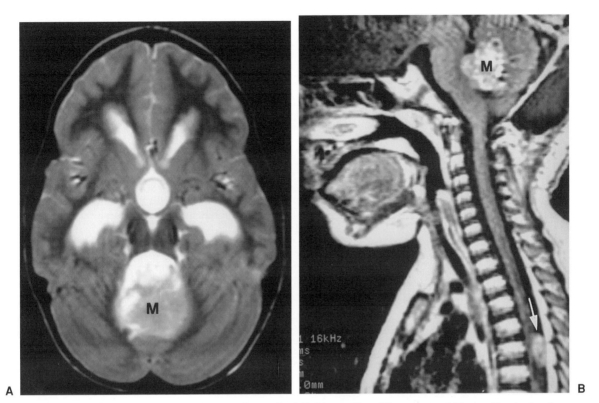

FIG. 2-87. Medulloblastoma with cerebrospinal fluid seeding. Three-year-old boy with ataxia. **A:** Axial T2 MRI. Hypointense tumor *(M)* in the fourth ventricle producing obstructive hydrocephalus. **B:** Gadolinium-enhanced sagittal T1 MRI. Enhancing midline posterior fossa tumor *(M)* within the fourth ventricle. Note the large thoracic intraspinal metastasis *(arrow)* that enhances with contrast.

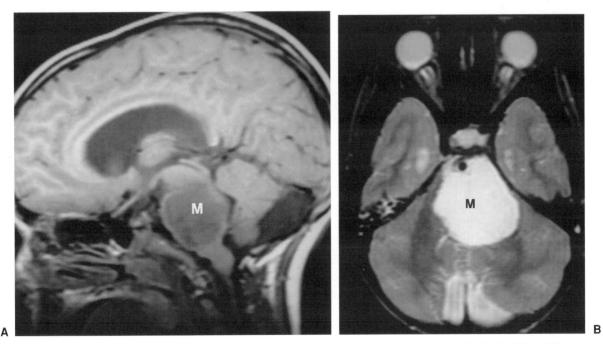

FIG. 2-88. Pontine glioma. A 7-year-old boy with multiple cranial nerve palsies. **A:** Sagittal T1 MRI. Hypointense mass *(M)* expanding the pons, extending into the midbrain, and elevating the floor of the fourth ventricle. **B:** Axial T2 MRI. Large brainstem mass *(M)*.

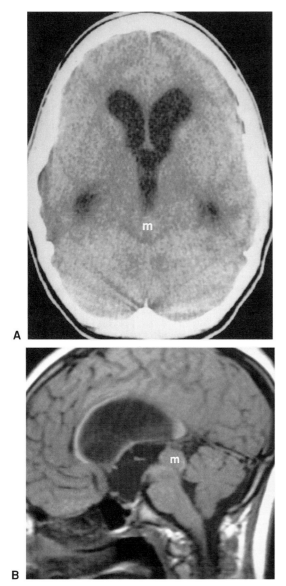

A

B

FIG. 2-89. Tectal glioma. A 14-year-old girl with severe headaches. **A:** Axial CT. Third and lateral ventricular dilation with an isodense fullness in the tectal region *(m)*. **B:** Sagittal T1 MRI. Tectal mass *(m)* with associated aqueductal stenosis causing obstructive hydrocephalus.

cisterns (202). Approximately 10% of brainstem gliomas have a significant cystic component that permits surgical drainage with improvement in clinical symptomatology.

The imaging modality of choice to show tumor extent and characteristics is MRI (203–205). Most brainstem gliomas have a homogeneous appearance and are hypointense on T1-weighted and isointense to hyperintense on T2-weighted sequences (see Fig. 2-88). Gadolinium enhancement is variable and may be diffuse, nodular, or ring-like along the margins of a cyst or about an area of necrosis. Enhancement is common in exophytic portions of brainstem gliomas and after radiation therapy; it is less common in untreated brainstem gliomas.

Patients with cervicomedullary brainstem tumors may have recurrent vomiting; these tumors may be detectable only by MRI (Fig. 2-90). MRI distinguishes brainstem tumors from other abnormalities such as infarction, encephalitis, demyelination, and vascular malformation more accurately than CT.

For most patients, complete surgical resection is not possible, so surgery is limited to resection of exophytic tumor and drainage of cystic components. Radiation therapy, often in hyperfractionated doses, remains the primary method of treatment; radiation therapy is sometimes reserved for those tumors demonstrating growth or those associated with specific neurologic symptoms or signs.

Ependymoma

Ependymomas, neoplasms of the ciliated ependymal cells, are considered paragangliomas of the CNS. They arise from the ependymal lining of the ventricles, are relatively slow-growing neoplasms, are usually benign, and account for approximately 10% of pediatric intracranial neoplasms (5,6). There may be considerable histologic diversity, and it is

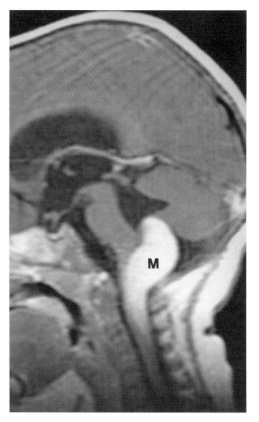

FIG. 2-90. Cervicomedullary astrocytoma. A 2-year-old girl with persistent vomiting. Gadolinium-enhanced sagittal T1 MRI. Enhancing mass *(M)* involving the upper cervical spinal cord and medulla with a dorsal exophytic component extending into the cisterna magna and caudal fourth ventricle. There is associated hydrocephalus.

occasionally difficult to distinguish these tumors from astrocytomas and oligodendrogliomas. The tumors are often strikingly circumscribed. They may contain areas of calcification, thrombosis, hemorrhage, focal necrosis, vascular hyperplasia, and even dysplastic cartilage or bone formation. Anaplastic forms rarely occur. The term ependymoblastoma is best reserved for a variant of PNET showing primitive ependymal differentiation.

Ependymomas usually present with hydrocephalus due to fourth ventricular obstruction. Two thirds of ependymomas are infratentorial, the usual site of origin being the midline in the floor of the fourth ventricle (Fig. 2-91). They may eventually fill the fourth ventricle and project through the outlet foramina into the cisterna magna (Fig. 2-92) or cerebellopontine angle (Fig. 2-93); there may also be extension through the foramen magnum into the cervical spinal canal (6). Seeding of ependymoma into the subarachnoid space occurs in 10% of patients; this frequency is exceeded only by that of medulloblastoma (5,6).

Plain skull radiographs show sutural diastasis in 70% and calcification in 15% (5). CT demonstrates a mass in the region of the fourth ventricle associated with obstructive hydrocephalus (208). Calcification within the mass is frequent (70%). The tumor mass is usually of slightly greater density than surrounding cerebellar tissue. There is some contrast enhancement, usually inhomogeneous (Fig. 2-91)

(208). Ependymomas frequently show a lobular contour with a wide-based attachment along the fourth ventricular floor.

MRI confirms the presence of the tumor in the fourth ventricle (6,209). The tumor is typically inhomogeneous in MRI signal and shows variable hypointensity on T1-weighted and hyperintensity on T2-weighted sequences (Fig. 2-92) (6,209). The density and intensity heterogeneity is characteristic of ependymomas and is due to variability in the solid, cystic, necrotic, edematous, calcified, and hemorrhage components (Fig. 2-93). Hemorrhage within the tumor may produce hyperintensity on T1-weighted images. Signal voids, best seen by gradient-echo sequences, indicate calcifications within the tumor or enlarged vessels in or around the mass.

Other Posterior Fossa Tumors

Choroid plexus tumors, including papilloma and carcinoma, occasionally arise within the posterior fossa, usually in the fourth ventricle, infrequently in the cerebellopontine angle (7). Mixed gliomas and neuronal or mixed neuronal-glial tumors may also arise in the posterior fossa. A classic type of gangliocytoma may be confined to the cerebellum as a malformative or dysplastic gangliocytoma (Lhermitte-Duclos disease) (210).

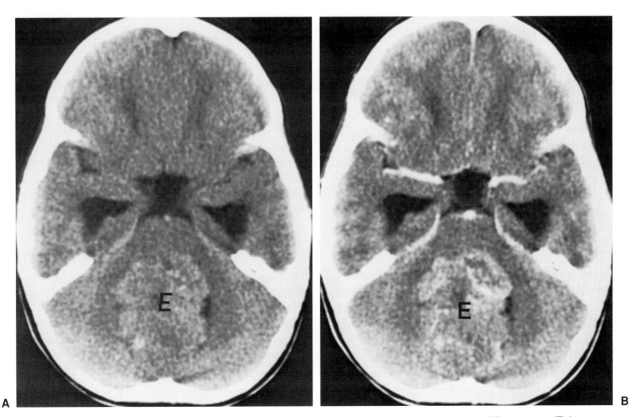

FIG. 2-91. Ependymoma. A: On a noncontrast CT section, the posterior fossa midline mass *(E)* is hyperdense due to calcification. **B:** There is minimal contrast enhancement with inhomogeneity due to necrosis of the tumor *(E)*.

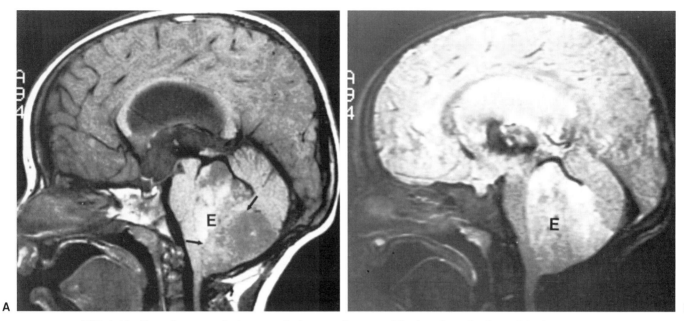

FIG. 2-92. Ependymoma. A: Intraventricular ependymoma *(E)* arises from the floor of the fourth ventricle and grows through outlet foramina *(arrows)* into the cisterna magna. Hyperintensity on T1-weighted MRI is due to previous hemorrhage. **B:** Inhomogeneous signal intensity within the mass *(E)* is seen on T2-weighted MRI.

Tumors arising from cranial nerves are rare in the posterior fossa in childhood. They include schwannomas (neurilemmoma or neurinoma), neurofibromas, and malignant peripheral nerve sheath tumors. The most common intracranial schwannoma arises from the vestibular branch of the VIIIth cranial nerve and is usually referred to as an acoustic neuroma (211–213). Acoustic neuroma accounts for only 1.4% of intracranial neoplasms in children; bilateral acoustic neuromas are pathognomonic of neurofibromatosis type 2, but unilateral tumors are not associated with neurofibromatosis. Plexiform neurofibromas are characteristically seen in neurofibromatosis type 1.

Epidermoid/dermoid tumors arise as a result of entrapment of epidermis or mesoderm at the time of anterior neural tube closure. This rest of embryonic tissue may enlarge with time, producing a dermocutaneous sinus, infection and abscess, aseptic meningitis due to chemical irritation, or increased intracranial pressure due to obstruction of CSF pathways. Epidermoids and dermoids may arise in infratentorial or supratentorial locations. In the posterior fossa, epidermoids most commonly arise in the cerebellopontine angle cisterns; dermoids more commonly arise in the midline adjacent to the cerebellar vermis, brainstem, fourth ventricle, or cisterna magna (Fig. 2-94) (214–217). Epidermoids are typically lobulated in appearance, do not enhance with contrast material, and have CSF density on CT and CSF intensity on MRI. Dermoids, on the other hand, almost always have fat-like densities or intensities, and may be calcified.

Hemangioblastomas are rare in children, accounting for only 1% to 2% of all intracranial neoplasms. They are more common in males and frequently occur in association with

von Hippel-Lindau disease, transmitted as an autosomal dominant trait with variable penetrance. These tumors are considered benign and contain abundant vascular stroma as well as pseudoxanthoma cells. Production of erythropoietin in the tumor may cause polycythemia. These tumors most commonly arise in the cerebellar hemisphere; other less common sites are the brainstem, fourth ventricle, and spinal canal. Approximately 60% are cystic with an enhancing mural nodule. The remainder are solid, are isodense on unenhanced CT, and have marked contrast enhancement. The cyst of hemangioblastoma is usually hypointense on T1-weighted and hyperintense on T2-weighted MRI. If there is T1 hyperintensity, it usually due to shortening of T1 relaxation secondary to hemorrhage within the cyst. The mural nodule is often isointense on T1-weighted and slightly hyperintense on T2-weighted images; the mural nodule markedly enhances following gadolinium administration (see Fig. 2-161) (218–220).

Tumors About the Third Ventricle

Tumors about the third ventricle may be subdivided into suprasellar or anterior third ventricular tumors, pineal region or posterior third ventricular tumors, intraventricular tumors, and paraventricular tumors (Table 2-19) (6,7). Common manifestations are hydrocephalus, a neuroendocrine disorder (growth failure, hypopituitarism, precocious puberty, amenorrhea, galactorrhea, diabetes insipidus, diencephalic syndrome), and optic pathway or other cranial nerve involvement (221). In childhood, common neoplasms in this region

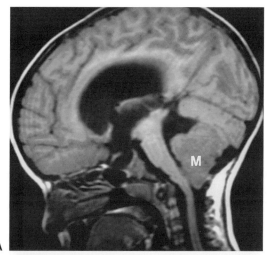

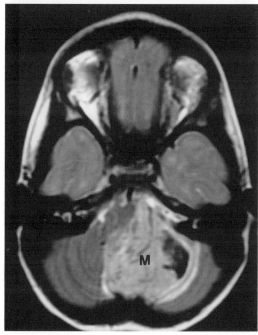

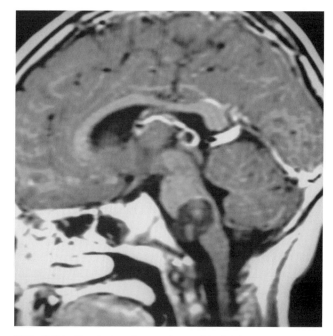

FIG. 2-94. Posterior fossa dermoid. Adolescent girl with recurrent aseptic meningitis. Sagittal T1 MRI demonstrates a mixed-intensity, pontomedullary mass with some intrinsic high intensities.

FIG. 2-93. Ependymoma. A 4-year-old girl with ataxia. **A:** Sagittal T1 MRI. Large midline posterior fossa tumor *(M)* within fourth ventricle producing hydrocephalus. **B:** Axial T2 MRI. Left paramedian posterior fossa mass *(M)* with cavitation and extension into the left cerebellopontine angle.

origin may invade the midline brain structures; these include neuroblastoma, PNET, histiocytosis, esthesioneuroblastoma, sarcoma, chordoma, angiofibroma, carcinoma, mucocele, plasmacytoma, granulomatous processes (aspergillosis), and metastatic disease.

are optic glioma, hypothalamic glioma, craniopharyngioma, and germ cell tumor. Less common tumors include pituitary adenoma, dermoid/epidermoid, choristoma, histiocytosis, pineal cell tumor (pinealoma, pineoblastoma), third ventricular glioma, ganglioglioma, ependymoma, meningioma, choroid plexus papilloma, paraganglioma, schwannoma, and neoplastic seeding. Nonneoplastic masses and processes confused with neoplasms include arachnoid cyst, sphenoidal encephalocele, colloid cyst, Rathke pouch cyst, hamartoma (glial, neuronal, or mesenchymal), ectopic posterior pituitary bright spot, aneurysm, Galenic varix, cavernous malformation, granuloma, arachnoiditis, hypophysitis, and sarcoidosis. Extracranial (parameningeal) processes of bone or sinus

TABLE 2-19. *Tumors about the third ventricle*

Glioma
  Optic nerve
  Hypothalamic
  Other
Germ cell tumors
  Germinoma
  Embryonal carcinoma
  Endodermal sinus tumor
  Choriocarcinoma
  Teratoma
Pineal parenchymal tumors
  Pineoblastoma
  Pineocytoma
Malformative tumors
  Craniopharyngioma
  Rathke cleft cyst
  Colloid cyst
  Arachnoid cyst
  Lipoma
  Neuroepithelial hamartomas
  Meningioangiomatosis
  Dermoid/epidermoid
Pituitary adenoma
Meningioma

Hypothalamic Glioma

Hypothalamic gliomas are usually low-grade astrocytomas. Tumors in this location are less frequent than astrocytomas of the cerebral hemisphere, brainstem, and optic pathways. In infants a hypothalamic glioma may cause the diencephalic syndrome with marked emaciation in the presence of alertness and euphoria. Radiographs of the extremities of patients with the diencephalic syndrome show a complete absence of subcutaneous fat. Other symptoms of hypothalamic gliomas include visual loss, diabetes insipidus, gait or motor disturbance, short stature, delayed puberty, congenital nystagmus, and gelastic seizures (222).

Hypothalamic gliomas rarely calcify, but skull radiographs may show sutural diastasis, sellar erosion, or thinning of the clinoids. CT demonstrates a suprasellar mass, which may be isodense with the surrounding brain tissue or increased or decreased in density. On MRI, the tumor is usually slightly hypointense on T1-weighted and markedly hyperintense on T2-weighted images. Enhancement after gadolinium administration is usually inhomogeneous and may be marked. The tumor frequently extends to extraaxial regions, e.g., the prepontine cistern of the posterior fossa. There is distortion or obliteration of the third ventricle with hydrocephalus in approximately 50% of patients. There is almost always marked contrast enhancement on CT or MRI.

Optic Glioma

Optic pathway gliomas are astrocytic tumors that arise from the optic nerve alone, the optic nerve and chiasm, or the chiasm alone with secondary involvement of the hypothalamus. They sometimes co-exist with neurofibromatosis. Optic gliomas account for 7% of all intracranial neoplasms in children. Depending on the site of origin, presenting signs and symptoms include decreased visual acuity, exophthalmos, optic atrophy, papilledema, nystagmus, increased intracranial pressure, and visual field deficits. Proptosis is almost always present when the glioma is orbital. There may be signs and symptoms of increased intracranial pressure if there is a large intracranial component causing hydrocephalus. Disturbances of hypothalamic function (precocious puberty, increased growth, panhypopituitarism, obesity, diabetes insipidus) can occur if there is a large chiasmatic lesion.

Astrocytomas arising from the optic pathway constitute one of the common perisellar tumors of childhood. They are frequently associated with neurofibromatosis type 1 (223,224). Exclusively intraorbital lesions include hamartomas, arachnoidal hyperplasia, and low-grade astrocytomas. Tumors arising from the chiasm and optic tracts may range from hamartomas and low-grade astrocytomas to anaplastic astrocytomas. Often there is intraorbital, intracanalicular, and intracranial optic nerve involvement. Glial neoplasms arising primarily within the hypothalamus also range from low-grade astrocytomas to anaplastic forms. When a large

intracranial suprasellar mass is present, it may be difficult to decide whether it is chiasmatic or hypothalamic in origin. Occasionally, differentiation from germinoma and hypothalamic hamartoma is also not possible.

The sella turcica is abnormal in three fourths of children with optic gliomas. These abnormalities include thinning of the clinoids, enlargement of the chiasmatic sulcus, flattening of the tuberculum sellae, and blunting of the posterior clinoids. Anterior sellar changes suggest chiasmatic involvement, and hypothalamic extension. Optic foramen views and particularly CT of the optic canals are usually abnormal. Sutures are split if there is associated hydrocephalus, which is usually due to obstruction at the level of the third ventricle. Calcification in an optic pathway glioma is unusual. CT or MRI demonstrates bulbous enlargement of the optic nerves if the glioma is confined to the orbit. Occasionally there is involvement of the posterior optic pathways (optic tracts, lateral geniculate bodies, optic radiations) by an optic chiasm glioma (Fig. 2-95; see Fig. 2-154).

It is difficult to differentiate a hypothalamic glioma from an optic chiasmatic glioma. Chiasmatic gliomas frequently invade the hypothalamus, and hypothalamic gliomas commonly extend to the chiasm. These two entities are best distinguished by the clinical presentation and the CT or MRI appearance. Enlargement of the optic nerves and chiasm is characteristic of optic nerve glioma. In addition, T2-weighted signal hyperintensity or involvement of the optic pathways posterior to the chiasm is most consistent with an optic glioma, especially in patients with type 1 neurofibromatosis. On occasion, hyperintense signal of the optic tracts

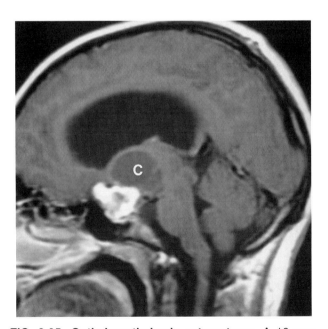

FIG. 2-95. Optic-hypothalamic astrocytoma. A 16-year-old boy with visual loss. Gadolinium-enhanced sagittal T1 MRI. Suprasellar tumor with an enhancing solid component involving the optic chiasm and hypothalamus; a cystic component *(C)* is adjacent to the third ventricle and produces hydrocephalus.

is noted with hypothalamic glioma; it is due to edema of the tracts rather than tumor extension. Miller et al. suggested that hypothalamic glioma and optic chiasm glioma should be considered together as hypothalamic-optic chiasm gliomas, as the origin may be difficult to establish (222).

Histiocytoma

A hypothalamic histiocytoma may be impossible to differentiate from a suprasellar glioma or germinoma. Children with hypothalamic histiocytomas usually have diabetes insipidus and skeletal lesions characteristic of Langerhans-cell histiocytosis. The MRI findings of a histiocytoma may be similar to and indistinguishable from those of a germ cell tumor (225,226). Findings of hypothalamic histiocytosis include enlargement of the pituitary stalk, a mass in the floor of the third ventricle, enlargement of the pituitary gland and absence of the posterior pituitary bright spot (see Fig. 2-112).

Pituitary Tumors

Pituitary adenoma, the most common tumor arising from the pituitary gland, is much more common in adults than children. Hormonally active pituitary adenomas (70% of the total) may produce and secrete prolactin, growth hormone, and adrenocorticotropic hormone (ACTH). Approximately 10% of pituitary adenomas produce more than one hormone.

Many of the tumors secreting prolactin or ACTH are microadenomas; they measure less than 1 cm in diameter, and cross-sectional imaging is critical for diagnosis (227). Prolactin-secreting pituitary adenomas may become hemorrhagic during adolescence. There is frequently suprasellar extension of a hemorrhagic pituitary adenoma; this appears hyperintense on T1 MRI and may be mistaken for craniopharyngioma or a Rathke cleft cyst. Hemorrhage into the tumor is not uncommon in adolescents (228).

Germ Cell Tumors

Germ cell tumors may arise in the pineal region, the hypothalamic region, or both (229–231). Germ cell tumors include germinoma, embryonal carcinoma, endodermal sinus tumor, choriocarcinoma, and teratoma. Germ cell tumors of mixed histology do occur. With the exception of mature teratomas, all germ cell tumors are classified as malignant neoplasms and may metastasize along CSF pathways. Most of the pure germinomas are highly radiosensitive. Elevated immunohistochemical markers, such as α-fetoprotein and human chorionic gonadotropin, are associated with embryonal carcinoma, endodermal sinus tumor (yolk sac tumor), and choriocarcinoma.

Germinoma. Germinoma is the most common of the germ cell tumors. Imaging demonstrates a midline or paramedian pineal region, hypothalamic (especially in females), or third periventricular mass (Figs. 2-96 and 2-97). The mass

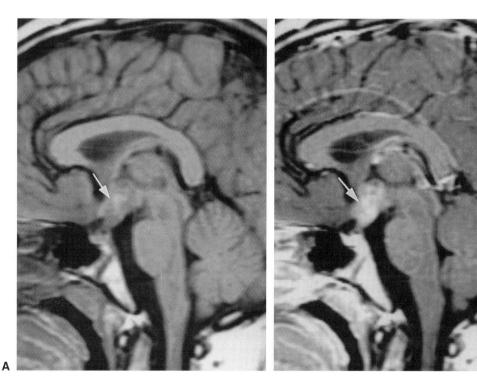

FIG. 2-96. Hypothalamic germinoma. A 13-year-old boy with diabetes insipidus. **A:** Sagittal T1 MRI. Mixed-intensity hypothalamic mass *(arrow)* and absence of the posterior pituitary bright spot. **B:** Gadolinium-enhanced sagittal T1 MRI. Moderate enhancement of the hypothalamic mass *(arrow)*.

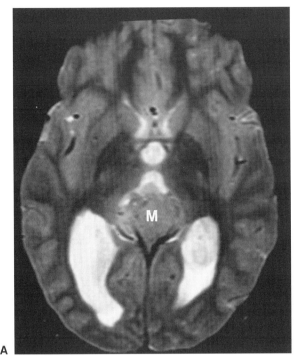

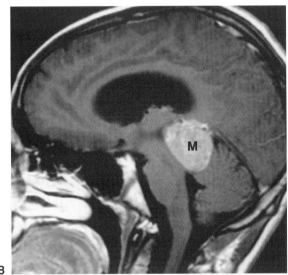

FIG. 2-97. Pineal germinoma. An 11-year-old boy with headaches. **A:** Axial T2 MRI. Low signal intensity pineal region mass *(M)*. **B:** Gadolinium-enhanced sagittal T1 MRI. Enhancing pineal region tumor *(M)* producing hydrocephalus.

noma may have an imaging appearance similar to that of pure germinoma. However, these three germ cell tumors usually have more variable tumor density, intensity, and enhancement characteristics. Primitive neuroectodermal tumors may also arise in the pineal region (Fig. 2-98) (234).

Teratoma. A teratoma is a mixture of differentiated tissues derived from all three embryonic germ layers (178). These masses are usually circumscribed, are often cystic, and may contain calcification, bone, cartilage, teeth, or fat (Fig. 2-99). Teratomas are divided into mature or immature types, depending on whether the tissue components resemble mature adult tissues or immature embryonic tissues. Mature teratomas grow slowly and are generally considered benign. Immature teratomas may behave in a benign or malignant fashion; abundant embryonic tissue suggests the potential for more rapid growth and metastases. Teratomas containing other germ cell tumor types, or areas of carcinoma or sarcoma, are referred to as teratocarcinomas, are considered malignant, and usually adopt the behavior of their most malignant components. Imaging of teratoma usually demonstrates heterogeneous CT densities and MRI intensities within a lobulated mass that contains fat, calcium, ossification, or cartilage. Contrast enhancement usually occurs, especially in the more malignant types of teratoma.

Pineal Parenchymal Tumors

Pineal parenchymal tumors include pineoblastoma, pineocytoma, and mixed pineal tumors (229,231,234–238). Tumors of the pineal region expand and eventually obstruct the aqueduct of Sylvius, producing hydrocephalus. There may also be paralysis of upward gaze due to pressure on the quadrigeminal plate, cerebellar signs, hypothalamic symptoms, and even pyramidal or thalamic symptoms. Precocious puberty is occasionally present. In contrast to germ cell tumors, tumors that arise from pineal cells have an equal sex distribution. Thus, a tumor in the pineal region in a male is probably of germ cell origin whereas in a female it should be considered a primary pineal cell tumor. There is commonly calcification in primary pineal cell tumors.

Pineoblastoma. Pineoblastomas occur primarily in childhood. Histologically, these embryonal tumors are similar to PNET (see Fig. 2-98); pineoblastomas are highly malignant neoplasms and frequently metastasize by seeding along CSF pathways. Imaging demonstrates a large lobulated mass with calcification in the pineal region. On CT, the tumor matrix is usually isodense or slightly more dense than brain tissue. On MRI, the tumor is usually isointense to hypointense on T1 images, and isointense on T2 images; it enhances markedly. There is almost always ventricular dilatation due to obstructive hydrocephalus.

Pineocytoma. Pineocytomas are usually well circumscribed and may be calcified. They may be indistinguishable from pineoblastoma by both CT and MRI.

is often associated with abnormal pineal calcification. The tumor is occasionally hemorrhagic but rarely cystic. CT usually demonstrates an isodense or hyperdense mass with tumor enhancement. Although variable, MRI usually shows isointensity to hypointensity on T1 images, isointensity to hyperintensity on T2 images, and contrast enhancement. Germinomas of the hypothalamic region frequently present with central diabetes insipidus with absence of the posterior pituitary bright spot (see Fig. 2-96) (232,233).

Embryonal carcinoma, yolk sac tumor, and choriocarci-

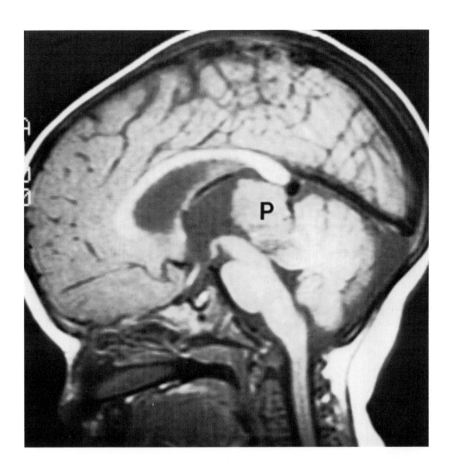

FIG. 2-98. Primitive neuroectodermal tumor. Sagittal MRI identifies a mass *(P)* in the pineal region.

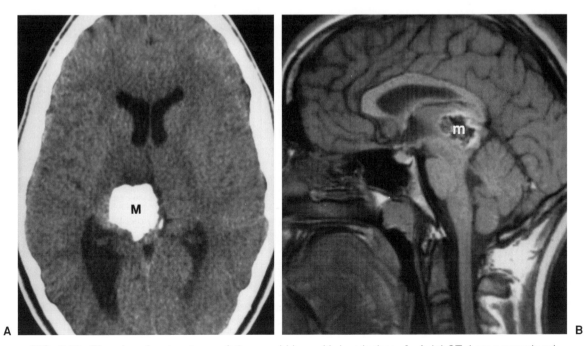

FIG. 2-99. Pineal region teratoma. A 9-year-old boy with headaches. **A:** Axial CT. Large parapineal calcified mass is shown *(M)*. **B:** Sagittal T1 MRI. Bone, cartilage, and fat elements are identified within the pineal region teratoma *(m)*.

Craniopharyngiomas

Craniopharyngioma is the most common brain tumor that arises from embryonal remnants. It is caused by the persistence and proliferation of squamous epithelial rests during the development of the pituitary gland and the pituitary stalk. The anterior adenohypophysis develops, in part, from the primitive buccal epithelium (Rathke pouch); the stalk and neurohypophysis develop from an outpouching in the floor of the third ventricle (craniopharyngeal duct). Thus, craniopharyngiomas are derived from both neural ectodermal and epithelial ectodermal elements. They can arise in any portion of the primitive buccal epithelium or craniopharyngeal duct that extends from the floor of the third ventricle near the tuber cinereum into the body of the sphenoid bone and retropharyngeal space.

Craniopharyngiomas account for 6% to 7% of all intracranial tumors of childhood (5,6). They are usually both intrasellar and suprasellar in location, although they may be purely intrasellar (10%) or purely suprasellar (20%). They often compress or displace the optic chiasm, hypothalamus, and anterior third ventricle. Craniopharyngiomas are benign and slow-growing. They induce a considerable arachnoid reaction, which causes adherence to surrounding structures including the carotid arteries and the base of the brain. They tend to compress, envelop, or infiltrate adjacent structures and produce a reactive gliosis. Presenting symptoms include increased intracranial pressure, visual impairment, growth retardation, diabetes insipidus, and, rarely, limb weakness.

Skull radiographs are rarely normal in children with craniopharyngioma. Calcification is visible in 80% of pediatric craniopharyngiomas. The sella turcica is eroded or enveloped in 75% of patients. Calcifications may be flocculent (Fig. 2-100A), curvilinear, coalescent, or mixed. CT demonstrates a suprasellar mass (Fig. 2-100B), usually large and calcified (200,239). In 85% of cases there is a low-density cystic area in the tumor that is of water or even fat density. The cyst may become large and extend into the anterior, middle, and posterior fossae. Cystic craniopharyngiomas frequently have calcification within the cyst wall. CT and MRI show contrast enhancement of the cyst wall or the entire mass (Fig. 2-100B).

MRI demonstrates a mass in the suprasellar region that may extend superiorly to efface the chiasmatic and infundibular recesses of the third ventricle (Fig. 2-101). Signal intensity for the cyst is variable on both T1- and T2-weighted sequences depending on the amount of lipid, protein, hemorrhage, cholesterol, and debris in the tumor (6,240). Solid tumors are usually isointense on T1-weighted and minimally to moderately hyperintense on T2-weighted images. Cystic lesions tend to be high intensity on all sequences because of hemorrhage, proteinaceous fluid, or cholesterol. Hypointensity on MRI may indicate keratin, calcium, or iron within the craniopharyngioma.

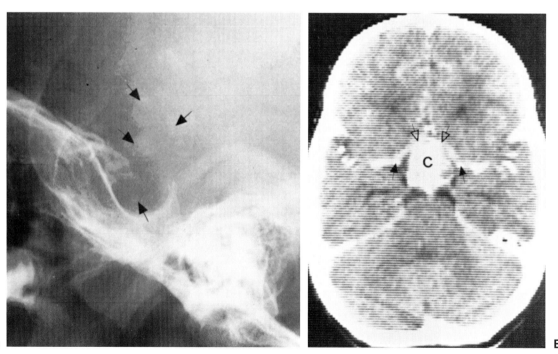

FIG. 2-100. Craniopharyngioma. A 2-year-old boy with vertical nystagmus. **A:** There is enlargement of the sella with amputation of the dorsum sellae. This is a type 3 (J-shaped) sella turcica with bony erosion of the tuberculum sellae and associated enlargement of the sellar fossa. There are flocculent intrasellar and suprasellar calcifications *(arrows)*. **B:** Computed tomography. There is marked contrast enhancement of the calcified mass *(C)*. Note the close approximation of the craniopharyngioma to the internal carotid arteries *(solid arrows)* and anterior cerebral arteries *(open arrows)*.

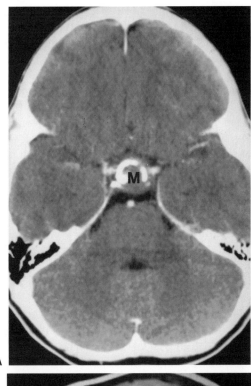

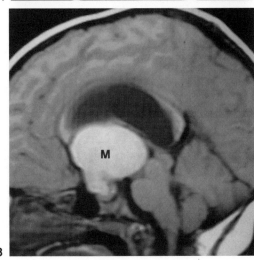

FIG. 2-101. Craniopharyngioma. A 7-year-old girl with short stature. **A:** Axial CT. Calcification within a suprasellar mass *(M)*. **B:** Sagittal T1 MRI. Large suprasellar mass *(M)* with cystic component; mass effect causes obstructive hydrocephalus.

A number of other tumors may arise in the region of the anterior third ventricle. The mnemonic of SATCHMO (Sellar tumor with superior extension; Aneurysm; Tuberculum sellae meningioma, teratoma-dermoid-germinoma; Craniopharyngioma; Hypothalamic glioma, hamartoma, histiocytoma; Metastatic disease; Optic glioma) is an easy way to remember the differential diagnosis of parasellar masses. Any child with a suspected parasellar mass should have an MRI exam (6,239,240). In addition to these more common suprasellar masses, the differential diagnosis also includes

other malformative tumors (see below). Calcifications within the mass or cyst wall, fat or fluid within the tumor, and contrast enhancement suggest the diagnosis of craniopharyngioma. When the diagnosis remains in doubt or stereotactic radiotherapy is contemplated, thin section CT may be required.

Other Malformative Tumors

In addition to craniopharyngioma, other malformative tumors that occur about the third ventricle are Rathke cleft cysts, colloid cysts, neuroepithelial cysts, pineal cysts, arachnoid cysts, lipomas, hamartomas, and dermoid/epidermoid cysts.

Rathke Cleft Cyst. The clinical presentation and imaging appearance of Rathke cleft cyst is usually similar to that of craniopharyngioma. However, calcification and contrast enhancement are rare (241–243). The cyst is round or lobulated, smaller than a craniopharyngioma, hyperintense to normal pituitary gland on precontrast MRI, and hypointense compared to the gland after contrast. When a well-demarcated mass located anterior to the pituitary stalk has these signal characteristics, Rathke cleft cyst should be strongly considered (6,241).

Colloid Cyst. Colloid cysts are probably of neuroepithelial derivation and occur much more frequently in the adult than in children (244). These epithelial-lined cysts have fibrous walls and proteinaceous content; they arise in the wall or roof of the third ventricle at the foramina of Monro. Hydrocephalus, which may be unilateral, is common. Hemorrhage occasionally occurs within the cyst. A colloid cyst is usually of high density on CT; there is usually no contrast enhancement. The lesion is of variable intensity on all MRI sequences. The most critical imaging characteristic for diagnosis of colloid cyst is its location at the foramen of Monro.

Neuroepithelial Cysts. Other neuroepithelial (glioependymal) cysts may arise in the choroid plexus and pineal gland. The small masses may be detected only by MRI; characteristically, they are hypointense on T1 sequences and hyperintense on proton density and T2 sequences. Gadolinium injection may show contrast enhancement of the cyst wall and filling in of the cyst with delayed scanning. A pineal cyst may deform the adjacent tectum and aqueduct. However, hydrocephalus is rare (245,246). Differential diagnosis includes other pineal region masses (234).

Arachnoid Cyst. Arachnoid cysts most commonly occur in the suprasellar and quadrigeminal plate regions. The cysts characteristically contain CSF and therefore follow CSF intensity throughout the MRI sequences (T1-hypointense, proton density-hypointense, T2-hyperintense) and do not enhance with contrast administration. They may have no identifiable wall. Hemorrhage or infection may alter their imaging appearance.

Lipoma. Lipomas are benign mesenchymal tumors that contain adipose tissue (neutral fat) alone or as the dominant component of a tumor containing other mesenchymal tissues such as muscle, fibrous tissue, and vascular elements. The most common intracranial locations are the hypothalamus, quadrigeminal plate region, and pericallosal region. Pericallosal lipomas are frequently associated with dysgenesis of the corpus callosum.

Lipomas are of fat density on CT and are occasionally calcified. MRI demonstrates the characteristics of neutral fat, including high intensity on T1 and proton density images, T2 isointensity or hypointensity, chemical shift artifact, and decrease in signal intensity with fat suppression techniques.

Ectopic Posterior Pituitary. An ectopic posterior pituitary, which mimics a mass, is usually associated with growth hormone deficiencies, appears as a hypothalamic or infundibular T1 hyperintensity, and is associated with absence of the normal intrasellar posterior pituitary bright spot. It must be distinguished from a hypothalamic or infundibular lipoma. With an ectopic posterior pituitary bright spot, there is frequently transsection or attenuation of the pituitary stalk. The hyperintensities of both lipomas and ectopic posterior pituitaries usually lie posterior to the pituitary stalk; this is in contrast to craniopharyngioma and Rathke cleft cyst, which are centered anterior to the pituitary stalk.

Neuroepithelial Hamartoma. Neuroepithelial hamartomas may be composed of disorganized mature neurons (neuronal hamartoma), disorganized glial elements with thickened blood vessels (glial hamartoma), or disorganized neuronal and glial elements (neuronoglial hamartoma). The most common of these hamartomatous conditions is hamartoma of the tuber cinereum (Fig. 2-102) (247–249). This may be associated with precocious puberty, partial complex seizures of the gelastic type, or neurofibromatosis 1. CT demonstrates a suprasellar mass of variable size, of low den-

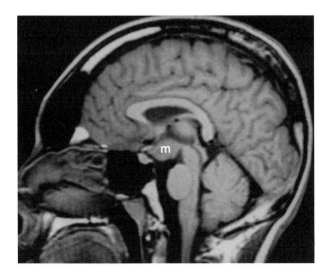

FIG. 2-102. Hypothalamic neuroepithelial hamartoma. A 14-year-old boy with gelastic seizures. Sagittal T1 MRI demonstrates an isointense mass *(m)* of the hypothalamus.

sity or isodense to brain tissue. The mass is T1 isointense and T2 hyperintense. Contrast enhancement is unusual.

Meningioangiomatosis. Meningioangiomatosis is a rare hamartomatous condition that consists of proliferation of arachnoid cells, vessels, and Schwann cells (250).

Epidermoid/Dermoid Tumors. Epidermoid and dermoid tumors, about the third ventricle or elsewhere, tend to be cystic and probably are caused by inclusion of epithelial elements at the time of neural tube closure (214). Epidermoid tumors are of ectodermal origin and are lined with keratinizing stratified squamous epithelium. They often contain desquamated cellular debris and cholesterol, the latter as a breakdown product of keratin. Dermoids are also of ectodermal origin; additional elements include hair, sebaceous glands, and sweat glands. They may contain breakdown products of these structures and secretions. Dermoids may also contain calcification, bone, cartilage, or, rarely, teeth.

Epidermoids commonly occur off the midline. They follow CSF densities and intensities on both CT and MRI. Occasionally, there is cyst wall calcification. Dermoid cysts are midline lesions, contain calcification or formed elements, have fat-like densities and intensities, and may be associated with a congenital dermal sinus and a bony defect (251). It may be impossible to distinguish an epidermoid/dermoid from a teratoma (see Figs. 2-94 and 2-99). Epidermoid/dermoid cyst rupture may be associated with aseptic meningitis and subsequent hydrocephalus.

Supratentorial Tumors

Cerebral tumors may present with seizures, hemiparesis, a movement disorder, headache, other sensory phenomena, increased intracranial pressure, or a cognitive disorder. In infancy, most supratentorial masses are nonneoplastic and ''cystic'' (porencephaly, arachnoid cyst, Galenic varix). Neoplasms, although rare in neonates and young infants, may be astrocytomas, embryonal tumors (PNET), germ cell tumors (teratoma), choroid plexus tumors (papilloma, carcinoma), or mesenchymal tumors (sarcoma, rhabdoid) (Table 2-20) (252–256). In older children and adolescents, most supratentorial tumors are of neuroepithelial origin, including gliomas (astrocytoma, oligodendroglioma, glioblastoma). Other less common tumors include neuronal or mixed neuronal and glial tumors (ganglioglioma, neurocytoma, dysembryoplastic neuroepithelial tumor), and embryonal tumors (PNET). Nonneoplastic supratentorial masses include arachnoid cyst, abscess or empyema, hamartoma, vascular malformation (cavernous malformation, venous anomaly), and hematoma. Extradural, calvarial, and scalp lesions that may encroach on the cerebral hemisphere include metastases, osteoma, dermoid, epidermoid, histiocytosis, hemangioma and other vascular anomalies, fibrous dysplasia, sarcomas, lymphoma, leukemia, neurofibroma, fibroma, fibromatosis, and infection.

TABLE 2-20. *Cerebral tumors*

Glial tumors
    Astrocytoma
    Glioblastoma
    Oligodendroglioma
    Ependymoma
Choroid plexus tumors
    Choroid plexus papilloma
    Choroid plexus carcinoma
Neuronal tumors
    Ganglioglioma
    Dysembryoplastic neuroepithelial tumor
    Central neurocytoma
    Desmoplastic ganglioglioma
Embryonal tumors
    PNET
Meningeal tumors
    Meningioma
Nonmeningothelial mesenchymal tumors
Lymphoma

PNET, primitive neuroectodermal tumor.

Cerebral Glioma

Astrocytic Tumors. Astrocytic tumors account for the majority of gliomas and primary cerebral tumors in childhood. The imaging findings of these supratentorial neoplasms are frequently nonspecific. It may be difficult to differentiate astrocytic tumors from other glial neoplasms as well as to distinguish high-grade from low-grade malignancies. Tumors may be well defined and circumscribed (pilocytic astrocytoma) or ill defined and infiltrating (fibrillary or diffuse astrocytoma). These supratentorial, astrocytic neoplasms may be cystic, solid, or mixed; they may occasionally contain calcification. The tumors are usually isodense or of low density on CT. The tumors are frequently isointense or of low intensity on T1 MRI and isointense to high intensity on T2 images. Contrast enhancement is variable (Fig. 2-103). A well-defined tumor in which contrast enhancement matches T2 hyperintensity suggests a pilocytic astrocytoma. Higher grades of malignancy are suggested by tumor heterogeneity, irregular shape, poor margination, mass effect, edema, hemorrhage, and nodular rim enhancement.

It must be emphasized that imaging characteristics do not correspond well to histologic diagnosis and grade of malignancy. Moreover, distinguishing tumor margin from surrounding edema is difficult. An attempt has been made to characterize these cerebral gliomas by imaging appearance into three categories: central tumor core only (pilocytic astrocytoma, pleomorphic xanthoastrocytoma); central tumor core with isolated peripheral tumor cells (glioblastoma); diffuse tumor cells only (fibrillary or diffuse astrocytoma) (257–261).

As with most other CNS neoplasms, total excision and tumor debulking are preferred to biopsy. Radiation therapy and chemotherapy are important in higher grade tumors as well as recurrent or symptomatic lower grade tumors. High-grade tumors tend to show a rapid response to therapy but recur early; low-grade malignancies demonstrate slower response rates and later recurrence. An increase in tumor volume due to edema may occur after radiation therapy, par-

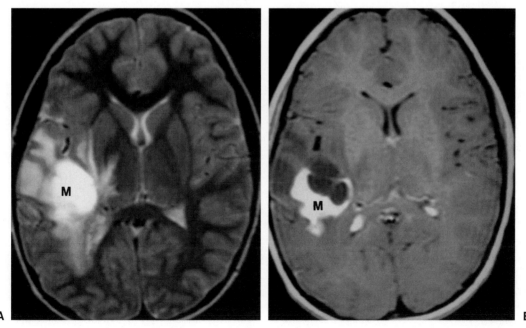

FIG. 2-103. Anaplastic astrocytoma. An 11-year-old boy with seizures. **A:** Axial T2 MRI. Note the hyperintense cystic and solid cerebral mass *(M)* with surrounding hyperintense edema. **B:** Axial gadolinium-enhanced T1 MRI. There is marked enhancement of solid tumor *(M)* components.

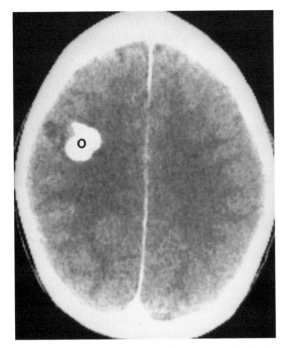

FIG. 2-104. Oligodendroglioma. A 13-year-old girl with seizure disorder. Axial CT demonstrates a right frontal calcified tumor *(O)* with adjacent low-density edema.

ticularly after stereotactic radiosurgery or fractionated radiotherapy.

Glioblastomatous Tumors. Glioblastomatous tumors are considered to be anaplastic forms of astrocytoma (178). They occur primarily in the cerebral hemispheres during adolescence and are the most malignant of the neuroepithelial tumors. They are characterized by CSF metastases and poor survival. Imaging findings are diverse and range from a circumscribed mass to a diffuse infiltrative process. These are usually large tumors with irregular nodular contrast enhancement, a necrotic center, and surrounding vasogenic edema;

calcification is occasionally also present. Glioblastoma may not be easily distinguished from other gliomas by imaging techniques (see Figs. 2-103 and 2-105). Variants include the giant cell glioblastoma and the gliosarcoma. The term *gliomatosis cerebri* refers to the rare entity of diffuse infiltrative glioma that involves multiple sites or large portions of the CNS, usually the cerebral hemispheres (262,263). This term should not be used as a synonym for diffuse leptomeningeal or intraventricular spread of malignant glioma. Imaging often underestimates the extent of tumor involvement in gliomatosis cerebri even with contrast enhancement.

Oligodendroglioma. Oligodendrogliomas are usually located in the white matter but may gradually extend to the periphery of the cortex. Oligodendrogliomas may contain other glial elements; an astrocytic component is most frequent, and the tumor is then referred to as an oligoastrocytoma. Well-differentiated oligodendrogliomas are slow growing and are usually circumscribed (Fig. 2-104) (264–266). Calcification is common (70%) and may be dense, clumped, or rim-like. There may be an associated thin-walled cyst. The tumor itself is usually an isodense or low-density mass on CT. Calcification, despite being obvious on CT, may go unnoticed on MRI (Fig. 2-105). Oligodendroglioma is usually isointense or of low intensity on T1 images and isointense to hyperintense on T2-weighted images.

Ependymoma

Although much less common, supratentorial ependyomas have imaging characteristics similar to those of the posterior fossa. These tumors may project from the ependymal surface of a lateral ventricle or arise from ependymal cell rests (178,209). Calcification and cyst formation are typical features. Differentiation from astrocytoma and oligodendroglioma is difficult (see Fig. 2-105).

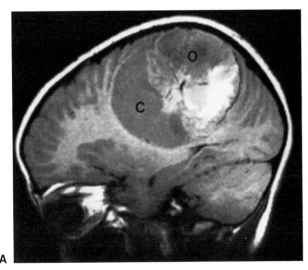
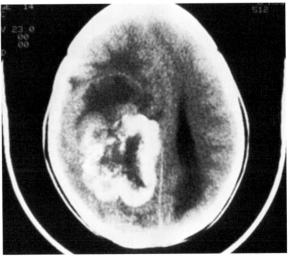

FIG. 2-105. Oligodendroglioma. A: Tumor *(O)* is isointense on T1-weighted MRI. Hyperintense signal represents previous hemorrhage. A hypointense cyst *(C)* lies anterior to the mass. **B:** Calcification demonstrated by CT was not appreciated by MRI.

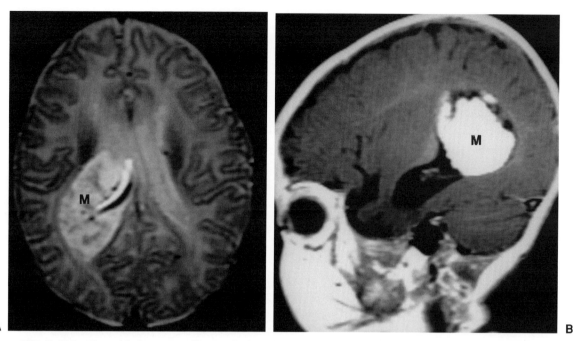

FIG. 2-106. Choroid plexus papilloma. A: Axial T2 MRI. There is high-intensity right lateral intraventricular mass *(M)* with vascular hypointensities. **B:** Gadolinium-enhanced sagittal T1 MRI. Marked enhancement of the intraventricular tumor *(M)* is shown.

Choroid Plexus Tumors

Choroid plexus tumors arise from epithelial cells of the choroid plexus and are considered by most to belong to the neuroectodermal group of neoplasms. They account for approximately 2% of all intracranial neoplasms in children. They can arise wherever choroid plexus is present (lateral ventricles, third ventricle, fourth ventricle, and lateral recesses of the fourth ventricle) but most frequently occur in a lateral ventricle, especially in the region of the trigone; 80% are benign and slow growing (267–269). Papillomas are usually circumscribed intraventricular tumors (270). Carcinomas are invasive, frequently extend beyond the ventricular margins, and are associated with mass effect as well as edema. The most common clinical presentation is hydrocephalus, which may be due to overproduction of CSF or ventricular obstruction or both (271).

These tumors are characterized by their marked vascularity and their frequent trigonal location. CT and MRI demonstrate an intraventricular mass with marked contrast enhancement (Fig. 2-106).

Neuronal Tumors

Common neuronal and mixed neuronal-glial tumors of the cerebrum include ganglioglioma, dysembryoplastic neuroepithelial tumor, and neurocytoma (272–276). Gangliogliomas are often circumscribed cystic or calcified, are frequently associated with focal seizures, and usually demonstrate contrast enhancement (273,276,277). CT shows isodense or hypodense tumor matrix, whereas MRI shows T1

isointensity or hypointensity with proton density and T2 isointensity to hyperintensity (Fig. 2-107). Desmoplastic gangliogliomas are often cystic and characteristically occur in infancy (278). Dysembryoplastic neuroepithelial tumors are typically associated with intractable seizures of the partial-complex type (275). These tumors are well defined and cause little or no edema. Mass effect and cortical effacement, if present at all, are usually subtle. Nodularity is characteristic, whereas focal contrast enhancement, calcification, and cystic change are present less frequently (Fig. 2-108). Focal erosion of the adjacent bony calvaria may be associated with cortical lesions. Central neurocytomas typically occur about the lateral ventricles, often in the region of the foramen of Monro (274). Calcification is common. The differential diagnosis includes oligodendroglioma, ependymoma, and cerebral neuroblastoma.

Embryonal Tumors

The common embryonal tumors arising within the cerebral hemispheres are PNETs and (less often) primary cerebral neuroblastoma (279–282). Imaging demonstrates a large hemispheric mass with calcification or cyst formation, sometimes hemorrhage, and variable edema (Fig. 2-109). CT shows an isodense or hyperdense homogeneous tumor or mixed-density tumor matrix. Contrast enhancement is common and may be either homogeneous or nonuniform. The MRI appearance is somewhat variable; tumor matrix is usually isointense or hypointense on T1-weighted images and isointense or hypointense with surrounding hyperintense

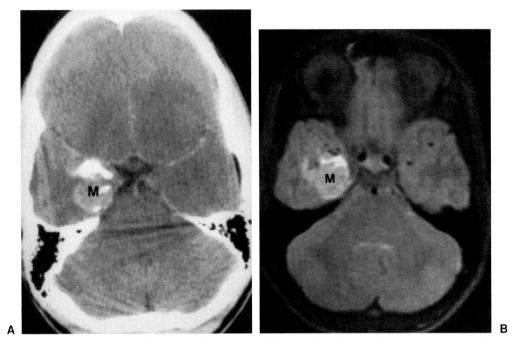

FIG. 2-107. Temporal ganglioglioma. A 12-year-old boy with seizures. **A:** Axial contrast-enhanced CT. There is calcified and enhancing right temporal lobe tumor *(M)*. **B:** Axial T2 MRI. The tumor mass *(M)* contains calcific hypointensities.

edema on proton density and T2-weighted images. The CT density and MRI intensity correlate with tumor cellularity. The CT and MRI appearances and the marked contrast enhancement are often characteristic (Fig. 2-109).

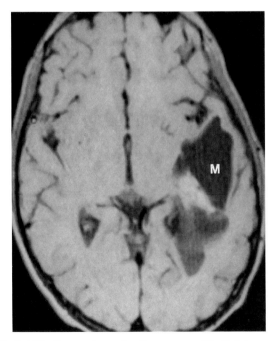

FIG. 2-108. Dysembryoplastic neuroepithelial tumor. A 13-year-old boy with seizures. Axial T1 MRI demonstrates a left temporal lobe tumor *(M)* containing solid and cystic components.

Meningeal Tumors

Meningiomas are the most common tumors of meningeal origin. They occur more commonly in adults than in children, are more frequent in females, are commonly associated with neurofibromatosis type 2, and may be induced by radiation (283–286). They most commonly occur in the parafalcine location but may arise anywhere in the meninges. Menngiomas arising in the brain substance and the ventricular system presumably arise from the perivascular meningeal tissues and the meningeal core of the choroid plexus. Meningiomas are frequently calcified and may be highly vascular. Imaging often demonstrates a well-defined extracerebral or intraventricular mass with calcification. If the tumor arises next to the skull, lytic or blastic (hyperostotic) bony involvement is usually present (287–289). The mass is often isodense or hyperdense on CT. MRI demonstrates T1 isointensity or hypointensity and proton density/T2 isointensity or hyperintensity. Marked contrast enhancement is common. Intrinsic punctate, nodular, or linear low intensities seen by MRI represent either calcification or vessels. A sharp interface with brain is often apparent by MRI; this may represent CSF, edema, vascularization, or dural thickening. Occasionally, there is striking edema or gliosis of the underlying brain.

Other nonmeningothelial mesenchymal tumors arising from the meninges include various benign and malignant neoplasms (see Table 2-17). Examples are meningeal sarcomatosis and rhabdoid tumor. The malignant mesenchymal or sarcomatous neoplasms of meningeal origin demonstrate a variety of findings including CT isodensity or hyperdensity

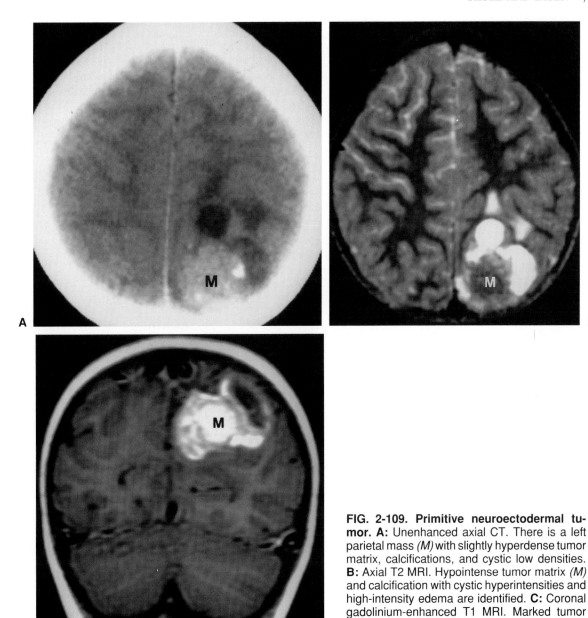

FIG. 2-109. Primitive neuroectodermal tumor. A: Unenhanced axial CT. There is a left parietal mass *(M)* with slightly hyperdense tumor matrix, calcifications, and cystic low densities. **B:** Axial T2 MRI. Hypointense tumor matrix *(M)* and calcification with cystic hyperintensities and high-intensity edema are identified. **C:** Coronal gadolinium-enhanced T1 MRI. Marked tumor *(M)* enhancement is shown.

and contrast enhancement. There is T1 isointensity or hypointensity and proton density/T2 isointensity, hyperintensity, or hypointensity; the neoplasms enhance with contrast. Cystic or necrotic components may have ring enhancement and edema.

Primary melanocytic lesions of the meninges include melanosis, melanocytoma, melanoma, and melanomatosis (290–292). Melanin-containing tumors may be suspected by CT hyperdensity and by T1 hyperintensity. Proton density/ T2 hypointensity depends on the concentration of melanin in the tumor and the presence or absence of hemorrhage.

Hematologic Malignancies

Secondary involvement of the CNS by lymphoid and other hematologic malignancies is extremely uncommon in childhood. It sometimes occurs in patients with congenital or acquired immunodeficiency disorders, including AIDS (293,294).

Parameningeal and Metastatic Tumors

Parameningeal tumors or tumor-like processes are those that arise just outside the dura (Table 2-21) (7). They may encroach on or invade the intracranial structures with or without producing specific neurologic symptoms or signs. Parameningeal tumors may arise from or involve the scalp, cranial vault, cranial base, sinuses or pharynx, orbits, petrous temporal structures, or soft tissues of the face or neck (295–297). Although invasive parameningeal processes are often histologically malignant, benign neoplasms and non-neoplastic processes occasionally resemble malignant tu-

TABLE 2-21. *Parameningeal tumors and metastatic disease*

Mesenchymal	Neural tumors
Rhabdomyosarcoma	Neuroblastoma
Histiocytosis	PNET
Fibromatosis	Plexiform neurofibroma
Angiofibroma	
Other sarcomas	

PNET, primitive neuroectodermal tumor.

mors in their aggressiveness. Dysplastic conditions may also be associated with bony defects or soft tissue masses and mimic neoplasms; neurofibromatosis type 1 is an example. The common parameningeal tumors of childhood are metastatic neuroblastoma (Fig. 2-110) (297), rhabdomyosarcoma (Fig. 2-111), histiocytosis (Fig. 2-112), plexiform neurofibroma, and angiofibroma. The presence and extent of intracranial involvement often affect therapy drastically. With recent advances in craniofacial and skull base surgery, ablation of the tumor may be possible without sacrificing function or appearance. In cases with intracranial involvement, surgery may serve primarily to establish the diagnosis and the extent of disease. Tumor debulking is sometimes done before chemotherapy and radiotherapy. Imaging often requires CT for bony involvement and calcification as well as MRI for soft tissue components and vascularity. Ultrasonography distinguishes cystic from solid masses of the head and neck, guides needle aspiration and biopsy, and may be used for follow-up.

The CNS may also be involved by metastases from primary CNS neoplasms or from neoplasms arising elsewhere. Some primary CNS neoplasms, especially embryonal tumors, malignant gliomas, and germ cell tumors, commonly metastasize via the subarachnoid space (298–301). Most metastatic neoplasms arising from non-CNS tumors are blood-borne, although the subarachnoid space provides a mechanism for further spread of tumors originally reaching the CNS originally by direct extension. Other than CNS involvement by systemic neoplasia such as leukemia, lymphoma, Langerhans cell histiocytosis, and neuroblastoma, hematogenous metastasis to the brain from a distant primary tumor occurs less frequently in children than in adults. CT or MRI may demonstrate single or multiple masses, often enhancing, sometimes with variable edema. Hemorrhage and calcification may also occur.

Trauma

Head trauma in childhood may be divided into parturitional and postnatal trauma. The immaturity of the brain and calvarium coupled with forces present during birth result in a unique set of injuries in the neonate. As brain and skull maturation progress, the manifestations of intracranial trauma become more like those encountered in the adult.

Parturitional Trauma

Extracranial hemorrhages associated with labor and delivery include caput succedaneum, subgaleal hemorrhage, and cephalohematoma (146). Caput succedaneum is a self-limited subcutaneous hemorrhage, with a large component of edema, frequently seen after vaginal delivery. Subgaleal hemorrhage occurs beneath the aponeurosis of the occipito-

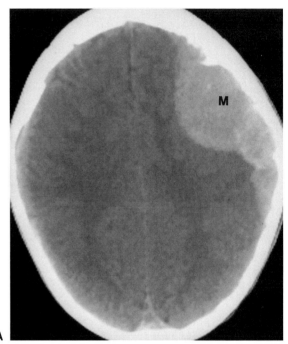

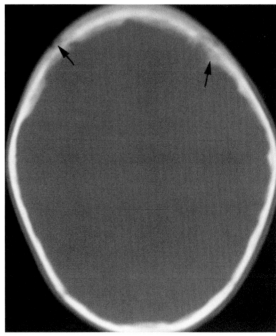

FIG. 2-110. Metastatic neuroblastoma. A 1-year-old girl with abdominal neuroblastoma. Axial contrast-enhanced CT **(A, B)**. Enhancing epidural intracranial masses *(M)* with associated bony calvarial permeative destruction *(arrows)* are shown.

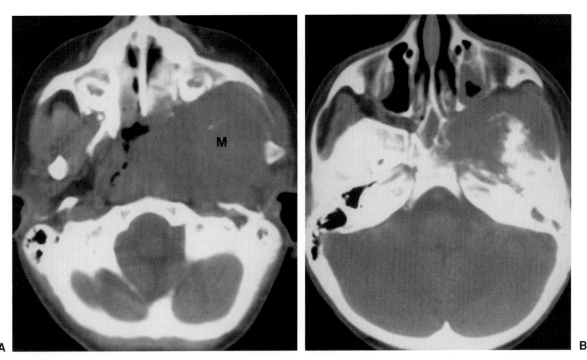

FIG. 2-111. Infratemporal rhabdomyosarcoma. Axial CT. There is a large left retromaxillary and infratemporal mass *(M)* with associated bony destruction, and intracranial extension through the floor of the middle cranial fossa.

frontalis muscle. The hemorrhage is usually asymptomatic unless very large. A cephalohematoma is a subperiosteal hemorrhage; it is very common and is seen most frequently with forceps deliveries and vacuum extractions. Because the hemorrhage is beneath the periosteum, a cephalohematoma

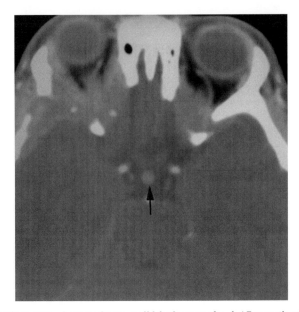

FIG. 2-112. Langerhans cell histiocytosis. A 15-month-old boy with proptosis and diabetes insipidus. Contrast-enhanced axial CT demonstrates bilateral enhancing orbital masses and bony destruction. There is nodular enhancement of the thickened pituitary stalk *(arrow)*.

typically does not cross a suture. The bleeding is usually self-limited and is very rarely associated with a skull fracture. A cephalohematoma may later calcify and present as a skull mass (Fig. 2-113); it may mimic a soft tissue tumor or a depressed skull fracture. Calcified cephalohematomas gradually disappear over a period of months or years.

Neonatal skull fractures may be linear or depressed. Linear fractures most frequently occur in the parietal bone. Cephalohematomas sometimes co-exist. Normal structures such as sutures and parietal fissures (see Fig. 2-11) can be confused with fractures. Linear fractures are treated conservatively. Depressed fractures readily occur during the neonatal period because of the thinness of the calvarial bones. There may be a broad area of depression in the ''ping-pong'' fracture. Depressed fractures are best evaluated with CT which demonstrates the depressed and angulated fragments of bone and their relationship to the brain. Occasionally, there are congenital depressions of the cranial vault secondary to prolonged, focal, in utero pressure on the skull; these may mimic a depressed fracture. These congenital depressions usually resolve spontaneously, whereas most depressed skull fractures may require elevation.

The trauma associated with birth occasionally produces intracranial hemorrhage. Posterior fossa subdural hemorrhage may result from tentorial laceration or traumatic occipital osteodiastasis. Tentorial tears may be associated with rupture of the vein of Galen or straight sinus. Massive posterior fossa bleeding may occur and cause brainstem compression or hydrocephalus. More commonly, tears in tentorial or infratentorial cortical veins produce only a small asymp-

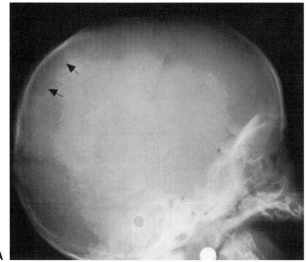

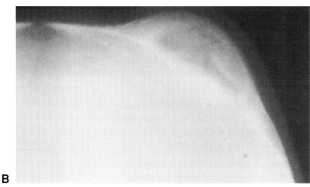

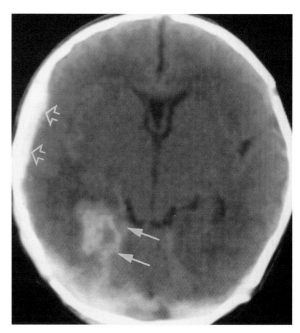

FIG. 2-114. Hemorrhage following vacuum extraction delivery. Newborn infant. Axial CT demonstrates high-density hemorrhage *(closed arrows)* along the tentorium on the right, and along the tentorium and dural venous sinuses posteriorly. A small right frontotemporal subdural hemorrhage is also noted *(open arrows)*.

FIG. 2-113. Calcified cephalohematoma. A 4-month-old boy with a palpable mass of the left parietal region. **A:** Curvilinear density *(arrows)* with posterior lucency is noted in the parietal bone. **B:** Coned-down Towne view shows the calcifying cephalohematoma. There is crescentic peripheral calcification with a central lucency.

tomatic posterior fossa subdural hematoma, discovered incidentally on US, CT, or MRI (Fig. 2-114). Occipital osteodiastasis is a traumatic separation of the occipital squamosa from the paired bones of the exocciput. Severe diastasis may cause a tear in the occipital sinus, massive posterior fossa bleeding, and cerebellar laceration. Infratentorial bleeding may be associated with supratentorial hemorrhage.

Supratentorial subdural hemorrhages in the neonate are usually the result of laceration of the falx or a superficial cerebral vein and may be associated with forceps delivery or vacuum extraction (Figs. 2-114 and 2-115). An adjacent fracture may be present. Lacerations of the falx are less common than tears of the tentorium. Rupture of the inferior sagittal sinus, which may also occur, produces an interhemispheric subdural hematoma near the genu of the corpus callosum (146). Laceration of a cortical vein produces a subdural hematoma over the cerebrum. Convexity subdurals in neonates are usually unilateral; those in older infants and children are more frequently bilateral (6). Parturitional intracerebral and intraventricular hemorrhage is unusual, particularly in the absence of extracerebral hemorrhage.

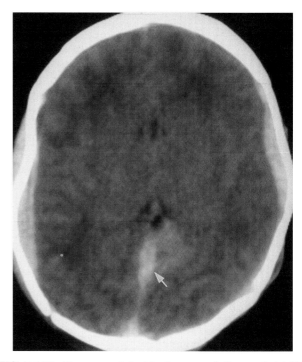

FIG. 2-115. Trauma related to forceps delivery. Axial CT. Depressed right temporal fracture and bilateral high-density subdural hemorrhages. High-density hemorrhage is also shown along the left tentorium and along the straight sinus *(arrow).*

Postnatal Trauma

Postnatal head trauma in children has a spectrum of imaging findings similar to that in adults. However, the clinical manifestations and the etiologies of trauma in childhood are very different. Loss of consciousness, a frequent presentation of adult head injury, is uncommon in children less than 1 year of age. At that age, nonaccidental trauma is 10–15 times as common as accidental head injury (302).

Skull Fractures

Head trauma involves sudden acceleration and immediate deceleration of the intracranial contents compared with the bony vault and dural edges (303). Trauma in the child may be associated with sufficient distortion of the cranial vault to produce a skull fracture, which merely confirms that a significant force was applied. The brain of the infant is surrounded by large amounts of CSF over the convexity and at the base separating it from the cranial vault. Movement of the brain within the bony vault may be therefore considerable (303). The morphology of cerebral injuries during infancy differ from those in the adult. Contrecoup injuries occur in only 10% of children under 3 years of age and in 25% of children 3–4 years of age, in contrast to the 85% incidence in adults (303). Skull fractures may occur at the inbending of the cranial vault due to direct local pressure or at the secondary peripheral outbending of the vault. Traumatic suture separation (Fig. 2-116) reflects the same type and degree of force applied to the cranial vault as a skull fracture (303).

Skull fractures, including simple linear fractures, diastatic fractures, and depressed fractures, are relatively common in children. Nine percent of children have serious sequelae (subdural hematoma, extradural hematoma, brain injury) to their head injuries (303). The incidence of serious sequelae is similar in patients with or without a skull fracture (304). The presence of a skull fracture does not necessarily indicate intracranial injury, and the absence of fracture does not preclude it (304–307). A child with a normal neurologic evaluation and a simple linear skull fracture has the same chance of serious intracranial sequelae as a child without a skull fracture, and they should be treated in the same manner (304).

Simple linear skull fractures tend to occur away from the point of impact along the area of outbending of the skull (303). Multiple comminuted linear fractures may occur, particularly in infants, without depression or sutural diastasis. Linear nondepressed fractures are more frequent in children less than 2 years of age (see Fig. 2-116), whereas depressed fractures are more common in older children (Fig. 2-117). Linear fractures may be straight or irregular. They may also be diastatic without being depressed. Healing of linear skull fractures requires only 3–6 months in an infant but up to a year in older children (303).

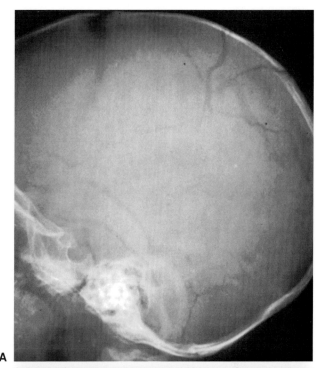

A

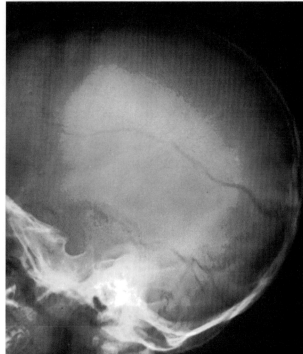

B

FIG. 2-116. Skull fractures. A: Stellate parietal skull fracture in a 7-month-old battered child. **B:** Long, linear, parietal skull fracture is due to a vehicular accident. There is associated bilateral coronal sutural diastasis.

Approximately 25% of skull fractures in children are depressed (303). Depressed fractures are usually due to birth trauma in the neonate and either automobile accidents or a direct blow to the head in older infants and children (see Fig. 2-117). The most frequent site of a depressed skull fracture in children is the parietal bone (46%) followed by the frontal

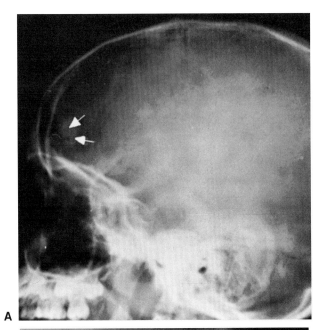

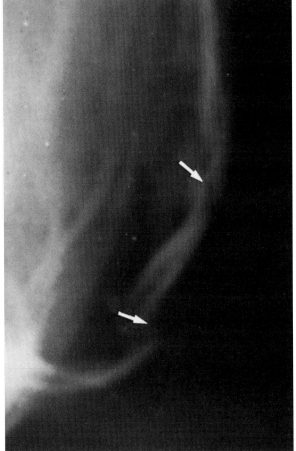

FIG. 2-117. Depressed skull fracture. An 8-year-old boy was struck above the left orbit by his father's golf club. **A:** Lateral skull radiograph shows an oval density *(arrows)* of the frontal bone. **B:** Tangential fluoroscopic spot film. Note the depressed fragment of bone with offsets of the cranial vault *(arrows).*

bone (33%), occipital bone (11%), and temporal bone (10%) (303). This distribution reflects the relative thickness of bone and bony buttressing in these regions. Dural tears are present in approximately one third of children with depressed fractures. There may be concomitant brain damage, but associated subdural or extradural hematomas are uncommon (303). A sclerotic line in the cranial vault on a radiograph after trauma should be considered a depressed fracture (see Fig. 2-117) and requires CT for evaluation of intracranial structures and to demonstrate the fracture fragments if surgery is contemplated. Surgical repair depends on the degree of deformity. If the outer table is not depressed beyond the border of the inner table, the depression is usually not serious unless it overlies a vital cortical area.

The gross overutilization of skull radiographs for evaluating children with head trauma contributes not only to the increasing costs of health care but also to unnecessary radiation exposure (305,306,308). The major clinical consideration in patients with head trauma is the extent of injury not of the skull but of the brain and cranial contents. The presence or absence of a fracture, without neurologic deficits, almost never affects therapy (303,304,306,308,309). Skull radiography should be based on medical considerations alone (310). If there are no medical considerations, no legal considerations exist. A skull fracture only verifies that there has been cranial trauma; the decision to obtain CT is based on neurologic findings and not on the presence or absence of a skull fracture.

If it is important that a skull fracture should not go undetected, application of the high-risk criteria of Bell and Loop (308) with modifications (303) should decrease the number of skull radiographs in pediatric head trauma by at least 50%. Valid clinical indications for skull radiography of pediatric patients with trauma include possible radiopaque foreign body, possible depressed skull fracture, suspicion of child abuse, possible CSF leak from the nose or ear, and objective neurologic findings. Strong clinical evidence of depressed skull fracture, CSF leak, or neurologic deficit is an indication for CT. Positive plain film findings as above or neurologic findings warrant the performance of cranial CT; most skull fractures can be verified on the scout view or on axial images. Neither radiography nor CT should be performed in low-risk situations. Prompt performance of CT is waranted in patients with high-risk criteria (306,308). These principles should decrease the number of unnecessary skull radiographs and imaging evaluations in children with head trauma.

Leptomeningeal Cyst

Leptomeningeal cysts (growing skull fractures) are infrequent, late complications of skull fractures in infants and children (15,303,304). These posttraumatic cysts are encapsulated fluid collections within the arachnoid space surrounded by adhesions. The initial skull fracture is usually

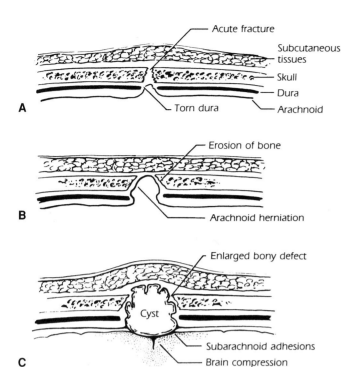

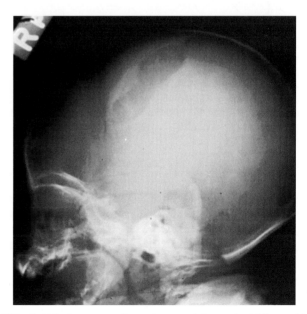

FIG. 2-118. Pathophysiology of leptomeningeal cyst. A: Dural tear associated with initial diastatic fracture. B: Dural defect allows herniation of arachnoid with subsequent erosion of bone due to transmitted cerebrospinal fluid pulsations. C: Subarachnoid adhesions produce a walled-off cyst with further bone erosion. There is compression of underlying brain with development of parenchymal injury and porencephaly.

linear and diastatic. Leptomeningeal cysts occur most frequently in children less than 3 years of age, presumably because of the close adherence of the dura to the skull during infancy and early childhood, which predisposes to a dural tear with fracture. The postulated mechanism for a growing skull fracture is a tear of the dura underneath an acute fracture and subsequent herniation of fluid-filled arachnoid tissue through the dural defect. The arachnoid fluid is surrounded by subarachnoid adhesions that form an encapsulated cyst (Fig. 2-118). The continuous, pulsatile pressure of CSF causes cyst enlargement toward the overlying skull fracture and the underlying brain parenchyma. This outward cyst extension not only prevents fracture healing but causes widening of the edges of the fracture through bone erosion (Fig. 2-119). The enlarging cyst also compresses underlying brain parenchyma and may cause occlusion of cerebrocortical vessels and subsequent porencephaly. There is always some encephalomalacia beneath a leptomeningeal cyst. Other complications of growing skull fractures are cerebral herniation through the bony defect and pseudoaneurysm formation.

This potential complication should be kept in mind in any infant or young child with a diastatic skull fracture. Erosion of the skull vault may begin as soon as 2 months after the fracture (5). Examination shows a soft, fluctuant, slowly enlarging pulsatile mass. A careful clinical evaluation should

be performed 4–6 weeks after a diastatic skull fracture in an infant and then again at 3–4 months. If this clinical follow-up shows enlargement of the fracture defect or a soft tissue mass, imaging evaluation is indicated. Prompt surgical removal of a leptomeningeal cyst may prevent serious, irreversible neurologic damage.

Radiography shows a soft tissue mass with an underlying smooth skull defect. The leptomeningeal cyst typically produces an oval area of bony erosion with scalloped margins (see Fig. 2-119). CT confirms the bony defect and the leptomeningeal cyst. MRI better evaluates the amount of herniated cerebral tissue in the bony defect, the presence or absence of ventricular dilatation, and the presence of encephalomalacia or porencephaly. There may also be subgaleal and subdural fluid collections. Angiography may be required to diagnose an associated pseudoaneurysm.

Intracranial Hemorrhage and Parenchymal Injury

As in adults, the most common imaging finding in acute intracranial injury in childhood is hemorrhage. Delineation of the anatomic compartment involved and the extent of the hemorrhage is critical. In the emergency setting, CT remains the imaging modality of choice (6,15,16). Extraparenchymal hemorrhages may be epidural, subdural, or subarachnoid (Fig. 2-120). Although hemorrhage in one compartment may predominate, all three may be involved. Traumatic parenchymal lesions include contusion, hematoma, shear injury, and edema.

Epidural Hematoma. An epidural or extradural hema-

FIG. 2-119. **Leptomeningeal cyst.** A 7-week-old boy with palpable left parietal scalp mass following a diastatic skull fracture at 1 week of age. Lateral skull film shows a left parietal bony lucency with scalloped margins. CT confirmed a leptomeningeal cyst.

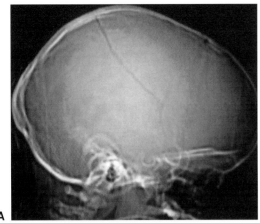

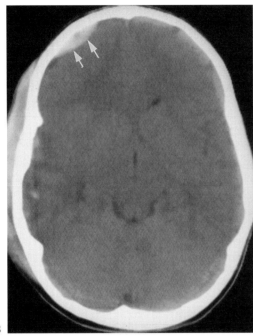

FIG. 2-120. Epidural hematoma. A 2-year-old girl with head trauma. **A:** CT scout projection image. Diastatic parietal skull fracture is well demonstrated. **B:** Axial CT. Right temporal lobe low densities with smaller high densities are due to contusions. There is a right frontal high-density epidural hematoma *(arrows)*. A scalp hematoma is also present on the right.

toma is a collection of blood between the cranial vault and the dura mater. Less than 1% of children with craniocerebral trauma have an epidural hematoma (5). Epidural hematomas are particularly uncommon in young infants. Most epidural hematomas in children are caused by a fall; there is blunt trauma to a limited area of the vault, which causes inbending of the skull, stripping of the dura from the inner table during rebound, and tearing of crossing vessels (303). Epidural hematomas in young children are due to torn meningeal arteries or veins. Rarely, ventricular shunting and decrease in intracranial volume cause an epidural hematoma.

Epidural hematomas usually involve the parietal or temporal regions; sometimes there is extension into the frontal or occipital area. There is an associated skull fracture in 40%

of children (see Fig. 2-120), compared to an 80% to 90% occurrence in adults (30). The most common source of bleeding is the posterior branch of the middle meningeal artery and its accompanying veins. Other potential bleeding sites include the main meningeal artery, anterior meningeal artery branch, dural sinus, and dural blood vessels. Posterior fossa epidural hematomas may be venous in origin.

As previously noted, most children with epidural hematoma do not have a skull fracture. An acute epidural hematoma contains fresh blood, which has a higher attenuation coefficient value than normal brain tissue (Fig. 2-120B). On CT, an acute epidural hematoma is seen as a zone of increased density between the cranial vault and brain with a medially convex contour; it is usually limited by the sutures. Infantile acute epidural hematomas, more often the result of a venous tear than an arterial laceration, are frequently of mixed density because of active hemorrhage.

The MRI signal characteristics of an epidural hematoma depend on the age of the hemorrhage. Hyperacute hemorrhage containing oxyhemoglobin will be hypointense on T1- and hyperintense on T2-weighted images. During the next several hours, the hemoglobin becomes deoxygenated, T2 shortening occurs, and the hematoma becomes hypointense on T2-weighted images. A fluid-fluid level may be identified.

In the subacute phase, deoxyhemoglobin is converted to methemoglobin. Initially, this methemoglobin is intracellular and causes T1 shortening (hyperintense signal) and T2 shortening (hypointense signal). Extracellular methemoglobin caused by later breakdown of red blood cell membranes decreases the susceptibility effect on T2-weighted images. Thus, during the late subacute and chronic phases, the hematoma is hyperintense on both T1- and T2-weighted images.

In contrast to an acute epidural hematoma, an acute subdural hematoma usually has a concave contour toward the brain. A shift of midline structures more than the thickness of the epidural hematoma indicates traumatic edema or contusion in the underlying brain. Although epidural hematomas in children are usually convex, they occasionally may be crescentic, especially in the posterior fossa. In addition to localized displacement of cerebral vessels away from the inner table, angiography, if performed, may show displacement of the dural sinus inward from the inner table, dural sinus rupture or thrombosis, displacement of meningeal arteries, extravasation from meningeal arteries, and meningeal arteriovenous fistulas.

Subdural Hematoma. A subdural hematoma is a posttraumatic collection of serosanguineous fluid between the arachnoid and dura mater. There is considerable pathologic overlap between subdural hematomas and subdural hygromas, which may occur after meningitis or trauma. If the subdural fluid contains hemosiderin, detected pathologically or by MRI, this indicates a posttraumatic subdural hematoma. Subdural hematomas are due to a tear of the veins bridging the subdural space; these veins are particularly vulnerable to injury in the young infant due to the softness of the underlying unmyelinated brain.

Subdural hematomas are more common in infants than older children. Child abuse is an increasing cause of subdural hematomas in children less than 1 year of age. The most common cause in older infants and children is also trauma, explained or unexplained. The frequent cause of subdural hematoma in the abused child is direct trauma or forceful shaking. In those patients MRI may identify subdural hematomas not previously detected by CT (48). Subdural hematomas may be clinically silent in young infants with open sutures; common presentations are an enlarging head in a young child or increased intracranial pressure in an older child. Subdural hemorrhage in the absence of a convincing clinical history should always raise the suspicion of child abuse.

Supratentorial subdural hematomas are usually extensive and involve the parietal, frontal, and temporal regions. Up to 85% are bilateral, and there is frequently an associated interhemispheric hematoma (6). Only 10% of subdural hematomas in children are located in the posterior fossa.

Subdural hematomas are second only to hydrocephalus as a cause of an enlarging head in infants and children (5). A skull fracture occasionally accompanies a subdural hematoma (303). If the hematoma is acute and contains fresh blood, it is seen by CT as a crescentic area of increased attenuation between the inner table of the skull and the cerebral cortex (see Fig. 2-115). After several weeks, subdural hematomas are isodense on noncontrast CT. Contrast enhancement will aid in the visualization of these isodense collections by enhancement of subdural membranes or septations as well as by the demonstration of inward displacement of cortical vessels. MRI is also extremely helpful in verifying subdural hemorrhages in this subacute phase, because the collections will have a different signal characteristic from CSF. Chronic subdural hematomas have density and signal characteristics similar to those of CSF.

On occasion, particularly by CT, it may be difficult to distinguish chronic subdural hematomas from benign external hydrocephalus in an infant with macrocephaly. The differentiation, however, is important because subdural hematomas are usually traumatic, and benign external hydrocephalus is a self-limited, often familial, condition resulting from immaturity of the arachnoid granulations. Benign external hydrocephalus typically resolves by 2 years of age. Features consistent with benign external hydrocephalus are mild dilatation of the ventricular system and extracerebral CSF spaces, especially over the frontal lobes. The gyri are not compressed, the fluid collection follows CSF on all pulse sequences, and the cortical vessels pass through the collection. By contrast, chronic subdural hematomas will have a signal intensity different from that of CSF, compress gyri, and displace cortical vessels toward the brain surface.

Rarely, calcification occurs in a chronic subdural hematoma. It is seen more frequently in subdural hematomas developing after shunting for hydrocephalus than in purely traumatic hematomas. This calcification may become dense and even progress to ossification. There may be an irregular focal calcific density, a diffuse and floccular density, or a localized, oval, calcified mass. Calcification may occur as soon as 6 months after a subdural hematoma but more frequently occurs after 1–2 years (5). Calcification usually involves the arachnoid as well as the organized hematoma.

Parenchymal Injury. The types of parenchymal injury caused by head trauma are similar in the child and the adult: laceration, contusion, shearing injury, hemorrhage, and focal edema. Many children with a subdural or epidural hematoma also have brain parenchymal contusion or hemorrhage. Contusion of the brain may be due to local inbending and deformity of the skull (coup injury), or the force may be transferred to the opposite pole of the brain (contracoup). The inferior surface and pole of the frontal lobe and the pole of the temporal and occipital lobes are frequently involved in contracoup injuries. Cortical contusions occur as the brain slides over the irregular internal surface of the cranium; the usual mechanism is an acceleration-deceleration injury. Diffuse axonal shear injury results from translational forces on the brain and is often located at the gray-white matter junctions, the corpus callosum, the deep white matter, and the dorsolateral midbrain (Fig. 2-121). Hemorrhage is usually found in these lesions, particularly if they are studied with gradient-echo MRI. The most frequent sites of intracerebral hematoma are the frontal (35%) and the parietal lobes (35%) with the temporal lobe, occipital lobe, and posterior fossa being involved much less commonly.

Unenhanced CT readily determines the presence of acute bleeding in the brain (Fig. 2-122). It can also identify associated skull fractures, midline shift, other hematomas, subarachnoid or intraventricular hemorrhage, and edema. Midline shift and mass effect are frequently much greater than

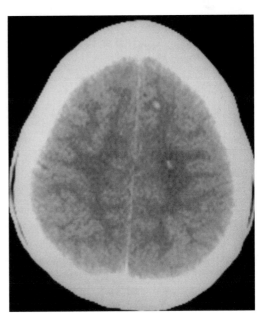

FIG. 2-121. Shear injury. A 14-year-old boy with head trauma. Axial CT. Small, punctate, high-density hemorrhages are present within the left cerebral white matter.

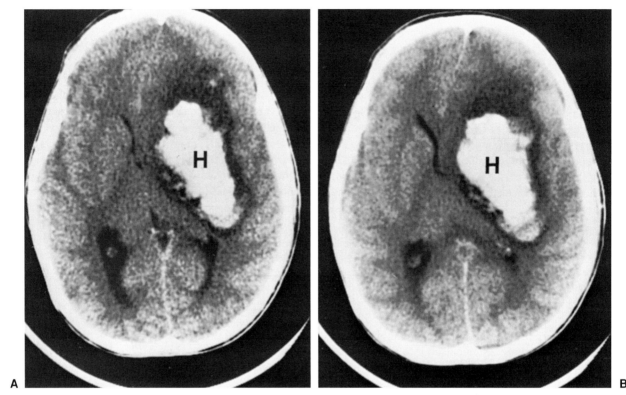

A B

FIG. 2-122. Intraparenchymal hematoma. High-density mass *(H)* in the region of the left basal ganglia with significant mass effect on the ventricular system is caused by a large hematoma.

the size of the hematoma itself because of the coexisting cerebral edema. Massive brain injury may cause severe generalized edema and nonvisualization of the ventricles and subarachnoid spaces on CT despite the paucity of focal brain abnormalities. MRI is more sensitive than CT to the subacute and chronic sequelae of head trauma.

Subarachnoid Hemorrhage. Subarachnoid hemorrhage is common after head injury and often accompanies parenchymal trauma. CT is more sensitive to acute subarachnoid hemorrhage than conventional MRI techniques, in which the signal intensity of oxygenated hemoglobin parallels that of CSF (311). CT demonstrates subarachnoid hemorrhage as high density extending into the sulci, fissures, and cisternas or layering along the tentorium.

Vascular Trauma

Vascular trauma resulting in dissection or a pseudoaneurysm is most frequently seen in young boys. The injury may be penetrating or nonpenetrating; sometimes there is no history of significant injury (312). Occasionally multiple vessels are involved. Dissections of the internal carotid artery typically involve the cervical or supraclinoid segments (313). Dissections of the vertebrobasilar system are most common in the vertebral artery at the level of C1–2. Dissections of intracranial vessels are uncommon but do occur. Dissections are usually diagnosed because of distal embolic

complications. Pseudoaneurysms may produce local hemorrhage.

The MRI and MRA appearances of dissections are described later in this chapter. By conventional angiography, dissections are recognized by tapering or occlusion of the involved vessel. A pseudoaneurysm may or may not be present. The parent vessel may rarely have a beaded appearance indicative of underlying fibromuscular dysplasia.

Child Abuse

Intracranial injury is the leading cause of death and disability in child abuse. The spectrum of lesions encountered is similar to those produced by accidental injury; subdural and subarachnoid hemorrhages, cortical contusions, axonal shear injury, and cerebral edema may all be found. Child abuse should be strongly suspected when the severity of the injury is out of proportion to the history or when injuries of varying ages are present. Intracranial lesions which are particularly suspicious for child abuse are interhemispheric subdural hematoma (shaken-impact injury) (15,16) and subdural hematoma associated with hypoxic-ischemic injury or infarction (strangulation/suffocation injury) (Fig. 2-123). When these findings are encountered, additional signs of nonaccidental trauma such as retinal hemorrhages, posterior rib fractures, metaphyseal fractures, and long bone fractures of varying ages should be sought (see Chapter 5).

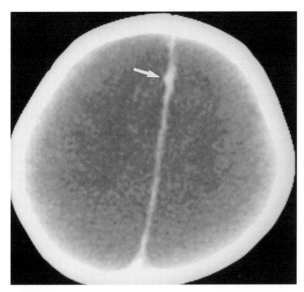

FIG. 2-123. Child abuse. Axial CT. A 6-month-old infant was found comatose. High-density interhemispheric subdural hemorrhage *(arrow)* and bilateral cerebral low densities with loss of gray-white matter differentiation are identified. This is consistent with severe hypoxic-ischemic brain injury.

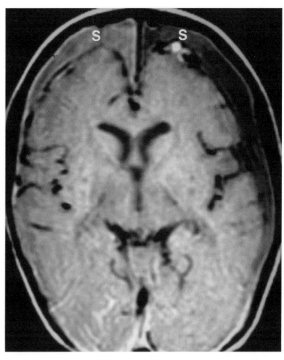

FIG. 2-124. Child abuse. Axial proton density MRI in a 7-month-old infant. Bilateral subdural hematomas *(S)* of differing ages are present.

Plain radiographs of the skull may be useful in diagnosing nonaccidental trauma. Stellate, multiple, bilateral, depressed, and diastatic fractures are all suspicious for child abuse (see Fig. 2-116A). CT reveals acute hemorrhages with excellent sensitivity. MRI will document subdural hematomas of different ages (Fig. 2-124), other injuries of varying ages, and shear injuries. Coronal imaging helps to demonstrate subdural collections along the tentorium. Gradient-echo MRI is of use in detecting hemorrhagic shear injury, which may not be evident on conventional or fast spin-echo images.

Cerebral Edema

Diffuse cerebral edema during childhood may be due to trauma, hypoxia, or infection. Focal cerebral edema is most commonly posttraumatic but may also be due to neoplasm, cerebritis, or infarction.

Early CT changes of cerebral edema may be subtle and are easily overlooked. The ventricles and extraaxial fluid spaces may be small because of an increase in brain volume. Obliteration of the quadrigeminal and ambient cisterns as well as the suprasellar CSF spaces is a particularly ominous finding. Poor delineation and margination between gray and white matter may be present but is easily overlooked. With time and increasing edema, differentiation between white and gray matter is lost, and the entire brain demonstrates low attenuation (Fig. 2-125). The reversal sign of diffuse cerebral edema is a serious prognostic indicator (314). MRI is more sensitive than CT in detecting early changes of cerebral edema.

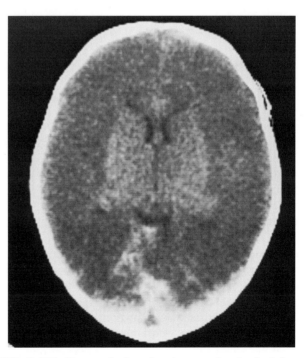

FIG. 2-125. Reversal sign due to massive brain injury. Diffuse low attenuation of peripheral brain with loss of gray-white matter differentiation is due to diffuse brain edema and necrosis. The low density of the peripheral brain and increased density centrally is a reversal of the normal CT appearance.

Vascular Abnormalities

Cerebral Hemiatrophy

Cerebral hemiatrophy is a condition that may result from a variety of disease processes causing atrophy of one of the cerebral hemispheres (315). Primary hemiatrophy is present at birth or shortly thereafter with no known etiology; the cerebral damage has presumably occurred during intrauterine life. Acquired or secondary cerebral hemiatrophy is due to CNS damage during the perinatal period or later. Possible causes include infection, trauma, vascular abnormality, hypoxia, ischemia, and hemorrhage. Intracranial hemorrhage in the premature infant is an increasingly frequent cause of cerebral hemiatrophy. Compensatory skull changes develop when damage to the brain occurs during the first 2 years of life.

Hemiatrophy presents clinically with seizures, hemiparesis, and mental retardation. Many months may pass between the first seizure and the onset of the hemiparesis. Either may occur first. Mental retardation is not always present.

Skull radiographic changes are unilateral and include calvarial thickening as well as loss of the normal convolutional markings on the inner table of the skull. There may be overdevelopment of the ipsilateral frontal sinuses, ethmoid sinuses, and mastoid air cells and elevation of the ipsilateral petrous ridge. These changes reflect the adaptation of the skull to a unilateral decrease in brain substance (315). The plain skull radiographic changes may be subtle, becoming apparent only retrospectively after diagnosis by CT or MRI. MRI may clarify the cause and specify the nature of the parenchymal brain abnormalities (see Fig. 2-139). Thinning of the cortical mantle on the side of involvement is best appreciated on T2-weighted images. In addition, the volume of white matter is often decreased, corresponding to unilateral enlargement of the lateral ventricle. Often there is a delay in myelination within the ipsilateral hemisphere resulting in increased signal of the white matter. The ipsilateral cerebral peduncle and contralateral cerebellum may be small due to Wallerian degeneration secondary to atrophy of the upper motor cortex.

Neonatal Intracranial Hemorrhage

The development of high-resolution neonatal intracranial imaging modalities (sonography, Doppler sonography, CT, MRI) has greatly increased our awareness of the frequency and potential complications of neonatal hypoxia-ischemia, intracranial hemorrhage, and infarction. Although intracranial bleeding can occur with birth trauma or coagulation defects, the most common predisposing factors are asphyxia (oxygen lack and acidosis), hypoxia (oxygen lack), and ischemia (decreased blood flow). Ischemia is probably more important than hypoxia since the newborn brain is relatively resistant to decreased oxygen concentration.

Germinal matrix-intraventricular hemorrhage (IVH) and leukomalacia are the most common nonrespiratory causes of death in the premature neonate. Approximately 90% of neonatal intracranial hemorrhage is intraparenchymal or intraventricular and 10% is subarachnoid. The morbidity and mortality of periventricular-intraventricular hemorrhage is considerably greater than that of subarachnoid hemorrhage. More than 90% of IVHs originate in the subependymal germinal matrix.

The residual germinal matrix of the late gestational fetus is a highly vascular structure adjacent to the lateral ventricles in the region of the caudothalamic groove (316,317). It is a source of both spongioblasts and neuroblasts, which subsequently migrate peripherally to form the cerebral cortex. The arterial supply to the subependymal germinal matrix is derived from the anterior cerebral artery, the lateral striate arteries, and the anterior choroidal artery (146,318). After flow through a rich capillary bed, blood drains into the deep cerebral venous system through thin-walled terminal branches of the terminal, medullary, choroidal, and thalamostriate veins. The germinal matrix decreases in size with increasing fetal maturity; it has almost completely involuted by 36 weeks of gestation. Germinal matrix hemorrhage probably originates from the thin-walled veins and capillary-venule junctions rather than from arterioles or arteries (146,318).

Several factors may be important in the etiology of IVH in any particular patient (316,317). The pathogenesis is related to intravascular factors (fluctuating cerebral blood flow; increase in cerebral blood flow; increase in cerebral venous pressure; decrease in cerebral blood flow followed by reperfusion; platelet and coagulation disturbances), vascular factors (tenuous capillary integrity of germinal matrix; particular vulnerability of the germinal matrix capillaries to hypoxic-ischemic injury), and extravascular factors (deficient vascular support; fibrinolytic activity; possible postnatal decrease in extravascular tissue pressure) (146).

Potential complications of germinal matrix-intraventricular hemorrhage include germinal matrix destruction, periventricular hemorrhagic infarction, and posthemorrhagic hydrocephalus. The destruction of glial precursor cells may have a deleterious effect on subsequent brain development. At least 15% of neonates with IVH develop hemorrhagic necrosis in the periventricular white matter adjacent to the lateral ventricle. This is in reality a venous infarction and should not be considered an extension of IVH. This venous infarction is probably due to obstruction of the terminal veins. It may be difficult by imaging to distinguish this periventricular hemorrhagic venous infarction from hemorrhagic periventricular leukomalacia (PVL); the latter is usually bilateral and symmetric. The third neuropathologic complication of IVH is posthemorrhagic ventricular dilatation. Obstructive hydrocephalus may be due to impaired CSF absorption, obliterative arachnoiditis in the posterior fossa, or aqueduct obstruction (146).

IVH usually occurs during the first 3 days of life in premature infants (319,320). Classic clinical signs are obtundation, hypotonia, low hematocrit, intractable metabolic acidosis,

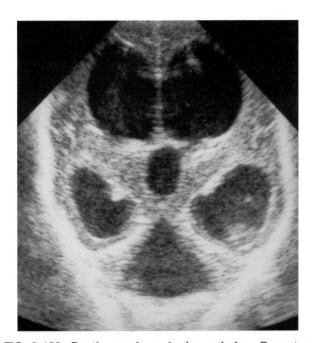

FIG. 2-126. Posthemorrhage hydrocephalus. Premature infant with a history of intraventricular and parenchymal hemorrhage. Coronal ultrasound shows marked dilatation of the lateral, third, and fourth ventricles.

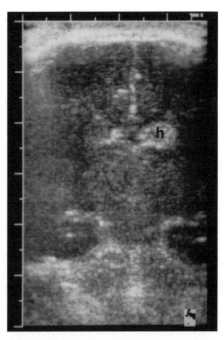

FIG. 2-127. Grade I germinal matrix hemorrhage. Premature infant. Coronal ultrasound shows an echogenic left subependymal hemorrhage (h).

and bloody CSF. The frequency of intraventricular hemorrhage in premature infants weighing less than 1500 g has been reported as high as 43% (320); recent studies have shown a declining but still high incidence (146). At least 80% of IVH detected by imaging is clinically silent. There may be associated periventricular leukomalacia (146,318). Survivors may develop hydrocephalus (Fig. 2-126), porencephaly, and mental retardation.

The sonographic appearance of IVH is characteristic. The increased echogenicity of blood is seen within the lateral, third, and occasionally fourth ventricles. The blood in the lateral ventricle usually has a crescentic shape. On sagittal or coronal sonography, the clot appears as an amorphous mass of increased echogenicity that may fill the ventricle, layer in the dependent part of the ventricle, or adhere to the choroid plexus. Germinal matrix hemorrhage produces an ovoid echogenic mass in the caudothalamic groove, as best seen on coronal and parasagittal images. The hemorrhage may remain confined to the subependymal germinal matrix, extend into the ventricular system, or involve the brain parenchyma. Germinal matrix-intraventricular hemorrhage has been divided into grades depending on extent, as follows: grade I hemorrhage is confined to the subependymal germinal matrix (Fig. 2-127); grade II hemorrhage has blood in nondilated ventricles; grade III hemorrhage shows hemorrhage within dilated ventricles; and grade IV is massive intraventricular and intraparenchymal hemorrhage, with marked dilatation of the ventricular system (Fig. 2-128) (319). As noted before, the parenchymal hemorrhage in

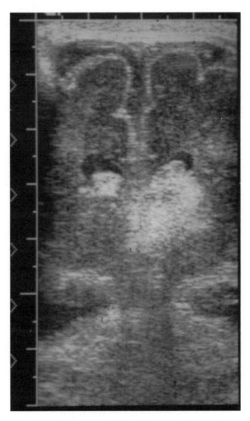

FIG. 2-128. Grade IV germinal matrix hemorrhage. Coronal ultrasound. Bilateral (left > right) subependymal germinal matrix hemorrhage. Hemorrhage extends into the dilated lateral ventricle and brain parenchyma on the left.

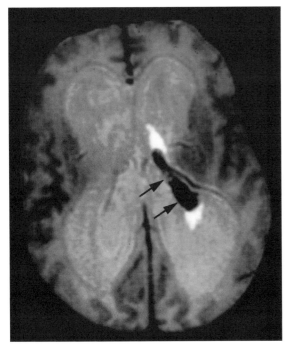

FIG. 2-129. Choroid plexus hemorrhage and hydrocephalus. Axial T2 MRI of neonate. Methemoglobin and hemosiderin intensities within the choroid plexus of the left lateral ventricle *(arrows)* are seen. There is marked lateral ventricular dilatation and associated periventricular edema.

grade IV IVH is probably due to venous thrombosis with infarction rather than parenchymal extension from the germinal matrix. The prognosis in patients with a grade I or II hemorrhage is good; there is a high frequency of neonatal death, neurologic morbidity, hydrocephalus, and porencephaly in patients with grade III or IV hemorrhage (146,320).

Approximately 90% of patients with grade IV IVH have neurologic impairment (321).

Sonography can detect subependymal germinal matrix hemorrhage, ventricular dilatation, intraventricular blood, and intraparenchymal hemorrhage (320). However, ultrasonography may not completely image the subarachnoid space or brain parenchyma, especially peripherally or in the posterior fossa. CT or MRI is often needed to confirm associated subarachnoid hemorrhage or hypoxic-ischemic encephalomalacia.

In contrast to premature infants, germinal matrix hemorrhage at term is rare. Possible sites of hemorrhage in the term infant include the choroid plexus (Fig. 2-129), subpial region, and thalamus. Venous thrombosis, particularly sagittal sinus thrombosis, is the most common cause of thalamic, choroid plexus, parasagittal, and temporal lobe hemorrhage in full-term neonates (322). Choroid plexus and thalamic hemorrhages usually occur in severely stressed infants. Neonates with thalamic hemorrhage have a relatively high frequency of neurologic sequelae including seizures, spastic paraparesis, and hydrocephalus (323).

Diffuse Hypoxic-Ischemic Brain Injury

Perinatal asphyxia is a common cause of morbidity and mortality and has significant medicolegal and economic implications. Severe asphyxia is fairly common, occurring in between 1 in 100 and 1 in 500 live births (324–330). It is estimated that between 20% and 30% of survivors have some long-term neurologic sequelae, including seizures, developmental delay, movement disorders, and spasticity.

The regions of the brain that are most susceptible to hy-

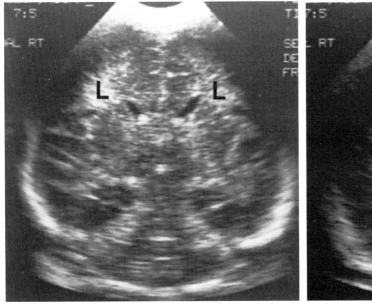
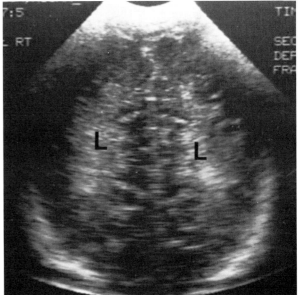

FIG. 2-130. Periventricular leukomalacia. The increased periventricular echogenicities *(L)* are due to ischemia.

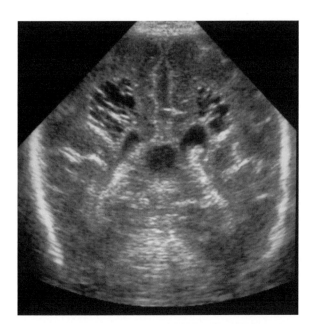

FIG. 2-131. Cystic periventricular leukomalacia. Premature neonate. Coronal ultrasound. Bilateral, periventricular sonolucencies with surrounding areas of increased echogenicity are shown.

poxic-ischemic injury encephalopathy (HIE), change as the infant matures. Thus, the type of parenchymal injury resulting from HIE depends not only on the duration and severity of the insult but also the gestational age at which it occurs (324–327).

In partial asphyxia, there is relative preservation of blood flow to the basal ganglia and brainstem, the ''watershed'' areas between the major arterial territories being most affected. Prior to 35–36 weeks gestational age, the border zone or ''watershed'' area between the major arterial territories (posterior choroidal branches and middle cerebral arteries) is in a periventricular location. Ischemic injury to the periventricular region produces necrosis of white matter resulting in periventricular leukomalacia (PVL). In addition to germinal matrix-intraventricular hemorrhage and periventricular hemorrhagic infarction, PVL in the premature infant may lead to severe neurologic deficits (146,318,331,332). Most commonly, it affects the white matter of the posterior trigone next to the atria of the lateral ventricles and the white matter adjacent to the frontal horns of the lateral ventricles. Ischemia causes edema, necrosis, cystic degeneration, and eventually diffuse loss of white matter volume. PVL is usually bilateral, symmetric, and nonhemorrhagic. It may be difficult to distinguish hemorrhagic PVL from periventricular venous infarction due to IVH. The latter is usually markedly asymmetric. In summary, periventricular hemorrhagic infarction is probably due to a venous circulatory disturbance, is almost always hemorrhagic, and is usually asymmetric. PVL is due to partial but prolonged ischemia in the premature infant. It is rarely hemorrhagic and usually symmetric (146,326).

Sonography of PVL demonstrates increased periventricu-

lar echogenicity, particularly next to the anterior frontal horns and the atria of the lateral ventricles (Fig. 2-130) (331). Severe PVL may progress to cystic encephalomalacia (Fig. 2-131) with subsequent loss of brain substance (Fig. 2-132); neurologic injury and sequelae may be severe. For follow-up evaluation, MRI most accurately assesses abnormalities of brain parenchyma and myelination due to PVL (see Fig. 2-132) and hypoxic encephalomalacia (332). Although ultrasonography is an excellent method for detecting hemorrhage and diagnosing PVL, a baseline MRI may be worthwhile approximately 4–8 weeks after sonographic detection of sig-

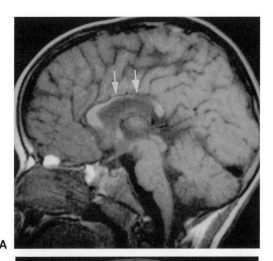

A

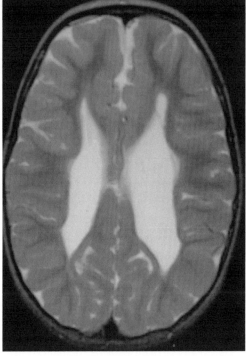

B

FIG. 2-132. Chronic periventricular leukomalacia. A 3-year-old girl with spastic diplegia. **A:** Sagittal T1 MRI. Marked thinning of the body of the corpus callosum *(arrows)* is shown. **B:** Axial T2 MRI. Irregular dilatation of the lateral ventricles, marked decrease in volume of periventricular white matter, and periventricular hyperintensity are demonstrated.

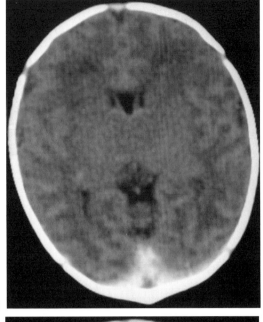

A

FIG. 2-133. **Hypoxic-ischemic encephalopathy (HIE).** Term infant with low Apgar score. **A:** Axial CT of acute phase. Subtle hypodensity and lack of gray-white matter differentiation of the basal ganglia and deep capsular tracts. **B:** Axial CT of subacute phase. Bilateral basal ganglia and thalamic mixed low densities with symmetric high densities. There is now marked low density of the cerebral white matter. **C:** Axial proton density MRI of chronic phase. Bilateral putaminal and thalamic hyperintensities. Note the large extraaxial fluid spaces anteriorly consistent with cerebral atrophy.

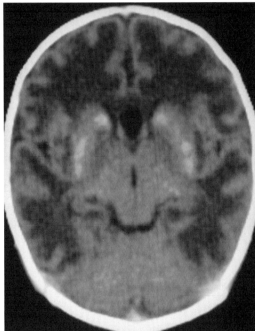

B

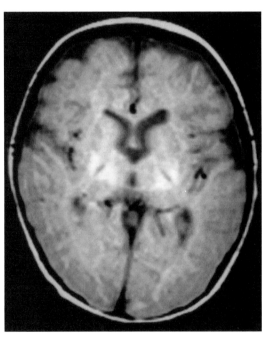

C

nificant hemorrhage or PVL and prior to any shunting for hydrocephalus (4,320).

At term, the border zones are typically in a parasagittal location. Partial HIE in the term infant leads to cortical and subcortical injury at the border zones between the anterior, middle, and posterior cerebral arteries (see Fig. 2-134A) (327). Due to the relatively poor vascularization in the depths of the sulci, the base of the gyrus is particularly vulnerable to hypoperfusion. Posthypoxic constriction of the gyrus at its base produces a pattern referred to as ulegyria, or "mushroom-shaped" gyri. In the chronic phase, encephalomalacia is noted in the parasagittal regions (see Fig. 2-134B).

Regions of high metabolic activity are at risk during profound asphyxia. Sites of active myelination, such as the posterior limbs of the internal capsule and perirolandic regions, are particularly vulnerable (326). When exposed to hypoxia-ischemia, the presence of excitatory neurotransmitters leads to cell death. High concentrations of these neurotransmitters are found in the thalami and basal ganglia of newborns. Imaging of preterm or fullterm neonates after profound asphyxia shows regions of increased water content in the basal ganglia, thalami, posterior limbs of the internal capsule, and perirolandic regions (Fig. 2-133) (326,328–330).

Early CT and sonographic evaluation of HIE may show

nonspecific cerebral edema. There is an increase in cortical echogenicity and a disorganized gyral-sulcal appearance (328,329). Subsequently, ventricular margins become indistinct, and there is decreased density of the periventricular white matter on CT. MRI will frequently demonstrate T1-shortening in corresponding locations indicating petechial hemorrhage, mineralization, or protein deposition.

Status marmoratus is a rare manifestation profound HIE that occurs in term infants. Hypermyelination, neuronal loss,

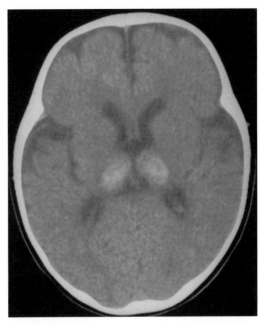

FIG. 2-135. Status marmoratus. Axial CT in a 6-month-old male. Bilateral thalamic high densities.

and gliosis occur in the thalami and basal ganglia (6). There may be hypodensity seen acutely on CT due to edema or necrosis (see Fig. 2-133A). Hyperdensity may develop due to hemorrhage or mineralization in these anatomic regions (Fig. 2-135). On MRI, T1 hypointensity and T2 hyperintensity indicate edema, necrosis, or gliosis; T1 or proton density hyperintensity and T2 hypointensity indicate hemorrhage or mineralization.

In older children with HIE or circulatory arrest as in near-drowning, the initial CT may demonstrate subtle hypodensity of the basal ganglia and insular cortex. Later, CT will show diffuse cerebral edema, with decreased gray matter/white matter differentiation, effacement of sulci and cisterns, and decreased attenuation of the basal ganglia and cortex. After several days, hemorrhage may be apparent in the basal ganglia or cortex. Late in the course of HIE, CT demonstrates patchy areas of decreased density throughout the brain (see Fig. 2-133B). MRI shows delayed myelination and loss of brain substance (atrophy) with ventricular dilatation and widening of cortical sulci (see Figs. 2-133C and 2-134B).

As previously noted, severe cerebral edema may produce the so-called reversal sign (314); the cerebral white matter has greater CT density than the gray matter. This reversal of density is felt to be due to accumulation of blood in the capillaries and veins of the white matter because of increased intracranial and venous pressure (314). In some cases, due to the relative preservation of perfusion of the posterior fossa and brainstem, these structures appear dense when compared with the rest of the brain producing the so-called white cerebellum sign. The reversal sign indicates an extremely poor prognosis; profound atrophy frequently follows this severe asphyxic injury and there may be cystic or cavitary changes, mineralization, and gliosis.

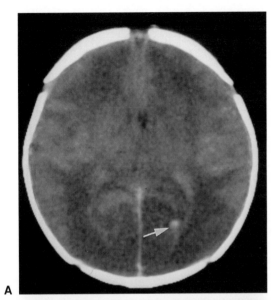

A

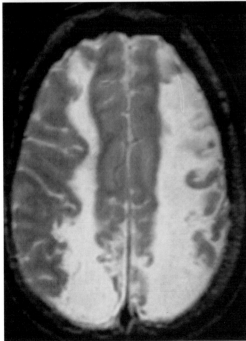

B

FIG. 2-134. Hypoxic-ischemic encephalopathy (HIE). Term infant with hypoxic injury. **A:** Axial CT in acute/subacute phase. Bilateral frontal and temporoparietal low-density abnormalities with a small left parietooccipital hemorrhagic focus *(arrow)* are shown. **B:** Axial T2 MRI in chronic phase. Frontoparietal parasagittal encephalomalacia is noted.

TABLE 2-22. *Causes of neonatal stroke*

Idiopathic[a]
Vascular maldevelopment
   Atresia
   Hypoplasia
Vasculopathy
   Proliferative
   Neonatal isoimmune
   Thrombocytopenia
Vasospasm
   Maternal cocaine use
   Other drugs
Vascular distortion
   Extreme head and neck motion
   Trauma
ECMO Therapy
Emboli
   Placental fragments or clots[a]
   Clots from involuting fetal vessels (umbilical vein, ductus arteriosus)[a]
   Congenital heart disease (especially cyanotic heart disease)[a]
   Clots from catheterized vessels[a]
Thrombosis
   Meningitis[a]
   HIE[a]
   Dehydration-hypernatremia
   Sepsis-disseminated intravascular coagulopathy (DIC)
   Polycythemia-hyperviscosity
   Protein S or C deficiency
   Antithrombin III deficiency
   Antiphospholipid antibodies
Thromboembolic
   Placental vascular anastamoses in twin gestation
   Fetal death of twin
   Fetofetal transfusion
HIE-asphyxia with thromboembolism

[a] More common.
HIE, hypoxic-ischemic encephalopathy.
Adapted from Blaser (19) and Volpe (146).

Vascular Occlusive Disease

Occlusive lesions affect one or more specific vascular distributions. Whether single (focal), or multiple (multifocal), it is the specific vascular distribution of arterial or venous occlusions that distinguishes vascular occlusive disease from generalized HIE discussed above.

Seizures and hypotonia are common presenting signs of acute cerebral infarction in the newborn (19,333). However, a stroke of prenatal or perinatal origin may manifest itself only later in infancy as a ''congenital hemiplegia'' with early onset (prior to 15 months of age) of hand preference or with focal seizures. Acute focal infarction in older children, as in adults, causes the abrupt onset of a neurologic deficit corresponding to the affected vascular territory.

Acute cerebral infarction (stroke) may be caused by ischemia or hemorrhage. In the neonate strokes are most often ischemic (Table 2-22). Stroke in the older child is usually due to arterial occlusion or hemorrhage (Table 2-23).

Focal cortical ischemic lesions most often involve the middle cerebral artery territory and less often the posterior or anterior cerebral arterial distribution (146). Emboli are flow-directed and principally occlude vessels in the middle cerebral artery territory. Multifocal involvement may occasionally be seen.

In addition to heart disease, extracranial and intracranial vascular abnormalities such as arterial dissection (313), moyamoya disease, vasculitis, and sickle cell disease are more common causes of stroke in older children than in infants. Other potential causes include hypercoagulable states, particularly dehydration, meningoencephalitis, effects of radiation therapy or drugs, and inborn errors of metabolism (6,19,49,146).

TABLE 2-23. *Causes of stroke in older infants and children*

Cardiac disease
   Congenital heart disease (especially cyanotic disease)
   Mitral valve prolapse
   Cardiomyopathies
   Endocarditis
   Cardiac tumors
Arterial dissection[a]
Arteriopathy
   Moyamoya[a]
   Vasculitis[a]
   Fibromuscular dysplasia
   Marfan syndrome
   Takayasu arteritis
   Kawasaki disease
   Polyarteritis nodosa
   Systemic lupus erythematosus
Hypercoagulable state
   Dehydration[a]
   Protein S deficiency
   Protein C deficiency
   Antithrombin III deficiency
   Antiphospholipid antibodies
   Heparin cofactor-II deficiency
   Nephrotic syndrome
   Oncologic disease
Infection[a]
Hemolytic uremic syndrome
Hemoglobinopathies
   Sickle cell disease[a]
Treatment of oncologic disease
   Radiation therapy
   Chemotherapy
Metabolic disease
   Homocystinuria
   Dyslipoproteinemia
   Fabry disease
   Mitochondrial disorders
Hemorrhage[a]
   Vascular malformation
   Aneurysm
   Tumor[a]

[a] More common.
Adapted from Blaser (19) and Volpe (146).

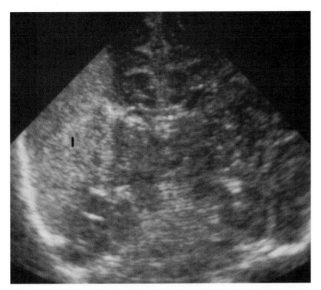

FIG. 2-136. Hemorrhagic infarction. Newborn on extracorporeal membrane oxygenation. Coronal ultrasound. Unilateral echogenic infarction *(I)* in the distribution of the right middle cerebral artery is shown.

Arterial Occlusive Disease

The neuroimaging findings of acute cerebral infarction due to arterial occlusive disease are often characteristic. A wedge-shaped, cortically based lesion with gyral swelling and edema is present in a specific vascular territory. Infarcts may be echogenic (Fig. 2-136) or hypoechoic (Fig. 2-137A). Doppler sonography is helpful in assessing arterial and venous blood flow as well as complications (Fig. 2-137B). Acute infarcts are usually hypodense by CT (Fig. 2-138A); gyriform enhancement may be present. Large infarcts may develop petechial hemorrhages or become frankly hemorrhagic, although this is less common in children than adults. Parenchymal injury following infarction may produce focal or generalized atrophy (Fig. 2-138), ventricular dilatation, porencephaly, and encephalomalacia (Fig. 2-139). Although spin-echo images may be normal for the first few hours after a stroke, MRI is more sensitive to early infarction than either sonography or CT. Perfusion and diffusion imaging offer earlier demonstration of ischemic lesions than conventional MRI. Intracranial MRA may demonstrate the site of vascular occlusion, intramural thrombus, and luminal narrowing due to dissection (334,335). Small vessel disease and vasculitis usually require conventional angiography for diagnosis.

SPECT imaging may be used to define perfusion deficits associated with arterial occlusions. In the critically ill patient with severely compromised cerebral blood flow due to increased intracranial pressure, flow and static imaging may be used to exclude or confirm brain death (Fig. 2-140).

Primary Cerebral Arterial Occlusive (Moyamoya) Disease. As previously noted, acute hemiplegia during childhood may be due to cerebral vascular occlusion or specific abnormalities of the brain parenchyma. Cerebral occlusions may be due to extracranial arterial emboli (congenital heart

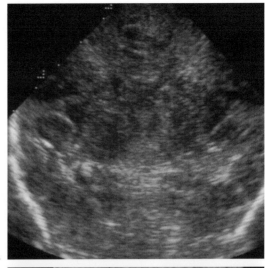

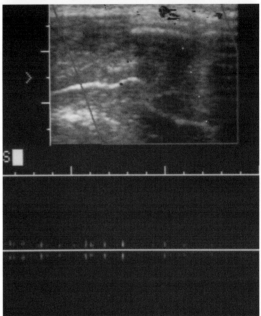

FIG. 2-137. Multiple cerebral infarctions. A: Coronal ultrasound. Multiple bilateral basal ganglia and deep cerebral sonolucent infarctions are shown. **B:** Doppler ultrasound. Only background noise can be found at the level of the superior sagittal sinus; this is consistent with absence of blood flow and brain death.

disease, endocarditis, left atrial myxoma, fat emboli, pulmonary septic emboli, air emboli, iatrogenic emboli), thrombosis (traumatic, infectious, hematologic), or abnormalities of the vascular wall (angiitis, sinusitis, dissection, neurocutaneous syndromes, homocystinuria, Menkes syndrome, irradiation, collagen vascular disease, neoplasm). Harwood-Nash (336) and Hilal (337,338) verified a group of children with cerebral arterial occlusive disease for which an etiology was not determined (339). Some investigators have noted a strong association between previous nasopharyngeal or tonsillar infection and subsequent cerebral arterial occlusive disease (5,336). However, an infectious etiology has never been proved, and it is probably better to consider this entity as a

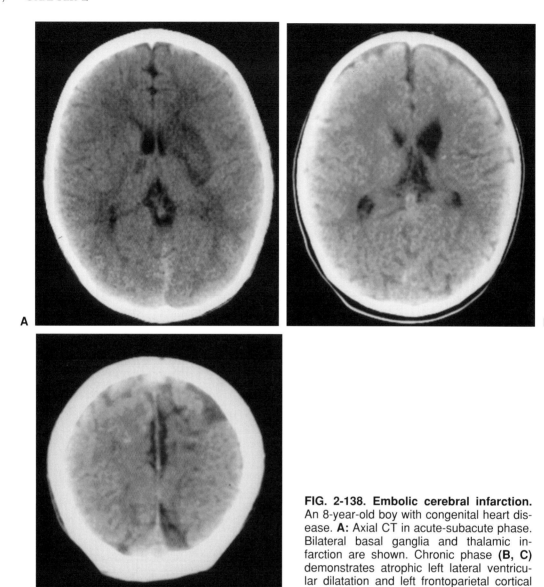

FIG. 2-138. Embolic cerebral infarction. An 8-year-old boy with congenital heart disease. **A:** Axial CT in acute-subacute phase. Bilateral basal ganglia and thalamic infarction are shown. Chronic phase **(B, C)** demonstrates atrophic left lateral ventricular dilatation and left frontoparietal cortical hypodensities.

primary cerebral arterial occlusive process, moyamoya disease (340).

Moyamoya disease is characterized by progressive occlusion of the internal carotid artery (ICA) bifurcation accompanied by the development of collaterals which may be basal (parenchymal), leptomeningeal, or transdural. Moyamoya is Japanese for "a puff of smoke" and has been used to describe the angiographic appearance of the basal collaterals which occur. Pathologically, intimal hyperplasia is identified at the ICA bifurcation (341). In the early stages of the disease only narrowing of the bifurcation is demonstrated. In advanced stages the occlusive process extends proximally to involve the entire supraclinoid ICA and ultimately may result in occlusion of both the intracranial and cervical ICA segments. The disease typically progresses during the first decade of life and then stabilizes (342).

Angiography shows stenosis or complete occlusion of the supraclinoid ICAs bilaterally. There may be involvement of the proximal segments of both anterior and middle cerebral arteries. There is associated telangiectasia ("puff of smoke") in the basal ganglia (Figs. 2-141 and 2-142). Vascular flow voids corresponding to lenticulostriate collaterals in the basal ganglia are demonstrated by MRI (Fig. 2-143A). MRA demonstrates ICA occlusion or stenosis as well as the extent of involvement of anterior and middle cerebral arteries (Fig. 2-143B).

In addition to primary cerebral arterial occlusive disease, the moyamoya pattern has been described in children with neurofibromatosis, sickle cell disease, and Down syndrome and after local radiation treatment. Childhood moyamoya differs from the adult disease in that ischemic complications are frequent, hemorrhagic complications are uncommon, basal collaterals are particularly prominent, and the disease is almost always bilateral (339,343,344).

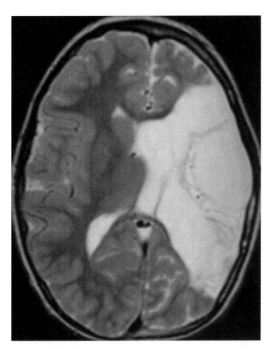

FIG. 2-139. Cerebral hemiatrophy. A 2-year-old girl with congenital hemiplegia. Axial T2 MRI demonstrates cystic encephalomalacia involving the left middle cerebral artery distribution. There is atrophic dilatation of the left lateral ventricle and cerebral cortical sulci.

Surgical revascularization is the treatment of choice for moyamoya disease. Some patients improve after synangiosis; this causes the development of transdural and transpial collaterals with revascularization of the middle cerebral artery (345,346). Conventional angiography is usually performed before this surgery in order to assess the extent of existing transdural collateral formation and the status of external carotid artery branches possibly usable for anastomosis. Angiography, perfusion imaging and MRA are often used after synangiosis for follow-up.

Venous Thrombosis

Thrombosis of the deep venous system, the cortical veins, a dural sinus, or a combination of these may occur in children. Although cerebral venous and dural sinus thrombosis may be idiopathic, they are frequently associated with infection (meningitis, encephalitis, abscess, subdural empyema, mastoiditis, cellulitis, septicemia, Tolosa-Hunt syndrome), dehydration, trauma (craniectomy, epidural hematoma, subdural hematoma, penetrating trauma), neoplasm (meninges, brain), or hematologic disorders (polycythemia, cardiac bypass, hemolysis, clotting abnormalities) (5,347). In children, venous thrombosis is most commonly due to infection or dehydration. Clinical signs and symptoms include leth-

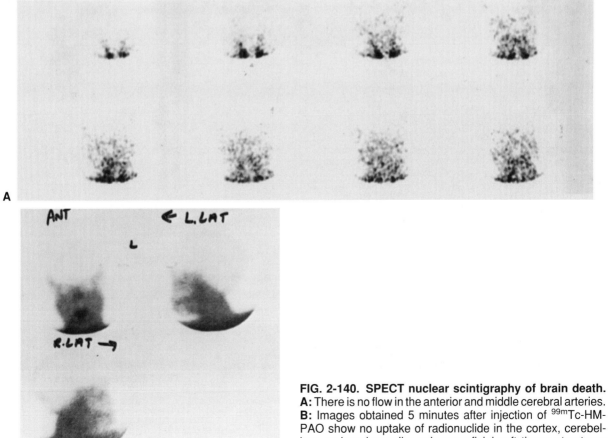

FIG. 2-140. SPECT nuclear scintigraphy of brain death.
A: There is no flow in the anterior and middle cerebral arteries.
B: Images obtained 5 minutes after injection of ^{99m}Tc-HM-PAO show no uptake of radionuclide in the cortex, cerebellum, or basal ganglia; only superficial soft tissue structures are perfused.

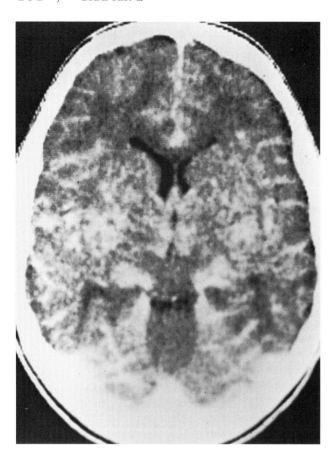

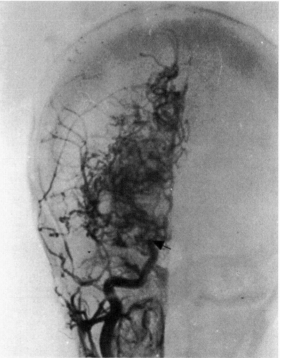

FIG. 2-141. Moyamoya disease. A 10-year-old girl with acute hemiplegia. Contrast-enhanced CT shows extensive parenchymal and leptomeningeal collateral circulation enhancement.

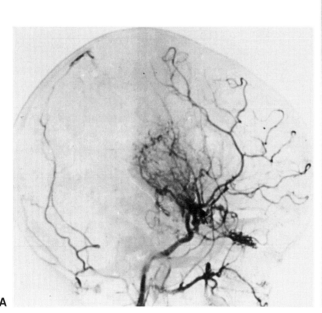

A

B

FIG. 2-142. Moyamoya disease. A 6-year-old boy with sudden onset of hemiplegia. Lateral **(A)** and frontal **(B)** views of a selective right internal carotid arteriogram. There is occlusion of the supraclinoid portion of the internal carotid artery *(arrow)*, with "puff of smoke" appearance due to extensive collaterals within the basal ganglia. Note the transdural collaterals arising from the ophthalmic artery and the external carotid artery.

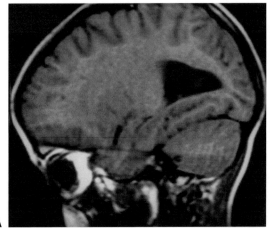

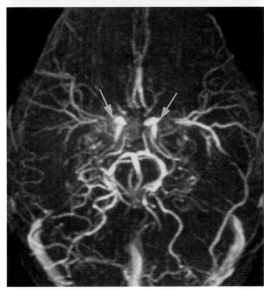

FIG. 2-143. Moyamoya disease. A 6-year-old boy with multiple strokes. **A:** Sagittal T1 MRI. Serpiginous flow signal voids are shown in basal ganglia and deep capsular structures (telangiectatic collateralization). **B:** Axial 3-D time-of-flight MR angiography. Bilateral ICA bifurcation stenoses *(arrows)* with involvement of the anterior and middle cerebral arteries are well demonstrated.

argy, vomiting, neck pain, headache, unconsciousness, seizures, hemiparesis, subarachnoid hemorrhage, cerebral edema, coma, and eventually even death.

The onset of seizures or a focal neurologic deficit in a pediatric patient with hemorrhagic lesions not corresponding to an arterial vascular territory should suggest venous thrombosis (Fig. 2-144A) (347). In addition to showing the parenchymal hemorrhagic infarctions, CT or MRI may directly demonstrate the venous sinus thrombosis (Fig. 2-144). Nonenhanced CT frequently demonstrates enlargement and increased density of the affected dural sinus (Fig. 144A). Following contrast administration, CT shows enhancement around the clot producing the "empty delta sign" (348). Thrombosis is directly visualized on MRI as increased signal within the venous sinus (Fig. 2-144B); lack of flow may be confirmed by Doppler sonography (see Fig. 2-137B) or MR

venography (Fig. 2-144C). Thrombosis of the veins of the cortex is extremely difficult to diagnose, even with conventional angiography.

Vascular Anomalies

Important vascular anomalies of the CNS in childhood include vascular malformations, vein of Galen malformations (Galenic arteriovenous malformations, or AVMs), aneurysms, and angiodysplasias (5–7,49,349,350).

Vascular Malformations

Vascular malformations of the CNS include AVMs, cavernous malformations, venous anomalies, and capillary telangiectasias (349–351). The clinical presentation and the significance of these malformations depends on their pathologic type and anatomic location (350,351).

Arteriovenous Malformations. An AVM is a high-flow lesion; multiple, dilated, thin-walled arterial structures communicate directly with draining veins without an intervening capillary bed. AVMs are due to persistent fistulous connections between primitive endothelial vessels. The malformation consists of enlarged arterial feeders, a vascular nidus, and draining veins.

Most CNS AVMs are supratentorial. Cerebral hemispheric AVMs (56%) are more common than galenic AVMs (24%). Infratentorial (16%) and dural (4%) AVMs are much less common than the supratentorial type (5,352). The most common locations of intracranial AVMs are the parietal (42%) and temporal (25%) lobes (5). Clinical symptomatology may include headaches, seizures, and hemiplegia. Symptoms are frequently due to spontaneous intracranial hemorrhage. Other potential complications include a mass effect from hemorrhage, subarachnoid hemorrhage, focal atrophy secondary to "vascular steal" and ischemia, vascular thrombosis, and calcification. Rupture of an AVM has a mortality rate of 10% and morbidity as high as 50% (353). The risk of hemorrhage is increased with dilatation of the component vessels, venous stenosis, and drainage of the malformation into the deep venous system.

The CT findings of AVM are variable but there is usually a mixed lesion of isodense and hyperdense tissue. The malformation enhances markedly after contrast injection. This enhancement is usually inhomogeneous and lobulated. There may be no mass effect unless the AVM has bled. If hemorrhage has occurred, CT will show a high-density lesion with mass effect and surrounding edema (Fig. 2-145A). MRI is a more sensitive modality for detecting AVMs and any associated parenchymal changes and shows the age(s) of the hemorrhage(s) (Fig. 2-145B, C). The nidus of the malformation itself is frequently identified as serpiginous areas of flow void, indicating high flow, inside the malformation. MRA may provide a noninvasive overview of the vascular components of the AVM (Fig. 2-145D). Angiography pre-

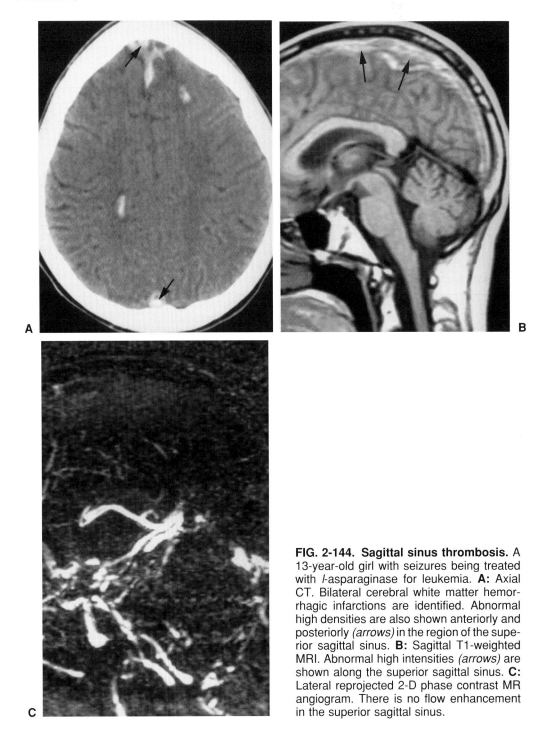

FIG. 2-144. Sagittal sinus thrombosis. A 13-year-old girl with seizures being treated with *l*-asparaginase for leukemia. **A:** Axial CT. Bilateral cerebral white matter hemorrhagic infarctions are identified. Abnormal high densities are also shown anteriorly and posteriorly *(arrows)* in the region of the superior sagittal sinus. **B:** Sagittal T1-weighted MRI. Abnormal high intensities *(arrows)* are shown along the superior sagittal sinus. **C:** Lateral reprojected 2-D phase contrast MR angiogram. There is no flow enhancement in the superior sagittal sinus.

cisely defines the feeding arteries, the size of the nidus, the venous drainage, and any high-flow vasculopathy (Fig. 2-145E). The precise anatomic detail given by selective angiography is required for appropriate therapy (Fig. 2-145E).

The treatment of AVMs includes surgical excision, endovascular ablation, radiation therapy, and a combination of these approaches (6,354). The nidus of the malformation must be completely obliterated for cure. Depending on location and access, small AVMs may be treated with either surgery or endovascular techniques. Deep AVMs are frequently not amenable to either surgical or endovascular approaches; they may be treated with stereotactic radiation or proton beam therapy. Larger AVMs are usually treated by a combination of surgery and embolization.

Cavernous Malformations. Cavernous malformations, also referred to as cavernomas or cavernous angiomas, are low-flow vascular malformations composed of clusters of endothelial-lined spaces without enlarged arterial feeders or intervening brain parenchyma (355). These are the most common CNS vascular malformations in childhood. Similar

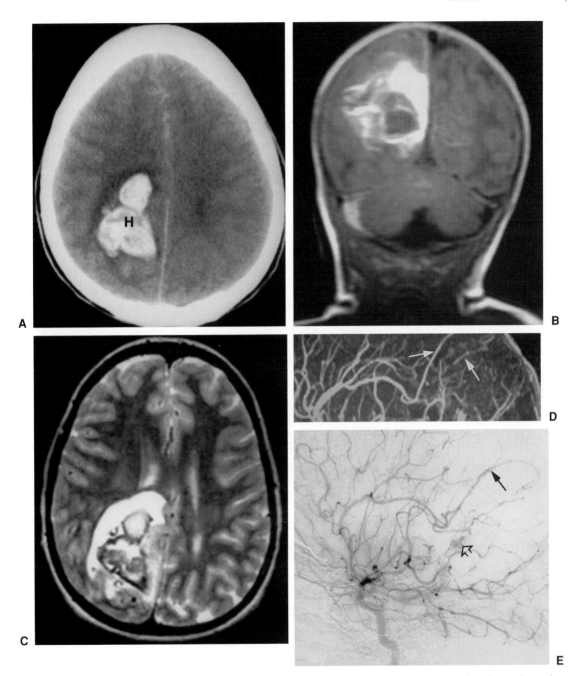

FIG. 2-145. Cerebral arteriovenous malformation. A 16-year-old boy with acute hemiparesis and cerebral hemorrhage. **A:** Axial CT. There is a large parietal high-density intracerebral hemorrhage *(H)* with surrounding low-density edema. **B:** Coronal T1 MRI. **C:** Axial T2 MRI. Intensity findings consistent with hemorrhage of varying ages. A few vascular signal flow voids are also noted. **D:** Lateral reprojected 3-D time-of-flight MRA. Abnormally enlarged artery pattern within the right parietal region *(arrows)* is demonstrated. **E:** Lateral internal carotid digital subtraction angiogram. Enlarged middle cerebral feeding artery *(closed arrow)* and vascular nidus *(open arrow)* are confirmed.

lesions have been reported after radiation therapy for intracranial neoplasms (356). Cavernomas may be asymptomatic or may cause headache, seizures, or intracranial hemorrhage. The lesions may be single or multiple and are often familial. Most cavernomas are supratentorial.

CT demonstrates a dense lesion with occasional punctate calcification (Fig. 2-146). Contrast enhancement is variable.

MRI shows a mixed-intensity lesion indicating hemorrhage of varying ages (Fig. 2-147). On T2-weighted images, a speckled focus of T2 hyperintensity is surrounded by a hypointense hemosiderin rim. Cavernomas are usually not apparent at angiography.

Venous Anomalies. Developmental venous anomalies (DVA) are congenital low-flow lesions in which an abnor-

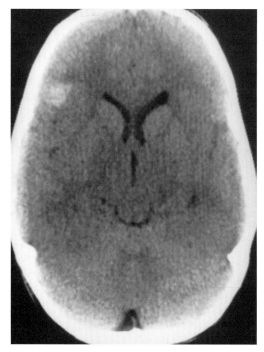

FIG. 2-146. Cavernous malformation. A 3-year-old boy with a seizure. Nonenhanced axial CT demonstrates a right frontal intracerebral high-density focus, part of which enhanced on a contrast-enhanced study.

mal collection of radially oriented veins drains either normal or dysplastic brain parenchyma. There is no arterial component or nidus. DVAs are most commonly located in the frontal lobes and cerebellum; they may be associated with cortical dysplasias or migrational anomalies. Although most

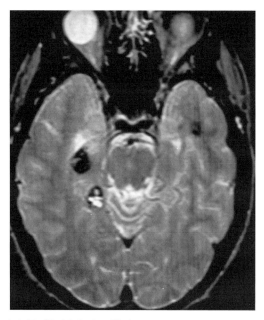

FIG. 2-147. Multiple familial cavernous malformations. A 20-year-old man. Axial T2 MRI. Multiple mixed intensity lesions are consistent with hemorrhages of varying age.

DVAs are asymptomatic and incidental, they rarely cause seizures or hemorrhage.

CT or MRI demonstrates a collection of dilated medullary veins which converge into a single transparenchymal vein that drains into either the superficial or deep venous system (357). They may be apparent on CT only after contrast enhancement. MRI shows signal voids converging to a single vessel; enhancement may be necessary to document the typical ''Medusa head'' appearance of the converging veins. Angiography confirms the presence of a venous anomaly and also excludes an AVM or aneurysm.

Capillary Telangiectasias. Capillary telangiectasias are clusters of small vessels that are anatomically similar to capillaries (355). These malformations occur in the ventral pons; because hemorrhage is rare, patients with capillary telangiectasias are usually asymptomatic. The lesions are seen on MRI only with contrast enhancement; angiography is normal.

Vein of Galen Malformation

A vein of Galen malformation (Galenic AVM; vein of Galen aneurysm) is a rare congenital vascular malformation characterized by a fistulous communication between cerebral arteries and a vein in the region of the vein of Galen (358). These connections can be large direct fistulas, numerous small connections, or a combination. Although the etiology is unknown, there is a strong association with anomalies of the dural sinuses such as absent straight sinus and persistent falcine sinus. This suggests that intrauterine straight sinus thrombosis with recanalization causes the malformation (359). Radiologic studies have shown that the large venous structure that receives the arteriovenous shunt is not the vein of Galen but the midline prosencephalic vein. A Galenic malformation must be differentiated from a parenchymal AVM with drainage into the deep venous system, which includes the vein of Galen and straight sinus; these latter malformations frequently present with hemorrhage in older children and adults (6). The treatment of a parenchymal AVM with deep venous drainage is the same as that of an AVM elsewhere in the brain (360).

Vein of Galen malformations are classified into choroidal and mural types. The choroidal type is an arteriovenous connection between the thalamoperforator, choroidal, pericallosal, or superior cerebellar arteries and the anterior wall of the midline prosencephalic vein (6,358). The choroidal type is more common (90%), usually presenting in the neonate with congestive heart failure and an intracranial bruit. Untreated, choroidal malformations are fatal. The mural type of Galenic malformation usually presents in later infancy with developmental delay, seizures, or increasing head circumference due to hydrocephalus. In this type, there are fewer but larger connections between the posterior choroidal or collicular arteries and the prosencephalic vein (6).

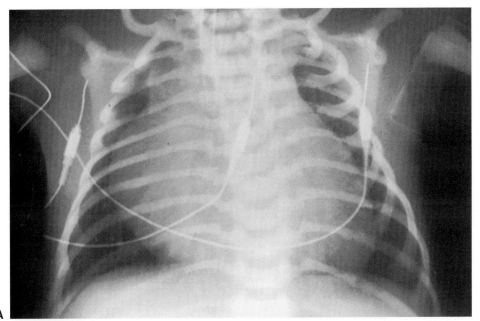

A

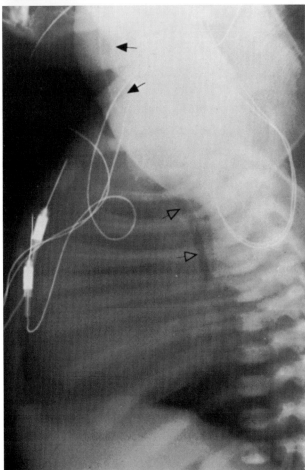

B

FIG. 2-148. Galenic arteriovenous malformation. A: A 1-day-old boy with cardiomegaly, right atrial enlargement, wide superior mediastinum, and normal or decreased pulmonary vascularity. **B:** Lateral chest radiograph confirms right ventricular enlargement as well as retrosternal fullness, posterior displacement of the intrathoracic trachea *(open arrows)*, and anterior displacement of the cervical trachea *(closed arrows)*.

A constellation of plain film findings is highly suggestive of a Galenic AVM in the neonate (361): cardiomegaly with right-sided chamber dominance, widening of the superior mediastinum, retrosternal fullness, posterior displacement of the upper trachea, and anterior displacement of the cervical trachea (Fig. 2-148). The cardiomegaly is due to left-to-right shunting of blood through the malformation with increased return to the heart, which enlarges the right atrium and right

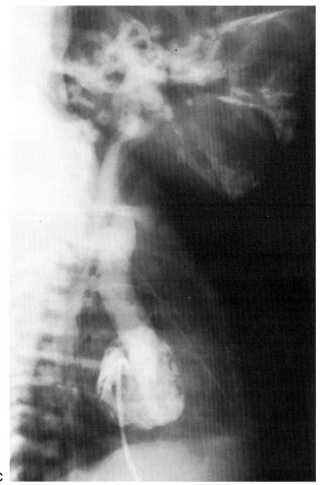

C

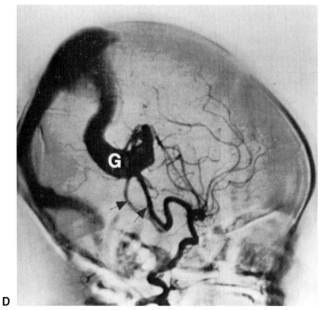

D

FIG. 2-148. *Continued.* **C:** Left ventriculogram shows that the wide superior mediastinum and posterior displacement of the thoracic trachea are due to enlargement of the aorta and other great vessels. The retropharyngeal soft tissue mass is due to dilatation of both the carotid arteries and jugular veins. **D:** Aneurysmal dilatation of the vein of Galen *(G)* is secondary to an arteriovenous malformation supplied primarily by posterior choroidal branches of the posterior cerebral artery *(arrows).*

ventricle. Because of physiologic elevation of pulmonary artery pressure in the newborn, with right-to-left shunting at the ductus arteriosus, pulmonary vascularity often remains normal or is decreased, which produces even more promi-

nence of the right-sided cardiac chambers (see Fig. 2-148). The wide superior mediastinum, retrosternal fullness, and posterior displacement of the intrathoracic trachea are due to dilatation and enlargement of the aorta, innominate artery,

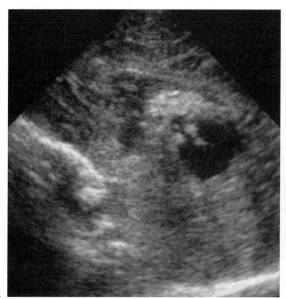

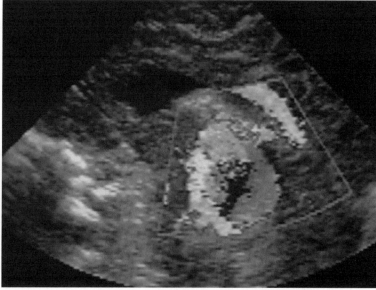

A   B

FIG. 2-149. Galenic arteriovenous malformation. Newborn infant with congestive heart failure. Sagittal ultrasound **(A)** and Doppler **(B)** demonstrate a mixed anechoic/echogenic mass in the pineal region with prominent vascular flow characteristics.

carotid arteries, jugular veins, innominate vein, and superior vena cava (see Fig. 2-148). Anterior displacement of the cervical trachea is due to dilatation of the carotid arteries and jugular vein (see Fig. 2-148C) (361).

Ultrasonography shows the hypoechoic and frequently pulsatile dilated prosencephalic vein (Fig. 2-149). Doppler sonography confirms the high flow within the malformation (see also Fig. 2-149). CT demonstrates a large mass of increased attenuation in the region of the posterior third ventricle; it has an attenuation coefficient of 35–40 Hounsfield units, presumably the density of flowing blood (362). Dilatation of the lateral and third ventricles is usually present, and there is marked contrast enhancement of the mass. MRI demonstrates the dilated prosencephalic vein in the quadrigeminal plate cistern (Fig. 2-150). Prominent feeding branches of the posterior cerebral and pericallosal arteries are well demonstrated; high flow is indicated by signal void in these vessels and in the dilated venous structures. MRA confirms the diagnosis of the malformation (Fig. 2-150C). Selective internal carotid and vertebral arteriography is required to evaluate all feeding vessels prior to any attempt at surgical or neuroradiologic intervention (see Fig. 2-148D). Pericallosal branches of the anterior cerebral artery also supply the malformation in 15% to 40% of cases (5).

Embolization techniques are useful in a few patients (359,360). Arterial embolization is performed after superselective catheterization of each feeding vessel. If congestive failure persists and further arterial embolization is considered too risky, a transvenous embolization may be performed (363). The overall cure rate for vein of Galen malformations ranges from 40% to 60% (359,360). The cure rate for the mural type of malformation is greater than that of the choroidal type.

Cerebral Aneurysms

A cerebral aneurysm is a localized arterial dilatation that consists only of anatomic components of the vessel wall. Aneurysms of the cerebral vasculature in infants in children are rare (1.3% of CNS aneurysms at all ages) and are associated with local vessel changes (364). Local arterial ectasias, venous vascular varices, false aneurysms, and AVMs should not be considered congenital cerebral aneurysms. Aneurysms in children may be congenital or idiopathic (77%), inflammatory or mycotic (11%), or traumatic (11%) (5,6,364). Congenital (idiopathic) cerebral aneurysms in children are presumably due to a defect in the media, complicated by an acquired lesion of the internal elastic lamina (Figs. 2-151A, B). Because no asymptomatic cerebral aneurysms have been detected by either angiography or autopsy in infants and children, it is assumed that pediatric aneurysms are due to an acquired abnormality of the arterial wall superimposed on a congenitally defective vessel (5,364). Mycotic aneurysms (Fig. 2-151C) may be secondary to congenital heart disease with septic emboli, cavernous sinus thrombophlebitis, osteomyelitis of the skull, or meningitis. Traumatic aneurysms (Fig. 2-151D) may be due to direct penetrating injury or severe generalized head trauma.

As previously noted, cerebral aneurysms and AVMs are rare in children. However, when they do occur, their most common clinical presentation is intracerebral or subarachnoid hemorrhage. Other causes of subarachnoid hemorrhage in children include arterial occlusive disease, venous occlusive disease, birth trauma, birth hypoxia, intracranial neoplasm, hematologic abnormality, hypersensitivity vasculopathy, infection, and trauma (5,6). Idiopathic cerebral hemorrhage is rare in children. Cerebral aneurysms are

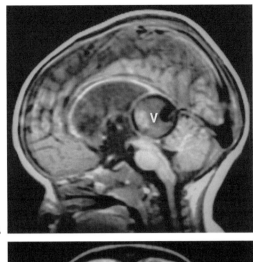

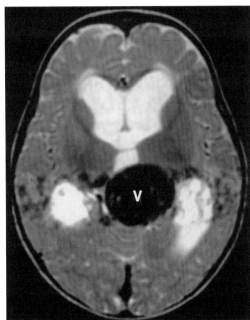

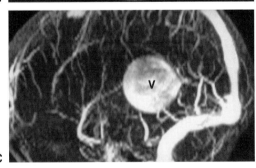

FIG. 2-150. Galenic arteriovenous malformation. A 9-day-old boy with enlarged head. **A:** Sagittal T1 MRI. Mixed intensity pineal region mass *(V)* causes obstructive hydrocephalus. **B:** Axial T2 MRI. Vascular signal flow voids *(v)* within the large mass with pulsatile vascular flow artifacts along the phase-encoding gradient are apparent. There is marked ventricular dilatation and periventricular edema. **C:** Lateral reprojected 3-D time-of-flight venous MR angiogram. Vascular flow enhancement of the enlarged median prosencephalic vein *(V)* is well demonstrated.

rarely diagnosed before 1 year of age. There is a higher frequency in males than in females. Approximately two thirds of pediatric cerebral aneurysms are in patients less than 10 years of age. Patients with certain conditions such as coarctation of the aorta, polycystic kidney disease, and neurofibromatosis have an increased risk of cerebral aneurysm formation, as do those with a positive family history.

Cerebral aneurysms in children differ in several ways from those in adults (see Fig. 2-151). Aneurysms in children are frequently large; at least half are greater than 1 cm in diameter (364). The sites of pediatric cerebral aneurysms vary; they include the supraclinoid internal carotid artery, internal carotid artery bifurcation, proximal middle cerebral artery, distal middle cerebral artery, proximal anterior cerebral artery, distal anterior cerebral artery, posterior cerebral artery, posterior communicating artery, tip of the basilar artery, and posteroinferior cerebellar artery. The only common site of congenital aneurysms is the internal carotid artery bifurcation (364). Mycotic aneurysms are frequently multiple and may change in size. The tip of the basilar artery (see Fig. 2-151C) is a common site for a mycotic aneurysm (6,364). The location of traumatic aneurysms is related to the path of the penetrating trauma, the vascular suspensory points of the brain, and the vascular contiguity with the edges of the dura (364). Traumatic aneurysms secondary to skull fracture or penetrating trauma may involve peripheral cortical vessels. Branches of the anterior cerebral artery (see Fig. 2-151D) may also be involved because of the close relationship of the pericallosal branches and the falx (364).

CT is currently the best initial imaging modality in the investigation of possible subarachnoid hemorrhage and cerebral aneurysm in children. Blood clot, mass effect, surrounding edema, leakage of contrast material, and blood within the subarachnoid space may be detected by CT in association with an aneurysm (see Fig. 2-152A). The distribution of hemorrhage frequently suggests the location of the aneurysm (Fig. 2-152). Conventional arteriography is essential to define the precise location and morphology of the aneurysm, identify other aneurysms, and plan surgical or interventional therapy (Fig. 2-152B).

Based on the experience in adults, MRI and MRA may also play a significant role in the evaluation of pediatric aneurysms. By MRI, aneurysms are rounded areas of signal void often accompanied by adjacent phase artifact due to vascular pulsations. Giant aneurysms (>2.5 cm) are usually laminated with regions of signal void and increased signal due to thrombus and flow distortion. Either TOF or phase contrast MRI may be used to verify the presence of an aneurysm. MRA is a useful technique for screening high-risk populations for aneurysms (365). CT angiography may also be used for screening but does require the use of intravenous contrast media.

The treatment of cerebral aneurysms depends on their size and location. Although surgical clipping of the aneurysm neck is the most common therapy, endovascular therapy with detachable coils is assuming a greater role. Follow-up MRI should always be performed with care; imaging is performed

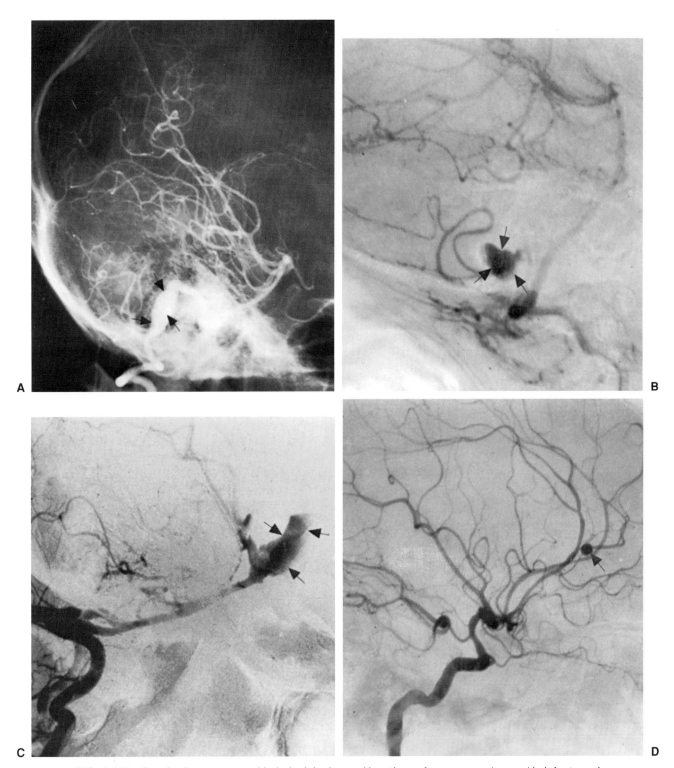

FIG. 2-151. Cerebral aneurysms. Varied etiologies and locations of aneurysms *(arrows)* in infants and children. **A:** Idiopathic aneurysm of the left vertebral artery. **B:** Idiopathic aneurysm of the posterior inferior cerebellar artery. **C:** Mycotic aneurysm of the tip of the basilar artery. **D:** Traumatic aneurysm of the pericallosal branch of the anterior cerebral artery. (Courtesy of Derek C. Harwood-Nash, M.B., Ch.B., Toronto, Ontario, Canada.)

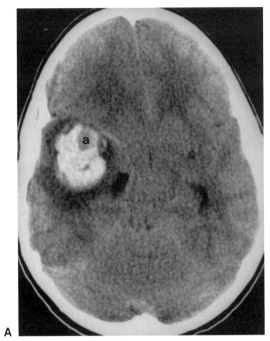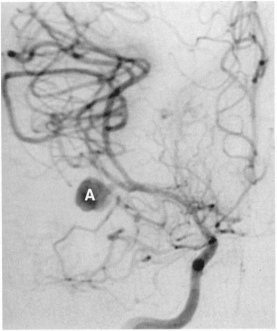

FIG. 2-152. Cerebral aneurysm. A 13-year-old boy with intracerebral hemorrhage. **A:** Axial CT. Large right temporal intracerebral high-density hemorrhage with surrounding low-density edema. There is mass effect on the adjacent brainstem. **B:** Frontal right internal carotid digital subtraction angiogram. Large middle cerebral artery trifurcation aneurysm *(A)* which is seen in retrospect as a relative hypodensity *(a)* within the hemorrhage on CT.

only after confirmation that the therapeutic material used is MRI-compatible (366).

Cerebral Angiodysplasias

Cerebral angiodysplasias are rare in children (5). They may produce irregularities of vessels, stenoses, or even occlusions. Angiodysplasias may be due to the phakomatoses or neurocutaneous syndromes (Sturge-Weber syndrome, neurofibromatosis, tuberous sclerosis, von Hippel-Lindau disease, ataxia-telangiectasia), connective tissue disease, sickle cell disease, fibromuscular dysplasia, inborn errors of metabolism (Menkes syndrome, homocystinuria), chronic infectious disease (moniliasis), and radiation injury (5,338,339,367).

Neurocutaneous Syndromes

The neurocutaneous syndromes or phakomatoses (Table 2-24) are a group of disorders primarily affecting tissues of ectodermal origin (nervous system, skin, retina, globe and its contents); visceral organs are also involved, but usually to a lesser extent. Neurologic symptoms are prominent features of these diseases. In this section, imaging characteristics of the most common of the neurocutaneous syndromes

as well as some less common entities are presented. More complete descriptions of the neurocutaneous syndromes are available in several excellent textbooks and review articles (6,38,39,368).

TABLE 2-24. *Neurocutaneous syndromes*

Neurofibromatosis
Tuberous sclerosis
Sturge-Weber syndrome
Other vascular phakomatoses
  Wyburn-Mason syndrome
  Ataxia-telangiectasia
  Osler-Weber-Rendu disease
  Klippel-Trenaunay-Weber syndrome
  Meningioangiomatosis
von Hippel-Lindau disease
Melanocytic phakomatoses
  Neurocutaneous melanosis
  Oculodermal melanosis
  Incontentinentia pigmenti
  Hypomelanosis of Ito
Basal cell nevus syndrome
Linear sebaceous nevus syndrome
Blue rubber bleb syndrome
Cowden syndrome

Adapted from Pont and Elster (38).

Neurofibromatosis

Neurofibromatosis (NF) is a hamartomatous disorder of neural or neural crest origin. It is an inherited autosomal dominant disease of both neural ectoderm and mesenchyme. It is the most common of the neurocutaneous disorders. Neurofibromatosis has been divided into seven types; an eighth type is for patterns of involvement not fulfilling the criteria of the other seven types. Neurofibromatosis type 1 (NF-1) and neurofibromatosis type 2 (NF-2) are the most common types; these are discussed separately in the following sections. The other types of neurofibromatosis are as follows: NF-3—overlap between NF 1 and NF 2; NF-4—diverse manifestations of neurofibromatosis; NF-5—segmental involvement; NF-6—café-au-lait spots without neurofibromas; NF-7—late-onset form of the disease.

Neurofibromatosis Type 1

Neurofibromatosis type 1 (NF-1) is the disorder initially described by von Recklinghausen in 1882 (6). NF-1 is one of the most common autosomal dominant CNS disorders, and the most common of the phakomatoses. The incidence in the general population is approximately 1 in 4000. It is autosomal dominant with variable penetrance. The genetic locus is on the long arm of chromosome 17 near the locus for the nerve growth factor receptor gene (369). A National Institutes of Health (NIH) consensus conference developed strict diagnostic criteria for NF-1 (Table 2-25) (370). CNS

TABLE 2-25. *Diagnostic criteria for NF-1*

Two or more of the following:
6 or more café-au-lait macules (>5 mm in a child, >15 mm in an adult)
2 or more neurofibromas of any type or 1 plexiform neurofibroma
Axillary or inguinal freckles
Bilateral optic nerve glioma
2 Lisch nodules (hamartomas of the iris)
Characteristic osseous dysplasia (sphenoid wing, occipital defect or tibia pseudoarthrosis)
Parent, sibling, or child with NF-1

NF, neurofibromatosis.
Adapted from the National Institutes of Health Consensus Development Conference (370).

manifestations are present in approximately 15% of affected patients with NF-1 (371). They include developmental delay, seizures, visual disturbances, and stroke (6).

NF-1 Spots. The most common CNS lesions of NF-1 are the "histogenetic foci" or "NF-1 spots." Two groups of these foci are distinguished: those found in the globus pallidus and those located elsewhere (372,373). NF-1 spots in the globus pallidus are characteristically slightly hyperintense on T1-weighted images, may exhibit minimal mass effect, and do not enhance (Fig. 2-153). The T1 shortening may be due to heterotopic Schwann cells or melanin (374,375). The second group of NF-1 spots causes foci of hyperintensity on proton density and T2-weighted MRI in the cerebellum, brainstem, internal capsule, splenium, and

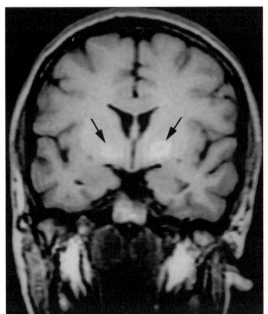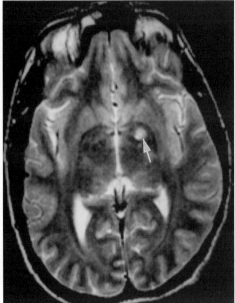

FIG. 2-153. Neurofibromatosis type 1 (NF-1) spots. A 5-year-old boy with neurofibromatosis type 1. **(A)** Coronal T1 MRI and **(B)** axial T2 MRI demonstrate characteristic hyperintensities, the NF-1 spots, *(arrows)* in the basal ganglia, including the globi pallidi.

thalamus. These lesions, seen in up to 75% of patients with NF-1, are first identified at approximately 3 years of age and increase in number and size until 10–12 years of age, after which they regress (6,375,376). Biopsy of these lesions has shown hamartomas or collections of atypical glial cells (377). These lesions are isointense on T1-weighted images and exhibit no mass effect or contrast enhancement.

Optic Glioma. The most common intracranial neoplasm in NF-1 is the optic pathway glioma (OPG). These tumors are most commonly of low histologic grade, particularly those involving only the optic nerves. Optic gliomas can be isolated to a single optic nerve or can extend to both optic nerves, the chiasm, and the optic tracts. Rarely, the tumor will extend beyond the lateral geniculate bodies into the optic radiations. Lesions involving the optic chiasm and other parts of the hypothalamus are most likely to behave in an aggressive manner.

CT provides excellent delineation of the intraorbital extent of these gliomas. However, MRI gives superior delineation of the intracanalicular and intracranial tumor extent. Optic nerve gliomas are hypo- or isointense on T1 sequences and hyperintense on T2 images (Fig. 2-154). Fat suppression sequences improve visualization of intraorbital tumors (24). The tumor is usually low density or isodense by CT with variable contrast enhancement that is frequently intense. Cavitation and cyst formation within the tumor mass occasionally occur. For further discussion, see also page 132.

Other Gliomas. Cerebral astrocytomas occur more commonly in NF-1 than in the general population. These astrocytomas are most commonly juvenile pilocytic astrocytomas. Although the optic system is the most common site, the mesencephalic tectum may also be involved by neoplasia; other common locations for astrocytomas in patients with NF-1 are the pons and the cerebellum. Enhancement of an NF-1 spot should always raise the possibilty of neoplasm.

Hydrocephalus. Hydrocephalus may develop in patients with NF-1. The site of obstruction of CSF flow is usually the aqueduct of Sylvius; this obstruction may be due to a tectal glioma or benign aqueductal stenosis (378). MRI can easily make the distinction.

Vascular Dysplasia. Cerebral angiodysplasia may occur in patients with NF-1. The dysplasia is usually due to intimal proliferation producing stenosis or occlusion of the common carotid, internal carotid, proximal middle cerebral, or anterior cerebral artery. The moyamoya phenomenon with marked enlargement of collateral lenticulostriate arteries is seen in 60% to 70% of these patients (6). Arterial ectasias and aneurysms also occur in patients with NF-1.

Dural Ectasia. Dural ectasia is a characteristic neuroradiologic feature of NF-1. Arachnoidal ectasia (hyperplasia) may involve the optic nerve sheath and mimick an optic nerve glioma or widen the internal auditory canal and simulate an acoustic neuroma. MRI or contrast-enhanced CT may distinguish hyperplasia from tumor.

Bone Dysplasia. Mesodermal abnormalities affecting the skull base include sphenoid wing dysplasia and calvarial

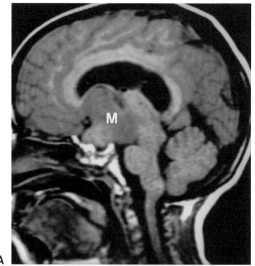

A

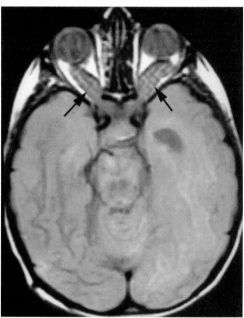

B

FIG. 2-154. Optic glioma in neurofibromatosis type 1. A 3-year-old boy with neurofibromatosis type 1. Sagittal T1 MRI **(A)** and axial proton density MRI **(B)**. Large suprasellar tumor *(M)* involving the optic chiasm, hypothalamus, and third ventricle with hydrocephalus. The tumor also involves the intraorbital and intracanalicular optic nerves bilaterally *(arrows)*.

dysplasia along the lambdoid suture. The orbital dysplasia is due to abnormal development and ossification of one or both greater wings of the sphenoid bone (5). This may be mistaken clinically and radiographically for a neoplasm unless its characteristic plain film findings are appreciated (129). These patients usually have pulsating exophthalmos. Radiography or CT shows hypoplasia of the greater and lesser sphenoid wings, elevation of the lesser sphenoid wing, widening of the superior orbital fissure, and lateral displacement of the oblique orbital line (129). Anterior protrusion of the pulsating temporal lobe and its coverings enlarges the bony defect and causes pulsating exophthalmos (Fig.

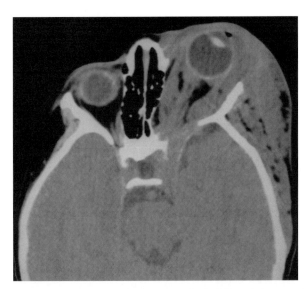

FIG. 2-155. Sphenoorbital dysplasia in NF-1. A 3-year-old boy with neurofibromatosis type 1 and severe left proptosis. Axial CT demonstrates left sphenoorbital bony defect, intraorbital and periorbital plexiform neurofibromas, and proptotic buphthalmos (congenital glaucoma).

2-155). Sphenoid wing dysplasia may be associated with plexiform neurofibromas in the orbit or periorbital regions (Fig. 2-155).

The dysplastic defect in the squamosal portion of the occipital bone near the lambdoid suture (Fig. 2-156) is more frequent on the left, but also occurs on the right (Fig. 2-156B). Only rarely is the defect of bone along the lambdoid suture associated with an overlying neurofibroma.

Plexiform Neurofibromas. Plexiform neurofibromas, the hallmark of NF-1 (Table 2-25), are locally aggressive congenital lesions composed of tortuous cords of Schwann cells, disorganized neurons, and collagen (6). They tend to extend along the nerve of origin into the cranium and cause distortion and compression of adjacent structures. Plexiform neurofibromas usually arise in the head and neck and frequently involve the scalp or orbit. Most commonly, in the orbit the neurofibromas act as masses, and cause impaired ocular movements and exophthalmos (6).

Tumors arising in the ciliary body or choroid of the globe may produce glaucoma and buphthalmos (see Fig. 2-155). Glaucoma in NF-1 may also be due to maldevelopment of the anterior chamber. Plexiform neurofibromas are irregular masses of low density on CT; they tend to be of low signal on T1 MRI and high signal intensity on T2 images (see Fig. 2-155). Contrast enhancement is variable (6).

Other Neuroradiologic Manifestations. Cranial nerve schwannomas are rare in NF-1. When they occur, they raise the possibility of the overlap syndrome (NF-3), the clinical and genetic implications of which are unknown (6). Spine manifestations of NF-1 include acute angle scoliosis, nerve sheath tumors, and lateral meningoceles. The scoliosis, usually minimal or mild but occasionally severe, is most commonly the result of dysplasia of the vertebral bodies. The paraspinous nerve sheath tumors in NF-1 are neurofibromas. Meningoceles occurring in NF-1 are probably a primary dys-

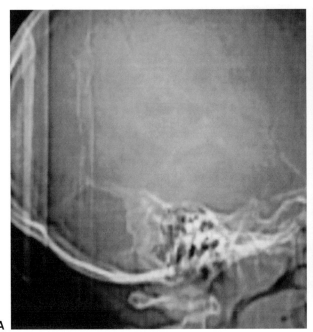

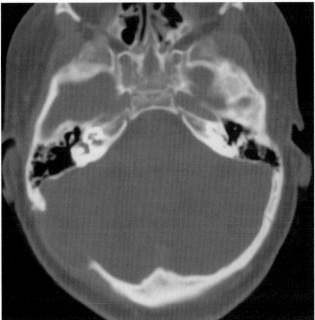

A   B

FIG. 2-156. Lambdoid defect in NF-1. A 7-year-old girl with neurofibromatosis type 1. **A:** Lateral CT scout projection image. **B:** Axial CT section demonstrates right occipital bony defect adjacent to the lambdoid suture.

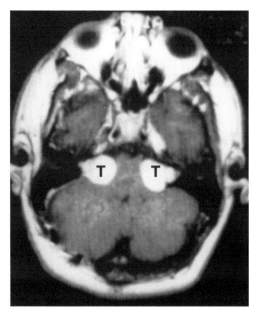

FIG. 2-157. Bilateral acoustic neuromas in NF-2. A 19-year-old boy with neurofibromatosis type 2. Gadolinium-enhanced axial T1 MRI demonstrates bilateral enhancing cerebellopontine angle tumors *(T)* with extension into the enlarged internal auditory canals.

plasia of the meninges, the same factor that causes scalloping of the posterior vertebral bodies (6).

Neurofibromatosis Type 2

Neurofibromatosis type 2 (NF-2) has also been called the central form or neurofibromatosis with bilateral acoustic schwannomas. However, it is actually a separate disease. NF-2 is associated with an abnormality of chromosome 22, has an overall frequency of approximately 1 in 50,000 in the population, and most commonly presents during adult life (370,379). The major feature of NF-2 is the presence in nearly all affected individuals of bilateral acoustic schwannomas (Fig. 2-157). Other tumors of the CNS, particularly meningiomas, may be present as well. The established diagnostic criteria for NF-2 are listed in Table 2-26 (370).

Schwannomas are tumors composed of abnormal Schwann cells surrounding neurons. The vestibular division of cranial nerve VIII is the most frequently involved cranial nerve in NF-2. Other cranial nerves that may be involved include V, IX, and X. The acoustic schwannomas may be unilateral or bilateral. They are typically hypodense on precontrast CT, hypointense on T1-weighted images, and markedly hyperintense on T2-weighted MRI images. Contrast enhancement is usually intense (see Fig. 2-157). Expansion of the internal auditory canal is common and can be appreciated on plain films, CT, or MRI. Contrast-enhanced MRI is required for the detection of small intracanalicular tumors.

Meningiomas present at an earlier age in NF-2 than in the general population; meningioma in a child should prompt a thorough investigation for other stigmata of NF-2. The imaging features and location of meningiomas in NF-2 are similar to those not associated with the syndrome. The tumors are dural based and usually parasagittal or juxtasellar in location. Intraventricular meningiomas may also occur in NF-2. Meningiomas are typically isointense with brain on precontrast T1-weighted images, mildly hyperintense or hypointense on T2-weighted images, and demonstrate intense enhancement. A "dural tail" of enhancement is frequently seen extending away from the center of the tumor. The hyperostosis that is often associated with meningiomas may be seen on plain films but is better demonstrated by CT.

Tuberous Sclerosis

Tuberous sclerosis (Bourneville disease), a dominantly inherited disease (with variable penetrance), is characterized by the abnormal proliferation of cells in the brain, skeletal system, skin, and viscera (Table 2-27) (380–382). The diagnosis is made with certainty if the triad of seizures (78%), mental retardation (71%), and facial adenoma sebaceum (27%) is present (380). Cerebral lesions may be present in the absence of any element of the triad (380–382). Myoclonic seizures frequently begin in infancy and are seen in up to 80% of affected patients (6,383). Patients who develop seizures prior to 5 years of age have a higher incidence of mental retardation than those whose seizures develop later (383). An adenoma sebaceum is an angiofibroma of the skin; these tumors first begin to appear between 1 and 5 years of age. Neuroimaging is important for the diagnosis of tuberous sclerosis because there are many possible causes for seizures and psychomotor retardation in infancy and because the characteristic skin lesions may not be present until later childhood.

Brain tubers are present in all patients with tuberous sclerosis and may be identified as early as the newborn period. These nodules consist of astrocytes, spindle cells, and glial tissue. Tubers are most commonly located beneath the ependyma of the lateral ventricles but may occur anywhere from this subependymal location out to the cortex (5,6,380,382, 384).

TABLE 2-26. *Diagnostic criteria for NF-2*

One or more of the following:
Bilateral acoustic schwannomas
NF-2 in a relative and a unilateral acoustic schwannoma
NF-2 in a relative and any two of the following:
    Neurofibroma
    Meningioma
    Glioma
    Schwannoma
    Juvenile posterior lens opacity

NF, neurofibromatosis.
Adapted from the National Institutes of Health Consensus Development Conference (370).

TABLE 2-27. *Abnormalities in tuberous sclerosis*

Brain
    Calcifications
    Tubers[a]: subependymal, cortical
    Tumors: gliomas
Skeletal system
    Skull
        Sclerotic lesions: inner table, diploë
        Calvarial thickening
    Long bones
        Metaphyseal cysts
        Cortical thickening
        Prominent trabeculation
        Periosteal nodules
    Spine and pelvis: sclerotic lesions
    Hands and feet
        Cortical thickening
        Cysts
Skin
    Adenoma sebaceum[a]
    Shagreen patches
    Subungual fibromas
    Achromic patches
    Subcutaneous nodules
    Hyperpigmentation[a]
    Café-au-lait spots
Viscera
    Cardiac rhabdomyoma and sarcoma
    Mixed embryonal hamartomas: kidney[a], duodenum, liver,
        thyroid, adrenal, ovary, pulmonary interstitium
    Renal cysts[a]
    Retinal phakoma

[a] More common.
Modified from Fitz et al. (380) and Medley et al. (381).

Subependymal tubers (hamartomas) almost always contain calcification in older patients and are seen by CT as punctate or larger areas of increased density in the subependyma or cortex (Fig. 2-158) (384). The MRI signal intensity of subependymal nodules varies with age. During infancy, because of the immaturity of myelination, the lesions are typically hyperintense to white matter on T1-weighted images and hypointense on T2-weighted images (Fig. 2-159). With increasing age, the lesions become isointense to white matter and are identified as masses of variable size projecting into the ventricles (385,386). There is usually only mild contrast enhancement on MRI.

Hamartomas, containing fibrous and cellular tissue, may occur in a variety of other organs and systems (see Table 2-27) (380,381,383). Cortical hamartomas consist of giant cells, disordered myelin, and gliosis. As with subependymal nodules, the imaging features of the cortical lesions vary with age. In early infancy, the lesions are hypodense on CT, slightly hyperintense on T1-weighted MRI, and hypointense to white matter on T2-weighted images. With increasing age, the lesions tend to become isodense to brain on CT, isointense to brain on T1-weighted MRI, and hyperintense to white matter on T2-weighted images (385–388). Contrast enhancement is not a feature unless there has been malignant

degeneration. By 10 years of age, at least half of patients with tuberous sclerosis will have one or more calcified cortical tubers (389).

White matter lesions are also found in tuberous sclerosis. Increase in white matter intensity on T2-weighted images is due to either clusters of abnormal glial or neuronal cells or linear bands of unmyelinated fibers radiating outward from the ventricles. Calcification may occur in these white matter lesions, but contrast enhancement should not be present.

Subependymal hamartomas near the foramen of Monro have a tendency to enlarge and are referred to as giant cell tumors (see Fig. 2-158). These tumors differ histologically from the subependymal nodules found elsewhere by the predominance of large giant cells in them. Giant cell tumors develop in 5% to 10% of patients with tuberous sclerosis (382,385,389); hydrocephalus due to foraminal obstruction is a frequent complication. Imaging of giant cell tumors reveals an enlarging, enhancing mass near the foramen of Monro. On rare occasions, these tumors undergo malignant degeneration and invade the brain parenchyma.

Sturge-Weber Syndrome

Sturge-Weber syndrome (encephalotrigeminal angiomatosis) is a neurocutaneous disorder characterized by low-flow vascular malformations of the face, globe, and leptomeninges (38,39,390,391). Most cases are sporadic. A typical ''port wine'' facial nevus is almost always present and is usually unilateral, most often in the distribution of the

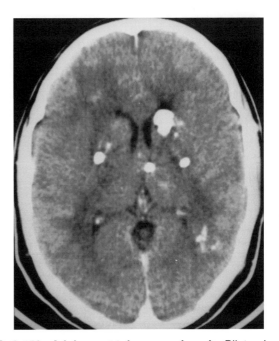

FIG. 2-158. Adolescent tuberous sclerosis. Bilateral periventricular and basal ganglia calcified tubers with a dominant tuber, or perhaps a giant cell tumor, in the left frontal periventricular region.

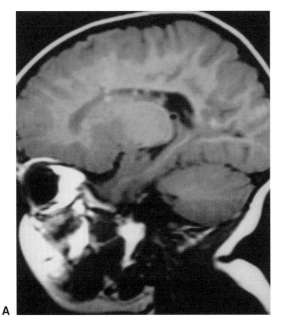

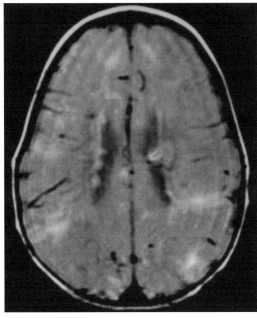

FIG. 2-159. Infantile tuberous sclerosis. (A) Sagittal T1 and **(B)** axial proton density MRI demonstrate bilateral periventricular, subcortical, and cortical white matter nodular hyperintensities. The findings represent the dysplastic neuroglial foci (tubers) of tuberous sclerosis.

ophthalmic division of the trigeminal nerve. Low-flow vascular malformations of the choroid of the globe are also present and can cause glaucoma or buphthalmos. The leptomeningeal capillary-venous malformation represents persistent primordial sinusoids and dysgenesis or thrombosis of the superficial venous system. Manifestations of the disease include seizures in up to 90% of patients, often presenting as infantile spasms. Mental retardation, hemiparesis, and hemianopia are also common. The visceral, truncal, or extremity low-flow vascular malformations of Klippel-Trenau-

nay syndrome may coexist with the typical findings of Sturge-Weber syndrome (39).

The leptomeningeal angiomas consist of thin-walled vessels in the pia of the cerebral convexities, usually in the posterior parietal, temporal, and lateral occipital lobes. The calcific deposits occur in a pericapillary distribution in the fourth layer of the cerebral cortex underneath the angioma; this dystrophic calcification is due to chronic ischemia.

Calcification is rarely seen on skull radiographs before 2 years of age. It typically starts in the posterior occipital region and progresses forward. The calcification follows the contours of the gyri to form serpiginous railroad-track or tram-track densities. CT may show extensive calcification prior to plain film changes (Fig. 2-160A). CT of Sturge-Weber syndrome shows superficial cortical calcification, ipsilateral cortical atrophy, and superficial contrast enhancement (6,38,39,390,391). There may be brain atrophy beneath the malformation with a thick cranial vault, small hemicranium, dilated ventricles, and wide subarachnoid spaces. Contrast-enhanced MRI is the most sensitive study for the extent of the pial malformation (392). Enlarged medullary and subependymal veins are frequently present because of the preferential shunting of blood to the deep venous system. The choroid plexus ipsilateral to the pial vascular malformation is often enlarged (Fig. 2-160C), more commonly because of hyperplasia than involvement with vascular malformation. Atrophy of the involved hemisphere is usually evident (Fig. 2-160B); the ipsilateral sinuses and mastoids are large and the calvaria is thick (5). Angiography, although rarely required for diagnosis in the MRI era, demonstrates absence of the superficial cortical veins in the region of the capillary-venous malformation and enlargement of the medullary and subependymal veins (393).

von Hippel-Lindau Disease

Von Hippel-Lindau disease (CNS hemangioblastamatosis) is an autosomal dominant disorder with incomplete penetrance and multisystem involvement. It is characterized by hemangioblastomas of the retina, cerebellum and spinal cord, renal cell carcinoma, pheochromocytoma, and cysts of abdominal viscera (6,368,390). It is associated with an abnormality on chromosome 3 (394). Males and females are affected equally. The onset of symptoms is usually in the third or fourth decade of life and is often due to a complication of a retinal lesion (intraocular hemorrhage, retinal detachment, glaucoma, cataract) or symptoms due to mass effect in the posterior fossa (headache, vomiting, vertigo). Symptoms referable to spinal cord tumors are less common.

Intracranial hemangioblastomas, most commonly found in the cerebellum, are present in up to half of patients. Hemangioblastomas of the brainstem are unusual, and supratentorial lesions are rare. Hemangioblastomas are typically cystic masses with intensely enhancing mural nodules (Fig. 2-161). Small lesions may be solid enhancing nodules without any cyst. Hemangioblastomas are highly vascular; en-

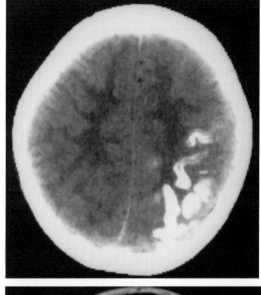

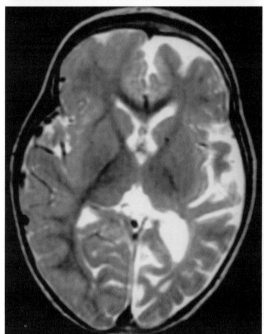

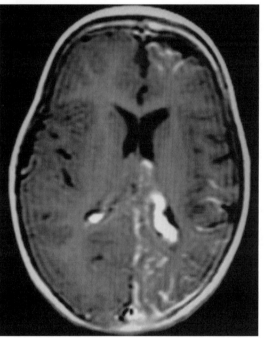

FIG. 2-160. Sturge-Weber syndrome. A 22-month-old boy with Sturge-Weber syndrome. **A:** Axial CT. Gyriform calcification involves the left parietal lobe. **B:** Axial T2 MRI. Atrophy causes sulcal and ventricular dilatation of the temporal, parietooccipital, and frontal cerebrum on the left. **C:** Axial gadolinium-enhanced T1 MRI. Left temporoparietal, occipital, and frontal leptomeningeal enhancement and marked enhancement of the choroid plexus of the left lateral ventricle are shown.

larged vessels are frequently seen in or near the nodular portion of the tumor (219,220). Preoperative angiography provides detailed vascular anatomy.

Ataxia-Telangiectasia

Ataxia-telangiectasia (Louis-Bar syndrome) is an autosomal recessive disorder characterized by capillary telangiectasias of the face, cerebrum, and conjunctiva; progressive cerebellar atrophy; immunodeficiencies; and an increased incidence of lymphoma, leukemia, and other malignancies (6,368). The genetic defect responsible for this disorder has not been elucidated; however, defects in DNA repair are known to occur (395). Ionizing radiation sometimes contrib-

utes to the development of malignancy in these patients. Ataxia is apparent when the child begins to walk. However, cutaneous telangiectasias may not be evident before 3–6 years of age (6). Imaging demonstrates progressive cerebellar degeneration and atrophy involving the cerebellar hemispheres and vermis. Pulmonary vascular malformations may lead to emboli with cerebral infarction. Intracranial hemorrhage can occur from the rupture of cerebral telangiectasias (368).

Basal Cell Nevus Syndrome

Basal cell nevus syndrome (Gorlin syndrome) is an autosomal dominant neurocutaneous syndrome in which multi-

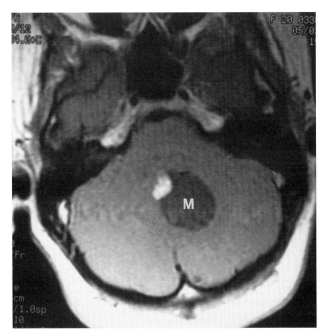

FIG. 2-161. von Hippel-Lindau disease with cerebellar hemangioblastoma. A 20-year-old woman with family history of von Hippel-Lindau disease. Axial gadolinium-enhanced T1 MRI. Low-intensity cyst and enhancing nodule of cerebellar hemangioblastoma *(M)*.

ple basal cell carcinomas of the skin develop. Neurologic findings include mental retardation, seizures, hydrocephalus, and an increased frequency of CNS malignancies (368); medulloblastoma, meningioma, craniopharyngioma, ameloblastoma, and astrocytoma have all been reported. Other radiologic findings include bifid ribs, agenesis of the corpus callosum, dural calcification, and odontogenic cysts of the maxilla and mandible.

Neurocutaneous Melanosis

Neurocutaneous melanosis is a disorder in which large pigmented cutaneous nevi are seen in association with abnormal meningeal pigmentation (6,368,396). The disorder may be related to aberrant melanoblast formation and migration from the neural crest. Melanocytes are normally found in the basal meninges; in neurocutaneous melanosis, they are found in markedly increased numbers throughout the meninges and can produce abnormal pigmentation as well as thickening (397). There may also be abnormal melanin-producing cells along the perivascular spaces. The regions of the brain parenchyma most often involved are the anterior temporal lobes (particularly the amygdala) and the cerebellum. The lesions of neurocutaneous melanosis produce focal areas of T1 and T2 shortening. This is probably due to the accumulation of free radicals within melanin. Leptomeningeal enhancement usually is present (398). Degeneration to melanoma with enlargement of the lesions develops in approximately 10% of patients (368).

Hypomelanosis of Ito

Hypomelanosis of Ito is characterized by regions of cutaneous hypopigmentation in association with scoliosis, skull defects, syndactyly, cleft palate, and ocular abnormalities (368). Seizures and mental retardation are common. Atrophy, porencephaly, white matter changes, and heterotopias have all been described in this entity.

Metabolic, Degenerative, and Toxic Disorders

Metabolic, degenerative, and toxic disorders are rare and are usually untreatable. Many are heredofamilial and due to specific enzymatic defects. Genetic counseling and prenatal screening are often important. These disorders are classified by metabolic defect (Table 2-28) and anatomic predilection (Table 2-29) (6). The diagnosis is usually based on metabolic testing or biopsy. MRI is superior to sonography and CT for evaluating disease distribution and extent. MR spectroscopy may someday permit specific *in vivo* characterization of these disorders.

Many of these disorders have radiologic manifestations outside the CNS and are discussed in other chapters.

Lysosomal Storage Disorders

The lysosomal storage disorders result from catabolic enzyme defects that cause the abnormal accumulation of metabolites within lysosomes. Depending upon the accumulations, lysosomal storage disorders are grouped into the lipidoses, mucopolysaccharidoses, the mucolipidoses, glycogenoses, and lysosomal leukodystrophies (399). Some of these storage diseases have mainly CNS manifestations; in others, the systemic manifestations predominate.

Lipidoses

Gaucher Disease. Gaucher disease, the most common lysosomal storage disease, is a deficiency of glucocerebrosidase, which results in the accumulation of cerebroside (400). Three variants are recognized. Type 1 (chronic) Gaucher disease is the most common variety and usually does not have CNS manifestations except for those occurring as a consequence of bone marrow failure (hemorrhage) or splenectomy (infection). Spinal complications include vertebral body collapse and extramedullary hematopoiesis (401). Type 2 (rapidly progressive infantile) and type 3 (juvenile) forms are extremely uncommon; their manifestations include demyelination of the brainstem, neuronal loss, and cerebral atrophy. The most frequent imaging finding is prominence of CSF spaces due to atrophy.

Niemann-Pick Disease. Niemann-Pick disease involves accumulation of sphingomyelin within the reticuloendothelial system (400). At least five different types, based on the enzymatic defect, are recognized. Imaging findings vary but include generalized or selective (isolated cerebellar) atrophy,

TABLE 2-28. *Classification of metabolic and degenerative disorder by defect*

Lysosomal storage disorders
  Lipidoses
    Gaucher disease (deficiency in glucocerebrosidase)
    Niemann-Pick disease
    GM_1 gangliosidosis
    GM_2 gangliosidosis (Tay-Sachs and Sandoff)
    Neuronal ceroid lipofuscinoses
  Mucopolysaccharidosis
    Hurler
    Hunter
    Sanfillipo
    Morquio
    Scheie
    Maroteaux-Lamy
    Sly
  Lysosomal leukodystrophies
    Metachromatic leukodystrophy
    Krabbe disease (globoid cell leukodystrophy)
Disorders of mitochondria
  Leigh disease (subacute necrotizing encephalomyelopathy)
  Kearns-Sayre syndrome
  MELAS (mitochondrial encephalomyelopathy with lactic acid and stroke)
  MERRF (myoclonic epilepsy and ragged red fibers)
  Menkes disease (kinky hair syndrome)
  Alper disease
  Glutaric acidurias
  Infantile bilateral striatal necrosis
Peroxisomal disorders
  Adrenoleukodystrophy complex
  Zellweger syndrome (cerebrohepatorenal syndrome)
Amino acid disorders
  Phenylketonuria
  Maple syrup urine disease
  Lowe syndrome (oculocerebrorenal syndrome)
  Methylmalonic aciduria
  Propionic aciduria
  Nonketotic hyperglycinemia
Miscellaneous metabolic/neurodegenerative disorders
  Canavan disease (spongiform leukodystrophy)
  Alexander disease (fibrinoid leukodystrophy)
  Pelizaeus-Merzbacher disease
  Hallervorden-Spatz disease
  Wilson disease (hepatolenticular degeneration)
  Fahr disease
  Cockayne syndrome
  Friedreich ataxia
  Olivopontocerebellar atrophies
Toxic injuries

Adapted from Barkovich (6), Wolpert and Barnes (7), Volpe (146), and Blaser (400).

TABLE 2-29. *Characterization of metabolic disorders by primary site of involvement*

Disorders Primarily Affecting Gray Matter
  Cortical gray matter
    Neuronal ceroid lipofuscinosis
    GM_1 gangliosidosis
    Mucolipidoses
  Deep gray matter
    Leigh disease
    MELAS
    Methylmalonic aciduria
    Propionic aciduria
    Carbon monoxide poisoning
    Kernicterus
    Hallervorden-Spatz disease
Disorders Primarily Affecting White Matter
  Peripheral white matter early
    Canavan disease
    Alexander disease
    Galactosemia
  Central white matter early
    Krabbe disease
    Peroxisomal disorders
    Metachromatic leukodystrophy
    Phenylketonuria
    Maple syrup urine disease
    Lowe syndrome
  Lack of myelination
    Pelizaeus-Merzbacher disease
    Trichothiodystrophy
  Nonspecific white matter pattern
    Nonketotic hyperglycinemia
    Urea cycle disorders
    Collagen vascular diseases
    Demyelinating disease
    End-stage white matter disease
Disorders Affecting Both Gray and White Matter
  Cortical gray matter plus white matter
    Generalized peroxysomal disorders
    Alper disease
    Menkes disease
    Mucopolysaccharidoses
    Lipid storage disorders
  Deep gray matter plus white matter
    Primarily thalamic involvement
      Krabbe disease
      GM_2 gangliosidosis
    Primarily globus pallidus involvement
      Canavan disease
      Kearns-Sayre disease
      Methylmalonic/propionic aciduria
      Carbon monoxide poisoning
      Maple syrup urine disease
    Primarily striatal involvement
      Leigh disease
      MELAS
      Wilson disease
      Cockayne disease
      Toxins

MELAS, mitochondrial encephalopathy with lactic acidosis and stroke.

Adapted from Barkovich (6), Wolpert and Barnes (7), Volpe (146), and Blaser (400).

demyelination, prominent periventricular lucencies on CT, and white matter hyperintensities on T2-weighted images throughout the brain parenchyma or in the periventricular region (400).

GM_1 Gangliosidosis. GM_1 gangliosidosis is an autosomal recessive condition resulting from a deficiency in β-galactosidase (400). Infantile, juvenile, and adult types are recognized; the different ages of onset probably reflect the percentage of normal activity of the enzyme. Children with the

infantile form, the most prominent, develop hypotonia and hypoactivity. Abnormal storage of GM_1 galactoside occurs in neurons and produces prominent neuronal loss. Secondary axonal degeneration with myelin loss results in central atrophic changes. Imaging reveals atrophy and white matter low attenuation or T2 hyperintensities. Putaminal hyperintensity on T2-weighted MRI has also been observed.

GM₂ Gangliosidoses. The GM_2 gangliosidoses (Tay-Sachs and Sandoff diseases) are caused by deficiencies in hexosaminidase (400). Tay-Sachs disease is the more common. Depending on the severity of the enzyme deficiency, presentation may be in infancy, later childhood, or even in adult life. In the most severe forms, death occurs within 3–5 years. Adults may present with severe psychiatric disorders. The abnormal metabolite is stored in neurons and may produce megalencephaly at first, although atrophic changes predominate later. Increased attenuation in the thalami on CT and T2 hypointensity on MRI have been noted (400,402). Demyelination may also occur. Adults may have selective but profound cerebellar atrophic changes.

Neuronal Ceroid Lipofuscinosis. Neuronal ceroid lipofuscinosis (NCL) is a storage disorder in which there is abnormal accumulation of subunit ''c'' of ATP synthase within lysosomes (400). The disorder is characterized by visual loss, seizures, and dementia. The age of onset is variable. NCL predominantly affects gray matter. Cortical thinning may be present on MRI as well as T1 hypointensity and T2 hyperintensity in the basal ganglia and thalami (6).

Mucopolysaccharidoses

The mucopolysaccharidoses (MPS) are a group of heritable storage disorders resulting from deficiencies in the lysosomal enzymes that degrade dermatan, heparan, and keratan sulfate (400). These include Hurler, Hunter, Sanfilippo, Morquio, Scheie, Maroteaux-Lamy, and Sly syndromes and their subtypes. The enzyme deficiencies allow mucopolysaccharides to accumulate in various tissues; their catabolites are excreted in the urine (6). With the exception of Hunter disease, which has an X-linked recessive inheritance, the mucopolysaccharidoses are autosomal recessive illnesses. The syndromes differ by the enzymatic defect, metabolites that accumulate and are excreted in the urine, and the clinical manifestations, many of which are nonneurological. Mental impairment, most marked with Hurler disease, may also be present in Hunter, Sanfilippo, and Sly syndromes. Vertebral subluxation and meningeal thickening in Morquio and Maroteaux-Lamy syndromes may result in spinal cord compression at the craniocervical junction.

Imaging commonly demonstrates macrocrania, calvarial thickening, meningeal thickening, megalencephaly, and hydrocephalus. White matter degeneration and volume loss are frequent (403–405). The white matter abnormalities include diffuse or patchy low attenuation by CT and T2 prolongation

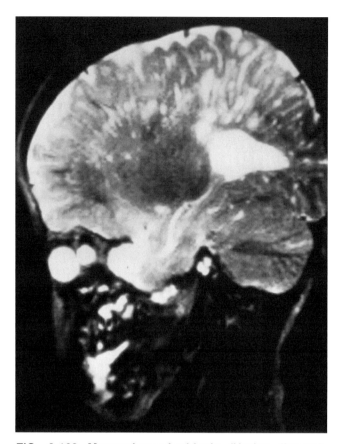

FIG. 2-162. Mucopolysaccharidosis (Hurler disease). Sagittal T2-weighted image. There is marked prominence of the perivascular spaces from the surface of the brain to the ventricular margin. This actually results from the deposition of mucopolysaccharide within perivascular histiocytes and surrounding demyelination.

(hyperintensity) by MRI (Fig. 2-162). Focal ovoid or rounded lesions are due to deposition of mucopolysaccharides in the perivascular spaces of the basal ganglia, corpus callosum, and hemispheric white matter (Fig. 2-162). Arachnoid cysts occasionally occur (406).

Lysosomal Leukodystrophies

Metachromatic Leukodystrophy. Metachromatic leukodystrophy (MLD) is an autosomal recessive disorder caused by variable deficiency in the enzyme arylsulfatase A (6,407). The age of onset of symptoms often depends on the degree of enzyme deficiency. Affected infants commonly present with abnormalities of gait, spasticity, impaired speech, and progressive intellectual decline beginning in the second year of life. Death typically occurs within the next 4 years. The less common juvenile and rare adult forms of MLD have a more chronic course.

Imaging demonstrates confluent regions of demyelination (low density by CT; T2 hyperintensity by MRI) in the deep cerebral white matter (Figs. 2-163 and 2-164). The periph-

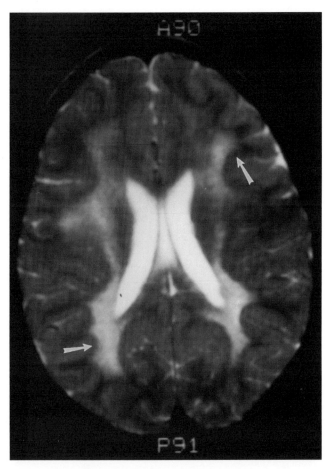

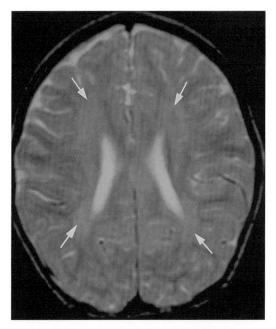

FIG. 2-164. Metachromatic leukodystrophy. A 3-year-old boy with developmental delay. Axial T2 MRI demonstrates periventricular and subcortical white matter hyperintensities *(arrows)* as well as delayed myelination *(arrows).*

FIG. 2-163. Metachromatic leukodystrophy. Axial T2-weighted image. Diffuse hyperintense signal is identified within the deep and periventricular white matter of both cerebral hemispheres as a result of abnormal myelination in this disorder. Note the sparing of the subcortical white matter tracts *(arrows)* ("U fibers"), which is an early characteristic of this and other lysosomal storage leukodystrophies.

eral (subcortical) white matter tracts (U fibers) are less affected until late in the course of the disease (Figs. 2-163 and 2-164) (50,399). There is usually no contrast enhancement. There is progressive development of diffuse atrophy.

Krabbe Disease. Krabbe disease (globoid cell leukodystrophy) is an autosomal recessive disease in which a deficiency in β-galactocerebrosidase activity causes a breakdown of the myelin sheath (400). The disease is divided into infantile, late infantile, and adult forms. Affected individuals develop psychomotor deterioration, irritability, seizures, optic atrophy, and gait disturbances. The basic pathology is demyelination of the brain and spinal cord. The demyelination of the supratentorial and infratentorial white matter is seen as zones of low attenuation on CT and of mildly decreased intensity on T1-weighted and increased signal on T2-weighted MR images. Areas of decreased density on CT and increased T2 intensity on MRI are often seen in the cerebellum, the heads of the caudate nuclei, and the posterior thalami (Fig. 2-165).

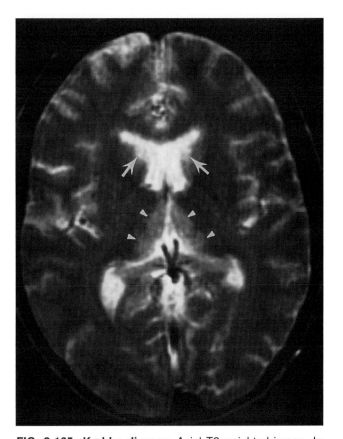

FIG. 2-165. Krabbe disease. Axial T2-weighted image. In this child presenting with progressive neurologic dysfunction, patchy increased signal is identified in both caudate heads *(arrows)* and in the posterior thalami *(arrowheads).*

Mitochondrial Disorders

The mitochondrial cytopathies are characterized by enzyme defects in the respiratory oxidative pathway that result in impaired adenosine triphosphate (ATP) production (6,408). The mitochondrial disorders include Leigh disease, Kearns-Sayre syndrome, mitochondrial encephalomyopathy with lactic acidosis and stroke (MELAS), myoclonic epilepsy and ragged red cell fibers (MERRF), Menkes disease, Alper disease, glutaric aciduria types 1 and 2, and infantile bilateral striatal necrosis. Manifestations of these illnesses overlap; seizures, muscle weakness, mental deterioration, sensorineural hearing loss, and short stature occur in many of them (6). The CNS abnormalities characteristically involve the deep gray matter structures and the white matter.

Leigh Disease

Leigh disease (subacute necrotizing encephalomyelopathy) is caused by several different mitochondrial enzyme defects (6,409). Affected individuals typically develop hypotonia and progressive psychomotor deterioration within the first 2 years of life. Death soon follows. Capillary proliferation and microcystic cavitation occur in the basal ganglia, brainstem, and dentate nuclei. The lesions most often shown by imaging involve the putamina and periaqueductal gray matter. Abnormalities of the cerebral and cerebellar peduncles, dentate nuclei, globi pallidi, and caudate nuclei may also be identified. Abnormalities in the caudate heads, putamina, and globi palladi are low density on CT; they are hypointense on T1-weighted and hyperintense on T2-weighted MRI (Fig. 2-166). MRS shows decreased N-acetyl aspartate (NAA) and elevated lactate levels in the brain (6).

Kearns-Sayre Syndrome

The Kearns-Sayre syndrome is an autosomal dominant disorder characterized by the triad of external ophthalmoplegia, pigmentary degeneration of the retina, and heart block (410). Muscle weakness, sensorineural hearing loss, short stature, and mental deterioration may also occur. The symptoms begin before 20 years of age (6). Elevations of serum pyruvate and CSF protein are present. Spongy degeneration develops in the deep gray matter nuclei, white matter, and brainstem.

Imaging studies show white matter low density on CT and T2 hyperintensity on MRI (50,408,411). The white matter findings affect the subcortical white matter preferentially and tend to spare the periventricular white matter. CT density and MRI intensity abnormalities caused by increased water content are also frequently identified in the basal ganglia,

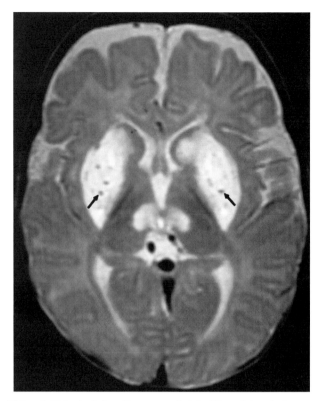

FIG. 2-166. Leigh disease. Axial T2-weighted image. Marked symmetric hyperintense signal is identified in the caudate heads, putamina, and globus pallidi. Prominent perivascular spaces *(arrows)* are also seen scattered throughout the basal ganglia.

thalami, and cerebellar nuclei. Calcifications are occasionally present in these deep gray matter structures.

Mitochondrial Encephalomyopathy with Lactic Acidosis and Stroke (MELAS)

MELAS is a group of disorders in which strokes or stroke-like episodes, nausea, and vomiting accompany systemic signs of mitochondrial dysfunction (6,408). The neurologic deficits may be permanent or reversible. The onset of symptoms is usually in the second decade.

Imaging demonstrates cortical foci of low density on CT and high intensity on T2-weighted MRI images; these abnormalities may not conform to vascular territories and are most frequent in the occipital and parietal lobes (Fig. 2-167A). The changes may disappear and reappear. Cortical enhancement may occur with contrast administration (412). Increased water content is also observed in the basal ganglia on both CT (low density) and MRI (T1 hypointensity; T2 hyperintensity) (Fig. 2-167B). MRS may show elevations in lactate content; however, acute and subacute infarctions not caused by mitochondrial disease may also exhibit elevated lactate levels (413).

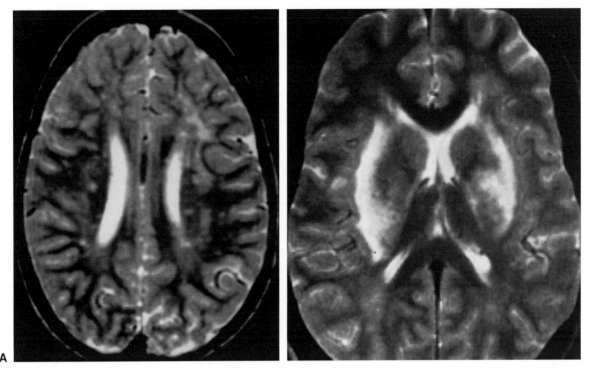

FIG. 2-167. MELAS. A: Axial T2 MRI. Asymmetric bilateral subcortical and periventricular white matter hyperintensities. **B:** Axial T2-weighted image. Bilateral symmetric hyperintense signal involves the basal ganglia and external capsules. The clinical presentation was that of an acute neurologic change indicative of stroke. Increased lactate was identified in both serum and cerebrospinal fluid. An evaluation revealed a cytochrome *c* oxidase deficiency.

Myoclonic Epilepsy and Ragged Red Fibers (MERRF)

MERRF primarily occurs in adulthood and is exceedingly rare in childhood (6). This mitochondrial disorder is characterized by myoclonic jerks and ataxia. Imaging may show basal ganglia calcification. Cerebral and cerebellar white matter degeneration also occur.

Menkes Disease

Menkes disease (kinky hair syndrome; trichopolydystrophy) is an X-linked recessive condition in which there is decreased absorption of copper from the gastrointestinal tract (6,367,414). Reduction in copper decreases cytochrome oxidase activity in the mitochondria. Failure to thrive, seizures, and hypotonia are common clinical manifestations. The hair is sparse, coarse, and lacks pigment. Most patients die during the first 2 years of life (415). The relative lack of copper results in vessel tortuosity and intimal irregularity in many body regions. The vascular abnormalities may produce infarctions. Typically, there is hypomyelination of the white matter. Rapidly progressive cortical atrophy is frequently present and may be accompanied by large subdural collections (6,408). Foci of T1 and T2 hypointensity are occasionally seen on MRI. The imaging findings in the CNS and the skeletal system may mimic those of child abuse.

Alpers Disease

Alpers disease is a rare autosomal recessive disease or group of diseases with marked cortical atrophy and liver dysfunction (6,416). Affected children develop seizures, failure to thrive, and developmental delay. Imaging reveals delayed myelination and atrophy of the cortical and deep gray matter.

Glutaric Acidurias

Glutaric aciduria type 1 is an autosomal recessive aminoacidopathy resulting from a defect in glutaryl-CoA dehydrogenase, a mitochondrial enzyme. The disorder produces progressive hypotonia, dystonia, and encephalopathy, usually beginning in the first year of life (6,417). Imaging shows delayed myelination and frontotemporal atrophy with widening of the Sylvian fissure.

Glutaric aciduria type 2 is the result of acyl-CoA deficiency. Hypoglycemia, hypotonia, and acidosis occur during early infancy. Imaging studies may reveal basal ganglia involvement with T2 hyperintensity in the corpus striatum and in the cerebral white matter (6).

Infantile Bilateral Striatal Necrosis

Infantile bilateral striatal necrosis is a mitochondrial disorder characterized clinically by dystonia, muscle weakness, and intellectual impairment. Imaging demonstrates bilateral low density within the putamina on CT with corresponding T1 hypointensity and T2 hyperintensity on MRI (418).

Peroxisomal Disorders

Peroxisomal disorders are due to enzyme defects in the processing of very long chain fatty acids. The disorders may be due to a single enzyme defect, as in X-linked adrenoleukodystrophy; may be the product of multiple enzyme deficiencies, as in neonatal adrenoleukodystrophy; or may be caused by absence of the peroxisome itself, as in Zellweger syndrome.

Adrenoleukodystrophy

Adrenoleukodystrophy (ALD) includes three X-linked variants, each resulting from a single peroxisomal enzyme defect and all occurring almost exclusively in males (6,419). The most common variant typically has its onset between 5 and 10 years of age. Neurologic manifestations include seizures, behavioral changes, gait disturbances, hearing impairment, and mild intellectual decline. Adrenal insufficiency is also present. The disease has a progressive course; death usually occurrs within 3 years.

A fourth form of the disease, with late onset and occurring in males and females, is referred to as adrenoleukomyeloneuropathy; this presents as peripheral neuropathy, impotence, and sphincter disturbances.

An even rarer type, neonatal ALD, involves multiple enzyme deficiencies, occurs in early infancy, and is autosomal recessive.

The pathologic findings in ALD consist of confluent zones of abnormal white matter, usually in the occipital and parietal lobes. Demyelination is frequently severe and bilateral; the corpus callosum is involved. Lymphocytes accumulate at the margins of the lesions. On imaging, regions of demyelination and astrogliosis exhibit increased water content as detected by CT (low density) and MRI (T1 hypointensity; T2 hyperintensity) in the parietal and occipital lobes (Fig. 2-168) (419,420). The peripheral white matter is often spared until late in the disease. Pontomedullary cortical spinal tract involvement may also be seen (421). Contrast enhancement in the zone of active myelination and thinning of the splenium of the corpus callosum are often seen. MRS demonstrates decreased levels of NAA and myoinositol with increased choline, glutamine, and glutamate (6,30).

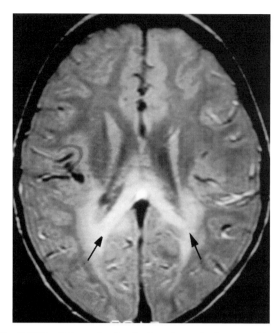

FIG. 2-168. Adrenoleukodystrophy. A 5-year-old boy. Axial proton density MRI. Bilateral temporoparietal periventricular and subcortical white matter hyperintensities along with hyperintensities of the posterior corpus callosum and forceps major *(arrows)* are shown.

Zellweger Syndrome

Zellweger syndrome (cerebrohepatorenal syndrome) results from a defect in peroxisome structure and consequent deficiencies of many enzymes. The disorder presents in infancy with dysmorphic features, seizures, mental retardation, stippled epiphyses, renal abnormalities, and liver dysfunction (6,420). Severe hypomyelination is present in addition to abnormalities of gray matter; these include neuronal heterotopia, polymicrogyria, and pachygyria (Fig. 2-169). Cortical dysplasias are associated with many of the infantile peroxisomal disorders, including Zellweger syndrome and neonatal adrenoleukodystrophy.

Amino Acid Disorders

Phenylketonuria

Phenylketonuria is an autosomal recessive disorder in which a defect in phenylalanine hydroxylase results in an inability to convert phenylalanine to tyrosine (6). The impaired enzymatic activity leads to the accumulation of neurotoxic metabolites. Treatment is dietary. Left untreated, affected individuals exhibit developmental delay, seizures, irritability, and vomiting. MRI of the brain in phenylketonuria shows delayed myelination and an increased signal in the periventricular white matter on T2-weighted images (Fig. 2-170) (422). The peripheral white matter is usually spared.

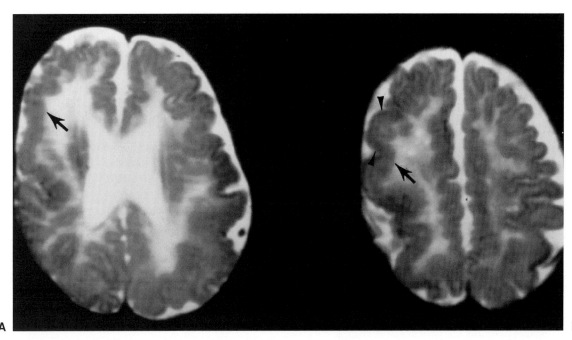

FIG. 2-169. Zellweger syndrome. A,B: Axial T2-weighted images. In this 3-month-old infant with diffuse hypotonia and developmental delay, the cortex appears disorganized and thickened *(arrows)* and several of the gyri are broad and coarse *(arrowheads).*

Maple Syrup Urine Disease

Maple syrup urine disease is an autosomal recessive disorder characterized by an inability to decarboxylate the

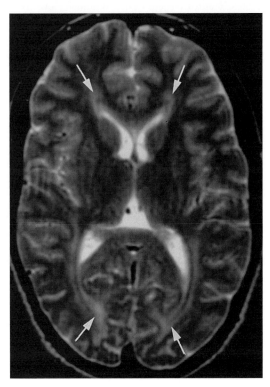

FIG. 2-170. Phenylketonuria. A 20-year-old man. Axial T2 MRI. Bilateral temporoparietal and frontal periventricular white matter hyperintensities *(arrows)* are demonstrated.

branched chain amino acids leucine, isoleucine, and valine (6,423). As a result, ketoacids accumulate in the serum and urine. The sweet smell of ketoacids in the urine gives the disease its name. Symptoms usually develop in the first few days of life and includes seizures, opisthotonos, and coma.

Imaging shows edema in white matter that is myelinated or being actively myelinated at birth (deep cerebellar white matter, dorsal parts of the brainstem, cerebral peduncles, and posterior limbs of the internal capsule). Generalized edema may also be present (423).

Lowe Syndrome

Lowe syndrome (oculocerebrorenal syndrome) includes congenital ocular abnormalities (glaucoma, cataracts), mental retardation, and renal tubular acidosis (6,424,425). Cranial imaging reveals scalloping of the calvaria. MRI shows focal and confluent areas of T2 prolongation in white matter with initial sparing of the subcortical U fibers (Fig. 2-171).

Miscellaneous Metabolic and Neurodegenerative Disorders

Canavan Disease

Canavan disease (spongiform leukodystrophy) is an autosomal recessive disorder in which a defect in *N*-acetylaspartylase results in the accumulation of *N*-acetyl aspartic acid

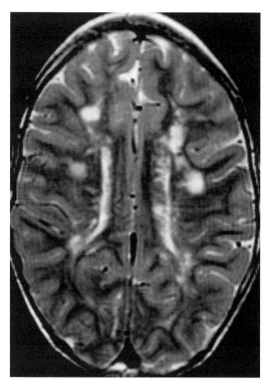

FIG. 2-171. Lowe syndrome. Axial T2 MRI of a 10-year-old boy. Bilateral nodular white matter hyperintensities are seen.

in the brain (6). The disease usually becomes apparent in the first few months of life. Manifestations include macrocrania, seizures, failure of intellectual development, optic atrophy, and spasticity. Death usually occurs between 2 and 5 years of age. As the name implies, there is spongiform degeneration of the white matter, early in the disease preferentially involving the peripheral white matter including the subcortical U-fibers. Imaging shows diffuse white matter edema (low density on CT; T1 hypointensity and T2 hyperintensity on MRI) (Fig. 2-172A). Density and intensity abnormalities may also involve the globi pallidi; the putamina are usually spared. MR proton spectroscopy shows increased *N*-acetyl aspartate in the brain (6).

Alexander Disease

Alexander disease (fibrinoid leukodystrophy) is a sporadically occurring disorder that usually presents during infancy. Affected infants exhibit macrocephaly, psychomotor retardation, seizures, and vomiting. Death typically occurs in the first few years of life (6,146). Imaging shows increased water (low density on CT; T1 hypointensity and T2 hyperintensity on MRI) starting in the frontal lobes and progressing toward the parietal region (6,426,427). The peripheral white matter is usually involved. White matter cysts may be present late in the disease. Contrast enhancement may occur near the frontal horns of the lateral ventricles.

Pelizaeus-Merzbacher Disease

Pelizaeus-Merzbacher disease is a rare X-linked disorder in which a deficiency in proteolipid protein, one of the primary components of myelin, results in the inability of the oligodendroglia to form and maintain myelin (6,428). Abnormal eye movements, psychomotor retardation, and cerebellar ataxia usually develop in infancy. Imaging typically shows complete or partial absence of myelination throughout the brain. This is demonstrated on CT as decreased attenuation and on T2-weighted MRI as diffuse high intensity of the white matter (Fig. 2-173) (428–430). Progressive sulcal enlargement ensues. Basal ganglia and thalamic T2 hypointensities, possibly representing iron, have also been observed.

Hallervorden-Spatz Disease

Hallervorden-Spatz disease, a rare metabolic disorder, usually causes progressive gait impairment, choreoathetoid movements, slowing of voluntary movements, and mental deterioration during the second decade of life (6). The disease is pathologically characterized by bilateral symmetric destruction of the globus pallidus, substantia nigra, and red nucleus. There may be deposition of iron-containing elements or calcification. Imaging may show changes associated with tissue destruction or may predominantly reflect the associated iron deposition. Iron deposition produces high density on CT and marked T2 hypointensity on MRI (Fig. 2-174) (431). A characteristic appearance on T2-weighted MRI is bilateral ring-like hypointensity and central hyperintensity of the globi pallidi.

Wilson Disease

Wilson disease (hepatolenticular degeneration) is an autosomal recessive condition in which diminished concentrations of ceruloplasmin (a copper-binding protein) lead to an increased concentration of copper in the liver, which causes cirrhosis (6). Affected individuals may present either with hepatic failure or with neurologic dysfunction. Neurologic findings include dystonia, impaired speech, gait disturbances, and tremors. Kayser-Fleischer rings (green rings in the corneas) are commonly present.

Imaging in Wilson disease usually shows low density on CT and T2 hyperintensity on MRI in the putamina and caudate nuclei (432). Similar density and intensity changes may also occur in the dorsal midbrain, pons, and cerebellum. The basal ganglia appear abnormally hyperintense, particularly in patients with liver failure; the thalami are typically spared (Fig. 2-175). Mild hyperintensity may be observed in the white matter, particularly in the frontal and temporal lobes. Brain atrophy is frequently present.

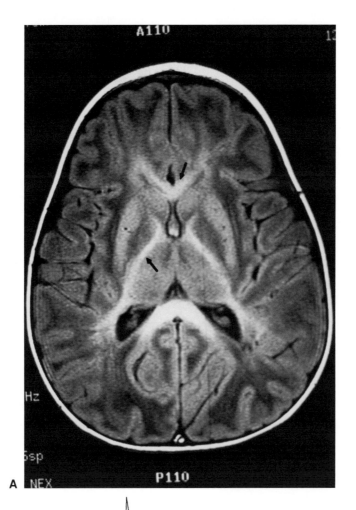

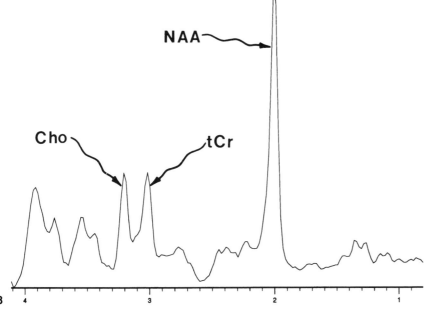

FIG. 2-172. **Canavan disease. A:** Axial T1-weighted image. In this 13-month-old child with macrocrania, myelin (hyperintense signal) is only seen within the deep white matter tracts such as the internal capsule and corpus callosum *(arrows)*. The peripheral white matter tracts including the subcortical tracts and optic radiations are devoid of myelin. **B:** Proton MRI spectroscopy from the superficial centrum semiovale reveals a marked elevation of the *N*-acetyl aspartate peak *(NAA)* compared to choline *(Cho)* and total creatine *(tCr)*, which is characteristic of this disorder.

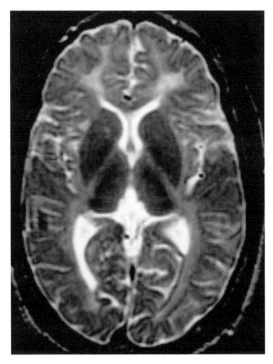

FIG. 2-173. Pelizaeus-Merzbacher disease. A 19-year-old boy. Marked white matter hyperintensity (hypomyelination) throughout the cerebrum.

Fahr Disease

Fahr disease, a group of heritable disorders rather than a single disease process, causes calcification in the walls of vessels in the basal ganglia, cortex, and dentate nuclei. Men-

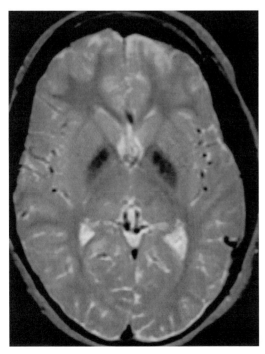

FIG. 2-174. Hallervorden-Spatz disease. A 9-year-old girl. There is marked hypointensity of the globus pallidus bilaterally.

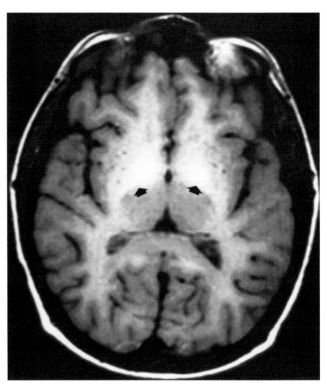

FIG. 2-175. Wilson disease. Axial T1-weighted image. The basal ganglia are abnormally hyperintense *(arrows)*. The thalami are spared. Basal ganglia involvement is characteristic of this disorder.

tal and growth retardation usually occur. CT demonstrates bilateral basal ganglia calcifications and severe cerebral atrophy (Fig. 2-176) (433). The mineralization of the basal ganglia and dentate nuclei usually leads to hypointensity on T1- and T2-weighted MRI; the white matter lesions may be hyperintense on T1-weighted images.

Cockayne Syndrome

Cockayne syndrome is an autosomal recessive disorder characterized by microcephaly, cutaneous photosensitivity, cachexia, dwarfism, and progressive encephalopathy (6). Calcification in the basal ganglia and dentate nuclei is seen on CT as high density and on MRI as T1 hyperintensity and T2 hypointensity (434,435). White matter intensity abnormalities similar to those in Pelizaeus-Merzbacher syndrome have also been described (435). Progressive atrophy is evident.

Friedreich Ataxia

Friedreich ataxia, a disorder of unknown etiology, causes demyelination and gliosis of the long tracts of the spinal cord and sometimes involvement of the cerebellum and brainstem. An increase in the volume of the fourth ventricle,

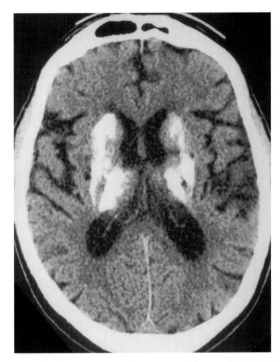

FIG. 2-176. Fahr disease. A 20-year-old man. Axial CT demonstrates bilateral basal ganglia calcifications and severe cerebral atrophy.

atrophy of the dentate nuclei, cerebellar hemispheres, and vermis may occur.

Olivopontocerebellar Atrophies

Olivopontocerebellar atrophies cause cerebellar ataxia, tremor, speech impairment, extrapyramidal signs, and cranial nerve palsies. Although these disorders usually develop in adult life, an infantile form has been described. Imaging shows cerebellar and brainstem atrophy reflecting the neuronal loss in the cerebellar cortex, pons, inferior olivary nucleus, and nuclei of cranial nerves X and XII (436).

Toxic Injuries

Exposure to toxic agents such as carbon monoxide, hydrogen sulfide, methanol, and cyanide commonly produces destructive lesions of the basal ganglia (6,437,438). The reasons for the relative susceptibility of the basal ganglia include the high metabolic demands of the corpus striatum and its border location between the major vascular territories. The lesions produced by these toxic insults are hypodense on CT, hypointense on T1 MRI, and hyperintense on T2 MRI.

Lead intoxication may cause cerebral edema with mass effect (439). Previously, this was the most common cause of toxic injury to the CNS. In severe cases there may be extensive intracranial calcification.

REFERENCES

General Information

1. Harwood-Nash DC. Pediatric neuroradiology: its evolution as a subspecialty. *AJR* 1993;160:5–14.
2. Chasler CN. *Atlas of Roentgen anatomy of the newborn infant skull.* St. Louis: Green, 1972.
3. Kirks DR, Harwood-Nash DC. Computed tomography in pediatric radiology. *Pediatr Ann* 1980;9:66–76.
4. Harwood-Nash DC, Flodmark O. Diagnostic imaging of the neonatal brain: review and protocol. *AJNR* 1982;3:103–115.
5. Harwood-Nash DC, Fitz CR. *Neuroradiology in infants and children.* St. Louis: CV Mosby, 1976.
6. Barkovich AJ. *Pediatric neuroimaging.* 2nd ed. New York: Raven Press, 1995.
7. Wolpert SM, Barnes PD, eds. *MRI in pediatric neuroradiology.* St. Louis: CV Mosby, 1992.

Techniques

8. Babcock DS, Han BK, LeQuesne GW, et al. B-mode gray scale ultrasound of the head in the newborn and young infant. *AJR* 1980;134: 457–468.
9. Grant EG, Schellinger D, Borts FT, et al. Real-time sonography of the neonatal and infant head. *AJR* 1981;136:265–270.
10. Naidich TP, Yousefzadeh DK, Gusnard DA. Sonography of the normal neonatal head. Supratentorial structures: state-of-the-art imaging. *Neuroradiology* 1986;28:408–427.
11. Slovis TL, Kuhns LR. Real-time sonography of the brain through the anterior fontanelle. *AJR* 1981;136:277–286.
12. Teele RL, Share JC. *Ultrasonography of infants and children.* Philadelphia: WB Saunders, 1991.
13. Buckley KM, Taylor GA, Estroff JA, et al. Use of the mastoid fontanelle for improved sonographic visualization of the neonatal midbrain and posterior fossa. *AJR* 1997;168:1021–1025.
14. Barnes PD, O'Tuama L, Tzika A. Investigating the pediatric central nervous system. *Curr Opin Pediatr* 1993;5:643–652.
15. Zimmerman RA. Pediatric head trauma. In: Kirks DR, ed. *Emergency pediatric radiology. A problem-oriented approach.* Reston, VA: American Roentgen Ray Society, 1995, 41–49.
16. Zimmerman RA, Bilaniuk LT. Pediatric head trauma. *Neuroimaging Clin North Am* 1994;4:349–366.
17. Glasier CM, Bates SR. Pediatric seizures: emergency imaging. In: Kirks DR, ed. *Emergency pediatric radiology. A problem-oriented approach.* Reston, VA: American Roentgen Ray Society, 1995, 7–12.
18. Barnes PD. Increased intracranial pressure. In: Kirks DR, ed. *Emergency pediatric radiology. A problem-oriented approach.* Reston, VA: American Roentgen Ray Society, 1995, 23–27.
19. Blaser SI. Pediatric stroke: radiologic evaluation of acute neurological deficit in childhood. In: Kirks DR, ed. *Emergency pediatric radiology. A problem-oriented approach.* Reston, VA: American Roentgen Ray Society, 1995, 13–22.
20. Tice HM, Jones KM, Mulkern RV, et al. Fast spin-echo imaging of intracranial neoplasms. *J Comput Assist Tomogr* 1993;17:425–431.
21. Tzika AA, Vigneron DB, Ball WS Jr, et al. Localized proton MR spectroscopy of the brain in children. *J Magn Reson Imaging* 1993; 3:719–729.
22. Tzika AA, Massoth RJ, Ball WS Jr, et al. Cerebral perfusion in children: detection with dynamic contrast-enhanced T2*-weighted MR images. *Radiology* 1993;187:449–458.
23. Tzika AA, Vajapeyam S, Barnes PD. Multivoxel proton MR spectroscopy and hemodynamic MR imaging of childhood brain tumors: preliminary observations. *AJNR* 1997;18:203–218.
24. Simon J, Szumowski J, Totterman S, et al. Fat-suppression MR imaging of the orbit. *AJNR* 1988;9:961–968.
25. Robertson RL Jr, Blaustein PA, Gonzalez RG. Intracranial magnetic resonance angiography. In: Yucel EK, ed. *Magnetic resonance angiography: a practical approach.* New York: McGraw-Hill, 1995, 36–52.
26. Podreka I, Suess E, Goldenberg G, et al. Initial experience with technetium-99m Hm-PAO brain SPECT. *J Nucl Med* 1987;28: 1657–1666.

27. Packard AB, Roach PJ, Davis RT, et al. Ictal and interictal technetium-99m-bicisate brain SPECT in children with refractory epilepsy. *J Nucl Med* 1996;37:1101–1106.

28. Barnes PD, Poussaint TY, Burrows PE. Imaging of pediatric central nervous system infections. *Neuroimaging Clin N Am* 1994;4:367–391.

29. Ryvlin P, Philippon B, Cinotti L, et al. Functional neuroimaging strategy in temporal lobe epilepsy: a comparative study of 18FDG-PET and 99mTc-HMPAO-SPECT. *Ann Neurol* 1992;31:650–656.

Imaging Guidelines

30. Tzika AA, Ball WS Jr, Vigneron DB, et al. Childhood adrenoleukodystrophy: assessment with proton MR spectroscopy. *Radiology* 1993;189:467–480.

31. Naidich TP, Altman NR, Braffman BH, et al. Cephaloceles and related malformations. *AJNR* 1992;13:655–690.

32. McLone DG, Naidich TP. Developmental morphology of the subarachnoid space, brain vasculature and contiguous structures, and the cause of the Chiari II malformation. *AJNR* 1992;13:463–482.

33. Fitz CR. Holoprosencephaly and septo-optic dysplasia. *Neuroimaging Clin N Am* 1994;4:263–281.

34. Altman NR, Naidich TP, Braffman BH. Posterior fossa malformations. *AJNR* 1992;13:691–724.

35. Elster AD. Radiologic screening in the neurocutaneous syndromes: strategies and controversies. Commentary. *AJNR* 1992;13:1078–1082.

36. Braffman B, Naidich TP. The phakomatoses: part I. Neurofibromatosis and tuberous sclerosis. *Neuroimaging Clin N Am* 1994;4:299–324.

37. Braffman B, Naidich TP. The phakomatoses: part II. von Hippel-Lindau disease, Sturge-Weber syndrome, and less common conditions. *Neuroimaging Clin N Am* 1994;4:325–348.

38. Pont MS, Elster AD. Lesions of skin and brain: modern imaging of the neurocutaneous syndromes. *AJR* 1992;158:1193–1203.

39. Smirniotopoulos JG, Murphy FM. The phakomatoses. *AJNR* 1992;13:725–746.

40. Barkovich AJ, Gressens P, Evrard P. Formation, maturation, and disorders of brain neocortex. *AJNR* 1992;13:423–446.

41. Naidich TP, Grant JL, Altman N, et al. The developing cerebral surface: preliminary report on the patterns of sulcal and gyral maturation—anatomy, ultrasound, and magnetic resonance imaging. *Neuroimaging Clin N Am* 1994;4:201–240.

42. Barkovich AJ, Lyon G, Evrard P. Formation, maturation, and disorders of white matter. *AJNR* 1992;13:447–461.

43. Fitz CR. Inflammatory diseases of the brain in childhood. *AJNR* 1992;13:551–567.

44. Edwards-Brown MK. Supratentorial brain tumors. *Neuroimaging Clin N Am* 1994;4:437–455.

45. Vezina LG, Packer RJ. Infratentorial brain tumors of childhood. *Neuroimaging Clin North Am* 1994;4:423–436.

46. Ball WS Jr, Prenger EC, Ballard ET. Neurotoxicity of radio/chemotherapy in children: pathologic and MR correlation. *AJNR* 1992;13:761–776.

47. Harwood-Nash DC. Abuse to the pediatric central nervous system. *AJNR* 1992;13:569–575.

48. Sato Y, Yuh WT, Smith WL, et al. Head injury in child abuse: evaluation with MR imaging. *Radiology* 1989;173:653–657.

49. Ball WS Jr. Cerebrovascular occlusive disease in childhood. *Neuroimaging Clin N Am* 1994;4:393–421.

50. Kendall BE. Disorders of lysosomes, peroxisomes and mitochondria. *AJNR* 1992;13:621–653.

51. Harwood-Nash DC, Fitz CR. Large heads and ventricles in infants. *Radiol Clin North Am* 1975;13:199–224.

52. Maytal J, Alvarez LA, Elkin CM, Shinnar S. External hydrocephalus: radiologic spectrum and differentiation from cerebral atrophy. *AJR* 1987;148:1223–1230.

53. Wilms G, Vanderschueren G, Demaerel PH, et al. CT and MR in infants with pericerebral collections and macrocephaly: benign enlargement of the subarachnoid spaces versus subdural collections. *AJNR* 1993;14:855–860.

54. Naidich TP, Schott LH, Baron RL. Computed tomography in evaluation of hydrocephalus. *Radiol Clin North Am* 1982;20:143–167.

55. Quencer RM. Intracranial CSF flow in pediatric hydrocephalus: evaluation with cine-MR imaging. *AJNR* 1992;13:601–608.

56. McLaurin R. Ventricular shunts: complications and results. In: McLaurin R, Schut L, Venes J, Epstein F, eds. *Pediatric neurosurgery.* 2nd ed. Philadelphia: WB Saunders, 1989, 219–229.

57. Lee FA, Gwinn JL. Complications of ventriculoperitoneal shunts. *Ann Radiol* 1975;18:471–478.

Normal Skull Radiology and Normal Variants

58. Swischuk LE. The normal pediatric skull: variations and artifacts. *Radiol Clin North Am* 1972;10:277–290.

59. Swischuk LE. The normal newborn skull. *Semin Roentgenol* 1974;9:101–113.

60. Swischuk LE. The growing skull. *Semin Roentgenol* 1974;9:115–124.

61. Momose KJ. Developmental approach in the analysis of roentgenograms of the pediatric skull. *Radiol Clin North Am* 1971;9:99–116.

62. Shapiro R, Robinson F. Embryogenesis of the human occipital bone. *AJR* 1976;126:1063–1068.

63. Franken EA Jr. The midline occipital fissure: diagnosis of fracture versus anatomic variants. *Radiology* 1969;93:1043–1046.

64. Capitanio MA, Kirkpatrick JA. Widening of the cranial sutures: a roentgen observation during periods of accelerated growth in patients treated for deprivation dwarfism. *Radiology* 1969;92:53–59.

65. Currarino G. Normal variants and congenital anomalies in the region of the obelion. *AJR* 1976;127:487–494.

66. Currarino G. Skull size in the roentgenogram. *Prog Pediatr Radiol* 1976;5:160.

67. Erasmie U, Ringertz H. Normal width of cranial sutures in the neonate and infant. An objective method of assessment. *Acta Radiol* 1976;17:565–572.

68. Swischuk LE. *Imaging of the newborn, infant, and young child.* 3rd ed. Baltimore: Williams and Wilkins, 1989.

69. Berger PE, Harwood–Nash DC, Fitz CR. The dorsum sellae in infancy and childhood. *Pediatr Radiol* 1976;4:214–220.

70. Silverman FN. Roentgen standards for size of the pituitary fossa from infancy through adolescence. *AJR* 1957;78:451–460.

71. Swischuk LE, Sarwar M. The sella turcica (some lesser known dynamic features). *Crit Rev Diagn Imaging* 1978;11:37–55.

72. Underwood LE, Radcliffe WB, Guinto FC. New standards for the assessment of sella turcica volume in children. *Radiology* 1976;119:651–654.

73. Babbitt DP, Tang T, Dobbs J, Berk R. Idiopathic familial cerebrovascular ferrocalcinosis (Fahr's disease) and review of differential diagnosis of intracranial calcification in children. *AJR* 1969;105:352–358.

74. Lourie GL. A mnemonic for intracranial calcifications. *AJR* 1981;136:225–227.

75. Ozonoff MB, Gooding CA. Intracranial calcification in children. *Prog Pediatr Radiol* 1978;6:84–111.

76. Schey WL. Intracranial calcifications in childhood. Frequency of occurrence and significance. *AJR* 1974;122:495–502.

77. Teele RL, Hernanz-Schulman M, Sotrel A. Echogenic vasculature in the basal ganglia of neonates: a sonographic sign of vasculopathy. *Radiology* 1988;169:423–427.

Congenital and Developmental Abnormalities

78. van der Knaap MS, Valk J. Classification of congenital abnormalities of the CNS. *AJNR* 1988;9:315–326.

79. Duggan CA, Keener EB, Gay BB Jr. Secondary craniosynostosis. *AJR* 1970;109:277–293.

80. Griscom NT. Craniosynostosis. *Prog Pediatr Radiol* 1978;6:3–38.

81. Rollins N, Sklar F. Factitious lambdoid perisutural sclerosis: does the "sticky suture" exist? *Pediatr Radiol* 1996;26:356–358.

82. Cremin BJ, Zeeman BJ. Three-dimensional reconstruction in coronal synostosis: pre- and post-operative appearances. *Pediatr Radiol* 1989;19:313–315.

83. Currarino G, Silverman FN. Orbital hypotelorism, arhinencephaly and trigonocephaly. *Radiology* 1960;74:206–217.

84. McRae DL. Observations of craniolacunia. *Acta Radiol* 1966;5:55–64.

85. Shopfner CE, Jabbour JT, Vallion RM. Craniolacunia. *AJR* 1965;93:343–349.

86. Diebler C, Dulac O. Cephaloceles: clinical and neuroradiological appearance. Associated cerebral malformations. *Neuroradiology* 1983;25:199–216.

87. Byrd SE, Naidich TP. Common congenital brain anomalies. *Radiol Clin North Am* 1988;26:755–772.
88. Barkovich AJ, Vandermarck P, Edwards MSB, Cogen PH. Congenital nasal masses: CT and MR imaging features in 16 cases. *AJNR* 1991;12:105–116.
89. Barkovich AJ, Wippold FJ, Sherman JL, Citrin CM. Significance of cerebellar tonsillar position on MR. *AJNR* 1986;7:795–799.
90. Mikulis DJ, Diaz O, Egglin TK, Sanchez R. Variance of the position of the cerebellar tonsils with age: preliminary report. *Radiology* 1992;183:725–728.
91. Elster AD, Chen MYM. Chiari I malformations: clinical and radiologic reappraisal. *Radiology* 1992;183:347–353.
92. Naidich TP, Pudlowski RM, Naidich JB. Computed tomographic signs of the Chiari II malformation. Part II: Midbrain and cerebellum. *Radiology* 1980;134:391–398.
93. Naidich TP, Pudlowski RM, Naidich JB, et al. Computed tomographic signs of the Chiari II malformation. Part I: Skull and dural partitions. *Radiology* 1980;134:65–71.
94. Naidich TP, Pudlowski RM, Naidich JB. Computed tomographic signs of the Chiari II malformation. Part III: Ventricles and cisterns. *Radiology* 1980;134:657–663.
95. Naidich TP, McLone DG, Fulling KH. The Chiari II malformation. Part IV: The hindbrain deformity. *Neuroradiology* 1983;25:179–197.
96. Wolpert SM, Anderson M, Scott RM, et al. The Chiari II malformation: MR imaging evaluation. *AJNR* 1987;8:783–792.
97. McLone DG, Knepper PA. The cause of Chiari II malformation: a unified theory. *Pediatr Neurosci* 1989;15:1–12.
98. Babcock DS, Han BK. Cranial sonographic findings in meningomyelocele. *AJR* 1981;136:563–569.
99. Scotti G, Musgrave MA, Fitz CR, Harwood-Nash DC. The isolated fourth ventricle in children: CT and clinical review of 16 cases. *AJR* 1980;135:1233–1238.
100. Kurlander GJ, DeMyer W, Campbell JA, Taybi H. Roentgenology of holoprosencephaly (arhinencephaly). *Acta Radiol* 1966;5:25–40.
101. DeMyer W, Zeman W, Palmer CG. The face predicts the brain: diagnostic significance of median facial anomalies for holoprosencephaly (arhinencephaly). *Pediatrics* 1964;34:256–263.
102. Barkovich AJ, Norman D. Anomalies of the corpus callosum: correlation with further anomalies of the brain. *AJNR* 1988;9:493–501.
103. Barkovich AJ. Apparent atypical callosal dysgenesis: analysis of MR findings in six cases and their relationship to holoprosencephaly. *AJNR* 1990;11:333–339.
104. Barkovich AJ, Fram EK, Norman D. Septo-optic dysplasia: MR imaging. *Radiology* 1989;171:189–192.
105. Brodsky MC, Glasier CM. Optic nerve hypoplasia: clinical significance of associated central nervous system abnormalities on magnetic resonance imaging. *Arch Ophthalmol* 1993;111:66–74.
106. Strand RD, Barnes PD, Poussaint TY, et al. Cystic retrocerebellar malformations: unification of the Dandy–Walker complex and Blake's pouch cyst. *Pediatr Radiol* 1993;23:258–260.
107. Barkovich AJ, Kjos BO, Norman D, Edwards MS. Revised classification of posterior fossa cysts and cystlike malformations based on the results of multiplanar MR imaging. *AJNR* 1989;10:977–988.
108. Kollias SS, Ball WS Jr, Prenger EC. Cystic malformations of the posterior fossa: differential diagnosis clarified through embryologic analysis. *RadioGraphics* 1993;13:1211–1231.
109. Barkovich AJ, Chuang SH. Unilateral megalencephaly: correlation of MR imaging and pathologic characteristics. *AJNR* 1990;11:523–531.
110. Cusmai R, Curatolo P, Mangano S, et al. Hemimegalencephaly and neurofibromatosis. *Neuropediatrics* 1990;21:179–182.
111. Hager BC, Dyme IZ, Guertin SR, et al. Linear nevus sebaceous syndrome: megalencephaly and heterotopic gray matter. *Pediatr Neurol* 1991;7:45–49.
112. Peserico A, Battistella PA, Bertoli P, Drigo P. Unilateral hypomelanosis of Ito with hemimegalencephaly. *Acta Paediatr Scand* 1988;77:446–447.
113. Sarwar M, Schafer ME. Brain malformations in linear nevus sebaceous syndrome: an MR study. *J Comput Assist Tomogr* 1988;12:338–340.
114. Barkovich AJ, Newton TH. MR of aqueductal stenosis: evidence of a broad spectrum of tectal distortion. *AJNR* 1989;10:471–476.
115. Byrd SE, Bohan TP, Osborn RE, Naidich TP. The CT and MR evaluation of lissencephaly. *AJNR* 1988;9:923–927.
116. Byrd SE, Osborn RE, Bohan TP, Naidich TP. The CT and MR evaluation of migrational disorders of the brain. Part I. Lissencephaly and pachygyria. *Pediatr Radiol* 1989;19:151–156.
117. Byrd SE, Osborn RE, Bohan TP, Naidich TP. The CT and MR evaluation of migrational disorders of the brain. Part II. Schizencephaly, heterotopia and polymicrogyria. *Pediatr Radiol* 1989;19:219–222.
118. Yakovlev PI, Wadsworth RC. Schizencephalies: a study of the congenital clefts in the cerebral mantle. I. Clefts with fused lips. *J Neuropathol Exp Neurol* 1946;5:116–130.
119. Yakovlev PI, Wadsworth RC. Schizencephalies: a study of the congenital clefts in the cerebral mantle. II. Clefts with hydrocephalus and lips separated. *J Neuropathol Exp Neurol* 1946;5:169–206.
120. Barkovich AJ, Norman D. MR imaging of schizencephaly. *AJNR* 1988;9:297–302.
121. Barkovich AJ, Chuang SH, Norman D. MR of neuronal migration anomalies. *AJR* 1988;150:179–187.
122. Wesenberg RL, Juhl JH, Daube JR. Radiological findings in lissencephaly (congenital agyria). *Radiology* 1966;87:436–444.
123. Motte J, Gomes H, Morville P, Cymbalista M. Sonographic diagnosis of lissencephaly. *Pediatr Radiol* 1987;17:362–364.
124. Babcock DS. Sonographic demonstration of lissencephaly (agyria). *J Ultrasound Med* 1983;2:465–466.
125. Heschl R. Gehirndefect und hydrocephalus. *Vierteljahrschrift Prakt Heilk* 1859;61:59.
126. Bresler NC. Klinische und pathologish-anatomische Beitraege zur Mikrogyrie. *Arch Psychiatry* 1899;31:566.
127. Barkovich AJ, Kjos BO. Normal postnatal development of the corpus callosum as demonstrated by MR imaging. *AJNR* 1988;9:487–491.
128. Aicardi J, Lefebre J, Lerrique-Koechlin A. A new syndrome: spasm in flexion, callosal agenesis, ocular abnormalities. *Electroencephalogr Clin Neurophysiol* 1965;19:609–610.
129. Taybi H, Lachman RS. *Radiology of syndromes, metabolic disorders, and skeletal dysplasias.* 4th ed. St. Louis: CV Mosby, 1996.
130. Rakic P, Yakovlev PI. Development of the corpus callosum and cavum septi in man. *J Comp Neurol* 1968;132:45–72.
131. Babcock DS. The normal, absent and abnormal corpus callosum: sonographic findings. *Radiology* 1984;151:449–453.
132. Barkovich AJ, Kjos BO, Jackson DE Jr, Norman D. Normal maturation of the neonatal and infant brain: MR imaging at 1.5 T. *Radiology* 1988;166:173–180.
133. Bird CR, Hedberg M, Drayer BP, et al. MR assessment of myelination in infants and children: usefulness of marker sites. *AJNR* 1989;10:731–740.
134. Dietrich RB, Bradley WG, Zaragoza EJ IV, et al. MR evaluation of early myelination patterns in normal and developmentally delayed infants. *AJNR* 1988;9:69–76.
135. Raybaud C. Destructive lesions of the brain. *Neuroradiology* 1983;25:265–291.
136. Naidich TP, McLone DG, Radkowski MA. Intracranial arachnoid cysts. *Pediatr Neurosci* 1985-1986;12:112–122.
137. Klucznik RL, Wolpert SM, Anderson ML. Congenital and developmental abnormalities of the brain. In: Wolpert SM, Barnes PD, eds. *MRI in pediatric neuroradiology.* St. Louis: CV Mosby, 1992, 83–120.
138. Naidich TP, Gado M. Hydrocephalus. In: Newton TH, Potts DG, eds. *Ventricles and cisterns.* Vol. 4., St. Louis: CV Mosby, 1978, 3764–3834.

Infection

139. Wolpert SM, Kaye EM. Intracranial inflammatory processes. In: Wolpert SM, Barnes PD, eds. *MRI in pediatric neuroradiology.* St. Louis: CV Mosby, 1992, 151–xxx.
140. Barkovich AJ, Lindan CE. Congenital cytomegalovirus infection of the brain: imaging analysis and embryologic considerations. *AJNR* 1994;15:703–715.
141. Bale JF, Jr., Murph JR. Congenital infections and the nervous system. *Pediatr Clin North Am* 1992;39:669–690.
142. Becker LE. Infections of the developing brain. *AJNR* 1992;13:537–549.
143. Desmonts G, Couvreur J. Congenital toxoplasmosis. A prospective study of 378 pregnancies. *N Engl J Med* 1974;290:1110–1116.
144. Sugita K, Ando M, Makino M, et al. Magnetic resonance imaging of the brain in congenital rubella virus and cytomegalovirus infections. *Neuroradiology* 1991;33:239–242.

145. Hutto C, Arvin A, Jacobs R, et al. Intrauterine herpes simplex virus infections. *J Pediatr* 1987;110:97–101.
146. Volpe JJ. *Neurology of the newborn.* 3rd ed. Philadelphia: WB Saunders, 1995.
147. Koch TK. AIDS in children. In: Berg BO, ed. *Neurologic aspects of pediatrics.* Boston: Butterworth-Heinemann, 1992, 531–549.
148. Balakrishnan J, Becker PS, Kumar AJ, et al. Acquired immunodeficiency syndrome: correlation of radiologic and pathologic findings in the brain. *RadioGraphics* 1990;10:201–215.
149. Kauffman WM, Sivit CJ, Fitz CR, et al. CT and MR evaluation of intracranial involvement in pediatric HIV infection: a clinical-imaging correlation. *AJNR* 1992;13:949–957.
150. Bell WE. Bacterial meningitis in children. Selected aspects. *Pediatr Clin North Am* 1992;39:651–668.
151. Han BK, Babcock DS, McAdams L. Bacterial meningitis in infants: sonographic findings. *Radiology* 1985;154:645–650.
152. Chang KH, Han MH, Roh JK, et al. Gd-DTPA-enhanced MR imaging of the brain in patients with meningitis: comparison with CT. *AJNR* 1990;11:69–76.
153. Enzmann DR, Britt RH, Yeager AS. Experimental brain abscess evolution: computed tomographic and neuropathologic correlation. *Radiology* 1979;133:113–122.
154. Enzmann DR, Britt RH, Placone R. Staging of human brain abscess by computed tomography. *Radiology* 1983;146:703–708.
155. Haimes AB, Zimmerman RD, Morgello S, et al. MR imaging of brain abscesses. *AJNR* 1989;10:279–291.
156. Weiner LP, Fleming JO. Viral infections of the nervous system. *J Neurosurg* 1984;61:207–224.
157. Shaw DW, Cohen WA. Viral infections of the CNS in children: imaging features. *AJR* 1993;160:125–133.
158. Neils EW, Lukin R, Tomsick TA, Tew JM. Magnetic resonance imaging and computerized tomography scanning of herpes simplex encephalitis. Report of two cases. *J Neurosurg* 1987;67:592–594.
159. Schroth G, Gawehn J, Thron A, et al. Early diagnosis of herpes simplex encephalitis by MRI. *Neurology* 1987;37:179–183.
160. Whiteman ML, Donovan Post MJ, Berger JR, et al. Progressive multifocal leukoencephalopathy in 47 HIV-seropositive patients: neuroimaging with clinical and pathologic correlation. *Radiology* 1993;187:233–240.
161. Rasmussen T. Further observations on the syndrome of chronic encephalitis and epilepsy. *Appl Neurophysiol* 1978;41:1–12.
162. Baum PA, Barkovich AJ, Koch TK, Berg BO. Deep gray matter involvement in children with acute disseminated encephalomyelitis. *AJNR* 1994;15:1275–1283.
163. Caldemeyer KS, Harris TM, Smith RR, Edwards MK. Gadolinium enhancement in acute disseminated encephalomyelitis. *J Comput Assist Tomogr* 1991;15:673-675.
164. Jamieson DH. Imaging intracranial tuberculosis in childhood. *Pediatr Radiol* 1995;25:165–170.
165. Wallace RC, Burton EM, Barrett FF, et al. Intracranial tuberculosis in children: CT appearance and clinical outcome. *Pediatr Radiol* 1991;21:241–246.
166. Chang KH, Han MH, Roh JK, et al. Gd-DTPA enhanced MR imaging in intracranial tuberculosis. *Neuroradiology* 1990;32:19–25.
167. Weinberg S, Bennett H, Weinstock I. Central nervous system manifestations of sarcoidosis in children. Case report and review. *Clin Pediatr* 1983;22:477–481.
168. Hayes WS, Sherman JL, Stern BJ, et al. MR and CT evaluation of intracranial sarcoidosis. *AJNR* 1983;8:841–847.
169. Seltzer S, Mark AS, Atlas SW. CNS sarcoidosis: evaluation with contrast-enhanced MR imaging. *AJNR* 1991;12:1227–1233.
170. Carbajal JR, Palacios E, Azar-Kia B, Churchill R. Radiology of cysticercosis of the central nervous system including computed tomography. *Radiology* 1977;125:127–131.
171. Byrd SE, Locke GE, Biggers S, Percy AK. The computed tomographic appearance of cerebral cysticercosis in adults and children. *Radiology* 1982;144:819–823.
172. Suh DC, Chang KH, Han MH, et al. Unusual MR manifestations of neurocysticercosis. *Neuroradiology* 1989;31:396–402.
173. Teitelbaum GP, Otto RJ, Lin M, et al. MR imaging of neurocysticercosis. *AJR* 1989;153:857–866.

Cranial and Intracranial Tumors

174. Pollack IF. Brain tumors in children. *N Engl J Med* 1994;331:1500–1507.

175. Davis P. Tumors of the brain. In: Cohen MD, Edwards MK, eds. *MR imaging of children.* Philadelphia: BC Decker, 1990, 155–220.
176. Dean BL, Drayer BP, Bird CR, et al. Gliomas: classification with MR imaging. *Radiology* 1990;174:411–415.
177. Rorke LB, Gilles FH, Davis RL, Becker LE. Revision of the World Health Organization classification of brain tumors for childhood brain tumors. *Cancer* 1985;56:1869–1886.
178. Kleihues P, Burger PC, Scheithauer BW. The new WHO classification of brain tumors. *Brain Pathol* 1993;3:255–268.
179. Johnson PC, Hunt SJ, Drayer BP. Human cerebral gliomas: correlation of postmortem MR imaging and neuropathologic findings. *Radiology* 1989;170:211–217.
180. Bronstein AD, Nyberg DA, Schwartz AN, et al. Soft tissue changes after head and neck radiation: CT findings. *AJNR* 1989;10:171–175.
181. Curnes JT, Laster DW, Ball MR, et al. Magnetic resonance imaging of radiation injury to the brain. *AJNR* 1986;7:389–394.
182. Davis PC, Hoffman JC Jr, Pearl GS, Braun IF. CT evaluation of effects of cranial radiation therapy in children. *AJR* 1986;147:587–592.
183. Dooms GC, Hecht S, Brant-Zawadski M, et al. Brain radiation lesions: MR imaging. *Radiology* 1986;158:149–155.
184. Duffner PK, Cohen ME, Thomas PR, Lansky SB. The long-term effects of cranial irradiation on the central nervous system. *Cancer* 1985;56:1841–1846.
185. Grossman RI, Hecht-Leavitt CM, Evans SM, et al. Experimental radiation injury: combined MR imaging and spectroscopy. *Radiology* 1988;169:305–309.
186. Hecht-Leavitt C, Grossman RI, Curran WJ Jr, et al. MR of brain radiation injury: experimental studies in cats. *AJNR* 1987;8:427–430.
187. Moss SD, Rockswold GL, Chou SN, et al. Radiation-induced meningiomas in pediatric patients. *Neurosurgery* 1988;22:758–761.
188. Ron E, Modan B, Boice JD Jr, et al. Tumors of the brain and nervous system after radiotherapy in childhood. *N Engl J Med* 1988;319:1033–1039.
189. Tsuruda JS, Kortman KE, Bradley WG, et al. Radiation effects on cerebral white matter: MR evaluation. *AJR* 1987;149:165–171.
190. Valk PE, Dillon WP. Radiation injury of the brain. *AJNR* 1991;12:45–62.
191. Young Poussaint T, Siffert J, Barnes PD, et al. Hemorrhagic vasculopathy after treatment of central nervous system neoplasia in childhood: diagnosis and follow-up. *AJNR* 1995;16:693–699.
192. Rosen BR, Aronen HJ, Kwong KK, et al. Advances in clinical neuroimaging: functional MR imaging techniques. *RadioGraphics* 1993;13:889–896.
193. Segall HD, Zee CS, Naidich TP, et al. Computed tomography in neoplasms of the posterior fossa in children. *Radiol Clin North Am* 1982;20:237–253.
194. Zimmerman RA, Bilaniuk LT, Bruno L, Rosenstock J. Computed tomography of cerebellar astrocytoma. *AJR* 1978;130:929–933.
195. Fulham MJ, Melisi JW, Nishimiya J, et al. Neuroimaging of juvenile pilocytic astrocytomas: an enigma. *Radiology* 1993;189:221–225.
196. Bourgouin PM, Tampieri D, Grahovac SZ, et al. CT and MR imaging findings in adults with cerebellar medulloblastoma: comparison with findings in children. *AJR* 1992;159:609–612.
197. Kingsley DP, Harwood-Nash DC. Radiologic features of the neuroectodermal tumours of childhood. *Neuroradiology* 1984;26:463–467.
198. Meyers SP, Kemp SS, Tarr RW. MR imaging features of medulloblastomas. *AJR* 1992;158:859–865.
199. Zimmerman RA, Bilaniuk LT, Pahlajani H. Spectrum of medulloblastomas demonstrated by computed tomography. *Radiology* 1978;126:137–141.
200. Berger PE, Kirks DR, Gilday DL, et al. Computed tomography in infants and children: intracranial neoplasms. *AJR* 1976;127:129–137.
201. Rollins N, Mendelsohn D, Mulne A, et al. Recurrent medulloblastoma: frequency of tumor enhancement on Gd-DTPA MR imaging. *AJNR* 1990;11:583–587.
202. Bilaniuk LT, Zimmerman RA, Littman P, et al. Computed tomography of brain stem gliomas in children. *Radiology* 1980;134:89–95.
203. Hueftle MG, Han JS, Kaufman B, Benson JE. MR imaging of brain stem gliomas. *J Comput Assist Tomogr* 1985;9:263–267.
204. Kane AG, Robles HA, Smirniotopoulos JG, et al. Radiologic-pathologic correlation. Diffuse pontine astrocytoma. *AJNR* 1993;14:941–945.
205. Lee BCP, Kneeland JB, Walker RW, et al. MR imaging of brainstem tumors. *AJNR* 1985;6:159–163.
206. Barnes PD, Kupsky WJ, Strand RD. Cranial and intracranial tumors. In: Wolpert SM, Barnes PD, eds. *MRI in pediatric neuroradiology.* St. Louis: CV Mosby, 1992, 234–260, 282–297.

207. May PL, Blaser SI, Hoffman HJ, et al. Benign intrinsic tectal "tumors" in children. *J Neurosurg* 1991;74:867–871.

208. Swartz JD, Zimmerman RA, Bilaniuk LT. Computed tomography of intracranial ependymomas. *Radiology* 1982;143:97–101.

209. Spoto GP, Press GA, Hesselink JR, Solomon M. Intracranial ependymoma and subependymoma: MR manifestations. *AJNR* 1990;11:83–91.

210. Smith RR, Grossman RI, Goldberg HI, et al. MR imaging of Lhermitte-Duclos disease: a case report. *AJNR* 1989;10:187–189.

211. Hernanz-Schulman M, Welch K, Strand R, Ordia JI. Acoustic neuromas in children. *AJNR* 1986;7:519–521.

212. Mulkens TH, Parizel PM, Martin J-J, et al. Acoustic schwannoma: MR findings in 84 tumors. *AJR* 1993;160:395–398.

213. Smirniotopoulos JG, Yue NC, Rushing EJ. Cerebellopontine angle masses: radiologic-pathologic correlation. *RadioGraphics* 1993;13:1131–1147.

214. Tampieri D, Melanson D, Ethier R. MR imaging of epidermoid cysts. *AJNR* 1989;10:351–356.

215. Gao PY, Osborn AG, Smirniotopoulos JG, Harris CP. Radiologic-pathologic correlation. Epidermoid tumor of the cerebellopontine angle. *AJNR* 1992;13:863–872.

216. Latack JT, Kartush JM, Kemink JL, et al. Epidermoidomas of the cerebellopontine angle and temporal bone: CT and MR aspects. *Radiology* 1985;157:361–366.

217. Yuh WTG, Barloon TJ, Jacoby CG, Schultz DH. MR of fourth-ventricular epidermoid tumors. *AJNR* 1988;9:794–796.

218. Filling-Katz MR, Choyke PL, Patronas NJ, et al. Radiologic screening for von Hippel-Lindau disease: the role of Gd-DTPA enhanced MR imaging of the CNS. *J Comput Assist Tomogr* 1989;13:743–755.

219. Ho VB, Smirniotopoulos JG, Murphy FM, Rushing EJ. Radiologic-pathologic correlation: hemangioblastoma. *AJNR* 1992;13:1343–1352.

220. Lee SR, Sanches J, Mark AS, et al. Posterior fossa hemangioblastomas: MR imaging. *Radiology* 1989;171:463–468.

221. Johnsen DE, Woodruff WW, Allen IS, et al. MR imaging of the sellar and juxtasellar regions. *RadioGraphics* 1991;11:727–758.

222. Miller JH, Pena AM, Segall HD. Radiological investigation of sellar region masses in children. *Radiology* 1980;134:81–87.

223. Pomeranz SJ, Shelton JJ, Tobias J, et al. MR of visual pathways in patients with neurofibromatosis. *AJNR* 1987;8:831–836.

224. Brown EW, Riccardi VM, Mawad M, et al. MR imaging of optic pathways in patients with neurofibromatosis. *AJNR* 1987;8:1031–1036.

225. Graif M, Pennock JM. MR imaging of histiocytosis X in the central nervous system. *AJNR* 1986;7:21–23.

226. Maghnie M, Arico M, Villa A, et al. MR of the hypothalamic-pituitary axis in Langerhans cell histiocytosis. *AJNR* 1992;13:1365–1371.

227. Chong BW, Kucharczyk W, Singer W, George S. Pituitary gland MR: a comparative study of healthy volunteers and patients with microadenomas. *AJNR* 1994;15:675–679.

228. Young Poussaint T, Barnes PD, Anthony DC, et al. Hemorrhagic pituitary adenomas of adolescence. *AJNR* 1996;17:1907–1912.

229. Chang T, Teng MM, Guo WY, Sheng WC. CT of pineal tumors and intracranial germ-cell tumors. *AJNR* 1989;10:1039–1044.

230. Mathews VP, Broome DR, Smith RR, et al. Neuroimaging of disseminated germ cell neoplasms. *AJNR* 1990;11:319–324.

231. Tien RD, Barkovich AJ, Edwards MSB. MR imaging of pineal tumors. *AJNR* 1990;11:557–565.

232. Appignani B, Landy H, Barnes P. MR in idiopathic central diabetes insipidus of childhood. *AJNR* 1993;14:1407–1410.

233. Gudinchet F, Brunelle F, Barth MO, et al. MR imaging of the posterior hypophysis in children. *AJNR* 1989;10:511.

234. Smirniotopoulos JG, Rushing EJ, Mena H. Pineal region masses: differential diagnosis. *RadioGraphics* 1992;12:577–596.

235. Ganti SR, Hilal SK, Stein BM, et al. CT of pineal region tumors. *AJR* 1986;146:451–458.

236. Nakagawa H, Iwasaki S, Kichikawa K, et al. MR imaging of pineocytoma: report of two cases. *AJNR* 1990;11:195–198.

237. Tien RD, Barkovich AJ, Edwards MSB. MR imaging of pineal tumors. *AJR* 1990;155:143–151.

238. Zimmerman RA, Bilaniuk LT, Wood JH, et al. Computed tomography of pineal, parapineal, and histologically related tumors. *Radiology* 1980;137:669–677.

239. Naidich TP, Zimmerman RA. Primary brain tumors in children. *Semin Roentgenol* 1984;19:100–114.

240. Pusey E, Kortman KE, Flannigan BD, et al. MR of craniopharyngiomas: tumor delineation and characterization. *AJNR* 1987;8:439–444.

241. Christophe C, Flamant-Durand J, Hanquinet S, et al. MRI in seven cases of Rathke's cleft cyst in infants and children. *Pediatr Radiol* 1992;23:79–82.

242. Kucharczyk W, Peck WW, Kelly WM, et al. Rathke cleft cysts: CT, MR imaging, and pathologic features. *Radiology* 1987;165:491–495.

243. Sumida M, Uozumi T, Mukada K, et al. Rathke cleft cysts: correlation of enhanced MR and surgical findings. *AJNR* 1994;15:525–532.

244. Maeder PP, Holtas SL, Basibuyuk LN, et al. Colloid cysts of the third ventricle: correlation of MR and CT findings with histology and chemical analysis. *AJNR* 1990;11:575–581.

245. Fleege MA, Miller GM, Fletcher GP, et al. Benign glial cysts of the pineal gland: unusual imaging characteristics with histologic correlation. *AJNR* 1994;15:161–166.

246. Mamourian A, Towfighi J. Pineal cysts: MR imaging. *AJNR* 1986;7:1081–1086.

247. Barral V, Brunelle F, Bauner R, et al. MRI of hypothalamic hamartomas in children. *Pediatr Radiol* 1988;18:449–452.

248. Boyko OB, Curnes JT, Oakes WJ, Burger PC. Hamartomas of the tuber cinereum: CT, MR, and pathologic findings. *AJNR* 1991;12:309–314.

249. Burton E, Ball WS Jr, Crone K, Dolan LM. Hamartoma of the tuber cinereum: a comparison of MR and CT findings in four cases. *AJNR* 1989;10:497–501.

250. Aizpuru RN, Quencer RM, Norenberg M, et al. Meningioangiomatosis: clinical, radiologic, and histopathologic correlation. *Radiology* 1991;179:819–821.

251. Shackelford GD, Shackelford PG, Schwetschenau PR, McAlister WH. Congenital occipital dermal sinus. *Radiology* 1974;111:161–166.

252. Ambrosino MM, Hernanz-Schulman M, Genieser NB, et al. Brain tumors in infants less than a year of age. *Pediatr Radiol* 1988;19:6–8.

253. Hanna SL, Langston JW, Parham DM, Douglass EC. Primary malignant rhabdoid tumor of the brain: clinical, imaging, and pathologic findings. *AJNR* 1993;14:107–115.

254. Radkowski MA, Naidich TP, Tomita T, et al. Neonatal brain tumors: CT and MR findings. *J Comput Assist Tomogr* 1988;12:10–20.

255. Buetow PC, Smirniotopoulos JG, Done S. Congenital brain tumors: a review of 45 cases. *AJNR* 1990;11:793–799.

256. Tadmor R, Harwood-Nash DCF, Savoiardo M, et al. Brain tumors in the first two years of life: CT diagnosis. *AJNR* 1980;1:411–417.

257. Lee YY, Van Tassel P, Bruner JM, et al. Juvenile pilocytic astrocytomas: CT and MR characteristics. *AJR* 1989;152:1263–1270.

258. Lipper MH, Eberhard DA, Phillips CD, et al. Pleomorphic xanthoastrocytoma, a distinctive astroglial tumor: neuroradiologic and pathologic features. *AJNR* 1993;14:1397–1404.

259. Strong JA, Hatten HP Jr, Brown MT, et al. Pilocystic astrocytoma: correlation between the initial imaging features and clinical aggressiveness. *AJR* 1993;161:369–372.

260. Tien RD, Cardenas CA, Rajagopalan S. Pleomorphic xanthoastrocytoma of the brain: MR findings in six patients. *AJR* 1992;159:1287–1290.

261. Yoshino MT, Lucio R. Pleomorphic xanthoastrocytoma. *AJNR* 1992;13:1330–1332.

262. Felsberg GJ, Silver SA, Brown MT, Tien RD. Radiologic-pathologic correlation. Gliomatosis cerebri. *AJNR* 1994;15:1745–1753.

263. Shin YM, Chang KH, Han MH, et al. Gliomatosis cerebri: comparison of MR and CT features. *AJR* 1993;161:859–862.

264. Lee YY, Van Tassel P. Intracranial oligodendrogliomas: imaging findings in 35 untreated cases. *AJR* 1989;152:361–369.

265. Shimizu KT, Tran LM, Mark RJ, Selch MT. Management of oligodendrogliomas. *Radiology* 1993;186:569–572.

266. Tice H, Barnes PD, Goumnerova L, et al. Pediatric and adolescent oligodendrogliomas. *AJNR* 1993;14:1293–1300.

267. Coates TL, Hinshaw DB Jr, Peckman N, et al. Pediatric choroid plexus neoplasms: MR, CT, and pathologic correlation. *Radiology* 1989;173:81–88.

268. Ellenbogen RG, Winston KR, Kupsky WJ. Tumors of the choroid plexus in children. *Neurosurgery* 1989;25:327–335.

269. Thompson JR, Harwood-Nash DC, Fitz CR. The neuroradiology of childhood choroid plexus neoplasms. *AJR* 1973;118:116–133.

270. Jelinek J, Smirniotopoulos JG, Parisi JE, Kanzer M. Lateral ventricular neoplasms of the brain: differential diagnosis based on clinical, CT, and MR findings. *AJNR* 1990;11:567–574.

271. Zimmerman RA, Bilaniuk LT. Computed tomography of choroid plexus lesions. *J Comput Tomogr* 1979;3:93–103.

272. Altman NR. MR and CT characteristics of gangliocytoma: a rare cause of epilepsy in children. *AJNR* 1988;9:917–921.

273. Castillo M, Davis PC, Takei Y, Hoffman JC Jr. Intracranial ganglioglioma: MR, CT, and clinical findings in 18 patients. *AJNR* 1990;11: 109–114.
274. Goergen SK, Gonzales MF, McLean CA. Intraventricular neurocytoma: radiologic features and review of the literature. *Radiology* 1992; 182:787–792.
275. Koeller KK, Dillon WP. Dysembryoplastic neuroepithelial tumors: MR appearance. *AJNR* 1992;13:1319–1325.
276. Tampieri D, Moumdjian R, Melanson D, Ethier R. Intracerebral gangliogliomas in patients with partial complex seizures: CT and MR imaging findings. *AJNR* 1991;12:749–755.
277. Dorne HL, O'Gorman AM, Melanson D. Computed tomography of intracranial gangliogliomas. *AJNR* 1986;7:281–285.
278. Martin DS, Levy B, Awwad EE, Pittman T. Desmoplastic infantile ganglioglioma: CT and MR features. *AJNR* 1991;12:1195–1197.
279. Altman N, Fitz CR, Chuang S, et al. Radiologic characteristics of primitive neuroectodermal tumors in children. *AJNR* 1985;6:15–18.
280. Davis PC, Wichman RD, Takei Y, Hoffman JC Jr. Primary cerebral neuroblastoma: CT and MR findings in 12 cases. *AJNR* 1990;11: 115–120.
281. Figueroa RE, El Gammal T, Brooks BS, et al. MR findings on primitive neuroectodermal tumors. *J Comput Assist Tomogr* 1989;13: 773–778.
282. Mirich DR, Blaser SI, Harwood-Nash DC, et al. Melanotic neuroectodermal tumor of infancy: clinical, radiologic, and pathologic findings in five cases. *AJNR* 1991;12:689–697.
283. Elster AD, Challa VR, Gilbert TH, et al. Meningiomas: MR and histopathologic features. *Radiology* 1989;170:857–862.
284. Darling CF, Byrd SE, Reyes-Mugica M, et al. MR of pediatric intracranial meningiomas. *AJNR* 1994;15:435–444.
285. Glasier CM, Husain MM, Chadduck W, Boop FA. Meningiomas in children: MR and histopathologic findings. *AJNR* 1993;14:237–241.
286. Hope JKA, Armstrong DA, Babyn PS, et al. Primary meningeal tumors in children: correlation of clinical and CT findings with histologic type and prognosis. *AJNR* 1992;13:1353–1364.
287. Buetow MP, Buetow PC, Smirniotopoulos JG. Typical, atypical, and misleading features in meningioma. *RadioGraphics* 1991;11: 1087–1106.
288. Sheporaitis LA, Osborn AG, Smirniotopoulos JG, et al. Radiologic-pathologic correlation. Intracranial meningioma. *AJNR* 1992;13: 29–37.
289. Spagnoli MV, Goldberg HI, Grossman RI, et al. Intracranial meningiomas: high-field MR imaging. *Radiology* 1986;161:369–375.
290. Barkovich AJ, Frieden IJ, Williams ML. MR of neurocutaneous melanosis. *AJNR* 1994;15:859–867.
291. Naul LG, Hise JH, Bauserman SC, Todd FD. CT and MR of meningeal melanocytoma. *AJNR* 1991;12:315–316.
292. Woodruff WW Jr, Djang WT, McLendon RE, et al. Intracerebral malignant melanoma: high-field-strength MR imaging. *Radiology* 1987;165:209–213.
293. Epstein LG, DiCarlo FJ Jr, Joshi VV. Primary lymphoma of the central nervous system in children with acquired immunodeficiency syndrome. *Pediatrics* 1988;82:355–363.
294. Haney PJ, Yale-Loehr AJ, Nussbaum AR, Gellad FE. Imaging of infants and children with AIDS. *AJR* 1989;152:1033–1041.
295. Arthur RJ, Brunelle F. Computerised tomography in the evaluation of expansile lesions arising from the skull vault in childhood—a report of 5 cases. *Pediatr Radiol* 1988;18:294–301.
296. Som PM, Dillon WP, Sze G, et al. Benign and malignant sinonasal lesions with intracranial extension: differentiation with MR imaging. *Radiology* 1989;172:763–766.
297. Armstrong EA, Harwood-Nash DCF, Fitz CR, et al. CT of neuroblastomas and ganglioneuromas in children. *AJR* 1982;139:571–576.
298. Davis PC, Friedman NC, Fry SM, et al. Leptomeningeal metastasis: MR imaging. *Radiology* 1987;163:449–454.
299. Krol G, Sze G, Malkin M, Walker R. MR of cranial and spinal meningeal carcinomatosis: comparison with CT and myelography. *AJR* 1988;151:583–588.
300. Rippe DJ, Boyko OB, Friedman HS, et al. Gd-DTPA-enhanced MR imaging of leptomeningeal spread of primary intracranial CNS tumor in children. *AJNR* 1990;11:329–332.
301. Sze G. Diseases of the intracranial meninges: MR imaging features. *AJR* 1993;160:727–733.

Trauma

302. Rivara FP, Kamitsuka MD, Quan L. Injuries to children younger than 1 year of age. *Pediatrics* 1988;81:93–97.
303. Harwood-Nash DC. Craniocerebral trauma in children. *Curr Probl Radiol* 1973;3:3–24.
304. Harwood-Nash DC, Hendrick EB, Hudson AR. The significance of skull fractures in children. A study of 1,187 patients. *Radiology* 1971; 101:151–155.
305. Thornbury JR, Campbell JA, Masters SJ, Fryback DG. Skull fracture and the low risk of intracranial sequelae in minor head trauma. *AJR* 1984;143:661–664.
306. Thornbury JR, Masters SJ, Campbell JA. Imaging recommendations for head trauma: a new comprehensive strategy. *AJR* 1987;149: 781–783.
307. Masters SJ, McClean PM, Arcarese JS, et al. Skull x-ray examinations after head trauma. Recommendations by a multidisciplinary panel and validation study. *N Engl J Med* 1987;316:84–91.
308. Bell RS, Loop JW. The utility and futility of radiographic skull examination for trauma. *N Engl J Med* 1971;284:236–239.
309. Roberts F, Shopfner CE. Plain skull roentgenograms in children with head trauma. *AJR* 1972;114:230–240.
310. Leonidas JC, Ting W, Binkiewicz A, et al. Mild head trauma in children: when is a roentgenogram necessary. *Pediatrics* 1982;69: 139–143.
311. Bradley WG Jr, Schmidt PG. Effect of methemoglobin formation on the MR appearance of subarachnoid hemorrhage. *Radiology* 1985; 156:99–103.
312. Schievink WI, Mokri B, O'Fallon WM. Recurrent spontaneous cervical-artery dissection. *N Engl J Med* 1994;330:393–397.
313. Klufas RA, Hsu L, Barnes PD, et al. Dissection of the carotid and vertebral arteries: imaging with MR angiography. *AJR* 1995;164: 673–677.
314. Han BK, Towbin RB, De Courten-Myers G, et al. Reversal sign on CT: effect of anoxic/ischemic cerebral injury in children. *AJNR* 1989; 10:1191–1198.

Vascular Abnormalities

315. Zilkha A. CT of cerebral hemiatrophy. *AJR* 1980;135:259–262.
316. Hambleton G, Wigglesworth JS. Origin of intraventricular haemorrhage in the preterm infant. *Arch Dis Child* 1976;51:651–659.
317. Wigglesworth JS, Pape KE. An integrated model for hemorrhage and ischemic lesions in the newborn brain. *Early Hum Dev* 1978;2: 179–199.
318. Volpe JJ. Current concepts of brain injury in the premature infant. *AJR* 1989;153:243–251.
319. Burstein J, Papile LA, Burstein R. Intraventricular hemorrhage and hydrocephalus in premature newborns: a prospective study with CT. *AJR* 1979;132:631–635.
320. Kirks DR, Bowie JD. Cranial ultrasonography of neonatal periventricular/intraventricular hemorrhage: who, how, why, and when? *Pediatr Radiol* 1986;16:114–119.
321. van de Bor M, Ens-Dokkum M, Schreuder AM, et al. Outcome of periventricular-intraventricular hemorrhage at five years of age. *Dev Med Child Neurol* 1993;35:33–41.
322. Flodmark O. Neuroradiology of selected disorders of the meninges, calvarium and venous sinuses. *AJNR* 1992;13:483–491.
323. Roland EH, Flodmark O, Hill A. Thalamic hemorrhage with intraventricular hemorrhage in the full-term newborn. *Pediatrics* 1990;85: 737–742.
324. Barkovich AJ, Truwit CL. Brain damage from perinatal asphyxia: correlation of MR findings with gestational age. *AJNR* 1990;11: 1087–1096.
325. Barkovich AJ. MR and CT evaluation of profound neonatal and infantile asphyxia. *AJNR* 1992;13:959–972.
326. Barkovich AJ, Westmark K, Partridge C, et al. Perinatal asphyxia: MR findings in the first 10 days. *AJNR* 1995;16:427–438.
327. Barkovich AJ. Perinatal brain injury. In: Kirks DR, ed. *Emergency pediatric radiology. A problem-oriented approach.* Reston, VA: American Roentgen Ray Society, 1995, 135–143.
328. Babcock DS, Ball W Jr. Postasphyxial encephalopathy in full-term infants: ultrasound diagnosis. *Radiology* 1983;148:417–423.

329. Martin DJ, Hill A, Fitz CR, et al. Hypoxic/ischaemic cerebral injury in the neonatal brain. A report of sonographic features with computed tomographic correlation. *Pediatr Radiol* 1983;13:307–312.

330. Siegel MJ, Shackelford GD, Perlman JM, Fulling KH. Hypoxic-ischemic encephalopathy in term infants: diagnosis and prognosis evaluated by ultrasound. *Radiology* 1984;152:395–399.

331. Flodmark O, Roland EH, Hill A, Whitfield MF. Periventricular leukomalacia: radiologic diagnosis. *Radiology* 1987;162:119–124.

332. Flodmark O, Lupton B, Li D, et al. MR imaging of periventricular leukomalacia in childhood. *AJNR* 1989;10:111–118.

333. Lanska MJ, Lanska DJ, Horwitz SJ, Aram DM. Presentation, clinical course, and outcome of childhood stroke. *Pediatr Neurol* 1991;7:333–341.

334. Levy C, Laissy JP, Raveau V, et al. Carotid and vertebral artery dissections: three-dimensional time-of-flight MR angiography and MR imaging versus conventional angiography. *Radiology* 1994;190:97-103.

335. Masaryk TJ, Modic MT, Ross JS, et al. Intracranial circulation: preliminary clinical results with three-dimensional (volume) MR angiography. *Radiology* 1989;171:793–799.

336. Harwood-Nash DC, McDonald P, Argent W. Cerebral arterial disease in children. An angiographic study of 40 cases. *AJR* 1971;111:672–686.

337. Hilal SK, Solomon GE, Gold AP, Carter S. Primary cerebral arterial occlusive disease in children. Part I. Acute acquired hemiplegia. *Radiology* 1971;99:71–86.

338. Hilal SK, Solomon GE, Gold AP, Carter S. Primary cerebral arterial occlusive disease in children. Part II. Neurocutaneous syndromes. *Radiology* 1971;99:87–94.

339. Taveras JM. Multiple progressive intracranial arterial occlusions: a syndrome of children and young adults. *AJR* 1969;106:235–268.

340. Takeuchi K, Shimizu K. Hypoplasia of the bilateral internal carotid arteries. *Brain Nerve* 1957;9:37–43.

341. Yamashita M, Oka K, Tanaka K. Histopathology of the brain vascular network in moyamoya disease. *Stroke* 1983;14:50–58.

342. Ezura M, Yoshimoto T, Fujiwara S, et al. Clinical and angiographic follow-up of childhood-onset moyamoya disease. *Childs Nerv Syst* 1995;11:591–594.

343. Satoh S, Shibuya H, Matsushima Y, Suzuki S. Analysis of the angiographic findings in cases of childhood moyamoya disease. *Neuroradiology* 1988;30:111–119.

344. Suzuki J, Kodama N. Moyamoya disease—a review. *Stroke* 1983;14:104–109.

345. Matsushima Y, Fukai N, Tanaka K, et al. A new surgical treatment of moyamoya disease in children: a preliminary report. *Surg Neurol* 1981;15:313–320.

346. Scott RM, Renkens KL Jr. Ischemic strokes and moyamoya syndrome. In: Cheek WR, ed. *Pediatric neurosurgery: surgery of the developing nervous system,* 3rd ed. Philadelphia: WB Saunders, 1994, 515–523.

347. Govaert P, Achten E, Vanhaesebrouck P, et al. Deep cerebral venous thrombosis in thalamo-ventricular hemorrhage of the term newborn. *Pediatr Radiol* 1992;22:123–127.

348. Virapongse C, Cazenave C, Quisling R, et al. The empty delta sign: frequency and significance in 76 cases of dural sinus thrombosis. *Radiology* 1987;162:779–785.

349. Baker LL, Dillon WP, Hieshima GB, et al. Hemangiomas and vascular malformations of the head and neck: MR characterization. *AJNR* 1993;14:307–314.

350. Barnes PD, Burrows PE, Hoffer FA, Mulliken JB. Hemangiomas and vascular malformations of the head and neck: MR characterization. *AJNR* 1994;15:193–195.

351. Mulliken JB, Glowacki J. Hemangiomas and vascular malformations in infants and children: a classification based on endothelial characteristics. *Plast Reconstr Surg* 1982;69:412–422.

352. Brunelle FOS, Harwood-Nash DCF, Fitz CR, Chuang SH. Intracranial vascular malformations in children: computed tomographic and angiographic evaluation. *Radiology* 1983;149:455–461.

353. Celli P, Ferrante L, Palma L, Cavedon G. Cerebral arteriovenous malformations in children. Clinical features and outcome of treatment in children and in adults. *Surg Neurol* 1984;22:43–49.

354. Martin NA, Edwards M, Wilson CB. Management of intracranial vascular malformations in children and adolescents. *Concepts Pediatr Neurosurg* 1983;4:264–290.

355. McCormick WF. The pathology of vascular (''arteriovenous'') malformations. *J Neurosurg* 1966;24:807–816.

356. Poussaint TY, Siffert J, Barnes PD, et al. Hemorrhagic vasculopathy after treatment of central nervous system neoplasia in childhood: diagnosis and follow-up. *AJNR* 1995;16:693–699.

357. Rothfus WE, Albright AL, Casey KF, et al. Cerebellar venous angioma: ''benign'' entity? *AJNR* 1984;5:61–66.

358. Horowitz MB, Jungreis CA, Quisling RG, Pollack I. Vein of Galen aneurysms: a review and current perspective. *AJNR* 1994;15:1486–1496.

359. Lasjaunias P, Ter Brugge K, Lopez Ibor L, et al. The role of dural anomalies in vein of Galen aneurysms: report of six cases and review of the literature. *AJNR* 1987;8:185–192.

360. Berenstein A, Lasjaunias P. Arteriovenous fistulas of the brain. In: *Surgical neuroangiography. Endovascular treatment of cerebral lesions.* Vol. 4. Berlin: Springer-Verlag, 1992.

361. Swischuk LE, Crowe JE, Mewborne EJ Jr. Large vein of Galen aneurysms in the neonate. A constellation of diagnostic chest and neck radiologic findings. *Pediatr Radiol* 1977;6:4–9.

362. Martelli A, Scotti G, Harwood-Nash DC, et al. Aneurysms of the vein of Galen in children: CT and angiographic correlations. *Neuroradiology* 1980;20:123–133.

363. Dowd CF, Halbach VV, Barnwell SL, et al. Transfemoral venous embolization of vein of Galen malformations. *AJNR* 1990;11:643–648.

364. Thompson JR, Harwood-Nash DC, Fitz CR. Cerebral aneurysms in children. *AJR* 1973;118:163–175.

365. Huston J III, Nichols DA, Luetmer PH, et al. Blinded prospective evaluation of sensitivity of MR angiography to known intracranial aneurysms: importance of aneurysm size. *AJNR* 1994;15:1607–1614.

366. Kanal E, Shellock FG. The value of published data on MR compatibility of metallic implants and devices. *AJNR* 1994;15:1394–1396.

367. Wesenberg RL, Gwinn JL, Barnes GR Jr. Radiological findings in the kinky-hair syndrome. *Radiology* 1969;92:500–506.

Neurocutaneous Syndromes

368. Barnes PD, Korf BR. Neurocutaneous syndromes. In: Wolpert SM, Barnes PD, eds. *MRI in pediatric neuroradiology.* St. Louis: CV Mosby, 1992, 299–327.

369. Seizinger BR, Rouleau GA, Ozelins LJ, et al. Genetic linkage of von Recklinhausen neurofibromatosis to the nerve growth factor receptor gene. *Cell* 1987;49:589–594.

370. Neurofibromatosis. Conference Statement. National Institutes of Health Consensus Development Conference. *Arch Neurol* 1988;45:575–578.

371. Huson SM, Harper PS, Compston DA. Von Recklinghausen neurofibromatosis. A clinical and population study in south-east Wales. *Brain* 1988;111:1355–1381.

372. Aoki S, Barkovich AJ, Nishimura K, et al. Neurofibromatosis types 1 and 2: cranial MR findings. *Radiology* 1989;172:527–534.

373. Van Es S, North KN, McHugh K, De Silva M. MRI findings in children with neurofibromatosis type 1: a prospective study. *Pediatr Radiol* 1996;26:478–487.

374. Mirowitz SA, Sartor K, Gado M. High-intensity basal ganglia lesions on T1-weighted MR images in neurofibromatosis. *AJNR* 1989;10:1159–1163.

375. Bognanno JR, Edwards MK, Lee TA, et al. Cranial MR imaging in neurofibromatosis. *AJNR* 1988;9:461–468.

376. Sevick RJ, Barkovich AJ, Edwards MSB, et al. Evolution of white matter lesions in neurofibromatosis type 1: MR findings. *AJR* 1992;159:171–175.

377. Rubinstein LJ. The malformative central nervous system lesions in the central and peripheral forms of neurofibromatosis: a neuropathological study of 22 cases. In: Rubenstein AE, Bunge RP, Housman DE, eds. *Neurofibromatosis.* New York: New York Academy of Sciences, 1986, 14–29.

378. Pou-Serradell A, Ugarte-Elola AC. Hydrocephalus in neurofibromatosis. Contribution of magnetic resonance imaging to its diagnosis, control, and treatment. *Neurofibromatosis* 1989;2:218–226.

379. Seizinger BR, Martuza RL, Gusella JF. Loss of genes on chromosome 22 in tumorigenesis of human acoustic neuroma. *Nature* 1986;322:644–647.

380. Fitz CR, Harwood-Nash DC, Thompson JR. Neuroradiology of tuberous sclerosis in children. *Radiology* 1974;110:635–642.

381. Medley BE, McLeod RA, Houser OW. Tuberous sclerosis. *Semin Roentgenol* 1976;11:35–54.

382. Bell DG, King BF, Hattery RR, et al. Imaging characteristics of tuberous sclerosis. *AJR* 1991;156:1081–1086.

383. Gomez MR. *Tuberous sclerosis.* 2nd ed. New York: Raven Press, 1988.

384. Altman NR, Purser RK, Donovan Post MJ. Tuberous sclerosis: characteristics at CT and MR imaging. *Radiology* 1988;167:527–532.

385. Braffman BH, Bilaniuk LT, Naidich TP, et al. MR imaging of tuberous sclerosis: pathogenesis of this phakomatosis, use of gadopentetate dimeglumine and literature review. *Radiology* 1992;183:227–238.

386. Martin N, de Brouker T, Cambier J, et al. MRI evaluation of tuberous sclerosis. *Neuroradiology* 1987;29:437–443.

387. Menor F, Marti-Bonmati L, Mulas F, et al. Neuroimaging in tuberous sclerosis: a clinicoradiological evaluation in pediatric patients. *Pediatr Radiol* 1992;22:485–489.

388. Martin N, Debussche C, De Broucker T, et al. Gadolinium-DTPA enhanced MR imaging in tuberous sclerosis. *Neuroradiology* 1990; 31:492–497.

389. Kingsley DP, Kendall BE, Fitz CR. Tuberous sclerosis: a clinicoradiological evaluation of 110 cases with particular reference to atypical presentation. *Neuroradiology* 1986;28:38–46.

390. Braffman BH, Bilaniuk LT, Zimmerman RA. The central nervous system manifestations of the phakomatoses on MR. *Radiol Clin North Am* 1988;26:773–800.

391. Coulam CM, Brown LR, Reese DF. Sturge-Weber syndrome. *Semin Roentgenol* 1976;11:55–60.

392. Elster AD, Chen MYM. MR imaging of Sturge-Weber syndrome: role of gadopentetate dimeglumine and gradient-echo techniques. *AJNR* 1990;11:685–689.

393. Probst FP. Vascular morphology and angiographic flow patterns in Sturge-Weber angiomatosis: facts, thoughts, and suggestions. *Neuroradiology* 1980;20:73–78.

394. Latif F, Tory K, Gnarra J, et al. Identification of the von Hippel-Lindau disease tumor suppressor gene. *Science* 1993;260:1317–1320.

395. Meyn MS. High spontaneous intrachromosomal recombination rates in ataxia-telangiectasia. *Science* 1993;260:1327–1330.

396. Sebag G, Dubois J, Pfister P, et al. Neurocutaneous melanosis and temporal lobe tumor in a child: MR study. *AJNR* 1991;12:699–700.

397. Rhodes RE, Friedman HS, Hatten HP Jr, et al. Contrast-enhanced MR imaging of neurocutaneous melanosis. *AJNR* 1991;12:380–382.

398. Byrd SE, Darling CF, Tomita T, et al. MR imaging of symptomatic neurocutaneous melanosis in children. *Pediatr Radiol* 1997;27:39–44.

Metabolic, Degenerative, and Toxic Disorders

399. Hatten HP, Jr. Dysmyelinating leukodystrophies: "LACK proper myelin." *Pediatr Radiol* 1991;21:477–482.

400. Blaser SI, Clarke JTR, Becker LE. Neuroradiology of lysosomal disorders. *Neuroimaging Clin N Am* 1994;4:283–298.

401. Hermann G, Wagner LD, Gendal ES, et al. Spinal cord compression in type I Gaucher disease. *Radiology* 1989;170:147–148.

402. Brismar J, Brismar G, Coates R, et al. Increased density of the thalamus on CT scans in patients with GM2 gangliosidoses. *AJNR* 1990; 11:125–130.

403. Lee C, Dineen TE, Brack M, et al. The mucopolysaccharidoses: characterization by cranial MR imaging. *AJNR* 1993;14:1285–1292.

404. Murata R, Nakajima S, Tanaka A, et al. MR imaging of the brain in patients with mucopolysaccharidosis. *AJNR* 1989;10:1165–1170.

405. Watts RW, Spellacy E, Kendall BE, et al. Computed tomography studies on patients with mucopolysaccharidoses. *Neuroradiology* 1981;21:9–23.

406. Neuhauser EBD, Griscom NT, Gilles FH, Crocker AC. Arachnoid cysts in the Hurler-Hunter syndrome. *Ann Radiol* 1968;11:453–469.

407. Wolpert SM, Anderson ML, Kaye EM. Metabolic and degenerative disorders. In: Wolpert SM, Barnes PD, eds. *MRI in pediatric neuroradiology.* St. Louis: CV Mosby, 1992, 121–150.

408. Barkovich AJ, Good WV, Koch TK, Berg BO. Mitochondrial disorders: analysis of their clinical and imaging characteristics. *AJNR* 1993; 14:1119–1137.

409. Savoiardo M, Uziel G, Strada L, et al. MRI imaging findings in Leigh's disease with cytochrome-c-oxidase deficiency. *Neuroradiology* 1991;33;507–508.

410. Kearns T, Sayre GP. Retinitis pigmentosa, external ophthalmoplegia, and complete heart block. *Arch Ophthalmol* 1958;60;280–289.

411. Demange P, Gia HP, Kalifa G, Sellier N. MR of Kearns-Sayre syndrome. *AJNR* 1989;10:S91.

412. Hasuo K, Tamura S, Yasumari K, et al. Computed tomography and angiography in MELAS (mitochondrial myopathy, encephalopathy, lactic acidosis, and stroke-like episodes): report of three cases. *Neuroradiology* 1987;29:393–397.

413. Duijn JH, Matson GB, Maudsley AA, et al. Human brain infarction: proton MR spectroscopy. *Radiology* 1992;183:711–718.

414. Menkes JH, Alter M, Steigleder GK, et al. A sex-linked recessive disorder with retardation of growth, peculiar hair, and focal cerebral and cerebellar degeneration. *Pediatrics* 1962;29:764–779.

415. Faerber EN, Grover WD, DeFilipp GJ, et al. Cerebral MR of Menkes kinky-hair disease. *AJNR* 1989;10:190–192.

416. Harding BN. Progressive neuronal degeneration of childhood with liver disease (Alpers-Huttenlocher syndrome): a personal review. *J Child Neurol* 1990;5:273–287.

417. Altman NR, Rovira MJ, Bauer M. Glutaric aciduria type I: MR findings in two cases. *AJNR* 1991;12:966–968.

418. Seidenwurm D, Novotny E Jr., Marshall W, Enzmann D. MR and CT in cytoplasmically inherited striatal degeneration. *AJNR* 1986;7: 629–632.

419. van der Knaap MS, Valk J. MR of adrenoleukodystrophy: histopathologic correlations. *AJNR* 1989;Suppl 10:S12–14.

420. van der Knaap MS, Valk J. The MR spectrum of peroxisomal disorders. *Neuroradiology* 1991;33:30–37.

421. Barkovich AJ, Ferriero DM, Bass N, Boyer R. Involvement of the pontomedullary corticospinal tracts: a useful finding in the diagnosis of x-linked adrenoleukodystrophy. *AJNR* 1997;18:95–100.

422. Shaw DW, Maravilla KR, Weinberger E, et al. MR imaging of phenylketonuria. *AJNR* 1991;12:403–406.

423. Brismar J, Aqeel A, Brismar G, et al. Maple syrup urine disease: findings on CT and MR scans of the brain in 10 infants. *AJNR* 1990; 11:1219–1228.

424. Carroll WJ, Woodruff WW, Cadman TE. MR findings in oculocerebrorenal syndrome. *AJNR* 1993;14:449–451.

425. O'Tuama LA, Laster DW. Oculocerebrorenal syndrome: case report with CT and MR correlates. *AJNR* 1987;8:555–557.

426. Trommer BL, Naidich TP, Dal Canto MC, et al. Noninvasive CT diagnosis of infantile Alexander disease: pathologic correlation. *J Comput Assist Tomogr* 1983;7:509–516.

427. Farrell K, Chuang S, Becker LE. Computed tomography in Alexander's disease. *Ann Neurol* 1984;15:605–607.

428. van der Knaap MS, Valk J. The reflection of histology in MR imaging of Pelizaeus-Merzbacher disease. *AJNR* 1989;10:99–103.

429. Penner MW, Li KC, Gebarski SS, Allen RJ. MR imaging of Pelizaeus-Merzbacher disease. *J Comput Assist Tomogr* 1987;11:591–593.

430. Journel H, Roussey M, Gandon Y, et al. MR imaging in Pelizaeus-Merzbacher disease. *Neuroradiology* 1987;29:403–405.

431. Savoiardo M, Halliday WC, Nardocci N, et al. Hallervorden-Spatz disease: MR and pathologic findings. *AJNR* 1993;14:155–162.

432. Kvicala V, Vymazal J, Nevsimalova S. Computed tomography of Wilson disease. *AJNR* 1983;4:429–430.

433. Scotti G, Scialfa G, Tampieri D, Landoni L. MR imaging in Fahr disease. *J Comput Assist Tomogr* 1985;9:790–792.

434. Demaerel P, Wilms G, Verdru P, et al. MRI in the diagnosis of Cockayne's syndrome. One case. *J Neuroradiol* 1990;17:157–160.

435. Boltshauser E, Yalcinkaya C, Wichmann W, et al. MRI in Cockayne syndrome type I. *Neuroradiology* 1989;31:276–277.

436. Ramos A, Quintana F, Diez C, et al. CT findings in spinocerebellar degeneration. *AJNR* 1987;8:635–640.

437. Aquilonius SM, Bergstrom K, Enoksson P, et al. Cerebral computed tomography in methanol intoxication. *J Comput Assist Tomogr* 1980; 4:425–428.

438. Finelli PF. Case report. Changes in the basal ganglia following cyanide poisoning. *J Comput Assist Tomogr* 1981;5:755–756.

439. Harrington JF, Mapstone TB, Selman WR, et al. Lead encephalopathy presenting as a posterior fossa mass. *J Neurosurg* 1986;65:713–715.

Practical Pediatric Imaging: Diagnostic Radiology of Infants and Children, Third Edition.
D. R. Kirks, editor and N. T. Griscom, associate editor.
Lippincott–Raven Publishers, Philadelphia © 1998.

CHAPTER 3

Head and Neck

Caroline D. Robson, Francine M. Kim, and Patrick D. Barnes

This chapter discusses imaging of the head (other than brain) and neck in infants and children. For discussions of imaging of the brain and cervical spine, see Chapters 2 and 4.

C. D. Robson and P. D. Barnes: Division of Neuroradiology, Department of Radiology, Children's Hospital, Harvard Medical School, Boston, Massachusetts 02115.

F. M. Kim: Department of Radiology, Le Bonheur Children's Medical Center, University of Tennessee at Memphis, Memphis, Tennessee 38103.

IMAGING TECHNIQUES AND GUIDELINES

Conventional Radiography

Advances over the past two decades have revolutionized imaging of the head and neck. As a result, routine radiography has largely been replaced by high-resolution computed tomography (CT) and magnetic resonance imaging (MRI). Plain films, however, are still used in a number of situations (1–9). Trauma and inflammatory disease are the most frequent indications for radiographs of the orbits, sinuses, and facial bones. Plain films usually include frontal (anteroposterior [AP] or posteroanterior [PA]), lateral, and Waters projections, obtained in the upright position when feasible to detect air-fluid levels. Trauma is the most frequent indication

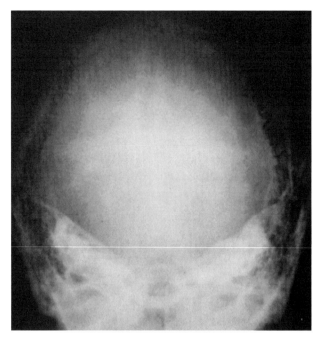

FIG. 3-1. Normal mastoids. Towne view of this 6-year-old girl permits comparison of the right and left mastoid air cells. There is no evidence of decreased aeration, bony demineralization, or bone destruction.

for radiographic (AP, Towne, oblique projections supplemented by Panorex tomography) assessment of the mandible. Plain films also allow preliminary assessment of focal bony lesions and malformations. Orbital views are obtained when radiopaque foreign bodies are suspected. Plain films are also important in the initial assessment of craniofacial anomalies.

Plain films of the petrous portion of the temporal bone help to evaluate mastoid pneumatization and gross bony involvement by large destructive lesions and to visualize the position and integrity of cochlear implant electrodes (1–5). Mastoid radiographs, though seldom obtained and technically difficult in children, should include frontal (AP or PA), Towne, and angled lateral (Laws or Owens) projections. In young children, the Towne projection is particularly useful for visualization of the mastoids and for direct comparison of symmetry of aeration, bony septation, and mineralization (Fig. 3-1). The Schüller projection is a lateral view of the mastoid with 30° cephalocaudad angulation of the x-ray beam. The transorbital projection (PA or AP) permits visualization of the whole length of the internal auditory canal (CT is usually employed instead), and the Stenvers projection displays the length of the petrous apex and mastoid.

Lateral plain films of the neck are often useful in upper airway abnormalities of children, particularly inflammatory conditions (1–5). Frontal views of the neck and chest films may also be helpful, particularly to evaluate foreign body ingestion and extension of an inflammatory process or tumor into the mediastinum.

Ultrasonography

Real-time ultrasonography (US) may be used to delineate the size, location, and tissue characteristics of soft-tissue masses of the head and neck (2,5–7,10). High frequency (7.5- or 10-MHz) transducers permit differentiation of solid from cystic masses and may detect calcifications. Doppler US provides important information about blood flow, particularly in vascular anomalies. US readily detects and characterizes cysts and masses of the thyroid gland.

Computed Tomography

Computed tomography has become the primary imaging modality for the head and neck (2,5–9,11). Axial and coronal contiguous sections are usually obtained. Sagittal, coronal, and oblique reformatting of thin axial sections is often useful, although the spatial resolution is less than with direct imaging. However, abnormalities of the cervical spine and upper airway may forbid direct coronal imaging, and axially acquired reformatting may then be used. All studies are planned from a lateral or frontal scout projection. Intravenous contrast enhancement is often not needed except in the neck but may be employed to demonstrate normal vessels, abnormal vascularity, or abnormal permeability from inflammation or neoplastic neovascularity, especially if intracranial extension is suspected.

Ophthalmologic assessment and US often suffice for the clinical evaluation of intraocular disease. CT is often indicated, however, in the assessment of a suspected mass (such as a retinoblastoma) and for treatment planning (5–9). Extraocular lesions are usually best evaluated first with high-resolution axial and coronal CT. This evaluation is often definitive, especially in trauma, infection, and pseudotumor. CT can also detect accompanying intracranial injury, inflammation, and hydrocephalus. Axial 1- to 3-mm sections are routine. Direct coronal sections are often added, particularly for injuries like blow-out fractures. Orbital involvement in craniofacial syndromes is often best delineated by 3-D CT, especially when reconstructive surgery is being planned.

Because it precisely demonstrates both bony and soft-tissue structures including intraorbital and intracranial contents (5–9), CT is preferred for evaluation of the facial bones and orbits in severe facial trauma and in complex craniofacial malformations. CT is also the most accurate method for examination of neoplastic and inflammatory involvement of the paranasal sinuses because of its precise delineation of the ostiomeatal complex, bone destruction, and soft-tissue changes such as mucosal thickening. CT imaging of the facial bones and mandible utilize axial or coronal 3- to 5-mm sections, occasionally supplemented by 1- to 3-mm sections of the temporomandibular joints. Unenhanced 5-mm axial sections are often performed to demonstrate sinusitis, whereas direct coronal 3- to 5-mm sections with supplementary 1-mm sections are used to evaluate the ostiomeatal complex. Evaluation of nasochoanal stenosis or atresia requires axial 1- to 3-mm sections and gantry angulation.

CT has replaced plain films and polytomography for the evaluation of developmental, inflammatory, traumatic, and neoplastic processes of the petrous portion of the temporal bone, e.g., in hearing loss and facial palsy (5–9,11). CT delineates bony destruction associated with cholesteatoma, mastoiditis, and tumors. Intracranial extension of disease can also be detected. Contiguous 1- to 3-mm axial sections are performed and are often followed by direct coronal 1- to 3-mm sections. For better delineation of intracranial involvement, a suppurative collection, or venous thrombosis, a contrast-enhanced series may be added or substituted.

CT imaging of the neck is usually done with bolus intravenous contrast enhancement to visualize the vessels and 5-mm axial sections from the clavicles to the skull base (5–9). Nonionic contrast agents are preferred and are used to visualize normal neck vessels and abnormal vascularity. Delayed imaging may demonstrate abnormal tissue enhancement of an abscess or neoplasm. To detect calcification and hemorrhage, 5- to 10-mm axial sections may be obtained before the enhanced study. Other contrast-enhanced techniques that have replaced conventional radiographic and fluoroscopic procedures include CT sialography and CT dacryocystography.

Magnetic Resonance Imaging

MRI is often complementary to CT in the assessment of head and neck lesions (5–9). However, in a number of situations (e.g., vascular anomalies), MRI may be the technique of choice. In general, MRI should be considered for specific delineation of soft-tissue elements, vascular components, and intracranial involvement. Abnormalities of the skull base are probably best evaluated with a combination of CT for bony involvement and MRI for neurovascular involvement. MR angiography-venography (MRA/MRV) may be added to confirm vascular occlusions (e.g., dural sinus thrombosis) or to show high-flow lesions such as arteriovenous malformations (AVMs) and hemangiomas. Doppler US is often preferred in young infants, however, and CT angiography may be better for vascular assessment in older children, especially in the diagnosis of venous thrombosis. In petrous bone abnormalities, MRI is generally reserved for the detection and delineation of tumors or complicated inflammatory conditions. Indications for MRI include retrocochlear sensorineural hearing loss, facial nerve paralysis, and vertigo.

MRI techniques for head and neck imaging include fast spin-echo (FSE), inversion recovery, fat suppression, and contrast-enhanced sequences (5–9). The volume head coil, or semivolume head and neck coil, is used to obtain sagittal T1-weighted images, axial proton density images, and axial T2-weighted images. Short tau inversion recovery (STIR) images may be preferred, however, for the additive T1 and T2 effects and the superb fat suppression provided. Contrast-enhanced T1-weighted images are often used in one or more planes, particularly for the evaluation of tumors and inflammation. A 5-mm slice thickness is routinely used, usually with a 1-mm gap. High-resolution 3-mm axial and coronal T1-weighted sections are often used with fat suppression and contrast enhancement, particularly to evaluate the orbits and internal auditory canals. Surface coils increase the signal-to-noise ratio and provide higher spatial resolution. Gradient-echo techniques are used to enhance vascular flow, cerebrospinal fluid (CSF) flow, and magnetic susceptibility effects due to mineralization or hemorrhage. Non-MRA vascular flow–enhanced studies may be done using multiple single-slice (SPGR) or multislice (FMPSPGR) gradient-echo techniques. A number of 2-D and 3-D time-of-flight (TOF) and phase contrast (PC) MRA techniques are available.

Nuclear Medicine

Probably the most important use of nuclear medicine in the evaluation of neck disease in childhood is the imaging of the thyroid (12). Two agents, iodine-123 (I-123) and technetium-99m (Tc-99m) pertechnetate, are currently used. I-123 is trapped and organified by the thyroid, whereas Tc-99m pertechnetate is trapped but not organified. I-123 is preferred because its biochemical behavior is identical to that of stable iodine and because it affords a higher thyroid-to-background ratio. Common indications for thyroid scintigraphy include identification of ectopic thyroid tissue in an extrathyroidal neck mass, assessment or detection of ectopic thyroid tissue in congenital hypothyroidism, and evaluation of a solitary thyroid nodule.

Angiography

Catheter angiography is the definitive modality for the diagnosis and treatment of vascular occlusive disease, vascular anomalies, and vascular trauma. It is an integral component of endovascular interventional therapy (5–9). Percutaneous injection of sclerosing agents is used to treat venous malformations.

ORBIT AND GLOBE

Normal

Embryology and Development

The eye develops from the neuroectoderm, the cutaneous ectoderm, and the neural crest cells (5,13–20). The optic primordium is identifiable at the 22nd day of embryonic life and gives rise to the optic vesicle and stalk; these become the eye, including the retina and the optic nerve. During its development, the eye briefly has a vascular system, the hyaloid artery and its branches, that is replaced by the primary vitreous. These vessels involute by the 35th gestational week.

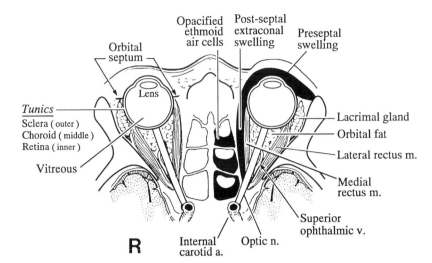

FIG. 3-2. Orbital anatomy. Line drawing showing normal anatomy of the right (R) orbit. Orbital cellulitis, with both preseptal and postseptal inflammation, and ethmoid sinusitis are present on the left.

Anatomy

The globe is embedded in the fat of the orbit (Fig. 3-2) (5,17,18,20,21) and is surrounded by a thin capsule. The sclera and cornea form the outer layer of the globe. The middle layer is formed by the choroid, the ciliary body, and the iris. The retina, the inner layer, is the neural membrane that receives visual images. The retina is continuous posteriorly with the optic nerve. The refracting media of the eye are the aqueous humor, the crystalline lens, and the vitreous of the globe. The lacrimal gland is situated in the upper outer angle of the orbit; its tears are conveyed by the excretory ducts to the surface of the eye. The tears are carried away by the lacrimal canals into the lacrimal sac medially and then into the nasolacrimal duct, which empties into the inferior meatus of the nasal cavity.

The orbit contains the orbital fascia, ocular muscles, globe and its appendages, and arteries, veins, nerves, and fat (see Fig. 3-2) (5,17,18,20,21). The orbital roof is formed by the frontal bone and the lesser wing of the sphenoid. The floor is formed by the maxilla, the zygomatic bone, and the orbital process of the palatine bone. The medial wall is formed by the maxilla, the lacrimal bone, the lamina papyracea of the ethmoid, and the body of the sphenoid. The lateral wall is formed by the zygomatic bone and the greater wing of the sphenoid. The optic foramen lies at the orbital apex and transmits the optic nerve and ophthalmic artery. The superior orbital fissure lies inferolateral to the optic foramen and transmits the IIIrd and IVth cranial nerves, the ophthalmic division of the Vth cranial nerve, the VIth cranial nerve, sympathetic nerves, and the ophthalmic vein.

The extraocular muscles are the levator palpebrae, superior rectus, inferior rectus, medial rectus, lateral rectus, superior oblique, and inferior oblique (5,17,18,20,21). The muscles, except the inferior oblique, originate at the orbital apex and insert on the globe forming a cone about the globe and optic nerve (see Fig. 3-2). The orbital fascia forms the periosteum of the orbit. Anteriorly it forms a circumferential reflection known as the orbital septum. The structures anterior to the or-

bital septum are termed preseptal; the posterior ones are postseptal (see Fig. 3-2). The postseptal space may be further subdivided by the cone of muscles into intraconal and extraconal compartments.

The orbital cavity grows passively in response to the growth of the globe (1–9). The globe is 75% of adult size at birth, and its growth is complete by age 7 years. The bony orbit and optic canal have almost reached adult size by age 10. The normal interorbital distance measured by CT for children at birth is 11 mm; at 1 year, 12.7–18.5 mm; 6 years, 17.4–23.1 mm; and 12 years, 22.5–28.1 mm. The infant optic canal averages 3.5 mm in diameter and reaches the normal adult measurement of 5.5 mm by 5 years. This diameter should never exceed 7 mm, nor should the two canal diameters differ by more than 1 mm.

General Abnormalities

Hypertelorism is the condition in which the interorbital distance is greater than normal (1–9). Causes include familial hypertelorism, median cleft face syndrome, trisomy 13, infantile hypercalcemia, Hurler disease, cleidocranial dysplasia, bilateral coronal craniosynostosis, Crouzon disease, hypothyroidism, cephalocele, and thalassemia. The condition in which the interorbital distance is less than normal is *hypotelorism* (1–9). Causes include arhinencephaly, holoprosencephaly, primary developmental abnormalities of the eyes, microcephaly, trigonocephaly, and sagittal craniosynostosis.

A *large orbit* may be caused by brain herniation through a mesenchymal bony defect (greater sphenoid wing in neurofibromatosis), cephalocele, or some other increase in orbital contents, as from optic glioma, neurofibroma, hemangioma, lymphatic malformation, dermoid, or teratoma (1–9). A *small orbit* is seen in congenital anophthalmia, microphthalmia, early orbital enucleation, irradiation, and hyperostotic lesions such as fibrous dysplasia, osteopetrosis, hypercalcemia, and severe anemia (1–9).

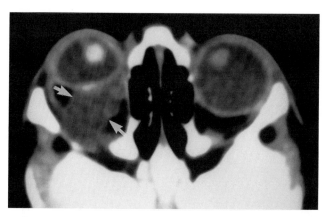

FIG. 3-3. Microphthalmia and coloboma. A 3-month-old girl with right exophthalmos. Unenhanced CT shows a small right globe and a retroocular multicystic mass *(arrows)*.

A *large optic canal* is almost always due to an intracanalicular optic glioma (1–9). Rare causes include other tumors (neurofibroma, meningioma, hemangioma, dermoid, teratoma) and dural ectasia (as in neurofibromatosis). A *small optic canal* is due to a small optic nerve (anophthalmia, microphthalmia, infantile optic atrophy, early orbital enucleation) or bony hyperostosis (fibrous dysplasia, osteopetrosis, severe anemia, hypercalcemia) (1–9).

Specific Abnormalities

Congenital and Developmental Abnormalities

Primary Ocular Abnormalities

Anophthalmia (congenital absence of the eye) results from failure of formation of the optic vesicle or from its degeneration (5,14,15,18,20). Anophthalmia is rare, occurs sporadically, and is often associated with trisomy 13, Klinefelter syndrome, and complex craniofacial malformations. Imaging demonstrates a poorly formed, shallow orbit containing only rudimentary tissue. Anophthalmia and a congenital cystic eye may coexist. It may be difficult to differentiate clinically and radiologically between true anophthalmia, severe microphthalmia (hypoplastic eye), and primary orbital hypoplasia. Ocular structures (the lens and the globe) can be identified in microphthalmia (Fig. 3-3) but are absent in primary anophthalmia. Although microphthalmia may exist alone, it is frequently associated with other abnormalities such as coloboma (Fig. 3-3), duplication cyst of the eye, glaucoma, cataracts, septooptic dysplasia, genetic syndromes (e.g., trisomy 13), and toxoplasmosis, rubella, cytomegalovirus, and herpes (TORCH) infections (5,14,15,18,20).

Coloboma refers to any inherited or acquired defect or fissure of the ocular structures (5,14,15,18,20). Typical colobomas result from failure of the embryonic choroidal fissure to close properly. These malformations are common and are usually bilateral. On imaging, a mass is found behind the globe at the head of the optic nerve (Fig. 3-3). Colobomas are usually inherited as an autosomal dominant trait. They may also be sporadic and unilateral. They need not be associated with any systemic abnormality.

Optic nerve hypoplasia, a subnormal number of axons (5,14,15,18,20), is a frequent anomaly, often an isolated one. Particularly when bilateral, it may be associated with ocular, facial, endocrine, or central nervous system (CNS) anomalies, among which are septooptic dysplasia and encephalocele. Imaging studies may demonstrate small optic nerves and a small chiasm.

Persistent hyperplastic primary vitreous (PHPV) represents persistence and hyperplasia of the embryonic hyaloid vascular system (5,14,15,18,20). PHPV is usually unilateral and associated with microphthalmia. The most typical clinical findings are leukocoria (white pupil), microphthalmia, and cataract in a term infant. PHPV is the second most common cause, after retinoblastoma, of leukocoria. The presence of microphthalmia and the absence of calcification by CT are important in differentiating PHPV from retinoblastoma. The latter usually contains calcifications and involves a normal or large globe. Glaucoma is a frequent complication of PHPV, and the affected eye may therefore be buphthalmic. Other complications include recurrent hemorrhage, retinal detachment, and phthisis bulbi. Imaging demonstrates a small globe with increased or decreased CT density and hyperintensity on T1-weighted MRI that extends from the lens to the back of the globe in a band-like, cone-shaped, or triangular or rounded configuration (Fig. 3-4).

Glaucoma is an abnormal elevation of intraocular pressure (5,14,15,18,20), usually caused by increased resistance to normal outflow of aqueous humor. Primary congenital glaucoma is bilateral in up to 80% of cases. It may occur with other disorders such as the phakomatoses. The increase in intraocular pressure causes enlargement of the entire eye (buphthalmos). Secondary congenital glaucoma refers to cases that result from intrauterine eye inflammation (e.g., rubella), trauma, or an ocular tumor such as retinoblastoma.

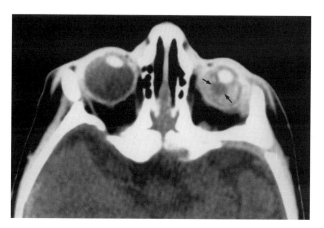

FIG. 3-4. Persistent hyperplastic primary vitreous. Unenhanced CT. A small, high-density left globe contains a central hypodensity *(arrows)*.

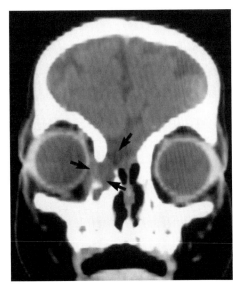

FIG. 3-5. Nasoorbital cephalocele. Unenhanced coronal CT. There is a bony defect in the right cribriform plate with extension of dysplastic frontal lobe tissue and CSF into the right nasal cavity and medial orbit *(arrows)*.

Coats disease is a primary retinal vascular anomaly characterized by telangiectasia and the accumulation of a lipoproteinaceous exudate in the retina and subretinal space (5,14,15,18,20). Retinal detachment, when present, may cause leukocoria and can be difficult to differentiate from retinoblastoma. The characteristic imaging findings of Coats disease include high CT density or increased intensity on T1-weighted MRI of the vitreous but no focal mass. Calcification sometimes occurs. The peak incidence of Coats disease is near the end of the first decade.

Retrolental fibroplasia or retinopathy of prematurity is seen in premature infants who receive prolonged oxygen therapy (5,14,15,18,20). It is usually bilateral but asymmetric. In severe cases, these infants develop leukocoria from retinal detachment. The prevalence of the abnormality has decreased dramatically because of greater caution in the use of oxygen. The retinal detachment it causes is usually easily diagnosed and differentiated from retinoblastoma by CT and MRI.

Ocular and Orbital Abnormalities Associated with CNS Malformations

Disorders of neural tube closure in which there may be orbital abnormalities include cephaloceles, dermal sinus and cyst, neuroglial heterotopia, holoprosencephaly, septooptic dysplasia, absence of the septum pellucidum, craniosynostosis, and craniofacial syndromes (19). Cephaloceles that commonly involve the orbit or optic pathways include sphenoidal, nasoorbital (Fig. 3-5), and frontoethmoidal cephaloceles (Fig. 3-6) (17,22–27). Dermal sinuses, dermoids, and epidermoids are discussed later (19,22,24). There may be associ-

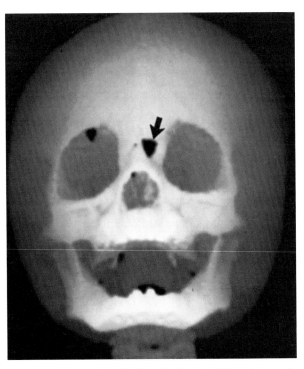

FIG. 3-6. Frontoethmoidal cephalocele. There is excellent anatomic demonstration on three-dimensional CT of the hypertelorism and bony defect *(arrow)* associated with a frontoethmoidal encephalocele.

ated widening of the nasal bridge, hypertelorism (see Fig. 3-6), or associated midline intracranial defects such as callosal agenesis or dysgenesis with a lipoma. Direct orbital involvement is unusual (see Fig. 3-5).

Midface hypoplasia and hypotelorism are commonly associated with the holoprosencephalies (19,23,28). The alobar form of holoprosencephaly is the most severe. Midface and orbital anomalies associated with alobar holoprosencephaly include cyclopia (single midline orbit with proboscis and absent nose), ethmocephaly (median proboscis between two hypoteloric orbits), cebocephaly (rudimentary nose with single aperture and orbital hypotelorism), median cleft lip with hypertelorism, and simple hypotelorism. Septooptic dysplasia (DeMorsier syndrome), also a disorder of ventral neural tube closure, has been considered a mild form of holoprosencephaly (19,28,29); the malformation includes partial or complete absence of the septum pellucidum and optic hypoplasia.

Unilaterally or bilaterally deformed orbits are commonly associated with the craniosynostoses, particularly those involving the metopic or coronal or many sutures (1,19,26). Orbital abnormalities are part of the craniofacial malformations associated with Apert syndrome (acrocephalosyndactyly), Crouzon disease (craniofacial dysostosis), Carpenter syndrome (acrocephalopolysyndactyly), and Pfeiffer syndrome (acrocephalosyndactyly). In these syndromes, reconstructive craniofacial surgery is often required to improve

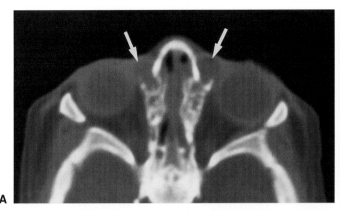
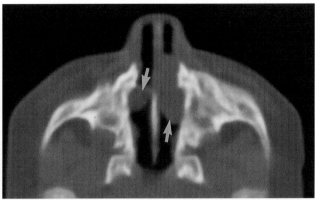

FIG. 3-7. Nasolacrimal mucoceles. A 3-month-old girl with bilateral orbital soft-tissue swelling. **A:** CT sections at the level of the orbits show bilateral medial canthal soft-tissue masses *(arrows)*. **B:** The nasolacrimal canals are enlarged and masses *(arrows)* are also seen in the inferior nasal cavity.

appearance and preserve vision. Treacher Collins syndrome (mandibulofacial dysostosis) is another craniofacial syndrome in which orbital and ocular abnormalities such as microphthalmia and coloboma may be seen.

Neuroophthalmologic involvement often occurs with the neurocutaneous syndromes of childhood. These include neurofibromatosis-1, (sphenorbital dysplasia, optic glioma), tuberous sclerosis (retinal neuroglial hamartoma), Sturge-Weber syndrome (choroidal venocapillary malformation with buphthalmos), and von Hippel-Lindau disease (retinal hemangioblastoma with retinal detachment and hemorrhage) (19).

Disorders of migration that are often associated with ocular, orbital, or optic pathway abnormalities include dysgenesis of the corpus callosum and the lissencephaly syndromes (19,30–33). Callosal agenesis and dysgenesis are seen in a wide array of anomalies including cephaloceles, dermal sinuses, septooptic dysplasia, cleft lip and palate, Apert syndrome, hypertelorism, coloboma, and Aicardi syndrome. Midface and orbital dysmorphia, as well as ocular anomalies, are frequently seen in the lissencephaly syndromes.

Malformative Lesions

Malformative abnormalities are neoplastic and nonneoplastic masses which arise from an aberration of development (14,15,18,19,34). These are usually of neuroectodermal origin (e.g., dermoid or epidermoid) or mesodermal origin (e.g., lipoma). The germ cell neoplasms (e.g., teratoma) (35) are also included in this category, as are the vascular anomalies. Malformative lesions are often cystic but may be solid or of mixed consistency. In the orbital region in childhood, these include colobomas, duplication cysts of the eye, nasolacrimal duct cysts, lacrimal ectopia, dermoids and epidermoids, teratomas, and (rarely) arachnoid cysts and lipomas. Coloboma has been discussed earlier. It may be difficult to differentiate a coloboma from a retrobulbar duplication cyst (14). Hydrops and arachnoid cysts of the optic

nerve sheath are exceedingly rare abnormalities in isolation (36) but are occasionally associated with suprasellar tumors or cysts.

Congenital nasolacrimal duct cyst and mucocele are the most common abnormalities of the infant lacrimal apparatus (37–40). These abnormalities probably result from incomplete canalization of the duct, a residual membrane persisting where the duct enters the nasal cavity. The obstruction produces cystic dilatation of the duct. The condition may be bilateral. It often resolves spontaneously in the early postnatal months. If persistent, there may be nasal airway obstruction, the mucocele may become infected, or there may be a complicating dacryocystitis. Imaging demonstrates a unilateral or bilateral cystic mass at the medial canthus in continuity with an enlarged nasolacrimal duct and canal and an intranasal submucosal cystic mass (Fig. 3-7). The latter differentiates the condition from other medial canthal cystic masses of early childhood such as dacryocystitis, choristoma, dermoid or epidermoid, and cephalocele (41).

Ectopic lacrimal gland tissue causes benign solid or cystic lesions of the orbit and may produce proptosis at any age (42). The ectopic tissue may be located intraconally. Neoplastic transformation to pleomorphic adenoma and adenocarcinoma has been reported.

The dermoid and epidermoid are the most common congenital lesions of the orbit (14,43–45). They may occur subcutaneously, subconjunctivally, or deeper in the orbit. Developmental sequestration of ectoderm in a suture line of the orbit is the probable cause. The most common location is the superior temporal quadrant at the frontozygomatic suture. They also arise from the frontoethmoidal suture as a medial cystic mass. The relatively slow growth of the dermoid or epidermoid erodes adjacent bone and displaces adjacent structures. CT hypodensity or fat-like hyperintensity on T1-weighted MRI may be seen, with or without calcification (Fig. 3-8). Notching of the bony site of origin and bony scalloping are characteristic. There may be a fat-fluid level within the mass.

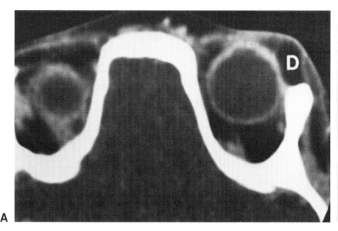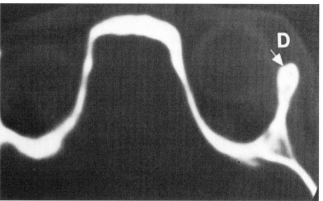

FIG. 3-8. Dermoid/epidermoid. Enhanced CT at soft-tissue window **(A)** and using a bone window **(B)**. A well-defined, low-density mass *(D)* causes adjacent bony erosion and remodeling *(arrow)*.

Orbital teratomas are usually benign. They cause severe, progressive proptosis in infancy (14,15,18,34). The tumors are usually multicystic but may be both cystic and solid or entirely solid. There is often marked expansion of the orbit and compressive displacement of the globe. As in dermoid or epidermoid, imaging may demonstrate fat, soft tissue, calcification, or ossification.

Mesodermal dysplasias affecting the orbit include NF-1 and skeletal dysplasias such as fibrous dysplasia, craniometaphyseal dysplasia, and osteopetrosis (19). Particularly with fibrous dysplasia, a characteristic ground-glass or sclerotic appearance is evident in the bones of the orbit, face (especially the maxillae), or skull base.

Inflammatory Lesions

The orbit may be the site of primary infectious or inflammatory processes or may be secondarily involved by spread from adjacent structures, especially the sinuses (16,18, 19,34). The infectious process is usually bacterial. Less often it is viral, mycotic, parasitic, or tuberculous. Noninfectious or postinfectious orbital inflammation may cause orbital pseudotumor with myositis. Infection may also be seen after penetrating trauma, especially if associated with a foreign body. Unusual inflammations include endophthalmitis, dacryoadenitis, and optic neuritis.

Suppurative Infections

Infections are the most common orbital diseases of childhood and are usually bacterial. *Hemophilus*, staphylococcal, streptococcal, and pneumococcal infections are particularly common (46,47). Preseptal (periorbital) cellulitis is an infection of the eyelid and often of the adjacent face (see Fig. 3-2). It is seen most often in infants after *Hemophilus influenzae* bacteremia, the incidence of which is declining with immunization. Postseptal (intraorbital) cellulitis is almost always associated with preseptal inflammation, and the orbital involvement is usually extraconal and subperiosteal (Figs. 3-9 and 3-10). Orbital cellulitis usually follows ethmoid sinusitis in younger children and maxillary or frontal sinusitis in older children and adolescents.

Intraorbital involvement may also occur as an extension from facial infection, particularly after trauma. Postseptal

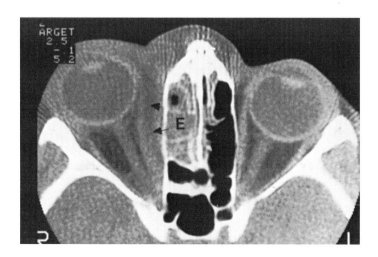

FIG. 3-9. Orbital cellulitis. There is both preseptal and postseptal soft-tissue swelling of the right orbit. An area of low attenuation medial to the right medial rectus muscle *(arrows)* represents a subperiosteal abscess secondary to extension of ethmoid sinusitis *(E)*.

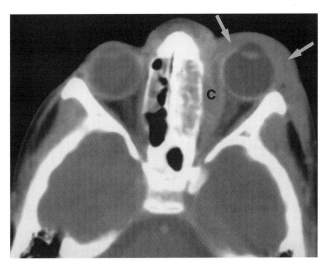

FIG. 3-10. Orbital cellulitis. A 6-year-old boy with left orbital swelling. Unenhanced CT shows ethmoid opacification, preseptal soft-tissue swelling *(arrows)*, subperiosteal inflammatory thickening *(C)* and lateral displacement of the medial rectus muscle.

(orbital) involvement may result from further extension of infection from the subperiosteal space into the extraconal or intraconal space. This is particularly common after penetrating trauma with a retained foreign body (48). Further spread may result in osteomyelitis, orbital thrombophlebitis, cavernous sinus thrombophlebitis, epidural abscess, subdural empyema, meningitis, cerebritis, or brain abscess. Orbital infection may also complicate an existing orbital abnormality (e.g., a cephalocele or nasolacrimal mucocele) or follow a fracture. Infections may also involve the lacrimal gland (dacryoadenitis).

Orbital infection may cause edema, cellulitis, or abscess (46,47). An abscess is indicated by central fluid or air and rim enhancement. The imaging findings in preseptal and subperiosteal infection tend to be localized and relatively discrete. Infection extending into the extraconal or intraconal

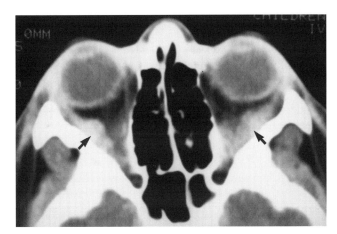

FIG. 3-11. Orbital pseudotumors. Unenhanced CT. Both lateral rectus muscles *(arrows)* are markedly thickened because of inflammation.

postseptal space produces increased density of the orbital fat; this may obscure the optic nerve, muscles, and other orbital landmarks. Antibiotic treatment may uncover an orbital cephalocele, neoplasm, or other primary abnormality.

Inflammatory Pseudotumors

The second most common inflammatory process of the pediatric orbit is an orbital pseudotumor (49–53). *Orbital pseudotumor* is the term for a group of idiopathic disorders with inflammatory (lymphoid) infiltration of the intraorbital tissues. By CT or MRI there may be unilateral or bilateral uveoscleral thickening with enhancement, an enhancing retroocular mass, or enlargement of the extraocular muscles and tendons and lacrimal gland (Fig. 3-11). The disease often responds to steroid treatment. Bony involvement is rare. In childhood, orbital pseudotumor is seldom due to Wegener granulomatosis or other systemic diseases. Inflammatory pseudotumor occasionally arises within the paranasal sinuses and secondarily causes orbital bony destruction and infiltration (54,55). In these cases, pseudotumor must be distinguished from infection and neoplasm, particularly lymphoma. Orbital pseudotumor is distinguished from Graves disease by the asymmetric muscular involvement, the painful proptosis, and the lack of thyroid abnormalities (56).

The *Tolosa-Hunt syndrome*, another type of inflammatory pseudotumor (57,58), is a painful, steroid-responsive ophthalmoplegia caused by idiopathic granulomatous inflammation of the orbital apex and cavernous sinus. It is often encountered in adolescence. There may be complicating orbital venous and cavernous sinus thrombosis. The clinical and imaging differential diagnosis includes fungal infection, meningioma, lymphoma, and sarcoidosis.

Other Inflammatory Processes

Orbital involvement may follow sinusitis due to an unusual pathogen (59,60), particularly aggressive fungal sinus infections such as mucormycosis and aspergillosis (60). These infections tend to invade the orbit, cavernous sinus, and neurovascular structures and may cause thromboses, infarctions, and hemorrhage. Fungal sinusitis is particularly aggressive in immunocompromised individuals.

Complications of sinusitis that may involve the orbit include mucoceles, retention cysts, papillomas, polyps, and granulomas (61–64). Other rare chronic inflammatory processes that may involve the sinuses and orbit include Wegener granulomatosis, tuberculosis, and sarcoidosis (15,18,34).

Sclerosing endophthalmitis is a granulomatous uveitis due to *Toxocara canis* infestation of the eye. Chorioretinitis is usually present bilaterally. Seizures and intracranial calcifications are common. An area of high attenuation or increased signal intensity without a discrete mass is usually seen in the vitreous by CT or MRI. The pattern, including the retinal

TABLE 3-1. *Masses of the orbit and optic pathways*

Congenital
  Cephalocele
  Neurofibromatosis type 1 (NF-1): sphenoid wing dysplasia
  Congenital glaucoma
Inflammatory
  Orbital cellulitis
  Orbital abscess
  Orbital pseudotumor
  Granulomatous disease
Neoplastic
  Benign tumor
    Hemangioma
    Dermoid/epidermoid
    Teratoma
    Optic nerve sheath meningioma
    Optic nerve sheath schwannoma
    Plexiform neurofibroma
  Malignant tumor
    Rhabdomyosarcoma
    Optic nerve glioma
    Retinoblastoma
    Lymphoma
    Leukemia
    Metastatic disease
    Langerhans cell histiocytosis
Vascular
  Arteriovenous malformation
  Carotid-cavernous fistula
  Venous varix
  Venous malformation
  Lymphatic malformation
Miscellaneous
  Hematoma
  Fibrous dysplasia
  Graves disease

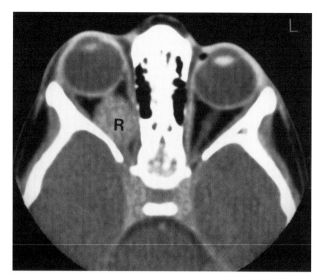

FIG. 3-12. Rhabdomyosarcoma. A 2-year-old girl with right exophthalmos. Enhanced CT shows an intraconal enhancing mass *(R)* surrounding the right optic nerve.

detachment, is similar to that of Coats disease. Chorioretinitis may also be seen with the TORCH infections, particularly cytomegalovirus.

Optic neuritis, rare in childhood, usually occurs as an acute central visual deficit and orbital pain. The neuritis may be viral or postviral, a manifestation of inflammatory pseudotumor, or due to leukemia, granulomatous disease, or juvenile multiple sclerosis (15,18,34). Imaging may demonstrate diffuse and irregular thickening of the optic nerve and sheath, and there may be marked enhancement.

Neoplasms

Tumors of the orbit and optic pathways in childhood (Table 3-1) can be classified by the site of primary involvement into ocular tumors, extraocular orbital tumors, sinus or craniofacial tumors with secondary orbital involvement, and tumors of the optic pathways (7,15,18,19,34,45). Tumors may also be classified pathologically according to the cell or tissue of origin, e.g., mesenchymal tumors, neural tumors, and malformative lesions.

The most common benign primary orbital masses of childhood are dermoid and epidermoid, hemangioma, lymphatic malformation, plexiform neurofibroma, and teratoma

(15,18,19,45). The most common malignant primary orbital tumors are retinoblastoma, optic nerve glioma, and rhabdomyosarcoma. The most common malignancies involving the orbit secondarily are acute and chronic leukemia (by infiltration or by a chloromatous mass), neuroblastoma, rhabdomyosarcoma, Langerhans cell histiocytosis, and lymphoma. Pediatric orbital tumors usually arising in the extraconal compartment include dermoid and epidermoid, hemangioma, lymphatic malformation, plexiform neurofibroma, teratoma, metastatic neuroblastoma, rhabdomyosarcoma, histiocytosis, and lymphoma. The most common intraconal orbital masses of childhood are optic nerve glioma and hemangioma.

Mesenchymal Tumors

Rhabdomyosarcoma is the most common malignant soft-tissue tumor of the head and neck region in childhood. The most common sites of origin are the orbits and the paranasal sinuses (7,15,18,19,34,45); other sites are the pharynx, temporal bone, and neck. These aggressive, invasive neoplasms are usually of the embryonal or alveolar subtypes. Like other small round-cell malignancies of childhood (neuroblastoma, Ewing sarcoma, primitive neuroectodermal tumor [PNET], lymphoma, leukemia, histiocytosis), these hypercellular tumors often form large soft-tissue masses (Fig. 3-12) that infiltrate along tissue planes and destroy bone in a permeative fashion. There may be intracranial extension, and regional or systemic metastases may occur. Rhabdomyosarcomas arising elsewhere may metastasize to the orbit. Like other small round-cell tumors, rhabdomyosarcomas often appear isodense or of high density on CT, and they frequently enhance after intravenous contrast administration (Fig. 3-12). MRI signal intensity relative to muscle tends to show nonspecific isointensity or hypointensity on T1-

weighted images, and isointensity to hypointensity, or occasional hyperintensity, on proton density and T2-weighted images. The degree and character of gadolinium enhancement varies.

Reticuloendothelial and lymphoreticular neoplasms of childhood which involve the orbit include histiocytosis, leukemia, and lymphoma (7,15,18,19,34,65,66). In Langerhans cell histiocytosis, solitary or multiple soft-tissue masses and bony destruction of the orbit, sinuses, cranial base, or cranial vault may be seen (Fig. 3-13). Intradural or extradural intracranial involvement may also occur. CT may demonstrate isodense or high-density masses, or occasionally low-density masses, usually with prominent enhancement. T1-weighted MRI shows masses of isointensity or hypointensity compared with muscle and enhancement after contrast administration (Fig. 3-13). On proton density and T2-weighted images, isointensity or hypointensity with occasional hyperintensity is seen. There may be marrow replacement with loss of the normal high signal intensity on T1-weighted images. There may also be pituitary-hypothalamic involvement with diabetes insipidus, absence of the posterior pituitary bright spot, and hypothalamic or stalk enhancement.

Leukemic infiltration or involvement of the orbit occurs in acute lymphoblastic leukemia. Chloromas (leukemic tumors) occur more often with the myeloblastic forms of leukemia (65,66). Non-Hodgkin lymphoma (e.g., Burkitt lymphoma) is more common than Hodgkin lymphoma (HL) of the orbit, primarily or secondarily. Juvenile angiofibroma is a histologically benign but aggressive and invasive fibrovascular mesenchymal tumor seen in adolescent males in the nasopharynx and paranasal sinuses (7,67,68). Occasionally there is extension into the orbit. Fibromas are mesenchymal tumors that may be isolated and relatively benign. When aggressive and malignant, they are usually termed fibrosarcomas or fibromatosis (7,69). They may invade the orbit primarily or secondarily. Benign and malignant osteochondral tumors rarely involve the orbit in childhood (7,70–72).

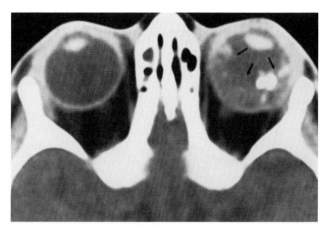

FIG. 3-14. Retinoblastoma. Multiple calcifications *(arrows)* within a left intraorbital mass.

Neural Tumors

Neural tumors of the orbit include retinoblastoma, medulloepithelioma, neuroblastoma, esthesioneuroblastoma, PNET, progonoma, schwannoma, neurofibroma, and plexiform neurofibroma (7,15,18,34).

Retinoblastoma is the only common primary intraocular malignant tumor of childhood (15,18,34). Ninety percent occur in children younger than 5 years of age. This neuroectodermal tumor of the retina is usually calcified and nodular. Retinoma (retinocytoma) is a benign variant. Ten percent of retinoblastomas are familial. Up to 25% are either multifocal or bilateral. Bilateral retinoblastoma is usually transmitted by autosomal dominant inheritance with incomplete penetrance. Bilateral hereditary retinoblastomas are occasionally associated with a pineal neuroectodermal tumor (trilateral retinoblastoma), or with pineal and hypothalamic neuroectodermal tumors (quadrilateral retinoblastoma). Approximately 1% of retinoblastomas undergo spontaneous regression. In hereditary retinoblastoma, there is an increased susceptibility to radiation-induced malignancies as well as second nonocular malignancies such as osteosarcoma, fibrosarcoma, and rhabdomyosarcoma.

Most children with retinoblastoma have leukocoria and strabismus (15,18,34). Although the differential diagnosis for leukocoria is lengthy, CT and MRI are usually able to differentiate retinoblastoma from its benign mimics. The distinction is crucial because mortality approaches 100% if retinoblastoma spreads beyond the eye. Calcification is identified by CT in more than 90% of cases. CT usually also shows a high-density intraocular mass with variable contrast enhancement (Fig. 3-14). MRI demonstrates variable signal intensity relative to the vitreous on T1-weighted MRI images, isointensity or hypointensity on T2-weighted images, and gadolinium enhancement. Spread may occur by direct extension along the optic nerve and perioptic subarachnoid space, or by the lymphatic or hematogenous route. Other lesions also causing leukocoria, intraocular calcification, ocular CT hyperdensity, and hyperintensity on T1-weighted

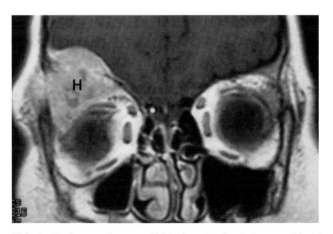

FIG. 3-13. Langerhans cell histiocytosis. A 9-year-old girl with right orbital mass. Coronal enhanced T1-weighted MRI. An enhancing superior orbital mass *(H)* causes bony destruction of the orbital roof and extends intracranially.

images include retinoma, Coats disease, PHPV, retrolental fibroplasia, chronic retinal detachment, sclerosing endophthalmitis, congenital cataract, coloboma, retinal hemangioblastoma, and choroidal or retinal hemangioma with detachment.

Medulloepithelioma, a rare tumor also causing leukocoria, arises from the primitive medullary epithelium of the ciliary body and is located anteriorly about the iris (15,18). Occasionally the tumor may arise next to the optic nerve. On CT and MRI, medulloepithelioma is usually a well-defined, markedly enhancing tumor that may erode the orbital wall or induce hyperostosis. The lack of calcification helps to differentiate it from retinoblastoma.

Neuroblastoma is the most common neural tumor that metastasizes to the orbit. It is usually a nodular infiltrating mass causing permeative bone destruction and occasionally blastic or spiculated bony changes (73). Esthesioneuroblastoma, PNET, and progonomas are other neural tumors which may have similar imaging findings. Nerve sheath tumors, which rarely involve the orbit in childhood, include schwannoma, neurofibroma, and plexiform neurofibroma (7). The last is commonly associated with the sphenorbital dysplasia of neurofibromatosis (NF-1).

Optic Pathway Tumors

Optic nerve tumors are the most common intraconal tumors of childhood (7,19,74). Exclusively intraorbital lesions include hamartomas, arachnoidal hyperplasia, and low-grade astrocytomas. Tumors arising from the chiasm and optic tracts range from hamartomas and low-grade astrocytomas to anaplastic astrocytomas. Optic pathway tumors are commonly associated with NF-1 and may be asymptomatic when discovered by routine screening (7). Gliomas limited to the intraorbital optic nerve are rare (Fig. 3-15). More often there is intraorbital, intracanalicular, and intracranial optic pathway involvement. Optic gliomas must be distinguished from tumors that arise extrinsically but may extend to the optic nerve, such as a schwannoma, neurofibroma, and meningioma (7).

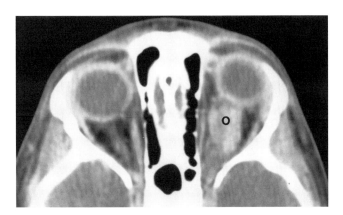

FIG. 3-15. Optic glioma. A 5-year-old girl with decreased visual acuity. Enhanced CT. There is an enhancing intraconal mass *(O)* that expands the left optic nerve.

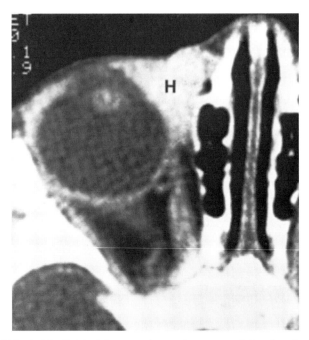

FIG. 3-16. Orbital hemangioma. Large medial epicanthal hemangioma *(H)*. There is remodeling of the orbital rim but no evidence of bony destruction. Note the intense contrast enhancement.

Trauma

Both penetrating and blunt injuries to the orbit are common during childhood (15,18,19,34). Orbital fracture may result from direct impact to the orbit or be part of other cranial or facial fractures. Classic craniofacial injuries associated with orbit fractures include blow-out orbital fractures, tripod fractures, and LeFort complex fractures (75–78). Orbital complications include hematoma, emphysema, CSF leak, traumatic cephalocele, growing fracture, retinal tear, intraocular hemorrhage, ocular rupture, optic nerve avulsion, and carotid-cavernous fistula (79). Penetrating orbital injury is more common in children than in adults, and often there is a retained foreign body and secondary infection (47). Orbital complications of cranial, sinus, or orbital surgery include infection, hematoma, pseudomeningocele or pseudoencephalocele, CSF leak, vascular occlusion, and pseudoaneurysm.

Vascular Abnormalities

According to the Mulliken-Glowacki biological classification, hemangiomas are congenital tumors characterized histologically by early endothelial proliferation and late involution. Vascular malformations, on the other hand, are endothelial-lined anomalies and are subclassified as capillary, arterial, venous, lymphatic, and combined (19,80–83). These abnormalities are distinguished both by clinical criteria and imaging characteristics.

In hemangioma, CT shows a soft-tissue mass with marked contrast enhancement (Fig. 3-16). MRI using spin-echo (SE)

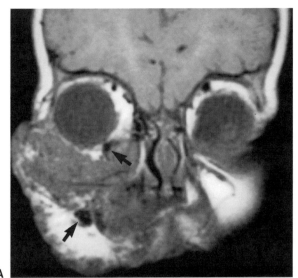

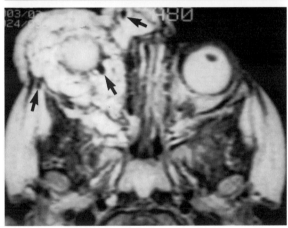

FIG. 3-17. Orbital hemangioma. A 1-year-old girl. Coronal T1 **(A)** and axial T2 **(B)** MRI. The mass in the inferior right orbit contains vascular high-flow signal voids *(arrows)*.

sequences with presaturation and gradient-echo (GE) sequences with gradient moment nulling is particularly helpful in assessing flow characteristics (82). Proliferating hemangiomas are high-flow benign neoplasms with SE vascular flow voids, GE vascular flow–related enhancement, and marked contrast enhancement of the tumor parenchyma (Fig. 3-17). Involuting hemangiomas demonstrate decreasing flow characteristics, decreasing tumor volume, and an increased proportion of fibrofatty tissue. A hemangioma usually completes its involution by age 7–8 years and may then have the appearance of a fibrofatty mass and mimic a lipoma or low-flow malformation. AVMs are also high-flow anomalies but have no solid parenchymal component. However, reactive tissue changes may be present.

Lymphatic and venous malformations are low-flow malformations (they have no SE vascular flow voids) that consist of cystic, septated, or cavernous channels. Often there is a fibrofatty stroma. Phleboliths and contrast enhancement of the blood-filled channels are typical of venous malformations. These malformations may also have prominent draining or anomalous veins demonstrated as high-intensity GE vascular flow–related enhancement. In lymphatic malformations, only the septa may show enhancement, and there may be hemorrhage or infection. Fluid-fluid levels are characteristic of lymphatic malformations (80). Combined anomalies such as lymphovenous malformations have features characteristic of their lymphatic and venous components.

Other vascular abnormalities of the orbit include varices and aneurysms or pseudoaneurysms associated with the angiodysplastic syndromes, and vascular occlusive disease (15,18,34,84–86). The Wyburn-Mason syndrome is a vascular malformation with orbital and intracranial components (19). Associated pituitary-hypothalamic and brainstem involvement is characteristic.

Primary orbital varices are venous malformations which drain into the cavernous sinus or into the face and scalp veins. Secondary varices are associated with arteriovenous shunting or major venous occlusive disease. Arteriovenous shunting into the orbital veins may occur with intracranial AVMs or with carotid-cavernous or dural AV fistulas (19). Large secondary varices may also be associated with proliferating hemangiomas. The varices may be associated with an angiodysplastic syndrome (e.g., Klippel-Trenaunay-Weber). Secondary orbital varices may also be seen with dural sinus or jugular venous occlusive disease, including stenosis or atresia (small or absent jugular foramina), and thrombosis. The varices appear as prominent, tortuous flow voids whose size may vary with respiration, the Valsalva maneuver, or arterial pulsation. Marked blood pool enhancement may be seen on CT or MRI due to venous obstruction and stasis. Hemorrhage is rare.

Also rare in childhood, aneurysms sometimes occur in association with proliferating hemangiomas or as pseudoaneurysms associated with carotid dissection (19). In moyamoya disease there may be involvement of the orbit, especially with prominent ophthalmic arterial collaterals. A moyamoya-like appearance and other vascular dysplasias have been observed in association with regional proliferating hemangiomas.

NASAL CAVITY, PARANASAL SINUSES, AND FACE

Normal

Embryology and Development

The mesenchymal primordia of the face appear about the stomodeum (primitive mouth) in the fourth week and include the frontonasal prominence, the paired maxillary prominences, and the paired mandibular prominences (6,13,21). The frontonasal prominence gives rise to the forehead, the nose and nasal septum, the philtrum of the upper lip, the premaxilla and its incisor teeth and gingiva, and the primary palate. The maxillary prominences form the lateral parts of the upper lip, most of the maxillae, and the secondary palate, which in turn give rise to the hard palate, soft palate, and

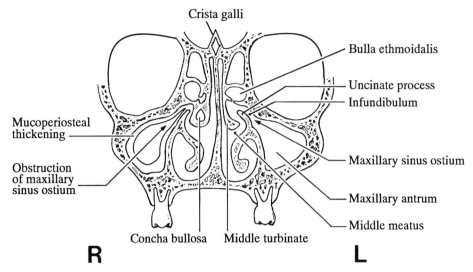

FIG. 3-18. Nasosinus anatomy. Normal anatomy of the left *(L)* ostiomeatal complex. Occlusion by mucoperiosteal swelling and distortion by the concha bullosa on the right *(R)*.

uvula. The mandibular prominences become the mandible, lower lip, chin, and lower cheek.

The developing nasal cavities ultimately communicate with the nasopharynx and oral cavity after rupture of the oronasal membrane at the level of the choanae. The paired turbinates form from the lateral walls of the nasal cavities. Specialized olfactory epithelium develops in the roof of each nasal cavity and connects with the olfactory bulbs of the prosencephalon. The paranasal sinuses form as outgrowths, or diverticula, of the walls of the nasal cavities and become pneumatized after birth.

Complete development of the face is slow and somewhat late. The small size of the face relative to the entire head at birth results from rapid development of the brain, relative to the development of the maxilla and mandible, the lack of erupted teeth, and the small size of the nasal cavities and sinuses. The size of the paranasal sinuses is influenced by brain growth. When brain growth is impaired, there is calvarial thickening and enlargement of the paranasal sinuses, the maxillary antra being affected least.

Anatomy

The nose and paranasal sinuses are not completely developed until puberty (6,13,21). The nose is the major portal of air exchange, especially in the newborn. The vestibule is the opening to each nasal cavity and is bound medially by the columella and nasal septum and laterally by the nasal alae. The nasal septum consists of an anteroinferior cartilaginous portion and a posterosuperior bony portion, the vomer and the perpendicular plate of the ethmoid. Three bony turbinates (superior, middle, and inferior) arise from each lateral nasal wall. The nasal cavity and paranasal sinuses are covered with respiratory epithelium.

The paranasal sinuses are located in the maxillary, ethmoid, sphenoid, and frontal bones (Fig. 3-18) (1–6,21). They communicate freely with the nasal cavity by ostia. There is considerable variation between individuals in the size of the paranasal sinuses. The maxillary sinus cavities are present at birth but usually are not radiographically visible until 2 or 3 months of age. At first they are small and project as triangles. The ethmoid cells are also present at birth and parallel the maxillary sinuses in development. However, the individual ethmoid air cells are much smaller and are usually not radiographically apparent until 3–6 months. The maxillary and ethmoid sinuses reach adult size by 10–12 years. The sphenoid sinuses may be visibly aerated as early as 1 or 2 years and reach adult size by 14 years. The frontal sinuses develop from anlagen shared with the anterior ethmoid cells. Although pneumatization of rudimentary frontal sinuses begins as early as 1 year of age, it is seldom possible to distinguish frontal sinuses as separate structures until they extend above the superior orbital rims at 8–10 years of age. Some individuals never develop frontal sinuses large enough to be distinguished from ethmoid cells.

The sinuses may be divided into two anatomic and functional groups (87–90). The frontal sinuses, anterior and middle ethmoidal air cells, and maxillary sinuses drain into the middle meatus via the ostiomeatal complex (OMC) and are frequently involved by inflammatory disease (see Fig. 3-18). The second group, the posterior ethmoidal air cells and sphenoidal sinuses, drain into the sphenoethmoidal recess and superior meatus of the nasal cavity and are less frequently involved.

General Abnormalities

Plain film interpretation of the paranasal sinuses is considerably more difficult in infants and children than in adults (1–6). The sinus cavities are smaller and their bony margins less distinct. During early infancy, there may be physiologic underaeration due to redundant but normal mucosa. The maxillary, ethmoid, sphenoid, and frontal sinuses should each be analyzed for the extent of aeration in the Waters, AP, and lateral projections. Paranasal sinus disease is characterized by opacification, mucosal thickening, soft-tissue masses (mucous retention cysts, polyps), air-fluid levels, and demineralization or frank bone destruction. Opacification and mucosal thickening are common in asymptomatic children, particularly less than 2 years of age. Correlation between sinus opacification and clinical sinus disease (infection) improves in children over 2 years of age.

Specific Abnormalities

Congenital and Developmental Abnormalities

Congenital Nasal Stenosis and Atresia

Obstruction of the nasal airway may cause respiratory distress and be life threatening in the infant. Prompt diagnosis and treatment are necessary (6,24,91). The obstruction becomes obvious when passage of a catheter is attempted. CT using an axial plane with caudal angulation of 10–15° to the hard palate displays the posterior nasal choanae and the nasopharynx optimally. The obstructive abnormalities include stenosis of the entire nasal passage, segmental nasal cavity stenosis or atresia, and stenosis or atresia of one or both choanae.

Stenosis of the entire nasal airway is usually bony and may be associated with the maxillary underdevelopment of prematurity or with maxillary hypoplasia as in Apert syndrome. These patients may not come to attention until rhinitis further compromises the airway. Some think that stenosis is a factor in the sudden infant death syndrome (SIDS).

Atresia, unilateral or bilateral, of the entire nasal passage is extremely rare. Segmental atresia or stenosis occasionally occurs at the anterior nasal opening (piriform aperture).

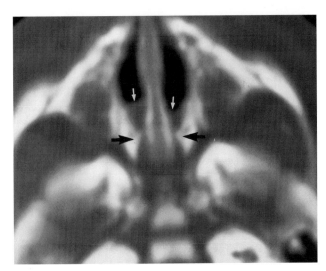

FIG. 3-19. Bilateral choanal atresia. An 8-day-old boy with respiratory distress. Bilateral posterior nasal cavity bony thickening *(black arrows)* and air-fluid levels *(white arrows)*.

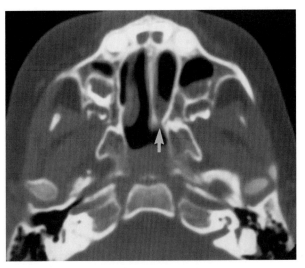

FIG. 3-20. Unilateral choanal atresia. A 6-month-old girl. Left posterior nasal cavity bony narrowing *(arrow)* and intranasal soft-tissue thickening.

There may be severe respiratory difficulty in the neonate simulating choanal atresia. In many such infants there is fusion of the upper central incisor teeth, and some patients also have abnormalities of the pituitary-adrenal axis or holoprosencephaly (24). Segmental stenosis of the nasal cavity may also result from local maxillary hypoplasia or from turbinate hyperplasia. Nasal septal deviation is another cause of nasal cavity stenosis and may coexist with other obstructions.

Choanal stenosis and atresia are characterized, respectively, by narrowing of the posterior nasal cavity and its obstruction by an atresia plate (6,24,91–93). The plate may be bony, membranous, or both. There may be coexisting stenosis or atresia of one or both nasal cavities and other anomalies. The anomaly, persistence of the oronasal membrane, develops around the seventh week of gestation. The more common bilateral form causes respiratory distress in the newborn infant (Fig. 3-19). The unilateral form may not be discovered until an older age (Fig. 3-20).

Although the majority of reported atresia plates are bony, combined bony and membranous atresia may be just as common (6,24,91–93). In bony atresia, there is commonly medial bowing and thickening of the lateral wall of the nasal cavity, enlargement of the vomer, and fusion of these bony elements. In patients with membranous atresia, the air passage between the lateral wall of the nasal cavity and the vomer is also small. In the combined bony and membranous atresia, the membranous component may be at the level of the pterygoid plates or lower. Nasal septal deviation and nasal cavity stenosis may coexist with choanal atresia. Other associations include cleft palate, cardiovascular and abdominal abnormalities, Treacher Collins syndrome, fetal alcohol syndrome, Apert syndrome, Crouzon disease, and the CHARGE association (coloboma; heart disease; atresia of choana; retarded growth and development; genital hypoplasia; ear anomalies and/or deafness).

Congenital Nasal Masses

Failure of canalization of the proximal nasolacrimal duct with mucocele of the lacrimal sac presents as a mass in the medial orbital canthus (6,24,37–39). Failure of canalization of the distal duct produces a mucocele that extends beneath the inferior turbinate into the nasal cavity. The two types may coexist (see Fig. 3-7) and bilateral involvement may simulate choanal atresia.

Congenital nasal masses resulting from anomalous neural tube closure include cephaloceles, neuroepithelial heterotopias (nasal gliomas), and dermoid or epidermoid (6,22,24). The fonticulus frontalis and prenasal space are transient nasofrontal structures appearing during the second gestational month. With normal involution, a fibrous foramen cecum remains as the only remnant of these structures. Persistence of the fonticulus with protrusion of intracranial contents results in a nasofrontal cephalocele. Persistence of a dural diverticulum in the prenasal space and protrusion of intracranial contents leads to a nasoethmoidal cephalocele. If the intracranial connection is partially or completely obliterated, the cephalocele becomes a sequestered neuroepithelial heterotopia (nasal glioma).

Cephaloceles and heterotopias at either the nasofrontal or nasoethmoidal site must be distinguished from dermoids and epidermoids. With regression of the dural diverticulum, surface ectoderm may be incorporated and result in the formation of a dermal sinus. The sinus is often seen in the nasal region as a skin dimple or mass. The distal opening of the sinus may be found at any point from the columella to the glabella, and there may be a nasal or frontal bony defect or an enlarged foramen cecum. A dermoid/epidermoid (Fig. 3-21), and lipoma often coexist. The mass is often of low density on CT but may be calcified. Fat-like hyperintensity may be seen on T1-weighted MRI. An intracranial communication is present in up to half of cases and may result in recurrent meningitis, abscess, or empyema (see Chapter 2).

Other rare congenital nasal masses include nasoalveolar (incisive canal) cysts, dentigerous cysts, mucous cysts, vascular anomalies, branchial cysts, hamartomas, and teratoid tumors (embryoma, epignathus) (6).

A cyst may arise within the pharyngeal bursa of Tornwaldt (6). The bursa lies in the nasopharyngeal midline and may be patulous at birth. A Tornwaldt cyst probably arises from a focal adhesion between the notochord and the pharyngeal mucosa. The lesion is most commonly observed as an asymptomatic, circumscribed, thin-walled cyst up to 1 cm in diameter and located at the midline in the nasopharyngeal raphe. CT and MRI appearances vary with the cyst contents. There is usually no contrast enhancement.

Other Nasal Anomalies

Congenital nasal deformity and obstruction may occur as part of various craniofacial syndromes. Examples are the Treacher Collins, Crouzon, and Apert syndromes (6,24,94).

There may be hypoplasia of the nose or nasal obstruction secondary to malar, maxillary, or palatal hypoplasia. Coronal craniosynostosis accompanied by brachycephaly may result in midface contracture and nasopharyngeal obstruction. Nasal and other median facial anomalies are often associated with microcephaly, trigonocephaly, or holoprosencephaly. Nasal deformity is also commonly associated with cleft lip and cleft palate.

Facial Anomalies

Cleft lip and cleft palate are the most common anomalies of the head and neck (6,24,94). Clefts may be partial or complete and unilateral or bilateral. The most severe deformities are found in unilateral or bilateral complete clefts (i.e., clefts involving the lip, alveolus, and palate) (Fig. 3-22). Maxillary hypoplasia and relative prognathism often accom-

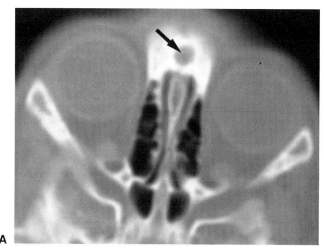

A

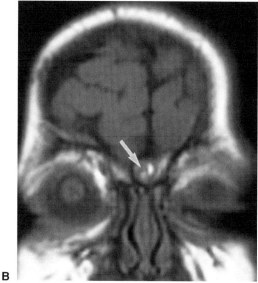

B

FIG. 3-21. Nasal dermoid/epidermoid. A 1-year-old boy with nasal mass. The mass *(arrows)* is isodense on CT **(A)** and hyperintense on coronal T1-weighted MRI **(B)**. There is enlargement of the foramen cecum.

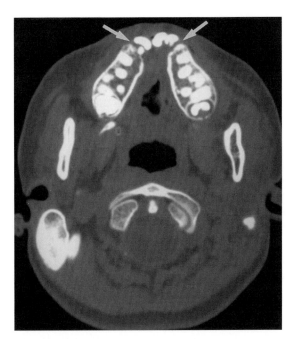

FIG. 3-22. Cleft lip and palate. CT demonstrates bilateral maxillary alveolar bony defects *(arrows)*.

pany bilateral clefts. A complete cleft disrupts facial growth and severely affects dentition, occlusion, speech, and eustachian tube function and contributes to upper respiratory infections.

Cranial and facial clefts, areas of tissue deficiency, were classified by Tessier (94) and extend along continuous axes through the eyebrows or eyelids, the maxilla, the nose, and the lip. Facial clefts extend caudally from the lower eyelid, whereas cranial clefts extend upward from the upper eyelid; craniofacial clefts do both. Anomalies associated with cranial or craniofacial clefts include orbital dystopia, microphthalmos, coloboma, cephalocele, and orbital hypertelorism. Syndromes associated with craniofacial clefting include median cleft syndrome, Treacher Collins syndrome, hemifacial microsomia, amniotic band syndrome, otomandibular syndrome, and Goldenhar syndrome (6,24,94).

The rare median cleft syndrome is accompanied by hypertelorism and may be divided into low and high groups. In the low group the clefts involve the upper lip, hard palate, and, occasionally, the nose. Associated anomalies include basal cephaloceles, agenesis of the corpus callosum, intracranial lipomas, and optic nerve dysplasias (e.g., colobomas). In the high group, the clefts involve the nose and forehead and, less commonly, the upper lip and hard palate. Associated anomalies include frontoethmoidal and intraorbital cephaloceles, cranium bifidum, frontonasal dysplasia, microphthalmia, anophthalmia, holoprosencephaly, intracranial lipoma, and occasionally callosal agenesis.

Craniofacial Syndromes

Craniofacial dysmorphia is often associated with synostosis of multiple sutures (6,24,94). Bilateral coronal craniosyn-

ostosis is associated with the craniofacial dysostosis syndromes (e.g., Crouzon disease) and the acrocephalosyndactyly syndromes (Apert, Pfeiffer, Carpenter, Saethre-Chotzen syndromes) (6,94). These disorders have abnormalities of the forehead, orbits (hypertelorism), midface, and anterior cranial base (Fig. 3-23). The orbits are shallow and there is exophthalmos.

Syndromes associated with craniofacial clefting and involvement of the whole face include amniotic band syndrome, hemifacial microsomia, Goldenhar syndrome, and Treacher Collins syndrome (6,94). Amniotic band syndrome is a sporadic disorder manifested by congenital extremity constrictions or amputations, facial clefts, calvarial defects, hydrocephalus, and, occasionally, anencephaly or cephaloceles (6,94).

Hemifacial microsomia is a sporadic disorder with facial asymmetry, microtia, macrostomia, and hypoplasia of the mandibular ramus and condyle (Fig. 3-24) (6,94). There is also hypoplasia or atresia of the external ear and middle ear, ipsilateral maxillary and malar hypoplasia, and in severe cases microphthalmia, congenital cystic eye, and coloboma.

Goldenhar syndrome (oculoauriculovertebral syndrome) is a mandibulofacial dysostosis with hemifacial microsomia, epibulbar dermoids or lipodermoids, and vertebral anomalies (6,94). Treacher Collins syndrome is a mandibulofacial dysostosis inherited as an autosomal dominant condition with variable expressivity. It is characterized by bilateral hypoplasia of the zygoma, malar bone, and mandible. Microtia and hypoplasia or atresia of the external ear and middle ear are common, as are colobomata and microphthalmia (6,94).

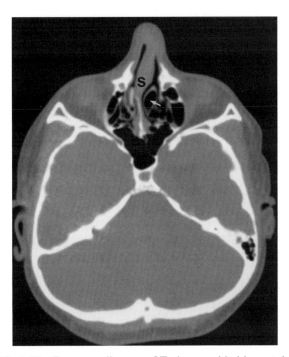

FIG. 3-23. Crouzon disease. CT shows orbital hypertelorism, nasal septum *(S)* deviation, and a pneumatized left middle turbinate *(arrow)*. Note that the orbits are extremely shallow.

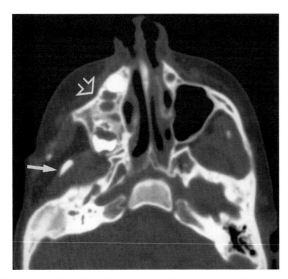

FIG. 3-24. Hemifacial microsomia. A 5-year-old boy with severe facial deformity. CT. The right maxilla *(open arrow)* is hypoplastic, the maxillary sinus is absent and the temporomandibular joint is hypoplastic *(arrow)*. There is atresia of the right external and middle ear.

Developmental Variants and Anomalies of the Paranasal Sinuses

Aplasia or hypoplasia of the maxillary sinus is almost always unilateral (59,95,96). The small sinus is often opacified on radiographs and CT (Fig. 3-25). There is lateral placement of the nasomaxillary partition, which leads to an enlarged nasal cavity. The opacification of a small sinus is usually due to noninflammatory mucosal thickening. When the sinus is nonexistent, the ''opacification'' is merely bone marrow. The orbital floor is depressed and rounded, the orbit looks large, and the orbital roof may be depressed.

Developmental variants and anomalies of the nose and sinuses predispose the patient to ostiomeatal obstruction

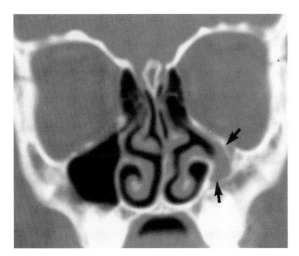

FIG. 3-25. Hypoplastic maxillary sinus. CT. The left maxillary sinus *(arrows)* is small and opacified. Note the lateral extension of the left nasal cavity.

when mucosal inflammation develops, and they influence the planning of endoscopic and open surgical procedures (5,6,88–90,97). They include primary bony variations and anomalies (e.g., of the septum and turbinates and extramural extensions of sinus air cells). Septal deviation is very common and is often associated with asymmetry or deformity of adjacent structures (see Fig. 3-23). Focal septal deviation usually accompanies an abnormally large middle turbinate. Septal spurs may occur with or without septal deviation. A middle turbinate with a laterally convex configuration is often large, is associated with generalized or focal nasal septal deviation, and may be pneumatized. Intrinsic anomalies of the middle and superior turbinates may also narrow the ostiomeatal complex and are commonly associated with anomalies of the nasal septum and inferior turbinates and with extramural sinus pneumatization. Abnormal orientation of the uncinate process commonly coexists with septal deviation, a large turbinate, or both.

Extramural extension of the ethmoid cells includes pneumatization of the supraorbital ridge, middle and superior turbinates, orbital plate of the maxilla, and the sphenoid bone (90). The agger nasi cells lie anterior to the upper end of the nasolacrimal duct. Haller cells originate from the anterior ethmoid group and are closely related to the infundibulum. Particularly when large, these cells may obstruct the infundibulum. They are often implicated in recurrent maxillary sinusitis. Pneumatization of the middle turbinate may be unilateral or, less commonly, bilateral (see Fig. 3-23). Pneumatization of the superior turbinate and uncinate process may also be encountered. Posterior ethmoid air cell extension into the anterior sphenoid bone (Onodi cells) may surround the optic nerve and reach the anterior wall of the sella turcica next to the internal carotid artery and cavernous sinus. Extramural extensions of the sphenoid sinus and maxillary sinus beyond the parent bone are common but rarely obstructive. Other anatomic anomalies include maxillary sinus septation and accessory maxillary sinus ostia.

Inflammatory Lesions

Rhinitis and Sinusitis

Upper respiratory tract inflammation, usually viral in etiology, is the most common disease of childhood (6,98). Bacterial rhinitis, generally a secondary infection, results from swelling, obstruction, and stasis. Acute and chronic sinusitis may subsequently develop because of ostiomeatal obstruction from persistent swelling or from disorders of the mucociliary apparatus. The challenge is to distinguish simple viral infections and allergic inflammation from secondary bacterial infection requiring antibiotics (6,98). Agents implicated in bacterial rhinitis and sinusitis include the group A streptococci, other streptococcal species (e.g., *S. pneumoniae*), *Hemophilus influenzae, Staphylococcus,* and *Moraxella catarrhalis* (6,98). Continued sinus ostial obstruction or mucociliary impairment allows anaerobic organisms to proliferate. Cultures obtained from sinus aspiration are more reliable than a culture of the nasal cavity. Although persistent nasal discharge suggests sinusitis, it may also be due to an intranasal foreign body or obstruction by nasochoanal stenosis or atresia, septal deviation, a polyp, or a tumor. Fungal infection of the paranasal sinuses tends to be seen in chronically ill, immunodeficient, or immunosuppressed children and is often fatal (6,98). Mucormycosis and aspergillosis are the most common fungal infections. Diagnosis may require both culture and biopsy.

Allergic rhinitis is another common cause of nasal or sinus obstruction and rhinorrhea in children (6,98). Allergic mucostasis and ostial obstruction are often followed by bacterial infection. With chronic mucosal hyperplasia and hypersecretion, polyps tend to form in the nose and sinuses. Adenoidal hyperplasia, another common cause of upper airway obstruction in children (6,90,98), may lead to purulent rhinorrhea and, if severe, to alveolar hypoventilation, cor pulmonale, and sleep apnea. Nasal obstruction and rhinorrhea may also be seen in children with cerebral palsy, familial dysautonomia, craniofacial syndromes and midface anomalies, and tumors.

Obstruction of the nose and sinuses is an important early manifestation of cystic fibrosis (6,98). The obstruction is produced by a combination of thick mucus, chronically thickened mucosa, and nasal polyps. Chronic sinusitis is very common. Inflammation of the sinuses and nasal passages also occurs in systemic lupus erythematosus, other rheumatoid or connective tissue diseases, Wegener granulomatosis, midline lethal granuloma, sarcoidosis, Churg-Strauss syndrome, and atrophic rhinitis (6,98). Nasal septal destruction often occurs in those conditions.

Sinus infection may occasionally be of dental origin (6). Periodontitis or a periapical abscess may extend into an antrum and cause maxillary sinusitis. Perforation may occur from minor dental trauma or during a dental procedure. If the perforation persists, the tract may epithelialize to form an oroantral fistula. Developmental bony defects and dental cysts may also provide a direct pathway to the sinus.

It is often impossible to differentiate acute rhinitis from sinusitis without imaging (6,98–103). However, in childhood a diagnosis of sinusitis is not justified by mucosal thickening or sinus opacification in the absence of supportive clinical findings (101). Sinusitis is often underdiagnosed or overdiagnosed in infants and children on the basis of plain film findings (100). Sinus CT frequently shows mucosal thickening in children without symptoms or signs of sinusitis or an upper respiratory infection. Furthermore, children with a recent upper respiratory infection and no clinical manifestations of sinusitis often have mucosal thickening on CT. Similar observations have been made with MRI (104). Therefore, in children mucosal thickening shown by plain films, CT, or MRI should not be attributed to sinusitis without appropriate clinical support. However, air-fluid levels are much more suggestive of true sinus disease.

In spite of the many false positives just described, the

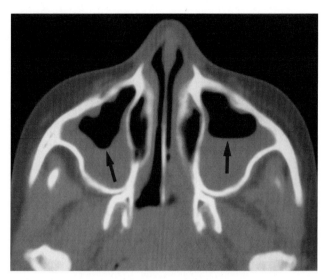

FIG. 3-26. **Acute maxillary sinusitis.** CT shows air-fluid levels *(arrows)* and mucosal thickening of both maxillary sinuses.

imaging hallmark of acute sinusitis is sinus opacification caused by mucosal edema and mucous secretions (5,59,60). An air-fluid level may be seen on plain radiographs or CT (Fig. 3-26). The maxillary sinus is most frequently involved. Sphenoid, frontal, and ethmoid sinusitis may require aggressive therapy including surgical drainage. Imaging findings of chronic sinusitis (Fig. 3-27) include (a) mucosal thickening, sometimes irregular because of retention cysts or polyps, (b) total sinus opacification from fluid, mucosal thickening, cysts, or polyps, and (c) loss of the sharp mucoperiosteal margins, obliteration of ostiomeatal landmarks, patchy osteopenia, or sclerosis (5,59,60,99).

Differentiation of infectious from allergic sinusitis may be impossible. They often coexist. Unilateral involvement

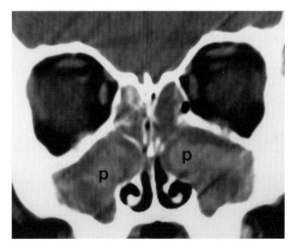

FIG. 3-27. **Chronic sinusitis and polyposis.** A 12-year-old girl with cystic fibrosis. Coronal CT. Bilateral isodense and high-density polyps *(p)* with expansion of the maxillary and ethmoid sinuses and obliteration of the ostiomeatal landmarks.

or an air-fluid level suggests an infectious process secondary to ostiomeatal obstruction. In allergic sinusitis, there is usually bilateral, general sinus involvement (59,60). Nodular mucosal thickening may be demonstrated, but air-fluid levels are unusual. The nasal turbinates are often thickened and edematous. Nasal or sinus polyps are commonly multiple in allergic disease but may be solitary.

CT of sinus disease shows soft-tissue density filling normally aerated spaces (5,60). The soft-tissue density represents mucosal thickening or edema, mucous secretions, or a combination of both (see Figs. 3-26 and 3-27). With inspissation, the secretions may become concretions in the mucosa or polyps and have a high density on CT (see Fig. 3-27). On MRI, sinonasal secretions are of low intensity on T1-weighted images and high intensity on proton density and T2-weighted images. Decreasing free water content and increasing protein content lead at first to hyperintensity on T1-weighted images. With further increases in protein content, the semisolid and solid secretions or concretions become hypointense initially on T2-weighted images and then on T1-weighted images (5,60,105–107). Mucosal inflammation characteristically is hypointense on T1-weighted images but of high intensity on proton-density and T2-weighted images. The hyperintensity on T2-weighted images may allow differentiation of mucosal inflammation from the intermediate signal intensity of tumor. Fibrosis is usually hypointense on all MRI pulse sequences.

Mucosal thickening due to active inflammation usually enhances by CT and MRI (5,60,105–107). Chronic, noninflamed, or fibrotic mucosal thickening lacks enhancement. Mucoid secretions and submucosal edema usually do not enhance. Therefore, the mucosal enhancement caused by mucosal inflammation may be ring-like, contrasting with the nonenhancing submucosal edema and mucosal secretions.

Radiographic loss of the mucoperiosteal line has been reported in prolonged active sinus infection and probably results from hyperemia (5,60,105–107). When sinus inflammation has been present for several months or years, thick, dense reactive bone may develop. Osteomyelitis is rarely secondary to sinonasal infection but is usually posttraumatic or iatrogenic. It causes an irregularly mottled appearance of the sinus wall (Fig. 3-28). A similar appearance may be caused by radiation osteitis.

Enlargement of a single turbinate is usually part of the normal nasal cycle, particularly in the absence of evidence of paranasal sinus disease (5,60,105–108). The normal or abnormally enlarged turbinate is hypointense on T1-weighted images and hyperintense on T2-weighted images and enhances on CT and MRI. Although air-fluid levels (usually in the maxillary sinuses) are most often due to acute bacterial sinusitis, levels may also be seen after sinus trauma (including barotrauma), after lavage, following nasotracheal or nasogastric intubation, with sinus hemorrhage, after rupture of a mucocele, and with CSF rhinorrhea (5,60, 105–107).

Inflammatory pseudotumors of the sinuses are chronic in-

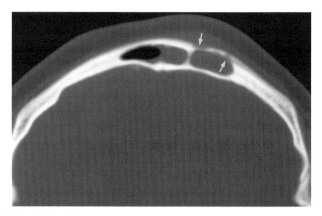

FIG. 3-28. Frontal sinusitis complicated by osteomyelitis. CT. Frontal sinus opacification due to sinusitis. The erosive bony changes *(arrows)* indicate osteomyelitis.

flammatory lesions and may result from an exaggerated immune response to an unidentified pathogen (5,55). They are histologically diverse tumoral masses of acute and chronic inflammatory cells with a variable fibrous response and often a pronounced plasmocytic component but no granulomatous elements. They often respond to steroid therapy. The imaging findings may suggest lymphoma or chloroma (55).

Complications of Sinusitis

The local sequelae of sinonasal inflammation include retention cyst, polyp, mucocele or pyocele, cellulitis, and osteomyelitis. Intracranial complications include meningitis, abscess or empyema, and thrombophlebitis (5,6,59,60).

The most frequent sequelae are retention cysts and polyps. Retention cysts, mucous or serous are more common and

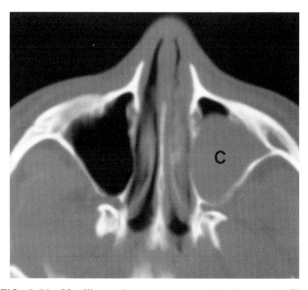

FIG. 3-29. Maxillary sinus mucous retention cyst. The mucous retention cyst *(C)* has a rounded anterior contour and partially fills the left maxillary sinus.

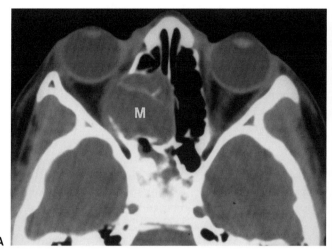
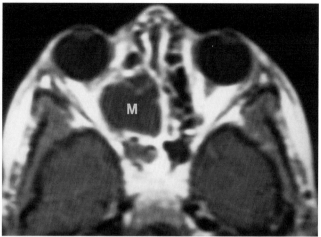

A   B

FIG. 3-30. Ethmoid mucocele. A: Axial CT. A soft-tissue mass *(M)* expands the right ethmoid air cells and distorts the lateral bony contours. **B:** Contrast-enhanced T1-weighted MRI. There is marked peripheral, ring-like enhancement of the mucocele *(M)*.

result from obstruction of submucosal mucinous glands or from a submucosal serous effusion. Although they may develop in any sinus, retention cysts usually occur in the maxillary sinus (Fig. 3-29). It may be impossible to distinguish a retention cyst from a polyp. Polyps are due to mucous membrane hyperplasia and arise in either the nasal cavity or paranasal sinuses (5,59,60). They are usually of allergic origin but commonly occur in the chronic sinusitis of cystic fibrosis (see Fig. 3-27). They may be solitary or multiple and are most common in the maxillary sinus (see Fig. 3-27). Antrochoanal polyps are usually solitary, arise from the antral mucosa (5,59,60), and extend through the ostium into the middle meatus, enlarging the sinus cavity. They may even extend through the choana into the nasopharynx.

On CT and MRI, retention cysts and polyps are homogeneous soft-tissue masses with smooth margins, part of which is usually outlined by air. Outlining by air distinguishes polyps and cysts, when they do not fill the entire chamber, from mucoceles. The upper surface of a large retention cyst may flatten and resemble an air-fluid level. Cysts and polyps usually have MRI characteristics similar to those of mucosal inflammation. The MR (5,59,60) intensity pattern of retention cysts, like that of sinus secretions, varies with the protein content. Imaging findings suggestive of polyposis include a rounded mass (sometimes more than one) within the nasal cavity, ostial enlargement, expansion of a sinus or of the nasal cavity, and erosive bony changes. It may be difficult to distinguish polyposis from a neoplastic process. Polyps are usually hyperintense on T2-weighted images and may enhance peripherally or throughout. Although polyps tend to be of mucoid density and intensity on CT and MRI, sometimes they are fibrous and have higher density on CT and lower intensity on T2-weighted MRI. Multiple polyps are associated with entrapped secretions and are often intermixed with mucoceles. This results in variable CT densities and MR signal intensities.

A mucocele develops within a sinus because of obstruc-

tion of its ostium, or within a compartment of a septated sinus, and is lined by sinus mucosa (5,6,59,60,64,109). There is total opacification and expansion of the sinus or compartment (Fig. 3-30). Mucoceles arise most commonly in the frontal sinuses and ethmoid cells but may be encountered elsewhere. They are usually uninflamed. Their signs and symptoms result from mass effect and expansion into adjacent structures. In the ethmoid complex, an air-fluid level may be due to rupture of an ethmoid mucocele and suggests a mucopyocele. On CT and MRI, the appearance of a mucocele varies with its water and protein content. The peripheral enhancement of a mucocele distinguishes it from a neoplasm (Fig. 3-30B) (110).

The CT appearance of central high density within a sinus surrounded by a zone of mucoid density may be seen with chronic inspissated secretions, mycetoma (usually aspergillosis), and hemorrhage. On MRI, these may be of low intensity, or void of signal, as is also true of a sinolith or tooth in the sinus. The MRI appearance of sinus hemorrhage varies with its state of evolution.

Orbital complications of sinusitis include preseptal periorbital cellulitis, postseptal orbital cellulitis, and orbital abscess (5,59,60). Thrombophlebitis may occur with sinusitis but less commonly than in otomastoiditis (60). Cavernous sinus thrombosis may be associated with sphenoid sinusitis. Superior sagittal sinus thrombosis occasionally follows frontal sinusitis.

Sinonasal mucormycosis and aspergillosis are aggressive and fulminant fungal infections with a tendency to invade the orbit, cavernous sinus, and neurovascular structures (5,60,111). This may result in thrombosis, infarction, hemorrhage, or abscess. These infections tend to be even more aggressive in the immunocompromised patient. Extramucosal (intraluminal) sinonasal fungal infections (including aspergillosis) may cause polypoid lesions or fungus balls in patients with atopy. Relative CT hyperdensity and hypointensity on T2-weighted MRI are seen, along with marked enhancement.

TABLE 3-2. *Sinonasal masses*

Congenital
  Nasal glioma
  Nasal dermoid/epidermoid
  Cephalocele
Inflammatory
  Mucous retention cyst
  Mucocele
  Polyps
  Fungal disease
  Granulomatous disease
Neoplastic
  Benign tumor
    Hemangioma
    Juvenile angiofibroma
    Fibrous dysplasia
    Antrochoanal polyp
    Osteoma
    Odontogenic cyst
  Malignant tumor
    Rhabdomyosarcoma
    Neuroblastoma
    Langerhans cell histiocytosis
    PNET
    Progonoma
    Esthesioneuroblastoma
    Odontogenic tumor
    Osteogenic sarcoma
    Other sarcomas
    Lymphoma
    Leukemia
    Carcinoma
    Lymphoepithelioma
    Metastatic disease
Vascular
  Arteriovenous fistula
  Venous malformation
  Lymphatic malformation
Miscellaneous
  Pseudomass due to "redundant mucosa" in infants
  Pseudomass due to turbinate swelling
  Idiopathic midline granuloma
  Cocaine nose

Osteomyelitis may affect the bony wall of any sinus but most often involves the frontal sinus (5,59,60). It may arise from hematogenous spread, direct trauma, surgery, or, rarely, from adjacent sinusitis. Osteopenia progresses to bone destruction (see Fig. 3-28). With chronic infection there is irregular thickening, sclerosis, and sequestrum formation.

Neoplasms

Masses arising in the nasal cavity, sinuses, and face in childhood may be neoplastic and benign, neoplastic and malignant, or nonneoplastic (Table 3-2). They may be circumscribed and contained or more aggressive and expanding or infiltrating. There may be invasion of the orbit and cranium. Neoplasms may be mimicked by the bony abnormalities and soft-tissue masses associated with dysplastic conditions. Their origin may be mesenchymal, neural, or from the cutaneous or mucosal epithelium (5–7,59,112). The delineation

of regional involvement is critical. A combination of surgery, chemotherapy, and radiotherapy is often required. With recent advances in craniofacial and skull base surgery, tumor ablation may be possible without the sacrifice of function or appearance.

Mesenchymal tumors of the head and neck in childhood are of vascular, soft tissue, reticuloendothelial, osteochondroid, dental, and notochordal origin (5–7,59,112). Neural tumors include those of neuroepithelial, neural crest, and nerve sheath origins. Neoplastic lesions of cutaneous or mucosal epithelial origin are rare. The most common tumors arising in the sinonasal region are juvenile angiofibroma, rhabdomyosarcoma, neuroblastoma, histiocytosis, chondrosarcoma, osteosarcoma, leukemia, lymphoma, and fibrous dysplasia. Hemangiomas and vascular malformations are discussed later. Tumors and cysts of dental origin are presented in the last section of this chapter.

Vascular Tumors

Juvenile angiofibroma, the most common benign nasopharyngeal tumor of childhood, occurs primarily in adolescent boys (6). It is a histologically benign but locally aggressive fibrovascular tumor. It usually arises from the posterolateral nasal cavity near the pterygopalatine fossa and sphenopalatine foramen. Nasal obstruction and recurrent epistaxis are the common manifestations. Large tumors cause facial swelling, proptosis, otitis media, and headache. On CT these are isodense or low-density masses that enhance markedly (5,7). Bony expansion and erosion are common (Fig. 3-31). In most cases the pterygopalatine fossa is widened and there is anterior bowing of the posterolateral wall of the maxillary sinus. Extension into the sphenoid, maxillary, and ethmoid sinuses, orbit, middle cranial fossa, and parasellar region is common (Fig. 3-31A). The MR characteristics depend on the relative combination of vascularity (flow-related signal voids), fibrous components (hypointensity), and tumor edema (hypointensity on T1-weighted images and hyperintensity on proton density and T2-weighted MRI) (5,7,67). Cysts, cavitation, and hemorrhage may develop. Sinus obstruction, mucosal edema, and retained secretions are frequent. Marked gadolinium enhancement is usually observed (Fig. 3-31B). Vascular and neural involvement and intracranial extension are best evaluated by MRI. Angiography and preoperative embolization are critical adjuncts to surgical resection.

An angiomatous polyp is occasionally histologically mistaken for an angiofibroma but is rare in childhood and usually has a quite different imaging appearance (5,68). Hemangiopericytoma, an extremely rare vascular tumor of the nasal cavity or paranasal sinuses in childhood (5), is generally considered only a low-grade malignancy, but recurrence and metastasis have been reported. These are expansile lesions of homogeneous CT density and MRI intensity; enhancement is variable.

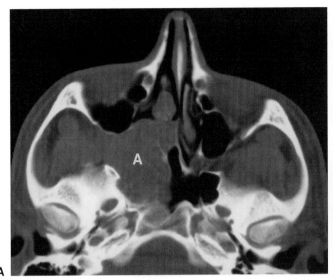
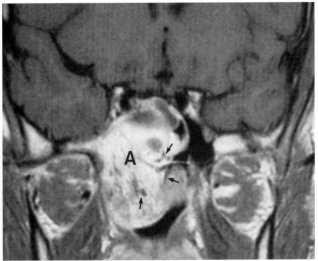

FIG. 3-31. Angiofibroma. A 17-year-old boy with epistaxis. **A:** CT. The right nasal cavity is expanded by a nasopharyngeal soft-tissue mass *(A)*. This mass extends through the pterygomaxillary fissure and sphenopalatine foramen into the infratemporal space and inferior orbit. **B:** Contrast-enhanced T1-weighted MRI. There is marked contrast enhancement of the mass *(A)* and multiple vascular flow-related signal voids *(arrows)*.

Soft-Tissue and Reticuloendothelial System Tumors

Rhabdomyosarcoma is the most common malignant soft-tissue tumor of the head and neck region in childhood (5–7,59,112). Other soft-tissue malignancies include lymphoma, Ewing sarcoma, histiocytosis, leukemia, neural origin tumors (neuroblastoma, PNET), and fibromatous tumors. The orbit and paranasal sinuses are the most common sites of origin of rhabdomyosarcoma. Like the other small round-cell malignancies listed above, these hypercellular tumors often present as large infiltrating soft-tissue masses that destroy bone (5,7). Regional and systemic metastasis may occur. They are isodense to high density or occasionally low density by CT. They frequently show contrast enhancement (Fig. 3-32A). On MRI these lesions are isotense or hypointense on T1-weighted MRI and isointense or hypointense on T2-weighted images, or occasionally hyperintense on T2-weighted MRI. There is variable contrast enhancement (Fig. 3-32B).

Fibromatous tumors are mesenchymal neoplasms that

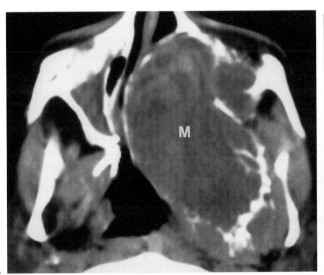
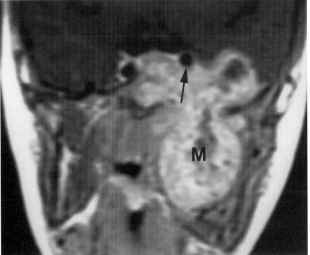

FIG. 3-32. Rhabdomyosarcoma. A: Contrast-enhanced CT. The large mass *(M)* of the left nasal cavity extends into the maxillary sinus, orbit, and masticator space. Part of it enhances. **B:** Contrast-enhanced T1-weighted MRI. The markedly enhancing infratemporal component of the mass *(M)* extends intracranially to involve the temporal lobe and cavernous sinus. The left internal carotid artery *(arrow)* is encased by tumor.

may be isolated and benign in behavior (solitary fibroma) or aggressive and malignant with invasion and extensive involvement (fibromatosis, fibrosarcoma) (5,7,69). Fibromatosis is a locally infiltrating pseudoneoplastic process characterized by fibroelastic proliferation. The congenital form has widespread visceral and bone lesions but usually no metastases. The less aggressive juvenile form usually involves musculoskeletal structures but not the viscera. Imaging shows fibromatosis as infiltrating soft-tissue masses that obliterate tissue planes and secondarily involve bone.

A desmoid tumor is a well-differentiated childhood form of fibromatosis with no tendency to metastasize. However, extensive infiltration often makes complete resection impossible. Recurrence is common, and progression to fibrosarcoma may occur even after radiotherapy. CT and MRI usually reveal isodensity or hypodensity and relative hypointensity throughout the sequences. There is little or no enhancement in lesions with a large mature fibrous component. CT hypodensity and hyperintensity on proton density and T2-weighted MRI may be seen in the more aggressive and malignant forms.

Common reticuloendothelial neoplasms in childhood include histiocytosis, lymphoma, and leukemia (5–7). Langerhans cell histiocytosis is a reticuloendothelial disorder histologically characterized by tissue infiltration with reticulum cells, histiocytes, plasmocytes, and leukocytes (113). The involvement may be isolated (usually termed eosinophilic granuloma), or there may be dissemination with cutaneous, visceral, and bony involvement.

In some series, lymphoma is the most common malignant solid tumor of the head and neck region in childhood (5–7). Hodgkin disease often presents with cervical lymphadenopathy and usually spreads contiguously along nodal chains. The more common non-Hodgkin lymphoma is often widespread at diagnosis initially and involves noncontiguous nodes. Extranodal non-Hodgkin lymphomas occasionally occur in children in the nasopharynx, sinuses, adenotonsillar region, and salivary glands. Head and neck lymphomas may be associated with childhood AIDS. Leukemia involves the nasal cavity and paranasal sinuses only rarely (5–7). More often, nasal or sinus abnormalities in leukemia are due to infection or hemorrhage. Occasionally, a leukemic chloroma (granulocytic sarcoma) is seen as an osseous or soft-tissue lesion of the nasal cavity, paranasal sinuses, nasopharynx, or some other sinonasal site (Fig. 3-33) (114). Chloromas more commonly complicate myeloblastic than lymphoblastic leukemia. On CT and MRI they are bulky soft-tissue masses and show moderate or marked enhancement (5–7). They are isodense or hyperdense on CT, and isointense or hypointense on proton density and T2-weighted images. Occasionally there is marked hyperintensity on T2-weighted MRI. There may also be bony expansion, remodeling, or erosion.

Osseous and Chondroid Tumors

Osteochondral tumors of the nasal cavity, paranasal sinuses, and face usually arise from the skull base and second-

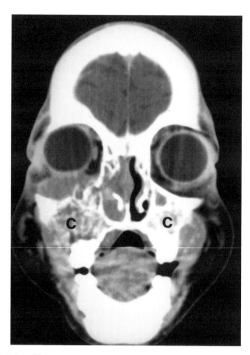

FIG. 3-33. Chloroma. A 2-year-old boy with acute myelogenous leukemia in relapse. Contrast-enhanced coronal CT. There are bilateral enhancing maxillary sinus masses *(C)* with adjacent bony reaction. The lower part of the right orbit is also involved.

arily involve the nasal cavity, sinuses, and nasopharynx (5–7). Occasionally, they are primary in the facial bones or paranasal sinuses.

Osteoma, a benign osseous neoplasm, may be of the cortical, cancellous, or fibrous histologic subtype. Rare in childhood and adolescence, osteomas most often arise in a frontal or ethmoid sinus at the junction of membranous and enchondral bone formation. The appearance on plain films and CT depends on the histologic subtype and varies from a sclerotic lesion to a soft-tissue density (5). Although often incidental, an osteoma may be associated with headache, frontal sinus obstruction, or CSF rhinorrhea. Multiple osteomas are part of the Gardner syndrome.

An osteochondroma (benign osteocartilaginous exostosis) contains mature cancellous, cortical, and cartilaginous elements that are continuous with the mature elements of the parent bone (5,7). Although rare in the facial bones in childhood, they may arise from the mandible, maxilla, sphenoid bone, zygoma, or nasal septum. Multiple lesions occur in familial cases. Osteochondromas also arise after radiation therapy. Growth is slow, and malignancy is rare in nasofacial osteochondromas except in familial cases. The CT and MRI appearance is that of a miniature metaphysis, growth plate, and cartilaginous cap, with marrow and cortical elements in continuity with the bone of origin (5,7). Malignant degeneration to osteosarcoma or chondrosarcoma is indicated by a disorganized appearance, cap disruption, an unexpected soft-tissue mass, and involvement of the marrow of the parent bone.

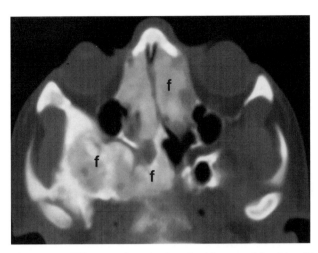

FIG. 3-34. Fibrous dysplasia. A 12-year-old girl with McCune-Albright syndrome. The thickened and sclerotic bone *(f)* of the sphenoid body and right sphenoid wing encroaches on the right orbit and obliterates the nasal cavities.

Fibrous dysplasia, an idiopathic benign fibroosseous disorder, may be monostotic, polyostotic, or part of the McCune-Albright syndrome (polyostotic fibrous dysplasia, cafe-au-lait pigmentation, and sexual precocity in a female) (Fig. 3-34) (5,7). Involvement of the facial bones and skull is more common in the polyostotic form and may be unilateral or bilateral. The maxilla and mandible are most frequently involved, especially the former. There may be encroachment on the neurovascular foramina, orbit, nasal structures, or sinuses. Ostiomeatal obstruction may lead to a mucocele. Growth of the lesion may continue after skeletal maturation. Transformation to osteosarcoma, fibrosarcoma, or chondrosarcoma is rare. The CT and plain film appearance ranges from an inhomogeneous soft-tissue density to a ground glass appearance with sclerotic bony thickening (Fig. 3-34) (5,7). On MRI there may be soft tissue, bony, or combined intensities, often with enhancement marked enough to suggest a neoplasm.

Other benign fibroosseous tumors include ossifying fibroma and cementifying fibroma (5,7,115). Ossifying fibroma is a circumscribed fibrous neoplasm that undergoes progressive ossification. On CT and MRI, the lesion is expansile and has prominent areas of nonossified fibrous tissue. In some cases the imaging appearance is indistinguishable from that of fibrous dysplasia, although ossifying fibroma tends to grow faster and recur after resection. Cementifying fibroma is also aggressive and tends to recur.

Giant cell tumor, giant cell reparative granuloma, aneurysmal bone cyst, and osteoblastoma are benign osseous tumors rarely arising in this region in childhood (5,7,72). Often with overlapping pathologic findings, these tumors are covered in detail in Chapter 5. Combined lesions with elements of giant cell tumor, osteoblastoma, and aneurysmal bone cyst have been reported. CT and MRI show lytic, expansile-appearing lesions containing bony matrix or calcification with cortical erosion, a soft-tissue mass, and a thin calcified rim

(Fig. 3-35) (5,7). Cavitation, cyst formation, and hemorrhage may be observed. Moderate enhancement is common. A multiloculated appearance with fluid-fluid levels suggests aneurysmal bone cyst (Fig. 3-35); however, the finding has also been reported with lymphatic malformations, venolymphatic malformations, and telangiectatic osteosarcoma.

Cherubism is a benign autosomal dominant disorder with progressive fibroosseous lesions of the mandible and maxilla in childhood. It has often been mislabeled as congenital fibrous dysplasia (5,6).

Chondrosarcoma is a malignant bone neoplasm of cartilage origin that may arise de novo or from a preexisting osteochondroma or may follow radiation therapy. In childhood the tumor is occasionally found in the sphenoid bone or at the sphenooccipital synchondrosis (5,7). On CT and MRI, the mass is often of nonspecific soft-tissue density and intensity. Chondroid matrix calcifications are often not evident. The lesion tends to be expansile and produce bony thinning. Enhancement may be seen.

Chordoma is a rare tumor of childhood arising from intraosseous notochordal remnants in the skull base and often centered at the synchondroses. Chordomas are locally invasive tumors that destroy bone, and metastasis has been observed. The chondroid form of chordoma may be radiologically indistinguishable from chondrosarcoma by plain films, CT, and MRI.

Osteosarcoma, fibrosarcoma, and Ewing sarcoma are other mesenchymal neoplasms, rare in this region, that arise de novo or after radiation therapy (e.g., for retinoblastoma) (5,7). These highly invasive tumors may give rise to regional and distant lymphatic and hematogenous metastases. The mandible and maxilla are the most common locations in the head and neck region. The imaging appearance of osteosarcoma depends upon the degree of osteoid matrix; it is seen

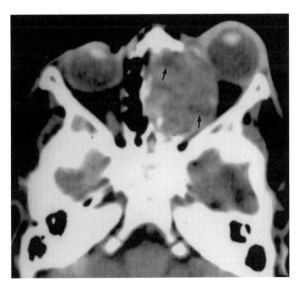

FIG. 3-35. Aneurysmal bone cyst. A 2-year-old boy with left exophthalmos. Axial CT. The left nasoorbital mass contains multiple fluid-fluid levels *(arrows)*.

as either a soft-tissue mass with aggressive bony destruction and a spiculated periosteal bone reaction or a partially calcified or ossified mass. Fibrosarcoma and Ewing sarcoma are usually soft-tissue masses with permeative bony destruction but without osteoid or chondroid matrix elements. Bony fibrosarcomas tend to be more aggressive than soft-tissue fibrosarcomas.

Neural Tumors

Tumors of neuroepithelial or neural crest origin which may involve the nasosinus region include neuroblastoma, PNET, esthesioneuroblastoma, retinoblastoma, and progonoma (5–7,59). Neuroblastoma, the most common of these tumors, may involve the skull base, nose, sinuses, or orbit, usually as part of metastatic disease. Esthesioneuroblastoma (olfactory neuroblastoma) is a very rare tumor that arises from the olfactory groove, produces extensive destruction of the sinuses, orbit, and adjacent skull base, and extends intracranially. Primitive neuroectodermal tumors (PNETs), rare malignancies of primitive neuroepithelial origin arising outside of the central nervous system, are characterized by small round cell infiltrations similar to those of neuroblastoma and other round-cell tumors. Progonomas, rare retinal anlage tumors that often contain melanin, tend to arise from the cranial base and invade the adjacent nasosinus structures or orbit. These tumors all tend to have a similar appearance on CT and MRI: soft-tissue mass effect, permeative bone destruction, and calcification (Fig. 3-36) (5,7). Tumor hyper-

cellularity is characteristically demonstrated as CT isodensity or hyperdensity and isointensity or hypointensity on T2-weighted MRI. Prominent contrast enhancement is characteristically seen.

Schwannomas, neurofibromas, and plexiform neurofibromas rarely arise in the nasal cavity, paranasal sinuses, or nasopharynx.

Tumors of Cutaneous and Mucosal Epithelial Origin

Nasal cavity papillomas are benign mucosal tumors and are subclassified as fungiform, inverted, and cylindric cell papillomas (5,116,117). Extension into the maxillary and ethmoid sinuses is common, and involvement of the sphenoid and frontal sinuses has also been reported. Malignant transformation is extremely rare in childhood. CT often demonstrates a polypoid mass, small or large, in the nasal cavity. Often there is remodeling of the nasal wall and septum and extension into the sinuses resulting in ostiomeatal obstruction. Cylindric cell and inverted papillomas tend to be more aggressive than the fungiform papillomas. Complete surgical excision may be difficult, and recurrence is common.

Squamous cell carcinoma and adenocarcinoma of the nasal cavity and sinuses are extremely rare in childhood (5,6,63,116–119). Undifferentiated carcinoma may be the most common type. The maxillary sinus is usually involved, primarily or secondarily. These tumors may also originate in the nasal cavity, ethmoid complex, or sphenoid or frontal sinus. Imaging demonstrates a mass within a sinus, with bone destruction in the majority of cases. The tumors are often of homogeneous density and intensity, but enhancement is uncommon. Necrosis and hemorrhage develop in large tumors. Regional extension may occur, along with nodal and distant metastases.

Trauma

Nasal Foreign Body

Insertion of foreign material into the nose is common in young children (6,120). Vomiting or coughing of an ingested or aspirated foreign body occasionally results in posterior choanal entry. Commonly inserted foreign bodies include beans, seeds, plastic or metal objects, toy parts, buttons, beads, and so forth. Intrinsic ''foreign'' bodies—a misnomer—are rare and usually result from chronic inflammation or infection. They include inspissated mucosal secretions, bony sequestra, and mineralized concretions (rhinoliths) (120). Infection superimposed on any of these objects results in a purulent rhinitis or sinusitis. Secondary adenoiditis or otitis media due to nasopharyngeal or eustachian tube reflux may develop. Imaging is rarely required but plain films or CT may be needed to identify the radiopaque object or to delineate the extent and nature of infection. Complications

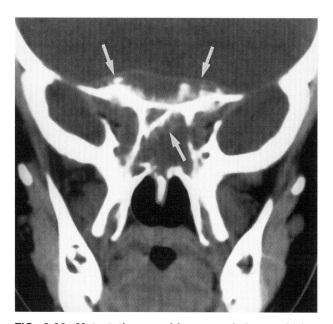

FIG. 3-36. Metastatic neuroblastoma. A 3-year-old boy with stage 4 neuroblastoma. Coronal CT. A soft-tissue mass involves the sphenoid sinus and sphenoid ridge bilaterally. There is bony destruction and spiculated reactive bone formation (arrows).

of nasal foreign bodies and attempts at their removal include aspiration and ingestion.

Nasosinus and Facial Injury

Facial fractures are infrequent under the age of 12 years (6,120,121). Most are related to vehicular accidents and falls; others are caused by recreational events, altercations, and child abuse. Adult-type injuries begin to emerge at age 10–12 years (5). The young child has a relatively large cranial vault and prominent frontal region and small midface and mandible. As a result, frontal fractures and cranial and intracranial injuries are much more common than midfacial or mandibular fractures in infants and children. Facial fractures in younger children tend to be of the greenstick type. With maturation there is increased pneumatization of the facial bones, and an adult fracture pattern including comminution and fragment displacement becomes more common.

Nearly half of pediatric facial fractures involve the nasal bones, 30% the mandible, and 20% the orbit and zygomaticomaxillary structures. Maxillary fractures are unusual and suggest severe injury. Nearly three fourths of children with facial trauma have other injuries, and management priorities must be established quickly. Although plain films may be used initially, CT with axial and coronal sections or reformatted images is the definitive imaging procedure.

Nasal Fractures

Because the nasal pyramid is variably cartilaginous in childhood and the internasal suture is unfused, greenstick fractures are common after a frontal impact (5,6). As a result, there is traumatic splaying of the nasal bones over the intact frontal processes of the maxillae. In adolescence, frontal impact usually results in bilateral fractures of the distal thirds of the nasal bones. The cartilaginous nasal septum is often fractured and displaced. With more severe trauma, the entire nasal pyramid and the frontal processes of the maxilla are fractured, and there are lacrimal and ethmoid fractures and severe nasal septal injuries extending into the cribriform plate and orbital roof (Fig. 3-37) (5,6). There may be a major hemorrhage or a CSF leak. Nasal septal cartilage injury may result in a subperichondrial hematoma. Septal hematoma is suggested on imaging studies by local septal thickening. If the hematoma is not recognized and promptly drained, ischemic septal necrosis, septal abscess, or septal perforation may result in a permanent saddle nose deformity.

Mandible Injury

Condylar fractures are more common in children than fractures of the angle, body, or parasymphyseal region (121,122). Fracture of the mandibular condyle in a young

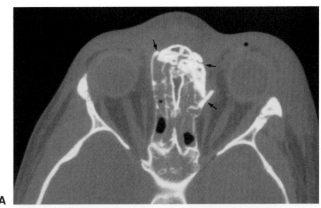
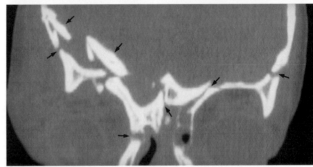

FIG. 3-37. Complex nasoethmoidal and orbitofrontal fractures. A 6-year-old boy struck by an automobile. Axial **(A)** and coronal **(B)** CT. There are multiple fractures *(arrows)* of the nasal bones, ethmoids, cribriform plate, and frontal bone. Several bony fragments are displaced into the orbit and intracranially.

child often results from a fall with impact on the chin. The injury is often bilateral and may be associated with a parasymphyseal fracture (Fig. 3-38A). There is frequently a severe crush injury of the condylar head. The condylar injury may result in decreased mandibular growth or ankylosis. The risk of permanent deformity lessens with age. In older children and adolescents, fractures typically occur at the condylar neck (5). Although rare in childhood, injury of the temporomandibular joint may occur with other mandibular fractures (5). CT readily demonstrates the osseous components, whereas MRI demonstrates disk abnormalities better.

Other Midface Injuries

Maxillary and zygomatic fractures are rare in children under 10 years (6,121,123). In young children maxillary fractures may extend bilaterally or superiorly to involve the frontal region, and associated CNS injury and CSF leaks are common (Fig. 3-38B). In older children and adolescents, adult fracture patterns (isolated maxillary alveolar fractures, partial fractures of the maxilla, palatal fractures, LeFort fractures, and lateral midface or trimalar fractures) become more common (5).

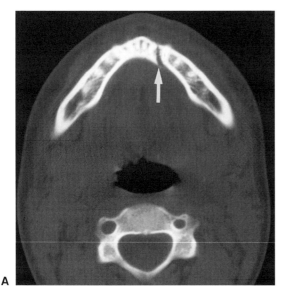

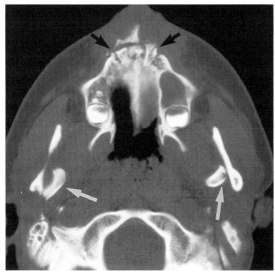

FIG. 3-38. Mandibular and maxillary fractures. A: Axial CT of the mandible. A left parasymphyseal fracture *(white arrow)* is well demonstrated. **B:** Maxillary CT. There are bilateral maxillary alveolar fractures *(black arrows)* and bilateral mandibular condylar fractures *(white arrows)*.

Orbital Injury

Orbital floor and rim fractures are infrequent until substantial pneumatization of the maxillary sinus has occurred (6,121,123). A nonpenetrating frontal blow to the orbit may result in a blow-out fracture of the orbital floor into the maxillary sinus near the infraorbital canal (5). Herniation of orbital fat or displacement of the inferior rectus or inferior oblique muscle into or through the fracture line is readily demonstrated by direct coronal CT (Fig. 3-39). Rarely, there is upward displacement of the orbital floor fracture fragments (blow-in fracture) and impingement upon the inferior extraocular muscles or globe (5). A depressed orbital roof or superior orbital rim fracture occasionally impinges upon

the globe and impairs upward gaze. Coronal CT easily differentiates these types of injury.

Orbital roof fractures may be associated with CSF leakage or herniation of brain tissue or meninges into the orbit (see Fig. 3-37) (5). Orbital emphysema is unusual in orbital floor and orbital roof fractures. Medial orbital wall fractures into the ethmoid sinuses may occur alone or be associated with an orbital floor fracture. Orbital emphysema is common in ethmoid fractures and orbital fat may herniate into the fracture defect although muscle entrapment is rare. Orbital emphysema is seldom associated with frontal or sphenoid sinus fractures except in severe injuries and complex fractures. Orbital emphysema may become apparent or dramatically increase with nose blowing. Significant enophthalmos with displacement of the globe into the maxillary sinus or ethmoid sinus may occur acutely or after an interval following an orbital floor or medial orbital wall fracture.

Frontal and Sphenoid Injury

Frontal fractures are most common in children less than 6 years of age (6,121,123). Since the frontal sinus is not pneumatized until about 5 years of age or older, frontal region fractures in younger children tend to be of the greenstick type. These fractures often extend through the skull or orbital roof. In older children, frontal sinus fractures result from direct trauma or extension of a skull fracture into the sinus. Associated intracranial injury is common. With fractures involving the posterior wall of the frontal sinus, CSF leakage occurs and pneumocephalus or CNS infection may develop (5).

Sphenoid sinus fractures, exceedingly rare in childhood, are associated with severe trauma and skull base fractures

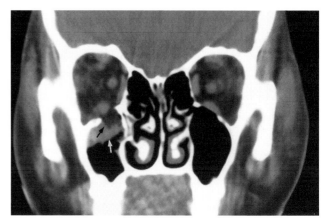

FIG. 3-39. Orbital floor blow-out fracture. An 18-year-old girl with trauma to the right eye. Coronal CT shows a fracture defect of the right orbital floor with displacement of orbital fat *(black arrow)* into the maxillary sinus with surrounding hemorrhage *(white arrow)*.

(6,121,123). Imaging demonstrates sinus opacification or an air-fluid level and may show pneumocephalus (5). There may be carotid arterial or cavernous sinus injury and a carotid-cavernous fistula.

Vascular Abnormalities

Vascular abnormalities of the nasal cavity, paranasal sinuses, and face include vascular anomalies and vascular tumors (6,7,82,83). Vascular tumors were discussed earlier. Vascular abnormalities may present with epistaxis, obstruction of the sinuses or nose, or a cosmetic deformity (6). The nose and nasal cavity are vascularized by terminal branches of the internal and external carotid arteries. These include the anterior and posterior ethmoidal branches of the ophthalmic artery, the sphenopalatine and descending palatine branches of the internal maxillary artery, and the superior labial branch of the facial artery. The veins of the nasal cavity drain into the pterygoid and ophthalmic venous plexus and intracranially into the cavernous sinus.

More than 90% of pediatric epistaxis arises from the anterior nasal cavity, where the most exuberant arterial coalescence (the Kiesselbach plexus) is found (6). Common causes of epistaxis in childhood are infections, allergic rhinitis, and trauma. Specific examples of injury include fracture, foreign body, dry air, pollution, and injury by the patient or his or her physician. Uncommon causes suggested by recurrent epistaxis include bleeding disorders, neoplasia, and vascular anomalies such as Reuder-Osler-Weber. In recurrent epistaxis, imaging should begin with CT. MRI may follow, or angiography if embolization for control of the epistaxis is a consideration (6).

Vascular Anomalies

The Mulliken and Glowacki biological classification of vascular anomalies distinguishes hemangiomas from vascular malformations (7,82,83). Hemangiomas are the most common and most rapidly growing vascular tumors of the head and neck in childhood. They evolve from a cellular proliferative phase into an involuting phase and appear to be sensitive to angiogenic factors. Vascular malformations, on the other hand, are anomalies of vascular development. These two types of abnormality can be distinguished on clinical and imaging criteria, especially using MRI.

Several syndromes are associated with vascular anomalies (6,7,82,83). These include Sturge-Weber syndrome (capillary or telangiectatic malformation of the skin of the face in the distribution of the trigeminal nerve), Beckwith-Wiedemann syndrome (facial capillary or telangiectatic malformation), Klippel-Trenaunay-Weber syndrome (capillary, venous, and lymphatic malformations), Maffucci syndrome (multiple venous malformations), Rendu-Osler-Weber syndrome (capillary or telangiectatic malformation), and the blue rubber bleb nevus syndrome.

TEMPORAL BONE AND EAR

Normal

Embryology and Development

The external ear and middle ear are derived from the branchial apparatus. The internal ear is derived from the neuroectoderm (6,13). The auricle and external ear begin development at the cranial end of the neck and move to the side of the head as the mandible is formed. The middle ear (tympanic) cavity expands to contain the auditory ossicles, their tendons and ligaments, and the chorda tympani nerve. During the late fetal period, extension of the tympanic cavity gives rise to the mastoid antrum in the petromastoid part of the temporal bone. The mastoid bone (not including the mastoid process) is almost of adult size at birth. Mastoid air cell development and pneumatization take place primarily during the first 2 years of life. The middle ear continues to grow until puberty. The formation of the inner ear begins during the fourth embryonic week, when the otic vesicle gives rise to the membranous labyrinth. The bony labyrinth (otic capsule) arises from mesenchyme surrounding the otic vesicle. The inner ear reaches adult size and shape by 20–22 fetal weeks (6,13), one of the earliest body parts to reach adult dimensions.

Anatomy

The temporal bone has five parts: the squamous, mastoid, petrous, and tympanic portions and the styloid process (Fig. 3-40). The mastoid portion contains air cells that communicate with the mastoid antrum (6). The petrous portion separates the middle cranial fossa from the posterior fossa, contains the inner ear (otic capsule), and transmits the internal carotid artery, jugular vein, cochlear and vestibular aqueducts and cranial nerves (CNs) VII to XI (Fig. 3-40) (124). The crista falciformis is a horizontal bony septum in the lateral part of the IAC. It separates the facial nerve (CN VII) and superior vestibular nerve (CN VIII) above from the inferior vestibular nerve (CN VIII) and cochlear nerve (CN VIII) below. The superior ridge of the petrous bone is grooved by the superior petrosal sinus and provides attachment for the tentorium cerebelli.

The tympanic portion of the temporal bone forms much of the bony external auditory canal and provides attachment for the tympanic membrane (Fig. 3-40F). The styloid process develops after birth from the inferior surface of the petrous bone and lies anterior to the stylomastoid foramen, which transmits the facial nerve. The external auditory canal (EAC) is predominantly fibrocartilaginous in its lateral third and bony in its medial two thirds. The EAC terminates at the tympanic membrane, which is attached to the tympanic annulus and scutum. The middle ear consists of the tympanic membrane, the middle ear cavity (MEC), three ossicles, two

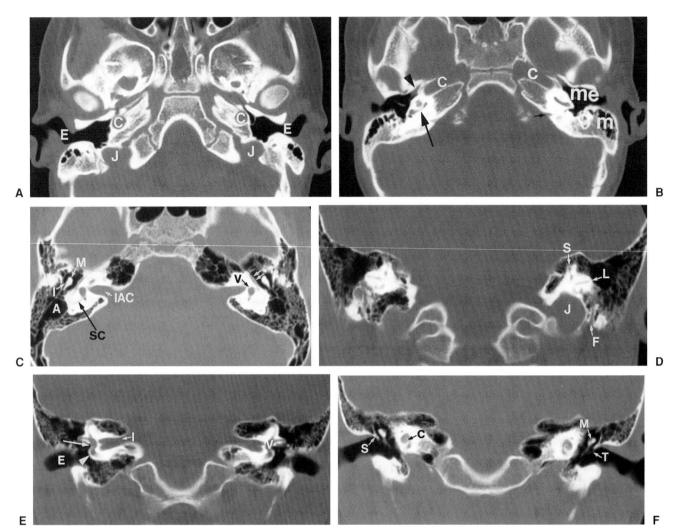

FIG. 3-40. CT of normal temporal bone. Axial **(A–C)** and coronal **(D–F)** CT of a 6-year-old child. **A:** Most inferior axial image. *E*, external auditory meatus; *C*, carotid canal; *J*, jugular foramen. **B:** More superior image. *m*, mastoid air cells; *me*, middle ear cavity and its posterior recesses; *large arrow*, cochlea; *small arrow*, cochlear aqueduct; *c*, carotid canal; *arrowhead*, canal for tensor tympani muscle. **C:** Most superior axial image. *M*, malleus; *I*, incus within the attic; *A*, mastoid antrum; *small arrows*, tympanic segment of the facial nerve canal; *IAC*, internal auditory canal; *V*, vestibule: *SC*, lateral semicircular canal. **D:** Most posterior coronal image. *S*, superior semicircular canal; *L*, lateral semicircular canal; *F*, descending mastoid segment of facial nerve canal; *J*, jugular foramen. **E:** More anterior image. *I*, internal auditory canal; *V*, vestibule; *arrow*, oval window; *arrowhead*, promontory overlying basal turn of cochlea; *E*, external auditory canal. **F:** Most anterior coronal image. *C*, cochlea; *M*, malleus; *S*, bony scutum; *T*, tympanic membrane.

muscles and their tendons, and the chorda tympani nerve (6). The otic capsule forms the medial wall. On it are several important landmarks: from top to bottom, the prominence of the lateral semicircular canal, the horizontal portion of the facial nerve canal, the oval window, the promontory over the cochlea, and the round window. The jugular wall separates the MEC from the internal jugular vein inferiorly, and a thin plate of bone separates the MEC from the internal carotid artery anteriorly. The eustachian tube connects the MEC with the nasopharynx and runs in the petrous bone parallel and lateral to the carotid canal. The middle ear cavity includes three regions: the attic or epitympanum above the

tympanic membrane; the mesotympanum opposite the tympanic membrane; and the hypotympanum below the level of the tympanic membrane. Prussak's space is an important recess between the scutum and the ossicles (11). The posterior MEC contains the pyramidal eminence, which separates the recess of the sinus tympani anteromedially from the facial nerve recess posterolaterally (11,125).

The auditory ossicles are the malleus, incus, and stapes. These are suspended by the malleolar ligaments and by the stapedius and tensor tympani muscles and their tendons. The short process and manubrium of the malleus are embedded in the tympanic membrane. On axial CT, the articulation of the body of the incus with the head of the malleus is seen within the attic. On coronal images the long process of the incus extends downward, and its medial extension (lenticular process) articulates with the head of the stapes (5,11). The foot plate of the stapes rests on the oval window.

The inner ear consists of the membranous labyrinth and is composed of the utricle, saccule, three semicircular ducts, the endolymphatic sac and duct, and the cochlear duct. The fluid in the labyrinth appears bright on T2-weighted MR images. The membranous labyrinth contains endolymph, is surrounded by perilymph, and is enclosed within the bony labyrinth. The bony labyrinth consists of the vestibule, cochlea, and semicircular canals (see Fig. 3-40). Seen well on axial and coronal CT, the normal cochlea consists of 2 1/2 spirals. The vestibule, containing the utricle and saccule, is found posterolaterally together with the lateral, posterior, and superior semicircular canals (5).

The facial nerve leaves the anterosuperior compartment of the IAC, travels anteriorly in its labyrinthine segment, widens slightly to form the geniculate ganglion, then forms an anterior genu in the petrous bone. The nerve then courses posteriorly as the tympanic segment, travelling beneath the lateral semicircular canal. Just lateral to the pyramidal eminence the nerve forms a second genu posterior to the facial recess. In its mastoid segment, the nerve turns downward to exit through the stylomastoid foramen.

General Abnormalities

There is considerable variation in the size, contour, and aeration of the human temporal bone (1,4). The mastoid antrum is present at birth. Computed tomographically visible aeration of it is frequently present in the newborn and is usually present by 2–3 months of age. Pneumatization of the mastoid process occurs rapidly, and the cells are visible by 4–6 months of age. These cells continue to proliferate and aerate into puberty. Chronic otitis media may cause decreased pneumatization.

Because of variation in aeration and the technical difficulties of the examination, mastoid films are challenging to interpret and are often foregone in favor of CT. The importance of views that permit direct side-to-side comparison of the mastoids (Towne, AP, and basal projections) should be stressed (see Fig. 3-1). Mastoid disease is characterized by decreased aeration, mucosal thickening, edema, accumulation of fluid, bony demineralization, and bone destruction (1–6).

Specific Abnormalities

Congenital and Developmental Abnormalities

Anomalies of the External Auditory Canal and Middle Ear

Development of the outer ear and middle ear is independent of inner ear development (5). As a result, dysplasia of

the EAC is commonly associated with a malformed auricle and anomalies of the middle ear and mastoid but only rarely with inner ear anomalies. External and middle ear dysplasia may be isolated or be associated with hemifacial microsomia and syndromes such as Treacher Collins, Crouzon, and Goldenhar. Nearly one third of cases of EAC atresia are bilateral. A coexisting mandibular deformity usually implies a complicated atresia (11). EAC atresia may be partial or complete. Complete, or osseous, atresia consists of a bony plate in the location of the tympanic membrane and fusion of the neck of the malleus to the atresia plate (Fig. 3-41) (126,127). Partial or membranous atresia consists of a soft-

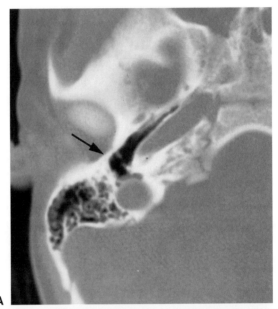

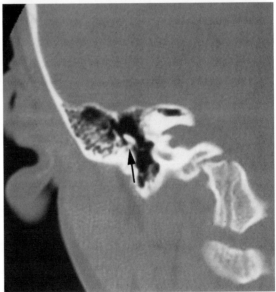

FIG. 3-41. External auditory canal atresia. A 4-year-old boy with malformation of the right ear. A: Axial CT. There is microtia, absence of an aerated external auditory canal, and a bony atresia plate *(arrow)*. B: Coronal CT. The dysplastic ossicles are fused to the bony atresia plate *(arrow)*.

tissue plug in the location of the tympanic membrane with or without fusion of the neck of the malleus to it. When EAC atresia is associated with a congenital cholesteatoma (primary epidermoid) of the middle ear, CT may show an abnormally formed and nonaerated middle ear cavity or opacity plus erosion of the walls of the tympanic cavity.

Surgical repair is indicated in bilateral EAC atresia, provided that the inner ear, oval window, and round window are normal (9,126). Poor prognostic factors for surgical correction include a thick bony atresia plate, small tympanic cavity, poorly pneumatized mastoid bone, severe ossicular anomaly, anterior course or dehiscence and protrusion of the facial nerve, and posterosuperior position of the mandibular condyle.

Middle ear cavity hypoplasia may be mild (occurring with or without EAC atresia) or so severe as to amount to virtual agenesis of the middle ear cavity (see Fig. 3-41). Anomalies of the ossicles include absence, rotation, fusion, and dysplasia. The severity ranges from mild dysplasia with morphologically normal ossicles fused to the atresia plate or epitympanum, to severe dysplasia with only an amorphous mass of ossicular bone. First (mandibular) branchial arch dysplasia results in unilateral (hemifacial microsomia) or bilateral (Treacher Collins) mandibulofacial dysostosis with anomalies of the mandible, EAC, MEC, malleus, and incus. Second (hyoid) branchial arch dysplasia results in anomalies of the hyoid bone, styloid process, stylohyoid ligament, and stapes. The facial nerve is often thickened and usually has an aberrant course lying exposed on the floor of the tympanic cavity (5). Congenital, or primary, cholesteatoma may be associated with EAC or MEC anomalies.

Anomalies of the Inner Ear

In approximately 20% of patients with congenital sensorineural hearing loss, imaging shows anomalies of the inner ear (128). Abnormalities of the membranous labyrinth are radiologically occult if the bony labyrinth is normal. The most common inner ear anomaly is malformation of the lateral semicircular canal (128). It is unusual to see anomalous posterior and superior semicircular canals when the lateral canal is normal (5). The semicircular canals may be absent or malformed, either too narrow or too short and wide. With severe malformation the vestibule may be dilated. Anomalies of the vestibule, which seldom occur in isolation, commonly consist of some degree of malformation of the semicircular canals.

Anomalies of the cochlea may be classified according to the stage of developmental arrest (5,6,11). Complete labyrinthine aplasia (Michel deformity) is extremely rare and results in a single small cystic cavity. Other anomalies of the cochlea include a large common cavity (cochlea and vestibule), cochlear aplasia, and cochlear hypoplasia. Incomplete partition (Mondini malformation) results in an ''empty shell'' appearance with a small cochlea with incomplete septation and less than 2 1/2 turns (Fig. 3-42). This is the most common radiographically detectable form of genetic deafness.

Malformations of the internal auditory canal consist of stenosis and atresia. Isolated dilatation has also been described and is of unknown significance (129). Malformations of the vestibular aqueduct range from obliteration to dilatation (>1.5 mm diameter). Approximately 60% of patients with aqueduct malformations also have radiographically

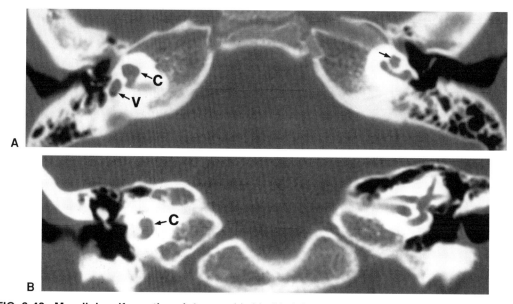

FIG. 3-42. Mondini malformation. A 6-year-old girl with right sensorineural hearing loss. **A:** Axial CT. The right cochlea *(C)* and vestibule *(V)* are dysplastic. Note the normal left cochlea *(arrow)*. **B:** Coronal CT. The right cochlea *(C)* is small, lacks normal septation, and has fewer turns than normal.

identifiable malformations of the cochlea (usually of the Mondini type), vestibule, or semicircular canals (130).

Facial Nerve Anomalies

The two most common anomalies of the facial nerve are aberrant position and partial absence or dehiscence of the bony canal. An aberrant course of the facial nerve is usually associated with an anomaly of the external, middle, or inner ear (6). Lateral and anterior displacement of the descending portion of the facial nerve is common in anomalies of the external and middle ear. The anomalous facial nerve may be directly involved in the production of ossicular malformations (6). Dehiscence of the facial nerve canal most often occurs in its tympanic portion. Hypoplasia of the facial nerve has been described in some trisomies, in the VATER association, and in the Goldenhar and other syndromes (6). Absence of the facial nerve is rare but has been described as a thalidomide-induced anomaly and in the Möbius syndrome (6).

Inflammatory Lesions

Otitis Media and Mastoiditis

Acute and chronic otitis media (OM) characteristically produce a conductive hearing loss but usually require no radiologic evaluation (6). The acute effect is mucosal edema, effusion, and stasis. Rupture of the tympanic membrane with otorrhea and atelectasis of the middle ear (collapse of the tympanic membrane) also occur. Although the initial process may be viral or allergic, secondary bacterial infection with such agents as *Hemophilus influenzae, Streptococcus pneumoniae,* and *Moraxella catarrhalis* is common. Serous and purulent acute otitis media both produce CT opacification of the middle ear cavity and mastoid air cells. This is usually the result of eustachian tube dysfunction or obstruction and is most common in infants and young children.

Mastoiditis (due to blockage of the aditus ad antrum) may be a complication of otitis media or may follow some other chronic disease of the middle ear such as cholesteatoma (131). In mastoiditis, CT shows patchy opacification of the mastoid air cells (5) due to mucoperiosteal swelling and mucus or mucopurulent secretions. CT is required when coalescent mastoiditis or its complications are suspected. Continued mucopurulent discharge from the middle ear, pain, and mastoid tenderness suggest coalescent mastoiditis, which causes demineralization and destruction of bony septa and the formation of a large cavity in the mastoid bone. The triad of mastoiditis, VIth cranial nerve palsy, and deep pain in the distribution of the trigeminal nerve is referred to as Gradenigo syndrome and indicates petrous apicitis.

Other complications of coalescent mastoiditis include suppurative labyrinthitis, facial nerve palsy, perforation of the external mastoid cortex to form a subperiosteal abscess (Fig. 3-43A), osteomyelitis (Fig. 3-43B), and spread of infection from the mastoid tip to form a neck abscess (Bezold abscess) (131). While CT detects many of the complications

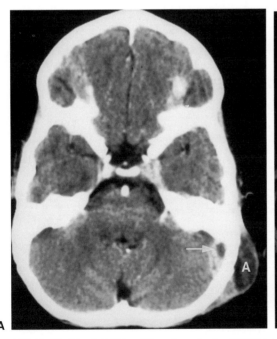 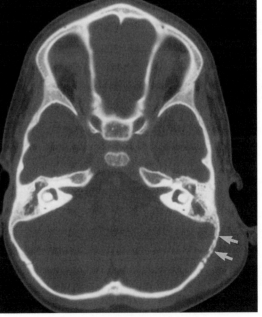

FIG. 3-43. Mastoiditis with subperiosteal abscess. A 3-year-old girl with otitis media and a left postauricular mass. **A:** Contrast-enhanced CT. There is a left subperiosteal abscess *(A)* and a small posterior fossa epidural abscess *(arrow)*. **B:** CT using bone algorithm. There is bilateral opacification of the attic, antrum, and mastoid air cells. Note the mottled destruction of the left temporal bone *(arrows)*.

of mastoiditis, MRI with intravenous contrast administration may demonstrate enhancement of the membranous labyrinth due to labyrinthitis or enhancement of the facial nerve due to inflammatory involvement. Meningeal irritation and cerebellar symptoms in coalescent mastoiditis suggest intracranial complications due to bony erosion or septic thrombophlebitis. In childhood the lateral part of the tegmen tympani may be unossified and may permit direct extension of infection from the middle ear to the epidural space of the middle cranial fossa (5). CNS complications of mastoiditis include epidural abscess (Fig. 3-43A), subdural abscess, meningitis, cerebritis, cerebellitis, brain abscess (usually in the temporal lobe or cerebellum), and thrombosis of a dural venous sinus. Although contrast enhanced CT usually diagnoses these complications accurately, MRI is more sensitive.

Chronic Otitis Media, Acquired Cholesteatoma, and Cholesterol Granuloma

Persistent atelectasis or perforation of the tympanic membrane, recurrent infection, and chronic middle ear effusion are associated with chronic otitis media (6). Granulation tissue is common in chronic otitis media and appears as a nonspecific CT density or MRI intensity. The tissue usually enhances, especially on MRI (132). Granulation tissue may be soft, fibrous, or composed of cholesterol, and may coexist with a cholesteatoma (133). It is friable, and bleeding with hemotympanum may occur.

Cholesteatomas may be congenital (2%) or acquired (98%). They consist of sacs of stratified squamous epithelium containing exfoliated keratin (133). Primary acquired cholesteatoma, the most common type, is thought to arise

from retraction of the superior pars flaccida of the tympanic membrane. This results in an epithelial pocket that becomes sealed and then expands (5). Pars flaccida retractions may be due to eustachian tube dysfunction or attic block. Superimposed bacterial infection may develop (5). Secondary acquired cholesteatoma is thought to arise in association with chronic otitis media, with perforation of the pars tensa of the tympanic membrane and with subsequent trapping of epithelium in the middle ear. Pars flaccida (attic) cholesteatomas characteristically begin in Prussak's space and extend posteriorly through the aditus ad antrum to the antrum and mastoid air cells. Often there is medial displacement of the ossicles. In children there is also a tendency for extension to the posterior tympanic recesses. Pars tensa cholesteatomas commonly involve the posterior recesses and may displace the ossicular chain laterally. Cholesteatomas may also extend along the petrous apex.

Complications of cholesteatoma are invariably related to erosion of bone (11). Erosion of the scutum and ossicles is most common. Other complications include destruction of the mastoid, tegmen tympani, and sigmoid sinus plate; erosion of the facial nerve canal; and erosion of bone around the lateral semicircular canal with the formation of a labyrinthine fistula. Intracranial complications are rare but include meningitis, abscess, venous sinus thrombosis, and CSF rhinorrhea (133).

On CT, a cholesteatoma appears as a nondependent, homogeneous mass. The tympanic membrane bulges. Displacement and erosion of the ossicles, bony erosion with blunting of the scutum, and expansion of the attic are often seen (Figs. 3-44 and 3-45). Involvement of the posterior recesses, invisible to otoscopy, is frequently found. MRI

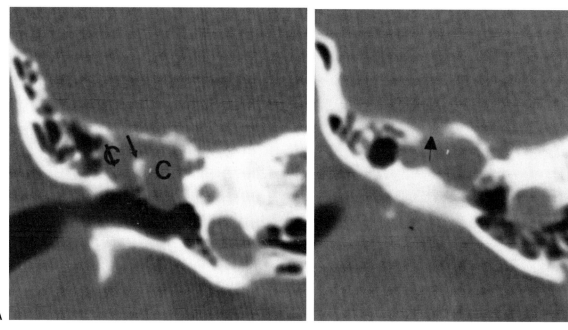

A   **B**

FIG. 3-44. Cholesteatoma. A: Soft-tissue mass *(C)* fills Prussak's space and upper middle ear cavity; the cholesteatoma displaces the ossicles medially *(arrow)*. **B:** There is minimal erosion of the tegmen tympani *(arrow)* by the cholesteatoma.

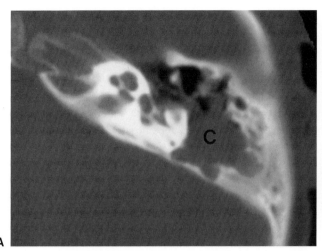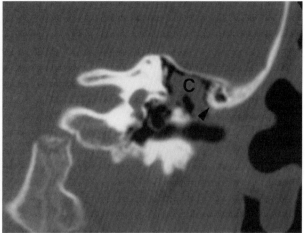

A   B

FIG. 3-45. Cholesteatoma. A 5-year-old boy with chronic otitis media and left conductive hearing loss. **A:** Axial CT. An epitympanic and mastoid mass *(C)* erodes and destroys adjacent bone. **B:** Coronal CT. The cholesteatoma *(C)* within the attic and Prussak's space displaces and destroys the ossicles. There is erosion of the bony scutum *(arrowhead)*.

may be useful if the middle ear cavity is completely opacified. It usually reveals an isointense lesion on T1-weighted images with moderate hyperintensity on T2-weighted images. Labyrinthitis or facial nerve involvement may result in enhancement in the otic capsule or facial nerve canal (11,134).

Cholesterol granulomas are rare in childhood but may arise anywhere from the middle ear cavity to the petrous apex; they consist of brownish hemorrhagic fluid containing cholesterol crystals. The lesion is thought to result from obstruction of the middle ear cavity, mastoid, or both. It can also occur in a mastoidectomy cavity. Cholesterol granulomas must be distinguished from cholesteatomas. On CT a cholesterol granuloma appears as a nonspecific, nonenhancing soft-tissue mass with sharply marginated bone destruction (135). On MRI the appearance is characteristic, high signal on both T1 and T2 images due to hemoglobin breakdown products.

Conductive hearing loss is common in association with cholesteatoma and usually results from ossicular erosion. When it occurs with chronic otitis media in the absence of a cholesteatoma, possible causes include ossicular erosion, ossicular fixation, and tympanosclerosis. Ossicular erosion may be visible on both axial and coronal CT and most commonly involves the long and lenticular processes of the incus (5). Ossicular fixation may be due to fibrosis, tympanosclerosis, or ossification. Fibrous tissue appears as a nonspecific density on CT. Tympanosclerosis results from hyalinized collagen deposition in the middle ear cavity and produces a punctate or web-like calcific density on CT.

Otitis Externa

Otitis externa usually requires no radiologic evaluation. Immunocompromised patients, however, may develop a se-

vere necrotizing form of otitis externa that spreads to the middle ear cavity and mastoid. This disease, usually caused by *Pseudomonas aeruginosa*, is rare in childhood. CT demonstrates the extent of bony erosion, and MRI may be used to detect intracranial complications (5).

The Postoperative Middle Ear and Mastoid

The aim of surgery for chronic otitis media and cholesteatoma is the removal of diseased tissue with preservation of as many normal structures as possible (5). Mastoid surgery may be broadly divided into simple and radical procedures. A simple (cortical) mastoidectomy consists of removal of mastoid air cells with preservation of the EAC wall and ossicular chain. Radical and modified radical mastoidectomy, performed for atticoantral cholesteatoma, entail removal of the EAC wall. Modified radical mastoidectomy permits preservation of the ossicular chain, the bulk of which is removed in radical mastoidectomy. The surgical defect, bony defects along the cavity margins, residual debris, and the integrity of the ossicular chain can be assessed with CT. The inner ear is evaluated for fistula formation, and the course of the facial nerve canal and its relation to the cavity are noted (5).

Neoplasms

Tumors of the ear and temporal bone are rare in childhood. Only the more frequently encountered lesions will be described.

Congenital Cholesteatoma

A cholesteatoma is classified as congenital if there is no prior history of inflammation, trauma, or surgery and the

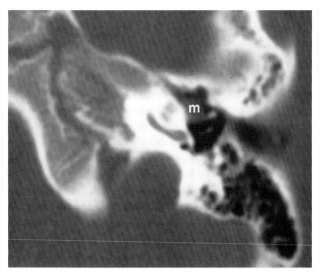

FIG. 3-46. Congenital cholesteatoma. A 4-year-old girl with a mass visible behind an intact left tympanic membrane. No history of infection, trauma, or surgery. Axial CT. The anterior hypotympanic mass *(m)* is adjacent to the promontory and malleus.

tympanic membrane is intact. Believed to originate from displaced epithelial rests present at birth, they are identical to epidermoid cysts (5,6). Growth of the mass occurs as debris accumulates and the sac enlarges. Congenital cholesteatomas of the temporal bone may occur in the petrous apex, the mastoid, the middle ear, or the external auditory canal. Congenital cholesteatoma may also form medial to a bony atresia plate. The commonest location is within the antero-superior and anteroinferior parts of the middle ear cavity (5,6). The usual presentation is conductive hearing loss. Otoscopy may show a whitish mass behind the intact tympanic membrane (5,6). Congenital cholesteatoma is a homogeneous mass on CT (Fig. 3-46), sometimes associated with bony erosion similar to that seen in acquired cholesteatoma (136). The MR appearance of both forms of cholesteatoma is nonspecific: low intensity on T1-weighted images, high intensity on T2-weighted images (11).

Fibrous Dysplasia

About one fifth of patients with fibrous dysplasia of the skull have temporal bone involvement. The disease is usually monostotic and results in expansion of bone due to deposition of fibroosseous tissue (11). Findings include painless temporal bone enlargement, progressive hearing loss, and external canal narrowing. A canal cholesteatoma may develop secondary to obstruction (137). CT demonstrates characteristic expansion of the bone and alteration in its density with either a ground glass appearance, sclerosis, or lytic destruction. The differential diagnosis includes other benign and malignant fibroosseous lesions such as ossifying fibroma.

Bony Exostoses

Exostoses are probably the most common benign bony proliferation found in the external canal and are typically associated with cold exposure. They are seldom symptomatic before the age of 10 years (6). They are localized bony hyperplasias, are usually bilateral, and arise in the tympanic ring in the region of the tympanic sutures. Symptoms include hearing loss, pain, ear infection, and tinnitus (138). CT demonstrates nodular bony thickening encroaching on the canal. Exostoses should be differentiated from osteomas, uncommon benign bony tumors that are usually unilateral and arise more laterally in the bony canal (11).

Nerve Sheath Tumors

Subcutaneous neurofibromas are not uncommon in the auricle and external canal (139). However, nerve sheath tumors in the temporal bone, including schwannomas, are rare in childhood (6). Acoustic schwannomas are one of the causes of retrocochlear hearing loss (6). An acoustic schwannoma in a child, even if unilateral, suggests neurofibromatosis type 2. Changes in the bony contour of the internal auditory canal depend on the site and size of the lesion. Widening of 2 mm or more of any portion of the IAC or shortening of the posterior wall by 3 mm or more compared to the opposite side should raise the suspicion of a tumor (9).

Although the bony alteration is best appreciated on CT, MRI is the best study for the diagnosis of acoustic schwannoma. The tumor has high signal intensity on T2-weighted images and enhances with gadolinium on T1-weighted images. Unenhanced T1-weighted images should also be performed to differentiate a schwannoma from other hyperintense lesions such as a lipoma (9). Schwannomas of other cranial nerves traversing the temporal bone are rare in children. Smoothly marginated facial canal or jugular foraminal enlargement by an enhancing mass is characteristic.

Glomus Tumor

Glomus tumor, although the most common middle ear tumor in adults, is rare in childhood (140). The disease may be hereditary and may be multicentric, especially if familial. These slow-growing, vascular tumors arise from paraganglionic chemoreceptor cells in the glomus bodies of the jugular bulb along the tympanic branch of the glossopharyngeal nerve and the auricular branch of the vagus nerve. The most common symptoms are conductive hearing loss and pulsatile tinnitus. On otoscopy a reddish retrotympanic mass may be seen (140). Differentiation from anomalies of the internal carotid artery and jugular bulb, as discussed later, is critical. Glomus tumors in children may be masked by otitis media. They are more likely than adult tumors to be hormonally active (140).

Contrast-enhanced CT will show an enhancing mass in the region of the jugular foramen (glomus jugulare) or in the mesotympanum (glomus tympanicum). On MRI, multiple areas of flow-related signal loss within the tumor correspond to prominent tumor vascularity. There is a characteristic "salt-and-pepper" appearance on T2-weighted images (141). Preoperative angiography and embolization are used for surgical planning and hemostasis.

Metastases

The most common metastatic neoplasms involving the temporal bone are leukemia and neuroblastoma (5,6). The symptomatology depends on the location of the lesion. CT usually shows permeative, lytic bone destruction. In the mastoid, differentiation from coalescent mastoiditis may be difficult. Intracranial spread of disease is best assessed with contrast-enhanced MRI.

Rhabdomyosarcoma

Rhabdomyosarcoma, the most common malignancy of the temporal bone, is a highly aggressive lesion (5,6). The mass is usually visible in the external canal or in the postauricular area. Extensive local disease, meningeal invasion, and metastatic disease are common. Tumor may spread via the eustachian tube to the nasopharynx. Contrast-enhanced CT demonstrates the enhancing soft-tissue mass, bony destruction, and vascular complications such as occlusion of the internal jugular vein by thrombosis, compression, or direct invasion. MRI is also useful for demonstrating intracranial and vascular involvement.

Langerhans Cell Histiocytosis

The temporal bone is occasionally involved in histiocytosis, and the disease may be bilateral (5,6,142). Radiographs may show punched-out lytic lesions. On contrast-enhanced CT, bony destruction is sharply marginated and there is enhancement of any soft-tissue masses (Fig. 3-47). Contrast-enhanced MRI also exquisitely delineates the soft-tissue masses and any intracranial disease.

Trauma

Temporal bone trauma may cause bleeding from the external auditory canal, hemotympanum, CSF otorrhea, hearing loss, vertigo, and facial nerve palsy. As the mastoid process develops only postnatally, the facial nerve is susceptible to trauma in the neonate (e.g., during forceps delivery) and young infant (143). CT is the best method for evaluating fractures of the temporal bone, including delineation of fracture orientation and alignment and detection of bony fragments, ossicular disruption, and fracture of the facial nerve canal or bony labyrinth. Indications for surgery include hear-

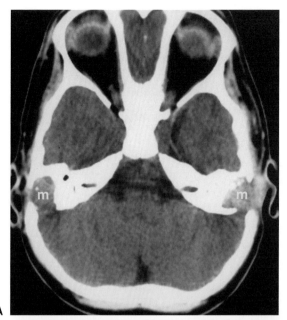

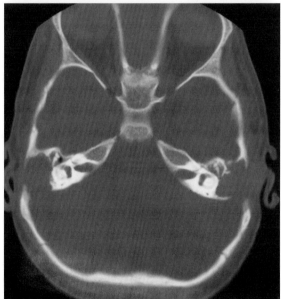

FIG. 3-47. Langherhans cell histiocytosis. A 2 1/2-year-old boy with bilateral postauricular swelling. Axial CT **(A)** with bone algorithm **(B)** shows bilateral soft-tissue masses *(m)*, mastoid opacification, and temporal bone destruction.

ing loss, facial paralysis, and persistent CSF leak. Fractures are classified according to their course relative to the long axis of the petrous bone. Longitudinal fractures, parallel to the long axis (posterolateral to anteromedial), are most common (Fig. 3-48). Transverse fractures are perpendicular to that axis. Combined (longitudinal and transverse) fractures usually cause fragmentation of the petrous bone (144).

Longitudinal fractures usually result from a moderate or severe temporoparietal impact, commonly involve the tympanic portion of the temporal bone, and frequently rupture the tympanic membrane (6). Ossicular disruption may occur, but

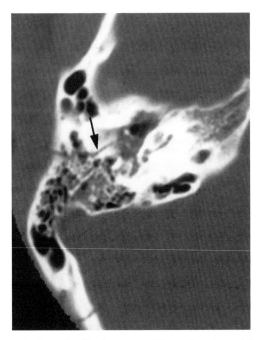

FIG. 3-48. Longitudinal temporal bone fracture. A 6-year-old boy with blood in the right external auditory canal after trauma. Axial CT. A longitudinal fracture *(arrow)* extends through the right mastoid air cells and into the epitympanum. Opacity due to hemorrhage surrounds the ossicles and fills some of the mastoid air cells.

the bony labyrinth is usually spared. Facial nerve paralysis may ensue, is often incomplete and delayed, and usually results from injury to the proximal tympanic segment of the canal just distal to the geniculate ganglion (145). CSF otorrhea usually results from perforation of the tympanic membrane, is associated with fracture of the tegmen tympani, and is more common in longitudinal than transverse fractures.

Transverse fractures usually result from a severe blow to the occiput or frontal region and tend to involve the labyrinth and internal auditory canal. The bony labyrinth and auditory ossicles are relatively avascular, are extremely hard, and have a poor osteogenic response (143). As a result, labyrinthine fractures may heal only by fibrous union (5). Severe sensorineural hearing loss and vertigo often result (6). Facial nerve paralysis is common, is usually immediate and permanent, and is often due to injury of the labyrinthine segment just proximal to the geniculate ganglion.

CT features of petrous fractures include demonstration of the fracture line and secondary opacification of the mastoid air cells, sphenoid sinus, external auditory canal, and middle ear cavity (see Fig. 3-48). Local pneumocephalus is characteristic (145). Intracranial hemorrhage and brain injury may also occur.

Vascular Abnormalities

Anomalies of the internal carotid artery (ICA) include an aberrant course and partial or complete absence. An aberrant course is thought to be the result of absence of the hypotympanic bony plate of the carotid canal; the ICA runs a more posterolateral course than usual in the hypotympanum and may rest against the tympanic membrane (5). This anomaly usually becomes symptomatic only in later life as the vessel dilates. In childhood there is the danger of inadvertent puncture of the anomalous ICA during a middle ear procedure. Partial absence of the ICA most often involves the vertical petrous segment, and the vertical portion of the carotid canal is missing. Aberrant flow through an enlarged inferior tympanic artery reconstitutes the ICA. Both anomalies on CT appear as a densely enhancing soft-tissue mass in the hypotympanum. Agenesis of the ICA may be an incidental finding or may cause neurologic symptoms. CT shows no carotid canal. Angiography readily shows the collaterals reconstituting for the ICA.

High postition of the jugular bulb, above the annulus of the tympanic bone, is the most common vascular anomaly of the temporal bone (146). The hypotympanic bony covering is thin, and the mastoid is poorly pneumatized. With dehiscence of the floor of the middle ear there is protrusion of the jugular bulb through the defect. Symptoms include pulsatile tinnitus, headache, and conductive hearing loss. On CT an enhancing mass is seen in the middle ear at the bony defect. The anomalous vein is vulnerable to trauma and to puncture during myringotomy and other middle ear procedures. Atresia and stenosis of the jugular vein may be found alone but also occur in Crouzon disease, achondroplasia, and a few other similar conditions. The jugular foramen is absent or small, and venous collaterals are easily seen.

Hemangiomas and vascular malformations may involve the auricle and EAC but are uncommon in the temporal bone itself.

NECK, ORAL CAVITY, AND MANDIBLE

Normal

Embryology and Development

The branchial apparatus contributes to the formation of the ectodermal, mesodermal, and endodermal structures of the head and neck (Table 3-3) (6,13). This development begins during the fourth and fifth weeks of embryonic life. The branchial apparatus consists of six paired branchial arches, five paired pharyngeal pouches, and four pairs of branchial grooves and branchial membranes (Fig. 3-49). The fifth branchial arch and pouch are vestigial. Derivatives of the fourth, fifth, and sixth arches are grouped together (Table 3-3). The bar-like branchial arches form along the sides of the primitive pharynx and consist of a mesenchymal core covered externally by surface ectoderm and internally by endoderm. The mesenchymal core of each arch contains neural crest cells that have migrated from the neuroectoderm. Each branchial arch also contains an artery, a nerve, and

TABLE 3-3. *Structures derived from branchial apparatus*

Cleft (Ectoderm)	Arch (Mesoderm)	Pouch (Endoderm)
First (A) External auditory canal Tympanic membrane	First (Mandibular; Meckel cartilage) Mandible Malleus Incus Muscles of mastication Anterior belly digastric m. Mylohyoid m. Tensor tympani m. Tensor veli palatini m. Cranial nerves V_2 and V_3 Mucosa of mouth Anterior tongue	First Eustachian tube Tympanic cavity Mastoid air cells Tympanic membrane
Second (B) Cervical sinus of His	Second (hyoid; Reichert cartilage) Stapes Styloid process Lesser horns of hyoid Upper hyoid body Stylohyoid ligament Stapedius muscle Muscles of facial expression Stylohyoid muscle Posterior belly digastric m. Cranial nerve VII	Second Palatine tonsil Supratonsillar fossa
Third (C) Cervical sinus of His	Third Greater horn of hyoid Lower hyoid body Stylopharyngeus muscle Cranial nerve IX Posterior tongue	Third Inferior parathyroid Thymus reticulum Pyriform fossa
Fourth (D) Cervical sinus of His	Fourth, Fifth, and Sixth Thyroid cartilage Arytenoid cartilage Laryngeal cartilage Cricoid cartilage Laryngeal muscles Pharyngeal muscles Cranial nerve X Cranial nerve XI Aortic arch Right subclavian artery Part of epiglottis Pulmonary arteries	Fourth and Fifth Superior parathyroid Parafollicular "C" cells of thyroid gland

cartilage and muscular components. Externally the arches are separated by branchial grooves and internally by pharyngeal pouches. Branchial membranes form segmentally between the arches at the contact between the ectodermally lined grooves and the endodermally lined pouches. A number of anomalies may result from abnormal development of the branchial apparatus (Table 3-4).

The primitive mouth arises from the surface ectoderm as the stomodeum, is in contact with the amniotic cavity externally, and communicates with the primitive gut internally via the esophagus after rupture of the primitive buccopharyngeal membrane (6,13). The tongue buds are proliferations of mesenchyme derived from the first pair of branchial arches. These form the anterior two thirds (oral part) of the tongue. The posterior third (pharyngeal part) of the tongue is formed from the hypobranchial eminence of the third branchial arch. The salivary glands begin as solid proliferations from epithe-

TABLE 3-4. *Anomalies of the branchial apparatus*

Branchial sinus
Branchial fistula
Branchial cyst
Aberrant cervical thymus
Thymic cysts
Aberrant parathyroid glands
Parathyroid cysts
Thyroglossal duct anomalies
Ectopic thyroid
Heterotopic salivary gland tissue
DiGeorge syndrome (third and fourth branchial pouch syndrome)
Otocraniofacial syndromes (first and second branchial arch dysplasias)
    Treacher Collins
    Hemifacial microsomia

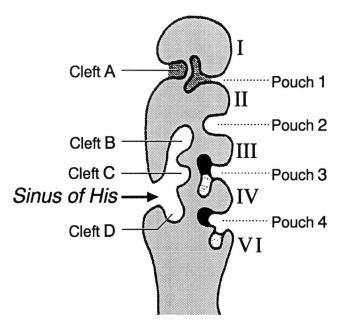

FIG. 3-49. Branchial apparatus. See text for embryology and Table 3-3 for structures derived from clefts *(capital letters)*, arches *(Roman numerals)*, and pouches *(Arabic numerals)* of the branchial apparatus. The fifth arch and pouch are rudimentary.

lial buds that arise during the sixth and seventh weeks. The parotid glands arise from the ectodermal lining of the stomodeum, the submandibular glands from the endoderm of the stomodeum, and the sublingual glands develop as multiple endodermal buds in the paralingual sulcus.

The developing thyroid gland is a diverticulum connected to the growing tongue by the thyroglossal duct, which opens into the tongue at the foramen cecum (6,13). The diverticulum descends in the neck passing ventral to the developing hyoid bone and laryngeal cartilages. It becomes solid and divides into right and left lobes connected by an isthmus. By the seventh week it lies anterior to the developing second and third tracheal rings. The thyroglossal duct normally involutes except for a small blind pit at the foramen cecum and a caudal remnant that may persist as the pyramidal lobe extending superiorly from the thyroid isthmus. The thymic and inferior parathyroid primordia originate from the third pharyngeal pouch, become disconnected from the pharynx, and migrate caudally. Thereafter, the inferior parathyroid glands separate from the thymus and come to rest on the dorsal part of the thyroid gland. The superior parathyroid glands arise from the fourth pharyngeal pouch and lie on the upper and dorsal surface of the thyroid.

TABLE 3-5. *Contents of suprahyoid neck and oral cavity compartments*

Suprahyoid neck	Retropharyngeal space
Parapharyngeal space	Fat
Prestyloid	Lateral (Rouviere) and medial retropharyngeal
Fat	lymph nodes
Branches of cranial nerve V_3	Perivertebral space
Internal maxillary artery	Prevertebral and paraspinal muscles
Ascending pharyngeal artery	Vertebral artery and vein
Pharyngeal venous plexus	Scalene muscles
Retrostyloid (carotid)	Brachial plexus
Internal carotid artery	Phrenic nerve
Internal jugular vein	Vertebrae
Cranial nerves IX–XII	Posterior cervical space
Sympathetic plexus	Fat
Deep cervical lymph nodes	Lymph nodes
Pharyngeal mucosal space	Oral cavity
Adenoids	Mylohyoid muscle
Tonsils	Genioglossus muscle
Constrictor muscles	Geniohyoid muscle
Salpingopharyngeal muscle	Mucosa of oral cavity
Pharyngobasilar fascia	Mucosal area
Levator palatini muscle	Sublingual space
Torus tubarius (pharyngeal opening of eustachian tube)	Hyoglossus muscle
Masticator space	Lingual nerve
Pterygoid muscles	Cranial nerves IX and XII
Masseter muscle	Lingual artery and vein
Temporalis muscle	Sublingual glands and ducts
Inferior alveolar nerve	Deep portion of submandibular gland and Wharton
Ramus and body of mandible	duct
Parotid space	Submandibular space
Parotid gland	Submandibular and submental lymph nodes
Facial nerve	Facial artery and vein
Retromandibular vein	Cranial nerve XII
External carotid and internal maxillary arteries	Anterior belly of digastric muscle
Intraparotid lymph nodes	Superficial portion of submandibular gland
	Fat

During the fourth week of development, a median laryngotracheal groove appears at the caudal end of the ventral wall of the primitive pharynx (6,13). The groove deepens and forms a diverticulum ventral to the primitive pharynx and becomes separated from this portion of the foregut by longitudinal tracheoesophageal folds. These folds subsequently fuse to form the tracheoesophageal septum, which divides the foregut into a ventral laryngotracheal tube and a dorsal esophagus.

Anatomy

Neck

The neck is divided at the hyoid bone into the suprahyoid and infrahyoid regions (Figs. 3-50 and 3-51; Table 3-5) (6,8). The suprahyoid portion extends up to the skull base; the infrahyoid portion extends down to the clavicles. Knowledge of the anatomy (Figs. 3-50 and 3-51) and content of each

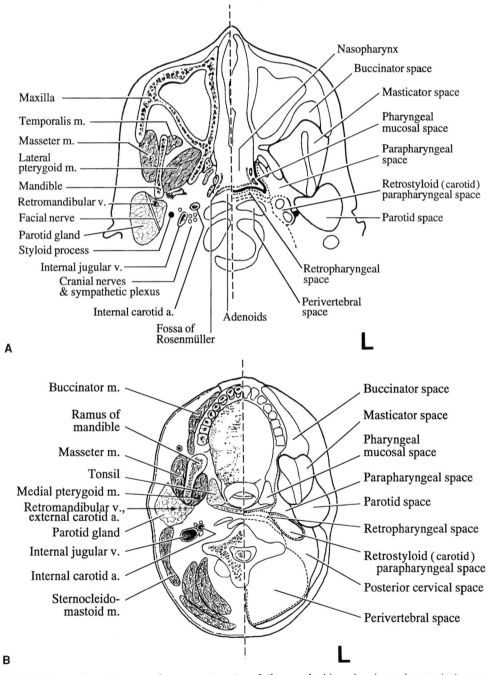

FIG. 3-50. Normal anatomy and compartments of the neck. Line drawings demonstrate normal cross-sectional anatomic structures of the right neck and fascial planes of the left *(L)* neck. **A:** Suprahyoid neck at the level of the nasopharynx. **B:** Suprahyoid neck at the level of the oropharynx. Adapted from Harnsberger (8).

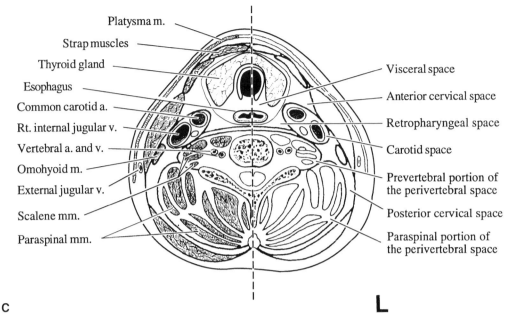

Platysma m.
Strap muscles
Thyroid gland
Esophagus
Common carotid a.
Rt. internal jugular v.
Vertebral a. and v.
Omohyoid m.
External jugular v.
Scalene mm.
Paraspinal mm.

Visceral space
Anterior cervical space
Retropharyngeal space
Carotid space
Prevertebral portion of the perivertebral space
Posterior cervical space
Paraspinal portion of the perivertebral space

C   L

FIG. 3-50. *Continued.* **C:** Infrahyoid neck at the level of the thyroid gland.

compartment (Tables 3-5 and 3-6) is important in the diagnosis of head and neck lesions.

Three layers of deep cervical fascia divide the suprahyoid neck into eight compartments. The parapharyngeal space is subdivided into the prestyloid and retrostyloid (carotid) compartments (Table 3-5). The pharyngeal mucosal space contains muscles, as well as the adenoids and tonsils, which form part of Waldeyer's ring (Table 3-5) (147). The adenoids become conspicuous within the nasopharynx by 2–3 years of age and regress during adolescence. If no adenoidal tissue is seen in a young child, immunodeficiency should be considered. On CT the adenoids are similar in density to muscle. Their signal intensity on MRI is similar to muscle on T1-weighted images but higher on T2-weighted images. Other spaces of the suprahyoid neck include the masticator, parotid, retropharyngeal, perivertebral, and posterior cervical spaces (Table 3-5).

The sternocleidomastoid muscle divides the infrahyoid neck into anterior and posterior triangles (5,8). The layers of the deep cervical fascia permit further subdivision of the infrahyoid neck on axial imaging into five major spaces which are continuous with corresponding spaces in the suprahyoid neck. These are the visceral, carotid, posterior cervical, retropharyngeal, and perivertebral spaces (Table 3-6).

The lymph nodes of the neck are in contiguous groups and may be classified by various systems (Table 3-7). One system describes a collar of nodes by location encircling the junction of the head and neck (Table 3-7) (148). Anterior and lateral cervical chains descend from this collar along the front and sides of the neck. A second system divides the cervical lymph nodes into seven groups by levels (Table 3-7) (148). Nodes in the upper part of the neck tend to be larger than those lower down. On nonenhanced CT, normal

nodes are usually homogeneous, of similar density to muscle, and oval or flat (148,149). Contrast enhancement of lymph nodes is abnormal; it may be seen in a variety of inflammatory and neoplastic processes (5).

The major arteries of the head and neck include the right

TABLE 3-6. *Contents of infrahyoid neck compartments*

Visceral space
 Hypopharynx
 Larynx
 Trachea
 Esophagus
 Thyroid gland
 Parathyroid glands
 Recurrent laryngeal nerves
 Paratracheal lymph nodes
Carotid space
 Common carotid artery
 Internal jugular vein
 Cranial nerve X
 Sympathetic chain
 Deep cervical lymph nodes
Posterior cervical space
 Fat
 Spinal accessory nerve
 Preaxillary brachial plexus
 Lymph nodes
Retropharyngeal space
 Fat
Perivertebral space
 Prevertebral and paraspinal muscles
 Scalene muscles
 Brachial plexus nerve roots
 Phrenic nerve
 Vertebral artery and vein
 Vertebrae

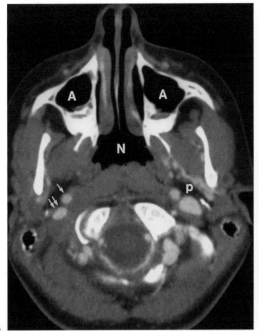

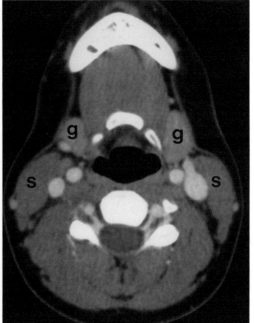

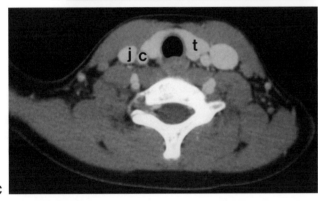

FIG. 3-51. Normal contrast-enhanced CT of the neck. A: Suprahyoid neck at level of nasopharynx. *A*, maxillary antra; *N*, nasopharynx; *single arrow*, internal carotid artery; *double arrows*, internal jugular vein; *p*, parapharyngeal space. B: Neck at the level of the hypopharynx and hyoid bone. *g*, submandibular salivary gland; *s*, sternocleidomastoid muscle. C: Infrahyoid neck at the level of the thyroid gland. *t*, left lobe of thyroid gland; *c*, common carotid artery; *j*, internal jugular vein.

TABLE 3-7. *Lymph nodes of the neck*

Location:
  Jugulodigastric ("sentinel") of internal jugular chain
  Internal jugular/deep cervical chain
  Virchow ("signal") of internal jugular chain
  Intraparotid nodes
  Submandibular nodes
  Submental nodes
  Transverse cervical/supraclavicular chain
  Spinal accessory/posterior triangle chain
  Anterior cervical: prelaryngeal, pretracheal, and paratracheal nodes
  Pretracheal/Delphian nodes
  Retropharyngeal/lateral (Rouviere) and medial groups
  Mastoid nodes
  Occipital nodes
Level:
  I: Submental and submandibular nodes
  II: Upper deep cervical nodes
  III: Middle deep cervical nodes
  IV: Lower deep cervical nodes
  V: Spinal accessory and transverse cervical nodes
  VI: Prelaryngeal, pretracheal, and paratracheal nodes
  VII: Upper mediastinal nodes

and left common carotid arteries, which bifurcate into internal and external carotid arteries at approximately the level of the hyoid bone (6). The external carotid artery (ECA) is smaller than the ICA and initially lies anteromedial to the ICA before coursing posterolaterally as it ascends and branches. There is considerable variation in the course and size of the major veins of the head and neck, which include the external jugular veins, the anterior jugular veins, and the internal jugular veins. The right internal jugular vein is usually larger than the left. At the skull base the internal jugular veins lie posterior to the internal carotid arteries. Within the neck they course lateral to the internal and common carotid arteries. The internal jugular veins join the subclavian veins to form the innominate (branchiocephalic) veins.

The major nerves traversing the neck include cranial nerves VII and IX through XII and the sympathetic chains. Cranial nerves IX, X, and XII descend between the ICA and internal jugular vein, XI lies between and then lateral to the vessels, and the sympathetic chain is posterior and medial to the vascular bundle (9). The facial nerve (cranial nerve

VII) exits the skull at the stylomastoid foramen, courses laterally around the styloid process and posterior belly of the digastric muscle, and then enters the posterior part of the parotid gland. Within the gland the facial nerve lies lateral to the posterior facial vein and external carotid artery before dividing into several branches.

Oral Cavity, Tongue, and Salivary Glands

The oral cavity contains muscles, mucosa, the sublingual space, and the submandibular space (see Table 3-5) (8).

The major salivary glands consist of the paired parotid, submandibular, and sublingual glands (5). The parotid gland lies on the outer surface of the masseter muscle and the ascending ramus of the mandible. The plane of the facial nerve is used surgically to demarcate the superficial and deep parts of the parotid gland. The angle of the mandible and retromandibular vein are imaging landmarks that correspond to this plane. Stensen's duct emerges from the parotid gland and travels to its mucosal orifice lateral to the second upper molar tooth. Lymph nodes and fat are located in the substance of the parotid gland and superficial to it. The submandibular gland is about half the size of the parotid gland and is located within the submandibular triangle of the neck along the dorsal free edge of the mylohyoid muscle. Wharton's duct emerges from the gland to open in the anterior part of the floor of the mouth on the sublingual papilla. The sublingual gland is about half the size of the submandibular gland and lies beneath the mucosa in the floor of the mouth close to the symphysis of the mandible. The small ducts of Rivinus open individually into the floor of the mouth along the sublingual papilla and fold. Minor salivary glands lie beneath the mucosa of the oral cavity, palate, paranasal sinuses, pharynx, and larynx (5).

Mandible

The parts of the mandible include the symphysis, body, angle, ramus, and condyle, and bony projections named the coronoid processes and genial tubercles (8). The mylohyoid sling attaches to the inner surface of the mandible, and the mandibular and mental foramina allow entrance and egress of nerves. Most muscles of the suprahyoid neck attach to the mandible. The maxilla contains the maxillary sinuses. The alveolar margins of the maxilla and the mandible constitute the jaw.

General Abnormalities

The neck, mouth, and mandible are well shown by a lateral radiograph; the structures of the neck are better shown in extension and inspiration. Frontal plain films may also be obtained. A high-kilovoltage technique using selective filtration enhances soft-tissue/air interfaces (1–6). Radiographic evaluation of the mandible often includes PA or AP, Towne, and both oblique projections or a Panorex tomogram. Abnormalities readily detected on plain films include lytic or sclerotic bony lesions, bony deformities, calcifications, foreign bodies, soft-tissue masses, airway encroachment, and extraluminal air or air-fluid collections. Abnormalities of the upper airway itself are presented in Chapter 7.

Specific Abnormalities

Congenital and Developmental Abnormalities

Branchial Anomalies

Branchial anomalies arise from incomplete evolution of the branchial apparatus or from buried epithelial rests (150,151). These anomalies are therefore classified according to the cleft or pouch of origin (see Table 3-4) (152,153). Defects of the branchial apparatus consist of sinuses, fistulas, cysts, and aberrant tissue. A branchial sinus is an incomplete tract, usually opening externally, that may communicate with a cyst. A branchial fistula is an epithelial tract with both external (skin) and internal (foregut) openings. Branchial cysts usually have no external or internal opening but may communicate with a sinus or fistula.

Fistulas and sinuses are usually visible at birth or soon after because of drainage. In general, sinuses and fistulas are identified in infants and children; cysts are more commonly diagnosed in older children and adults and are far more common than sinuses and fistulas overall (5). These anomalies are rarely bilateral but may be familial (153). A branchial cyst usually presents as a soft-tissue mass that may enlarge after an upper respiratory tract infection. Sonography reveals a cystic or complex mass that often contains echogenic debris (154). Contrast-enhanced CT shows an oval or round cystic mass. Wall thickness, enhancement, and surrounding soft-tissue edema depend on the presence and extent of inflammatory changes. An uncomplicated cyst is of low density and has a thin, smooth wall. An infected cyst is of higher density because of increased protein content and has a thick, irregular, enhancing wall. By MRI the appearance of the cyst varies with protein content (5). The best initial procedure to image a branchial sinus or fistula without a mass is a fistulogram (153).

A first branchial cyst is rare. It may arise anywhere along the potential tract of a first branchial fistula, i.e., in the submandibular triangle above the hyoid bone, the nasopharynx, the parotid region, the cartilage-bone junction of the external auditory canal, anterior or posterior to the pinna, or within the middle ear cavity (152,153). It usually presents as an enlarging mass near the lower pole of one parotid gland. On imaging the mass may appear to lie inside or just outside of the gland (153). The differential diagnosis includes an inflammatory parotid cyst, a lymphatic malformation, and necrotic adenopathy.

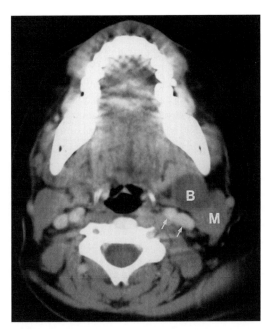

FIG. 3-52. Branchial cleft cyst. Contrast-enhanced CT. There is a left low-density mass *(B)* just anteromedial to the sternocleidomastoid muscle *(M)* and anterolateral to the carotid artery and jugular vein *(arrows)*. This cyst arises from the second branchial cleft.

Second branchial cysts are the most common of these anomalies and usually present as masses at the angle of the mandible (Fig. 3-52). However, they can occur anywhere along the potential tract of a second branchial fistula from the tonsillar fossa to the supraclavicular region (153). A cephalad prolongation may reach as far as the skull base (147,152). The differential diagnosis includes vascular anomaly, paramedian thyroglossal duct cyst, external laryngocele, and metastatic or suppurative adenopathy. A second branchial sinus often opens into the tonsillar fossa. Injection of iodinated contrast medium may demonstrate the tract descending along the anterior border of the sternocleidomastoid muscle. A sinus or fistula may open on the skin at any point along this path.

Third and fourth branchial sinuses, fistulae, and cysts are rare. The third branchial sinus arises from the lowest point of the pyriform sinus and extends between the common carotid artery and vagus nerve to the lower lateral neck. The fourth branchial sinus also arises from the lowest point of the pyriform sinus, usually on the left, runs downward to loop under the aortic arch (or subclavian artery if right-sided), then travels upward through the carotid bifurcation to end in the lateral neck. Recurrent neck abscess in an appropriate location or suppurative thyroiditis should raise the possibility of a pyriform sinus fistula (155). Radiographic fistulography is best delayed until after treatment of inflammation, as edema may prevent the tract from filling (5).

The remaining branchial anomalies are exceedingly rare but include anomalies of the thymus, thyroid, and parathyroid glands. The thymus develops from the third and, to a lesser extent, fourth branchial pouch. Anomalies of the thymus may result from incomplete descent of the thymus into the chest, sequestration of foci of thymic tissue along the path of descent, and failure of involution of the embryonic thymopharyngeal duct. Resultant anomalies include aberrant cervical thymus and thymic cysts (5). Parathyroid cysts and aberrantly located parathyroid tissue may be located anywhere about the thyroid gland but usually lie below it.

Anomalies of the Thyroid

Thyroglossal duct cysts arise from remnants of the thyroglossal duct. This is the most common midline developmental lesion of the neck in childhood. It occurs at any site from the base of the tongue to the suprasternal region. Nearly 75% of thyroglossal duct cysts are midline. Most of the off-midline cysts occur near the outer surface of the thyroid cartilage and deep to the neck muscles (5). On sonography the typical cyst is circumscribed and anechoic or hypoechoic and has good through-transmission (154,156,157). Sonographically heterogeneous lesions also occur, particularly if there has been infection (Fig. 3-53) (154,156). Demonstration of a sinus tract extending cephalad from the cyst supports the diagnosis of thyroglossal duct cyst (157). On CT and MRI, uncomplicated cysts are circumscribed lesions of uniform density and intensity (Fig. 3-54). The differential diagnosis for midline lesions includes dermoid or teratoma, vallecular cyst or mucous retention cyst, and laryngocele. For off-midline lesions, lymphatic malformation and branchial anomalies should be considered.

Other anomalies of the thyroid gland include complete or unilateral agenesis and ectopia. Ectopic thyroid tissue is most frequent in the midline of the tongue near the foramen cecum (lingual thyroid). In children with congenital hypothyroidism and absence of a normal thyroid gland, ultrasound examination should include a search for ectopic thyroid tissue. Confirmation requires thyroid scintigraphy, but the ectopic tissue may be nonfunctional and the scan there-

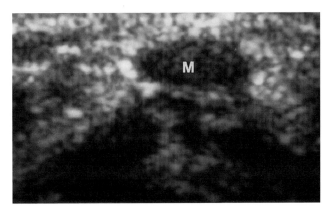

FIG. 3-53. Thyroglossal duct cyst. Transverse ultrasonography. There is a midline mass *(M)* of mixed echogenicity just anterior to the trachea.

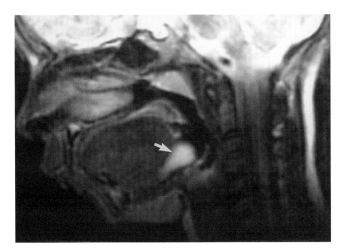

FIG. 3-54. Thyroglossal duct cyst. Sagittal T2 MRI. The high-intensity mass *(arrow)* arises from the base of the tongue.

fore falsely negative. In 70% of cases of absence of a normally positioned thyroid gland with hypothyroidism, the ectopic gland is the only functioning thyroid tissue (157). While I-123 scintigraphy readily shows both ectopic and normally located thyroid tissue, it may be less reliable in differentiating athyrosis from markedly impaired thyroid function (158).

Laryngocele

A laryngocele results from obstruction and dilatation of the appendix of the laryngeal ventricle (9). It may be filled with air or fluid. An internal laryngocele is totally within the larynx and produces a submucosal supraglottic mass. A combined laryngocele protrudes through the thyrohyoid membrane and has intralaryngeal and extralaryngeal components. Purely external laryngoceles are rare (9). Complications of laryngoceles include infection (laryngopyocele) and airway compromise. Plain films, CT, and MRI are all useful in the diagnosis of laryngocele. The attenuation or intensity of the fluid varies with its protein content. There may be slight enhancement of the cyst wall (5,9). Other cystic lesions found near or in the larynx are the thyroglossal duct cyst and the laryngeal mucosal cyst.

Anomalies of the Oral Cavity, Tongue, and Salivary Glands

Congenital and developmental abnormalities of the oral cavity include many lesions described in the preceding section, including lingual ectopic thyroid, thyroglossal duct cyst, and second branchial cleft cyst. Other common lesions include dermoid/epidermoid and vascular anomalies; these are discussed later.

Agenesis of the major salivary glands is rare, may be associated with absence of the lacrimal glands, and causes xerostomia. The diagnosis can be confirmed by radionuclide imaging or MRI (6,9). Congenital cystic lesions of the salivary glands are uncommon and usually involve the parotid gland. These include branchial cysts and dermoid cysts. Presentation may be late in childhood or in adulthood with painless swelling or with signs of inflammation if infected. Nonobstructive sialectasis is one of the more common congenital abnormalities of the salivary glands (6). Saccular dilatation involves small ducts of both parotid glands. Superimposed bacterial infection may exacerbate the ectasia. The clinical presentation is that of parotitis, often unilateral. These cysts must be differentiated from lymphoepithelial cysts, most commonly seen in patients with AIDS.

Fibroosseous Dysplasias

Fibrous dysplasia is of unknown etiology and occurs more often in the maxilla than the mandible (5), as discussed earlier. Radiologically fibrous dysplasia appears as a unilocular or multilocular, ill-defined, expansile lesion, radiolucent when fibrous tissue predominates. Admixture of bony matrix increases the density of lesions, which may appear homogeneously radiopaque with bony expansion.

Inflammatory Lesions

Inflammatory processes of the mouth, throat, and neck are very common in childhood (6). Clinical symptoms may include fever, sore throat, dysphagia, trismus, decreased appetite, drooling, voice change, and torticollis. On physical examination it may be difficult to differentiate between abscess, cellulitis, and adenitis. Inflammation of the airway itself (epiglottitis, croup, and the like) is discussed and illustrated in Chapter 7.

Retropharyngeal Cellulitis and Abscess

In young children acute tonsillitis is usually self-limited (6). However, spread of infection may lead to cellulitis or abscess in the peritonsillar space. Infection may also spread to the parapharyngeal and retropharyngeal spaces. The retropharyngeal space extends from the skull base to the mediastinum and is divided by a median raphe into two halves containing chains of lymph nodes in the suprahyoid neck. These nodes drain the nose, paranasal sinuses, pharynx, and eustachian tube. Infection of this space causes unilateral posterior pharyngeal swelling, although CT may also show inflammation in the contralateral retropharyngeal space. Infection of the perivertebral space sometimes follows vertebral osteomyelitis or epidural abscess and presents as a bulging mass in the midline of the pharynx.

Plain film findings of cellulitis and abscess include thickening of the retropharyngeal soft tissues and anterior displacement of the airway. There is often doubt about whether

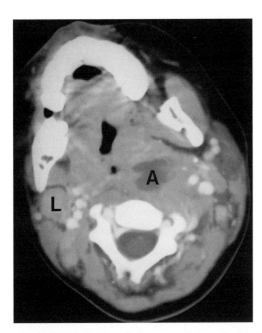

FIG. 3-55. Retropharyngeal abscess. A 6-year-old girl with sore throat and fever. Contrast-enhanced CT shows a low-density mass *(A)* in the left retropharyngeal and parapharyngeal space. There is displacement and extrinsic compression of the airway. Anterior cervical lymphadenopathy *(L)* is noted on the right.

the retropharyngeal tissues are truly pathologically thickened. This doubt can be reduced or eliminated by a lateral film in inspiration and extension or by fluoroscopy in that position; pathologic thickening persists, but factitious thickening varies or disappears. The presence of gas in the abscess, although uncommon, is diagnostic in the absence of acute trauma, foreign body ingestion, and recent surgery. There may be anteroposterior, rotary, or transverse displacement of C1 on C2, or C2 on C3, caused by intense muscle spasm or direct inflammatory ligamentous involvement (3).

Ultrasound examination will often distinguish adenitis from retropharyngeal cellulitis and abscess; it also provides guidance for aspiration and drainage. Despite CT findings compatible with abscess, US may show swelling without actual fluid. This retropharyngeal cellulitis usually responds to a course of antibiotics alone without drainage (159). Contrast-enhanced CT will demonstrate the location and extent of the disease (Fig. 3-55). Complications include airway encroachment, osteomyelitis, sinus or orbital involvement, internal jugular vein thrombosis, carotid artery rupture, intracranial sepsis, and mediastinal spread. The source of infection may be apparent on CT; examples are dental infection, penetrating foreign body, and sialolithiasis (160).

Differentiation of cellulitis from abscess determines which patients need surgery. Prompt diagnosis and, in most cases, drainage of abcesses are important to prevent airway obstruction, rupture with aspiration, dissection in the mediastinum, and involvement of the great vessels (159). Celluli-

tis has heterogeneous echogenicity at sonography. On CT, cellulitis appears as soft-tissue swelling with obliteration of fat planes but without a discrete mass (159). Abscesses are demonstrated by sonography as complex, lobulated masses with partially anechoic centers (159). Hypoechoic fluid collections represent abscesses and should be drained. Rarely, ultrasonography may be falsely negative for abscess if it contains echogenic solid-appearing proteinaceous material. On contrast-enhanced CT, an abscess appears as a discrete, low attenuation mass with variable peripheral enhancement and adjacent edema (Fig. 3-55). Gas bubbles in the abscess, although diagnostic, are uncommon (160). CT differentiation of abscesses from necrotic adenitis may be difficult. On MRI, an abscess appears as a focal encapsulated mass with low-signal intensity on T1-weighted images, high-signal intesity on T2-weighted images, and peripheral enhancement following gadolinium administration.

Lymphadenopathy

Cervical lymphadenitis is common in children and often follows tonsillar, pharyngeal, or dental infection. Acute bilateral adenitis is usually due to systemic infection or a localized viral pharyngitis, whereas acute unilateral adenitis is more commonly represents local streptococcal or staphylococcal infection (6). The persistence of acute adenitis despite antibiotic therapy suggests infectious mononucleosis in older children and Kawasaki disease in very young children. The most common causes of subacute or chronic adenitis are mycobacterial infections, cat-scratch disease, toxoplasmosis, and AIDS. Nontender adenopathy raises the possibility of malignancy.

Imaging studies will show the size, number, and location of enlarged lymph nodes and may indicate their composition. The typical sonographic appearance of adenitis is multiple, discrete, oval, relatively hypoechoic masses along the cervical lymphatic chain (156). On CT or MRI lymph nodes greater than 1.0–1.5 cm in diameter are considered to be abnormal (Fig. 3-55) (6). Uniform enhancement of nodes is usually seen with viral inflammatory processes. Bacterial infection may result in abscess formation. In cat-scratch disease, caused by the coccobacillus *Rochalimaea henselae,* the lymph nodes are markedly enlarged and may become necrotic with surrounding edema; the appearance may simulate neoplasm (161). A conglomerate nodal mass with central lucency, thick enhancement of node margins, and minimal effacement of fascial planes suggests mycobacterial adenitis (162). Late calcification is common in tuberculous adenopathy but may be seen in other granulomatous infections, treated lymphoma, and metastatic disease. The association of lymphadenopathy with salivary gland enlargement and multiple parotid cysts is characteristic of AIDS. Lymphadenopathy and parotid enlargement may also be seen in sarcoidosis.

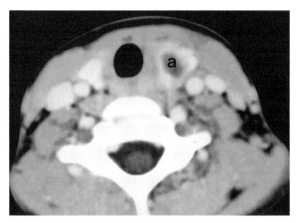

FIG. 3-56. Thyroid abscess due to pyriform sinus fistula. A 10-year-old boy with left neck swelling. Contrast-enhanced CT shows a low-density mass *(a)* within the left lobe of the thyroid gland. An esophagogram demonstrated a left pyriform sinus fistula.

Inflammatory Diseases of the Thyroid

Hashimoto thyroiditis, a nonsuppurative inflammation of the thyroid gland, is the most common cause of juvenile hypothyroidism and is the most common acquired thyroid disorder in children and adolescents (158). Sonographically, it causes homogeneous enlargement of the thyroid gland but no discrete mass. Acute suppurative thyroiditis and thyroid or perithyroid abscess are rare in children and suggest the presence of a congenital pyriform sinus fistula (Fig. 3-56) (155). Thyroid abscess is sonographically variable but usually causes a hypoechoic or anechoic mass. Sonography of multinodular goiter shows masses of mixed echogenicity, sometimes leading to confusion with inflammatory disease (156).

Inflammatory Diseases of the Salivary Glands

Acute salivary gland inflammation is usually viral or bacterial in etiology. Acute suppurative bacterial sialadenitis, most common in the parotid gland is usually due to decreased salivary flow and ascending spread of organisms from the mouth. Other predisposing factors include prior infections, dehydration, trauma, surgery, prior radiation therapy, certain medications, and obstruction by stone or tumor (5,6). The illness causes acute, painful, diffuse swelling of the gland and lymphadenopathy. Although most cases of acute parotitis respond to rehydration and antibiotics, an undiagnosed or untreated case may progress to an intraglandular abscess. Neonatal suppurative parotitis sometimes occurs in dehydrated premature infants and presents approximately 1–2 weeks after delivery with erythema of the skin over the parotid gland. Acute suppurative submandibular sialadenitis is less common than suppurative parotitis and is often related to sialolithiasis. Sialodochitis refers to inflammation of the ducts of Wharton or Stensen and is usually due to obstruction.

During acute infection, sialography is usually contraindicated, as it may cause exacerbation or recurrence (5). On nonenhanced CT the infected gland is large and has increased attenuation. A calcified stone may be identified in a duct. Contrast-enhanced CT often shows enhancement of the gland and duct walls and ductal dilatation. Thickened, enhancing duct walls indicate sialodochitis. An abscess appears as a region of low attenuation with a rim of enhancement (Fig. 3-57). On MRI sialadenitis results in glandular enlargement and enhancement. The signal intensity on T2-weighted images may be higher or lower than normal depending on the relative amounts of edema and cellular infiltrate (5).

Most salivary gland stones occur in Wharton's duct and are solitary; bilaterality is rare. Complications of sialolithiasis include obstruction, infection, stricture, mucocele, and glandular swelling that may progress to atrophy. A Küttner tumor is palpable firm enlargement of the submandibular gland due to chronic inflammation caused by sialolithiasis, autoimmune disease, or unknown factors (5). Most submandibular gland stones but fewer than half of parotid gland stones are radiopaque enough to be seen on plain films. Nearly all calcified stones are visible on noncontrast CT (Fig. 3-58). Noncalcified stones cause filling defects on sialography. Larger noncalcified stones may be visible on contrast-enhanced CT (5,6). On CT the involved gland is usually large, dense, and enhancing and may contain scattered calcifications. On MRI the gland is enlarged and inhomogeneous, with low intensity on T1-weighted images, and intermediate to high intensity on T2-weighted images (5).

Obstruction of one of the sublingual ducts or an accessory duct results in an accumulation of fluid known as a ranula. Extension of fluid below the mylohyoid muscle and anterior to the submandibular gland is called a plunging ranula. The lesion is usually hypodense on CT (Fig. 3-59).

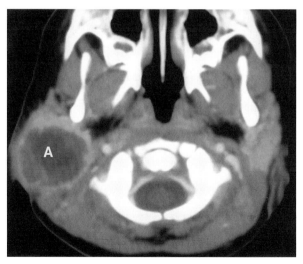

FIG. 3-57. Parotid abscess. A 17-year-old boy with swelling of the right parotid gland. Contrast-enhanced CT. There is a low-density mass *(A)* within the right parotid salivary gland.

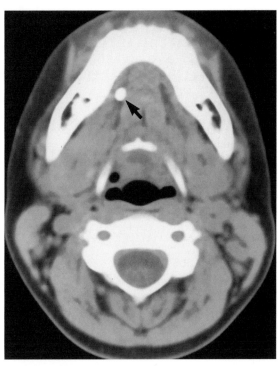

FIG. 3-58. Salivary gland stone. Calcification *(arrow)* in the right submandibular duct.

Chronic inflammation of the salivary glands may be due to recurrent bacterial infection, granulomatous disease, prior irradiation, or autoimmune disease or may be of unknown cause (6). There may be repeated episodes of acute sialadenitis and either fluctuating size or progressive enlargement of the gland. Sometimes tumor is suggested by progressive, painless enlargement of the gland. Nonobstructive causes

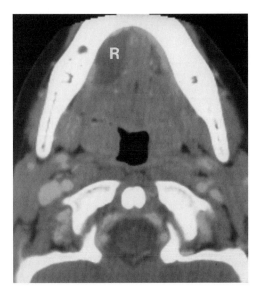

FIG. 3-59. Plunging ranula. CT demonstrates a low-density mass *(R)* in the right submandibular space.

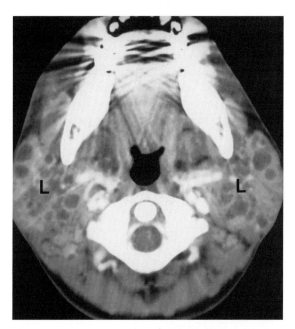

FIG. 3-60. Parotid swelling in AIDS. A 9-year-old girl who is HIV-positive. Contrast-enhanced CT. There are many low-density lymphoepithelilal cysts *(L)* in the parotid glands.

are more common in the parotid gland, obstructive disorders in the submandibular gland.

Autoimmune disease occasionally involves the salivary glands. It is referred to as primary Sjögren syndrome when limited to the salivary or lacrimal glands and secondary Sjögren syndrome when associated with systemic connective tissue disease. The peak incidence in childhood is from 3 to 6 years of age. Most cases resolve spontaneously at puberty (5). On CT the involved gland is large and dense. Sialectasis may occur, and dilated ducts may be shown by sialography. A small number of cases may develop lymphoma in the affected gland or elsewhere (6).

Other conditions such as AIDS, tuberculosis, and sarcoid cause salivary gland enlargement and dysfunction or enlargement of lymph nodes adjacent to or inside the parotid gland. Up to 30% of human immunodeficiency virus (HIV)-infected children have parotid enlargement due to lymphocytic infiltration and lymphoepithelial cysts (6). On cross-sectional imaging the cysts are multiple, bilateral, and of varying size (Fig. 3-60). They are often associated with diffuse cervical adenopathy. Other causes of salivary gland enlargement in patients with HIV infection are intraglandular adenopathy, other infections, and HIV-related neoplasms such as lymphoma. Ultrasound, CT, or MRI will often distinguish between lymphadenopathy and salivary gland enlargement.

Sialosis is chronic or recurrent salivary gland enlargement, nonneoplastic and noninflammatory. It predominantly affects the parotid glands (6). It is associated with diabetes, nutritional deprivation, and certain medications. On CT the affected glands are enlarged and either hyperdense or fatty. Sialography reveals normal ducts, splayed by the increased volume of the gland.

Osteomyelitis

Osteomyelitis of the mandible results from hematogenous dissemination, direct inoculation, or contiguous spread from adjacent soft-tissue infection (163). Predisposing factors include persistent or neglected infection of the teeth or paranasal sinuses, an indwelling intravascular catheter, and a distant focus of infection (163). Imaging demonstrates a permeative destructive process. There is often adjacent soft-tissue edema, cellulitis, or abscess. Dense periosteal reaction, sequestrum formation, and bony sclerosis indicate chronicity.

Caffey Disease

Caffey disease (infantile cortical hyperostosis) which often involves the mandible, is discussed in Chapter 5.

Tumors and Neoplasms

Benign and malignant masses of the neck may be congenital, inflammatory, neoplastic, or vascular in etiology. They may be suprahyoid (Table 3-8) or infrahyoid (Table 3-9).

Benign tumors of the neck may be developmental or inflammatory. Developmental lesions include branchial cysts, thyroglossal duct cysts, thyroid ectopia, vascular anomalies, salivary gland cysts, fibromatosis colli, dermoid/epidermoid, teratoma, lipoma, and nerve sheath tumors. Inflammatory masses such as lymphadenopathy, cellulitis, and abscess have already been discussed.

Approximately 5% of primary malignant tumors in children and adolescents originate in the head and neck (6). The age of the child is an important guide to the diagnosis. Malignant teratomas are primarily congenital tumors. Neuroblastomas are characteristically found in infants and young children. Sarcomatous neoplasms may span the entire age range but rhabdomyosarcomas typically occur in the preschool years. Non-Hodgkin lymphoma occurs in a broad age range but particularly in later childhood and adolescence. Hodgkin disease, thyroid carcinoma, nasopharyngeal carcinoma, and salivary gland neoplasms occur in adolescents. Predisposing conditions include a family history of childhood cancer, a previous primary neoplasm, an illness known to be complicated by cancer, and exposure to ionizing radiation or carcinogenic or immunosuppressive drugs.

The most common malignancies of the head and neck present as painless masses (6). Early signs and symptoms such as lymphadenopathy, otalgia, otorrhea, rhinorrhea, nasal obstruction, and headache are shared with benign conditions. Voice change, hoarseness, stridor, dysphagia, and hemoptysis typically occur late in the disease. Findings suggestive of malignancy include onset in the neonatal period, rapid or progressive growth of the mass, firmness, skin ulceration, fixation to underlying structures, and diameter greater than 3 cm.

TABLE 3-8. *Suprahyoid neck masses*

Congenital
  Tornwaldt cyst
  Thyroglossal duct cyst
  Branchial cleft cyst
  Lingual thyroid tissue
  Dermoid/epidermoid
Inflammatory
  Adenoidal or tonsillar hypertrophy
  Adenoidotonsillitis
  Odontogenic infection
  Reactive or suppurative adenopathy
  Cellulitis
  Abscess
  Benign lymphoepithelial cysts (AIDS)
  Sialadenitis
  Salivary duct calculus
  Salivary gland mucocele
  Ranula
  Osteomyelitis
  Caffey disease
  Postinflammatory dystrophic calcification
  Postinflammatory retention cyst
Neoplastic
  Benign
    Hemangioma
    Lipoma
    Nerve sheath tumor
    Pleomorphic adenoma
  Malignant
    Rhabdomyosarcoma
    Lymphoma
    Osteogenic sarcoma
    Carcinoma
    Salivary gland malignancy
    Metastatic disease
Vascular
  Venous malformation
  Lymphatic malformation
  Venolymphatic malformation
  Arteriovenous malformation
  Jugular vein thrombosis/thrombophlebitis
  Internal carotid or vertebral artery aneurysm or pseudoaneurysm
  Internal carotid or vertebral artery thrombosis or dissection
Miscellaneous
  Hematoma

Pseudotumors

One must be aware of pseudotumors that may involve the orbit, nasal cavity, paranasal sinuses, temporal bone, neck, and mandible (Table 3-10). These lesions are normal variants or benign masses that do not require surgical intervention. Most have characteristic clinical features or imaging findings.

Fibromatosis Colli

Fibromatosis colli is an uncommon benign mass of the neonatal sternocleidomastoid muscle. Torticollis with tilting of the head toward the same side and rotation of the chin toward the opposite side often coexist. Suggested causes

TABLE 3-9. *Infrahyoid neck masses*

Congenital
  Thyroglossal duct cyst
  Branchial cyst
  Dermoid-epidermoid
Inflammatory
  Reactive or suppurative adenopathy
  Cellulitis
  Abscess
  Thyroiditis
Neoplastic
  Benign
    Hemangioma
    Lipoma
    Teratoma
    Nerve sheath tumor
  Malignant
    Lymphoma
    Rhabdomyosarcoma
    Thyroid carcinoma
    Metastasis
Vascular
  Lymphatic malformation
  Venous malformation
  Lymphovenous malformation
  Arteriovenous malformation
  Jugular vein thrombosis/thrombophlebitis
  Carotid artery pseudoaneurysm
Miscellaneous
  Hematoma
  Laryngocele
  Thymic cyst
  Thyroid cyst
  Goiter

TABLE 3-10. *Pseudotumors of the head and neck*

Orbit
  Graves ophthalmopathy
  Increased fat due to steroid usage
  Inflammatory pseudotumor
Nasal cavity
  Foreign body
  Inflammatory mucosal thickening
  Inflammatory pseudotumor
  Turbinate engorgement
Paranasal sinuses
  Inflammatory mucosal thickening
  Redundant mucosa in infants
Temporal bone
  Aberrant internal carotid artery
  Dehiscent jugular bulb
Neck
  Aberrant thymus
  Asymmetric pterygoid venous plexus
  Accessory parotid gland
  Benign masseteric hypertrophy
  Normal muscle opposite muscle atrophy
  Ectatic or asymmetric vessels
  Fibromatosis colli
  Large or asymmetric transverse process
  Cervical rib
  Pyramidal lobe of thyroid gland
  Prominent thyroid isthmus
Mandible
  Caffey disease
  Stafne cyst

include venous occlusion leading to fibrosis, birth trauma, and in utero torticollis (6,69,164). A firm, nontender, fibrous mass is usually palpated in the muscle. Enlargement often occurs during the first month and then is followed by resolution of the mass, a contracted muscle, and torticollis. Mild ipsilateral hemifacial microsomia and plagiocephaly develop in some untreated patients (6).

Sonography shows a focal mass in, or diffuse enlargement of, the sternocleidomastoid muscle, the echogenicity of which is increased, decreased, or similar to that of the normal muscle (157). On CT, fibromatosis colli appears as an isodense or calcified enlargement of the sternocleidomastoid muscle (Fig. 3-61) (157). MRI may show a mass that contains hemorrhage or mineralizations. Frequently no imaging is done. Treatment usually consists of stretching exercises, but surgical division or partial excision of the muscle is occasionally required (6).

Dermoid and Epidermoid

Dermoid and epidermoid cysts are of ectodermal origin. In the neck, they usually occur as midline or near-midline upper neck lesions in asymptomatic patients under the age of 3 years. Sonography shows them as circumscribed, thin-walled echogenic masses (157). CT and MRI show an encapsulated mass, similar in appearance to a thyroglossal duct

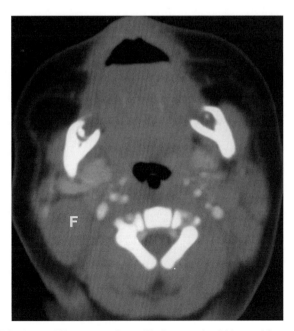

FIG. 3-61. Fibromatosis colli. A 6-week-old boy with torticollis. Contrast-enhanced CT. There is an isodense mass *(F)* within the right sternocleidomastoid muscle.

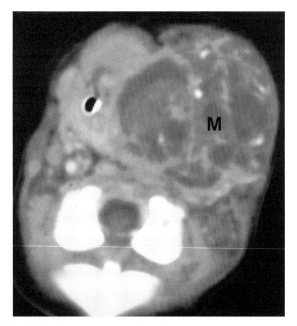

FIG. 3-62. Teratoma. A 1-day-old boy with a large left neck mass. Contrast-enhanced CT. The large, lobular left neck mass *(M)* contains soft tissue, areas of low density, and calcifications. An endotracheal tube is in place.

cyst. If focal regions of fatty density or signal intensity are seen in a midline cyst, then the lesion is probably a dermoid or teratoma rather than a thyroglossal duct cyst.

Teratoma

Teratomas, thought to arise from pluripotential cells, occur in the head and neck region. The incidence of malignancy is approximately 20% (6). Neck teratomas usually present at birth as large anterior masses causing respiratory distress and dysphagia. There is an increased incidence of polyhydramnios, stillbirth, and prematurity (6). Imaging reveals a heterogeneous mass containing cystic areas, calcification, and variable amounts of fat (Fig. 3-62).

Lipoma

Lipomas are soft, mobile, encapsulated collections of fat cells that tend to grow with age (5). On imaging, including fat-suppressed MRI, a lipoma is isoechoic, isodense, and isointense with subcutaneous fat. The presence on CT of areas isodense with muscle suggests hemorrhage or liposarcoma (5).

Nerve Sheath Tumors

Nerve sheath tumors (neurofibromas and schwannomas), arising from peripheral cranial or somatic nerves may be sporadic or occur in patients with neurofibromatosis. Plexiform neurofibromas are pathognomonic of neurofibromatosis and consist of several masses or fusiform enlarge-

ments of peripheral nerves that often entrap contiguous soft tissue. The tumors are isodense to hypodense on CT, have low to intermediate signal intensity on T1-weighted MRI, intermediate to high intensity on T2-weighted MRI, and enhance irregularly. Malignant degeneration occurs in 15% to 30% of cases (157). Paragangliomas are exceedingly rare in childhood (7).

Lymphoma

Non-Hodgkin lymphoma (NHL) is more common than Hodgkin lymphoma (HL). NHL frequently involves extranodal sites in the head and neck such as the adenoids and tonsils, the paranasal sinuses, and the nasal cavity. HL involves contiguous groups of lymph nodes, extranodal disease being uncommon (165). Congenital or acquired immunodeficiency predisposes to NHL. Asymptomatic lymphadenopathy is the most common mode of presentation of lymphoma of the neck. Imaging findings include lymphadenopathy in several locations, usually with a dominant larger node or group of nodes. Involvement of the tonsils and adenoids is usually bilateral and may obstruct the airway. Necrosis and mineralization are rare but may be seen in treated lymphoma (5,157). On CT these tumors are isodense with muscle. On MRI these tumors are isointense with muscle on T1-weighted MRI and usually of higher intensity than muscle on T2-weighted MRI. Local bone destruction may occur. A facial mass originating from the maxilla or mandible is characteristic of the African type of Burkitt lymphoma, a disease linked to infection with Epstein-Barr virus.

Rhabdomyosarcoma and Other Sarcomas

Rhabdomyosarcoma, typically the embryonal subtype, often originates in the head and neck, especially in the orbit, nasopharynx, mastoid region, and sinonasal cavities (166). Other sarcomas include fibrosarcoma, Ewing sarcoma, chondrosarcoma, osteosarcoma, malignant schwannoma, hemangiopericytoma, and Kaposi sarcoma. Fibrosarcoma, the most common sarcoma after rhabdomyosarcoma, usually occurs as a slowly enlarging, painless, firm mass (6,167).

Thyroid Carcinoma

Thyroid carcinoma in childhood is sometimes associated with previous irradiation of the head and neck or multiple endocrine neoplasia type 2. Three major types occur in childhood: papillary (70%), follicular (20%), and medullary (10%) (157). Presentation is usually that of an asymptomatic, firm, movable thyroid mass. Rapid growth, hoarseness, dysphagia, and fixation of the mass increase the suspicion of malignancy (6). Palpable cervical lymph node metastases are present in more than 50% at presentation. Ultrasound is used to show the size, location, and number of masses and to differentiate between solid and cystic masses. Thyroid carcinoma is usually hypoechoic relative to normal thyroid tissue but may be isoechoic.

Children with solitary thyroid nodules are usually scanned using Tc-99m or I-123. A thyroid nodule that takes up radioiodine is very unlikely to be malignant (158). Open biopsy is advocated if there is no uptake. Cystic masses are usually aspirated. The management of nodules with varying degrees of uptake remains controversial; some recommend fine needle aspiration and cytologic study (6).

Tumors of the Salivary Glands

Hemangiomas are the most common benign neoplasms of the salivary glands. The most common benign nonvascular tumor is the pleomorphic adenoma (6).

Malignant tumors of the salivary glands usually occur in older children and adolescents. Up to 50% of reported salivary gland tumors (excluding vascular neoplasms) are malignant. Mucoepidermoid carcinoma is the most common low-grade salivary gland malignancy in children. The usual location is the parotid gland. The tumor causes an asymptomatic, solitary, slow-growing, firm mass in the preauricular region (6). Rapid growth, facial weakness, pain, and cervical adenopathy suggest a higher grade of malignancy. Imaging plays only a minor role in the evaluation of parotid tumors; excisional biopsy is usually performed. Ultrasound may be used to localize a mass and to differentiate solid from cystic lesions. MRI is the best imaging procedure for evaluating the extent of salivary tumors. Most salivary neoplasms are of low signal on T1-weighted images and high signal on T2-weighted images. Relatively low signal intensity on T2-weighted MRI suggests a highly cellular lesion. Invasion of adjacent structures suggests malignancy (9).

Cysts and Tumors of the Jaws

Cysts and tumors of the mandible and maxilla are classified as odontogenic or nonodontogenic and benign or malignant (Table 3-11). Odontogenic cysts arise from tooth derivatives and include radicular cysts, dentigerous cysts, odontogenic keratocysts, and calcifying odontogenic cysts (5,9,168).

A radicular cyst is a circumscribed radiolucent lesion arising from the apex of a tooth and surrounded by a thin rim of cortical bone. In plain film and CT appearance it resembles a periapical granuloma.

A dentigerous cyst is a sharply defined unilocular or multilocular radiolucency related to the crown of an unerupted tooth, usually in the mandible (Fig. 3-63).

An odontogenic keratocyst is a unilocular or multilocular radiolucent cyst that contains keratin and is most common in the body or ramus of the mandible. Marked cortical thinning and expansion of bone may occur. Multiple keratocysts occur in the basal cell nevus syndrome.

Nonodontogenic cysts are developmental and include fis-

TABLE 3-11. *Cysts and tumors of the maxilla and mandible*

Odontogenic cysts
   Dentigerous cyst
   Odontogenic keratocyst
   Radicular cyst
   Calcifying odontogenic cyst
Nonodontogenic cysts
   Fissural cyst
   Hemorrhagic bone cyst
Benign odontogenic tumors
   Ameloblastoma
   Adenomatoid odontogenic tumor
   Ameloblastic fibroma
   Cementoma
   Myxoma
   Odontoma
Benign nonodontogenic tumors and fibroosseous lesions
   Exostosis
   Osteoma
   Osteoblastoma
   Giant cell granuloma
   Aneurysmal bone cyst
   Langerhans cell histiocytosis
   Melanotic neuroectodermal tumor of infancy
   Fibrous dysplasia
   Cherubism
   Ossifying fibroma
   Hyperparathyroidism
   Caffey disease
Malignant tumors
   Osteogenic sarcoma
   Ewing sarcoma
   Burkitt lymphoma
   Metastases

sural cysts, hemorrhagic bone cysts, and Stafne cysts. Fissural cysts occur along lines of fusion of bone and are named according to their location. Most of these fissural cysts cause small, circumscribed, corticated radiolucencies (5,9).

Hemorrhagic bone cysts occur predominantly in the man-

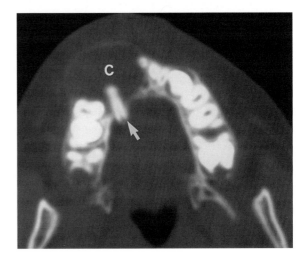

FIG. 3-63. Dentigerous cyst. A 7-year-old boy. CT shows a cystic area of low density *(c)* of the maxillary alveolus containing an unerupted tooth *(arrow)*.

dible and are unilocular and scalloped with a slightly indistinct border.

The Stafne cyst, an anatomic variant representing a deep fossa for the submandibular gland (169), is seen as a well-defined round or oval radiolucency close to the angle of the mandible.

Many different benign odontogenic tumors may be partially cystic. They include ameloblastomas and a variety of mixed epithelial odontogenic tumors such as odontoma and cementoma (5,9). Ameloblastomas are benign but locally aggressive lesions of teenagers and young adults in the mandible or maxilla. Radiographically, ameloblastoma appears as a radiolucent and unilocular or multilocular lesion with distinct borders. Additional features may include slight marginal sclerosis, expansion of bone, a soap bubble appearance, and cortical disruption with a soft-tissue mass. On CT the tumor usually consists of cystic low-density areas interspersed with areas of density similar to muscle. On MRI the tumor is usually of heterogeneous signal intensity. On T1-weighted images the usual high signal intensity of marrow fat is replaced by low-signal-intensity tumor; T2-weighted images show areas of both low and high intensity.

Benign nonodontogenic tumors, which also may be partially cystic, include exostoses, osteomas, giant cell tumors, aneurysmal bone cysts, and fibroosseous lesions (5,9).

Malignant tumors involve the jaw in three ways: primary bony origin in the jaw, contiguous spread from an adjacent soft-tissue tumor, and metastasis. Examples are osteogenic sarcoma, Ewing sarcoma, Langerhans cell histiocytosis, neuroblastoma, leukemia, and lymphoma.

Trauma

Injuries to the head and neck are common in childhood and are usually accidental. Mechanisms of injury include motor vehicle accidents, bite wounds, injuries from knives, guns and endoscopic instruments, burns, and intraoral penetration by foreign bodies and compressed gases (6). Child abuse is sometimes a factor.

Trauma to the soft tissues may result in soft-tissue swelling, laceration, hematoma, or emphysema. Acute complications include compromise of the airway, contusion, laceration or perforation of the airway or esophagus, and vascular injury. Infection may develop later. Imaging is often required to demonstrate the extent of injury, locate foreign bodies (Fig. 3-64), and detect complications. Although the nature of the injury may be apparent from plain films, CT is usually needed. Intravenous contrast enhancement is often used to delineate vessels or to evaluate infection. Upper GI contrast studies are used to show hypopharyngeal or esophageal penetrating injuries.

Vascular injuries include laceration, transection, contusion, and dissection. Complications include false aneurysm, arteriovenous fistula, and distal embolization. If the carotid artery is forcefully compressed against the cervical trans-

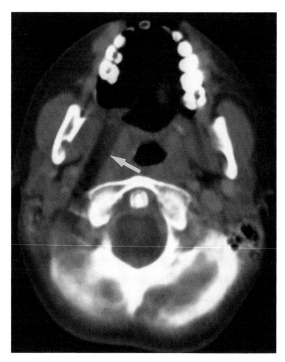

FIG. 3-64. Penetrating trauma. A 7-year-old girl fell with a popsicle stick in her mouth. The low-density foreign body *(arrows)* in the right oropharyngeal space extends to the region of the internal carotid artery and internal jugular vein. Angiography demonstrated thrombosis of the internal jugular vein.

verse processes, intimal disruption and thrombosis may follow. These rare complications usually develop within 48 hours of injury and are suggested by neurologic dysfunction without any other identifiable cause (6). CT with CT angiography or MR with MRA may be used for noninvasive imaging of arterial dissection, but conventional arteriography is often required for detailed demonstration.

Salivary gland trauma may cause hematoma, stricture or transection of the duct, fistula formation, and sialocele. Infection may later develop. Insufflation of the parotid ductal system with air has been reported in association with trumpet playing and as a form of malingering (9). Trauma to the jaw was discussed and illustrated earlier in this chapter.

Vascular Abnormalities

Vascular Variants

The internal jugular veins are almost always asymmetric, right usually larger than left. Occasionally they are multiple. The external and anterior jugular veins are also asymmetric and may be multiple or absent. Phlebectasia is a term used to describe a normal vein which may dilate in the supine position and may cause soft-tissue fullness. It grows smaller in the erect position (5). The pterygoid venous plexus, located along the medial border of the lateral pterygoid muscle, may be asymmetric and appears on CT and MRI as a pseudomass in the parapharyngeal space. The internal carotid artery sometimes has a tortuous course, swings medially, and causes a pulsatile submucosal retropharyngeal mass. An aberrant medial course is also found in the velocardiopalatal syndrome and must be documented before corrective surgery for the palatal abnormality.

Vascular Anomalies

The Mulliken and Glowacki biological classification distinguishes hemangiomas from vascular malformations (82,83), as was previously discussed. In the neck, lymphatic malformations and hemangiomas are common. They may be small and localized or large and extensively involve many compartments including the mediastinum. Venous, venolymphatic, and arteriovenous malformations occur less often. Although present at birth, they usually become clinically manifest only in older children.

Lymphatic malformations, once referred to as lymphangiomas or cystic hygromas, are low-flow vascular anomalies (82). These cystic or septated masses contain proteinaceous fluid (Fig. 3-65). They often change in size with time and commonly enlarge because of infection or hemorrhage. Fluid-fluid levels are characteristic on US, CT, and MRI. The septations often enhance. A fibrofatty matrix is commonly present. Enhancement of the cyst spaces is suggestive of a combined venolymphatic malformation. Hemangiomas demonstrate marked tumor enhancement and prominent vascularity (Fig. 3-66) (82). These high-flow anomalies show flow voids on spin-echo sequences and flow related enhancement on gradient echo MRI. With involution there is de-

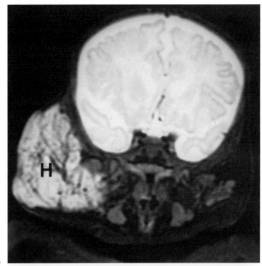

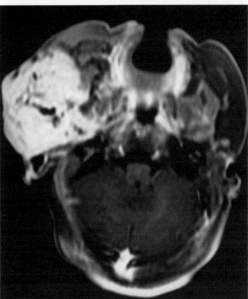

FIG. 3-66. Facial hemangioma. A 7-month-old girl with right facial mass. **A:** Coronal T2-weighted MRI. The hyperintense mass *(H)* contains many high-flow signal voids. **B:** Contrast-enhanced axial T1-weighted MRI. There is intense contrast enhancement of the right facial hemangioma. Again noted are the high-flow signal voids in vascular channels.

creasing enhancement and vascularity and replacement with fibrofatty tissue.

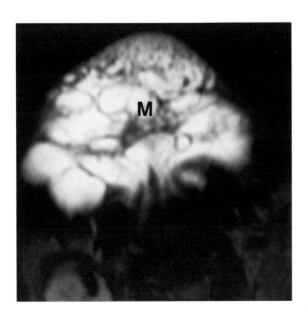

FIG. 3-65. Lymphatic malformation. A 13-year-old boy with large neck mass. Axial T2-weighted MRI. The large, high-intensity mass *(M)* has low-intensity septations and a few fluid-fluid levels.

REFERENCES

General Information

1. Harwood-Nash DC, Fitz CR. *Neuroradiology in infants and children.* St. Louis: Mosby, 1976.
2. Swischuk LE. *Imaging of the newborn, infant, and young child.* 3rd ed. Baltimore: Williams and Wilkins, 1989.
3. Swischuk LE. *Emergency imaging of the acutely ill or injured child.* 3rd ed. Baltimore: Williams and Wilkins, 1994.

4. Silverman FN, Kuhn JP. *Essentials of Caffey's pediatric X-ray diagnosis.* Chicago: Year Book, 1990.
5. Som PM, Curtin HD, eds. *Head and neck imaging.* St. Louis: Mosby–Year Book, 1996.
6. Bluestone CD, Stool SE, Kenna MA, eds. *Pediatric otolaryngology.* 3rd ed. Philadelphia: WB Saunders, 1996.
7. Wolpert SM, Barnes PD, eds. *MRI in pediatric neuroradiology.* St. Louis: Mosby–Year Book, 1992.
8. Harnsberger HR. *Handbook of head and neck imaging.* 2nd ed. St. Louis: Mosby–Year Book, 1995.
9. Valvassori GE, Mafee MF, Carter BL, eds. *Imaging of the head and neck.* New York: Thieme, 1995.
10. Teele RL, Share JC. *Ultrasonography of infants and children.* Philadelphia: WB Saunders, 1991.
11. Swartz JD, Harnsberger HR, eds. *Imaging of the temporal bone.* 2nd ed. New York: Thieme, 1992.
12. Treves ST. *Pediatric nuclear medicine.* New York: Springer-Verlag, 1995.
13. Moore KL. *The developing human: clinically oriented embryology.* 4th ed. Philadelphia: WB Saunders, 1988.

Orbit and Globe

14. Bilaniuk LT, Farber M. Imaging of developmental anomalies of the eye and the orbit. *AJNR* 1992;13:793–803.
15. Hopper KD, Sherman JL, Boal DKB. Abnormalities of the orbit and its contents in children: CT and MR imaging findings. *AJR* 1991;156: 1219–1224.
16. Hopper KD, Sherman JL, Boal DK, Eggli KD. CT and MR imaging of the pediatric orbit. *RadioGraphics* 1992;12:485–503.
17. Lustrin ES, Robertson RL, Tilak S. Normal anatomy of the skull base. *Neuroimaging Clin N Am* 1994;4:465–478.
18. Wells RG, Sty JR, Gonnering RS. Imaging of the pediatric eye and orbit. *RadioGraphics* 1989;9:1023–1044.
19. Barnes PD, Robson CD, Robertson RL, Young Poussaint T. Pediatric orbital and visual pathway lesions. *Neuroimaging Clin N Am* 1996; 6:179–198.
20. Mafee MF, Ainbinder D, Afshani E, Mafee RF. The eye. *Neuroimaging Clin N Am* 1996;6:29–59.
21. Pick TP, Howden R, eds. *Gray's anatomy: the classic collector's edition, by Henry Gray.* New York: Bounty Books, 1977.
22. Barkovich AJ, Vandermarck P, Edwards MS, Cogen PH. Congenital nasal masses: CT and MR imaging features in 16 cases. *AJNR* 1991; 12:105–116.
23. Byrd SE, Naidich TP. Common congenital brain anomalies. *Radiol Clin North Am* 1988;26:755–772.
24. Castillo M. Congenital abnormalities of the nose: CT and MR findings. *AJR* 1994;162:1211–1217.
25. Downey EF Jr, Weinstein ZR. Unusual case of orbital encephalocele. *AJNR* 1984;5:199–200.
26. Koch BL, Ball WS Jr. Congenital malformations causing skull base changes. *Neuroimaging Clin N Am* 1994;4:479–498.
27. Levy RA, Wald SL, Aitken PA, Dorwart RH. Bilateral intraorbital meningoencephaloceles and associated midline craniofacial anomalies: MR and three-dimensional CT imaging. *AJNR* 1989;10: 1272–1274.
28. Fitz CR. Holoprosencephaly and septo-optic dysplasia. *Neuroimaging Clin N Am* 1994;4:263–281.
29. Barkovich AJ, Fram EK, Norman D. Septo-optic dysplasia: MR imaging. *Radiology* 1989;171:189–192.
30. Barkovich AJ, Norman D. Anomalies of the corpus callosum: correlation with further anomalies of the brain. *AJR* 1988;151:171–179.
31. Byrd SE, Bohan TP, Osborn RE, Naidich TP. The CT and MR evaluation of lissencephaly. *AJNR* 1988;9:923–927.
32. Hall-Craggs MA, Harbord MG, Finn JP, et al. Aicardi syndrome: MR assessment of brain structure and myelination. *AJNR* 1990;11: 532–536.
33. Osborn RE, Byrd SE, Naidich TP, et al. MR imaging of neuronal migrational disorders. *AJNR* 1988;9:1101–1106.
34. Sobel DF, Kelly W, Kjos BO, et al. MR imaging of orbital and ocular disease. *AJNR* 1985;6:259–264.
35. Appignani BA, Jones KM, Barnes PD. Primary endodermal sinus tumor of the orbit: MR findings. *AJR* 1992;159:399–401.
36. Jinkins JR. Optic hydrops: isolated nerve sheath dilation demonstrated by CT. *AJNR* 1987;8:867–870.
37. Rand PK, Ball WS Jr, Kulwin DR. Congenital nasolacrimal mucoceles: CT evaluation. *Radiology* 1989;173:691–694.
38. Castillo M, Merten DF, Weissler MC. Bilateral nasolacrimal duct mucocele, a rare cause of respiratory distress: CT findings in two newborns. *AJNR* 1993;14:1011–1013.
39. John PR, Boldt D. Bilateral congenital lacrimal sac mucoceles with nasal extension. *Pediatr Radiol* 1990;20:285–286.
40. Meyer JR, Quint DJ, Holmes JM, Wiatrak BJ. Infected congenital mucocele of the nasolacrimal duct. *AJNR* 1993;14:1008–1010.
41. Friedman DP, Rao VM, Flanders AE. Lesions causing a mass in the medial canthus of the orbit: CT and MR features. *AJR* 1993;160: 1095–1099.
42. Guy JR, Quisling RG. Ectopic lacrimal gland presenting as an orbital mass in childhood. *AJNR* 1989;10(5 Suppl):S92.
43. Nugent RA, Lapointe JS, Rootman J, et al. Orbital dermoids: features on CT. *Radiology* 1987;165:475–478.
44. Hesselink JR, Davis KR, Dallow RL, et al. Computed tomography of masses in the lacrimal gland region. *Radiology* 1979;131:143–147.
45. Lallemand DP, Brasch RC, Char DH, Norman D. Orbital tumors in children. Characterization by computed tomography. *Radiology* 1984; 151:85–88.
46. Towbin R, Han BK, Kaufman RA, Burke M. Postseptal cellulitis: CT in diagnosis and management. *Radiology* 1986;158:735–737.
47. Zimmerman RA, Bilaniuk LT. CT of orbital infection and its cerebral complications. *AJR* 1980;134:45–50.
48. Roberts CF, Leehey PJ III. Intraorbital wood foreign body mimicking air at CT. *Radiology* 1992;185:507–508.
49. Bencherif B, Zouaoui A, Chedid G, et al. Intracranial extension of an idiopathic orbital inflammatory pseudotumor. *AJNR* 1993;14: 181–184.
50. Dresner SC, Rothfus WE, Slamovits TL, et al. Computed tomography of orbital myositis. *AJNR* 1984;5:351–354.
51. Harr DL, Quencer RM, Abrams GW. Computed tomography and ultrasound in the evaluation of orbital infection and pseudotumor. *Radiology* 1982;142:395–401.
52. Lexa FJ, Galetta SL, Yousem DM, et al. Herpes zoster ophthalmicus with orbital pseudotumor syndrome complicated by optic nerve infarction and cerebral granulomatous angiitis: MR–pathologic correlation. *AJNR* 1993;14:185–190.
53. Nugent RA, Rootman J, Robertson WD, et al. Acute orbital pseudotumors: classification and CT features. *AJNR* 1981;2:431–436.
54. Maldjian JA, Norton KI, Groisman GM, Som PM. Inflammatory pseudotumor of the maxillary sinus in a 15-year-old boy. *AJNR* 1994;15: 784–786.
55. Som PM, Brandwein MS, Maldjian C, et al. Inflammatory pseudotumor of the maxillary sinus: CT and MR findings in six cases. *AJR* 1994;163:689–692.
56. Hosten N, Sander B, Cordes M, et al. Graves ophthalmopathy: MR imaging of the orbits. *Radiology* 1989;172:759–762.
57. Yousem DM, Atlas SW, Grossman RI, et al. MR imaging of Tolosa-Hunt syndrome. *AJNR* 1989;10:1181–1184.
58. Kwan ESK, Wolpert SM, Hedges TR III, Laucella M. Tolosa-Hunt syndrome revisited: not necessarily a diagnosis of exclusion. *AJNR* 1987;8:1067–1072.
59. Towbin R, Dunbar JS. The paranasal sinuses in childhood. *RadioGraphics* 1982;2:253–279.
60. Yousem DM. Imaging of sinonasal inflammatory disease. *Radiology* 1993;188:303–314.
61. Ferris NJ, Tien RD. Ethmoid mucocele in an infant with a benign fibroosseous lesion. *AJNR* 1995;16:473–475.
62. Som PM, Lawson W, Lidov MW. Simulated aggressive skull base erosion in response to benign sinonasal disease. *Radiology* 1991;180: 755–759.
63. Som PM, Shapiro MD, Biller HF, et al. Sinonasal tumors and inflammatory tissues: differentiation with MR imaging. *Radiology* 1988; 167:803–808.
64. Van Tassel P, Lee Y-Y, Jing BS, De Pena CA. Mucoceles of the paranasal sinuses: MR imaging with CT correlation. *AJR* 1989;153: 407–412.
65. Banna M, Aur R, Akkad S. Orbital granulocytic sarcoma. *AJNR* 1991; 12:255–258.
66. Morimura T, Hayashi H, Kohchi N, et al. MR appearance of intraorbital granular cell tumor: a case report. *AJNR* 1991;12:714–716.

67. Bryan RN, Sessions RB, Horowitz BL. Radiographic management of juvenile angiofibromas. *AJNR* 1981;2:157–166.
68. Som PM, Cohen BA, Sacher M, et al. The angiomatous polyp and the angiofibroma: two different lesions. *Radiology* 1982;144:329–334.
69. Patrick LE, O'Shea P, Simoneaux SF, et al. Fibromatoses of childhood: the spectrum of radiographic findings. *AJR* 1996;166:163–169.
70. Lee Y-Y, Van Tassel P. Craniofacial chondrosarcomas: imaging findings in 15 untreated cases. *AJNR* 1989;10:165–170.
71. Lee Y-Y, Van Tassel P, Nauert C, et al. Craniofacial osteosarcomas: plain film, CT, and MR findings in 46 cases. *AJNR* 1988;9:379–385.
72. Rhea JT, Weber AL. Giant-cell granuloma of the sinuses. *Radiology* 1983;147:135–137.
73. David R, Lamki N, Fan S, et al. The many faces of neuroblastoma. *RadioGraphics* 1989;9:859–882.
74. Swenson SA, Forbes GS, Younge BR, Campbell RJ. Radiologic evaluation of tumors of the optic nerve. *AJNR* 1982;3:319–326.
75. Hammerschlag SB, Hughes S, O'Reilly GV, et al. Blow-out fractures of the orbit: a comparison of computed tomography and conventional radiography with anatomical correlation. *Radiology* 1982;143:487–492.
76. Unger JM. Orbital apex fractures: the contribution of computed tomography. *Radiology* 1984;150:713–717.
77. Unger JM. Fractures of the nasolacrimal fossa and canal: a CT study of appearance, associated injuries, and significance in 25 patients. *AJR* 1992;158:1321–1324.
78. Unger JM, Gentry LR, Grossman JE. Sphenoid fractures: prevalence, sites, and significance. *Radiology* 1990;175:175–180.
79. Seigel RS, Williams AG, Hutchison JW, et al. Subperiosteal hematomas of the orbit: angiographic and computed tomographic diagnosis. *Radiology* 1982;143:711–714.
80. Barnes PD, Burrows PE, Hoffer FA, Mulliken JB. Hemangiomas and vascular malformations of the head and neck: MR characterization. *AJNR* 1994;15:193–195.
81. Graeb DA, Rootman J, Robertson WD, et al. Orbital lymphangiomas: clinical, radiologic, and pathologic characteristics. *Radiology* 1990;175:417–421.
82. Mulliken JB, Glowacki J. Hemangiomas and vascular malformations in infants and children: a classification based on endothelial characteristics. *Plast Reconstr Surg* 1982;69:412–422.
83. Meyer JS, Hoffer FA, Barnes PD, Mulliken JB. Biological classification of soft-tissue vascular anomalies: MR correlation. *AJR* 1991;157:559–564.
84. Klufas RA, Hsu L, Barnes PD, et al. Dissection of the carotid and vertebral arteries: imaging with MR angiography. *AJR* 1995;164:673–677.
85. Tech KE, Becker CJ, Lazo A, et al. Anomalous intracranial venous drainage mimicking orbital or cavernous arteriovenous fistula. *AJNR* 1995;16:171–174.
86. Williams DW III, Elster A. Cranial CT and MR in the Klippel–Trenaunay-Weber syndrome. *AJNR* 1992;13:291–294.

Nasal Cavity, Paranasal Sinuses, and Face

87. Mafee MF. Endoscopic sinus surgery: role of the radiologist. *AJNR* 1991;12:855–860.
88. Zinreich SJ, Kennedy DW, Rosenbaum AE, et al. Paranasal sinuses: CT imaging requirements for endoscopic surgery. *Radiology* 1987;163:769–775.
89. Laine FJ, Smoker WRK. The ostiomeatal unit and endoscopic surgery: anatomy, variations, and imaging findings in inflammatory diseases. *AJR* 1992;159:849–857.
90. Earwaker J. Anatomic variants in sinonasal CT. *RadioGraphics* 1993;13:381–415.
91. Chinwuba C, Wallman J, Strand R. Nasal airway obstruction: CT assessment. *Radiology* 1986;159:503–506.
92. Tadmor R, Ravid M, Millet D, Leventon G. Computed tomographic demonstration of choanal atresia. *AJNR* 1984;5:743–745.
93. Slovis TL, Renfro B, Watts FB, et al. Choanal atresia: precise CT evaluation. *Radiology* 1985;155:345–348.
94. Hoffman HJ, Epstein F, eds. *Disorders of the developing nervous system: diagnosis and treatment.* Boston: Blackwell Scientific, 1986.
95. Modic MT, Weinstein MA, Berlin AJ, Duchesneau PM. Maxillary sinus hypoplasia visualized with computed tomography. *Radiology* 1980;135:383–385.
96. Som PM, Sacher M, Lanzieri CF, et al. The hidden antral compartment. *Radiology* 1984;152:463–464.
97. Mafee MF, Chow JM, Meyers R. Functional endoscopic sinus surgery: anatomy, CT screening, indications, and complications. *AJR* 1993;160:735–744.
98. Wald ER. Sinusitis in children. *N Engl J Med* 1992;326:319–323.
99. Swischuk LE, Hayden CK Jr, Dillard RA. Sinusitis in children. *RadioGraphics* 1982;2:241–252.
100. McAlister WH, Lusk R, Muntz HR. Comparison of plain radiographs and coronal CT scans in infants and children with recurrent sinusitis. *AJR* 1989;153:1259–1264.
101. Glasier CM, Ascher DP, Williams KD. Incidental paranasal sinus abnormalities on CT of children: clinical correlation. *AJNR* 1986;7:861–864.
102. Kovatch AL, Wald ER, Ledesma-Medina J, et al. Maxillary sinus radiographs in children with nonrespiratory complaints. *Pediatrics* 1984;73:306–308.
103. Phillips CD, Platts-Mills TA. Chronic sinusitis: relationship between CT findings and clinical history of asthma, allergy, eosinophilia, and infection. *AJR* 1995;164:185–187.
104. Rak KM, Newell JD II, Yakes WF, et al. Paranasal sinuses on MR images of the brain: significance of mucosal thickening. *AJR* 1991;156:381–384.
105. Som PM, Dillon WP, Fullerton GD, et al. Chronically obstructed sinonasal secretions: observations on T1 and T2 shortening. *Radiology* 1989;172:515–520.
106. Som PM, Dillon WP, Curtin HD, et al. Hypointense paranasal sinus foci: differential diagnosis with MR imaging and relation to CT findings. *Radiology* 1990;176:777–781.
107. Dillon WP, Som PM, Fullerton GD. Hypointense MR signal in chronically inspissated sinonasal secretions. *Radiology* 1990;174:73–78.
108. Lidov M, Som PM. Inflammatory disease involving a concha bullosa (enlarged pneumatized middle nasal turbinate): MR and CT appearance. *AJNR* 1990;11:999–1001.
109. Siegel MJ, Shackelford GD, McAlister WH. Paranasal sinus mucoceles in children. *Radiology* 1979;133:623–626.
110. Lanzieri CF, Shah M, Krauss D, Lavertu P. Use of gadolinium-enhanced MR imaging for differentiating mucoceles from neoplasms in the paranasal sinuses. *Radiology* 1991;178:425–428.
111. Zinreich SJ, Kennedy DW, Malat J, et al. Fungal sinusitis: diagnosis with CT and MR imaging. *Radiology* 1988;169:439–444.
112. Allbery SM, Chaljub G, Cho NL, et al. MR imaging of nasal masses. *RadioGraphics* 1995;15:1311–1327.
113. Meyer JS, Harty MP, Mahboubi S, et al. Langerhans cell histiocytosis: presentation and evolution of radiologic findings with clinical correlation. *RadioGraphics* 1995;15:1135–1146.
114. Freedy RM, Miller KD Jr. Granulocytic sarcoma (chloroma): sphenoidal sinus and paraspinal involvements evaluated by CT and MR. *AJNR* 1991;12:259–262.
115. Han MH, Chang KH, Lee CH, et al. Sinonasal psammomatoid ossifying fibromas: CT and MR manifestations. *AJNR* 1991;12:25–30.
116. Woodruff WW, Vrabec DP. Inverted papilloma of the nasal vault and paranasal sinuses: spectrum of CT findings. *AJR* 1994;162:419–423.
117. Yousem DM, Fellows DW, Kennedy DW, et al. Inverted papilloma: evaluation with MR imaging. *Radiology* 1992;185:501–505.
118. Vogl T, Dresel S, Bilaniuk LT, et al. Tumors of the nasopharynx and adjacent areas: MR imaging with Gd-DTPA. *AJNR* 1990;11:187–194.
119. Som PM, Dillon WP, Sze G, et al. Benign and malignant sinonasal lesions with intracranial extension: differentiation with MR imaging. *Radiology* 1989;172:763–766.
120. Baker MD. Foreign bodies of the ears and nose in childhood. *Pediatr Emerg Care* 1987;3:67–70.
121. Cummings CW, ed. *Otolaryngology—head and neck surgery.* 2nd ed. St. Louis: Mosby–Year Book, 1993.
122. Thoren H, Iizuka T, Hallikainen D, Lindqvist C. Different patterns of mandibular fractures in children. An analysis of 220 fractures in 157 patients. *J Craniomaxillofac Surg* 1992;20:292–296.
123. McGraw BL, Cole RR. Pediatric maxillofacial trauma. Age-related variations in injury. *Arch Otolaryngol Head Neck Surg* 1990;116:41–45.

Temporal Bone and Ear

124. Howard JD, Elster AD, May JS. Temporal bone: three-dimensional CT. Part I. Normal anatomy, techniques, and limitations. *Radiology* 1990;177:421–425.

125. Swartz JD. High-resolution computed tomography of the middle ear and mastoid. Part I. Normal radioanatomy including normal variations. *Radiology* 1983;148:449–454.
126. Swartz JD, Faerber EN. Congenital malformations of the external and middle ear. High-resolution CT findings of surgical import. *AJNR* 1985;6:71–76.
127. Jahrsdoerfer R. Congenital malformations of the ear. Analysis of 94 operations. *Ann Otolaryngol* 1980;89:348–352.
128. Jackler RK, Luxford WM. Congenital malformations of the inner ear. *Laryngoscope* 1987;97:1.
129. Jensen J. Congenital anomalies of the inner ear. *Radiol Clin North Am* 1974;12:473–482.
130. Valvassori GE, Clemis JD. The large vestibular aqueduct syndrome. *Laryngoscope* 1978;88:723–728.
131. Mafee MF, Singleton EL, Valvassori GE, et al. Acute otomastoiditis and its complications: role of CT. *Radiology* 1985;155:391–397.
132. Martin N, Sterkers O, Nahum H. Chronic inflammatory disease of the middle ear cavities: Gd-DTPA-enhanced MR imaging. *Radiology* 1990;176:399–405.
133. Swartz JD. Cholesteatomas of the middle ear. Diagnosis, etiology, and complications. *Radiol Clin North Am* 1984;22:15–35.
134. Daniels DL, Czervionke LT, Pojunas KW, et al. Facial nerve enhancement in MR imaging. *AJNR* 1987;8:605–607.
135. Lo WW, Solti-Bohman LG, Brackmann DE, Gruskin P. Cholesterol granuloma of the petrous apex: CT diagnosis. *Radiology* 1984;153:705–711.
136. Swartz JD, Glazer AU, Faerber EN, et al. Congenital middle-ear deafness: CT study. *Radiology* 1986;159:187–190.
137. Brown EW, Megerian CA, McKenna MJ, Weber A. Fibrous dysplasia of the temporal bone: imaging findings. *AJR* 1995;164:679–682.
138. Turetsky DB, Vines FS, Clayman DA. Surfer's ear: exostoses of the external auditory canal. *AJNR* 1990;11:1217–1218.
139. Cunningham MJ, Myers EN. Tumors and tumorlike lesions of the ear and temporal bone in children. *Ear Nose Throat J* 1988;67:726–749.
140. Bartels LJ, Gurucharri M. Pediatric glomus tumors. *Otolaryngol Head Neck Surg* 1988;99:392–395.
141. Olsen WL, Dillon WP, Kelly WM, et al. MR imaging of paragangliomas. *AJNR* 1986;7:1039–1042.
142. Cunningham MJ, Curtin HD, Butkiewicz BL. Histiocytosis X of the temporal bone: CT findings. *J Comput Assist Tomogr* 1988;12:70–74.
143. Shambaugh GE, Glasscock ME. Developmental anatomy of the ear. In: Shambaugh GE, Glasscock ME, eds. *Surgery of the ear.* 3rd ed, vol 1. Philadelphia: WB Saunders, 1980, 5–29.
144. Harwood-Nash DC. Fractures of the petrous and tympanic parts of the temporal bone in children: a tomographic study of 35 cases. *AJR* 1970;110:598–607.
145. Holland BA, Brant-Zawadzki M. High-resolution CT of temporal bone trauma. *AJNR* 1984;5:291–295.
146. Overton SB, Ritter FN. A high placed jugular bulb in the middle ear: a clinical and temporal bone study. *Laryngoscope* 1973;83:1986–1991.

Neck, Oral Cavity, and Mandible

147. Harnsberger HR, Osborn AG. Differential diagnosis of head and neck lesions based on their space of origin. 1. The suprahyoid part of the neck. *AJR* 1991;157:147–154.
148. Som PM. Lymph nodes of the neck. *Radiology* 1987;165:593–600.
149. Mancuso AA, Harnsberger HR, Muraki AS, Stevens MH. Computed tomography of cervical and retropharyngeal lymph nodes: normal anatomy, variants of normal, and applications in staging head and neck cancer. Part I: Normal anatomy. *Radiology* 1983;148:709–714.
150. Maran AGD, Buchanan DR. Branchial cysts, sinuses and fistulae. *Clin Otolaryngol* 1978;3:77–92.
151. Chandler JR, Mitchell B. Branchial cleft cysts, sinuses, and fistulas. *Otolaryngol Clin North Am* 1981;14:175–186.
152. Benson MT, Dalen K, Mancuso AA, et al. Congenital anomalies of the branchial apparatus: embryology and pathologic anatomy. *RadioGraphics* 1992;12:943–960.
153. Harnsberger HR, Mancuso AA, Muraki AS, et al. Branchial cleft anomalies and their mimics: computed tomographic evaluation. *Radiology* 1984;152:739–748.
154. Wadsworth DT, Siegel MJ. Thyroglossal duct cysts: variability of sonographic findings. *AJR* 1994;163:1475–1477.
155. Lucaya J, Berdon WE, Enriquez G, et al. Congenital pyriform sinus fistula: a cause of acute left-sided suppurative thyroiditis and neck abscess in children. *Pediatr Radiol* 1990;21:27–29.
156. Kraus R, Han BK, Babcock DS, Oestreich AE. Sonography of neck masses in children. *AJR* 1986;146:609–613.
157. Vazquez E, Enriquez G, Castellote A, et al. US, CT, and MR imaging of neck lesions in children. *RadioGraphics* 1995;15:105–122.
158. Paltiel HJ, Summerville DA, Treves ST. Iodine-123 scintigraphy in the evaluation of pediatric thyroid disorders: a ten year experience. *Pediatr Radiol* 1992;22:251–256.
159. Glasier CM, Stark JE, Jacobs RF, et al. CT and ultrasound imaging of retropharyngeal abscesses in children. *AJNR* 1992;13:1191–1195.
160. Nyberg DA, Jeffrey RB, Brant-Zawadzki M, et al. Computed tomography of cervical infections. *J Comput Assist Tomogr* 1985;9:288–296.
161. Dong PR, Seeger LL, Yao L, et al. Uncomplicated cat-scratch disease: findings at CT, MR imaging, and radiography. *Radiology* 1995;195:837–839.
162. Reede DL, Bergeron RT. Cervical tuberculous adenitis: CT manifestations. *Radiology* 1985;154:701–704.
163. Wald ER. Risk factors for osteomyelitis (Review). *Am J Med* 1985;78:206–212.
164. Crawford SC, Harnsberger HR, Johnson L, et al. Fibromatosis colli of infancy: CT and sonographic findings. *AJR* 1988;151:1183–1184.
165. Lee Y-Y, Van Tassel P, Nauert C, et al. Lymphomas of the head and neck: CT findings at initial presentation. *AJR* 1987;149:575–581.
166. Latack JT, Hutchinson RJ, Heyn RM. Imaging of rhabdomyosarcomas of the head and neck. *AJNR* 1987;8:353–359.
167. Kransdorf MJ. Malignant soft-tissue tumors in a large referral population: distribution of diagnosis by age, sex, and location. *AJR* 1995;164:129–134.
168. Regezi JA. Oral pathology in children and young adults. *Oral Maxillofacial Surg Clin North Am* 1994;6:21–36.
169. Resnick D. *Diagnosis of bone and joint disorders.* 3rd ed. Philadelphia: WB Saunders, 1995.

*Practical Pediatric Imaging: Diagnostic Radiology of
Infants and Children, Third Edition.*
D. R. Kirks, editor and N. T. Griscom, associate editor.
Lippincott–Raven Publishers, Philadelphia © 1998.

CHAPTER 4

Spine and Spinal Cord

Tina Young Poussaint, Patrick D. Barnes, and William S. Ball, Jr.

A discussion of the pediatric spine and its contents forms a natural link between pediatric neuroradiology (spinal cord and coverings) and pediatric skeletal radiology (the vertebral column and the rest of the skeletal system) (1–3). Abnormal-ities of the spine and its contents are relatively uncommon in infants and children. Congenital malformations are much more frequent than infections, tumors, trauma, and other abnormalities (1,2,4). Back pain in children is important and unusual and requires an ordered imaging approach (1,2,5–8).

 T. Y. Poussaint and P. D. Barnes: Division of Neuroradiology, Department of Radiology, Children's Hospital, Harvard Medical School, Boston, Massachusetts 02115.
 W. S. Ball, Jr.: Department of Radiology, Section of Neuroradiology, Children's Hospital Medical Center, University of Cincinnati, Cincinnati, Ohio 45229.

TECHNIQUES

 Many conventional radiologic techniques and more modern imaging modalities are now available for the evaluation of the spine and its contents (Fig. 4-1). The initial examina-

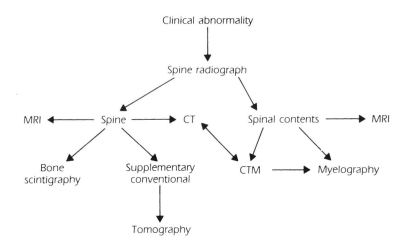

FIG. 4-1. Potential imaging of spine and contents. Computed tomography *(CT)*; computed tomographic myelography *(CTM)*; magnetic resonance imaging *(MRI)*. MRI is critical for imaging of the spinal cord.

tion remains conventional anteroposterior (AP) and lateral radiography. If an abnormality is shown in the bony spine, supplementary conventional radiography (obliques, tomography), nuclear scintigraphy, computed tomography (CT), or magnetic resonance imaging (MRI) is usually required. The spinal cord and its coverings are best evaluated with MRI and, rarely, myelography or CT myelography.

Conventional Radiography

Spine radiography should include both AP and lateral views. Collimation to the precise area of interest often helps. Because of radiation concerns, oblique views of the spine are not routinely obtained in children. Supplemental oblique views of the cervical spine are valuable for confirming enlargement of vertebral foramina and are occasionally used in trauma and other difficult cases. Spondylolysis and other abnormalities of the lumbar articulating facet, pars interarticularis, and pedicle are well visualized on oblique projections. Oblique views of the thoracic spine are rarely of any value (9).

Initial radiographs in patients with scoliosis should include AP and lateral views, preferably in the erect position, from the external auditory meatus to the iliac crest (see Appendix 2). Lateral bending films are less important but may be obtained prior to surgery. Follow-up scoliosis films are obtained in the AP erect position.

Tomography

Conventional tomography has yielded to CT (especially with thin sections, 2-D reformation, and 3-D reconstruction) and MRI for the evaluation of spinal dysraphism, congenital scoliosis and many other problems. In their absence, linear or pluridirectional tomography in the frontal or lateral plane may help clarify abnormalities of the bony spine such as osteomyelitis, discitis, osteoid osteoma, fracture, and formation-segmentation anomalies such as hemivertebra and pedicle bar.

Nuclear Scintigraphy

Bone scintigraphy, especially single photon emission computed tomography (SPECT), is frequently helpful in children with lesions of the bony spine. Vague back pain, painful scoliosis, loss of normal spinal curvature, hip pain, knee pain, fever of unknown etiology, and limp may be caused by spinal infection, trauma, or tumor; the correct diagnosis is often first suggested by scintigraphy (5,10).

Spinal Sonography

Ultrasonography, or ultrasound (US), is often helpful for evaluating the spine and its contents in newborns and young infants (11). The bedside capability of US and the infrequent need for sedation make it the ideal modality for the premature or unstable infant. Scanning is performed with high-resolution, linear array transducers (5 or 7.5 MHz) in the sagittal and axial planes. Patients are studied while prone but may be scanned while supine, as well, if cord tethering is a consideration. Visualization of the cord, cauda equina, and dura can be facilitated by spinal flexion to widen the interspinous acoustic window.

Computed Tomography

CT imaging of the spine after trauma is usually done without intravenous or intrathecal contrast enhancement. Contiguous 5-mm axial sections may be used to survey the spine in spinal stenosis. Contiguous 3- to 5-mm axial sections are performed for trauma, spondylolysis, spondylolisthesis, disc protrusion, and planning for neurosurgical (dysraphism, diastematomyelia) or orthopedic (bone tumor, infection) procedures. Axial 5- to 10-mm sections without intravenous or cerebrospinal fluid (CSF) contrast enhancement may also be done to evaluate the spine after orthopedic instrumentation and fusion. More often than not, spinal CT is an adjunct to spinal MRI. Contiguous 1-mm axial imaging or spiral CT, with reformatting (coronal, sagittal, oblique) and 3-D reconstruction, is often important in the preoperative evaluation of spine trauma, craniocervical anomalies, and congenital scoliosis.

Myelography

The multiplanar imaging capabilities and considerable tissue specificity of MRI have made it the modality of choice for most spinal cord imaging. Myelography, however, still plays a role in the evaluation of patients whose severe scoliosis precludes adequate evaluation with MRI. Myelography is also indicated for patients who are unable to have an MRI examination because of an implanted ferromagnetic device, a pacemaker or neurostimulator, an internal spinal fixation device, or claustrophobia.

Water-soluble, low osmolar, nonionic contrast material approved for myelography is used because of its low toxicity. Imaging is done by conventional radiography, digital radiography, or CT (see below). A 90° tilting table with television image amplification is used for fluoroscopy. Because the examination is prolonged and accurate positioning is required, sedation or anesthesia is often necessary in children below the age of 15 years. A short-beveled 22- or 25-gauge needle is used in infants and younger children. This type of needle permits the radiologist to feel the dural ''pop,'' which verifies subarachnoid placement (2).

The skin is prepared with an antiseptic solution, and the puncture is performed away from the level of symptoms in the prone position with a pillow beneath the abdomen. A midline puncture is performed between the lumbar spinous processes, the tip of the needle angled cephalad toward the center of the vertebral body. The needle tip is monitored by intermittent fluoroscopy during the entire procedure. A cervical puncture at C1–2 may be required for clarification of a complete block of CSF flow or when caudal pathology precludes a safe lumbar puncture. Small samples of CSF are obtained for culture, measurement of protein and glucose, counting of cells, and other tests. The amount of contrast material injected should cover at least three lumbar vertebral interspaces with the patient prone; this requires approximately 5 ml in a 1-year-old, 7 ml in a 6-year-old, and 10 ml in a 12-year-old. Maximum concentrations of water-soluble contrast material range from 180 mg/dl in the neonate to 240 mg/dl in young children to 300 mg/dl in older children. Although the entire subarachnoid space may be imaged, the primary focus is on the level of suspected pathology. The subarachnoid space from the sacrum to the clivus is visualized in the prone position. Subsequently, contrast material is pooled in the lumbar region and the patient is placed supine to evaluate the lumbar region, conus medullaris, and lower thoracic region. Cross-table decubitus filming may be warranted.

CT Myelography

The indications for CT myelography (CTM) are similar to those for conventional myelography. However, CTM is easier and safer in children, precisely demonstrates the relation between intrathecal anatomy and the adjacent vertebral column, and requires lower concentrations and smaller volumes of contrast material (12). However, this examination often requires sedation or anesthesia. The scan levels are determined by a frontal or lateral CT scout projection image or by fluoroscopy or radiography with the placement of a radiopaque marker for subsequent CT sections. A small volume (2–5 ml) of nonionic water-soluble contrast material (180 mg/dl) is injected into the lumbar subarachnoid space. The needle is then removed, the patient's head flexed, and the body placed in a mild Trendelenburg position for a few minutes. Patients are almost always examined supine. CT sections 1.0–10.0 mm in thickness are obtained through the area of interest. CT sections are viewed at a high window level and a wide window width (bone technique). The images are frequently magnified for improved display.

Magnetic Resonance Imaging

Spinal and craniospinal MRI techniques for children differ from those used for adults (1,13). In general, for most developmental spinal neuraxis anomalies, sagittal and coronal T1-weighted conventional spin-echo (CSE) images are obtained for screening, whereas axial CSE T1-weighted images are used for more definitive evaluation and surgical planning. In infants less than 1 year of age, contiguous 3-mm sections are performed. For the older child, a 3-mm section thickness with a 1-mm interslice gap is employed. All spinal and craniospinal MRI is done using a surface coil or combined volume head and surface spine coils.

In the evaluation of lumbar dysraphism, rapid sagittal CSE T1-weighted images are obtained for localization with the field-of-view (FOV) including the entire sacrum. Following that, thinner sections (3–4 mm) and smaller FOV (20–24 cm) sagittal CSE T1-weighted images are obtained with anterior presaturation to eliminate motion artifact and better define the conus medullaris. Coronal CSE T1-weighted images are obtained to confirm normal conus morphology. Axial CSE T1-weighted images are usually required to confirm normality of the conus level, to rule out a thickened filum or a filar lipoma, and to evaluate for the presence and extent of a dermal sinus. If the conus medullaris is at a lower than normal position (i.e., below L1–2), then axial CSE T1-weighted images must be done from the distal conus down through the caudal dural sac termination to evaluate for a cause of tethering such as a thickened filum or filar lipoma. Axial images are imperative for surgical planning, particularly when a lipoma is present. More cephalad imaging of the spinal neuraxis is rarely indicated unless there are neurologic signs or plain film indications of abnormalities at higher levels. If cord splitting (diastematomyelia) is demonstrated, then axial sections through the split are necessary using a technique that highlights or enhances CSF, either a T2-fast spin echo (FSE) sequence or a T2/T2* gradient echo acquisition, in order to demonstrate or rule out a septum. Diastematomyelia and other rare neurenteric spectrum anomalies must be ruled out when congenital scoliosis is the indication for spinal MRI.

In patients with atypical scoliosis, sagittal CSE T1-weighted imaging of the lumbosacral spine is done to confirm a normal conus level. If the conus is in normal position, sagittal and coronal CSE T1-weighted images of the thoracic and cervical spine are done to evaluate for hydrosyringomyelia and Chiari I malformation. Gadolinium enhancement is important if there is cord expansion or hydrosyringomyelia and a possible intramedullary lesion. Craniospinal imaging evaluates complications and sequelae of repair of myelomeningocele and Chiari II malformation; these include fourth ventricular isolation and hydrosyringomyelia. Also, scarring and formation of a dermoid-epidermoid may occur at the original repair site. Craniospinal MRI should include sagittal and coronal CSE T1-weighted images of the brain and cervical spine followed by sagittal CSE T1-weighted images of the thoracic and lumbosacral spine. Axial CSE T1-weighted images are done at the original placode/repair site and at other levels if necessary.

When evaluating extradural neoplastic, inflammatory, or traumatic processes such as neuroblastoma, sarcoma, osteomyelitis, spondylolysis, and disc protrusion, sagittal CSE T1-weighted images are initially performed. Sagittal proton density and T2-FSE images, or, preferably, short T1 inversion recovery (STIR) images, are then performed. Axial CSE T1-weighted images are often done, especially for spondylolysis (CT is even better) and disc protrusion. Additional gadolinium-enhanced CSE T1-weighted images may occasionally be important for demonstrating neoplastic and inflammatory processes, and for evaluating disc protrusion after surgery. In the evaluation of intradural and intramedullary neoplastic or inflammatory processes, sagittal CSE T1-weighted images are done first. Gadolinium enhancement is particularly helpful for intramedullary tumors, intradural tumors such as neurofibromas and schwannomas, and metastatic CSF seeding.

For emergency cord compression studies, gadolinium enhancement and proton density/T2-FSE images are only occasionally necessary if the CSE T1-weighted images are negative. Axial CSE T1-weighted images may occasionally be needed to confirm cord atrophy. Contrast-enhanced craniospinal MRI is also used to evaluate central nervous system (CNS) tumors with a tendency for CSF seeding. Sagittal CSE T1-weighted images of the brain and cervical spine are performed initially. Then, after gadolinium injection, sagittal and coronal CSE T1-weighted craniocervical images are obtained, and then sagittal CSE T1-weighted images of the thoracic and lumbosacral spine to the tip of the sacrum. Occasionally, coronal or axial CSE T1-weighted images are also performed.

A combination of sagittal and coronal CSE T1-weighted images and PD-weighted and T2-FSE images is done for patients with a possible spinal vascular malformation. Gadolinium-enhanced imaging is occasionally needed to rule out other abnormalities. Magnetic resonance angiography (MRA) is rarely helpful; conventional angiography is still preferred. Spinal trauma patients are evaluated with MRI if there is a partial or changing myelopathy or radiculopathy. Sagittal CSE T1-weighted images and PD plus T2-weighted FSE or STIR imaging are usually done to evaluate for cord compression by a fragment of bone or disc and for intraspinal hematoma. Cord injury and ligamentous injury are also assessed with MRI.

IMAGING GUIDELINES

General Guidelines

MRI is now established, along with CT and US, as an excellent method for structural evaluation of the pediatric CNS. MRI has largely replaced more costly and invasive procedures such as conventional angiography and myelography (13,14). US is the screening procedure of choice for fetal and infant craniospinal abnormalities, whereas plain films, CT, and SPECT continue to be excellent modalities for bony spine abnormalities such as fracture. MRI is now considered the definitive modality for evaluating the spinal neuraxis.

Imaging Approaches

Developmental Malformations

Disorders of neural tube closure include open spinal dysraphism (meningocele, myelomeningocele), the Chiari malformations, and hydrosyringomyelia. Less common abnormalities are skin-covered spinal dysraphic disorders such as tethered cord and lipoma, dermal sinus, diastematomyelia, the caudal dysplasia spectrum, and developmental tumors.

Developmental disorders of the bony spine and spinal neuraxis include anomalies at the craniocervical junction, spinal vascular anomalies, developmental bony malformations, and the Klippel-Feil syndrome. US is the screening procedure of choice for spinal neuraxis malformations in the fetus and young infant and often serves as an effective intraoperative guide. MRI, however, is the definitive modality for diagnosis, surgical planning, and follow-up. Myelography or CT myelography is occasionally needed in patients with metallic spinal instrumentation because artifacts compromise MR image quality. Unenhanced spinal CT, however, is often used for evaluating bony anatomy; an example is the use of 3-D reconstruction and 2-D reformatting for the preoperative evaluation of craniocervical anomalies and congenital scoliosis. Angiography and interventional techniques are important in the management of spinal vascular anomalies (1,2,14).

Infection

Plain films, SPECT, and MRI are recommended for the evaluation of osteomyelitis, sacroiliac pyarthrosis, discitis, and epidural abscess. MRI is the best procedure for spinal neuraxis infections. Gadolinium enhancement is critical. Recurrent infectious or noninfectious meningitis may require investigation for a parameningeal focus such as a dermal sinus, a primitive neurenteric connection, or a dermoid-epidermoid.

Neoplastic Disease

Neoplastic diseases of the spine and spinal neuraxis may be classified as extradural, intradural-extramedullary, or intramedullary. Extradural tumors may be benign (aneurysmal bone cyst, osteoid osteoma, osteochondroma), or malignant and invasive (neuroblastoma, primitive neuroectodermal tumor, sarcoma, histiocytosis) (1,2,13). SPECT imaging is a good way of detecting multiple lesions. Common intradural extramedullary neoplasms of childhood include metastatic CSF seeding, neurofibromas, and schwannomas. Astrocytomas and ependymomas, the majority of intramedullary tumors in children, are often associated with cysts or hydrosyringomyelia.

Although CT may be indicated for single-level bony lesions (osteoid osteoma), MRI is recommended for the definitive evaluation of all spinal column and spinal neuraxis tumors. Spinal MRI is particularly indicated in children with atypical scoliosis when hydrosyringomyelia is suspected or a developmental cause (Chiari I malformation) must be distinguished from a neoplastic cause (astrocytoma).

Trauma

Plain films and CT are best for emergency imaging of spine trauma (1,2,15). US is the primary modality for screening the newborn with perinatal trauma such as spinal cord transection. After the initial evaluation with plain films or CT, radiologic abnormality or clinical signs of spinal cord dysfunction are indications for MRI. Neurologic symptoms and signs out of proportion to the history of trauma suggest an existing spinal anomaly (hydrosyringomyelia and craniocervical anomalies are examples), tumor, or child abuse. MRI obviates the need for myelography in acute trauma for patients with progressive myelopathy or radiculopathy due to intraspinal hemorrhage, cord contusion, and hematoma (16). MRI is also the procedure of choice for evaluating the sequelae of spinal cord trauma such as syrinx and myelomalacia. SPECT imaging of the spinal column is particularly effective in delineating traumatic lesions not apparent at radiography, such as spondylolysis or stress fracture (6,14,17,18).

Vascular Disease and Hemorrhage

Acute myelopathy due to spontaneous vascular occlusion or spontaneous hemorrhage is extremely rare in childhood. Spinal MRI is the primary and often the definitive procedure for evaluation of spinal cord infarction or hemorrhage. Spinal angiography is necessary for complete evaluation of any vascular abnormality, in anticipation of surgery or interventional therapy. The muscular and cutaneous vascular anomalies of childhood, including hemangiomas and vascular malformations, frequently involve the head, neck, and paraspinal regions. These are definitively evaluated by MRI.

SYSTEMATIC APPROACH TO THE PEDIATRIC SPINE

One should develop a systematic, ordered approach to radiographs of the pediatric spine (Table 4-1). A thorough evaluation of every radiographic examination of the spine decreases the possibility of overlooking significant pathology. It should be emphasized that conventional radiographs may be normal despite severe abnormalities of the underlying spinal cord and coverings. In the proper clinical setting, radiologic evaluation of spinal contents by MRI, CTM or conventional myelography is mandatory even when radiographs of the spine are negative.

The spine, except in difficult-to-position infants, is normally straight in the AP projection. Lateral films normally show cervical and lumbosacral lordoses and a thoracic kyphosis. These normal curvatures of the spine are much more pronounced in the older child and adult, after an upright posture is assumed, than in the neonate. Although the midthoracic to midlumbar area is the straightest segment of the spine in the lateral projection, a completely straight segment of any portion of the spine suggests abnormality. Such straightening may be due to soft-tissue abnormality, muscle spasm, bony abnormality, or intraspinal tumor (2). Malformations of the vertebral column frequently cause abnormal bony alignment.

The density of the bony structures is usually symmetric. Abnormal density may be due to sclerotic lesions or lytic defects. Abnormalities of the subcutaneous tissues or paravertebral soft tissues may provide a clue to underlying abnor-

TABLE 4-1. *Ordered approach to spine radiography*

General examination
  Alignment
  Bony density
Specific examination
  Soft tissues
  Vertebral bodies
  Intervertebral discs
  Vertebral arches
    Pedicles
    Laminae
    Facets
      Superior
      Inferior
    Processes
      Transverse
      Spinous

malities of the spine or its contents. The location (vertebral body, intervertebral disc, neural arch) of a spinal abnormality is an important clue to its etiology.

NORMAL SPINE AND SPINAL CORD

Embryology and Development

Vertebral Column

The bony spine (spinal column) develops in three stages: membrane development, chondrification, and ossification (18). The notochord separates from the primitive gut and dorsal neural tube at the 25th gestational day, to create zones filled with mesenchyme. This mesenchyme, located lateral to the closing neural tube, forms a series of somites or segments. These subsequently form the myotomes, precursors of the paraspinous muscles, and the sclerotomes, precursors of the spinal column (19). After resegmentation, the vertebral bodies are formed (20). Chondrification of the vertebral bodies occurs from 6 to 8 weeks; ossification begins at about 9 weeks of gestation. Remnants of the notochord persist between the developing vertebral bodies and become part of the nucleus pulposus of the discs. The craniocervical junction (the occipital bone, the atlas [C1], the axis [C2], and multiple ligaments of the atlantooccipital and atlantoaxial articulations) arises from the first five primordial vertebrae (21).

Spinal Cord

The spinal cord develops through the process of neurulation (neural tube closure). At the 15th day of gestation, embryonic ectodermal cells proliferate and form the primitive streak along the surface of the embryo. A nodule of proliferating cells (Hensen node) and migration of these cells into a neural pit leads to formation of the notochord. The notochord induces the formation of the neural plate, which is composed of neural ectoderm continuous with cutaneous ectoderm. The neural plate is the origin of the neural tube, from which the CNS forms, and the neural crest, from which the peripheral nervous system is derived. At 17 days of gestation, the neural plate thickens and neural folds develop. This leads to cephalic closure of the neural groove by 24–27 days to form the upper end of the craniospinal neural tube. At closure, the overlying ectoderm is separated from the neural tissue. The dorsal root ganglia, cranial and spinal nerves, and sympathetic chain form from the neural crest. The distal conus medullaris, associated nerve roots, and filum terminale form from the process of canalization and differentiation of the caudal neural tube (caudal cell mass origin), which begins at 30–38 days of gestation (20). Early in fetal life the spinal cord extends to the end of the spinal canal. There is rapid longitudinal growth of the spinal column so that by 3 months of age the tip of the conus is usually at or above the middle of the L2 vertebral body level (22–24). There is evidence, based on both in utero and neonatal spinal sonography, that the tip of the conus medullaris is at its final position of L2 or higher by late fetal life (22,25,26).

Normal Bony Spine

There are two centers in each half of each vertebral body, separated in the midline by the dorsoventral sheath of the notochord, and a center for each half of the posterior arch (Fig. 4-2) (18). As these chondrification centers form and join, the notochordal cells are squeezed out of the vertebral body into the disc space where they expand slightly to become the nucleus pulposus of the disc. The two chondrification centers fuse into a cartilaginous vertebral body and are joined to the cartilaginous centers for the arch, which have fused dorsally behind the neural tube.

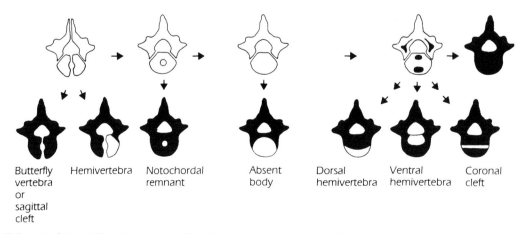

Butterfly vertebra or sagittal cleft Hemivertebra Notochordal remnant Absent body Dorsal hemivertebra Ventral hemivertebra Coronal cleft

FIG. 4-2. Chondrification and ossification of a vertebral body. Upper row, left to right shows appearance of chondrification centers *(white)*, appearance of ossification centers *(black)*, and complete normal ossification of vertebra. **Lower row**, left to right, shows congenital malformation of vertebrae due to abnormalities of chondrification or ossification. Modified from Harwood-Nash and Fitz (2).

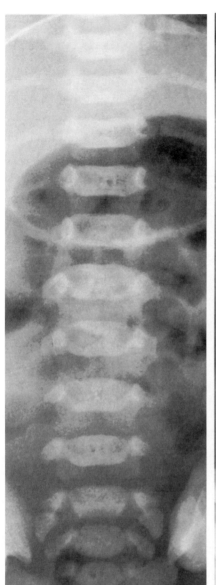
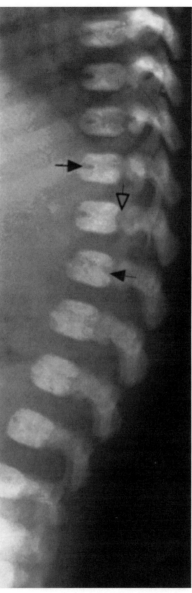

A,B

FIG. 4-3. Normal neonatal spine. A: AP view of the thoracolumbar spine shows only slight widening of the inter-pediculate distance of the lower lumbar vertebrae. **B:** The thoracic vertebral bodies are rectangular and the lumbar vertebral bodies are oval on the lateral view. Note the anterior and posterior vascular grooves *(solid arrows)* and the neurocentral synchondrosis *(open arrow)*.

Ossification of the neural arches occurs first in the cervical region, whereas ossification of the vertebral bodies occurs first in the lower thoracic and upper lumbar areas. Contrary to the chondrification pattern, the vertebral body ossifies from anterior and posterior centers, which quickly fuse to form a single center. Ossification centers appear in each half of the posterior arch during the third fetal month (Fig. 4-2).

Vertebral bodies of the neonate tend to be rectangular, as seen on lateral views, in the thoracic region and oval in the lumbar region (Fig. 4-3). A "bone-within-bone" appearance is often present from 3 to 6 weeks of life and represents a normal stage of growth and development (27). Anterior and posterior vascular channels are prominent in normal neonates and young infants (Fig. 4-3). The anterior channels usually disappear during infancy but are occasionally visible in adults. The posterior channels are more frequently visible in adulthood (2). At birth, the synchondroses between the

vertebral body and the posterior neural arches are quite visible.

The first cervical vertebra (atlas) has a separate center in its anterior portion (body), which is ossified in 20% of normal newborns (Fig. 4-4) and in most individuals by 1 year of age. The odontoid process is attached to the body of the axis by a cartilaginous segment (synchondrosis) which may make it look separated (Fig. 4-4). This synchondrosis usually disappears late in childhood. In the AP projection, the odontoid process may appear split vertically because of the normal side-by-side ossification centers (Fig. 4-4).

The neurocentral synchondroses, between the vertebral bodies and the posterior neural arches, begin to disappear in the cervical region at approximately 3 years of age, and this fusion reaches the lumbar region by 6 years of age. Conversely, fusion of the two halves of the posterior neural arches begins in the lumbar region during the first year of

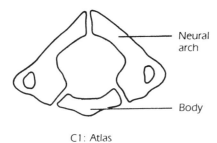

C1: Atlas

Neural
arch

Body

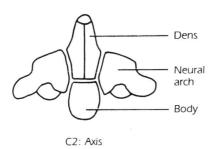

C2: Axis

Dens

Neural
arch

Body

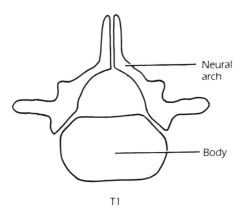

T1

Neural
arch

Body

FIG. 4-4. Normal ossification centers for C1 (axial view), C2 (frontal view), and T1 (axial view).

life. This fusion progresses cephalad; the cervical laminae are the last to fuse, during the third year (2). During late childhood, the vertebral bodies begin to assume their adult shape.

Ring apophyses appear in the middle and lower thoracic and upper lumbar areas at approximately 6 years of age. They are prominent throughout later childhood, completely ossify, and fuse with the vertebral bodies by age 18. They occasionally appear as early as 2 years of age (28). Secondary ossification centers appear at the tips of the spinous processes, transverse processes, and articulating facets just before (females) or after (males) puberty.

Normal Spinal Sonography

Sagittal spine sonography in the newborn or young infant readily demonstrates alternating echogenic vertebral bodies, ventral epidural fat, ventral dura, spinal cord with central echo complex, dorsal dura, and posterior spinous processes (Fig. 4-5) (11). Below the level of the conus medullaris, the cauda equina can be seen to be dependent within the thecal sac. Axial images show dorsal laminae and neurocentral synchondroses, spinal cord and central echo complex, dorsal and ventral nerve root bundles below the level of the conus medullaris, and occasionally the filum terminale. Sagittal and axial imaging is required to delineate the relation of subcutaneous or epidural masses to spinal contents.

Normal Conventional Myelography

In the lumbar region, the subarachnoid space varies considerably in size from one patient to another. The lumbar nerve root sleeves are well visualized and bilaterally symmetric. With water-soluble contrast material, individual nerve roots are exquisitely demonstrated in both the prone and supine positions. The conus medullaris and its tip must be visualized in every pediatric myelogram. The normal conus

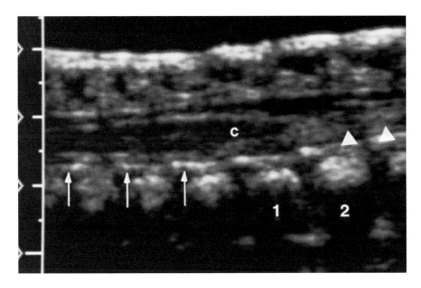

FIG. 4-5. Normal spinal sonography. Sagittal spinal US shows the hypoechoic conus medullaris *(c)* with its tip at the level of L1–2. Ventral dura-arachnoid interface *(arrows)* produces an echogenic band just posterior to alternating echogenic vertebral bodies. The cauda equina and its nerve roots *(arrowheads)* lie in the dependent, ventral portion of the thecal sac.

C7 level. The dentate ligaments divide the cervical cord into dorsal and ventral halves. Irregular arachnoid veils are also noted in the supine position in the cervical subarachnoid space. The normal cisterna magna may be extremely large in children and may fill with contrast material in the supine position. The margins of the cerebellar tonsils are shown, and the fourth ventricle is frequently filled.

Normal CT Myelography

CTM provides excellent visualization of the spinal cord, conus medullaris, cauda equina, and subarachnoid space. This technique requires less radiation and less time, carries less risk to the patient, and provides greater anatomic definition than conventional myelography (2). The size, shape, and position of the cord, clearly outlined by CTM, vary with anatomic level (Fig. 4-7) and age. The cervical cord is round in infants and somewhat oval in older children (Fig. 4-7). The cervical cord is usually central to slightly dorsal in location within the spinal

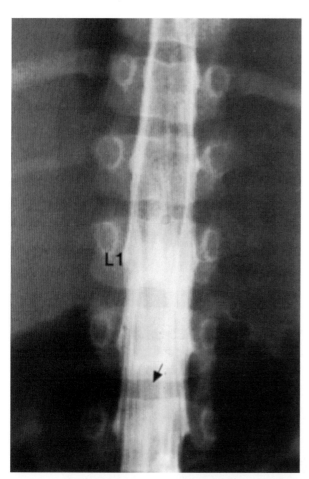

FIG. 4-6. Normal myelography. Normal water-soluble contrast myelogram in a 1-year-old girl. The tip of the conus medullaris is above the L2-L3 interspace *(arrow).*

widens in its transverse and AP diameters and terminates in the filum terminale, readily visible with water-soluble contrast material. The tip of the conus is normally at or above the middle of the body of L2 by age 3 months (Fig. 4-6).

In the thoracic region, the intraarachnoid portions of the nerve roots extend laterally and somewhat caudally. The anterior spinal artery is thin in the upper thoracic canal but becomes larger and tortuous in the lower canal. Its tortuosity must not be mistaken for a spinal arteriovenous malformation (AVM). The artery of Adamkiewicz, seen between T9 and T11, is usually on the left. The lateral margins of the subarachnoid space are only slightly irregular in the thoracic region. The distance between the subarachnoid space and the thoracic pedicles is small and symmetric. Flow of contrast material may produce an artifact that mimics an extradural mass, so any such finding must be confirmed by decubitus views. In the supine position, the dorsal arachnoid veils produce irregular lucencies in the central subarachnoid space.

In the upper cervical region, on conventional myelography, the nerve roots are almost perpendicular to the axis of the spinal cord. They gradually angle more caudally to form an angle of approximately 60° to the perpendicular at the

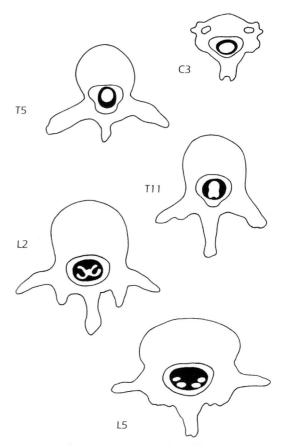

FIG. 4-7. Normal CT myelogram. The contrast opacified subarachnoid space is depicted in black surrounding the spinal cord and nerve roots in white. Axial CT demonstrates the oval spinal cord in the cervical region *(C3)*, a more rounded or sagittally oval cord in the thoracic region *(T5, T11)*, the conus medullaris *(T11)*, conus termination with anterior and posterior nerve roots *(L2)*, and intradural nerve roots below the spinal cord termination *(L5)*. Modified from Resjo et al. (12).

canal, the subarachnoid space being slightly broader ventrally. The thoracic cord is round in infants and children. It is located centrally within the spinal canal in infants, whereas it is normally located ventrally in older children. This positioning causes the subarachnoid space to be wider dorsally than ventrally in older children (Fig. 4-7). The sagittal and transverse diameters of the normal conus increase and the emerging lumbar nerve roots make the cord almost square (Fig. 4-7). The tip of the conus (origin of the filum terminale) is seen as the center of an ''X'' with angled arms (Fig. 4-7). The dural sac is oval in the lumbar area and caudally becomes triangular with a dorsal tip (12). Separate nerve roots are usually seen within the contrast-filled root sleeves in the cauda equina (Fig. 4-7).

Normal Magnetic Resonance Imaging

Bony Spine

At birth, the vertebral bodies are ovoid in shape; their height equals the height of the disc spaces. With progressive ossification, they become more rectangular in lateral profile and significantly increase in height by approximately 2 years of age (13). The spinal column is initially composed of red marrow and incompletely ossified cartilage. There is conversion from red marrow to yellow marrow with increasing age. Red marrow contains 40% water, 20% protein, and 40% fat and is more highly vascularized than yellow marrow, which contains 15% water, 5% protein, and 80% fat (29). At birth, the spinal marrow is T1-hypointense, but each vertebral body has a horizontal band of high intensity, the basivertebral plexus. The cartilaginous endplates are hyperintense whereas the intervening nucleus pulposus is hypointense. Progressive T1 shortening begins at the superior and inferior borders of the vertebral bodies and proceeds centrally to involve the entire vertebral body by 2 years of age (Figs. 4-8 and 4-9) (30).

Spinal Neuraxis

Sagittal T1-weighted images show a tapering, slightly bulbous conus medullaris ending at the level of mid-L2 or above (Fig. 4-8A). Parasagittal images often reveal discrete ventral and dorsal nerve root bundles. The distal thecal sac usually terminates at S1 or S2 but may end as low as S5. Axial

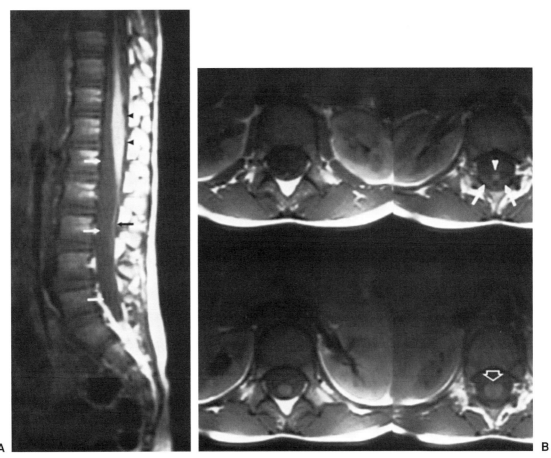

FIG. 4-8. Normal spine MRI of 4-year-old child. A: Sagittal T1 MRI demonstrates the conus medullaris *(arrowheads)* terminating at the mid-L2 level, cauda equina nerve roots *(black arrow)*, and the CSF intensity dural sac *(white arrows).* **B:** Axial T1 MRI sections demonstrate the spinal cord *(open arrow)* at and above the termination of the conus medullaris *(arrowhead).* The dorsal and ventral nerve roots are also shown *(arrows).*

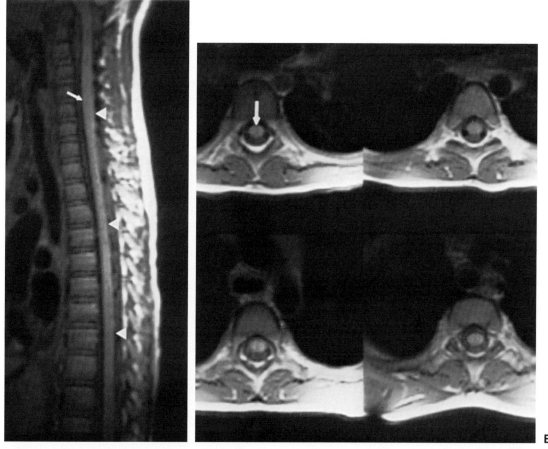

FIG. 4-9. Normal spine MRI of 4-year-old child. A: Sagittal T1 MRI of the cervical and thoracic spine shows the thoracic spinal cord *(arrowheads)* and the normal cervical enlargement *(arrow)*. **B:** Contiguous axial T1 MRI sections show an oval-to-round appearance of the thoracic spinal cord *(arrow)*.

images through the cauda equina reveal discrete dorsal and ventral nerve root groups; this may be mistaken for diastematomyelia (Fig. 4-8B). The filum terminale may contain high signal due to fat, often a normal variant if the diameter of the filum is less than 2 mm.

Sagittal images of the thoracic spine show uniform cord diameter and homogeneous signal intensity (Fig. 4-9A). Frequently, turbulent CSF flow dorsal to the cord creates inhomogeneous signal in the posterior subarachnoid space, whereas laminar flow ventral to the cord creates a homogeneous signal void in the anterior subarachnoid space. Axial images provide additional information about the diameters of the cord and vertebral canal (Fig. 4-9B).

The cervical spine and craniocervical junction are well demonstrated with MRI. Sagittal images show the anatomy of the craniovertebral junction, cervical spinal cord, medulla, and skull base particularly well.

COMMON NORMAL VARIANTS

Variants of the Atlas and Axis

The atlas is formed from three ossification centers, which give rise to the anterior arch and the two lateral masses. At birth, the occiput is ossified, as are the lateral masses and posterior arch of the atlas. The anterior arch is ossified in only 20% of newborns, but is almost always seen by 1 year of age, and it unites with the lateral masses by 3 years. The posterior arch centers fuse in the midline by 5–6 years.

The axis is composed of the odontoid process, body, and two neural arches. The odontoid, or dens, forms from two lateral ossification centers, visible and already fused at birth. The "summit" ossification center of the dens (ossiculum terminale) ossifies at 3–6 years of age and fuses with the dens by 12 years (31,32). The synchondroses between the dens and neural arches (see Fig. 4-4), and the subdental synchondrosis between the dens and body (Fig. 4-10) fuse at 3–6 years of age. Prior to ossification and fusion, these normal structures are sometimes misinterpreted as fractures or lytic defects (33). The dens may be tilted posteriorly (34); this should not be misinterpreted as a congenital or traumatic abnormality.

The os odontoideum is a hypertrophied remnant of the proatlas (31,32) and is associated with hypoplasia of the dens and atlantoaxial instability. The third condyle is a fragment of bone attached to the inferior edge of the anterior border of the foramen magnum and is a common normal variant (Table 4-2).

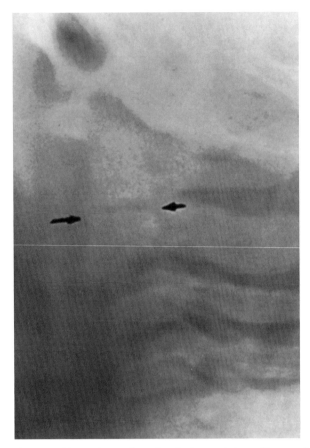

FIG. 4-10. Normal synchondrosis. Lateral view of the cervical spine in a 7-month-old girl. The normal synchondrosis between the dens and vertebral body of C2 *(arrows)* is well visualized.

Posterior Cleft or Spina Bifida Occulta

As previously described, the posterior neural arches are normally separated by a midline cartilaginous cleft early in life. It appears as a narrow vertical lucency on AP projections and should not be mistaken for a defect in the vertebral body (35,36). This cleft ossifies and disappears between 3 and 5 years of age, starting in the lumbosacral region and proceeding cephalad. The cervical clefts are usually the last to close. Occasionally, one of these clefts persists to adulthood, most frequently at S1. Other sites in decreasing order of frequency are L5, C1, C7, and T1. The reason for this predilection for the boundaries between the major spinal regions is not known. The lucent cleft is 1 or 2 mm wide and vertical or slightly oblique in orientation. There may be some asymmetry of the adjacent laminae. When isolated and not associated with other deformities of the vertebra, cutaneous lesions, or a neurologic abnormality, this defect of the posterior arch is a benign condition and is termed spina bifida occulta.

Cervical Pseudosubluxation

The fulcrum for flexion and extension of the cervical spine in infants and children is roughly at the C2–3 or C3–4 level

but at the C5–6 level in the adult. Therefore on lateral cervical spine radiographs in children obtained with flexion, it appears that the upper cervical spine is subluxed forward (Fig. 4-11). This appearance is thought to be due to a normal generalized laxity of ligaments as well as the horizontal orientation of the apophyseal joints (37). On films taken in mild flexion, there is frequently also anterior buckling of the trachea and distortion of the prevertebral soft tissues; this may mimic soft-tissue swelling. If another normal variant (wedging of C3 vertebral body) is present, differentiation of pseudosubluxation from a real abnormality (subluxation, fracture) may be even more difficult (37,38). Swischuk advocates the use of the posterior cervical line to differentiate physiologic from pathologic anterior displacement of C2 on C3 in flexion (39). With physiologic displacement of C2 on C3 (pseudosubluxation), the posterior cervical line passes through or comes within 1 mm of the anterior cortex of the arch of C2 (Fig. 4-11). If there is a pathologic dislocation or true subluxation of C2 on C3, the posterior cervical line misses the posterior arch of C2 by 2 mm or more (39). The posterior cervical line is occasionally well anterior to C2 even in the absence of subluxation (Fig. 4-12), a condition termed "pseudo-pseudosubluxation" (39).

TABLE 4-2. *Common normal variants*

Cervical spine
Third condyle
Pseudospread of atlas
Cleft anterior arch of atlas
Ossiculum terminale[a]
Bifid odontoid[a]
Odontoid dysplasia
Mach band of dens
Dens-arch synchondrosis
Dens-body synchondrosis
Neurocentral synchondrosis
Posterior tilted dens
Pseudoatlantoaxial subluxation
Absent or hypoplastic posterior arches
Cleft in posterior neural arches[a]
Pseudonotch of axis
Ponticulus posticus[a]
Pseudosubluxation[a]
Pseudowidening of interpediculate distance[a]
Absent or hypoplastic pedicle
Wedging of vertebral bodies[a]
Transverse processes overlying disc spaces
Spina bifida occulta[a]
Thoracic and lumbosacral spine
Neurocentral synchondroses[a]
Cleft in posterior neural arches[a]
Absent or hypoplastic pedicle[a]
Wedging of vertebral bodies[a]
Posterior scalloping of vertebral bodies
Spina bifida occulta[a]
Coronal clefts
Vascular grooves[a]
Posterior widening of S1–2 disc interspace
Ring apophyses[a]
Pediculate thinning[a]
"Bone-within-bone"[a]

[a] More common.

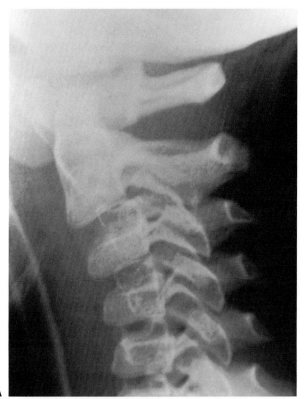

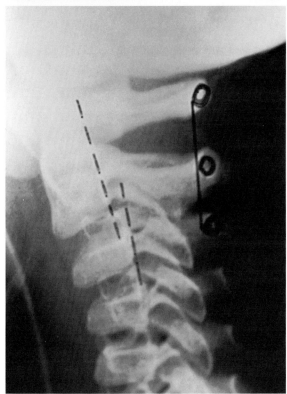

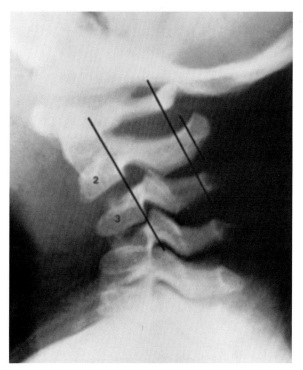

FIG. 4-12. Cervical pseudo-pseudosubluxation. This 2-year-old child had a stiff neck after minor trauma. The posterior cervical line is anterior to C2, but there is no offset (subluxation) of C2 on C3.

Pseudowidening of Cervical Interpediculate Distances

The diameter of the spinal canal in infants is relatively wider than in older children or adults, particularly in the cervical spine, where the interpediculate distances appear prominent (40). This normal widening of the cervical spinal canal is accentuated by slight obliquity in positioning.

Absent or Hypoplastic Cervical Pedicle

The radiologic features of congenital absence of a cervical pedicle include absence of the pedicle with a double (conjoint) vertebral foramen, an abnormally small transverse process, and a displaced lateral articular mass (41). Many of these patients have symptoms (pain, limb weakness, numbness) referable to the cervical spinal cord, and so the condition may not truly be a normal variant. MRI shows an abnormal outpouching of dura containing two nerve roots at the level of the absent pedicle. This entity should not be confused with a transforaminal neurogenic tumor; in the latter, the articular masses are intact and not displaced (41).

Absent or Hypoplastic Lumbar Pedicle

Unilateral aplasia or hypoplasia of a lumbar pedicle is unusual. In contrast to comparable cervical lesions, these

FIG. 4-11. Cervical pseudosubluxation. A: Lateral radiograph of the cervical spine obtained in moderate flexion. Distortion of the prevertebral soft tissues mimics edema. There is apparent subluxation of C2 on C3. **B:** Posterior cervical line of Swischuk (39) passes through the anterior cortex of the arch of C2 *(solid line)*. Therefore the displacement of C2 on C3 *(broken lines)* is physiologic pseudosubluxation.

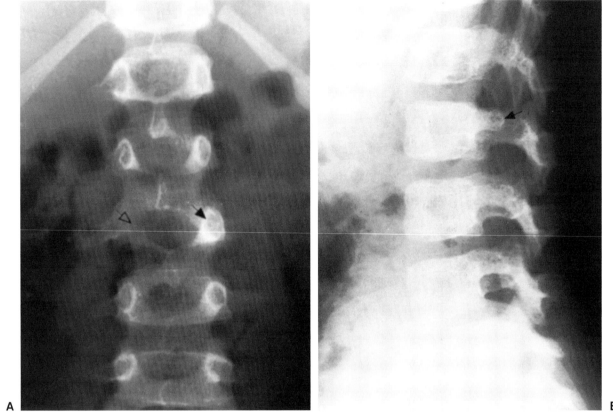

FIG. 4-13. Hypoplastic lumbar pedicle. An asymptomatic 6-year-old boy. **A:** Pedicle of L3 on the right is absent *(open arrow)* with compensatory hypertrophy and sclerosis of the contralateral pedicle *(solid arrow)*. **B:** Lateral radiograph shows round margin *(arrow)* of the hypoplastic pedicle.

patients are usually asymptomatic (42–44). Radiographs show absence or hypoplasia of a pedicle (Fig. 4-13). There may be enlargement of the adjacent neural foramina, mimicking an intraspinal tumor, or compensatory hypertrophy with sclerosis of the contralateral pedicle, mimicking a primary bony abnormality (Fig. 4-13A). The ipsilateral transverse process is always in an abnormal position.

Coronal Clefts

Coronal clefts are common anomalies of the vertebral bodies. They are usually incidental, may be single or multiple, and are more common in the lumbar region, and may extend into the thoracic spine. Radiographically, vertical lucencies are seen in one or more vertebral bodies (Fig. 4-14). These clefts are composed of cartilage, are contiguous with the cartilaginous endplates, and completely divide the ventral and dorsal halves of the vertebral bodies. They represent failure of fusion of the anterior and posterior ossification centers (see Fig. 4-2). Although coronal cleft vertebrae may be seen in association with imperforate anus, meningomyelocele, and chondrodystrophia calcificans congenita, they may also be seen in normal infants (45,46). They are more common in males and usually disappear by 6 months of age.

Pediculate Thinning

The pedicles at the thoracolumbar junction are flattened medially in up to 7% of normal children (47). This normal pediculate thinning should not be confused with erosion by a spinal tumor (40,48). With pediculate thinning the flattened pedicle is usually concave laterally and convex medially, the interpediculate distance at the level of the flattened pedicle is within normal limits, and there is no erosion of the vertebral body or posterior elements (47). This normal variant probably represents an intrinsic anatomic variation in the shape of the pedicles (48).

"Bone-Within-Bone"

Lateral radiographs of normal infants frequently display a "bone-within-bone" appearance of the thoracic and lumbar vertebral bodies (27). Because the superior and inferior bony surfaces of the vertebral body are the counterpart of the zone of provisional calcification of a long bone, it is thought that the bone-within-bone appearance is simply a normal stage in the growth and development of the infantile vertebral body without clinical significance (27).

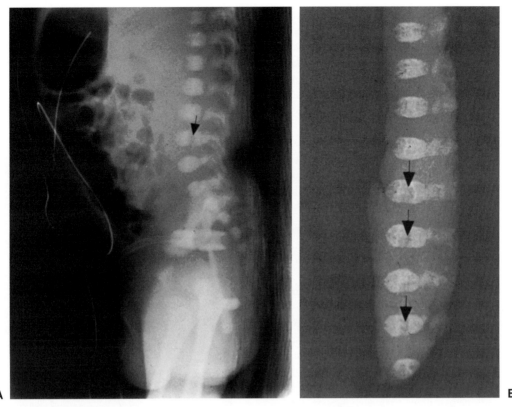

FIG. 4-14. Coronal clefts. A: Lateral film of the abdomen obtained for placement of umbilical venous catheter shows a coronal cleft of L4 *(arrow)*. **B:** Autopsy specimen of a different patient. Coronal cleft vertebrae at L1, L2, and L4 *(arrows)*. (Specimen courtesy of Derek C. Harwood-Nash, M.D., Toronto, Ontario, Canada.)

GENERAL ABNORMALITIES

Abnormal Density

Conventional radiographs are excellent for demonstrating either increased or decreased bony density of the spine. Increased or sclerotic density of the pediatric spine represents increased osteoblastic activity. It may be physiologic (neonatal sclerosis), hereditary, or reactive (Table 4-3). Reactive increased density of the spine may be caused by infectious, neoplastic, traumatic, or other insults. Sclerotic lesions of the spine are unusual, and the radiologic features in conjunction with clinical information are usually diagnostic.

Decreased density of the pediatric spine is due to increased osteoclastic activity, which may be congenital or reactive (Table 4-3). The differential diagnosis is based on the clinical history as well as on radiologic features (number of vertebrae involved, portion of vertebra involved, margins of lytic defect, other abnormalities).

Congenital Bony Malformations

Most malformations of the vertebral column are readily explained if the normal processes of chondrification and ossification are understood (see Fig. 4-2). Abnormal formation

TABLE 4-3. *Abnormal density of spine*

Increased or sclerotic density	Decreased or lytic density
Congenital disorders	Congenital disorders
Neonatal sclerosis	Osteogenesis imperfecta
(a normal finding)[a]	Gaucher disease
Osteopetrosis	Niemann-Pick disease
Tuberous sclerosis	Neurofibromatosis
Infections: osteomyelitis[a]	Homocystinuria
Neoplasms	Hypophosphatasia
Lymphoma	Infections: osteomyelitis[a]
Osteoid osteoma[a]	Neoplasms
Osteoblastoma	Leukemia[a]
Metastases	Lymphoma
Osteosarcoma	Metastases[a]
Ewing sarcoma	Hemangioma
Hemangioma	Aneurysmal bone cyst
Trauma	Osteoid osteoma
Fracture[a]	Osteoblastoma
Irradiation	Trauma: irradiation
Miscellaneous disorders	Miscellaneous disorders
Renal osteodystrophy[a]	Rickets
Sarcoidosis	Renal osteodystrophy[a]
Fluorosis	Hyperthyroidism
Hypervitaminosis A	Histiocytosis
or D	Steroids[a]
Myelosclerosis	Osteoporosis[a]
Hypercalcemia	Hyperparathyroidism
Mastocytosis	Cushing disease
Sickle cell disease[a]	Anemia[a]

[a] More common.

and abnormal segmentation and persistence of the notochord are responsible for most malformations of vertebral bodies. These may occur with or without intraspinal or systemic abnormalities. Malformations include hemivertebra, butterfly vertebra, and block vertebra. Spinal dysraphism is splaying of the pedicles and laminae associated with nonfusion of the spinous processes plus varying defects in organization of the spinal neuraxis (1,2). Abnormalities of formation and segmentation (hemivertebrae) frequently coexist (1,2).

Agenesis of the sacrum and coccyx may be either partial or complete. The defect is usually associated with severe lower spinal and sacral root abnormalities. There may be associated rectal and genitourinary malformations and lower limb anomalies. Sacrococcygeal segmental defects also occur.

Abnormal Curvature

The normal spine is straight on upright, well-positioned AP radiographs. As discussed previously, normal postinfancy spines have a cervical lordosis, a thoracic kyphosis, and a lumbar lordosis. Abnormal curvatures of the spine include *scoliosis* (lateral curvature) and *kyphosis* (abnormal posterior curvature). These two conditions may occur in association, producing *kyphoscoliosis*. Abnormal curvatures of the spine may be idiopathic or due to underlying abnormalities of the bony spine (congenital malformation, bony dysplasia, infection, tumor, trauma), or neuromuscular disorders (muscular dystrophy, cerebral palsy, spinal cord tumor, hydrosyringomyelia). Radiology plays an important role in evaluating abnormal curvatures of the spine (6). Appropriate radiologic examination confirms the presence, extent, and severity of the deformity. The etiology of the abnormal curvature may be apparent. Sequential radiologic examinations are also important for evaluating progression and the effect of therapy.

Platyspondyly

Platyspondyly (''flat spine'') is a decrease in the distance between the intact upper and lower vertebral body endplates (Fig. 4-15). The cause of platyspondyly is usually easily determined. A skeletal survey is often useful (49). Platyspondyly may affect all vertebral bodies (generalized platyspondyly), some vertebral bodies (multiple platyspondyly), or one vertebral body (localized platyspondyly or vertebra plana). The differential diagnosis of platyspondyly is presented in Table 4-4 (49). Important differentiating features include the age of the patient, the density and shape of the vertebrae, the number of affected vertebrae, and the severity of platyspondyly (49).

Increased Vertebral Body Height

Vertebral bodies change shape with age. In the neonate, the thoracic vertebral bodies are nearly rectangular in profile

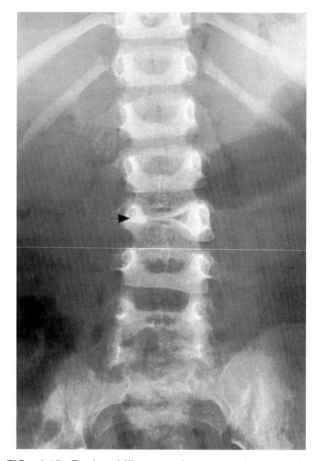

FIG. 4-15. Eosinophilic granuloma causing vertebra plana. The markedly asymmetric flattening of the L3 vertebral body *(arrow)* is somewhat unusual.

whereas the lumbar vertebral bodies are oval, with the AP diameter of the vertebral body being greater than the vertical diameter (see Fig. 4-3). Growth of the vertebral body in the vertical direction occurs at the cartilaginous layers of the superior and inferior endplates. Decrease in the normal effect of gravity and weight bearing on these surfaces causes longitudinal overgrowth of the vertebral body (50,51). Tall vertebrae in older infants or children may be due to neuromuscular disease (Fig. 4-16) (51).

Tall vertebral bodies may also be seen in neonates with Down syndrome or, rarely, other trisomy conditions (51). Vertebral bodies with a slightly increased vertical height are occasionally seen in normal individuals (2,35,50,52).

Abnormal Intervertebral Disc

The intervertebral disc consists of an external annulus fibrosus attached to the adjacent vertebral body and a central nucleus pulposus; the latter is a remnant of the notochord. The intervertebral disc appears large at birth, and its apparent height approximates that of the vertebral body. With progressive vertebral body ossification and after the child sits and

TABLE 4-4. *Causes of platyspondyly*

Generalized platyspondyly
  Osteochondrodysplasias
    Thanatophoric dwarfism
    Metatropic dwarfism
    Spondyloepiphyseal dysplasia
    Spondylometaphyseal dysplasia
    Spondyloepimetaphyseal dysplasia
    Mucopolysaccharidoses (e.g., Morquio syndrome, Hurler syndrome, Hunter syndrome)
    Dyggve disease
    Osteogenesis imperfecta
    Kniest disease
    Geroderma osteodysplastica
    Achondrogenesis
    Achondroplasia[a]
    Pseudoachondroplasia
    Diastrophic dwarfism
    Metaphyseal dysplasia (Pyle disease)
    Parastremmatic dwarfism
    Homocystinuria
  Endocrine disorders
    Cushing syndrome[a]
    Hypoparathyroidism
    Hyperparathyroidism
    Hypothyroidism
  Metabolic disorders
    Osteoporosis
      Idiopathic
      Steroids[a]
      Hepatic neoplasm
    Therapy
      Steroids[a]
      Adrenocorticotropic hormone (ACTH)
    Rickets
    Hypophosphatasia
  Hematologic disorders
    Leukemia[a]
    Lymphoma
    Anemia[a]
  Trauma
    Fractures[a]
    Irradiation[a]
    Tetanus
Localized platyspondyly: vertebra plana
  Histiocytosis[a]
  Infection
    Bacterial[a]
    Tuberculosis
  Trauma: fracture[a]
  Tumors
    Leukemia[a]
    Lymphoma
    Hemangioma
    Metastasis[a]
  Miscellaneous
    Gaucher disease
    Neurofibromatosis

[a] More common

Source: Modified from Kozlowski (49).

stands, the relative height of the intervertebral disc gradually decreases until in the young adult it is approximately one third the height of the vertebral body. The intervertebral disc may be secondarily involved by infection (discitis) or trauma of the vertebral body. This often leads to narrowing of the disc space. Idiopathic intervertebral disc calcification and discitis are two primary abnormalities that are unique to infants and children.

Atlantoaxial Instability

The first and second cervical vertebrae are functionally and anatomically different from the remainder of the cervical spine (see Fig. 4-4). Flexion and extension of the head on the neck occurs primarily at the articulation between the occipital condyles and the lateral masses of the atlas. Rotation occurs primarily at the atlantoaxial articulation. The atlantoaxial articulation is stabilized by the cruciate, alar, and apical ligaments. The transverse ligament, a portion of the cruciate ligament, arises from the lateral masses of the atlas and crosses dorsal to the odontoid process (dens). It is the main ligament that holds the odontoid process close to the anterior arch of the atlas.

Atlantoaxial subluxation leads to an increase in distance

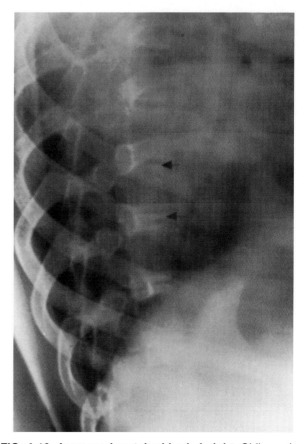

FIG. 4-16. Increased vertebral body height. Oblique view of the thoracic spine of a 12-year-old girl with severe cerebral palsy shows tall vertebral bodies *(between arrows).*

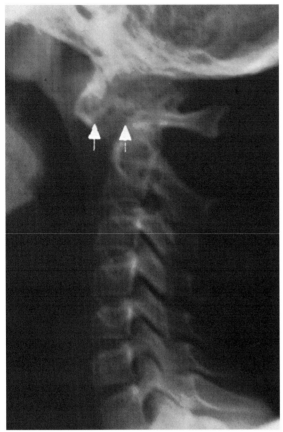

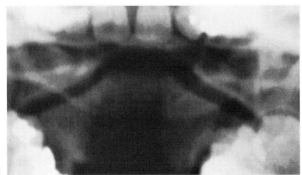

FIG. 4-17. Atlantoaxial subluxation due to odontoid dysplasia. A: Atlas-dens interval *(arrows)* measures 6 mm. The tip of the hypoplastic odontoid does not extend above a line connecting the most cephalad margin of the vertebral body and the vertebral arch of C1. **B:** Hypoplasia of the odontoid is confirmed on open-mouth AP view.

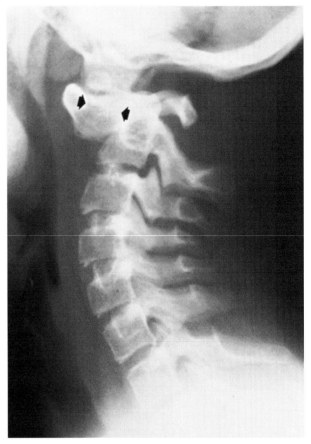

FIG. 4-18. Atlantoaxial dislocation in Down syndrome. Lateral radiographs of a 16-year-old Down syndrome patient with increasing lower extremity weakness. In the neutral position, there is 11 mm of atlantoaxial dislocation *(arrows)*. Note that the vertebral canal width (distance from the posterior margin of the odontoid to the anterior cortex of the posterior ring of C1) is markedly decreased. MRI confirmed marked spinal cord compression.

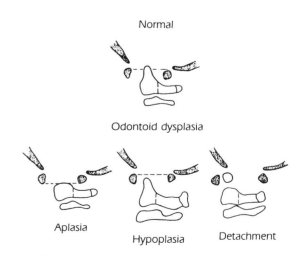

FIG. 4-19. Odontoid dysplasia. Occipitocervical junction: normal *(above)* and odontoid dysplasia *(below)*. Congenital dysplasia of the odontoid includes aplasia, hypoplasia, and detached odontoid (os odontorideum). Modified from Perovic et al. (53).

between the dens and the anterior arch of the atlas (Figs. 4-17 and 4-18); as a result, the vertebral canal is narrowed at that level. Subluxation may be due to trauma, inflammatory disease, developmental abnormalities, skeletal dysplasia, or Down syndrome (Table 4-5). Developmental anomalies of the odontoid may be isolated or a local expression of a generalized skeletal dysplasia (53). Congenital abnormalities of the odontoid include aplasia, hypoplasia, and os odontoideum (Fig. 4-19) (53). Each of these conditions may produce atlantoaxial subluxation and instability (see Fig. 4-17).

TABLE 4-5. *Atlantoaxial subluxation*

Congenital factors
    Atlantooccipital fusion
    Absent anterior arch of atlas
    Odontoid dysplasia (aplasia, hypoplasia, detached odontoid)
    Down syndrome (trisomy 21)[a]
    Morquio syndrome
    Chondrodysplasia punctata
    Diastrophic dwarfism
    Cartilage hair hypoplasia (metaphyseal chondrodysplasia)
    Winchester-Grossman syndrome
    Spondylometaphyseal dysplasia
    Spondyloepiphyseal dysplasia
    Pseudoachondroplastic dysplasia
Infection
    Rhinopharyngitis
    Retropharyngeal abscess
Trauma
    Fracture[a]
    Ligamentous injury
Miscellaneous disorders
    Rheumatoid arthritis[a]
    Ankylosing spondylitis
    Systemic lupus erythematosus
    Psoriatic arthritis

[a] More common.

The atlas-dens interval is measured from the bony cortex of the posteroinferior portion of the anterior arch of the atlas to the adjacent anterior border of the dens (54). This measurement tends to increase during flexion and decrease during extension; therefore, the neutral position is recommended for measurement. The atlas-dens interval is usually less than 3 mm, although a measurement of 5 mm can occasionally be found in a normal infant (54). A measurement of greater than 3 mm should alert one to the possibility of atlantoaxial subluxation. The sagittal dimension of the vertebral canal at that level should not be less than 13 mm (55–58).

TABLE 4-6. *Enlarged cervical intervertebral foramina*

Congenital abnormalities
    Absent or hypoplastic pedicle[a]
    Lateral meningocele
    Neurofibromatosis
Neoplasms
    Neurogenic tumor
        Neuroblastoma
        Ganglioneuroblastoma
        Ganglioneuroma[a]
        Neurofibroma[a]
    Dermoid
    Lipoma
    Lymphoma-leukemia

[a] More common.

TABLE 4-7. *Scalloped vertebral bodies*

Posterior scalloping
    Normal variant—mild scalloping[a]
    Congenital skeletal abnormalities
        Achondroplasia
        Mucopolysaccharidoses (Hurler syndrome, Morquio syndrome)
        Neurofibromatosis[a]
        Metatropic dwarfism
        Osteogenesis imperfecta
    Dural ectasia
        Neurofibromatosis
        Marfan syndrome
        Ehlers-Danlos syndrome
    Increased intraspinal pressure
        Local
            Intradural neoplasm or cyst
            Syringomyelia or hydromyelia
        General
            Severe communicating hydrocephalus
Anterior scalloping
    Neurofibromatosis
    Lymphadenopathy
        Infection
        Metastases
    Leukemia-lymphoma

[a] More common.

Enlarged Cervical Intervertebral Foramina

Enlargement of one or more cervical intervertebral foramina is much less common in children than in adults. Such enlargement may be congenital or due to neoplasia (Table 4-6). Neoplasms that produce this enlargement are usually neurogenic in origin.

Scalloped Vertebral Bodies

Scalloping of a vertebral body is an exaggeration of the normal slight concavity of its dorsal or ventral surface (59). Posterior scalloping is well known and occurs more frequently than anterior scalloping. Slight posterior scalloping is normal in children. Abnormal posterior scalloping may be due to increased intraspinal pressure, dural ectasia, or congenital skeletal abnormalities (Table 4-7) (59). Anterior scalloping in children is usually due to the mesodermal dysplasia of neurofibromatosis-1 but rarely is secondary to intrinsic bone destruction or extrinsic bony erosion (Table 4-7) (59).

SPECIFIC ABNORMALITIES

Congenital Abnormalities

Developmental Bony Malformations

Developmental abnormalities of the bony spine are common. Such abnormalities may involve the vertebral body

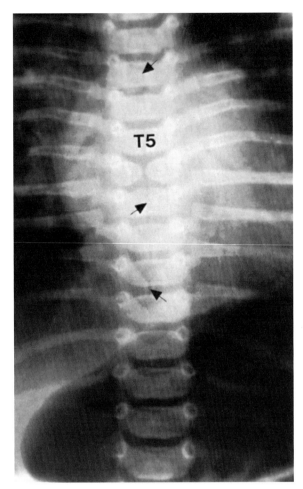

FIG. 4-20. Butterfly vertebra. There is a butterfly vertebra at T6. Note also the vertical lucencies due to cartilaginous clefts in the posterior vertebral arches *(arrows)*. These posterior clefts overlie vertebral bodies as well as intervertebral discs at several levels.

or the posterior neural arches. Coronal cleft vertebrae have already been discussed. Segmentation anomalies may be isolated or seen in association with spinal dysraphism.

Butterfly Vertebra

Lack of fusion of the two cartilaginous centers of the vertebral body produces a sagittal cleft (see Fig. 4-2). There may be asymmetric ossification of the two lateral centers with hypoplasia near this sagittal cleft, producing a butterfly vertebra (Fig. 4-20).

Lateral Hemivertebra

If one of the two lateral chondrification centers fails to develop, a lateral hemivertebra is formed (see Fig. 4-2). Hemivertebrae may be single or multiple, and there is usually a secondary lateral spinal curvature. There are often

ipsilateral rib anomalies at that level and, rarely, hypoplasia of the lung and pulmonary artery.

Anterior or Posterior Hemivertebra

If there is a failure to form either the ventral or dorsal ossification center of the vertebral body, an anterior or posterior hemivertebra is formed (see Fig. 4-2). A posterior hemivertebra is more common and may lead to a serious gibbus deformity. If there is associated underdevelopment of the posterior arches, there may be marked posterior displacement of the hemivertebra and extrinsic compression of the spinal cord (Fig. 4-21, see Fig. 4-73). This condition has been referred to as posterior vertebral slippage (2). Posterior slippage of a hemivertebra may be isolated or associated with a tethered cord or myelomeningocele (2). This posterior slippage usually occurs at the thoracolumbar junction but also may occur at the lower lumbar and cervicothoracic junction regions.

Block Vertebrae

Block vertebrae are due to a lack of segmentation. This may occur alone or with posterior arch defects (dysraphism). Block vertebrae have fusion of one or more vertebral bodies with an absent or rudimentary intervertebral disc. In contrast to acquired fusion due to disc abnormality, there is no loss of segmental height of the vertebral bodies themselves in block vertebrae. There may be fusion of a portion of the posterior neural arches. Complex vertebral arch anomalies and dysraphism are frequently present.

Craniocervical Anomalies

Craniocervical anomalies occurring in childhood and adolescence include the Klippel-Feil anomaly, basilar invagination, occipitalization of the atlas, odontoid abnormalities, and craniocervical instability. Craniocervical junction anomalies lead to signs and symptoms of torticollis, craniofacial or craniocervical dysmorphism, limitation of motion, headache or neck pain, neck mass, or clicking. Kyphosis and scoliosis may also be present. Patients may also have hindbrain, cervical cord, or vertebrobasilar compromise (13,60,61).

Anatomy of the Craniocervical Junction

The craniocervical junction consists of the basiocciput, the atlas, the axis, and the ligaments of the atlantooccipital and atlantoaxial articulations. Imaging of this region includes frontal and lateral plain films of the cervical spine and skull base, flexion-extension lateral radiographs or fluoroscopy, CT, conventional tomography, and MRI (62–64).

The McGregor and McRae lines are helpful in distinguishing normal from abnormal relationships at the craniocervical

space (vertebral canal width), the distance from the posterior cortex of the dens to the posterior arch of the atlas or to the posterior margin of the foramen magnum, is at least 13 mm in children and up to 19 mm in adults (13,55,56). The vertebral canal space (distance from anterior arch to posterior arch of C1), according to the Steel rule of thirds, includes one third dens, one third cord, and one third "safe zone." The dens tip should line up with the cortex of the clivus; "if a marble rolled down the clivus, it would hit the tip of the dens." Finally, the vertical distance between the inferior margins of the foramen magnum and the anterior and posterior arches of C1 should never be more than 5 mm. A distance over 5 mm indicates atlantooccipital dislocation (65–67). The distance between the dens and clivus should never be more than 1 cm.

Klippel-Feil Anomaly

The Klippel-Feil anomaly is a congenital bony fusion of cervical vertebrae at one or more levels (Figs. 4-22 and 4-23) (68). The anomaly probably results from abnormal seg-

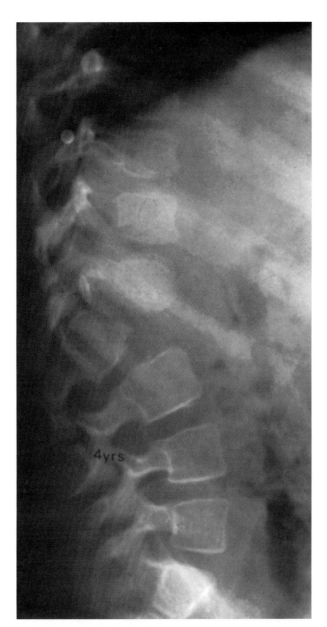

FIG. 4-21. **Posterior hemivertebra.** A 4-year-old girl. Lateral radiograph demonstrates a congenital lumbar kyphosis due to posterior slippage of a posterior hemivertebra at L3. (Courtesy of Derek C. Harwood-Nash, M.D., Toronto, Ontario, Canada.)

junction. The *McGregor line* is drawn from the posterior hard palate to the lowest point of the occiput of the posterior margin of the foramen magnum. The tip of the dens is normally not more than 4.5 mm above this line. The *McRae line* connects the anterior and posterior margins of the foramen magnum; the dens tip should always be below this line.

As previously noted, the predental space (interval between the anterior arch of the atlas and the dens) varies in infants and young children from 3 mm to a maximum of 5 mm in flexion; it may normally increase 2 mm from extension to flexion. The predental space is normally less than 3 mm in the neutral position in adolescents and adults. The postdental

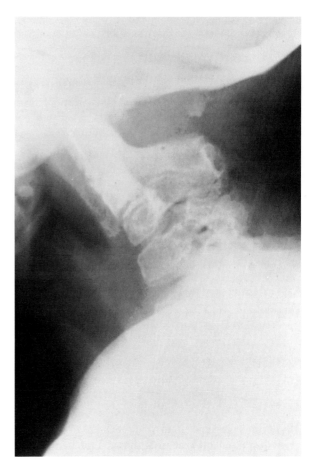

FIG. 4-22. **Klippel-Feil anomaly.** A 4-year-old boy with ataxia. Lateral radiograph demonstrates fusion of upper cervical segments both anteriorly and posteriorly. Also, there is occipitalization of the atlas anteriorly and basilar invagination with a high-placed odontoid.

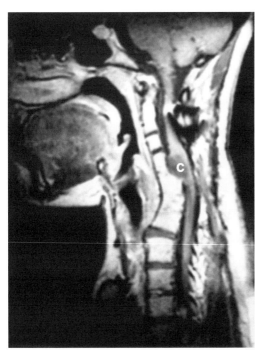

FIG. 4-23. Klippel-Feil anomaly and neurenteric cyst. A 20-year-old woman with neck pain. Sagittal T1 MRI shows multiple bony segmentation anomalies of the cervical spine. A hypointense neurenteric cyst *(c)* is located anterior to the spinal cord.

mentation of the cervical somites between the third and eighth weeks of gestation. The triad of low posterior hairline, short webbed neck, and limitation of neck motion classically seen in the Klippel-Feil anomaly actually occurs in fewer than 50% of cases. A Sprengel deformity of the scapula and a bridging omovertebral bone are present in 25% of patients (69). Genitourinary anomalies, congenital heart disease, and abnormalities of the limbs and digits may also be present (69–71). Bony spine findings may include abnormalities of the posterior elements, occipitalization of the atlas, basilar impression, anomalies of the dens, and scoliosis. The Chiari I malformation, a neurenteric cyst (Fig. 4-23), hydrosyringomyelia (Fig. 4-24), and diastematomyelia may also be associated. These patients may have hypermobility or instability because of unfused vertebral segments. They develop early degenerative disease of the spine, which leads to foraminal or spinal canal stenosis, osteophytic spurs, subluxation, facet arthropathy, and disc herniation (72).

Basilar Invagination

Basilar invagination refers to an occipital dysplasia with upward displacement of the margins of the foramen magnum (73). The odontoid is superiorly displaced relative to the McGregor and McRae lines. The posterior fossa may be small and have an irregularly shaped foramen magnum and a short clivus. Basilar invagination may be primary as part of more extensive craniocervical anomalies or syndromes

(see Fig. 4-22). Secondary basilar invagination is due to bone softening. Possible causes include Paget disease, rickets, fibrous dysplasia, achondroplasia, mucopolysaccharidoses, osteogenesis imperfecta, osteomalacia, and cleidocranial dysplasia (74). Basilar invagination may lead to neural, CSF flow, or vascular compromise. Chiari I malformation, hydrocephalus, and hydrosyringomyelia may also be present.

Occipitalization of the Atlas

Fusion of the atlas to the occipital bone may be bony or fibrous and complete or incomplete (21). It may involve the anterior or posterior arches or one of the lateral masses. The most common type of occipitalization is assimilation of the anterior arch into the anterior rim of the foramen magnum. Occipitalization of the atlas may coexist with hypoplasia of the dens, basilar invagination, atlantoaxial instability, and the Klippel-Feil anomaly (see Fig. 4-22). Symptoms and signs are due to compromise at the level of C1 or the foramen magnum.

Odontoid Abnormalities

Major congenital malformations of the odontoid process include aplasia, hypoplasia, and the presence of an os odontoideum (see Fig. 4-19) (32,75,76). Odontoid abnormalities,

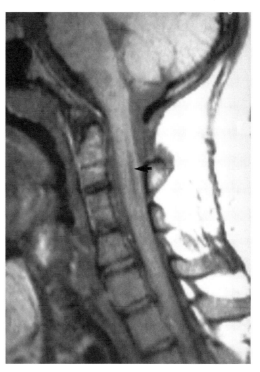

FIG. 4-24. Klippel-Feil anomaly. A 15-year-old girl with known Klippel-Feil anomaly. Sagittal T1 MRI shows failure of segmentation (fusion) of several upper cervical vertebral bodies. A small upper cervical hypointense syrinx *(arrow)* is also demonstrated.

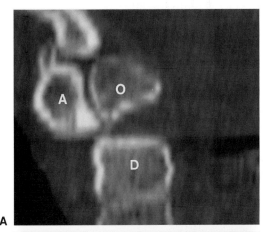

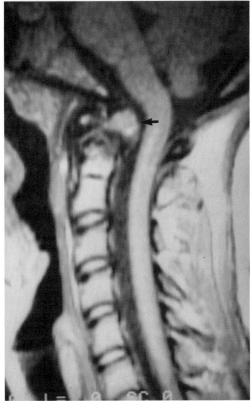

FIG. 4-25. Down syndrome and craniocervical instability. A 14-year-old girl with Down syndrome. **A:** Sagittally reformatted CT shows a hypoplastic dens *(D)*, os odontoideum *(O)*, and hypertrophied anterior arch of the atlas *(A)*. **B:** Sagittal T1 MRI. Atlantoaxial subluxation and extrinsic compression of the cervicomedullary spinal cord *(arrow)* by the os odontoideum are demonstrated.

including absence, can also be acquired (77). Aplasia of the odontoid process is rare; when present, there is severe atlantoaxial dislocation. In hypoplasia of the odontoid process, the tip of the short dens lies just above the C1–2 articulation. The os odontoideum may either be a remnant of the proatlas or may be caused by hypertrophy of the ossiculum terminale. There is usually associated hypoplasia of the dens with the os odontoideum located near its tip or at the basion (Fig. 4-

25). The ossiculum terminale is often round, has a thick cortex, and lacks a normal fusion line (21). There is hypertrophy of the anterior arch of C1 and hypoplasia or midline clefting of the posterior arch. Atlantoaxial or occipitoaxial instability commonly occurs.

Odontoid abnormalities may be idiopathic but are often important components of skeletal dysplasias such as Morquio syndrome, Down syndrome, spondyloepiphyseal dysplasia, and Klippel-Feil anomaly. Odontoid abnormalities are often detected after trauma but should not be confused with fracture (75,78).

Craniocervical Instability

Craniocervical instability includes atlantoaxial instability, atlantooccipital instability, and rotatory atlantoaxial displacements. Atlantoaxial instability results from absence or insufficiency of the transverse ligament holding the odontoid close to the anterior arch of C1 (79). Subluxation may occur in the rotary or anteroposterior directions. As previously noted, neither the predental distance should be increased nor the vertebral canal distance decreased; abnormal distances, particularly if associated with neurologic symptoms or signs, are indications for MRI (55). Severe instability may require surgical stabilization. Atlantoaxial instability and atlantooccipital instability are commonly found in patients with Down syndrome (see Figs. 4-18 and 4-25) (13,80–82). The association of hypoplasia of the posterior arch of C1 and atlantoaxial instability in Down syndrome increases the likelihood of spinal cord injury and necessitates MRI (55,82). Other common causes of atlantoaxial instability are rheumatoid arthritis and trauma.

Rotary atlantoaxial displacement is a common cause of torticollis. It may be associated with trauma, infection, or skeletal dysplasia or may be spontaneous (7). Evaluation is done using plain films, one lateral to the skull and one lateral to the cervical spine. The extent of displacement is confirmed by axial CT images (Fig. 4-26) (7,83).

Spinal Dysraphism

Spinal dysraphism is a spectrum of disorders in which there is defective midline closure of neural, bony, and other mesenchymal tissues. There is separation of the pedicles and laminae and disorganization of spinal elements (2). This group of spinal column and neuraxis malformations is the most common congenital central nervous system abnormality (1,2,13,84,85). Spina bifida aperta (cystica) is the term for open neurulation defects in which neural tissue is exposed through a dorsal bony spinal and cutaneous defect (Table 4-8). These include myelocele, myelomeningocele, hydromyelia, Chiari II malformation, hemimyelocele, myeloschisis, and cranioschisis (73). Occult spinal dysraphism, in which the myelodysplasia lies deep to intact skin, includes dermal sinus, lipoma, diastematomyelia, split-notochord syndrome,

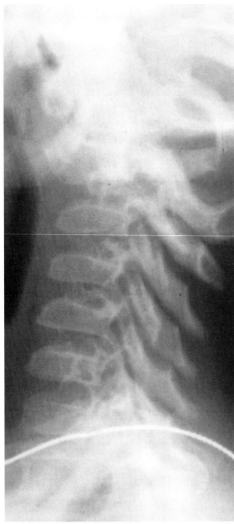

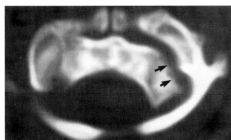

FIG. 4-26. Rotary atlantoaxial subluxation. A 5-year-old girl with skeletal dysplasia. **A:** Lateral radiograph. Platyspondyly of the mid-to-lower cervical segments and poor visualization of the craniocervical junction because of torticollis. **B:** Axial CT. Hypoplastic dens, bifid anterior and posterior arches of C1, and rotary articular offset on the left of the atlas relative to the axis *(arrows).*

neurenteric fistula, lipomyelomeningocele, and tethered cord syndrome (Table 4-8) (1,2,86).

Patients with spinal dysraphism almost always have cutaneous stigmata, including exteriorized placodes associated with the myelocele and myelomeningocele or skin-covered lesions such as subcutaneous lipoma, hairy patch (hyper-

trichosis), nevus, hemangioma, or sinus tract. Plain films may show anomalous formation or segmentation, congenital scoliosis or kyphosis, canal widening, and spinolaminal defects (Fig. 4-27). CT is extremely helpful for preoperative definition of bony anomalies. Sonography is useful for screening the fetus and young infant (87,88); it is also used for intraoperative surgical guidance (89). MRI is the definitive modality for diagnosis, surgical planning, and follow-up (90,91). Some of the more important aspects of the various entities in the spectrum of spinal dysraphism will be discussed separately.

Myelomeningocele and Meningocele

Myelomeningocele and meningocele, two of the more common abnormalities of the spinal cord and meninges, are the result of nondisjunction of the cutaneous ectoderm from the neural ectoderm and failure of neural tube closure. *Meningocele* is herniation of distended spinal meninges but not neural tissue through a dysraphic spine. In *myelomeningocele*, portions of the spinal cord and nerve roots lie within the sac. Myelomeningocele (including myelocele) (85%) is a much more common form of spina bifida cystica than meningocele (15%). If only the placode is at the skin surface, the anomaly is referred to as a *myelocele*. These abnormalities commonly occur at the lumbar and sacral levels (Fig. 4-28);

TABLE 4-8. *Spinal dysraphism*

Spina bifida aperta (open spinal dysraphism)
    Myeloschisis
    Cranioschisis
    Dorsal meningocele
    Myelomeningocele[a]
    Myelocele
    Hemimyelocele
    Chiari II malformation[a]
    Hydromyelia
Spina bifida occulta (occult spinal dysraphism)
    Lipomyelomeningocele
    Lipoma[a]
    Congenital dermal sinus[a]
    Tethered-cord syndrome[a]
    Myelocystocele
    Meningocele
        Anterior
        Lateral
    Split-notochord syndrome
        Neurenteric cyst
        Diastematomyelia
        Neurenteric fistula
Associations
    Hydromyelia-hydrobulbia
    Hemimyelocele
    Hemimyelomeningocele
    Developmental tumor[a]
    Hydrocephalus[a]
    Chiari II malformation[a]
    Brainstem compression and dysfunction[a]

[a] More common.

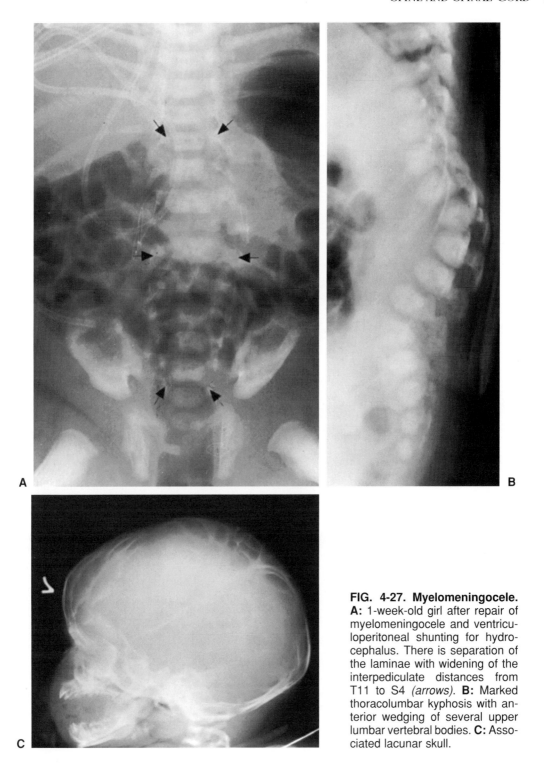

**FIG. 4-27. Myelomeningocele.
A:** 1-week-old girl after repair of
myelomeningocele and ventriculoperitoneal shunting for hydrocephalus. There is separation of
the laminae with widening of the
interpediculate distances from
T11 to S4 *(arrows).* **B:** Marked
thoracolumbar kyphosis with anterior wedging of several upper
lumbar vertebral bodies. **C:** Associated lacunar skull.

70% are below the level of L2 (2). They may also occur in
the lower thoracic spine and, rarely, in the cervical region.
Involvement at several separate levels is rare.

Myelomeningocele, meningocele, and myelocele are
readily apparent on physical examination. Associated abnormalities include rib anomalies, lacunar skull (see Fig. 4-
27C), Chiari II malformation, segmentation anomalies, kyphoscoliosis, club foot, hip dislocation, hydronephrosis with

reflux, anorectal malformation, congenital heart disease, and
sacral agenesis (2,92,93). Occasionally, there is an associated diastematomyelia (hemimyelomeningocele) and dermal
sinus (94).

Radiographs show widening of the spinal canal and interpediculate distances, usually at four to six vertebral levels
(see Fig. 4-27A). There may be a number of associated abnormalities of the bony spine, including hemivertebrae, ab-

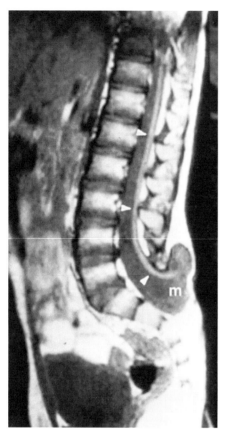

FIG. 4-28. Myelomeningocele. Sagittal T1 MRI shows a low-lying, tethered spinal cord *(arrowheads)* extending posteriorly to a placode. Meningocele *(m)* is at the L5–S1 level.

sent vertebral bodies, fused vertebral bodies, fused pedicles, posterior arch fusions, and posterior arch distortions. Occasionally, the neural arch structures are so deformed that a bony density mimicking diastematomyelia is seen overlying the widened spinal canal in the AP projection. There may also be scoliosis due to vertebral abnormalities. At least 25% of thoracolumbar and lumbar spinal dysraphism is associated with a fixed kyphosis (see Fig. 4-27B). This kyphosis is associated with a classic wedge shape of the vertebral bodies on lateral radiographs and is presumably due to more rapid growth of neuroectodermal tissue in the open primitive neural tube than of mesodermal tissue forming the vertebral bodies.

MRI defines the abnormality precisely. It may also show widening of the spinal cord due to hydromyelia (95). Lipomas may coexist with meningocele. Intraabdominal structures such as the aorta and kidneys are frequently displaced posteriorly and toward the midline; this displacement of the kidneys produces a ''pseudo-horseshoe'' kidney appearance. The Chiari II malformation is rarely present in patients with meningocele but is essentially always associated with myelomeningocele and myelocele. Hydrocephalus occurs in 60–90% of these patients.

The dysraphic defect is usually closed surgically within 24–48 hours of birth. Hydrocephalus is shunted early. Patients may subsequently be referred for neuroimaging to evaluate changes in neurologic status due to the Chiari II malformation and associated anomalies, the sequelae of myelomeningocele closure, or hydrocephalus and its shunting (Fig. 4-29; Table 4-9). Imaging of the Chiari II malformation

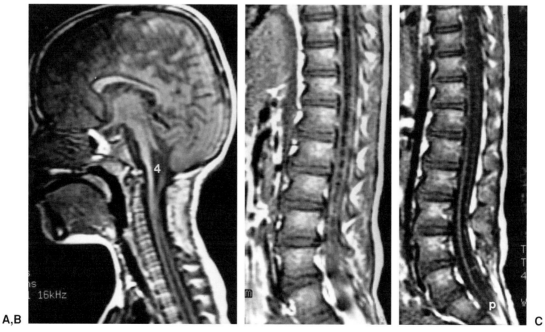

FIG. 4-29. Chiari II malformation with syringohydromyelia. An 8-year-old girl after repair of a myelomeningocele. Sagittal T1 MRI **(A)** demonstrates Chiari II malformation with dilated fourth ventricle *(4)* and **(B)** an intramedullary low intensity expansion extending the entire length of the spine down to **(C)** the sacral placode *(p)*.

TABLE 4-9. *Complications of spinal dysraphism*

Hydromyelia-hydrobulbia
Syringohydromyelia
Cord ischemia
Cord compression
Cord constriction
Progressive kyphoscoliosis
Scarring and retethering at operative site[a]
Dural sac stenosis[a]
Implant dermoid-epidermoid
Isolated (trapped, encysted) fourth ventricle
Hydrocephalus
Brainstem compression and dysfunction[a]
Shunt malfunction
Arachnoid cyst

[a] More common.

has been presented in detail in Chapter 2. Associations and complications of spinal dysraphism include hydrocephalus, shunt malfunction, encystment of the fourth ventricle, hydrosyringomyelia, brainstem compression or dysfunction, cervical cord compression or constriction, hemimyelocele or hemimyelomeningocele, lipoma, dermoid or epidermoid, arachnoid cyst, scarring and retethering at the operative site, dural sac stenosis, progressive scoliosis, and cord ischemia and infarction (Tables 4-8 and 4-9) (90,96–99).

Hydrosyringomyelia

Hydromyelia refers to dilatation of the central canal of the spinal cord. Syringomyelia refers to a cavity within the spinal cord. However, the term hydrosyringomyelia is commonly used because hydromyelia and syringomyelia may be indistinguishable and may coexist (13,100). Hydrosyringomyelia is most commonly associated with the Chiari malformations (see Fig. 4-29), spinal dysraphism, and craniocervical anomalies (100–102). MRI is the best modality for evaluation and may demonstrate focal, segmental, or total involvement of the cord (102–104). MRI shows intramedullary CSF intensities, sometimes sacculated or septated. The cord may be diffusely enlarged. An intramedullary syrinx or cyst may also occur with a spinal cord neoplasm or develop after trauma, infection, or arachnoiditis.

Lipomyelomeningocele

Lipomyelomeningocele, the most common of the occult myelodysplasias, represents from 20% to 50% of cases (1,105–108). Affected children may be asymptomatic, present with a subcutaneous mass; or have motor or sensory loss, bladder dysfunction, or orthopedic deformities of the legs or feet. Lipomyeloceles and lipomyelomeningoceles probably result from faulty disjunction, as do myeloceles and myelomeningoceles (1,106). However, the skin is intact and a lipoma is present. The lipoma typically extends from the in-

completely fused cord caudally or dorsally through a dural and bony defect to become continuous with the subcutaneous fat (Fig. 4-30). The tip of the conus medullaris is usually located below L3. Lipomyeloceles are within the vertebral canal, and lipomyelomeningoceles have expansion of the subarachnoid space and protrude beyond the vertebral canal. In both, the vertebral canal is usually enlarged. Spina bifida or segmentation anomalies of the vertebral column may be present (109). MRI demonstrates the relationship of the T1-hyperintense lipoma and the neural elements for surgical planning (Fig. 4-30). There may be associated thickening of the filum or a filar lipoma (Fig. 4-31).

Congenital Dermal Sinus

A congenital dermal sinus is an epithelial tract that extends from the skin surface to the deeper tissues (1,2,13). These abnormalities result from incomplete disjunction of the cutaneous ectoderm from neuroectoderm during neurulation (1). Dermal sinuses most commonly occur in the lumbosacral or cervicooccipital regions (110). There is often a midline dimple or ostium with hairy nevus, hemangioma, or hyperpigmented patch. The sinus extends from the skin through the deeper tissues to enter the spinal canal in as many as two thirds of cases (1). The sinus may extend to the dura, penetrate the dura and terminate in the subarachnoid space, or insert into the filum terminale or conus medullaris. Approximately 50% of sinuses end in a dermoid, epidermoid, or lipoma (111,112). These patients often present with infection secondary to meningitis or with an abscess in the vertebral canal (113,114). The dermal sinus is usually hypointense on MRI (Fig. 4-32). Associated dermoid or epidermoid tumors may also be hypointense to CSF on MRI sequences. Contrast enhancement is helpful for better delineation if infection is present (Fig. 4-33) (115,116).

Tethered Cord Syndrome

The tethered cord syndrome is a clinical and radiologic entity in which neurologic symptoms are due to an abnormally low position of the spinal cord. This tethering of the cord may be primary (tethered or tight filum terminale, tethered conus) (117), secondary to other dysraphic entities (diastematomyelia, internal meningocele, neurenteric cyst, dermoid cyst, lipomeningocele) and after meningomyelocele repair (99). Tethering of the cord either secondary to the dysraphic state or primary, leads to clinical abnormalities: neurologic symptoms (gait disturbance, weakness, muscle atrophy, bowel or bladder dysfunction), orthopedic symptoms (scoliosis, foot deformities, painful or numb lower extremities, low back pain), or urologic symptoms (urinary incontinence, recurrent urinary tract infection) (117). External signs of spinal dysraphism, including hypertrichosis, subcutaneous lipoma, dermoid, and sinus tract, are present in approximately 50% of patients (117). Plain radiographs

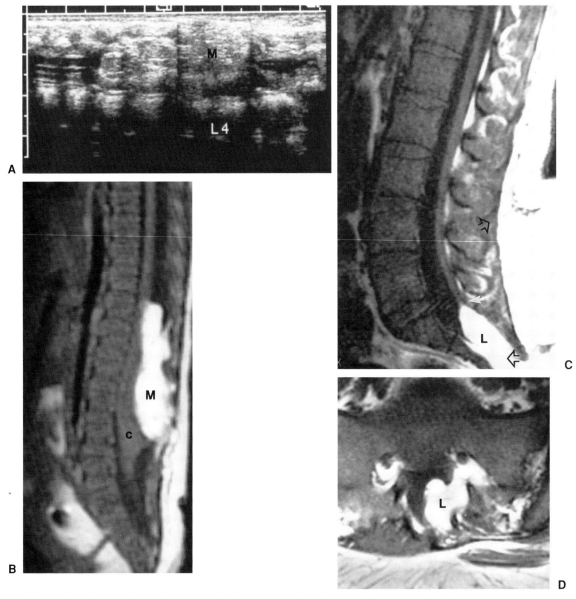

FIG. 4-30. Lipomyelomeningocele. A, B: A 3-month-old infant. Ultrasound **(A)** demonstrates echogenic intradural mass *(M)*. Sagittal T1-weighted MRI **(B)** shows low conus *(c)* and dorsal high-intensity mass *(M)*. **C, D:** A 20-year-old woman. Sagittal **(C)** and axial **(D)** T1-weighted MRI. Low position of the spinal cord with placode-like termination of the conus medullaris *(arrow)*, which is attached to a high-intensity intraspinal lipoma *(L)*. The lipoma is continuous with dorsal subcutaneous fat *(open arrows)*.

may show only spina bifida occulta. If the tethered cord is due to other dysraphic states (meningomyelocele, lipomyelocele, diastematomyelia), radiologic features of these particular entities will be present.

A definitive diagnosis depends on demonstration of a low position of the conus (below the middle of the body of L2) associated with a short, thick filum terminale (117–119). This low position may result from incomplete differentiation and failure of involution of the caudal neural tube or from failure of lengthening of the nerve fibers that form the filum (1). The thickening of the filum (diameter greater than 2 mm at the L5 or S1 level) is usually fibrous but may be fatty or

cystic. The tethered cord syndrome is commonly associated with other types of spinal dysraphism such as a lipomyelomeningocele (see Fig. 4-31), dermal sinus (see Fig. 4-32), and diastematomyelia (Fig. 4-34). Occasionally, the thickened filum terminates in a developmental tumor such as a lipoma, dermoid, or epidermoid (73). The filar abnormality is best demonstrated by MRI.

The goal of neurosurgery is removal of the cause of tethering in order to prevent progression of symptoms. Appropriate surgical therapy of the dysraphic state is performed in patients with secondary tethered cord syndrome. In those with primary tethered cord syndrome, the thickened filum

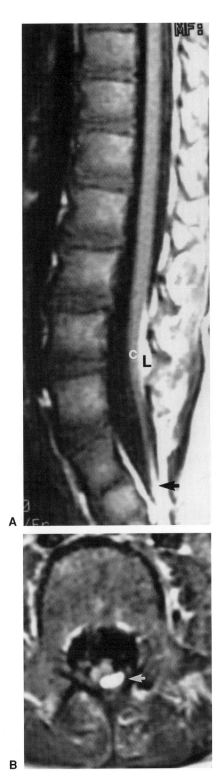

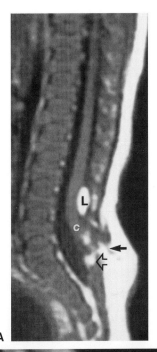

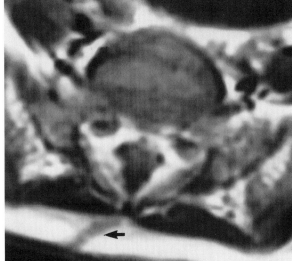

FIG. 4-31. Lipoma and tethered cord. A 9-year-old girl with cloacal exstrophy. **A:** Sagittal T1-weighted MRI. Low placement of conus medullaris *(c),* dorsal high-intensity lipomatous mass *(L),* and lipoma of the filum *(arrow).* **B:** Axial T1 MRI confirms the dorsal lipoma *(arrow).*

FIG. 4-32. Dermal sinus with lipoma. A 1-month-old boy. Sagittal **(A)** and axial **(B)** T1-weighted MRI. A hypointense dermal sinus tract *(closed arrows)* extends from the skin to attach to a low conus medullaris *(c).* High-intensity dorsal *(L)* and caudal *(open arrow)* lipomas are shown.

terminale is transected and the conus medullaris freed from surrounding adhesions.

Myelocystocele

Myelocystocele is the least common type of occult myelodysplasia associated with posterior spina bifida (120,121). Myelocystoceles usually occur at the lumbosacral level but occasionally at the cervical level. They may be associated with other malformations of caudal cell mass origin. The "terminal" myelocystocele consists of hydromyelia and a dilated terminal ventricle of the conus-placode which is continuous with a dorsal, ependymal-lined cyst within or adjacent to a meningocele (Fig. 4-35) (1,13). There is sometimes a lipomatous component (lipomyelocystocele).

Anterior and Lateral Meningoceles

Anterior sacral or presacral meningoceles may be associated with dysraphic lumbosacral defects and anorectal or urogenital anomalies in the caudal dysplasia spectrum (Fig. 4-36). Presacral meningoceles extending through the sacral foramina may occur in neurofibromatosis (NF-1) (122–124). In the cervical, thoracic, and lumbar regions, anterior meningocele is considered an anomaly in the

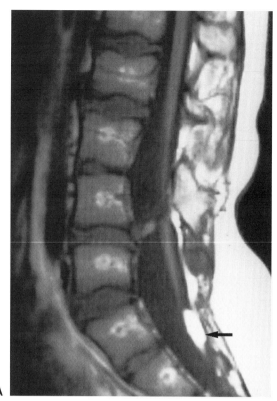

A

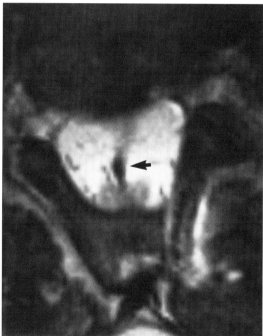

B

FIG. 4-34. Diastematomyelia and filar lipoma. A 20-year-old woman with hairy patch on her lower back. **A:** Sagittal T1-weighted MRI. Spinal cord is tethered in a low position by a high-intensity filar lipoma *(arrow)* and bony septum. **B:** Axial T2-weighted MRI. The bony septum *(arrow)* divides the spinal cord into two hemicords.

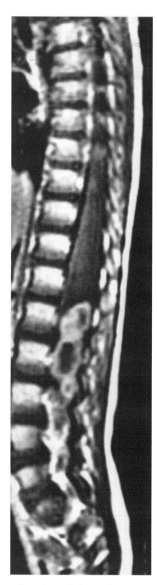

FIG. 4-33. Complication of dermal sinus. An 18-month-old girl with fever and difficulty walking. Gadolinium-enhanced sagittal T1-weighted MRI shows an edematous, low-placed spinal cord. The ring-enhancing masses are intradural abscesses.

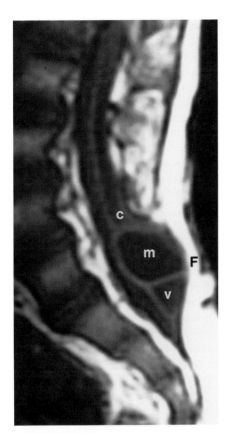

FIG. 4-35. Myelocystocele. A 5-year-old girl. Sagittal T1-weighted MRI shows low placement of spinal cord *(c)* with hydromyelia, dilated terminal ventricle *(v)*, and large meningocele sac *(m)* adherent to dorsal subcutaneous fat *(F)*.

neurenteric spectrum. Lateral meningoceles extending through the intervertebral foramina may be seen in NF-1 and Marfan syndrome (125).

Split Notochord Syndrome

The occurrence of posterior spina bifida cystica (meningocele, myelomeningocele) and anterior spina bifida (neurenteric fistula) is well recognized. Occasionally, there are complete clefts of the vertebral column with combined anterior and posterior spina bifida. This has been called the split notochord syndrome and is due to abnormal separation of the endoderm and ectoderm during the formation of the notochord (126–128). The malformation results from complete or partial failure of obliteration of the primitive neurenteric (ectodermal-endodermal) connection (13). The most severe form of this anomaly is the dorsal enteric fistula, the fistula extending from the gut through the prevertebral soft tissues, vertebral bodies, meninges, spinal cord, and posterior elements to the skin surface (127,128). Any part of such a fistula may become obliterated; the components of the split notochord syndrome may include a dorsal enteric sinus, dorsal enterogenous cyst, or dorsal enteric diverticulum. Severe malformations of the central nervous system and gastrointes-

tinal tract are usually associated with the complete clefts of the split notochord syndrome. Most cases involve the spine above the diaphragm; the entity is rare in the lumbosacral spine.

Plain films show a complete defect of the bony spine involving the posterior neural arches as well as the anterior vertebral bodies. This total rachischisis may be associated with dorsal herniation of the gastrointestinal tract into the defect, a neurenteric cyst extending anteriorly, hamartomas of the spine or deformed extremities (52).

Neurenteric Cyst. A neurenteric cyst is one component of the split notochord spectrum (1,126). Associated vertebral segmentation anomalies include butterfly vertebrae, hemivertebrae, and block vertebrae (13). A classic plain film finding is that of a posterior mediastinal mass associated with vertebral segmentation anomalies. Neurenteric cysts usually arise in the lower cervical or thoracic region. The intraspinal lesions are usually intradural but extramedullary. The cyst may be lined by gastrointestinal or respiratory epithelium. The cyst fluid may be similar in MRI intensity to CSF (see Fig. 4-23) or may be mucoid and appear hyperintense on T1-weighted MRI (129–131).

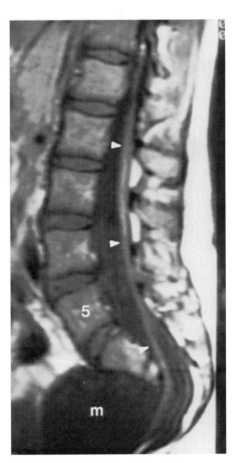

FIG. 4-36. Presacral meningocele. Sagittal T1-weighted MRI demonstrates sacral hypoplasia with a presacral CSF-hypointensity meningocele *(m)*. The low-lying, tethered spinal cord *(arrowheads)* extends anteriorly to the meningocele sac.

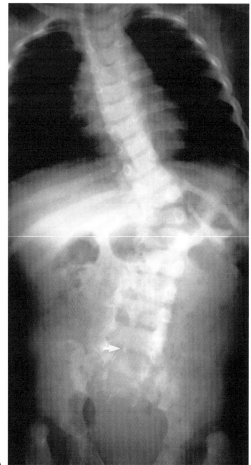

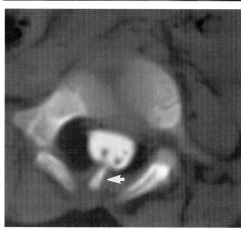

FIG. 4-37. Diastematomyelia. A 3-year-old girl with scoliosis. **A:** Conventional radiography. Thoracolumbar scoliosis is convex to the left and associated with vertebral body segmentation anomalies. A small bony spicule *(arrow)* is identified at the L5–S1 level. Note widening of the lumbar interpediculate distances. **B:** Axial CT myelogram. Two hemicords are identified within the opacified dural sac. A component of the bony spur is seen posteriorly *(arrow)*.

Diastematomyelia. Diastematomyelia is the most common anomaly in the split notochord spectrum (1,13, 103,132). It consists of sagittal clefting of the cord into symmetric or asymmetric hemicords, with each half having the dorsal and ventral nerve roots for that side (133). In 50–60% of cases, the hemicords are contained in a single dural sac (134,135). In the remaining cases, the split is traversed by a septum, and at that level each hemicord has its own pial, arachnoid, and dural sheath. The septum may be composed of bony, cartilaginous, fibrous, vascular, or neuroglial tissue. The hemicords usually join above and below the cleft (132,135,136). The malformation is more common in females, usually occurs in the lumbar or thoracolumbar region, and is associated with cutaneous stigmata overlying the spine. Plain films may show spina bifida, intersegmental laminar fusion, anomalies of the vertebral bodies, and kyphoscoliosis (Fig. 4-37). There is local widening of the vertebral canal (interpediculate distances) and interspace narrowing. For definition of the septum, axial spin-echo T2-weighted MRI, axial T2* gradient echo MRI, CT, or CTM is often necessary (see Figs. 4-34 and 4-37). Other commonly associated anomalies include a thickened filum, developmental tumor (lipoma, dermoid-epidermoid), hydromyelia, and tethering bands (meningocele manque) (94, 137,138).

Caudal Dysplasia Spectrum

Caudal dysplasia is a spectrum of malformations of caudal cell mass origin that includes lumbosacral, anorectal, urogenital, and lower limb anomalies (1,2,13,139–141). The caudal regression syndrome, part of this spectrum, consists of one or more of the following: fusion of the lower extremities (sirenomelia), lumbosacral agenesis, anal atresia, abnormal genitalia, renal aplasia, and pulmonary hypoplasia. The syndrome may be associated with Potter syndrome. There is an increased incidence in infants of diabetic mothers. The spinal anomalies range from partial sacral agenesis to total agenesis of the lumbar and sacral vertebrae (Fig. 4-38) (142,143). MRI demonstrates a high-positioned and blunted or wedge-shaped conus termination (Fig. 4-39) (140). There is stenosis of the spinal canal and the dural sac. Other abnormalities that may be seen include anterior (presacral) meningocele (see Fig. 4-36), cord tethering with filar thickening or developmental tumor, lipomyelomeningocele, and myelocystocele (see Fig. 4-35). In children with urogenital and anorectal malformations such as high imperforate anus, cloacal malformation, and cloacal exstrophy, there is a high prevalence of spinal dysraphism (Fig. 4-39; see Chapter 9) (143,144).

Infection

Infections of the spine may involve the vertebral body, intervertebral disc, paravertebral soft tissues, epidural space, leptomeninges, or spinal cord. Inflammatory processes arising during childhood include vertebral osteomyelitis, sacro-

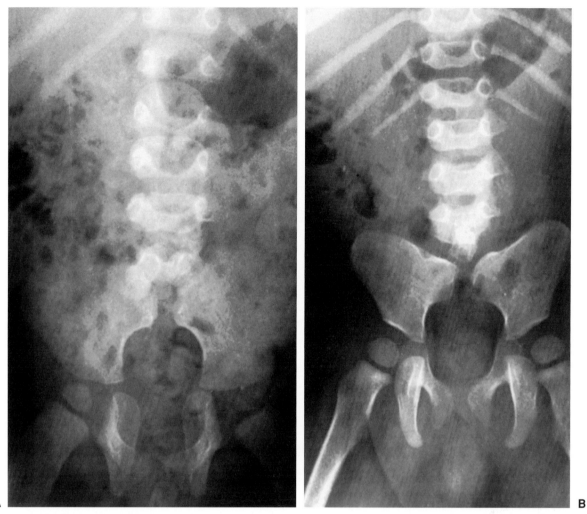

A

B

FIG. 4-38. Sacral agenesis. A: There is total sacral agenesis, with the ilia articulating with the sides of L5. **B:** There is agenesis of the sacrum as well as of L4 and L5. The caudal portion of L3 articulates with an iliac arthrosis.

iliac pyarthrosis, discitis, epidural abscess, meningitis, arachnoiditis, myelitis, and spinal cord abscess.

Osteomyelitis

In infants and children, osteomyelitis of the spine is less common in the spine than in the long bones. Possible infectious organisms include bacterial, tuberculosis, coccidioidomycosis, blastomycosis, and actinomycosis (145). Infection usually begins in the subchondral bone and leads to bony destruction, cortical penetration, and involvement of the intervertebral disc. A decrease in the vertical height of the vertebral body as well as narrowing of the intervertebral disc space may occur, especially the latter. Extension into the soft tissues frequently produces a paravertebral mass. Eventually, a bony fusion of vertebral bodies may occur. Calcification in a paraspinal mass is particularly common with tuberculous vertebral osteomyelitis, and the disc may be spared.

Osteomyelitis may be difficult to differentiate from leukemia-lymphoma or metastatic disease. The latter entities usually affect several noncontiguous vertebral bodies, do not involve the disc space, and may not produce a paraspinal mass.

Occasionally, infection involves the pedicles and posterior neural arches. There may be a sclerotic or lytic reaction to osteomyelitis. If there is sclerosis of a pedicle (Fig. 4-40), differential diagnostic considerations include osteoid osteoma, osteoblastoma, Brodie abscess, and bony reaction opposite a defect in the contralateral posterior spinal elements.

Sacroiliac Pyarthrosis

Pyogenic arthritis of the sacroiliac joint is uncommon, usually occurs during late childhood, is difficult to diagnose, and may result in joint ankylosis. The most frequently responsible organism is *Staphylococcus aureus*. Involvement is either primary (hematogenous) or extends from osteomye-

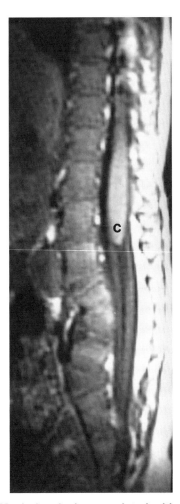

FIG. 4-39. Myelodysplasia associated with high imperforate anus. A 1-year-old girl with anorectal malformation. Sagittal T1 MRI demonstrates sacral dysgenesis, congenital lumbar kyphosis, lumbosacral dural sac stenosis, and blunted, wedge-shaped hypoplasia of the caudal spinal cord (c).

litis of the adjacent sacrum or ilium (146). This infection is more common in boys and has a subacute onset in at least two thirds of cases (147). The history and physical findings are frequently nonspecific, and the condition is often not considered for several weeks. Symptoms include low back pain, hip discomfort, limp, and lower limb pain (146).

Radiographs of the sacroiliac joints are negative in two thirds of patients at the time of diagnosis. Subsequent radiographic changes include widening of the joint space, sclerosis or lytic destruction of adjacent bony margins, and, much later, synostosis. Bone scintigraphy shows increased activity at the affected joint; this examination may be positive as early as 2 days after the onset of symptoms (147), with strikingly increased accumulation of bone-seeking radionuclide at the abnormal joint. Fluoroscopically guided joint aspiration and culture are performed to establish the specific etiologic agent, which is usually *S. aureus*. Scintigraphy allows the delay in diagnosis to be reduced from 4.8 weeks to 1.7 weeks (146).

Discitis

Discitis is an inflammatory process of the intervertebral disc space. Although the exact etiology is unknown, it is considered by most to be a low-grade viral or bacterial infection (148). There is probably a spectrum of disorders, including nonspecific discitis, intervertebral disc space infection, and vertebral osteomyelitis with a proven bacterial etiology. The lumbar region is frequently involved, particularly in young children. The most common site is L3–4 or L2–3 with other common sites being L1–2, L4–5, and L5–S1. The lower thoracic region may occasionally be involved, particularly in teenagers.

Discitis occurs most frequently in children from 6 months to 4 years of age; there is a second peak at age 10–14 years (149). The symptoms are highly variable. Children tend to refer pain away from the primary anatomic site of location; this may make the diagnosis extremely difficult. Symptoms and signs include fever, irritability, abdominal pain, back pain, hip pain, knee pain, limp, malaise, and refusal to walk or sit up. The discomfort is frequently decreased when the patient is lying flat. There is usually a mild leukocytosis and elevated erythrocyte sedimentation rate. There may be point tenderness over the spine.

At first radiographs of the spine are normal. Bone scintigraphy shows increased uptake in the vertebral bodies on each side of the involved disc space and may be positive as early as 1–2 days after the onset of symptoms (Fig. 4-41A) (5,149).

Radiographic evaluation of the spine several weeks after the onset of symptoms shows narrowing of the intervertebral disc space and irregularity and erosions of the adjacent vertebral body endplates. The shortest interval between the onset of symptoms and plain film changes has been 12 days (150). Follow-up radiographs after several weeks or months show persistent narrowing of the intervertebral disc space and sclerosis of adjacent vertebral bodies (Fig. 4-42). Characteristic MRI findings include disc space narrowing with vertebral T1 hypointensity and T2 hyperintensity reflecting marrow edema (Fig. 4-41B) (150–154). There may be contrast enhancement of the disc and adjacent vertebral body (154). There is frequently poor delineation of the involved intervertebral disc (155). There may be disc extrusion and the formation of an epidural or paraspinal abscess (13).

Cultures of blood or biopsy material are positive in one third to one half of patients (149). The organism is almost always *S. aureus*. There is controversy regarding the proper treatment of discitis. Wenger et al. recommended bed rest and intravenous antibiotic therapy after confirmation of the diagnosis by blood cultures, although antibiotics are continued even if blood cultures are negative (149,156). Others believe that an open surgical or percutaneous needle biopsy of the abnormal disc should be obtained for culture and sensitivity testing prior to the institution of antibiotic therapy. There is usually a decrease in symptoms within 2–3 days

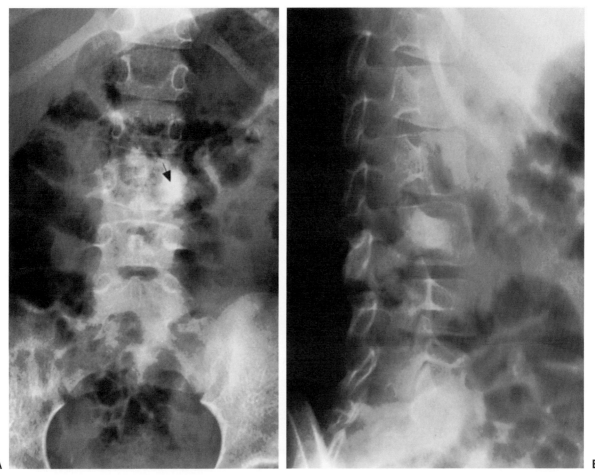

FIG. 4-40. Chronic osteomyelitis. A 5-year-old girl with a 7-month history of low back pain. **A:** There is sclerosis of the pedicle of L3 on the left *(arrow)*. **B:** Left posterior oblique view demonstrates that the sclerosis also involves the superior articulating facet, pars interarticularis, inferior articulating facet, and left lamina.

in response to antibiotic therapy. This supports the impression that the disorder usually has a bacterial etiology (149). Immobilization is usually not advocated for the young child who has responded to antibiotics and who moves comfortably. However, immobilization may be required in older children, who tend to have more protracted symptoms (149).

Epidural Abscess

Epidural abscess, although uncommon in childhood, may arise from hematogenous spread or by direct extension, usually from discitis or osteomyelitis (157). Any level of the spine may be affected. The most common organism is *S. aureus* (158). MRI, the imaging modality of choice, demonstrates an extradural soft-tissue mass that may extend over several segments. The collection is often T1-isointense or hypointense and T2-hyperintense. Diffuse homogeneous enhancement may occur during the phlegmon stage. An enhancing rim surrounding a low-signal collection indicates an abscess with a necrotic center

(159). Infection may be present in an adjacent disc or vertebral body (see Fig. 4-41B).

Meningitis

Meningitis may be caused by bacterial, fungal, viral, or parasitic organisms. However, most cases are bacterial. MRI may demonstrate gadolinium enhancement of the meninges, spinal cord, or nerve roots; the enhancement may be linear or nodular (160).

Arachnoiditis

Arachnoiditis may follow infection, trauma, nontraumatic subarachnoid hemorrhage, intraspinal anesthetic or myelographic agents, and surgery. MRI shows clumping and thickening of the nerve roots, often with mild enhancement. Occasionally there is associated dural or meningeal thickening, with the clumped nerve roots appearing as intradural, adher-

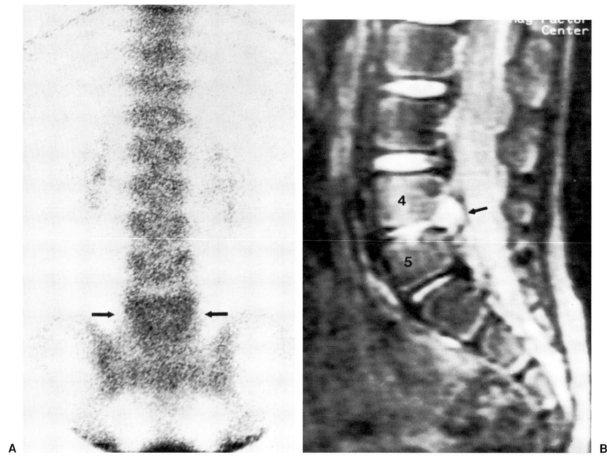

FIG. 4-41. Discitis. A: Posterior bone scintigraphy shows increased uptake *(arrows)* at the L4–5 level. **B:** Sagittal T2-weighted MRI shows increased signal intensity within the L4 and L5 vertebral bodies, decreased height of the L4–5 disc, and a hyperintense epidural collection *(arrow)* presumably due to posterior disc extrusion and/or an epidural abscess.

ent soft-tissue masses (161). Syringohydromyelia or arachnoid cysts may also be present.

Myelitis

Myelitis refers to inflammatory disease of the spinal cord. It may be an active viral infection or a sequela to a viral infection. Viruses associated with myelitis include herpes, coxsackie, polio, and human immunodeficiency virus (HIV). It may also occur after vaccination or after a viral infection as in acute disseminated encephalomyelitis (ADEM) (13). In acquired immunodeficiency syndrome (AIDS)-related myelopathy there is a vacuolar myelopathy and demyelination of the posterior and lateral columns of the spinal cord (162). Other rare causes of acute myelopathy in childhood include autoimmune demyelination related to multiple sclerosis or systemic lupus erythematosus; demyelination may also be a complication of systemic malignancy. *Devic syndrome* is the association of transverse myelitis with optic neuritis. Myelitis can also occur after irradiation. MRI find-

ings in myelitis include intramedullary T2 hyperintensity, cord expansion, and contrast enhancement (Fig. 4-43) (163).

Spinal Cord Abscess

Spinal cord abscess is rare. However, it may occur by direct extension, spread from a dermal sinus, or a hematogenous, or lymphatic spread. It may occur in the immunosuppressed child and is often associated with meningitis and myelopathy (13).

Neoplasms of the Bony Spine

Primary and secondary neoplasms of the bony spine are rare in children. Secondary neoplasms that may involve the spine include leukemia-lymphoma, neuroblastoma, soft-tissue sarcoma, carcinoma, and teratoma (2). Primary neoplasms of the spine are even less common than secondary neoplasms. Differential diagnostic considerations of a pri-

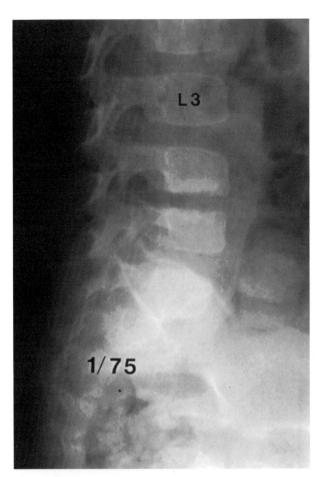

FIG. 4-42. Healed discitis. Lateral radiograph 8 months after acute discitis. There is narrowing of the L4–5 disc space with vertebral endplate sclerosis and irregularity.

mary neoplasm of the vertebral column in a child include osteoid osteoma, osteoblastoma, aneurysmal bone cyst, giant cell tumor, chordoma, osteogenic sarcoma, Ewing sarcoma, and osteochondroma (2,160).

Osteoid Osteoma

Osteoid osteoma is a benign process of unknown etiology that contains an osteoid matrix and a stroma of loose vascular connective tissue (164,165). This osteoid nidus may contain calcification. No convincing histologic or microbiologic evidence of infection has been found in osteoid osteomas.

Children with osteoid osteoma of the spine tend to present with backache that is worse at night and is relieved by small doses of aspirin, mild scoliosis due to paravertebral muscle spasm, and localized vertebral or paravertebral tenderness (166). The age range is 3 years and up. Most affected children are 10–12 years old at the time of diagnosis (166). Pain is seldom present in children with idiopathic scoliosis; if a child presents with painful scoliosis, a vertebral lesion such as osteoid osteoma, osteoblastoma, histiocytosis, osteomye-

litis, or aneurysmal bone cyst should be considered (5,167). The painful scoliosis is due to persistent muscle spasm caused by an osseous lesion of the vertebra or posterior rib. This scoliosis is convex away from the lesion; muscle spasm predominates on the concave side of the curvature (Fig. 4-44).

Radiologic features of osteoid osteoma of the spine are similar to those in other parts of the skeletal system. There is a radiolucent nidus, which may contain calcification, surrounded by sclerotic bone (Fig. 4-44). The nidus usually involves the neural arch or its appendages; involvement of a vertebral body is rare (166). There is usually sclerosis of the pedicle, transverse process, and lamina adjacent to the nidus (Fig. 4-44A). Although bony sclerosis is readily apparent on conventional radiography, the lucent nidus is best visualized by conventional tomography or CT (Fig. 4-44C). There is an associated mild scoliosis with the convexity of the curve away from the lesion. Nuclear scintigraphy, which shows marked uptake of bone tracer agents by osteoid osteoma, is helpful for confirming the diagnosis or clarifying subtle and confusing cases (Fig. 4-44B). The differential diagnostic considerations for sclerosis of the posterior neural arches include osteomyelitis and an acquired defect in the pars interarticularis of the other side (168).

MRI, although rarely used, shows extensive bone mar-

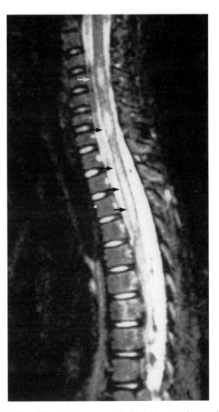

FIG. 4-43. Myelitis. A 4-year-old girl with previous viral infection. Sagittal T2-weighted MRI. Patchy intramedullary hyperintensities in the cervical and thoracic spinal cord *(arrows).*

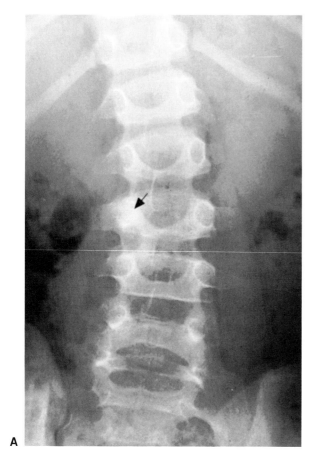

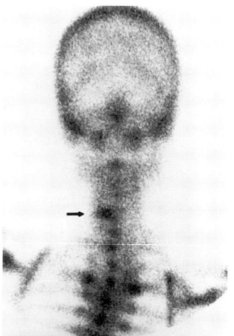

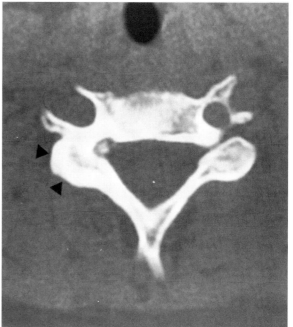

FIG. 4-44. Osteoid osteoma. A: A 5-year-old boy with painful scoliosis. Lumbar scoliosis with convexity to the left. Sclerosis of the right pedicle of L3 is seen *(arrow).* There is an inferior rounded lytic lesion. **B, C:** A 12-year-old boy with neck pain. Anterior bone scintigraphy **(B)** shows increased uptake in right C6 pedicle *(arrow).* Axial CT **(C)** through C6 vertebral body demonstrates a small sclerotic nidus *(arrow)* with a lucent collar and reactive sclerosis *(arrowheads).*

row edema with T1 hypointensity and T2 hyperintensity (169). There is usually contrast enhancement of the nidus.

Although spontaneous regression of osteoid osteoma of the spine has been reported, surgical excision of the nidus is the treatment of choice. Because there may be difficulty identifying the nidus at operation, precise preoperative localization by CT is critical. Intraoperative localization with nuclear scintigraphy may be helpful. Percutaneous removal or cautery of the nidus for definitive therapy is more difficult in the spine than other skeletal sites; CT

is critical in this type of percutaneous therapy. Removal of the nidus relieves pain and either improves or corrects the secondary scoliosis.

Osteoblastoma

Osteoblastoma, also known as giant osteoid osteoma, contains a fibrovascular matrix and sclerotic mesenchyme with giant cells and rich vascularization. Osteoblastoma has a

TABLE 4-10. *Intraspinal masses in infants and children*

Mass	%
Developmental masses	37.5
Dermoid-epidermoid[a]	
Teratoma	
Syringohydromyelia[a]	
Lipoma[a]	
Neurenteric cyst	
Intraspinal meningocele	
Primary neural neoplasms	30.0
Astrocytoma[a]	
Neuroblastoma[a]	
Neurofibroma[a]	
Ependymoma[a]	
Ganglioneuroma	
Miscellaneous intraspinal masses	14.0
Herniated intervertebral disk	
Hematoma	
Abscess	
Posterior slippage of vertebral body	
Other	
Cerebrospinal fluid metastases[a]	10.5
Spine neoplasms	8.0
Metastatic disease[a]	
Primary vertebral neoplasm	

[a] More common.

Source: Modified from Harwood-Nash and Fitz (2).

larger number of giant cells and osteoblasts than osteoid osteoma; moreover, it is usually greater than 2 cm in diameter. Forty percent of all osteoblastomas occur in the spine (170). The majority are solitary and arise in the posterior elements. Plain films and CT usually show an expansile lytic lesion containing flecks of calcification. MRI shows T1 isointensity or hypointensity with heterogeneous signal on T2-weighted imaging because of hemorrhage (171). Treatment is excision; preoperative embolization may be extremely helpful.

Intraspinal Tumors

In children, intraspinal tumors occur much less frequently than intracranial tumors. Clinical signs of an intraspinal mass may be subtle, and plain radiography of the spine frequently is normal. Complete radiologic evaluation requires imaging of the paravertebral region, bony spine, and intraspinal contents. The specific site of an intraspinal mass is difficult to establish without cross-sectional imaging; MRI is the best method for diagnosis, staging, preoperative planning, and follow-up.

Intraspinal mass lesions in children may be developmental, inflammatory, neoplastic, or traumatic. In a few cases it may be difficult to determine the specific anatomic site of a mass within the spinal canal (1,2,13). Intraspinal mass lesions may be classified by their histology (Table 4-10) and by their radiologic location (Table 4-11).

Location of Intraspinal Tumors

Intraspinal mass lesions may be intramedullary (within the spinal cord), intradural-extramedullary (within the dura but outside the spinal cord), or extradural (outside of the

TABLE 4-11. *Location of intraspinal masses in infants and children*

Intramedullary (22%)
Astrocytoma[a]
Ependymoma[a]
Ganglioglioma
Mixed glioma
Hemangioblastoma
Syringohydromyelia[a]
Epidermoid-dermoid[a]
Teratoma[a]
Lipoma
Neurenteric cyst
Intradural-extramedullary (44%)
Cerebrospinal fluid metastatic seeding[a]
Developmental tumors
Dermoid-epidermoid[a]
Lipoma[a]
Teratoma[a]
Hamartoma
Ependymoma[a]
Neurofibroma
Schwannoma
Astrocytoma
Meningeal tumor
Arteriovenous malformation
Arachnoid cyst
Neurenteric cyst
Extradural (34%)
Tumors of neural crest origin
Neuroblastoma[a]
Ganglioneuroblastoma
Ganglioneuroma
Vertebral neoplasm
Osteoid osteoma[a]
Osteoblastoma
Osteochondroma[a]
Aneurysmal bone cyst
Giant cell tumor
Chordoma
Osteogenic sarcoma
Ewing sarcoma
Leukemia-lymphoma[a]
Histiocytosis[a]
Metastases
Sarcoma and carcinoma
Herniated disc[a]
Primitive neuroectodermal tumor[a]
Neurofibroma
Hematoma
Abscess
Dermoid
Teratoma
Lipoma
Posterior slippage of vertebral body

[a] More common.
See Fig. 4-45.

Source: Modified from Harwood-Nash and Fitz (2).

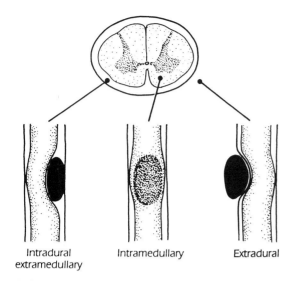

Intradural
extramedullary   Intramedullary   Extradural

FIG. 4-45. Anatomic locations of spinal tumors.

dura); they may involve two or all of these compartments (Fig. 4-45). Fortunately, the last combination is unusual.

Determining whether a mass is extradural or intradural may be difficult. An intradural lesion must be further classified as to whether it originates within the spinal cord (intramedullary) or within the subarachnoid space (intradural-extramedullary). MRI has made this distinction much easier, as its orthogonal images show the spinal cord, subarachnoid space, and dural margins in multiple planes.

Intramedullary Tumors

Intramedullary tumors comprise approximately one fourth of intraspinal neoplasms in childhood (2) (Table 4-11). Astrocytomas constitute approximately 55% of intramedullary tumors in childhood, and ependymomas constitute 25% (2). Intramedullary lesions widen the spinal cord in all projections (172).

Intradural-Extramedullary Tumors

Intradural-extramedullary tumors include tumors of the nerve roots (schwannoma, neurofibroma), meningiomas, ependymomas, dermoids, lipomas, teratomas, and CSF metastases (Table 4-11). At the junction of the conus and cauda equina, the two types of intradural lesions may not be distinguished from each other. Lower lumbar intradural lesions are simply intraarachnoidal, and the differential diagnosis is the same for intradural-extramedullary lesions. If CSF or MRI or contrast material on myelography caps an abnormality, the lesion is intradural-extramedullary (see Fig. 4-45). The half-cap adjacent to a displaced spinal cord is diagnostic of an intradural-extramedullary lesion.

Extradural Tumors

Extradural tumors arise in the spinal column or paraspinal soft tissues and are capped by epidural fat (170). These tu-

mors can extend directly into the vertebral canal or spread by hematogenous, lymphatic, or epidural venous extension. Extradural masses in infants and young children most frequently represent extension of a paravertebral neuroblastoma. Other extradural masses include benign and malignant tumors of the bony spine, sarcoma, carcinoma, herniated disc, ganglioneuroma, neurofibroma, and extensions of some lesions arising in one of the other two intraspinal compartments (see Table 4-11).

Diagnostic Considerations

Intraspinal masses may also be classified according to their histology. They may also be classified by their origin as a developmental abnormality, benign neoplasm, malignant neoplasm, or nonneoplastic mass. Although definitive diagnosis requires histologic examination, the pathology of an intraspinal mass may be predicted from its level, anatomic location, and imaging appearance. An *intramedullary* mass lesion in the cervical or cervicothoracic region is most likely to be hydrosyringomyelia, astrocytoma, or ganglioglioma, and rarely, an ependyoma, dermoid-epidermoid, or teratoma in the thoracolumbar or lumbar region with a dysgraphic spine, dermoid-epidermoid, lipoma, or teratoma; and in the thoracolumbar or lumbar region without spinal dysraphism, astrocytoma, ependymoma, or dermoid-epidermoid (2,13). An *intradural-extramedullary* mass lesion in the cervical region is most likely to be a schwannoma or neurofibroma, in the thoracic region CSF metastatic seeding, in the lumbar region with dysraphia a dermoid or lipoma, and in the lumbar region without dysraphia a schwannoma, neurofibroma, ependyoma, or CSF metastatic seeding (2,13). An *extradural* mass lesion of the cervical region is most likely to be a neurofibroma, in the upper thoracic region a paravertebral or metastatic vertebral neoplasm, and in the lower thoracic and lumbar regions a neuroblastoma or extradural sarcoma. A herniated disc is a common extradural mass in the lumbar region of an older child and adolescent (2,13).

Because of the frequency of developmental lesions in infants, intraspinal mass lesions are most common in early childhood. Primary neural neoplasms usually present after 8 years of age, whereas herniated discs are frequent only in teenagers. There is an equal incidence of intraspinal neoplasms in boys and girls, with the exception of dermoids, which are more frequent in boys, and astrocytomas, ganglioneuromas, and neuroblastomas, which are more frequent in girls (2).

Symptoms of an intraspinal mass include leg weakness, limp, back pain, scoliosis, torticollis, urinary incontinence, abdominal pain, arm weakness, rectal incontinence, orthopedic foot problems, and genitourinary problems. Signs include pathologic reflexes, flaccid paralysis, decreased sensation, spastic paralysis, sphincter disturbance, scoliosis, and spinal tenderness (1,2).

Radiographic abnormalities are seen in only 50% of patients with intraspinal mass lesions. There are frequently plain film abnormalities in patients with developmental mass lesions associated with dysraphism; there may be no abnormalities in patients with primary neural neoplasms, CSF metastatic seeding, or a herniated disc. Radiographic findings include loss of normal lordosis or kyphosis, scoliosis, paraspinal mass, spinal dysraphism, spinal canal enlargement, acquired abnormality of the vertebra or disc, and soft-tissue calcification (2).

Developmental Mass Lesions

Developmental tumors of the spinal neuraxis include lipoma, dermoid-epidermoid, teratoma, arachnoid cyst, neurenteric cyst, and hamartoma (see Table 4-10). Neurenteric cysts have been previously discussed.

Lipoma

A lipoma is a localized mass lesion in the spinal canal that contains fibrous and fatty tissue. It is the most common developmental tumor of childhood. Lipomas are divided into intradural lipomas (4%), lipomyeloceles/lipomyelomeningocele (84%), and filar lipomas (12%) (1,13). Lipomas are due to embryonic rests and metaplasia of fatty tissue attached to the leptomeninges or spinal cord. Intradural lipomas are rare subpial masses found in the cervical or thoracic region along the dorsal aspect of the spinal cord (173,174).

Intraspinal lipomas frequently have an associated subcutaneous lipoma or skin dimple. These lesions are usually diagnosed during childhood and are almost always in the lower lumbar or upper sacral region. Spinal dysraphism and segmentation anomalies are usually present. Partial sacral agenesis may be associated with lipomas of the sacral canal. Lipomas usually involve the intradural extramedullary space. Because they occur in the lower lumbosacral region below the level of the conus, they present simply as an intra-arachnoidal mass. There is often a large, irregular, dural sac; incorporation of an enlarged filum by the mass; and a low conus medullaris. The mass is lobular and may be either small or large. MRI demonstrates the intraarachnoidal location of the mass and confirms the diagnosis of a lipoma by the T1 shortening; it shows that the lobulated hyperintense mass is adherent to or occupies the cleft of an incompletely neurulated cord (see Figs. 4-30, 4-31, and 4-34).

Dermoid-Epidermoid

The broad category of dermoid-epidermoid (ectodermal origin) includes epidermoids derived from epidermus alone and dermoids derived from both epidermus and dermis. Dermoids may contain skin, hair, sweat glands, sebaceous glands, and squamous epithelium. Epidermoids are composed entirely of epidermal elements. Dermoids and epidermoids may also contain the products of squamous epithelial desquamation, such as keratin and cholesterol.

Dermoids/epidermoids are most commonly caused by abnormal closure of the neural tube and sequestration of epithelium or dermis. There is a dermal sinus in 20% of patients (112). Most children are 2–8 years of age at the time of diagnosis, and there is a marked male predominance. The lumbar region, particularly the cauda equina, is the most frequent location (2). These tumors occasionally arise from implants after surgery or spinal puncture using a nonstyleted needle (1).

Plain films show spinal dysraphism in one third of patients, evidence of an intraspinal mass without dysraphism in one third, and a normal spine in one third (2). The dermoid is frequently lobulated and usually contiguous with a portion of the conus medullaris; it occurs most frequently in the intradural extramedullary compartment; intramedullary and extradural locations are less frequent (2,175). Complications include spinal cord tethering, abscess formation, and chemical meningitis. These lesions are usually low in CT attenuation and are frequently difficult to distinguish from CSF. They are of low to intermediate intensity on T1-weighted and high intensity on T2-weighted MR images. Occasionally, there is T1 hyperintensity because of fat or calcification. Contrast enhancement suggests superimposed inflammation.

Teratoma

Teratomas are neoplasms containing derivatives of ectoderm, mesoderm, and endoderm. They are composed of tissues that are foreign to the anatomic region in which they arise. In contrast to dermoids, intraspinal teratomas usually present in young infants. They are large lesions that frequently involve several vertebral levels, occurring in the thoracic, lumbar, and sacral regions (2).

Almost all infants with teratomas have abnormal radiographs; they show dysraphism or enlargement of the spinal canal. There is usually marked bony erosion or even destruction. Teratomas are usually intramedullary but may also be intradural-extramedullary.

Arachnoid Cyst

Arachnoid cysts are either primary or secondary to previous inflammation (13). Primary arachnoid cysts may be intradural or extradural. Secondary cysts usually are intradural and are associated with arachnoiditis. Although they may be seen at any level, arachnoid cysts usually occur in the thoracic or lumbar region. There may be scoliosis, spinal canal widening, and thinning of the pedicles. MRI demonstrates a CSF intensity cyst that displaces the cord, nerve roots, or epidural fat (Fig. 4-46).

Hamartoma

A hamartoma may contain tissue of either neuroectodermal (neuroglial or meningeal) or mesodermal (bone, fat, car-

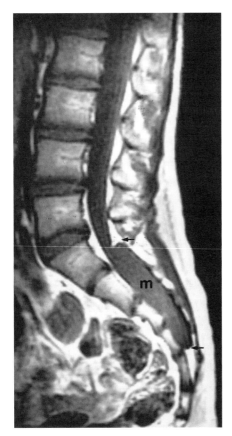

FIG. 4-46. Sacral arachnoid cyst. A 4-year-old boy with low back pain. Sagittal T1-weighted MRI. The sacral CSF intensity mass *(m)* is capped by fat both rostrally and caudally *(arrows)*. This confirms the extradural location of the arachnoid cyst.

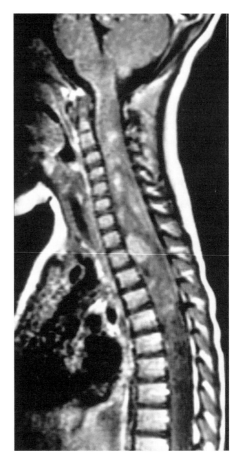

FIG. 4-47. Spinal cord ganglioglioma. A 3-year-old girl. Gadolinium-enhanced sagittal T1-weighted MRI. There is diffuse expansion of the cervical and thoracic spinal cord and several areas of nodular enhancement.

tilage, or muscle) origin. Hamartomas are solid or cystic subcutaneous masses in the midthoracic, thoracolumbar, or lumbar regions; they are frequently associated with cutaneous vascular anomalies (1,13). Spina bifida and spinal canal widening are also usually present (176).

Primary Neural Neoplasms

Aproximately one third of all intraspinal tumors are of neural tube or neural crest origin (see Table 4-11) (1,2). Because most of these lesions are slow growing, there is frequently (75%) evidence of spinal canal or foraminal enlargement on conventional radiographs. MRI should always be performed.

Astrocytoma

Astrocytoma is the most common tumor of neural tube origin arising within the spinal cord in children. Others include ependymoma and ganglioglioma. Affected children are usually over 8 years of age (2,13). The cervical cord is the most common location, with the lower thoracic cord also commonly involved. Conventional radiographs may show widening of the spinal canal, which in the cervical region

is best detected by an increase in the sagittal diameter. The mass is almost always intramedullary, although exophytic components can be seen. There is occasionally a complete block at myelography. MRI demonstrates spinal cord widen-

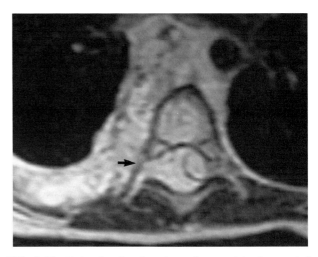

FIG. 4-48. Extradural extension of neuroblastoma. A 2-year-old boy with a thoracic neuroblastoma. Axial proton density MRI demonstrates a right paraventebral, high-intensity mass. Foraminal and extradural extension *(arrow)* produces spinal cord compression and displacement.

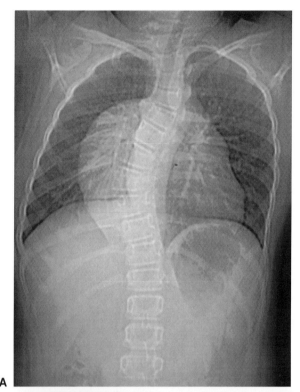

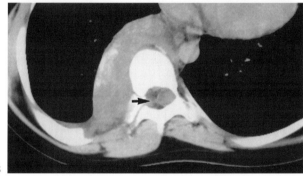

FIG. 4-49. Extradural extension of ganglioneuroblastoma. An 8-year-old girl with scoliosis. **A:** Frontal CT scout projection image demonstrates a large right mediastinal mass and scoliosis. **B:** Axial CT confirms right posterior mediastinal mass with calcification and extradural tumor extension *(arrow)*.

ing and prolonged T1 and T2 relaxation times (Fig. 4-47). There may be cyst formation, tumor necrosis, or hydrosyringomyelia. Contrast enhancement helps separate solid tumor from regions of cyst formation, necrosis, or edema. Astrocytomas in children are often histologically of low grade but nevertheless are infiltrative (177).

Ependymoma

Ependymomas are common primary neural neoplasms in infants and children. Spinal ependymomas usually arise from ependymal cells within the spinal cord or filum terminale but may also secondarily seed from a primary brain tumor. The most frequent age at presentation is 10–14 years (2). The lum-

bar region is the most frequent site of involvement, with the thoracic region being involved somewhat less frequently.

Plain films in children with intraspinal ependymomas are usually normal, although there may be subtle interpediculate widening or posterior vertebral scalloping. MRI shows a large, smooth-surfaced, mildly lobulated mass lesion that is usually located within the conus medullaris or filum terminale. If the tip of the conus or the filum is involved, the mass appears to be simply intraarachnoidal rather than intramedullary. The absence of spinal dysraphism suggests ependymoma rather than teratoma, dermoid, or lipoma.

It is difficult to distinguish an ependymoma from an astrocytoma. Ependymomas tend to be more sharply circumscribed, particularly after contrast enhancement, than astrocytomas; ependymomas also tend to have areas of hemorrhage at their inferior and superior margins (1,180). Other less common intramedullary masses of childhood include ganglioglioma (see Fig. 4-47), mixed glioma, hemangioblastoma, syringohydromyelia, dermoid-epidermoid, teratoma, lipoma, and neurenteric cyst (1,2).

Neurogenic Tumors

Neurogenic tumors are of neural crest origin and arise from the adrenal glands or sympathetic chain, anywhere

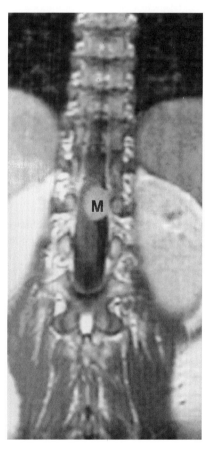

FIG. 4-50. Lumbar schwannoma. A 4-year-old girl with lower back stiffness. Gadolinium-enhanced coronal T1-weighted MRI demonstrates an intradural extramedullary enhancing mass *(M)* compressing the spinal cord at the T12–L1 level.

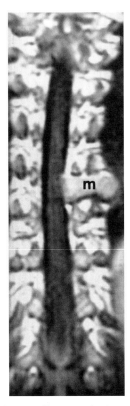

FIG. 4-51. **Spinal neurofibroma.** An 8-year-old girl with neurofibromatosis type 1. Gadolinium-enhanced coronal T1-weighted MRI. The enhancing mass *(m)* of the midthoracic region has foraminal and intraspinal components that produce a dumbbell appearance. There is extrinsic compression of the spinal cord.

from the base of the skull to the pelvis but commonly in the thorax or abdomen. There is a pathologic spectrum that extends from malignant neuroblastoma to ganglioneuroblastoma to benign ganglioneuroma. Neuroblastomas (Fig. 4-48) tend to occur in infants and young children, whereas ganglioneuromas (Fig. 4-49) occur in older children and young adults. Other neurogenic tumors, much less common in children than adults, include schwannomas and neurofibromas. Extradural extension of paravertebral neurogenic tumors may occur without neurologic symptoms or bone erosion (see Figs. 4-50 and 4-51) (178,179). For this reason, MRI should be performed in any pediatric patient with a paravertebral mass regardless of the absence of neurologic symptoms (1,13).

Plain radiographs show a paraspinal mass that may cause bone erosion or destruction. The intraspinal component is almost always extradural. MRI shows displacement of the cord away from the extradural tumor and accurately delineates tumor extent.

CSF Metastases

Some intracranial neoplasms, most commonly medulloblastoma, may cause spinal cord signs and symptoms due to subarachnoid metastatic seeding. Other neoplasms that

metastasize by the CSF route are germ cell tumors, ependymomas, astrocytomas, pineoblastomas, other pineal neoplasms, primitive neuroectodermal tumors (PNETs), choroid plexus carcinomas, lymphomas, leukemias, retinoblastomas, rhabdomyosarcomas, other sarcomas, and rhabdoid tumors.

CSF metastases are usually multiple, the most frequent location being the lumbosacral and lower thoracic region, perhaps because of gravitational effects of the erect position (181). Lesions are usually intradural-extramedullary in location. Plain films are normal, but myelography shows nodules of different sizes scattered throughout the subarachnoid space. Spinal metastases may be detected at the time of initial diagnosis or, more commonly, at the time of recurrence (1,181). MRI with gadolinium enhancement is the best modality for demonstrating CSF spread of tumor (Fig. 4-52) (182,183). MRI patterns of CSF spread include single or multiple nodules, diffuse sheets or plaques of tumor, thicken-

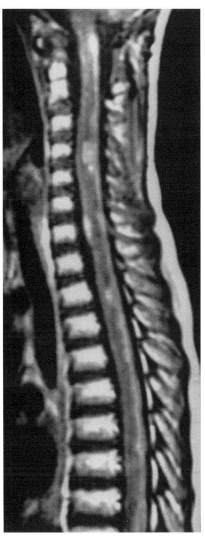

FIG. 4-52. **Spinal seeding of medulloblastoma.** A 7-year-old boy treated for medulloblastoma. Gadolinium-enhanced sagittal T1-weighted MRI. There are many nodular and laminar-enhancing intradural lesions along the cervical and thoracic spinal cord.

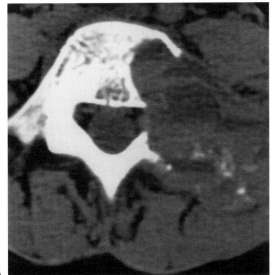

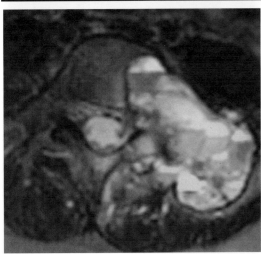

FIG. 4-53. Aneurysmal bone cyst. A 14-year-old girl with low back pain. **A:** Axial CT through L5 shows extensive bony destruction of the vertebral body and neural arch on the left. The soft-tissue mass contains low-density areas and calcification. **B:** Axial T2-weighted MRI. Fluid-fluid levels are identified in the aneurysmal bone cyst.

ing of nerve roots with irregular crowding or clumping, and scalloping of the subarachnoid space. Hemorrhagic or enhancing postoperative subdural or subarachnoid collections are sometimes confused with CSF spread of tumor (13,184).

Intraspinal Extension of Bony Neoplasms

Bony spinal neoplasms may secondarily affect the intraspinal contents. These neoplasms may be primary (osteoid osteoma, osteoblastoma, isolated osteochondroma, multiple exostoses, aneurysmal bone cyst [Fig. 4-53], giant cell tumor, chordoma, osteogenic sarcoma, Ewing sarcoma, chondroblastoma, fibrosarcoma, chondrosarcoma, PNET, histiocytosis [Fig. 4-54], other small cell tumor) or second-

ary to contiguous spread (neuroblastoma, ganglioneuroblastoma, ganglioneuroma, teratoma, sarcoma) and distant metastases (leukemia, lymphoma, rhabdomyosarcoma, teratoma, Ewing's sarcoma, renal cell carcinoma, Wilms tumor, reticulum cell sarcoma) (1,2,160,164,165,169, 185–191). This type of intraspinal extension usually produces an extradural mass that is most accurately imaged by MRI.

Vascular Anomalies

Vascular anomalies may involve the paraspinal soft tissues, bony spine, spinal cord, neural elements, meninges, or any combination of these. The Mulliken and Glowacki biological classification of vascular anomalies includes vascular tumors (hemangiomas), vascular malformations, and the angiodysplastic syndromes (13,192).

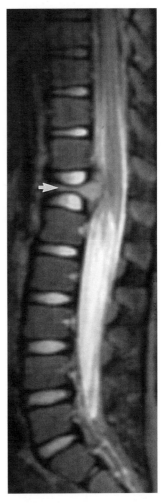

FIG. 4-54. Langerhans cell histiocytosis and spinal cord compression. A 3-year-old girl with eosinophilic granuloma. Sagittal T1-weighted MRI demonstrates high-intensity involvement *(arrow)* of the T12 vertebral body with platyspondyly. Extradural extension causes mild spinal cord displacement and compression.

Hemangiomas are common benign neoplasms characterized by endothelial proliferation in infancy and later involution (73). MRI shows enhancing tumor parenchyma with high-flow vascular characteristics.

Vascular malformations are characterized by normal endothelial turnover; these include capillary, arterial, venous, lymphatic, and combined subtypes. Lymphatic and venous malformations are slow-flow anomalies. MRI shows septated masses without any high-flow vascular intensities. There may be associated fibrofatty stroma. Lymphatic malformations may have fluid-fluid levels. Phleboliths and prominent veins are characteristic of venous malformations. Gadolinium enhancement of septations is characteristic of lymphatic malformations; enhancement of vascular channels is typical of venous malformations. AVMs are high-flow anomalies without tumor parenchyma; reactive changes may be identified.

Vascular anomalies of the CNS have traditionally been classified as AVMs, venous malformations, cavernous malformations, telangiectasias, and aneurysms. Intradural spinal vascular anomalies are often AVMs and are further classified by the anatomic site of origin or involvement. They may also be classified as spinal cord AVMs (intramedullary), dural arteriovenous fistulas, and metameric AVMs (Cobb syndrome). The latter involve any or all layers of a spinal segment from the spinal cord to the skin. MRI of spinal AVMs, which are high-flow malformations, may show nodular or serpiginous signal voids (Fig. 4-55) without evidence of tumor parenchyma. There may be associated hemorrhage, cord edema, infarct, myelomalacia, syrinx, or atrophy (193,194). Spinal angiography is required for complete diagnostic evaluation prior to surgery or interventional therapy. Cavernous malformations of the spinal cord are rare causes of hemorrhage (subarachnoid or intramedullary) or myelopathy.

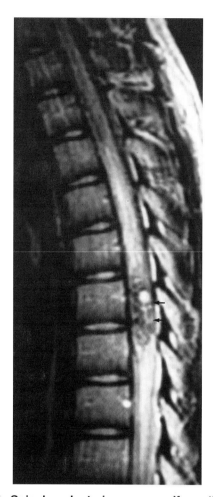

FIG. 4-55. Spinal cord arteriovenous malformation. A 16-year-old boy with lower extremity weakness. Sagittal T2-weighted MRI shows intramedullary vascular flow signal voids due to feeding vessels *(arrows)*. Adjacent hyperintensities are caused by hemorrhage and edema.

Sacrococcygeal Teratoma

Teratomas are rare (1 per 35,000 live births) congenital tumors derived from all three germinal layers (195). The sacrococcygeum is the most frequent site. Sacrococcygeal teratomas are the most frequent tumors of the caudal region during childhood (196–199). The tumor develops from multipotential cells that arise in Hensen's node and migrate caudally to lie within the coccyx (200).

Sacrococcygeal teratomas are more common in girls than in boys (4:1), but tumors identified at birth are more often malignant in boys than in girls (18,200). Most sacrococcygeal teratomas are benign and are obvious at birth. However, tumors beyond the neonatal age have a high incidence of malignancy; the older the patient, the more likely are malignant elements. The size of the mass does not correlate well with the presence of malignancy. Because there is malignant transformation with increasing age, any delay in treatment of these tumors should be avoided (195,200). If the tumor is completely presacral, the patient may be asymptomatic until, at an older age, urinary tract or bowel symptoms become apparent.

The usual presentation is a large soft-tissue sacrococcygeal mass detected in utero or at birth (Fig. 4-56). Type I tumors are primarily external in location and distort the buttocks. Type II tumors have some intrapelvic component that may displace or invade pelvic structures, but the external part of the mass dominates. Type III tumors have a larger intrapelvic component and only a small external component; this type profoundly displaces or invades surrounding structures. Type IV tumors are presacral without clinical evidence of external mass. They may displace the rectum and bladder. Any type of sacrococcygeal teratoma may have an intraspinal component (195,199,200). If there are signs of neurologic deficit or radiographic findings suggestive of intraspinal extension, preoperative MRI is mandatory (18,201).

The hereditary type of this tumor includes a presacral teratoma, a specific sacrococcygeal bony defect, and autosomal dominant inheritance (202). Many of these patients also have

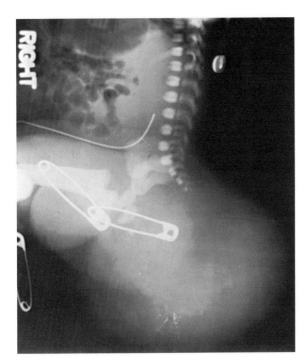

FIG. 4-56. **Sacrococcygeal teratoma.** Newborn girl with a huge soft-tissue mass containing fat and calcium. There is elevation of the umbilical artery and internal iliac artery (outlined by the umbilical artery catheter) and mass effect on the sacrum.

vesicoureteral reflux, skin dimples, a retrorectal abscess, and anorectal stenosis (202). Calcification in the teratoma is rare. The developmental deformity of the sacrum and coccyx with this hereditary presacral teratoma may be difficult to distinguish from that seen with anterior sacral meningocele, but MRI makes the distinction. Hereditary presacral teratomas are benign, regardless of age at diagnosis (202).

Radiographs show a soft-tissue mass that arises from the ventral surface of the coccyx (Fig. 4-56); the mass may be extrapelvic, intrapelvic, or both. Calcifications are present in at least 60% of sacrococcygeal teratomas and occur more frequently in benign lesions. The calcifications may be amorphous, punctate, spiculated, flocculent, and even ossified. Fatty density due to lipomatous tissue may be seen in the mass. Ultrasonography confirms the cystic, solid, or mixed character of the mass. Completely cystic or partially cystic lesions are usually benign, whereas solid lesions are frequently malignant (200). Ultrasonography shows the extent of the mass well and also shows any secondary hydronephrosis. MRI demonstrates the content of a sacrococcygeal teratoma as well as its extent; these tumors often have heterogeneous signal characteristics (Fig. 4-57).

The therapy is prompt surgical removal of the mass and the entire coccyx. Only 10% of sacrococcygeal teratomas are malignant at birth, whereas 91% of those removed after 2 months of age contain malignant tissue (196,197). This emphasizes the possibility of malignant transformation and the importance of prompt removal.

Many other masses may occur in the presacral region in infants and children (Table 4-12). The primary differential diagnostic considerations in a newborn with a presacral mass are sacrococcygeal teratoma, germ cell tumor, meningocele, lipoma, neuroblastoma, and rectal duplication (196,198, 203). More common presacral masses in older infants and children are neuroblastoma, sacrococcygeal teratoma, germ cell tumors, abscess, ovarian tumor, ectopic kidney, and anterior meningocele (Table 4-12) (196,198,203).

Trauma

Spinal Fractures

Spinal fractures are much less common in infants and children than in teenagers and adults (7,15,204,205). Most nonpathologic fractures are due to motor vehicle accidents. Other causes include bicycle accidents, moped or motorcycle accidents, lap-belt injuries (206), falls, diving accidents, other sports and recreational injuries, traumatic delivery, and child abuse. In infants and young children, the injuries are

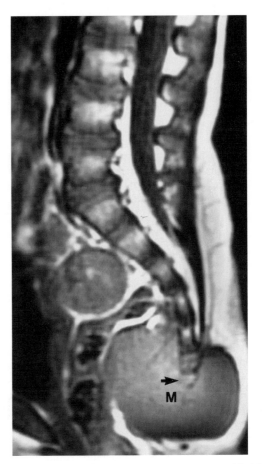

FIG. 4-57. **Sacrococcygeal teratoma.** A 2-year-old girl with palpable soft-tissue mass. Sagittal T1-weighted MRI shows a soft-tissue mass (M) surrounding and partially destroying the coccyx (arrow). Note that the presacral component of the teratoma extends into the pelvis.

TABLE 4-12. *Presacral masses in infants and children*

Congenital lesions	Inflammatory etiology	Miscellaneous lesions
Anterior meningocele	Abscess[a]	Fibroma
Chordoma	Granulomatous colitis	Fibrosarcoma
Dermoid	Osteomyelitis of	Fibrous dysplasia
Ectopic kidney	sacrum	Hemangioma
Hamartoma	Ulcerative colitis	Hemangioendothelioma
Neurenteric cyst	Osteocartilaginous tumors	Hematoma
Rectal duplication	Aneurysmal bone cyst	Hydrometrocolpos
Sacrococcygeal teratoma[a]	Chondroma	Leiomyoma
Neurogenic lesions	Chondrosarcoma	Leiomyosarcoma
Ependymoma	Ewing sarcoma	Lipoma
Ganglioneuroblastoma	Giant cell tumor	Lymphatic malformation
Ganglioneuroma	Osteosarcoma	Lyphoma, leukemia
Neurilemmoma	Osteoma	Meconium plug
Neurinoma		Metastaic disease
Neuroblastoma[a]		Omental cyst
Neurofibroma		Ovarian tumor
Paraganglioma		Yolk sac tumor[a]
		Germ-cell tumor[a]

[a] More common.

Source: Modified from Werner and Taybi (196).

usually upper cervical in location because of the large head size, the immaturity of the spinal column, and the higher effective fulcrum for flexion and extension (13,204,207). Injuries include fractures of the synchondroses of the atlas, axis, and dens as well as atlantoaxial and occipitoatlantal dislocations. After closure of the major synchondroses by 8–10 years of age, cervical injuries tend to be centered at lower levels of the cervical spine as in adults (204).

The radiologist must first determine if a fracture is present. One must then establish whether a spinal injury is stable or unstable. The spine should be considered as anterior (vertebral bodies) and posterior (vertebral arches and appendages) bony columns (208–211). If there is potential movement between these columns, the injury is unstable. If the patient is not ambulatory, initial cross-table lateral and occasionally vertical beam AP views of the spine should be obtained while the patient remains immobilized. Questionable cases may require views with the tube angled (trauma obliques, angled pillar views) while the patient remains supine. If the patient is ambulatory or these initial views are completely normal, erect lateral, frontal, open-mouth odontoid (this may be impossible in infants and young children), oblique, and even flexion-extension lateral views may be required. Oblique views are only occasionally needed. Conventional tomography or CT may help in questionable cases of bony spinal injuries.

One should always use an ordered radiologic approach (see Table 4-1) to the pediatric spine after injury (211). In general, lateral views are the most informative. Abnormalities include loss of the normal cervical or lumbar lordosis, loss of the thoracic kyphosis, thickening of the prevertebral soft tissues, increase in the predental space, displacement of vertebral bodies, abnormal width of intervertebral disc spaces, abnormal configuration of apophyseal joints, abnormality of the joints of Luschka, increase in the distance be-

tween spinous processes, lateral deviation of spinous processes, widening of interpediculate distances, offset of the lateral masses of the atlas, compression of a vertebral body and frank fracture (15).

There are basically six mechanisms of spinal injury (7,13,211,212). *Flexion injuries* apply compressive force to the vertebral bodies and a distracting force to the posterior ligaments and neural arches, which cause compression or vertical fractures of the vertebral body and separation of the vertebral arches and spinous processes (Table 4-13). Hyperflexion may lead to posterior ligamentous sprains, bilateral or unilateral facet dislocations, compression fractures, clay shoveler's fractures, flexion tear-drop fractures, fractures of the dens, and Chance fractures (15,206,213). Lap-belt injuries may be difficult to diagnose by CT; plain films or lateral scout-view CT is critical (206).

Extension injuries cause compressive forces posteriorly and distracting forces anteriorly (Table 4-13), these produce fractures of the neural arches and widening of the intervertebral disc spaces and sometimes tear-drop fractures of the anterosuperior aspects of the vertebral body (15). Hyperextension leads to anterior ligamentous sprains, avulsion fractures of the anterior arch of C1, C1 posterior arch fractures, extension tear-drop fractures of C2, laminar fractures, hangman's fractures (traumatic spondylolistheses), pillar fractures, pedicle fractures, and laminae fractures. Hyperextension injuries may also produce the central cord syndrome due to compression of the spinal cord by the ligamentum flavum, sometimes with few or no radiologic abnormalities.

Lateral flexion injuries cause ipsilateral vertebral body compressions, contralateral fractures of the uncinate and transverse processes, brachial plexus avulsion and widening of the joints of Luschka (Table 4-13). A fracture of the lateral mass of C1 or C2 is an uncommon lateral flexion injury.

TABLE 4-13. *Spinal fractures: mechanisms and possible radiologic findings*

Flexion injury
 Dens: fracture and anterior displacement
 Isolated atlantoaxial dislocation
 Soft tissues: prevertebral swelling
 Vertebral body
  Anterior compression
  Teardrop fracture of anteroinferior margin
  Limbus fracture
  Vertical fracture of body
  Posterior dislocation
 Disc space
  Narrow
  Wide
 Apophyseal joint
  Wide
  Narrow
  Subluxation
 Vertebral arch and spinous process
  Separation
  Avulsion fracture (clay shoveler's)
 Seatbelt fracture of lumbar spine
Extension injury
 Atlas
  Transverse fracture of anterior arch
  Vertical fracture of posterior arch
 Axis
  Fracture of dens
  Hangman's fracture
 Isolated atlantoaxial dislocation
 Vertebral arch and spinous process
  Wide
  Narrow
  Fracture
 Apophyseal joint
  Narrow
  Wide
  Subluxation
 Central cord syndrome
 Disc space
  Wide
  Narrow

 Vertebral body: teardrop fracture of anterosuperior
  margin
 Soft tissues: prevertebral swelling
Lateral flexion injury
 Dens: fracture of base
 Vertebral body: ipsilateral compression fracture
 Uncinate process: contralateral fracture
 Brachial plexus: contralateral avulsion
 Joint of Luschka
  Wide
  Narrow
 Rotation injury
  Atlantoaxial
   Subluxation
   Dislocation
   Fixation
  Vertebral arch and spinous process
   Wide
   Narrow
   Shifted
   Fracture
  Apophyseal joint
   Wide
   Narrow
   Subluxation
   Locked facet
  Joint of Luschka
   Wide
   Narrow
   Dislocation
  Disc space
   Narrow
   Wide
   Subluxation
  Vertebral body: anterior displacement
 Axial compression injury
  Atlas: Jefferson fracture
  Vertebral body: expansion and bursting

Source: Modified from Swischuk (15).

Rotational injuries are usually associated with flexion and may be difficult to diagnose. These rotational or translational injuries may cause subluxation or even dislocation between the anterior (vertebral body) and posterior (vertebral arch) bony structures. The anatomic site of maximal rotational displacement may be at the disc space, joint of Luschka, or apophyseal joint (Table 4-13). Translational injuries include atlantoaxial or atlantooccipital subluxations and dislocations, unilateral or bilateral facet subluxations, and fracture dislocations.

Axial compression injuries cause bursting and distraction of the vertebral body. A specific type of vertical compression injury is the Jefferson fracture of C1.

Distraction injuries cause severe ligamentous and soft-tissue injuries in addition to bony damage. Examples include atlantoaxial dislocation, atlantooccipital dislocation, and the Chance fracture.

Flexion Injuries of the Atlas and Axis

Flexion injuries of the atlas and axis usually cause a fracture through the base of the dens. In infants and young children this fracture is through the synchondroses between the dens and the body of C2 (Fig. 4-58). There is usually anterior displacement of C1 and associated prevertebral soft tissue swelling. Occasionally, severe bony resorption occurs at this synchondrosis, leading to acquired absence of the dens (15).

Extension Injuries of the Atlas and Axis

Extension injuries of the atlas and axis occur fairly frequently. They may cause fractures of the posterior arch of C1, fractures of the dens, and a "hangman's fracture" of C2. A congenital defect in the posterior arch of the atlas

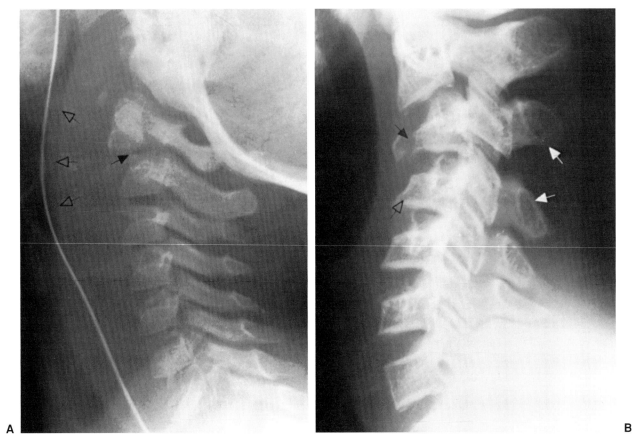

FIG. 4-58. Flexion fractures of cervical spine. A: A 2-year-old girl with right arm weakness following an automobile accident. There is a fracture through the synchondrosis between the dens and the body of C2 *(solid arrow)*. Anterior displacement of C1 and associated prevertebral soft-tissue swelling *(open arrows)* are apparent. **B:** A 13-year-old boy who suffered a hyperflexion injury during a fall from his bicycle. A compression fracture of the vertebral body of C3 *(black arrow)*, linear fracture of the vertebral body of C4 *(open arrow)*, and slight widening of the C4 intervertebral disc are present. There is also separation of the vertebral arches and spinous processes of C3 and C4 *(white arrows)*, indicating posterior ligamentous injury due to the distracting force.

should not be confused with a fracture. Defects are frequently wide and have tapered, well-defined medial cortices. The "hangman's fracture" is due to hyperextension causing lateral fractures of the posterior vertebral arches (214). If there is a question of "hangman's fracture" (see Fig. 4-60) versus physiologic subluxation of C2 on C3 (see Fig. 4-11), the posterior cervical line should be used for clarification (15,214).

Jefferson Fracture of C1

The Jefferson bursting fracture of the atlas is due to axial compression of the upper cervical spine (215). This fracture is unstable, with outward displacement of the anterior ring, posterior ring, and lateral masses of C1. The lateral cervical spine may show overlap of the posterior arches of C1 due to the comminution (Fig. 4-59A). Frontal views show outward displacement of the lateral masses of C1 in relation to the

dens and body of C2 (Fig. 4-59). CT verifies the fracture and its extent (215).

Compression Fractures of the Spine

Traumatic compression fractures of the vertebral body are due to flexion injuries. They are most common in the thoracolumbar spine (216). Causes include a fall, vehicular accident, direct trauma, or tetanus (216). Pathologic compression fractures may occur in patients with osteopenia due to a variety of causes (steroid therapy, malignancy, rheumatoid arthritis, osteoporosis, renal osteodystrophy). The symptoms and signs of these fractures may be insignificant or atypical. These fractures occur throughout childhood and have no particular age or sex predominance (216).

Lateral films of the spine show anterior compression of one or more vertebral bodies. There is usually a wedge-shaped deformity, occasionally with an associated beak-shaped prominence (216). It should be noted that there may

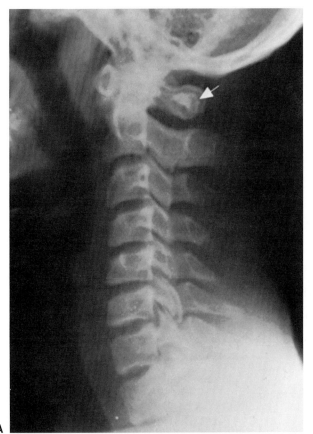

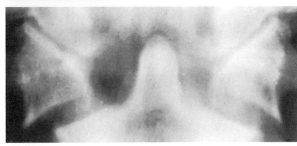

FIG. 4-59. Jefferson fracture of C1. A 15-year-old boy with neck pain following a diving injury. **A:** Lateral view of the cervical spine shows overlap of the posterior arches of C1 *(arrow)*. **B:** AP tomogram demonstrates marked outward displacement of the lateral masses of C1 in relation to the dens and body of C2.

be slight wedging of vertebral bodies in normal children. However, if the height of the ventral portion of the vertebral body divided by the height of the dorsal portion of the vertebral body is less than 95% in the thoracic or lumbar spine, wedging is considered to be due to fracture. These compression fractures commonly occur between T4 and L2, the most common sites being T4, T5, and L2 (216).

Spinal Fractures in the Neonate and Young Infant

In the neonate and young infant, spinal injury may occur during delivery or from an accident or child abuse (15). Occurring chiefly in the cervical spine, the injuries are likely to be fractures of the neurocentral synchondroses or dens or

dislocations of the atlantooccipital or atlantoaxial articulations. Epidural, subdural, or subarachnoid hemorrhage may co-exist.

Spinal Fractures in Older Infants and Children

In older infants and in children up to 8 years of age, injuries to the cervical spine often result in fractures of the epiphyses and synchondroses and avulsions and apophyseal separations at the level of the dens, axis, and atlas. The Jefferson fracture was described previously. Less common fractures of C1 include posterior arch fractures and avulsion injuries of the anterior arch. Odontoid fractures often occur at the subdental synchondrosis.

"Hangman's fracture" is a bilateral fracture of the pars interarticularis of C2 caused by hyperextension (Fig. 4-60) leading to acute, severe spondylolisthesis and severe narrowing of the spinal canal. Atlantoaxial or atlantooccipital instability is often associated with these fractures. Atlantoaxial and atlantooccipital dislocations may also occur without obvious fracture (Fig. 4-61) (65–67). Dislocation at the atlantoaxial junction is four times as common as at the craniocervical junction; both usually have associated severe spinal cord injury (7).

In children over the age of 12 years, cervical spine fractures are similar to those seen in adults (204,209,217). Thoracolumbar fractures are less common in childhood than cervical fractures. They include compression fractures and Chance fractures (horizontal fractures of the body and neural arch) caused by hyperflexion, as from a lap seat belt. Burst fractures, from axial compression, may also occur.

Brachial Plexus Injuries

Brachial plexus injuries are due to excessive lateral flexion, frequently in association with some rotation. They are due to birth trauma in the neonate or to a vehicular (motorcycle) accident in the teenager. Duchenne-Erb palsy (usually from a birthing injury) occurs with C5–7 nerve root injuries, causing paralysis of the shoulder and upper arm. Klumpke palsy due to C7-T1 nerve root injury causes paralysis of the hand.

Brachial plexus injury is a clinical diagnosis. In the newborn, there may be diaphragmatic paralysis due to phrenic nerve injury. There may be a dural tear and CSF leakage. Plain radiographs of the cervical spine are usually normal. Traumatic pseudomeningoceles along avulsed nerve roots may be shown by myelography or MRI (Fig. 4-62).

Spinal Cord Injury

Spinal cord injury in the neonate is presumably associated with transient, undetected vertebral dislocation (218). Types of injury include cord contusion, edema, necrosis, and transection (7,217–222).

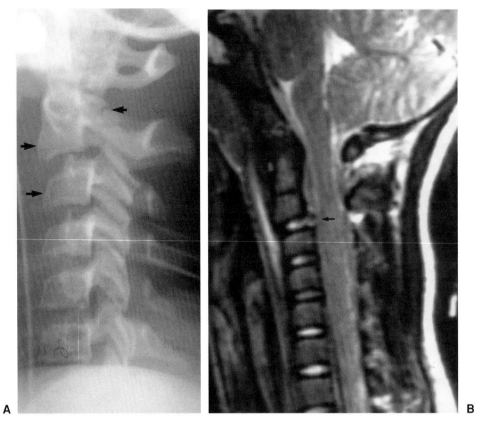

FIG. 4-60. "Hangman's fracture" with spinal cord injury. A 9-year-old girl in a motor vehicle accident. **A:** Lateral radiograph shows subluxation of C2 on C3 *(left arrows)* and fracture of neural arch of C2. **B:** Sagittal T2-weighted MRI. Extensive edema and swelling of the cervical spinal cord. The C2 disc is displaced posteriorly *(arrow)*.

Spinal cord injury is best assessed with MRI (223–226). Vertebral malalignment, bony fragments, disc herniation, cord compression or transection, ligamentous abnormality, and intraspinal hematoma are readily demonstrated (162). Cord contusion and complete transection have been associated with birth trauma, particularly breech delivery (219,227). Cord contusion is isointense on MR T1-weighted images and is of mixed intensity on T2-weighted images. MRI of cord transection shows cord disruption and, in chronic cases, mixed-intensity cystic changes (Fig. 4-63). In the patient with progressive myelopathy or radiculopathy, MRI detects and differentiates hematomyelia, cord edema, and contusion. MRI is also the procedure of choice for assessing the chronic sequelae of spinal cord trauma, such as posttraumatic spinal cord cyst or syringomyelia, myelomalacia, arachnoiditis, arachnoid cyst, and neuroarthropathy (228).

Irradiation Injury

Irradiation may cause iatrogenic abnormalities of the spine. The spine may be included in the field of radiation for thoracic lymphoma, abdominal lymphoma, neuroblastoma, Wilms tumor, brain neoplasms, or spine neoplasms. Irradia-

tion causes growth disturbances in the spine; the disturbance is directly related to dosage and inversely related to the age when irradiated (229). Irradiation with less than 1000 cGy (1000 rads) does not cause deformity of vertebrae regardless of age, whereas dosages over 2000 cGy cause growth disturbances at any age below maturity (229).

Radiologic changes include osteopenia, post-growth arrest lines adjacent to the vertebral endplates, irregularity and scalloping of the vertebral endplates, platyspondyly, abnormal contour of vertebral bodies, and scoliosis (Fig. 4-64). Occasionally, bony exostoses arise from the spine in the field of irradiation (229). An effort should always be made to minimize radiation dosage to the developing spine.

Miscellaneous Abnormalities

Spondylolysis and Spondylolisthesis

Spondylolysis is a defect in or an interruption of the pars interarticularis of the vertebral arch. It is bilateral in 75% to 85% of cases (230). *Spondylolisthesis* is overt slippage of one vertebral body on the one beneath it. The amount of this slippage is graded by measuring the amount of superior vertebral body that protrudes over the anterior margin of the

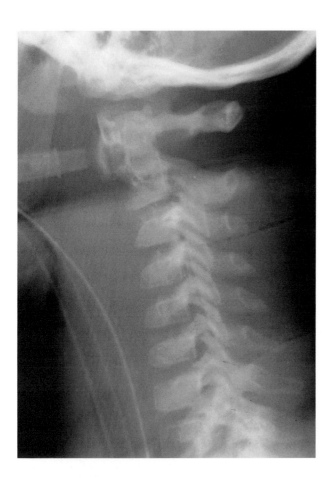

FIG. 4-61. Atlantooccipital dissociation. A 1-year-old girl with trauma. Lateral radiograph shows marked prevertebral soft-tissue swelling, separation of the occipital condyles from the atlas, and malalignment of the dens relative to the basion.

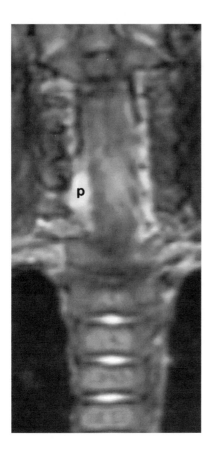

lower vertebral body. Grade I represents anterior displacement of up to one third of the superior vertebral body, grade II up to two thirds, grade III up to the entire vertebral body, and grade IV complete anterior (and often inferior) displacement. Spondylolysis and spondylolisthesis are acquired lesions that probably have a congenital predisposition. The age distribution suggests that spondylolysis and therefore spondylolisthesis are acquired traumatic lesions (231). Moreover, patients who have previously had normal radiographs of the lumbar spine sometimes develop spondylolysis and spondylolisthesis (232). An underlying congenital predisposition explains the strong familial tendency of this abnormality (231,232).

The incidence of spondylolysis in young adults is as high as 7.1% and may be as high as 5% in asymptomatic children (231). The sex distribution among children is equal, whereas in adults there is a strong male predominance. The youngest reported patient with spondylolysis was 10 months old (231). Approximately one third of patients are diagnosed by 9 years

FIG. 4-62. Brachial plexus injury. A 4-month-old boy with history of difficult delivery. Coronal T2-weighted MRI demonstrates a right C4–5 pseudomeningocele *(p)* and nonvisualization of the adjacent nerve roots. (Courtesy of Paul Chandler, M.D., Macon, Georgia.)

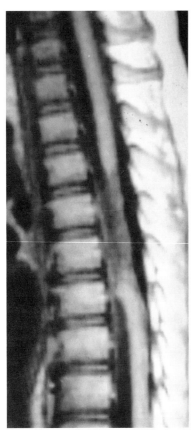

FIG. 4-63. Chronic spinal cord changes following transection. A 3-year-old girl struck by an automobile three months earlier. Sagittal T1-weighted MRI shows variable intensity and decreased size of the thoracic spinal cord.

of age; the prevalence slowly increases into young adulthood. Half of patients have lumbar or sciatic pain, and half are asymptomatic (231).

Spondylolysis is often and spondylolisthesis is usually apparent on lateral views of the lumbosacral spine in children (230). In older children and young adults, supplementary oblique views may be required. SPECT nuclear imaging may suggest abnormalities not seen on any other imaging studies (17,233). CT is preferred to conventional tomography if confirmation is required (Fig. 4-65). MRI may rarely be performed to exclude other causes of back pain. Spondylolysis may be extremely difficult to demonstrate by MRI (234).

The abnormality is at L5–S1 in 93% of cases, L4–5 in 5%, and other sites in 2% (231). Spondylolysis and spondylolisthesis occur together in 74.5%. Spondylolysis occurs alone in only 17.5% of children. Eight percent have spondylolisthesis without spondylolysis, a condition usually due to a congenital defect of the facets (231).

Disc Herniation

Intervertebral disc herniation in infants and children is uncommon (1,2). It is presumably due to trauma superimposed on early degenerative changes of the disc (235). In adolescence, disc herniation is usually due to trauma, extreme exertion, or athletic activities. The age of symptom onset is usually between 11 and 16 years; there is a slight male predominance (236). Usually there is low back pain that progresses to sciatica, but the classic symptoms of nerve root compression may not be recognized in children as due to intervertebral disc herniation. This diagnostic difficulty is due partly to the rarity of the lesion in children. Because disc herniations are frequently large in children, they may present as a cauda equina lesion that mimics an ependymoma of the filum terminale (2).

There may be loss of the normal lumbar lordosis because of muscle spasm, mild to moderate scoliosis, and mild disc space narrowing. Frequently, plain films are completely normal. Disc herniations are almost always in the lower lumbosacral region at either the L4–5 or L5–S1 level.

The diagnosis may be confirmed by CT or MRI. MRI shows an extradural mass usually contiguous with the parent disc, which has similar signal characteristics (Fig. 4-66). The associated loss of intervertebral disc height and decreased signal intensity within the parent disc help to differentiate extruded disc material from other extradural masses. Occasionally, a calcified intervertebral disc herniates anteriorly or posteriorly (see later discussion).

Disc herniations in childhood and adolescence may be associated with a slipped vertebral apophysis (Fig. 4-66). The posteroinferior apophysis may be displaced into the spinal canal; this type of avulsion is most common at the L4 level (13,237).

Anterior Intervertebral Disc Herniation

Anterior intervertebral disc herniation is not uncommon in children (238). This entity is most frequent in teenage boys who participate in vigorous activities and is presumably traumatic. They usually complain of minor or moderate back pain.

Lateral radiographs of the lumbar spine show irregular defects with sclerotic margins in the upper and anterior portions of the vertebral bodies. There may be a decrease in the height of the associated vertebral bodies, presumably due to long-standing trauma, abnormal chronic stress, and anterior nucleus pulposus protrusion or herniation. This anterior herniation of the nucleus pulposus may cause separation of a triangular smooth bony fragment, which presumably represents the ring apophysis. This apophysis then remains separate from the body, producing a limbus vertebra (239,240).

The radiologic appearance of a well-marginated defect or a triangular limbus bone involving the anterosuperior margin of a midlumbar vertebral body is fairly characteristic (240). Differential diagnostic considerations include Scheuermann disease, osteomyelitis, fracture, and bone tumor. MRI may

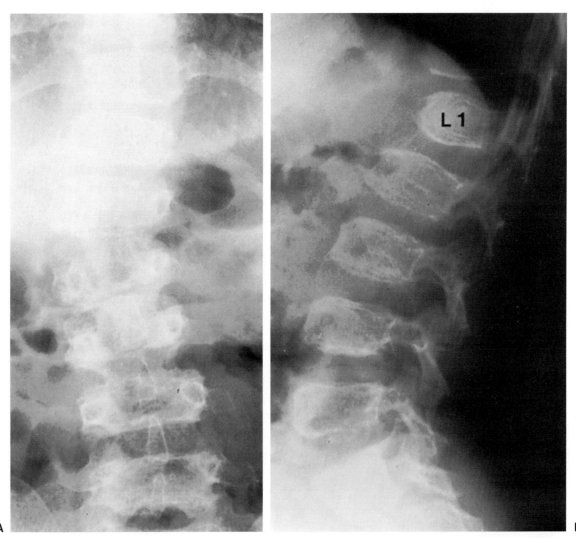

FIG. 4-64. Radiation injury. An 8-year-old girl who received abdominal irradiation at 5 years of age for bilateral Wilms tumors. **A:** AP view of the lumbar spine shows osteopenia and scoliosis with convexity to the right. The changes are limited to the irradiation portal, which did not include the lower thoracic spine. **B:** Lateral lumbar spine shows osteopenia, platyspondyly localized to the lumbar region, and a beaked L1 vertebral body.

be used to confirm the diagnosis and to avoid further diagnostic procedures such as biopsy (239).

Disc Calcification

Intervertebral disc calcification during childhood has a characteristic radiologic appearance (Fig. 4-67). The etiology is unknown, but it probably represents deposition of calcified material in the nucleus pulposus of a disc after inflammation. Trauma has also been implicated as a causative factor (241–243).

Patients with disc calcification may be symptomatic or asymptomatic. Symptoms include pain, stiffness, decreased range of motion, muscle spasm, tenderness, and torticollis (243,244). These symptoms are frequently present in chil-

dren with cervical disc calcification but rarely present in those with thoracic and lumbar disc calcification. The symptoms seem to appear when the calcification, for some unknown reason, begins to resorb or herniate (241). There is an increased frequency of these calcifications in boys. The predominant site of calcification in boys is the cervical region, whereas in girls there is a uniform distribution throughout the spine (241). The mean age at the time of diagnosis is 8 years.

The radiologic appearance is characteristic, with calcification within the intervertebral disc (Fig. 4-67) (243). The calcification may be round, oval, flattened, or fragmented. There may be anterior (245) or posterior (245,246) herniation of calcified intervertebral disc material. The anteroposterior herniation seems to be part of the pathologic process rather than a rare complication (241). Such herniations

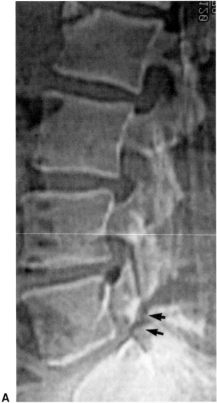

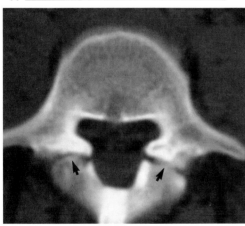

FIG. 4-65. Spondylolysis and spondylolisthesis. A 16-year-old girl with chronic low-back pain. **A:** Lateral CT scout projection. Pars interarticularis defects at the L5 level *(arrows)* with anterior displacement of the L5 vertebral body relative to S1. An incidental limbus deformity of the anterosuperior portion of the L2 vertebral body is also demonstrated. **B:** Axial CT. Bilateral pars defects *(arrows)* with adjacent bony sclerosis is shown.

undergo spontaneous resorption with conservative therapy, and symptoms disappear (245).

Conditions associated with disc calcification include block vertebrae, vitamin D poisoning, degenerative disease, and alkaptonuria. These conditions are readily distinguished by the clinical history, age of the patient, and radiologic appearance. Treatment of intervertebral disc calcification is conservative, with bed rest and analgesics used as needed.

The calcified material is resorbed or herniated within weeks to months from the onset of clinical symptoms. MRI or CT may be used to assess the extent of any associated disc herniation. MRI may show disc changes even when calcification is not visible on plain radiographs (247).

Scheuermann Disease

Scheuermann disease is one of the most confusing and poorly understood abnormalities of the pediatric spine. It consists of primary irregularity of ossification of one or more vertebral endplates (18,248). This entity may or may not be associated with clinical symptomatology, wedging, kyphosis, and Schmorl nodes (249). This definition of Scheuermann disease excludes wedging and kyphosis without irregularity of endplates as well as Schmorl nodes without associated endplate ossification disturbance (248).

The etiology of Scheuermann disease remains unknown. There is evidence that central Schmorl nodes, marginal Schmorl nodes, and the irregular ossification of Scheuermann disease result from different mechanisms. Marginal Schmorl nodes are due to trauma, whereas central Schmorl

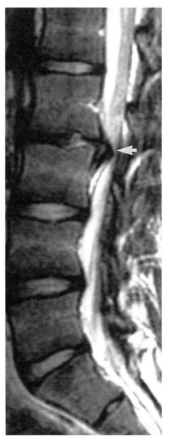

FIG. 4-66. Disc herniation. A 16-year-old girl with back pain after heavy lifting. Sagittal T2-weighted MRI. Narrowing and hypointensity of the L2 disc. Protrusion of the disc and apophyseal bony fragment causes extradural compression of the cauda equina nerve roots *(arrow)*.

central Schmorl nodes, marginal Schmorl nodes, kyphosis, narrowing of intervertebral disc spaces, hypertrophic degenerative changes, and scoliosis (249). Three or more contiguous vertebral bodies are usually involved, and the angle of kyphosis is usually greater than 35°. Bone scintigraphy may be helpful in patients with atypical Scheuermann disease (251,252).

Scoliosis

Types of Scoliosis

Spinal curvatures require careful radiologic evaluation. *Scoliosis* is lateral curvature of the spine; *kyphosis* is in-

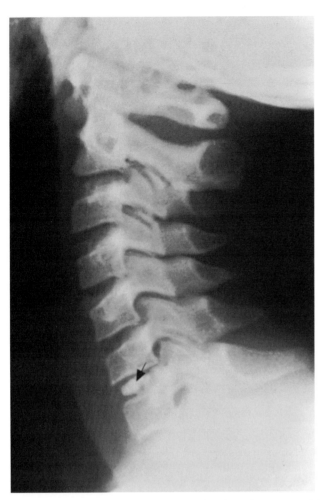

FIG. 4-67. Intervertebral disc calcification. A 10-year-old boy with neck pain and stiffness. Lateral radiograph demonstrates calcification in the C6 intervertebral disc *(arrow)*.

nodes correlate with dynamic stress in the erect position (248). Alexander postulated that Scheuermann disease differs from both of these entities in cause and distribution. He suggested that Scheuermann disease is a stress spondylodystrophy due to traumatic growth arrest and endplate fractures occurring with the heightened vulnerability of the spine during the adolescent growth spurt (248). The irregular ossification and frequently associated wedging and kyphosis are probably due to a static load applied to the flexed spine in the sitting position (248). The irregular endplates are caused by disturbed cell vectoring, traumatic growth arrest, and microfractures (18,248). In summary, Scheuermann disease is probably the result of trauma (hyperflexion, axial loading) on the growing spine.

Scheuermann disease is the commonest cause of thoracic kyphosis in older children and adolescents (250). It may occur anywhere from T4 to L4 but is most common in the midthoracic spine; the apex is usually at T7–10 (248). There is a 1.5:1 male predominance. Using the definition above, the sine qua non for the radiologic diagnosis of Scheuermann disease is irregularity of vertebral endplates (Fig. 4-68) (248). There may be associated wedging of vertebral bodies,

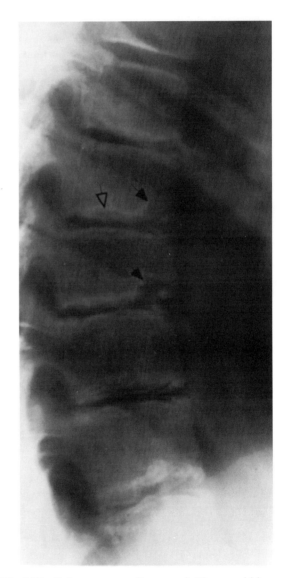

FIG. 4-68. Scheuermann disease. A 15-year-old boy with back pain. Lateral radiograph demonstrates thoracic kyphosis, irregularity of multiple vertebral endplates, slight vertebral body anterior wedging, a central Schmorl node *(open arrow)*, marginal Schmorl nodes *(solid arrows)*, and irregular narrowing of intervertebral disc spaces.

TABLE 4-14. *Classification of scoliosis in infants and children*

Idiopathic scoliosis[a]	Myopathies
Infantile	Friedreich ataxia
Juvenile	Polymyositis
Adolescent[a]	Muscular dystrophy
Congenital anomaly	Spinocerebellar degeneration
Abnormal bone development	Skeletal dysplasias: osteochondrodysplasias[a]
Failure of formation	Ectodermal or mesodermal defects
Complete unilateral: hemivertebra[a]	Neurofibromatosis[a]
Partial unilateral: wedge[a]	Marfan syndrome
Failure of segmentation	Ehlers-Danlos syndrome
Partial or unilateral: bar	Arthrogryposis
Complete or bilateral: block	Homocystinuria
Syndromes	Contractural arachnodactyly
Spondylocostal dysostosis	Posttraumatic scoliosis
Oculovertebral syndrome	Vertebral: fracture, irradiation, postoperative[a]
Klippel-Feil syndrome	Extravertebral: burns, thoracoplasty, irradiation
Caudal regression syndrome	Inflammatory and neoplastic causes
Miscellaneous: Sprengel deformity	Tuberculosis
Abnormal neural or bone development	Rheumatoid arthritis
Myelodysplasia[a]	Histiocytosis
Miscellaneous	Osteoid osteoma: osteoblastoma
Diastematomyelia	Intraspinal lesions
Tethered-cord syndrome	Astrocytoma
Neurenteric cyst	Ependymoma
Anterior or lateral meningocele	Cyst or lipoma
Extravertebral abnormalities	Neurofibroma
Rib fusion	Osteopenia: bone softening
Hypoplastic lung	Osteoporosis
Myositis ossificans progressiva	Osteomalacia
Neuromuscular disorders[a]	Rickets
Poliomyelitis	Hyperparathyroidism
Syringohydromyelia	Cushing disease
Cerebral palsy[a]	Steroid therapy
Duchenne muscular dystrophy	Miscellaneous disorders: Larsen syndrome; familial dysau-
Spinal muscular atrophy	tonomia

[a] More common.

Source: Modified from McAlister and Shackelford (253).

creased posterior angulation of the spine; and *lordosis* is increased anterior angulation of the spine. An angulation of more than 40° is considered abnormal kyphosis in the thoracic region or abnormal lordosis in the lumbar region (18,253).

Scoliosis may be structural or nonstructural. With structural scoliosis, lateral-bending films show an asymmetric loss of normal mobility of the primary curve. Individual vertebrae in the curve are frequently rotated. There are compensatory, secondary curves above and below the primary structural curvature. The spine has normal mobility and no rotational deformity in nonstructural scoliosis; the curve is usually either lumbar or thoracolumbar without associated compensatory curves. A classification of spinal curvatures is presented in Table 4-14 (253).

Idiopathic Scoliosis. Idiopathic scoliosis, lateral curvature of the spine without known cause, is by far the most common spinal curvature abnormality of childhood (254). Most cases occur in adolescence; there are also infantile and juvenile types of idiopathic scoliosis (18,253).

Nonprogressive infantile idiopathic scoliosis is more com-

mon in boys, has a curve that is convex to the left in the thoracic region, and may be secondary to intrauterine molding. These curves do not increase beyond 30°; they resolve spontaneously and require no therapy.

Progressive infantile idiopathic scoliosis is more frequent in boys, is convex to the left in the mid- and lower thoracic regions, and has a poor prognosis. The usual patient has a curve of approximately 30° when diagnosed, usually before 2 years of age. The curvature is particularly likely to progress if greater than 35° or if diagnosed early (253,255). When progressive, the curvature increases at the rate of approximately 5° per year (253). There may be cardiorespiratory insufficiency due to the severe scoliosis.

Juvenile idiopathic scoliosis occurs most commonly in girls between 4 and 9 years of age with thoracic curves that are convex to the right. The prognosis is poor, and progression is frequent.

Adolescent idiopathic scoliosis is much more frequent, especially in girls. The curvature is usually convex to the right in the thoracic region. There is a positive family history for scoliosis in 15% to 20% of patients. Moreover, 28% of male siblings and 43% of female siblings of patients with adolescent idiopathic scoliosis will have scoliotic curvatures of more than 10° (253). The major complications or sequelae of idiopathic scoliosis include curve progression, cosmetic deformity, back pain in older patients, neurologic dysfunction, degenerative joint disease, and (in severe cases) respiratory compromise. Progression of the curve characteristically occurs during accelerated linear growth, i.e., between birth and 2 years and just before puberty. Progressive curvatures tend to occur more often in females and when large amounts of skeletal growth remain prior to epiphyseal closure. Also, curves in excess of 40–50° tend to progress after skeletal maturity. Pain may occur as a result of curvature progression, or may be due to associated degenerative disc or facet disease. The higher the level of structural curve, the worse is the prognosis. The shape and type of the structural curve and compensatory secondary curves are present from the onset of the deformity.

The most frequent patterns of idiopathic scoliosis, in decreasing order of frequency, are a convex right thoracic curve, a convex right thoracic and left lumbar curve, a convex right thoracolumbar curve, and a convex right lumbar curve (256).

Adolescent idiopathic scoliosis occurs in approximately 7% of patients with congenital heart disease and up to 15% of patients with cyanotic congenital heart disease. There is no female predominance in this group of patients. The convexity of the thoracic curve is always opposite the side of the aortic arch. Chest roentgenograms in patients with congenital heart disease should be closely monitored for the possible development of scoliosis.

Atypical Idiopathic Scoliosis. Atypical manifestations of idiopathic scoliosis include early onset (prior to age 10 years), rapid progression, back pain, unusual curve patterns, abnormal neurologic symptoms or signs, and unusual plain radiographic findings, such as spinal canal widening, pedicle thinning, and an unusual degree of kyphosis (6,256). Some of these atypical signs and symptoms may be due to rapid curve progression, disc protrusion, nerve root impingement, or cord thinning. Rarely, a neoplasm or hydrosyringomyelia is an unsuspected neuropathologic finding. Rare or ''atypical'' curvature patterns include a convex left thoracic curve, a convex left thoracolumbar curve (Fig. 4-69), a convex left cervical curve, and a convex left cervicothoracic scoliosis. Exaggerated thoracic kyphosis is unusual in typical idiopathic scoliosis, except in the progressive infantile form and in adults after many years of involvement.

Patients with presumed idiopathic scoliosis who have atypical clinical or radiographic features should have MRI. MRI findings in patients with atypical idiopathic scoliosis include hydrosyringomyelia, Chiari I malformation, dural ectasia, disc protrusion, and spinal cord tumor (256).

Congenital Scoliosis. Congenital scoliosis is due to abnormal neural or bone development or extravertebral abnormalities (see Table 4-14). Many patients with congenital scoliosis have a progressive curve and require close follow-up and, often, early operation. Genitourinary anomalies occur in 20% of these patients. The most common site of curvature is the thoracic region; congenital thoracic curves are often associated with cardiac anomalies. The likelihood of progression increases with the number of vertebral segments involved (253). The average congenital scoliosis progresses by 5° per year, and the curve must be monitored carefully. Diastematomyelia is present in 5% of all patients with congenital scoliosis (253). If vertebral anomalies and scoliosis are noted, the possibility of unilateral failure of segmentation (bony bar) should be considered.

Common abnormalities causing congenital scoliosis are wedge vertebrae, hemivertebrae, butterfly vertebrae, pedicle fusion bars, block vertebrae, and block hemivertebrae. Spinal dysraphism is present in 20% of patients with congenital scoliosis (13,253).

Neuromuscular Scoliosis. A variety of entities produce neuromuscular scoliosis (see Table 4-14). The classic curve of neuromuscular scoliosis is in the shape of a ''C'' in contrast to the ''S'' shape of idiopathic scoliosis.

Skeletal Dysplasia. Osteochondrodysplasias may cause abnormal spinal curvatures. Some of the more important skeletal dysplasias causing scoliosis include osteogenesis imperfecta, diastrophic dwarfism, metatropic dwarfism, spondyloepiphyseal dysplasia, spondylometaphyseal dysplasia, cleidocranial dysplasia, enchondromatosis, and Kniest syndrome.

Ectodermal or Mesodermal Scoliosis. Neurofibromatosis type 1 (NF-1), a mesodermal and ectodermal dysplasia, is one of the most common skeletal dysplasias of childhood. Characteristic spinal abnormalities may include scoliosis or kyphosis involving only a short segment, posterior vertebral body scalloping, vertebral body wedging, dural ectasia, lateral thoracic meningocele (Figs. 4-70 and 4-71), or a neurofibroma (123,257,258). Cervical kyphosis, hypoplasia of the posterior elements (spinous processes, transverse processes, pedicles), dysplasia of the vertebral bodies, and rib deformities (twisted ribbon appearance) may also occur.

Posttraumatic Scoliosis. Posttraumatic scoliosis may be due to injury to the vertebrae or extravertebral tissues (see Table 4-14). Scoliosis following radiation has become less common with new techniques and inclusion of the entire vertebral bodies in the therapy field. Soft-tissue muscle and muscle damage, in addition to damage to the growth plates, must also play a role in scoliosis due to irradiation.

Radiologic Evaluation of Scoliosis

The type and frequency of radiologic evaluation depends on the age and likely etiology of the curvature. Initial radiologic examination includes a minimum of erect (standing if possible, seated if necessary) frontal and lateral radiographs from the external auditory meatus to the iliac crest (see Appendix 2). To reduce irradiation of the breast, the frontal

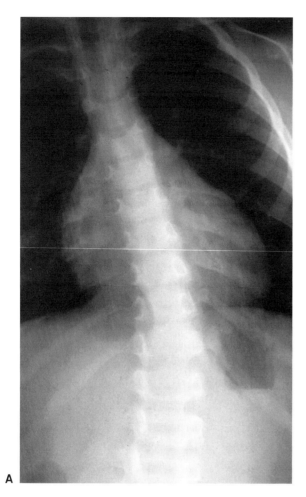

A

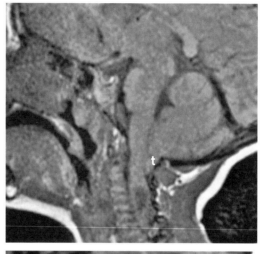

B

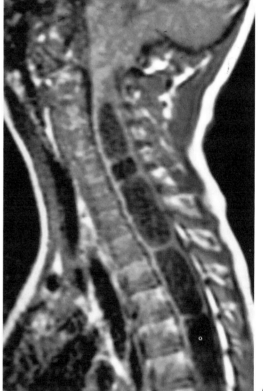

C

FIG. 4-69. Atypical scoliosis with Chiari I malformation and syringohydromyelia. A 5-year-old boy with atypical thoracolumbar scoliosis. **A:** Frontal radiograph demonstrates thoracolumbar scoliosis that is convex to the left. **B:** Sagittal T1-weighted MRI shows caudal projection of the cerebellar tonsils *(t)* and cervicomedullary junction below the foramen magnum. **C:** The low-intensity saccular expansion of the cervicothoracic spinal cord is due to syringohydromyelia.

film should be PA rather than AP. Right and left lateral-bending films are frequently obtained to determine whether the scoliosis is structural or nonstructural. 14 × 17 in. cassettes are usually satisfactory in younger children, although 14 × 36 in. cassettes are usually required in older children and adults (259). Skeletal maturation is determined by hand and wrist radiography during the initial evaluation in patients with adolescent idiopathic scoliosis. Conventional tomography may be helpful if there may be a bony bar.

MRI is performed in patients with atypical clinical or radiologic findings (256,260). Skeletal surveys are obtained in patients with chondrodysplasias and dysmorphic syndromes. Asymmetry of the positions of the iliac crests on the erect

frontal film should raise the question of leg length discrepancy. Lower extremity scanograms as well as an erect film with a foot lift in place are indicated.

Measurement of Scoliosis

Although there is a variety of techniques for the measurement of scoliosis, the Lippman-Cobb method is the most widely used and is recommended by the Scoliosis Research Society. Lines are drawn tangential to the superior endplate of the top vertebra of the curve and the inferior endplate of the bottom vertebra of the curve (Fig. 4-72). The angle of

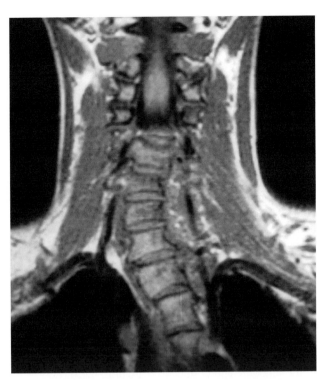

FIG. 4-70. Neurofibromatosis type 1 and scoliosis. A 17-year-old girl with NF-1. Coronal T1-weighted MRI shows acute-angle, short segment cervicothoracic scoliosis with wedging and scalloping of multiple vertebral bodies.

20°; group II, 20–30°; group III, 31–50°; group IV, 51–75°; group V, 76–100°; group VI, 101–125°; and group VII, more than 126° (259).

The extent of vertebral rotation is a major indicator of the length of bony fusion necessary to produce stability. One determines rotation by noting the relation of the oval pedicles to the lateral margins of vertebral bodies in the frontal erect view. With rotation, the pedicles on the convex side of the curve shift toward the concave side and change their configuration (259). Rotation is graded from 0 to 100% and from the vertebra with the maximum rotation, which is usually located at the apex of the curve.

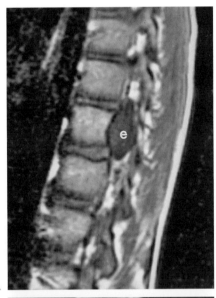

A

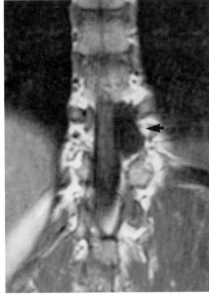

B

FIG. 4-71. Dural ectasia in neurofibromatosis type 1. A 14-year-old girl with known NF-1. Sagittal **(A)** and coronal **(B)** T1-weighted MRI show a CSF intensity expansion of the dural sac *(e)* at the lower thoracic level with localized extension of the dural ectasia into an adjacent intervertebral foramen *(arrow)*.

the curve may be measured directly either by extending the lines laterally until they intersect or by drawing perpendiculars to the lines. The angle formed is equal to the degree of curvature (Fig. 4-72). Kuhns and Martin have modified a standard goniometer so that scoliotic angles may be measured directly from the radiograph without placing marks on the film (261).

The top vertebra is the vertebra whose superior surface tilts maximally to the concavity of the curve. It is the last vertebra that shows widening of its inferiorly adjacent intervertebral disc space on the convex side of the curve. The inferior surface of the vertebra above the top vertebra of the curve begins to tilt in the opposite direction, and the intervertebral disc space above this top vertebra is wider on the concave side of the primary curve (Fig. 4-72). The bottom vertebra is also the one whose inferior surface tilts maximally to the concavity of the curve. The intervertebral disc space above this bottom vertebra is widened on the convex side of the curve, whereas the intervertebral disc space below this bottom vertebra is wider on the concave side of the primary curve (Fig. 4-72). The top and bottom vertebrae of the curve exhibit the least amount of rotation. The top or bottom vertebra of the curve sometimes shifts on follow-up studies, and remeasurement may be needed. The same method and same levels should be used for initial and follow-up examinations. The Lippman-Cobb method tends to magnify the curve as it progresses (259). The severity of the curve may be divided into seven groups: group I, less than

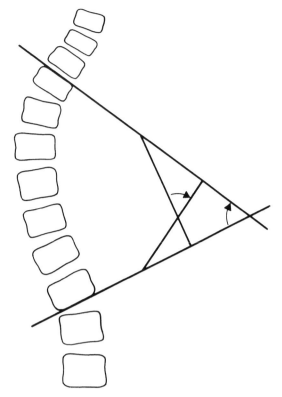

FIG. 4-72. Lippman-Cobb method for measuring scoliosis. Thoracic scoliosis with convexity to the right. Lines are drawn tangential to the superior vertebral endplate at the top of the curve and the inferior vertebral endplate at the bottom of the curve. The angle of the curve *(curved arrows)* may be measured by extending the lines laterally until they intersect or by drawing perpendiculars to the tangential lines, as illustrated.

Some idea of the torso balance may be determined by extending a perpendicular line from the midsacrum and determining the centimeters of deviation from the middle of the vertebral body of T1 (255). Scoliosis patterns are identified by the curves having the greatest angles. Curve patterns include cervicothoracic, double thoracic, main thoracic, thoracolumbar, main lumbar, and thoracic and lumbar curves (255).

Surgical Correction of Scoliosis

The natural history of scoliosis is frequently one of increasing deformity. The most rapid progression of curves occurs during the years of major linear growth, but curves over 35–40° can be expected to increase even after skeletal maturation. Scoliosis may be treated by bracing or by surgical intervention. Radiology is critical for posttherapy evaluation (262).

Current operative treatment of scoliosis includes internal fixation of the spine in addition to bony fusion. The Harrington rod (distracting and compression) fixation-and-fusion procedure is performed using a posterior approach to the spine. The Dwyer fixation-and-fusion procedure is performed using an anterior, retroperitoneal approach to the spine through a thoracoabdominal incision. Whereas the Harrington rod is rigid, the Dwyer cable remains flexible. Both devices are designed to maintain the correction of the curve until the bone graft becomes solid, which allows earlier postoperative ambulation. The appliances serve no function after the bony graft is solid, but they are left in place unless there is a complication. The Dwyer technique is difficult above the level of T5, so it is used more frequently for correction of lower curves. Because it is placed anteriorly, the Dwyer technique is particularly helpful in patients with deficient posterior elements, such as those with myelomeningocele. A number of other operative techniques and fixation devices (Texas Scottish Rite Hospital devices, Luque rods, Cotrell-Dubousset method, etc.) may also be used for the surgical treatment of scoliosis.

Because of the immobility of the patient during the early postoperative period, usually only AP films are obtained. Stable reduction of scoliosis usually suggests satisfactory fixation. The position and integrity of the metal appliances should be noted, as should any other early complications (pneumothorax, atelectasis, pleural fluid). The bony graft is not solid for approximately 9 months (262). Follow-up radiographic evaluation should include at least frontal and lateral radiographs. Oblique views are best for details of the posterior bone graft. Loss of correction of the scoliosis and failure of hardware position during the early postoperative months suggest nonunion. Pseudarthrosis usually occurs if motion of the spine inhibits normal fusion. Failure of solid bony union is assumed when there is demonstrated loss of correction or failure of hardware. The patient may have localized pain at the site of the pseudarthrosis. If pain persists or if significant loss of correction occurs, the hardware may have to be removed and regrafting performed.

Complications of surgical correction of scoliosis include pseudarthrosis formation, osteomyelitis, gallstone formation, body cast syndrome, hiatus hernia with reflux, aneurysm formation, renal atrophy due to vascular injury, and retroperitoneal fibrosis (262).

Kyphosis

Kyphosis is increased (over 40° in the thoracic spine) posterior angulation of the spine (263). It may be due to Scheuermann disease, failure of bony segmentation or formation (Fig. 4-73), neuromuscular disorder, osteopenia, chondrodysplasia, trauma, inflammation, arthritis, bony or intraspinal tumor, or the Stickler syndrome (253).

A Lippman-Cobb modification is used to measure kyphosis. Lines are drawn tangential to the superior endplate of the top vertebra and the inferior endplate of the bottom vertebra of the kyphotic curvature. The angle of kyphosis is the angle formed by intersecting perpendiculars to these two lines. In addition to standing AP and lateral views of the spine, the kyphosis evaluation should also include a hyperex-

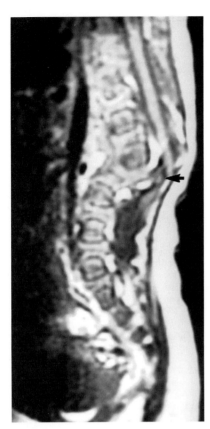

FIG. 4-73. Severe congenital kyphosis. A 3-month-old girl with severe kyphosis. Sagittal T1 MRI. Vertebral body aplasia with severe kyphosis and malalignment. Note compression of the spinal cord *(arrow)* just above the conus medullaris.

tension lateral view, to help evaluate instability or rigidity of the curvature (253,259).

Lordosis

Lordosis is increased (over 40° in the lumbar spine) anterior angulation of the spine. Lordosis may be congenital (failure of formation, failure of segmentation) or acquired (spondylolisthesis, neuromuscular defect, skeletal dysplasia).

Lordosis is measured by modifying the Lippman-Cobb technique. Again, perpendiculars are erected to lines drawn tangential to the superior endplate of the top vertebra and inferior endplate of the bottom vertebra of the lordotic curve. In addition to standing AP and lateral views of the entire spine, a hyperflexion lateral view should be obtained to evaluate instability or rigidity of the lordotic curve.

REFERENCES

1. Barkovich AJ. *Pediatric neuroimaging.* 2nd ed. New York: Raven Press, 1995.
2. Harwood-Nash DC, Fitz CR. *Neuroradiology in infants and children.* St. Louis: Mosby, 1976.
3. Harwood-Nash DC. Pediatric neuroradiology: its evolution as a subspecialty. *AJR* 1993;160:5–14.
4. Silverman FN, Kuhn JP, eds. *Caffey's pediatric x-ray diagnosis: an integrated imaging approach.* 9th ed. St. Louis: Mosby–Year Book, 1993.
5. Afshani E, Kuhn JP. Common causes of low back pain in children. *RadioGraphics* 1991;11:269–291.
6. Harcke HT. Acute back pain in children. In: Kirks DR, ed. *Emergency pediatric radiology. A problem-oriented approach.* Reston, VA: American Roengten Ray Society, 1995, 29–34.
7. Armstrong DC. Spine trauma. In: Kirks DR, ed. *Emergency pediatric radiology. A problem-oriented approach.* Reston, VA: American Roentgen Ray Society, 1995, 51–59.
8. Sty JR, Wells RG, Conway JJ. Spine pain in children. *Semin Nucl Med* 1993;23:296–320.
9. Roberts FF, Kishore PRS, Cunningham ME. Routine oblique radiography of the pediatric lumbar spine: is it necessary? *AJR* 1978;131: 297–298.
10. Treves ST. *Pediatric nuclear medicine.* 2nd ed. New York: Springer-Verlag, 1995.
11. Teele RL, Share JC. *Ultrasonography of infants and children.* Philadelphia: WB Saunders, 1991.
12. Resjo IM, Harwood-Nash DC, Fitz CR, Chuang S. Normal cord in infants and children examined with computed tomographic metrizamide myelography. *Radiology* 1979;130:691–696.
13. Wolpert SM, Barnes PD. *MRI in pediatric neuroradiology.* St. Louis: Mosby–Year Book, 1992.
14. Barnes PD, O'Tuama L, Tzika A. Investigating the pediatric central nervous system. *Curr Opin Pediatr* 1993;5:643–652.
15. Swischuk LE. *Emergency imaging of the acutely ill or injured child.* 3rd ed. Baltimore: Williams and Wilkins, 1994.
16. Davis PC, Reisner A, Hudgins PA, et al. Spinal injuries in children: role of MR. *AJNR* 1993;14:607–617.
17. Bellah RD, Summerville DA, Treves ST, Micheli LJ. Low-back pain in adolescent athletes: detection of stress injury to the pars interarticularis with SPECT. *Radiology* 1991;180:509–512.
18. Kirks DR. *Practical pediatric imaging: diagnostic radiology of infants and children.* 2nd ed. Boston: Little, Brown, 1991.
19. Sarwar M, Kier EL, Virapongse C. Development of the spine and spinal cord. In: Newton TH, Potts DG, eds. *Computed tomography of the spine and spinal cord.* San Anselmo: Clavedel Press, 1983, 15–30.
20. Naidich TP, McLone DG. Growth and development. In: Kricun ME, ed. *Imaging modalities in spinal disorders.* Philadelphia: WB Saunders, 1988, 1–19.
21. Dietemann J, Doyon D, Aubin M, Manelfe C. Cervico-occipital junction: normal and pathological aspects. In: Manelfe C, ed. *Imaging of the spine and spinal cord.* New York: Raven Press, 1992, 705–749.
22. DiPietro MA. The conus medullaris: normal US findings throughout childhood. *Radiology* 1993;188:149–153.
23. Wilson DA, Prince JR. MR imaging determination of the location of the normal conus medullaris throughout childhood. *AJNR* 1989;10: 259–262.
24. Barson AJ. The vertebral level of termination of the spinal cord during normal and abnormal development. *J Anat* 1970;106:489–497.
25. Rowland Hill CA, Gibson PJ. Ultrasound determination of the normal location of the conus medullaris in neonates. *AJNR* 1995;16:469–472.
26. Wolf S, Schneble F, Troger J. The conus medullaris: time of ascendence to normal level. *Pediatr Radiol* 1992;22:590–592.
27. Brill PW, Baker DH, Ewing ML. ''Bone-within-bone'' in the neonatal spine. Stress change or normal development. *Radiology* 1973;108: 363–366.
28. Hindman BW, Poole CA. Early appearance of the secondary vertebral ossification centers. *Radiology* 1970;95:359–361.
29. Vogler JB 3d, Murphy WA. Bone marrow imaging. *Radiology* 1988; 168:679–693.
30. Sze G, Baierl P, Bravo S. Evolution of the infant spinal column: evaluation with MR imaging. *Radiology* 1991;181:819–827.
31. Shapiro R, Youngberg AS, Rothman SLG. The differential diagnosis of traumatic lesions of the occipito-atlanto-axial segment. *Radiol Clin North Am* 1973;11:505–526.
32. Shapiro R, Robinson F. Anomalies of the craniovertebral border. *AJR* 1976;127:281–287.
33. Swischuk LE, Hayden CK Jr, Sarwar M. The dens-arch synchondrosis versus the hangman's fracture. *Pediatr Radiol* 1979;8:100–102.

34. Swischuk LE, Hayden CK Jr, Sarwar M. The posteriorly tilted dens. A normal variation mimicking a fractured dens. *Pediatr Radiol* 1979; 8:27–28.

35. Keats TE. *Atlas of normal roentgen variants that may simulate disease.* 5th ed. St. Louis: Mosby–Year Book, 1992.

36. Currarino G, Rollins N, Diehl JT. Congenital defects of the posterior arch of the atlas: a report of seven cases including an affected mother and son. *AJNR* 1994;15:249–254.

37. Swischuk LE. *Imaging of the newborn, infant, and young child.* 3rd ed. Baltimore: Williams and Wilkins, 1989.

38. Swischuk LE, Swischuk PN, John SD. Wedging of C-3 in infants and children: usually a normal finding and not a fracture. *Radiology* 1993; 188:523–526.

39. Swischuk LE. Anterior displacement of C2 in children: physiologic or pathologic? A helpful differentiating line. *Radiology* 1977;122: 759–763.

40. Hinck VC, Clark WM Jr, Hopkins CE. Normal interpediculate distances (minimum and maximum) in children and adults. *AJR* 1966; 97:141–153.

41. Oestreich AE, Young LW. The absent cervical pedicle syndrome: a case in childhood. *AJR* 1969;107:505–510.

42. Bardsley JL, Hanelin LG. The unilateral hypoplastic lumbar pedicle. *Radiology* 1971;101:315–317.

43. Morin ME, Palacios E. The aplastic hypoplastic lumbar pedicle. *AJR* 1974;122:639–642.

44. Wortzman G, Steinhardt MI. Congenitally absent lumbar pedicle: a reappraisal. *Radiology* 1984;152:713–718.

45. Cohen J, Currarino G, Neuhauser EBD. A significant variant in the ossification centers of the vertebral bodies. *AJR* 1956;76:469–475.

46. Fielden P, Russell JG. Coronally cleft vertebra. *Clin Radiol* 1970;21: 327–328.

47. Benzian SR, Mainzer F, Gooding CA. Pediculate thinning: a normal variant at the thoracolumbar junction. *Br J Radiol* 1971;44:936–939.

48. Charlton OP, Martinez S, Gehweiler JA Jr. Pedicle thinning at the thoracolumbar junction: a normal variant. *AJR* 1980;134:825–826.

49. Kozlowski K. Platyspondyly in childhood. *Pediatr Radiol* 1974;2: 81–88.

50. Gooding CA, Neuhauser EBD. Growth and development of the vertebral body in the presence and absence of normal stress. *AJR* 1965; 93:388–394.

51. Donaldson JS, Gilsanz V, Gonzalez G, et al. Tall vertebrae at birth: a radiographic finding in flaccid infants. *AJR* 1985;145:1293–1295.

52. Swischuk LE. *Radiology of the newborn and young infant,* 2nd ed. Baltimore: Williams and Wilkins, 1980.

53. Perovic MN, Kopits SE, Thompson RC. Radiological evaluation of the spinal cord in congenital atlanto-axial dislocation. *Radiology* 1973; 109:713–716.

54. Locke GR, Gardner JI, Van Epps EF. Atlas-dens interval (ADI) in children: a survey based on 200 normal cervical spines. *AJR* 1966; 97:135–140.

55. White KS, Ball WS, Prenger EC, et al. Evaluation of the craniocervical junction in Down syndrome: correlation of measurements obtained with radiography and MR imaging. *Radiology* 1993;186:377–382.

56. Hinck VC, Hopkins CE, Savara BS. Sagittal diameter of the cervical spinal canal in children. *Radiology* 1962;79:97–108.

57. Markuske H. Sagittal diameter measurements of the bony cervical spinal canal in children. *Pediatr Radiol* 1977;6:129–131.

58. Yousefzadeh DK, El-Khoury GY, Smith WL. Normal sagittal diameter and variation in the pediatric cervical spine. *Radiology* 1982;144: 319–325.

59. Mitchell GE, Lourie H, Berne AS. The various causes of scalloped vertebrae with notes on their pathogenesis. *Radiology* 1967;89:67–74.

60. Canale ST, Griffin DW, Hubbard CN. Congenital muscular torticollis. A long term follow-up. *J Bone Joint Surg* 1982;64A:810–816.

61. Dubousset J. Torticollis in children caused by congenital anomalies of the atlas. *J Bone Joint Surg Am* 1986;68A:178–188.

62. Calvy TM, Segall HD, Gilles FH, et al. CT anatomy of the craniovertebral junction in infants and children. *AJNR* 1987;8:489–494.

63. Lee BCP, Deck MDF, Kneeland JB, Cahill PT. MR imaging of the craniocervical junction. *AJNR* 1985;6:209–213.

64. Smoker WRK. Craniovertebral junction: normal anatomy, craniometry, and congenital anomalies. *RadioGraphics* 1994;14:255–277.

65. Kaufman RA, Carroll CD, Buncher CR. Atlanto-occipital junction: standards for measurement in normal children. *AJNR* 1987;8: 995–999.

66. Maves CK, Souza A, Prenger EC, Kirks DR. Traumatic atlanto-occipital disruption in children. *Pediatr Radiol* 1991;21:504–507.

67. Bulas DI, Fitz CR, Johnson DL. Traumatic atlanto-occipital dislocation in children. *Radiology* 1993;188:155–158.

68. Nguyen VD, Tyrrel R. Klippel-Feil syndrome: patterns of bony fusion and wasp-waist sign. *Skeletal Radiol* 1993;22:519–523.

69. Ramsey J, Bliznak J. Klippel-Feil syndrome with renal agenesis and other anomalies. *AJR* 1971;113:460–463.

70. Hensinger RN, Lang JE, MacEwen GD. Klippel-Feil syndrome: a constellation of associated anomalies. *J Bone Joint Surg* 1974;56A: 1246–1253.

71. Moore WB, Matthews TJ, Rabinowitz R. Genitourinary anomalies associated with Klippel-Feil syndrome. *J Bone Joint Surg* 1975;57A: 355–357.

72. Hall JE, Simmons ED, Danylchuk K, Barnes PD. Instability of the cervical spine and neurological involvement in Klippel-Feil syndrome. A case report. *J Bone Joint Surg Am* 1990;72A:460–462.

73. Barnes PD, Poussaint TY, Robertson RL. Imaging of the spine and spinal neuraxis in children. In: Lee RR, ed. *Spine: state of the art reviews.* vol 9. Philadelphia: Hanley and Belfus, 1995, 73–92.

74. Kao SCK, Waziri MH, Smith WL, et al. MR imaging of the craniovertebral junction, cranium and brain in children with achondroplasia. *AJR* 1989;153:565–569.

75. Fielding JW, Hensinger RN, Hawkins RJ. Os odontoideum. *J Bone Joint Surg Am* 1980;62A:376–383.

76. Harwood-Nash DC. Anomalies of the craniovertebral junction. In: Hoffman H, Epstein F, eds. *Disorders of the developing nervous system.* Boston: Blackwell Scientific, 1986, 423–447.

77. Gwinn JL, Smith JL. Acquired and congenital absence of the odontoid process. *AJR* 1962;88:424–431.

78. Wackenheim A, Burguet JL, Sick H. Section of the odontoid process by a shortened transverse ligament (a possible etiology for the mobile odontoid). *Neuroradiology* 1986;28:281–282.

79. Greenberg AD. Atlanto-axial dislocation. *Brain* 1968;91:655–684.

80. Rosenbaum DM, Blumhagen JD, King HA. Atlantooccipital instability in Down syndrome. *AJR* 1986;146:1269–1272.

81. Pueschel SM, Scola FH. Atlanto-axial instability in individuals with Down syndrome: epidemiologic, radiographic, and clinical studies. *Pediatrics* 1987;80:555–560.

82. Martich V, Ben-Ami T, Yousefzadeh DK, Roizen NJ. Hypoplastic posterior arch of C-1 in children with Down syndrome: a double jeopardy. *Radiology* 1992;183:125–128.

83. Kowalski HM, Cohen WA, Cooper P, Wisoff JH. Pitfalls in the CT diagnosis of atlantoaxial rotary subluxation. *AJNR* 1987;8:697–702.

84. Barnes PD, Lester PD, Yamanashi WS, Prince JR. MRI in infants and children with spinal dysraphism. *AJR* 1986;147:339–346.

85. van der Knaap MS, Valk J. Classification of congenital abnormalities of the CNS. *AJNR* 1988;9:315–326.

86. Scatliff JH, Kendall BE, Kingsley DPE, et al. Closed spinal dysraphism: analysis of clinical, radiological, and surgical findings in 104 consecutive patients. *AJR* 1989;152:1049–1057.

87. Naidich TP, Fernbach SK, McLone DG, Shkolnik A. Sonography of the caudal spine and back: congenital anomalies in children. *AJR* 1984;142:1229–1242.

88. Kollias SS, Goldstein RB, Cogen PH, Filly RA. Prenatally detected myelomeningoceles: sonographic accuracy in estimation of the spinal level. *Radiology* 1992;185:109–112.

89. Quencer RM, Montalvo BM, Naidich TP, et al. Intraoperative sonography in spinal dysraphism and syringohydromyelia. *AJNR* 1987;8: 329–337.

90. Altman NR, Altman DH. MR imaging of spinal dysraphism. *AJNR* 1987;8:533–538.

91. Barnes PD, Lester PD, Yamanashi WS, Prince JR. Magnetic resonance imaging in infants and children with spinal dysraphism. *AJNR* 1986;7:465–472.

92. Piggott H. The natural history of scoliosis in myelodysplasia. *J Bone Joint Surg Br* 1980;49B:54–58.

93. Hoppenfeld S. Congenital kyphosis in myelomeningocele. *J Bone Joint Surg Br* 1967;49B:276–280.

94. Pang D. Split cord malformation. Part II: clinical syndrome. *Neurosurgery* 1992;31:481–500.

95. Resjo IM, Harwood-Nash DC, Fitz CR, Chuang S. Computed tomographic metrizamide myelography in spinal dysraphism in infants and children. *J Comput Assist Tomogr* 1978;2:549–558.

96. McLone DG, Dias MS. Complications of myelomeningocele closure. *Pediatr Neurosurg* 1991–1992;17:267–273.

97. Nelson MD Jr, Bracchi M, Naidich TP, McLone DG. The natural history of repaired myelomeningocele. *RadioGraphics* 1988;8:695–706.

98. Samuelsson L, Bergstrom K, Thuomas K-A, et al. MR imaging of syringohydromyelia and Chiari malformations in myelomeningocele patients with scoliosis. *AJNR* 1987;8:539–546.

99. Heinz ER, Rosenbaum AE, Scarff TB, et al. Tethered spinal cord following meningomyelocele repair. Radiology 1979;131:153–160.

100. Harwood-Nash DC, Fitz CR. Myelography and syringohydromyelia in infancy and childhood. *Radiology* 1974;113:661–669.

101. Sherman JL, Barkovich AJ, Citrin CM. The MR appearance of syringomyelia: new observations. *AJR* 1987;148:381–391.

102. Hoffman HJ, Neill J, Crone KR, et al. Hydrosyringomelia and its management in childhood. *Neurosurgery* 1987;21:347–351.

103. Han JS, Benson JE, Kaufman B, et al. Demonstration of diastematomyelia and associated abnormalities with MR imaging. *AJNR* 1985;6:215–219.

104. Lee BCP, Zimmerman RD, Manning JJ, Deck MDF. MR imaging of syringomyelia and hydromyelia. *AJNR* 1985;6:221–228.

105. Villarejo FJ, Blazquez MG, Gutierrez-Diaz JA. Intraspinal lipomas in children. *Childs Brain* 1976;2:361–370.

106. Naidich TP, McLone DG, Mutluer S. A new understanding of dorsal dysraphism with lipoma (lipomyeloschisis): radiologic evaluation and surgical correction. *AJR* 1983;140:1065–1078.

107. Vade A, Kennard D. Lipomeningomyelocystocele. *AJNR* 1987;8:375–377.

108. Sutton LN, Lipomyelomeningocele. *Neurosurg Clin N Am* 1995;6:325–338.

109. Gold LHA, Kieffer SA, Peterson HO. Lipomatous invasion of the spinal cord associated with spinal dysraphism: myelographic evaluation. *AJR* 1969;107:479–485.

110. Wright RL. Congenital dermal sinuses. *Prog Neurol Surg* 1971;4:175–191.

111. Giuffre R. Intradural spinal lipomas: review of the literature (99 cases) and report of an additional case. *Acta Neurochir* 1966;14:69–95.

112. List CF. Intraspinal epidermoids, dermoids, and dermal sinuses. *Surg Gynecol Obstet* 1941;73:525–538.

113. Walker AE, Bucy PC. Congenital dermal sinuses: source of spinal meningeal infection and subdural abscesses. *Brain* 1934;57:401–421.

114. Mount LA. Congenital dermal sinuses as a cause of meningitis, intraspinal abscess and intracranial abscess. *JAMA* 1949;139:1263–1268.

115. Algra PR, Hageman LM. Gadopentetate dimeglumine-enhanced MR imaging of spinal dermal sinus tract. *AJNR* 1991;12:1025–1026.

116. Barkovich AJ, Edwards MSB, Cogen PH. MR evaluation of spinal dermal sinus tracts in children. *AJR* 1991;156:791–797.

117. Fitz CR, Harwood-Nash DC. The tethered conus. *AJR* 1975;125:515–523.

118. Sarwar M, Virapongse C, Bhimani S. Primary tethered cord syndrome: a new hypothesis of its origin. *AJNR* 1984;5:235–242.

119. Raghaven N, Barkovich AJ, Edwards M, Norman D. MR imaging in the tethered spinal cord syndrome. *AJNR* 1989;10:27–36.

120. McLone DG, Naidich TP. Terminal myelocystocele. *Neurosurgery* 1985;16:36–43.

121. Byrd SE, Harvey C, McLone DG, Darling CF. Imaging of the terminal myelocystoceles. *J Natl Med Assoc* 1996;88:510–516.

122. Braffman B, Naidich TP. The phakomatoses: Part I. Neurofibromatosis and tuberous sclerosis. *Neuroimag Clin N Am* 1994;4:299–324.

123. Holt JF. Neurofibromatosis in children. *AJR* 1978;130:615–639.

124. Kaufmann HJ. Anterior sacral meningocele. *Ann Radiol* 1967;10:121–128.

125. Edeiken J, Lee KF, Libshitz H. Intrathoracic meningocele. *AJR* 1969;106:381–384.

126. Burrows FGO, Sutcliffe J. The split notochord syndrome. *Br J Radiol* 1968;41:844–847.

127. Faris JC, Crowe JE. The split notochord syndrome. *J Pediatr Surg* 1975;10:467–472.

128. Hoffman CH, Dietrich RB, Pais MJ, et al. The split notochord syndrome with dorsal enteric fistula. *AJNR* 1993;14:622–627.

129. Geremia GK, Russell EJ, Clasen RA. MR imaging characteristics of a neurenteric cyst. *AJNR* 1988;9:978–980.

130. Brooks BS, Duvall ER, El Gammal T, et al. Neuroimaging features of neurenteric cysts: analysis of nine cases and review of the literature. *AJNR* 1993;14:735–746.

131. D'Almeida AC, Steward DH Jr. Neurenteric cyst: case report and literature review. *Neurosurgery* 1981;8:596–599.

132. Scatliff JH, Till K, Hoare RD. Incomplete, false, and true diastematomyelia: radiological evaluation by air myelography and tomography. *Radiology* 1975;116:349–354.

133. Neuhauser EBD, Wittenborg MH, Dehlinger K. Diastematomyelia. *Radiology* 1950;54:659–664.

134. Naidich TP, Harwood-Nash DC. Diastematomyelia: hemicord and meningeal sheaths; single and double arachnoid and dural tubes. *AJNR* 1983;4:633–636.

135. Scotti G, Musgrave MA, Harwood-Nash DC, et al. Diastematomyelia in children: metrizamide and CT metrizamide myelography. *AJR* 1980;135:1225–1232.

136. Hilal SK, Marton D, Pollack E. Diastematomyelia in children. Radiographic study of 34 cases. *Radiology* 1974;112:609–621.

137. Kaffenberger DA, Heinz ER, Oakes JW, Boyko O. Meningocele manque: radiologic findings with clinical correlation. *AJNR* 1992;13:1083–1088.

138. Gower DJ, Del Curling O, Kelly DL Jr, Alexander EJ Jr. Diastematomyelia—a 40-year experience. *Pediatr Neurosci* 1988;14:90–96.

139. Currarino G, Coln D, Votteler T. Triad of anorectal, sacral, and presacral anomalies. *AJR* 1981;137:395–398.

140. Nievelstein RAJ, Valk J, Smit LME, Vermeij-Keers C. MR of the caudal regression syndrome: embryologic implications. *AJNR* 1994;15:1021–1029.

141. Renshaw TS. Sacral agenesis. *J Bone Joint Surg* 1978;60A:373–383.

142. Barkovich AJ, Raghaven N, Chuang SH. MR of lumbosacral agenesis. *AJNR* 1989;10:1223–1231.

143. Appignani BA, Jaramillo D, Barnes PD, Poussaint TY. Dysraphic myelodysplasias associated with urogenital and anorectal anomalies: prevalence and types seen with MR imaging. *AJR* 1994;163:1199–1203.

144. Tunell WP, Austin JC, Barnes PD, Reynolds A. Neuroradiologic evaluation of sacral abnormalities in imperforate anus complex. *J Pediatr Surg* 1987;22:58–61.

145. Pinckney LE, Currarino G, Highgenboten CL. Osteomyelitis of the cervical spine following dental extraction. *Radiology* 1980;135:335–337.

146. Miller JH, Gates GF. Scintigraphy of sacroiliac pyarthrosis in children. *JAMA* 1977;238:2701–2704.

147. Schaad UB, McCracken GH Jr, Nelson JD. Pyogenic arthritis of the sacroiliac joint in pediatric patients. *Pediatrics* 1980;66:375–379.

148. Fischer GW, Popich GA, Sullivan DE, et al. Diskitis: a prospective diagnostic analysis. *Pediatrics* 1978;62:543–548.

149. Wenger DR, Bobechko WP, Gilday DL. The spectrum of intervertebral disc-space infection in children. *J Bone Joint Surg* 1978;60A:100–108.

150. Brass A, Bowdler JD. Non-specific spondylitis of childhood. *Ann Radiol* 1969;12:343–354.

151. Banna M, Gryspeerdt GL. Intraspinal tumours in children (excluding dysraphism). *Clin Radiol* 1971;22:17–32.

152. Heller RM, Szalay EA, Green NE, et al. Disc space infection in children: magnetic resonance imaging. *Radiol Clin North Am* 1988;26:207–209.

153. Thrush A, Enzmann D. MR imaging of infectious spondylitis. *AJNR* 1990;11:1171–1180.

154. du Lac P, Panuel M, Devred P, et al. MRI of disc space infection in infants and children. Report of 12 cases. *Pediatr Radiol* 1990;20:175–178.

155. Sharif HS. Role of MR imaging in the management of spinal infections. *AJR* 1992;158:1333–1345.

156. Ring D, Wenger DR. Pyogenic infectious spondylitis in children. The evolution to current thought. *Am J Orthop* 1996;25:342–348.

157. Jacobsen FS, Sullivan B. Spinal epidural abcesses in children. *Orthop* 1994;17:1131–1138.

158. Numaguchi Y, Rigamonti D, Rothman MI, et al. Spinal epidural abscess: evaluation with gadolinium-enhanced MR imaging. *RadioGraphics* 1993;13:545–559.

159. Nussbaum ES, Rigamonti D, Standiford H, et al. Spinal epidural abscess: a report of 40 cases and review. *Surg Neurol* 1992;38:225–231.

160. Osborne AG. *Diagnostic neuroradiology.* St. Louis: Mosby–Year Book, 1994.

161. Ross JS, Masaryk TJ, Modic MT, et al. MR imaging of lumbar arachnoiditis. *AJR* 1987;149:1025–1032.
162. Atlas SW, ed. *Magnetic resonance imaging of the brain and spine.* New York: Raven Press, 1991.
163. Awerbuch G, Feinberg WM, Ferry P, et al. Demonstration of acute post-viral myelitis with magnetic resonance imaging. *Pediatr Neurol* 1987;3:367–369.
164. Azouz EM, Kozlowski K, Marton D, et al. Osteoid osteoma and osteoblastoma of the spine in children. Report of 22 cases with brief literature review. *Pediatr Radiol* 1986;16:25–31.
165. Mahboubi S. CT appearance of nidus in osteoid osteoma versus sequestration in osteomyelitis. *J Comput Assist Tomogr* 1986;10:457–459.
166. Freiberger RH. Osteoid osteoma of the spine. A cause of backache and scoliosis in children and young adults. *Radiology* 1960;75:232–236.
167. Mehta MH, Murray RO. Scoliosis provoked by painful vertebral lesions. *Skeletal Radiol* 1977;1:223–230.
168. Wilkinson RH, Hall JE. The sclerotic pedicle: tumor or pseudotumor? *Radiology* 1974;111:683–688.
169. Glass RB, Poznanski AK, Fisher MR, et al. MR imaging of osteoid osteoma. *J Comput Assist Tomogr* 1986;10:1065–1067.
170. Kozlowski K, Beluffi G, Masel J, et al. Primary vertebral tumors in children. Report of 20 cases with brief view of the literature. *Pediatr Radiol* 1984;14:129–139.
171. Kroon HM, Schurmans J. Osteoblastoma: clinical and radiologic findings in 98 new cases. *Radiology* 1990;175:783–790.
172. Brunberg JA, DiPietro MA, Venes JL, et al. Intramedullary lesions of the pediatric spinal cord: correlation of findings from MR imaging, intraoperative sonography, surgery, and histologic study. *Radiology* 1991;181:573–579.
173. Chapman PH. Congenital intraspinal lipomas: anatomic considerations and surgical treatment. *Childs Brain* 1982;9:37–47.
174. Schroeder S, Lackner K, Weiand G. Lumbosacral intradural lipoma. *J Comput Assist Tomogr* 1981;5:274.
175. Guidetti B, Gagliardi FM. Epidermoid and dermoid cysts. Clinical evaluation and late surgical results. *J Neurosurg* 1977;47:12–18.
176. Tibbs PA, James HE, Rorke LB, et al. Midline hamartomas masquerading as meningomyeloceles or teratomas in the newborn infant. *J Pediatr* 1976;89:928–933.
177. Sandler HM, Papadopoulos SM, Thornton AF Jr, Ross DA. Spinal cord astrocytomas: results of therapy. *Neurosurgery* 1992;30:490–493.
178. Kirks DR, Berger PE, Fitz CR, Harwood-Nash DC. Myelography in the evaluation of paravertebral mass lesions in infants and children. *Radiology* 1976;119:603–608.
179. Kirks DR, Harwood-Nash DC. Computed tomography in pediatric radiology. *Pediatr Ann* 1980;9:66–76.
180. Nemoto Y, Inoue Y, Tashiro T, et al. Intramedullary spinal cord tumors: significance of associated hemorrhage at MR imaging. *Radiology* 1992;182:793–796.
181. Stanley P, Senac MO Jr, Segall HD. Intraspinal seeding from intracranial tumors in children. *AJR* 1985;144:157–161.
182. Kramer ED, Rafto S, Packer RJ, Zimmerman RA. Comparison of myelography with CT follow-up versus gadolinium MRI for subarachnoid metastatic disease in children. *Neurology* 1991;41:46–50.
183. Blews DE, Wang H, Kumar AJ, et al. Intradural spinal metastases in pediatric patients with primary intracranial neoplasms: Gd-DTPA enhanced MR vs CT myelography. *J Comput Assist Tomogr* 1990;14:730–735.
184. Wiener MD, Boyko OB, Friedman HS, et al. False-positive spinal MR findings for subarachnoid spread of primary CNS tumor in postoperative pediatric patients. *AJNR* 1990;11:1100–1103.
185. Albrecht S, Crutchfield JS, SeGall GK. On spinal osteochondromas. *J Neurosurg* 1992;77:247–252.
186. Munk PL, Helms CA, Holt RG, et al. MR imaging of aneurysmal bone cysts. *AJR* 1989;153:99–101.
187. Clough JR, Price CH. Aneurysmal bone cyst: pathogenesis and long term results of treatment. *Clin Orthop* 1973;97:52–63.
188. Boyko OB, Cory DA, Cohen MD, et al. MR imaging of osteogenic and Ewing's sarcoma. *AJR* 1987;148:317–322.
189. Erlemann R, Sciuk J, Bosse A, et al. Response of osteosarcoma and Ewing sarcoma to preoperative chemotherapy: assessment with dynamic and static MR imaging and skeletal scintigraphy. *Radiology* 1990;175:791–796.
190. Massad M, Haddad F, Slim M, et al. Spinal cord compression in neuroblastoma. *Surg Neurol* 1985;23:567–572.
191. Beltran J, Noto AM, Chakeres DW, Christoforidis AJ. Tumors of the osseous spine: Staging with MR imaging versus CT. *Radiology* 1987;162:525–569.
192. Mulliken JB, Glowacki J. Hemangiomas and vascular malformations in infants and children: a classification based on endothelial characteristics. *Plast Reconstr Surg* 1982;69:412–422.
193. Dormont D, Gelbert F, Assouline E, et al. MR imaging of spinal cord arteriovenous malformations at 0.5 T: study of 34 cases. *AJNR* 1988;9:833–838.
194. Minami S, Sagoh T, Nishimura K, et al. Spinal arteriovenous malformation: MR imaging. *Radiology* 1988;169:109–115.
195. Altman RP, Randolph JG, Lilly JR. Sacrococcygeal teratoma. American Academy of Pediatrics Surgical Section Survey-1973. *J Pediatr Surg* 1973;9:389–398.
196. Werner JL, Taybi H. Presacral masses in childhood. *AJR* 1970;109:403–410.
197. Noseworthy J, Lack EE, Kozakewich HPW. Sacrococcygeal germ cell tumors in childhood: an updated experience with 118 patients. *J Pediatr Surg* 1981;16:358–364.
198. Partlow WF, Taybi H. Teratomas in infants and children. *AJR* 1971;112:155–166.
199. Wells RG, Sty JR. Imaging of sacrococcygeal germ cell tumors. *RadioGraphics* 1990;10:701–713.
200. Schey WL, Shkolnik A, White H. Clinical and radiographic considerations of sacrococcygeal teratomas: an analysis of 26 new cases and review of the literature. *Radiology* 1977;125:189–195.
201. Dillard BM, Mayer JH, McAlister WH, et al. Sacrococcygeal teratoma in children. *J Pediatr Surg* 1970;5:53–59.
202. Hunt PT, Davidson KC, Ashcraft KW, Holder TM. Radiography of hereditary presacral teratoma. *Radiology* 1977;122:187–191.
203. Keslar PJ, Buck JL, Suarez ES. Germ cell tumors of the sacrococcygeal region: radiologic-pathologic correlation. *RadioGraphics* 1994;14:607–620.
204. Apple JS, Kirks DR, Merten DF, Martinez S. Cervical spine fractures and dislocations in children. *Pediatr Radiol* 1987;17:45–49.
205. Hadley MN, Zabramski JM, Browner CM, et al. Pediatric spinal trauma. Review of 122 cases of spinal cord and vertebral column injuries. *J Neurosurg* 1988;68:18–24.
206. Taylor GA, Eggli KD. Lap-belt injuries of the lumbar spine in children: a pitfall in CT diagnosis. *AJR* 1988;150:1355–1358.
207. Ehara S, el-Khoury GY, Sato Y. Cervical spine injury in children: radiologic manifestations. *AJR* 1988;:1175–1178.
208. Daffner RH, Deeb ZL, Rothfus WE. The posterior vertebral body line: importance in the detection of burst fractures. *AJR* 1987;148:93–96.
209. Gehweiler JA Jr, Clark WM, Schaaf RE, et al. Cervical spine trauma: the common combined conditions. *Radiology* 1979;130:77–86.
210. Denis F. The three column spine and its significance in the classification of acute thoracolumbar spinal injuries. *Spine* 1983;8:817–831.
211. Miller MD, Gehweiler JA, Martinez S, et al. Significant new observations on cervical spine trauma. *AJR* 1978;130:659–663.
212. Harris JH Jr, Mirvis SE. *The radiology of acute cervical spine trauma.* 3rd ed. Baltimore: Williams and Wilkins, 1996.
213. Kim KS, Chen HH, Russell EJ, Rogers LF. Flexion teardrop fracture of the cervical spine: radiographic characteristics. *AJR* 1989;152:319–326.
214. Elliott JM Jr, Rogers LF, Wissinger JP, Lee JF. The hangman's fracture. Fractures of the neural arch of the axis. *Radiology* 1972;104:303–307.
215. Wirth RL, Zatz LM, Parker BR. CT detection of a Jefferson fracture in a child. *AJR* 1987;149:1001–1002.
216. Hegenbarth R, Ebel K.-D. Roentgen findings in fractures of the vertebral column in childhood. Examination of 35 patients and its results. *Pediatr Radiol* 1976;5:34–39.
217. Bohn D, Armstrong D, Becker L, Humphreys R. Cervical spine injuries in children. *J Trauma* 1990;30:463–469.
218. Enriquez G, Aso C, Lucaya J, et al. Traumatic cord lesions in the newborn infant. *Ann Radiol* 1976;19:179–186.
219. Babyn PS, Chuang SH, Daneman A, Davidson GS. Sonographic evaluation of spinal cord birth trauma with pathologic correlation. *AJR* 1988;151:763–766.
220. Filippigh P, Clapuyt P, Debauche C, Claus D. Sonographic evaluation

of traumatic spinal cord lesions in the newborn infant. *Pediatr Radiol* 1994;24:245–247.
221. Fotter R, Sorantin E, Schneider U, et al. Ultrasound diagnosis of birth-related spinal cord trauma: neonatal diagnosis and follow-up and correlation with MRI. *Pediatr Radiol* 1994;24:241–244.
222. Franken EA Jr. Spinal cord injury in the newborn infant. *Pediatr Radiol* 1975;3:101–104.
223. Hackney DB, Asato R, Joseph PM, et al. Hemorrhage and edema in acute spinal cord compression: demonstration by MR imaging. *Radiology* 1986;161:387–390.
224. Mirvis SE, Geisler FH, Jelinek JJ, et al. Acute cervical spine trauma: evaluation with 1.5-T MR imaging. *Radiology* 1988;166:807–816.
225. Felsberg GJ, Tien RD, Osumi AK, Cardenas CA. Utility of MR imaging in pediatric spinal cord injury. *Pediatr Radiol* 1995;25:131–135.
226. Grabb PA, Pang D. Magnetic resonance imaging in the evaluation of spinal cord injury without radiographic abnormality in children. *Neurosurgery* 1994;35:406–414.
227. Byers RK. Spinal-cord injuries during birth. *Dev Med Child Neurol* 1975;17:103–110.
228. Quencer RM, Sheldon JJ, Donovan Post MJ, et al. MRI of the chronically injured cervical spinal cord. *AJR* 1986;147:125–132.
229. Neuhauser EBD, Wittenborg MH, Berman CZ, Cohen J. Irradiation effects of roentgen therapy on the growing spine. *Radiology* 1952;59:637–650.
230. Oakley RH, Carty H. Review of spondylolisthesis and spondylolysis in paediatric practice. *Br J Radiol* 1984;57:877–885.
231. McKee BW, Alexander WJ, Dunbar JS. Spondylolysis and spondylolisthesis in children: a review. *J Can Assoc Radiol* 1971;22:100–109.
232. Beeler JW. Further evidence on the acquired nature of spondylolysis and spondylolisthesis. *AJR* 1970;108:796–798.
233. Gelfand MJ, Strife JL, Kereiakes JG. Radionuclide bone imaging in spondylolysis of the lumbar spine in children. *Radiology* 1981;140:191–195.
234. Grenier N, Kressel HY, Schiebler ML, Grossman RI. Isthmic spondylolysis of the lumbar spine: MR imaging at 1.5T. *Radiology* 1989;170:489–493.
235. Salo S, Paajanen H, Alanen A. Disc degeneration of pediatric patients in lumbar MRI. *Pediatr Radiol* 1995;25:186–189.
236. Bradford DS, Garcia A. Herniations of the lumbar intervertebral disk in children and adolescents. A review of 30 surgically treated cases. *JAMA* 1969;210:2045–2051.
237. Banerian KG, Wang AM, Samberg LC, et al. Association of vertebral end plate fracture with pediatric lumbar intervertebral disk herniation: value of CT and MR imaging. *Radiology* 1990;177:763–765.
238. Kozlowski K. Anterior intervertebral disc herniations in children: unrecognised chronic trauma to the spine. *Australas Radiol* 1979;23:67–71.
239. Ghelman B, Freiberger RH. The limbus vertebra: an anterior disc herniation demonstrated by discography. *AJR* 1976;127:854–855.
240. Henales V, Hervas JA, Lopez P, et al. Intervertebral disc herniations (limbus vertebrae) in pediatric patients: report of 15 cases. *Pediatr Radiol* 1993;23:608–610.
241. Blomquist HK, Lindqvist M, Mattsson S. Calcification of intervertebral discs in childhood. *Pediatr Radiol* 1979;8:23–26.

242. McGregor JC, Butler P. Disc calcification in childhood: computed tomographic and magnetic resonance imaging appearances. *Br J Radiol* 1986;59:180–182.
243. Girodias JB, Azouz EM, Marton D. Intervertebral disk space calcification. A report of 51 children with a review of the literature. *Pediatr Radiol* 1991;21:541–546.
244. Melnick JC, Silverman FN. Intervertebral disk calcification in childhood. *Radiology* 1963;80:399–408.
245. Mainzer F. Herniation of the nucleus pulposus. A rare complication of intervertebral-disk calcification in children. *Radiology* 1973;107:167–170.
246. Sutton TJ, Turcotte B. Posterior herniation of calcified intervertebral discs in children. *J Can Assoc Radiol* 1973;24:131–136.
247. Swischuk LE, Stansberry SD. Calcific discitis: MRI changes in discs without visible calcification. *Pediatr Radiol* 1991;21:365–366.
248. Alexander CJ. Scheuermann's disease. A traumatic spondylodystrophy? *Skeletal Radiol* 1977;1:209–221.
249. Williams HJ, Pugh DG. Vertebral epiphysitis: a comparison of the clinical and roentgenologic findings. *AJR* 1963;90:1236–1247.
250. Sachs B, Bradford D, Winter R, et al. Scheuermann kyphosis. Follow-up of Milwaukee-brace treatment. *J Bone Joint Surg Am* 1987;69A:50–57.
251. Mandell GA, Morales RW, Harcke HT, Bowen JR. Bone scintigraphy in patients with atypical lumbar Scheuermann disease. *J Pediatr Orthop* 1993;13:622–627.
252. Cleveland RH, Delong GR. The relationship of juvenile lumbar disc disease and Scheuermann's disease. *Pediatr Radiol* 1981;10:161–164.
253. McAlister WH, Shackelford GD. Classification of spinal curvatures. *Radiol Clin North Am* 1975;13:93–112.
254. Benson DR. Idiopathic scoliosis. The last ten years and state of the art. *Orthopedics* 1987;10:1691–1698.
255. Young LW, Oestreich AE, Goldstein LA. Roentgenology in scoliosis: contribution to evaluation and management. *AJR* 1970;108:778–795.
256. Barnes PD, Brody JD, Jaramillo D, et al. Atypical idiopathic scoliosis: MR imaging evaluation. *Radiology* 1993;186:247–253.
257. Casselman ES, Mandell GA. Vertebral scalloping in neurofibromatosis. *Radiology* 1979;131:89–94.
258. Casselman ES, Miller WT, Lin SR, Mandell GA. Von Recklinghausen's disease: incidence of roentgenographic findings with a clinical review of the literature. *CRC Rev Diagn Imag* 1977;9:387–419.
259. McAlister WH, Shackelford GD. Measurement of spinal curvatures. *Radiol Clin North Am* 1975;13:113–121.
260. Nokes SR, Murtagh FR, Jones JD 3d, et al. Childhood scoliosis: MR imaging. *Radiology* 1987;164:791–797.
261. Kuhns LR, Martin AJ. A simple device for measuring angles without marking the radiographic film. *Radiology* 1975;115:220–221.
262. Wilkinson RH, Willi UV, Gilsanz V, Mulvihill D. Radiographic evaluation of the spine after surgical correction of scoliosis. *AJR* 1979;133:703–709.
263. Fon GT, Pitt MJ, Thies AC Jr. Thoracic kyphosis: range in normal subjects. *AJR* 1980;134:979–983.

Practical Pediatric Imaging: Diagnostic Radiology of Infants and Children, Third Edition.
D. R. Kirks, editor and N. T. Griscom, associate editor.
Lippincott–Raven Publishers, Philadelphia © 1998.

CHAPTER 5

Musculoskeletal System

Tal Laor, Diego Jaramillo, and Alan E. Oestreich

T. Laor and D. Jaramillo: Department of Radiology, Children's Hospital, Harvard Medical School, Boston, Massachusetts 02115.
A. E. Oestreich: Department of Pediatric Radiology, Children's Hospital Medical Center, University of Cincinnati College of Medicine, Cincinnati, Ohio 45229.

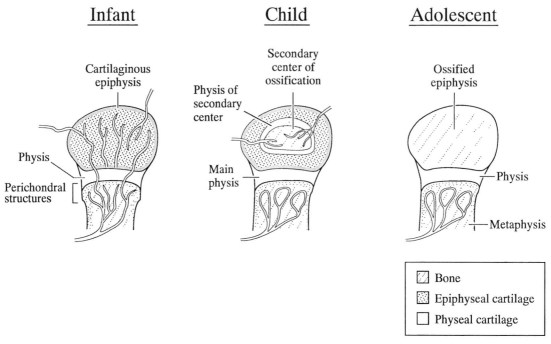

Infant   Child   Adolescent

FIG. 5-1. Age-related changes in the anatomy of a growing long bone. *Infant:* The epiphysis is completely or almost completely cartilaginous. Epiphyseal and metaphyseal vessels communicate across the physis. The perichondral metaphysis adjacent to the physis has a straight peripheral border, the collar of Laval-Jeantet. *Child:* The ossification center in the epiphysis is well formed. The physis acts as a barrier between epiphyseal and metaphyseal vessels. *Adolescent:* The epiphysis is ossified, but the physis remains cartilaginous. The epiphysis has fewer vessels than the metaphysis.

Imaging of skeletal disorders of children has changed significantly over the past decade. Radiography remains the most important diagnostic modality and should be the starting point for nearly every evaluation (1–13). With advances in cross-sectional imaging and scintigraphy, however, the focus of imaging has broadened beyond the bones to include structures such as the cartilaginous epiphysis and physis, bone marrow, tendons, ligaments, and muscles (14).

NORMAL ANATOMY AND DEVELOPMENT

The skeletal system undergoes dramatic changes during the first two decades of life. The structures for support and locomotion, initially cartilaginous, slowly grow and ossify. The bone marrow, initially hematopoietic, is mostly transformed into fatty marrow. The normal and abnormal aspects of these two transformations explain many of the imaging findings of skeletal diseases in children.

Cartilaginous, Vascular, and Osseous Structures

The skeletal system begins as a condensation of primitive mesenchymal cells. The primitive mesenchymal cells are then transformed into precursors of membranous bone or cartilage. The cranial vault and the facial bones originate directly from mesenchyme by the process of *intramembranous ossification.* The long bones, vertebrae, and skull base are initially cartilaginous; the cartilage is then transformed

into bone by a process known as *endochondral ossification.*

Most tubular bones of children have a similar structure (Fig. 5-1). At the ends are the epiphyses, each of which lies between a joint and a physis (growth plate) (Fig. 5-2). At birth, most of the epiphyses are still entirely cartilaginous. The secondary centers of ossification (epiphyseal ossification centers) appear at predictable ages. They are spherical at first but become hemispherical as they enlarge. The time of appearance and pattern of growth of the ossified epiphyses are part of the determination of skeletal maturation; this is discussed later. The epiphyseal margin adjacent to the joint surface is lined by articular cartilage. A secondary center of ossification that is not articular is termed an apophysis. Apophyses do not generally contribute to longitudinal growth and are usually located at the insertion of muscles. They share many of the characteristics and diseases of the epiphyses.

Normal growth of long bones includes elongation, increase in physeal and diaphyseal diameter, epiphyseal enlargement, and tubulation. Longitudinal growth of long bones occurs at the physis by endochondral ossification. The epiphysis enlarges and ossifies in a manner similar to the shaft, although much more slowly. In the diaphysis, transverse growth is due primarily to deposition of periosteal (intramembranous) new bone along the shaft. The physis and the juxtaphyseal metaphysis increase their diameter by membranous growth at the zone of Ranvier complex (15).

The physis is a flat disc at birth but becomes irregularly curved with age. It is composed of columns of cartilage cells (chondrocytes) (16). The chondrocytes undergo mitotic activity on the epiphyseal side of the physis in the germinal or resting zone. Growth occurs both from cellular division in the proliferative zone and from an increase in the size of the chondrocytes in the hypertrophic zone. The hypertrophied cells ultimately die, and the surrounding matrix mineralizes in the zone of provisional calcification, immediately adjacent to the metaphysis. As the child approaches skeletal maturity, the physis becomes progressively thinner and more undulating. Physeal curving can mimic premature fusion on radiographs and can look abnormal on cross-sectional imaging (Fig. 5-3). The pattern of physeal closure varies according to site. Knowledge of the normal patterns of closure allows differentiation of normal fusion from fusion due to disease (17). In the distal radius, the distal femur, and the proximal tibia, normal physeal closure first occurs centrally (18). In the distal tibia, physeal closure begins anteromedially, in an undulation called the Kump bump (19).

The junction of the physeal cartilage and metaphyseal bone is the weakest part of the growing skeleton. This junction is held together in the periphery by a ring of perichondrium, which resists shearing stresses. The strong perichondral attachments are also a barrier to the spread of subperiosteal disease. The recently formed bone of the metaphysis is remodeled primarily by osteoclastic resorption. The diameter of the bone decreases from a wide physeal region to a more narrowed tubular shaft (tubulation). The metaphyseal cortex of tubular bones in children is thin, porous, and breakable. The diaphyseal cortex is thicker and stronger.

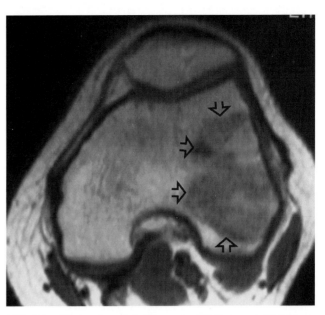

FIG. 5-3. Physeal undulation as a pitfall on axial images. Axial T1-weighted MR image of the distal femur of a 13-year-old boy shows an area of decreased signal intensity in the lateral part of the bone *(arrows)*. Only a portion of the curved physis is included in the axial section, and the appearance falsely suggests a lesion in the marrow.

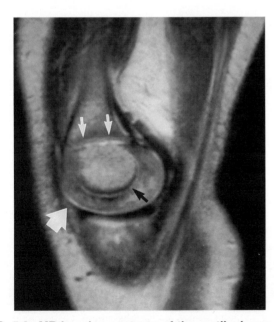

FIG. 5-2. MR imaging anatomy of the cartilaginous epiphysis. Sagittal T2-weighted image of the medial part of the distal femoral epiphysis in a 5-year-old shows the physis *(double white arrows)*, articular cartilage *(large white arrow)*, and physis of the secondary center of ossification *(black arrow)*. Epiphyseal cartilage of heterogeneous signal intensity lies deep to the articular cartilage and surrounds the ossification center. From Jaramillo and Hoffer (340).

The diaphysis is a structurally important but metabolically less active region of the pediatric skeleton. The periosteum is loosely attached to the diaphysis. Infections, tumors, and hematomas can elevate the periosteum and spread through the subperiosteal space.

In children, vascular changes influence both normal bony development and skeletal disease manifestations. The earliest diaphyseal ossification occurs around the main nutrient vessel. The nutrient artery penetrates the diaphyseal cortex, and its branches course toward each metaphysis. The terminal branches form tight loops near the physis. Arterial blood subsequently empties into large venous sinusoids in the medullary portion of the metaphysis (see Fig. 5-1). The physiologic slowing of blood in these metaphyseal sinusoidal structures predisposes to lodgement and proliferation of circulating organisms. The epiphysis is invaded by vessels that stimulate the formation of the secondary center of ossification. During the first 18 months of life, the epiphyseal and metaphyseal vessels anastomose across the physis. These anastomoses disappear during childhood. The physis becomes an avascular structure that serves as a barrier, but only an imperfect one, to the spread of infections and tumors.

During childhood, the physis lies between two vascular beds, one epiphyseal and the other metaphyseal. Oxygen and nutrients are supplied by the epiphyseal vessels. The epiphyseal vasculature must be intact to sustain the chondrocytes. The metaphyseal vessels interact with the physeal chondrocytes of the hypertrophic zone and may contribute to the death of these cells, a necessary step during endochondral ossification. The metaphyseal vasculature must be intact to sustain normal ossification.

Bone Marrow

Bone marrow can be hematopoietic or fatty. At birth, the entire skeleton contains hematopoietic marrow. From infancy to early adulthood, fatty marrow replaces hematopoietic marrow in a fixed pattern of transformation (Fig. 5-4). In each extremity, this transformation begins at the periphery in the fingers and toes, and moves centrally to the shoulder girdle and hips (20–24). Within each bone, the transformation to fatty marrow begins in the epiphyses. Epiphyseal marrow conversion is nearly complete 6 months after the radiographic appearance of the epiphyseal ossification center (25). In the tubular bones, marrow conversion in the shaft begins in the diaphysis and moves as a front toward the metaphyses. Thus, the last areas to convert in the appendicular skeleton are the proximal humeral and femoral metaphyses, which contain hematopoietic marrow into adult life. Marrow transformation in the axial skeleton is much slower, occurring in the spine and pelvis throughout adult life.

Hematopoietic marrow has a rich vascularity and therefore is prone to blood-borne diseases such as infections and metastases. Fatty marrow is poorly vascularized and is often the site of ischemic disease such as avascular necrosis. To a great extent the distribution of marrow at a particular age determines the distribution of bony diseases (26).

Magnetic resonance imaging (MRI) is very sensitive to the relative concentrations of fat and water. On T1-weighted images, hematopoietic marrow is of low signal intensity whereas fatty marrow is of high signal intensity (Fig. 5-4). On short tau inversion recovery (STIR) images, fatty marrow is of very low signal intensity and hematopoietic marrow is of intermediate to high signal intensity. These images are fat-suppressed and predominantly T1-weighted, but they visually resemble T2-weighted images. On conventional spin echo T2-weighted images, both fatty and hematopoietic marrow are of intermediate signal intensity, reflecting magnetic susceptibility effects and the fact that even hematopoietic marrow is partly fatty. Hematopoietic marrow usually can be distinguished from lesions invading the marrow on T2-weighted images. Figure 5-5 summarizes the changing marrow appearance on T1-weighted images in different anatomic regions.

TECHNIQUES

Radiography

Adequate evaluation of any portion of the skeletal system, especially for trauma, requires radiographic views in at least two projections, preferably at a right angle to each other. The two views are usually frontal and lateral. Certain anatomic regions (foot, ankle, wrist) may require a third, oblique projection. Comparison views are not routinely obtained, except for the hip, but may be required if there is a question of a normal variant or of a joint effusion. In the elbow, shallow obliques are particularly helpful in demonstrating subtle fractures. Im-

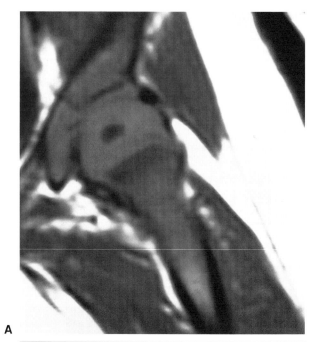

A

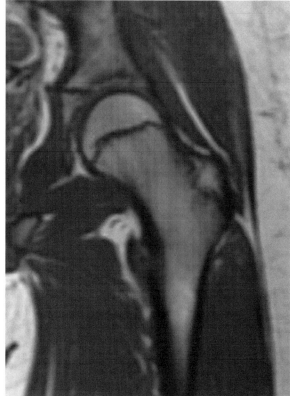

B

FIG. 5-4. Hematopoietic and fatty marrow on T1-weighted MR images. A: Coronal image of the hip in an infant shows hematopoietic marrow (lower signal intensity than the epiphyseal cartilage) in the metaphysis and epiphyseal ossification center. **B:** Coronal image of the hip in a 9-year-old girl shows that the marrow of the epiphysis and the diaphysis has almost reached isointensity with the subcutaneous fat. From Laor and Jaramillo (63).

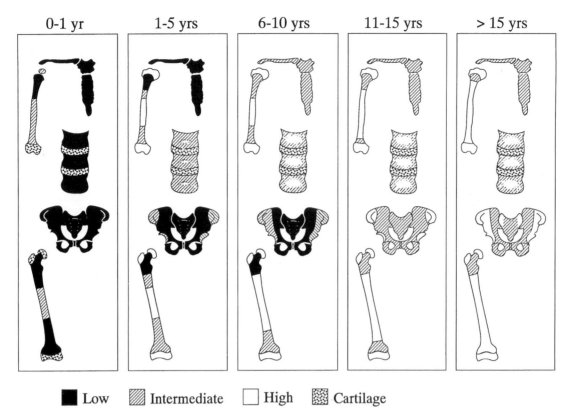

| 0-1 yr | 1-5 yrs | 6-10 yrs | 11-15 yrs | > 15 yrs |

■ Low ▨ Intermediate ☐ High ▦ Cartilage

FIG. 5-5. Marrow transformation as depicted on T1-weighted MR images (20–26). In the young infant most of the bones contain hematopoietic marrow rather than fat and are therefore of low signal intensity. The vertebral bodies are less intense than the discs. In early childhood (1–5 years), the epiphyses and diaphyses of long bones are of high signal intensity and the vertebral bodies are isointense with the discs. During late childhood and early adolescence, the spine, iliac wings, and distal metaphyses continue to become more fatty. In late adolescence, there is residual hematopoietic marrow of intermediate signal intensity in the axial skeleton and in the proximal metaphysis of each limb; the rest of the marrow is fatty and of high signal intensity.

aging of the hip should include frontal and frog-lateral views. Gonadal shielding should be removed for one of the views, in order to evaluate the sacrum and nearby structures.

Estimation of Gestational Age

A knowledge of the approximate gestational age of a neonate is important for radiologic diagnosis. Although the gestational age may be obtained by history or physical and neurologic examination, this information is not always available to the radiologist. Occasionally the gestational history is inaccurate and the neonate is too ill for neurologic evaluation. Considerable information about estimating gestational age is available from chest radiographs. It is derived from the images of the humeral epiphyses, coracoid apophyses, teeth, and thoracic spine (27–29).

The *proximal humeral ossification center* normally does not appear before 36 weeks gestation; therefore, its presence indicates that the neonate is near or at term. An ossified coracoid suggests the same. Although seen in 40% of patients between 40 and 41 weeks and in 82% of patients over 42 weeks gestation (29), the 95th percentile of age for pres-

ence (in boys) is 4 months, so that absence at birth does not imply prematurity. *Tooth mineralization* is also useful. It is less affected than epiphyseal maturation by intrauterine disorders and is therefore a better radiologic indicator of gestational age. The presence or absence of tooth mineralization within the cusps of the tooth buds of the first and second deciduous molars (27), often shown on a lateral view of the chest, is determined. If the first deciduous molar is mineralized, the neonate is of at least 33 weeks gestation, and if the second deciduous molar is mineralized, the neonate is of at least 36 weeks gestation (Fig. 5-6). *Thoracic spine length* is a relatively good guide to gestational age except in small-for-gestational-age infants and infants of a diabetic mother. The thoracic spine length is measured from the superior endplate of the first thoracic vertebra to the inferior endplate of the twelfth thoracic vertebra in the anteroposterior (AP) projection. Gestational age is estimated by thoracic spine length and correlates within 2 weeks of gestational age as determined by the Dubowitz physical examination in more than 90% of cases (28). The chart of Kuhns and Holt (28) (Fig. 5-7) shows mean thoracic length (in millimeters) to equal 2.54 times gestational age (in weeks) minus 6.271.

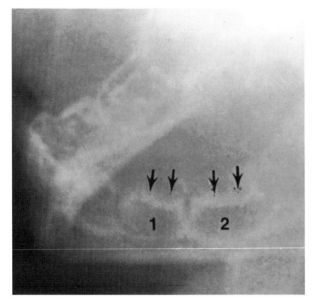

FIG. 5-6. Gestational age. There is mineralization of the cusps *(arrows)* of the first *(1)* and second *(2)* molars.

Skeletal Maturation

Radiographic evaluation of the skeleton for determination of maturity constitutes nearly 1% of pediatric imaging examinations. This "bone age" determination is important in endocrine disorders, particularly those involving the thyroid, pituitary, and gonads. Skeletal maturation is also determined in children who are too short or too tall for their chronological age. Maturation and growth are accelerated or decreased in many syndromes, malformations, nutritional abnormalities, and bone dysplasias. The child's ultimate height as well as the optimal time for surgical intervention to correct scoliosis or limb length discrepancies also can be predicted from the bone age. Evaluating skeletal maturation is complex, partly due to interobserver and intraobserver error as well as the wide range of variation in normal children. Some

ethnic groups mature earlier than others (30). In general, bone age should be at least 2 standard deviations (SD) from the mean before it is considered abnormal.

There are several methods for determining skeletal maturation in children. The usual procedure over the age of 12 months is to obtain a posteroanterior (PA) radiograph of the left hand and wrist. Skeletal maturity is estimated by comparing the patient's bones with known standards. The standards of Greulich and Pyle (31) are the most widely used. In younger children, the evaluation begins by assessing the number of secondary centers of ossification. These epiphyseal ossification centers are round at first but later become more oval in shape. As the ossification centers enlarge, it is important to determine how much of the metaphysis is covered by the epiphysis. Once the epiphyseal ossification reaches the diameter of the metaphysis, the degree of undulation of the physis becomes a useful indicator. Finally, physeal closure occurs, marking the beginning of skeletal maturity. In general, evaluation of the phalangeal epiphyses provides more accurate assessment of maturation than analysis of carpal and metacarpal bones. The more distal, the better (31)!

The thumb undergoes peculiar changes that are easily recognizable and therefore useful. For example, the sesamoid seen adjacent to the distal end of the first metacarpal appears at about 11 years in girls and 13 in boys. The first metacarpal secondary center is another convenient index for beginning the comparison to the standards. The transformation of the epiphysis from rounded to oval to a complex shape is more easily recognizable than that of the more distal centers. This epiphysis also undergoes progressive notching with increasing maturity. The thickness of the physis is more an indicator of growth rate than of maturity (31). In general, carpal bones are used only as broad indicators of bone age. Determinations of maturity based primarily on the carpal bones tend to have greater variation and consistently underestimate skeletal age (32). In fact, patients with abnormal skeletal maturation usually show exaggerated retardation or accelera-

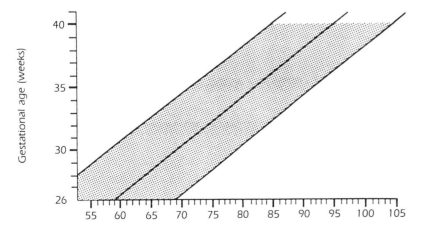

FIG. 5-7. Estimating gestational age from thoracic length. Thoracic length is measured from the top of the vertebral body of T1 to the bottom of T12 on the AP projection. The mean thoracic spine length *(central solid line)* and 2 SD above and below this mean *(hatched area)* are plotted versus gestational age. Modified from Kuhns and Holt (28).

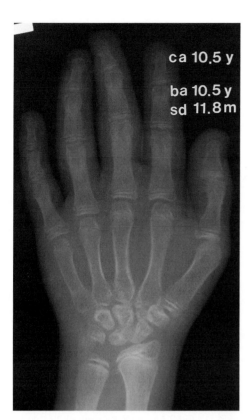

ca 10.5 y

ba 10.5 y
sd 11.8 m

FIG. 5-8. Bone age determination in a patient with Turner syndrome. The chronological age is 10 years and 6 months. According to the standards of Greulich and Pyle (31), the bone age is 10 years and 6 months, coinciding with the chronological age. One standard deviation for a patient of this chronological age is 11.8 months according to the Brush foundation study (31). The carpal bones are small and deformed and there is medial angulation of the distal radial articular surface, as is typical of Turner syndrome.

tion in the carpal bones. For more unbiased estimation, the bone age should be decided with knowledge of the subject's gender but without knowledge of the chronological age.

If the child's skeletal age falls between two bone age standards in the atlas (31), the radiologist should interpolate. If the skeletal age seems to be halfway between two standards, it should be reported as such. The chronological age, bone age or skeletal maturation according to Greulich and Pyle (31), and 2 SD for the patient's chronological age according to the Brush Foundation Study (31) are written on each radiograph (Fig. 5-8). The same information is provided in the written report, together with a statement that the bone age is normal, advanced, or delayed according to the calculations.

The Tanner-Whitehouse method, based on assigning an individual maturity score to each of several bones of the hand and wrist, is a more comprehensive approach (33). It is used mostly for research purposes, because it is time-consuming and more difficult to learn and apply. Computerized approaches to evaluation of skeletal maturity may result in greater speed, ease, and reliability (34).

If the chronological age is 1 year or less, other methods are necessary. Bone age in newborns and young infants can be determined by comparing radiographs of the knee and foot with published standards. A simpler although less reliable method involves counting the number of carpal, tarsal, and secondary ossification centers in the left upper and lower extremities, using the method of Sontag (35,36). Frontal radiographs are obtained of the left upper extremity from shoulder to fingertips and the left lower extremity from mid-thigh to toes. The shafts of the long bones, metacarpals, metatarsals, and phalanges are not counted. The capital femoral epiphysis, which appears at approximately 3 months of age in girls and 4 months of age in boys, is assumed to be present and is counted even though not shown. The secondary centers of the shoulder (including coracoid, even if not shown), elbow, wrist, hand, hip, knee, ankle (excluding talus and body of calcaneus), and foot are counted, and this number is compared with a chart of normals for age and gender (Table 5-1). The chronological age, number of hemiskeletal ossification centers, mean expected number of centers ± 2 SD, and closest calculated bone age are written on the radiograph (Fig. 5-9). The same information is included in the written report.

Computed Tomography and Conventional Tomography

Computed tomography (CT) helps define the relationship between osseous structures. Musculoskeletal applications of CT are expanding due to the ease of performing 2-D and 3-D reconstructions with superb spatial resolution. General indications for CT (or conventional tomography, less frequently used) include evaluation of difficult anatomic regions such as the sternum, verification and precise localization of bony abnormalities (osteoid osteoma, sequestrum, stress fracture), confirmation of a questionable radiographic finding (cervical spine fracture), preoperative planning (including 3-D reconstruction), and anatomic definition of an area obscured by a cast (dislocation of the hip, spinal fusion).

Helical CT can be used to image the hips with greater

TABLE 5-1. *Normal hemiskeletal ossification centers[a]*

Age (mo)	Number of centers			
	Boys		Girls	
	Mean	2 SD	Mean	2 SD
1	4.11	2.82	4.58	3.52
3	6.63	3.72	7.78	4.32
6	9.61	3.90	11.44	5.06
9	11.88	5.32	15.36	9.84
12	13.96	7.92	22.40	13.86
18	19.27	13.22	34.10	16.88

[a] Talus and body of calcaneus are not counted even if present. Shafts of long bones, metacarpals, metatarsals, and phalanges are also not counted. Coracoid and proximal femoral centers are counted even if not shown.

Source: Modified from Sontag et al. (36). See also Keats (563).

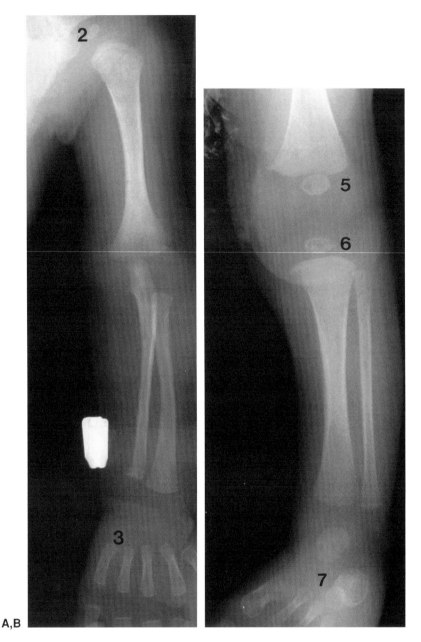

FIG. 5-9. Evaluation of bone age by the Sontag method in a 6-week-old boy. Using the method of Greulich and Pyle (31), the bone age was found to be less than 1 year. AP radiographs of the left upper extremity from the shoulder to the fingers **(A)** and of the left lower extremity from the midthigh to the toes **(B)** were obtained. Using the method of Sontag et al. (36,563), there are seven secondary ossification centers in the hemiskeleton. The coracoid center is counted as present although not visualized in this image, and the proximal femoral ossification center is counted although not included on the film. The counting is as follows: coracoid *1*, proximal humeral center *2*, hamate *3*, proximal femur *4*, distal femur *5*, proximal tibia *6*, cuboid *7*, total *7*. The calcaneus and talus are not counted. The mean number of hemiskeletal ossification centers for this patient's chronological age is 4.11 with 2 SD being 2.82 centers. The seven centers correspond to a skeletal age of just over 3 months (see Table 5-1). Incidentally noted is a fracture of the distal ulnar metaphysis.

A,B

efficiency and less radiation than conventional CT (37). However, conventional CT remains a better technique for evaluation of subtle fractures (38). Helical CT is limited because of increased volume averaging, decreased spatial resolution, and decreased signal-to-noise ratio (39).

Magnetic Resonance Imaging

Magnetic resonance imaging (MRI) is of major importance when evaluating bone marrow, joints, cartilage, soft tissues, and, increasingly, cortical bone itself. Its role in examining tumors, avascular necrosis, joint disease, infection, and certain injuries and in orthopedic planning is rapidly becoming standard practice. It is the main modality for evaluation of cartilaginous and ligamentous disorders of the knee.

Ultrasonography

Ultrasonography is the initial modality of choice for evaluation of the neonatal hip (40) and for confirmation of joint effusions, especially at the hip. It is increasingly relevant to tendon abnormalities, osteomyelitis, muscle diseases, foreign bodies, and soft-tissue tumors.

Skeletal Scintigraphy

Skeletal scintigraphy is important in the detection and evaluation of osteomyelitis, other inflammation, trauma, marrow vascularity, tumors (especially osteoid osteoma), and metabolic disorders. The standard bone-imaging agents are technetium-99m (^{99m}Tc) complexes such as ^{99m}Tc-methylene diphosphonate. ^{99m}Tc-sulfur colloid is usually used for marrow imaging. Inflammation and other disorders may be evaluated by gallium-67 citrate, indium-111-labeled white blood cells, or ^{99m}Tc-HMPAO (hexamethylpropylene aminoxide)-labeled white blood cells.

Arthrography

Arthrography is the injection of air or water-soluble contrast material into a joint followed by fluoroscopy, radiography, or CT. General anesthesia is usually required in patients under 10 years of age. In children, the joints most frequently evaluated by arthrography are the hip and elbow. Arthrography allows dynamic evaluation in varied positions (e.g., films of an injected hip in abduction, adduction, etc.), which is often difficult with MRI or CT. After conventional radiographic arthrography, CT or MRI may also be obtained; diagnostic CT arthrograms can be obtained up to several hours after contrast injection.

Hip arthrography is usually performed for preoperative evaluation of the shape and the contour of the cartilaginous femoral head and joint space (Fig. 5-10). The normal cartila-

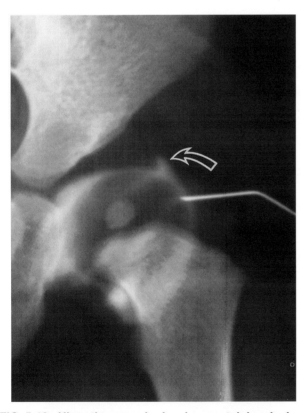

FIG. 5-10. Hip arthrogram in developmental dysplasia of the hip. In this radiograph of a 2-year-old girl, there is contrast in the left hip joint, outlining the articular cartilage of the femoral head and acetabulum. The bony acetabulum is markedly deficient. The cartilaginous acetabulum is also deficient, but there is coverage of nearly half of the femoral head. There is medial pooling of contrast, indicating that the distance between the medial femoral head and the deepest part of the acetabulum is increased. The arrow indicates the recess at the junction of the capsule and the labrum, the so-called rose thorn.

ginous femoral head should be outlined by contrast material to a uniform thickness in all projections. The surface of the acetabular cartilage is smooth and adjacent to that of the femoral head. The margin of the acetabular cartilage extends laterally as a prominent fibrocartilaginous triangular structure, the acetabular labrum (4). The labrum is outlined by contrast material and normally helps to hold the femoral head in the acetabulum. The ligamentum teres may be seen medial to the femoral head extending from the inferior part of the acetabulum. The orbicular ligament is seen usually as a prominent constriction between the upper and lower recesses. Ideally, contrast material is injected into the larger upper recess (4).

CONGENITAL AND DEVELOPMENTAL VARIANTS

In pediatric skeletal radiology, variation in normal anatomy is compounded by dynamic growth changes. Recognition of the abnormal requires knowledge of the normal, so that a variant does not lead to inappropriate treatment. One of the outstanding features of Caffey's classic textbook (2,3) is the emphasis on normal variants of the skeletal system.

Osteosclerosis of the Newborn

The long bones often appear unusually dense in the neonate. This apparent sclerosis is due to relative thickness of the cortex, narrowness of the medullary cavity, and increase in the bony spongiosa. The medullary cavities may be almost completely obliterated by the marked thickening of the cortex (Fig. 5-11). Prominent nutrient canals within this sclerotic bone should not be mistaken for fractures. Chronic intrauterine or postnatal stress leads to thinner trabecula and decreased metaphyseal density; when present, this makes the diaphysis look even more sclerotic. The sclerotic appearance gradually disappears during the first few weeks of life.

Physiologic Periosteal New Bone Formation

Periosteal new bone can be seen paralleling the cortices of long bones during the first few months of life. This finding involves at least one third of infants and presumably is somehow due to rapid bone growth during early infancy (41). This physiologic periosteal new bone formation is not seen before 1 month of age and usually peaks at 6 months of age (4). It may involve the femur, humerus, and tibia, and usually is bilaterally symmetric. If it is present in one of these three bones, it is often present in the other two as well (4). Radiologically, there is one or more thin lines that closely parallel the cortex of the underlying diaphysis, a lucency separating them from the normal bony cortex (Fig. 5-12). With increasing age, this periosteal new bone is incorporated into the bony cortex. Periosteal new bone formation also occurs in osteomyelitis, trauma, syphilis, infantile cortical hyperosto-

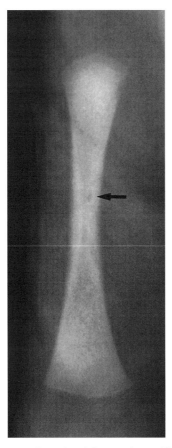

FIG. 5-11. Osteosclerosis of the newborn. There is relative cortical thickening and narrowing of the medullary cavity in the diaphysis of the femur of this normal newborn. The rounded lucency *(arrow)* is a nutrient foramen.

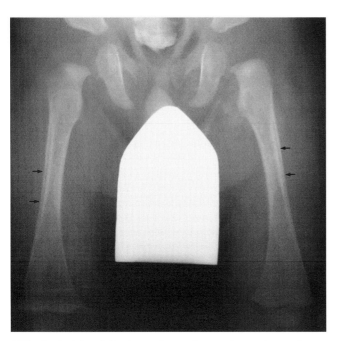

FIG. 5-12. Physiologic periosteal new bone formation. Note the bilateral symmetric periosteal reaction *(arrows)* along the diaphyses of both femurs in this 4-month-old boy. (Courtesy of Robert H. Cleveland, M.D., Boston, Massachusetts.)

sis, vitamin A intoxication, prostaglandin therapy (42), leukemia, and neuroblastoma (41). The distinguishing features of physiologic periosteal new bone formation are the age of the infant, the classic benign radiologic appearance, and the bilateral symmetry.

Dense Transverse Metaphyseal Bands

Radiopaque transverse lines across the width of the metaphyses of long bones and next to the physes of other bones can be seen in normal children. They are found most often in children between the ages of 2 and 6 years. The density and width of the transverse bands generally approximate that of the adjacent cortex. Unlike growth recovery lines, dense metaphyseal bands are not progressively left behind by the physis. Their formation is thought to be due to a relative flattening of the rate of bone growth at this time (2) (Fig. 5-13).

The physiologic dense transverse bands are formed at the zone of provisional calcification. The normal zone of provisional calcification also may appear as a dense thin line when the adjacent metaphysis is relatively lucent due to leukemia or scurvy, for example.

Similar dense metaphyseal bands are due to heavy metal

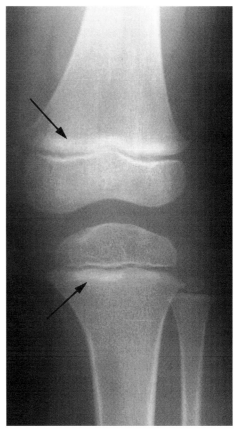

FIG. 5-13. Dense transverse metaphyseal bands. There are dense transverse bands across the metaphyses of the distal femur and proximal tibia *(arrows)* of a toddler. A similar band is not seen in the proximal fibula.

intoxication, most commonly lead. However, lead-poisoned children tend to be under 2 years of age. Their pathologic dense bands are generally thicker than the normal developmental bands, and this indicates a longer period of formation. With time and bone growth, lead bands are left behind by the physis. The sclerosis of lead poisoning tends to involve all metaphyses and somtimes the epiphyses about the knee (Fig. 5-14), whereas normal physiologic sclerosis generally does not affect the proximal fibula (43).

It should be stressed that the diagnosis of lead poisoning rests on the serum lead levels more than the radiologic findings. Patients with lead poisoning have stippling of red blood cells long before lead lines appear in bone. Some patients with lead poisoning also have signs of increased intracranial pressure; and occasionally opaque lead-containing material is present in the gastrointestinal tract. Any dense transverse band in a child with unexplained encephalopathy should be provisionally considered lead intoxication.

Vacuum Phenomenon

When traction is placed on a joint, negative pressure is created in that joint so that nitrogen, normally in solution, becomes gaseous in the joint space. This phenomenon is

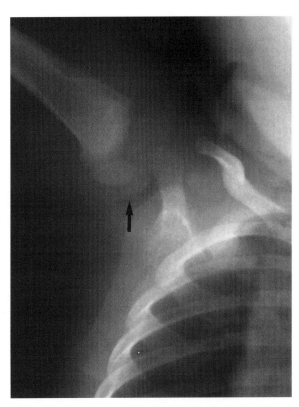

FIG. 5-15. Vacuum phenomenon. Traction placed on the arms of this infant produces a vacuum phenomenon in the shoulder joint *(arrow)*. The lucency outlines the cartilaginous margin of the proximal humeral epiphysis.

commonly seen in children's shoulders when the arms are immobilized above the head for a chest radiographs (Fig. 5-15). If the patient is immobilized and traction is placed on the joint, this phenomenon also may be seen in the elbow, wrist, hip, knee, and ankle. Traction may be applied to the lower extremity with the intent of creating this vacuum phenomenon to assess the cartilaginous margins of the hip joint (6). The vacuum phenomenon does not fully exclude a joint effusion (44). If the lucency of a vacuum phenomenon overlaps a bone, it may mimic a linear fracture.

Proximal Humeral Pseudofracture

One side of the proximal humeral physis frequently projects below the other. This linear lucency is sometimes mistakenly interpreted as a fracture line (Fig. 5-16). A comparison view of the contralateral humerus or an oblique radiograph of the side in question proves that this finding is normal. A similar lucency is seen, although less frequently, in the femur and other bones.

Ischiopubic Synchondrosis

The ossification of the cartilage between the ischium and pubis is highly variable in both rate and radiologic appearance. Bilateral bony fusion at the inferior ischiopubic syn-

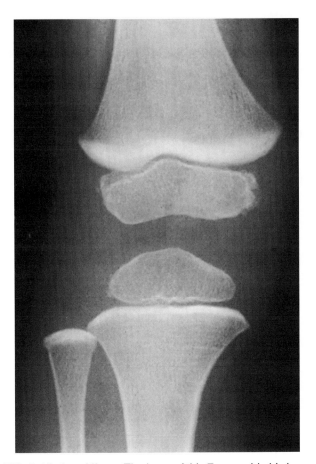

FIG. 5-14. Lead lines. The knee of this 7-year-old girl shows dense metaphyseal bands in the distal femur and, to a lesser extent, the proximal tibia and fibula. Normal physiologic sclerosis usually does not affect the proximal fibula.

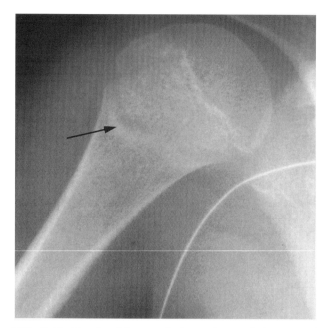

FIG. 5-16. Proximal humeral physeal pseudofracture. A linear lucency is projected across the proximal humerus of a 9-year-old girl *(arrow)*. The lucency is actually the intersection of the physis with the other cortex of the humerus. It should not be mistaken for a fracture.

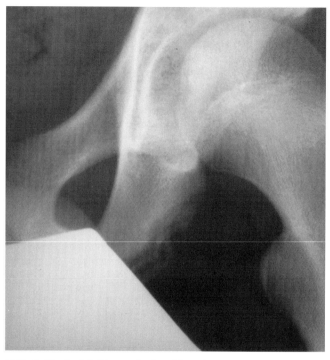

FIG. 5-18. Ischial irregularity. Note the marked irregularity along the descending ramus of the ischium. A normal finding. (Courtesy of George A. Taylor, M.D., Boston, Massachusetts.)

chondroses is complete in only 6% of children at 4 years of age but in 83% of children at 12 years of age (45). There frequently is irregular ossification and expansion at this synchondrosis in prepubertal children (Fig. 5-17). The finding may be asymmetric. Bony fusion often is preceded by an intermittent increase in the size of the lucent cartilaginous component, and this leads to a swollen or bubbly appearance (45). Bony closure and reopening may occur. This morphologic variation makes recognition of osteomyelitis and fracture difficult. Unfortunately, the ischiopubic synchondrosis is one of the most frequent pelvic sites of osteomyelitis.

Skeletal scintigraphy in normals shows variable degrees of increased uptake, often asymmetric, in the ischiopubic synchondroses (46). MR imaging can be helpful if infection or fracture are still suspected.

Ischial Irregularities

Irregularities are occasionally noted in the ischia of preadolescents and adolescents (Fig. 5-18). These irregularities may involve the cortical margin, tuberosity, or descending

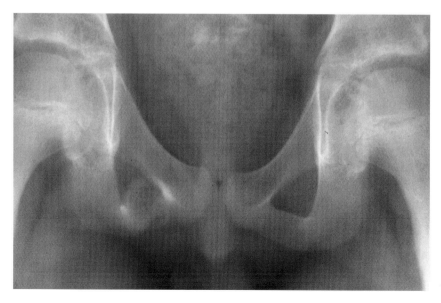

FIG. 5-17. Prominent ischiopubic synchondrosis. There is an asymmetric expansile ischiopubic synchondrosis on the right in this 8-year-old boy. A normal finding.

ramus (47). The inferior ischium next to its apophysis is the equivalent of a metaphysis and therefore is subject to insults like those seen at the metaphyses of long bones, such as hematogenous osteomyelitis (48). This also is a common site of avulsion injury. As with the ischiopubic synchondrosis, clinical information and, in selected cases, MRI can help to differentiate normal from abnormal.

Distal Femoral Epiphyseal Irregularity

During the period of rapid growth, the ossification of the distal femoral bony epiphysis can be irregular. Caffey and coauthors (49) described this appearance in 66% of boys and 41% of girls between the ages of 3 and 13 years. It was observed in both condyles in 44% of cases, in only the lateral condyle in 44%, and in only the medial condyle in 12%. It often disappears by 12 years of age. When the irregularity is bilateral, it is not necessarily symmetric. It most commonly is located posteriorly. Multiple small ossification centers separate from the main osseous epiphysis may be seen (Fig. 5-19).

Differentiating the normal ossific irregularity from traumatic lesions, either acute or chronic, is difficult. In fact, there may be a spectrum of stress-related alterations, from the clearly abnormal to indistinguishable from normal. MRI of the knees in children (performed for unrelated indications) may show signal alterations of the adjacent bone marrow or overlying epiphyseal cartilage. There is decreased T2 signal along the weight-bearing areas and increased signal posteriorly in the cartilaginous femoral condyles (Fig. 5-20).

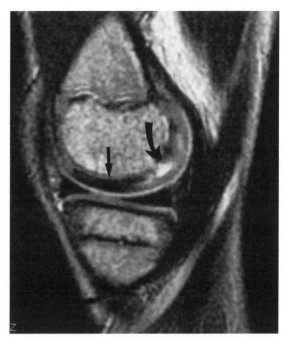

FIG. 5-20. Distal femoral epiphyseal cartilage. This T2-weighted sagittal MR image of the knee of a 9-year-old boy obtained for unrelated reasons shows heterogeneity of the distal unossified femoral epiphysis. There is decreased signal *(straight arrow)* in the weight-bearing portion. In the more posterior part of the unossified epiphysis, there is high T2-weighted cyst-like signal *(curved arrow)*. These findings presumably are stress-related, but there were no symptoms.

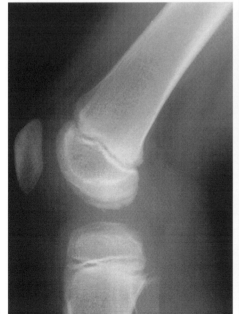 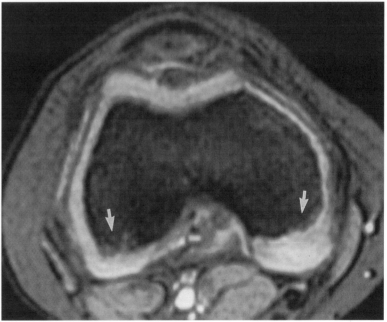

A B

FIG. 5-19. Irregular ossification of distal femoral epiphysis. An 8-year-old boy with knee trauma. **A:** Irregular ossification is seen in the distal femoral bony epiphysis. **B:** An axial gradient recalled echo MRI sequence of the distal femur shows irregularity of the posterior parts of both bony femoral condyles *(arrows)*. The overlying unossified epiphyseal cartilage is smooth.

These alterations seem to be more common in young children as they become active.

Benign Cortical Defect

Benign cortical defect, fibrous cortical defect, fibrous metaphyseal defect, fibroxanthoma, and *nonossifying fibroma* are all terms that are used to describe lesions that histologically and clinically are similar. Fibrous cortical defect often refers to a small lesion based in the cortex. Nonossifying fibroma is a larger lesion that intrudes into the medullary canal (50). The term fibroxanthoma includes both entities (51). In this discussion, all lesions in this group will be referred to as a benign cortical defect.

Benign cortical defects are rarely identified prior to 18 months of age. The incidence is highest at 5–6 years of age (2). They are seen in at least 40% of boys and 30% of girls at some time during normal growth (2). They typically are discovered when a radiograph is performed for some other reason. Because of their frequency, they should be considered normal developmental variants that require no treatment unless of an extremely large size or complicated by a pathologic fracture. They are rarely seen in adults, suggesting that they resolve with normal bone growth.

The radiologic appearance is usually characteristic. They most frequently involve the distal femur (especially the posteromedial aspect) but also can involve other bones, such as the tibia and fibula. They initially are located eccentrically, near the perichondrium of the physis, at sites of ligamentous or tendinous insertions (52). They extend farther into the metaphysis with bone growth. They are rounded, oval, or polycyclic and have thin cortical rims (Fig. 5-21). With time, they become more distant from the physis and develop a more sclerotic border, usually beginning at the diaphyseal margin and proceeding toward the physis. They may enlarge. The sclerosis becomes more homogeneous, and the defects eventually are replaced by normal bone (52). There is an equal incidence of unilateral and bilateral defects. An epiphyseal location has not been reported (4). Since the radiographic appearance is usually very characteristic, additional imaging is not required.

A benign cortical defect is often seen incidentally on MRI. It has a variable appearance, depending on its stage of evolution. The decreased T2-weighted signal seen in many of the

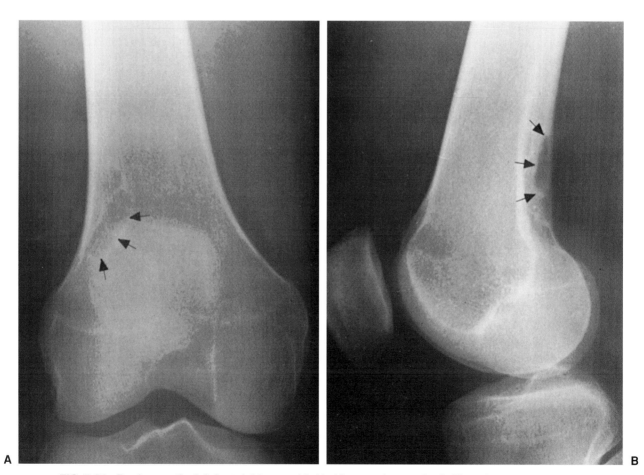

FIG. 5-21. Benign cortical defect. A 14-year-old girl with vague knee pain. **A:** There is an oval, multicystic, well-marginated lucency involving the lateral part of the distal right femoral metaphysis *(arrows)*. **B:** This benign cortical defect also involves the posterior cortex *(arrows)*.

lesions has been attributed to both collagen and to hemosiderin deposition in the center. Following gadolinium enhancement, the lesion usually shows a ring-like peripheral zone of hyperintensity. The center generally shows little or no enhancement (53).

Multiple, bilateral, nonossifying fibromas have been associated with neurofibromatosis and may be another manifestation of the mesodermal defect associated with that disease (54). Multiple nonossifying fibromas associated with café-au-lait spots is termed the Jaffe-Campanacci syndrome.

Avulsive Cortical Irregularity

Avulsive cortical irregularity is one name for a finding in the distal femur in the region of the posterior medial condyle, with a characteristic location and radiologic appearance (55). It has been variously termed *periosteal desmoid, subperiosteal desmoid, cortical desmoid, subperiosteal abrasion, cortical abrasion, medial distal metaphyseal femoral irregularity, subperiosteal cortical defect,* and *benign cortical irregularity of the distal femur.* Most cases are free of symptoms.

Avulsive cortical irregularity is an appropriate term because it describes the general location, radiologic appearance, and presumed origin of the finding. The avulsive cortical irregularity is almost always identified along the posterior aspect of the medial femoral condyle just above the adductor tubercle. It is frequently next to a benign cortical defect. The lesion is best demonstrated in a slight external oblique projection. It is located approximately 1–2 cm from the physis (4,55). When found incidentally on a lateral projection, the lesion appears as a localized area of cortical roughening of the distal metaphysis or a shallow, concave, irregular lucency in the surface of the cortex (Fig. 5-22A). The irregularity may be as long as 4 or 5 cm. Small cortical fragments may be seen in the soft tissues adjacent to the lesion.

Resnick and Greenway differentiate the *distal femoral cortical irregularity* (near but not at the insertion of the adductor magnus tendon) from the *femoral cortical excavation* (at the origin of the medial head of the gastrocnemius muscle) (56). Both probably represent traction-related lesions. In a small study using MRI, all avulsive cortical irregularities imaged were identified at or near the origin of the medial head of the gastrocnemius muscle (Fig. 5-22B) (57).

The avulsive cortical irregularity is seen between the ages of 3 and 17 years but is most frequent at 10–15 years of age (55,58). It is more common in boys and is often bilateral; a view of the other side may be helpful if a similar finding

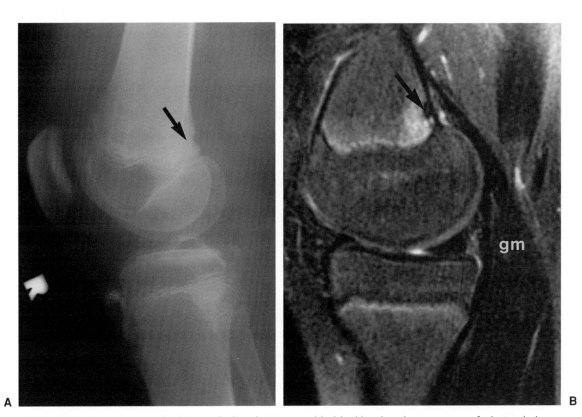

A   **B**

FIG. 5-22. Avulsive cortical irregularity. A 12-year-old girl with minor knee trauma. **A:** Lateral view of the knee shows irregularity of the posterior cortex of the femoral metaphysis *(arrow)*. No soft-tissue mass is seen. **B:** A T2-weighted MR image shows high signal in the posterior femoral metaphysis. This area is adjacent to the origin of the medial head of the gastrocnemius muscle *(gm)*. A small area of dark T2 signal *(arrow)* is consistent with a healing fibrous cortical defect.

is identified. The characteristic patient age, radiologic appearance, and anatomic location are important for correct diagnosis.

If there are acute symptoms, evaluation with skeletal scintigraphy or MRI is appropriate. The lesion has a dark rim and typically is of low signal intensity on T1-weighted images and high signal intensity on T2-weighted images. MRI may also show marrow edema adjacent to the lesion (57). There may be slightly increased bone uptake on skeletal scintigraphy, which supports the idea that it represents avulsion. If the lesions are bilaterally symmetric, they may be less obvious on skeletal scintigraphy. More frequently, the bone scan is normal, which helps confirm the diagnosis and exclude a malignancy. This lesion, despite the presence of a bony defect and periosteal reaction (Fig. 5-23), is fairly easy to distinguish from malignancy and infection. Biopsy of an active lesion may result in the erroneous histologic diagnosis of osteosarcoma.

Irregularity of the Tibial Tubercle

The tibial tubercle, an anteroinferior extension of the proximal tibial cartilaginous epiphysis, frequently ossifies from numerous small centers. Ossification generally occurs between 8 and 12 years of age in girls and 9 and 14 years

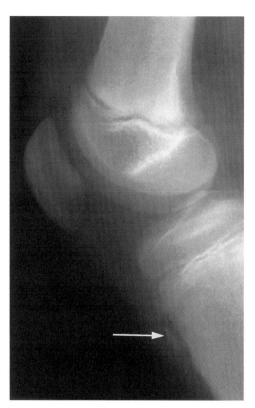

FIG. 5-24. Irregularity of the tibial tubercle. Lateral view of the knee in this 10-year-old girl shows a separate ossicle *(arrow)*, simulating an avulsion fragment.

of age in boys (4). Prior to bony fusion with the proximal tibial epiphysis, the separate ossicles may simulate avulsed fragments (Fig. 5-24). The appearance need not be symmetric. When only the anterior portion of the tibial physis remains unossified, a radiolucency can be seen on a frontal radiograph (2). Soft-tissue edema and patellar tendon thickening anterior to the tibial tubercle in a peripubertal child with pain suggests the diagnosis of the Osgood-Schlatter lesion, which is discussed later. However, isolated multiplicity of bony centers in the tibial tubercle is usually a normal developmental stage or the remaining sign of prior avulsion.

Calcaneal Apophyseal Sclerosis

Sclerosis of the apophysis of the calcaneus is a normal anatomic finding. The calcaneal apophysis, behind the main calcaneus, ossifies from several nuclei that first appear between the ages of 4 and 6 years in girls and 5 and 7 years in boys. These multiple ossification sites coalesce to form a single apophyseal center, which usually has an irregular outline and often is crossed by several linear lucencies. The normal calcaneal apophysis is more sclerotic than the body of the calcaneus (Fig. 5-25). This sclerosis occurs with normal weight bearing and requires approximately one month to disappear with inactivity or reappear with resumed activity (59). The apophysis fuses with the body of the calcaneus

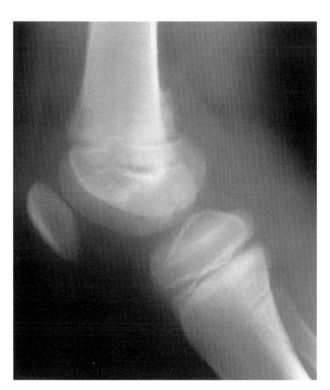

FIG. 5-23. Avulsive cortical irregularity. Lateral view of the knee in an 8-year-old boy immediately after a twisting injury. There is prominent cortical irregularity of the posteromedial aspect of the distal femoral metaphysis; this could be mistaken for a malignancy. No soft-tissue mass is seen. There also is irregularity of the distal femoral condyle.

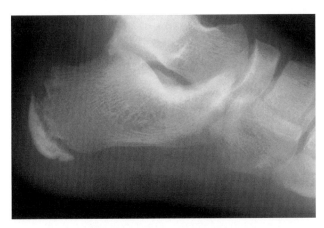

FIG. 5-25. Normal calcaneal apophysis. On the lateral projection, the calcaneal apophysis of this asymptomatic 11-year-old girl is sclerotic, is slightly irregular, and is partly crossed by a linear lucency.

at approximately 12–15 years of age and assumes the same density as the remainder of the bone at that time (4).

A true symptomatic overuse syndrome (Sever disease) of the apophysis is supported by positive skeletal scintigraphy (60), although the radiographs do not deviate from the normal appearance described here.

Calcaneal Pseudocyst

The calcaneal pseudocyst, a normal lucency of the calcaneus just anterior and inferior to the posterior calcaneal facet,

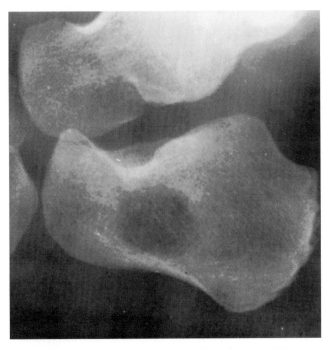

FIG. 5-26. Calcaneal pseudocyst. There is an oval lucency of the midportion of the calcaneus of this asymptomatic 2-year-old boy. A similar pseudocyst was present in the opposite calcaneus.

may radiographically resemble a true pathologic cyst (4). It is due to thinning of the trabeculae in the midportion of the calcaneus (Fig. 5-26). A similar radiolucency in the opposite calcaneus is a useful clue that one is dealing with a pseudocyst rather than a true cyst, which also occurs in this bone. A nutrient foramen, if seen in the lucency, indicates a calcaneal pseudocyst rather than a true cyst (61).

GENERAL ABNORMALITIES

Bone Density

Decreased Bone Density

Bone is formed by the impregnation of calcium salts on an organic matrix of collagen fibers and a ground substance. Almost all of these salts are in the form of calcium hydroxyapatite crystals. These crystals contain calcium, phosphate, and hydroxide ions. Normal bone formation involves induction and mineralization (62). *Osteopenia* (poor bone or bone lack) is a general term meaning decreased radiologic density of bone. It may be localized or generalized (Table 5-2). Osteopenia includes both osteomalacia (rickets in children) and osteoporosis.

Localized osteopenia in growing bones often occurs in the metaphysis (63). Metaphyseal lucencies extend to the physis if the zone of provisional calcification is absent or partially disrupted. This is seen with rickets, hypophosphatasia, and as a sequela of metaphyseal insults such as infections (syphilis, rubella, and cytomegalovirus infections), trauma (accidental, child abuse), or ischemia (Legg-Calvé-Perthes disease [LCP], radiation therapy, vasculitis). A well-defined horizontal radiolucent band on the metaphyseal side of an intact zone of provisional calcification can be seen in a neonate under stress and in infants with systemic disease or malnutrition. In children older than 2 years, these lucencies suggest leukemia, particularly if they are widespread and symmetric.

Generalized osteopenia may be due to deficiency of organic matrix (osteoporosis) or minerals and salts (rickets in children, osteomalacia in adults). Osteopenia may be caused by congenital abnormality, infection, tumor, trauma, disuse, weightlessness, medication, or endocrine abnormality (Table 5-2). In addition to abnormal formation, a decrease in bone density may be secondary to increased turnover of bone or bone destruction.

Increased Bone Density

Sclerotic lesions of bone may be either localized or generalized (Table 5-3). Causes of osteosclerosis include congenital abnormalities and syndromes, infection, tumor, trauma, and miscellaneous metabolic or developmental etiologies (Table 5-3).

Increased bony density may be due to cortical thickening or increased thickening of the medullary trabeculae, which

TABLE 5-2. *Causes of osteopenia*

Localized osteopenia	Widespread or generalized osteopenia
Congenital and developmental factors	Congenital factors
Metaphyseal lucent bands of early infancy	Osteochondrodysplasias
Bone-in-bone vertebrae of early infancy	Dysostosis multiplex
Infection	Hypophosphatasia
Acute hematogenous osteomyelitis	Osteogenesis imperfecta
Tuberculosis	Osteopenia of prematurity
Neoplasm	Deficiencies
Benign	Calcium or phosphorus deficiencies
Malignant	Copper deficiency
Trauma	Rickets
Injury to metaphyseal vasculature	Scurvy
Child abuse	Disuse
Sports injuries	Cerebral palsy
Myelodysplasia	Immobilization
Fracture healing	Neuromuscular disease
Frostbite	Spinal cord abnormality
Reflex sympathetic dystrophy	Myelomeningocele
Burn	Endocrine Disorders
Miscellaneous	Adrenocortical
Arthritis	Gonadal
Disuse	Parathyroid
Immobilization	Miscellaneous
Paralysis	Collagen vascular diseases
Metaphyseal lucent bands	Drugs (steroids, heparin)
Leukemia	Idiopathic juvenile osteoporosis
Stress	Hemophilia
	Leukemia

TABLE 5-3. *Causes of osteosclerosis*

Localized osteosclerosis	Generalized osteosclerosis
Congenital factors	Congenital factors
Tuberous sclerosis	Engelmann disease
Infection	Mastocytosis
Sclerosing osteomyelitis	Melorheostosis
Syphilis	Osteopathia striata
Neoplasm	Osteopetrosis
Benign	Osteopoikilosis
Healed nonossifying fibroma	Pycnodysostosis
Osteoblastoma	Tuberous sclerosis
Ossifying fibroma	Neoplasm
Osteofibrous dysplasia	Leukemia
Osteoid osteoma	Lymphoma
Osteoma	Osteosarcomatosis
Malignant	Miscellaneous
Ewing sarcoma	Healing rickets
Lymphoma	Hypervitaminosis D
Metastatic disease (medulloblastoma)	Physiologic sclerosis of the newborn
Osteogenic sarcoma	Renal osteodystrophy
Trauma	Sickle cell disease
Callus	Hypercalcemia
Compression fracture, overlapping fragments	Hypothyroidism
Radiation injury	
Stress fracture	
Miscellaneous	
Aseptic necrosis	
Bone island	

in turn may be due to increased deposition of mineral in the matrix or decreased resorption. Moreover, dead bone appears relatively dense in comparison to adjacent osteoporotic bone.

Disorders of Shape and Symmetry

Body Asymmetry

Although minor asymmetry of the two halves of the body is common, gross asymmetry is rare. Body asymmetry may be due to hemihypertrophy, hemiatrophy, or hemidystrophy. It also may result from damage to or stimulation of physes. It is important to distinguish these various types of body asymmetry because only patients with hemihypertrophy have a predisposition to develop intraabdominal and other neoplasms. Somatic overgrowth varies in severity and distribution, affecting a whole body side (hemihypertrophy), a limb (macromelia), or a single digit (macrodactyly) (64). Overgrowth may be of all tissues in a given area or only of certain structures.

TABLE 5-4. *Congenital disorders associated with asymmetry (localized or generalized)*

Idiopathic
Primary disorders of the lymphatic vessels
    Lymphedema
    Lymphangiomatosis
Other vascular disorders or tumors
    Malformations
        Arteriovenous malformations and fistulas
        Venous malformations
        Klippel-Trenaunay and Parkes-Weber syndromes
    Hemangiomas
Phakomatoses
    Neurofibromatosis
    Tuberous sclerosis
    Von Hippel-Lindau syndrome
    Sturge-Weber syndrome
Lipomatosis and macrodystrophia lipomatosa
Beckwith-Wiedemann syndrome
Proteus syndrome
Neoplasia associated with asymmetry
    Renal
    Adrenal
    Hepatic
    Gonadal
    Retroperitoneal sympathetic chain
    Heart
    Muscle
    Brain
    Appendix
Bone dysplasias
    Fibrous dysplasia
    Multiple enchondromatoses
    Dysplasia epiphysealis hemimelica
    Maffucci syndrome
    Progressive diaphyseal dysplasia
    Melorheostosis

Modified from Levine (64).

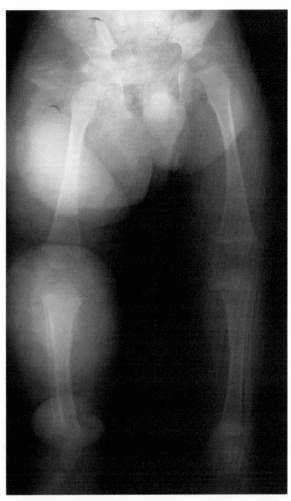

FIG. 5-27. Hemihypertrophy. Frontal radiograph of a 6-year-old boy with Klippel-Trenaunay syndrome shows enlargement of the right lower extremity. The soft tissues are increased due to the diffuse capillary-lymphatic-venous malformation. From Laor (568).

Hemiatrophy is a postnatal process with onset usually during preadolescence. It is an acquired loss of body structures that usually involves fat and subcutaneous tissue. It is associated with neurologic disorders or muscular diseases and is therefore easy to recognize.

Hemidystrophy and *hemihypotrophy* are terms for the failure of growth of one side of the body, rather than loss of previously developed structures. It is associated with various chromosomal abnormalities and syndromes such as the Russell-Silver syndrome (65). Hemidystrophy may be associated with intrauterine growth retardation. With hemidystrophy and hemiatrophy, the larger half of the body is more normal in size than the smaller half.

Hemihypertrophy is the overgrowth of half of, or portions of half of, the body (64). Localized enlargement may be secondary to acquired processes such as neoplasia, trauma, and infection. Congenital abnormalities, frequently detectable at birth, also result in asymmetry. Hemihypertrophy may be total (involving neurologic, muscular, skeletal, vascular, and lymphatic systems) or limited to a single system or combination of systems of the body, and unilateral or crossed (overgrowth of contralateral limbs); the last is rare. The most important orthopedic problem in children with hemihypertrophy is the development of a leg length discrepancy with consequent pelvic obliquity and scoliosis (4). Several syndromes and disorders are associated with progressive disproportion (Table 5-4; Figs. 5-27 and 5-28).

Many congenital anomalies and neoplastic diseases have been documented in patients with congenital hemihypertrophy. Congenital anomalies include urogenital malformations (hypogonadism, hypospadias), renal abnormalities (polycystic disease, medullary sponge kidney, benign nephromegaly), and sporadic aniridia. The neoplastic abnormalities may be benign or malignant. The side of the hypertrophy is not related to the side of the neoplasm. Benign neoplasms in-

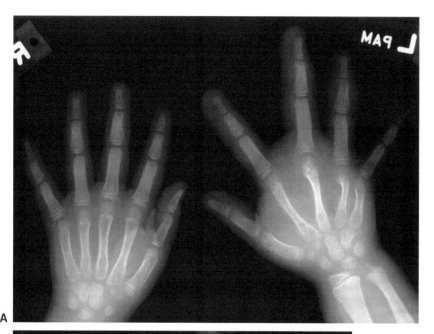

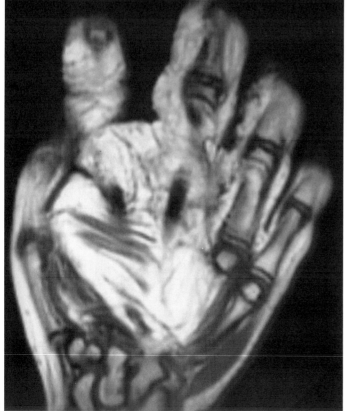

FIG. 5-28. Macromelia. This 6-year-old boy has macrodystrophia lipomatosa involving the left hand and distal forearm. A: Frontal radiograph shows enlargement, primarily of the soft tissues, of the left hand and distal forearm. This is due to hypertrophy of the mesodermal tissues, with dramatic overgrowth of fat. The metacarpals are thinned, and the second and third are slightly elongated. B: Coronal T1-weighted MR image of the left hand shows extensive high signal from the increased fat.

clude nephroblastomatosis, retroperitoneal ganglioneuroma, adrenal adenoma, cardiac hamartoma, atrial myxoma, hepatic hemangioendothelioma, and focal nodular hyperplasia of the liver (66–69). Common malignant neoplasms include Wilms tumor (especially those associated with deletion of the short arm of chromosome 11), adrenocortical carcinoma, rhabdomyosarcoma, hepatoblastoma, and glioma.

Children with hemihypertrophy are at chronic risk for abdominal neoplasms. These children should undergo frequent

TABLE 5-5. *Causes of abnormal tubulation of long bones*

Overtubulation
Neuromuscular disorders
  Myelomeningocele
  Cerebral palsy
Disuse syndromes
  Osteogenesis imperfecta
Epiphyseal and metaphyseal dysplasias
Miscellaneous
  Rheumatoid arthritis

Undertubulation
Osteochondrodysplasias
  Osteopetrosis
  Pyle disease
  Enchondromatosis
  Multiple exostoses
Tumors
  Fibrous dysplasia
  Exostoses
Storage diseases
  Gaucher
  Niemann-Pick
  Mucopolysaccharidoses
  Mucolipidoses
Miscellaneous
  Severe anemia, often hemolytic
  Healing fracture
  Heavy metal poisoning (e.g., lead)

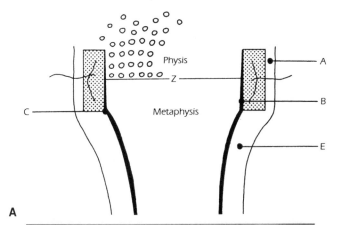

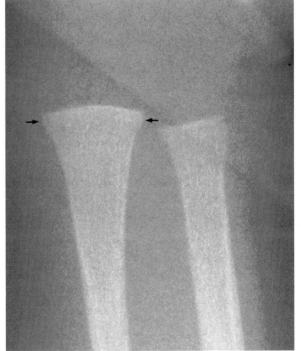

FIG. 5-29. Normal metaphyseal contour. A: Longitudinal section to illustrate the zone of Ranvier *(shaded)* of the metaphysis in children. This zone and its central bone cortex *(B)* maintain a longitudinally straight contour for a few millimeters (collar of Laval-Jeantet) to the junction with the curved metaphyseal cortex *(C)*. Periosteum *(E)*; perichondrium *(A)*; zone of provisional calcification *(Z)*. **B:** The distal forearm of a normal newborn shows the straight contour of the zone of Ranvier *(arrows)*. This joins with the relatively curved metaphysis.

abdominal physical examination by the parents and the primary care physician. Imaging by ultrasonography and other modalities as necessary is also an important part of the long-term follow-up. Screening abdominal ultrasonography for the young child with hemihypertrophy should be performed as frequently as three or four times a year, through age 5 (peak onset of Wilms tumor is 4 years of age) (70).

Abnormal Tubulation of Long Bones

Normal tubulation of long bones is due to concurrent diametric transverse widening at the physis, longitudinal endochondral lengthening at the physis, and osteoclastic remodeling of the cortex of the metaphysis. Tubulation may be described as the amount of concavity of the lateral bony contours of the metaphysis. In the young child, tubulation begins 1–3 mm shaftward from the physis. The first few millimeters have longitudinally straight margins bounded by the zone of Ranvier (Fig. 5-29) (71). Appositional bone growth occurs at the periosteum of the diaphysis (not the metaphysis, which is being cut away by osteoclasts), to allow circumferential growth of the shaft.

Because normal motor activity is a stimulus for diaphyseal bone growth, neuromuscular disorders and disuse are associated with thin shafts (Fig. 5-30A). Overtubulation (excessive tubulation, increased concavity of the outer margins of the metaphyses) may also be noted in certain syndromes and miscellaneous conditions when the rate of endochondral bone production is slowed relative to circumferential growth

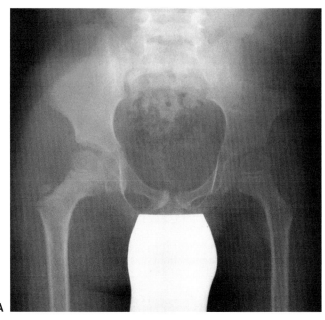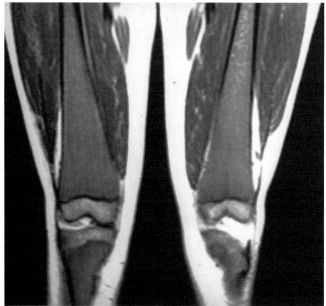

A

B

FIG. 5-30. Abnormal tubulation. A: Overtubulation. A 6-year-old boy with prior poliomyelitis of the left lower extremity. In addition to excessive tubulation of the proximal left femur, there is decreased muscle mass on the left. **B:** Undertubulation. T1-weighted MR image of the femurs of a 16-year old girl with Gaucher disease. The distal femurs are undertubulated, and the normal fatty marrow signal is lost because of diffuse marrow replacement by Gaucher cells.

or circumferential growth at the physis is increased relative to that of the shaft.

Undertubulation (decreased concavity of the outer margins of the metaphyses) results in an expanded bone, particularly in the metaphyseal region. The common mechanisms for this modeling abnormality are marrow packing or storage disorders, bone dysplasias, bone tumors, and osteoclastic or osteocytic dysfunction and consequent lack of normal osteolysis (63). The Erlenmeyer flask deformity of Gaucher disease is a classic example of undertubulation (underconstriction) (Fig. 5-30B). Table 5-5 summarizes the more common causes of abnormal tubulation of the long bones.

SPECIFIC ABNORMALITIES

Constitutional Diseases of Bone

Constitutional diseases of bone affect the growth, histology, and morphology of the entire skeleton or selected portions thereof. These conditions may be due to genetic abnormalities or intrauterine factors. Metabolic and endocrine diseases sometimes show similar patterns. Some abnormalities are recognized at birth, whereas others become evident during infancy, childhood, or adolescence. Rarely are constitutional skeletal diseases first recognized in an adult. The clinical clues to a dysplasia include history, stature (short trunk or limbs), nonbony features (e.g., findings in the ears or teeth), joint morphology, gait, and abnormalities of the hands and feet (72).

There have been several attempts to classify constitutional skeletal diseases. The most satisfactory nomenclature of constitutional skeletal diseases was devised in 1969 and revised in 1977 (73). A modification developed in 1992 focused on the osteochondrodysplasias (74). The classification divides the skeletal dysplasias into the following five major groups:

1. Osteochondrodysplasias
2. Dysostoses
3. Idiopathic osteolysis
4. Chromosomal aberrations or bony disorders due to abnormalities of other organ systems
5. Primary metabolic abnormalities

Osteochondrodysplasias are abnormalities of growth and development of bone or cartilage that systematically affect their structure. *Dysostoses* are malformations of an individual bone that may be noted alone or in combination with other malformations. *Idiopathic osteolysis* involves conditions associated with the resorption of bone. The fourth group is self-explanatory. In the fifth group, *primary metabolic abnormalities,* the pathogenetic mechanism is known or a biochemical defect (such as a complex carbohydrate, lipid, or amino acid disorder) has been demonstrated (9,62,75).

Osteochondrodysplasias

The osteochondrodysplasias may be subgrouped into those involving abnormal growth of bones (recognizable at birth or later in life), those characterized by disorganized development of cartilaginous and fibrous components of the skeleton, and those characterized by abnormalities of bone density, diaphyseal cortical thickness, or metaphyseal shape.

The nomenclature, genetic significance, clinical features, and radiologic features of the osteochondrodysplasias are complex. The conditions themselves are numerous but uncommon or rare. However, one should develop an understanding of the basic aspects of the skeletal dysplasias to provide a radiologic evaluation and differential diagnosis. The excellent textbooks by Maroteaux (62), Spranger et al. (75), and Taybi and Lachman (9) give more detailed discussions of the various osteochondrodysplasias.

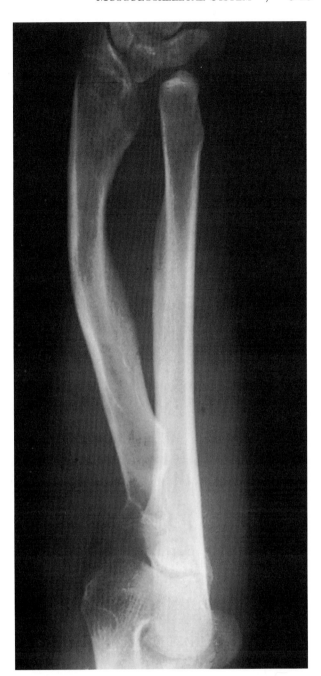

FIG. 5-32. Mesomelic dwarfism. There is marked shortening of the ulna and radius, bowing of the radius, and a Madelung deformity in this 14-year-old girl with dyschondrosteosis.

Abnormal Growth of Bones

Osteochondrodysplasias that affect the growth of the tubular bones and the spine may be grouped into those evident at birth (often diagnosed by prenatal ultrasonography) (Fig. 5-31) and those first recognized during late childhood or early adulthood. Congenital dwarfism (shortening of the limbs or spine below the third percentile for normal newborns) may be due to a number of conditions with characteristic genetic and radiologic features (Table 5-6). Some of

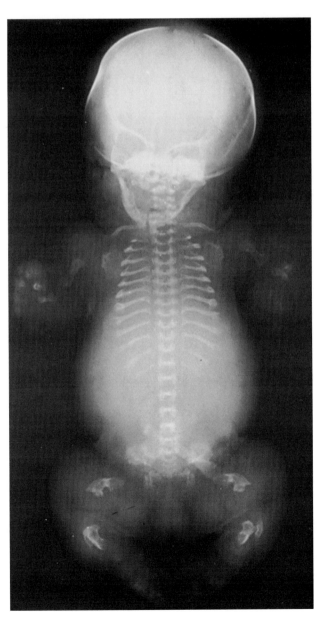

FIG. 5-31. Neonatal short-limbed dwarfism. Newborn girl with thanatophoric dwarfism.

TABLE 5-6. *Neonatal*

| Disease | Inheritance | Skull | | Chest: short ribs | Spine | | Distal narrowing of interpediculate distance |
		Enlarged cranium	Short base		Short	Vertebrae	
Achondrogenesis I & II	Aut. recess.	+	−	+	+	Poorly or not mineralized	−
Achondroplasia	Aut. dom.	+	+	+	+	Small canal, decreased height, increased disk space	+
Asphyxiating thoracic dystrophy	Aut. recess.	−	−	+	−	Normal	−
Camptomelic dysplasia	Aut. recess.	+	+	−	−	± Ossification defects	−
Cartilage hair hypoplasia	Aut. recess.	−	−	−	−	Normal	−
Chondrodysplasia punctata	Aut. recess., aut. dom.	−	+	−	−	Stippling	−
Chondroectodermal dysplasia	Aut. recess.	−	−	±	−	Normal	−
Cleidocranial dysplasia	Aut. dom	+	−	−	−	Abnormal ossification	−
Diastrophic dysplasia	Aut. recess.	−	−	−	−	Scoliosis	+
Mesomelic dysplasias	Aut. recess., aut. dom.	−	−	−	−	Normal	−
Metatropic dysplasia	Aut. recess., aut. dom.	−	−	+	−	Platyspondyly, increased intervertebral space	−
Osteogenesis imperfecta	Aut. dom., aut. recess.	+	−	−	±	Osteoporosis	−
Spondyloepiphyseal dysplasia congenita	Aut. dom.	−	−	−	+	Platyspondyly, ovoid shape; dens hypoplasia	−
Thanatophoric dysplasia	Aut. dom., lethal	+	+	+	±	Platyspondyly	+

Source: Spranger et al. (75), Cremin and Beighton (76), and Taybi and Lachman (9).
Courtesy of William H. McAlister, M.D., St. Louis, Missouri.

these disorders may be lethal (9,76). Adequate radiologic evaluation of osteochondrodysplasias requires examination of the skull, thorax, spine, pelvis, and extremities. Diseases affecting the growth of tubular bones may be categorized according to the part of the extremity that is maximally shortened. *Rhizomelic* shortening predominantly affects the proximal (humerus and femur) portions of the extremities (Table 5-7). Achondroplasia is the prototype of rhizomelic dwarfism and is discussed at length below. *Mesomelic* shortening affects the middle portions (forearm or leg) of the extremities (Table 5-7). Dyschondrosteosis is a classic example of mesomelic dwarfism (Fig. 5-32). *Acromelic* shortening primarily affects the distal portions (hands and feet) of the extremities (Table 5-7) and is characteristic of the acrodysostoses.

The dysplasias may also be classified by the site affected primarily (epiphyses, metaphyses, diaphyses, spine) (Table 5-8). Prototypes of each of these groups are reviewed below.

More complete discussions, are given by the texts referenced previously.

Disorders Recognizable at Birth Affecting Growth of Tubular Bones and Spine.

Achondroplasia. The heterozygous (usual) form of achondroplasia is the most common short-limbed dwarfism. It is transmitted with an autosomal dominant inheritance mode but often arises sporadically. It is manifested at birth by rhizomelic micromelia, more marked in the upper extremities (77), and by craniofacial abnormalities.

Clinical examination of patients with heterozygous achondroplasia shows a disproportionately large cranial vault, a depressed nasal bridge, a prominent forehead, and mild hypoplasia of the midface. There may be muscular hypotonicity, which can mimic psychomotor retardation. This hypotonicity can accentuate the invariable neonatal kyphosis at the thoracolumbar junction. After infancy, when the child stands

short-limbed dwarfism

Pelvis, Iliac wings	Acetabular roof	Extremities		Other anomalies
		Maximal shortening	Radiographic appearance	
Poorly mineralized	Poorly ossified	Both	Poorly ossified, metaphyseal enlargement	Early death
Squared, small sacroiliac notch	Horizontal	Proximal	Metaphyseal margin concavity	± Hydrocephalus, hypotonia
Reduced height	Trident	Distal	Metaphyseal irregularity, beaking	Cone-shaped epiphyses of hands, respiratory distress
Tall and narrow	Steep	Both	Bowing of femurs, tibias, fibulas, radii, and ulnas	Hypertelorism, micrognathia, cleft palate, narrow trachea
Normal	Normal	Both	Metaphyseal flaring, irregularity	Fine hair, megacolon
Normal	Normal	Proximal	Stippled epiphyses, asymmetry	Cataracts, erythroderma
Reduced height	Trident	Distal	Metaphyseal irregularity	Congenital heart disease, polydactyly, abnormal nails
Hypoplasia	Horizontal	Both (slight)	Hypoplasia of distal phalanges, metacarpal pseudoepiphyses	Abnormal ossification of skull, clavicles, vertebrae, and pubis
Normal	Normal	Proximal or mesomelic	Metaphyseal enlargement	Swelling of ears, clubfeet, hitchhiker thumb
Normal	Normal	Mesomelic	Shortening of tibias, fibulas, radii, and ulnas	Bowing, ± mandibular hypoplasia
Short, small sacroiliac notch	Horizontal	Both	Club-like metaphyses	Tail-like appendage
May be deformed	Normal	Variable	Thin cortex, fractures	Blue sclerae (types I, II, ± III, ± IV)
Retarded ossification	Normal	Both (slight)	Epiphyses irregular, ossification delayed	± Myopia
Squared	Horizontal	Proximal	Metaphyseal flaring, "telephone receiver" femurs	Early death

TABLE 5-7. *Examples of extremity-shortening dysplasias in infants and children*

Rhizomelic shortening
  Achondroplasia
  Chondrodysplasia punctata
  Thanatophoric dwarfism
  Hypochondroplasia
  Pseudoachondroplasia
  Diastrophic dysplasia

Mesomelic shortening
  Dyschondrosteosis (Léri-Weill disease)
  Other mesomelic dwarfisms
    Langer syndrome
    Nievergelt syndrome
    Acromesomelic dwarfism
    Cornelia de Lange syndrome

Acromelic shortening
  Asphyxiating thoracic dystrophy (Jeune syndrome)
  Chondroectodermal dysplasia (Ellis-van Creveld syndrome)
  Peripheral dysostosis
  Trichorhinophalangeal syndrome
  Acrodysostosis

and walks, the buttocks are prominent. The hands are short and there is separation of the middle digits from each other. This trident hand is due to the similar length of the second, third, and fourth digits (Fig. 5-33). There may be limitation of elbow extension and excessive sweating.

The radiologic manifestations of achondroplasia show little variability. They include craniofacial disproportion due to a relatively large calvaria, and prominence of the frontal, parietal, and occipital regions. In contrast, there is decreased size of the base of the skull (i.e., the part formed in cartilage), foramen magnum, and jugular foramina. The ossified sella turcica is frequently small and may have an abnormal shape. The basal angle is reduced (77). The small jugular foramina, small foramen magnum, and a small spinal canal can have severe neurologic consequences such as compression of the lower brainstem, spinal cord, cauda equina, and nerve roots (77,78). This abnormal anatomy is delineated readily with MRI (79). MRI also may show dilatation of the lateral and third ventricles and prominent bifrontal subarachnoid spaces (79).

TABLE 5-8. *Examples of skeletal dysplasia in infants and children, by site*

Epiphyseal
  Multiple epiphyseal dysplasia
  Chondrodysplasia punctata (stippled epiphyses)
  Cretinism
Epimetaphyseal
  Asphyxiating thoracic dystrophy
  Diastrophic dwarphism
  Chondroectodermal dysplasia
Metaphyseal
  Achondroplasia
  Metaphyseal chondrodysplasia
    Type Jansen
    Type Schmid
    Type McKusick
    Schwachman syndrome
  Hypophosphatasia
Diaphyseal
  Fibrous dysplasia
  Osteogenesis imperfecta
  Diaphyseal dysplasia
  Pyknodysostosis
  Osteopetrosis
Spondyloepiphyseal
  Spondyloepiphyseal dysplasia
Spondyloepimetaphyseal
  Morquio disease
  Metatropic dysplasia
Spondylometaphyseal
  Spondylometaphyseal dysplasia

The ribs are short and have cup-shaped anterior ends. There is a decrease in the anteroposterior diameter of the chest. The interpediculate distances decrease from the upper to the lower lumbar spine, which is abnormal, and there is shortening of the pedicles as seen on the lateral view. Absence of the normal increase in the interpediculate distances downward in the lumbar spine may be less apparent in the newborn (Fig. 5-34) than in older infants and children (77). There is an absolute as well as a relative increase in intervertebral disc space height, and both the height and anteroposterior diameter of vertebral bodies are decreased. An exaggerated lumbar lordosis is present after infancy. The posterior surfaces of the vertebral bodies are concave (Fig. 5-35). Undergrowth of the vertebral arch results in a small vertebral canal. Thus, even a minor disc protrusion is likely to cause neurologic symptoms and signs.

The iliac bones have decreased vertical height, producing a nearly square shape. The acetabular angles are decreased, whereas the iliac angles are large (Figs. 5-36 and 5-37). The sacrosciatic notches are small or narrow, and there is beaking of the medial edges of the ilia. The pelvic inlet is wide and shallow and the femoral necks are short.

Rhizomelic shortening of the tubular bones due to slowed endochondral ossification is present at all ages. Metaphyseal flaring is also due to the decreased endochondral bone

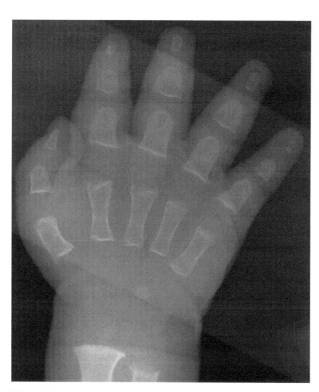

FIG. 5-33. Achondroplasia. Frontal hand radiograph of an infant boy shows the trident configuration. There is shortening of the bones, especially of the metacarpals and proximal and middle phalanges.

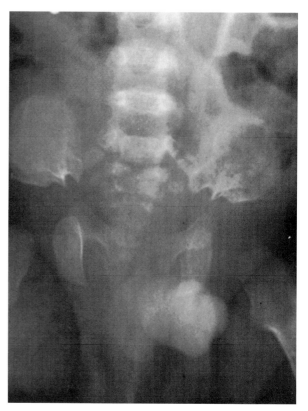

FIG. 5-34. Achondroplasia. Frontal radiograph of a 3-month-old boy shows platyspondyly, flaring of proximal femoral metaphyses, and flat acetabular angles. The interpediculate distances do not increase distally in the lower lumbar spine.

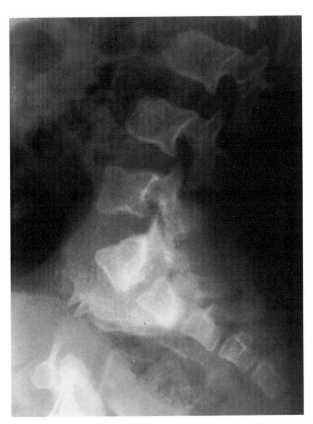

FIG. 5-35. Achondroplasia. Lateral view of the lumbosacral spine of a 6-month-old boy shows platyspondyly and posterior vertebral body scalloping. There is marked shortening of the pedicles, and the spinal canal is very shallow from front to back.

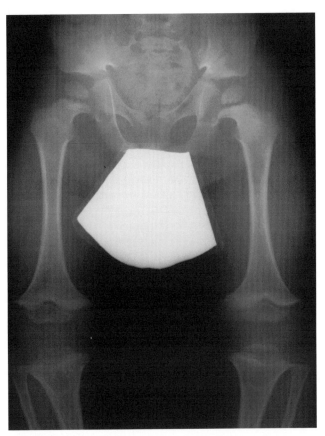

FIG. 5-36. Achondroplasia. Frontal view of the lower extremities in a 5-year-old boy shows shortening of both femurs. There is metaphyseal flaring at the knees and an inverted V configuration of the distal femoral physes. The iliac wings are square and the acetabular angles are flattened.

growth in length with normal periosteal and perichondral (zone of Ranvier) intramembranous bone formation. This discrepancy may subsequently lead to cone-like or ball-and-socket distal femoral physes, which take an inverted V configuration (Fig. 5-36). The disproportion between normal width and shortened length makes the tubular bones look stocky. There also is shortening of the bones of the hands and feet, most evident in the proximal and middle phalanges. The trident deformity of the digits is frequently present in infants (see Fig. 5-33) as is a square or oval radiolucent area in the proximal femur (Fig. 5-37) and humerus on frontal films. Langer et al. suggest that this relative lucency is due to an abnormally narrowed anteroposterior diameter of the proximal femur (77). Muscle attachments are prominent and normal bony curvatures are exaggerated (77). The contour of the epiphyseal ossification centers is smooth but ossification is slowed.

Heterozygous achondroplasia is one form of dwarfism in which leg lengthening techniques have shown promising results. The radiologist should be aware of the radiologic evaluation of these procedures (80,81). With callotasis, for example, medical distraction is begun only after callus is identified on radiographs (80). The homozygous form of achondroplasia is very rare and uniformly lethal. The radio-

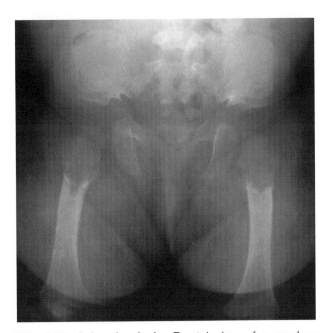

FIG. 5-37. Achondroplasia. Frontal view of a newborn shows oval radiolucent areas in both proximal femurs. The femurs are short, the iliac bones are squared, and the acetabular roofs are flattened.

graphic findings are much more severe than those seen with the heterozygous form and may be indistinguishable from thanatophoric dysplasia.

Camptomelic dysplasia. Camptomelic ("bent limb") dysplasia has an autosomal recessive or sporadic inheritance pattern. It is characterized by anterior bowing of the long bones of the lower extremities, pretibial skin dimples (Fig. 5-38), hypoplastic scapulae, abnormalities of the cervical and thoracic spine, small face with a large and elongated skull, and dysplastic pelvic bones. Neonatal death is frequent, because of respiratory distress from a small thoracic cage, narrow larynx, and hypoplastic cartilaginous tracheal rings (82).

Diastrophic dysplasia. Diastrophic dysplasia (diastrophic dwarfism) is an autosomal recessive dysplasia identifiable at birth. The name refers to the characteristic twisted extremities and vertebral column (78). A marked cervical kyphosis usually develops. Other clinical findings include short stature, abduction of a hypermobile thumb with a short first metacarpal ("hitchhiker's thumb") (Fig. 5-39), symphalangism, progressive scoliosis, deformed earlobes ("cauliflower ear"), limited mobility and dislocation of peripheral joints, and a cleft or high-arched palate (9,83). The dysplastic changes are thought to be due to abnormal collagen formation (82).

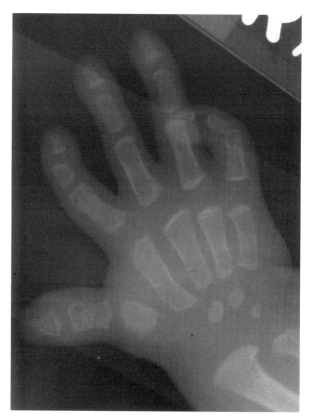

FIG. 5-39. Diastrophic dysplasia. Frontal view of a hand in a 7-month-old girl shows abduction of the thumb and a short first metacarpal ("hitchhiker's thumb"). Epiphyseal ossification is delayed.

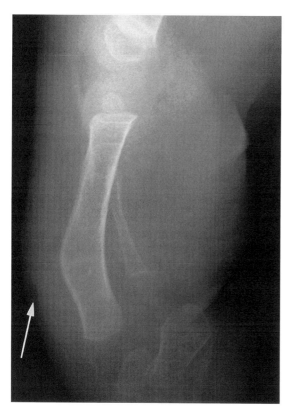

FIG. 5-38. Camptomelic dysplasia. Lateral view of the leg in a 2-year-old girl shows anterior bowing of the distal half of the tibia. There is a skin dimple *(arrow)* at the apex of the curve.

The skull is radiographically normal. The vertebral body contours are irregular and the odontoid may be hypoplastic. As in achondroplasia, the lumbar interpediculate distance decreases distally. The tubular bones are short and the metaphyses widened. The epiphyses are flattened and may ossify late.

Disorders Recognized Later in Life Affecting Growth of Tubular Bones and Spine.

Multiple epiphyseal dysplasia. Multiple epiphyseal dysplasia is a heterogeneous group of abnormalities, most commonly with an autosomal dominant inheritance mode and complete penetrance but variable expression. The primary defect is thought to be within the chondrocytes of the unossified epiphyses (9,78). Although "stippled epiphyses" may be noted during infancy, these dysplasias often are not recognized until later in life, sometimes not until adulthood. The disease usually causes restricted mobility, difficulty walking, a waddling gait, moderately short stature, and thoracic kyphosis with back pain.

The *Fairbanks type* is the classic severe disorder that causes distal shortening of both long and short tubular bones. There is delayed appearance of the epiphyses of the hands and feet, which when present are small and irregular. The metaphyses and diaphyses of the tubular bones are usually normal. In some cases, mild metaphyseal flaring is seen.

The spine may be normal or show moderate flattening of vertebral bodies with irregular endplates and Schmorl nodes. Occasionally, the patella is sagittally duplicated.

The *Ribbing type* is mild and is often detected incidentally on radiographs. This type can be confined to the spine, with nearly normal extremities except for the proximal portions of the long tubular bones. The spine shows irregularity of vertebral endplates, many Schmorl nodes, slight decrease in vertebral body height, and some vertebral body wedging. There may be irregularity and deformity of the epiphyses of the femurs and humeri, the hips being most severely affected. Degenerative changes may develop in the hips.

The differential diagnosis of these disorders includes spondyloepiphyseal dysplasia, the juvenile arthritides, progressive pseudorheumatoid dysplasia, osteonecrosis, hypothyroidism, and the mucopolysaccharidoses (78).

Spondyloepiphyseal dysplasia. The many forms of spondyloepiphyseal dysplasia (SED) are distinguishable by clinical, genetic, and radiologic differences. In most varieties, the characteristic abnormalities of the spine and epiphyses become more evident with age.

SED congenita is a short trunk dysplasia with mildly shortened limbs. It is evident at birth. It may have an autosomal dominant inheritance pattern, although most cases are sporadic. In the infant spine, the vertebrae are short and have a pear-shaped configuration in the lateral projection. This

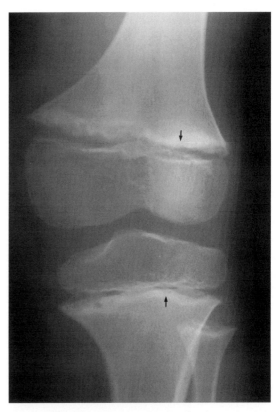

FIG. 5-41. Metaphyseal chondrodysplasia, type Schmid. There is metaphyseal irregularity and growth plate widening at the knee of a 10-year-old boy. The distal femoral metaphysis is mildly flared. Unlike rickets, the density of the zone of provisional calcification *(arrows)* and metaphyseal collar of Laval-Jeantet are normal.

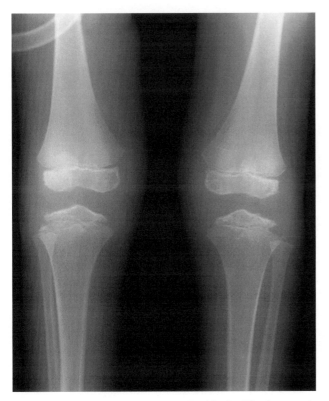

FIG. 5-40. Spondyloepiphyseal dysplasia. The knees of a 7-year-old boy show small, irregularly ossified epiphyses of the distal femurs, proximal tibias, and proximal fibulas.

shape is due to underdevelopment of the posterior portion of the vertebral bodies. With age, a severe thoracolumbar kyphoscoliosis and lumbar lordosis develop with universal flattening of the vertebral bodies. The odontoid is often hypoplastic, and there is atlantoaxial instability. The chest is bell-shaped. Ossification of the tubular bones is delayed, and the femurs may be bowed with a coxa vara configuration. The radiographic appearance resembles that of Morquio disease (see below), but the morphology of the metacarpal and metatarsal bones is relatively normal (9,75,78).

The tarda forms of SED usually do not become evident until 5–10 years of age. The children have short trunks as a manifestation of relatively flattened and posteriorly bulbous vertebral bodies. The disc spaces are widened anteriorly and narrowed posteriorly. The appendicular epiphyses are dysplastic (Fig. 5-40), and arthritic changes may be seen in the hips and shoulders. This abnormality is usually inherited as an X-linked recessive, but autosomal dominant and autosomal recessive forms also occur (78).

Metaphyseal chondrodysplasia. Metaphyseal chondrodysplasia (metaphyseal dysostosis) is a group of disorders characterized by significant metaphyseal changes in the long tubular bones. There is short stature of variable degree. The most common form is the *type Schmid*. This autosomal dominant disorder is characterized by flaring and irregularity of the metaphyses. The physes are wider than usual. The vertebral bodies are ovoid on lateral views, and there may be a triangular fragment of bone at the medial and inferior aspect of the femoral neck (84). The metaphyseal changes are somewhat suggestive of hypophosphatemic rickets; in metaphyseal chondrodysplasia type Schmid the zone of provisional calcification and the metaphyseal collar are usually normal (Fig. 5-41) (63,85). *Type Jansen,* a very rare form of metaphyseal chondrodysplasia, is characterized by severe dwarfism. *Type McKusick,* also known as cartilage hair hypoplasia, has more prominent metaphyseal changes than type Schmid, and radiographs also show cone-shaped phalangeal epiphyses. The patients have sparse hair (84). Metaphyseal chondrodysplasia associated with exocrine pancreatic insufficiency and bone marrow dysfunction (Schwachman-Diamond syndrome) may present as failure to thrive and malabsorption in a young child (86).

Disorders of Development of the Cartilaginous and Fibrous Components of the Skeleton.

Cleidocranial dysplasia. Cleidocranial dysplasia (cleidocranial dysostosis) is a relatively common abnormality of mesenchymal development and is manifest at birth. It has an autosomal dominant type of genetic transmission, but one third of cases are spontaneous mutations. There is great phenotypic variability. Clinical features include a coronally enlarged head, wide sutures, delayed closure of the anterior fontanel, small face, drooping shoulders with increased mobility, dental dysplasia including supernumerary teeth and failure of eruption of teeth, abnormal gait, muscular hypotonia, joint hypermobility, short distal phalanges, and hypoplastic nails.

There is retarded ossification of the membranous part of the skull with bossing, delayed closure of sutures and fontanels, and many wormian bones. (Fig. 5-42A). The metopic suture usually fails to close (87). Deformity of the foramen magnum has also been described (88). The paranasal sinuses

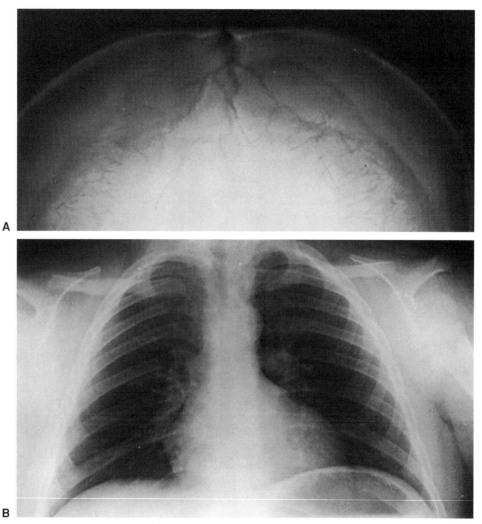

FIG. 5-42. Cleidocranial dysplasia. A: Multiple wormian bones. **B:** Aplasia of the outer ends of the clavicles.

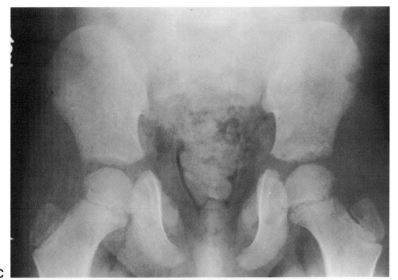

C

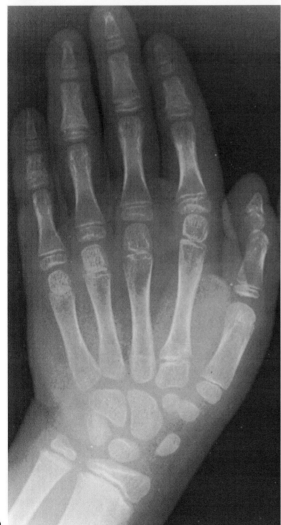

D

FIG. 5-42. *Continued.* **C:** Wide symphysis pubis and hypoplasia of the iliac wings. The proximal femoral epiphyses are rounded and there are characteristic notches along the lateral epiphyseal margins. **D:** Proximal pseudoepiphysis of a long second metacarpal. Several cone epiphyses are noted in the middle phalanges.

and mastoids are underpneumatized. Hypertelorism is present. Irregular ossification of the spine and undertubulation of the metaphyseal long bones also may be present (88). Often there is delayed fusion of the posterior elements of the spine.

Normally, the clavicles are formed from three centers by membranous ossification. There may be total or partial aplasia of one or both clavicles in cleidocranial dysplasia. The most common defect is loss of the outer end of the clavicle (Fig. 5-42B) The next most frequent abnormality is loss of part of the middle ossification center leaving two unfused, separated medial and lateral fragments (87). It is rare to lose just the inner third of the clavicle. In 10% of patients, the clavicles are normal. The scapulas are small and winged.

There invariably is abnormal ossification of the pelvis (Fig. 5-42C). This disorder therefore is sometimes referred to as pelvicocleidocranial dysplasia. The pubic bones are unossified during early infancy and underdeveloped during childhood. A seemingly wide symphysis pubis is present with apparent widening of the sacroiliac joints and the triradiate cartilages of the acetabula. Hypoplasia of the iliac wings and a valgus deformity of the femoral necks are usually present. A lateral notch in the proximal femoral epiphyses has been described (87).

There are characteristic large pseudoepiphyses (accessory proximal epiphyses) of the metacarpals and metatarsals, and the second metacarpal is often long (Fig. 5-42D). There may be shortening of the distal phalanges and retarded ossification of both carpal and tarsal bones. The terminal phalangeal tufts may be pointed (87,88). The distal phalanges of the fingers may have remarkably large epiphyses, and cone epiphyses are common (Fig. 5-42D).

Hereditary multiple exostoses. Hereditary multiple exostoses (osteochondromatosis, diaphyseal aclasis) is an autosomal dominant disorder with variable penetrance that usually presents in the first two decades of life. Multiple subcutaneous masses formed by cartilage-capped exostoses develop bilaterally. Microscopic organization of each exostosis is identical to that of the primary and secondary spongiosa of the metaphysis. In the long bones, metaphyseal modeling is altered and bone growth may be asymmetric. The lesions often lead to secondary shortening of limb bones, bowing, and limited joint movement (9). The bones of the knee are affected most commonly (Fig. 5-43), with the distal ulna and radius next. The proximal femur develops a short, broad neck and typically a valgoid configuration. Valgus deformity of the tibia at the knee and valgus deformity of the ankle due to a short fibula are also common. The limbs are involved more than the spine, and this leads to a mild skeletal disproportion (89).

Surgical osteotomies, lesional resections, and epiphysiodeses to correct leg length discrepancies may be required (90). Complications of multiple exostoses include mass effects from the lesions leading to neurovascular compromise, popliteal artery aneurysm, bursa formation, fracture, and malignant degeneration (89). Depending on the series and the

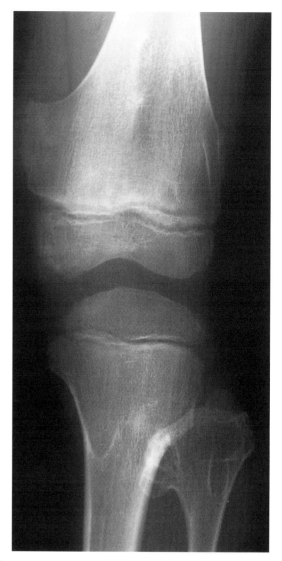

FIG. 5-43. Hereditary multiple exostoses. Knee of a 7-year-old girl shows several exostoses arising from the metaphyses of the femur, tibia, and fibula. They point away from the physes. From Laor and Jaramillo (63).

ages of patients included, the reported lifetime incidence of malignant transformation into a chondrosarcoma ranges from 5% to 27% of patients (89,91). The true incidence of malignancy is likely to be at the lower end of this range, but it is greater than with a solitary osteochondroma. Centrally located exostoses (i.e., in the pelvis, scapula, proximal humerus and femur, and spine) have a higher incidence of degeneration than do peripherally located exostoses. However, malignant transformation is very rare in childhood.

Multiple enchondromatoses. Enchondromatosis (Ollier disease) is an uncommon, nonhereditary disorder. It is characterized by multiple asymmetric intrametaphyseal cartilaginous foci that persist in a linear pattern perpendicular to the physis (Fig. 5-44). Growth at the physis leaves these lesions behind, and they often extend into the diaphysis. Calcification of the matrix is less common in the child than in the

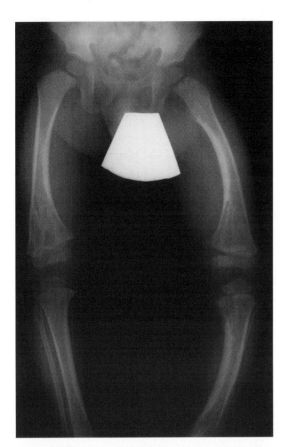

FIG. 5-44. Multiple enchondromas. Lower extremities in a 2-year-old boy show mildly expanded metaphyseal contours and longitudinally oriented irregular lucent areas. There is bilateral lower extremity bowing, greater on the left (the more affected side).

adult. The lesions are found bilaterally, although one side tends to dominate. There is shortening of the long tubular bones and widening of the metaphyses. Angular deformities and leg length discrepancies develop with time. Enchondromatosis can also affect the flat endochondral bones, especially the pelvis (89). The incidence of multiple enchondromas is less than that of a single enchondroma. Single enchondromas usually occur in the hands and feet, but the lesions of enchondromatosis are distributed throughout the enchondral skeleton.

The precise incidence of malignancy (chondrosarcoma) in multiple enchondromatoses is unknown but probably is about 30% (92). Reports of malignant degeneration range from 11% to 50% (93). However, malignant degeneration is rare until adulthood.

The combination of multiple enchondromas and soft-tissue venous malformations is known as Maffucci syndrome. Radiographs may show phleboliths in soft-tissue masses in addition to the bony deformities. The rate of malignancy is higher than with Ollier disease, and some authors consider Maffucci syndrome a premalignant condition. These patients are also at risk for malignant neoplasms of the abdomen and central nervous system (94).

Polyostotic fibrous dysplasia. Fibrous dysplasia is a developmental abnormality of mesenchyme in which osteoblasts fail to differentiate and mature. It can be monostotic or polyostotic. Twenty to thirty percent of patients with fibrous dysplasia have the polyostotic form (95). The lesions are composed of varying amounts of fibrous and osseous tissue, and, less commonly, cartilage. Some lesions may have fluid-filled components resulting from degeneration and necrosis.

Half of patients with polyostotic fibrous dysplasia have abnormal cutaneous pigmentation due to increased melanin in the epidermis. Two to three percent also have endocrine dysfunction (especially precocious puberty in girls) in addition to cutaneous pigmentation; this is termed the McCune-Albright syndrome (95). The skin changes frequently parallel the distribution of the bony changes. However, they may precede the development of bony or endocrine abnormalities. These flat lesions are often fewer, darker, and much more irregularly contoured than the café-au-lait spots of neurofibromatosis (95).

The skeletal findings of polyostotic fibrous dysplasia usually involve the facial bones, pelvis, spine, and shoulders. The findings may be unilateral or bilateral, albeit asymmetric

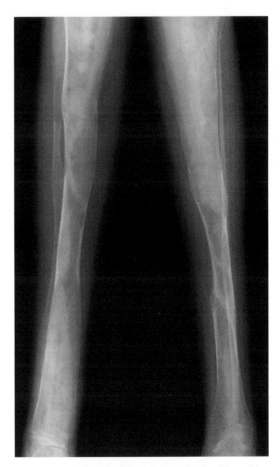

FIG. 5-45. Polyostotic fibrous dysplasia. The tibias and fibulas of this 15-year-old boy show extensive expansile deformities with undertubulation. There is irregular lucency throughout the bones with a hazy ground glass matrix. The cortices are thin and the metaphyses wide.

(95). The proximal femurs develop a coxa vara deformity, known as the shepherd's crook. When the long weight-bearing bones are involved, they are expanded in a fusiform fashion and are frequently bowed, which can result in a leg length discrepancy. The lesions are typically intramedullary and diaphyseal. They may be central or eccentric. The well-defined lucencies are hazy, or ground glass-like, and often have a sclerotic rim. Calcification and ossification may be present in the lesion. The osseous changes in the polyostotic form are more pronounced than in single bone involvement (Fig. 5-45) (95). Malignant degeneration is rare.

Patients with polyostotic fibrous dysplasia present with pain or spontaneous fracture, usually before the age of 10 years. CT and MRI help to show the extent of disease within a bone. The signal intensity on T1-weighted images usually is low. The appearance on T2-weighted images is more variable; this variability is due to the heterogeneous composition of the lesions, with even true cysts or fluid-fluid levels being present in some instances (96). The signal is variable after gadolinium enhancement.

Neurofibromatosis. Neurofibromatosis type 1 (NF-1) is a hereditary, hamartomatous disorder involving the neuroectoderm, mesoderm, and endoderm of any organ system of the body (97). It is inherited as an autosomal dominant trait with variable penetrance. Half of the cases probably represent new mutations. It occurs in approximately 1 in 3000 births (98). There is no sex or racial predominance.

There are at least two distinct forms of neurofibromatosis. Type 1 (an abnormality of chromosome 17), by far the more common, is the peripheral form. Type 2 (an abnormality of chromosome 22) is the central form, characterized by acoustic neuromas and other intracranial tumors. (For further discussion, especially of common central nervous system [CNS] abnormalities, see Chapter 2.)

TABLE 5-9. *Radiologic spectrum of neurofibromatosis*

Skull	Extremities
Macrocranium	Soft tissues
Dysplastic defects	Neurofibroma
Orbit	Bone
Lambdoidal suture	Overgrowth
Parietal	Bowing
Enlarged foramina	Overtubulation
Enlarged internal auditory canals	Sclerosis
Sellar abnormalities	Cortical defect
Brain	Hematoma
Megalencephaly	Intramedullary lesion
Neoplasms	Vascular system
Optic glioma	Renal system
Acoustic neuroma (neurofibromatosis type 2)	Stenosis
Meningioma	Coarctation
Astrocytoma	Cardiac system
Ependymoma	Congenital heart disease
Hamartoma	Pulmonary stenosis
Glioblastoma	Coarctation
Calcifications	Cerebral: occlusive disease
Spine and spinal cord	Gastrointestinal system
Kyphoscoliosis	Neurofibromas
Idiopathic type	Plexiform neurofibromatosis
Sharp angle type	Associated
Vertebral dysplasia	Carcinoid
Dural ectasia	Benign tumor
Lateral meningocele	Endocrine abnormalities
Neurofibroma	Pheochromocytoma
Syringohydromyelia	Hyperparathyroidism
Chest	Sipple syndrome
Ribs	Carcinoid of bowel
Twisted ribbon	Multiple endocrine adenomatosis
Notched	Precocious sexual development
Mediastinal mass	Miscellaneous problems and complications
Meningocele	Neurilemmoma of choroid
Neurofibroma	Airway involvement
Interstitial pulmonary fibrosis	Sarcomatous degeneration
Urinary tract	Osteopenia
Bladder neurofibroma or rhabdomyosarcoma	
Retroperitoneal tumor	
Neurofibroma	
Sarcoma	

Source: Modified from Casselman et al. (567), Holt (97), and Klatte et al. (98).

The classic clinical signs of neurofibromatosis type 1 include café-au-lait spots, multiple soft cutaneous tumors (fibroma molluscum), Lisch spots of the iris, and palpable neurofibromas of peripheral nerves (97,98). There may be dysfunction of any organ system. In neurofibromatosis, the café-au-lait spots are tan, macular, and smoothly marginated. The presence of five or more such café-au-lait spots, generally 0.5 cm or larger in diameter, is considered to indicate neurofibromatosis until proven otherwise (97). Like syphilis, neurofibromatosis has been considered a great imitator of other diseases (98).

The radiologic spectrum of neurofibromatosis-1 may involve every organ system (Table 5-9). The musculoskeletal manifestations of neurofibromatosis are protean. Most are thought to be due to a mesodermal dysplasia. In the skull, the manifestations include hypoplasia of the greater wing of the sphenoid bone and a bony defect at the lambdoid suture (usually on the left side) associated with mastoid underdevelopment. The spinal canal commonly is enlarged, usually over several thoracic or lumbar segments. The posterior aspects of the vertebral bodies are scalloped and the pedicles may be eroded, probably because of dural ectasia. The neural foramina may be enlarged, due to a meningocele, dural ectasia, or a neurofibroma. Kyphoscoliosis is seen in up to 10% of patients with neurofibromatosis. It typically involves only a short segment (fewer than six vertebrae), and is mid- to lower thoracic, angular, and rapidly progressive. However,

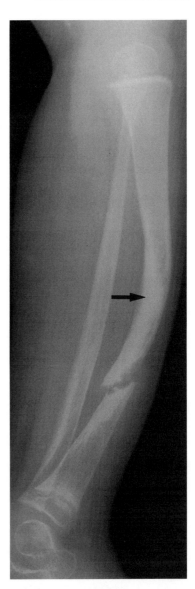

FIG. 5-47. Neurofibromatosis type 1. Anterior tibial bowing and pseudarthrosis of the distal third of the tibia of a 4-year-old boy. The medullary cavity is narrowed *(arrow)*. The distal fibula is minimally bowed.

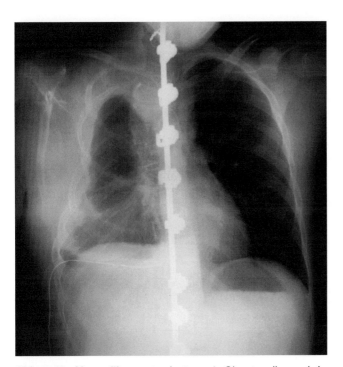

FIG. 5-46. Neurofibromatosis type 1. Chest radiograph in a 10-year-old boy shows many manifestations of neurofibromatosis. A spinal fixation rod was placed to stabilize a short-segment, upper thoracic scoliosis. There are marked dysplastic changes of the right ribs, scapula, humerus, and clavicle. A large plexiform neurofibroma involves the right axillary region and apex of the chest.

idiopathic (not short segment, not angular) is a more common form of scoliosis in neurofibromatosis.

Notching and thinning of ribs secondary to the mesodermal defect, and rib erosion by intercostal neurofibromas, may be seen (Fig. 5-46). Extremity findings may include increase in bone length, anterolateral bowing of the tibia (frequently with pseudoarthrosis) (Fig. 5-47), multiple non-ossifying fibromas, and subperiosteal hematomas (98). The bone shafts may be thinned (98).

Schwannomas (neurilemmomas), often present in neurofibromatosis-1, are well-circumscribed encapsulated lesions that lie on the surface of the nerve. They are more common than the more infiltrative neurofibromas (95). Neurofibromas tend to be fusiform, and they have a target appearance on T2-weighted MR images. This signal pattern correlates with their different geographic histologic zones; these zones are absent in schwannomas, neurofibrosarcomas, and atypical neurofibromas (99). Benign plexiform neurofibromas are seen only in neurofibromatosis. They are interdigitating, tortuous soft-tissue masses that arise along the axis of a large nerve (Fig. 5-48). They can recur following surgery and may become malignant.

Disorders of Density and Modeling.

Osteogenesis imperfecta. Osteogenesis imperfecta (OI) is a group of disorders caused by a disturbance in the formation of type I collagen, the most common form of collagen. The pathologic changes are consistent with a primary defect of the extracellular bone matrix. OI classically has been divided into a potentially lethal recessive congenital form with thick tubular bones (from the healing of repeated healed fractures) and a dominant tarda form with thin tubular bones (75). This distinction not entirely satisfactory, as there is frequently an overlap between the two forms, and multiple genetic loci causing abnormal type I collagen have been identified in both forms. A classification based on distinct genetic types had been proposed by Sillence and coworkers (100,101) (Table 5-10). All forms are characterized by osteopenia due to osteoporosis on radiographs and a propensity to fracture.

The clinical features depend on the subtype of OI. They include short-limbed dwarfism, a poorly ossified calvaria, ligamentous laxity, muscular hypotonia, blue sclerae, increased bone fragility, increased susceptibility to caries, dis-

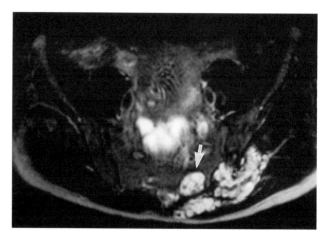

FIG. 5-48. Neurofibromatosis type 1. Axial T2-weighted MR image of the pelvis in a 16-year-old boy shows lobular high signal from a plexiform neurofibroma involving the left sacral foramen *(arrow)* and gluteal muscles.

coloration of teeth, otosclerosis, thin skin, bleeding tendency, and respiratory distress.

Periosteal and endosteal bone formation is disturbed. The lack of normal collagen causes osteoporosis, which leads to an increased tendency to fracture (Fig. 5-49). The more severe forms of osteogenesis imperfecta have thickening and shortening of the long bones because of multiple fractures

TABLE 5-10. *Classification of osteogenesis imperfecta*

Type	Inheritance	Bone fragility	Bone deformity	Teeth	Stature	Sclerae	Other comments
I	AD*	Variable	Mild or moderate	IA: Normal IB: DI***	Normal or short	Blue	Most common form, conductive hearing loss, fractures present at birth, large or normal skull, wormian bones, kyphoscoliosis, bleeding diatheses
II	AD* (new mutation) AR** (rare)	V. extreme (crumbled)	Accordion	Unknown	Lethal	Blue	Most AD as new mutations, <10% AR poor skull mineralization, wormian bones, multiple fractures
		II A Broad long bones, beaded ribs II B Broad long bones, but discontinuous/absent rib beading II C Thin long bones and ribs (rare)					
III	AD* (new mutation) AR** (rare)	Severe	Severe (bowing)	±DI***	Very short	Blue at birth, white in adolescence	Rare, many fractures at birth, triangular facies
IV	AD*	Moderate	Moderate	IV A: Normal IV B: DI***	Short	Normal/blue at birth, white in adolescence	25% fractures at birth (less than type I)

* AD, autosomal dominant, **AR, autosomal recessive, ***DI, dentinogenesis imperfecta.
Source: Modified from Sillence (100,101), Taybi (9), and Ablin (104).

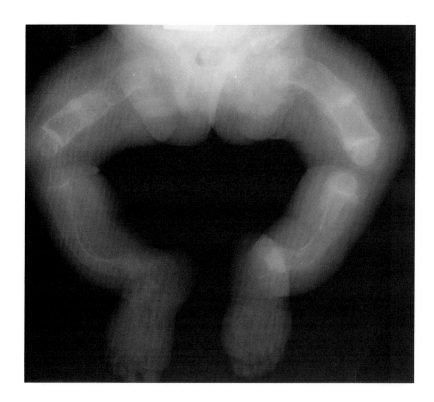

FIG. 5-49. Osteogenesis imperfecta. Lower extremities in this 18-month-old girl show severe osteoporosis. The bones are bowed and widened because of the many healing and healed fractures.

and hyperplastic callus formation. The callus is occasionally so hyperplastic as to suggest malignancy. The milder forms are characterized by thin bones with thin cortices and fewer fractures. The short tubular bones are similarly affected but less frequently fractured. There is thinning of the cortices of the carpal and tarsal bones. ''Popcorn calcifications'' of the metaphyses and epiphyses are presumably related to traumatic fragmentation of the physes. These usually resolve with skeletal maturation (102).

On chest examination, the ribs are thinned, particularly posteriorly. There may be multiple healing rib fractures, resulting in a beaded appearance. Aortic insufficiency and cystic medial necrosis can develop in patients with the less severe forms of osteogenesis imperfecta.

Radiographs of the skull reveal poor mineralization and many wormian bones, although milder forms may show normal skull development. Basilar invagination may lead to a tam-o'shanter skull, characterized by an ascending clivus and severe occipital protrusion. After many years, some cervical vertebrae may become intracranial. Radiographic findings in the spine include collapsed vertebrae with biconcave endplates and scoliosis. There may be kyphosis and scalloping of the dorsal aspects of the vertebral bodies.

The differential diagnosis for osteogenesis imperfecta varies with age. In the newborn the differential possibilities include achondrogenesis, thanatophoric dwarfism, and asphyxiating thoracic dystrophy (103), although the neonatal appearance of osteogenesis imperfecta is usually characteristic. In an infant with multiple fractures, child abuse must be excluded. During childhood and adolescence, the radio-

graphic appearance of osteogenesis imperfecta can resemble idiopathic juvenile osteoporosis and Cushing disease. In these cases, clinical correlation is needed for differentiation (103).

The history, physical exam, and radiographic findings are paramount in differentiating osteogenesis imperfecta from child abuse. Characteristics such as blue sclerae and abnormal dentition as well as radiographic findings such as poor skull mineralization and wormian bones strongly suggest OI. Metaphyseal corner fractures, skull fractures, posterior rib fractures, sternal fractures, and scapular fractures suggest child abuse (104).

Progressive diaphyseal dysplasia. Diaphyseal dysplasia (Camurati-Engelmann disease) is an autosomal dominant disease with marked variability in expression. It is characterized by abnormal intramembranous bone formation. The age of onset is variable, but patients usually are not diagnosed until after 2 years of age (75). Presenting complaints include leg pain, lower extremity weakness, failure to thrive, muscle atrophy, and an abnormal, waddling gait. The intelligence is normal.

Films show marked cortical thickening and progressive sclerosis of the diaphyses of tubular bones, due principally to periosteal and endosteal bone proliferation (Fig. 5-50). CT has shown that the endosteal changes are more prominent than the periosteal thickening (105). This condition causes a reduced size of the medullary cavity and an increased diameter of the shaft of the bone. The metaphyses and epiphyses are spared, and there is only minimal hand and foot involvement. There may be sclerosis of the base of the skull

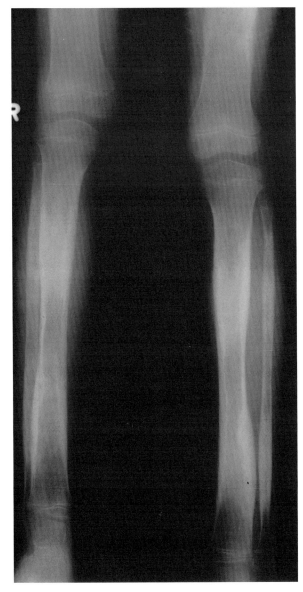

FIG. 5-50. Progressive diaphyseal dysplasia. In this 9-year-old girl there is marked cortical thickening and sclerosis of the diaphyses of the lower extremities. The metaphyses and epiphyses are normal.

and hyperostosis of the calvaria. Complications occur from increased intracranial pressure and cranial nerve encroachment (78). Spinal sclerosis is usually minimal.

Skeletal Disorders Due to Chromosomal Abnormalities

Trisomy 21 (Down Syndrome)

Chromosomal abnormalities may involve either the sex chromosomes or the autosomes. Chromosomal abnormalities of the autosomes include trisomies (three chromosomes of the same pair), deletions (lack of all or part of a chromosome), and translocations (transfer of a part of one chromosome to another). The most common live-born chromosomal abnormality is trisomy 21, also known as Down syndrome. Table 5-11 lists the abnormalities in Down syndrome and also those of two much rarer trisomies, trisomy 13 and trisomy 18.

The child with trisomy 21 usually has brachycephalic microcephaly. This is not present at birth but is evident by age 3 months. Hypoplasia of the paranasal sinuses, nasal bones, maxillae, and sphenoid is frequently present. The sutures may be wide, closure may be delayed, and the metopic suture persists beyond 10 years in 40% to 70% of affected patients. There may be hypotelorism and sagittal shortening of the hard palate.

There is an increased height and a decreased anteroposterior (AP) diameter of the vertebral bodies, especially in children less than 2 years of age. Atlantoaxial dislocation, perhaps due to ligamentous laxity, is eventually present in up to 25% of trisomy 21 patients, but it is seldom symptomatic. There may also be hypoplasia of the posterior arch of C1 or of the odontoid. Eleven pairs of ribs are seen in 15% to 40% of children with Down syndrome. Double manubrial

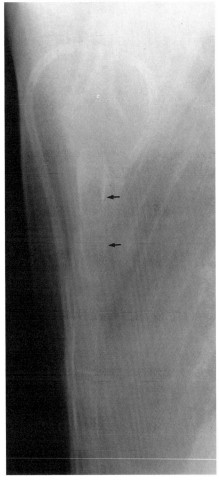

FIG. 5-51. Down syndrome. Lateral view of the sternum shows a double manubrial ossification center *(arrows)*.

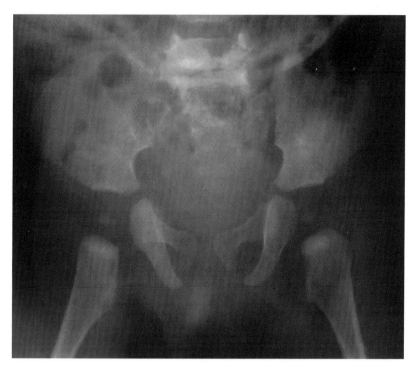

FIG. 5-52. Down syndrome. Pelvis in this infant with trisomy 21 shows flared iliac wings and decreased acetabular angles.

ossification centers are present in 90% of Down syndrome children under 4 years of age (Fig. 5-51) but also in 10% of normals (106); therefore, if the finding turns up unexpectedly, the child usually does not have Down syndrome.

Characteristic radiographic features of trisomy 21 involve the pelvis and are most pronounced in patients under 1 year of age. There are widened and flared iliac wings, which produce a Mickey Mouse ears appearance. The acetabular angles are decreased and the acetabular roofs are flattened (Fig. 5-52). The ischia are tapered and elongated. Coxa valga frequently is present. The proximal femoral ossification centers often appear late. Forty percent of infants with trisomy 21 have developmental hip dysplasia (78), despite the flattening of the acetabular roofs.

The hands are short and the digits stubby. Clinodactyly is seen in approximately 50% of trisomy 21 children but in only 1% of normal children. There may be increased space between the first and second toes. Double ossification centers for the body of the calcaneus may be present. Although skeletal maturation is usually retarded, it may be normal or even advanced.

Approximately 40% of Down syndrome children have clinically recognized congenital heart disease, and slightly over 50% have autopsy evidence of congenital heart disease. The most common lesions at autopsy are ventricular septal defect, atrial septal defect, patent ductus arteriosus, and endocardial cushion defect. The most common clinically detected types of congenital heart disease are endocardial cushion defect and ventricular septal defect. An aberrant right subclavian artery is present in approximatley 20% of those with Down syndrome but in only 1% of normals (107).

Infants with trisomy 21 may have duodenal atresia, duo-

denal stenosis, annular pancreas, Hirschsprung disease, anorectal malformation, and umbilical hernia. Few genitourinary anomalies have been reported with trisomy 21 (Table 5-11). Leukemia is 3–20 times as common with trisomy 21 as in the normal population.

Triploidy

In triploidy there are 69 chromosomes, not 46. Live births of this lethal disorder are increasingly reported. Characteristic radiographic manifestations include harlequin orbits (steep greater sphenoid wings), small anterior fontanel, narrow iliac bones with steep iliac angles, gracile ribs and long bones, and lateral clavicle hooks (9,108).

Skeletal Disorders Due to Primary Metabolic Abnormalities

Mucopolysaccharidoses and Mucolipidoses

Mucopolysaccharidoses (MPSs) and mucolipidoses (MLs, more recently termed glycoproteinoses or oligosaccharidoses) are hereditary disorders caused by deficiencies of specific lysosomal enzymes (109). The skeletal findings in most types of mucopolysaccharidoses, mucolipidoses, and other heteroglycanoses are somewhat similar and have been termed dysostosis multiplex (75) (Table 5-12). Because the radiographic findings can be similar, a specific diagnosis must often be based on clinical and biochemical features, such as age, intelligence, and the presence or absence of

TABLE 5-11. *Radiologic features of trisomies*

Area	Trisomy 13	Trisomy 18	Trisomy 21 (Down syndrome)
Skull	Holoprosencephaly Wide sutures and fontanels Cleft palate Micrognathia	Microcrania Wormian bones Cleft palate Small maxilla	Microcrania Brachycephaly Small maxilla and nasal bones Short palate
Spine	Increased cervical interpediculate distance Errors of segmentation	Usually normal Fusions, hemivertebrae	Increased vertebral body height Atlantoaxial dislocation
Chest	Poorly formed ribs Asymmetry Diaphragmatic hernias	Increased AP diameter Hypoplastic sternum Thin ribs and clavicles Eventration	11 pairs of ribs Double manubrial ossification Sternal abnormalities
Heart	VSD, PDA, ASD, PS Transposition, truncus Dextroversion	VSD, PDA PS, bicuspid aortic valve	ECD, VSD PDA, aberrant subclavian artery
Pelvis	Normal	Increased iliac angles Normal acetabular angles Hip dislocation	Decreased iliac angles Decreased acetabular angles Developmental hip dysplasia Coxa valga
Extremities	Polydactyly and syndactyly Narrow terminal phalanges Increased soft tissues Flexion contractures Delayed skeletal maturation	Flexion deformities of hands and feet Rocker-bottom foot Poor ossification of phalanges Hypoplastic thumbs Delayed skeletal maturation	Clinodactyly Delayed skeletal maturation
Miscellaneous	Malrotation Meckel diverticulum Hernias Situs inversus	GI: Meckel diverticulum, hernia, malrotation, TEF GU: horseshoe kidney, hydronephrosis, polycystic kidneys	Duodenal obstruction Hirschsprung disease TEF Anorectal malformation Hypothyroidism Dental caries

ASD, atrial septal defect; ECD, endocardial cushion defect; GI, gastrointestinal; GU, genitourinary; PDA, patent ductus arteriosus; PS, pulmonary stenosis; TEF, tracheoesophageal fistula; VSD, ventricular septal defect.

TABLE 5-12. *Dysostosis multiplex and other storage disorders*

Mucopolysaccharidoses:
I-H:	Hurler syndrome
I-S:	Scheie syndrome
I-H/S:	Hurler-Scheie syndrome
II:	Hunter syndrome
III:	Sanfilippo syndrome
IV:	Morquio syndrome
V:	None designated (formerly Scheie)
VI:	Maroteaux-Lamy syndrome

Mucolipidoses:
I:	Juvenile form of sialidosis
II:	I-Cell disease
III:	Pseudo-Hurler polydystrophy
Other:	Gangliosidosis
	Fucosidosis
	Mannosidosis
	Sialidosis
	Gaucher disease
	Niemann-Pick disease

increased urinary excretion of acid mucopolysaccharides and other substances.

Radiographic features found in these disorders include osteoporosis, prominent trabeculae, macrocephaly, thick calvaria, wide clavicles and ribs (but narrow near the costovertebral junction, canoe paddle appearance), anteriorly (mid- or inferior) beaked oval vertebral bodies, constricted iliac bones, dysplasia of the femoral heads (Fig. 5-53A), coxa valga, irregular diaphyseal modeling, an acute angle between the axes of the distal radius and ulna, submetaphyseal overconstriction, shortening of short tubular bones, and proximal tapering of the second to fifth metacarpal bones (Fig. 5-53C). In Hurler syndrome, these findings are particularly marked. The skeletal changes of mucolipidosis may be present at birth, whereas they are visible only later in mucopolysaccharidosis (84). ML-II (I-cell disease) in utero and infancy may resemble the pattern of hyperparathyroidism.

There are some relatively distinctive clinical and radiographic features of MPS-IV (Morquio disease). Children with MPS-IV excrete keratan sulfate in their urine, whereas children with the other forms of MPS excrete dermatan and/or heparan sulfate. The radiographic findings in MPS-IV

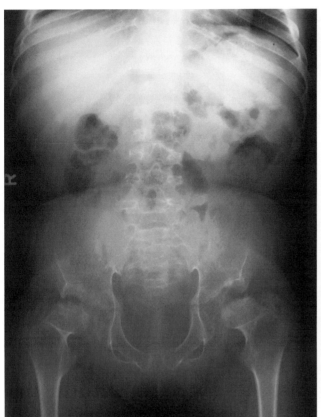

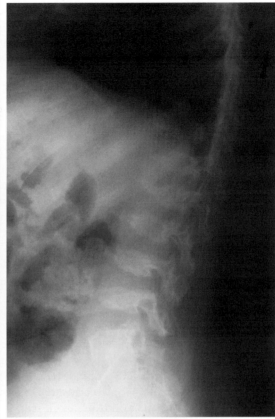

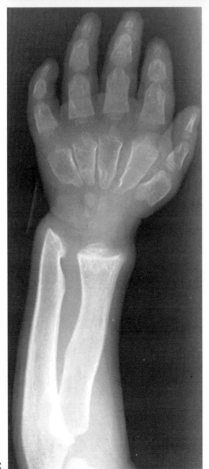

FIG. 5-53. Mucopolysaccharidoses. A: Pelvis of this 11-year-old girl with Morquio disease (MPS IV) shows underdevelopment of the superior acetabular region and constricted iliac bones. Both proximal femurs are irregularly ossified. The vertebral bodies are flattened and the ribs are relatively widened. **B:** Lateral view of the spine in another child with Morquio disease shows generalized platyspondyly and beaking of the anterior part of the vertebral bodies. **C:** The film of this child with Maroteaux-Lamy disease (MPS VI) shows osteoporosis, submetaphyseal overconstriction, shortening of short tubular bones, and proximal tapering of the second to fifth metacarpals, with the distal ulna inclined toward the radius.

include irregular epiphyses resembling those of spondylo-epiphyseal dysplasia, midanterior vertebral body beaking (Fig. 5-53B), generalized platyspondyly that results in short stature, odontoid hypoplasia, and anterior protrusion of the sternum (3).

Miscellaneous Constitutional Diseases of Bone

Arthrogryposis

Arthrogryposis is a term that describes a heterogeneous group of conditions that result in multiple joint contractures at birth. The common factor is restriction of movement in utero. This limitation of motion may be neurogenic or myogenic or may result from extrinsic restriction, such as occurs in oligohydramnios.

The findings often involve the distal segments of the limb. There may be muscular atrophy, flexion or extension contractures, and joint ankylosis (4). The lesions are usually bilateral but are not necessarily symmetric. They are present at birth and may progress with age.

The lower extremities are invariably involved, and over half of patients have upper extremity involvement. The limbs typically lack subcutaneous fat and skin creases (Fig. 5-54), and there may be joint swelling (4). Associated skeletal abnormalities include equinovarus deformities of the feet, tarsal and carpal fusions, clubhand, and hip dislocation (110). Fractures and scoliosis may develop; a limb fracture may occur during delivery.

Amniotic Band Syndrome

Amniotic band syndrome (Streeter dysplasia, congenital constriction band syndrome) is a sporadic disorder that presents with a wide spectrum of clinical abnormalities. The findings include asymmetric constriction bands of soft tissues, intrauterine amputations, syndactyly, acrosyndactyly (distal fusion of digits), and craniofacial and visceral defects (111).

Streeter initially described 16 fetuses with constriction bands and suggested focal defects in germ plasm development (111,112). Of the presently proposed etiologies, the most widely accepted is mechanical constriction of appendages that become entangled in bands that form following a tear in the amniotic membrane. The earlier in utero the membrane is torn, the more severe the deformities, such as craniofacial and abdominal wall defects. Later in the gestation, the effects may be limited to limb abnormalities. The cause of the bands is not known, but there is often prematurity and low birth weight (113).

Radiographs show the soft-tissue constrictions and amputations, resultant lymphedema, and variable bony deformities. Several limbs are usually affected (Fig. 5-55), the upper limbs more commonly. Acrosyndactyly probably is related to the tying together of digits distally by amniotic bands (111). Clubfoot and leg length discrepancies also are com-

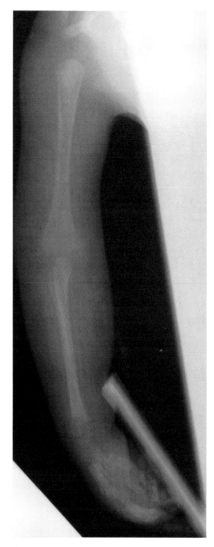

FIG. 5-54. Arthrogryposis. Upper extremity of this newborn shows absence of the normal skin creases. There are flexion deformities at the wrist and fingers. The muscles are atrophic.

mon findings. Therapy for amniotic bands is aimed at optimizing early function and cosmesis (113). Often this includes relief of the resultant lymphedema by staged excision of the constrictions.

Infection

Acute Osteomyelitis

Acute osteomyelitis continues to be a significant cause of childhood morbidity despite earlier diagnosis and appropriate antibiotic therapy. Osteomyelitis occurs in 1 in 5000 children (114). One third of these patients are under 2 years of age, and more than half are under 5 years of age (115). Most pediatric infections are hematogenous and arise from transient, asymptomatic bacteremia or from acute sepsis with bacterial, viral, or other infectious agents. Thirty percent of

The development of antibiotics was followed by a dramatic decrease in the overall incidence of osteomyelitis. Recently, however, the disease has become more common. There has been a particular increase in the frequency of the subacute variety of hematogenous osteomyelitis (which accounts for 10% to 15% of all new cases) (117) and of chronic multifocal osteomyelitis (118). The changing patterns of osteomyelitis are presumably due to the too frequent use of short-term antibiotics, the changing virulence of organisms, and the increasing survival of patients on immunosuppressive drug therapy.

Pathophysiology

Acute hematogenous osteomyelitis originates in the metaphyses or metaphyseal equivalents of bones. Circulating organisms tend to lodge and proliferate in the metaphysis because of local slowing of blood flow in the looping arterial vessels and sinusoidal venous structures (Fig. 5-56A). Absence of phagocytic cells lining these venous sinusoids probably also plays a role. Infecting organisms often seed recently injured bones (119); a history of recent local trauma can be obtained in one third of cases (120). The relatively avascular physeal cartilage serves as a barrier to the extension of infection into the epiphysis. In children younger than 18 months of age, however, transphyseal vessels still exist; this allows spread of the infection to the physis, the epiphysis, and the adjacent joint (Fig. 5-56A) (121). The metaphyseal infection causes an acute exudative reaction that can be likened to a boil. As this inflammatory reaction continues, there is localized increased intraosseous pressure that leads to further stasis of blood and eventual thrombosis of adjacent arterial and venous structures and necrosis of bone.

In summary, the pathogenesis of hematogenous osteomyelitis includes bacteremia, metaphyseal lodging of organisms, inflammatory response, exudate, increased intraosseous pressure, stasis of blood flow, thrombosis, bone necrosis, and, somewhat later, bone resorption (48,117, 121–124).

Because the bony trabeculae do not accommodate swelling of the marrow, the increased intraosseous pressure also forces organisms, reactive cells, and their lytic enzymes through the interstices of endosteal bone (48). This action permits extension of infection in various directions. Transverse extension occurs through the cortex, with elevation of the periosteum and invasion of adjacent soft tissues (Fig. 5-56B) (125). Infection also spreads readily to the medullary cavity and diaphysis (Fig. 5-56B). In the proximal femur and proximal radius, the joint capsule attaches along the neck of the bone, and most of the metaphysis is intracapsular. In these areas, infections readily extend from the metaphysis to the articular space (Fig. 5-56B). Septic arthritis can occur also from direct extension from an epiphyseal focus; this pattern is most common in the knee.

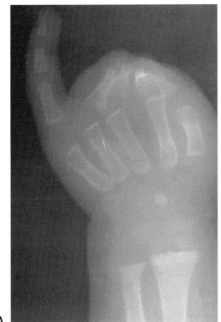

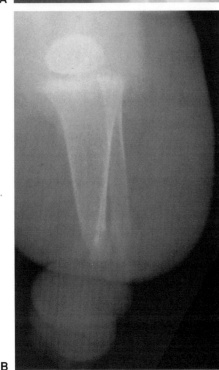

FIG. 5-55. Amniotic band syndrome. A: The hand of this infant shows amputation of the first through fourth digits. The residual phalanges are severely deformed. **B:** The lower extremity of the same infant shows soft-tissue constriction bands and distal amputations of the tibia and fibula.

patients have a history of upper respiratory infection, otitis media, or some other infection from which the hematogenous spread arises (116). Infection of bone also may follow a direct penetrating wound or may spread to bone by extension from adjacent structures such as skin, paranasal sinuses, or pleura, but these are all uncommon.

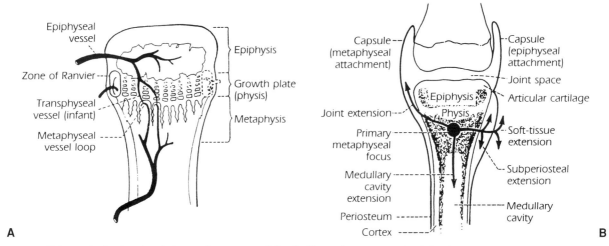

FIG. 5-56. Pathophysiology of osteomyelitis. A: Normal anatomy of epiphysis-metaphysis in infants less than 18 months of age. Modified from Ogden and Lister (121). **B:** Potential extension of osteomyelitis. Modified from Nixon (48).

Etiology

Staphylococcus aureus, the most frequent cause of acute hematogenous osteomyelitis, is responsible for up to 71% (126) of pediatric cases. In neonates, group B *β-hemolytic Streptococcus* accounts for one third of the cases (127). *Salmonella,* other gram-negative bacteria, mycobacteria, virulent bacillus Calmette-Guérin, syphilis, fungi, and viral agents are less frequent causes of osteomyelitis. *Pseudomonas* sometimes causes infections secondary to penetrating foot wounds.

Sites of Involvement

Three fourths of cases of acute hematogenous osteomyelitis involve the tubular bones (117). The most rapidly growing and largest metaphyses are usually affected. The sites of involvement in order of decreasing frequency are the distal femur, proximal femur, proximal tibia, distal tibia, proximal humerus, distal humerus, fibula, and other tubular bones (117). Flat and irregular bones and juxtaapophyseal metaphyses are involved in about one fourth of cases of acute hematogenous osteomyelitis. The sites of involvement in these bones, in order of decreasing frequency, are the ilium, vertebra, calcaneus, femur adjacent to the trochanter, ischium, tibia adjacent to the tubercle, scapula, talus, pubis, patella, tarsal navicular, and sternum (117). In these bones, areas adjacent to bone-forming cartilage are metaphyseal-equivalent locations until growth ceases (48,117). The vascular anatomy of these areas predisposes them to acute hematogenous osteomyelitis. For example, in children, most cases of pelvic osteomyelitis occur in the vicinity of the triradiate cartilage.

Clinical Features

The frequency of osteomyelitis increases during infancy and then stabilizes for the remainder of childhood. The gender ratio is equal during infancy, but older boys are affected twice as frequently as older girls (117).

Infections are difficult to diagnose and localize in the first years of life (128). Osteomyelitis is usually silent in newborns and infants and is often detected only 2–4 weeks after the infection has begun (127). The usual findings are regional edema, tenderness, and pseudoparalysis of the affected extremity. Young children may only develop limping or the refusal to bear weight. Older children have more localized symptoms and signs including tenderness localized to the metaphysis of the affected bone, pain aggravated by motion, limitation of use of the affected extremity, localized swelling, muscle spasm, and joint flexion for comfort. Systemic signs and symptoms include fever, chills, vomiting, malaise, and dehydration.

The erythrocyte sedimentation rate is elevated in 90% of cases, but only 30% of children have leukocytosis (126). Blood cultures are positive in only 40% of children, so cultures from aspirations of the affected bone are very important (115). Aspirated pus is culture-positive in up to 70% of cases (116). Even with operative drainage, 20% of cases do not yield a positive culture, often because of previous antibiotic therapy (117).

Radiography

The main reason to obtain radiographs in the first week after the onset of the disease is to exclude pathology such as tumor or fracture that may resemble osteomyelitis. Radiographs are insensitive to destruction of less than about 30%

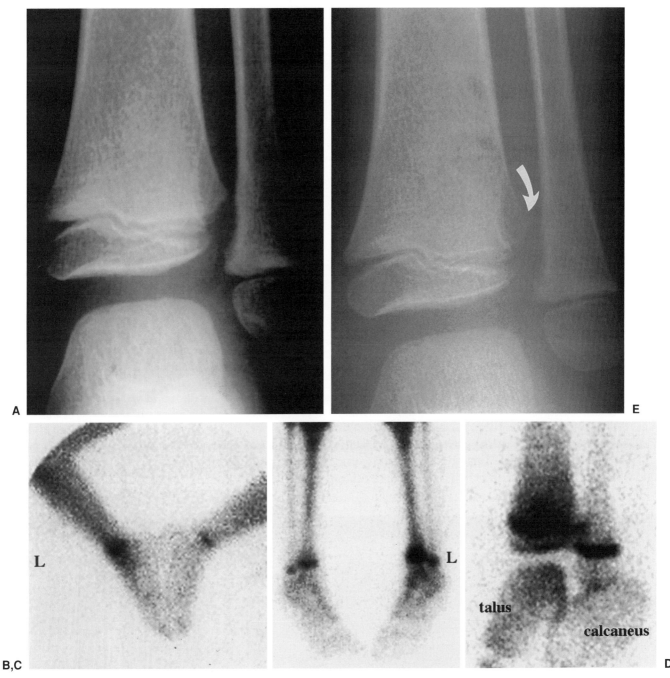

FIG. 5-57. Ankle osteomyelitis. A: The initial radiograph is normal. **B–D:** Bone scintigraphy shows increased tracer localization that is most pronounced in the distal left tibial metaphysis in the tissue phase image **(B)** and skeletal phase image **(C)**. An extended pattern of uptake of the tibial diaphysis and talus is also noted. A pinhole magnification skeletal scintigram **(D)** confirms that the predominant abnormality is in the distal tibial metaphysis. **E:** Radiograph obtained seven days later shows early destruction of the lateral part of the tibial metaphysis *(arrow)*.

of the bone mass (126), and therefore bone destruction is not recognizable until 7–10 days after the beginning of symptoms (Fig. 5-57A). The soft-tissue abnormalities, however, are detectable much earlier. Radiographs can show deep soft-tissue swelling and loss or displacement of adjacent muscle planes as early as 48 hours after the beginning of symptoms (125). These local areas of swelling are adja-

cent to the metaphysis and usually do not extend to the joint region. By the third or fourth day of an acute osteomyelitis, the radiographs show soft-tissue swelling extending a considerable distance away from the metaphysis, blurring of the interface between muscle and subcutaneous fat, and thickening and increased visualization of subcutaneous vessels and lymphatics (125).

Absence of these findings cannot exclude osteomyelitis in a child with fewer than 10 days of symptoms. Prompt therapy may even prevent the development of radiographic bone changes (125). Skeletal scintigraphy, cross-sectional imaging, and the judicious use of needle biopsy are more sensitive at this phase of the disease (Fig. 5-57B–D).

Destructive bone changes of acute osteomyelitis are visible first as focal and later as confluent radiolucencies in bone (Fig. 5-57E). This destructive process proceeds more rapidly in the neonate because of the rapid spread of infection through the spongiosa and cortex. The localized metaphyseal rarefaction soon progresses to irregular bony destruction. There is frequently extension into the metaphyseal cortex and subperiosteal region. Early periosteal new bone formation is identified after about 10 days have elapsed. Because of early diagnosis and treatment, extensive bone destruction and the formation of involucra and sequestra are seldom seen.

Skeletal Scintigraphy

Three-phase skeletal scintigraphy with technetium-99m (^{99m}Tc)–labeled phosphate compounds (e.g., methylene diphosphonate) has a major role in the diagnosis of acute hematogenous osteomyelitis (Fig. 5-57), particularly during the first week of the process (129). The three phases include radionuclide angiography (RNA), static imaging immediately following RNA to depict tracer in the extravascular compartment (tissue phase imaging), and static imaging 2 or more hours after tracer administration to depict skeletal radionuclide localization (skeletal phase imaging). High- or ultrahigh-resolution collimation should be used routinely, and pinhole magnification is frequently required. Because osteomyelitis may be multifocal, particularly in neonates (127) but also in older children (115), and because pathologic conditions such as Ewing sarcoma, leukemia (130), and metastatic neuroblastoma (131) clinically mimic osteomyelitis, skeletal phase images of the entire skeleton must be obtained.

Skeletal scintigraphy of osteomyelitis typically shows a well-defined focus of increased tracer localization on the angiographic, tissue phase, and skeletal phase images (132,133). Occasionally, the focal increase is superimposed on a more diffuse increase due to hyperemia. Skeletal scintigraphy may be positive as early as 24 hours after the onset of symptoms, before any radiographic changes of deep soft-tissue edema or bone destruction are evident (123,133,134). Cellulitis and septic arthritis may produce a diffuse increase in tracer localization, primarily affecting the soft tissues but also bone, on all three phases (133). A focal abnormality on skeletal phase images indicates a bony abnormality. Nonfocal, periarticular increased activity may be present in arthropathy. A focus of decreased or absent tracer localization is occasionally noted with osteomyelitis, particularly in its early stages. This finding, which reflects localized ischemia, is often seen with subperiosteal collections (135). When a region of decreased tracer localization is next to an area of

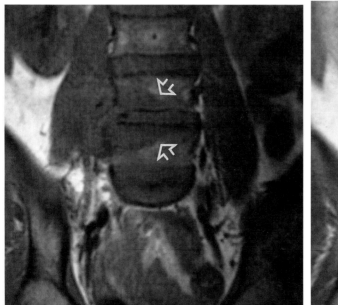
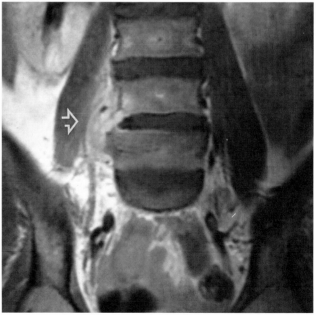

A **B**

FIG. 5-58. Spinal osteomyelitis. A 13-year-old boy with history of pain in the right lower pelvis and lower lumbar region and fever of 40°C of 5 days duration. **A:** Coronal T1-weighted MR image of the lumbar spine shows decreased signal intensity of the paraspinal fat, disc, and vertebral marrow *(arrows)*. **B:** Coronal T1-weighted MR image following the intravenous administration of gadolinium shows enhancement of the involved vertebral bodies and adjacent paraspinal region *(arrow)*. There is no abscess.

increased uptake, devitalized bone is suggested and the need for urgent surgical drainage is implied (132).

The pathogenesis of acute hematogenous osteomyelitis explains the spectrum of scintigraphic findings. Osteomyelitis is a dynamic process. In the early avascular or thrombotic phase, one may see decreased uptake suggesting local bone ischemia (136), or even a normal scintigram (137). The latter may represent a balance between impaired but not absent tracer delivery and relatively increased osteoblastic activity. Later as the process continues, locally increased blood flow and increased osteoblastic activity result in focally increased uptake, providing that vascular compromise does not persist. In addition to the patterns of focally increased or decreased uptake, one may also see increased uptake in the adjacent or more distal long bones, particularly in the high-flow metaphyseal regions (extended uptake) (136). This extended pattern is due to reflex hyperemia in the affected limb (Fig. 5-57) (136). It is commonly seen with osteomyelitis in the feet.

In rare cases where skeletal scintigraphy is interpreted as normal but the clinical suspicion of osteomyelitis persists, further imaging with gallium-67 (^{67}Ga) citrate or leukocytes labeled with either indium-111 (^{111}In) or ^{99m}Tc may be considered. When sufficient symptom localization is present, such cases are more often evaluated with MRI.

MRI

MRI demonstrates increased fluid due to the infectious process and the surrounding reactive edema. It detects abnormalities of the bone marrow and soft tissues within a day or two of the beginning of symptoms. Osteomyelitis is typically seen as a well-defined focal lesion in the metaphysis or metaphyseal equivalent with a large halo of edema extending into the marrow and soft tissues (Figs. 5-58 to 5-60). The lesion and halo are of low signal intensity on T1-weighted

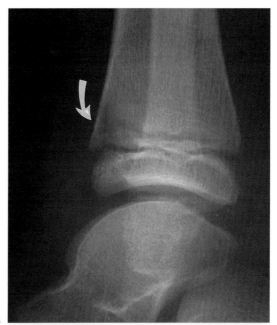

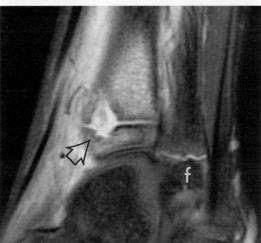

FIG. 5-60. Ankle osteomyelitis with physeal involvement. An 11-year-old boy with a history of pain in the ankle and fever for 2 days. **A:** Lateral radiograph of the distal tibia shows an ill-defined metaphyseal lucency adjacent to the distal tibial physis *(arrow)*. **B:** Sagittal fat-suppressed T1-weighted MR image following the intravenous administration of gadolinium shows a lesion crossing the tibial physis *(arrow)*. The center of the lesion is hypointense, indicating central necrosis. The abscess was drained, and the patient did not develop growth arrest. *f,* Secondary fibular ossification center.

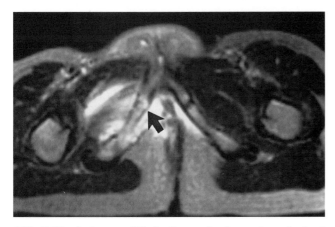

FIG. 5-59. Osteomyelitis in the metaphyseal equivalent adjacent to the ischiopubic synchondrosis. A 5-year-old girl with pain and fever. Axial T2-weighted MR image shows increased signal intensity in the bone adjacent to the synchondrosis *(arrow)* and in the adjacent fat and musculature.

images and high signal intensity on T2-weighted images. Gadolinium administration detects nonenhancing areas of necrosis. MRI is especially valuable in cases of osteomyelitis of the spine (Fig. 5-58) and pelvis (Fig. 5-59), where extension into the epidural space or pelvic soft tissues may be the main cause of morbidity (138). MRI also is useful in infections extending into the physis, where it can help to focus surgical treatment and decrease the risk of growth arrest (Fig. 5-60).

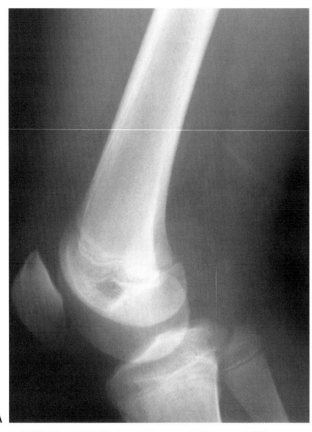

A

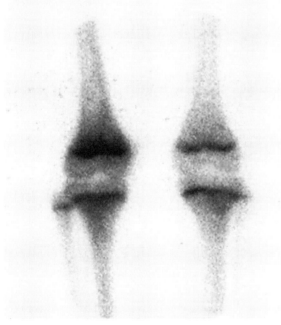

B

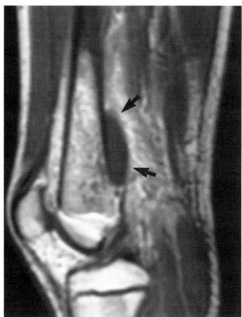

C

FIG. 5-61. Osteomyelitis of the distal femur not responding to antibiotics. A 13-year-old with osteomyelitis of the distal femur and persistence of fever after two days of intravenous antibiotics. **A:** Lateral radiograph of the distal femur shows no abnormality. **B:** Skeletal scintigraphy shows increased uptake in the right distal femoral metaphysis. **C:** Sagittal T1-weighted MR image obtained after the intravenous administration of gadolinium shows a nonenhancing subperiosteal abnormality compatible with an abscess *(arrows)*. This collection was drained percutaneously; the patient improved after the procedure and continued antibiotic therapy.

Ultrasonography and CT

Ultrasonography permits recognition of periosteal elevation due to osteomyelitis quite early. Superiosteal fluid is seen as a hypoechoic region next to bone, and the elevated periosteum is a more echogenic interface with adjoining soft tissues. Increased echogenicity in the deep soft tissues corresponds to edema (139). The main limitation of this modality is its inability to image intraosseous disease. There are also false negatives when purulent collections are similar in echogenicity to adjacent soft tissues. Although often helpful, ultrasonography should not be used in place of MRI or skeletal scintigraphy (140).

CT has a very limited role in the evaluation of acute hematogenous osteomyelitis if skeletal scintigraphy and MRI are available.

Suggested Use of Imaging to Guide Therapy

MRI is slightly more sensitive and specific (138,141) than scintigraphy, but both techniques are useful for the detection of infection. In cases where symptoms are poorly localized, skeletal scintigraphy will identify the site of infection. When the site of the abnormality is already clear, MRI characterizes the extent of the lesion to better advantage. The choice between the two modalities is partly governed by cost and availability.

Radiographs should be obtained at presentation to guide further imaging or therapy and to exclude other pathology such as fracture or tumor. Skeletal scintigraphy should be performed to image the entire skeleton and exclude multifocal osteomyelitis. MRI should be used initially in all patients suspected of having spinal osteomyelitis and in patients with pelvic and physeal infections in whom the clinical presentation is atypical or surgery is considered. In patients who fail to respond to 48 hours of antibiotic therapy, MRI can exclude complications such as subperiosteal, medullary, or soft-tissue abscesses (Fig. 5-61) (138). MRI should be performed with gadolinium enhancement because this is the only way to detect drainable collections (142).

Special Forms of Acute Osteomyelitis

Neonatal Osteomyelitis. Transphyseal vessels, present until 18 months of age (see Fig. 5-56A), allow passage of bacteria across the physis into the epiphysis in neonates and young infants. There also may be direct infectious destruction of the physis (Fig. 5-62) (121). Neonatal osteomyelitis involves more than one bone in 22% of cases (127) and one or more joints. Decreased or increased longitudinal growth often leads to a skeletal deformity (121). Osteomyelitis and septic arthritis frequently coexist (Figs. 5-62, 5-63). Streptococcal skeletal infection in the neonate may produce relatively mild clinical signs despite advanced osseous destruction of one or several bones (117). If radiographs are normal, skeletal scintigraphy may detect a focus of infection. While

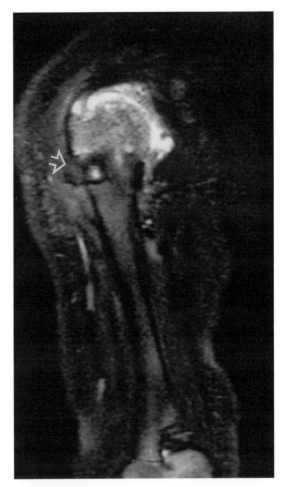

FIG. 5-62. Osteomyelitis of the proximal humerus with physeal involvement and septic arthritis. A 2-month-old infant with fever. Coronal fast spin-echo T2-weighted MR image of the proximal humerus shows extensive irregularity in the region of the physis *(arrow)*. No normal growth plate can be seen; it apparently has been destroyed. There is an adjacent effusion.

these foci usually cause increased uptake, osteomyelitic areas of decreased uptake suggesting ischemia are more common in the neonate than in the older child.

The sensitivity of skeletal scintigraphy to neonatal osteomyelitis has been the subject of controversy. Early studies reported a lower sensitivity to osteomyelitis in neonates than older ages (143,144). Although others have achieved excellent results with more modern instrumentation (145), a study that seems to be normal should be viewed with particular caution in a neonate. The sensitivity of MRI for diagnosing neonatal osteomyelitis has not been established. MRI can demonstrate extension into unossified epiphyses (146), which is particularly common in newborns.

Osteomyelitis in the Infant. The systemic response to bone infection is diminished or frequently absent in infants. There may be nothing more than localized swelling, tenderness, and failure to move a limb, and this may delay diagnosis and appropriate therapy. Osteomyelitis in the infant often

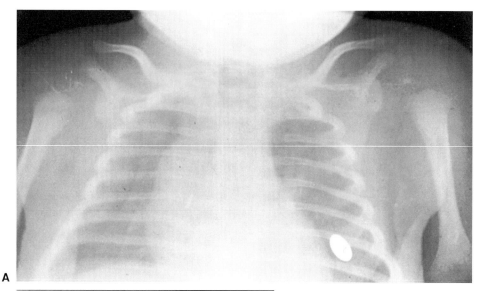

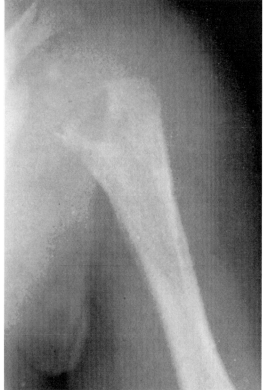

FIG. 5-63. Streptococcal osteomyelitis and septic arthritis. A 3-week-old boy with failure to move the left upper extremity. **A:** There is increased distance between the humerus and the glenoid of the scapula on the left. Aspiration confirmed pus within the joint. **B:** Film 2 weeks later shows destruction of the proximal metaphysis despite appropriate antibiotic therapy.

leads to extensive bony involvement rather than the narrow metaphyseal localization seen in the older child. Infection is allowed to spread from its metaphyseal focus by the loose attachment of the periosteum, the thin metaphyseal cortex (though the periphery of the most recently formed 2 mm of the metaphysis is relatively strong), the decreased number of trabeculae in the medullary cavity, and the transphyseal arteries. These anatomic features also lead to much more frequent joint and epiphyseal involvement.

Osteomyelitis in Flat and Irregular Bones. As was previously discussed, approximately 25% of cases of acute hema-togenous osteomyelitis involve the metaphyseal-equivalent regions. Patients with involvement of the bony pelvis are challenging diagnostic problems, as their symptoms and signs may mimic acute appendicitis, urinary tract infection, pelvic abscess, and vertebral disease (48). Radiographs may remain normal or equivocal for longer than 10 days; skeletal scintigraphy or MRI is critical for early, accurate diagnosis.

Vertebral Osteomyelitis. Acute osteomyelitis may involve the vertebral body or the intervertebral disc (see Fig. 5-58). Vertebral osteomyelitis and discitis are discussed in Chapter 4.

Antibiotic-Modified Osteomyelitis. Prediagnosis antibiotic therapy may modify or suppress the clinical and radiologic features of osteomyelitis. This explains why some children are ill for long periods before it is realized that they have subacute or chronic osteomyelitis.

Subacute and Chronic Osteomyelitis. The radiologic appearance of subacute osteomyelitis differs considerably from that of acute osteomyelitis. There are two forms. Brodie abscess, a localized small area of bone destruction surrounded by extensive reactive bone formation, is the more common form of subacute osteomyelitis. There is a well-defined, usually oval, longitudinally oriented cavity within the metaphysis that may extend through the physis into the epiphysis. A rim of surrounding sclerosis with a fading halo of abnormality is present, but there is little or no periosteal reaction.

Subacute osteomyelitis may also cause irregular resorption of the cortex and spongiosa of the metaphysis with extension into the diaphysis or epiphysis. Periosteal reaction is frequently present in this form. The reaction may be thicker but less laminated than that of acute osteomyelitis. There may be associated bony sclerosis, but a soft-tissue mass is not identified and local soft-tissue swelling is minimal. Irregularly destructive chronic osteomyelitis may be difficult to distinguish on radiographs from Ewing sarcoma.

Spread of the infectious process to the cortex of the bone can result in a sequestration of a fragment of avascular bone within the pus. This fragment, a sequestrum, is eventually surrounded by a thick rim of periosteal new bone, the involucrum. Further spread of the infection may lead to the formation of a draining sinus known as a cloaca (Latin for sewer) (Fig. 5-64).

The chronic forms of osteomyelitis described above may be present for months or years (122). Dense chronic osteomyelitis is also known as Garré sclerosing osteomyelitis. Another type of chronic osteomyelitis, chronic multifocal osteomyelitis (see below), is characterized by multiple lucent sites that eventually heal and do not harbor culturable organisms. The features of subacute and chronic osteomyelitis are usually well demonstrated by MRI. Because the main abnormalities (Brodie abscess, sequestrum, involucrum, and draining sinus) are primarily bony, they also can be clearly depicted by CT.

Epiphyseal Osteomyelitis. Infection of the epiphysis usually spreads from a focus of metaphyseal osteomyelitis. In infants, this occurs through transphyseal vessels, whereas in older children, the infection spreads to the epiphysis by direct extension across the physis. Less commonly, the infection reaches the epiphysis hematogenously or from a septic arthritis (147). Epiphyseal infections are usually subacute. They are most frequent in the distal femurs of older children and almost always cause or follow infection in the joint. They commonly cause small areas of destruction surrounded by bony reaction. Epiphyseal osteomyelitis usually does not lead to a growth disturbance.

Chronic Multifocal Osteomyelitis. This is a poorly understood disease in which the metaphyses of multiple bones are

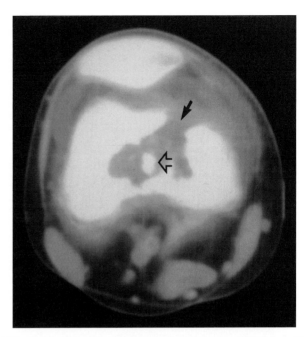

FIG. 5-64. Chronic osteomyelitis. A 14-year-old boy with chronic osteomyelitis involving the distal femoral metaphysis. Image from CT scan shows sequestrum *(open arrow)* and cloaca *(closed arrow)* with inflammatory tissue draining into surrounding soft tissues.

affected. Marrow aspirates show a large number of plasma cells, but no organisms can be cultured (118). It is more common in girls and is usually seen in older children. There are few symptoms of infection, and the lesion can be confused with a tumor. These metaphyseal lesions do not appear radiographically to be aggressive. There is a mixture of destruction and sclerotic reaction but little or no periosteal reaction. MRI can demonstrate adjacent soft-tissue abnormality such as edema or mass. There is an association with skin infections, such as plantopalmar pustulosis (118). Chronic multifocal osteomyelitis does not respond to antibiotics but tends to improve gradually without specific treatment. Not all patients have complete resolution of disease (148).

Complications. The complications of acute osteomyelitis are less common and less severe than during the preantibiotic era. They include septic emboli, growth disturbance (shortening, angulation, overgrowth), chronic osteomyelitis, pathologic fracture, avascular necrosis, septic arthritis (Fig. 5-65), and death due to overwhelming sepsis. Early diagnosis and proper treatment of acute osteomyelitis decreases the frequency of these complications.

Disseminated intravascular coagulation complicating meningococcemia and other severe septicemias of infancy leads to multiple areas of ischemia in epiphyses, physes, and metaphyses (149). The consequent growth disturbance results in tethering of part of the epiphysis, physeal coning, or even complete physeal closure.

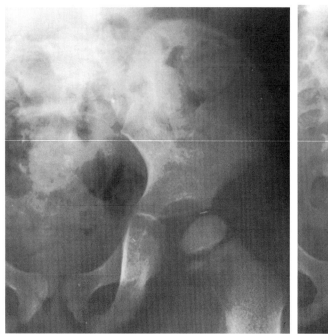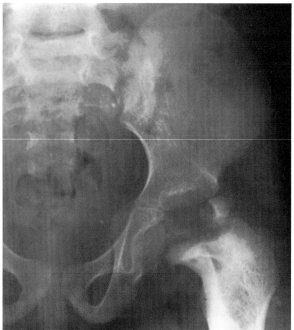

A

B

FIG. 5-65. Complication of osteomyelitis and septic arthritis. A: 1-year-old girl with staphylococcal osteomyelitis of the proximal left femoral metaphysis with associated purulent arthritis. **B:** AP view of the pelvis 2 years later. There is sclerosis and transverse widening of the proximal left femoral metaphysis and resorption of most of the left capital femoral epiphysis. Deformity and abnormal modeling of the left acetabulum are also apparent.

Septic Arthritis

Pathophysiology

Septic arthritis is an infection, usually due to pyogenic organisms, of a joint. In the neonate and young infant, the usual route of bacterial spread is from the metaphysis through transphyseal blood vessels to the epiphysis and joint space. In the child, most cases of septic arthritis occur as direct spread from an adjacent focus of osteomyelitis. Less frequently, septic arthritis is secondary to sepsis with direct bacterial seeding of the synovium or direct implantation (penetrating trauma, attempted venipuncture) into the joint. Bacterial embolization of the proximal femoral metaphysis due to septicemia also may produce septic arthritis, as this portion of the femoral neck is intraarticular. Septic arthritis of the hip also may originate from infections in metaphyseal equivalents at the triradiate cartilage.

In septic arthritis, lytic enzymes in the purulent articular fluid destroy the articular and epiphyseal cartilages. The prognosis is therefore governed by the duration of symptoms, which reflects the time over which these cartilages are exposed to destructive enzymes. The prognosis is worse in younger patients, in cases where there is adjacent osteomyelitis, and in patients with infections due to *Staphylococcus aureus* (150). Increased intracapsular pressure reduces blood flow to the epiphysis. This epiphyseal ischemia, if more than transient, leads to infarction. Other complications of septic

arthritis include dislocation, malalignment, or destruction of the femoral head and neck, or deformity of the epiphysis, physis, or metaphysis (151,152).

Etiology

In septic arthritis, precise bacteriologic diagnosis is essential for optimal therapy. A combination of joint fluid culture, blood culture, and vaginal or urethral culture in adolescents when indicated identifies the etiologic agent in at least 75% of cases (153). Potential organisms include *Staphylococcus, Streptococcus, Gonococcus, Pneumococcus, Pseudomonas, Enterobacter, Meningococcus, Salmonella, Klebsiella, Hemophilus, Candida,* other fungi, viruses, and *Mycobacterium.* Coliforms and gram-positive cocci predominate during the neonatal period. In infants, *Hemophilus* influenza type B was once predominant, but with widespread use of infant conjugate vaccines, this infection is now responsible for fewer than 14% of joint infections (154,155). In older infants and children, most cases are due to *S. aureus* (56%) and group A streptococci (22%).

Anatomic Sites

Septic arthritis usually involves the large joints. The joints most commonly affected are the knee (35%), the hip (35%), and the ankle (10%) (154,155). The anatomic site of involvement does not differentiate between the etiologic agents (153). Septic arthritis is monoarticular in 90% of cases.

Radiography

Evaluation of the paraarticular soft tissues is critical for diagnosing acute joint problems in children (156). The radiologic assessment of soft tissues varies from joint to joint. The assessment includes determination of the presence of an effusion, displacement of fat pads, and obliteration of soft-tissue planes because of edema. These changes are not specific for infection and may result from other inflammations and trauma. Ultrasonography can play a major role in demonstrating radiographically occult joint fluid, especially a hip effusion. MRI and CT demonstrate joint fluid, bone, and bone marrow space; MRI also shows cartilage well.

Knee. The normal fat pads around the knee include the suprapatellar fat pad, the triangular posterior fat pad group, the infrapatellar fat pad (of Hoffa), and the fat pad behind the proximal tibial epiphysis (156). Fluid accumulation in the knee joint occurs first in the suprapatellar bursa. One first sees soft-tissue widening of the neck of the suprapatellar bursa and, then distention of the entire bursa. Subsequently, fluid accumulates in the popliteal bursal extension (156).

Hip. Three perimuscular fat pads are normally seen around the hip: the gluteus medius, obturator internus, and iliopsoas (156). None of these fat pads lies directly against the joint capsule; however, the gluteus medius fat pad can be displaced laterally by intraarticular fluid, and with greater accumulations and edema the other fat pads are also displaced or become invisible. These fat pad signs are late and insensitive. Fluid also displaces the capsule anteriorly, as is demonstrated early by ultrasonography (Fig. 5-66A, B). The effusion later displaces the femur laterally and widens the joint space, as is shown by radiographs. Radiographic evaluation should always include AP views of the pelvis with hips in neutral and frog-lateral positions, to allow comparison with the uninvolved hip. The distance from the teardrop of the acetabulum to the medial metaphysis of each femoral neck should be measured (Fig. 5-66C). On a nonrotated frontal view of the pelvis and hips, asymmetry of 1–2 mm suggests joint effusion, and asymmetry of more than 2 mm is pathologic. The absence of asymmetry does not exclude a hip joint effusion demonstrable by ultrasonography. Apparent asymmetry often is due to abduction of the involved hip. Nonrotated, symmetrical positioning is necessary for these measurements to be reliable. Visualization of intraarticular gas, the vacuum phenomenon, does not exclude joint fluid (44), nor do normal radiographs and measurements.

Although joint fluid is readily demonstrated by MRI and CT, ultrasonography remains the imaging modality of choice for detecting hip effusion (Fig. 5-66A, B).

Ankle. The normal fat pads about the ankle include the pre-Achilles, anterior juxtacapsular, and posterior juxtacapsular. The anterior juxtacapsular fat pad is valuable for diag-

nosing an effusion; on the lateral radiograph, a teardrop of soft-tissue density (the effusion) displaces this fat pad anteriorly. A comparison lateral view of the normal ankle may be helpful.

Elbow. Septic arthritis of the elbow usually causes joint fluid. It is manifested by displacement of both anterior and posterior fat pads. The fat pads are intracapsular and thus are sensitive indicators of joint infection. The posterior fat pad, normally not visible on a 90° flexed lateral film, is pushed up and back and becomes visible with a joint effusion. The anterior fat pad, often visible in normals, is displaced by an effusion

Shoulder. Fluid within the shoulder joint may produce lateral displacement of the humerus (see Fig. 5-63A). If joint sepsis is a consideration in a young child, an AP view should include both shoulders. The distances from the glenoid labra to the proximal metaphyses of the humeri should be symmetric. As in the hip, a difference of 1–2 mm suggests joint effusion and a difference of more than 2 mm is pathologic. Again, ultrasonography is far more sensitive and specific than radiography for shoulder effusions.

Ultrasonography and Ultrasonographically Guided Aspiration

A hip effusion is seen ultrasonographically as an anechoic area between the proximal femoral metaphysis and the joint capsule (Fig. 5-66). This finding is not specific for infection and can be seen with other causes of effusion such as toxic synovitis, LCP disease, and noninfectious arthritis. The thickness of the capsule and the echogenicity of the fluid are not good predictors of infection in the joint. The absence of fluid, however, excludes septic arthritis (157). Ultrasonographically guided aspiration of the hip should be performed in any patient suspected of having septic arthritis (138), as the only reliable means of diagnosis is examination of the joint fluid.

Skeletal Scintigraphy and MRI

Skeletal scintigraphy and MRI are mostly useful for excluding associated osteomyelitis. In cases of acute septic arthritis, skeletal scintigraphy may be normal. Often, however, angiographic, tissue phase, and skeletal phase images demonstrate increased periarticular tracer uptake. Diminished or absent radionuclide uptake in the femoral capital epiphysis and physis indicates tamponade of the intracapsular epiphyseal vessels; this generally normalizes after arthrocentesis. Osteomyelitis must be suspected when a focal area of increased localization is centered not on the joint but on the adjacent bone (10,158). In septic arthritis, MRI shows increased enhancement of the synovium. The findings from both tests merely suggest articular inflammation, and the diagnosis of infection can be confirmed only by direct analysis of the joint fluid (138).

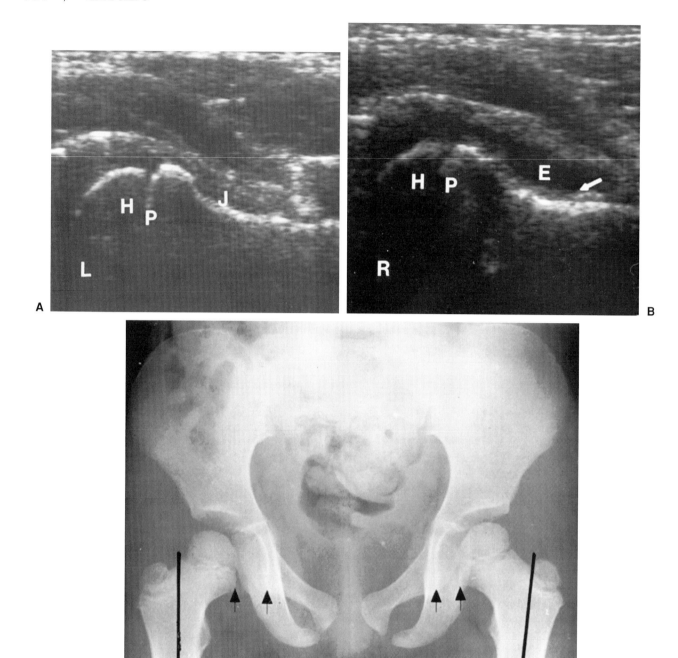

FIG. 5-66. Septic arthritis. A, B: Sonographic demonstration of hip joint effusion. Longitudinal anterior ultrasonographic sections of the left hip **(A)** and the right hip **(B)**. Both hips are shown as cranial to the viewer's left and caudal to the viewer's right. Echogenic line *(P)* is the junction of the physis with the metaphysis. Head of femur *(H)*; normal joint space with concave anterior margin along the femoral neck *(J)*. The wider anechoic joint space of the right hip *(E)*, with a convex anterior margin and thickened synovium *(arrow)*, represents a confirmed joint effusion. **C:** Radiographic demonstration of hip joint effusion. A 4-year-old girl with fever and a limp. There is widening of the distance from the acetabular teardrop to the medial femoral metaphysis on the right *(arrows)* compared to that on the left *(arrows)*. Note that the right femur is slightly more abducted than the left. Cultures of pus from the right hip joint grew out *Hemophilus influenzae*.

Differential Diagnosis

If blood is aspirated from the joint, an intraarticular physeal fracture should be considered. This type of fracture has been reported in the battered child syndrome (159). Widening of the hip and shoulder joints also occurs with epiphyseal-metaphyseal fractures and brachial plexus injuries. In the latter, there usually is no soft-tissue swelling about the shoulder. Rotation also causes apparent widening of the joint space.

Toxic Synovitis. Transient synovitis (toxic synovitis, observation hip, irritable hip) is a symptom complex of pain (in the hip or referred to the knee), limp, and spasm, generally of acute onset. The child is usually less than 10 years of age and has no history of illness or trauma. There is a slight male predominance. Joint aspiration shows no bacterial or viral etiology. Symptoms usually subside with rest, and usually there are no complications (4). However, in a small number of children, LCP disease develops, or perhaps the symptoms were a prodrome of that illness. Differential diagnostic considerations include septic arthritis, trauma, juvenile rheumatoid arthritis, LCP disease, and leukemia.

On radiologic evaluation of toxic synovitis, joint space widening is minimal, and there is no osteopenia or soft-tissue swelling. Ultrasonography demonstrates joint fluid. Hip aspiration, to decrease intraarticular pressure and exclude septic arthritis, is necessary. Synovial swelling is also noted on ultrasonography, but there is usually no particulate debris in the anechoic fluid. Increased joint pressure due to synovial fluid may interfere with perfusion of the femoral head (Fig. 5-67).

Complications

Complications of acute septic arthritis during childhood include true dislocation, epiphyseal separation (160), contracture of the joint capsule, joint destruction, subsequent osteomyelitis, and, rarely, destruction of the epiphyseal ossification center (161). Cross-sectional imaging may be required to diagnose these complications.

Transplacentally Acquired Infections

Viral Infections

The congenital rubella syndrome is the most common transplacentally acquired viral infection producing skeletal changes. Congenital rubella infection also may cause intrauterine growth failure, thrombocytopenic purpura, cataracts and other eye abnormalities, deafness, anemia, hepatosplenomegaly, skin rash, patent ductus arteriosus, aortic stenosis, and peripheral systemic or pulmonic stenosis.

Bone changes have been reported in 20% to 50% of cases. These bone changes are secondary to trophic disturbances rather than a local viral infection. Similar changes in cytomegalovirus infection presumably are also nonspecific trophic disturbances of endochondral bone formation (162). The differential diagnosis of bone changes due to transplacentally acquired infection should include TORCHS (*to*xoplasmosis, *r*ubella, *c*ytomegalovirus, *h*erpes, *s*yphilis). Congenital syphilis usually has associated periostitis and bone destruction, as will be described later.

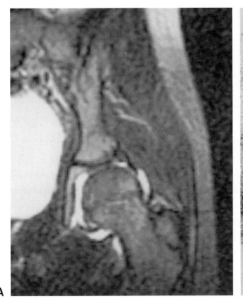
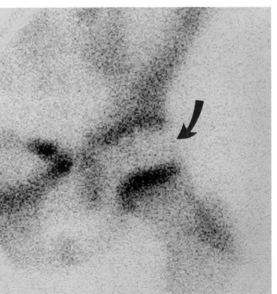

A   **B**

FIG. 5-67. Toxic synovitis. Decreased hip perfusion due to hip effusion. A 7-year-old boy with limp and painful left hip. **A:** Coronal T2-weighted MR image of the hip shows evidence of a high signal intensity joint effusion. **B:** Anterior pinhole image shows absence of tracer uptake in the entire femoral head *(arrow).*

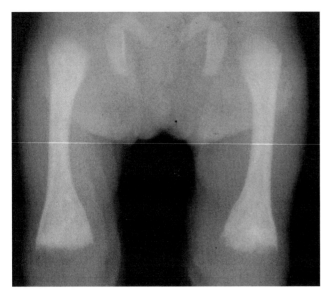

FIG. 5-68. Congenital cytomegalovirus infection. Newborn girl with cytomegalovirus infection. There is fraying and undertubation of the metaphyses.

The radiologic features of transplacentally acquired viral infections (Fig. 5-68), especially rubella, include irregular fraying of the metaphyses of the long bones. There is a generalized lucency of the metaphyses, often with alternating longitudinal relatively radiodense lines. This celery stalk appearance is most pronounced at the knees but may be seen in any of the long bones. Occasionally the bones are sclerotic. With congenital rubella, the medullary cavities of the long bones tend to be narrower than usual at birth. Skeletal maturation is usually delayed with congenital rubella but is more normal with cytomegalovirus infection (163). Periosteal reaction is unusual with congenital viral bone disease.

Although bony lesions may be present at birth, they become more apparent during the first few weeks of life. Then the trophic changes heal rapidly, and the bones return to normal by 3–6 months of age. Occasionally, the bone changes fail to resolve and actually progress. These chronic changes, which occur in infants who have continued poor growth and development, include osteopenia of the metaphyses, dense, irregular zones of provisional calcification, and metaphyseal cupping.

Although congenital infection with human immunodeficiency virus (HIV) has become increasingly frequent, skeletal manifestations are seldom reported. Musculoskeletal abnormalities in HIV infection are related primarily to superinfections (including osteomyelitis, septic arthritis, and bacterial myositis) and to malignancies such as Burkitt lymphoma (164).

Congenital Syphilis

Congenital syphilis is due to transplacental infection, usually during the second or third trimester of gestation. Its incidence has been increasing in the United States. It is associated with maternal drug abuse, particularly with crack cocaine (165). Clinical manifestations include rhinorrhea, rash, anemia, hepatosplenomegaly, ascites, and the nephrotic syndrome. Skeletal involvement occurs in 95% of cases with overt disease (166) but is infrequent in infants without symptoms. There is usually a latent period of 6–8 weeks between the time of infection and the appearance of skeletal lesions. If infection is acquired late in pregnancy, skeletal changes may not develop until 6–8 weeks of age. The blood serology may also be negative for the first week or two of life.

The first radiologic changes in the long bones are found in the metaphyses. These abnormalities include nonspecific trophic metaphyseal lucent bands and fragmentation and destruction (Fig. 5-69). The Wimberger corner sign is metaphyseal destruction in the upper medial tibia, usually sparing the most recently formed few millimeters of metaphysis (Laval-Jeantet collar). Although the Wimberger sign also may be seen with bacterial osteomyelitis, fibromatosis, hyperparathyroidism, and other conditions, it strongly suggests congenital syphilis. Pathologic fractures sometimes occur in the regions of metaphyseal destruction. They are associated with abundant callus formation and may present as a pseudoparalysis. There is usually periosteal new bone formation bilaterally involving the diaphyses and the metaphyses. Destructive lesions occasionally involve the diaphyses.

There usually is widespread involvement of the skeletal system, although occasionally single-bone involvement is noted. Involvement of the skull and flat bones usually causes well-marginated lytic lesions. The Centers for Disease Control recommends obtaining long bone radiographs in all newborns suspected of having congenital syphilis. The usefulness of this recommendation has been questioned recently in a study in which only 5 of 93 newborns had findings suggesting the disease (165,166).

Noninfectious Inflammation

Juvenile Rheumatoid Arthritis

Juvenile rheumatoid arthritis (JRA), one of the juvenile chronic polyarthritides, is a systemic disease of unknown etiology that primarily affects the connective tissues, particularly the joints (167–169). The pathologic process is similar to that of rheumatoid arthritis in adults. However, juvenile rheumatoid arthritis has unique clinical features, distribution of joint involvement, and radiologic manifestations.

Juvenile rheumatoid arthritis (167,169) may be divided into adult-type seropositive rheumatoid arthritis and seronegative disease. The seronegative disease, which accounts for the majority of cases in children, is in turn divided into a systemic form known as Still disease (with only mild joint involvement), a polyarticular form, and a pauciarticular or monoarticular form (170).

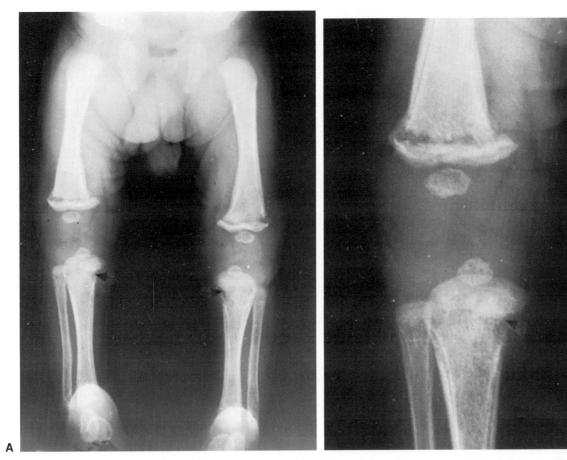

A   B

FIG. 5-69. Congenital syphilis. Lower extremities **(A)** and coned-down view of the right knee **(B)** show metaphyseal lucencies and periosteal new bone formation. Wimberger sign is present bilaterally *(arrows)*. The newest several millimeters of metaphysis (collar of Laval-Jeantet) are characteristically spared.

Only 15% of cases of rheumatoid arthritis in children are seropositive. There is a distinct female preponderance. The usual age of onset is after 10 years. The disease is polyarticular, with early involvement of the interphalangeal and metacarpophalangeal joints of the hand, frequently accompanied or followed by involvement of the wrist and knee. Early films show swelling of and around the joints, particularly of the hands. There may be periosteal reaction near an affected joint (167). The growth centers, particularly in the wrists, become abnormal in shape. Many patients develop erosions of the bones of the hands or feet within a few years of the onset of disease. Sites of involvement, in order of decreasing frequency, are hands, wrists, feet, knees, and hips.

The remaining 85% of children with rheumatoid arthritis have seronegative disease. This seronegative JRA remains primarily a clinical diagnosis, as the immunoglobulin M rheumatoid factor is not present and there are no other specific tests to confirm the diagnosis. In approximately half of the cases, the disease is pauciarticular, in which four or fewer joints are involved. Less commonly a single joint is affected, usually the knee (4). The polyarticular form (30–40% of childhood JRA) most frequently affects the knee, wrist,

ankle, and hindfoot (168). These patients are also prone to disease in the temporomandibular joints and in the cervical spine and to develop synovial cysts. Children with the systemic form of JRA (Still disease) usually have no or few skeletal abnormalities.

Radiologic abnormalities in JRA occur in the knee (90%), ankle (70%), wrist (70%), hand (55%), elbow (40%), hip (35%), shoulder (25%), cervical spine (21%), sacroiliac joint (5%), and sternoclavicular joint (3%) (168). Splenomegaly and thoracic changes (e.g., pleural effusion) are frequent. Antegonial notching (a concave undersurface) of the mandible is characteristic of JRA. Radiologic changes of the hands and wrists include soft-tissue swelling, accelerated skeletal maturation, squaring and small size of the epiphyses and carpal bones, joint space narrowing, and ultimately ankylosis (Figs. 5-70 and 5-71). Diaphyseal periosteal reaction is frequent. In the knee and elbow, radiographic abnormalities are initially subtle. There may be accelerated maturation and overgrowth of the epiphyses. Coarsening of trabeculae and, later, erosive changes are frequently present. The hip commonly shows osteopenia, coxa valga deformity due to lack of weight bearing, overgrowth of the capital epiphysis with

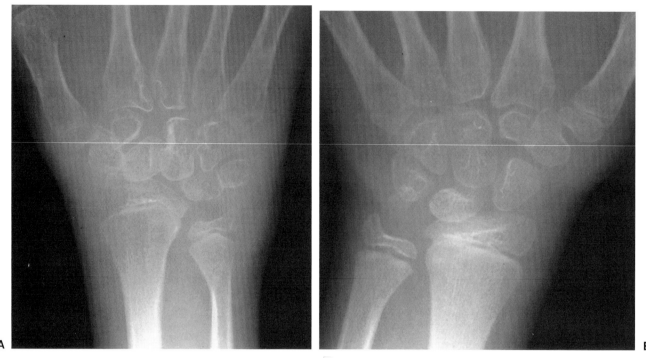

A

B

FIG. 5-70. Polyarticular juvenile rheumatoid arthritis. A 10-year-old girl with chronic arthritis. **A:** PA radiograph of the right wrist shows squaring of the carpal bones, soft-tissue swelling, and slightly short ulna. **B:** The left wrist shows much less advanced changes with only mild carpal irregularity and soft-tissue swelling.

premature closure of its physis, and abnormal growth of the femoral neck. Changes in the cervical spine include ankylosis of the apophyseal joints (Fig. 5-71), abnormal development of the adjacent vertebral bodies, narrowing of the intervertebral disc spaces, osteopenia, and atlantoaxial subluxation.

MRI, particularly after gadolinium enhancement, can accurately show cartilage loss and erosions, hypoplasia or atrophy of the menisci, inflammation and hypertrophy of the synovium (Fig. 5-72), joint effusions, and avascular necrosis caused by corticosteroids (171,172). It can also define the extent of temporomandibular disc disease, which is seen in 40% of these patients (173). Sonography can detect joint fluid and increased thickness of the synovium (174).

The differential diagnosis of JRA includes the other types of chronic juvenile polyarthritis. The juvenile spondyloarthropathies (ankylosing spondylitis, psoriatic arthritis, arthritis associated with inflammatory bowel disease, and Reiter syndrome) commonly involve the sacroiliac joints. When these spondyloarthropathies occur in children, they present with dactylitis, tenosynovitis, and enthesitis (175). Other rare causes of polyarthritis in childhood include Farber disease (lipogranulomatosis) (Fig. 5-73), lipoid dermatoarthritis (multicentric reticulohistiocytosis), and polyarthropathies associated with disorders such as systemic lupus erythematosus and familial Mediterranean fever (167,169). These entities can usually be distinguished by

their clinical and radiologic features. In the large joints, the radiographic appearance of hemophilia often mimics that of juvenile rheumatoid arthritis. Leukemia occasionally presents with articular symptoms suggestive of JRA.

Dermatomyositis

Dermatomyositis is an inflammatory disease of the striated muscle and skin. In children, the diagnosis is based on clinical findings (weakness, rash, systemic signs), elevated muscle enzymes, and electromyography or biopsy. Radiographs in the initial stages of disease and in patients who are well controlled with steroid treatment are usually normal. Patients who are not treated can develop calcification in the muscles and subcutaneous tissues (Fig. 5-74). MRI has been used to determine the extent of involvement of the disease, to guide biopsy for diagnosis, and to monitor the response to therapy (176). Patients with active disease show increased signal in affected muscles on fat-suppressed T2-weighted images, perimuscular edema, and abnormalities in the subcutaneous fat (Fig. 5-75). Usually the thighs and pelvis are examined. The muscles in the anterior compartment of the thigh and those around the hip tend to be most severely affected.

Abnormalities in the signal intensity of muscles are also present in patients with rhabdomyolysis and in patients with infectious myositis.

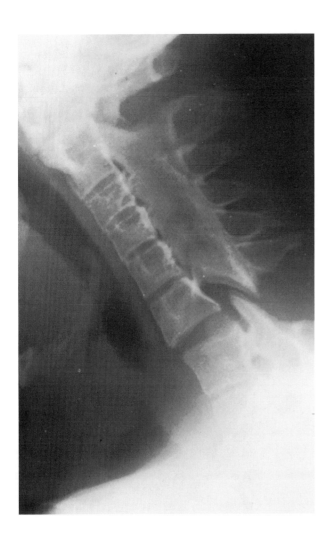

FIG. 5-71. Juvenile rheumatoid arthritis. Ankylosis of apophyseal joints of the upper cervical spine. The C6 disc and joint space are abnormally wide; this is where most of the motion of the neck must occur.

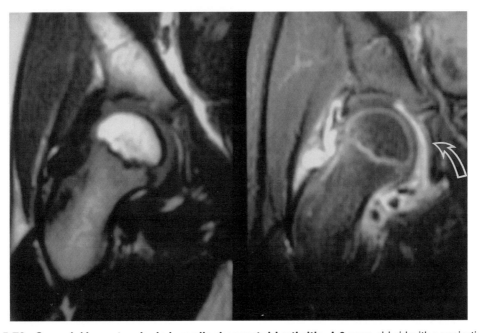

FIG. 5-72. Synovial hypertrophy in juvenile rheumatoid arthritis. A 6-year-old girl with pauciarticular juvenile rheumatoid arthritis. T1-weighted MR images before *(left)* and after the administration of gadolinium *(right)* show that there is abundant enhancing synovium *(arrow)* surrounding the femoral head and neck.

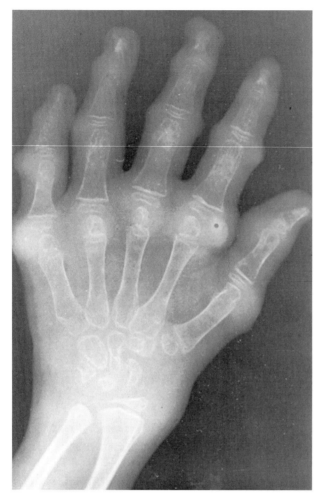

FIG. 5-73. Farber disease. A 5-year-old girl with Farber lipogranulomatosis. The bones are osteopenic, and there are carpal irregularities and crowding, as with juvenile rheumatoid arthritis. However, multiple, large, soft-tissue masses are also noted.

Caffey Disease

Caffey disease (infantile cortical hyperostosis) is a disease of unknown etiology that occurs during the first few months of life, although it has been detected prenatally (177). It is characterized by irritability, fever, and soft-tissue swelling and radiologic evidence of periosteal new bone and cortical thickening (178–183). Although its precise etiology is not known, Caffey disease shows many clinical, radiologic, and histologic features of inflammation. A viral etiology would explain its tendency to cluster in time and geographic location. It would also explain the cases that present prenatally or during the first months of life and its familial predisposition (183). A causative role of prostaglandins is also hypothesized, as high repeated doses of prostaglandin E during infancy create the same clinical and radiographic pattern as classic Caffey disease (181). There has been a marked decrease in the frequency of Caffey disease since the 1970s (179).

The triad of irritability, swelling of soft tissues, and underlying cortical thickening is usually present. Other clinical features include fever, pallor, and pseudoparalysis. There may be a family history of Caffey disease. Laboratory findings include anemia, thrombocytosis, leukocytosis with a shift to the left, and elevation of the erythrocyte sedimentation rate.

The bones involved, in order of decreasing frequency, are the mandible, ribs, clavicles, humerus, ulna, femur, scapula, radius, tibia, fibula, metatarsals, metacarpals, hands, feet, and skull (180). When Caffey disease is intrauterine, polyhydramnios is usually present (perhaps the fetus does not swallow because of jaw pain). Radiographs show periosteal new bone formation, sclerosis, and a soft-tissue mass (Fig. 5-76). Periosteal reaction is mostly diaphyseal and occurs early in the disease. (Fig. 5-77) Subsequently, there may be a dense laminated appearance in and underneath the periosteum or a considerable increase in the diameter of the bone due to subperiosteal new bone formation (180). This striking cortical hyperostosis may produce a cast of the involved bone. Congenital and familial cases have frequent involvement of the extremities bilaterally but less marked involvement of the

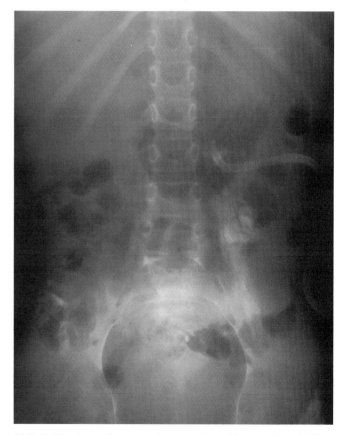

FIG. 5-74. Juvenile dermatomyositis with muscle calcifications. A 14-year-old girl not complying with therapy for long-standing dermatomyositis. Frontal radiograph of the abdomen shows linear calcifications in the region of the left psoas muscle, compatible with calcified myositis. There are smaller calcifications in the right iliacus muscle and around the left hip.

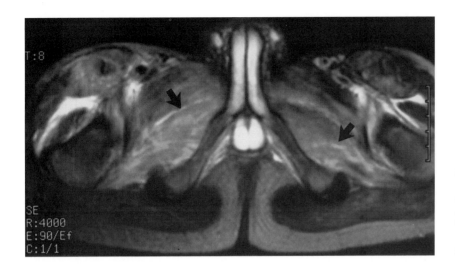

FIG. 5-75. MRI findings in dermatomyositis. A 15-year-old boy with generalized myalgia. An axial fat-suppressed fast spin-echo T2-weighted image shows extensive areas of muscle edema involving the adductor muscles *(arrows)*. The gluteal muscles remain hypointense, indicating that they are spared.

ribs and mandible (Fig. 5-77). There may be late recurrences (182). MRI can show the periosteal abnormalities when the radiographic findings are not characteristic (184).

Neoplasms

Introduction

The current role of imaging in malignant bone tumors in children includes (a) formulating a presumptive diagnosis, (b) determining the extent, (c) evaluating response to therapy, and (d) evaluating complications. Radiographs remain the best modality for making a specific diagnosis prior to biopsy. Determination of tumor extent is paramount in order to perform surgery that will maximize function. This is best established with MRI. Response of a tumor to chemotherapeutic agents is difficult to evaluate precisely. Response is defined histologically as more than 95% tumor necrosis, a determination that is nearly impossible with current imaging techniques. Indicators suggesting response (185) include greater maturity of tumor bone on radiographs, decrease in

size of the soft-tissue component of the mass on radiographs or MR images, decreased enhancement on dynamic and static gadolinium-enhanced MR images (186, 187), and decreased uptake on ^{201}Tl scintigraphic studies (188). The imaging of complications depends largely on the amount and type of hardware placed during surgery; hardware gravely limits MRI and CT. Radiographs often are the most reliable means of diagnosing failure of the graft, local recurrence, or development of a postradiation sarcoma.

General Principles

The incidence of tumors varies with age and location (Table 5-13). Metastatic neuroblastoma is the most frequent cause of tumoral destruction of bone in children under 5 years of age. Ewing sarcoma is the leading primary bone malignancy in children 5–10 years of age. Osteogenic sarcoma is the most common malignant bone tumor in adolescents. There are two main types of bone neoplasms in children: round cell tumors that infiltrate the marrow, and

TABLE 5-13. *Location of musculoskeletal tumors or tumor-like lesions in children*

Location	Central	Eccentric	Cortical	Periosteal	Soft tissue
Epiphysis	Chondroblastoma Histiocytosis		Trevor disease		PVNS
Metaphysis	Enchondroma Osteosarcoma[a] Ewing[a] UBC[a]	ABC Osteosarcoma[a] Ewing[a]	Osteochondroma[a] Osteosarcoma[a] Ewing[a]	Osteosarcoma[a] Ewing[a]	Osteosarcoma[a] Ewing[a]
Metadiaphysis	Fibrous dysplasia	Chondromyxoid fibroma	Nonossifying fibroma		Myositis ossificans
Diaphysis	Histiocytosis Ewing[a]		Osteoid osteoma[a] Osteofibrous dysplasia Adamantinoma		Neurofibromatosis Rhabdomyosarcoma

PVNS, pigmented villonodular synovitis; UBC, unicameral bone cyst; ABC, aneurysmal bone cyst.
[a] More common.

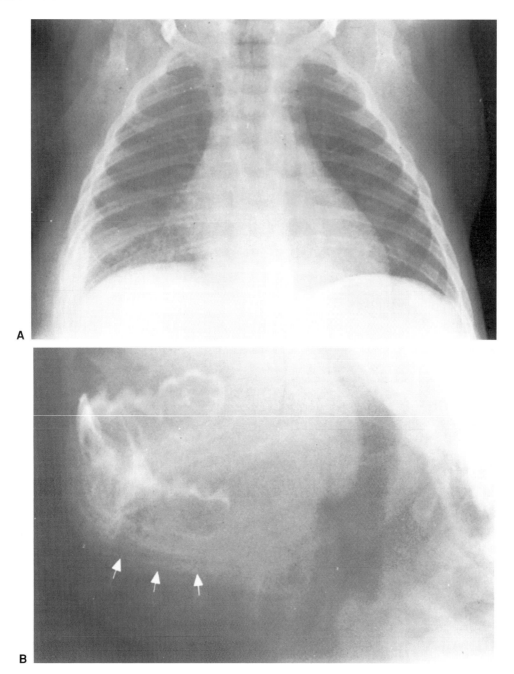

FIG. 5-76. Caffey disease. A 3-month-old boy with irritability and swelling of the right jaw. **A:** AP chest radiograph shows periosteal reaction involving the posterolateral parts of the right seventh and eighth ribs. **B:** Oblique view shows periosteal reaction in the body of the right mandible *(arrows).*

mesenchymal tumors, related to ossification of cartilage and formation of new bone. Marrow-infiltrating tumors include metastatic neuroblastoma, Ewing sarcoma, lymphoma, and Langerhans cell histiocytosis. These tumors follow the distribution of hematopoietic bone marrow and do not produce tumor matrix. They are recognizable radiographically by bone destruction and by the response of bone to the tumor (periosteal bone deposition, reactive bone formation). Tumors associated with production of cartilage and bone in-

clude osteogenic sarcomas and benign cartilaginous tumors (enchondromas, osteochondromas, chondroblastomas). These tumors tend to occur near the fastest growing physes (distal femur, proximal tibia, proximal humerus) and often produce a characteristic tumor matrix.

The skeleton of children reacts aggressively to tumors. Bone is deposited rapidly along the margins of the tumor, in the invaded bone, and along the periosteum. The loose periosteal attachments allow extensive subperiosteal spread

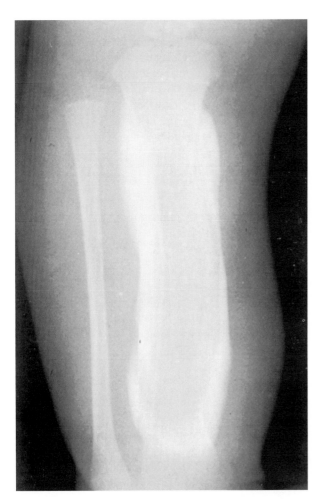

FIG. 5-77. Familial Caffey disease. An 8-day-old girl with swelling of the right leg. The patient's mother and maternal aunt had Caffey disease diagnosed during the neonatal period. There is marked periosteal new bone formation and abnormal modeling of the right tibia, indicating intrauterine onset of the condition.

of tumor, which typically stops at the perichondrium. The physis acts as a partial barrier to the spread of tumor, but only a temporary one.

Radiologic Evaluation

There are only a few ways in which bone can react to tumor. Bone may be destroyed if it is invaded and replaced by the growing tumor. Alternatively, there may be bony reaction and bone formation, due either to osteoblastic stimulation within bone and periosteum or to calcification within tumor matrix. Osteolytic and osteogenic reactions often occur together.

Osteolytic lesions are recognizable when they involve compact cortical bone (Fig. 5-78) and are much less visible if limited to trabecular bone. *Geographic osteolysis* has clearly defined borders and is sharply distinguished from the neigh-

boring bone. The defect frequently has a polycyclic contour. This type of osteolysis may be seen in benign or slowly invading malignant primary bone tumors, some metastatic tumors, subacute infection, and Langerhans cell histiocytosis (62). *Moth-eaten osteolysis* denotes small confluent areas of cortical destruction with edges that are less well defined. This type of osteolysis is frequently noted with early primary malignant tumors, some infections, and metastatic disease. *Permeative osteolysis* has small defects in the cortex of bone that produce decreased density and are frequently associated with marked periosteal reaction. The margins of the lesions are poorly defined. This pattern is most frequently seen with highly malignant, rapidly growing lesions and with acute osteomyelitis, but it may occasionally be seen with Langerhans cell histiocytosis. *Mixed osteolysis* is common and usually consists of central geographic osteolysis and a peripheral permeative pattern. It generally indicates the presence of a rapidly growing tumor or infection with extensive involvement (189). These descriptors were codified by Lodwick (190) and have proved to be very useful radiographic clues to the aggressiveness of a bone lesion.

Involvement of the periosteum by any process, usually arising from underlying bone but occasionally from adjacent

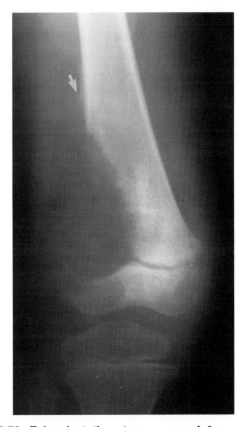

FIG. 5-78. Telangiectatic osteosarcoma. A 6-year-old girl with knee pain. Frontal view shows a large, mainly lytic metaphyseal lesion that penetrates through the physis into the epiphysis. The borders are ill defined, and there is a soft-tissue mass. Thin periosteal reaction is also seen *(arrow)*.

soft tissues, causes reaction by subperiosteal osteoblasts. It requires at least 10 days to produce a periosteal reaction visible on radiographs (62). With MRI, and sometimes with ultrasonography, the periosteal membrane can be seen as a well-defined structure that is peeled from the bone shaft by the tumor and that converges with the bone at the tight perichondral attachments of the physis.

The pattern of periosteal reaction depends on the duration of the stimulus and the rapidity of growth of the underlying process. A *sunburst appearance* indicates cortical destruction with rapid elevation of the periosteum and reaction of bone along Sharpey fibers to produce bony spicules perpendicular to the long axis of the bone. Such a reaction is frequently noted with sarcomas, especially osteogenic sarcoma (Fig. 5-79). *Parallel layering* of the periosteum (laminated periosteal reaction) is due to repeated periosteal stimulation

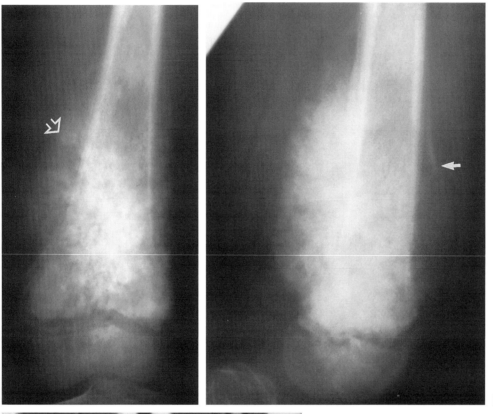

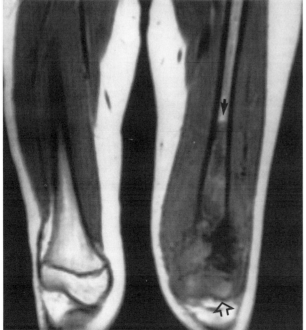

FIG. 5-79. **Osteosarcoma of the distal femur**. An 11-year-old boy with history of pain in the knee and a limp. The frontal **(A)** and lateral **(B)** views show a large lesion involving the distal femur with cloud-like density compatible with tumor bone *(open arrow)*. There is spiculated periosteal reaction giving the "sunburst" appearance. There is a soft-tissue mass. On the lateral view, a Codman triangle *(closed arrow)* results from bone formation along the periosteum at the periphery of the lesion. **C:** Coronal T1-weighted MR image shows a large mass with inhomogeneous low-signal-intensity-areas destroying the cortex and extending into the soft tissues. The tumor invades the epiphysis *(open arrow)*. There is a sharp transition between the tumor and the normal marrow *(closed arrow)*.

without time for incorporation into the cortex. The series of bony layers gives an onion-skin appearance. Although it indicates a rapidly progressive local lesion and is often seen with Ewing sarcoma or other primary or secondary malignant neoplasms, it is not specific and may be seen with osteomyelitis, Langerhans cell histiocytosis, periosteal hematoma, and Caffey disease. *Solid periosteal reaction* is due to a slowly progressive underlying lesion that is usually benign. It is usually thin and smooth when seen in association with Langerhans cell histiocytosis, osteoid osteoma, subperiosteal hematoma, subperiosteal fracture, hypertrophic pulmonary osteoarthropathy, and osteomyelitis. Thick solid periosteal reaction may be wavy when seen in conjunction with vascular disturbances such as varicose veins. It may be smooth when seen with osteoid osteoma, Langerhans cell histiocytosis, Caffey disease, and nonimmobilized fractures. Solid periosteal reaction may be thick but interrupted when seen with treated sarcomas, osteomyelitis, and storage diseases. *Periosteal remodeling* produces cortical expansion due to slowly growing lesions originating in the medulla or deeper layers of the cortex. This type of bony expansion is often due to a benign tumor. The *Codman triangle* is ossification along and below the elevated periosteum at the periphery of an underlying lesion (Figs. 5-79 and 5-80). A triangle is formed at the transition between normal periosteum and adjacent elevated periosteum. The top of this triangle is adjacent to the normal cortex, and the periosteum is maximally displaced away from the bone shaft at its base. A Codman triangle simply indicates that there is periosteal elevation by mass effect. Although it is commonly seen in malignant lesions, it may also be caused by osteomyelitis and benign, slow-growing tumors such as aneurysmal bone cysts, periosteal hematomas, and Langerhans cell histiocytosis (62).

Chondroid or osteogenic tumors may produce calcification in tumor matrix. The radiologic appearance of the calcification is related to the type of cells. Punctate, ring-like, or flocculent calcifications usually indicate cartilaginous matrix, benign or malignant. Calcification in osteogenic matrix usually has a homogeneous density with ill-defined margins and a cloud appearance (Fig. 5-79).

In general, round cell tumors cause a permeative pattern of destruction indicative of very diffuse infiltration of the marrow and frequently produce a laminated periosteal reaction (189). Malignant tumors with bone and cartilage production have moth-eaten margins and tend to have a sunburst type of periosteal reaction. In children, however, some of the most severe instances of marrow infiltration and subperiosteal spread of tumor are associated with nearly normal radiographs; this happens when tumor invasion is too fast to elicit visible bone reaction (190). Certain tumors, notably aneurysmal bone cysts but also the aneurysmal component of a giant cell tumor or telangiectatic osteosarcoma, can show fluid-fluid levels on CT or MRI (191).

The differentiation between benign and malignant bone tumors depends on the clinical information, radiologic appearance, presence of metastases, and histology. Important considerations include the age of the patient, overall incidence of various neoplasms, duration of symptoms, type of bone reaction, nature of any periosteal reaction, character of calcification within the tumor matrix, extent of involvement including marrow and soft tissues, site of the lesion, relation to the physis, and rapidity of progression. Benign lesions usually have no soft-tissue mass and have well-defined margins, limited extent, homogeneous internal structure, lack of periosteal reaction in the absence of fracture, and deformity of bone due to remodeling. Some benign lesions, such as Langerhans cell histiocytosis, chondroblastoma, and osteoid osteoma, can elicit considerable inflammatory response in the marrow, cortex, periosteum, and adjacent soft tissues. They can resemble a malignant lesion on both radiographs and MRI. Malignant lesions usually have rapid growth, aggressive behavior, indistinct radiographic borders, marked extension from the medullary cavity through the cortex, cortical destruction, a soft-tissue mass, large diameter, moth-eaten and permeative internal texture, aggressive periosteal reaction, and absence of deformity due to remodeling.

Periosteal abnormalities due to neoplasms are well demonstrated by MRI. In cases of aggressive neoplasms, MR images readily identify tumor under the hypointense line of periosteum and penetration of the periosteum by the mass.

Radiographic concepts are not always applicable to MRI. The margins of signal abnormality on MR images reflect the tumor plus peritumoral edema. The most ill-defined margins on MRI usually are related to diseases that elicit prominent inflammatory responses, such as infection, osteoid osteoma, Langerhans cell histiocytosis, and chondroblastoma. Very aggressive tumors, such as Ewing sarcoma, can have very well-defined margins on MR images, particularly on T1-weighted sequences.

Imaging Principles. Plain radiography, the modality most likely to lead to a specific diagnosis, should always be performed. The goal of the radiographs is to decide whether the lesion is aggressive and requires further imaging or biopsy, or can be observed or ignored. Arriving at a specific radiographic diagnosis is relatively unimportant. Ninety percent of all malignant bone tumors in children are either Ewing sarcoma or osteogenic sarcoma (185), and their radiographic characteristics overlap.

If the radiographs suggest an aggressive lesion, MRI should be the next study. MRI can address most issues of tumor extent better than CT (89) and usually obviates the use of CT except when there are specific questions about cortical destruction, tumor calcification, or the risk of fracture. Skeletal scintigraphy and CT of the chest are always obtained to search for metastatic disease in children with malignant bone tumors.

In most children with malignant bone tumors, MRI should begin with coronal T1-weighted images that include as much of the length of the bone as possible (Fig. 5-79C and 5-80B). The most common mistake in MRI of bone tumors is not to study the entire lesion. T1-weighted images with a large field of view best depict the intramedullary extent of the tumor, show skip metastases when present, and serve as a localizer for prescription of oblique sequences (192). Extension of the tumor through the cortex, into the subperiosteal space, and into the soft tissues is readily seen with axial proton density and T2-weighted images (Fig. 5-80C). Most

malignant bone tumors are of low signal intensity on T1-weighted images and of high signal intensity on T2-weighted images. STIR sequences (for further evaluation of marrow abnormality) (Fig. 5-80D) and gradient echo images (for evaluation of vascular involvement) can provide supplemen-

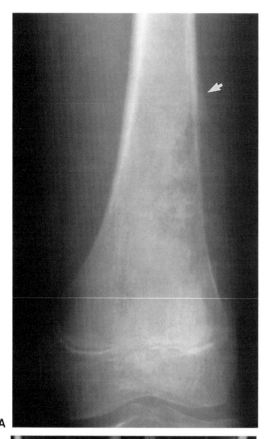

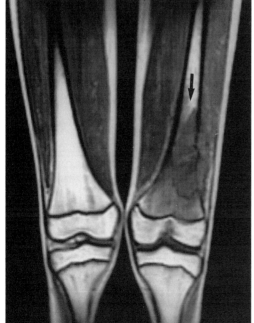

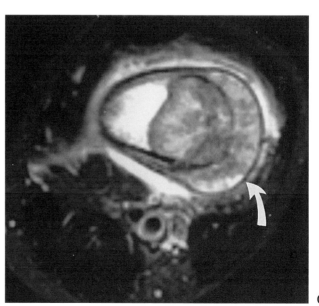

FIG. 5-80. Osteosarcoma of the distal femur. A 14-year-old-boy with left knee pain. **A:** Frontal radiograph demonstrates a lesion in the lateral portion of the metadiaphyseal region with a mixed lytic and sclerotic pattern. There is evidence of elevation of the periosteum at the periphery of the lesion (Codman triangle) *(arrow).* **B:** Coronal T1-weighted MR image with a wide field-of-view (FOV) shows loss of normal marrow signal in the left femoral diametaphysis, depicting clearly the transition between normal and abnormal marrow *(arrow).* **C:** Axial fat-suppressed fast spin-echo T2-weighted MR image demonstrates penetration of the tumor through the cortex and extension beneath the periosteum *(arrow).* There is significant peritumoral edema but no evidence of vascular involvement.

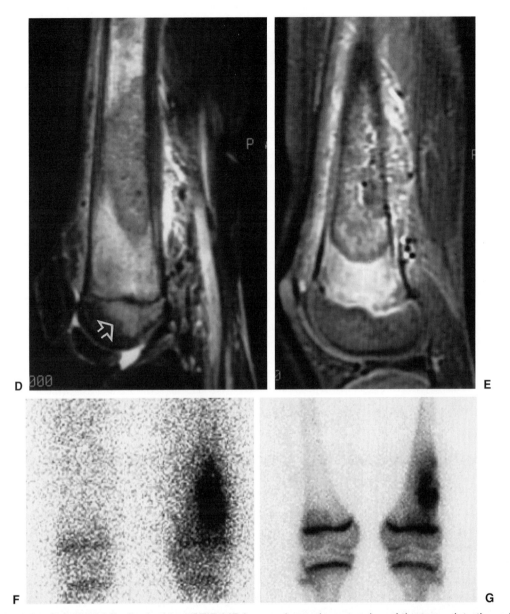

FIG. 5-80. *Continued.* **D:** Sagittal fast STIR MR image shows the extension of the tumor into the epiphysis *(arrow)*. Because of the increased sensitivity of this sequence to peritumoral edema, the transition of normal marrow signal to abnormal signal is not as well defined as on the T1-weighted image. **E:** Sagittal fat-suppressed gadolinium-enhanced T1-weighted image shows enhancement of signal intensity in the tumor. The enhancement has a radiating pattern similar to the sunburst pattern seen radiographically. **F:** Scintigraphy. There is marked thallium-201 uptake in the left distal femoral osteosarcoma. **G:** Skeletal scintigraphy demonstrates intense but heterogenous tracer localization in the tumor.

tary information. Gadolinium-enhanced images (Fig. 5-80E), usually in the sagittal plane for femoral, tibial, and humeral lesions, are best for evaluating extension into the joint (193), tumor necrosis, and, when performed dynamically, the differentation of tumor from edema (194–196), and the response of tumor to chemotherapy. MR angiography, spectroscopy, and positron emission tomography (PET) have been used to assess tumor activity, but they remain experimental.

Malignant Lesions

Osteogenic Sarcoma

Osteogenic sarcoma, or osteosarcoma, is a malignant tumor that arises from bone or its coverings and rarely from connective tissue. It forms neoplastic osteoid and bone during its evolution as well as some chondroid or fibroid cellular material. The tumor usually arises within the medullary space (intraosseous osteosarcoma), but it may arise on the surface of the bones (periosteal and parosteal forms). The tumor is classified as high grade or low grade according to its aggressiveness on histologic examination. Osteogenic sarcoma includes osteoblastic, chondroblastic, and fibroblastic types, depending on the predominating tissue.

Pathology. Osteogenic sarcoma, as the name says, is a bone-producing tumor. In children it is found in the areas of fastest skeletal growth. It arises in the metaphyses of long bones in 80% to 90% of cases. The sites, in decreasing order of frequency, are the distal femur (40%), proximal tibia (20%), and proximal humerus (15%) (89,197). Flat bones are involved in 10% of cases, particularly the ilium and mandible; mandibular osteosarcomas are usually of low histologic grade.

The tumor is usually eccentric in the metaphysis. It often extends through the physis into the epiphysis. Epiphyseal extension is detectable by MRI in 80% of osteosarcomas (198). Extension into the joint is rare and is almost always extrasynovial; in the knee, it is along the cruciate ligaments (193). The tumor spreads along the medullary cavity, penetrates the cortex, and enters the subperiosteal space, elevating the periosteum. When the tumor extends into the soft tissues it may involve the nerves or vessels, particularly the popliteal vessels, or major muscle groups such as the quadriceps. Involvement of these structures may preclude limb salvage surgery (199).

The microscopic appearance of osteosarcoma is highly variable. Two essential criteria for the diagnosis of osteogenic sarcoma are the presence of sarcomatous stroma and the formation of malignant osteoid or tumor bone from this malignant connective tissue stroma (197). In addition to tumor osteoid and bone, neoplastic cartilaginous tissue and fibrous tissue are frequently present.

Clinical Features. Osteogenic sarcoma is the most common primary malignant tumor of bone in childhood. It is somewhat more common in boys than girls. The peak incidence is between the ages of 10 and 20. Sixty-eight percent develop in patients 15 years of age or younger and 21% in those under age 10 (200). The etiology is unknown, but viral and genetic factors may be involved. Osteogenic sarcoma can develop years after radiation therapy, generally given for a Ewing sarcoma. Children with hereditary retinoblastoma have a strong predisposition to osteogenic sarcoma, and the risk is increased by exposure to radiation (201). Osteosarcoma may develop in preexisting benign lesions, but this is rare.

Pain and local swelling are the most frequent symptoms. A pathologic fracture, occurring in approximately 5% of patients, disturbs normal barriers to tumor spread and worsens the prognosis. Laboratory tests are usually negative, with the exception of elevation of the alkaline phosphatase in approximately 50% of patients.

Radiologic Findings. Osteogenic sarcomas are usually large at presentation, and the radiographic findings are dramatic (Figs. 5-78, 5-79, and 5-80). Tumor bone, the distin-

guishing feature of osteosarcoma, is seen in 90% of cases (197) and appears as cloud-like densities that usually extend beyond the normal contours of the bone. Approximately half of the cases show a mixture of bone destruction and sclerosis due to bone production (Figs. 5-79 and 5-80). There is usually a soft-tissue mass. Periosteal reaction is usually irregular, with interrupted spicules that are perpendicular or radial to the cortex of the involved bone and to the center of the tumor mass. A Codman triangle may be produced by the advancing tumor mass as it elevates the periosteum and then destroys the new bone subsequently formed (Figs. 5-78, 5-79, and 5-80).

The radiographic appearance of osteogenic sarcoma depends on the amount of destruction and production of bone. In very aggressive lesions, and especially in telangiectatic tumors, the appearance may be predominantly lytic. The margins can be ill defined and mottled, with a wide transition zone from abnormal to normal bone. Rarely, there may be a sharp transition zone, falsely suggesting a benign lesion, between malignant tumor and normal bone (202). Occasionally, younger children present with uniform sclerosis of the affected bone, without periosteal reaction, a soft-tissue mass, or destruction of cortex (200).

On skeletal scintigraphy, osteosarcomas typically demonstrate marked tracer localization corresponding to tumor bone formation (Fig. 5-80G). Regions of decreased tracer localization in either viable but nonossifying tumor or necrotic tumor are often present. Due to hyperemia or medullary reactive bone formation, the pattern of increased tracer localization frequently extends beyond the pathologic confines of the tumor (203–205). This extended pattern, which typically involves bone directly contiguous with the tumor or immediately across the joint from it but may affect the entire extremity, limits the utility of skeletal scintigraphy in defining the tumor's margins.

Skeletal scintigraphy is most useful in detecting distant skeletal metastases. These lesions, which appear as areas of increased tracer localization, are often radiographically occult or asymptomatic (206,207). Skip lesions may also be demonstrated, although their incidence is probably underestimated because of concealment by falsely extended patterns of increased uptake. Skeletal scintigraphy occasionally shows unsuspected mediastinal metastases or confirms questionable pulmonary parenchymal lesions (208).

Skeletal scintigraphy with ^{99m}Tc-methylene diphosphonate has not proven reliable in assessing chemotherapeutic response; some studies have shown a good correlation between reduction in skeletal tracer localization and tumor response (209,210) whereas others have not (186,211). Scintigraphy with ^{201}Tl may, however, be useful in this assessment (188,211–213) (Fig. 5-80F). Tumoral uptake of this potassium analog reflects tumor mass, cellular viability, metabolic activity, and tumor vascularity (214). Osteosarcomas are highly ^{201}Tl-avid tumors. A significant reduction in ^{201}Tl uptake after chemotherapy suggests an excellent therapeutic response; uptake that does not diminish suggests a poor response. Other tracers with potential use in assessing osteosarcoma are ^{99m}Tc-methoxyisobutylisonitrile (^{99m}Tc-MIBI) and fluorine-18 deoxyglucose (FDG).

MRI is the most useful modality for evaluating the extent of osteogenic sarcoma in both bone and soft tissue. The MRI pattern typical of most bone tumors (low signal intensity on T1-weighted images and high intensity on T2-weighted images) is usually present throughout most of the tumor mass. Areas with abundant tumor osteoid formation are of low signal intensity on all sequences. The medullary component of the tumor, destruction of cortex, and soft-tissue mass are readily identified. Differentiation between tumor and normal marrow is difficult when there is significant peritumoral edema, which is most evident on STIR and gadolinium-enhanced images. Since tumor and adjacent marrow reaction cannot be distinguished reliably, it is prudent to assume during surgical planning that any area with abnormal signal intensity is involved by the neoplasm. Telangiectatic osteosarcomas sometimes can be recognized by their blood-filled spaces, making them resemble aneurysmal bone cysts. Chondroblastic osteosarcomas have a septal-like pattern of enhancement typical of cartilaginous lesions (197). Tumor response to therapy results in decrease in the soft-tissue mass and peritumoral edema. MRI appears to identify failure of response to therapy (typically recognized as increase in soft-tissue mass, peritumoral edema, and bone destruction) (215,216) more reliably than positive response to therapy. CT of the primary lesion is very seldom necessary. The multiplanar capability of MRI evaluates the medullary cavity for skip lesions better than CT (217). MRI defines the relation of extraosseous tumor mass to muscles, nerves, and vessels and demonstrates invasion of growth and articular cartilage better than CT (218). Precise determination of local tumor extent is mandatory before limb salvage procedures. On conventional and MR angiography, osteogenic sarcomas are usually highly vascular with irregular tumor vessels, arteriovenous shunting, and tumor staining (219).

CT is used to monitor pulmonary metastatic disease. A baseline CT scan of the chest is obtained at diagnosis, followed by reexamination at 3- to 6-month intervals. When feasible, patients undergo resection of all pulmonary metastases to maximize the chance for long-term survival (220). Any nodule, regardless of size, in a child with osteosarcoma is presumed to be metastatic until proven otherwise with follow-up imaging or at thoracotomy.

Treatment. Surgery and adjuvant chemotherapy remain the primary treatment combination for osteogenic sarcoma of the appendicular skeleton. Limb sparing is currently performed in 80% of patients with osteosarcomas (221). Accurate preoperative staging by MRI helps determine when local resection or limb salvage procedure is appropriate. Chemotherapy has prolonged average survival. The response to preoperative chemotherapy is evaluated by follow-up MRI, which should include T1-weighted gadolinium-enhanced images.

Prognosis. In the past, surgery (amputation or disarticula-tion) resulted in a 20% survival rate at 5 years. The advent of adjuvant chemotherapy changed the prognosis drastically. In a review of the Memorial Hospital experience, survival 5 and 10 years after diagnosis was 77% and 73%, respectively (222). Death usually results from pulmonary metastases. Aggressive surgical management has improved the prognosis for patients with lung metastases, as long as the metastases do not abut the pleura (201). Skeletal metastases now develop in up to 15% of patients, usually involving flat bones such as ribs, skull, and vertebrae (223).

Ewing Sarcoma

Ewing sarcoma is the second most common primary bone malignancy of childhood. It is composed of small, round cells, perhaps of neural origin (224). It is closely related to the primitive neuroectodermal tumor (PNET) of bone, which has identical imaging characteristics (225). Ewing sarcoma can be radiographically confused with other round cell tumors of childhood such as metastatic neuroblastoma and lymphoma and with osteomyelitis.

Sites of Involvement. Sixty percent of Ewing sarcomas arise in the extremities, but any bone may be involved. The sites of involvement, in order of decreasing frequency, are the femur, pelvis, tibia, humerus (Fig. 5-81), rib, vertebra, fibula, and scapula. Two thirds involve the lower extremities and pelvis (Fig. 5-82) (200). The tumor may develop in the diaphysis but more commonly occurs in the metaphysis. Epiphyseal origin is rare. The lesions in the diaphysis are usually central, whereas those in the metaphysis are eccentric (200,226). In patients under 20 years of age, the tumor usually involves long bones, whereas flat bones predominate in older patients.

Clinical Features. Most patients complain of pain and local swelling. Tenderness, warmth, and a palpable mass are frequently present. There may be anemia, elevated erythrocyte sedimentation rate, leukocytosis, and fever, which along with local symptoms sometimes suggest osteomyelitis.

Most patients are between 5 and 25 years of age at the time of diagnosis. Approximately half develop the tumor during the second decade of life. If the patient is under 5 years of age, the possibility of metastatic neuroblastoma must be considered. Ewing sarcoma has a predilection for Caucasians (89) and a slightly greater incidence in boys.

Pathology. Ewing sarcomas are grayish white and contain areas of necrosis, hemorrhage, and cyst formation (227). Tumor tends to spread along the marrow cavity, through the cortex, and beyond the periosteum. Neoplastic tissue is frequently mixed with proliferative bone and fibrous tissue. Although its origin is usually metaphyseal in a tubular bone, the lesion tends to involve a long segment of the bone.

The tumor is highly cellular and has little intercellular stroma except for strands of fibrous tissue. Within the round tumor cells are relatively large oval or round nuclei surrounded by scanty cytoplasm. Light microscopy shows

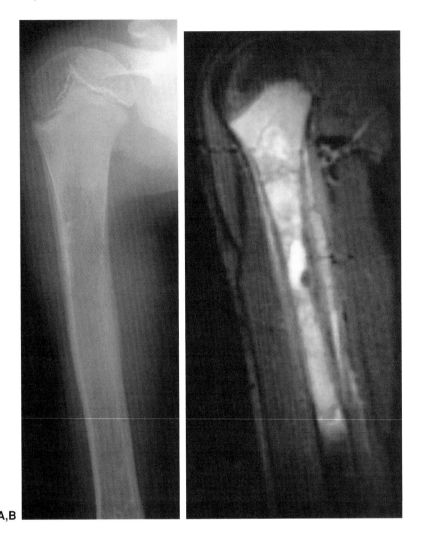

A,B

FIG. 5-81. Ewing sarcoma of the humeral shaft. A 7-year-old boy with arm pain. **A:** Radiograph of the proximal humerus shows laminated periosteal reaction and ill-defined metadiaphyseal destruction. **B:** Sagittal STIR MR image of the humerus shows extensive involvement of the marrow and subperiosteal space. The lesion abuts the physis.

abundant glycogen-containing cytoplasmic granules. In contrast to PNET, electron microscopy shows no neurosecretory granules. The microscopic features of Ewing sarcoma may be difficult to distinguish from those of other small, round cell tumors, such as lymphoma-leukemia and neuroblastoma. Ewing sarcoma and PNET of bone express a chromosomal translocation (t11:22), which suggests that oncogenes contribute to their development (224).

Radiologic Features. The appearance of Ewing sarcoma is highly variable. The tumor tends to involve a large portion of the diaphysis (Fig. 5-81), although the focus of bone destruction or bone production is usually in the metaphysis. The lesion is purely lytic in 62% of patients, lytic with minimal reactive bone formation in 23%, and predominantly sclerotic in 15% (200). This sclerosis, unlike that of the osteosarcomas, is not cloud-like and is usually confined to the bone. Poorly marginated bone destruction, seen in 96% of cases (228,229), is characteristically seen near the junction of the metaphysis and diaphysis of a large tubular bone; the transition to normal bone is gradual. Areas of lucency due to rapid spread and permeation may be seen in the cortex. There also may be an irregular underlying endosteal contour (scalloping) due to medullary spread of the neoplasm.

There can be extensive destruction of bone despite sharply demarcated margins. More frequently, there is highly aggressive destruction combined with permeative reaction. Reactive bone formation is common in flat bones, ribs, and the cancellous bone of the metaphysis of long bones.

When tumor spreads to the periosteal surface, it usually stimulates periosteal new bone formation, seen in nearly 60% of patients (228,229). This formation may be laminated parallel to the cortex ("onion skin") (Fig. 5-81A) or spiculated perpendicular to the cortex. This laminated and spiculated new bone is characteristically thin in Ewing sarcoma. Soft-tissue masses are seen in 80% of cases (Fig. 5-82B). Infrequently (6%), the tumor is solely within the soft tissues or erodes the bone from the outside (cortical saucerization) (230).

Skeletal scintigraphy usually shows increased uptake of bone tracers and is useful for the evaluation of metastatic disease. MRI is valuable for assessing medullary extension and the soft-tissue component of the tumor (Figs. 5-81 and 5-82) (231). The soft-tissue component of the tumor decreases after therapy, but the medullary abnormality remains (232,233). Although these tumors are usually hypervascular, angiography is not specific and is rarely indicated. Dynamic

Ewing sarcoma is 50% to 70% but is less than 30% when the disease has metastasized (224). Long-term survival is more common with primary lesions of the long bones than in lesions of the axial skeleton, thoracic cage, and shoulder girdle. The tumor sometimes recurs 3 or more years after diagnosis (130).

Leukemia and Lymphoma

Bone marrow involvement by leukemia or lymphoma is demonstrated most effectively by MRI (234–236). Acute lymphoblastic leukemia infiltrates the marrow diffusely (Fig. 5-83), whereas acute myelocytic leukemia produces a more patchy involvement. In leukemia, however, osteomyelitis and osteonecrosis are common complications that can similarly disturb the MRI pattern. Leukemia and lymphomas may be aggressive and destroy cortex, usually in the metaphyseal region. The nonspecific lucent metaphyseal bands called leukemic lines represent interference with endochondral ossification rather than infiltration by tumor. They suggest leukemia if there is no other cause for trophic bone changes (63). Quantitative MR methods sometimes distinguish leukemic children who will respond to therapy from those who

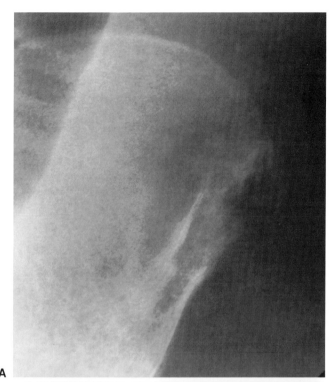

A

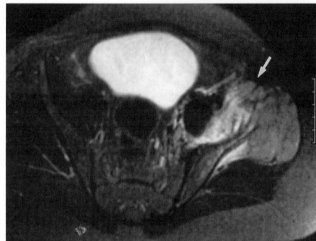

B

FIG. 5-82. Ewing sarcoma of the left iliac wing. A 10-year-old boy with hip pain. **A:** Oblique coned down radiograph of the iliac wing shows permeative destruction in the region of the anterosuperior iliac spine. **B:** Axial fast spin-echo T2-weighted MR image of the iliac wing shows marrow replacement in much of the ilium and a large mass in the gluteal region and left iliac fossa *(arrow).*

enhanced MRI has been used to assess tumor response, as was described in the discussion of osteosarcoma. CT is used for assessment of pulmonary metastases.

Treatment and Prognosis. Ewing sarcoma usually is treated with radiation therapy and multidrug-multicycle chemotherapy. In the long bones, resection of the tumor with limb salvage procedures is performed with increasing frequency (221). The 5-year survival rate for patients with

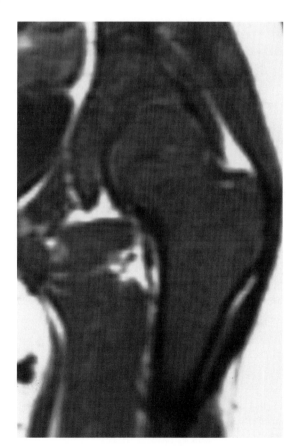

FIG. 5-83. Diffuse marrow infiltration in acute lymphoblastic leukemia. Coronal T1-weighted MR image of the proximal femur shows very low signal intensity throughout the entire visualized marrow. From Laor and Jaramillo (63).

will not, but these methods have not achieved widespread use (237,238).

Soft-Tissue Malignancies

Malignant tumors of the soft tissues are age-related. In the neonate and young infant, fibrosarcoma is the most common soft-tissue malignancy. This soft-tissue mass has large feeding vessels and contains many areas of necrosis. The MRI appearance can resemble that of a hemangioma. The adjacent bones are often splayed rather than destroyed. In the older child, rhabdomyosarcomas usually are more common (Fig. 5-84). These most commonly arise from the muscles of the extremities; peripheral rhabdomyosarcomas are of the alveolar variety, in contrast to the rhabdomyosarcomas of the genitourinary tract, which usually are of the embryonal type. Other soft-tissue malignancies in children include primitive neuroectodermal tumors, synovial sarcomas, and neurofibrosarcomas.

Metastatic Disease

The most common lesions metastatic to the bones of children are small round cell tumors. These metastases may be from leukemia, lymphoma, or neuroblastoma (Figs. 5-85, 5-86, and 5-87). Most metastatic skeletal lesions are osteolytic and produce a moth-eaten appearance. Metastases frequently involve the proximal metaphyses of the proximal long bones of the extremities (Fig. 5-86). If metastases are generalized, there is a tendency toward bilaterality and relative symmetry. Diffuse metastatic disease may be difficult to differentiate from normal marrow on MRI. Diastasis of cranial sutures in patients with metastatic neuroblastoma is due to bulky extradural metastatic deposits rather than focal destruction or hydrocephalus.

Metastatic skeletal lesions may also be due to osteogenic sarcoma, Ewing sarcoma, primitive neuroectodermal tumor, rhabdomyosarcoma, retinoblastoma, and cerebellar medulloblastoma. Except in osteogenic sarcoma and medulloblastoma, these metastatic lesions are almost always osteolytic. Vertebral involvement in leukemia or neuroblastoma may result in partial collapse. Skeletal metastases occur in fewer than 5% of Wilms tumors (62).

Scintigraphy in the Evaluation of Skeletal Metastases in Children. In many pediatric malignancies, skeletal scintigraphy is more useful than plain film radiography for staging and follow-up. These malignancies include neuroblastoma, osteosarcoma, Ewing sarcoma, rhabdomyosarcoma, retinoblastoma, medulloblastoma, PNET, and the clear cell variant

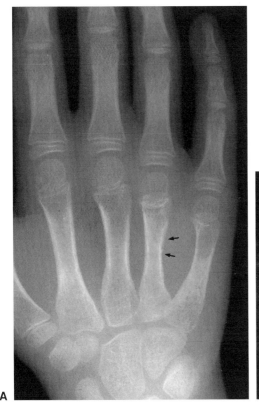
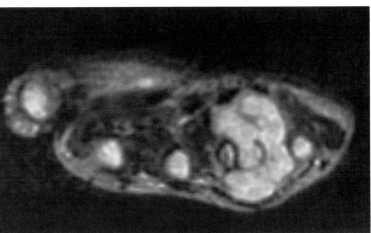

A   B

FIG. 5-84. Alveolar rhabdomyosarcoma of the hand. An 8-1/2-year-old boy with a painless mass in his hand. **A:** Frontal radiograph demonstrates erosion and scalloping of the ulnar cortex of the fourth metacarpal *(arrows).* **B:** Axial T2-weighted MR image shows that the mass, which is hyperintense with respect to the adjacent musculature, extends ventrally and dorsally between the fourth and fifth metacarpals.

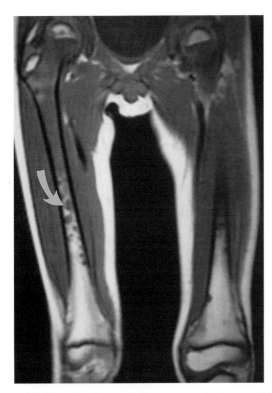

FIG. 5-85. Metastatic neuroblastoma. A 4-year-old boy with a large neuroblastoma of the retroperitoneal sympathetic chain. Coronal T1-weighted MR image shows many lesions of intermediate signal intensity in the proximal metaphysis and shaft of the right femur corresponding to metastases *(curved arrow).*

of Wilms tumor. Neuroblastoma, the most frequent source of bone metastases in childhood, deserves special consideration.

Skeletal metastases (i.e., metastases involving the cortical bone, the bone marrow, or both) are frequently present at diagnosis or develop later in children with neuroblastoma (239). Cortical bone metastases are considered prognostically more ominous than metastases limited to the marrow (130,240). Skeletal scintigraphy is more sensitive to neuroblastoma metastases in cortical bone than radiography (240). The metastases appear as areas of increased or, occasionally, decreased tracer uptake (241–243). Any bone can be affected. Characteristic sites of involvement are the calvaria, periorbital facial bones, spine, pelvis, and the metaphyses of long bones (158). Since scintigraphic diagnosis depends heavily on asymmetry, symmetrically distributed metaphyseal lesions may escape detection.

Skeletal scintigraphy demonstrates the primary mass in 40% to 85% of neuroblastomas. Skeletal tracer localization in the primary tumor site may reflect calcium metabolism by viable tumor (240). Uptake may occur without identification of calcification by radiography or CT (243). The likelihood of skeletal tracer localization may increase with the size of the primary (244). Skeletal scintigraphy may detect an occult primary in children with neuroblastoma and symptoms due to skeletal metastases (131).

Scintigraphy with metaiodobenzylguanidine (MIBG) labeled with iodine-131 or iodine-123 is also useful for identifying metastatic neuroblastoma. Skeletal neuroblastoma may be somewhat easier to identify with MIBG imaging than with skeletal scintigraphy because the normal distribution of MIBG does not include bone or bone marrow (245); cortical and marrow metastases therefore are visible as areas of abnormal MIBG localization (Fig. 5-87). MIBG uptake occurs in 85% of primary tumors (246).

The optimal use of skeletal scintigraphy and MIBG imaging in children with neuroblastoma is controversial (247). Because the tracers localize by different mechanisms, either study may reveal metastases when the other does not. In neuroblastoma patients whose skeletal and MIBG scintigrams both reveal metastases, MIBG imaging often reveals more sites of disease (248), but it does not distinguish cortical from marrow involvement. Due to its specificity for viable tumor, MIBG is more useful than skeletal scintigraphy for evaluating therapeutic response (249).

The somatostatin analog, octreotide, labeled with ^{111}In also localizes to neuroblastoma with a reported sensitivity

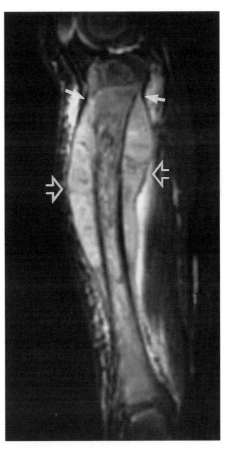

FIG. 5-86. Metastatic neuroblastoma. A 15-month-old boy with an abdominal neuroblastoma. STIR MR image of the tibia shows extensive involvement of the marrow. There is tumor elevating the periosteum *(open arrows).* The periosteum is elevated in the diaphyseal region but approaches the physis in the region of the perichondral attachments *(closed arrows).*

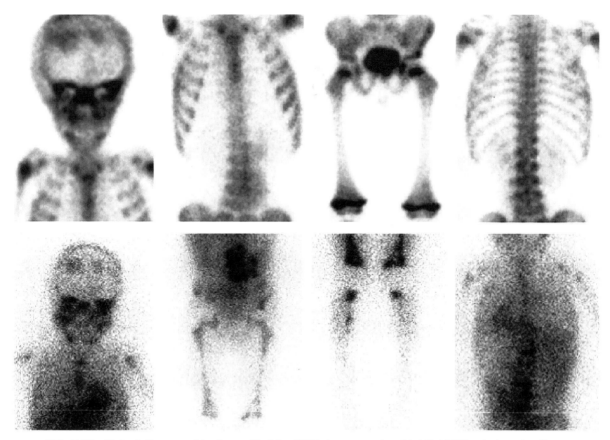

FIG. 5-87. Metastatic neuroblastoma. Tc-99m MDP *(upper row)* and I-123 MIBG scintigraphy *(lower row)*. Anterior images of the head, trunk, and extremities and posterior images of the spine demonstrate a lumbar paravertebral neuroblastoma and metastatic disease involving the calvaria, periorbital facial bones, ribs, spine, pelvis, and extremities. Renal and bladder Tc-99m MDP localization and myocardial and hepatic I-123 MIBG localization reflect the normal distribution of these tracers.

of greater than 80% (250). Experience with this tracer is still too limited to allow its role relative to ^{99m}Tc-MDP or MIBG to be assessed accurately.

Musculoskeletal Abnormalities Due to Antineoplastic Treatment

Radiation Therapy Injury. In children, musculoskeletal abnormalities due to radiation therapy include diminished or disordered growth, muscle atrophy, bone marrow depletion, and development of secondary neoplasms. Radiation injury usually results from local high-dose therapy, but it has also been recently described in patients undergoing total body irradiation prior to bone marrow transplantation (251). Radiation changes due to local therapy are confined to the radiation port. These changes have sharply defined and straight margins, sometimes at 90 degree angles, and do not follow ordinary anatomic boundaries.

Radiation of growing bone may produce changes in the epiphysis, physis, metaphysis, and diaphysis (252,253). In general, the greater the growth potential of the bone (the younger the child) and the higher the radiation dosage, the greater the probability and extent of skeletal damage

(252,253). Whenever possible, epiphyses and physes should be excluded from the treatment field. Radiation therapy to physes of long bones produces physeal widening, metaphyseal fraying, metaphyseal sclerosis, abnormal tubulation, and premature epiphyseal fusion (254,255) as well as occasional exostosis formation. Physeal widening is due to arrest of ossification of the cartilage of the physis, with an increased number of cell layers, and swelling of cartilage cells. Metaphyseal sclerosis is due to increased mineral deposition as well as deficient chondroclasis and osteoclasis (253). Metaphyseal fraying presumably results from persistence of unossified cartilage in the metaphysis due to impaired endochondral ossification (254) co-existing with relatively unimpaired membranous ossification in the perichondral zone of Ranvier.

On MR images, radiation therapy changes during the first months after treatment include edema of the marrow and adjacent musculature (256). Fatty transformation of the marrow and muscle atrophy later develop (Fig. 5-88).

Long-term complications of radiation therapy to growing long bones include limb shortening and deformity, angulation, bony exostosis (Fig. 5-89), epiphyseal destruction, slipped capital femoral epiphysis, hypoplasia (Fig. 5-90),

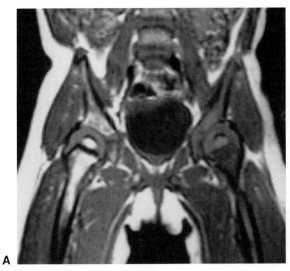
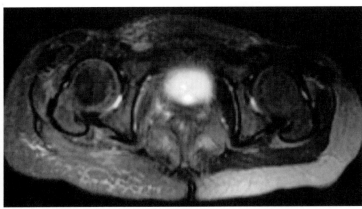

A

B

FIG. 5-88. Postradiation changes in the marrow on MRI. A 2-year-old girl with rhabdomyosarcoma of right hip and thigh. **A:** T1-weighted MR image shows fatty transformation of the marrow of the right iliac wing and femur. Left side shows red marrow of normal low signal intensity. **B:** Axial T2-weighted image shows increased signal intensity in the marrow and subcutaneous tissues of the right hip. Note that the border of the abnormality is sharp and geometric, rather than anatomic.

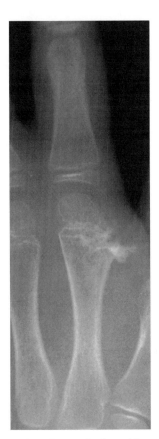

FIG. 5-89. Osteochondroma induced by total body irradiation. A 6-year-old girl with leukemia who had been irradiated prior to bone marrow transplantation. An osteochondroma of the metacarpal of the index finger developed after therapy.

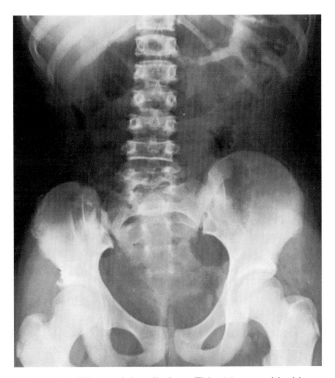

FIG. 5-90. Effect of irradiation. This 11-year-old girl received irradiation to the right abdomen for neuroblastoma. There is platyspondyly and hypoplasia of the right iliac wing.

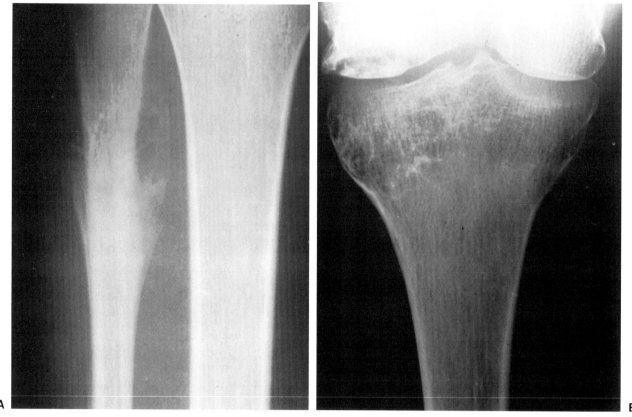

FIG. 5-91. Complication of irradiation. A: This 13-year-old boy was treated for Ewing sarcoma of the proximal right fibula. **B:** Follow-up radiograph 4 years after surgical resection and radiation. Osteopenia involves the lateral aspect of the distal right femur and proximal right tibia. Osteochondritis dissecans has developed in the lateral condyle of the distal femur.

osteochondritis dissecans (Fig. 5-91), and radiation-induced sarcoma (257).

Changes Due to Chemotherapy. Changes due to chemotherapy include diffuse marrow depletion, abnormalities of bone formation (osteopathy, rickets), growth retardation, and osteonecrosis. Methotrexate produces a form of osteopathy that resembles scurvy, with marked osteoporosis, radiodense lines in the metaphyses and surrounding the epiphyses, and metaphyseal fractures (258). Hypophosphatemic rickets and renal tubular disorders can result from administration of ifosfamide, particularly during therapy for Wilms tumor (259). Growth recovery lines develop after each cycle of chemotherapy, resulting in a striped appearance of the metaphysis. Marrow changes on MR images include fatty transformation and osteonecrosis, particularly if the patient is also receiving steroids.

Granulocyte colony-stimulating factor (GCSF) is used as an adjunct to chemotherapy in order to reduce the marrow depletion associated with antineoplastic agents. GCSF results in a striking reconversion to hematopoietic marrow; this must be differentiated on MR images from metastasis and recurrent tumor (260,261). The reconverted marrow is initially metaphyseal, has a patchy distribution, and contains fat, like normal marrow (Fig. 5-92).

Benign Lesions

Cystic Lesions

Unicameral Bone Cyst. Unicameral bone cyst (simple or solitary bone cyst) is a relatively common lesion (262). Approximately 75% of unicameral bone cysts are found in children. They are approximately three times as common in boys. Eighty percent of childhood cysts are located in the metaphyses of the proximal humerus or femur, much more commonly in the humerus, and they also occur in the proximal tibia. In patients over 17 years of age, approximately half of the lesions are located in the pelvis or calcaneus. The lesions usually come to attention incidentally on a chest film or after a pathologic fracture. This complication occurs in 50% of identified cases (262). Bone cysts are usually 2–3 cm in diameter. They consist of an intramedullary cavity lined by a thin layer of connective tissue filled with serous or serosanguineous fluid.

The etiology is uncertain. Stasis of interstitial fluid secondary to trauma or venous obstruction has been proposed. The cyst fluid is similar to serum but it can be clear or hemorrhagic, depending on the age of the cyst and the degree of blood content (4). The cyst may undergo spontaneous

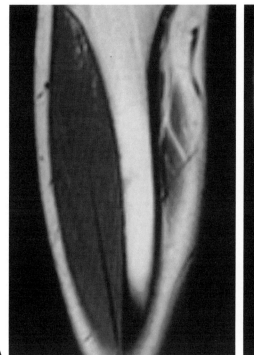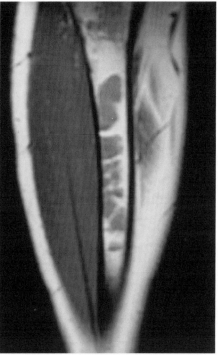

A   B

FIG. 5-92. Effect of granulocyte colony-stimulating factor (GCSF) on marrow. A 16-year-old after chemotherapy for synovial sarcoma of the right calf. **A:** Coronal T1-weighted MR image obtained at the beginning of chemotherapy shows fatty marrow throughout the entire tibial shaft. **B:** Coronal T1-weighted MR image of the tibial shaft after the administration of GCSF shows many intermediate signal intensity patches within the marrow, indicating hematopoietic transformation.

regression and fill in with bone; this probably happens frequently. However, the larger cysts may result in growth disturbances, limb length discrepancy, and deformity.

The lesions usually can be diagnosed with radiographs alone, which makes biopsy unnecessary. The characteristic radiologic appearance is a unicentric, intramedullary, lucent, expansile lesion surrounded by an attenuated but intact cortex. Unlike an aneurysmal bone cyst, the lesion tends to have a transverse width no greater than that of the adjacent physis (263). Occasionally septations are suggested, but they probably represent bony ridges in the cyst wall rather than true loculations (4). The cyst is usually found in the metaphysis, immediately adjacent to the physis. With bone growth, the physis leaves the cyst behind, in the diaphysis. Extension into the epiphysis is infrequent. A pathologic fracture causes periosteal reaction. Occasionally, a fragment of cortex falls to the bottom of the lesion after a pathologic fracture (the "fallen fragment") (264) (Fig. 5-93). This sign proves that the lesion contains fluid, which offers no resistance to the fragment and allows it to fall freely to the bottom of the cyst (264).

The MRI signal characteristics suggest a fluid-filled structure. After gadolinium administration, only the walls of the lesion enhance, which confirms its cystic nature (265). Fluid-fluid levels due to prior hemorrhage may be seen on both CT and MRI (191,262,265).

Treatment, for the large lesions that compromise bony

integrity and for those in high-stress anatomic sites, is aimed at the prevention of a pathologic fracture (266). The initial treatment of choice is intracyst corticosteroid injection to stimulate healing (263). Aspiration of yellow or slightly bloody fluid prior to corticosteroid injection confirms the diagnosis. Contrast injection into the lesion confirms that all loculated areas have been injected. Several injections may be needed, over months. Lesions that do not heal after injection may be treated with curettage and bone packing or with subtotal diaphyseal resection with bone grafting, but this is seldom necessary (266).

The differential diagnosis is limited. Aneurysmal bone cysts and fibrous dysplasia have some radiographic similarity.

Aneurysmal Bone Cyst. The cause of aneurysmal bone cysts (ABCs) is not fully settled. They are thought to be the result of trauma in some cases; other cases are attributed to tumor-induced abnormal vascular processes, such as an intraosseous vascular malformations. Some ABCs may represent primary bone abnormalities. One third of ABCs develop in a preexisting lesion, such as giant cell tumor (the most common), osteoblastoma, chondroblastoma, fibrous dysplasia, nonossifying fibroma, chondromyxoid fibroma, unicameral bone cyst, eosinophilic granuloma, and osteosarcoma. More than 80% of aneurysmal bone cysts thought to arise de novo are found in patients less than 20 years of age. They are rare in children under 5 years of age. The lesion

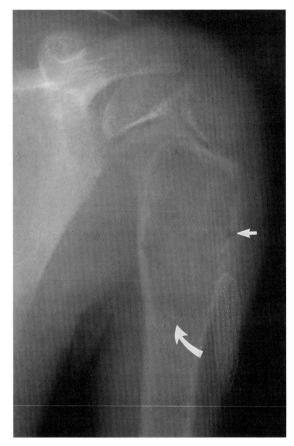

FIG. 5-93. **Unicameral bone cyst.** This frontal view of the proximal humerus shows a central lucent metaphyseal lesion. A pathologic fracture is seen through the lateral cortical margin *(arrow)*. An osseous density ("fallen fragment") is seen at the base of the lesion *(curved arrow)*.

is slightly more common in girls. More than half occur in the long bones. Other common locations include the posterior spinal elements and the pelvis. Patients often have a history of pain and swelling, usually of less than 6 months duration (267). On pathologic examination, the underlying bone is replaced by cavities of various sizes filled with blood or sometimes with proteinaceous material. There is a variable amount of fibrous and osseous structure within the lesion (268).

In the long bones, the typical radiographic appearance of an ABC is one of a lytic, eccentric metaphyseal lesion. In the smaller tubular and flat bones, the ABC may be central (Fig. 5-94). The lesion may go through the following stages: initial—well-defined osteolysis with periosteal elevation; active growth—a "blown-out" appearance with an expanded outer cortex that is so thinned as to appear absent, somewhat suggesting malignancy; stabilization—maturation of the bony shell giving a "soap bubble" appearance, with a distinct bony shell and osseous septa; and healing—progressive calcification and ossification (268). The delicate trabeculated appearance seen in the stabilization

stage may be formed by periosteal ridges rather than true bony septa (267).

An ABC typically appears as a well-defined lesion with lobular contours on both CT and MRI. Multiple fluid-fluid levels from the various components of blood and cellular debris, separated by fibrous septae, suggest this diagnosis (Fig. 5-94B). The fluid levels are readily seen on T1-weighted, T2-weighted, and STIR MRI sequences (269). Following gadolinium administration there is enhancement of the septa, which helps to delineate them from the fluid they contain (Fig. 5-95). Fluid-fluid levels are nonspecific and can be seen in unicameral bone cysts, fibrous dysplasia, osteosarcomas (especially the telangiectatic form), malignant fibrous histiocytomas, soft-tissue sarcomas, and vascular malformations (191).

An ABC can heal spontaneously, after curettage and bone grafting, or after surgical removal. Up to 44% of lesions recur within 2 years of surgical excision. An even higher percentage recur after curettage; one series found a 100% recurrence rate in young children with aggressive lesions treated with curettage and grafting (270). If a coexistent lesion is identified, treatment of that lesion is mandatory. Selective arterial embolization has proven useful, both as a primary treatment and preoperatively (especially for lesions of the spine, and pelvis) to minimize blood loss (271).

Cartilaginous Lesions

Osteochondroma. Osteochondroma (osteocartilaginous exostosis) is a very common benign lesion in children. It is derived from aberrant growth cartilage that separates from the edge of the physis, proliferates, and subsequently undergoes endochondral ossification (272). The presenting complaint is typically a hard, slowly enlarging mass near a joint. These children may have pain due to irritation of an adjacent muscle or neurovascular bundle or to inflammation of an overlying bursa (266). The lesions may enlarge into the third decade of life. Removal is indicated if there is damage to adjacent muscles or neurovascular structures, limitation of motion, sufficient discomfort or deformity, or suspicion of malignant degeneration.

The radiographic appearance is very characteristic: an ossified mass projecting out from a broad (sessile osteochondroma) or narrow (pedunculated osteochondroma) base. Pedunculated osteochondromas point away from the adjacent joint. There is an overlying cartilaginous cap, usually radiographically invisible, which may be greater than 1 cm thick in a growing child (91). The medullary cavity and cortices of the osteochondroma are in continuity with of the parent bone. Both CT and MRI help to assess complications from the mass effect, such as neurovascular bundle compromise (273). The lifetime incidence of malignant degeneration of a single lesion is low—probably less than 1% or 2%. Radiographic clues to degeneration include an indistinct bony mar-

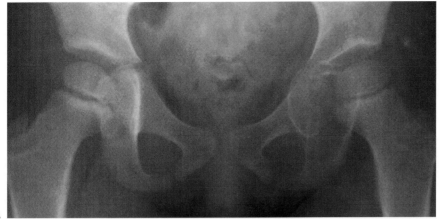

A

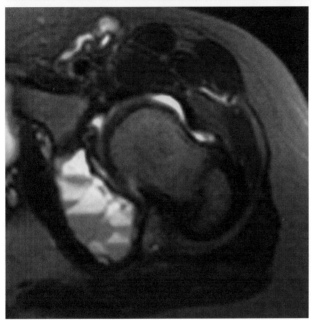

B

FIG. 5-94. Aneurysmal bone cyst. A: Frontal view of the pelvis of a 4-year-old girl with left hip pain. There is an expansile, lucent lesion of the left ischium. **B:** An axial T2-weighted MR image of the left hip shows many fluid-fluid levels within the expanded left ischium. The dependent layer contains red blood cells and the supernatant represents plasma.

gin, especially near the cap, an enlarging soft-tissue mass, and an area of lucency within the osteochondroma (91). MRI with gadolinium enhancement may help to determine the histopathologic characteristics of the cartilaginous cap. Peripheral enhancement suggests benignity (Fig. 5-96), whereas septal enhancement in fibrovascular bundles is suggestive of a low-grade chondrosarcoma. Inhomogeneous or homogenous enhancement of the cartilaginous cap suggests a higher grade chondrosarcoma (274).

The development of an osteochondroma following therapeutic radiation is well documented (see Fig. 5-89). Radiation results in either disorganization or growth arrest of the physis. The development of an osteochondroma and subsequent sarcomatous degeneration is directly related to the dose of radiation (275). Other osteochondromas follow skeletal trauma.

Enchondroma. An enchondroma is a central metaphyseal lesion that probably arises from actively proliferating physeal cartilage that has failed to undergo normal endochondral

ossification (272). Residual cartilage from the original cartilaginous anlage of the bone may also be responsible for the formation of an enchondroma (266). Solitary enchondromas are usually found in the small tubular bones of the hand and feet. Other sites include the femur and humerus.

On radiographs, the lesion usually is radiolucent. As the patient ages, the lesion may develop ring-like areas of calcification. Periosteal reaction is absent. An enchondroma may be noted incidentally or at the time of a pathologic fracture. Although sarcomatous degeneration in children is rare, especially in the bones of the hand and foot, it must be suspected if a lesion is progressively destructive, becomes painful, or enlarges after normal bone growth ceases (266). The typical gadolinium-enhanced MRI appearance of an enchondroma is one of rings and arcs, which reflect the lobular growth pattern. However, this enhancement pattern does not necessarily differentiate benignity from malignancy (276).

Chondroblastoma. A chondroblastoma (Codman tumor) is a benign tumor that is typically found in the second decade

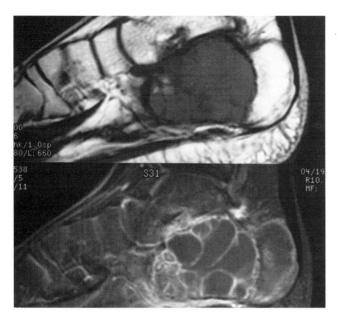

FIG. 5-95. Aneurysmal bone cyst. Sagittal pre- *(top)* and post- *(bottom)* gadolinium-enhanced MR images of the foot of a 13-year-old boy show an expansile mass in the anterior part of the calcaneus. Following gadolinium administration (T1-weighted fat suppressed image), there is enhancement of the lobular septa. The central nonenhancing cavities are fluid-filled.

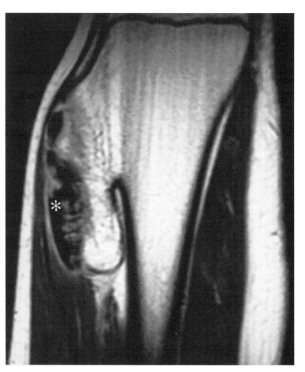

FIG. 5-96. Osteochondroma. Sagittal T1-weighted MR image of the tibia of a 14-year-old girl following gadolinium enhancement shows a large osteochondroma projecting from the proximal tibial metaphysis. The enhancement of the cartilaginous cap *(asterisk)* is predominantly peripheral.

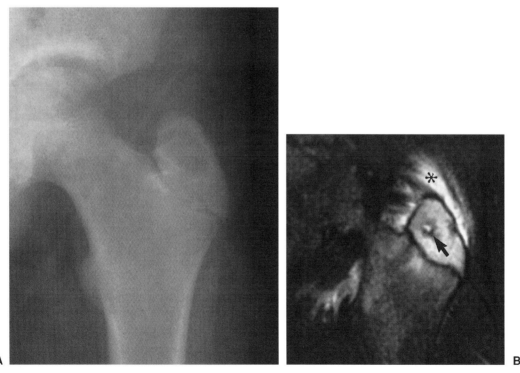

FIG. 5-97. Chondroblastoma. A: This 11-year-old girl developed left hip pain. There is an ovoid well-marginated lucent lesion in the greater trochanter. **B:** Coronal T2-weighted fat-suppressed MR image of the greater trochanter shows high signal in the lesion *(arrow)* and the surrounding gluteal muscles *(asterisk)*.

of life when the physes are still open. It usually occurs in the epiphyses of long bones, especially in the proximal humerus or femur or in epiphyseal equivalents (Fig. 5-97A). There may be extension into the adjacent metaphysis in older patients. On radiographs, it is a well-defined lucent lesion that sometimes expands the adjacent cortex. There may be stippled calcification of the chondroid matrix. A thick solid or layered periosteal reaction is present in approximately 50% of chondroblastomas found at sites with periosteum (277). The differential diagnosis of this radiographic appearance includes chronic infection, eosinophilic granuloma, osteoblastoma, giant cell tumor, and aneurysmal bone cyst. The preferred treatment is curettage and bone grafting; however, recurrences do occur, necessitating further surgery (266).

The MRI appearance of chondroblastoma may be misleading because of variable amounts of soft tissue and bone marrow edema that can simulate a more aggressive lesion (Fig. 5-97B). These changes presumably are due to inflammation and hyperemia. Other benign lesions with MRI demonstration of prominent surrounding edema include osteomyelitis, osteoblastoma, eosinophilic granuloma, and osteoid osteoma (278). The lesion itself has a heterogeneous intermediate T2-weighted signal with a lobular architecture. Gadolinium enhancement is more pronounced in the surrounding soft tissues than in the lesion itself (278).

Chondromyxoid Fibroma. Chondromyxoid fibroma is an infrequent benign tumor of the second or third decade of life. Patients typically complain of dull pain over the affected bone (266). Most lesions occur in the long bones; half are located about the knee. On radiographs, chondromyxoid fibroma is an eccentric metaphyseal lucency. It may be lobulated and septated, often expanding and attenuating the cortex (Fig. 5-98). The pattern of destruction is geographic and well circumscribed, and the rim may be sclerotic. Internal calcification is rare, as is periosteal reaction. The appearance is not specific, and the differential diagnosis for a chondromyxoid fibroma should include more common lesions such as nonossifying fibroma and aneurysmal bone cyst. If there is epiphyseal involvement, chondroblastoma and, in older children or young adults, giant cell tumor should also be considered (279).

Osseous Lesions

Osteoid Osteoma and Osteoblastoma. Osteoid osteoma is a relatively common small benign bone lesion with a variable radiographic appearance. Debate persists as to whether it is a neoplasm or an inflammatory lesion. It is found most often in boys in their second decade. Pain becoming more severe and constant with time is usually the presenting symptom. The pain frequently is worse at night. In three quarters of patients, it is relieved by aspirin. Histologically, an osteoid osteoma is composed of osteoid and woven bone with an osteoblastic rim (280).

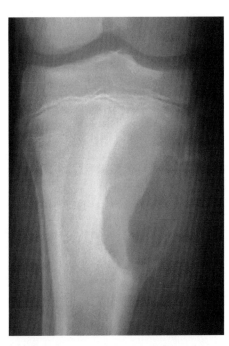

FIG. 5-98. Chondromyxoid fibroma. There is an eccentric, bubbly, lucent, expansile lesion of the medial part of the proximal tibial metaphysis in this 12-year-old girl. From Jaramillo and Cleveland (564).

The lesions are usually found in the cortices of the diaphyses or metadiaphyses of the long bones of the lower extremities. An osteoid osteoma typically does not exceed 1.5 cm in diameter (280). A radiolucent area representing the lesion itself is surrounded by a dense area of reactive sclerosis (Fig. 5-99A). Once the lucent nidus is removed or ablated, the sclerosis should resolve. Less often, the lesion is in a cancellous or intramedullary location. A cancellous osteoid osteoma often is intraarticular, especially within the hip joint, and incites a less intense sclerotic reaction than do lesions of compact cortical bone. The sclerosis may be distant from the lesion. When the lesion is intraarticular, synovitis and joint fluid may also be present. Other locations of cancellous osteoid osteomas include the small bones of the hands and feet and the posterior elements of the spinal column. In rare instances, an osteoid osteoma is located subperiosteally, where it produces almost no reactive sclerosis (280).

For the cortical lesions conventional radiography is usually diagnostic. Symptoms often develop well before the radiographs become positive, however, and in cases with referred pain, the lesion may not be included on the radiograph (280).

If the nidus is intramedullary, intraarticular, or subperiosteal, and is subtle or difficult to locate, scintigraphy and CT are useful (Figs. 5-99B,C and 5-100). Skeletal scintigraphy is useful in patients thought to have osteoid osteomas when the radiographs are negative or confusing. Osteoid osteomas show marked tracer localization on skeletal scintigraphy. While this is often apparent on all three phases of a three-phase study, the sensitivity of skeletal phase imaging to

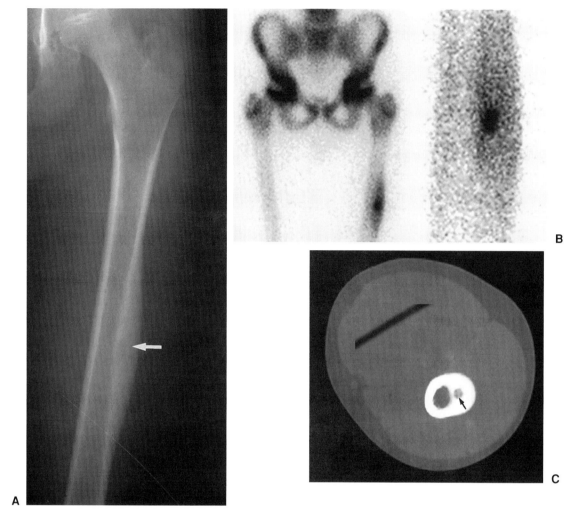

FIG. 5-99. Osteoid osteoma. A: Frontal view of the left femur of a 9-year-old boy shows fusiform thickening of the lateral cortex of the femoral diaphysis. A small lucent focus is barely visible in the midportion of the lesion *(arrow).* **B:** Skeletal scintigraphy *(left)* with pinhole magnification *(right)* shows a focal area of intense tracer uptake in the cortex of the middiaphysis of the left femur. **C:** Axial CT image shows extensive cortical thickening with a small rounded predominantly lucent nidus *(arrow).*

symptomatic lesions approaches 100% (281). Intense uptake in the nidus surrounded by less prominently increased uptake in reactive bone, the so-called ''double-density sign'' (282), is commonly seen with osteoid osteomas of the appendicular skeleton, particularly when pinhole magnification images are obtained (283). Although not entirely specific for osteoid osteoma, the pattern is highly suggestive and probably reflects the presence of a cortical nidus.

Scintigraphy is also valuable in planning and guiding the excision of osteoid osteomas. The nidus can be localized and its complete excision immediately confirmed with intraoperative pinhole magnification (284). The surgeon can thereby minimize the amount of bone removed, an important consideration in the weight-bearing bones and vertebrae (285).

Thin section CT helps to define the nidus, especially in areas of anatomic complexity (286). This localization facili-

tates the removal or curettage of the nidus, obviating the need for an en bloc resection of the entire sclerotic area (282). CT also locates the lesion precisely for percutaneous therapy. Approximately half of the lesions imaged with CT show mineralization of the nidus. MRI may be misleading, as it may show extensive edema of the marrow and surrounding soft tissues (286). Complete removal or ablation of the nidus, either surgically (266) or percutaneously, is curative (287,288).

The differential diagnosis of an osteoid osteoma includes a Brodie abscess. However, in this form of chronic osteomyelitis, the nidus is avascular and a sinus tract may be seen. A stress fracture (e.g., of the anterior tibial cortex) and chronic osteomyelitis without an abscess also may lead to sclerosis, but no lucent nidus is identified in these entities. Early stages of malignant neoplasms (such as Ewing sarcoma and osteosarcoma) occasionally appear similar on ra-

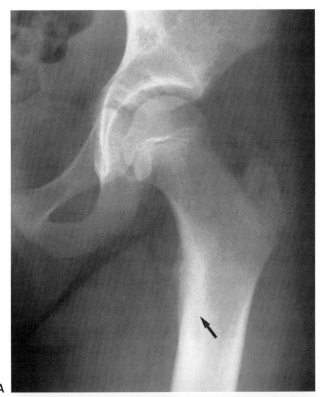

A

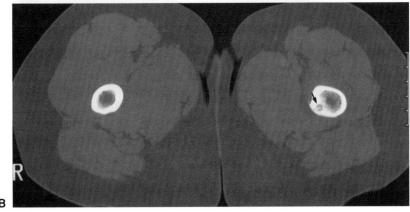

B

FIG. 5-100. Osteoid osteoma. A: 9-year-old girl with left hip pain. There is ill-defined sclerosis of the medial aspect of the proximal left femur *(arrow)*. **B:** Axial CT image of the thighs shows a small lucent nidus *(arrow)* within cortical sclerosis of the left proximal femur.

diographs. An intraarticular osteoid osteoma also can mimic inflammatory arthritis, septic arthritis, and nonspecific synovitis.

Although the histology of osteoid osteoma is similar to that of an osteoblastoma, the latter lesion is less painful and the pain does not respond to aspirin. An osteoblastoma exhibits progressive growth and is larger than 1.5 cm when seen (280). It is more commonly located in the axial skeleton, exhibits less sclerosis, and may have a more expansive, blown-out appearance (289).

Fibrous Lesions

Osteofibrous Dysplasia, Adamantinoma, and Monostotic Fibrous Dysplasia. Osteofibrous dysplasia is known also as *ossifying fibroma, congenital osteitis fibrosa, congenital fibrous dysplasia, fibroosseus dysplasia, congenital fibrous defect of the tibia,* and *Campanacci disease.* It is distinct from polyostotic fibrous dysplasia (discussed previously) and monostotic fibrous dysplasia (discussed below). Osteofibrous dysplasia is a proliferation of fibrous tissue that produces a well-defined, lucent or ground-glass uni- or multilocular lesion. It usually is located in the anterior diaphyseal cortex of the tibia or fibula (Fig. 5-101). It generally involves only one bone but can be bilateral. A sclerotic margin is common. Osteofibrous dysplasia is strictly cortical and does not invade the surrounding soft tissues. Boys and girls in the first decade are affected equally. Two thirds present before the age of 5 years, usually because of anterior tibial bowing or a pathologic fracture (290) but sometimes with a slowly growing painless mass over the anterior surface of

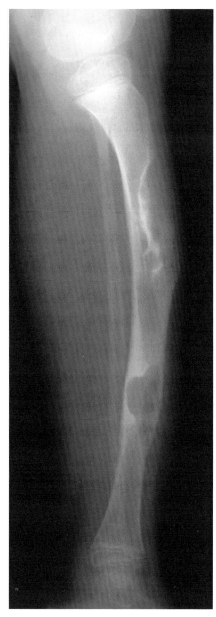

FIG. 5-101. Osteofibrous dysplasia. Lateral view of the tibia of an 8-year-old boy shows a multifocal, multilocular, relatively lucent lesion in the anterior aspect of the diaphyseal cortex of the tibia. There is anterior tibial bowing.

the tibia. The lesion may remain stable, regress spontaneously, or progress until skeletal maturity. Therapy is conservative unless a pathologic fracture or pseudarthrosis develops. Osteofibrous dysplasia is histologically benign but locally aggressive. It usually recurs after resection (266).

Osteofibrous dysplasia should be differentiated from adamantinoma. This rare malignant lesion usually occurs in female patients between 10 and 30 years of age. The tibia is affected almost exclusively. The radiographic appearance may be identical to that of osteofibrous dysplasia. It is recommended that skeletally immature patients who have a lesion with this appearance in the anterior tibial cortex have

radiographs at least every six months (266). If there is progression, biopsy is indicated. If the lesion presents after the physes have fused, resection is suggested because of the risk of adamantinoma (266).

Monostotic fibrous dysplasia also may radiographically resemble osteofibrous dysplasia on radiographs. However, monostotic fibrous dysplasia is typically intramedullary and tends not to be seen until the second decade of life (290). Histologically, active osteoblasts surround scattered bony trabeculae. There is woven bone centrally and lamellar bone peripherally. This pattern is referred to as "zonal architecture" (290).

Soft-Tissue Lesions

Fibromatosis. The fibromatoses are a group of histologically benign but locally aggressive tumors of proliferating fibrous tissue that occur in both the superficial and deep tissues of the body. Their typical infiltrative growth pattern can grossly and microscopically mimic malignancy. They can involve subcutaneous tissues, muscles, nerves, vascular channels, and (rarely) bone (291). The superficial lesions can be diagnosed by physical examination, whereas the deeper lesions require imaging to determine their extent. The infantile desmoid-type fibromatosis usually originates in skeletal muscle or in adjacent fascia, aponeuroses, or periosteum. It almost always is found before the fifth year of life, typically in the first or second year (292). Treatment of fibromatosis is wide surgical excision. Although the lesions do not metastasize, they may recur locally.

The lesions are formed by various amounts of myofibroblasts and collagen. A soft-tissue mass without distinguishing features is seen on radiographs. The rare intraosseous lesions tend to be medullary, multilobulated, well-defined lucencies. On ultrasonography the lesions are homogeneous and hypoechoic. The MRI appearance of fibromatosis reflects its diversity in composition. On T1-weighted images, the lesions usually are of low signal intensity. On T2-weighted images the lesions range from hypointensity, presumably due to abundant collagen and little cellularity, to hyperintensity, from greater cellularity and less collagen. In general, early fibromatosis is more hyperintense on T2-weighted images than more mature fibromatosis (291,293). The lesions usually enhance after gadolinium administration, which distinguishes them from the adjacent muscles.

Hemangiomas and Vascular Malformations. The confusing nomenclature of vascular lesions has led to a poor understanding of the pathophysiology, natural history, and therapy of these abnormalities. Mulliken and Glowacki (294) have devised a classification system for these lesions based on their endothelial characteristics. There are two major types of vascular lesions: those with rapid neonatal growth (characterized by hypercellularity) and eventual involution (diminished cellularity and increasing fibrosis) known as *hemangiomas*; and those that are present at birth, have a normal

TABLE 5-14. *Characteristics of hemangiomas and vascular malformations*

Hemangioma	Vascular malformation
Rapid endothelial cell proliferation and slow involution	Normal cellular turnover
30% present at birth	90% recognized at birth
Rapid postnatal growth	Grows commensurately with child
Female/male, 3:1	Female/male, 1:1
	Venous, capillary, lymphatic, arterial, combined

Modified from Mulliken (294, 565).

rate of endothelial turnover, and grow commensurately with the child, known as *vascular malformations.* The former are tumors; the latter are anomalies. Hemangiomas are the most common vascular tumors of infancy. They are present at birth but typically are not recognized until several weeks of life. These benign endothelial neoplasms grow rapidly and then, months or years later, usually regress. Vascular malformations, however, are developmental abnormalities and fail to regress. They may be composed of any combination of vascular channels: venous, capillary, lymphatic, and arterial, with or without fistulas (295). They may be superficial or deep and may involve the soft tissues, bones, or both. The two types of lesion can usually be differentiated by the history and physical examination (Table 5-14).

The aim of radiologic evaluation is to define tissue characteristics and to show extent. Involvement can be central, appendicular, or both (296). Conventional radiography is used to find and evaluate osseous abnormalities such as leg length discrepancy. Although ultrasonography and CT can show extent, MRI is used for more complete evaluation. MRI can define the type of channel in a vascular malformation (Table 5-15). For example, it can show high-flow feeding vessels typically seen with hemangiomas or arterial lesions (296).

Venous malformations are the most common vascular anomaly. Radiographs show areas of soft-tissue enlargement and occasionally small phleboliths (Fig. 5-102A). The lesions appear cystic on MRI and enhance throughout with intravenous gadolinium. Fluid-fluid levels can be seen (Fig. 5-102B). No high-flow vessels should be identified on gradient recalled echo sequences. Lymphatic malformations are also cystic but show only septal enhancement on MRI (Table 5-15). The differential diagnosis of vascular lesions includes hematomas and soft-tissue sarcomas.

Therapy for those rare hemangiomas that do not involute includes corticosteroids and α-interferon. Hemorrhage from severe thrombocytopenia in association with a large hemangioma is known as the *Kasabach-Merritt syndrome.* This has a mortality rate of 30% to 40% (295). Unlike hemangiomas, vascular malformations do not respond to pharmacologic therapy. Depending on the type and extent, they are treated with excision, embolization, or sclerotherapy (295).

Soft-Tissue Calcification; Myositis Ossificans. Calcification, somtimes progressing to ossification, may occur in skin, subcutaneous tissues, muscles, cartilage, joints, and vascular structures. Dystrophic soft-tissue calcification occurs in a number of the collagen vascular diseases, particularly in poorly controlled dermatomyositis (see Fig. 5-74). Other causes of soft-tissue calcification include trauma to the soft tissues (e.g., burns, foreign body, chronic infection), myositis ossificans (see below), tumoral calcinosis, renal osteodystrophy, hypercalcemic states, hypervitaminosis D, and a variety of syndromes.

The occurrence of heterotopic calcification and ossification in the soft tissues is termed *myositis ossificans.* It may be generalized as in fibrodysplasia ossificans progressiva (a very uncommon familial disorder) or localized to one region, often after trauma. The latter entity is referred to as *myositis ossificans circumscripta, heterotopic ossification,* and *pseudomalignant osseous tumor of soft tissue* (297).

Myositis ossificans circumscripta, a tumor-like soft-tissue mass, is a benign, self-limiting condition. Twenty-five to forty percent of patients give no history of trauma (4). Although myositis ossificans can be an incidental finding, patients usually present with pain, tenderness, and a palpable mass in or near the large skeletal muscles.

On pathologic examination, the lesions are well circumscribed with a distinct zonal architecture. The center is a nonossified cellular focus, with hemorrhagic cystic spaces. Maturation—progression to osteoid and then to mature lamellar bone—increases toward the periphery of the lesion.

TABLE 5-15. *MRI evaluation of vascular anomalies*

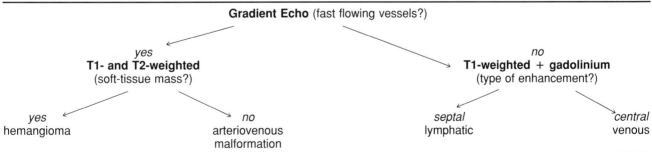

Modified from Meyer (296).

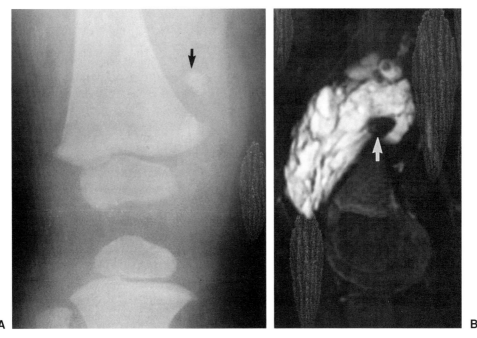

FIG. 5-102. Venous malformation. A: 13-month-old girl with a left knee mass. There is soft-tissue fullness and a large phlebolith *(arrow)*. **B:** Sagittal T2-weighted MR image of the thigh shows a multilocular lesion of high signal containing fluid-fluid levels. The phlebolith *(arrow)* is seen again.

As the lesion ages, the center is eventually replaced by mature bone (298).

Within 2–6 weeks of the onset of symptoms, feathery calcification can be detected on radiographs. By 6–8 weeks a well-demarcated bony mass is present (Fig. 5-103A). It decreases in size over the next 5–6 months. The lesion is usually adjacent to bone but separated from it by a thin area of radiolucency. Periosteal reaction can be seen (297). The process is self-limited. Further injury to the involved tissues should be avoided. Excision is rarely required.

Skeletal scintigraphy shows intense tracer uptake at first, but this decreases as the lesion matures. The CT appearance is very characteristic, with a well-defined rim of mineralization seen at several weeks. The center may be of low attenuation because of inflammation or hemorrhage. Occasionally fluid-fluid levels from hemorrhage are identified (Fig. 5-103B). The typical zonal pattern of more mature and sharply defined mineralization in the periphery is seen on both radiographs and CT; this helps to differentiate myositis ossificans from parosteal and extraskeletal osteosarcoma (297).

MRI, like CT, can show fluid-fluid levels. The more active lesions enhance after intravenous contrast administration. Extensive surrounding edema and a mass effect are most evident on MRI and can erroneously suggest soft-tissue malignancy (297). In cases of myositis, CT is the imaging modality of choice.

Langerhans Cell Histiocytosis

Langerhans cell histiocytosis (LCH; histiocytosis X) is a disease group characterized by an abnormal proliferation of Langerhans cell histiocytes. LCH manifests itself focally or systemically (299). The etiology remains unknown, although abnormal immune regulation with proliferation of histiocytes and granuloma formation has been suggested. No infectious organism has been isolated from LCH lesions (299). Recent work has suggested a neoplastic process, as a clonal proliferation of cells has been isolated from some lesions (300). Boys are affected about twice as often as girls. The disorder is rare in non-Caucasian patients (299). The disease process causes a broad spectrum of pathologic changes. The course ranges from benign to highly malignant. The numerous sites of involvement reflect the widespread distribution of the reticuloendothelial system. The osseous findings are dependent on the phase of the disease and may mimic infection, benign neoplasm, and malignant neoplasm.

Classification. Lichtenstein (301) first proposed the term histiocytosis X to include eosinophilic granuloma, Letterer-Siwe disease, and Hand-Schüller-Christian disease. Although there are sizable overlaps in these diseases and many difficulties with the classification, radiologists should be familiar with some of the pertinent features of these subgroups. As many as 50% of cases of histiocytosis cannot easily be placed in one of the syndromes. Moreover, there may be evolution from one syndrome into another. The extent of disease and age at presentation are important prognostic indicators.

Letterer-Siwe disease. Letterer-Siwe disease, the acute, disseminated form of histiocytosis throughout the reticuloendothelial system, usually has its onset during the first year of life. It accounts for approximately 10% of LCH cases (299). Clinical and laboratory features include hepatospleno-

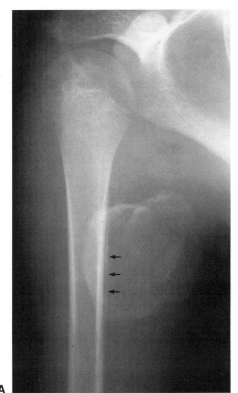

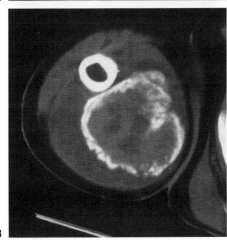

FIG. 5-103. Myositis ossificans. An 11-year-old girl presented with an upper arm mass 2 weeks after beginning field hockey practice. **A:** In the soft tissues of the upper arm, there is a well-demarcated, lobular density with peripheral mineralization. There is periosteal reaction *(arrows)* along the medial humeral shaft. **B:** Axial CT image through the upper arm shows a well-defined rim of mineralization at the periphery of the lesion, which is in the triceps muscle. Internal low attenuation fluid-fluid levels are probably due to hemorrhage.

megaly, lymphadenopathy, cutaneous lesions, purpura, otitis media, pulmonary involvement, anemia, leukopenia, and thrombocytopenia (200). There is rapid progression of soft tissue and visceral involvement. There may be no radiographically evident skeletal abnormality, except for diffuse osteopenia, despite extensive bone marrow involvement. Death usually occurs within 1 or 2 years (299).

Hand-Schüller-Christian disease. Hand-Schüller-Christian disease is the chronic, recurrent form of disseminated histiocytosis. It affects bone and extraosseous sites and accounts for approximately 20% of the patients with LCH (299). Most of these patients are between 3 and 6 years of age. Symptoms include bone pain, diabetes insipidus, exophthalmos, growth retardation, dermatitis, draining ears, lymphadenopathy, hepatosplenomegaly, anemia, and pulmonary involvement (200). The classic triad, which occurs in only 10% of patients with Hand-Schüller-Christian disease, is composed of areas of cranial destruction, exophthalmos (due to a mass effect on the globe), and diabetes insipidus (from involvement of the base of the skull or neurohypophysis). Skeletal lesions are detectable radiographically in more than 80% of patients, particularly in the skull. The prognosis is related to the extent of involvement. Dysfunction and morbidity are usually high.

Eosinophilic granuloma. Eosinophilic granuloma is the localized osseous or pulmonary form of LCH. It is a disease of children and young adults, the average age of onset being 10–14 years. The disease is usually monostotic and has an excellent prognosis (200). The patients develop local pain, tenderness, decreased motion, and soft-tissue swelling (200). Mastoid involvement may result in a draining ear. Back pain and scoliosis suggest a spinal lesion. The occasional clinical presentation of fever, elevated erythrocyte sedimentation rate, mild leukocytosis, and anemia may suggest infection (299).

In patients with disseminated disease, the symptoms of weakness, weight loss, anorexia, fever, irritability, lethargy, diarrhea, and failure to thrive may reflect direct involvement of organs or simply the presence of a chronic debilitating disease. Patients with monostotic involvement may be totally asymptomatic.

Laboratory studies are frequently normal. The diagnosis of LCH is based on consistent clinical features, radiologic abnormalities, pathologic changes, and exclusion of similar entities. Therapy varies with the extent of disease. It may involve observation without intervention, intraosseous steroid administration, low-dose radiation, or chemotherapy. In general, chemotherapy is not used for isolated skeletal disease (299). The prognosis for patients with skeletal disease without organ dysfunction is excellent (302).

Radiologic Features.

Skeletal findings. Skeletal involvement is the most common radiographic abnormality in histiocytosis (302). The extensive distribution of reticuloendothelial cells accounts for the numerous sites of bony involvement (Table 5-16). The radiologic appearance depends on the bone involved and the stage of the disease (299). Widespread dissemination of disease manifests as diffuse osteopenia, prominence of trabeculae, and decreased cortical thickness. More commonly, there are well-defined areas of cortical or medullary rarefaction, with or without sclerotic margins. There may be bone expansion, periosteal reaction, soft-tissue masses, and pathologic fractures. In the tubular bones of the young child,

TABLE 5-16. *Sites of skeletal involvement in Lagerhans cell histocytosis*

Site	Incidence (%)
Skull	27.8
Ribs	13.5
Femur	13.2
Pelvis	9.9
Spine	6.9
Mandible	6.5
Humerus	6.3
Scapula	4.4
Tibia	3.6
Clavicle	2.8
Radius	1.5
Maxilla	1.3
Fibula	1.1
Ulna	0.5
Hands and feet	0.5
Sternum	0.2
Total	100.0

Source: Modified from Kirks and Taybi in Parker and Castellino (200).

the characteristic pattern of a lytic lesion with a benign-appearing thick periosteal reaction may be seen. With healing and bone regeneration, there is sclerosis (especially above the orbits), prominence of the trabecular pattern, thickening of the cortex secondary to periosteal reaction, or complete return to normal (200).

Skull. The skull is the most common site of skeletal involvement in histiocytosis (Table 5-16). Uneven destruction of the inner and outer tables of the skull gives the lesions a beveled edge (Fig. 5-104A). Extension into the soft tissues or epidural space may occur. A button sequestrum is a round, radiolucent skull defect with a central nidus or sequestrum of intact bone; LCH is a common cause of this peculiar calvarial lesion in children. The calvaria, sella turcica, mastoids, orbits, and the mandible are frequently involved (Fig. 5-104B). Histiocytosis is the most common cause of multiple "floating teeth" in children (Fig. 5-104C), but this finding may also occur in infection, fibrous dysplasia, hyperparathyroidism, familial dysproteinemia, primary neoplasm, and metastatic neoplasm.

Ribs. Ribs are the second most common site of bony involvement (Table 5-16), and the lesions are frequently multiple. The ribs frequently become expanded and multilocular. Extrapleural masses may develop from extension into the soft tissues. There may be pathologic fractures.

Pelvis and scapula. Lytic lesions of pelvis and scapula are common (Fig. 5-104D–F; Table 5-16). These lesions are well defined. Periosteal reaction is infrequent. Sclerotic margins are common in the pelvis. Any supraacetabular lytic lesion in a child raises the possibility of histiocytosis (200).

Long bones. Long bone involvement is less frequent than flat bone involvement. The femur is the most commonly involved long bone, followed by the humerus, tibia, radius, fibula, and ulna (Table 5-16; Fig. 5-104F). These bones often

show a long area of mottled destruction. Unlike lesions of flat bones, there is often reactive sclerosis and periosteal reaction as the lesion matures (Fig. 5-104G). The diaphysis is more commonly involved than the metaphysis; although unusual, the epiphysis may also be involved (Fig. 5-104D,E).

Spine. The spine is frequently involved in histiocytosis. Radiologic findings include lytic destruction, extreme vertebral collapse ("vertebra plana") (Fig. 5-104F), and a soft-tissue paravertebral mass. Vertebra plana is highly suggestive of histiocytosis in countries where tuberculosis and tropical fungi are not prevalent. It may partly be a result of painless weakening of a vertebral body, which remains subject to normal vigorous childhood weight bearing. Considerable reconstitution of vertebral body height can occur over years.

Extraskeletal lesions. LCH may involve the mediastinum, pulmonary parenchyma, pleura, gastrointestinal tract, liver, spleen, and central nervous system (200). The radiologic evaluation is based on the child's symptoms. Although LCH is an uncommon disease, radiology is critical in its recognition, the determination of extent of disease, and the localization of lesions for biopsy.

The basic evaluation in any patient with histiocytosis includes chest radiography and a complete skeletal survey. Skeletal scintigraphy may be performed to identify lesions that are not evident on radiographs. However, the scintigraphic manifestations of LCH lesions vary. Particularly in the calvaria, the lesions frequently cause decreased tracer localization with or without surrounding circumferential increased localization. Some lesions cause increased tracer localization only. LCH lesions may escape scintigraphic detection when they are small or fail to incite a significant osteoblastic response (299,303). These are the reasons why skeletal scintigraphy should be obtained only as a complementary procedure in LCH (304).

The extent of bony destruction can be evaluated with CT. MRI also is used to delineate an osseous lesion, especially in areas of complex anatomy (e.g., skull, facial bones, and pelvis), and to better delineate extension into the adjacent soft tissue (305). It is particularly helpful for evaluation of the brain and spinal canal (306). On MRI, the area of abnormal signal intensity is typically greater than conventional radiography suggests. The lesions usually are hypointense on T1-weighted images, hyperintense on T2-weighted and STIR MR images, and hyperintense on gadolinium-enhanced images (Fig. 5-104E). Abnormal signal in the soft tissue and bone marrow is a prominent feature, but MRI cannot reliably differentiate actual LCH involvement from edema. Decreased T2-weighted signal intensity and decreased gadolinium enhancement may reflect response to therapy (307).

The differential diagnosis for the osseous lesions of LCH depends on the area and extent of involvement. The lesions may resemble fibrous dysplasia, unicameral and aneurysmal bone cysts, chondromyxoid fibroma, enchondroma, hemo-

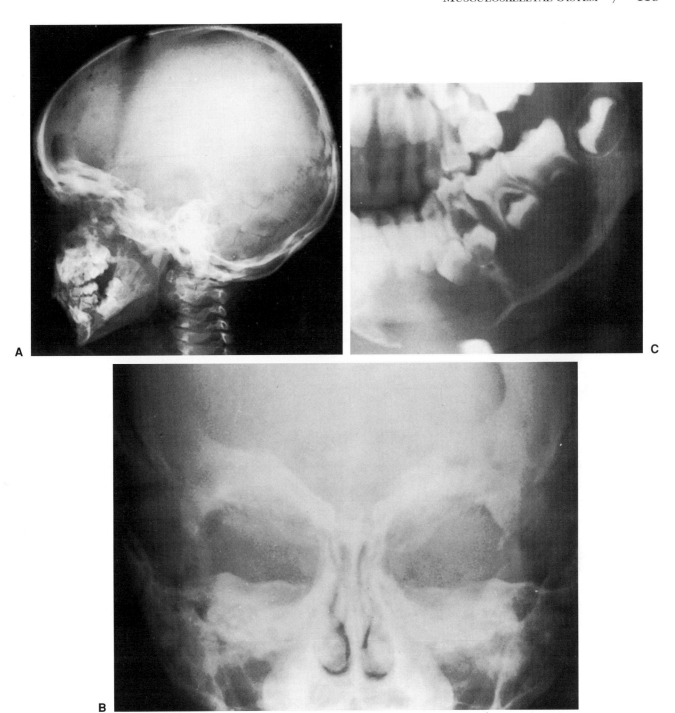

FIG. 5-104. Various radiographic manifestations of Langerhans cell histiocytosis. A: Many geographic lytic lesions of the calvaria and sutural diastasis. **B:** Thickening and sclerosis of orbits produce a raccoon appearance. **C:** A 5-year-old boy with swelling of the left jaw. Panorex view of the mandible shows two lytic lesions of the alveolar ridge, producing "floating teeth."

philiac pseudotumor, and more aggressive lesions such as Ewing sarcoma, lymphoma, and leukemia (299). Lesions that involve the epiphyses should be differentiated from infection (including tuberculosis) and chondroblastoma. Calvarial lesions may mimic osteomyelitis, vascular malformations, fibrous dysplasia, epidermoid or dermoid cysts, and metastatic lesions such as neuroblastoma.

Fractures and Other Injuries in Children

Regarding pediatric fractures, there is both good news and bad news. The good news is that healing is usually prompt, and growth and remodeling can correct most traumatic deformities. The bad news is that fractures involving growing bone (particularly the physis) may cause

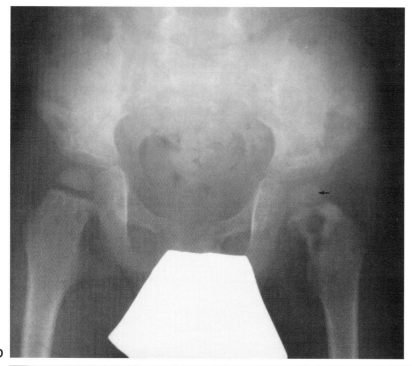

D

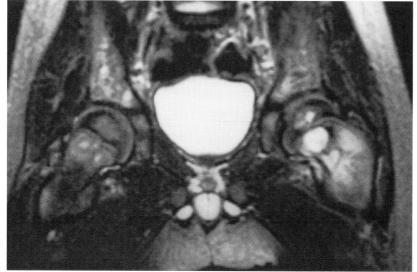

E

FIG. 5-104. *Continued.* **D:** There are multiple osteolytic lesions within the proximal femoral metaphyses and ilia. There also is a lucent lesion of the left femoral epiphysis *(arrow).* **E:** Coronal T2-weighted MR image of the pelvis in the same boy shows multiple rounded high signal lesions within the ilia, proximal femoral metaphyses, and left femoral epiphysis. There is edema in the left femoral neck, distal to the lesions.

subsequent deformity (308), often irremediable without surgery.

General Principles

Fractures in children differ from those in adults in regard to pattern, diagnosis, and treatment. These distinctions are due to differences in anatomy, biomechanics, and physiology (309).

Anatomic Differences

The important anatomic differences between children and adults relate to the physis, the regional blood supply, the cortex, and the periosteum. A critical part of a child's skeleton is nonradiopaque growth cartilage. Acute injury to this physeal cartilage can be diagnosed with radiography only by changes in its width or by findings in adjacent bone. The physis is avascular after infancy, but it maintains a delicate interaction with the blood vessels of the epiphysis and metaphysis (17,310). The supply of oxygen and nutrients to the epiphysis and most of the layers of the physis comes from the epiphyseal vessels. These usually originate from vessels in the adjacent joint capsule. The diaphysis is supplied by periosteal vessels and by nutrient vessels that enter the bone in the midshaft, at the site of the earliest ossification of the bone, and branch toward the metaphyses. Metaphyseal vessels interact with the chondrocytes of the hypertrophic zone of the physis as part of the process of chondrocyte death

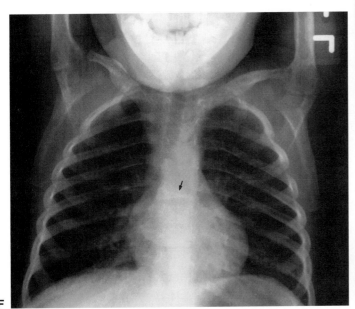
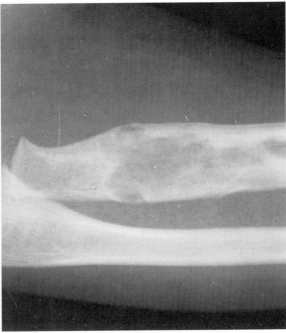

F

G

FIG. 5-104. *Continued.* **F:** Radiograph of the chest shows multiple lytic lesions in the proximal humeri, left clavicle, and both scapulas. The T6 vertebral body *(arrow)* is compressed (vertebra plana). **G:** Lateral view of the forearm in a 3-1/2-year-old girl shows an expansile, lytic lesion of the proximal left radius with associated thick periosteal reaction.

and ossification. Injury to the epiphyseal vessels results in ischemic injury to the physeal chondrocytes and ultimately in growth arrest. Injury to the metaphyseal vessels results in blockage of endochondral ossification and persistence of cartilage within the metaphysis. Small vessels cross from the metaphysis into the epiphysis only during the first 18 months of life (308) and after physeal closure at maturity.

The periosteum is thicker and stronger in a child than in an adult, and it can rapidly produce exuberant callus. However, the attachments of periosteum to the shaft of bone are less firm in children than in adults (308). The firmest periosteal attachments are at the ends of long tubular bones at the physeal-metaphyseal junctions. Subperiosteal collections are thus common in children, but they typically stop at the zone of Ranvier.

Biomechanical Differences

A child's bone is more porous and can tolerate a greater deformation than the bone of an adult. To a certain extent, pediatric bones bend without breaking. The large Haversian canals in children retard extension of a fracture line. Compact adult bone fails only with tension, whereas more porous pediatric bone fails with compression as well as with tension (309). As the child matures, trabecular (woven) bone is transformed into dense, lamellar bone. This transformation begins in the diaphysis and progressively extends into the metaphysis (17).

The physeal region is the weakest part of the growing skeleton. Experimentally, because the physeal cartilage is not as strong as the periarticular ligaments (309), it is easier to produce separation at the physis than dislocation at the adjacent joint. The physis is most resistant to traction and least resistant to torsion. Considerable force is required to separate the epiphysis from the metaphysis unless there is division of the periosteum. Medial and lateral forces loosen the periosteum and cause separation at the physis rather than rupture or detachment of a ligament (309).

Transition points in the growing skeleton are particularly breakable. Buckle fractures occur at the metaphyseal transition of woven to lamellar bone. During the periods of fastest growth (infancy and puberty), fractures occur at the transition between the physeal cartilage and the metaphyseal bone (17,311). The periosteum is thicker, stronger, and less frequently torn in a child than in an adult, acts as a stabilizing force during trauma, and (unless torn) resists displacement at a fracture.

Physiologic Differences

Fracture healing is much faster in children than in adults. The injury hastens further the already fast osteosynthesis of the immature skeleton. A diaphyseal fracture in a newborn heals in about 2 weeks; a similar fracture in an adult heals in 3 or 4 months. Nonunion is rare in children (309). Fracture remodeling is also fast because of rapid bone turnover. Remodeling usually restores normal alignment in the plane of motion of the adjacent joint. It is less adequate when the angular deformity is not in the plane of the joint and when there is rotational deformity. For example, most supracondylar fractures initially have posterior angulation of the distal humeral fragment. The most common residual deformity, however, is varus angulation of the distal humerus, which is not corrected by the hinge motion of the elbow. Fracture healing results in longitudinal overgrowth during childhood, so that fractures of long bone shafts are usually allowed to heal with 1–2 cm of overriding. Fractures involving the physis can result in arrest of growth or angular deformity. This is usually due to the formation of a bony bridge across the injured physis (312).

Radiologic Evaluation

Fractures should be immobilized for comfort prior to radiographic examination. At least two orthogonal views of the affected bony structures should be obtained—frontal (AP or PA) and lateral views, if possible (308). For acetabular fractures, the second plane is optimally provided by axial CT (Fig. 5-105). The proximal and distal ends of the in-

volved bone should usually be included on the radiographs. Supplementary and comparison views may be required, but comparison views of the other side should not be routine, except in the hips.

Types of Pediatric Fractures

Complete Diaphyseal Fractures. Complete diaphyseal fractures (Fig. 5-106) involve the shaft of a tubular bone. Usually "union will occur so long as the fracture fragments are in the same room" (308). Remodeling overcomes most deformities if there are 2 years or more of remaining growth, if the fracture is near the end of a bone, and if the deformity is in the plane of motion of the adjacent joint. Remodeling cannot correct a displaced intraarticular fracture, a grossly deformed fracture in the middle of the shaft of a bone, a displaced fracture when the axis of displacement is at right angles to the plane of movement, a fracture in which the distal fragment is rotated with respect to the proximal, or a displaced fracture crossing the physis at right angles (309).

Reactive overgrowth after a femoral fracture can correct

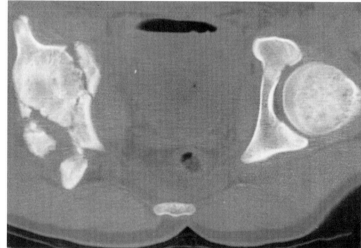

A

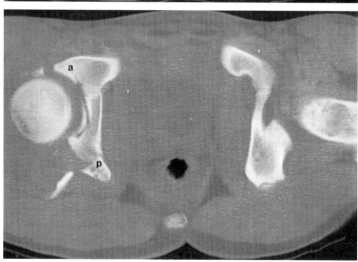

B

FIG. 5-105. Acetabular fracture. A 15-year-old boy with blunt trauma. **A, B:** Axial sections demonstrate unstable fractures involving both the anterior *(a)* and posterior *(p)* columns of the right acetabulum.

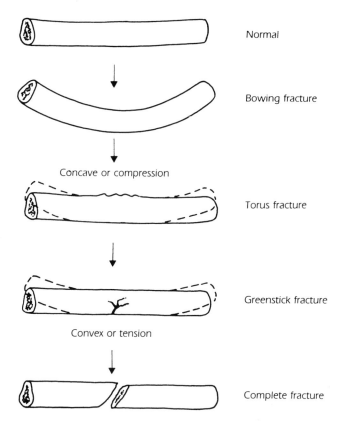

Normal

Bowing fracture

Concave or compression

Torus fracture

Greenstick fracture

Convex or tension

Complete fracture

FIG. 5-106. Types of pediatric fractures. Modified from Rang (309).

up to 2 cm of overriding. Any rotational deformity is bothersome, which is why joints proximal and distal to the fracture should be included in the radiograph. If the transverse widths of proximal and distal fragments are unequal, beyond inequality due to radiographic magnification, rotation may well be present.

After fracture, proximity of the radius to the ulna or the tibia to the fibula may lead to interosseous fusion and loss (in the forearm) of normal rotation. A fracture of one bone in the forearm or leg may be associated with a dislocation of the companion bone. Monteggia reported the association of proximal ulnar fracture and radial head dislocation. This should be suspected whenever an ulnar fracture is seen without an accompanying radial fracture. In children, isolated complete fractures of the ulna are rare (309). A line through the long axis of the radius should pass through the bone or cartilage of the capitellum in all views; failure to do so suggests dislocation of the radius. Galeazzi noted the association of fractures of the radius with dislocation of the distal radioulnar joint. Galeazzi fracture dislocations are much less common than Monteggia injuries (313).

The fracture site always should be carefully examined for predisposing pathology, such as a local bone lesion (unicameral bone cyst [see Fig. 5-93], nonossifying fibroma, osteogenic sarcoma, Ewing sarcoma, fibrous dysplasia, osteomyelitis) or generalized osseous weakness (spinal dysraphism, cerebral palsy, poliomyelitis, muscular dystro-

phy, cerebral palsy, osteoporosis, hyperparathyroidism, osteogenesis imperfecta, certain osteochondrodysplasias).

Vascular injury may complicate any fracture. In children, the incidence of vascular damage is highest with supracondylar fractures of the elbow and fractures of the distal third of the femur (308).

Bowing Fractures. Traumatic bowing is due to an acute plastic deformation of bone, a response to longitudinal stress (Fig. 5-106). If one applies longitudinal compression to bone, at first the bone goes through a range of elastic deformation in which curvature appears but then it disappears as the force is released (Fig. 5-107). With greater force, microfractures appear on the concave side of the bowed bone, and there is a defined zone of plastic deformation (Fig. 5-107). A bowing fracture is produced if the force is removed at this point; the bone's capacity to rebound elastically has been exceeded. Continued force produces a frank fracture (Fig. 5-107). Porous pediatric bone is particularly susceptible to this sequence, which helps explain the various types of childhood fractures shown in Fig. 5-106. Increasing longitudinal compression of bone in children produces traumatic bowing, then a torus fracture, then a greenstick fracture, and eventually complete fracture.

Although acute traumatic bowing most frequently involves a forearm, similar deformities have been described in the femur (314) and fibula (315). Radiologically, one sees bowing of a long tubular bone (Fig. 5-108). Comparison views of the unaffected limb are often warranted, as the findings may be subtle. Scintigraphy demonstrates increased uptake of tracer along the concave margin of the bowed bone. There are usually fractures in the companion bone (316). Occasionally, there is dislocation of the unbowed companion bone at the wrist or elbow, or both bones are bowed. Plastic bowing of a fibula may prevent healing of a companion tibial fracture.

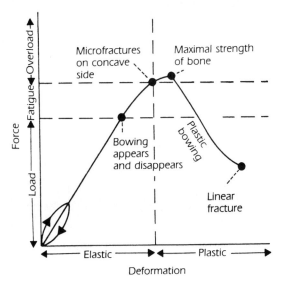

FIG. 5-107. Biomechanics of plastic bowing fractures. Modified from Borden (316).

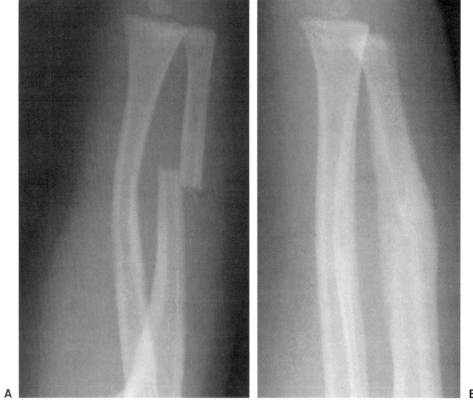

FIG. 5-108. Plastic bowing fracture. A 14-month-old girl who fell on her right wrist. **A:** There is a transverse fracture of the ulna and plastic bowing of the radius. **B:** Two months later there is periosteal reaction and remodeling of both bones.

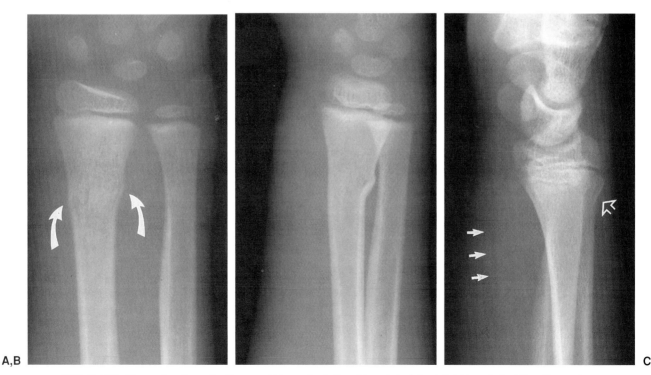

FIG. 5-109. Torus fracture. An 8-year-old boy who fell on his outstretched right hand. **A:** AP radiograph shows a buckle fracture involving the medial and lateral cortices of the distal radius *(arrows)*. This is a typical torus fracture. **B:** Lateral radiograph shows that the buckle is mostly dorsal. **C:** The same boy fell on the same hand at age 15 years. Lateral radiograph shows a dorsal buckle fracture *(open arrow)*. There is elevation of the pronator quadratus fat pad *(closed arrows)*.

Bowed forearm bones limit pronation and supination. A bowed bone remains bowed, resists attempts at reduction, holds an adjacent fracture in angulation, and prevents relocation of an adjacent dislocation (316). Vigorous manipulative force and general anesthesia may be required but may not suffice; occasionally the deformity requires surgical correction. Bowing deformities of less than 20° may remodel spontaneously, particularly in younger children (17).

Incomplete Linear Fractures. Compression failure, i.e., failure on the concave side of a bending bone (see Fig. 5-106), produces a buckle or torus fracture. *Torus* is a Latin word meaning protuberance, bulge, or round swelling. In architecture, a torus is an outward-bulging convex molding at the base of a classical column. The cortex of a bone is normally a smooth, curved line (down to the longitudinally straight 1- to 3-mm collar at the end of a young child's metaphysis). A torus fracture is an outward buckling of the cortical margin (Fig. 5-109). Torus fractures usually occur near the metaphysis, where the bone is most porous and the cortex thinnest. They are most frequent in the distal radial metaphysis and are best seen along the dorsal surface. These injuries usually occur in children who fall on an outstretched hand. There may be exquisite local tenderness. If AP and lateral views are equivocal, oblique projections should be obtained.

Greenstick Fractures. If a bone is angulated slightly beyond its limits of bending, a greenstick fracture is produced (Fig. 5-110). This fracture represents complete failure on the tension side of the bone but only bending on the compression side (see Fig. 5-106). The fracture occurs on the convex side of the bend. Subsequent marked elastic recoil, may improve the position (309). The fracture is often more nearly complete than the radiograph shows. It may later hinge open because of muscle pull.

Greenstick fractures are less common than torus fractures. One sees bending of the bone and an incomplete linear fracture extending from the convex side of the curvature. Because complete closure of the fracture may be prevented by spicules of bone, the treatment of midshaft greenstick fracture may be to convert it to a complete fracture, overcorrect the angulation, and then correctly position the bone for immobilization and healing.

Physeal Fractures

The understanding of physeal injuries has increased significantly since the publication of the classic article by Salter and Harris (311,317). The epiphyseal-metaphyseal complex, which consists of the epiphysis, physis, zone of Ranvier, and metaphysis, is involved in 6% to 18% of fractures of the long bones in children. Because in children the joint capsule and ligamentous structures are two to five times as strong as the physis (318), forces that produce a sprain or dislocation in the adult are more likely to cause a physeal fracture in the child.

If a joint dislocation or ligamentous injury is suspected, a physeal fracture must also be considered. The child with a physeal fracture usually complains of local pain and limitation of motion. If a child has point tenderness over the physis or localized soft-tissue swelling centered over the physis, the injury should be treated as a physeal fracture regardless of the radiographic appearance. Although the physis is weaker than the adjacent bone, fractures of osseous structures remain more common than demonstrable physeal fractures. The types of stress that cause physeal injuries are shearing or avulsion (80%) and splitting or compression (20%).

In a group of more than 1500 children with physeal injuries (319), the most frequent sites of fracture were the distal radius (28%), phalanges of the fingers (26%), distal tibia (less than 10%), distal humerus (7%), and phalanges of the toes (7%). Physeal injuries, like most fractures, are more common in boys; many occur during athletics. More than 75% of physeal fractures occur between the ages of 10 and 16 years; the median age is 13 years (317,318). An exception to this generalization is injury to the distal humerus (lateral condylar fracture), which usually occurs between the ages of 3 and 6 years. Preadolescent gymnasts may injure the distal radial physis from repeated trauma (320,321). The

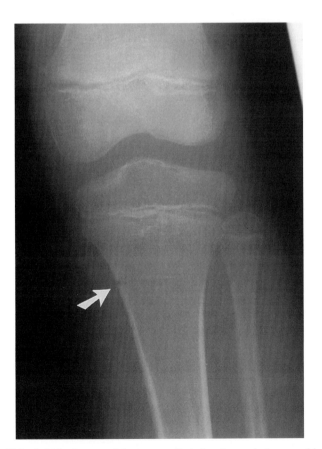

FIG. 5-110. Incomplete greenstick fracture. A 6-year-old girl with a linear incomplete fracture of the left proximal tibia after a fall. The greenstick fracture involves the medial cortex of the proximal left tibial metaphysis *(arrow)*. This fracture may result in tibia valga deformity.

physes of the knee (distal femur and proximal tibia) account for 3% of physeal injuries but are responsible for 53% of the cases of posttraumatic growth arrest (322).

Anatomy

The physis (growth plate, epiphyseal plate) consists of an ordered array of parallel columns of cartilage cells surrounded by the fibroosseous zone of Ranvier (323). Histologically, the three distinct zones identifiable in longitudinal section are the germinal or resting zone (stem cells adjacent to the epiphysis), proliferating zone (flattened cells arranged in columns), and hypertrophic zone (swollen and vacuolated cells). The zone of provisional calcification (dying chondrocytes with calcification of the matrix, adjacent to the metaphysis) is usually included as part of the hypertrophic zone (16) (Fig. 5-111). Following a fracture through the physis, there is rapid repair if there has been no damage to the germinal layer of cartilage cells or to the vascular supply. A transient increase in the thickness of the physis reaches its maximum in 10 days. The fracture is filled with fibrin, which is gradually resorbed; normal growth resumes in approximately 3 weeks.

Most epiphyses of long bones are partly extraarticular. The epiphyseal vessels, which supply the ossification center, the epiphyseal cartilage, and the physis, course directly from their origin into the epiphysis. A physeal injury usually does not compromise the epiphyseal vessels. In the proximal femur and radial head, however, the physes are wholly intraarticular. The epiphyseal vessels in these two regions must pass next to the physis en route to the epiphyseal centers, and injuries to the physis may involve the epiphyseal vessels as well. The vessels may be damaged before they enter the epiphysis, or the damage may occur intraepiphyseally with a crushing injury.

Pathophysiology

The cartilaginous matrix of the physis resists shearing forces. This strong matrix is abundant in the juxtaepiphyseal side of the physis, but the matrix becomes weaker (and more calcified) as the chondrocytes approach the metaphysis (hypertrophic zone and zone of provisional calcification). The more common shearing or avulsion forces are directed parallel to or away from the epiphyseal center. The hypertrophic zone is the most vulnerable to shearing injuries (311,317,324) (Figs. 5-111 and 5-112). Fractures through the hypertrophic zone usually cause no growth disturbance because the involved chondrocytes are already dying. In these injuries, the physis remains as an avascular barrier between epiphyseal and metaphyseal vessels (324). There is growing evidence, however, that in physeal injuries the fracture line may wander through the cartilage, particularly in areas of physeal undulation (322,325). Fractures extending into the epiphyseal side of the physis (germinal zone), although radiographically unimpressive, may result in growth arrest. This may explain why Salter-Harris fractures types 1 and 2 can lead to bony bridges in areas of physeal irregularity such as the intercondylar notch of the femur and the medial part of the distal tibia (326).

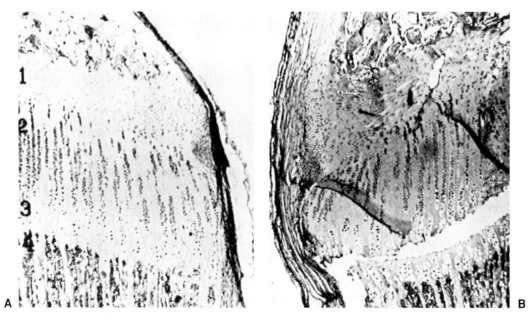

FIG. 5-111. Physeal and anatomy fractures. A: Normal physis consists of germinal or resting cartilage *(1)*, proliferating cartilage *(2)*, hypertrophying cartilage *(3)*, and zone of provisional calcification *(4)*. **B:** Experimental shearing forces produce a fracture through the zone of hypertrophying cartilage. The epiphysis is at the top in both **A** and **B**; the metaphysis is at the bottom. From Rogers (318).

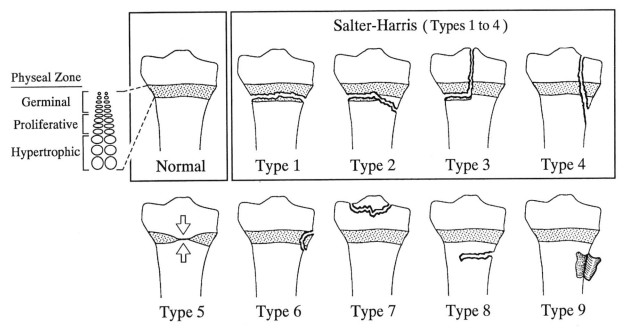

FIG. 5-112. Classification of fractures affecting the physis. Salter-Harris types 1–4 are commonly seen and represent injuries of progressive severity. Type 5 fracture results from compressive damage to the physis. Type 6 is an injury to the perichondral structures. Type 7 is an isolated epiphyseal injury. Type 8 is an isolated juxtaphyseal metaphyseal injury with potential damage to endochondral ossification. Type 9 is a periosteal injury potentially interfering with membranous growth.

Classification

The standard classification for physeal injuries is that of Salter and Harris (311). This classification divides the common injuries (types 1–4) according to the course of the fracture through the physis and the adjacent epiphyseal and metaphyseal bone (Fig. 5-112). A rare, radiographically occult type 5 injury is due to compression of the physeal cartilage. Subsequently, several additions to this classification (types 6–9) have been made (4,309,327). The importance of classification is that it relates the radiologic appearance of physeal injuries to their incidence, anatomic sites, and, most importantly, late morbidity (Fig. 5-112) (Table 5-17).

Type 1 injuries (Fig. 5-112) involve only the physis and usually result from a shearing or avulsion stress (Fig. 5-111B). They are common in children under 5 years of age. In the proximal humerus, they are seen in the neonatal period (Fig. 5-113) and in the 10- to 12-year group. Most apophyseal avulsions and slipped capital femoral epiphyses are type 1 injuries. Supination-inversion injuries of the ankle in puberty can result in a type 1 injury of the distal fibula, the most common fracture of the pediatric ankle (328). Usually these have already reduced themselves at the time of radiographic examination and are recognizable only because of soft-tissue swelling centered at the physis or mild physeal widening. Type 1 fractures have a good prognosis (Fig. 5-114A).

Type 2 injuries (Fig. 5-114B) are the most common physeal fractures (Table 5-17). The shearing or avulsion force

fractures the physis, and the fracture extends into the metaphysis. Radiographs show a triangular metaphyseal fragment of variable size (Thurston-Holland fragment) (Fig. 5-114B). The fracture spares the perichondrium on the side of the metaphyseal fracture, but it disrupts the perichondrium on the side of its physeal extension. One third to one half of the type 2 injuries occur in the distal radius (317). Reduction is usually uncomplicated (except at the posterior distal femur), and the prognosis is usually excellent.

Type 3 injuries are partly intraarticular with longitudinal

TABLE 5-17. *Common sites of physeal fractures*

Type	% Incidence	Common locations
1	6	Proximal humerus
		Distal humerus
		Proximal femur
		Distal tibia
		Distal fibula
2	75	Distal radius
		Distal tibia
		Distal fibula
		Distal femur
		Distal ulna
		Phalanges
3	8	Distal tibia
		Proximal tibia
		Distal femur
4	10	Distal humerus
		Distal tibia

Modified from Rang (309), Rogers (317), and Silverman (308).

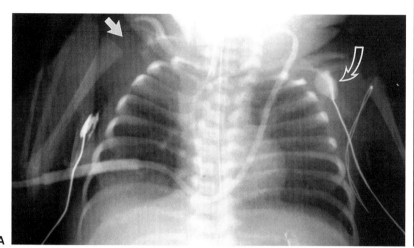
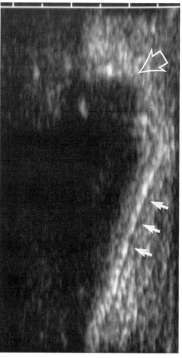

A

B

FIG. 5-113. Salter-Harris type 1 fracture-separation of the proximal humeral epiphysis. Newborn girl with arthrogryposis. The delivery was traumatic because of her contractures. **A:** Frontal radiograph of the chest shows increased distance between the humeral metaphysis and the glenoid of the left scapula *(curved open arrow)*. The proximal humeral ossification center, faintly visible on the right *(closed arrow)*, is not seen on the left. **B:** Coronal sonogram of the left proximal humerus, oriented to correspond with the radiograph. The metaphysis is well seen *(closed arrows)*, but the epiphysis is not visualized in its expected position *(open arrow)*. Transverse sonogram at the level of the metaphysis showed that the humeral epiphysis was displaced posteromedially upon its metaphysis; the joint was intact. From Jaramillo (329).

or oblique splitting of the epiphysis as well as a transverse fracture through part of the physis (see Fig. 5-112). These fractures are significant for two reasons: they are intraarticular; and they violate all the layers of the physis, which predisposes to growth arrest. They usually occur about the knee and ankle (for example, the juvenile Tillaux fracture). Type 3 injuries occur in early adolescence, near the time of physeal closure. Many of these fractures require operative reduction and fixation to prevent displacement (322).

Type 4 injuries cross the epiphysis, physis, and metaphysis. They are due to a longitudinally oriented splitting force, most common at the distal humerus or distal tibia (see Fig. 5-112). These fractures frequently require open reduction to bring the bony fragments into satisfactory apposition. There may be morbidity due to resultant angulation and limb shortening (Fig. 5-115).

Type 5 injuries are usually diagnosed retrospectively, when growth arrest develops in patient with normal radiographs at the time of injury. They are due to a severe compression force that injures the vascular supply and germinal cells of the physis (see Fig. 5-112). Although very

uncommon as an isolated injury, physeal crushing may occur in conjunction with other types of fracture, particularly in areas of physeal undulation like the distal femur (324). Most isolated type 5 fractures have been described in the ankle and knee.

Type 6 injury affects the perichondrium. The first radiographs may show a tiny sliver of bone at the periphery of the epiphysis or metaphysis. The acute radiographs are often negative, however, and the injury may be suspected later because of reactive bone formation external to the physis (see Fig. 5-112). This rare injury, usually due to a glancing injury (327,329), causes osseous bridging (Fig. 5-116). Since the tethering is peripheral, angular deformity occurs rapidly.

The next three types, although not directly affecting the physis, can result in growth disturbances. *Type 7 injury* is a relatively important fracture; it involves the epiphysis but not the physis. It occurs commonly in avulsions of the malleoli and of the humeral condyles and is also seen in osteochondral fractures of the distal femur (326). This type includes avulsion fractures of the intercondylar tibial eminence in prepubertal and pubertal patients who, if older, would have suffered a tear of the anterior cruciate ligament (330).

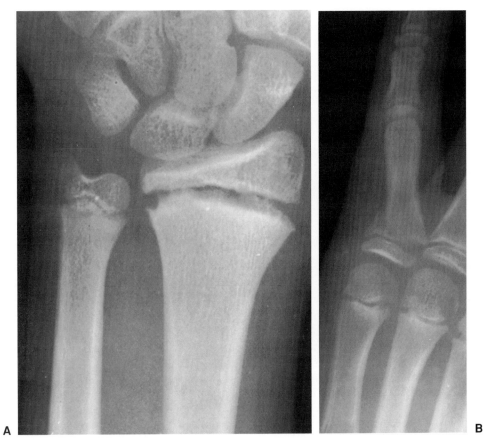

FIG. 5-114. Physeal fractures. A: Salter-Harris type I physeal fracture of the distal left radius. Note the widened and irregular physis. **B:** Salter-Harris type 2 fracture of the proximal phalanx of the little finger.

Type 8 injury involves the metaphysis only but blocks normal endochondral ossification, apparently because of metaphyseal vascular damage. *Type 9 injury* involves the periosteum of the diaphysis or metaphysis and interferes with appositional bone growth.

Physeal Fractures in Specific Locations

Distal Humerus. Lateral condylar fractures will be discussed below, under elbow injuries.

Distal Femur. Physeal fractures of the distal femur account for nearly 40% of cases of bony bridging of the physis, although they constitute only 1% or 2% of all physeal injuries (322). This contrasts sharply with the distal radius, which accounts for 45% of all physeal fractures but only 12% of disturbances. Growth arrest develops in more than half of the distal femoral physeal fractures, regardless of the Salter-Harris type (331). Hence, fractures of the distal femur (and to a lesser extent those of the proximal and distal tibia) should be considered at high risk for causing abnormal growth.

Distal Tibia. The Tillaux and triplane fractures will be discussed below.

Posttraumatic Growth Arrest

Growth disturbance occurs after as many as 30% of physeal fractures. However, only a minority of these (2%) result in growth arrest in a location or of a severity to require treatment (318). Growth arrest results from two mechanisms. The first is direct physeal disruption resulting in posttraumatic communication between the epiphyseal and metaphyseal vessels. Osteoprogenitor cells deposit bone along the vessels and form a bridge across the physeal cartilage (312, 323). The second is disruption of the epiphyseal vessels that supply the physeal chondrocytes (332,333), which causes bony bridge formation or disorganization of the physeal architecture. Growth arrest can be diagnosed on imaging studies by detecting the bridge across the physis. It can also be recognized by epiphyseal and metaphyseal ("cone" or "ball-and-cup") deformities, and by abnormalities of the growth recovery lines. Growth recovery lines (also known as growth arrest, Harris, or Park lines) (334–336) are seen after immobilization for fracture. They are normally parallel to the physis. With local growth arrest, the line will converge with the physis at the site of physeal tethering. To plan surgery, it is necessary to map accurately the extent and location

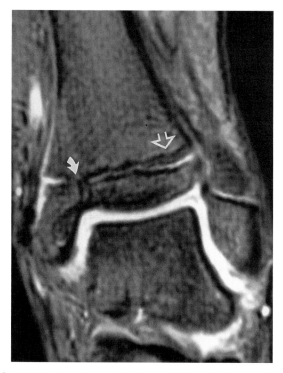

FIG. 5-115. Posttraumatic bony bridge. A 9-year-old girl who developed leg-length discrepancy after a Salter-Harris type 4 fracture. Coronal gradient-recalled-echo MR image shows a 6-mm area of decreased signal intensity *(curved arrow)* interrupting the normal high-signal-intensity physis. It is located in the region of the distal tibial irregularity (Kump bump). A growth recovery line is beginning to form *(straight arrow)*.

of the bony bridge. A bridge is resected if it involves less than 50% of the area of the physis and 2 or more years of skeletal growth are anticipated (337).

Leg Lengthening Procedures. A discrepancy in the length of the legs after a fracture may be due to overgrowth during healing, but more severe cases result from damage to the physis. One treatment is to staple one or more physes of the longer limb, reducing further growth of that bone. Estimation of further growth is based on the bone age. Other techniques treat asymmetry by lengthening the shorter limb (80,81). Several techniques (Ilizarov, Wagner) involve a diaphyseal osteotomy leaving an intact periosteal sleeve. Gradual distraction of the ends of the bones creates a gap between the fragments. Bone formation occurs fairly quickly in the periosteum-lined gap (338). These methods require precise imaging during planning and follow-up. Ultrasonography generally shows callus formation considerably earlier than radiography (339).

Imaging of Physeal Injuries and Growth Arrest. Most fractures require only radiographs at the time of injury and at varying intervals until skeletal maturity. Stress views probably should not be used to diagnose occult physeal fractures; experimental work suggests that the fracture can become more extensive or complex if force is applied to the physis. MRI is useful in evaluating complex physeal injuries

in high-risk areas such as the distal femur and in further defining the anatomy of fractures lying mostly in cartilage (317,340). Conventional tomography, scintigraphy, CT, and MRI have been used to evaluate growth arrest (341). Because MRI can image the cartilaginous abnormality directly and map the configuration of any bony bridge in several planes, it is preferred for preoperative evaluation (Figs. 5-115 and 5-116) (317).

Injuries at Specific Locations

Clavicular Fractures

The double curve of the clavicle resists stress so poorly that the clavicle is the most frequently broken bone in children (309). Occasionally, this normal double curvature of the clavicle mimics a fracture on the straight AP view. The 15° or 30° upshot view (beam angled toward the head) clarifies clavicular anatomy well. Fractures may involve the medial end, midshaft, or outer end.

The *medial end* of the clavicle has an epiphysis that ossifies between late adolescence and early adulthood and is the last in the body to close. Medial epiphyseal separation is the usual injury there before the age of 18 years and sternoclavicular dislocation after the age of 25 years. In sternoclavicular dislocation, pain and swelling are present at the sternoclavicular joint, but the AP radiograph of the clavicle may be normal. Although angled views can sometimes show the injury, CT is a more expeditious and sensitive diagnostic procedure. *Midshaft* fractures of the clavicle are the most common, being of either the greenstick or complete type. These fractures unite quickly, and complete remodeling oc-

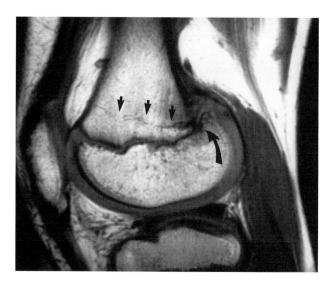

FIG. 5-116. Posttraumatic bony bridge. An 11-year-old with posttraumatic bony bridge due to a type 6 injury of the distal femur. Sagittal T1-weighted MR image of the distal femur shows posterior bridge involving the perichondral region. There is a growth recovery line *(small arrows)* which converges with the physis in the region of the bridge *(large arrow)*.

curs within 1 year. Malunion (309) and other complications are very rare unless open reduction is needed. Fracture of the *distal clavicle* is rare in children. There may be marked anteroposterior instability despite intact coracoclavicular ligaments (309). Dislocations at the acromioclavicular joints are rare in young children.

Shoulder Injuries

Except in the context of child abuse (342), fracture of the scapula and acute dislocation of the shoulder are primarily adult injuries.

Fractures of the proximal humerus are usually either type 1 or type 2 Salter-Harris physeal fractures (see Fig. 5-113). Birth injury may separate the proximal epiphysis and mimic Erb palsy. Visibility of callus on the follow-up radiographs depends on whether the fracture is intraarticular and, if extraarticular, whether the periosteum was raised. If the proximal humeral epiphysis is unossified, as is true in half of newborns, the only radiographic finding is an increased distance between the humeral metaphysis and the glenoid. This appearance mimics shoulder effusion. The diagnosis is established by ultrasonography (343). Proximal humeral epiphyseal separation has also been reported in the battered child syndrome. Type 1 or 2 humeral physeal injuries also occur in the 10- to 12-year-old range (317).

Elbow Injuries

Anatomy. The distal humeral shaft broadens to form the medial and lateral condyles. There are two depressions between these condyles, termed the coronoid fossa anteriorly and the (much deeper) olecranon fossa posteriorly. Four ossification centers develop in the distal humerus. The first to appear is the capitellum at age 1–2 years or sooner. The medial (internal) epicondyle appears at an average age of 4 years, the trochlea at about 8 years of age, and the lateral (external) epicondyle at an average age of 10 years (344,345). There is considerable variability in these times. The centers appear earlier in girls than in boys (346). The radial head appears at age 3–6 years, and the olecranon center of the ulna at 6–12 years (345). The ossification centers of the distal humerus fuse with each other and then with the parent bone between the ages of 14 and 16 years, except for the medial epicondyle, which may not fuse until age 18 or 19. The ossification centers are usually oval and smooth with the exception of the trochlea, which is fragmented initially and irregular later. Although one should be aware of the approximate times of normal ossification of the growth centers of the distal humerus, it is more important to know the sequence. It is "critoeical" [sic] (*c*apitellum, *r*adial head, *i*nternal or medial epicondyle, *t*rochlea, *o*lecranon, *e*xternal or lateral epicondyle) to be familiar with this normal ossification sequence.

Elbow fat pads. The anterior fat pad is a summation of radial and coronoid fat pads, which are enveloped by two thick leaflets of fibrous joint capsule (Fig. 5-117A). These extrasynovial, intracapsular, anterior fat pads are normally pressed into the shallow radial and coronoid fossae by the brachialis muscle. In the lateral view with 90° of flexion, the anterior fat pad is normally seen as a faint, dark line, parallel to the anterior humerus. An abnormal anterior fat pad sign results when intrasynovial fluid or tissue displaces the fat pads superiorly and anteriorly (347), making them more visible (Fig. 5-117A).

The posterior fat pad is also extrasynovial and is invested by capsular leaflets. The posterior fat pad, pressed into the deep olecranon fossa by the triceps tendon and anconeus muscle, is invisible on the normal 90° flexed lateral radiograph (347). With abnormal joint fluid or tissue, the posterior fat is displaced posteriorly and superiorly and becomes visible on the lateral radiograph (Fig. 5-117A). A visible posterior fat pad is a more reliable index of joint effusion than an abnormal anterior fat pad sign (346).

The elbow fat pad signs are not specific for trauma. The joint can be distended by various fluids—blood, pus (exudate), water (transudate), cells—and for various reasons (trauma, hemorrhage, infection, inflammation, neoplasia). Traumatic joint distention is due to a dislocation or fracture of the radius, ulna, or humerus extending into the synovial cavity, allowing blood and marrow to expand the joint. More than 90% of children and adolescents with a traumatic posterior fat pad sign have a fracture, demonstrable at follow-up if not initially (346). Although radial fractures are the most frequent occult elbow injuries in adults, other injuries (supracondylar or lateral condylar fractures, and a jerked elbow or dislocated radial head, often reduced by the time of the examination) should be considered in the differential diagnosis of subtle elbow injuries in children. The fat pad sign may be falsely negative when the capsule is disrupted (4). Oblique or angled views may be helpful in demonstrating occult injuries. Horizontal beam radiographs may show a fat-fluid level in the joint at the time of injury, which increases the likelihood of fracture. In difficult cases, particularly if the history of trauma is unclear, ultrasonography can demonstrate joint fluid readily and guide aspiration of the joint.

Radiologic lines. Three lines help interpret elbow radiographs in children. The *anterior humeral line* (Fig. 5-117B), drawn tangential to the anterior humeral cortex, normally passes through the middle third of the ossified capitellum (348). With a supracondylar fracture and dorsal angulation of the distal humeral fragment, this line usually passes through in front of the anterior third of the capitellum. The *radiocapitellar line* (Fig. 5-117B), drawn along the center of the radial shaft normally passes through the capitellum on all radiographic views (347), although not necessarily through the middle of the ossification center. This line confirms articulation between the radial head and the capitellum. If the line fails to pass through the capitellum, dislocation of the radial head is likely. However, before the epiphysis

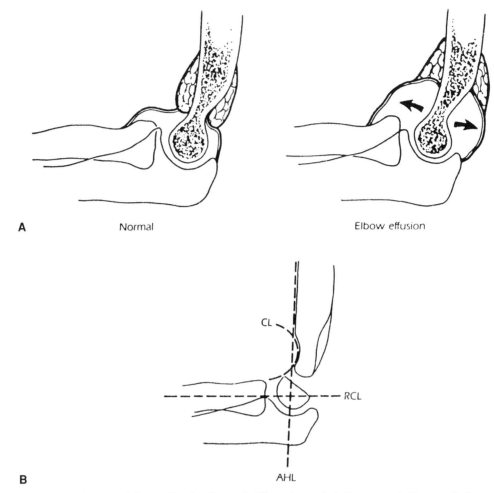

A Normal Elbow effusion

B CL RCL AHL

FIG. 5-117. Radiology of the pediatric elbow. A: Elbow fat pads in the normal elbow and elbow when effusion is present. **B:** Radiologic lines. Anterior humeral line *(AHL)*; coronoid line *(CL)*; radiocapitellar line *(RCL)*. See text for further description.

of the radial head ossifies, this line may appear to project somewhat laterally on the AP view; the lateral radiograph will show normal alignment (Fig. 5-117B). The *coronoid line* (Fig. 5-117B) is drawn along the distal portion of the humerus on the lateral view; it outlines the coronoid fossa and is concave anteriorly. An extension of this line just touches or projects anterior to the developing capitellum. The coronoid line helps to demonstrate anterior or posterior displacements of the capitellum in supracondylar fractures.

Frequency of Injuries. Supracondylar fractures account for 60% of all elbow fractures in children. Fractures of the lateral condyle account for 15%, and separation of the medial epicondylar ossification centers account for 10% (346). Fractures of the olecranon and coronoid process, fractures of the radial neck, separations of the proximal radial epiphysis, and Monteggia fractures account for the remainder. An awareness of the most common sites of injury aids in the search for fractures.

Supracondylar Fractures. Supracondylar fracture is the most common fracture of the elbow in children. It is a fracture occurring during the latter half of the first decade and is usually caused by a hyperextension injury while falling

on an outstretched hand. During this period, the newly deposited bone in the thin area between the coronoid and olecranon fossae is weak and susceptible to breakage (349). The distal fragment is displaced posteriorly. Seventy-five percent are complete fractures, 25% incomplete (348). Radiologic diagnosis in the incomplete type (bowing, torus, greenstick) may be difficult. A positive posterior fat pad sign is almost always present, and the fracture eliminates or reduces the normal volar angulation of the distal articular surface. Loss of this angulation causes the anterior humeral line to pass through or anterior to the anterior third of the capitellum (Fig. 5-118A). The fracture line may be difficult to identify on the AP projection (Fig. 5-118B), but disruption of the humeral cortex is usually present on the lateral view. Oblique views may help to confirm the fracture.

Cubitus varus is the most common complication of supracondylar fractures. Its incidence varies considerably, but it has been reported to be as high as 60% (349). It is generally believed that cubitus varus is the result of residual angulation of the distal fragment after reduction rather than of growth disturbance. The degree of varus angulation is estimated using the Bauman angle (Fig. 5-119A), the angle between

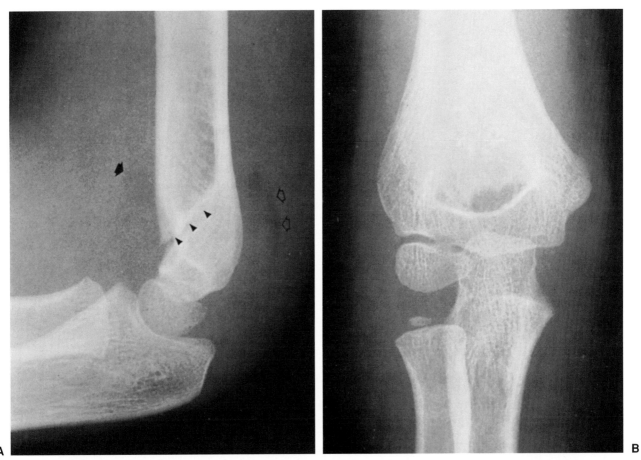

FIG. 5-118. Supracondylar fracture. A 6-year-old girl with trauma to the right elbow. **A:** Lateral radiograph shows displacement of the anterior and posterior fat pads *(arrows)*. Anterior humeral line passes through the anterior third of the capitellum. The supracondylar fracture is seen *(arrowheads)*. **B:** Frontal view does not reveal any abnormality. This emphasizes the importance of the lateral (orthogonal) view.

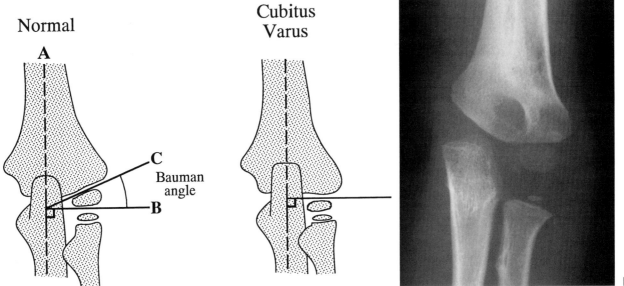

FIG. 5-119. Cubitus varus after supracondylar fracture. **A:** Left diagram shows the normal (Bauman) angle between the shaft of the humerus and the distal humeral physis. Right diagram shows that in cubitus varus, the distal humeral physis and the shaft are nearly perpendicular. **B:** A 5-year-old boy with cubitus varus that developed after a supracondylar fracture 6 months earlier. The distal humeral physis is nearly perpendicular to the shaft.

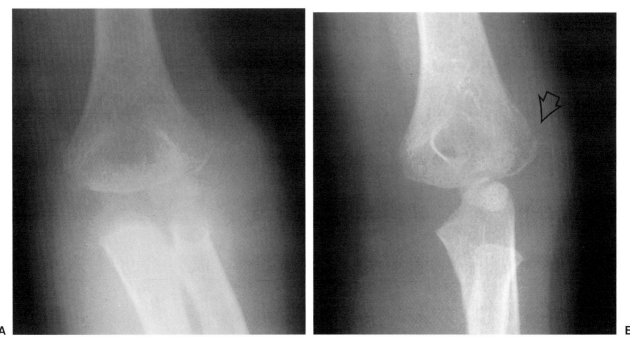

FIG. 5-120. Subtle lateral condylar fracture. A 4-year-old girl with a subtle lateral condylar fracture after falling on an outstretched arm. **A:** AP radiograph suggests soft-tissue swelling and an irregularity along the lateral aspect of the distal humeral metaphysis. The patient was not able to extend the elbow fully for the radiograph. **B:** The internal oblique projection shows that there is a fracture extending from the metaphysis into the capitellar ossification center *(arrow)*.

the physeal line (a line between the capitellum and the distal humeral metaphysis) and the long axis of the humerus. The angle is normally 75°, but with varus angulation it may increase to 90° or more (Fig. 5-119B). An acceptable reduction results in a Bauman angle within 4° of that of the contralateral side (350).

Lateral Condylar Fractures. The second most common fracture of the elbow in children is the lateral condylar fracture (346) (Fig. 5-120). It is usually a Salter-Harris type 4 injury, involving a small fragment of metaphysis and extending into the mostly unossified epiphysis of the lateral humeral condyle (Fig. 5-121A). Open reduction and internal fixation are necessary when there is radiographic evidence of extension into the joint and displacement of the distal fragment (type 3). The extensor muscles of the forearm pull the fragment posteriorly and distally. Nondisplaced fractures may extend through the epiphysis but not into the joint (type 1, stable injury) (Fig. 5-121A) or they may reach the joint (type 2, potentially unstable injury). A lateral condylar fracture may be difficult to detect on the frontal view; shallow oblique radiographs can confirm the diagnosis (see Fig. 5-120). Further imaging with arthrography or MRI helps define the extension into the unossified epiphysis and joint. It is particularly important to detect potentially unstable injuries (type 2) (Fig. 5-121B). Inadequate treatment of unstable injuries can result in nonunion (335).

Medial Epicondylar Injuries. The medial epicondyle is the insertion site of the ulnar collateral ligament and of the forearm flexor muscles. This insertion site is vulnerable to valgus stress and to excessive pull by the muscles (351), usually during throwing. An avulsion of the medial epicondyle can develop due to repeated insults or as a result of a single sudden force. Whereas adults usually tear the ligament, children usually injure the medial epicondylar ossification center. Injuries of the medial epicondyle account for 10% of elbow fractures in children (352). These injuries include minimal avulsion, moderate to severe avulsion, Little League elbow, isolated entrapment, and avulsion associated with dislocation.

Minimal avulsions are best identified on the AP view, as the first medial epicondylar displacement is almost always distal (352). Avulsions with separation greater than 5 mm on the AP view may require open reduction and pin fixation (350), particularly if there is valgus instability. Little League elbow is a tension stress injury of the medial epicondyle in young baseball pitchers (353). It is produced by violent contraction of the flexor and pronator groups of muscles during the acceleration phase of throwing. This separation is usually chronic, and leads to fragmentation, enlargement, and roughening of the medial epicondyle and widening and irregularity of the adjacent physis (349). MRI recently has been used to study the medial epicondylar region of normal and symptomatic children. There is normally an area of high signal intensity at the insertion of the ulnar collateral ligament. In children with symptomatic elbows, there may be evidence of osteochondral fragmentation (351).

Type 1   Type 2   Type 3

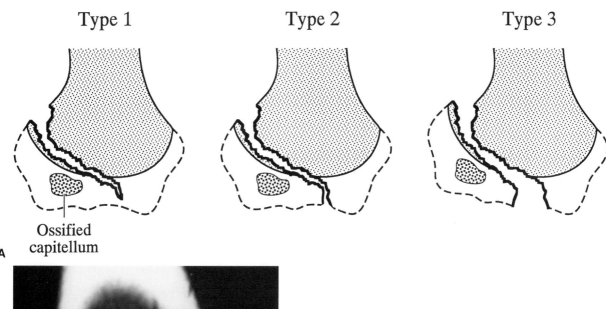

Ossified capitellum

A

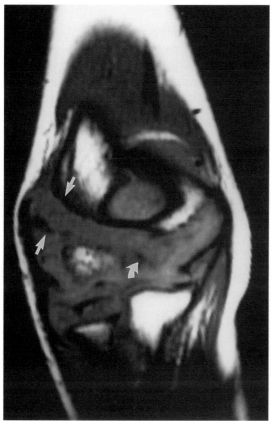

B

FIG. 5-121. Lateral condylar fracture. A: Diagram illustrates three types of lateral condylar injuries. The fracture can stop short of the joint, it can extend into the joint without displacement, or the fragment can be displaced. **B:** Coronal T1-weighted MR image of the distal humerus shows a fracture extending from the distal metaphysis *(straight arrows)* to the cartilaginous epiphysis but stopping just short of the articular surface *(curved arrow)*.

Isolated entrapment of the medial epicondyle is caused by valgus stress, frequently in the context of a posterolateral dislocation with temporary opening of the elbow joint space medially (Fig. 5-122). The epicondyle is avulsed and then drawn into the joint by traction from the attached flexor-pronator muscle group and the ulnar collateral ligament, which is tightly attached to the ulna (Fig. 5-123A). Nearly half of medial epicondyle separations are associated with elbow dislocations (352). The entrapped medial epicondylar ossification center may be mistaken for the trochlear ossification center and the true severity of the injury overlooked

(Fig. 5-123B). Therefore it is important to radiograph the elbow after reduction of posterolateral dislocations *before* the cast is applied, with careful attention to the location of all secondary centers. Comparison views of the other side sometimes help.

Olecranon and Coronoid Process Fractures. Fracture of the olecranon can occur at any age and seldom poses a diagnostic problem. The physis of the normal ossification center of the olecranon is sometimes mistaken in adolescents for a fracture. Fracture of the coronoid process is relatively uncommon and may require oblique views for diagnosis (353).

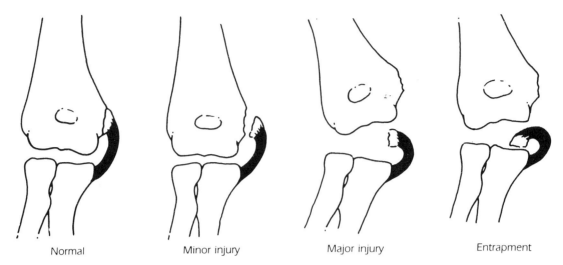

FIG. 5-122. **Injuries of the medial epicondylar ossification center.** Modified from Rogers (346).

The avulsed tip may be superimposed on the head of the radius on the lateral view.

Distal Humeral Epiphyseal Separation. Separation of the entire distal humeral epiphysis may be confused with elbow dislocation. The radius and ulna are displaced medially; in dislocation the characteristic displacement is lateral. The relationship of the capitellum and radius (radiocapitellar line) is normal, which means that the distal humeral epiphysis is displaced along with the bones of the forearm (354). This fracture usually occurs in children less than 3 years of age and may be due to birth trauma (Fig. 5-124) or child abuse (159).

Jerked Elbow (Nursemaid Elbow). The jerked elbow or nursemaid elbow occurs in toddlers and preschoolers as a

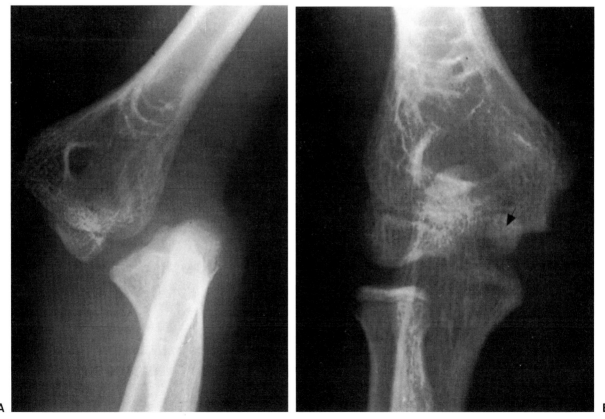

FIG. 5-123. **Entrapment of medial epicondylar ossification center.** A 7-year-old boy after an automobile accident. **A:** Elbow dislocation. **B:** Postreduction film. Note the entrapment of the medial epicondylar ossification center *(arrow),* which must not be mistaken for the trochlear ossification center.

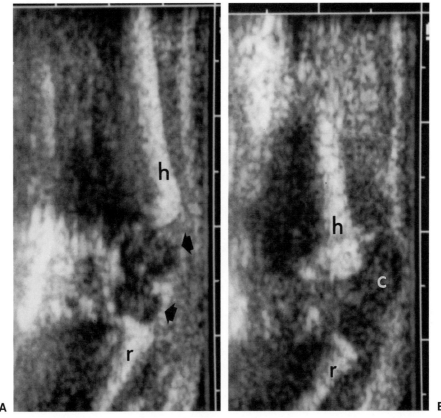

FIG. 5-124. Distal humeral epiphyseal separation. Premature baby with a difficult delivery. **A:** Sagittal ultrasonogram of the contralateral normal elbow from a posterior approach shows the unossified radial and capitellar epiphyses *(arrows)*, which are well aligned with the shafts of the humerus *(h)* and radius *(r)*. **B:** Sagittal posterior view of the injured side shows a normal radius *(r)* in normal relation to the capitellum *(c)*. However, the capitellum is posteriorly displaced from the humeral shaft *(h)*.

result of a sudden pull on the hand, usually by an impatient adult. It is the most common injury to the elbow in children. The clinical picture is characteristic: a child between 1 and 4 years of age refuses to move the arm and holds it slightly flexed and pronated. When longitudinal traction is applied to the arm with the forearm in pronation, the annular ligament tears at its attachment to the radius and the head of the radius escapes distally. When traction is released, the ligament becomes impacted between the radius and capitellum (309). The annular ligament can be returned to its normal position by slight flexion and supination. The reduction is frequently accomplished by the radiologic technologist when the forearm is supinated for a true AP radiograph of the elbow. The radiologic examination is almost always normal, but a joint effusion can be detected in some cases.

Wrist; Pronator Quadratus Fat Pad Sign

The pronator quadratus muscle is attached to the distal one-sixth of the radius and ulna. Its principal function is to prevent separation of the distal end of the radius and ulna when force is transmitted from the wrist (355). The normal pronator fat pad between the pronator quadratus muscle and the tendons of the flexor digitorum profundus muscle is seen on a lateral radiograph of the wrist as a thin line of fat that has a gentle ventral convexity (see Fig. 5-109C). This fat pad sign should be evaluated in every lateral radiograph of the wrist after trauma, as it is an indirect indicator of bony injury. A positive pronator quadratus fat pad sign, showing anterior displacement (increased convexity) or blurring or obliteration of the pronator fat pad plane, suggests a fracture (355). Oblique views may be required for clarification.

MacEwan reviewed 600 children with trauma to the lower forearm. Of 300 children with fractures at the level of the pronator quadratus attachment, only 5 had a normal fat pad (355), and they were always seen with fractures involving the dorsal surface of the radius or ulna (see Fig. 5-109C). Of 300 patients without fractures at the level of the pronator quadratus attachment, there were 19 abnormal fat pad signs, all due to direct trauma or muscle strain (355).

Pelvic Fractures

Pelvic fractures are not common in children and account for less than 5% of pediatric fractures (356). Although not as serious a problem in children as in adults, these fractures

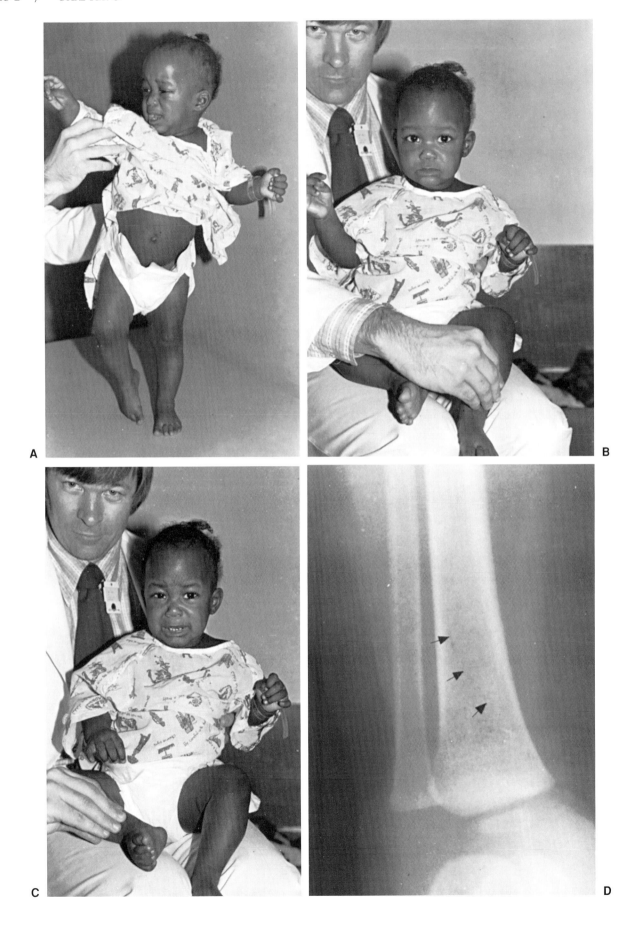

A

B

C

D

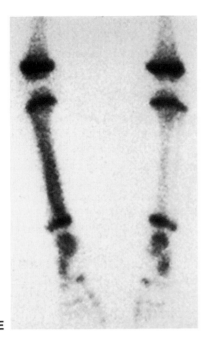

E

FIG. 5-125. Toddler's fracture. This 10-month-old girl had been walking for approximately 1 month but suddenly refused to bear weight. **A:** The child refuses to bear weight on the right leg. **B:** There is no tenderness over the left leg. **C:** There is marked point tenderness over the right leg. **D:** Oblique view demonstrates spiral fracture *(arrows)* of the distal right tibia. **E:** In another toddler refusing to bear weight, the skeletal scintigram shows diffusely increased radiotracer uptake in the midtibia, due to a toddler's fracture.

are still associated with a mortality rate of 2% (356), but death is almost always due to other injuries. The child's pelvis has abundant cartilage in the apophyses and triradiate cartilages. The joints (including the pubic symphysis and the sacroiliac joints) are more lax and elastic than in the adult, and the periosteum is thick. For these reasons, in childhood the pelvis can absorb more energy without breaking than in adult life. Unlike the adult, one fracture in a child's pelvic ring does not imply that a second fracture must be present. The cartilaginous areas are weaker than the bones, and thus fractures frequently occur through or partly through the cartilage (357). Pelvic fractures may be unstable, in which a large segment of the pelvic ring is isolated, or stable, with only a localized fracture. More than half (61%) of the pelvic fractures in children are stable, including unilateral or bilateral pubic and ischial rami fractures and simultaneous anterior and posterior fractures (356). Isolated fractures and avulsion fractures are also stable. Few pelvic fractures in children are significantly displaced.

Unstable fractures commonly include the combination of a posterior fracture (iliac fracture, sacral fracture, or sacroiliac separation) and a pubic fracture on either the same or the opposite side. Other unstable fractures include acetabular fractures and separations of the symphysis pubis combined with sacroiliac separations. Pelvic hemorrhage, a major complication of acetabular fractures in adults, is much less common in children (356). CT is very useful in evaluating these

fractures (see Fig. 5-105). The acetabular region should be evaluated with thin sections and three-dimensional reconstructions with special attention to the weight-bearing columns (358).

Most pelvic fractures in children are due to motor vehicle accidents, particularly of the car versus pedestrian type. One third of children with pelvic fractures have fractures of other bones, usually the femur or skull. Up to 80% of children with multiple pelvic fractures also have injuries of the lower urinary tract or intraabdominal organs (359). Most of these patients undergo CT of the abdomen for evaluation of visceral injury. It is important always to review the examination at settings for bones, which will show most significant pelvic fractures.

Proximal Femoral Epiphyseal Separation

Separation of the proximal femoral epiphysis occurs in traumatic births (proximal femoral epiphysiolysis), in child abuse, after radiation therapy, in renal osteodystrophy, in hypothyroidism, in hypopituitarism, and in myelomeningocele. Neonatal proximal femoral epiphysiolysis is a rare fracture resulting from hyperextension, abduction, and rotation of a lower extremity during a traumatic breech delivery. It may be misinterpreted clinically and radiographically as a dislocation of the hip, septic arthritis, or proximal focal femoral dysplasia. Early diagnosis and treatment can prevent persistent coxa vara, aseptic necrosis, and early closure of the physis (360). The infant keeps the involved extremity limp in flexion, abduction, and external rotation and resists motion (360). Radiographs show superolateral displacement of the proximal femoral metaphysis. Sonography shows normal articular relationships but loss of continuity between the unossified epiphysis and the metaphysis (361). In contrast, neonates with hip dislocation are usually asymptomatic but the acetabulum is already abnormal. Ultrasonography, arthrocentesis, and analysis of the aspirated fluid distinguish these conditions. After 2 weeks, periosteal reaction and callus are usually apparent. Treatment of neonatal proximal femoral epiphysiolysis includes traction and splinting.

Toddler's Fractures

The toddler's fracture is a nondisplaced spiral or oblique fracture of the distal tibia that occurs in children between the ages of 9 months and 3 years, when weight bearing is just beginning (362). Subtle stress fractures also occur in the calcaneus in the same age group (363) and cuboid (364,365). These fractures may go unrecognized by both the clinician and the radiologist. Although there are no known complications from missing these fractures, the child's pain and the parent's concern can be abbreviated and unnecessary diagnostic studies can be avoided with a correct diagnosis.

These patients usually are seen in the emergency room with failure to walk or refusal to bear weight on an extremity (Fig. 5-125A). There may be a history of minimal trauma.

The child is irritable but may otherwise be asymptomatic. There is a slight increase in temperature over the lower anterior leg of the affected side, and local tenderness is present (Fig. 5-125).

Because of the nonspecific clinical history, the patient may be referred to the radiologist for examination of any part of the lower extremities (362). The fracture is spiral or oblique and therefore it may not be shown by the AP and lateral films. Oblique films usually demonstrate the fracture (Fig. 5-125D); internal rotation oblique views are particularly helpful. There may be only soft-tissue swelling and edema at first, with the fracture line being apparent only after days or weeks. The fibula is normal. The lateral radiograph should include the hindfoot in order to exclude stress fractures in the calcaneus and cuboid. Skeletal scintigraphy or follow-up radiographs should be performed when the diagnosis is suspected but the initial radiographs are negative. In positive cases, there is focal, diffuse, or linear increase in uptake in the tibia (Fig. 5-125E), calcaneus, or cuboid (365).

Tillaux and Triplane Fractures

The physis of the distal tibia begins to fuse at the Kump bump, an undulation in the anteromedial part of the growth plate. In early adolescence the medial distal tibia therefore has the features of an adult bone, whereas the lateral tibia remains immature. This predisposes the distal tibia to complex injuries, the juvenile Tillaux fracture and the triplane fracture (366). These injuries usually do not cause significant growth disturbances, as they occur in patients with little remaining growth. Radiologic evaluation is aimed at defining the number of fragments and the separation of the articular components of the injury. More than 2–3 mm of diastasis in any plane at the articular surface requires open reduction (367). The juvenile Tillaux injury is due to avulsion of the anterolateral corner of the distal tibial epiphysis by the anterior tibiofibular ligament. Typically, the fracture extends sagittally through the epiphysis and transversely through the lateral part of the physis. The triplane, a more complex but closely related injury, has a metaphyseal coronal extension. On radiographs, the Tillaux fracture is a Salter-Harris type 3 fracture, whereas the triplane fracture (actually a Salter-Harris type 4 fracture) appears as a type 3 fracture on the frontal radiograph and a type 2 fracture on the lateral radiograph (Fig. 5-126). CT with thin sections and multiplanar reconstruction is the best modality for evaluation of these injuries (Fig. 5-127) (366).

Ankle Effusions

Ankle effusions may be due to infection, trauma, hemorrhage, primary or reactive arthritis, or neoplasia. The radio-

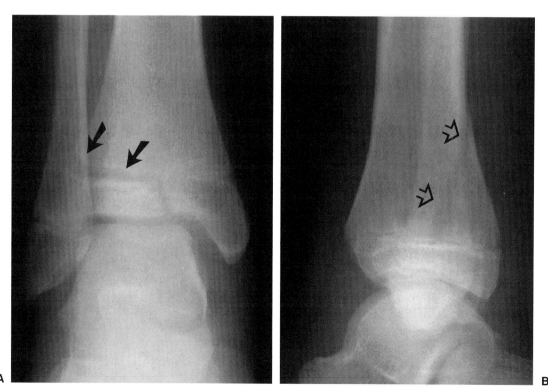

FIG. 5-126. Triplane fracture. A 15-year old boy who jumped from a tree and hurt his ankle. **A:** Frontal view shows a vertical fracture extending sagittally through the epiphysis and horizontally along the lateral physis *(arrows)* and suggests a Salter-Harris type 3 fracture. The medial part of the physis is closed. **B:** Lateral view shows a fracture that extends through the metaphysis along the coronal plane *(arrows)* and suggests a Salter-Harris type 2 fracture. The findings are typical of a triplane fracture.

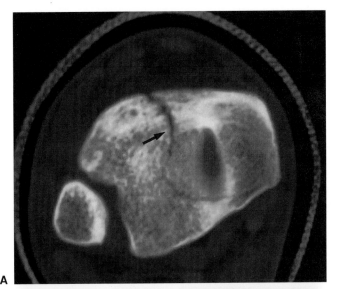

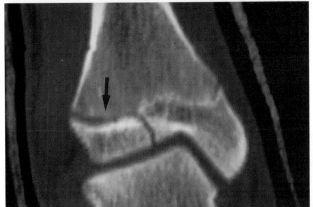

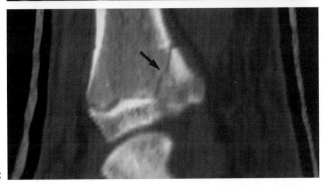

FIG. 5-127. A 13-year-old boy with triplane fracture. A: Axial 1.5-mm-thick CT image shows the sagittal component of the fracture in the distal tibial epiphysis *(arrow).* **B:** Coronal reconstruction shows the fracture extending sagittally through the epiphysis and propagating horizontally along the physis *(arrow).* **C:** Sagittal reconstruction shows the fracture extending anteriorly along the physis and coursing into the metaphysis posteriorly *(arrow).*

graphic diagnosis of ankle effusion may be difficult, and comparison views are occasionally of value (see Appendix 2), although ultrasonography, MRI, and CT readily demonstrate joint fluid.

The synovial cavity of the ankle joint has an anterior recess that extends anteriorly along the neck of the talus. There

is also a posterior recess, which has the shape of the number 3 (368). The fat pads of the ankle are often visualized on lateral radiographs. Anteriorly, the pretalar fat pad is crescentic and lies against the neck of the talus. Posteriorly, the thin juxtaarticular fat pad is closely opposed to the posterior recess. There is also a larger triangular pre-Achilles fat pad.

Towbin described the teardrop sign of ankle effusion seen on lateral radiographs (368). A teardrop-shaped soft-tissue density displaces the normal pretalar fat pad (Fig. 5-128). Occasionally, there is also curvilinear displacement of the posterior juxtaarticular fat pad. As little as 5 ml of fluid within the ankle joint may be detected using these signs (368). In patients who have suffered acute trauma demonstration of an ankle effusion has a sensitivity of greater than 80% and a specificity of greater than 90% for underlying fracture (369). The significance of the teardrop sign is thus similar to that of the fat pad sign in the elbow.

Stubbed Toe Fractures

Stubbing of the great toe is a hyperflexion injury (370). It may produce a Salter-Harris type 1, 2, or 3 physeal fracture of the distal phalanx. Because the skin above this physis consists only of a thin layer of dermis and the germinal matrix of the toe nail, the fracture extends to the skin between the cuticle and root of the nail or proximal to the root of the nail (370). There may be signs of bleeding from the nail bed. A fracture of the distal phalangeal physis of any toe (or finger) caused by stubbing (or thumping) and leading to a flexion deformity should be considered compound (Fig. 5-129) and treated with antibiotics to prevent infectious complications (370).

Injury to the Trabecular Bone: Stress and Insufficiency Fractures and Bone Contusions

Injuries producing microfractures involving only the trabeculae of bone result in marrow edema but often no radiographic evidence of fracture. They fall into two categories: bone contusions (bruises) and stress fractures (371). A bone bruise usually occurs from a single direct blow. It is usually found incidentally on MR images performed for evaluation of ligamentous and meniscal injuries. Bone bruises do not require therapy, but they are important as signs of injury nearby. For example, bruises in the lateral femoral condyle and posterolateral portion of the tibia (kissing contusions) are frequently seen when the anterior cruciate ligament has been torn. Tibial bruises may be found deep to a torn medial collateral ligament.

A stress fracture, on the other hand, results from repetitive trauma. Stress fractures occur in many bones but at sites predictable from the predisposing activity (372). A stress fracture is an osseous disruption due to repetitive pull or muscular action on bone unaccustomed to it, often during

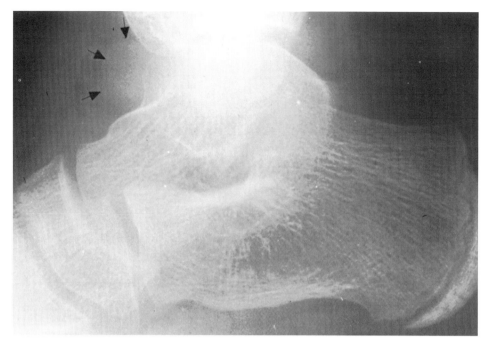

FIG. 5-128. Ankle effusion. "Teardrop" sign *(arrows)* is due to fluid in the anterior recess of the ankle joint displacing the normal pretalar fat pad (368).

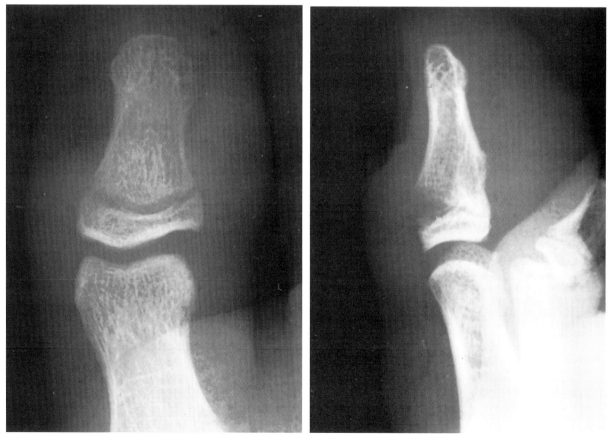

FIG. 5-129. Stubbed toe fracture. This 15-year old girl peeled off the base of the nail of her great toe during a stubbing injury. **A, B:** Salter 2 fracture of the distal phalanx of the great toe with associated soft-tissue swelling.

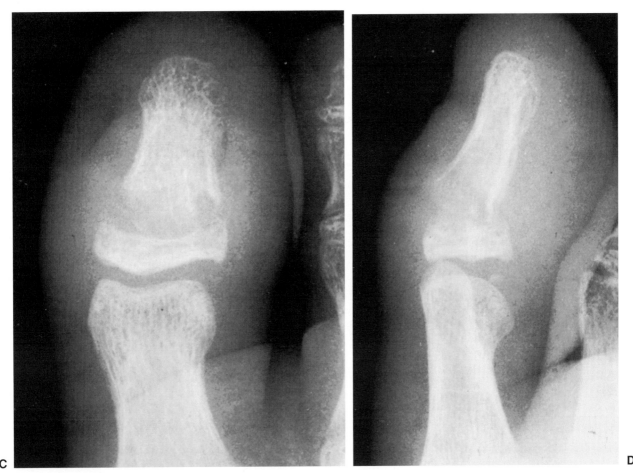

C   D

FIG. 5-129. *Continued.* **C, D:** Two weeks later bone destruction due to osteomyelitis is clearly evident.

vigorous activity the individual is not accustomed to performing.

Insufficiency fractures are stress fractures produced by normal or physiologic stresses placed on bone with deficient elastic resistance, that is, the application of normal stress to abnormal bone (Figs. 5-130 and 5-131). Pediatric conditions that predispose to insufficiency stress fractures include osteopenia related to prematurity, juvenile rheumatoid arthritis, rickets, osteoporosis, nonossifying fibroma (Fig. 5-132), fibrous dysplasia, osteogenesis imperfecta, osteopetrosis, hyperparathyroidism, osteopathy due to chemotherapy, and radiation injury (372,373). A common insufficiency fracture is a reambulation fracture of a hindfoot bone or distal tibia at a site of disuse osteoporosis.

Fatigue fractures are stress fractures that result from the application of abnormal stress to normal bone (Fig. 5-133). Most fatigue fractures are due to new or different activity, strenuous activity, or repeated activity. It is important to identify stress fractures so that the injuring activity can be stopped; continued activity results in a complete fracture of the injured bone or of the contralateral extremity only infrequently (374).

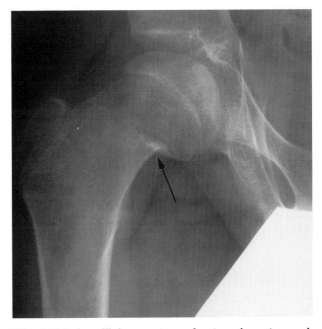

FIG. 5-130. Insufficiency stress fracture in osteopenic bone. A 12-year-old girl with juvenile osteoporosis. There is a buckle fracture *(arrow)* of the femoral neck.

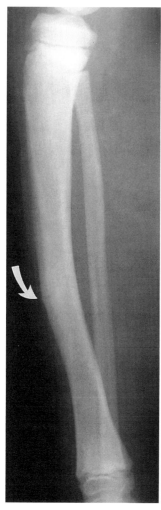

FIG. 5-131. Insufficiency stress fracture in sclerotic bone. A 9-year-old with pyknodysostosis. The lateral radiograph of the tibia shows increased bony sclerosis and anterior tibial bowing. There is an insufficiency fracture in the anterior tibial cortex *(arrow).*

Biomechanics

A stress fracture begins as a small cortical infraction that progresses as the stress increases or continues. Stress fractures do not result from jarring injuries but are related to muscular activity on bone. In children most stress fractures are fatigue rather than insufficiency fractures.

Clinical Features

Patients with stress fractures usually complain of pain that is relieved by rest. There may be the history of an unusual activity that accentuates the pain. There is localized tenderness, usually accompanied by a palpable mass due to hematoma over the fracture. The physical examination may suggest an underlying tumor such as osteogenic sarcoma or Ewing sarcoma.

In a child the tibia is the most frequent site of stress fracture, followed by the fibula. Other sites include the metatarsals, calcaneus, talus, cuboid, patella, femur, pelvis, cervical spine, ribs, distal humerus, and ulna. Toddler's fractures of the tibia, calcaneus, and cuboid are actually stress fractures of the fatigue variety.

Radiologic Features

Most stress fractures in children are of the compression type rather than the distraction type (372). These compression fractures generally occur in the cancellous bone and are most common in the proximal tibia. They may be transverse, oblique, or longitudinal. In cortical bone, the earliest sign is an area of resorption or infraction. After about two weeks, there is usually adjacent periosteal reaction, which may be the initial radiographic sign. In cancellous metaphyseal bone, the earliest sign is osteoblastic repair following microfractures. This usually produces a transverse osseous condensation that involves a part of or crosses the entire shaft of a long bone. In many cases, a fracture line is not seen on the first radiographs or may be detected only with conventional tomography or CT. Stress fractures of the upper third of the tibia characteristically involve the posterior part of that bone. Healing results in a thick lamellar or solid periosteal

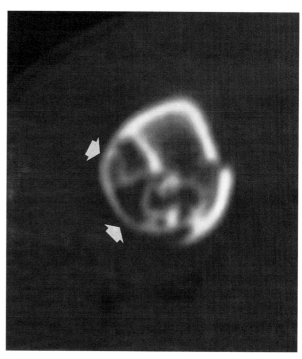

FIG. 5-132. Pathologic insufficiency fracture. A 13-year-old boy with arm pain after minor trauma. Radiograph showed a fracture through a well-defined lucent lesion with sclerotic borders. Axial CT scan of the proximal humerus shows a cortically based, well-marginated lucent lesion of the proximal humeral metadiaphyseal region compatible with a nonossifying fibroma *(arrows).* There is a fracture through the lesion.

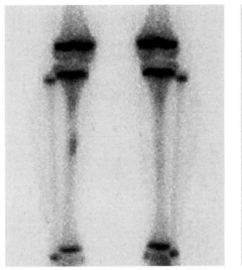 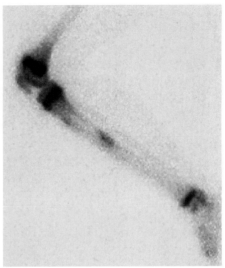

FIG. 5-133. Stress injury. A, B: Track athlete with leg pain. Radiographs were normal. Focally increased radionuclide localization is demonstrated in a stress injury of the posterior tibial diaphysis.

reaction. Stress injury may progress to a complete, displaced fracture, but this is rare.

Skeletal scintigraphy detects stress fractures days or weeks before radiographs (Fig. 5-133). In many patients, the skeletal scintigram is positive when conventional radiographs are normal (4). Radiographic findings usually lag 2 or 3 weeks behind positive skeletal scintigraphy. If the offending activity is stopped, radiographs may never become abnormal. Both focally and diffusely increased tracer localization may result from skeletal stress. A focal abnormality is more likely to progress to a radiologically visible fracture. A particularly common region of diffusely increased localization is the posterior tibial cortex at the origin of the soleus muscle (375). Common sites of focal abnormalities are the metatarsals, the posterior tibia, the medial concavity of the femoral neck, and the pars interarticularis. Demonstration of stress changes in the pars often requires single photon emission computed tomography (SPECT) (376). In all cases of suspected stress injuries, close correlation with symptoms and physical examination is required.

MRI is necessary only for the evaluation of difficult cases (377). There are only diffuse, nonspecific changes at first; later, the abnormality becomes linear across the bone. The abnormality is hypointense on T1-weighted MR images. On T2-weighted images, STIR images, and gadolinium-enhanced T-1 weighted images, there is high signal within the cortex and marrow consistent with edema. The fracture line and the adjacent callus are of decreased signal intensity.

When the exuberant periosteal reaction and inflammation of pediatric injuries renders radiographs and MR confusing, CT may be helpful in establishing the diagnosis. CT demonstration of endosteal bone formation indicates a stress fracture (378). If ultrasonography is performed, it may demonstrate periosteal elevation before radiographs (374).

Differential Diagnosis

The correct diagnosis of a stress fracture is more difficult in a child than in an adult because, especially in young children, the history of a causative activity frequently cannot be elicited. The radiologic appearance of a lesion compatible with stress fracture, in a location common for this entity, should prompt the radiologist to suggest the diagnosis and question the patient or parent.

The differential diagnosis of stress fractures in children includes chronic osteomyelitis, osteogenic sarcoma, and osteoid osteoma. Chronic osteomyelitis may produce a densely sclerotic lesion without apparent radiolucency; serial radiographs show little or no change over a week or two. Osteogenic sarcoma is usually metaphyseal. The sclerotic linearity of a stress fracture is not present in either lesion. Increasing abnormality rather than maturation of findings will be seen on follow-up examination. Osteoid osteoma produces a dense area of sclerosis surrounding a lucent nidus sometimes containing a central calcification. This lesion is usually eccentric, whereas a stress fracture tends to involve much or all of the shaft.

Apophyseal Avulsion Fractures

The apophyses are growth centers like epiphyses, but they do not contribute directly to longitudinal growth. They have been referred to as traction epiphyses because of their muscular attachments. Avulsion of an apophysis does not cause overall longitudinal growth disturbance. Apophyseal avulsion fractures are usually Salter-Harris type 1 physeal fractures, although types 2 (extension of the fracture into the metaphyseal equivalent) and 3 (extension through the ossified secondary center) occasionally occur. Apophyseal avul-

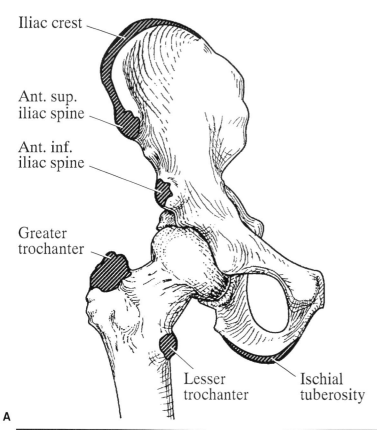

Iliac crest

Ant. sup.
iliac spine

Ant. inf.
iliac spine

Greater
trochanter

Lesser
trochanter

Ischial
tuberosity

A

FIG. 5-134. Avulsion fractures. A: Common sites of pelvic avulsion fractures. **B:** Bilateral avulsions at the insertions of the sartorius muscles and tensor fasciae latae muscles. This 15-year-old male sprinter had acute right hip pain, with similar pain of the left hip 1 year ago. There is an acute avulsion fracture *(solid arrows)* of the right anterosuperior iliac spine. Sclerosis and bony reaction on the left *(open arrows)* indicate a previous but similar injury on the opposite side.

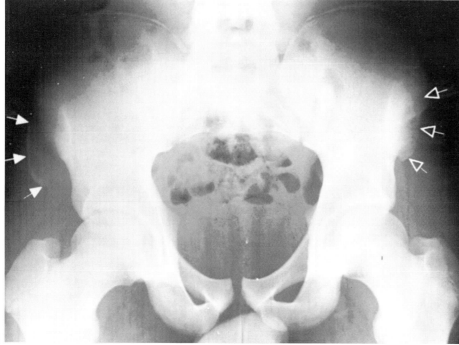

B

sions are frequently athletic injuries, as the apophyses are points of attachment for the muscles that do the avulsing (Fig. 5-134A). Characteristically, avulsion results from sudden muscular pull during vigorous athletic activity.

Potential sites of avulsion fracture (and the avulsing muscles) include the anterosuperior iliac spine (sartorius and tensor fasciae latae) (Fig. 5-134B), anteroinferior iliac spine (rectus femoris component of the quadratus femoris), lesser trochanter (iliopsoas), greater trochanter (gluteus medius, other external rotators), ischial apophysis (hamstrings and adductors), iliac crest apophysis (abdominal wall musculature), and medial epicondyle of the humerus (flexors and rotators of the forearm) (379,380). These avulsions occur in sprinters, football players, ballet dancers, jumpers, and baseball pitchers. The apophyseal center is pulled away from its normal position. There may be a large amount of callus; its irregular outline next to the bone may mimic a malignant lesion. These fractures may cause significant functional impairment, particularly in athletic children (379). The radiographic findings usually are characteristic, but occasionally CT or MRI is necessary to define further the separation of the fragments or to differentiate the lesion from a neoplasm. In some cases skeletal scintigraphy, by demonstrating increased tracer localization next to an apophysis, will first suggest the diagnosis of an avulsion injury.

Battered Child Syndrome

The battered child syndrome (child abuse, child abuse and neglect, nonaccidental injury, parent-infant traumatic stress syndrome, trauma X, the syndrome of Silverman, the syndrome of Ambroise Tardieu) is the abuse or neglect of a child by a parent or some other authority figure. It is an increasingly important problem. More than 1 million children are seriously abused each year in the United States, and 5000 of these children are killed (381). Boys and girls are affected nearly equally. Almost all cases occur before the age of 6 years, and more than half occur in the first year of life (382). Accidental injuries, on the other hand, are relatively rare in infants. Approximately two thirds of battered children have positive radiologic findings, and more than half have detectable fractures (4).

Clinical Features

When the child is first evaluated, there may be evidence of malnutrition and neglect. The abused child, if old enough to show these signs, is usually quiet, withdrawn, and fearful. The parents may be overly concerned about a child who shows no evidence of injury or disturbingly unconcerned about a child who appears critically ill (383). The child fails to seek the parent's reassurance and support. Physical examination may show cutaneous lesions (ecchymoses, abrasions, lacerations, genital lesions, human bites, alopecia, burns, scars), mucosal lesions (lacerations, hematomas), and ocular lesions (retinal detachment, hemorrhage) (383).

Radiologic Evaluation

The skeletal survey (see Appendix 2) remains the primary imaging study when child abuse is suspected. This survey should include AP and lateral views of the skull and thorax, a lateral view of the spine, AP views of the abdomen and pelvis, and AP views of each of the three segments of the extremities, with additional views of any suspicious site after review of the films (384). Meticulous attention must be paid

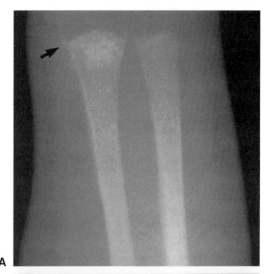

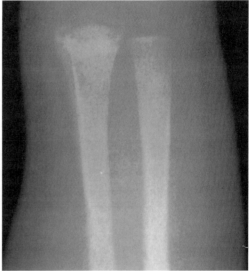

FIG. 5-135. Child abuse. A 1-month-old child with swelling of wrist. **A:** Metaphyseal fracture. The corner fracture *(arrow)* is obvious. There is the suggestion of a bucket handle fracture extending medially. **B:** One-week follow-up. Periosteal reaction (early healing) is now evident at the bucket handle fracture.

to technical details, and high-detail film screen combinations should be used. Many of the fractures are subtle and can easily escape detection without proper exposure and collimation (342). A limited survey after 2 weeks sometimes demonstrates injuries that were inapparent earlier (Fig. 5-135) (384).

Skeletal scintigraphy is particularly valuable for detecting diaphyseal injuries (which often appear as diffusely, rather than focally, increased tracer localization) and rib fractures that are not apparent on radiographs (Fig. 5-136) (385). However, classic epiphyseal-metaphyseal fractures and skull fractures identified on a skeletal survey may not be detected with scintigraphy (386).

If child abuse is suspected in a patient less than 6 years

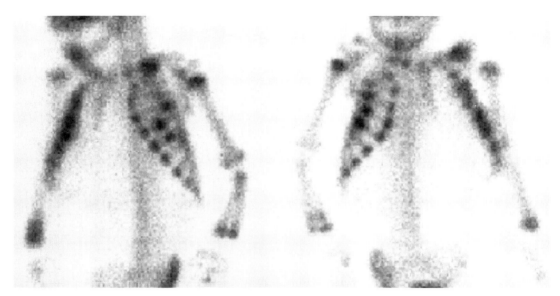

FIG. 5-136. Child abuse. Skeletal scintigraphy shows focal areas of increased tracer uptake in the ribs bilaterally, left clavicle, proximal humeri, and distal forearms.

old, the initial examination should be a skeletal survey as outlined above. If this study is negative and the history is suggestive, skeletal scintigraphy should be performed. CT, when indicated, will define skull, meningeal, cerebral, and abdominal organ injury (387,388). Ultrasonography is also useful for abdominal screening. MRI is even more sensitive than CT to cerebral injuries and can help date them (389).

The radiologic examination may be the first to suggest the diagnosis of battered child syndrome or may provide diagnostic support when the condition is already suspected (384). The radiologist should always consider abuse in any infant with a fracture, as 30% of fractures in infants are inflicted by adults (381). Once the possibility of battering is raised, it is important to confirm or refute the diagnosis. Failure to convey the suspicion of child abuse may return a child to an abusive environment, which can be fatal. Suggesting the diagnosis on insufficient grounds, however, may result in a false accusation, recrimination and distrust between the parents and perhaps in the unwarranted separation of the child from the parents. The radiographic picture is highly suggestive whenever the findings suggest more than one episode of trauma, particularly when the history is not consistent with the injuries observed. Many skeletal injuries in infant abuse are probably caused by grasping the baby about the torso and violently shaking, or by very forceful pulling of an extremity. A direct blow is a less common mechanism of injury.

It is useful to think of injuries in terms of their specificity for child abuse (Table 5-18). A fracture through the primary spongiosa of the metaphysis (Fig. 5-135) (the weakest, newly formed bone adjacent to the physis) is the most specific injury for child abuse (384). It accounts for almost 90% of the long bone fractures in infants who die of abuse (390). The fracture plane is close to the physis centrally, but periph-erally it deviates into the metaphysis incorporating the subperiosteal collar of Laval-Jeantet into the epiphyseal fragment (391). This metaphyseal bony rim will be seen as a crescent (bucket-handle) fracture when the epiphyseal fragment is imaged obliquely, or as two peripheral triangles (corner fractures) if imaged tangentially (Fig. 5-137) (384,392). The bones most frequently so injured are the femur, humerus, and tibia (393).

Fractures of the ribs constitute more than half of the fractures in child abuse and also are highly specific (Fig. 5-136).

TABLE 5-18. *Specificity of radiologic findings in child abuse*

High Specificity
  Metaphyseal lesions, especially corner or bucket-handle fractures
  Posterior rib fractures
  Scapular fractures
  Spinous process fractures
  Sternal fractures
Moderate specificity
  More than one fracture, especially bilateral fractures and fractures remote from each other
  Fractures of different ages
  Epiphyseal separations in infants and young children
  Vertebral body fractures and subluxations
  Digital fractures in infants and young children
  Complex skull fractures
Common in child abuse, but of low specificity
  Clavicular fractures
  Long bone shaft fractures
  Linear skull fractures

Note: Moderate- and low-specificity lesions become high-specificity lesions when a history of trauma is absent or the history is inconsistent with the injuries.
Source: Modified from Kleinman (342).

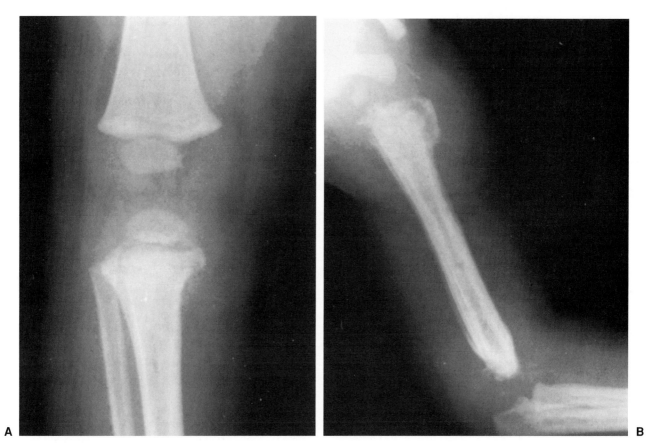

A   B

FIG. 5-137. Child abuse. A 9-month-old girl with failure to thrive. There are classic bucket handle fractures of the metaphyses of the proximal right tibia **(A)** and proximal left humerus **(B)**. There is also periosteal new bone formation indicative of repetitive trauma.

They are difficult to diagnose radiographically until callus appears. Posterior rib fractures, near the costovertebral joints, are particularly characteristic. The rib fractures, however, can occur in any location. They are very unusual in children who have not suffered major trauma, and they should always raise the suspicion of inflicted injury. Other highly specific but less common lesions include fractures of the scapula, spinous process, and sternum.

The coexistence of two or more fractures is a moderately specific sign, particularly if they are remote from each other and particularly if they show different stages of healing. Separations of the cartilaginous epiphyses are significant because they may be radiographically silent and require arthrography, ultrasonography, or MRI for diagnosis (159,394). They also can lead to abnormal growth, which is unusual for the more common metaphyseal fractures. Other injuries of moderate specificity include fractures of the vertebral bodies, fractures of the hands and feet in nonambulatory children, and complex skull fractures.

Low-specificity—but common—injuries include fractures of the long bones, seen in approximately a third of the cases (384,390). Femoral diaphyseal fractures are seldom due to abuse. Spiral diaphyseal fractures are not more specific than transverse ones for child abuse (395). Other low-

specificity injuries include clavicular and linear skull fractures. Occasionally, transverse lucent bands across metaphyses (just shaftward from the zone of provisional calcification) may be a sign of many weeks of neglect. Skeletal lesions are not detected radiographically in at least one third of infants with the battered child syndrome.

Analysis of the healing of the fractures helps determine whether there has been more than one episode of trauma. In infancy, periosteal reaction often becomes detectable radiographically about a week after the injury (396). Repetitive injury disrupts the normal sequential healing process (383). Hemorrhage is increased by repeated injury and lack of treatment, so that callus formation may be exaggerated. There may be a large, traumatic involucrum due to hemorrhage and subperiosteal productive changes. Metaphyseal lucencies due to persistence of unossified physeal cartilage in the metaphyseal spongiosa are also evidence of a healing fracture (397). Thin periosteal new bone can occur with abuse in the absence of fracture. However, periosteal new bone may be seen in normal infants until about 6 months of age (41,382); this normal variant is usually only diaphyseal, is most commonly seen along the medial aspect of the femurs, and is smooth and symmetric.

Although the skeleton most frequently shows the signs

of child abuse, extraskeletal manifestations have received increasing attention in recent years. A common craniocerebral injury in the abused child is acute parietooccipital interhemispheric subdural hematoma associated with parenchymal injury, which may lead to atrophy and infarction. Other craniocerebral findings include acute subdural hematoma, chronic subdural hematoma or hygroma, intracerebral hematoma, and cerebral edema (387,389). Lung contusions and lacerations may be associated with rib fractures. Subcutaneous fat is frequently reduced, and skeletal maturation is often delayed because of malnutrition. Trauma may produce a hematoma of the duodenum, jejunum, or mesentery, sometimes with obstruction. There may be lacerations and contusions of solid abdominal organs (398,399). Pneumoperitoneum due to perforation has also been described. Traumatic pancreatitis may lead to pseudocyst formation and to multifocal osteolysis due to release of pancreatic enzymes (388). There may be acute gastric distention after the patient is admitted to the hospital and allowed to eat; deprivation produces malnutrition, hypoproteinemia, and gastric atony. Sudden resumption of brain growth may cause alarming (but actually reassuring) sutural separation.

Fractures in varying stages of healing indicate more than one episode of injury. If there are fractures that are highly specific for child abuse (Table 5-18), multiple fractures, traumatic lesions of different ages, or fractures out of proportion to the history, a detailed social and medical investigation should follow. In most jurisdictions, laws require the physician to report suspected abuse to an appropriate authority or agency; the radiologist discharges this legal responsibility by communicating the possibility of child abuse to the referring physician and documenting this communication.

Differential Diagnosis

There are only a few pertinent considerations in the battered child syndrome. The history, physical examination, and radiologic features are usually adequate to establish the diagnosis. Entities that produce metaphyseal abnormalities or subperiosteal reaction, however, sometimes cause diagnostic difficulties. The battered child syndrome should be differentiated from diseases producing metaphyseal bone destruction (congenital syphilis, multifocal osteomyelitis, leukemia, metastatic neuroblastoma, meningococcemia); other metaphyseal abnormalities (rickets, metaphyseal chondrodysplasia [particularly the Schmid type]); diseases resulting in multiple fractures (neuromuscular disorders, congenital insensitivity to pain, osteogenesis imperfecta, Menkes syndrome); other traumatic injuries of the bones (frostbite, electrical burns [which also may be the result of abuse]); and causes of prominent periosteal bone formation (infantile cortical hyperostosis [Caffey disease], normal periosteal new bone formation of infancy, hypervitaminosis A). Rarer metabolic bone disorders such as scurvy, osteopetrosis, pyknodysostosis, and hypophosphatasia are occasionally confused with child abuse. In infants, the normal junction between the straight 1- to 3-mm metaphyseal collar (at the most immature metaphysis) and the more mature smoothly curved metaphysis is sometimes mistaken for an abuse fracture (see Fig. 5-29) (71,400). Simulators of child abuse also include birth trauma and traumatic injuries inflicted in the course of rescue of a subject from real or perceived danger (rescued child syndrome).

The entities the radiologist must always keep in mind and make a particular effort to exclude are osteogenesis imperfecta, Menkes syndrome (in boys), other causes of copper or trace mineral deficiency, and congenital insensitivity to pain. The former two diagnoses are associated with an excessive number of wormian bones and osteopenia (5). Osteogenesis imperfecta is a differential consideration frequently raised by defense lawyers (384). Of the types of osteogenesis imperfecta, only type IV (mild to moderate osseous fragility and normal sclerae) can be confused with child abuse (104). Only a few cases of this form, however, have ever been reported.

Neuropathic Injuries

Neuropathic injuries occur in children with impaired perception of pain. These injuries include fractures, epiphyseal separations, neuropathic arthropathy, and soft-tissue ulcers. Because the injuries often go unrecognized and untreated, marked disability can result. The most common cause of neuropathic abnormalities in children is an anomaly of the spinal cord (4). Other etiologies include familial dysautonomia, congenital insensitivity to pain, peripheral nerve damage, and congenital amniotic bands.

Metaphyseal and diaphyseal fractures of the lower extremities can occur because of severe or moderately severe osteoporosis from lack of normal activity. Fractures of the lower extremities occur in up to 20% of children with an anomaly of the spinal cord (usually myelodysplasia), often before 9 years of age (401). Minor trauma, often routine physical therapy, may produce a fracture, most commonly about the knee. Impaired sensation may leave the injury unnoticed; nonunion and pseudarthrosis eventually develop. The child may present with redness and warmth at the site, a low-grade fever, leukocytosis, and an elevated erythrocyte sedimentation rate. The signs may suggest septic arthritis, child abuse, osteomyelitis, cellulitis, or neoplasm. Acute fractures frequently have a transverse orientation and are located in the metaphysis (Fig. 5-138). The fractures heal quickly if they are recognized; casting is often required for only 4 weeks. There may be evidence of previous injury with malalignment, abnormal modeling and widened metaphyses (Erlenmeyer flask deformity) (402).

Physeal fractures are less common. They often occur in children with lower lumbar neurologic involvement who remain ambulatory. Minor repetitive trauma to a physis may cause irregular widening of the physis and epiphyseal separation (Fig. 5-139). Similar physical injuries are sometimes seen in budding atheletes who ignore their symptoms; proximal humeral physeal injuries in baseball pitchers may be the most common. Repeated injury produces subperiosteal hemorrhage. Healing is much slower than with the metaphyseal and diaphyseal fractures, and casting therapy often extends for 8–12 weeks (401). There may be subsequent deformity due to premature fusion of the physis.

The development of neuropathic arthropathy (Charcot joint) requires decreased pain sensation or indifference to pain and vigorous physical activity (403,404). The radiologic features of neuropathic joint disease in children include the four D's: density (sclerosis), debris, disorganization, dislocation. Fragmentation of the articular surfaces is associated with synovial hypertrophy and reactive bone sclerosis. Neuropathic joint changes in children also include physeal widening and metaphyseal fragmentation. Many of the changes are reactions to repetitive physeal disruption (405).

Soft-tissue ulcers usually occur in areas of pressure due to weight bearing or over bony prominences (403). If activity or pressure is continued and there is repeated trauma, the ulcer is deepened, the skin and subcutaneous tissues degenerate, and the ulcer penetrates bone to produce osteomyelitis.

Other congenital or acquired musculoskeletal abnormali-

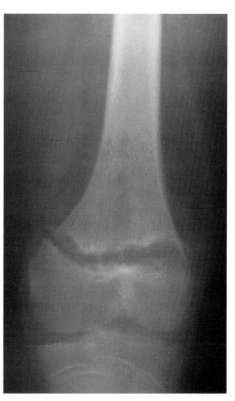

FIG. 5-139. Physeal fracture. There is a physeal fracture of the distal femur in this 10-year-old girl with myelodysplasia. The physis is widened. There is only a small amount of callus.

ties in children with neurologic impairment and resultant muscle imbalance include kyphosis, lordosis, scoliosis, subluxation and dislocation of the hips, coxa valga, contracture deformities of the proximal femurs, femoral and tibial torsion abnormalities, and ankle and foot malalignments (401). Unexplained cavus foot and unexplained resistant clubfoot deserve neurologic workup for a possible spinal cord lesion.

MISCELLANEOUS DISORDERS

Metabolic Disorders

Rickets

Rickets is a group of diseases of infants and children caused by a relative or absolute insufficiency of vitamin D (Table 5-19) or its hormonal derivative, 1,25-dihydroxycholecalciferol. This insufficiency causes a failure to transform growing cartilage into mineralized cartilage and then mineralized osteoid (bone).

Vitamin D is synthesized in the human by the endogenous conversion of dihydrocholesterol in the skin. If there is inadequate exposure to sunlight, additional vitamin D must be present in the diet. Vitamin D is hydroxylated first in the liver and then a second time in the kidneys to the most active form, 1,25-dihydroxycholecalciferol. There are many causes

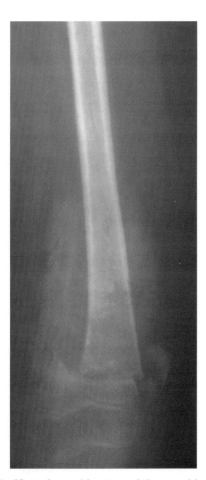

FIG. 5-138. Metaphyseal fracture. A 5-year-old girl with myelodysplasia. A distal femoral metaphyseal fracture developed during physical therapy. There is considerable callus formation, but the fracture is still evident.

TABLE 5-19. *Causes of rickets*

Dietary deficiency of vitamin D
  Prematurity[a]
  Hyperalimentation
  Prolonged nonsupplemented breastfeeding
  Starvation
  Unusual diet
Malabsorption of vitamin D
  Liver disease[a]
  Biliary obstruction
  Pancreatic insufficiency
    Cystic fibrosis
    Pancreatitis
  Small bowel abnormality
    Crohn disease
    Lymphoma
    Postsurgical state
Renal disease
  Renal glomerular failure[a]
  Renal tubular disorders
    Inherited
      Vitamin D-resistant rickets[a]
      Cystinosis
      De Toni-Fanconi syndrome
      Renal tubular acidosis
  Heavy metal intoxication
Increased requirements of vitamin D
  Vitamin D-dependent rickets (inherited)[a]
  Anticonvulsant therapy
Miscellaneous
  Aluminum toxicity
  Deficient vitamin D synthesis: lack of sunlight
  Tumor-dependent disorders

[a] More common.

of rickets (Table 5-19). All types eventually cause inadequate mineralization of and disorganization of the chondrocytes of the hypertrophic zone of the physis and failure to mineralize osteoid into bone. Rickets is associated with osteomalacia (inadequate or delayed mineralization of osteoid of mature trabeculae and cortical bone) (406,407). Rickets may be due to a pathologic deficiency of or resistance to vitamin D. An absolute deficiency of vitamin D may be due to nutritional lack or malabsorption of the vitamin, whereas relative deficiency may be secondary to increased requirements and other rare states (Table 5-19). The resistant form includes congenital and acquired renal diseases (Table 5-19).

Dietary rickets usually develops at 3–6 months of age. It is occasionally present during the neonatal period, particularly in premature infants (373), and is seldom diagnosed after 2 years of age. Clinical features include enlarged and distorted bones (rachitic rosary due to the widened costochondral junctions, widened ends of extremity bones), muscle weakness, chest deformities, kyphoscoliosis, growth failure, tetany, craniotabes (ping-pong ball sensation on palpation of the skull), delayed closure of the fontanels and sutures, and frontal bone thickening with bossing (408).

The radiologic findings of rickets often precede the clinical manifestations. At least a third of cases of radiologically diagnosed rickets are found serendipitously on studies done for other indications. The classic radiologic appearance of rickets occurs at the metaphyses of the most rapidly growing bones (Figs. 5-140, 5-141, and 5-142). Failure to ossify the

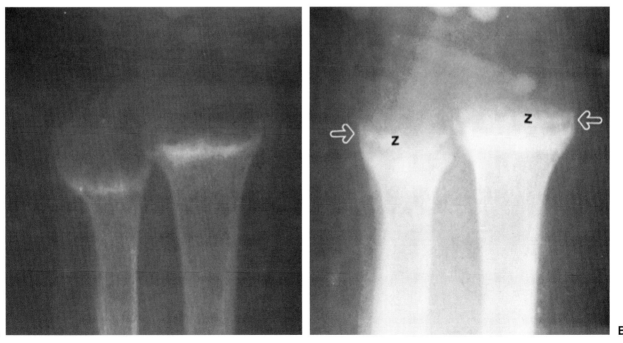

FIG. 5-140. Dietary rickets with prompt recovery. A 6-month-old infant with dietary rickets. **A:** Florid rickets with absence of the Laval-Jeantet ring (the straight area at the metaphyseal margins). **B:** Seventeen days after treatment began, the Laval-Jeantet ring *(arrows)* has reappeared, as the cartilage ossifies, beginning at the zone of provisional calcification *(z)*. Ossification around growth centers (hamate, capitate, and distal radius) has also progressed in the interim. From Oestreich and Crawford (5).

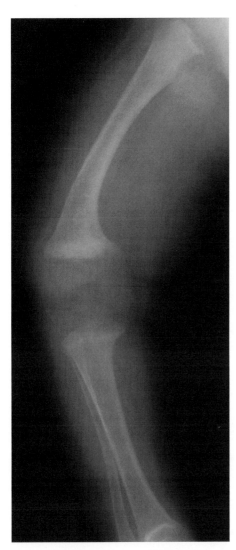

FIG. 5-141. Hypophosphatemic rickets. A 2-year-old-boy with hypophosphatemic rickets. There is cupping and fraying of the metaphyses and marked bowing of the femur. The distal femoral physis is more severely affected than the proximal because of its greater rate of growth.

physeal cartilage results in loss of the radiopaque fine line representing the zone of provisional calcification. Persistence of unossified cartilage in the metaphyseal new bone results in cupping, fraying, and irregularity of the physeal surface. In infants, there is a lack of mineralization of the longitudinally straight, most recently formed (1–3 mm) metaphyseal margin (Laval-Jeantet collar) (Fig. 5-140) (71,373). Coexistent osteomalacia, with osteoid being produced but not mineralized, results in unsharp, coarse, bony trabecula. There is loss of normal cortical distinction, perhaps due in part to secondary hyperparathyroidism. There is loss of definition of the margins of the epiphyses. Apparent longitudinal widening of the physis is due to the abnormal accumulation of unmineralized osteoid, persistence of uncalcified cartilage, and loss of the zone of provisional calcifi-

cation. Ossification centers are small radiographically because their periphery is unmineralized osteoid instead of bone. The apparently delayed bone age may show a remarkably rapid increase when the osteoid calcifies after treatment (Fig. 5-140). There often is bowing of the femoral and tibial shafts. In advanced cases, there may be insufficiency fractures (Looser zones), seen as bilateral, usually symmetric linear lucencies perpendicular to the cortex. Rickets is occasionally suggested from chest radiographs by the frayed, widened anterior rib ends, proximal humeral metaphyseal changes, and irregular concavity of the inferior scapular angle (373,409). There may be demineralization of the skull (410) and loss of the lamina dura about erupted and unerupted teeth. The teeth and petrous pyramids may be remarkably prominent because of the poor mineralization elsewhere. These patients may present with pathologic fractures. Secondary hyperparathyroidism tends to occur in all rachitic diseases except with phosphaturic causes of rickets.

The radiographic evaluation can be confined to the knees and wrists, or even the knees alone, which are the areas most severely affected because greatest linear growth is occurring there. Radiographs suggest the etiology of rickets only occasionally. If the infant is less than 6 months of age at presentation, the probable causes include biliary atresia, dietary deficiency, and rickets associated with prematurity. Resistance to treatment suggests renal tubular disorders and rickets-producing tumors. Children with X-linked hypophosphatemic rickets have only mild rachitic changes and nearly normal bone density. Evidence of severe hyperparathyroidism suggests renal osteodystrophy (407).

Renal Osteodystrophy

Renal osteodystrophy, a general term, includes a variety of skeletal and soft-tissue changes in patients with end-stage renal disease. These changes are rickets, osteomalacia, secondary hyperparathyroidism, osteosclerosis, and soft-tissue calcification.

Classification

There is considerable overlap in the manifestations of renal osteodystrophy (411–416). End-stage renal disease results from glomerular diseases or, less frequently, from tubular disorders. The glomerular disease may be due to chronic pyelonephritis, obstructive nephropathy, glomerulonephritis, collagen vascular disease, polycystic kidney disease, and extensive renal parenchymal loss. Patients with glomerular disease are azotemic; the radiologic findings are predominantly those of secondary hyperparathyroidism. Bone biopsy, however, frequently shows the coexistence of rickets or osteomalacia. There also may be osteosclerosis and soft-tissue calcification.

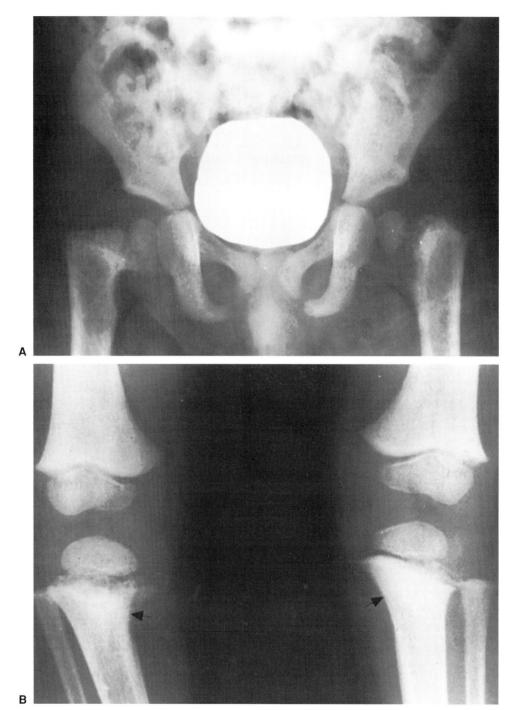

FIG. 5-142. Rickets due to renal tubular disease. A 3-year-old boy with renal tubular acidosis and the radiologic changes of rickets and secondary hyperparathyroidism. **A:** The bones are osteopenic. Loss of the normal zone of provisional calcification is due to rickets. Bony resorption along the medial femoral necks and coxa vara is due to secondary hyperparathyroidism. **B:** The subperiosteal bony resorption due to secondary hyperparathyroidism is most pronounced along the medial aspect of the proximal tibial metaphyses and produces a bite defect *(arrows)*.

Pathophysiology

The pathophysiology of renal osteodystrophy is complex and is still incompletely understood. Rickets results from several alterations of vitamin D metabolism in renal failure.

The first hydroxylation of vitamin D occurs in the liver; the second hydroxylation depends on renal mass and is impaired in chronic renal disease. Hyperphosphatemia, a consequence of glomerular failure, also impairs vitamin D production (407). Osteomalacia in renal osteodystrophy does not appear to be related to vitamin D, but rather to metal (especially aluminum) toxicity (411). Secondary hyperparathyroidism results from hypocalcemia, which in turn is due mainly to phosphate retention. Secondary hyperparathyroidism and local cytokines cause osteitis fibrosa. The classic pathologic lesion in renal osteodystrophy, osteitis fibrosa, is characterized by marrow fibrosis, increased production of bone, and focal areas of resorption of bone. Osteosclerosis is related to the effects of increased parathyroid hormone and may be due to stimulation of osteoblastic activity and increased production of trabecular bone (413,417). Soft-tissue calcification is primarily the result of an increase in the calcium-phosphate product in extracellular fluid.

Radiologic Changes

The length of time renal dysfunction is present prior to the radiologic detection of skeletal changes (rickets, osteomalacia, secondary hyperparathyroidism, osteosclerosis, and soft-tissue calcification) depends on the age of the patient. Skeletal changes may occur after only 1 or 2 months of renal dysfunction in the young infant (Fig. 5-143 and 5-144), but they usually require several years in the older child or adult.

Renal Rickets

Rickets in renal osteodystrophy is distinguishable from rickets of other causes only if hyperparathyroidism and osteosclerosis coexist (Fig. 5-143). There may be epiphyseal

separations, particularly involving the femoral head; these seem to be due to physeal weakening from the combined effects of rickets and hyperparathyroidism (418).

Secondary Hyperparathyroidism

The bone resorption and osteopenia seen in secondary hyperparathyroidism are similar to those phenomena in primary hyperparathyroidism but are much more common. Osteosclerosis, periostitis, and soft-tissue calcification, rare in the primary form, occur frequently in end-stage renal disease (417). Brown tumors, however, are unusual in secondary hyperparathyroidism, occurring in less than 2% of cases (413).

In children, subperiosteal bone resorption frequently involves the femoral necks (Fig. 5-143), proximal humeri, and medial aspects of the proximal tibias (Fig. 5-144B), producing a bite defect. In older children and adults, subperiosteal resorption is most commonly detected along the radial aspects of the middle and proximal phalanges of the second and third digits (Fig. 5-144A and 5-145B). These sites are affected because of tendinous insertions and their pull during apposition of the second and third digits toward the thumb. There may also be resorption of the phalangeal tufts (Fig. 5-145B). Other sites of subperiosteal bone resorption include the distal radius, the ends of clavicles, the superior aspects of ribs, the symphysis pubis, and the sacroiliac joints. The normal sharp cortical line is replaced by a toothbrush border (Fig. 5-145). Osteopenia or bony demineralization may ac-

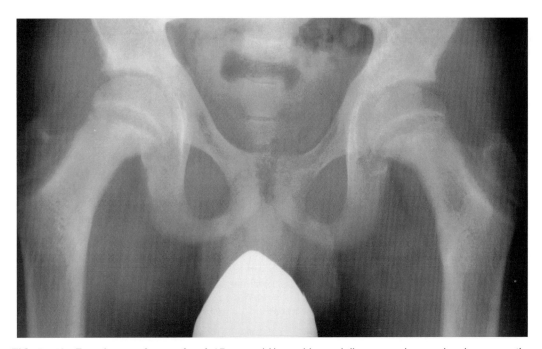

FIG. 5-143. Renal osteodystrophy. A 15-year-old boy with renal disease and secondary hyperparathyroidism. AP radiograph of the pelvis shows rachitic changes of the proximal femoral growth plates. The changes also involve the growth plates of the greater trochanters. There is coarsening of the trabeculae and irregularity of the pubic symphysis and femoral necks, indicating secondary hyperparathyroidism.

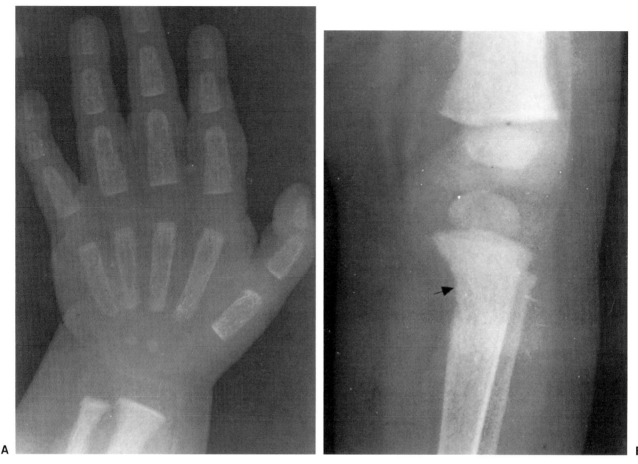

FIG. 5-144. Renal osteodystrophy. This 1-month-old girl had secondary hyperparathyroidism due to renal dysplasia. There is generalized osteopenia and subperiosteal resorption of all the cortices including the radial aspect of the phalanges **(A)**, the medial proximal tibia *(arrow)*, and the distal femur **(B)**.

centuate and smudge the trabecular pattern. Eventually, all cortices appear washed out or become invisible, in contrast to the sharply defined but thinned cortex of osteopenia due to osteoporosis (5).

Osteosclerosis

Diffuse osteosclerosis produces an overall increase in bone density and indistinct (smudged) trabeculae. Osteosclerosis (Fig. 5-146A) frequently involves the vertebral endplates (''rugger jersey'' spine) and occasionally even produces cortical thickening of the tubular bones. Nearly 40% of children with end-stage renal disease have sclerosis, probably due to a similar mechanism, in the metaphyses next to the physes (419).

Soft-Tissue Calcification

Soft-tissue calcifications occasionally develop in patients with secondary hyperparathyroidism. They may be subcutaneous, periarticular, visceral, or vascular (Fig. 5-146B). Cal-

cifications can produce pressure erosions on the adjacent bone.

Scurvy and Copper Deficiency

Ascorbic acid (vitamin C) and ascorbic acid oxydase, a copper-dependent enzyme, are essential for the synthesis of normal collagen (420). For this reason, ascorbic acid deficiency and copper deficiency are closely related and share radiographic and clinical features. Thanks to improved nutrition, scurvy is now extremely uncommon.

Scurvy almost always occurred in patients over 6 months of age, although there are documented cases in the neonate (421). The bones are demineralized, but the zone of provisional calcification is preserved. There is a lucent band, the scurvy line, on the metaphyseal side of the zone of provisional calcification. There can be pathologic fractures through the metaphyses; these heal to produce spurs. The epiphyses are outlined by a fine sharp white line, the ring of Wimberger (quite different from the corner sign of Wimberger in congenital syphilis), that represents mineral deposition in the peripheral zone of provisional calcification of

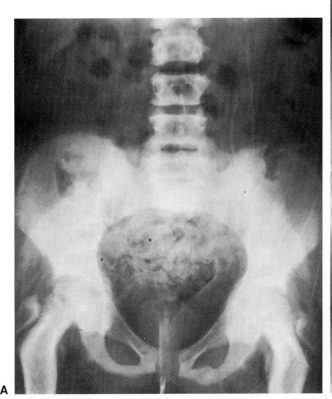

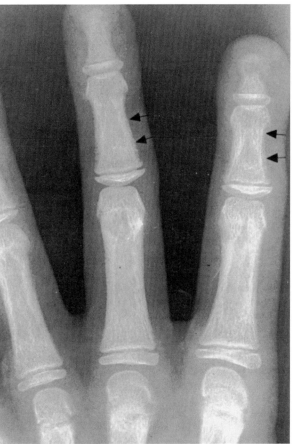

A

B

FIG. 5-145. Renal osteodystrophy. An 11-year-old girl with azotemia, hypertension, and secondary hyperparathyroidism due to chronic pyelonephritis. **A:** Generalized osteosclerosis and smudging of the trabecular pattern are evident. There is subperiosteal resorption at the femoral necks. **B:** Subperiosteal resorption of the cortices of the middle and proximal phalanges of the second and third digits produces a "toothbrush" cortical margin *(arrows)*. Note the resorption of phalangeal tufts.

the secondary ossification center. There can be extensive subperiosteal bleeding. This leads to cloaking of bone by periosteal ossification during healing. Epiphyseal slipping, such as at the distal femur and proximal humerus, may occur (3,5).

Copper deficiency is due to nutritional deficiency in premature infants, or to abnormal intestinal transport of copper, such as in Menkes disease. The radiographic findings are similar to those of scurvy (osteoporosis, prominent zones of provisional calcification, metaphyseal spurs), but the lucent band under the zone of provisional calcification is usually not present in copper deficiency (422). Copper deficiency and scurvy can mimic the metaphyseal fractures of battered child syndrome (Fig. 5-147). The cerebrovascular abnormalities of Menkes disease distinguish it from other entities.

Hypothyroidism and Hyperthyroidism

Hypothyroidism in the newborn (cretinism) is usually due to congenital absence or hypoplasia (often with ectopia) of the thyroid gland. Most cases are detected by neonatal screening. Rarely, cretinism is due to maternal ingestion of propylthiouracil. In older infants and children, hypothyroidism may be congenital or secondary to thyroiditis, autoimmune disease, or thyroid-stimulating hormone deficiency. Congenital hypothyroidism is usually sporadic but is occasionally inherited in an autosomal recessive pattern. The disease is up to three times as common in girls as in boys.

The most striking clinical features include retarded growth, persistence of infantile proportions, and lethargy. The height of the child is not nearly as retarded as the skeletal maturation, and, in fact, the neonate may even be large. Other clinical features include constipation, umbilical hernia, large tongue, difficulty feeding, anemia, prolonged neonatal jaundice, and prolonged neonatal cyanosis.

The most important radiologic finding is the retarded skeletal maturation. The retardation is usually marked. The bone age may be much more than 2 SD below the mean. Epiphyseal ossification centers for the distal femur, proximal tibia, cuboid, and proximal humerus, which appear normally at

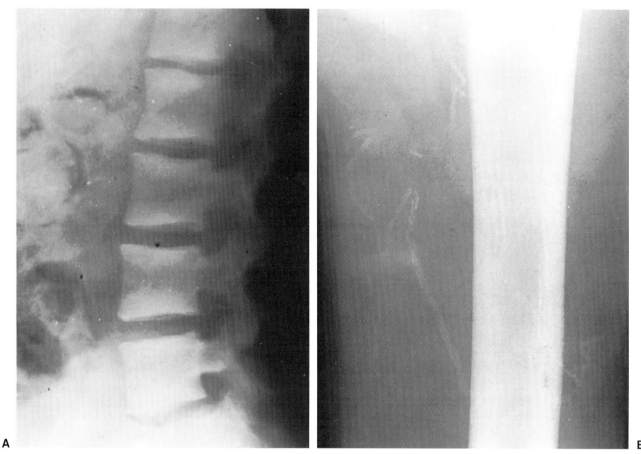

A   B

FIG. 5-146. Renal osteodystrophy. A 16-year-old boy with azotemia secondary to chronic renal failure.
A: Sclerosis of vertebral endplates produces a "rugger jersey" spine. **B:** Vascular calcifications.

the 34th, 36th, 38th, and 40th gestational weeks, are usually absent at birth in cretinism (423). Metaphyseal irregularities become prominent when the child's bone age is 1–3 years. Retarded skeletal maturation and irregularity and fragmentation of the epiphyses (epiphyseal dysgenesis) are noted in older infants and children (Fig. 5-148).

There is delay in closure of cranial sutures. The number of wormian bones is increased. In the infant, the sella often appears immature and bowl-like (424). In the older child, the sella appears round and slightly enlarged (''cherry'' sella) because of feedback hypertrophy of the pituitary gland (424). Tooth maturation is normal at birth and is less affected than skeletal maturation thereafter. The base of the skull may be unusually dense.

The vertebral bodies maintain their infantile features, including large central vascular grooves and an ovoid shape. The anterosuperior parts of the vertebral bodies are hypoplastic, and there is inferoanterior beaking. There is often a kyphosis at the thoracolumbar junction. The intervertebral disc spaces are wide, and the vertebral endplates are sclerotic.

In the newborn, apparent increased sclerosis results from failure of development of cancellous bone. The most recently ossified metaphyses may be broad and dense. Small,

dense projections are noted extending from the midmetaphyses into the physes of the distal phalanges (425). Epiphyseal dysgenesis results from disordered endochondral bone formation (Fig. 5-148). Occasionally, the epiphyses of the proximal femurs are sclerotic and mimic LCP disease; however, epiphyseal involvement in hypothyroidism is symmetric. The capital femoral epiphyses may slip, even before age 10 (426).

Conditions associated with hypothyroidism include trisomy 21, multiple endocrine deficiencies due to autoimmune processes, cystinosis, precocious thelarche, hypercalcemia with vitamin D therapy, and the association of congenital heart disease and spinal anomalies. Normal skeletal maturation resumes within 2–4 months of thyroid replacement therapy. Catch-up growth and skeletal maturation are particularly rapid prior to 1 year of age. Because growth is needed for rickets to be evident, it can be unmasked with the institution of hormonal therapy.

Hyperthyroidism is infrequent in children, and its effects on the skeleton are less pronounced. Radiographic manifestations include accelerated skeletal maturation, premature sutural closure, osteopenia (hyperthyroid osteopathy), and thymomegaly. The osteopenia can be very severe and affect the appendicular as well as the axial skeleton (427).

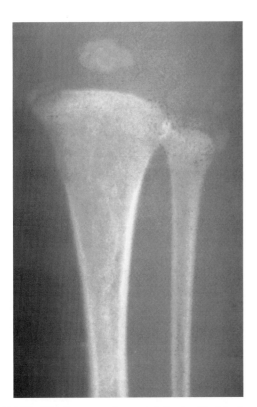

FIG. 5-147. Menkes syndrome. Infant with Menkes syndrome (congenital copper deficiency). There are subtle metaphyseal fractures of the "bucket handle" type, similar to those of child abuse. The zone of provisional calcification is well defined.

Systemic Disorders

Anemia: Sickle Cell Anemia and Thalassemia

Radiologic changes associated with anemias are related to marrow hyperplasia and, in sickle cell conditions, infarction and other effects of sludging of red blood cells (428–431). With bone marrow imaging (e.g., T1-weighted MRI), the first consequence of marrow hyperplasia during childhood is an increased volume and more widespread distribution of hematopoietic marrow, simulating that of a younger patient (236).

On radiographs, the more severe and long-lasting the anemia, the greater the effects of marrow hyperplasia. Thalassemia major usually has the most pronounced radiologic findings (430). Without relief of the anemia, the marrow cavities are expanded, the cortex is thin, and the trabeculae are coarse (Fig. 5-149). The ribs are broad. Both the ribs and the vertebral bodies have coarse trabeculae. The diploic space may be markedly widened, particularly in thalassemia ("hair-on-end" pattern; Fig. 5-150) and severe, chronic iron deficiency anemia. Rarely, a weakened vertebral body in a thalassemic child will collapse and become a vertebra plana. Extramedullary hematopoiesis leads to masses at the costovertebral junctions. Gallstones may occur in children with excessive hemolysis. Splenomegaly and, less often, nephromegaly are seen in many anemias; in sickle cell disease, however, the spleen becomes infarcted, small, and some-

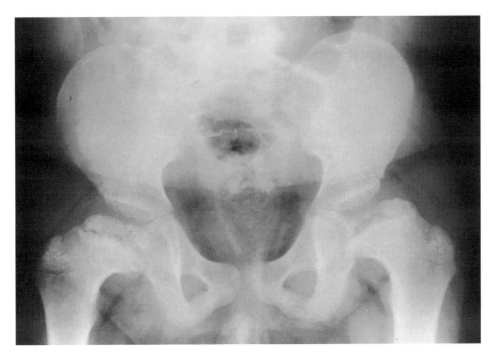

FIG. 5-148. Hypothyroidism. An 8-year-old boy with short stature and mental retardation. There is epiphyseal dysgenesis (delayed maturation, granular irregularity, and fragmentation) of the capital femoral epiphyses. Skeletal maturation was approximately 8 SD below the mean.

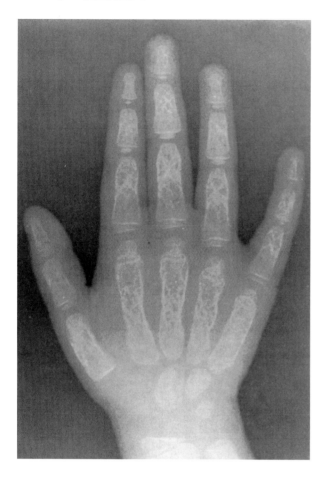

FIG. 5-149. Thalassemia. Typical pattern of coarse trabeculae, thin cortices, and expanded shaft contours in a 6-year-old girl with thalassemia major.

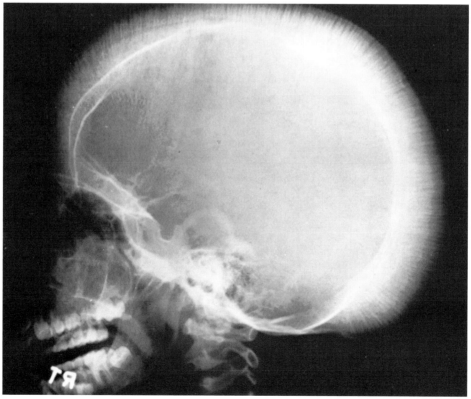

FIG. 5-150. Severe anemia. "Hair-on-end," widened diploic space in a 6-year-old child with thalassemia major.

times calcified. Cardiomegaly is typical of severe anemia, regardless of the etiology; in patients with sickle cell disease this may be complicated by cardiomyopathy.

The hand-foot syndrome of sickle cell disease is seen in children under 2 years of age; this swelling of fingers or toes may be the first indication of the disease. Radiographically, there is periosteal reaction along one or more small tubular bone shafts, with soft-tissue swelling that gradually resolves (5,428). The cause is probably infarction, not infection. However, older children with sickle cell disease have a high incidence of both osteomyelitis and bone infarction, which are difficult to distinguish by radiographs, skeletal scintigraphy, CT, or MRI. Gadolinium-enhanced MRI helps to identify abscesses, but there is considerable overlap between the appearances of acute osteomyelitis and acute infarction (432). Combined scintigraphy, subtracting ^{99m}Tc-labeled scintigraphic images from gallium-67 images, can sometimes make this distinction. Gallium-67 should therefore be the initial scintigraphic study in children with sickle cell disease and the suspicion of osteomyelitis. The definitive diagnosis of infection is made by aspirating pus from the lesion.

Both infarction and infection, as seen in sickle cell disease, begin with bone destruction (lucency) and periosteal reaction; infarction may also have areas of dense ossification. Infarction may affect epiphyses (leading to the pattern of avascular necrosis; Fig. 5-151) or physes (leading to coned epiphyses and short metacarpals). Often a characteristic flat indentation of the upper and lower vertebral endplates develops during childhood, sparing the most anterior and posterior

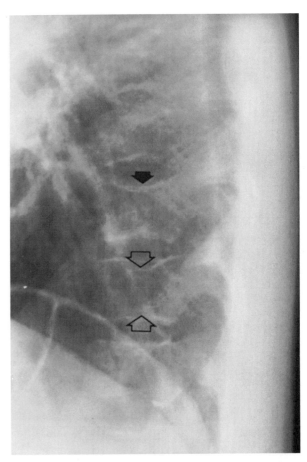

FIG. 5-152. Sickle cell anemia. This 16-year-old boy was known to have sickle cell anemia. Central portions of the affected endplates are flat (rather than concave as in osteoporosis) but indented *(arrows)*.

portions (Fig. 5-152). This configuration is variously referred to as H-shaped, Lincoln log, elevator, codfish vertebra, or the canoe sign; it differs from the concave endplates (fishmouth) of osteoporosis. The step-off probably results from impairment of the vascular supply to the centers of the physes. Infarctions or infections in children with sickle cell disease also affect the signal intensity of the marrow. The marrow becomes heterogeneous on T1-weighted, T2-weighted, and STIR MR images. It is characteristic for the bones of sickle cell patients to show mixed serpiginous marrow patterns (132,433) (Fig. 5-153). Bone age is often delayed in sickle cell disease and other severe anemias.

Other radiographic findings characteristic of specific anemias include the radial reduction deformities and lateral clavicle hook in Fanconi pancytopenia, and the triphalangeal thumb of the pure red blood cell anemia of Blackfan and Diamond (430). Thalassemia major occasionally causes rib notching (430).

Therapy with transfusion leads to regression of the changes of marrow expression. Patients who undergo repeated transfusions for hemolytic anemia may develop severe iron deposition. This can be detected on MRI as areas

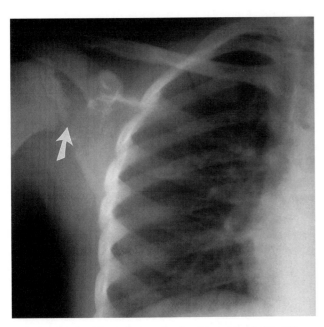

FIG. 5-151. Sickle cell anemia. An 11-year-old girl with arm pain. There is increased density of the ribs and avascular necrosis of the right humeral epiphysis *(arrow)*. In patients with sickle cell anemia, one should look for evidence of osteonecrosis of the humeral heads on chest radiographs.

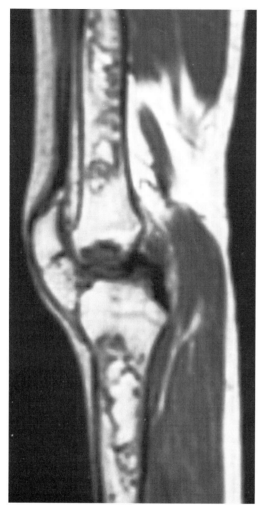

FIG. 5-153. Sickle cell anemia with multiple infarctions. Teenager with sickle cell anemia and recurrent bone pain. Sagittal T1-weighted MR image shows the characteristic serpiginous areas of abnormal signal intensity in the marrow of the femur and tibia.

of very low signal intensity on T1- and T2-weighted images (Fig. 5-154). Initially, the low signal intensity is confined to areas of active phagocytosis such as the liver, spleen, and bone marrow (secondary hemosiderosis). Further deposition of iron in the pituitary gland, thyroid, myocardium, and pancreas may result in tissue damage (hemochromatosis) and carries a much graver prognosis. Children treated with desferoxamine, a chelating agent, sometimes develop characteristic metaphyseal irregularities (434).

Hemophilia

The hemophilias are disorders of coagulation caused by a functional or absolute deficiency of a clotting factor. Classic hemophilia (hemophilia A) is due to factor VIII deficiency, and Christmas disease (hemophilia B) is due to factor IX deficiency. Both disorders have an X-linked recessive in-

heritance pattern and consequently are carried by females but manifested in males. Christmas disease is usually less severe than hemophilia A, although the clinical and radiologic features may be indistinguishable (435). The incidence of classic hemophilia is approximately 1 case per 10,000 newborn boys. It is five times as frequent as Christmas disease. Detecting joint involvement is of utmost importance in hemophilia, as repeated hemarthroses can result in severe disability. Radiographs rarely suggest the diagnosis until the patient has been aware of it for years. Radiography and cross-sectional imaging are important for demonstrating progressive deformity, revealing unsuspected complications, and excluding other conditions (435–437).

Recurrent bleeding into joints, spontaneous or traumatic, is characteristic of hemophilia. In order of decreasing frequency, the joints most often involved are the knee, elbow, and ankle. The wrist, shoulder, hand, foot, and hip are also sometimes involved (435). The fact that hinge articulations are more frequently involved than ball-and-socket joints suggests that weight bearing is less important than the type of stress applied to the joint. Bleeding into the joints presumably arises from the subsynovial vascular plexus. With *acute hemarthrosis*, radiographs show only joint capsule distention. After a single hemarthrosis, the joint may return to normal. Recurrent hemarthroses produce hemosiderin deposition within the synovium, which leads to synovial hypertrophy and fibrosis within a year. Synovial changes and pannus formation lead to *chronic hemophilic arthropathy*. The

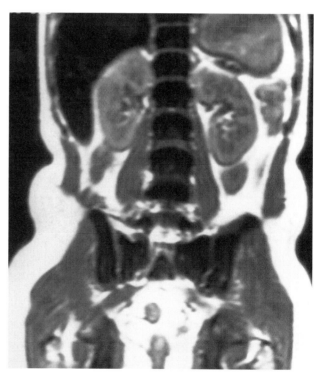

FIG. 5-154. Iron deposition. A 29-year-old man with thalassemia. Coronal T1-weighted MR image shows markedly hypointense liver and marrow because of extensive iron deposition.

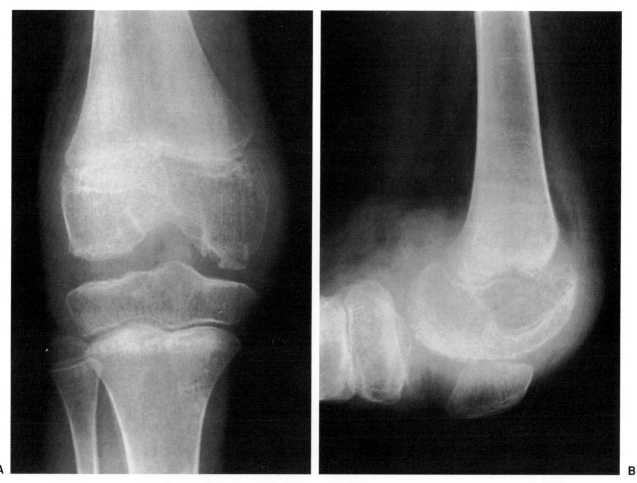

A
B

FIG. 5-155. Hemophilia. AP **(A)** and lateral **(B)** views of the right knee show osteopenia, epiphyseal enlargement, deepening and widening of the intercondylar notch, distention of the joint capsule, and increased synovium density due to hemosiderin deposition. There is also narrowing of the joint cartilage space, subarticular cyst formation, and subchondral sclerosis.

early radiographic changes of chronic arthropathy include increased density of the synovium due to hemosiderin deposition. On MRI, hemophilic arthropathy may appear as either focal or generalized destruction of the articular cartilage and synovial hypertrophy. The synovium is of low to intermediate signal intensity on T1- and T2-weighted images because of deposition of hemosiderin, an appearance similar to that of pigmented villonodular synovitis and synovial vascular malformations with repeated hemarthroses (438). Late changes of chronic hemophilic arthropathy include diffuse osteopenia (Fig. 5-155), joint space narrowing, subarticular cyst formation, subchondral sclerosis and collapse, loss of congruity of joint surfaces, and osteophyte formation. Most of these features indicate secondary degenerative joint disease (435).

Repeated hemarthroses are associated with increased blood flow to the epiphyses. The epiphyseal *and* physeal changes include premature ossification of epiphyses, epiphyseal overgrowth (Fig. 5-155), premature physeal fusion with limb shortening, and avascular necrosis of epiphyseal

centers. The latter is presumably due to occlusion of epiphyseal vessels by hemarthrosis. In addition to the increased epiphyseal size, certain bones undergo characteristic alteration in shape due to chronic synovitis. Abnormalities of epiphyseal contour include widening and deepening of the intercondylar notch of the femur at the cruciate ligament insertions (Fig. 5-155A) and squaring of the inferior margin of the patella due to appositional new bone formation. The carpal bones have a squared-off appearance. Occasionally, there is calcification of cartilage. These radiographic changes can resemble those of other chronic arthritides in children such as juvenile chronic arthritis and tuberculous arthritis.

Pseudotumor formation after a local hemorrhage is a potentially serious complication of hemophilia and other bleeding disorders. These pseudotumors may involve the soft tissues, periosteum, or bone (437,439). Most pseudotumors develop in patients who have antibodies to the replaced factor and whose bleeding is therefore difficult to control (440). Repeated episodes of bleeding, usually within a muscle, result in progressive enlargement of the hematoma and secondary compression necrosis of bone. Subperiosteal hemorrhage and intraosseous hemorrhage also may occur. The sites of hemophilic pseudotumor of bone in order of decreasing frequency are the femur, pelvis, tibia, calcaneus, small bones of the hands and feet, humerus, olecranon, and radius. Characteristic radiologic features include soft-tissue mass with or without coarse calcifications, periosteal elevation, new bone formation with bony struts, and varying degrees of

bone destruction (Fig. 5-156). MRI shows a mass with signal heterogeneity due to blood products of different ages (440). Treatment is usually conservative (immobilization and administration of factor VIII transfusions or factor IX concentrates); occasionally surgery may be necessary, or radiation therapy may be used. Patients with hemophilia require many transfusions and, if transfused before modern screening of donated blood, are at risk for hepatitis and acquired immunodeficiency syndrome (AIDS).

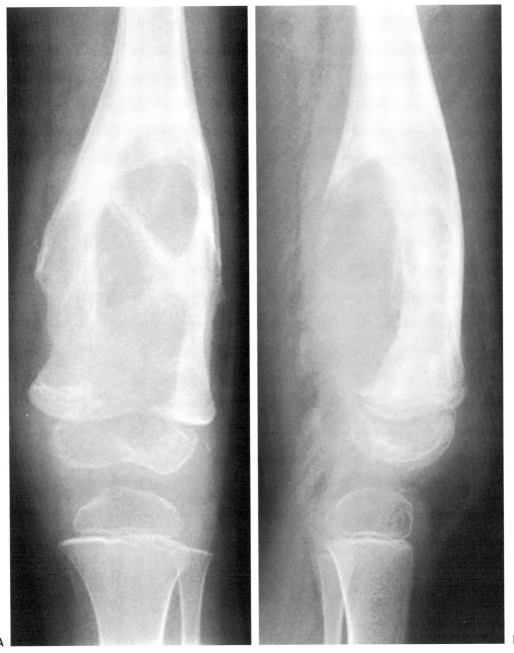

A   B

FIG. 5-156. Pseudotumor of hemophilia. This 2-year-old child with known hemophilia had previously been injured. AP **(A)** and lateral **(B)** views of the femur show a distal femoral lucency with bony struts, bony remodeling with undertubulation, periosteal reaction, and a soft-tissue mass. (Courtesy of Herman Grossman, M.D., Durham, North Carolina.)

DISORDERS LOCALIZED TO A SPECIFIC BODY AREA

Disorders of the Upper Extremity

Disorders of the Clavicle and Shoulder

Congenital Pseudarthrosis of the Clavicle

Congenital pseudarthrosis of the clavicle, which is rare, is characterized by a lack of bony continuity in the middle third of the bone. The anomaly is significant for cosmetic reasons and because it should be differentiated from trauma and other abnormalities. Approximately half of the patients present in the first month of life. Almost all cases occur on the right side. The medial segment is displaced superiorly and anteriorly and the lateral segment is displaced posteriorly and inferiorly (441). The borders of the bone are smooth and often bulbous (4), and there is no evidence of callus (Fig. 5-157). Cleidocranial dysostosis sometimes has a similar appearance.

Congenital Undescended Scapula (Sprengel Deformity)

Sprengel deformity results from failure of descent of the scapula from its cervical site of origin (442). In up to one third of cases, there is a residual bony connection with the spine, the omovertebral bone (4). This bone extends from the medial angle or medial border of the scapula to the spinous process, lamina, or transverse process of one or more of the lower cervical or upper thoracic vertebrae. The connection may be fibrous rather than bony. The scapula is elevated medially and rotated as seen from the front, the glenoid is at the normal level, and the humeral head articulates with

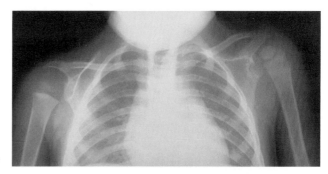

FIG. 5-158. Shoulder changes in Erb palsy. In this 3-year-old boy, the right humeral head and glenoid are hypoplastic, the scapula is winged, and the acromion is curved.

the glenoid. Seventy percent of patients have associated anomalies (441). The most frequent are scoliosis (40%) and rib anomalies (25%), but cardiac and renal anomalies also sometimes coexist. The Sprengel deformity is sometimes part of the Klippel-Feil anomaly.

Sequelae of Brachial Plexus Palsy

Obstetric trauma can produce brachial plexus injuries, particularly when the baby is large or in a breech presentation. The clinical manifestations depend on the level of the injured nerve roots. The fifth and sixth cervical nerve roots are most commonly affected. This results an Erb palsy, with the arm adducted and internally rotated, the elbow extended, and the forearm pronated. The right side is affected more commonly than the left (338).

MRI has been used in the first few weeks of life, to assess for nerve root avulsion (443). As the child grows, the lack of normal muscular support results in a progressive developmental dysplasia of the glenohumeral joint, a pattern similar to that of dysplasia of the hip. The proximal humeral epiphysis and its ossification centers are small, and the glenoid is shallow (Fig. 5-158). There is posterior dislocation or subluxation of the humeral head. Progressive deformity of the glenoid develops; it loses its normal concavity, and its posterior lip disappears (444). Delineation of these changes is difficult on plain radiographs and usually requires cross-sectional imaging (445).

Disorders of the Elbow and Forearm

Congenital Radial Dislocation and Radioulnar Synostosis

Congenital dislocation of the radial head can be anterior or posterior. The radial head is dome-shaped rather than concave and the capitellum is hypoplastic, which differentiates this condition from traumatic dislocation. The most common association of radial dislocation is with the nail-patella syndrome (Fong's osteo-onychodysostosis) (4).

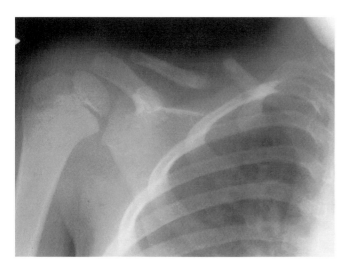

FIG. 5-157. Pseudarthrosis of the clavicle. A 4-year-old girl with chronic clavicular pain. AP radiograph of the clavicle shows a central gap in the clavicle with well-defined, rounded borders.

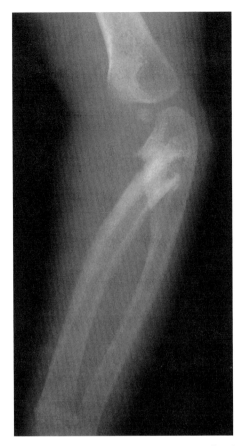

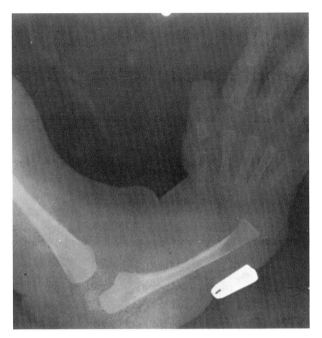

FIG. 5-160. Thrombocytopenia-absent radius syndrome. In this 6-week-old girl with a deformed forearm, there is complete absence of the radius but presence of a hypoplastic first metacarpal and thumb. A bleeding tendency due to thrombocytopenia developed at 18 months of age.

FIG. 5-159. Congenital radioulnar synostosis. A 1-year-old boy with limitation of motion at the elbow. The proximal radius and ulna are fused, and the proximal radius is dislocated posteriorly with respect to the capitellum.

Congenital radioulnar fusion (synostosis) is almost always proximal (Fig. 5-159), this being the last area of separation of the two bones during embryologic development. The radial head is dislocated posteriorly. When the bridge is unossified, the fusion is not evident radiographically and must be inferred from the dysplastic changes in the proximal radius.

Radial Dysplasia

Radial dysplasia includes all degrees of hypoplasia and aplasia. Frequently there is also absence or severe hypoplasia of the first metacarpal and thumb. An exception to this generalization is the thrombocytopenia-absent radius (TAR) syndrome in which there may be complete absence of the radius, yet presence of the first metacarpal and thumb (Fig. 5-160). The ulna tends to be short when there is absence or hypoplasia of the radius. Reduction deformities of the radius may be idiopathic or may be part of osteochondrodysplasias, various syndromes (most notably Holt-Oram cardiomelic syndrome and Fanconi pancytopenia), several chromosomal disorders, and phocomelia. Radial dysplasia may also be part of the VATER association (Table 5-20).

TABLE 5-20. *Conditions associated with radial dysplasia*

Idiopathic local dysplasia
Osteochondrodysplasias
  Dyschondrosteosis
  Mesomelic dwarfism
Syndromes
  Cornelia de Lange
  Holt-Oram
  Poland
  Seckel
Chromosomal abnormalities
  Ring D
  Trisomy 13q
  Trisomy 18 syndrome
Phocomelia
Associations
  VATER association
    Vertebral
    Vascular (congenital heart disease)
    Anorectal
    Tracheoesophageal fistula
    Esophageal atresia
    Renal
    Radial ray
Hematopoietic disorders
  Blackfan-Diamond disease
  Fanconi syndrome
  Thrombocytopenia-absent radius syndrome

Disorders of the Hand and Wrist

Fusion or Abnormal Number of Bones

Carpal fusion occurs as a normal variant in slightly more than 0.1% of the population (446). The most common carpal fusion (lunate to the triquetrum) occurs more frequently in African-Americans than in Caucasians; it causes no symptoms. When bones of the proximal row fuse with those of the distal row, a congenital malformation syndrome is usually present (7). Congenital carpal fusion is commonly seen in arthrogryposis and chondroectodermal dysplasia. Acquired fusion is most frequent in juvenile rheumatoid arthritis.

Fusions between the digits (syndactyly) can occur in isolation or be associated with congenital malformation syndromes. These fusions, bony or only of the soft tissues, are commonly seen in craniofacial syndromes and craniosynostoses such as acrocephalosyndactyly (Apert syndrome) and acrocephalopolysyndactyly (Carpenter syndrome). Fusion between phalanges of the same digit (symphalangism) is usually a familial, autosomal dominant trait, but it can also be associated with other anomalies.

Polydactyly, an increased number of digits, is classified as preaxial, when the extra digit is on the radial (thumb) side, or postaxial, when it is on the ulnar side of the hand (7). Preaxial polydactyly is more common and is associated with numerous syndromes including those with radial dysplasia (Fanconi anemia, Holt-Oram syndrome, VATER association) and some of the acrocephalosyndactyly syndromes.

Cone-Shaped Epiphyses

A cone-shaped epiphysis is as an apparent indentation of the epiphysis into the center of the adjacent metaphysis (447). Cone-shaped epiphyses usually occur in the middle and proximal phalanges. They develop when central physeal growth is slowed relative to peripheral growth or when the physis is fused centrally. Cone-shaped epiphyses are seen in the hands and feet (or both) of 1% to 2% of normal children, usually girls, but they are much more common in various osteochondrodysplasias and other constitutional abnormalities. Epiphyseal coning in the normal child is isolated and relatively inconspicuous; in the child with genetic disease, it is widespread and more pronounced (448). Cone-shaped epiphyses also can develop after vascular thrombosis, trauma, infection, in association with hereditary renal disease, and with anorchia.

Cone-shaped epiphyses are more typically associated with pathologic conditions when found in the hands rather than in the feet. Giedion has extensively analyzed and classified cone-shaped epiphyses (447). Only a few of the 38 types he described are specific for dysplasias (7). Some of the more common diseases associated with cone-shaped epiphyses are trichorhinophalangeal syndromes I and II (Fig. 5-161),

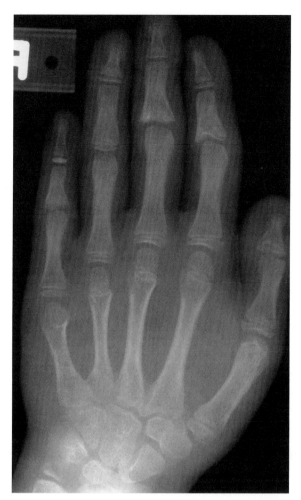

FIG. 5-161. **Cone-shaped and ivory epiphyses.** A 12-year-old girl with trichorhinophalangeal syndrome type I. The epiphyses of the middle phalanges of the index, middle, and little finger are coned. There is also central indentation of the metaphyses by the epiphyses, more noticeable in the index finger. This coning is typical of the trichorhinophalangeal syndrome. There is also an ivory epiphysis in the distal phalanx of the little finger.

achondroplasia, cleidocranial dysplasia, chondroectodermal dysplasia, asphyxiating thoracic dystrophy, and peripheral dysostosis.

Ivory Epiphyses

Ivory epiphyses are small and uniformly dense but have a normal contour. They have no radiologic evidence of any marrow space. They are usually found in the distal phalanges of digits 2–5. Kuhns et al. reported ivory epiphyses in 1 of 300 clinically well children (449); there was usually some delay in skeletal maturation.

Markedly dense epiphyses also occur with increased frequency in Cockayne syndrome, trichorhinophalangeal syndrome type I (Fig. 5-161), and various types of multiple epiphyseal dysplasia. The association of ivory epiphyses and cone-shaped epiphyses strongly suggests the trichorhinophalangeal type I syndrome. Accelerated skeletal maturation associated with ivory epiphyses suggests the rare Cockayne syndrome. The occurrence of ivory epiphyses in the hand other than in the distal phalanges of digits 2–5 and middle phalanx of digit 5 suggests generalized epiphyseal dysplasia. Finally, in epiphyseal acrodysplasia ivory epiphyses in the distal phalanges are commonly associated with fragmented epiphyses in other phalanges.

Curved Fingers

Abnormal curving of the fingers is fairly common. Clinodactyly, camptodactyly, Kirner deformity, and delta phalanx are varieties of curved fingers (4,9,450). The presence of curved fingers should alert the physician to the possibility of a more general abnormality.

Factitious Curved Fingers. The most common cause of curved fingers in children, particularly in uncooperative infants and younger children, is the position that is produced when the fingers do not lie flat against the x-ray cassette. Positioning artifact may be suspected when the adjacent phalanges are also bent and there are associated soft-tissue folds. Confirmation is by physical examination.

Clinodactyly. Clinodactyly is a curvature of the finger in a mediolateral plane. The curve may be radial or ulnar in direction and may involve any finger (450). It usually refers to a radial deviation of the fifth finger at the distal interphalangeal joint and is usually associated with a short middle phalanx, shorter on its radial than on its ulnar side. The distal phalangeal region is best shown by a coned-down AP film, to supplement the usual PA hand film.

Isolated clinodactyly occurs as a sporadic variant in over 1% of some populations, but it may be inherited as an autosomal dominant trait. It is frequently seen in Down syndrome (Fig. 5-162), but it has been reported in more than 30 other hand-foot abnormalities, chromosomal disorders, craniofacial syndromes, bone dysplasias, bone dysostoses, posttraumatic deformities, and miscellaneous conditions (450).

Camptodactyly. Camptodactyly is a permanent flexion contracture of one or more fingers. It may be congenital or acquired. Flexion deformities are typically located at the proximal interphalangeal joint. They usually involve the fifth finger but may also affect the ring, middle, or index finger (451).

Although unknown, the cause is probably a fascial abnormality or a contracture of the flexor digitorum sublimis (450). Camptodactyly is often an isolated sporadic or familial abnormality. It may be inherited as an autosomal dominant trait with variable penetrance (450). Occasionally, it is associated with clinodactyly in a chromosomal disorder, bone dysplasia, or craniofacial or other syndrome (450).

Kirner Deformity. Kirner deformity is a palmar bending of the terminal phalanx of the fifth finger (452). It is usually

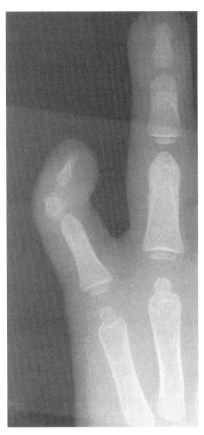

FIG. 5-162. Clinodactyly. A 3-year-old boy with trisomy 21. PA radiograph shows that the middle phalanx of the little finger is hypoplastic and there is radial angular displacement of the distal phalanx.

bilateral and symmetric. It affects more girls than boys (450) and is almost always an isolated anomaly. It may be sporadic or transmitted in an autosomal dominant fashion. The shaft of the distal phalanx is bent toward the palm, with enlargement of the normally directed epiphysis and increased width of the physis (Fig. 5-163). This deformity may be preceded by soft-tissue swelling (450). The widening of the physis is thought to be due to separation (450).

Delta Phalanx. Delta phalanx or longitudinally bracketed epiphysis/diaphysis is a triangular deformity of bones of the hands and feet. It is restricted to the short tubular bones with proximal epiphyses, i.e., the phalanges, first metacarpals, and first metatarsals (Fig. 5-164). It is most common in the thumb. Digital anomalies frequently coexist (4). There is anomolous physeal fusion, so the physis assumes a proximal-to-distal longitudinal orientation rather than the customary transverse position, and this causes angulation of the thumb, finger, or toe. The epiphysis frequently also is enlarged and deformed, so the involved bone has a trapezoidal or delta shape. When the thumb or great toe is involved, Rubinstein-Taybi syndrome and fibrodysplasia ossificans progressiva should be considered.

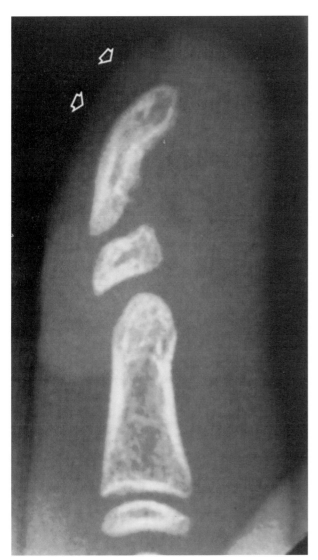

FIG. 5-163. Kirner deformity. This 3-year-old girl has a classic Kirner deformity of the distal phalanx of the little finger. Note the convex fingernail *(arrows)*. From Oestreich and Crawford (5).

Disorders of the Lower Extremity

Disorders of the Hip

Developmental Dysplasia of the Hip

Although predisposing factors are present in utero, most hip dislocations occur after birth. The term *congenital hip dislocation (CHD)* is therefore being replaced by the more appropriate term *developmental dysplasia of the hip (DDH)*. The term refers to an abnormal femoral head-acetabular relationship and development. The most common cause for DDH is now believed to be abnormal ligamentous laxity, accentuated by high levels of maternal estrogens. Abnormal position in utero and hereditary factors may be responsible for the remaining cases.

Clinical Features. Female infants with hip instability or dislocation outnumber affected male infants by 5:1 to 9:1. DDH is more common in Caucasian than African-American newborns. A particularly high incidence is reported in native American groups who papoose their neonates with the legs in adduction. Patients born by breech delivery (the hips presumably flexed and adducted in utero) have an incidence of DDH six times as high as those born by vertex. DDH is bilateral in about a third of affected children.

Examination of the hips for dysplasia is part of the routine clinical evaluation of the newborn. The Ortolani maneuver will reduce a dislocated hip by femoral abduction and flexion. A palpable jerk or audible click or clunk is noted as the femoral head suddenly slides back into the acetabulum. The Barlow maneuver determines if a hip is dislocatable. The femur is flexed and adducted while posterior pressure is applied. This will displace an unstable hip from the acetabulum. Both techniques should be used. The neonatal hip may be classified as normal (stable with full abduction), unstable (subluxable, dislocatable, or reducibly dislocated), or pathologic (irreducible dislocation). Pathologic (teratologic) hip dislocations are those that occur prenatally in association with congenital disorders such as meningomyelocele, arthrogryposis, and caudal regression syndrome (4). Proper diagnosis and treatment in the newborn period depend heavily on the expertise of the examining physician. If the hip is

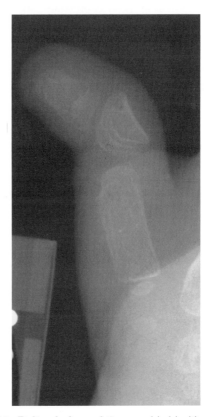

FIG. 5-164. Delta phalanx. A 2-year-old girl with a deformity of the right thumb. The proximal phalanx has a triangular shape. The lateral part of the physis is fused.

TABLE 5-21. *Findings suggesting developmental dysplasia of the hip*

Abnormal clinical examination
   Asymmetric gluteal folds
   Limited abduction
   Positive maneuvers ("click" or "clunk")
     Ortolani (relocation)
     Barlow (dislocation)
   Asymmetric knees (when supine)
   Foot deformities (e.g., metatarsus adductus, clubfoot)
   Torticollis
   Sacral agenesis
   Arthrogryposis
Positive family history
Breech presentation

Source: Modified from Harcke and Jacobs (453,555).

merely lax and not dislocatable, the infant is not treated but is reexamined at regular intervals.

Radiologic Evaluation.

Ultrasonography in the neonate. If physical examination suggests that a hip is abnormal, or if other risk factors are present, ultrasonography of both hips should be performed (453) (Table 5-21). The study is used to determine whether the hip is subluxable, dislocatable, or dislocated and to assess acetabular development (454). During the first few days of life, there is physiologic ligamentous laxity due to the persisting effect of maternal hormones. Therefore, the hips of a newborn may feel loose. It is preferable to wait until at least 2 weeks of age for screening ultrasonography. Ultrasonography is readily performed on infants under approximately 6 months of age, provided the ossification of the proximal femoral epiphyses is not too far advanced. Normally the epiphysis ossifies at about 2–6 months in girls and 3–7 months in boys.

Neonatal hip instability does not invariably lead to dislocation. However, which hips will progress to dislocation cannot yet be predicted. Therefore, sequential ultrasonography provides a safe, reliable way to follow the hip until it is clearly normal, without therapy in very mild cases or with a harness. It also identifies patients who do not improve

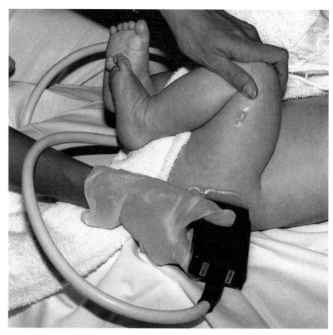

FIG. 5-165. Coronal hip sonographic technique. Ultrasonography of the hip is performed with a high-frequency linear transducer. The infant's hip may be flexed for the entire examination. The coronal image is obtained with the transducer held in a plane parallel to the baby's back.

sufficiently with a harness and who need other treatment (455). Recent work questions the efficacy of universal screening ultrasonography and advocates treatment based on an abnormal physical exam plus supplemental radiographs (456).

The static ultrasonographic method developed by Graf (457) is aimed at morphologic assessment of the femoral head and acetabulum. The hip can be classified according to the degree of development of the bony and cartilaginous components of the hip (457). This is a valuable classification, but some feel that it should not be used routinely. A simplified table summarizes this classification (Table 5-22). Dy-

TABLE 5-22. *Sonographic classification of types of infant hips*

Type		Bony roof	Rim	Alpha angle[a] (degrees)	Beta angle[b] (degrees)
Ia:	mature hip	Good	Angular	≥60	<55
Ib:	transitional form	Good	Blunt	≥60	>55
IIa:	physiologically immature (<3 mo of age)	Sufficient	Round	50–59	>55
IIb:	delayed ossification (>3 mo of age)	Deficient	Round	50–59	>55
IIc:	critical range (any age, normal labrum)	Deficient	Round or flat	43–49	70–77
IId:	subluxed hip	Severely def.	Round or flat	43–49	>77
IIIa:	dislocated hip (no structural alteration)	Poor	Flat	<43	>77
IIIb:	dislocated hip (with structural alteration)	Poor	Flat	<43	>77
IV:	severely dislocated hip	Poor	Flat	<43	>77

[a] Measure of bony acetabular development.
[b] Measure of cartilaginous acetabular (labral) development.

Source: Modified from Graf (457) and Schlesinger (566).

namic ultrasonography as performed by Harcke and Grissom involves stress maneuvers (454) and allows one to determine the stability of the hip. A combination of the static and dynamic approaches may be best (453).

The examination is performed with a high-frequency linear array transducer. The infant is placed with the side of interest slightly elevated or in a lateral decubitus position. The hips may remain flexed for the entire exam. Coronal and transverse planes are evaluated, both in neutral and stressed positions (Fig. 5-165). Stressing the hip is achieved by a modified Barlow (dislocating) maneuver (454). If the hip is already subluxed or dislocated, is being treated, or has been treated, stress imaging is not performed.

In the static coronal view, which simulates an AP radiograph (Fig. 5-166), the iliac bone should be imaged to form a straight line. The unossified femoral head should rest within the concavity of the acetabulum. The lateral edge of the bony acetabular rim should be sharply angulated. When dysplasia is present, this edge is rounded or even flattened. A line drawn along the iliac bone normally bisects the appropriately seated femoral head. A dislocated femoral head usually is displaced in a lateral, superior, and posterior direction

(Fig. 5-167). The α angle, as described by Graf (457), is the geometric complement of the acetabular angle (see below) drawn on an AP radiograph (Fig. 5-168). It is created by two lines drawn on the coronal ultrasonogram: one along the straight edge of the iliac bone, and one along the bony acetabular roof. The normal α angle is 60° or greater (Figs. 5-166 and 5-168). In the newborn, angles of approximately 55° are still considered normal. The β angle, less commonly used, is formed by the axis of the iliac bone and a line through the axis of the echogenic fibrocartilaginous labrum (the outer portion of the acetabular roof). This angle characterizes the development of the cartilaginous portion of the acetabulum (457). The normal β angle is less than 55°. The contour and thickness of the cartilaginous acetabulum should be assessed, as patients with normal angles can have dysplastic, poorly ossified acetabular contours (458). Ossification of the femoral epiphysis will be evident earlier on ultrasonography than on radiographs. Factors to be evaluated during an ultrasonographic examination of the hips are listed in Table 5-23.

Radiographs in the neonate. In newborn infants, AP radiography of the hips for DDH is no longer widely used except to evaluate for associated abnormalities or to exclude other congenital anomalies, such as a generalized bone dysplasia. However, once the femoral head has ossified sufficiently to hinder a complete ultrasonographic evaluation, imaging evaluation should begin with an AP radiograph. Positioning for the frog-lateral radiograph reduces an unstable hip; that projection therefore provides no useful information regarding displacement and is seldom used. Nevertheless, the hips must be evaluated on any pelvic or abdominal film obtained in a child. Therefore, one must be familiar with the radiographic signs of developmental dysplasia of the infant hip.

The *acetabular angle (acetabular index)* is derived from the anteroposterior view of the pelvis. In the newborn, the hips should be adducted to neutral and symmetrically positioned. The horizontal *Y-Y line (Hilgenreiner line)* is drawn between the two triradiate cartilages. A line connecting the most inferiomedial and the most superolateral bony corners of the (iliac) acetabular roof is then drawn. These two lines form the acetabular angle (Fig. 5-169). This angle is only an estimate only, as the true articulating surfaces of the acetabulum are still cartilaginous.

The acetabular angle as measured from AP radiographs

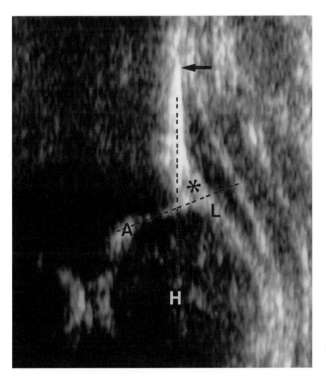

FIG. 5-166. Normal coronal sonography of the neonatal left hip. The coronal image is photographed to simulate the appearance of the hip on a traditional AP radiograph. The lateral bony margin of the ilium *(arrow)* is straight and vertical. The cartilaginous femoral head *(H)* of the hip is seated within the bony acetabulum *(A)*. A line along the iliac bone bisects the cartilaginous femoral head. The femoral head is also covered by the cartilaginous labrum *(L)*. The alpha angle *(asterisk)* is formed by a line drawn along the ilium and a line drawn across the bony acetabular roof.

TABLE 5-23. *Sonographic evaluation of the hip with ultrasonography*

Size and symmetry of cartilaginous femoral heads
Size and symmetry of ossific femoral nuclei
Shape of acetabular roof (should be concave, not straight or wavy)
Femoral head coverage by the bony acetabular roof
Configuration of the labrum and cartilaginous acetabulum
Stability of the joint

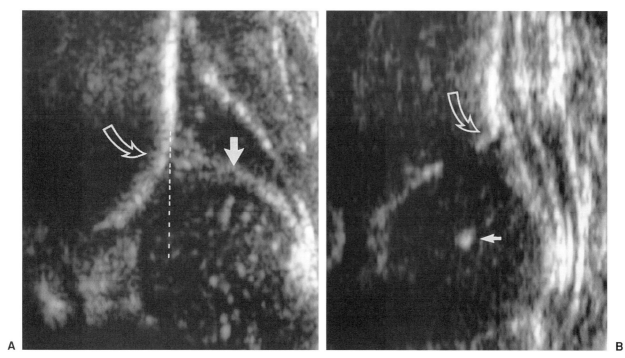

A   **B**

FIG. 5-167. Developmental dysplasia of the hip. A: Coronal image of the hip of a 3-week-old girl shows lateral displacement of the femoral head. The bony acetabular roof is shallow, and its rim is curved *(curved arrow)*. A line drawn along the ilium covers approximately 20% of the diameter of the femoral head. The labrum *(straight arrow)* is elevated. **B:** The same child after treatment with a Pavlik harness for 6 weeks. A coronal image shows an increase in the *(α)* angle and the interval development of a sharp bony acetabular rim *(curved arrow)*. The labrum is no longer elevated, and a femoral ossification center has developed *(straight arrow)*.

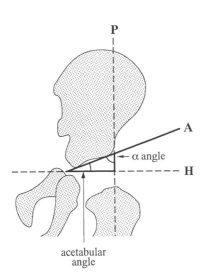

FIG. 5-168. Acetabular and α angles. The radiographic acetabular angle is formed by the horizontal line of Hilgenreiner *(H)* and a line along the acetabular roof *(A)*. It is the geometric complement (i.e., the two angles add up to 90°) of the α angle measured on ultrasonographic images. The α angle is formed by a line equivalent to the iliac line (Perkins line, *P*) and the line along the bony acetabular roof *(A)*.

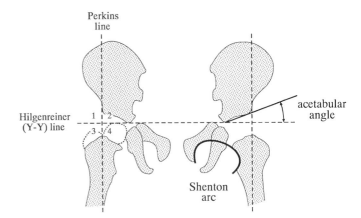

FIG. 5-169. The infant hip. Hilgenreiner *(Y-Y)* line is drawn through the triradiate cartilages. A second line is drawn tangential to the inferomedial and superolateral margins of the acetabular roof. The angle formed is the acetabular angle. The Perkins line is drawn perpendicular to the Hilgenreiner line, at the outer acetabular bony margin. The Shenton arc is a smooth curve formed by the inferior edge of the superior pubic ramus and the medial femoral neck metaphysis; these two components are actually skew lines lying in different planes, and a slightly rotated film will distort their relationship greatly. The Perkins and Hilgenreiner lines divide the hip into quadrants. The unossified femoral head should normally be centered in the inferomedial quadrant *(4)*.

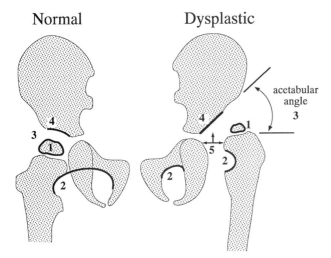

Normal   Dysplastic

acetabular angle 3

FIG. 5-170. Developmental dysplasia of the hip. The femoral ossification center *(1)* is small. There is disruption of the arc of Shenton's line *(2)*, and the acetabular angle is increased *(3)*. The bony acetabular roof is straightened *(4)*. The proximal femur is displaced superolaterally *(5)*.

was initially employed by Hilgenreiner for evaluation of hip dysplasia (459). There is a gradual decrease in the acetabular angle with age, presumably because of modeling of the acetabulum by the femoral head with normal motion and weight bearing plus progressive ossification of the acetabular carti-

lage. The normal acetabular angle is approximately 28° at birth and gradually decreases to 22° by 1 year of age (460). The standard deviation for these normal acetabular angles is approximately 4–5°, and this gives a relatively wide range of normal values.

The acetabular angle is often increased with congenital hip dislocation (Fig. 5-170) and neuromuscular disorders, perhaps because the normal stimulus for acetabular development is not present. There may be no acetabular roof at all in severe congenital dislocation or in proximal focal femoral deficiency.

Decreased acetabular angles are found during the first year of life in Down syndrome and may be used to suggest that diagnosis. The acetabular angle may also be decreased in various skeletal dysplasias (e.g., achondroplasia, Ellis-van Creveld syndrome, asphyxiating thoracic dystrophy, spondyloepiphyseal dysplasia). Decreased acetabular angles are also seen in several seemingly unrelated conditions such as osteogenesis imperfecta, hypophosphatasia, sacral agenesis, and arthrogryposis (460).

The *vertical line of Perkins* (see Fig. 5-169) is placed perpendicular to the line of Hilgenreiner at the outer edge of the acetabulum (461). The junction of the Perkins and Hilgenreiner lines divides the hip into quadrants. The ossification center of the femur—or, in its absence, the metaphyseal beak along the proximal medial femoral edge—and the center of the extrapolated outline of the cartilaginous femoral

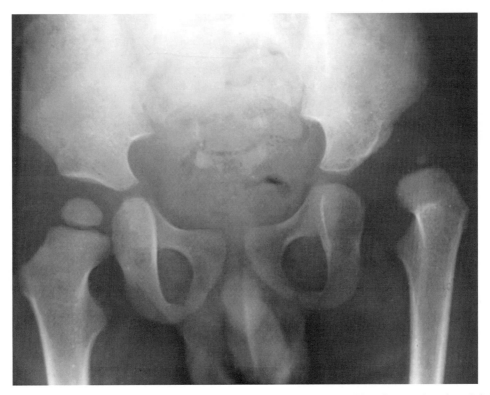

FIG. 5-171. Developmental dysplasia of the hip. A 2-year-old boy with a limp and a short left leg. There is superolateral displacement of the proximal femur and an increase in the acetabular angle, and the proximal femoral epiphysis on the left is small.

epiphysis should lie in the inferomedial quadrant. On radiographs, the dislocated femoral head typically is displaced superiorly and laterally (Fig. 5-170). In the normal hip, the Shenton line forms a smooth, unbroken arc bridging the medial femoral metaphyseal contour with the inferior edge of the superior pubic ramus. In a dysplastic hip, this arc is discontinuous (Fig. 5-170).

Radiographs in the older infant and child. The radiographic diagnosis of DDH becomes easier with increasing age, as the treatment becomes more and more difficult. Progressive ossification of the femur and pelvis demonstrates the alignment of the femur with the acetabulum and acetabular dysplasia more and more readily. By 2–4 months of age, lateral displacement of the femoral head and an increased acetabular angle are usually easily seen. In DDH, there is delayed ossification of the affected proximal femoral epiphysis. Older infants demonstrate superolateral displacement of the proximal femur, an increased acetabular angle, and a relatively small capital femoral epiphysis (Fig. 5-171). Other changes in the acetabulum include lack of its normal concavity, poor development of its lateral margin, lateral displacement of its concavity, and formation of a false acetabulum (Fig. 5-171). The normal acetabular concavity resembles an eyebrow. The area of maximum acetabular sclerosis should be at the apex of this concavity. The ossification center should rest within the acetabular cup. The dysplastic acetabulum has a decreased or absent concavity and a more vertical slant. Its lateral border is often curved cephalad.

In the older child, the *center-edge (CE) angle* is also used to evaluate the relationship of the ossified femoral head to the acetabulum (4). On an AP film, a horizontal baseline is drawn connecting the centers of the femoral heads. A line is then drawn through each center, perpendicular to the baseline. The intersection of this line with a line from the center to the outer bony edge of the acetabulum is the CE angle. The smaller the angle, the less is the femoral head coverage. In the infant, the angle should be greater than 18–20°, and in the adolescent, greater than 26–30° (4).

Physeal and epiphyseal abnormalities can develop as a result of ischemic damage to the proximal femur. Subsequent growth dysfunction caused by physeal closure in these dysplastic hips can be detected by analysis of the growth recovery lines formed in the proximal femur after therapy (462). In infancy the proximal femoral physis serves both the femoral head and the greater trochanter. It can be divided into a medial portion that contributes to longitudinal growth at the proximal end of the femoral neck and a lateral portion that contributes to growth of the greater trochanter. The femoral neck grows more rapidly than the greater trochanter and thus any growth recovery line should be farther from the proximal femoral physis than from the greater trochanteric physis. If the distance between a growth recovery line and the femoral neck physis is equal to or smaller than its distance from the greater trochanteric physis, femoral neck physeal dysfunction is implied (Fig. 5-172). Eventually, there may be broadening of the femoral neck and relative trochanteric overgrowth with varus deformation of the hip. Degenerative changes may develop later (4).

Arthrography, CT, and MRI in the older infant and child. A dislocatable or dislocated hip is usually treated by a

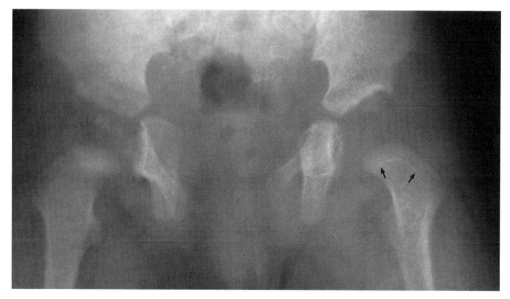

FIG. 5-172. **Developmental dysplasia of the hip.** An 8-month-old girl treated for developmental dysplasia of the left hip. There is deformity of the left acetabulum. The proximal left femur is displaced superolaterally. The growth recovery line in the proximal left femur is almost equidistant from the physes of the femoral neck and of the greater trochanter *(arrows)*. This suggests relative lack of growth of the subcapital part of the proximal femoral physis. The right hip shows the expected greater distance of the growth recovery line from the femoral neck physis than from the greater trochanteric physis.

flexion-abduction-external rotation brace (such as the Pavlik harness), splint, or cast. With this therapy, most children achieve and maintain a normal relationship between the acetabulum and proximal femur. If this does not occur, intraoperative arthrography or preoperative cross-sectional imaging is indicated prior to further intervention. Closed or open surgical reduction performed prior to the age of 4 years leads to a normal hip relationship in more than 95% of children (4).

A diagnostic arthrogram using fluoroscopy is often performed at the time of surgical reduction. In the *subluxed* hip, the labrum may be displaced superiorly by the femoral head. Contrast pools medially due to a laterally displaced femoral head and a capacious joint capsule. A stretched ligamentum teres can be identified. Reduction is usually readily accomplished at fluoroscopy. The subluxation of the femoral head may be apparent only during lateral stress (4). With *complete dislocation,* the femoral head is located superior and lateral to the cartilaginous labrum (4). An accordion-like compressed (or "inverted") labrum may lie interposed between the femoral head and acetabulum (Fig. 5-173). The capsule, which is adherent to the labrum, lies medial to the femoral head and is constricted, producing an hourglass configuration (4). In cases where the capsular isthmus and interposed labrum prevent complete reduction, open surgical reduction

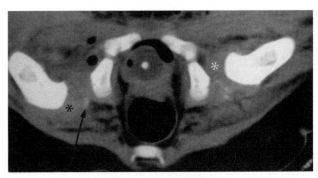

FIG. 5-174. Developmental dysplasia of the hip: CT. Axial image of a 6-month-old girl was obtained 2 hours after open reduction of a dislocated right hip. There is residual arthrographic contrast within the hip joint *(arrow)*. Air from the procedure is seen within the acetabulum and soft tissues. The cartilaginous femoral head remains posteriorly displaced *(black asterisk)*. The left proximal femur is located normally *(white asterisk)*. The configuration of the bony proximal femur has been likened to a Dutch clog (465); the cartilaginous femoral head normally sits at the end of the clog. A second surgical reduction was required.

is needed. MRI can also delineate these important soft tissue and cartilaginous structures (463); however, its capacity for dynamic evaluation is limited at present.

If a child undergoes surgical reduction and casting, a CT scan is performed, usually within 24 hours, to ensure adequate reduction (Fig. 5-174). This examination can be performed with 4–6 slices (spaced 3–5 mm apart), a low-dose technique (as low as 30 mAs), and a total ovarian dose of 112 mrad (1.12 mGy) (464). As in arthrography, CT can also detect obstacles to complete reduction (465). These include infolding or accordioning of the joint capsule or labrum, invagination of the iliopsoas tendon, and a hypertrophied ligamentum teres or pulvinar (fibrofatty tissue in the concavity of the acetabulum).

Any overly vigorous method of treatment with extreme abduction may lead to avascular necrosis of the femoral epiphysis. The children who undergo surgical reduction are especially at risk. Hyperabduction of both femurs during treatment compromises the vascular supply of the femoral heads. The incidence of avascular necrosis in patients treated with spica casts ranges from 25% to 47% (466). Recent studies suggest that ultrasonography and gadolinium-enhanced MRI may help in the early detection of vascular compromise caused by abduction (466–468). Continuing lack of ossification of the femoral head after therapy suggests ischemic injury.

In the older child, CT is useful in the management of advanced cases and in long term postoperative follow-up. Three-dimensional reconstruction clarifies the anatomy of the dysplastic proximal femur and pelvis (Fig. 5-175) (469). CT is also useful for measuring femoral anteversion (see below) (465). It should be stressed that surgical reconstruction is usually performed only in long-standing cases with marked soft-tissue contracture and acetabular dysplasia.

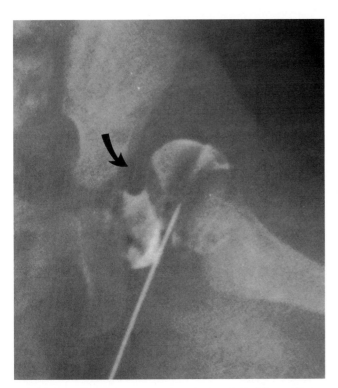

FIG. 5-173. Developmental dysplasia of the hip: arthrography. Contrast within the left hip joint in this 6-week-old girl with developmental dysplasia shows interposition of the cartilaginous labrum *(curved arrow)* between the femoral head and acetabular cavity. The joint capsule has an hour-glass constriction at the infolded labrum. The femoral head is dislocated superolaterally. This child required an open reduction.

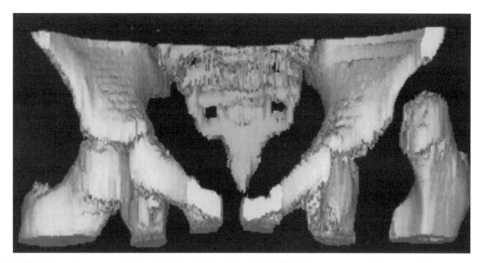

FIG. 5-175. Developmental dysplasia of the hip: 3-D CT. Reconstructed image of this 4-year-old boy shows a dislocated left proximal femur. The femur is displaced superolaterally. The left acetabulum is shallow. The right hip is normally aligned.

Differential Diagnosis. Developmental dysplasia of the hip should not be confused with inadequate acetabular coverage in cerebral palsy, hip subluxation due to neuromuscular disease, septic arthritis in the infant, epiphyseal fracture, congenital coxa vara, or abnormal joint laxity (4). Ultrasonography and joint aspiration (perhaps plus arthrography, MRI, or CT) may be required to diagnose septic arthritis, physeal fracture, and congenital coxa vara.

Surgical Treatment. Surgical reconstruction is reserved for those patients, a small minority, in whom acetabular development and hip stability have not been achieved by other methods. The purpose of these surgical procedures

is to provide better acetabular coverage, improve femoral head-acetabular congruence, restore normal biomechanics of the hip, prevent pain and degenerative joint disease, and increase the efficiency of the hip musculature (4,470). These objectives may be achieved with a variety of operative methods. The most common surgical procedures now used are the Salter innominate bone osteotomy (Fig. 5-176), Pemberton circumacetabular osteotomy, and Chiari median displacement pelvic osteotomy. Other procedures include augmented innominate osteotomy, acetabuloplasty, Steele triple osteotomy, Colonna arthroplasty, and femoral osteotomy (4).

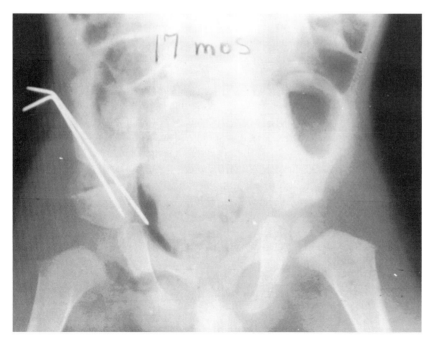

FIG. 5-176. Salter innominate osteotomy. This 17-month-old boy had a Salter osteotomy on the right for developmental dysplasia of the hip. The right femoral head ossification center is now well covered by the reconstructed acetabulum.

Legg-Calvé-Perthes Disease

Legg-Calvé-Perthes disease (LCP), or Legg-Perthes disease, or simply Perthes disease, is idiopathic avascular necrosis of the immature proximal femoral epiphysis. The cause of the interruption of blood supply to the femoral epiphysis is unknown, although the disease sometimes follows trauma or joint effusion. There is widespread disagreement regarding how best to assess the severity of disease. The significance of the radiologic findings also remains controversial, as does the most effective therapy (471). All these uncertainties make it difficult to specify the role for imaging in LCP disease.

Clinical Features. Common symptoms are groin, thigh, or knee pain; limp; muscular spasm; and limitation of internal rotation. Thigh and buttock atrophy may be seen late in the disease. These symptoms usually develop gradually, often with no history of trauma, hip effusion, or hip pain. If pain is present, it usually occurs during activity and subsides with rest.

The disease typically occurs in young, Caucasian boys. There is a boy-to-girl ratio of 4 : 1. It is uncommon in African-Americans. Bilateral but asymmetric disease occurs in as many as 13% of cases (472). The age at onset is 3–12 years, usually 5–8 years. The age at diagnosis is slightly younger for girls. There is striking retardation of skeletal maturation in both sexes, the bone age is almost always less than the chronologic age and frequently is at least 2 SD low (473).

Pathologic and Radiologic Appearance. Nearly all patients have abnormalities on their initial radiographic exami-

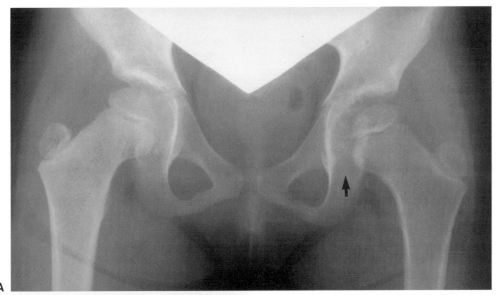

A

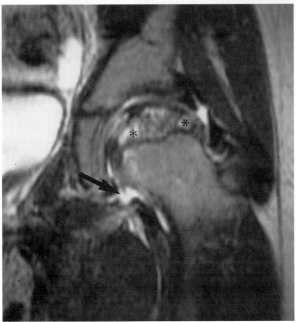

B

FIG. 5-177. **Legg-Calvé-Perthes disease. A:** A 7-year-old girl with left hip pain. The femoral epiphyses are symmetric. There is an increase in the left teardrop distance *(arrow)*, which suggests a joint effusion. **B:** Coronal T2-weighted MR image of the left hip obtained shortly thereafter shows heterogeneous signal in the femoral head. The high T2-weighted signal *(asterisks)* is consistent with marrow edema. There is a small joint effusion *(arrow)*.

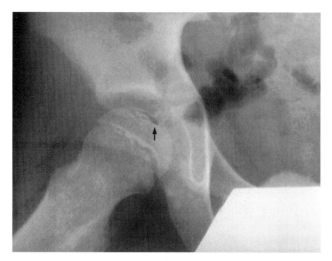

FIG. 5-178. Legg-Calvé-Perthes disease. Frog-lateral view of the right hip of an 11-year-old boy with right hip pain. There is a curvilinear lucency in the proximal femoral epiphysis (crescent sign) *(arrow)*.

nation. The identifiable radiographic stages of the disease include (a) initial or devascularization; (b) collapse and fragmentation; (c) reparative or reossification; and (d) remodeled or healed.

Initial stage. Radiographic findings at this stage include relative smallness of the ossified femoral epiphysis due to lack of growth from devascularization and an effusion. The medial part of the joint space may be widened because of synovial overgrowth and femoral and acetabular cartilage hypertrophy (Fig. 5-177) (474). Sonography can differentiate the simple effusion of transient synovitis from thicken-

ing of the joint capsule and cartilage (475). A characteristic subchondral fissure-fracture may be seen along the anterolateral aspect of the epiphysis on frog-lateral radiographs (Fig. 5-178). This lucency or crescent sign is the result of stress changes in the epiphysis. The lucency indicates the extent of the necrotic zone, which in turn determines the prognosis (476). There may be gas, the vacuum phenomenon, in this fracture. Later in this stage, the physis may be poorly delineated and the metaphysis relatively lucent, while the femoral head is relatively dense (Fig. 5-179). At this stage, histologic examination shows dead bone and disappearance of osteocytes from their lacunae (4).

If the radiographic findings are not convincing, MRI and scintigraphy may help. Marrow edema, an early, perhaps reversible sign on MRI, is manifested as low signal on T1-weighted images and high signal on T2-weighted images (Fig. 5-177B) (477,478). Other alterations in the MRI signal are seen as the disease progresses. Lack of gadolinium enhancement of the marrow supports the diagnosis of avascular necrosis (479,480).

Skeletal scintigraphy, particularly with pinhole magnification, also helps detect LCP early by lack of radionuclide uptake in the femoral capital epiphysis, the earliest scintigraphic finding in LCP (481–483). The size of this scintigraphic defect correlates with the eventual extent of femoral head deformity. "Shine-through" from tracer localization in the acetabulum, however, should not be confused with uptake in the femoral head when estimating the extent of initial involvement (Fig. 5-180).

Collapse and fragmentation stage. Some revascularization occurs during this stage, and changes due to repair are evident. The femoral head is fragmented, and radiographs

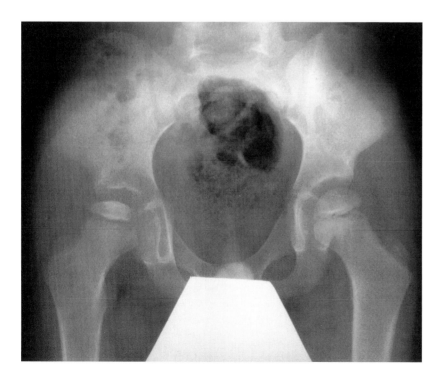

FIG. 5-179. Legg-Calvé-Perthes disease. A 7-year-old boy with right hip pain. Frontal radiograph shows a small, dense right proximal femoral epiphysis. The physis is widened and irregular, and the proximal metaphysis, especially medially, is relatively lucent.

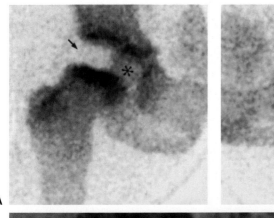
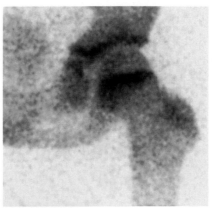

A

B

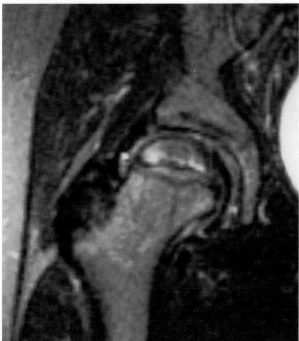

C

FIG. 5-180. Legg-Calvé-Perthes disease: skeletal scintigraphy and MRI. Pinhole magnification views of both hips in this 5-year-old boy with right hip pain show lack of tracer uptake in the right femoral epiphysis. **A:** The apparent tracer uptake in the medial aspect of the femoral head *(asterisk)* is actually from tracer localization in the acetabulum. **B:** There is normal tracer uptake in the left hip. **C:** Coronal T2-weighted image of the right hip in the same patient shows heterogeneous signal in much of the proximal femoral head, consistent with edema. (See also Fig. 5-181.)

show areas of both lucency and density. The increased density may be due to new bone production and thickening of the existing trabeculae (476). The resorptive process is most prominent anterolaterally but may involve most of the epiphysis. The resorption and reossification are usually mixed, so that there is a granular or fragmented appearance to the epiphysis (Fig. 5-181A). There may be apparent lateralization of the ossification center. Cyst-like areas of demineralization are seen on radiographs in the anterior metaphysis in approximately one third of patients (4). These are readily shown by MRI and correspond to persistence of cartilage in the metaphysis (484). MRI using gadolinium enhancement can also demonstrate early healing in this phase of the disease (480). If the epiphysis is unprotected from above during this phase, there may be gradual flattening and lateral extrusion of cartilage. A concave gouge in the upper epiphyseal contour is the impression of the lateral acetabular margin.

Reparative or reossification stage. Normal bone density begins to develop in the femoral head during this stage.

Changes in the shape of the proximal femur become evident. These deformities include *coxa magna, physeal arrest, irregular contour of the femoral head,* and *osteochondritis dissecans* (476). Coxa magna results from ossification of the cartilaginous hypertrophy (Fig. 5-181B). Physeal arrest results in a short femoral neck. When the arrest is lateral there is an externally tilted proximal femur. The femoral head subsequently impinges on the lateral edge of the acetabulum and causes a hinge type of deformity. Local physeal arrest and incomplete containment of the femoral head in the acetabulum may give the epiphysis an irregular contour. The femoral neck broadens and the femoral head widens. Overgrowth of the greater trochanter also may be seen. Osteochondritis dissecans, a less common complication, usually occurs in cases of late onset or incomplete healing (476). In this stage of LCP, there is histologic slowing of the resorption process and a predominance of immature-bone deposition (4).

Remodeled or healed stage. Residual shape alterations may be seen at this stage. The epiphysis has already ossified

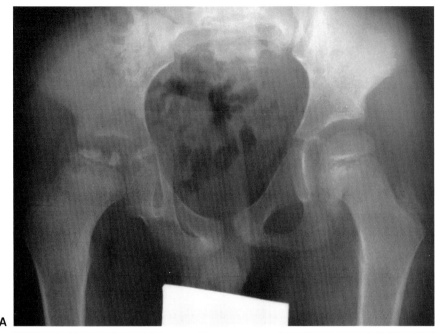

A

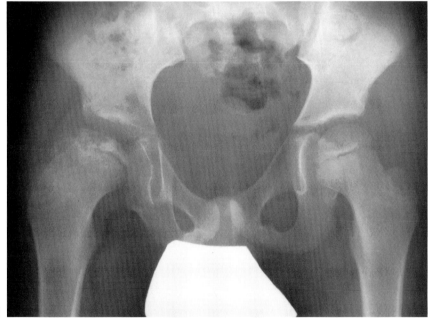

B

FIG. 5-181. Legg-Calvé-Perthes disease. A: Same patient as in Fig. 5-180. One year later, the right proximal femoral epiphysis is fragmented and irregularly ossified. There is widening of the femoral neck, and the metaphysis is lucent. The contralateral hip remains normal. **B:** Two years after presentation, the right proximal femur shows extensive deformity. A coxa magna deformity of the femoral head, a widened femoral neck, incomplete coverage (containment) of the head, and evidence of physeal growth arrest are seen.

into a pattern determined by the cartilaginous mold, and now the immature bone has been replaced by remodeled trabecular bone. The final size and shape of the bony epiphysis depend on the original amount of avascular necrosis, the effects of surgical or orthotic treatment, and abnormal forces that affect the reossifying epiphysis (4). There may be complete restoration to normal architecture; alternatively, the final state may be a flattened, misshapen femoral head, a short femoral neck, and coxa magna (Fig. 5-182).

Mature Haversian systems form at this stage. Congruency or incongruency of the femoral head to its acetabulum, the degree of femoral head containment, the smoothness of the cartilaginous surfaces, and the biomechanics of the hip components determine the eventual health of the hip.

Radiologic Evaluation. The initial radiologic evaluation usually includes AP and frog-lateral views of the pelvis and both hips. Because bony resorption and subchondral fracture are usually located anterolaterally, the frog-lateral projection is particularly valuable (see Fig. 5-178). The gonads can be shielded for both AP and frog-lateral views in a boy and at least for the frog-lateral view in a girl. At the time of initial diagnosis, bone age is determined using the method of Greulich and Pyle. The degree of skeletal maturation at the time of presentation is used to guide management (see below). If there is bilateral involvement in LCP disease, the two hips are almost always at different stages. This difference is presumably due to avascular insults at different times. If the patient is African-American or if there is bilateral, symme-

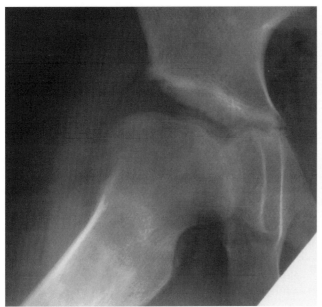
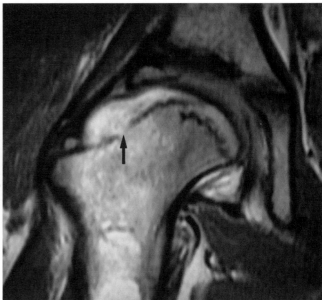

A

B

FIG. 5-182. Legg-Calvé-Perthes disease. A: Frog-lateral view of the right hip in a 14-year-old boy shows a coxa magna deformity, physeal arrest, and incomplete femoral head coverage. **B:** Proton density coronal MR image of the right hip in the same boy shows disruption of the proximal femoral physis, where a bony bridge has formed *(arrow)*. This growth arrest contributes to the deformity of the proximal femur, which is incompletely covered by the acetabulum.

tric femoral head involvement, other diagnoses should be considered (4).

The indications for MRI in the evaluation of LCP have increased. In the early detection of ischemia, MRI is at least as sensitive as scintigraphy (158). It can lead to prompt diagnosis in a child with no radiographic findings. In more established cases, MRI can determine the extent of physeal and marrow involvement and thus help with prognosis and treatment planning. In advanced disease, MRI can help with preoperative assessment of femoral head coverage and articular integrity.

Like MRI, skeletal scintigraphy can be used to evaluate patients with suspected LCP but negative radiographs. However, absence of tracer uptake in the femoral head is not quite specific for LCP, as it may also be seen with vascular tamponade from hip effusion (158). With an effusion, however, tracer uptake in the physis may also be relatively reduced, whereas in LCP it will be normal or increased (10).

Scintigraphy is also useful during the stages of revascularization, reossification, and repair. Normal tracer uptake gradually returns to the femoral head. Sometimes this is first seen as a column of tracer localization in the posterolateral epiphysis (the "lateral column sign") whereas the remainder of the epiphysis remains void of uptake. This pattern suggests a more favorable prognosis than does either the persistent complete absence of femoral head tracer uptake or the return of uptake along a broad physeal base. Differing revascularization mechanisms may account for these differences in scintigraphic patterns and prognosis (483).

Treatment. Most patients with LCP do well with no treatment (476). In the others, the purpose of treatment is to

keep the femoral head contained by the acetabulum, prevent lateral subluxation, protect the cartilage, reduce stress on the femoral head until the head reossifies, prevent pain, and minimize later degenerative joint disease (476). The head must be contained within the acetabulum to allow correct reciprocal molding and to prevent extrusion of the lateral part of the epiphyseal cartilage (4). Containment may be achieved with or without surgery. The literature regarding the best treatment for LCP is inconclusive (471). Treatment options include bracing in abduction, femoral varus-derotation osteotomy, and innominate osteotomy (4).

Prognosis. The final shape of the femoral head is governed by many factors. A poor result is more common in older onset patients and in those with persistent lateral subluxation (incomplete containment), large areas of metaphyseal cartilaginous foci ("cysts"), and lateral extrusion of part of the cartilaginous epiphysis (4). Physeal interruption on MR images predicts subsequent growth arrest with a sensitivity and specificity of over 90% (484). Maintaining a good range of motion with physical therapy is very important (485).

There also is good evidence that the final result correlates with the amount of femoral head involvement on the initial radiographs. Caterall divided patients into four prognostic groups based on seven radiographic features. The vast majority of patients with good results were in groups 1 and 2 (incomplete femoral head involvement). Those with poor outcomes were predominantly in groups 3 and 4 (more extensive femoral head involvement) (486). Salter and Thompson proposed a simpler classification system dividing the patients into two groups; group A have involvement of less than half of the femoral head, and group B more than half. Herring suggests that the presence or absence of lateral pillar involvement may be the major prognostic factor (487,488). Regardless of the final shape of the femoral head, one study has suggested that at least 60% of patients will be symptom-free 30–40 years later (4).

Differential Diagnosis. The radiographic differential diagnosis of LCP disease includes normal variants and avascular necrosis of known etiology. The femoral head dysplasia of Meyer should be considered in patients less than 4 years of age, as is discussed below. Femoral head avascular necrosis may be secondary to Gaucher disease, sickle cell disease, other hemoglobinopathies, endogenous or exogenous steroids, trauma, osteomyelitis, hypothyroidism, irradiation, surgery, and excessive traction. Bilaterality suggests a generalized disorder. Femoral head deformity is also seen in the epiphyseal dysplasias and mucopolysaccharidoses and after developmental dysplasia of the hip.

Meyer Dysplasia

Meyer dysplasia, or *dysplasia epiphysealis capitis femoris,* is a poorly defined femoral head dysostosis that has some of the characteristics of a normal variant but sometimes seems to progress to LCP disease. Meyer dysplasia is frequently detected incidentally on radiographs that include the pelvis (Fig. 5-183). It is seen almost exclusively in boys less than 5 years of age (489). There usually is delayed appearance of the femoral head ossification center; when it does become visible (frequently after 2 years of age), it is multipartite and granular. There is neither epiphyseal sclerosis nor subchondral fracture. Almost half of patients have bilateral changes at presentation (489,490).

Serial radiographs show progression to normal ossification. There is coalescence of the granular centers and growth of the epiphysis without resorption or sclerosis. The proximal femoral ossification center usually assumes a normal appearance within 3 years (4). However, LCP disease develops in as many as 20% of patients thought to have Meyer dysplasia.

Slipped Capital Femoral Epiphysis

Clinical Features. Slipped capital femoral epiphysis (SCFE) is analogous to a Salter-Harris type I physeal fracture involving the proximal femur. The cause of the fracture is unknown, although its occurrence during the pubertal growth spurt suggests that the hormone-mediated processes (including vascularity) that induce closure of the physis may play a role. Shearing forces, accentuated by obesity, applied to the vulnerable growth plate produce a physeal fracture. Slippage subsequently occurs. Although most cases of SCFE are idiopathic, it has been reported in association with hypothyroidism (491), treated or untreated hypopituitarism, renal osteodystrophy (418), and in children who have undergone irradiation for malignancy (251,492). These associations are

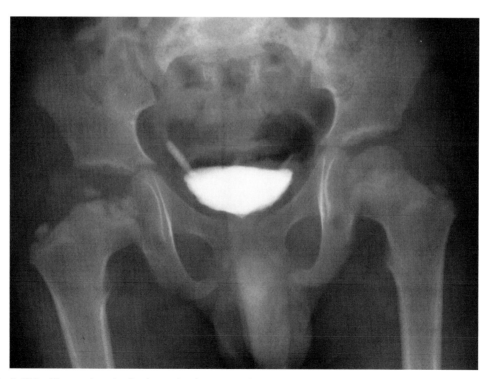

FIG. 5-183. Meyer dysplasia. Irregular fragmentation and ossification of the right proximal femoral epiphysis was discovered incidentally on a frontal film during intravenous urography. The patient was asymptomatic and remained so.

particularly common in SCFE developing prior to 10 years of age. Prophylactic pinning of the contralateral as-yet-uninvolved hip should be considered in patients with prior radiation therapy or a known metabolic or endocrinologic predisposition.

The boy-to-girl ratio is 2.5:1. In boys SCFE occurs most frequently between 12 and 15 years of age, and in girls between 10 and 13 years of age (493). African-Americans are more commonly affected than Caucasians; the incidence is 7.8 per 100,000 in African-American boys, 6.7 in African-American girls, 4.7 in Caucasian boys, and 1.6 in Caucasian girls (493). There are familial cases of SCFE. Although the reason is unknown, members of low socioeconomic groups are more frequently affected. Children with SCFE are usually overweight, are slightly tall for their age, and tend to have some delay in skeletal maturation. Proximal femoral retroversion or decreased anteversion may be a predisposing condition (494). Perhaps the mechanical forces across the proximal femoral epiphysis are altered enough by this rotational deformity to cause increased shear stresses on the physis; the forces generated by an overweight child may be within the range of those needed to fracture the physis.

Approximately half of patients give a history of significant trauma. The most common presenting symptoms are hip pain and limp, but 25% of patients have knee pain (4). The incidence of bilateral involvement ranges from 20% to 32%; both hips are affected more frequently in girls than in boys. Only half of patients with eventual bilateral SCFE have bilateral radiologic changes at presentation. The changes are rarely symmetric, as the slippages do not occur simultaneously. Slips may be considered chronic (the most common form), acute, or acute-on-chronic (495).

Radiologic Evaluation. The left hip is affected more frequently than the right in boys but not in girls. The usual initial displacement of the epiphysis is posterior (496). Because 99% of SCFE cases have major posterior displacement whereas only 75% have major medial displacement, the lateral view is critical. CT is used in selected cases to demonstrate the degree of posterior slippage and the width of the physis (Fig. 5-184).

Signs of slippage may be subtle on the AP projection. There is usually osteopenia of the femoral head and neck. The physis may be wide, and there is frequently blurring of its metaphyseal margin. A line drawn tangential to the lateral border of the femoral neck normally intersects the epiphyseal ossification center, so that approximately one sixth of the diameter of the femoral head lies lateral to this line. If there is medial slippage, less femoral head lies lateral to this line than on the normal side (Fig. 5-185). There frequently is displacement of the metaphysis from the acetabulum and a reduction in apparent epiphyseal height (496) (Fig. 5-185). Normally, on a true lateral or frog-lateral view, the anterior and posterior margins of the epiphysis and metaphysis match each other closely, and their junction is smooth (like a dip of ice cream on a cone). With SCFE, the lateral film shows a metaphyseal-epiphyseal discontinuity due to posterior dis-

placement of the epiphysis (Fig. 5-185) (like a dip of ice cream slipping backward off its cone).

If the epiphyseal slip is chronic, reactive bone formation is present at the medial and posterior aspects of the femoral neck, apparently an effort to buttress the displaced epiphysis (4,5). Premature fusion of the physis, a late complication, may result in slight femoral shortening.

Treatment. The purpose of fixation is to prevent further slippage, not to reposition the capital femoral epiphysis, and to promote physeal closure. Pinning in situ is thought to provide the best long-term functional outcome. There is a higher incidence of subsequent degenerative changes, acute cartilage necrosis (chondrolysis), and avascular necrosis when realignment is attempted in the presence of severe slippage (497). Since the pin may be closer to the curved surface of the femoral head than the radiographic projections at first suggest, the distance from any part of the pin to the peripheral cortex should be more than 15% of the overall diameter of the head on both views (4). The metallic pins are usually removed after physeal fusion has occurred.

Complications. The most significant complications are chondrolysis and avascular necrosis. Chondrolysis is defined as acute articular cartilage necrosis of the femoral head. The frequency of chondrolysis ranges from about 2% to 40% (498). Racial predilection for African-Americans, Hawaiian, and Hispanic patients has been cited (371). The incidence of chondrolysis is less in acute and mild epiphyseal displacement (498). Symptoms such as pain, limitation of motion, and flexion contracture usually develop within a year of the acute slippage. Chondrolysis can be detected radiographically by the rapid onset of periarticular osteoporosis, joint space narrowing, and osseous erosion. If this complication is suspected, one should exclude penetration of a fixating pin; this can be accomplished by computed or conventional tomography or fluoroscopy in various rotations. Treatment for chondrolysis is aimed at reduction of the presumed hip inflammation with antiinflammatory medications. Traction and physical therapy to restore motion are also employed (495).

The complication of avascular necrosis is most common after the acute development of epiphyseal slippage. This may be due to rapid, excessive stretch of epiphyseal vessels (495). An increased incidence is noted with more severe slips (495). It seldom occurs in untreated cases. Iatrogenic injury to the blood supply of the femoral head may be caused by manipulation and placement of fixation pins. When avascular necrosis is identified, the fixation pins should be removed or repositioned to prevent subsequent penetration into the joint and resultant chondrolysis (495).

Although SCFE is a radiographic and not a scintigraphic diagnosis, skeletal scintigraphy may be useful. An uncomplicated acute slip typically appears as increased tracer uptake in the physis and adjacent metaphysis and normal uptake in the epiphysis (499). Femoral head ischemia complicating untreated SCFE or pin fixation results in absence of tracer localization in the femoral head, a pattern which identifies

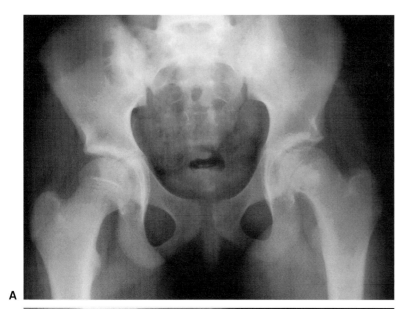

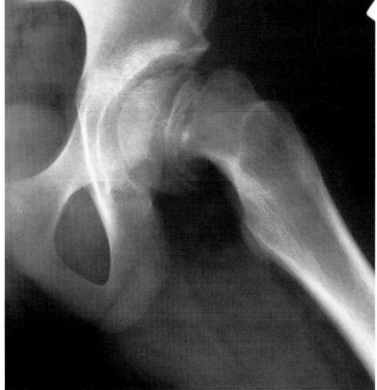

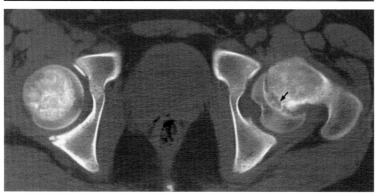

FIG. 5-184. Slipped capital femoral epiphysis. This 11-year-old girl had had left hip pain for 6 weeks. **A:** The proximal left femoral physis is less well demarcated than the physis of the right hip. There is loss of the medial triangular density (Capener triangle). A cortical line drawn along the femoral neck does not intersect the lateral margin of the epiphysis, and the apparent epiphyseal height is reduced. **B:** A frog-lateral view of the left hip shows medial, inferior, and posterior displacement of the epiphysis. **C:** Axial CT scan demonstrates the posterior component of the epiphyseal slip better. The physis is widened *(arrow)*.

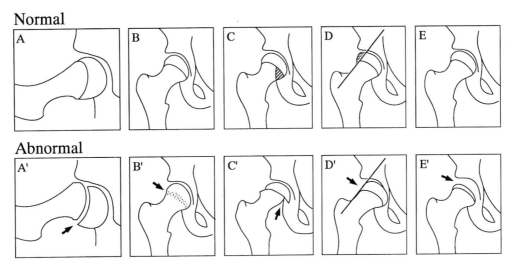

FIG. 5-185. Slipped capital femoral epiphysis: radiographic signs. A: The femoral epiphysis normally sits upon the metaphysis like a scoop of ice cream on a cone. **A′:** The scoop (the femoral head) has slipped part way off the cone (the femoral neck). **B:** The normal femoral physis is sharply marginated. **B′:** There is blurring of the proximal femoral physis. **C:** The medial femoral neck normally overlaps the posterior part of the acetabulum forming a dense triangle (Capener triangle). **C′:** This triangular density is lost by the lateral displacement of the femoral neck. **D:** A line drawn along the femoral neck normally intersects at least the lateral sixth of the femoral epiphysis. **D′:** With displacement, no part of the epiphysis lies lateral to the line. **E:** The femoral epiphysis is of normal height. **E′:** With posterior slippage, there is apparent decrease in the height of the epiphysis. Modified from Bloomberg (496).

children at risk for avascular necrosis (AVN) (499,500). Chondrolysis is suggested scintigraphically when there is prominent periarticular tracer uptake especially involving the acetabular roof. In patients with continued pain after treatment, scintigraphic assessment of the femoral neck physis bears on the recurrence of slippage; when scintigraphy demonstrates closure of the proximal femoral physis, recurrence is unlikely (501).

Proximal Focal Femoral Deficiency

Proximal focal femoral deficiency (PFFD) ranges from simple shortening and minor hypoplasia to total absence of major components of the proximal femur. Children with PFFD usually are identified in infancy because of a short lower extremity. Several classification systems, based on the osseous integrity of the proximal femur and acetabulum, have been proposed; these categories have prognostic and therapeutic implications. The most commonly used classification, by Aitken, divides PFFD into four groups, according to the degree of deformity (502). Aitken type A represents the least severe form; the femur is short, but a femoral head and adequate acetabulum are present (Fig. 5-186A). A pseudarthrosis may be present between the head and the rest of the femur, and there is varus alignment. Type D is the most severe form. Both the femoral head and acetabulum are absent. The femur is very short and deformed. Classifications that include congenital coxa vara and femoral bowing have also been proposed (503). Approximately 15% of abnormalities are bilateral, and up to two thirds of patients

have ipsilateral fibular hemimelia and a deformity of the foot (504).

For children with a femoral head and acetabulum (Aitken types A and B), surgery is generally not necessary and can result in loss of function. Patients with more severe deficiencies (types C and D) have markedly abnormal or absent acetabula and proximal femurs, severe leg length discrepancies, and poor supporting musculature. These patients usually benefit from a Syme amputation of the foot and arthrodesis of the knee. This treatment yields a stable stump for a prosthesis.

Radiographic classification of patients is difficult before hip structures ossify, and reclassification may be necessary as the patient matures. Ultrasonography (505) and MRI can be used to evaluate the extraosseous structures, which govern treatment and prognosis in the young child (Fig. 5-186B) (506).

Abnormalities of Orientation

Coxa Vara and Coxa Valga. The angle between the femoral neck and the femoral shaft as measured in the coronal plane is approximately 150° at birth but decreases to 120–130° in the adult. Coxa vara is a smaller than normal neck-shaft angle; coxa valga is a larger than normal angle (507).

Coxa vara present at birth (congenital coxa vara) is presumably due to a developmental abnormality of the limb bud. There is minimal progression after birth. It is associated with other musculoskeletal abnormalities, such as proximal

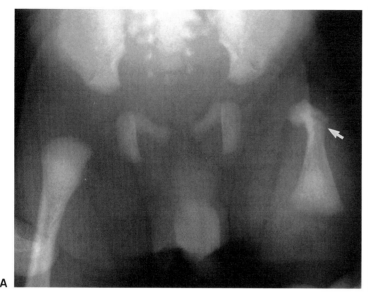
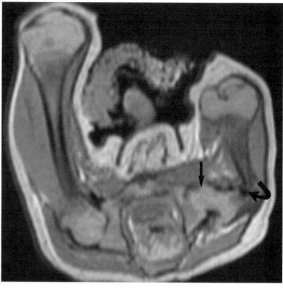

FIG. 5-186. Proximal focal femoral deficiency. A: This infant boy has a very short left femur. There is a pseudarthrosis *(arrow)* of the proximal femur. The acetabulum is well formed. **B:** Axial proton density MR image shows the cartilaginous femoral head *(arrow)* seated in a well-formed acetabulum (Aitken type A). The pseudarthrosis *(curved arrow)* is also seen.

focal femoral deficiency, congenital short femur, and congenital bowed femur (508).

Trauma, tumors, dysplasias (e.g., spondyloepiphyseal dysplasia and metaphyseal chondrodysplasia), and metabolic abnormalities may result in an acquired coxa vara (Fig. 5-187). Examples include coxa vara secondary to a slipped

capital femoral epiphysis, rickets, and fibrous dysplasia (508).

Developmental coxa vara (infantile coxa vara) develops in early childhood and progresses during growth. Aside from a minimal leg length discrepancy, other significant musculoskeletal abnormalities are usually absent. Boys and girls are

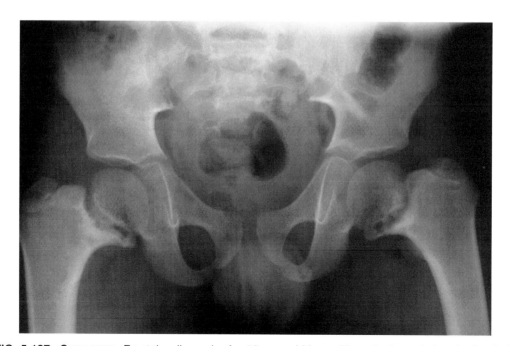

FIG. 5-187. Coxa vara. Frontal radiograph of a 10-year-old boy with metaphyseal chondrodysplasia type Schmid shows bilateral coxa vara deformities. The greater trochanters are at the level of the femoral epiphyses.

affected equally. Thirty to 50 percent of cases are bilateral. Histologic samples from the femoral necks of these children, like biopsy specimens of the proximal tibia in children with infantile Blount disease, show abnormal physeal cartilage production and metaphyseal bone formation. There is more physeal growth laterally than medially, and the orientation of the physis becomes progressively more oblique (508). The most effective treatment for advanced coxa vara is surgical derotational valgus osteotomy.

Coxa valga, or an increased neck-shaft angle, usually is the result of absence of normally balanced muscular or gravitational influences on the bones. Examples of this include neuromuscular disorders such as cerebral palsy, myelodysplasia, and poliomyelitis. It is less commonly associated with skeletal dysplasias (2).

Femoral Anteversion. Femoral anteversion (femoral torsion) is the projected angle between a line drawn through the long axis of the femoral neck and the dicondylar coronal plane of the distal femur (4). The average angle of anteversion at birth is 32° and decreases to 16° for children at 16 years of age (509). An increased angle of anteversion (also known as lateral femoral torsion) is found in children with developmental hip dysplasia and cerebral palsy. Increased anteversion may be the cause of intoeing in a child, as the affected child internally rotates the abnormally anteverted femur to achieve an acceptable gait. This angle can be evaluated with selected CT images for approximately the same dose as an AP radiograph (Fig. 5-188) (510,511). Knowledge of this angle is critical for planning hip reconstruction. Retroversion or diminished anteversion apparently predisposes to slippage of the capital femoral epiphysis (494).

Disorders of the Leg

Physiologic Bowing and Physiologic Knock-Knee

Localized congenital bowing of the tibia is common in newborns. Bow-leggedness and knock-knee alignment are common in infants and children, bow-leggedness at an earlier age, and are usually considered normal (Fig 5-189). However, continued severe malalignment is pathologic and is termed varus deformity or valgus deformity (512). Physiologic lateral bowing centered at the knee is present in later infancy and early childhood (Fig. 5-189A). There presumably is a continuum from slight bowing of the lower extremities when held in the neutral position to marked separation of the knees. Lower extremity bowing in the early years is more severe in girls and African-Americans and is associated with medial tibial torsion.

Radiographically, physiologic bowing of the lower extremities is characterized by prominent medioposterior metaphyseal beaks of the distal femur and proximal tibia and thickening of the medial femoral and tibial cortices. The medial parts of the epiphyses of the distal femur and proxi-

Proximal Femur

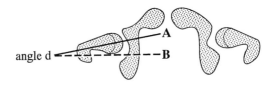

Distal Femur

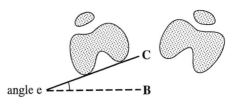

FIG. 5-188. Femoral anteversion: CT measurement. Axial image at the level of the femoral necks: *Line A* is drawn through the femoral neck. *Line B* is drawn along the horizontal plane. *Angle d* is formed by the intersection of these two lines. Distal femur: *Line C* is drawn along the posterior femoral condyles (some authors use a line bisecting the femur at this level). *Line B* is drawn along the same horizontal plane. *Angle e* is formed by these two lines. If the knee is externally rotated, angle e is subtracted from angle d to obtain an angle of anteversion. If the knee is internally rotated, angle e is added to angle d.

mal tibia ossify more slowly than the lateral parts, and this results in a wedge-like configuration. However, there is none of the epiphyseal fragmentation seen in Blount disease The distal tibial physes slant down laterally (4).

During the second year of life, varus alignment begins to disappear. By 3–4 years of age, slight valgus (physiologic knock-knees) develops in most children. Valgus alignment is especially evident in girls and obese children (Fig. 5-189B). The tibia is now abducted in relation to the femur. The cortical thickening and metaphyseal beaking are evident no longer. The valgus configuration generally diminishes over time from 4 to 12 years of age.

The angle of varus or valgus is calculated from the intersection of lines drawn through the longitudinal axes of the midshafts of the neutral-positioned femur and tibia. The average varus angle of 17° in the newborn decreases to about 9° by 1 year of age and then changes to a valgus angle of 2° at 2 years, 11° at 3 years, and 6° at 13 years (4). Thus, there is normal bowing in the newborn and infant, knock-knees in the young child, and a decrease in the valgus angle during later childhood. However, there is a group of children with markedly bowed legs in whom the transition from varus to valgus occurs late. Varus reaches a peak, rather than diminishes, in this group at 18–24 months of age. These children are at an increased risk for Blount disease.

The more common causes of varus and valgus alignment at the knee are summarized in Table 5-24.

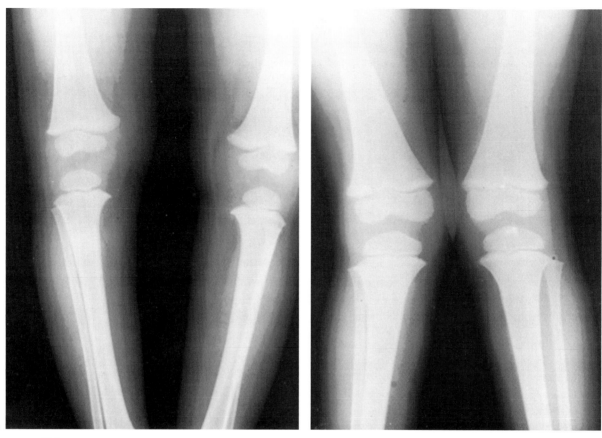

FIG. 5-189. Physiologic bowing. A: 1-1/2-year-old girl with slightly bowed legs. **B:** By 3 years of age, the same girl developed knock-knees.

Tibial Bowing

A bowed tibia in the neonate may be isolated or part of a generalized abnormality (513). With isolated bowing, there frequently is no other clinical abnormality and no genetic predisposition. In early infancy, isolated tibial bowing is a common finding and probably is due to intrauterine position-

TABLE 5-24. *The more common causes of genu varum (bowlegs) and genu valgum (knock knees)*

Physiologic
Lateral tibial bowing (early infancy)
Bow-legged (into late infancy, 2 years)
Knock-knees (beginning early childhood, 3–4 years)
Pathologic
Varus
Blount disease
Unresolved physiologic bowing
Varus (and less commonly valgus)
Posttraumatic (physeal arrest, malunion)
Metabolic (rickets, renal disease)
Osteopenia (osteogenesis imperfecta, juvenile arthritis)
Valgus
Medial tibial metaphyseal fracture
Lateral condylar hypoplasia
Unresolved physiologic valgus

Source: Modified from Tolo (512).

ing. However, children with multiple bowed limbs frequently have a genetic disorder (513). Abnormalities such as a bone dysplasia (e.g., neurofibromatosis and fibrous dysplasia), neurovascular insufficiency, or a cartilage disorder may be responsible for the bowing (4). One of the more common dysplasias with limb bowing, camptomelic dysplasia, receives its name from the bent long tubular bones.

Posterior Bowing. Tibial bowing can be present at birth and frequently is bilateral. The apex of the deformity is usually posterior, but it may be medial or lateral. The etiology is unknown, although Caffey postulated that fetal positioning, uterine constraints, and extrauterine pressure may be responsible (2). Cutaneous dimples may be present over the apex of the bow. The posterior angulation is at the distal portion of the middle third of the tibia, with thickening of the cortex on the concave side and thinning on the convex side (Fig. 5-190). There may be shortening of the affected tibia and ipsilateral fibula as well as a calcaneus deformity of the ipsilateral foot. This posterior bowing almost always resolves satisfactorily without fracture or pseudarthrosis. Protective bracing, however, is used in selected patients.

Anterior Bowing. Anterior bowing of the tibia can occur with a normal medullary canal, a cystic medullary canal, or a narrow sclerotic medullary canal and also in association with fibular hemimelia (513). Anterior bowing with a normal

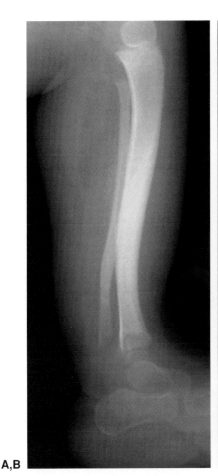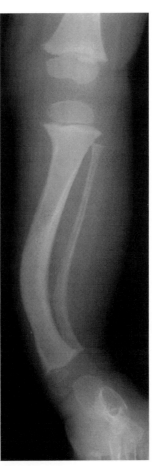

A,B

FIG. 5-190. Posterior tibial bowing. A: Lateral view of the lower extremity of a 2-year-old boy shows posterior bowing of both the tibia and fibula. The concave (anterior) cortex is thicker than the cortex (posterior) cortex. The fibula is short. **B:** Frontal view shows a medial component to the tibial and fibular bowing, with cortical thickening along the concave margins. From Jaramillo and Cleveland (564).

medullary canal has no hereditary predisposition. There is localized deformity of the tibia and occasionally of the femur. The skin overlying the convex surface of the affected bone is rarely dimpled. The cortex of the bowed bones is thickened along both the convex and concave surfaces, with greatest thickening along the concave margin. There may also be a lateral or medial component. Bowing usually resolves without treatment, and pseudarthrosis rarely occurs.

Anterior bowing with a cystic or narrowed sclerotic medullary canal usually progresses to pseudarthrosis within 2 years. There is an association with neurofibromatosis and, less frequently, with fibrous dysplasia. The limb is angulated anterolaterally or anteromedially. The most common site of bowing is the distal half of the tibia. Skin dimpling usually is not present. Both the tibia and fibula may be bowed, with a decrease in the diameter of the tibia in its distal half (see Fig. 5-47). The tibia is sclerotic or cystic with partial or complete obliteration of the medullary cavity. The prognosis for obtaining a functional extremity is poor. Finally, anterior bowing may also occur in association with fibular hemimelia (Fig. 5-191) (513) and with osteofibrous dysplasia (see Fig. 5-101).

Generalized bowing of the limbs may occur in the neonate with osteogenesis imperfecta, hypophosphatasia, fibrous dysplasia, camptomelic dysplasia (see Fig. 5-38), thanatophoric dwarfism, and other syndromes.

Blount Disease

Blount disease (tibia vara, historically termed *osteochondrosis deformans tibiae*) is an idiopathic illness that causes bowing of the lower extremities (514). It is divided into infantile and late onset forms, depending on the patient's age and associated conditions. The deformity in Blount disease is thought to be due to disturbed endochondral ossification resulting from abnormal pressure and force on the proximal medial tibial physis (4). *Infantile Blount disease* may be physiologic bowing that fails to undergo the normal valgoid change as the child becomes heavier and begins to walk. The findings are frequently bilateral but can be unilateral or much more severe on one side than the other. There is a high prevalence of obesity among children with infantile Blount disease (515). *Late onset (adolescent) Blount disease* affects children mainly between the ages of 6 and 15 years. It is much less common than the infantile type and is usually unilateral. The cause of this adolescent type is uncertain. There may be segmental arrest of physeal function secondary to trauma or infection.

Radiographic findings of Blount disease include medial tibial metaphyseal beaking similar to but often more marked than that seen with physiologic bowing. The beak is markedly depressed, irregular, and fragmented (Fig. 5-192A). MRI or arthrography demonstrates enlargement of the epi-

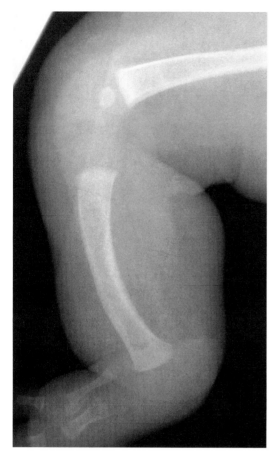

FIG. 5-191. **Complete fibular hemimelia.** The tibia is short-ened and bowed anteriorly. The fibula and two metatarsopha-langeal rays are completely absent.

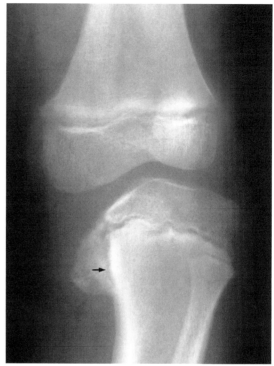

A

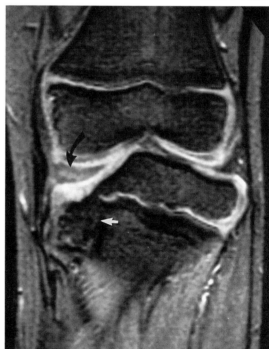

B

FIG. 5-192. **Blount disease. A:** Frontal view of the lower extremity in a 7-year-old boy shows depression and irregular-ity of the medial part of the proximal tibia. There is varus angulation at the knee. The medial tibial physis *(arrow)* is poorly defined. **B:** Coronal gradient recalled echo MR se-quence shows interruption of the medial proximal tibial physis *(straight arrow)*. There is downsloping of the medial part of the articulating surface of the tibia. Diffuse high signal *(curved arrow)* is seen in the medial meniscus.

physeal cartilage and medial meniscus. As weight-bearing pressure continues, the physis becomes narrowed medially, and the physeal cartilage decreases in height. Premature fu-sion of the physis occurs medially (Fig. 5-192B). There may be lateral widening of the physis of the distal femur or proxi-mal tibia (516). Evaluation of the integrity of the physis, including the detection of bony bridges, is possible with MRI. The medial meniscus may be abnormally large and of abnormal signal, which suggests degenerative changes (517).

The varus configuration of the tibia is due to angulation between the axis of the proximal epiphysis and that of the metadiaphyses (518). A *metaphyseal-diaphyseal angle* (Fig. 5-193), determined by a line drawn through the proximal tibial metaphysis and a line perpendicular to the long axis of the tibia on standing radiographs, exceeding 11° is associated with Blount disease (518). A measurement less than 11° suggests physiologic bowing. The *tibial-femoral angle* made by the longitudinal axes of those bones is not significantly different in Blount disease and physiologic bowing (518).

Although improvement may occur spontaneously or with bracing, severe infantile Blount disease requires tibial osteot-omy. The deformity in the adolescent type is usually milder

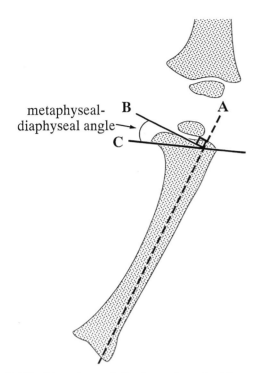

metaphyseal-diaphyseal angle→

FIG. 5-193. Metaphyseal-diaphyseal angle. The angle is formed by a line *(B)* perpendicular to the long axis of the tibia *(A)*, and a line through the tibial metaphysis *(C)*. This angle normally should not exceed 11°.

than in the infantile form, but surgical osteotomy and, in some patients, physeal bony bridge excision may be needed for correction. Differential diagnostic considerations for the radiographic appearance of Blount disease include severe physiologic bowing and vitamin D-resistant rickets (519).

Leg Length Discrepancy

Discrepancy in the lengths of the legs may be congenital or acquired. A difference of less than 2.5 cm generally can be treated with orthotics. Surgery is needed for the larger discrepancies (520). Measurements of the lower extremities can be made with radiographic scanograms or using the scout view (topogram) capability of CT. The scanogram uses a radiopaque ruler, a moving tube, and three separate exposures at the hips, knees, and ankles on a single 14 × 17 inch film (Fig. 5-194). CT is especially helpful in patients with joint contractures, in whom accurate measurement in the neutral position is difficult (521). Decisions to treat are based on the size of the discrepancy, the degree of skeletal maturity, and the estimated further growth of the child, which can be calculated from bone age radiographs.

Causes of length discrepancy include trauma (i.e., from physeal arrest or from overgrowth during healing), hemiatrophy, hemihypertrophy, slipped capital femoral epiphysis, LCP disease, vascular malformations, infection, melorheostosis, tumors, and arthritides. Treatment includes os-

seous epiphysiodesis or physeal stapling of the longer limb, effectively shortening that bone (or bones) over time. Other techniques treat the asymmetry by lengthening the shorter limb (520). These methods require precise imaging during planning and follow-up.

Problems associated with a leg length discrepancy include unacceptable appearance, increased energy expenditure in gait, equinus contracture at the ankle of the shorter limb, scoliosis and other lower back problems, and late degenerative changes at the hip (522).

Tibial Torsion

Tibial version, which is normal, is the rotation of the tibia at the ankle joint with respect to the tibia at the knee joint. When this is abnormal in either direction, it is termed tibial torsion. Medial or internal tibial torsion (as well as abnormal femoral anteversion) can result in intoeing. An excessive degree of internal rotation is associated with other congenital

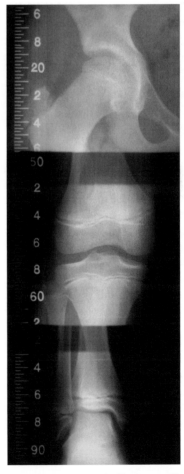

FIG. 5-194. Scanogram. A single film is used for three separate exposures taken at the level of the hip, the knee, and the ankle. Using the radiopaque ruler, measurement of the lengths (femur, tibia, total) can be made and compared to the opposite lower extremity.

abnormalities such as clubfoot, genu varum, and genu valgum. It can also be seen in trauma, Blount disease, and rickets (523). Patients with patellofemoral instability or Osgood-Schlatter disease (see below) may have an increase in lateral tibial torsion (524). The degree of torsion may correct itself, especially during the first several years of life. In cases severe enough to cause physical or cosmetic difficulties, derotational osteotomies are performed.

Measurement of the angle of rotation can be made clinically. As the child grows, there is relatively more external rotation (approximately 4° at birth and 14° at 10 years of age) (525,526). By adulthood, external rotation is approximately 20° (524). In children who are difficult to examine preoperatively, CT is used. Single 10-mm images are taken at the widest part of the proximal tibial condyles and at the level of the malleoli. The angle subtended between the transverse axis through the proximal tibia and a line drawn between the lateral and medial malleoli is measured (Fig. 5-195). Both legs should be imaged simultaneously (527).

Congenital Lower Limb Deficiencies

Congenital limb deficiencies are much more common than acquired amputations in children. They seem to occur as a result of abnormal limb bud development or an intrauterine destructive process. Most classification systems are based on the original work done by Frantz and O'Rahilly (528,529).

Fibular hemimelia (Greek for "half a limb") refers to partial or complete absence of the fibula. This is the most common long bone deficiency (529). It is often associated with absence of the lateral rays of the foot, a shortened and anteromedially bowed tibia, and proximal focal femoral deficiency (see Fig. 5-191). The clinical problems are the resultant leg length discrepancy and the abnormal foot alignment, often due to the tethering effect of the fibular remnant. Foot amputation at an early age and a prosthesis is currently the preferred therapy in most cases (504,530).

As with fibular hemimelia, *tibial hemimelia* may be partial or complete. It is bilateral in up to one third of patients and is often associated with other skeletal abnormalities such as lobster-claw hand and developmental dysplasia of the hip (504). The leg is markedly shortened, the foot is turned toward the perineum, and the medial foot rays are frequently absent. Depending on the functional capacity of the knee joint, a below-knee or above-knee amputation and a prosthesis are recommended (504).

Evaluation of congenital deformities of the lower extremities begins with radiography. However, only the bones are thus visualized. As therapy and prognosis are considered, additional information may be necessary. MRI can identify cartilaginous remnants of the tibia or fibula, cartilaginous tarsal coalitions, insufficient musculature (especially of the quadriceps mechanism, which is necessary for adequate function at the knee), and anomalies of the arterial branching pattern (531).

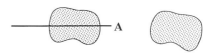

Proximal Tibia

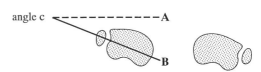

Distal Tibia

FIG. 5-195. Tibial torsion. The degree of tibial rotation *(angle c)* is determined by a line along the transverse axis of the proximal tibia *(A)* and a line between the lateral and medial malleoli *(B)* at the distal tibia. Both right and left tibias are shown.

Trauma to the Knee

Acute Trauma.

Meniscal injuries. The menisci acquire their characteristic morphology before birth and do not change shape significantly with age. They are highly vascular in early childhood. The intrameniscal vessels slowly regress from the inner to the outer meniscal edge. By approximately 12 years of age, they are present in only the outer third of the meniscus (532). On MRI, a horizontal linear high signal in the peripheral one third of the meniscus may well represent a nutrient vessel and should not be mistaken for a tear (Fig. 5-196).

Meniscal tears in children with open physes are uncommon, because the physes, which are weaker than the surrounding ligaments and menisci, tend to absorb trauma and give way to it first. The intraarticular structures are thus relatively well-protected in the younger child. The grading of meniscal and ligamentous injuries in children is similar to that used in adults. In adults, medial meniscal injuries are significantly more common than lateral meniscal tears, which in turn are more common than anterior cruciate ligament (ACL) tears. This trend is also seen in children, but

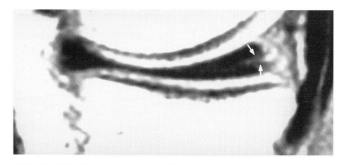

FIG. 5-196. Normal meniscal vessel. Sagittal proton density MR image of the medial meniscus of a 12-year-old boy shows a horizontal high-signal vessel *(arrows)* entering the posterior horn. This should not be mistaken for a meniscal tear.

only medial meniscal tears are significantly more common than ACL tears (533).

Young children. The majority of meniscal tears in children under 10 years of age are due to a lateral discoid meniscus. A discoid meniscus lacks the normal tapering from the periphery to the center and is a large, disc-shaped structure. The normal developing meniscus never has a discoid configuration (532). The discoid shape may be the result of instability from partial or complete absence of the normal meniscofemoral attachments. Because of abnormal fixation, the meniscus is drawn into the intercondylar notch with knee extension. Innumerable repetitions of this motion may cause a characteristic degenerative thickening (534). A discoid meniscus is occasionally associated with other deformities, such as hypoplasia of the lateral femoral condyle, hypoplasia of the tibial spines, a widened lateral joint space, high-riding fibular head, muscular defects, and abnormal vasculature.

As in MRI in adults, the discoid meniscus assumes a continuous bow-tie or slab appearance on three or more consecutive sagittal images (3–4 mm thick). On the midcoronal image where the meniscus should be at its smallest, the discoid meniscus occupies more than the usual one third of the width of the femoral-tibial articulation. The meniscus usually contains a band of high signal on all MRI sequences (535) (Fig. 5-197).

Adolescents. Most meniscal injuries in adolescents occur during sports, such as football, soccer, and basketball. The most common type of meniscal lesions are vertical tears and peripheral detachments (Fig. 5-198). Bucket-handle tears

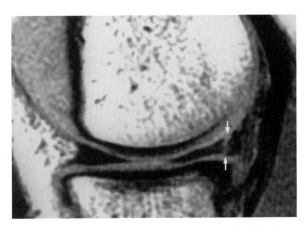

FIG. 5-198. Meniscal tear. Proton density sagittal MR image of the knee of a 16-year-old boy. A vertical tear *(arrows)* is present in the posterior horn of the medial meniscus.

(vertical longitudinal disruptions, in which the inner fragments are displaced toward the intercondylar notch) are frequent in the older child (536). Horizontal tears are much less common than in adults. The sensitivity (80% to 85%) and specificity (88% to 100%) of MRI for meniscal tears is similar to that in adults (533). Given the high vascularity and presumed greater reparative ability of the pediatric menisci, every effort should be made to preserve traumatized menisci and to repair peripheral detachments.

Ligamentous injuries. The capsular and cruciate ligaments, except for the tibial collateral ligament, originate from and insert on the epiphyses of the femur and tibia (537). In children, the strength of the ligaments concentrates the stress of the trauma at the physeal plates and usually produces physeal separation rather than ligamentous failure. Therefore, under 12 years of age, ligamentous problems about the knee are probably congenital rather than traumatic. Ligamentous injury becomes more common in older children. With age, the physes fuse, the bones become stronger, the children suffer sports injuries, and the incidence of motor vehicle accidents increases.

Medial collateral ligament injury usually is due to valgus or external rotational stress to the knee with the foot held stationary. Since the insertion of the major component of the medial collateral ligament, the tibial collateral ligament, is extraarticular in location, an associated large effusion implies an accompanying intraarticular injury. Isolated lateral collateral ligament injuries are uncommon. They usually are due to varus or hyperextension stress and are associated with injuries to the arcuate ligamentous complex and the popliteal tendon.

Isolated ACL disruption is unusual, especially in children under 14 years of age. The distal end of the ACL attaches anteriorly and laterally to the anterior tibial spine. Injuries that disrupt the ACL in adults tend to avulse the tibial eminence when the proximal tibial physis is open. This results in a type VII injury (see Fig. 5-112) which may be an epiphyseal or osteochondral (Fig. 5-199). If there is an ACL tear,

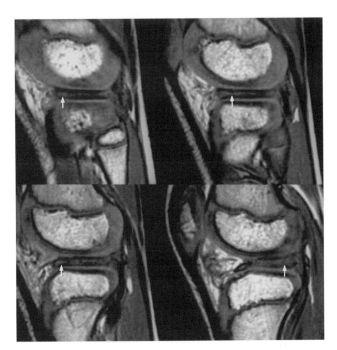

FIG. 5-197. Discoid meniscus. Four sequential sagittal proton density MR images (4 mm thick, 1 mm apart). The lateral meniscus in this 8-year-old boy with knee pain has a slablike configuration on four contiguous images. The high signal *(arrow)* within the discoid meniscus is due to trauma.

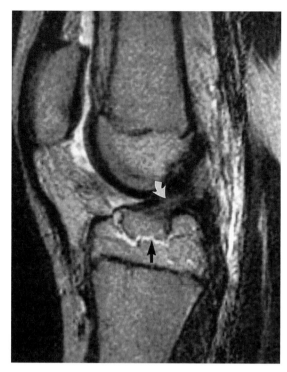

FIG. 5-199. Tibial eminence fracture. Sagittal T2-weighted MR image of the knee in this 8-year-old girl shows a fracture of the tibial intercondylar eminence *(arrow)*. The anterior cruciate ligament is intact *(curved arrow)*.

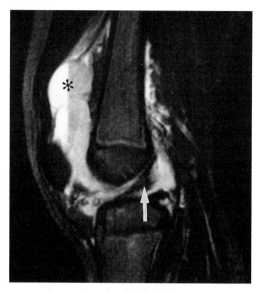

FIG. 5-200. Hemarthrosis. Sagittal T2-weighted MR image of the knee in a 5-year-old boy who sustained a soccer injury. A fluid-fluid level is seen in the suprapatellar bursa *(asterisk)*. The anterior cruciate ligament is partially torn *(arrow)*.

it most commonly occurs at its tibial insertion. However, the injury also can occur at the femoral attachment or elsewhere. As in adults, ACL injury frequently is associated with collateral ligament and meniscal injuries and bone bruises. The current treatment of ACL tears is prompt repair of avulsions at the tibial or femoral attachment, but nonoperative therapy for midsubstance tears if there is little joint laxity. Some surgeons prefer to delay surgery until the physes are nearly fused in order to avoid iatrogenic physeal injury (537).

Hemarthrosis. Acute hemarthrosis after trauma has a high association with intraarticular injury in children and adolescents (Fig. 5-200). The most common lesions associated with acute bleeding are meniscal and ACL tears. A few hemarthroses are due to osteochondral fractures (538), sometimes too minor to be radiographically evident.

Patellar injury. Patellar ossification usually begins around 3 years of age in girls and 5 or 6 years of age in boys. MRI can detect injuries to the ossified patella and its cartilaginous precursor that are difficult to see on radiographs (539). The patellar *"sleeve fracture"* refers to a cuff of cartilage that has been avulsed from the patella. The patient typically is 9–12 years of age and has an acute hyperflexion or deceleration movement that results in rapid quadriceps muscle contraction. This is a more extensive injury than is suggested by the small ossific fragments or the local soft-tissue swelling seen on radiographs. The radiographic appearance of a patellar sleeve fracture can be confused with a multipartite patella. Many linear osseous or calcific densi-

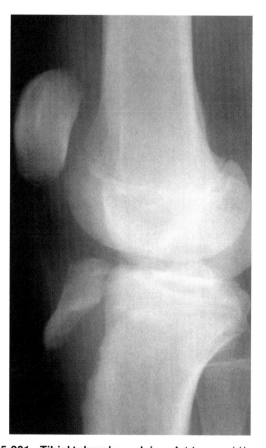

FIG. 5-201. Tibial tubercle avulsion. A 14-year-old boy with trauma to the knee. The fracture of the tibial tubercle extends into the articular surface of the tibia. The tibial tubercle is completely ossified, and the horizontal part of the tibial physis is almost closed.

ties shown paralleling the cortex of the lower pole of the patella probably represent prior chondral fractures.

Tibial tubercle avulsion. Although the tibial tubercle is anatomically part of the proximal tibial epiphysis, it behaves as an apophysis. It may be fractured acutely or be injured repeatedly and chronically. At first it is a strong inferior fibrocartilaginous extension of the proximal tibial epiphysis. During adolescence the tubercle is transformed into weaker hyaline cartilage, prior to ossification. It eventually forms a distinct ossification center, which then fuses with the rest of the ossified proximal epiphysis of the tibia (540).

The tibial tubercle is susceptible to chronic avulsion injury (Osgood-Schlatter disease; see below) during the stage when it is formed of hyaline cartilage, and the entire proximal tibial physis is still patent (540). As the tibial tubercle ossifies acute avulsions (Fig. 5-201), usually through the plane of its physis, are more common. Fractures occur after sudden acceleration or deceleration of the extensor mechanism of the knee (540). Tibial tubercle avulsions typically are seen in boys 14–16 years of age. Most of the proximal tibial physis is closing or closed, but the more distal physis of the tibial tubercle is still open. The fracture can be localized or extend into the articulating surface at the knee.

Chronic Injuries.

Osgood-Schlatter disease. Osgood-Schlatter disease (OSD) is an overuse-induced, posttraumatic abnormality probably involving tears of the deep fibers of the patellar tendon at its insertion into the tibial tuberosity (4,541). There is no histologic evidence of infection, osteochondritis, or avascular necrosis. A large powerful muscle group, the quadriceps femoris, inserts by the patellar tendon upon a small area of the tibial tuberosity. Tension applied to this area in active children produce ligamentous tears, hemorrhages, and avulsions of cartilage (4).

The disorder is characterized by localized pain, swelling, and tenderness. The condition occurs between the ages of 8 and 13 years in girls and between 10 and 15 years in boys (542). There is a boy-to-girl incidence of 3 : 1 to 7 : 1 (4,542). Approximately 25% to 33% of cases are bilateral.

The diagnosis of OSD is almost always clinical; radiologic confirmation is usually not necessary. Radiographs should be obtained when similar entities, such as osteomyelitis, primary bone tumor, and stress fracture, must be excluded.

Radiographic changes in OSD always involve the soft tissues and may involve the bony structures. The soft-tissue changes are best appreciated by a low-kilovoltage, soft-tissue lateral radiograph of the knee (Fig. 5-202). Soft-tissue changes of OSD include obliteration or loss of sharpness of the inferior angle of the infrapatellar fat pad and loss of definition and thickening of the prearticular soft tissues of the knee (542). Other soft-tissue changes include swelling anterior to the tibial tubercle, thickening of the patellar liga-

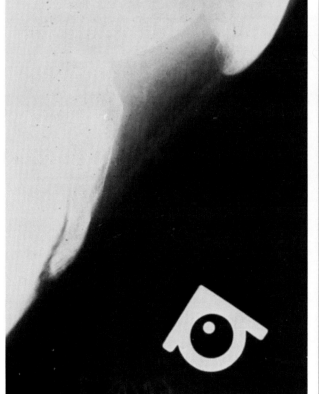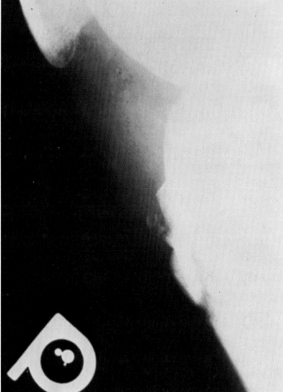

A   B

FIG. 5-202. Osgood-Schlatter disease. This 13-year-old boy had point tenderness over the right tibial tubercle. **A:** Normal left tibial tubercle and infrapatellar fat pad. **B:** Edematous obliteration of the inferior angle of the infrapatellar fat pad and swelling anterior to the irregularly mineralized tibial tubercle on the right.

ment, and loss of homogeneity of the infrapatellar fat pad. Bony changes in the tibial tubercle are highly variable. It may be difficult to decide whether irregularity or multiplicity of bony densities represents normal variations in ossification or abnormal fragmentation. Radiologic support for the diagnosis of OSD depends on soft-tissue changes due to traumatic edema and the associated inflammatory reaction rather than on bony abnormalities (542). Ultrasound also shows the tendinous involvement nicely (543).

MRI findings in OSD include high T2-weighted signal in the patellar tendon at its insertion on the tibial tuberosity and in the surrounding soft tissues. Adjacent bone marrow edema also may be present (541). However, in most cases MRI is not needed for diagnosis.

Sinding-Larsen-Johansson disease. Sinding-Larsen-Johansson disease is irregular calcification and ossification of the immature inferior patellar pole, thought to result from persistent or repeated minor traction injury there. Unlike the acute patellar sleeve fracture, Sinding-Larsen-Johansson disease results from chronic injury. The typical patient is a preteen boy, 10–12 years of age, who experiences anterior knee pain that increases with activity. It is the inferior patellar equivalent of Osgood-Schlatter disease. Infrequently, an equivalent injury can occur at the superior patellar-quadriceps tendon junction. Older children are likely to develop chronic patellar tendinitis of the adult type, which usually has no osseous radiographic findings (544).

Osteochondritis dissecans of the distal femur. Osteochondritis (osteochondrosis) dissecans (OCD) of the distal femur is an osteochondral fracture of the joint surface (545). The fracture may involve only the cartilage, in which case it is visible on MRI but not radiographs. Its etiology remains controversial. However, in children it is usually assumed to be due to repeated microtrauma, with possibly a superimposed acute traumatic event. A history of significant trauma is present in only 50% of patients.

OCD is three times as common in boys as in girls and is seen most often between the ages of 4 and 15 years (4). The most common site for OCD of the distal femur is the posterolateral nonweight-bearing portion of the medial femoral condyle. The lesion usually extends into the intercondylar notch and is bilateral in approximately 33% of children (4). A similar abnormality occasionally involves the patella, the talar dome, and the capitellum of the humerus.

Radiographs show a lucent crescentic defect in or fragmentation of subchondral bone of variable depth. There may be both radiodense and radiolucent zones that correspond to new bone formation and resorption of bone with replacement by granulation tissue or fibrocartilage (545). The defect can have irregular, slightly sclerotic edges (546) (Fig. 5-203).

MRI is used to assess the integrity of the overlying articular cartilage, the size of the subchondral bony fragment or fragments, and the stage of healing (546) (Fig. 5-204A). A stable fragment is in continuity with the underlying bone (546). The fragment is considered unstable if there is fluid between the fragment and the parent bone, as suggested by

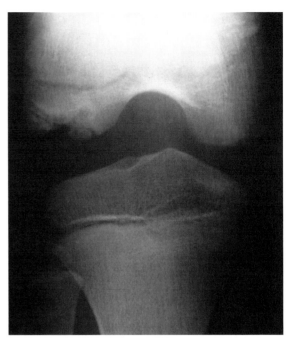

FIG. 5-203. Osteochondritis dissecans. An intercondylar notch (tunnel) view of the right knee of a 10-year-old boy complaining of knee pain shows several osseous fragments of the lateral condyle of the distal femur.

high signal on T2-weighted or gradient echo images. This finding implies disruption of the overlying hyaline cartilage (Fig. 5-204B). Once the underlying bone is exposed to synovial fluid, the bony fragment becomes unstable, spontaneous resolution is unlikely, and the fragment may become a loose body.

There is a higher rate of spontaneous resolution of stable OCD in children than in adults. They are often treated conservatively, whereas most patients over 20 years old need surgical intervention.

It may be difficult to differentiate OCD from an acute osteochondral fracture after an obvious traumatic episode or from the developmental condylar irregularities of the distal femur commonly seen in children 2–12 years of age. Developmental irregularities are usually lateral and do not involve the intercondylar notch on the AP view. On the lateral projection with the knee in extension, they are located posterior to the intercondylar eminence of the tibia, whereas OCD is usually more anterior (4). In fact, however, the developmental irregularities and OCD may be different points on a continuum of stress-related lesions.

Disorders of the Foot and Ankle

Congenital and acquired abnormalities of the foot are common. The physical and radiologic evaluation may be difficult, even confusing, particularly in infants and young children. Many foot abnormalities are recognizable at birth; others develop later because of neuromuscular disease. Some

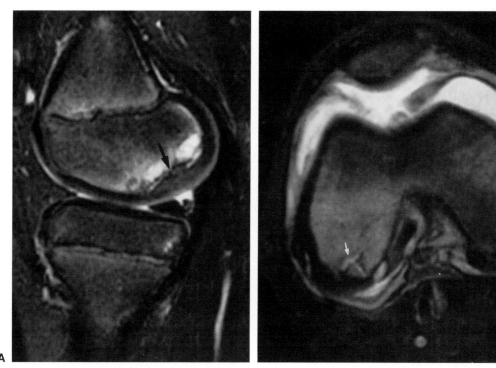

FIG. 5-204. Osteochondritis dissecans. A: An 8-year-old boy with knee pain. A sagittal T2-weighted MR image of the knee shows irregularity of the posterior part of the lateral femoral condyle *(arrow)*. The overlying epiphyseal cartilage and articular cartilage are intact. High signal, presumably from marrow edema, is seen adjacent to the lesion. **B:** An axial T2-weighted MR image of the distal femur in a boy shows high signal outlining a bony defect of the posterior medial condyle *(arrow)*. This bony defect should be considered unstable because of the fluid between the fragment and the donor bone.

abnormalities are hereditary and others are congenital malformations, such as tarsal coalitions, which are often discovered in the second decade. Prompt, correct diagnosis and treatment minimize growth disturbance and secondary osseous malformation (4).

Terminology

The radiologist must be able to correlate the radiologic appearance with the clinical findings. For this, definition of terms is required (5,507,547–549):

Talipes: a generic term for any congenital foot deformity.

Pes: (Latin for ''foot'') a generic term for any acquired foot deformity, such as a paralytic deformity associated with cerebral palsy.

Adduction: displacement of a bone or part toward the axis of the body.

Abduction: displacement away from the axis of the body.

Valgus: bending outward of a distal part from the midline of the body, distal to the point or joint of reference, relative to normal. In the foot, the term is equivalent to eversion.

Varus: bending inward toward the midline of the body, distal to the point or joint of reference, relative to normal. In the foot, the term is equivalent to inversion.

Heel or hindfoot valgus: significant outward slant of the heel increased over the normal 5–10°. The midtalar line (axis) lies medial to the line of the first metatarsal. The midtalar-midcalcaneal angle is increased on the lateral projection. The talus may be plantarflexed.

Heel or hindfoot varus: significant decrease in the normal 5–10° valgus angle; the heel slants inward. The midtalar line (axis) lies lateral to the line of the first metatarsal, and the midtalar and midcalcaneal lines become more parallel.

Equinus: fixed plantar flexion of the hindfoot at the ankle so that the calcaneus is plantar-flexed (anterior end down) on the lateral view, its long axis making an anterior angle of more than 90° with the axis of the tibia.

Calcaneus deformity: abnormal dorsiflexion of the calcaneus (anterior end up) so the calcaneus begins to approach a vertical position.

Cavus deformity: abnormally high longitudinal arch of the foot.

Planus deformity: flattened longitudinal arch.

Radiologic Evaluation

Radiologic evaluation is important for initial diagnosis and requires high-quality, reproducible technique (547). AP and lateral weight-bearing or simulated weight-bearing views of the feet are mandatory. Nonweight-bearing films do not portray the important relationships. A supplementary AP weight-bearing view of the ankle, a dorsiflexed or plantarflexed lateral view of the foot, and a tangential (Harris) view of the calcaneus may be required for complete evaluation of the hindfoot.

Weight-bearing AP and lateral views of the feet are relatively simple to obtain in the older child. However, these radiographs are a technical challenge in the infant, uncooperative child, or paralyzed child. For an AP weight-bearing view, the infant is erect, the tibia is placed perpendicular to the cassette, and downward pressure is applied on the foot. The vertical beam may be directed a few degrees posteriorly for this AP weight-bearing view. For the lateral view, a nonopaque block should be used to dorsiflex the foot maximally and simulate weight bearing, the infant being supine.

Radiologic interpretation of the foot is generally an analysis of the relationship between the talus and calcaneus, and then of those bones to the ankle joint, the remaining tarsal bones, and the metatarsals. The talus, calcaneus, and metatarsals are ossified in the newborn and can be used as reference points (548).

Normal Anatomy. On the AP view, the long axis of the talus passes through the base of the first metatarsal and along its axis, or close to this (Fig. 5-205A). The long axis of the calcaneus points to the head of the fourth metatarsal. The angle formed by the intersection of these lines is the *talocalcaneal angle*. The talocalcaneal angle on the AP view averages about 40° (range 25–55°) in the newborn. By 9 years of age, it decreases to the adult value of 25° (range 15–35°) (549). The axes of the metatarsal shafts are roughly parallel or fan out slightly on the AP view (548).

With the foot in neutral position, in the weight-bearing lateral projection, the long axis of the talus is plantarflexed and is continuous with the axis of the first metatarsal, except in children under age 5, in whom it normally passes inferior to the first metatarsal. The talocalcaneal angle on the lateral

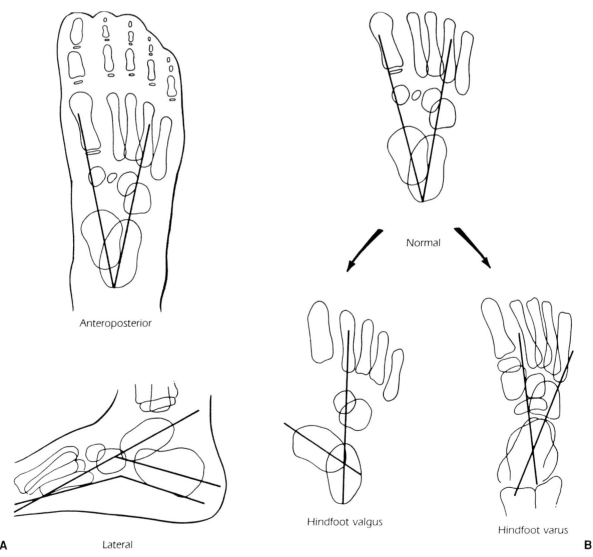

Normal

Hindfoot valgus

Hindfoot varus

Anteroposterior

Lateral

A

B

FIG. 5-205. Foot abnormalities. A: Normal AP and lateral weight-bearing views of the foot. **B:** Representations of normal and abnormal AP radiographs of the hindfoot. From Freiberger et al. (547).

projection (Fig. 5-205A) averages 40°, with the normal range being 25–55° (548). This talocalcaneal angle is increased by dorsiflexing the foot. The anterior angle formed by the longitudinal axes of the tibia and the calcaneus is normally 60–80°.

The normal heel, as seen from the rear, slants slightly outward to a 5–10° valgus position. The position of the heel cannot be determined directly from AP and lateral weight-bearing foot radiographs but must be inferred from the talocalcaneal angle on the AP view. The tangential view (Harris view) may also, because of minor rotation, be unsatisfactory for determining the varus or valgus position of the heel. Young children often relax into planovalgus positions, flattening their longitudinal arches (548).

Mechanics of Foot Deformities

When analyzing foot deformities, it is useful to think that the talus is part of the leg, the ankle being a hinge joint and allowing little lateral motion. No muscles arise from or insert on the talus; it may therefore be considered fixed at the ankle joint. The rest of the foot moves beneath and relative to the talus. Any alteration in the talocalcaneal angle is considered to be due to calcaneal motion. The midfoot is tightly attached to the calcaneus by ligaments, and these bones move together as a unit (550). If the tibia is positioned perpendicular to the cassette for an accurate weight-bearing AP view of the foot, the position of the talus is standardized. When the anterior portion of the calcaneus is abducted (the talocalcaneal angle is increased on both AP and lateral views), the calcaneus is in valgus position. When the anterior portion of the calcaneus is adducted (decreased talocalcaneal angle), the calcaneus is in varus. Therefore the talocalcaneal angle is an indication of the valgus or varus tilt of the hindfoot (Fig. 5-205B). Moreover, the midfoot generally maintains its relationship to the anterior end of the calcaneus.

To judge valgus or varus position of the hindfoot, one may simply extend the long axis of the talus on the AP view and note its relation to the base of the first metatarsal. In hindfoot valgus, this axis is considerably medial to the first metatarsal (Fig. 5-205B). In hindfoot varus, the long axis of the talus falls lateral to the first metatarsal (Fig. 5-205B). Almost all significant congenital abnormalities of the foot are hindfoot abnormalities rather than forefoot abnormalities. Therefore the radiologist must be thoroughly familiar with the diagnosis of hindfoot valgus and hindfoot varus, as the classification and prognosis of most foot deformities (Table 5-25) are based on these terms (547).

Foot abnormalities should be analyzed first at the level of the ankle. Equinus is present when, on the weight-bearing lateral view, the midshaft axis of the tibia forms an obtuse angle with the calcaneus axis. Calcaneus is present when the anterior angle formed by the midshaft axis of the tibia and the calcaneal axis line is significantly below normal (normally 10–30° less than a right angle). The second level of analysis

TABLE 5-25. *Classification of foot abnormalities*

Normal hindfoot
Normal foot
Metatarsus adductus
Pes planus
Hindfoot valgus
Metatarsus adductus
Planovalgus
Flexible flatfoot
Rigid flatfoot (tarsal coalition)
Congenital vertical talus
Talipes calcaneovalgus
Pes cavus
Pes valgus
Hindfoot varus
Talipes equinovarus (clubfoot)
Rocker-bottom deformity (treated clubfoot)
Flat-top talus (treated clubfoot)
Pes cavus
Pes varus

is the hindfoot, where there may be hindfoot varus or hindfoot valgus, as was discussed. Finally, there is analysis of the midtarsal joints and forefoot. Cavus is an accentuation of the arch producing upward angulation in the normally straight midtalar-first metatarsal line on the lateral view. Planus is present when the midtalar-first metatarsal line is angled more downward than normal on the lateral view. Forefoot adductus causes the midshaft axis of the metatarsals to angle toward the midline of the body so that the midcalcaneal line points lateral to the fourth metatarsal (548). Forefoot inversion causes a loss of toe parallelism so that the metatarsals converge posteriorly with overlapping of the bases. Forefoot abductus causes the midshaft axis of the metatarsals to angle away from the midline. Forefoot eversion causes an increase of toe parallelism on the frontal radiograph.

Specific Foot Deformities

Congenital Talipes Equinovarus (Congenital Clubfoot). Talipes, from the Latin talus, meaning ''ankle,'' and pes, ''foot,'' refers to any congenital foot deformity. Clubfeet fall into four main groups: congenital (also termed idiopathic), teratologic, syndromal, and positional. The congenital club foot is the most common form; the incidence is approximately 1.2 per 1000 live births, but double this figure in first-degree relatives of probands (551). It affects more boys than girls. Unilateral involvement is slightly more common than bilateral (551). Physical examination shows variable rigidity of the foot, mild calf atrophy, and mild hypoplasia of the tibia and fibula (552). Associations with clubfoot include myelomeningocele, arthrogryposis, dysplasias such as diastrophic dysplasia, and tibial hemimelia (4). Therapy generally begins with manipulation and casting of the foot. Surgery is reserved for children who require restoration of the bony architecture and balancing of the muscular forces by soft-tissue releases and tendon transfers (551).

If the clubfoot is very mild and correctable it is probably

related to the position of the foot in utero. The etiology of the more severe degrees of congenital clubfoot is unknown. Factors responsible for an abnormal talus, thought to be the central deformity, include a primary germ plasm defect that leads to a defective cartilaginous anlage, hypoplasia of the arterial supply, muscle imbalance, and soft-tissue contractures with subsequent growth in an abnormal position (547).

Radiographic evaluation. Because much of the foot is still cartilaginous in the infant, conclusions must be drawn from the ossified structures and the angles they form. In clubfoot, on AP radiographs, there is a decrease in the normal talocalcaneal angle and often complete superimposition of the talus on the calcaneus. The long axis of the talus passes lateral to the first metatarsal, which indicates metatarsus adductus (forefoot varus) (Fig. 5-206A). The navicular, which is unossified at birth, lies medial to the axis of the talus.

The ankle, not the forefoot, should be used as a point of reference for the lateral weight-bearing radiograph. The lateral radiograph demonstrates equinus of the hindfoot and a decrease in the talocalcaneal angle, often to 0° (Fig. 5-206B). The metatarsals do not overlap but are in stepwise alignment, with the fifth metatarsal being the most inferior. In summary, there is equinus at the ankle, hindfoot varus, and forefoot varus (metatarsus adductus). Depending on the severity, there also may be a cavus deformity.

Radiology is also important in the follow-up evaluation of clubfoot. The plantar arch may be convex downward (rocker bottom deformity) if dorsiflexion is applied before the equi-

nus and varus deformities are corrected. This abnormality is easy to differentiate from other forms of flatfoot because of the varus and equinus position of the heel. There is a decrease in the talocalcaneal angle on the AP projection. Another serious complication of the treatment of clubfoot is the development of a flat-top talus, which occurs with forced attempts to correct equinus. There is compression of the superior articular surface of the talus and subsequent ischemic necrosis, growth disturbance, and flattening (547).

Flexible Flatfoot (Pes Planovalgus). Infants and young children generally have little or no longitudinal arch. Persistent arch flattening beyond the early years is usually asymptomatic and may even be considered a developmental variant. A child with flexible flatfoot has a longitudinal arch when the foot hangs free (553). Hereditary factors may account for the generally lax ligamentous structures and the underdevelopment of the anterior end of the calcaneus.

On radiographs, the long axis of the talus falls well medial to the first metatarsal, which indicates hindfoot valgus. The talocalcaneal angle is increased on an AP view (Fig. 5-207A). On the lateral view, the foot dorsiflexes normally, and the talocalcaneal angle is increased (Fig. 5-207B). There is hindfoot valgus and abductus of the forefoot.

The patient is often asymptomatic, in which case no treatment is indicated. Shoe orthoses may help those children with mild pain. Surgery is reserved for patients who have more severe pain and disability.

Rigid Flatfoot. Less common than flexible flatfoot, rigid flatfoot is associated with limitation of pronation and supina-

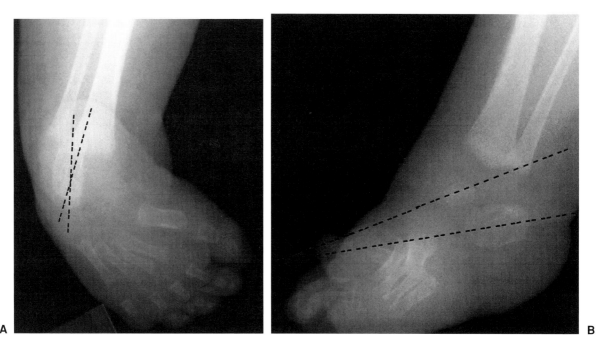

FIG. 5-206. Congenital talipes equinovarus (club foot). A: AP view of the foot in an infant. There is hindfoot varus with overlap of the talus and calcaneus. There is a decrease in the talocalcaneal angle. The forefoot is in varus. **B:** Lateral view shows equinus alignment, decrease in the talocalcaneal angle (hindfoot varus) and a stepwise configuration of the metatarsals.

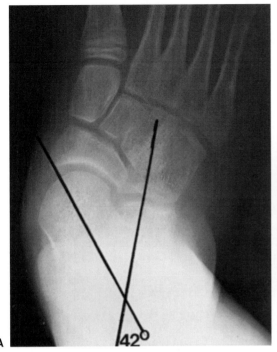
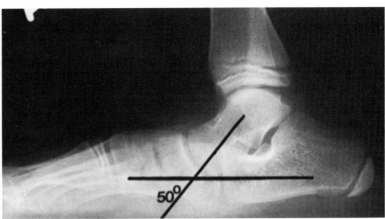

FIG. 5-207. Flexible flatfoot. AP **(A)** and lateral **(B)** views of the right foot of an 11-year-old girl. There is hindfoot valgus and planus of the forefoot.

tion and pain in the foot and calf (553). This abnormality is usually seen in older children and young adults. It is due to a long-standing deformity that has led to adaptive and even degenerative changes. Other associations include rheumatoid arthritis and prior osteochondral fracture. Surgical therapy usually involves a triple arthrodesis (551).

Congenital Vertical Talus. Congenital vertical talus (also referred to as *congenital convex pes planus, congenital flatfoot with talonavicular dissociation,* and *congenital rigid rocker-bottom foot*) is a serious, disabling foot deformity characterized by fixed dorsal dislocation of the navicular on the talus. It is the most severe form of congenital flatfoot and requires complex surgery (554). The etiologies proposed are similar to those of clubfoot: forced abnormal positioning in utero due to crowding and subsequent tendon contracture, and arrest in the normal embryologic development of the lower limb buds (554). Congenital vertical talus is associated with other congenital abnormalities, especially disorders of the central nervous system (551).

The radiographic findings include severe hindfoot valgus and, on both AP and lateral views, an increased talocalcaneal angle. The talar axis passes far medial to the first metatarsal. On the lateral view, the heel is in equinus position, the talus is in extreme plantar flexion, and the talocalcaneal angle is markedly increased. There is talonavicular dislocation causing the plantar surface of the foot to be convex (Fig. 5-208). When it ossifies, the navicular is shown to be deformed and dorsally dislocated and to lie anterosuperior to the neck of the talus. In extreme cases, the axis of the talus is parallel

to that of the tibia. Because the soft tissues are contracted, the foot does not respond to manipulation (551).

This condition should not be confused with pes planus, which has a vertical talus but neither equinus alignment nor talonavicular dislocation, nor with the rocker-bottom deformity of treated clubfoot, which has persistent heel equinus but neither a plantar-flexed talus nor hindfoot valgus (547). The lateral view in plantar flexion is essential for differentiation of true vertical talus from the less severe "oblique" talus. With true vertical talus, the navicular remains anterior to the dorsal surface of the talus even in plantar flexion (5). Before the navicular ossifies (usually after 2 years of age), ultrasonography or MRI will identify its relation to the talus and confirm or exclude the diagnosis of congenital vertical talus. MRI can also assess the musculature if muscle imbalance is thought to play a role in the deformity (554).

Talipes Calcaneovalgus. One of the more common congenital foot abnormalities, talipes calcaneovalgus is usually bilateral. It has a strong hereditary pattern but no sex predilection. In the newborn, the foot is extremely dorsiflexed, and its dorsum lies against the lower leg. The foot is generally flexible, and correction is readily obtained. The lateral view demonstrates a calcaneus deformity at the ankle and hindfoot valgus. The forefoot is in abductus and planus alignment (548).

Metatarsus Adductus. Most examples of metatarsus adductus and simple varus feet, which are probably due to intrauterine deformation, correct quickly and easily. There is as high as a 10% incidence of developmental hip dysplasia

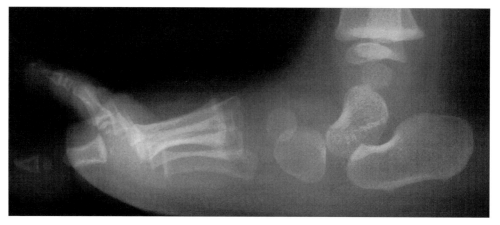

FIG. 5-208. Congenital vertical talus. Lateral view of the foot in an older child shows the talus in extreme plantar flexion and an increased talocalcaneal angle. The navicular is unossified. Talonavicular dislocation causes the plantar surface of the foot to be convex.

with metatarsus adductus (555). No sex predilection has been found. Slightly more than half of the abnormalities are bilateral. In true metatarsus adductus, the hindfoot and midfoot are in normal position. The forefoot is adducted as evidenced by overlapping of the metatarsals on the AP film. The first metatarsal usually is more deviated than the fifth. The talocalcaneal angle is normal. The infant with metatarsus adductus and a normal hindfoot usually can be corrected without surgery. Mild and moderate degrees of simple metatarsus adductus do not require radiographic evaluation, which is reserved for those children who have severe deformities or are undergoing serial cast therapy (551).

Skewfoot. Skewfoot, or ''Z foot,'' is an uncommon, severe, complex deformity that is usually inflexible (553). The metatarsals are adducted and medially subluxed, the navicular is laterally subluxed on the talus (valgus midfoot), and there is hindfoot valgus. On the lateral view, the talocalcaneal angle may be slightly increased because of plantar flexion of the talus. As with metatarsus adductus, the therapy can be conservative or operative (553).

Pes Cavus. Pes cavus is an abnormally high longitudinal arch of the foot. The anterior part of the calcaneus is dorsiflexed, but the metatarsals are plantarflexed. If the deformity is associated with a heel varus alignment, it is usually the result for treatment of clubfoot. If it coexists with heel valgus, it is probably due to weakness of the flexors of the foot because of a neurologic disorder (4) (Fig. 5-209). Spinal MRI is advised when surgery is contemplated or if pes cavus is otherwise unexplained.

Hallux Valgus. Hallux valgus is often used interchangeably with bunion and metatarsus primus varus (551). The deformity may be idiopathic or secondary to another foot malalignment or may have a neuromuscular basis. Hallux valgus is more common in girls and has a hereditary component (556). The deformity is present when there is an angle of 10° or more between the shafts of the first and second metatarsals, and greater than 15° of valgus alignment of the

first phalanx of the great toe relative to the first metatarsal (551). The bunion is formed by the medial prominence of the head of the first metatarsal and the associated soft-tissue swelling. Adolescents usually present with pain and cosmetic difficulties. Shoe orthotics are used for the only mildly symptomatic deformities, surgery for those that are persistently painful (551). The deformity can lead to degenerative arthritis in the adult.

Tarsal Coalition

Tarsal coalition refers to abnormal fusion between tarsal bones, motion thereby being prevented or restricted. Approximately 1% of the population has some sort of tarsal coalition. It is a common cause of pain in the active adolescent. The diminished mobility of the foot can result in fre-

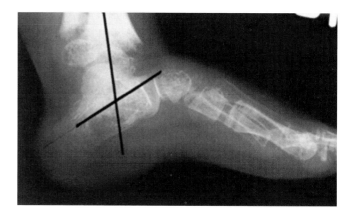

FIG. 5-209. Pes cavus. This 6-year-old boy had severe muscle weakness, rickets, and hyperparathyroidism due to untreated renal disease. There is decrease in muscle mass, osteopenia, high longitudinal arch (cavus) of the foot, and heel valgus. The lines show the axes of the calcaneus and tibia.

quent ankle sprains and strains. The postulated etiology is failure of differentiation and segmentation of primitive mesenchyme in the fetus (557). There may be a complete fibrous (syndesmosis), cartilaginous (synchondrosis), or bony (synostosis) bridge. These fusions become rigid, and therefore more painful, during the adolescent years, presumably because of progression from a more mobile fibrous union to a more rigid cartilaginous or bony bar. Up to 90% of coalitions are calcaneonavicular and talocalcaneal. Other types (talonavicular, calcaneocuboid, cuboid-navicular, navicular-cuneiform) are rare. Between 50% and 60% of coalitions are bilateral (558). Tarsal coalition may be isolated but is also associated with other congenital anomalies and syndromes such as tibial and fibular hemimelia, proximal focal femoral deficiency, and Apert syndrome.

Most cases of talocalcaneal coalition occur at the middle talocalcaneal joint, at the sustentaculum tali of the calcaneus. Coalition of the posterior and anterior joints is less common. Symptoms usually occur at the time of ossification of the fusion, usually around 12–14 years of age. This coalition is difficult to evaluate with conventional radiographs, but secondary signs are often present on both AP and lateral views. The signs include dorsal talar beaking, broadening and rounding of the lateral process of the talus, narrowing of the posterior talar joint, concavity of the undersurface of the neck of the talus, and rounding of the tibial articulation of the ankle joint (547). These signs are nonspecific and may be seen with any cause of limited talar motion. The talar beak associated with a coalition tends to terminate near the margin of the talonavicular joint, whereas the beak associated with neuromuscular or sports-related changes is more proximal (557). A 45° posterior axial (Harris) projection of the calcaneous may show the bony talocalcaneal coalition itself. The "C sign," an outline formed by the posteroinferior continuation of the medial talar dome to the sustentaculum tali, has been described as reliable radiographic indicator of a subtalar coalition (559).

Coronal CT can readily display hindfoot anatomy and delineates talocalcaneal coalition much better than radiographs. When suspicion is high but radiographs are negative, CT is suggested (560). Positioning for CT imaging requires flexion at the hips and knees. Both feet are placed flat on the gantry. Thin coronal slices (usually 3 mm) are obtained of both feet from the posterior subtalar joint to the navicular bone. Careful attention to symmetry of positioning is very helpful. CT findings include osseous bars, irregular and sclerotic joint surfaces, and abnormal alignment of the subtalar joints (Fig. 5-210). Nonosseous coalitions are more difficult to detect, and in those cases MRI may be useful (561). Imaging studies should include both feet, so subtle contralateral abnormalities may also be assessed.

Calcaneonavicular coalition, which usually presents between 8 and 12 years of age, is often less symptomatic than talocalcaneal coalition, and secondary signs are present less regularly. This coalition will not be shown directly on the AP and lateral projections unless the fusion is advanced, but one should be alerted by an anterior-superior prolongation

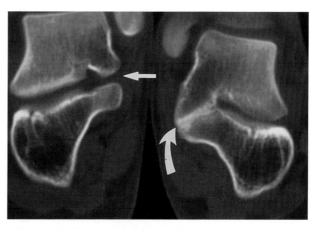

FIG. 5-210. Talocalcaneal coalition: CT. Direct coronal image through the hindfoot of a 13-year-old girl shows an osseous talocalcaneal coalition of the middle facet of the subtalar joint on the left *(curved arrow)*. The middle facet of the right foot is normal *(straight arrow)*.

of the calcaneus on the lateral projection ("anteater nose") (507). To diagnose calcaneonavicular fusion, a 30° to 45° oblique projection of the foot is necessary (Fig. 5-211). CT is usually not needed unless an additional coalition or other subtalar facet anomaly is suspected (557).

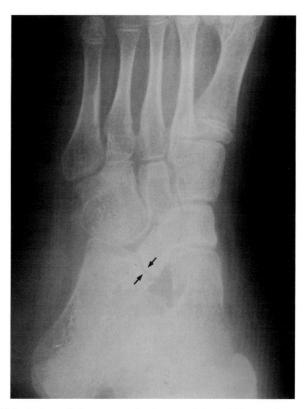

FIG. 5-211. Calcaneonavicular coalition. Oblique view in an 11-year-old girl with foot pain. There is abnormally close approximation of the calcaneus and navicular, the opposing surfaces of which are irregular *(arrows)*. The fusion is incompletely ossified.

For most patients, the initial therapy is generally conservative, and consists of rest, orthotics, or walking casts. The goal is to alleviate the pain. Surgical excision of the bar is reserved for persistent pain and stiffness in cases when the coalition does not involve more than half of the articular surface. If the coalition is large and is deemed unresectable, if pain and limited motion persist, and if degenerative changes are present, triple arthrodesis is performed (551).

Peroneal Spastic Flatfoot

Peroneal spastic flatfoot is a syndrome associated with tarsal coalition, especially talocalcaneal fusion (562). It is characterized by painful valgus hindfoot, contracture of the peroneus longus tendon, pronation (eversion) of the foot, and loss of the longitudinal arch. These deformities may occur when the foot is persistently held in valgus position at the subtalar joint to mitigate the discomfort of a tarsal coalition (558). The symptoms can be intermittent or continuous (562). The findings should make one suspect a coexistent coalition. Additional causes of a peroneal spastic flatfoot include other mechanisms of subtalar irritation, such as juvenile rheumatoid arthritis, osteoarthritis, infection, and trauma.

Ball-and-Socket Ankle

The combination of a domed talus (convex upper margin as seen from both front and side) and matching concavity of the articulating surfaces of the articulating fibula and tibia is found in children and young adults after a surgical talar fusion, or it may be a sign of one or more talar coalitions (5). Up to 65% of patients with ball-and-socket ankles have tarsal coalitions, usually isolated talocalcaneal fusions (558). Other associations include deficiency deformities of the tibia, fibula, and femur, and delayed maturation of the talus, calcaneus, or both.

REFERENCES

General

1. Resnick D. *Diagnosis of bone and joint disorders.* 3rd ed. Philadelphia: WB Saunders, 1995.
2. Silverman FN, Kuhn JP. *Caffey's pediatric x-ray diagnosis.* 9th ed. St. Louis: CV Mosby, 1993.
3. Silverman FN, Kuhn JP. *Essentials of Caffey's pediatric x-ray diagnosis.* Chicago: Year Book, 1990.
4. Ozonoff MB. *Pediatric orthopedic radiology.* 2nd ed. Philadelphia: WB Saunders, 1992.
5. Oestreich AE, Crawford AH. *Atlas of pediatric orthopedic radiology.* Stuttgart: Thieme, 1985.
6. Poznanski AK. *Practical approaches to pediatric radiology.* Chicago: Year Book, 1976.
7. Poznanski AK. *The hand in radiologic diagnosis.* 2nd ed. Philadelphia: WB Saunders, 1984.
8. Carty H, Brunelle F, Shaw D, Kendall B, eds. *Imaging children.* New York: Churchill Livingstone, 1994.
9. Taybi H, Lachman RS. *Radiology of syndromes, metabolic disorders, and skeletal dysplasias.* 4th ed. St. Louis: CV Mosby, 1996.
10. Sty JR, Wells RG, Starshak RJ, Gregg DC. The musculoskeletal system. In: Sty JR, Wells RG, Starshak RJ, Gregg DC, eds. *Diagnostic imaging of infants and children.* Gaithersburg, MD: Aspen Publishers, 1992, 233–405.
11. Mandell GA, Harcke HT, Kumar SJ. *Imaging strategies in pediatric orthopaedics.* Gaithersburg, MD: Aspen Publishers, 1990.
12. Reed MH, ed. *Pediatric skeletal radiology.* Baltimore: Williams and Wilkins, 1992.
13. Morrissy RT, Weinstein SL, eds. *Lovell and Winter's pediatric orthopaedics.* 4th ed. Philadelphia: Lippincott–Raven, 1996.

Normal Anatomy and Development

14. Laor T, Chung T, Hoffer FA, Jaramillo D. Musculoskeletal magnetic resonance imaging: how we do it. *Pediatr Radiol* 1996;26:695-700.
15. Oestreich AE. *Pediatric radiology.* 3rd ed. New Hyde Park, NY: Medical Examination, 1984.
16. Brighton CT. The growth plate. *Orthop Clin North Am* 1984;15: 571–595.
17. Ogden JA. Anatomy and physiology of skeletal development. In: *Skeletal injury in the child.* 2nd ed. Philadelphia: WB Saunders, 1990, 23–65.
18. Harcke HT, Snyder M, Caro PA, Bowen JR. Growth plate of the normal knee: evaluation with MR imaging. *Radiology* 1992;183: 119–123.
19. Chung T, Jaramillo D. Normal maturing distal tibia and fibula: changes with age at MR imaging. *Radiology* 1995;194:227–232.
20. Moore SG, Dawson KL. Red and yellow marrow in the femur: age-related changes in appearance at MR imaging. *Radiology* 1990;175: 219–223.
21. Sebag GH, Dubois J, Tabet M, et al. Pediatric spinal bone marrow: assessment of normal age-related changes in the MRI appearance. *Pediatr Radiol* 1993;23:515–518.
22. Dawson KL, Moore SG, Rowland JM. Age-related marrow changes in the pelvis: MR and anatomic findings. *Radiology* 1992;183:47–51.
23. Ricci C, Cova M, Kang YS, et al. Normal age-related patterns of cellular and fatty bone marrow distribution in the axial skeleton: MR imaging study. *Radiology* 1990;177:83–88.
24. Zawin JK, Jaramillo D. Conversion of bone marrow in the humerus, sternum, and clavicle: changes with age on MR images. *Radiology* 1993;188:159–164.
25. Jaramillo D, Laor T, Hoffer FA, et al. Epiphyseal marrow in infancy: MR imaging. *Radiology* 1991;180:809–812.
26. Kricun ME. Red-yellow marrow conversion: its effect on the location of some solitary bone lesions. *Skeletal Radiol* 1985;14:10–19.

Techniques

27. Kuhns LR, Sherman MP, Poznanski AK. Determination of neonatal maturation on the chest radiograph. *Radiology* 1972;102:597–603.
28. Kuhns LR, Holt JF. Measurement of thoracic spine length on chest radiographs of newborn infants. *Radiology* 1975;116:395–397.
29. Kuhns LR, Poznanski AK. Radiological assessment of maturity and size of the newborn infant. *CRC Crit Rev Diagn Imag* 1980;12: 245–308.
30. Loder RT, Estle DT, Morrison K, et al. Applicability of the Greulich and Pyle skeletal age standards to black and white children of today. *Am J Dis Child* 1993;147:1329–1333.
31. Greulich WW, Pyle SI. *Radiographic atlas of skeletal development of the hand and wrist.* 2nd ed. Stanford: Stanford University Press, 1959.
32. Carpenter CT, Lester EL. Skeletal age determination in young children: analysis of three regions of the hand/wrist film. *J Pediatr Orthop* 1993;13:76–79.
33. Tanner JM, Whitehouse RH, Cameron N, et al. *Assessment of skeletal maturity and prediction of adult height (TW2 method).* 2nd ed. London: Academic Press, 1983.
34. Tanner JM, Gibbons RD. A computerized image analysis system for estimating Tanner-Whitehouse 2 bone age. *Horm Res* 1994;42: 282–287.
35. Keats TE. *Atlas of normal roentgen variants that may simulate disease.* 5th ed. St. Louis: Mosby–Year Book, 1992.

36. Sontag LW, Snell D, Anderson M. Rate of appearance of ossification centers from birth to the age of five years. *Am J Dis Child* 1939;58:949–956.

37. Conway WF, Totty WG, McEnery KW. CT and MR imaging of the hip. *Radiology* 1996;198:297–307.

38. Link TM, Meier N, Rummeny EJ, et al. Artificial spine fractures: detection with helical and conventional CT. *Radiology* 1996;198:515–519.

39. Kasales CJ, Mauger DT, Sefczek RJ, et al. Multiplanar image reconstruction and 3D imaging using a musculoskeletal phantom: conventional versus helical CT. *J Comput Assist Tomogr* 1997;21;162–169.

40. Graf R. *Guide to sonography of the infant hip.* New York: Thieme, 1987.

Congenital and Developmental Variants

41. Shopfner CE. Periosteal bone growth in normal infants. A preliminary report. *AJR* 1966;97:154–163.

42. Gardiner JS, Zauk AM, Donchey SS, McInerney VK. Prostaglandin-induced cortical hyperostosis. Case report and review of the literature. *J Bone Joint Surg Am* 1995;77:932–936.

43. Blickman JG, Wilkinson RH, Graef JW. The radiologic "lead band" revisited. *AJR* 1986;146:245–247.

44. Middleton WD, McAlister WH. Hip joint fluid in the presence of the vacuum phenomenon. *Pediatr Radiol* 1986;16:171–172.

45. Caffey J, Ross SE. The ischiopubic synchondrosis in healthy children: some normal roentgenologic findings. *AJR* 1956;76:488–494.

46. Cawley KA, Dvorak AD, Wilmot MD. Normal anatomic variant: scintigraphy of the ischiopubic synchondrosis. *J Nucl Med* 1983;24:14–16.

47. Eklof O, Hugosson C, Lindham S. Normal variations and posttraumatic appearances of the tuberosity of ischium in adolescence. *Ann Radiol* 1979;22:77–84.

48. Nixon GW. Hematogenous osteomyelitis of metaphyseal-equivalent locations. *AJR* 1978;130:123–129.

49. Caffey J, Madell SH, Royer C, Morales P. Ossification of the distal femoral epiphysis. *J Bone Joint Surg Am* 1958;40:647–654.

50. Brower AC, Culver JE Jr, Keats TE. Histologic nature of the cortical irregularity of the medial posterior distal femoral metaphysis in children. *Radiology* 1971;99:389–392.

51. Kransdorf MJ, Utz JA, Gilkey FW, Berrey BH. MR appearance of fibroxanthoma. *J Comput Assist Tomogr* 1988;12:612–615.

52. Ritschl P, Karnel F, Hajek P. Fibrous metaphyseal defects—determination of their origin and natural history using a radiomorphological study. *Skeletal Radiol* 1988;17:8–15.

53. Ritschl P, Hajek PC, Pechmann U. Fibrous metaphyseal defects. Magnetic resonance imaging appearances. *Skeletal Radiol* 1989;18:253–259.

54. Schwartz AM, Ramos RM. Neurofibromatosis and multiple nonossifying fibromas. *AJR* 1980;135:617–619.

55. Keats TE, Joyce JM. Metaphyseal cortical irregularities in children: a new perspective on a multi-focal growth variant. *Skel Radiol* 1984;12:112–118.

56. Resnick D, Greenway G. Distal femoral cortical defects, irregularities, and excavations. *Radiology* 1982;143:345–354.

57. Yamazaki T, Maruoka S, Takahashi S, et al. MR findings of avulsive cortical irregularity of the distal femur. *Skeletal Radiol* 1995;24:43–46.

58. Young DW, Nogrady MB, Dunbar JS, Wiglesworth FW. Benign cortical irregularities in the distal femur of children. *J Can Assoc Radiol* 1972;23:107–115.

59. Shopfner CE, Coin CG. Effect of weight-bearing on the appearance and development of the secondary calcaneal epiphysis. *Radiology* 1966;86:201–206.

60. Lawson JP. Symptomatic radiographic variants in extremities. *Radiology* 1985;157:625–631.

61. Keats TE, Harrison RB. The calcaneal nutrient foramen: a useful sign in the differentiation of true from simulated cysts. *Skeletal Radiol* 1979;3:239–240.

Disorders of Bone Density, Shape, and Symmetry

62. Maroteaux P. *Bone diseases of children.* Philadelphia: JB Lippincott, 1979.

63. Laor T, Jaramillo D. Metaphyseal abnormalities in children: pathophysiology and radiologic appearance. *AJR* 1993;161:1029–1036.

64. Levine C. The imaging of body asymmetry and hemihypertrophy. *Crit Rev Diagn Imag* 1990;31:1–80.

65. Beals RK. Hemihypertrophy and hemihypotrophy. *Clin Orthop* 1982;166:199–203.

66. Wood BP, Putnam TC, Chacko AK. Infantile hepatic hemangioendotheliomas associated with hemihypertrophy. *Pediatr Radiol* 1977;5:242–245.

67. Kirks DR, Shackelford GD. Idiopathic congenital hemihypertrophy with associated ipsilateral benign nephromegaly. *Radiology* 1975;115:145–148.

68. Pfister RC, Weber AL, Smith EH, et al. Congenital asymmetry (hemihypertrophy) and abdominal disease: radiological features in 9 cases. *Radiology* 1975;116:685–691.

69. Ritter R, Siafarikas K. Hemihypertrophy in a boy with renal polycystic disease: varied patterns of presentation of renal polycystic disease in his family. *Pediatr Radiol* 1976;5:98–102.

70. Green DM, Breslow NE, Beckwith JB, Norkool P. Screening of children with hemihypertrophy, aniridia, and Beckwith-Wiedemann syndrome in patients with Wilms tumor: a report from the National Wilms Tumor Study. *Med Pediatr Oncol* 1993;21:188–192.

71. Oestreich AE, Ahmad BS. The periphysis and its effect on the metaphysis. II. Application to rickets and other abnormalities. *Skeletal Radiol* 1993;22:115–119.

Constitutional Diseases of Bone

72. Kozlowski K. The radiographic clues in the diagnosis of bone dysplasias. *Pediatr Radiol* 1985;15:1–3.

73. Anonymous. International nomenculture of constitutional diseases of bone. *J Pediatr* 1978;93:614–616.

74. Spranger J. International classification of osteochondrodysplasias. The International Working Group on Constitutional Diseases of Bone. *Eur J Pediatr* 1992;151:407–415.

75. Spranger JW, Langer LO Jr, Wiedemann HR. *Bone dysplasias.* Philadelphia: WB Saunders, 1974.

76. Cremin BJ, Beighton P. Dwarfism in the newborn: the nomenclature, radiological features, and genetic significance. *Br J Radiol* 1974;47:77–93.

77. Langer LO Jr, Baumann PA, Gorlin RJ. Achondroplasia. *AJR* 1967;100:12–26.

78. McAlister WH, Herman TE. Osteochondrodysplasias, dyostoses, chromosomal aberrations, mucopolysaccharidoses, and mucolipidoses. In: Resnick D. *Diagnosis of bone and joint disorders.* 3rd ed. Philadelphia: WB Saunders, 1995, 4163–4244.

79. Kao SC, Waziri MH, Smith WL, et al. MR imaging of the craniovertebral junction, cranium, and brain in children with achondroplasia. *AJR* 1989;153:565–569.

80. Aldegheri R, Renzi-Brivio L, Agostini S. The callotasis method of limb lengthening. *Clin Orthop* 1989;241:137–145.

81. Aldegheri R, Trivella G, Lavini F. Epiphyseal distraction. Chondrodiatasis. *Clin Orthop* 1989;241:117–127.

82. Sillence DO, Horton WA, Rimoin DL. Morphologic studies in the skeletal dysplasias. *Am J Pathol* 1979;96:813–870.

83. Lachman R, Sillence D, Rimoin D, et al. Diastrophic dysplasia: the death of a variant. *Radiology* 1981;140:79–86.

84. Thomas PS, Renton P, Hall C, et al. The musculoskeletal system. In: Carty H, Brunelle F, Shaw D, Kendall B, eds. *Imaging children.* New York: Churchill Livingstone, 1994, 845–1032.

85. Miller SM, Paul LW. Roentgen observations in familial metaphyseal dysostosis. *Radiology* 1964;83:665–673.

86. Berrocal T, Simon MJ, Al-Assir I, et al. Schwachman-Diamond syndrome: clinical, radiological, and sonographic findings. *Pediatr Radiol* 1995;25:356–359.

87. Jarvis JL, Keats TE. Cleidocranial dysostosis. A review of 40 new cases. *AJR* 1974;121:5–16.

88. Keats TE. Cleidocranial dysostosis. Some atypical roentgen manifestations. *AJR* 1967;100:71–74.

89. Resnick D, Kyriakos M, Greenway GD. Tumors and tumor-like lesions of bone: imaging and pathology of specific tumors. In: Resnick D. *Diagnosis of bone and joint disorders.* 3rd ed. Philadelphia: WB Saunders, 1995, 3662–3697.

90. Shapiro F, Simon S, Glimcher MJ. Hereditary multiple exostoses. Anthropometric roentgenographic and clinical aspects. *J Bone Joint Surg Am* 1979;61:815–824.

91. Garrison RC, Unni KK, McLeod RA. Chondrosarcoma arising in osteochondroma. *Cancer* 1982;49:1890–1897.

92. Liu J, Hudkins PG, Swee RG, Unni KK. Bone sarcomas associated with Ollier's disease. *Cancer* 1987;59:1376–1385.

93. Kricun ME. *Imaging of bone tumors.* Philadelphia: WB Saunders, 1993.

94. Schwartz HS, Zimmerman NB, Simon MA, et al. The malignant potential of enchondromatosis. *J Bone Joint Surg Am* 1987;69:269–274.

95. Feldman F. Tuberous sclerosis, neurofibromatosis, and fibrous dysplasia. In: Resnick D. *Diagnosis of bone and joint disorders.* 3rd ed. Philadelphia: WB Saunders, 1995, 4353–4398.

96. Utz JA, Kransdorf MJ, Jelinek JS, et al. MR appearance of fibrous dysplasia. *J Comput Assist Tomogr* 1989;13:845–851.

97. Holt JF. Neurofibromatosis in children. *AJR* 1978;130:615–639.

98. Klatte EC, Franken EA, Smith JA. The radiographic spectrum in neurofibromatosis. *Semin Roentgenol* 1976;11:17–33.

99. Suh JS, Abenoza P, Galloway HR, et al. Peripheral (extracranial) nerve tumors: correlation of MR imaging and histologic findings. *Radiology* 1992;183:341–346.

100. Sillence D. Osteogenesis imperfecta: an expanding panorama of variants. *Clin Orthop* 1981;159:11–25.

101. Sillence DO, Senn A, Danks DM. Genetic heterogeneity in osteogenesis imperfecta. *J Med Genet* 1979;16:101–116.

102. Goldman AB, Davidson D, Pavlov H, Bullough PG. ''Popcorn'' calcifications: a prognostic sign in osteogenesis imperfecta. *Radiology* 1980;136:351–358.

103. Stoltz MR, Dietrich SL, Marshall GJ. Osteogenesis imperfecta. Perspectives. *Clin Orthop* 1989;242:120–136.

104. Ablin DS, Greenspan A, Reinhart M, Grix A. Differentiation of child abuse from osteogenesis imperfecta. *AJR* 1990;154:1035–1046.

105. Kaftori JK, Kleinhaus U, Naveh Y. Progressive diaphyseal dysplasia (Camurati-Engelmann): radiographic follow-up and CT findings. *Radiology* 1987;164:777–782.

106. Currarino G, Swanson GE. A developmental variant of ossification of the manubrium sterni in mongolism. *Radiology* 1964;82:916.

107. Laurin S, Björkheur G. Aberrant subclavian artery in Down syndrome and in A-V canal defects. *Pediatr Radiol* 1982;12:314.

108. Silverthorn KG, Houston CS, Newman DE, Wood BJ. Radiographic findings in liveborn triploidy. *Pediatr Radiol* 1989;19:237–241.

109. Eggli KD, Dorst JP. The mucopolysaccharidoses and related conditions. *Semin Roentgenol* 1986;21:275–294.

110. Poznanski AK, La Rowe PC. Radiographic manifestations of the arthrogryposis syndrome. *Radiology* 1970;95:353–358.

111. Askins G, Ger E. Congenital constriction band syndrome. *J Pediatr Orthop* 1988;8:461–466.

112. Streeter GL. Focal deficiencies in fetal tissues and their relation to intrauterine amputation. *Contrib Embryol* 1930;22:1–44.

113. Foulkes GD, Reinker K. Congenital constriction band syndrome: a seventy-year experience. *J Pediatr Orthop* 1994;14:242–248.

Infection

114. Syriopoulou VP, Smith AL. Osteomyelitis and septic arthritis. In: Feigin RD, Cherry JD, eds. *Textbook of pediatric infectious diseases.* 3rd ed. Philadelphia: WB Saunders, 1992, 727–746.

115. Nelson JD. Acute osteomyelitis in children. *Infect Dis Clin North Am* 1990;4:513–522.

116. Scott RJ, Christofersen MR, Robertson WW Jr, et al. Acute osteomyelitis in children: a review of 116 cases. *J Pediatr Orthop* 1990;10:649–652.

117. Nixon GW. Acute hematogenous osteomyelitis. *Pediatr Ann* 1976;5:64–81.

118. Pelkonen P, Ryoppy S, Jaaskelainen J, et al. Chronic osteomyelitis–like disease with negative bacterial cultures. *Am J Dis Child* 1988;142:1167–1173.

119. Morrissy RT. Bone and joint infections. In: Morrissy RT, Weinstein SL, eds. *Lovell and Winter's pediatric orthopaedics.* 4th ed. Philadelphia: Lippincott–Raven, 1996, 579–624.

120. Nelson JD, Norden C, Mader JT, Calandra GB. Evaluation of new anti-infective drugs for the treatment of acute hematogenous osteomyelitis in children. Infectious Diseases Society of America and the Food and Drug Administration. *Clin Infect Dis* 1992;15:S162–166.

121. Ogden JA, Lister G. The pathology of neonatal osteomyelitis. *Pediatrics* 1975;55:474–478.

122. David R, Barron BJ, Madewell JE. Osteomyelitis, acute and chronic. *Radiol Clin North Am* 1987;25:1171–1201.

123. Majd M. Radionuclide imaging in early detection of childhood osteomyelitis and its differentiation from cellulitis and bone infarction. *Ann Radiol* 1977;20:9–18.

124. Trueta J. The three types of acute haematogenous osteomyelitis. *J Bone Joint Surg Br* 1959;41:671–680.

125. Capitanio MA, Kirkpatrick JA. Early roentgen observations in acute osteomyelitis. *AJR* 1970;108:488–496.

126. Faden H, Grossi M. Acute osteomyelitis in children. Reassessment of etiologic agents and their clinical characteristics. *Am J Dis Child* 1991;145:65–69.

127. Asmar BI. Osteomyelitis in the neonate. *Infect Dis Clin North Am* 1992;6:117–132.

128. Aronson J, Garvin K, Seibert J, et al. Efficiency of the bone scan for occult limping toddlers. *J Pediatr Orthop* 1992;12:38–44.

129. Gupta NC, Prezio JA. Radionuclide imaging in osteomyelitis. *Semin Nucl Med* 1988;18:287–299.

130. Cohen MD. *Imaging of children with cancer.* St. Louis: Mosby–Year Book, 1992.

131. Applegate K, Connolly LP, Treves ST. Neuroblastoma presenting clinically as hip osteomyelitis: a ''signature'' diagnosis on skeletal scintigraphy. *Pediatr Radiol* 1995;25:S93–S96.

132. Mahboubi S, ed. *Pediatric bone imaging: a practical approach.* Boston: Little, Brown, 1989.

133. Gilday DL, Paul DJ, Paterson J. Diagnosis of osteomyelitis in children by combined blood pool and bone imaging. *Radiology* 1975;117:331–335.

134. Duszynski DO, Kuhn JP, Afshani E, et al. Early radionuclide diagnosis of acute osteomyelitis. *Radiology* 1975;117:337–340.

135. Allwright SJ, Miller JH, Gilsanz V. Subperiosteal abscess in children: scintigraphic appearance. *Radiology* 1991;179:725–729.

136. Handmaker H. Acute hematogenous osteomyelitis: has the bone scan betrayed us? *Radiology* 1980;135:787–789.

137. Sullivan DC, Rosenfield NS, Ogden J, Gottschalk A. Problems in the scintigraphic detection of osteomyelitis in children. *Radiology* 1980;135:731–736.

138. Jaramillo D, Treves ST, Kasser JR, et al. Osteomyelitis and septic arthritis in children: appropriate use of imaging to guide treatment. *AJR* 1995;165:399–403.

139. Abiri MM, Kirpekar M, Ablow RC. Osteomyelitis: detection with US. *Radiology* 1989;172:509–511.

140. Harcke HT. Role of imaging in musculoskeletal infections in children. *J Pediatr Orthop* 1995;15:141–143.

141. Mazur JM, Ross G, Cummings RJ, et al. Usefulness of magnetic resonance imaging for the diagnosis of acute musculoskeletal infections in children. *J Pediatr Orthop* 1995;15:144–147.

142. Morrison WB, Schweitzer ME, Bock GW, et al. Diagnosis of osteomyelitis: utility of fat-suppressed contrast-enhanced MR imaging. *Radiology* 1993;189:251–257.

143. Mok PM, Reilly BJ, Ash JM. Osteomyelitis in the neonate. Clinical aspects and the role of radiography and scintigraphy in diagnosis and management. *Radiology* 1982;145:677–682.

144. Ash JM, Gilday DL. The futility of bone scanning in neonatal osteomyelitis: concise communication. *J Nucl Med* 1980;21:417–420.

145. Bressler EL, Conway JJ, Weiss SC. Neonatal osteomyelitis examined by bone scintigraphy. *Radiology* 1984;152:685–688.

146. Connolly SA, Connolly LP, Treves ST, Jaramillo D. *MRI of epiphyseal osteomyelitis.* Washington, DC: Society for Pediatric Radiology, 1995 (abstract).

147. Azouz EM, Greenspan A, Marton D. CT evaluation of primary epiphyseal bone abscesses. *Skeletal Radiol* 1993;22:17–23.

148. Brown T, Wilkinson RH. Chronic recurrent multifocal osteomyelitis. *Radiology* 1988;166:493–496.

149. Grogan DP, Love SM, Ogden JA, et al. Chondro-osseous growth abnormalities after meningococcemia. A clinical and histopathological study. *J Bone Joint Surg Am* 1989;71:920–928.

150. Bennett OM, Namnyak SS. Acute septic arthritis of the hip joint in infancy and childhood. *Clin Orthop* 1992;281:123–132.

151. Betz RR, Cooperman DR, Wopperer JM, et al. Late sequelae of septic arthritis of the hip in infancy and childhood. *J Pediatr Orthop* 1990;10:365–372.

152. Choi IH, Pizzutillo PD, Bowen JR, et al. Sequelae and reconstruction after septic arthritis of the hip in infants. *J Bone Joint Surg Am* 1990;72:1150–1165.

153. Nelson JD, Koontz WC. Septic arthritis in infants and children: a review of 117 cases. *Pediatrics* 1966;38:966–971.
154. Barton LL, Dunkle LM, Habib FH. Septic arthritis in childhood. A 13-year review. *Am J Dis Child* 1987;141:898–900.
155. Welkon CJ, Long SS, Fisher MC, Alburger PD. Pyogenic arthritis in infants and children: a review of 95 cases. *Pediatr Infect Dis* 1986; 5:669–676.
156. Hayden CK Jr, Swischuk LE. Paraarticular soft-tissue changes in infections and trauma of the lower extremity in children. *AJR* 1980; 134:307–311.
157. Zawin JK, Hoffer FA, Rand FF, Teele RL. Joint effusion in children with an irritable hip: US diagnosis and aspiration. *Radiology* 1993; 187:459–463.
158. Treves ST, Connolly LP, Kirkpatrick JA, et al. Bone. In: Treves ST, ed. *Pediatric nuclear medicine.* 2nd ed. New York: Springer-Verlag, 1995, 233–301.
159. Merten DF, Kirks DR, Ruderman RJ. Occult humeral epiphyseal fracture in battered infants. *Pediatr Radiol* 1981;10:151–154.
160. Kaye JJ, Winchester PH, Freiberger RH. Neonatal septic ''dislocation'' of the hip: true dislocation or pathological epiphyseal separation? *Radiology* 1975;114:671–674.
161. Wood BP. The vanishing epiphyseal ossification center: a sequel to septic arthritis of childhood. *Radiology* 1980;134:387–389.
162. Merten DF, Gooding CA. Skeletal manifestations of congenital cytomegalic inclusion disease. *Radiology* 1970;95:333–334.
163. Kuhns LR, Hernandez R, Poznanski AK. Knee maturation as a differentiating sign between congenital rubella and cytomegalovirus infections. *Pediatr Radiol* 1977;6:36–38.
164. Harty MP, Markowitz RI, Rutstein RM, Hunter JV. Imaging features of human immunodeficiency virus infection in infants and children. *Semin Roentgenol* 1994;29:303–314.
165. Greenberg SB, Bernal DV. Are long bone radiographs necessary in neonates suspected of having congenital syphilis? *Radiology* 1992; 182:637–639.
166. Dunn RA, Zenker PN. Why radiographs are useful in evaluation of neonates suspected of having congenital syphilis. *Radiology* 1992; 182:639–640.

Noninfectious Inflammation

167. Ansell BM, Kent PA. Radiological changes in juvenile chronic polyarthritis. *Skeletal Radiol* 1977;1:129–144.
168. Martel W, Holt JF, Cassidy JT. Roentgenologic manifestations of juvenile rheumatoid arthritis. *AJR* 1962;88:400–423.
169. Wilkinson RH, Weissman BN. Arthritis in children. *Radiol Clin North Am* 1988;26:1247–1265.
170. Resnick D, Niwayama G. Juvenile chronic arthritis. In: Resnick D. *Diagnosis of bone and joint disorders.* 3rd ed. Philadelphia: WB Saunders, 1995, 971–1007.
171. Senac MO Jr, Deutsch D, Bernstein BH, et al. MR imaging in juvenile rheumatoid arthritis. *AJR* 1988;150:873–878.
172. Herve-Somma CMP, Sebag GH, Prieur AM, et al. Juvenile rheumatoid arthritis of the knee: MR evaluation with Gd-DOTA. *Radiology* 1992;182:93–98.
173. Taylor DB, Babyn P, Blaser S, et al. MR evaluation of the temporomandibular joint in juvenile rheumatoid arthritis. *J Comput Assist Tomogr* 1993;17:449–454.
174. Sureda D, Quiroga S, Arnal C, et al. Juvenile rheumatoid arthritis of the knee: evaluation with US. *Radiology* 1994;190:403–406.
175. Azouz EM, Duffy CM. Juvenile spondyloarthropathies: clinical manifestations and medical imaging. *Skeletal Radiol* 1995;24:399–408.
176. Hernandez RJ, Sullivan DB, Chenevert TL, Keim DR. MR imaging in children with dermatomyositis: musculoskeletal findings and correlation with clinical and laboratory findings. *AJR* 1993;161:359–366.
177. Turnpenny PD, Davidson R, Stockdale EJ, et al. Severe prenatal infantile cortical hyperostosis (Caffey's disease) (Review). *Clin Dysmorphol* 1993;2:81–86.
178. Caffey J. Infantile cortical hyperostoses. *J Pediatr* 1946;29:541–559.
179. Harris VJ, Ramilo J. Caffey's disease: a case originating in the first metatarsal and review of a 12 year experience. *AJR* 1978;130: 335–337.
180. Padfield E, Hicken P. Cortical hyperostosis in infants: a radiological study of sixteen patients. *Br J Radiol* 1970;43:231–237.
181. Poznanski AK, Fernbach SK, Berry TE. Bone changes from prostaglandin therapy. *Skeletal Radiol* 1985;14:20–25.
182. Swerdloff BA, Ozonoff MB, Gyepes MT. Late recurrence of infantile cortical hyperostosis (Caffey's disease). *AJR* 1970;108:461–467.
183. Yousefzadeh DK, Brosnan P, Jackson JH Jr. Infantile cortical hyperostosis, Caffey's disease, involving two cousins. *Skeletal Radiol* 1979; 4:141–147.
184. Saatci I, Brown JJ, McAlister WH. MR findings in a patient with Caffey's disease. *Pediatr Radiol* 1996;26:68–70.

Neoplasms

185. Fletcher BD. Response of osteosarcoma and Ewing sarcoma to chemotherapy: imaging evaluation. *AJR* 1991;157:825–833.
186. Erlemann R, Sciuk J, Bosse A, et al. Response of osteosarcoma and Ewing sarcoma to preoperative chemotherapy: assessment with dynamic and static MR imaging and skeletal scintigraphy. *Radiology* 1990;175:791–796.
187. van der Woude HJ, Bloem JL, Verstraete KL, et al. Osteosarcoma and Ewing's sarcoma after neoadjuvant chemotherapy: value of dynamic MR imaging in detecting viable tumor before surgery. *AJR* 1995;165:593–598.
188. Menendez LR, Fideler BM, Mirra J. Thallium-201 scanning for the evaluation of osteosarcoma and soft-tissue sarcoma. A study of the evaluation and predictability of the histological response to chemotherapy. *J Bone Joint Surg Am* 1993;75:526–531.
189. Resnick D. Tumors and tumor-like lesions of bone: radiographic principles. In: Resnick D. *Diagnosis of bone and joint disorders.* 3rd ed. Philadelphia: WB Saunders, 1995, 3613–3627.
190. Lodwick GS. *The bones and joints.* Chicago: Year Book, 1971.
191. Tsai JC, Dalinka MK, Fallon MD, et al. Fluid-fluid level: a nonspecific finding in tumors of bone and soft tissue. *Radiology* 1990;175: 779–782.
192. Berquist TH. Magnetic resonance imaging of primary skeletal neoplasms. *Radiol Clin North Am* 1993;31:411–424.
193. Schima W, Amann G, Stiglbauer R, et al. Preoperative staging of osteosarcoma: efficacy of MR imaging in detecting joint involvement. *AJR* 1994;163:1171–1175.
194. Lang P, Honda G, Roberts T, et al. Musculoskeletal neoplasm: perineoplastic edema versus tumor on dynamic postcontrast MR images with spatial mapping of instantaneous enhancement rates. *Radiology* 1995;197:831–839.
195. Hanna SL, Parham DM, Fairclough DL, et al. Assessment of osteosarcoma response to preoperative chemotherapy using dynamic FLASH gadolinium-DTPA-enhanced magnetic resonance mapping. *Invest Radiol* 1992;27:367–373.
196. Mirra JM. *Bone tumors.* Philadelphia: Lea and Febiger, 1989.
197. Bloem JL, Kroon HM. Osseous lesions. *Radiol Clin North Am* 1993; 31:261–278.
198. Norton KI, Hermann G, Abdelwahab IF, et al. Epiphyseal involvement in osteosarcoma. *Radiology* 1991;180:813–816.
199. Springfield DS. Introduction of limb-salvage surgery for sarcomas. *Orthop Clin North Am* 1991;22:1–17.
200. Parker BR, Castellino RA, eds. *Pediatric oncologic radiology.* St. Louis: CV Mosby, 1977.
201. Link MP, Eilber F. Osteosarcoma. In: Pizzo PA, Poplack DG, eds. *Principles and practice of pediatric oncology.* Philadelphia: JB Lippincott, 1993, 841–866.
202. Huvos AG, Rosen G, Bretsky SS, Butler A. Telangiectatic osteogenic sarcoma: a clinicopathologic study of 124 patients. *Cancer* 1982;49: 1679–1689.
203. Chew FS, Hudson TM. Radionuclide bone scanning of osteosarcoma: falsely extended uptake patterns. *AJR* 1982;139:49–54.
204. Goldman AB, Braunstein P. Augmented radioactivity on bone scans of limbs bearing osteosarcomas. *J Nucl Med* 1975;16:423–424.
205. Thrall JH, Geslien GE, Corcoran RJ, Johnson MC. Abnormal radionuclide deposition patterns adjacent to focal skeletal lesions. *Radiology* 1975;115:659–663.
206. McKillop JH, Etcubanus E, Goris ML. The indications for and limitations of bone scintigraphy in osteogenic sarcoma: a review of 55 patients. *Cancer* 1981;48:1133–1138.
207. Rees CR, Siddiqui AR, duCret R. The role of bone scintigraphy in osteogenic sarcoma. *Skeletal Radiol* 1986;15:365–367.
208. Goldstein H, McNeil BJ, Zufall E, et al. Changing indications for bone scintigraphy in patients with osteosarcoma. *Radiology* 1980;135: 177–180.

209. Knop J, Delling G, Heise U, Winkler K. Scintigraphic evaluation of tumor regression during preoperative chemotherapy of osteosarcoma. Correlation of ^{99m}Tc-methylene diphosphonate parametric imaging with surgical histopathology. *Skeletal Radiol* 1990;19:165–172.

210. Sommer HJ, Knop J, Heise U, et al. Histomorphometric changes of osteosarcoma after chemotherapy. Correlation with ^{99m}Tc methylene diphosphonate functional imaging. *Cancer* 1987;59:252–258.

211. Ramanna L, Waxman A, Binney G, et al. Thallium-201 scintigraphy in bone sarcoma: comparison with gallium-67 and technetium-MDP in the evaluation of chemotherapeutic response. *J Nucl Med* 1990;31:567–572.

212. Rosen G, Loren GJ, Brien EW, et al. Serial thallium-201 scintigraphy in osteosarcoma. Correlation with tumor necrosis after preoperative chemotherapy. *Clin Orthop* 1993;293:302–306.

213. Ohtomo K, Terui S, Yokoyama R, et al. Thallium-201 scintigraphy to assess effect of chemotherapy in osteosarcoma. *J Nucl Med* 1996;37:1444–1448.

214. Sehweil AM, McKillop JH, Milroy R, et al. Mechanism of ^{201}Tl uptake in tumours. *Eur J Nucl Med* 1989;15:376–379.

215. Lawrence JA, Babyn PS, Chan HS, et al. Extremity osteosarcoma in childhood: prognostic value of radiologic imaging. *Radiology* 1993;189:43–47.

216. Holscher HC, Bloem JL, Vanel D, et al. Osteosarcoma: chemotherapy-induced changes at MR imaging. *Radiology* 1992;182:839–844.

217. O'Flanagan SJ, Stack JP, McGee HM, et al. Imaging of intramedullary tumour spread in osteosarcoma. A comparison of techniques. *J Bone Joint Surg Br* 1991;73:998–1001.

218. Sundaram M, McGuire MH, Herbold DR. Magnetic resonance imaging of osteosarcoma. *Skeletal Radiol* 1987;16:23–29.

219. Lang P, Grampp S, Vahlensieck M, et al. Primary bone tumors: value of MR angiography for preoperative planning and monitoring response to chemotherapy. *AJR* 1995;165:135–142.

220. Goorin AM, Shuster JJ, Baker A, et al. Changing pattern of pulmonary metastases with adjuvant chemotherapy in patients with osteosarcoma: results from the Multi-Institutional Osteosarcoma Study. *J Clin Oncol* 1991;9:600–605.

221. McDonald DJ. Limb-salvage surgery for treatment of sarcomas of the extremities. *AJR* 1994;163:509–513.

222. Glasser DB, Lane JM, Huvos AG, et al. Survival, prognosis, and therapeutic response in osteogenic sarcoma. The Memorial Hospital experience. *Cancer* 1992;69:698–708.

223. McCarten KM, Jaffe N, Kirkpatrick JA. The changing radiographic appearance of osteogenic sarcoma. *Ann Radiol* 1980;23:203–208.

224. Horowitz ME, DeLaney TE, Malawer MM, Tsokos MG. Ewing's sarcoma family of tumors: Ewing's sarcoma of bone and soft tissue and the peripheral primitive neuroectodermal tumors. In: Pizzo PA, Poplack DG, eds. *Principles and practice of pediatric oncology.* Philadelphia: JB Lippincott, 1993, 795–821.

225. Eggli KD, Quiogue T, Moser RP Jr. Ewing's sarcoma. *Radiol Clin North Am* 1993;31:325–337.

226. Sherman RS, Soong KY. Ewing's sarcoma: its roentgen classification and diagnosis. *Radiology* 1956;66:529–539.

227. Kissane JM, Askin FB, Foulkes M, et al. Ewing's sarcoma of bone: clinicopathologic aspects of 303 cases from the Intergroup Ewing's Sarcoma Study. *Hum Pathol* 1983;14:773–779.

228. Reinus WR, Gilula LA. Radiology of Ewing's Sarcoma: Intergroup Ewing's Sarcoma Study (IESS). *RadioGraphics* 1984;4:929–944.

229. Reinus WR, Gilula LA, Donaldson S, et al. Prognostic features of Ewing sarcoma on plain radiograph and computed tomography scan after initial treatment. A Pediatric Oncology Group study (8346). *Cancer* 1993;72:2503–2510.

230. Mueller DL, Grant RM, Riding MD, Coppes MJ. Cortical saucerization: an unusual imaging finding of Ewing sarcoma. *AJR* 1994;163:401–403.

231. Frouge C, Vanel D, Coffre C, et al. The role of magnetic resonance imaging in the evaluation of Ewing sarcoma. A report of 27 cases. *Skeletal Radiol* 1988;17:387–392.

232. Lemmi MA, Fletcher BD, Marina NM, et al. Use of MR imaging to assess results of chemotherapy for Ewing sarcoma. *AJR* 1990;155:343–346.

233. MacVicar AD, Olliff JFC, Pringle J, et al. Ewing sarcoma: MR imaging of chemotherapy-induced changes with histologic correlation. *Radiology* 1992;184:859–864.

234. Benz-Bohm G, Gross-Fengels W, Bohndorf K, et al. MRI of the knee region in leukemic children. Part II. Follow up: responder, nonresponder, relapse. *Pediatr Radiol* 1990;20:272–276.

235. Bohndorf K, Benz-Bohm G, Gross-Fengels W, Berthold F. MRI of the knee region in leukemic children. Part 1. Initial pattern in patients with untreated disease. *Pediatr Radiol* 1990;20:179–183.

236. Vogler JB III, Murphy WA. Bone marrow imaging. *Radiology* 1988;168:679–693.

237. Moore SG, Gooding CA, Brasch RC, et al. Bone marrow in children with acute lymphocytic leukemia: MR relaxation times. *Radiology* 1986;160:237–240.

238. Gerard EL, Ferry JA, Amrein PC, et al. Compositional changes in vertebral bone marrow during treatment for acute leukemia: assessment with quantitative chemical shift imaging. *Radiology* 1992;183:39–46.

239. Wilson LM, Draper GJ. Neuroblastoma, its natural history and prognosis: a study of 487 cases. *Br Med J* 1974;3:301–307.

240. Bousvaros A, Kirks DR, Grossman H. Imaging of neuroblastoma: an overview. *Pediatr Radiol* 1986;16:89–106.

241. Baker M, Siddiqui AR, Provisor A, Cohen MD. Radiographic and scintigraphic skeletal imaging in patients with neuroblastoma: concise communication. *J Nucl Med* 1983;24:467–469.

242. Heisel MA, Miller JH, Reid BS, Seigel SE. Radionuclide bone scan in neuroblastoma. *Pediatrics* 1983;71:206–209.

243. Podrasky AE, Stark DD, Hattner RS, et al. Radionuclide bone scanning in neuroblastoma: skeletal metastases and primary tumor localization of 99m Tc-MDP. *AJR* 1983;141:469–472.

244. Martin-Simmerman P, Cohen MD, Siddiqui A, et al. Calcification and uptake of Tc-99m diphosphonates in neuroblastomas: concise communication. *J Nucl Med* 1984;25:656–660.

245. Parisi MT, Greene MK, Dykes TM, et al. Efficacy of metaiodobenzylguanidine as a scintigraphic agent for the detection of neuroblastoma. *Invest Radiol* 1992;27:768–773.

246. Farahati J, Mueller SP, Coennen HH, Reiners C. Scintigraphy of neuroblastoma with radioiodinated m-iodobenzylguanidine. In: Treves ST, ed. *Pediatric nuclear medicine.* 2nd ed. New York: Springer-Verlag, 1995, 528–545.

247. Gilday DL, Greenberg M. The controversy about the nuclear medicine investigation of neuroblastoma. *J Nucl Med* 1990;31:135.

248. Shulkin BL, Shapiro B, Hutchinson RJ. Iodine-131-metaiodobenzylguanidine and bone scintigraphy for the detection of neuroblastoma. *J Nucl Med* 1992;33:1735–1740.

249. Englaro EE, Gelfand MJ, Harris RE, Smith HS. I-131 MIBG imaging after bone marrow transplantation for neuroblastoma. *Radiology* 1992;182:515–520.

250. Krenning EP, Kwekkeboom DJ, Bakker WH, et al. Somatostatin receptor scintigraphy with (111In-DTPA-D-Phe1)- and (123I-Tyr3)-octreotide: the Rotterdam experience with more than 1000 patients. *Eur J Nucl Med* 1993;20:716–731.

251. Fletcher BD, Crom DB, Krance RA, Kun LE. Radiation-induced bone abnormalities after bone marrow transplantation for childhood leukemia. *Radiology* 1994;191:231–235.

252. Rubin P, Casarett GW. *Clinical radiation pathology.* Philadelphia: WB Saunders, 1968.

253. Rutherford H, Dodd GD. Complications of radiation therapy: growing bone. *Semin Roentgenol* 1974;9:15–27.

254. De Smet AA, Kuhns LR, Fayos JV, Holt JF. Effects of radiation therapy on growing long bones. *AJR* 1976;127:935–939.

255. Mullen LA, Berdon WE, Ruzal-Shapiro C, et al. Soft-tissue sarcomas: MR imaging findings after treatment in three pediatric patients. *Radiology* 1995;195:413–417.

256. Stevens SK, Moore SG, Kaplan ID. Early and late bone-marrow changes after irradiation: MR evaluation. *AJR* 1990;154:745–750.

257. Probert JC, Parker BR. The effects of radiation therapy on bone growth. *Radiology* 1975;114:155–162.

258. Ecklund K, Laor T, Goorin AM, et al. Methotrexate osteopathy in patients with osteosarcoma. *Radiology* 1997;202:543–547.

259. Silberzweig JE, Haller JO, Miller S. Ifosfamide: a new cause of rickets. *AJR* 1992;158:823–824.

260. Ryan SP, Weinberger E, White KS, et al. MR imaging of bone marrow in children with osteosarcoma: effect of granulocyte colony-stimulating factor. *AJR* 1995;165:915–920.

261. Fletcher BD, Wall JE, Hanna SL. Effect of hematopoietic growth factors on MR images of bone marrow in children undergoing chemotherapy. *Radiology* 1993;189:745–751.

262. Norman A, Schiffman M. Simple bone cysts: factors of age dependency. *Radiology* 1977;124:779–782.
263. Campanacci M, Capanna R, Picci P. Unicameral and aneurysmal bone cysts. *Clin Orthop* 1986;204:25–36.
264. Reynolds J. The ''fallen fragment sign'' in the diagnosis of unicameral bone cysts. *Radiology* 1969;92:949–953.
265. Burr BA, Resnick D, Syklawer R, Haghighi P. Fluid-fluid levels in a unicameral bone cyst: CT and MR findings. *J Comput Assist Tomogr* 1993;17:134–136.
266. Springfield D. Bone and soft-tissue tumors. In: Morrissy RT, Weinstein SL, eds. *Lovell and Winter's pediatric orthopaedics.* 4th ed. Philadelphia: Lippincott–Raven, 1996, 423–468.
267. Kransdorf MJ, Sweet DE. Aneurysmal bone cyst: concept, controversy, clinical presentation and imaging. *AJR* 1995;164:573–580.
268. Dabska M, Buraczewski J. Aneurysmal bone cyst. Pathology, clinical course and radiologic appearance. *Cancer* 1969;23:371–389.
269. Hudson TM, Hamlin DJ, Fitzsimmons JR. Magnetic resonance imaging of fluid levels in an aneurysmal bone cyst and in anticoagulated human blood. *Skeletal Radiol* 1985;13:267–270.
270. Freiberg AA, Loder RT, Heidelberger KP, Hensinger RN. Aneurysmal bone cysts in young children. *J Pediatr Orthop* 1994;14:86–91.
271. De Cristofaro R, Biagini R, Boriani S, et al. Selective arterial embolization in the treatment of aneurysmal bone cyst and angioma of bone. *Skeletal Radiol* 1992;21:523–527.
272. Brien EW, Mirra JM, Kerr R. Benign and malignant cartilage tumors of bone and joint: their anatomic and theoretical basis with an emphasis on radiology, pathology, and clinical biology. I. The intramedullary cartilage tumors. *Skeletal Radiol* 1997;26:325–353.
273. Shore RM, Poznanski AK, Anandappa EC, Dias LS. Arterial and venous compromise by an osteochondroma. *Pediatr Radiol* 1994;24:39–40.
274. Geirnaerdt MJ, Bloem JL, Eulderink F, et al. Cartilaginous tumors: correlation of gadolinium-enhanced MR imaging and histopathologic findings. *Radiology* 1993;186:813–817.
275. Katzman H, Waugh T, Berdon W. Skeletal changes following irradiation of childhood tumors. *J Bone Joint Surg Am* 1969;51:825–842.
276. Aoki J, Sone S, Fujioka F, et al. MR of enchondroma and chondrosarcoma: rings and arcs of Gd-DTPA enhancement. *J Comput Assist Tomogr* 1991;15:1011–1016.
277. Brower AC, Moser RP, Kransdorf MJ. The frequency and diagnostic significance of periostitis in chondroblastoma. *AJR* 1990;154:309–314.
278. Weatherall PT, Maale GE, Mendelsohn DB, et al. Chondroblastoma: classic and confusing appearance at MR imaging. *Radiology* 1994;190:467–474.
279. Wilson AJ, Kyriakos M, Ackerman LV. Chondromyxoid fibroma: radiographic appearance in 38 cases and in a review of the literature. *Radiology* 1991;179:513–518.
280. Kransdorf MJ, Stull MA, Gilkey FW, Moser RP Jr. Osteoid osteoma. *RadioGraphics* 1991;11:671–696.
281. Lisbona R, Rosenthall L. Role of radionuclide imaging in osteoid osteoma. *AJR* 1979;132:77–80.
282. Helms CA. Osteoid osteoma. The double density sign. *Clin Orthop* 1987;222:167–173.
283. Roach PJ, Connolly LP, Zurakowski D, Treves ST. Osteoid osteoma: comparative utility of high-resolution planar and pinhole magnification scintigraphy. *Pediatr Radiol* 1996;26:222–225.
284. Simons GW, Sty J. Intraoperative bone imaging in the treatment of osteoid osteoma of the femoral neck. *J Pediatr Orthop* 1983;3:399–402.
285. Taylor GA, Shea N, O'Brien T, et al. Osteoid osteoma: localization by intraoperative magnification scintigraphy. *Pediatr Radiol* 1986;16:313–316.
286. Assoun J, Richardi G, Railhac JJ, et al. Osteoid osteoma: MR imaging versus CT. *Radiology* 1994;191:217–223.
287. Towbin R, Kaye R, Meza MP, et al. Osteoid osteoma: percutaneous excision using a CT-guided coaxial technique. *AJR* 1995;164:945–949.
288. Rosenthal DI, Springfield DS, Gebhardt MC, et al. Osteoid osteoma: percutaneous radio-frequency ablation. *Radiology* 1995;197:451–454.
289. Greenspan A. Benign bone-forming lesions: osteoma, osteoid osteoma, and osteoblastoma. Clinical, imaging, pathologic, and differential considerations. *Skeletal Radiol* 1993;22:485–500.
290. Resnick CS, Young JWR, Levine AM, Aisner SC. Case Report 604: osteofibrous dysplasia. *Skel Radiol* 1990;19:217–219.
291. Liu P, Thorner P. MRI of fibromatosis: with pathologic correlation. *Pediatr Radiol* 1992;22:587–589.
292. Cintora E, del Cura JL, Ruiz JC, et al. Case report 807: infantile desmoid-type fibromatosis. *Skeletal Radiol* 1993;22:533–535.
293. Quinn SF, Erickson SJ, Dee PM, et al. MR imaging in fibromatosis: results in 26 patients with pathologic correlation. *AJR* 1991;156:539–542.
294. Mulliken JB, Glowacki J. Hemangiomas and vascular malformations in infants and children: a classification based on endothelial characteristics. *Plast Reconstr Surg* 1982;69:412–423.
295. Fishman SJ, Mulliken JB. Hemangiomas and vascular malformations of infancy and childhood. *Pediatr Clin N Am* 1993;40:1177–1200.
296. Meyer JS, Hoffer FA, Barnes PD, Mulliken JB. Biological classification of soft-tissue vascular anomalies: MR correlation. *AJR* 1991;157:559–564.
297. Kransdorf MJ, Meis JM, Jelinek JS. Myositis ossificans: MR appearance with radiologic-pathologic correlation. *AJR* 1991;157:1243–1248.
298. Kransdorf MJ, Meis JM. Extraskeletal osseous and cartilaginous tumors of the extremities. *RadioGraphics* 1993;13:853–884.
299. Stull MA, Kransdorf MJ, Devaney KO. Langerhans cell histiocytosis of bone. *RadioGraphics* 1992;12:801–823.
300. Willman CL. Detection of clonal histiocytes in Langerhans cell histiocytosis: biology and clinical significance. *Br J Cancer* Suppl 1994;23:S29–S33.
301. Lichenstein L. Histiocytosis X. Integration of eosinophilic granuloma of bone, ''Letterer-Siwe disease,'' and ''Schüller-Christian disease,'' as related manifestations of single nosologic entity. *Arch Pathol* 1953;84:56–102.
302. Meyer JS, Harty MP, Mahboubi S, et al. Langerhans cell histiocytosis: presentation and evolution of radiologic findings with clinical correlation. *RadioGraphics* 1995;15:1135–1146.
303. Schaub T, Ash JM, Gilday DL. Radionuclide imaging in histiocytosis X. *Pediatr Radiol* 1987;17:397–404.
304. Parker BR, Pinckney L, Etcubanas E. Relative efficacy of radiographic and radionuclide bone surveys in the detection of the skeletal lesions of histiocytosis X. *Radiology* 1980;134:377–380.
305. David R, Oria RA, Kumar R, et al. Radiologic features of eosinophilic granuloma of bone. *AJR* 1989;153:1021–1026.
306. Rosenfield NS, Abrahams J, Komp D. Brain MR in patients with Langerhans cell histiocytosis: findings and enhancement with Gd-DTPA. *Pediatr Radiol* 1990;20:433–436.
307. George JC, Buckwalter KA, Cohen MD, et al. Langerhans cell histiocytosis of bone: MR imaging. *Pediatr Radiol* 1994;24:29–32.

Trauma

308. Silverman FN. Problems in pediatric fractures. *Semin Roentgenol* 1978;13:167–176.
309. Rang M. *Children's fractures.* 2nd ed. Philadelphia: JB Lippincott, 1983.
310. Trueta J. *Studies of the development and decay of the human frame.* Philadelphia: WB Saunders, 1968, 90–118.
311. Salter RB, Harris WB. Injuries involving the epiphyseal plate. *J Bone Joint Surg Am* 1963;45:587–622.
312. Jaramillo D, Shapiro F, Hoffer FA, et al. Posttraumatic growth-plate abnormalities: MR imaging of bony-bridge formation in rabbits. *Radiology* 1990;175:767–773.
313. Swischuk LE. *Emergency imaging of the acutely ill or injured child.* Baltimore: Williams and Wilkins, 1994, 398–421.
314. Cail WS, Keats TE, Sussman MD. Plastic bowing fracture of the femur in a child. *AJR* 1978;130:780–782.
315. Martin W III, Ridderold HO. Acute plastic bowing fractures of the fibula. *Radiology* 1979;131:639–640.
316. Borden S IV. Roentgen recognition of acute plastic bowing of the forearm in children. *AJR* 1975;125:524–530.
317. Rogers LF, Poznanski AK. Imaging of epiphyseal injuries. *Radiology* 1994;191:297–308.
318. Rogers LF. The radiography of epiphyseal injuries. *Radiology* 1970;96:289–299.
319. Mizuta T, Benson WM, Foster BK, et al. Statistical analysis of the incidence of physeal injuries. *J Pediatr Orthop* 1987;7:518–523.
320. Chang CY, Shih C, Penn IW, et al. Wrist injuries in adolescent gymnasts of a Chinese opera school: radiographic survey. *Radiology* 1995;195:861–864.

321. Shih C, Chang CY, Penn IW, et al. Chronically stressed wrists in adolescent gymnasts: MR imaging appearance. *Radiology* 1995;195: 855–859.

322. Peterson HA. Physeal and apophyseal injuries. In: Rockwood CA Jr, Wilkins KE, Beaty JH, eds. *Fractures in children.* 4th ed. Philadelphia: JB Lippincott, 1996, 103–166.

323. Shapiro F. Epiphyseal disorders. *N Engl J Med* 1987;317:1702–1710.

324. Shapiro F, Rand F. Traumatic fracture-separations of the epiphyses: a pathophysiologic approach. *Adv Orthop Surg* 1992;15:175–203.

325. Johnston RM, Jones WW. Fractures through human growth plates. *Orthop Trans* 1980;4:295.

326. Ogden JA. Injury to the growth mechanisms. In: Ogden JA. *Skeletal injury in the child.* 2nd ed. Philadelphia: WB Saunders, 1990, 97–174.

327. Ogden JA. Injury to the growth mechanisms of the immature skeleton. *Skeletal Radiol* 1981;6:237–253.

328. Dias LS, Tachdjian MO. Physeal injuries of the ankle in children: classification. *Clin Orthop* 1978;136:230–233.

329. Jaramillo D. Advanced musculoskeletal imaging in pediatric trauma. In: Kirks DR, ed. *Emergency pediatric radiology. A problem-oriented approach.* Reston, VA: American Roentgen Ray Society, 1995, 253–258.

330. Tolo V. Fractures and dislocations around the knee. In: Green NE, Swiontkowski MF, eds. *Skeletal trauma in children.* Philadelphia: WB Saunders, 1994, 369–395.

331. Riseborough EJ, Barrett IR, Shapiro F. Growth disturbances following distal femoral physeal fracture-separations. *J Bone Joint Surg Am* 1983;65:885–893.

332. Shapiro F. Epiphyseal growth plate fracture-separations: a pathophysiologic approach. *Orthopedics* 1982;5:720–736.

333. Jaramillo D, Laor T, Zaleske DJ. Indirect trauma to the growth plate: results of MR imaging after epiphyseal and metaphyseal injury in rabbits. *Radiology* 1993;187:171–178.

334. Hynes D, O'Brien T. Growth disturbance lines after injury of the distal tibial physis. Their significance in prognosis. *J Bone Joint Surg Br* 1988;70:231–233.

335. Jaramillo D, Hoffer FA, Shapiro F, Rand F. MR imaging of fractures of the growth plate. *AJR* 1990;155:1261–1265.

336. Ogden JA. Growth slowdown and arrest lines. *J Pediatr Orthop* 1984; 4:409–415.

337. Kasser JR. Physeal bar resections after growth arrest about the knee. *Clin Orthop* 1990;255:68–74.

338. Mandell GA, Harcke HT, Kumar SJ. Extremity trauma. In: Mandell GA. *Imaging strategies in pediatric orthopaedics.* Gaithersburg, MD: Aspen Publishers, 1990, 199–244.

339. Young JW, Kostrubiak IS, Resnik CS, Paley D. Sonographic evaluation of bone production at the distraction site in Ilizarov limb-lengthening procedures. *AJR* 1990;154:125–128.

340. Jaramillo D, Hoffer FA. Cartilaginous epiphysis and growth plate: normal and abnormal MR imaging findings. *AJR* 1992;158: 1105–1110.

341. Borsa JJ, Peterson HA, Ehman RL. MR imaging of physeal bars. *Radiology* 1996;199:683–687.

342. Kleinman PK. Diagnostic imaging in infant abuse. *AJR* 1990;155: 703–712.

343. Zieger M, Dörr U, Schulz RD. Sonography of slipped humeral epiphysis due to birth injury. *Pediatr Radiol* 1987;17:425–426.

344. Ogden JA. Humerus. In: Ogden JA. *Skeletal injury in the child.* Philadelphia: WB Saunders, 1990:325–425.

345. Brodeur AE, Silberstein MJ, Graviss ER. *Radiology of the pediatric elbow.* Boston: GK Hall, 1981.

346. Rogers LF. Fractures and dislocations of the elbow. *Semin Roentgenol* 1978;13:97–107.

347. Murphy WA, Siegel MJ. Elbow fat pads with new signs and extended differential diagnosis. *Radiology* 1977;124:659–665.

348. Rogers LF, Malave S, Jr., White H, Tachdjian MO. Plastic bowing, torus and greenstick supracondylar fractures of the humerus: radiographic clues to obscure fractures of the elbow in children. *Radiology* 1978;128:145–150.

349. Chambers HG, Wilkins KE. Fractures and dislocations of the elbow region. In: Rockwood CA Jr, Wilkins KE, Beaty JH, eds. *Fractures in children.* 4th ed. Philadelphia: JB Lippincott, 1996, 653–904.

350. Green NE. Fractures and dislocations about the elbow. In: Green NE, Swiontkowski MF, eds. *Skeletal trauma in children.* Philadelphia: WB Saunders, 1994, 369–395.

351. Sugimoto H, Ohsawa T. Ulnar collateral ligament in the growing elbow: MR imaging of normal development and throwing injuries. *Radiology* 1994;192:417–422.

352. Chessare JW, Rogers LF, White H, Tachdjian MO. Injuries of the medial epicondylar ossification center of the humerus. *AJR* 1977;129: 49–55.

353. John DS, Wherry K, Swischuk LE, Phillips WA. Improving detection of pediatric elbow fractures by understanding their mechanics. *Radiographics* 1996;16:1443–1460.

354. Rogers LF, Rockwood CA, Jr. Separation of the entire distal humeral epiphysis. *Radiology* 1973;106:393–400.

355. MacEwan DW. Changes due to trauma in the fat plane overlying the pronator quadratus muscle: a radiologic sign. *Radiology* 1964;82: 879–886.

356. Reed MH. Pelvic fractures in children. *J Can Assoc Radiol* 1976;27: 255–261.

357. Canale ST, Beaty JH. Pelvic and hip fractures. In: Rockwood CA Jr, Wilkins KE, Beaty JH, eds. *Fractures in children.* 4th ed. Philadelphia: JB Lippincott, 1996, 992–1046.

358. Magid D, Fishman EK, Ney DR, et al. Acetabular and pelvic fractures in the pediatric patient: value of two- and three-dimensional imaging. *J Pediatr Orthop* 1992;12:621–625.

359. Bond SJ, Gotschall CS, Eichelberger MR. Predictors of abdominal injury in children with pelvic fracture. *J Trauma* 1991;31:1169–1173.

360. Towbin R, Crawford AH. Neonatal traumatic proximal femoral epiphysiolysis. *Pediatrics* 1979;63:456–459.

361. Diaz MJ, Hedlund GL. Sonographic diagnosis of traumatic separation of the proximal femoral epiphysis in the neonate. *Pediatr Radiol* 1991; 21:238–240.

362. Dunbar JS, Owen HF, Nogrady MB, et al. Obscure tibial fracture of infants—the toddler's fracture. *J Can Assoc Radiol* 1964;15:136–144.

363. Starshak RJ, Simons GW, Sty JR. Occult fracture of the calcaneus—another toddler's fracture. *Pediatr Radiol* 1984;14:37–40.

364. Blumberg K, Patterson RJ. The toddler's cuboid fracture. *Radiology* 1991;179:93–94.

365. Englaro EE, Gelfand MJ, Paltiel HJ. Bone scintigraphy in preschool children with lower extremity pain of unknown origin. *J Nucl Med* 1992;33:351–354.

366. Feldman F, Singson RD, Rosenberg ZS, et al. Distal tibial triplane fractures: diagnosis with CT. *Radiology* 1987;164:429–435.

367. Crawford AH. Fractures and dislocations of the foot and ankle. In: Green NE, Swiontkowski MF, eds. *Skeletal trauma in children.* Philadelphia: WB Saunders, 1994, 449–516.

368. Towbin R, Dunbar JS, Towbin J, Clark R. Teardrop sign: plain film recognition of ankle effusion. *AJR* 1980;134:985–990.

369. Clark TW, Janzen DL, Ho K, et al. Detection of radiographically occult ankle fractures following acute trauma: positive predictive value of an ankle effusion. *AJR* 1995;164:1185–1189.

370. Pinckney LE, Currarino G, Kennedy LA. The stubbed great toe: a cause of occult compound fracture and infection. *Radiology* 1981; 138:375–377.

371. Resnick D. Physical injury: concepts and terminology. In: Resnick D. *Diagnosis of bone and joint disorders.* 3rd ed. Philadelphia: WB Saunders, 1995, 2561–2692.

372. Daffner RH. Stress fractures: current concepts. *Skeletal Radiol* 1978; 2:221–229.

373. Koo WW, Oestreich AE, Sherman R, et al. Osteopenia, rickets, and fractures in preterm infants. *Am J Dis Child* 1985;139:1045–1046.

374. Daffner RH, Pavlov H. Stress fractures: current concepts. *AJR* 1992; 159:245–252.

375. Michael RH, Holder LE. The soleus syndrome. A cause of medial tibial stress (shin splints). *Am J Sports Med* 1985;13:87–94.

376. Bellah RD, Summerville DA, Treves ST, et al. Low-back pain in adolescent athletes: detection of stress injury to the pars interarticularis with SPECT. *Radiology* 1991;180:509–512.

377. Meaney JEM, Carty H. Femoral stress fractures in children. *Skeletal Radiol* 1992;21:173–176.

378. Anderson MW, Greenspan A. Stress fractures. *Radiology* 1996;199: 1–12.

379. Sundar M, Carty H. Avulsion fractures of the pelvis in children: a report of 32 fractures and their outcome. *Skeletal Radiol* 1994;23: 85–90.

380. Fernbach SK, Wilkinson RH. Avulsion injuries of the pelvis and proximal femur. *AJR* 1981;137:581–584.

381. Green NE. Child abuse. In: Green NE, Swiontkowski MF, eds. *Skeletal trauma in children.* Philadelphia: WB Saunders, 1994, 517–531.

382. Carty HM. Fractures caused by child abuse. *J Bone Joint Surg Br* 1993;75:849–857.

383. Silverman FN. Unrecognized trauma in infants, the battered child syndrome, and the syndrome of Ambroise Tardieu. *Radiology* 1972; 104:337–353.

384. Kleinman PK. Imaging of child abuse: an update. In: Kirks DR, ed. *Emergency pediatric radiology. A problem-oriented approach.* Reston, VA: American Roentgen Ray Society, 1995, 189–195.

385. Sty JR, Starshak RJ. The role of bone scintigraphy in the evaluation of the suspected abused child. *Radiology* 1983;146:369–375.

386. Carty H. Radionuclide bone scanning. *Arch Dis Child* 1993;69: 160–165.

387. Cohen RA, Kaufman RA, Myers PA, Towbin RB. Cranial computed tomography in the abused child with head injury. *AJNR* 1985;6: 883–888.

388. Slovis TL, Berdon WE, Haller JO, et al. Pancreatitis and the battered child syndrome. Report of 2 cases with skeletal involvement. *AJR* 1975;125:456–461.

389. Harwood-Nash DC. Abuse to the pediatric central nervous system. *AJNR* 1992;13:569–575.

390. Kleinman PK, Marks SC Jr, Richmond JM, Blackbourne BD. Inflicted skeletal injury: a postmortem radiologic-histopathologic study in 31 infants. *AJR* 1995;165:647–650.

391. Kleinman PK, Marks SC Jr. Relationship of the subperiosteal bone collar to metaphyseal lesions in abused infants. *J Bone Joint Surg Am* 1995;77:1471–1476.

392. Kleinman PK, Marks SC, Blackbourne B. The metaphyseal lesion in abused infants: a radiologic-histopathologic study. *AJR* 1986;146: 895–905.

393. Kogutt MS, Swischuk LE, Fagan CJ. Patterns of injury and significance of uncommon fractures in the battered child syndrome. *AJR* 1974;121:143–149.

394. Nimkin K, Kleinman PK, Teeger S, Spevak MR. Distal humeral physeal injuries in child abuse: MR imaging and ultrasonography findings. *Pediatr Radiol* 1995;25:562–565.

395. Thomas SA, Rosenfield NS, Leventhal JM, Markowitz RI. Long-bone fractures in young children: distinguishing accidental injuries from child abuse. *Pediatrics* 1991;88:471–476.

396. O'Connor JF, Cohen J. Dating fractures. In: Kleinman PK. *Diagnostic imaging of child abuse.* Baltimore: Williams and Wilkins, 1987, 103–113.

397. Kleinman PK, Marks SC Jr, Spevak MR, et al. Extension of growth-plate cartilage into the metaphysis: a sign of healing fracture in abused infants. *AJR* 1991;156:775–779.

398. Sivit CJ, Taylor GA, Eichelberger MR. Visceral injury in battered children: a changing perspective. *Radiology* 1989;173:659–661.

399. Nimkin K, Teeger S, Wallach MT, et al. Adrenal hemorrhage in abused children: imaging and postmortem findings. *AJR* 1994;162: 661–663.

400. Oestreich AE. The periphysis and its effect on the metaphysis: I. Definition and normal radiographic pattern. *Skeletal Radiol* 1992;21: 283–286.

401. Westcott MA, Dynes MC, Remer EM, et al. Congenital and acquired orthopedic abnormalities in patients with myelomeningocele. *Radio-Graphics* 1992;12:1155–1173.

402. Hyre HM, Stelling CB. Radiographic appearance of healed extremity fractures in children with spinal cord lesions. *Skeletal Radiol* 1989; 18:189–192.

403. Schneider R, Goldman AB, Bohne WHO. Neuropathic injuries to the lower extremities in children. *Radiology* 1978;128:713–718.

404. Silverman FN, Gilden JJ. Congenital insensitivity to pain: a neurologic syndrome with bizarre skeletal lesions. *Radiology* 1959;72:176–190.

405. Gyepes MT, Newbern DH, Neuhauser EBD. Metaphyseal and physeal injuries in children with spina bifida and meningomyeloceles. *AJR* 1965;95:168–177.

Metabolic and Systemic Disorders

406. Pitt MJ. Rickets and osteomalacia are still around. *Radiol Clin North Am* 1991;29:97–118.

407. Pitt MJ. Rickets and osteomalacia. In: Resnick D. *Diagnosis of bone and joint disorders*, 3rd ed. Philadelphia: WB Saunders, 1995, 1885–1922.

408. Lovinger RD. Rickets. *Pediatrics* 1980;66:359–365.

409. Weiss A. The scapular sign in rickets. *Radiology* 1971;98:633–636.

410. Swischuk LE, Hayden CK Jr. Seizures and demineralization of the skull. A diagnostic presentation of rickets. *Pediatr Radiol* 1977;6: 65–67.

411. Hruska KA, Teitelbaum SL. Renal osteodystrophy. *N Engl J Med* 1995;333:166–174.

412. Kirkwood JR, Ozonoff MB, Steinbach HL. Epiphyseal displacement after metaphyseal fracture in renal osteodystrophy. *AJR* 1972;115: 547–554.

413. Murphey MD, Sartoris DJ, Quale JL, et al. Musculoskeletal manifestations of chronic renal insufficiency. *RadioGraphics* 1993;13: 357–379.

414. Shapiro R. The biochemical basis of the skeletal changes in chronic uremia. *AJR* 1971;111:750–761.

415. Teitelbaum SL. Progress in pathology. Renal osteodystrophy. *Hum Pathol* 1984;15:306–323.

416. Tigges S, Nance EP, Carpenter WA, Erb R. Renal osteodystrophy: imaging findings that mimic those of other diseases. *AJR* 1995;165: 143–148.

417. Resnick D. Parathyroid disorders and renal osteodystrophy. In: Resnick D. *Diagnosis of bone and joint disorders*. 3rd ed. Philadelphia: WB Saunders, 1995, 2012–2076.

418. Goldman AB, Lane JM, Salvati E. Slipped capital femoral epiphysis complicating renal osteodystrophy: a report of three cases. *Radiology* 1978;126:333–339.

419. Young W, Sevcik M, Tallroth K. Metaphyseal sclerosis in patients with chronic renal failure. *Skeletal Radiol* 1991;20:197–200.

420. Herman TE, McAlister WH. Inherited diseases of bone density in children. *Radiol Clin North Am* 1991;29:149–164.

421. Swischuk LE. *Imaging of the newborn, infant, and young child.* Baltimore: Williams and Wilkins, 1989.

422. Grunebaum M, Horodniceanu C, Steinherz R. The radiographic manifestations of bone changes in copper deficiency. *Pediatr Radiol* 1980; 9:101–104.

423. Chew FS. Radiologic manifestations in the musculoskeletal system of miscellaneous endocrine disorders. *Radiol Clin North Am* 1991; 29:135–147.

424. Swischuk LE, Sarwar M. The sella in childhood hypothyroidism. *Pediatr Radiol* 1977;6:1–3.

425. Hernandez RJ, Poznanski AK. Distinctive appearance of the distal phalanges in children with primary hypothyroidism. *Radiology* 1979; 132:83–84.

426. Puri R, Smith CS, Malhorta D, et al. Slipped upper femoral epiphysis and primary juvenile hypothyroidism. *J Bone Joint Surg Br* 1985;67: 14–20.

427. Resnick D. Thyroid disorders. In: Resnick D. *Diagnosis of bone and joint disorders*. 3rd ed. Philadelphia: WB Saunders, 1995, 1995–2011.

428. Bohrer SP. Bone changes in the extremities in sickle cell anemia. *Semin Roentgenol* 1987;22:176–185.

429. Gaston MH. Sickle cell disease: an overview. *Semin Roentgenol* 1987; 22:150–159.

430. Moseley JE. Skeletal changes in the anemias. *Semin Roentgenol* 1974; 9:169–184.

431. Reynolds J. The skull and spine. *Semin Roentgenol* 1987;22:168–175.

432. Bonnerot V, Sebag G, de Montalembert M, et al. Gadolinium-DOTA enhanced MRI of painful osseous crises in children with sickle cell anemia. *Pediatr Radiol* 1994;24:92–95.

433. Cohen MD. *Pediatric magnetic resonance imaging.* Philadephia: WB Saunders, 1986.

434. Brill PW, Winchester P, Giardina PJ, Cunningham-Rundles S. Deferoxamine-induced bone dysplasia in patients with thalassemia major. *AJR* 1991;156:561–565.

435. Stoker DJ, Murray RO. Skeletal changes in hemophilia and other bleeding disorders. *Semin Roentgenol* 1974;9:185–193.

436. Pettersson H, Gilbert M. *Diagnostic imaging in hemophilia.* New York: Springer-Verlag, 1985.

437. Wilson DA, Prince JR. MR imaging of hemophilic pseudotumors. *AJR* 1988;150:349–350.

438. Nuss R, Kilcoyne RF, Geraghty S, et al. Utility of magnetic resonance imaging for management of hemophilic arthropathy in children. *J Pediatrics* 1993;123:388–392.

439. Brant EE, Jordan HH. Radiologic aspects of hemophilic pseudotumors in bone. *AJR* 1972;115:525–539.

440. Gaary E, Gorlin JB, Jaramillo D. Pseudotumor and arthropathy in the knees of a hemophiliac. *Skeletal Radiol* 1996;25:85–87.

Disorders of the Upper Extremity

441. Bayne LG, Costas BL, Lourie GM. The upper limb. In: Morrissy RT, Weinstein SL, eds. *Lovell and Winter's pediatric orthopaedics.* 4th ed. Philadelphia: Lippincott–Raven, 1996, 781–848.
442. Leibovic SJ, Ehrlich MG, Zaleske DJ. Sprengel deformity. *J Bone Joint Surg Am* 1990;72:192–197.
443. Miller SF, Glasier CM, Griebel ML, Boop FA. Brachial plexopathy in infants after traumatic delivery: evaluation with MR imaging. *Radiology* 1993;189:481–484.
444. Hernandez RJ, Dias L. CT evaluation of the shoulder in children with Erb's palsy. *Pediatr Radiol* 1988;18:333–336.
445. Gudinchet F, Maeder P, Oberson JC, Schnyder P. Magnetic resonance imaging of the shoulder in children with brachial plexus birth palsy. *Pediatr Radiol* 1995;25:S125–S128.
446. Carlson DH. Coalition of the carpal bones. *Skeletal Radiol* 1981;7:125–127.
447. Giedion A. Cone-shaped epiphyses of the hands and their diagnostic value. The tricho-rhino-phalangeal syndrome. *Ann Radiol* 1967;10:322–329.
448. Giedion A. Genetic bone disease: radiologic sight and insight. *AJR* 1988;151:651–657.
449. Kuhns LR, Poznanski AK, Harper HA, Garn SM. Ivory epiphyses of the hands. *Radiology* 1973;109:643–648.
450. Poznanski AK, Pratt GB, Manson G, Weiss L. Clinodactyly, camptodactyly, Kirner's deformity and other crooked fingers. *Radiology* 1969;93:573–582.
451. Currarino G, Waldman I. Camptodactyly. *AJR* 1964;92:1312–1321.
452. Blank E, Girdany BR. Symmetric bowing of the terminal phalanges of the fifth fingers in a family (Kirner's deformity). *AJR* 1965;93:367–373.

Disorders of the Lower Extremity

453. Harcke HT. Screening newborns for developmental dysplasia of the hip: the role of sonography. *AJR* 1994;162:395–397.
454. Harcke HT, Grissom LE. Performing dynamic sonography of the infant hip. *AJR* 1990;155:837–844.
455. Boeree NR, Clark NM. Ultrasound imaging and secondary screening for congenital dislocation of the hip. *J Bone Joint Surg Br* 1994;76:525–533.
456. Hernandez RJ, Cornell RG, Hensinger RN. Ultrasound diagnosis of neonatal congenital dislocation of the hip. A decision analysis assessment. *J Bone Joint Surg Br* 1994;76:539–543.
457. Graf R, Schuler P. *Sonography of the infant hip: an atlas.* Weinheim: VCH Verlagsgesellschaft, 1986.
458. Soboleski DA, Babyn P. Sonographic diagnosis of developmental dysplasia of the hip: importance of increased thickness of acetabular cartilage. *AJR* 1993;161:839–842.
459. Thieme WT, Thiersch JB. Hilgenreiner on congenital hip dislocation. *J Pediatr Orthop* 1986;6:202–214.
460. Taybi H, Kane P. Small acetabular and iliac angles and associated diseases. *Radiol Clin North Am* 1968;6:215–221.
461. Perkins G. Signs by which to diagnose congenital dislocation of the hip. *Clin Orthop* 1992;274:3–5.
462. O'Brien T, Millis MB, Griffin PP. The early identification and classification of growth disturbances of the proximal end of the femur. *J Bone Joint Surg Am* 1986;68:970–980.
463. Johnson ND, Wood BP, Jackman KV. Complex infantile and congenital hip dislocation: assessment with MR imaging. *Radiology* 1988;168:151–156.
464. Eggli KD, King SH, Boal DK, Quoigue T. Low-dose CT of developmental dysplasia of the hip after reduction: diagnostic accuracy and dosimetry. *AJR* 1994;163:1441–1443.
465. Hernandez RJ. Evaluation of congenital hip dysplasia and tibial torsion by computed tomography. *J Comput Tomogr* 1983;7:101–108.
466. Jaramillo D, Villegas-Medina OL, Doty DK, et al. Gadolinium-enhanced MR imaging demonstrates abduction-caused hip ischemia and its reversal in piglets. *AJR* 1996;166:879–887.
467. Bearcroft PW, Berman LH, Robinson AHN, Butler GJ. Vascularity of the neonatal femoral head: in vivo demonstration with power Doppler US. *Radiology* 1996;200:209–211.
468. Sebag G, Ducou le Pointe H, Klein I, et al. Dynamic gadolinium-enhanced subtraction MR imaging—a simple technique for the early diagnosis of Legg-Calvé-Perthes disease: preliminary results. *Pediatr Radiol* 1997;27:216–220.

469. Conway WF, Totty WG, McEnery KW. CT and MR imaging of the hip. *Radiology* 1996;198:297–307.
470. Weinstein SL. Developmental hip dysplasia and dislocation. In: Morrissy RT, Weinstein SL, eds. *Lovell and Winter's pediatric orthopaedics.* 4th ed. Philadelphia: Lippincott–Raven, 1996, 903–950.
471. Herring JA. The treatment of Legg-Calvé-Perthes disease. A critical review of the literature. *J Bone Joint Surg Am* 1994;76:448–458.
472. Fisher RL. An epidemiological study of Legg-Perthes disease. *J Bone Joint Surg (Am)* 1972;54:769–778.
473. Girdany BR, Osman MZ. Longitudinal growth and skeletal maturation in Perthes' disease. *Radiol Clin North Am* 1968;6:245–251.
474. Rush BH, Bramson RT, Ogden JA. Legg-Calvé-Perthes disease: detection of cartilaginous and synovial changes wth MR imaging. *Radiology* 1988;167:473–476.
475. Dörr U, Zieger M, Hauke H. Ultrasonography of the painful hip. Prospective studies in 204 patients. *Pediatr Radiol* 1988;19:36–40.
476. Weinstein SL. Legg-Calvé-Perthes disease. In: Morrissy RT, Weinstein SL, eds. *Lovell and Winter's pediatric orthopaedics.* 4th ed. Philadelphia: Lippincott–Raven, 1996, 951–992.
477. Bos CF, Bloem JL, Bloem RM. Sequential magnetic resonance imaging in Perthes' disease. *J Bone Joint Surg Br* 1991;73:219–224.
478. Pinto MR, Peterson HA, Berquist TH. Magnetic resonance imaging in early diagnosis of Legg-Calvé-Perthes disease. *J Pediatr Orthop* 1989;9:19–22.
479. Sebag G, Ducou le Point H, Klein I, et al. Dynamic gadolinium-enhanced subtraction MR imaging—a simple technique for the early diagnosis of Legg-Calvé-Perthes disease: preliminary results. *Pediatr Radiol* 1997;27:216–220.
480. Ducou le Pointe H, Haddad S, Silberman B, et al. Legg-Calvé-Perthes disease: staging by MRI using gadolinium. *Pediatr Radiol* 1994;24:88-91.
481. Calver R, Venugopal V, Dorgan J, et al. Radionuclide scanning in the early diagnosis of Perthes' disease. *J Bone Joint Surg Br* 1981;63:379–382.
482. Cavailloles F, Bok B, Bensahel H. Bone scintigraphy in the diagnosis and follow-up of Perthes' disease. *Eur J Nucl Med* 1982;7:327–330.
483. Conway JJ. A scintigraphic classification of Legg-Calvé-Perthes disease. *Semin Nucl Med* 1993;23:274–295.
484. Jaramillo D, Kasser JR, Villegas-Medina OL, et al. Cartilaginous abnormalities and growth disturbances in Legg-Calvé-Perthes disease: evaluation with MR imaging. *Radiology* 1995;197:767–773.
485. Hubbard AM, Dormans JP. Evaluation of developmental dysplasia, Perthes disease, and neuromuscular dysplasia of the hip in children before and after surgery: an imaging update. *AJR* 1995;164:1067–1073.
486. Catterall A. The natural history of Perthes' disease. *J Bone Joint Surg Br* 1971;53:37–53.
487. Salter RB, Thompson GH. Legg-Calvé-Perthes disease. The prognostic significance of the subchondral fracture and a two-group classification of the femoral head involvement. *J Bone Joint Surg Am* 1984;66:479–489.
488. Farsetti P, Tudisco C, Caterini R, et al. Herring lateral pillar classification for prognosis in Perthes disease: late results in 49 patients treated conservatively. *Radiology* 1995;198:592.
489. Meyer J. Dysplasia epiphysealis capitis femoris. *Acta Orthop Scand* 1964;34:183–197.
490. Khermosh O, Wientroub S. Dysplasia epiphysealis capitis femoris. Meyer's dysplasia. *J Bone Joint Surg Br* 1991;73:621–625.
491. Zubrow AB, Lane JM, Parks JS. Slipped capital femoral epiphysis occurring during treatment for hypothyroidism. *J Bone Joint Surg Am* 1978;60:256–258.
492. Wolf EL, Berdon WE, Cassady JR, et al. Slipped femoral capital epiphysis as a sequela to childhood irradiation for malignant tumors. *Radiology* 1977;125:781–784.
493. Kelsey JL. Epidemiology of slipped capital femoral epiphysis: a review of the literature. *Pediatrics* 1973;51:1042–1050.
494. Gelberman RH, Cohen MS, Shaw BA, et al. The association of femoral retroversion with slipped capital femoral epiphysis. *J Bone Joint Surg Am* 1986;68:1000–1007.
495. Kehl DK. Slipped capital femoral epiphysis. In: Morrissy RT, Weinstein SL, eds. *Lovell and Winter's pediatric orthopaedics.* 4th ed. Philadelphia: Lippincott–Raven, 1996, 993–1022.
496. Bloomberg TJ, Nuttall J, Stoker DJ. Radiology in early slipped femoral capital epiphysis. *Clin Radiol* 1978;29:657–667.

497. Carney BT, Weinstein SL, Noble J. Long-term follow-up of slipped capital femoral epiphysis. *J Bone Joint Surg Am* 1991;73:667–674.

498. Ingram AJ, Clarke MS, Clark CS Jr, Marshall WR. Chondrolysis complicating slipped capital femoral epiphysis. *Clin Orthop* 1982;165:99–109.

499. Gelfand MJ, Strife JL, Graham EJ, Crawford AH. Bone scintigraphy in slipped capital femoral epiphysis. *Clin Nucl Med* 1983;8:613–615.

500. Gelfand MJ, Ball WS, Oestreich AE, et al. Transient loss of femoral head Tc-99m diphosphonate uptake with prolonged maintenance of femoral head architecture. *Clin Nucl Med* 1983;8:347–354.

501. Smergel EM, Harcke HT, Pizzutillo PD, Betz RR. Use of bone scintigraphy in the management of slipped capital femoral epiphysis. *Clin Nucl Med* 1987;12:349–353.

502. Aitken GT. Proximal focal femoral deficiency definition, classification and management. In: Aitken GT, ed. *Proximal focal femoral deficiency: a congenital abnormality*. Washington, DC: National Academy of Sciences, 1969, 1–22.

503. Kalamchi A, Cowell HR, Kim KI. Congenital deficiency of the femur. *J Pediatr Orthop* 1985;5:129–134.

504. Herring J, Cummings D. The limb-deficient child. In: Morrissy RT, Weinstein SL, eds. *Lovell and Winter's pediatric orthopaedics*. 4th ed. Philadelphia: Lippincott–Raven, 1996, 1137–1180.

505. Grissom LE, Harcke HT. Sonography in congenital deficiency of the femur. *J Pediatr Orthop* 1994;14:29–33.

506. Pirani S, Beauchamp RD, Li D, Sawatzky B. Soft-tissue anatomy of proximal femoral focal deficiency. *J Pediatr Orthop* 1991;11:563–570.

507. Oestreich AE. *How to measure angles from foot radiographs*. New York: Springer-Verlag, 1990.

508. Kehl D. Developmental coxa vara, transient synovitis, and idiopathic chondrolysis of the hip. In: Morrissy RT, Weinstein SL, eds. *Lovell and Winter's pediatric orthopaedics*. 4th ed. Philadelphia: Lippincott–Raven, 1996, 1023–1046.

509. Ruby L, Mital MA, O'Connor J, Patel U. Anteversion of the femoral neck. *J Bone Joint Surg Am* 1979;61:46–51.

510. Murphy SB, Simon SR, Kijewski PK, et al. Femoral anteversion. *J Bone Joint Surg Am* 1987;69:1169–1176.

511. Tomczak RJ, Guenther KP, Rieber A, et al. MR imaging measurement of the femoral antetorsional angle as a new technique: comparison with CT in children and adults. *AJR* 1997;168:791–794.

512. Tolo V. The lower extremity. In: Morrissy RT, Weinstein SL, eds. *Lovell and Winter's pediatric orthopaedics*. 4th ed. Philadelphia: Lippincott–Raven, 1996, 1047–1076.

513. Thompson W, Oliphant M, Grossman H. Bowed limbs in the neonate: significance and approach to diagnosis. *Pediatr Ann* 1976;5:50–62.

514. Langenskiöld A. Tibia vara. A critical review. *Clin Orthop* 1989;246:195–207.

515. Dietz WH Jr, Gross WL, Kirkpatrick JA Jr. Blount disease (tibia vara): another skeletal disorder associated with childhood obesity. *J Pediatr* 1982;101:735–737.

516. Currarino G, Kirks DR. Lateral widening of the epiphyseal plates in knees of children with bowed legs. *AJR* 1977;129:309–312.

517. Ducou le Pointe H, Mousselard H, Rudelli A, et al. Blount's disease: magnetic resonance imaging. *Pediatr Radiol* 1995;25:12–14.

518. Levine AM, Drennan JC. Physiological bowing and tibia vara. The metaphyseal-diaphyseal angle in the measurement of bowleg deformities. *J Bone Joint Surg Am* 1982;64:1158–1163.

519. Tapia J, Stearns G, Ponseti IV. Vitamin D-resistant rickets: a long-term clinical study of eleven patients. *J Bone Joint Surg Am* 1964;46:935–958.

520. Siffert RS. Lower limb-length discrepancy. *J Bone Joint Surg Am* 1987;69:1100–1106.

521. Huurman WW, Jacobsen FS, Anderson JC, Chu WK. Limb-length discrepancy measured with computerized axial tomographic equipment. *J Bone Joint Surg Am* 1987;69:699–705.

522. Moseley CF. Leg-length discrepancy. *Pediatr Clin North Am* 1986;33:1385–1394.

523. Mandell GA, Harcke HT, Kumar SJ. Developmental disorders of the extremities. *Top Magn Reson Imaging* 1991;4:21–30.

524. Turner MS, Smillie IS. The effect of tibial torsion on the pathology of the knee. *J Bone Joint Surg Br* 1981;63:396–398.

525. Ritter MA, DeRosa GP, Babcock JL. Tibial torsion? *Clin Orthop* 1976;120:159–163.

526. Staheli LT, Engel GM. Tibial torsion: a method of assessment and a survey of normal children. *Clin Orthop* 1972;86:183–186.

527. Jakob RP, Haertel M, Stussi E. Tibial torsion calculated by computerised tomography and compared to other methods of measurement. *J Bone Joint Surg Br* 1980;62:238–242.

528. Frantz CH, O'Rahilly R. Congenital skeletal limb deficiencies. *J Bone Joint Surg Am* 1961;43:1202–1224.

529. O'Rahilly R. Morphologic patterns in limb deficiencies and duplications. *Am J Anat* 1951;89:135–193.

530. Achterman C, Kalamchi A. Congenital deficiency of the fibula. *J Bone Joint Surg Br* 1979;61:133–137.

531. Laor T, Jaramillo D, Hoffer FA, Kasser JR. MR imaging in congenital lower limb deformities. *Pediatr Radiol* 1996;26:381–387.

532. Clark CR, Ogden JA. Development of the menisci of the human knee joint. Morphological changes and their potential role in childhood meniscal injury. *J Bone Joint Surg Am* 1983;65:538–547.

533. Zobel MS, Borrello JA, Siegel MJ, Stewart NR. Pediatric knee MR imaging: pattern of injuries in the immature skeleton. *Radiology* 1994;190:397–401.

534. Stanitski C. Meniscal lesions. In: DeLee JC, Drez D Jr, eds. *Orthopaedic sports medicine: principles and practice*. Vol. 3. *Pediatric and adolescent sports medicine*. Philadelphia: WB Saunders, 1994, 371–386.

535. Stark JE, Siegel MJ, Weinberger E, Shaw DW. Discoid menisci in children: MR features. *J Comput Assist Tomogr* 1995;19:608–611.

536. Busch MT. Meniscal injuries in children and adolescents. *Clin Sports Med* 1990;9:661–680.

537. DeLee JC. Ligamentous injury of the knee. In: DeLee JC, Drez D Jr, eds. *Orthopaedic sports medicine: principles and practice*. Vol. 3. *Pediatric and adolescent sports medicine*. Philadelphia: WB Saunders, 1994, 406–432.

538. Stanitski CL, Harvell JC, Fu F. Observations on acute knee hemarthrosis in children and adolescents. *J Pediatr Orthop* 1993;13:506–510.

539. Bates DG, Hresko MT, Jaramillo D. Patellar sleeve fracture: demonstration with MR imaging. *Radiology* 1994;193:825–827.

540. Jaramillo D, Wilkinson RH. Avulsing injuries of the tibial tubercle. *Contemp Diagn Radiol* 1989;13:1–6.

541. Rosenberg ZS, Kawelblum M, Cheung YY, et al. Osgood-Schlatter lesion: fracture or tendonitis? Scintigraphic, CT and MR imaging features. *Radiology* 1992;185:853–858.

542. Scotti DM, Sadhu VK, Heimberg F, O'Hara AE. Osgood-Schlatter's disease, an emphasis on soft tissue changes in roentgen diagnosis. *Skeletal Radiol* 1979;4:21–25.

543. De Flaviis L, Nessi R, Scaglione P, et al. Ultrasonic diagnosis of Osgood-Schlatter and Sinding-Larsen-Johansson diseases of the knee. *Skeletal Radiol* 1989;18:193–197.

544. Stanitski CL. Sinding-Larsen-Johansson disease. In: DeLee JC, Drez D Jr, eds. *Orthopaedic sports medicine: principles and practice*. Vol. 3. *Pediatric and adolescent sports medicine*. Philadelphia: WB Saunders, 1994, 325–328.

545. Milgram JW. Radiological and pathological manifestations of osteochondritis dissecans of the distal femur. A study of 50 cases. *Radiology* 1978;126:305–311.

546. De Smet AA, Fisher DR, Graf BK, Lange RH. Osteochondritis dissecans of the knee: value of MR imaging in determining lesion stability and the presence of articular cartilage defects. *AJR* 1990;155:549–553.

547. Freiberger RH, Hersh A, Harrison MO. Roentgen examination of the deformed foot. *Semin Roentgenol* 1970;5:341–353.

548. Ritchie GW, Keim HA. Major foot deformities: their classification and x-ray analysis. *J Can Assoc Radiol* 1968;19:155–166.

549. Vanderwilde R, Staheli LT, Chew DE, Malagon V. Measurements on radiographs of the foot in normal infants and children. *J Bone Joint Surg Am* 1988;70:407–415.

550. Greenspan A. *Orthopedic radiology: a practical approach*. 2nd ed. New York: Gower Medical Publishing, 1992.

551. Sullivan J. The child's foot. In: Morrissy RT, Weinstein ST, eds. *Lovell and Winter's pediatric orthopaedics*. 4th ed. Philadelphia: Lippincott–Raven, 1996, 1077–1136.

552. Thompson G, Simons GI. Congenital talipes equinovarus (clubfeet) and metatarsus adductus. In: Drennan JC, ed. *The child's foot*. New York: Raven Press, 1992, 97–134.

553. Mosca V. Flexible flatfoot and skewfoot. In: Drennan JC, ed. *The child's foot*. New York: Raven Press, 1992, 355–376.

554. Drennan JC. Congenital vertical talus. In: Drennan JC, ed. *The child's foot*. New York: Raven Press, 1992, 155–168.

555. Jacobs JE. Metatarsus varus and hip dysplasia. *Clin Orthop* 1960;16:203–213.

556. Koop S. Adolescent hallux valgus. In: Drennan JC, ed. *The child's foot.* New York: Raven Press, 1992, 417–424.

557. Olney B. Tarsal coalition. In: Drennan JC, ed. *The child's foot.* New York: Raven Press, 1992, 169–182.

558. Morgan RC, Crawford AH. Surgical management of tarsal coalition in adolescent athletes. *Foot Ankle* 1986;7:183–193.

559. Lateur LM, Van Hoe LR, Van Ghillewe KV, et al. Subtalar coalition: diagnosis with the C sign on lateral radiographs of the ankle. *Radiology* 1994;193:847–851.

560. Stoskopf CA, Hernandez RJ, Kelikian A, et al. Evaluation of tarsal coalition by computed tomography. *J Pediatr Orthop* 1984;4: 365–369.

561. Wechsler RJ, Schweitzer ME, Deely DM, et al. Tarsal coalition: depiction and characterization with CT and MR imaging. *Radiology* 1994; 193:447–452.

562. Mosier KM, Asher M. Tarsal coalitions and peroneal spastic flat foot. *J Bone Joint Surg Am* 1984;66:976–984.

563. Keats TE. *Atlas of roentgenographic measurement.* 6th ed. St. Louis: CV Mosby, 1990.

564. Jaramillo D, Cleveland RH. Osteofibrous dysplasia. In: Siegel MJ, Bisset GS III, Cleveland RH, et al, eds. *Pediatric disease (fourth series) test and syllabus.* Reston, VA: American College of Radiology, 1993, 791–817.

565. Mulliken JB, Young AE. *Vascular birthmarks.* Philadelphia: WB Saunders, 1988.

566. Schlesinger AE, Hernandez RJ. Diseases of the musculoskeletal system in children: imaging with CT, sonography, and MR. *AJR* 1992; 158:729–741.

567. Casselman ES, Miller WT, Shu Ren L, Mandell GA. Von Recklinghausen's disease: incidence of roentgenographic findings with a clinical review of the literature. *CRC Crit Rev Diagn Imag* 1977;9: 387–419.

568. Laor T, Burrows PE, Hoffer FA. Magnetic resonance venography of congenital vascular malformations of the extremities. *Pediatr Radiol* 1996;26:371–380.

Practical Pediatric Imaging: Diagnostic Radiology of Infants and Children, Third Edition.
D. R. Kirks, editor and N. T. Griscom, associate editor.
Lippincott–Raven Publishers, Philadelphia © 1998.

CHAPTER 6

Cardiovascular System

Janet L. Strife, George S. Bisset III, and Patricia E. Burrows

Imaging plays a critical role in the diagnosis and therapy of cardiovascular disease in children. Its role has been strengthened even more by the development of percutaneous techniques for the treatment of both congenital and acquired abnormalities. The differential diagnosis of congenital heart disease was formerly made on the basis of plain films and esophagography. Cardiac catheterization and angiography were used for definitive diagnosis and precise depiction of cardiovascular anatomy. Developments in cardiac imaging during the 1980s and 1990s included the emergence of non-invasive and semi-invasive imaging techniques such as echocardiography, color flow Doppler sonography, ultrafast computed tomography (CT), and magnetic resonance imaging (MRI). Echocardiography has become indispensable in diagnosing and managing newborns, infants, and young adults with cardiac disease. These new techniques provide anatomic information and can also assess myocardial function, blood flow, myocardial tissue characteristics, and myocardial metabolism.

   The purpose of this chapter is to present an overview of general and specific abnormalities in the framework of an ordered approach to conventional radiography, angiography, and MRI. First, cardiac anatomy and physiology are reviewed. Then an ordered approach to plain film interpretation is discussed. Finally, specific cardiovascular abnormali-

   J. L. Strife: Department of Radiology, Children's Hospital Medical Center, University of Cincinnati College of Medicine, Cincinnatti, Ohio 45229-3039.
   G. S. Bisset III: Department of Radiology, Duke University Medical Center, Duke University School of Medicine, Durham, North Carolina 27710.
   P. E. Burrows: Division of Cardiovascular/Interventional Radiology, Department of Radiology, Children's Hospital, Harvard Medical School, Boston, Massachusetts 02115.

ties are discussed and illustrated. Supplementary imaging modalities are presented for some of the congenital and acquired cardiovascular abnormalities. Schematic drawings, radiographs, angiograms, echocardiograms, and magnetic resonance images illustrate many of the common abnormalities of infants and children.

There are several excellent textbooks devoted to clinical recognition, radiographic diagnosis, and treatment of congenital heart disease in children (1–10).

TECHNIQUES

Diagnostic Evaluation

The diagnosis of congenital abnormalities of the heart and great vessels is sometimes perceived as difficult or even impossible. However, when conclusions are based on accurate clinical, laboratory, and radiologic observations, correct diagnoses follow. Although echocardiography is the modality of choice for the diagnosis of specific congenital heart lesions, the preliminary diagnosis depends on the age, the history, the physical examination, electrocardiography (ECG), and chest radiography.

Pertinent clinical information includes age, sex, symptoms and their time of onset, presence or absence of cyanosis, blood pressure, presence or absence of peripheral pulses, and type of murmur. Important laboratory data include hemoglobin, hematocrit, electrolytes, blood urea nitrogen (BUN), creatinine, calcium, and glucose. The ECG provides information about specific chamber size, hypertrophy, electrophysiologic activity, conduction, and cardiac axis. Echocardiography demonstrates anatomy and dynamic function. Although the chest radiograph is a static image of the heart and lungs, it provides important physiologic as well as anatomic information. An example of this physiologic information is pulmonary vascularity, one basis for the classification of congenital heart disease. Nuclear scintigraphy depicts and quantifies certain pulmonary vascular abnormalities, shunts, and myocardial dysfunctions. Cardiac catheterization provides information regarding pressure and oxygenation within selected chambers and great vessels. Angiocardiography demonstrates the anatomy and function of individual cardiac chambers and great vessels. Interventional procedures are increasingly used to treat specific congenital lesions. Magnetic resonance demonstrates the anatomy of the heart and great vessels without ionizing radiation. Developments include magnetic resonance angiography (MRA) and magnetic resonance spectroscopy (MRS). These functional imaging techniques show promise for tissue characterization, measurement of blood flow, and assessment of tissue metabolism and perfusion.

Cardiac Radiography

Chest Radiography

The conventional chest radiograph, though still important, has become less critical for the evaluation of congenital heart disease as newer imaging modalities, particularly echocardiography, have emerged. Routine evaluation of congenital heart disease includes posteroanterior (PA) or anteroposterior (AP) and lateral views of the chest. An understanding of the pathophysiology of congenital cardiovascular lesions is critical for accurate interpretation of the chest radiograph. Cardiac fluoroscopy and supplementary oblique radiography of the heart are rarely necessary in children.

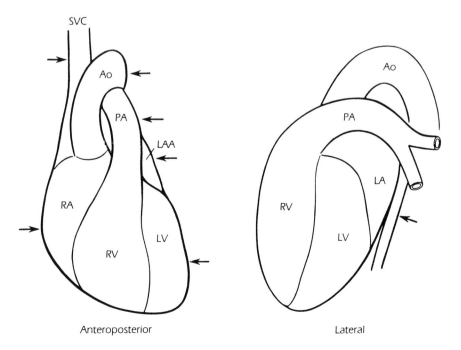

FIG. 6-1. Normal cardiac anatomy. The right heart border on the anteroposterior view *(left)* is formed by the superior vena cava and right atrium *(arrows)*. The left heart border is formed by the aortic arch, main pulmonary artery, left atrial appendage, and left ventricle *(arrows)*. In infants and young children, these structures are frequently not visualized because of overlying normal thymus. On the lateral view *(right)*, the anterior cardiac border is formed by the right ventricle and the root of the main pulmonary artery. The upper half of the posterior cardiac border is formed by the left atrium, which is in direct contact with the esophagus *(arrow)*. *Ao*, aorta; *LA*, left atrium; *LAA*, left atrial appendage; *LV*, left ventricle; *PA*, pulmonary artery; *RA*, right atrium; *RV*, right ventricle; *SVC*, superior vena cava.

Anteroposterior

Lateral

Normal Anatomy

The chest radiograph provides information about the situs, soft tissues, bony thorax, great vessels, heart, and pulmonary vascularity. The overall cardiac size and, in older children, certain specific types of chamber enlargement may be determined. Normally, the right mediastinal border, if the thymus is ignored, includes the superior vena cava (upper one third) and the right atrium (lower two thirds) (Fig. 6-1). The left mediastinal border consists of the transverse and descending portions of the thoracic aorta, main pulmonary artery, left atrial appendage, and left ventricle. It should be stressed that the right ventricle and ascending aorta do not normally form mediastinal borders on the PA projection. Moreover, the left atrial appendage is usually not convex laterally. Visualization of the margins of the heart chambers and great vessels may be impossible in infants because of an overlying normal thymus.

The lateral view is particularly helpful for assessing the right ventricle, left atrium, and left ventricle (Fig. 6-1). The right ventricle lies just behind the sternum and forms the lower one half to two thirds of the anterior cardiac border. The upper one third of this anterior cardiac border consists of the right ventricular outflow tract and the root of the pulmonary artery. There is a triangular lucency, made by the two lungs, behind the upper portion of the sternum unless the thymus gland is large, as it often is in infancy. The posterior cardiac border is made up of the left atrium in its upper half and the left ventricle in its lower half. Normally, in older children, the posterior wall of the inferior vena cava can be seen as it enters the right atrium.

Cardiac Catheterization and Angiocardiography

Cardiac catheterization is now less frequently performed for diagnosis because of the excellent noninvasive imaging of the heart with echocardiography and MRI. However, the number of catheterizations for interventional cardiac procedures has increased dramatically. During cardiac catheterization, pressures and oxygen saturation are measured in the heart chambers and great vessels. These data can be used to calculate cardiac output, volume of shunts, severity of obstruction, and cardiac indices.

Oxygen saturations in the superior vena cava, right atrium, right ventricle, and pulmonary artery should be similar (Fig. 6-2). Saturations in the pulmonary veins, left atrium, left ventricle, aorta, and peripheral arteries should also be the same. Small variations in saturation may be due to sampling difficulties, streaming of venous blood, valvular insufficiency, pulmonary parenchymal disease, or changes in physiology during the study.

After oximetry is measured and pressure measurements are performed, angiography is usually performed. Cardiac angiography provides information about atrial situs, atrial-ventricular-great artery connections, and the spatial relations

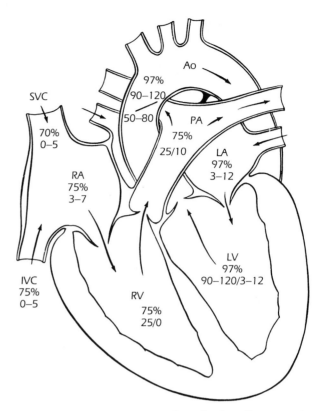

FIG. 6-2. Normal cardiac catheterization. Oxygen saturation is in percentages; pressure is in mm Hg. *Ao,* aorta; *IVC,* inferior vena cava; *LA,* left atrium; *LV,* left ventricle; *PA,* pulmonary artery; *RA,* right atrium; *RV,* right ventricle; *SVC,* superior vena cava.

between the ventricles and great vessels. Frontal and lateral views have now been replaced by axial imaging, as reported by Elliott, Bargeron, and colleagues in 1977 (11). Current cine angiographic equipment permits rotation from the midline and cranial or caudal angulation (12). Digital equipment is now an integral part of both diagnostic imaging and interventional procedures.

Nonionic contrast is used in most pediatric cardiac catheterization laboratories. In controlled studies, rise in left ventricular systolic and end-diastolic pressures, increase in serum osmolality, and bradycardia are significantly less with nonionic contrast than with ionic agents (12–14). Nonionic contrast media induce less hypocalcemia and are therefore less likely to produce ECG changes. The total volume of contrast media is limited to 2–3 ml/kg when possible, with 4 ml/kg the upper limit of safety in a sick neonate.

Sequential Analysis

The correct interpretation of angiocardiography, like any other radiologic or imaging examination, requires systematic analysis. This analysis should be both segmental and sequential in order to simplify the evaluation and diagnosis of complex congenital heart anomalies (15). Each vascular and car-

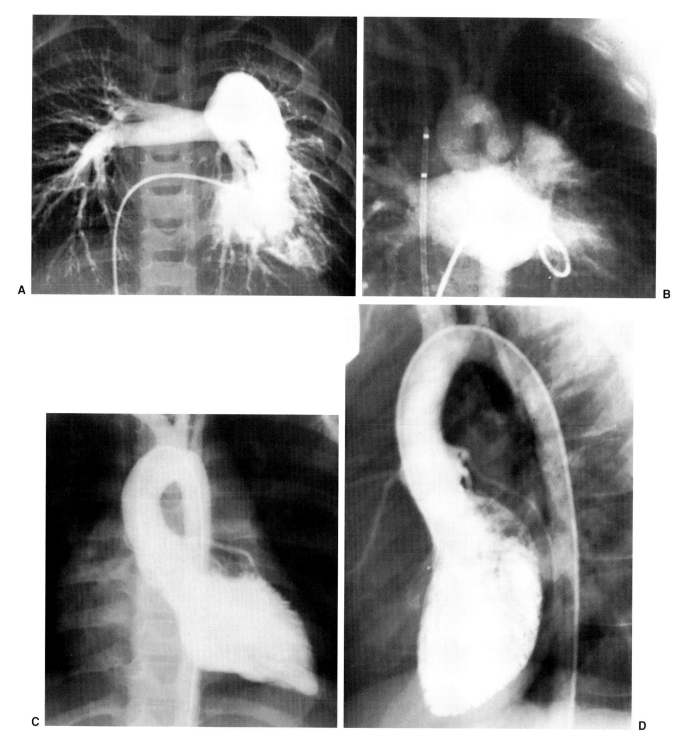

FIG. 6-3. Normal angiocardiography. A: Normal anatomy of the right ventricle and pulmonary arteries. **B:** On the levophase of the study, the pulmonary veins are seen entering the left atrium. **C:** Normal left ventriculogram demonstrating a smooth-walled chamber, aortic valve, and ascending aorta. **D:** Left ventriculography in the long axis view demonstrating an intact ventricular septum, aortic-mitral valve continuity, and normal coronary arteries and aorta.

diac segment is analyzed sequentially with regard to morphology, connections, size, and relations.

Normal

The normal long axis (cardiac axis) of the heart passes through the ventricular apex. This axis is usually to the left, termed *levocardia*. The location of the heart is almost always in the left chest; its location coincides with the cardiac axis. The normal flow of blood is from the systemic veins to the right atrium, right ventricle, pulmonary arteries, pulmonary capillaries, pulmonary veins, left atrium, left ventricle, and aorta.

The normal connections of the superior vena cava and inferior vena cava are to the right atrium. The pressure in these systemic veins is usually 0–5 mm Hg, and there is an oxygen saturation of 70% to 75% (Fig. 6-2). Morphologic identification of the right atrium is based on the appearance of the right atrial appendage, which has a triangular shape, a broad base of attachment to the body of the right atrium, and a blunt vertex. The normal pressure in the right atrium is 3–7 mm Hg, and the oxygen saturation is 75% (Fig. 6-2). Contrast flows from the right atrium across the tricuspid valve into the right ventricle. The right ventricle has a smooth inlet segment that supports the tricuspid valve (Fig. 6-3A). The musculature of the body of the right ventricle has a coarse, prominent trabecular pattern, apparent during both systole and diastole. The outflow tract of the right ventricle is elongated and has a prominent muscular ridge, the crista supraventricularis, which forms part of the posterior wall and separates the tricuspid valve from the pulmonary valve. The right ventricle is located anterior to and to the right of the left ventricle. Contrast flows from the right ventricle across the pulmonary valve into the pulmonary artery (Fig. 6-3A). The pulmonary valve is anterior, superior, and to the left of the aortic valve. Contrast then flows from the pulmonary artery into the pulmonary capillaries.

The four pulmonary veins drain into the posterior aspect of the left atrium (Fig. 6-3B). The left atrial appendage forms part of the left heart border and communicates with the main atrial cavity by a narrow orifice. Pressure in the left atrium is 3–12 mm Hg, and the oxygen saturation is 97% to 98%. Contrast flows from the left atrium across the mitral valve into the left ventricle. The left ventricle has a short, smooth-walled inflow tract that supports the mitral valve. The musculature of the body of the left ventricle has fine trabeculations, best visualized during diastole. The outflow tract is short compared with that of the right ventricle, and there is continuity between the aortic valve and atrioventricular mitral valve (Fig. 6-3C, D). The left ventricle is supplied by two anatomically distinct coronary arteries, the left anterior descending artery and the circumflex artery. Normal left ventricular pressure is 90–120/3–12 mm Hg, and its oxygen saturation is 97% to 98% (see Fig. 6-2). Contrast material flows from the left ventricle across the aortic valve into the

aorta. It should be noted that the ventricle-great artery connections cross each other (see Fig. 6-2) because the normal left ventricle is to the left of the right ventricle and the normal aortic valve is posterior and to the right of the pulmonary valve. The pressure in the thoracic aorta is 90–120/50–80 mm Hg, and the oxygen saturation is 97% to 98% (see Fig. 6-2).

Catheter Positions

Cardiac catheterization and angiocardiography may be performed by either the venous or the arterial approach. A venous catheter is readily positioned in the inferior vena cava, right atrium, or superior vena cava (Fig. 6-4A). The catheter may pass from the inferior vena cava to the right atrium and across the tricuspid valve to the right ventricle (Fig. 6-4B). The tip of the catheter may remain in the right ventricle or pass superiorly across the pulmonary valve into

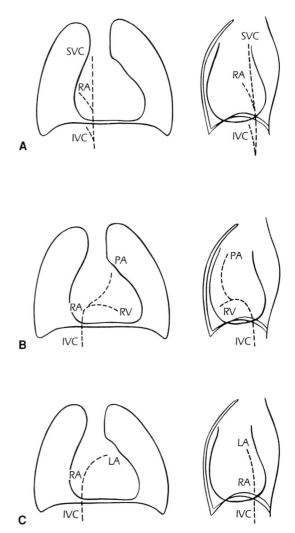

FIG. 6-4. A–C: Normal catheter positions. *IVC,* inferior vena cava; *LA,* left atrium; *PA,* pulmonary artery; *RA,* right atrium; *RV,* right ventricle; *SVC,* superior vena cava.

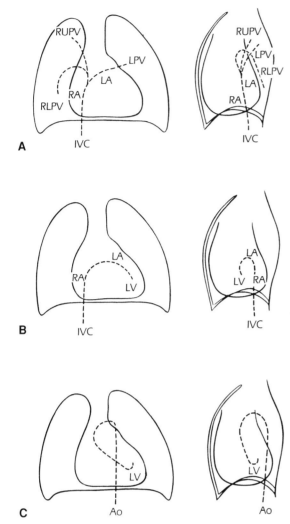

FIG. 6-5. A–C: Normal catheter positions. *Ao*, aorta; *IVC*, inferior vena cava; *LA*, left atrium; *LPV*, left pulmonary vein; *LV*, left ventricle; *RA*, right atrium; *RLPV*, right lower pulmonary vein; *RUPV*, right upper pulmonary vein.

the pulmonary artery (Fig. 6-4B). In infants and young children, the venous catheter may also pass from the inferior vena cava to the right atrium and across an atrial septal defect or, more commonly, across a patent foramen ovale into the left atrium (Figs. 6-5A and 6-5C) and subsequently through the mitral valve into the left ventricle (Fig. 6-5B). In the normal heart, an arterial catheter may pass retrograde from the descending aorta into the aortic arch and then down the ascending aorta, across the aortic valve, and into the left ventricle (Fig. 6-5C).

ORDERED APPROACH

Chest Radiography

One should develop an ordered approach to the evaluation of the chest radiograph (Table 6-1). This ordered repetitious

analysis ensures complete examination and simplifies the diagnosis of cardiovascular abnormalities.

Technique

The chest radiograph should be checked for proper technique. The patient and tube should be properly positioned with no rotation or angulation. Films should be adequately penetrated to show the intervertebral disk spaces through the heart but not so overpenetrated as to prevent evaluation of the pulmonary vascularity. In infants, the frontal chest radiograph is frequently obtained recumbent and AP. In older patients, the film is obtained with the patient upright, and the projection is PA. Correct techniques and proper immobilization usually prevent inadequacy of examination due to patient or respiratory motion. Respiratory motion during the exposure is usually best detected by blurring of the diaphragm and vessels. If the radiograph is exposed during adequate inspiration, the domes of the diaphragm should be approximately at the level of the sixth ribs anteriorly and the eighth ribs posteriorly. The trachea should be visualized just to the right of the midline; it deviates away from the side of the aortic arch during expiration.

Pulmonary Vascularity

The most important step, and usually the most difficult one, in the interpretation of any heart lesion is the radiologic

TABLE 6-1. *Approach to chest radiographs in congenital heart disease*

Technique	Heart size and chamber
Centering	enlargement
Augulation	Right atrium
Penetration	Right ventricle
Motion	Left atrium
Degree of inspiration	Left ventricle
Pulmonary vascularity	Extracardiac structures
Pulmonary arterial flow	Rib notching
Normal	Soft tissues and bony
Shunt vascularity	thorax
Decreased	Previous surgery
Bronchial	Scoliosis
Asymmetric	Vertebral anomalies
Pulmonary arterial	Sternal anomalies
hypertension	Situs
Pulmonary venous	Position of the stomach
hypertension	Position of liver and
Kerley A, B, C lines	spleen
Redistribution of	Tracheobronchial
pulmonary blood flow	anatomy
Great vessel anatomy	Cardiac apex
Main pulmonary artery	Aortic arch
Size	Evaluation of anomalies
Position	of venous return
Aorta	(systemic or pulmonary)
Size	Pericardium
Position	

Modified from Elliott and Schiebler (2).

analysis of the pulmonary vascularity; this is the basis of categorizing patients with congenital heart disease (2,5,7, 10,16). The pulmonary vascularity may be normal, decreased, or increased. Increased or prominent pulmonary vascularity may be due to shunt vascularity (active congestion), pulmonary venous hypertension (passive congestion), pulmonary arterial hypertension, or systemic (bronchial or aortic) pulmonary collaterals (16).

Normal Pulmonary Vascularity

The normal pulmonary vascular markings taper gradually toward the periphery of the lung. The vessels of the lower lobes tend to be more prominent when the film is obtained with the patient upright. When the patient is recumbent, there is even distribution of pulmonary vascular markings on frontal films. Most hilar shadows are caused by the right and left main pulmonary arteries. The right pulmonary artery is seen as a circular density on the lateral chest radiograph just anterior to the trachea. The left pulmonary artery is a crescentic opacity that courses posteriorly over the left main stem bronchus.

The radiographic assessment of pulmonary blood flow is difficult, even for an experienced observer. One method for assessing flow is to compare the diameter of the right descending pulmonary artery and the diameter of the trachea at the level of the aortic arch (Fig. 6-6). Tracheal diameter in normal children increases directly with age; the tracheal diameter equals the diameter of the right descending pulmonary artery throughout childhood (17). Most pediatric radiologists do not actually measure the artery/trachea ratio with a ruler but estimate it by eye. Children with a shunt have a right descending pulmonary artery diameter greater than the tracheal diameter (17). One may also compare the diameter of a pulmonary artery seen end-on to that of an adjacent bronchus; in normal patients, they are the same. This arterial-bronchial index is independent of age and sex. Therefore, by comparing an artery to the adjacent bronchus, an assessment can be made of artery size and, by inference, of pulmonary blood flow.

Decreased Pulmonary Arterial Flow

Diminished pulmonary blood flow is usually caused by a right-to-left cardiac shunt. Blood is diverted from the right side of the heart and pulmonary arteries to the left, which results in diminished blood flow to the lungs.

When the pulmonary blood flow is diminished, the main pulmonary artery segment is decreased in size. The peripheral arteries are also small; they appear thinned, and it is difficult to identify pulmonary arteries in the periphery of the lung. The right descending pulmonary artery is smaller than the trachea (Fig. 6-6); the diameter of a pulmonary artery end-on is less than that of the adjacent bronchus. The

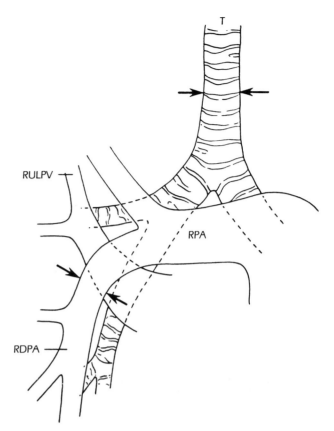

FIG. 6-6. Objective assessment of shunt vascularity. The diameter of the right descending pulmonary artery *(RDPA)* at the point where it crosses the right upper lobe pulmonary vein *(RULPV) (arrows)* is normally the same diameter as the trachea *(T) (arrows)*. RPA, right pulmonary artery. Modified from Coussement and Gooding (17).

sparseness of vessels may give the appearance of hyperlucency of the lung.

Shunt Vascularity

Increased pulmonary artery flow is characterized by uniform prominence of hilar and intrapulmonary arteries and veins. Although the vessels are increased in size, their margins remain sharp and distinct unless there is superimposed interstitial edema due to pulmonary venous hypertension. Maintenance of sharp vascular margination is important in the difficult distinction between shunt vascularity (active) and pulmonary venous hypertension and congestive failure (passive). With increased pulmonary blood flow, the main pulmonary arteries are enlarged and the right and left pulmonary arteries and their branches are bigger and appear to extend farther out from the hilum. The diameter of the right descending pulmonary artery is greater than the tracheal diameter. A pulmonary artery seen end-on is larger than the adjacent bronchus. If there is increase in pulmonary arterial flow, the main pulmonary artery is invariably dilated to accommodate the greater volume.

Pulmonary Venous Hypertension

Pulmonary venous hypertension (passive congestion) causes vascular redistribution, interstitial edema, and alveolar edema. The normal pulmonary venous wedge pressure is 12 mm Hg or less. Mild pulmonary venous hypertension (13–15 mm Hg) increases the resistance to blood flow in dependent lower vessels. In the erect older child, it produces equalization of the size of the lower lobe and upper lobe vessels. With moderate pulmonary venous hypertension (15–18 mm Hg), the upper lobe vessels are more dilated than the lower lobe vessels; this is difficult to detect in young children because the pressure head from the upper chest to the lower chest is small. With increasing pulmonary venous hypertension (18–25 mm Hg), interstitial edema forms in the peribronchial spaces, perivascular sheaths, interlobular septa, and subpleural spaces. This produces hazy, indistinct vessel margins. With severe pulmonary venous hypertension (usually over 30 mm Hg), there is an outpouring of edema fluid into alveoli to produce air space opacity (alveolar pulmonary edema). Hemosiderosis and ossification of the lung, radiologic signs of long-standing and severe pulmonary venous hypertension, rarely occur in children.

Pulmonary Arterial Hypertension

In infants and children with pulmonary arterial hypertension, the pulmonary arteries are prominent centrally. If there

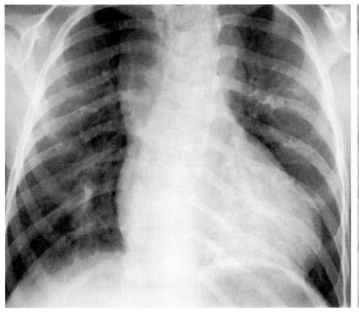

A

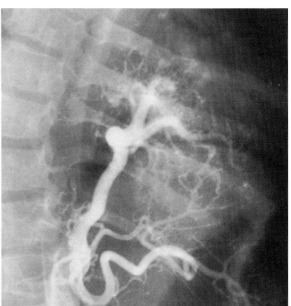

B

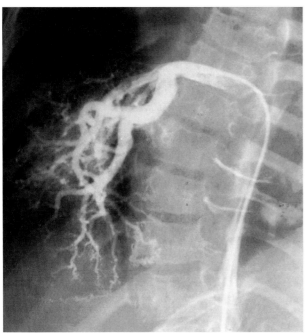

C

FIG. 6-7. Systemic collaterals in a patient with pulmonary atresia and VSD. A: Major aortic-pulmonary collaterals. Note the concave pulmonary artery segment and large aorta. **B, C:** Selective injections of bronchial collaterals arising from the descending aorta. There is increased tortuosity and abnormal branching of these vessels.

is a large left-to-right shunt, hyperinflation of the lungs may reflect abnormal pulmonary compliance. Pulmonary arterial hypertension in adolescents and young adults is characterized by prominent and well-defined central pulmonary arteries in association with tortuosity, deviation, and diminution in size of arteries in the middle and distal third of the lung (2). It produces the classic ''pruned tree'' appearance of pulmonary vessels. Fortunately, this late stage of disease is rare in children.

Systemic Collateral Arteries

In conditions of severe right ventricular outflow tract obstruction, such as pulmonary atresia with a ventricular septal defect, there may be large pulmonary collaterals originating from the descending aorta. These large collaterals often have a bizarre pattern of branching (Fig. 6-7). Although collateral vessels are prominent, they are disorganized, frequently nonuniform in distribution, and have a stringy or reticulated appearance. They may be stenotic, branch abnormally, and take an abnormal direction. Because the pressure in the aorta is at systemic level, there may be significant flow in these vessels; this gives the false impression of increased pulmonary vascularity.

Asymmetric Pulmonary Artery Blood Flow

In addition to the size and position of the pulmonary arteries, one should assess the symmetry of pulmonary blood flow. Asymmetric pulmonary blood flow has several causes. Patients may have unilateral stenosis or absence of a pulmonary artery. There may be a unilateral increase in pulmonary arterial flow in children who have had a palliative systemic-to-pulmonary anastomosis such as Blalock-Taussig shunt. With pulmonary valve stenosis, flow may preferentially enter the left pulmonary artery, causing its enlargement due to the jet phenomenon. Unequal arterial size is also seen in patients with transposition of the great vessels, in which the right pulmonary artery is often slightly larger than the left. Unequal blood flow may occur in patients with truncus arteriosus, some of whom have stenosis of the origin of the left or right pulmonary artery.

Main Pulmonary Artery

After evaluating the right and left pulmonary arteries and their branches, one should assess the position and size of the main pulmonary artery. The main pulmonary artery should be border forming along the left superior mediastinum, at least after the thymus has lost its infantile prominence. When it is dilated, it becomes more convex. During infancy, it may be mistaken for the transverse aorta (aortic knob). A dilated main pulmonary artery is occasionally seen higher than or at the same level as the aortic arch (Fig. 6-8). The main pulmonary artery is dilated in left-to-right

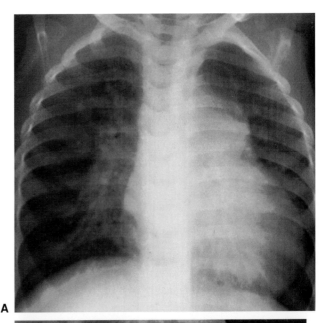

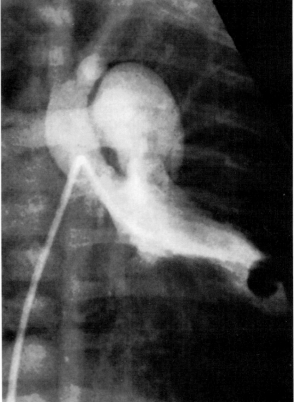

FIG. 6-8. Ventricular septal defect. A: Anteroposterior chest radiograph demonstrates cardiomegaly, increased flow, and marked enlargement of main pulmonary artery. **B:** Left ventriculography in RAO position demonstrates filling of both aorta and pulmonary artery. There is marked enlargement of the main pulmonary artery, which extends up to the level of the aortic arch.

shunts and in intracardiac mixing lesions such as single ventricle. Poststenotic dilatation is also seen in patients with pulmonary valvular stenosis. Patients who have pulmonary valve insufficiency also have a dilated pulmonary artery, as the regurgitant blood in the right ventricle adds to its normal output and increases the ejection (stroke) volume, which causes dilatation of the pulmonary artery in systole.

A small, concave pulmonary artery segment suggests that the pulmonary artery carries diminished flow or is malpositioned or absent. In patients with diminished blood flow, the main pulmonary artery may be absent (pulmonary atresia with ventricular septal defect) or small (tetralogy of Fallot) (see Fig. 6-7). In patients with transposition of the great vessels, the main pulmonary artery is rotated medially and the mediastinum is narrow because of the malposition of the great vessels.

Aorta

The position and size of the aorta should be carefully evaluated. In older patients the transverse portion of the aorta (aortic knob) is readily identified. Radiographic findings for determination of the side of the aorta include (a) an impression on the trachea by the aortic knob, (b) visualization of the arch itself, and (c) visualization of the descending aorta

(Fig. 6-9). In infants, the aortic arch and descending aorta are frequently poorly visualized, often because of the thymus. The side of the aortic arch is occasionally inferred from the position of the trachea. In infants, however, the trachea is sometimes in a normal position (slightly to the right of the midline), and yet the patient has a right arch (18). As the child becomes older the aortic knob is much more easily recognized. In older children with a right aortic arch, the trachea is almost always displaced to the left.

A right aortic arch suggests cyanotic congenital heart disease. The lesions commonly having a right aortic arch are truncus arteriosus (35%), tetralogy of Fallot (25%), pulmonary atresia with ventricular septal defect (30%), double-outlet right ventricle (20%), transposition of the great vessels (3% to 5%), and tricuspid atresia (3% to 5%) (19). Most children with vascular rings have right aortic arches or, in double aortic arches, a larger right arch. In patients with a right arch, the distinction between congenital heart disease and vascular ring frequently can be made on the lateral plain film; patients with vascular rings usually have anterior displacement of the trachea, whereas those with congenital heart disease do not (19,20).

The size of the aorta reflects physiology. The aorta may be normal, enlarged, or small. When the ascending aorta is large, one should consider poststenotic dilatation due to aor-

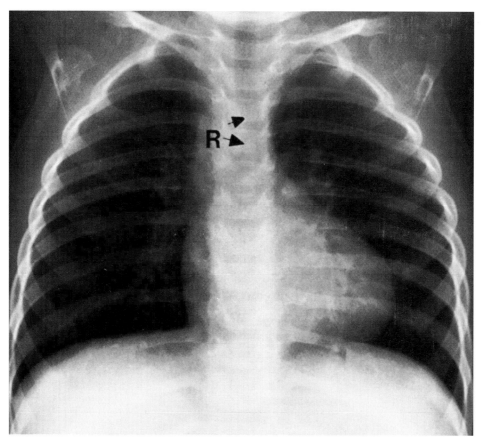

FIG. 6-9. Right aortic arch. Note the right lateral tracheal indentation *(arrows)*, displacement of trachea to the left, right aortic knob *(R)*, and the right-sided descending aorta.

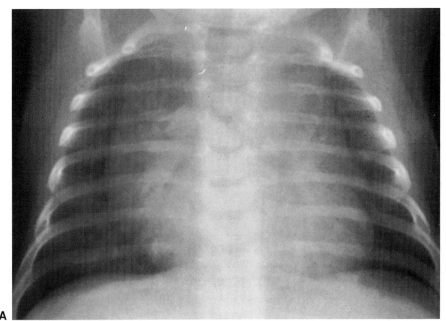

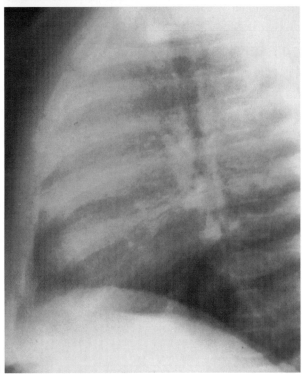

FIG. 6-10. Normal chest. A: The anteroposterior chest radiograph shows a prominent cardiothymic silhouette. However, nearly all of the silhouette is due to the thymus. **B:** The lateral film demonstrates normal heart size.

tic valvular stenosis, aortic valve insufficiency, and conditions with increased aortic blood flow. In patients who have severe pulmonary valvular obstruction and a ventricular septal defect (tetralogy of Fallot), the ascending aorta is large because the output of both the right and left ventricles enters the aorta. The ascending aorta may be prominent in patients who have extracardiac left-to-right shunts caused by patent ductus arteriosus, aortopulmonary window, or persistent truncus arteriosus. The aortic knob may also be large in patients who have coarctation of the aorta or systemic hypertension.

Heart Size

In young infants, assessment of heart size is often difficult on the anteroposterior radiograph because of a large thymus (Fig. 6-10A). The lateral film is more useful. On the lateral projection, one draws an imaginary line down the anterior margin of the trachea. If there is no heart posterior to this line, the heart is not enlarged (Fig. 6-10B). In such cases, most of the density seen on the AP film merely represents a normal thymus.

Compounding the difficulty of assessing heart size is the

degree of inspiration at which the child was radiographed. Even when the thymus is small, the heart frequently looks big on a film taken in expiration. On the other hand, there are severe congenital heart lesions in which the heart is truly normal or small. Cardiothoracic ratios are not usually helpful in infants and children. Comparison with prior films is often valuable.

Specific Cardiac Chamber Enlargement

Specific chambers tend to enlarge because of volume overload or distal obstruction. The atria may enlarge rapidly. Ventricular enlargement is due to hypertrophy or, more commonly, dilatation. However, determination of which chamber(s) are enlarged is almost always difficult and is often impossible. It is somewhat less difficult in older children than in infants.

Right Atrium

Right atrial enlargement causes a bulge or prominence along the right heart border on a frontal radiograph. Right atrial enlargement without enlargement of the right ventricle is rare. In patients who have left-to-right shunting at the atrial level, or left ventricle-to-right atrium shunting due to

a common atrioventricular canal, the right atrium may dilate. In newborns, massive right atrial enlargement may occur in pulmonary atresia with an intact septum or as part of the Ebstein anomaly. Mild prominence of the right atrial contour may also be normal.

Right Ventricle

On the frontal film, the normal right ventricle does not contribute to the contour of the heart. When there is right ventricular dilatation, clockwise rotation of the heart occurs; there is slight straightening of the left cardiac border and slight upward displacement of the cardiac apex. Right ventricular hypertrophy tends to cause more striking uplifting of the apex. On the lateral view in older patients, right ventricular enlargement causes filling-in of the retrosternal clear space. In infants and young children, accurate evaluation of right ventricle size on lateral views is impossible because of the thymus.

Left Atrium

The right lateral border of the left atrium can be seen on AP radiographs of 30% of normal children (21). Occasion-

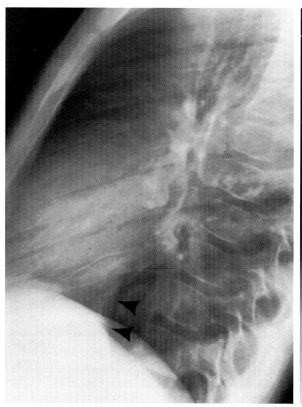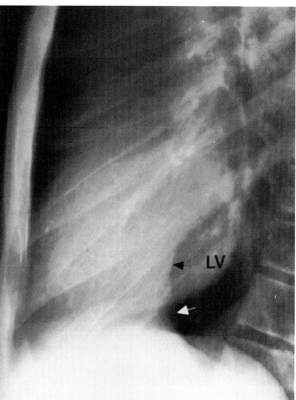

A   **B**

FIG. 6-11. Relationship of posterior heart border and inferior vena cava. A: Normal patient. The posterior border of the inferior vena cava *(arrows)* blends into the right atrium. The posterior margin of the left ventricle is not projected behind the inferior vena cava. **B:** Left ventricular enlargement. The left ventricular contour *(LV)* is seen behind the inferior vena cava *(arrows).*

ally, in young children, a normal left atrium is misdiagnosed as a mass.

Left atrial enlargement causes posterior displacement of the left mainstem bronchus and esophagus. On the frontal chest radiograph, left atrial enlargement may cause an extra bump or mogul in the left cardiac contour. In older children, it may produce a double density, a widened tracheal bifurcation, and elevation of the left mainstem bronchus. The causes of left atrial enlargement include mitral insufficiency, mitral stenosis, and left-to-right shunts (such as ventricular septal defects and patency of the ductus arteriosus) leading to volume overload of the left atrium. Prominence of the left atrial appendage may also be due to partial or complete absence of the pericardium.

Left Ventricle

Distinction between right ventricular and left ventricular enlargement is much more difficult in children than adults. Radiologic enlargement is almost always due to dilatation rather than hypertrophy. Left ventricular enlargement may produce a drooping or sagging appearance of the cardiac apex and increased convexity of the left cardiac border. The lateral film is useful; in normal children, there is little heart seen posterior to the inferior vena cava (Fig. 6-11A); however, with left ventricular dilatation or in cases of marked right ventricular enlargement with posterior displacement of the left ventricle, the left ventricle projects behind the inferior vena cava (Fig. 6-11B). Left ventricular hypertrophy is suggested if there is a left ventricular configuration (convex left heart border, downturned apex) in a child with normal pulmonary vascularity or evidence of pulmonary venous hypertension. Left ventricular dilatation may occur in cases of poor left ventricular function, mitral insufficiency, aortic insufficiency, and left-to-right shunts at the ductal level.

Extracardiac Structures

Rib Notching

Rib notching may involve either the superior or inferior margins of the ribs (Table 6-2). Superior rib notching is unusual in adults and extremely rare in children (22). Superior rib notching may be due to collagen vascular disease, resorption of bone in hyperparathyroidism, primary osseous abnormalities, neuroblastoma, neurofibromatosis, and previous surgery (22).

Inferior rib notching may be due to a primary abnormality of the rib or abnormalities of adjacent soft-tissue structures (arteries, veins, nerves). Occasionally, there is slight irregularity of the inferior aspects of several ribs in a normal child. The most common cause of rib notching in children, coarctation of the aorta, is caused by increased pulsations from

TABLE 6-2. *Rib notching in children*

Inferior rib notching (more common)
  Arterial
    High aortic obstruction: coarctation[a]
    Low aortic obstruction
      Abdominal coarctation
      Thrombosis
      Vasculitis
    Subclavian obstruction
      Blalock-Taussig shunt
      Vasculitis
      Pulseless disease
    Pulmonary oligemia
      Absent pulmonary artery
      Ebstein anomaly
      Tetralogy
      Pulmonary atresia
      Severe pulmonary stenosis
    Chronic lung disease
      Cystic fibrosis
  Venous
    Superior vena cava obstruction
  Arteriovenous
    Chest wall AV fistula
    Pulmonary AV fistula
    Neurogenic
      Neurofibromatosis
      Neurinoma
      Neurilemmoma
      Schwannoma
  Osseous
    Poliomyelitis
    Melnick-Needles syndrome
    Thalassemia
    Postoperative[a]
  Idiopathic
  Normal (minimal)
Superior rib notching (rare)
  Collagen vascular disease
    Rheumatoid
    Scleroderma
    Systemic lupus erythematosus
  Renal osteodystrophy
    Hyperparathyroidism (primary, secondary)
  Osseous
    Melnick-Needles syndrome
    Progeria
    Osteogenesis imperfecta
    Exostosis
    Poliomyelitis
    Radiation injury
    Marfan syndrome
  Neurogenic
    Neurofibromatosis
    Neuroblastoma
  Vascular: coarctation
  Postoperative[a]
  Idiopathic

[a] More common.

the posterior intercostal arteries, which run in the subcostal groove. In coarctation with high-grade obstruction, there is collateral flow from the internal mammary arteries to the intercostal arteries to the aorta below the obstruction.

Abnormalities of the Bony Thorax

Patients with congenital heart disease, particularly cyanotic disease, have an increased incidence of thoracic scoliosis (23). There may also be premature sternal fusion, resulting in a short sternum. A hypersegmented manubrial ossification center is seen in 90% of trisomy 21 patients under age 4 but also in 20% of normals (24). The VATER complex, which includes vertebral, cardiovascular, anorectal, tracheoesophageal, and radial or renal anomalies, is suggested by the association of congenital heart disease and thoracic vertebral abnormalities.

Previous Surgery

Bone and soft-tissue changes due to previous surgery are frequently a clue to the diagnosis of congenital heart disease. After thoracotomy, the ribs may be closer together, deformed, sclerotic, or fused. A left lateral thoracotomy is generally utilized for repair of coarctation, ligation of a patent ductus arteriosus, placement of a pulmonary artery band, and palliative shunting. In the past, the palliative shunt was always done opposite the side of the aortic arch; however, the use of a graft now permits performance of the shunt on either side. The presence of asymmetric pulmonary artery flow and postoperative rib changes on the side of the greater flow suggest the diagnosis of a palliative systemic-to-pulmonary shunt (Fig. 6-12).

Embryogenesis and Nomenclature

The simplified approach to cardiac embryogenesis and nomenclature presented here makes congenital lesions and terminology easier to understand (25–27). Initially, the primordia of various cardiac chambers are aligned in a primitive cardiac tube (Fig. 6-13). The primitive tube is fixed by the diaphragm inferiorly and by the thoracic inlet superiorly. The tube starts to elongate and bends either to the right or left side. When the tube bends to the right side, the right ventricle is on the right side of the left ventricle. This bulboventricular loop is called a D loop. When the tube bends to the left (an L loop), the ventricles are inverted and the right ventricle is to the left of the left ventricle (Fig. 6-13). In addition to bending to the right or left, the heart tube undergoes rotation on its axis. This rotation, clockwise or counterclockwise, positions the pulmonary artery either anterior or posterior to the aorta.

Situs

Situs refers to the relation of asymmetric organs (lungs, atria, liver, spleen, stomach) to the midline or sagittal plane. There are certain constant relationships between particular organs. Thus, the following four structures are normally located on one side of the body: the inferior vena cava, the liver, the right atrium, and a trilobed lung with its eparterial bronchus. The left atrium, descending aorta, stomach, and

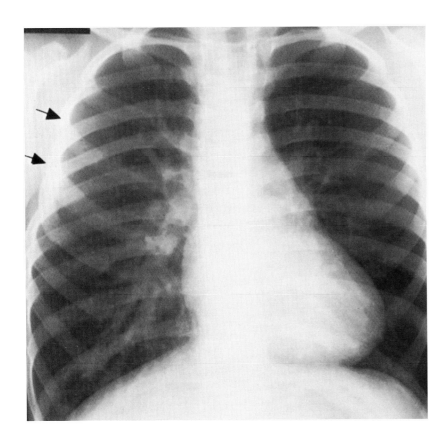

FIG. 6-12. Tetralogy of Fallot with right Blalock-Taussig shunt. The right pulmonary artery is larger than the left. Subtle postoperative rib changes *(arrows)* are due to a previous right thoracotomy.

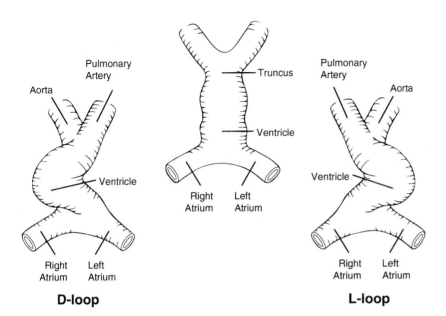

FIG. 6-13. Bulboventricular loop. The primitive tube *(center)* bends toward the right *(D loop)* or the left *(L loop)*. It then rotates in a clockwise or counterclockwise direction.

bilobed lung with its hyparterial bronchus are on the opposite side. Abdominal and chest radiographs suggest or indicate situs and provide insight into intrinsic cardiac anatomy and the probability of congenital heart disease (28–32). According to Van Praagh's definition of segmental anatomy of the heart (27), cardiovascular situs applies to the atria, the ventricles, and the great vessels. Situs may be solitus (normal), inversus, or ambiguus (Fig. 6-14). Plain films, scintigraphy, CT, ultrasonography, and MRI have been used to assess situs and associated cardiovascular anomalies.

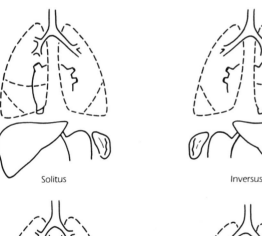

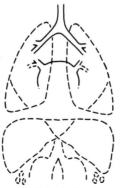

FIG. 6-14. Anatomic features of situs. The thoracic and abdominal organs are shown in situs solitus, situs inversus, and situs ambiguus (asplenia and polysplenia). The abdominal organs in *dotted outline* are variable in position.

Situs Solitus

Situs solitus is the normal situation in which the trilobed lung, inferior vena cava, systemic venous atrium, and liver are on the right, and the bilobed lung, pulmonary venous atrium, stomach, and spleen are on the left (Fig. 6-14). Although any cardiac anomaly may occur in situs solitus, the overall incidence of congenital heart disease is only 0.6% to 0.8%.

Situs Inversus

Situs inversus is the mirror image of normal. The trilobed lung, systemic venous atrium, and liver are on the left, and the bilobed lung, pulmonary venous atrium, stomach, and spleen are on the right (Fig. 6-14). This abnormality occurs in 0.01% of the population. The 3% to 5% incidence of congenital heart disease, although low, is much higher than in patients with situs solitus. The most common malformation is corrected transposition.

Situs Ambiguus

Situs ambiguus is an unusual condition in which the situs of the abdominal viscera and the atria are uncertain or indeterminate and the previously noted asymmetric structures tend to be symmetric (Fig. 6-14). Situs ambiguus suggests the presence of asplenia and polysplenia syndromes. In these situations, there is a tendency toward bilateral right-sidedness (asplenia) and bilateral left-sidedness (polysplenia). Although this tendency is a helpful teaching aid, it is not the actual biology. There is considerable overlap and variation between asplenia and polysplenia; they are two large subsets of anatomic arrangement among the many anatomic variations that can exist with situs ambiguus.

Patients may have bilateral left-sidedness (left-sided isomerism) or bilateral right-sidedness (right-sided isomerism). Remembering which side of the body normally has a spleen (the left side) reminds one that bilateral right-sidedness is associated with asplenia and bilateral left-sidedness is associated with polysplenia. Patients with bilateral right-sided isomerism or asplenia tend to have severe, complex cyanotic congenital heart disease characterized by decreased pulmonary blood flow. Polysplenia has less severe congenital heart disease characterized by increased pulmonary flow.

Tracheobronchial anatomy is one of the best indicators of situs (30,31). The elongated, hyparterial left main bronchus serves the bilobed lung; the shorter, eparterial bronchus leads to the trilobed lung. In many patients with situs ambiguus, there are associated anomalies of systemic and pulmonary venous return. The appearance of an enlarged azygous vein in the right superior mediastinum suggests the diagnosis of azygous continuation of the inferior vena cava.

Cardiac Malposition

Cardiac malposition is any inappropriate position of the heart, that is, any position other than left-sided in situs solitus. Cardiac malposition may represent cardiac displacement, developmentally abnormal cardiac position or rotation, or situs ambiguus.

Levocardia, dextrocardia, and mesocardia are general terms that indicate only the position of the heart in the thorax. They have nothing to do with situs or cardiac structure. Levocardia denotes a heart on the left side; dextrocardia denotes a heart on the right; and mesocardia denotes a midline heart. In situs solitus with dextrocardia and situs inversus with levocardia, there is discordance between the cardiac position and the situs. This discordance carries a 95% to 98% incidence of congenital heart disease, usually complex.

Cardiac displacement is a shifting of the heart by an extracardiac factor such as lung hypoplasia or lung mass. The displacement has been termed dextroposition, levoposition, or mesoposition, depending on the direction and amount of cardiac shift.

Inversion is an alteration in the normal lateral relations of asymmetric body structures so that a structure that normally lies on the right side (for example, an anatomic right ventricle) is situated on the left, or a normally left-sided structure (anatomic left ventricle) is on the right. This reversal of lateral relations (inversion) may involve the atria, the ventricles, the great vessels, or the entire body as in situs inversus.

If the morphologic right ventricle is on the right and the morphologic left ventricle is on the left, the ventricles are not inverted, and the heart has migrated from the right chest to the left chest in a D-bulboventricular loop (see Fig. 6-13). Conversely, if the morphologic right ventricle is on the left and the morphologic left ventricle is on the right, the ventricular inversion is due to an L-bulboventricular loop (see Fig. 6-13).

Heterotaxy indicates an abnormal arrangement of organs different from that of either situs solitus or situs inversus. It includes situs ambiguus. Abnormalities of bowel rotation and fixation are considered a particular type of heterotaxy limited to the intestines and have little to do with cardiac malposition. Malrotation should not be confused with the more generalized heterotaxy of asplenia and polysplenia, although malrotation may coexist with both these abnormalities.

A practical but simplified approach to the complex subject of cardiac malpositions is based on the classic works of Elliott et al. (25) and Van Praagh (27,33). Cardiac malposition due to extracardiac causes (cardiac displacement) such as skeletal anomalies, pulmonary parenchymal disease, or diaphragmatic abnormalities must be excluded. Dextroposition, levoposition, and mesoposition have an incidence of congenital heart disease that is the same as that of the general population.

Next, the possibility of asplenia should be considered. This entity is thought to be due to suppression of normal left-sided organ development resulting in bilateral right-sidedness. Asplenia should be suspected in any cyanotic infant with decreased pulmonary vascularity and a normal to slightly enlarged heart, particularly if there is malposition of the stomach, aortic arch, or cardiac apex. Hepatic symmetry or bilateral eparterial bronchi and minor fissures (see Fig. 6-14) in a cyanotic patient are diagnostic of asplenia.

The exclusion of situs ambiguus means that the right-left situs of the patient can be determined. The radiologic definition of situs should be confined to the position and type of the atria, the ventricles, and the great vessels. This method prevents confusing terms such as thoracic situs and abdominal situs. The liver and configuration of the tracheobronchial tree (see Fig. 6-14) may be used to determine the side of the right atrium (venous atrium) (25). The anatomy of the tracheobronchial tree is the best chest radiographic indicator of situs (2,25).

In summary, a practical approach to cardiac malpositions includes the following sequential analysis of the chest radiograph:

1. Determine the position of the apex of the heart. Exclude cardiac malposition due to extracardiac abnormality.
2. Evaluate the abdomen for position of the stomach, spleen, and liver. Consider the possibility of asplenia or polysplenia.
3. Determine the position of the atria (situs) by determining the anatomy of the mainstem bronchi and the position of abdominal organs (stomach, liver, spleen).
4. Evaluate for anomalies of systemic venous return or pulmonary venous return.

5. Predict the frequency and type of congenital heart disease based on situs and side of cardiac apex.

Echocardiography

Echocardiography is indispensable in diagnosing and treating newborns, infants, children, and young adults with congenital and acquired heart disease. This technique demonstrates anatomy, evaluates chamber size, assesses ventricular function, indirectly measures pressure gradients, and approximates ventricular afterload (34–37). Furthermore, its noninvasive nature allows for serial evaluation.

Two-dimensional echocardiography provides a real-time sector display of cardiac anatomy. It plays a key role in assessing global anatomy and ventricle-great artery relations. Although the M-mode echocardiogram is generally performed from a left parasternal location, two-dimensional echocardiography is performed in various projections: left parasternal, apical four-chamber, subxiphoid, and suprasternal notch. Each of these views is used for interrogating specific cardiac structures. As an example, the suprasternal notch view is most useful for evaluating aortic arch anomalies, such as coarctation.

A major role for echocardiography has been in evaluating newborns in whom the history and physical examination are often uninformative. Echocardiography at the bedside can establish the diagnosis of transposition of the great vessels and demonstrate the features of hypoplastic left heart syndrome. Major surgical repairs are often based on the information provided by echocardiography.

Doppler techniques provide hemodynamic data, measure gradients, and assess blood flow. Color Doppler sonography enhances diagnostic information. Contrast echocardiography is occasionally used to identify structures, detect intracardiac shunts, and assess flow patterns in the heart. Postoperatively, injecting contrast material into an existing left atrial line allows semiquantitative assessment of residual shunts and competence of atrioventricular valves. Although the pediatric patient has sonographic windows for imaging the heart, transesophageal echocardiography is being used increasingly as smaller transducers and miniprobes become available (38). Certain interventional procedures, such as placement of atrial septal closure devices, may be monitored by transesophageal echocardiography.

Intravascular ultrasound (IVUS) allows for in vivo imaging of vessel wall architecture with an ultrasound transducer mounted on a catheter tip. The technique helps to evaluate coronary vasculopathy after cardiac transplantation (39) and may be used to help define the pathophysiology of coronary artery lesions in Kawasaki disease (40,41). It is also used to evaluate the results of angioplasty and valvuloplasty.

Angiocardiography

The angiographic analysis of congenital heart malformation is based on the work of Arciniegas, Van Praagh, Elliott,

and others (15,33,42,43) whose contributions allow an orderly, sequential examination of the morphology, spatial relations, and connections of cardiac and vascular structures (Table 6-3). Connections, the linkage of one chamber or vessel to another, have physiologic implications for routing of blood flow through the heart. Relations refer to the spatial

TABLE 6-3. *Approach to angiocardiography*

Cardiac axis
  Dextrocardia
  Levocardia
  Mesocardia
Venous connections
  Systemic
  Pulmonic
Atrial morphology
  Right atrium
  Left atrium
  Atrial symmetry (isomerism)
Situs-atrial relationship
  Solitus
  Inversus
  Ambiguus (right isomerism, left isomerism)
Ventricular morphology
  Right ventricle
  Left ventricle
  Single ventricle with or without rudimentary chambers
Types of bulboventricular loops
  L-ventricular loop (inversion of ventricles)
  D-ventricular loop (noninversion of ventricles)
Atrioventricular connections
  Concordant
  Discordant
  Ambiguus
  Single ventricle—double inlet
  Single ventricle—single inlet (common AV valve)
  Single ventricle—absent right AV valve
  Single ventricle—absent left AV valve
Atrioventricular relations
  Parallel
  Criss-cross
Ventriculoarterial connections
  Concordant
  Discordant
  Double outlet
  Single outlet (aorta, pulmonary artery, or truncus arteriosus)
Ventriculoarterial relations
  Cross
  Parallel
Arterial relations
  Normal
  d-Transposition (complete)
  l-Transposition (corrected)
Additional cardiovascular abnormalities
  Shunt
  Stenosis
  Atresia
  Interruption
  Insufficiency
  Vascular anomaly

AV, atrioventricular.
Modified from Arciniegas et al. (15).

orientation and arrangement of cardiac and vascular structures. The use of axial views facilitates the identification of each of these components (Table 6-3).

Atrioventricular connections may be concordant (morphologic right atrium to right ventricle, morphologic left atrium to left ventricle), discordant (right atrium to left ventricle, left atrium to right ventricle), or ambiguus (atrial isomerism, atrioventricular [AV] connections neither concordant nor discordant). A single ventricle may have two atria and two AV valves connected to it (double inlet), an isolated connection through one AV valve (absent right or left AV valve), or a single AV connection through a common AV valve.

Ventriculoarterial connections may be concordant (right ventricle or outlet chamber to pulmonary artery, left ventricle or outlet chamber to aorta) or discordant (right ventricle or outlet chamber to aorta, left ventricle or outlet chamber to pulmonary artery). When the two great arteries, or one of them and more than half the circumference of the other, are supported by only one ventricle or rudimentary ventricular outflow chamber, the term double outlet is used. One great vessel (aorta in pulmonary atresia, pulmonary artery in aortic atresia, aortopulmonary trunk in truncus arteriosus) may be connected to the ventricular mass; this type of connection is known as a single outlet.

The spatial relationship of one great vessel to the other after they have emerged from the heart has poor correlation with underlying ventricular anatomy and relations (15). Associated cardiovascular abnormalities include (1) shunts, which may be at the atrial, ventricular, or great vessel level; (2) stenoses, atresias, or interruptions; (3) insufficiency of atrioventricular or arterial valve; and (4) vascular anomalies.

The first principle of axial angiocardiography is to align the heart in the axial plane (long axis of the heart perpendicular to the x-ray beam) (11,44). With rotation of AP and lateral radiographic equipment, this can readily be accomplished. The second principle is to rotate or angle the camera on its long axis so as to profile certain important morphologic and pathologic areas of the heart (11). Both axial alignment and rotation are accomplished by rotating and angling the angiographic cameras (12, 44).

The hepatoclavicular or four-chamber view profiles the posterior or inlet ventricular septum and the atrial septum (Fig. 6-15), separates the two atrioventricular valves, places the four cardiac chambers en face, and clarifies mitral valve-semilunar valve and outflow tract relations. The hepatoclavicular view involves angling the tube 40° to 45° left anterior oblique and angling it cranially 30° to 40° (Fig. 6-15). Lesions that are well demonstrated by the four-chambered view include posterior ventricular septal defects (as seen in atrioventricular canal), the AV valves, the atrial septum, and atrial septal defects. (Table 6-4).

A standard view to profile the interventricular septum is

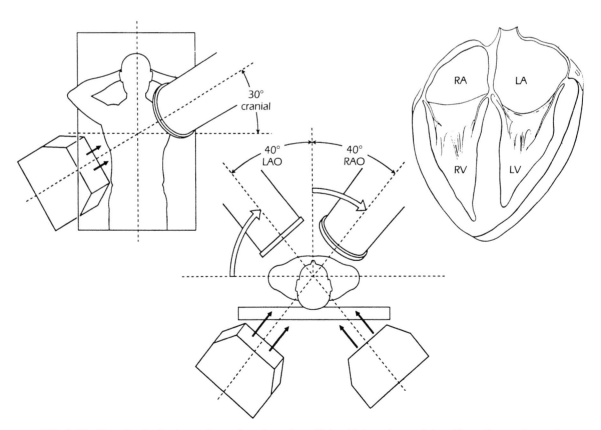

FIG. 6-15. Hepatoclavicular or four-chamber view. Using biplane image intensifiers, the posteroanterior tube is rotated 40° into the left anterior oblique *(LAO)* and 30° cranially. *LA*, left atrium; *LV*, left ventricle; *RA*, right atrium; *RV*, right ventricle; *RAO*, right anterior oblique.

TABLE 6-4. *Axial cineangiocardiography*

Anatomic view	Anatomic structures imaged	Specific indications
Four-chamber (hepatoclavicular)	Posterior ventricular septum	Posterior VSD
	Posterior leaflet mitral valve	
	Atrial septum	ASD
	Tricuspid valve ring	Straddling valve
	Pulmonary valve, annulus, trunk	Tetralogy of Fallot
Long axial oblique	Anterior ventricular septum	Conal VSD
	Left ventricular outflow tract	Perimembranous VSD
	Anterior leaflet mitral valve	Atrioventricular canal
	Muscular septum	Muscular VSD
	Left ventricle outflow tract	Transposition complexes
	Bifurcation of left coronary artery	
	Aortic valve cusps	Aortic stenosis
	Aortic arch	Aortic stenosis
	Right ventricular septum	Tetralogy of Fallot
Angled posterior view	Pulmonary valve and annulus	Pulmonary stenosis or atresia
	Pulmonary trunk	Tetralogy of Fallot
	Bifurcation of right and left PA	Aberrant left PA—sling

ASD, atrial septal defect; PA, pulmonary artery; VSD, ventricular septal defect
Modified from Bargeron et al. (11).

the long axial oblique view; the tube is angled 70° into the left anterior oblique and 20° cranially (Fig. 6-16). This view demonstrates ventricular septal defects, the outflow portion of the left ventricle, the aortic valve, coronary arteries, and the ascending aorta (Table 6-4).

Without cranial angulation, the main pulmonary artery is foreshortened and the origins of the right and left pulmonary arteries are not well seen. With 30° cranial angulation, the pulmonary trunk and branches are readily identified (Fig. 6-17). This angled view is used to assess pulmonary stenosis

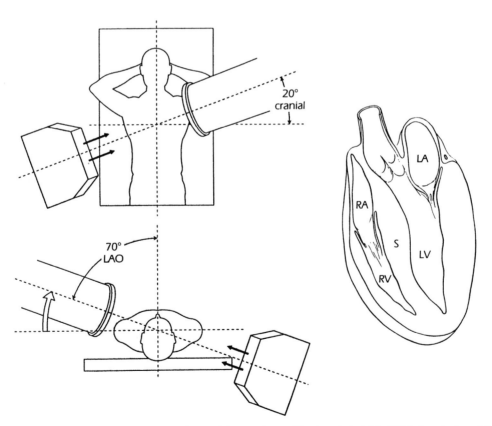

FIG. 6-16. Long axial oblique view. Lateral image intensifier is rotated 60–70° left anterior oblique *(LAO)* and 20° caudocranial angulation. This view profiles the ventricular septum *(S)*. *LA*, left atrium; *LV*, left ventricle; *RA*, right atrium; *RV*, right ventricle.

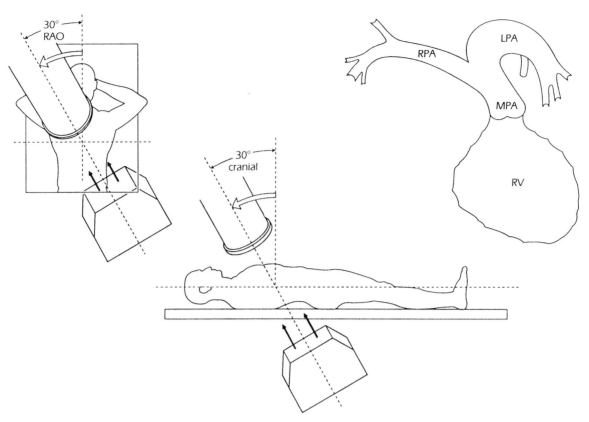

FIG. 6-17. Caudocranial angulation for main pulmonary artery and branches. The image intensifier is rotated 30° right anterior oblique *(RAO)* and 30° cranially. This view demonstrates the anatomy of the main pulmonary artery and its bifurcation. *LPA*, left pulmonary artery; *MPA*, main pulmonary artery; *RPA*, right pulmonary artery; *RV*, right ventricle.

or atresia, tetralogy of Fallot, pulmonary branch stenosis, and pulmonary sling (Table 6-4).

Magnetic Resonance Imaging

The role of MRI in evaluation of the pediatric cardiovascular system is evolving (45). Depicting the anatomy of simple extracardiac and complex intracardiac lesions is the most common indication for MRI of the heart (28,46–49). In some cases, MRI may replace echocardiography or cardiac catheterization. In other instances, MRI may add helpful information. In some patients, access to an adequate acoustic window is prevented by physical limitations such as obesity, chest wall deformities, hyperinflation of the lungs, sternotomy wires, and prosthetic valves; MRI may then be advantageous. Another advantage of MRI is inherent differentiation between flowing blood and the myocardium or vessel wall; this permits diagnosis without intravenous contrast material or ionizing radiation. Its multiplanar images provide three-dimensional information, which is particularly useful in demonstrating relationships of vessels and ventricular structures. Although cardiovascular MRI has focused on visualizing the anatomic components of specific lesions, there has been rapid development of techniques useful in evaluating physiology.

Current systems permit imaging with two basic pulse sequences: spin-echo (SE) and gradient-recalled acquisition (GRE) (50). Spin-echo techniques are used to assess anatomic structures. In this imaging sequence, flowing blood is depicted as signal void (dark signal), contrasting sharply with higher intensity vascular walls and myocardium. Gradient-recalled techniques generate images much faster. In these sequences, the cardiac blood pool is depicted as high signal intensity (bright blood) in areas of normal flow. Turbulent flow results in spin dephasing and loss of signal. Multiple images obtained throughout systole and diastole are interlaced to produce a cine-type movie. This technique is ideal for evaluating valve motion, flow phenomena, and ventricular function. Velocity-encoded cine MRI technique can provide simultaneous measurements of blood flow in the ascending aorta and pulmonary artery. Therefore, one can measure the difference between pulmonary arterial flow and aortic flow, and calculate the volume of left-to-right shunts (51). The role of MRS in evaluating myocardial metabolism is currently being investigated.

Cardiac imaging plane selection is best tailored to the individual patient and the information sought. In most cases of congenital heart disease the axial plane is optimal (46). To obtain adequate images one needs to gate the image acquisition to the patient's electrocardiogram. Echo-planar

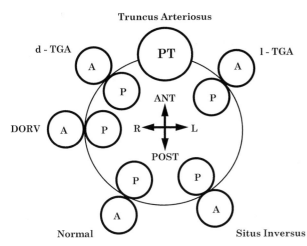

FIG. 6-18. Variations in conotruncal rotation depicted on axial MR images. Diagram demonstrating potential anatomic relationships between the aorta and pulmonary artery in variations of conotruncal rotation. *PT*, primitive truncus; *A*, aorta; *P*, pulmonary artery; *DORV*, double-outlet right ventricle; *TGA*, transposition of the great arteries. From Donnelly and Higgins (53).

MRI provides morphologic and functional data in a significantly shorter examination time than conventional spin-echo techniques.

Recognizing the position of the semilunar valves on axial MRI is key to distinguishing normal anatomy from conotruncal abnormalities. These abnormalities are related to abnormal division or rotation of the primitive truncus during embryologic development and include such abnormalities as truncus arteriosus, d-transposition of the great vessels, l-transposition of the great vessels, and double-outlet right ventricle (Fig. 6-18) (52–56). Developmentally, the primi-

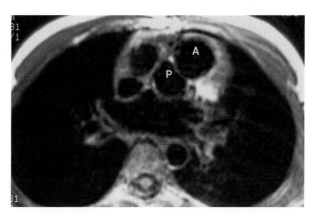

FIG. 6-20. l-TGA. The ascending aorta *(A)* is positioned anterior and to the left of the pulmonary artery *(P)*. From Donnelly and Higgins (53).

tive truncus is an anterior midline structure. With normal development, the primitive truncus first bends to the right; it then divides into aorta and pulmonary artery and then rotates in a counterclockwise direction. The normal pulmonary artery comes to lie anterior to and to the left of the aorta (Fig. 6-19). Variations in this rotation result in conotruncal abnormalities that are well depicted on axial MR images at the level of the semilunar valves (Fig. 6-18) (53,55). An abnormal relationship between the aorta and pulmonary artery is readily shown by axial imaging (Figs. 6-20 and 6-21). Because MRI is sometimes utilized in both the diagnosis and postsurgical assessment of complex congenital heart disease (45,46,55), an understanding of variations in aortopulmonary relationships is critical (53).

GENERAL ABNORMALITIES

The most common congenital heart anomalies, in decreasing order of frequency, are listed in Table 6-5 (2,7,9). The

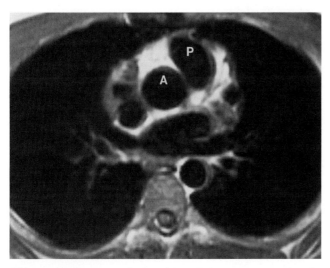

FIG. 6-19. Normal relationship of the great arteries in situs solitus. Axial image at the level of the semilunar valves demonstrates the pulmonary artery *(P)* to be positioned anterior to and to the left of the ascending aorta *(A)*. From Donnelly and Higgins (53).

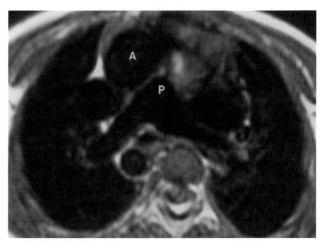

FIG. 6-21. d-TGA. The aorta *(A)* is positioned anterior and rightward in relation to the pulmonary artery *(P)*. From Donnelly and Higgins (53).

TABLE 6-5. *Incidence of congenital heart disease*

Diagnosis	Incidence (%)
Ventricular septal defect	29
Atrial septal defect	11
Secundum (7%)	
Atrioventricular canal (4%)	
Pulmonary stenosis	9
Patent ductus arteriosus	8
Tetralogy of Fallot	6
Aortic stenosis	5
Coarctation of aorta	5
Transposition of great arteries	4
Hypoplastic left ventricle	2
Total anomalous pulmonary venous return	2
Single ventricle	1
Tricuspid atresia	1
Truncus arteriosus	1
Hypoplastic right ventricle	1
Other	15
Total	100

TABLE 6-6. *Syndromes and chromosomal disorders with cardiac lesions*

Syndromes	Cardiac lesions
Alagille (arteriohepatic dysplasia)	Pulmonary stenosis (valvular/peripheral)
DiGeorge	Interrupted aortic arch, truncus, TOF
Ellis-van Creveld	ASD, VSD
Holt-Oram	ASD, VSD
Klinefelter	TOF, ASD
Marfan	Aortic aneurysm, vascular insufficiency
Mucolipidosis III	Valvular disease
Mucopolysaccharidosis	Myocardial infiltration, dysfunction
Noonan	Dysplastic pulmonary valve, hypertrophic cardiomyopathy
Osteogenesis imperfecta	Valvular insufficiency
Congenital rubella	Peripheral pulmonic stenosis, PDA
Sturge-Weber	Pulmonary arteriovenous malformation
Trisomy 13	VSD, double-outlet right ventricle (80%)
Trisomy 18	VSD, PDA
Trisomy 21	AV canal
Tuberous sclerosis	Rhabdomyosarcoma
Turner	Coarctation
VATER association	VSD, PDA, TOF, single ventricle
Williams	Supravalvar AS, peripheral pulmonary stenosis

TOF, tetralogy of Fallot; ASD, atrial septal defect; VSD, ventricular septal defect; PDA, patent ductus anteriosus; AV, atrioventricular; AS, aortic stenosis.

reported incidence of congenital heart disease, which will depend on the methods used for detection and diagnosis, has varied from a low of 3–5 per 1000 live births to 12 per 1000 live births (57). Children who are cyanotic or symptomatic come to medical attention and are promptly diagnosed, whereas asymptomatic patients with such lesions as minimal pulmonic stenosis or a bicuspid aortic valve may not be included in any series. Many newborns, especially prematures, have brief, self-limited patency of the ductus arteriosus. Echocardiography can detect small left-to-right shunts such as patent ductus arteriosus (PDA), ventricular septal defect (VSD), or atrial septal defect (ASD), many of which cause no symptoms and close spontaneously. In children shown to have congenital heart disease, 50% to 60% are diagnosed by 1 month of age (58). Left-to-right shunts account for nearly 50% of all lesions. The most common cyanotic disease is tetralogy of Fallot, although transposition of the great vessels is the most common cyanotic lesion of early infancy.

Many syndromes and chromosomal disorders have associated cardiovascular abnormalities (Table 6-6), and these are often quite significant. Occasionally, the cardiac lesion is the initial presentation of a syndrome or generalized illness. (Fig. 6-22).

Classification of Congenital Cardiac Malformations

Congenital cardiac malformations may be grouped into several pathologic, physiologic, radiologic, and clinical classifications. An important concept is that any malformation causes the heart to work against some sort of overload (Table 6-7). The overload may be caused by pressure, volume of flow, intrinsic myocardial disease, ischemic myocardial disease, or some combination of these categories. The most useful classification is a functional one that combines clinical, radiologic, and physiologic factors (Table 6-7). This

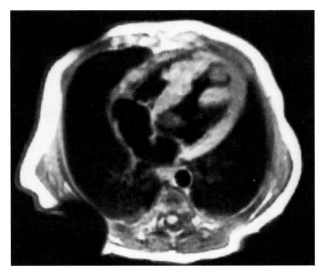

FIG. 6-22. Rhabdomyomas. Axial MR image shows several ventricular masses. A diagnosis of tuberous sclerosis was subsequently verified in this infant.

TABLE 6-7. *Classification of congenital cardiac malformations*

Overload classification
  Pressure
    Valvular stenosis
    Pulmonary arterial narrowing
    Systemic arterial narrowing
  Volume
    Shunt
    Valvular incompetence
  Myocardial disease
    Cardiomyopathy
    Myocarditis
    Infiltrative disease
    Ischemic myocardial disease
      Atherosclerosis
      Aberrant left coronary artery
    Combinations
Functional (clinical, radiologic, physiologic) classification
  Acyanotic with increased vascularity
  Acyanotic with normal vascularity
  Cyanotic with increased vascularity
  Cyanotic with decreased vascularity
  Pulmonary venous hypertension

Modified from Elliott and Schiebler (2).

classification, which combines the presence or absence of cyanosis and the radiologic appearance of the pulmonary vascularity, forms the basis for the differential diagnosis of congenital heart disease in children (Tables 6-8 to 6-11).

Cyanosis

Cyanosis—literally, blue skin—is an important clinical finding in patients with congenital heart disease. Desaturation is present when the arterial oxygen saturation is below normal (94% or less). However, cyanosis is not clinically

TABLE 6-8. *Acyanotic congenital heart disease with increased pulmonary blood flow*

Ventricular septal defect (VSD)
  Perimembranous VSD[a]
  Conal VSD
  VSD of AVC type
  Muscular VSD
Atrial septal defect (ASD)
  Secundum ASD[a]
  Sinus venosus ASD
  Ostium primum ASD
Patent ductus arteriosus (PDA)[a]
Atrioventricular canal (AVC)
  Partial AVC
  Complete AVC
Other shunts
  Aorticopulmonary window
  Coarctation syndrome (CA, PDA, VSD)
  Partial anomalous pulmonary venous return
  Coronary artery to right atrial fistula
  Anomalous left coronary artery from pulmonary artery

[a] More common.
PDA, patent ductus arteriosus; VSD, ventricular septal defect.

TABLE 6-9. *Acyanotic congenital heart disease with normal pulmonary blood flow*

Coarctation of the aorta (CA)
  Isolated coarctation[a]
Aortic stenosis
  Supravalvular
  Valvular[a]
  Subvalvular
    Muscular
    Membranous
Aortic insufficiency
Pulmonary stenosis[a]
Pulmonary insufficiency
Mitral stenosis
Mitral insufficiency

[a] More common.

TABLE 6-10. *Cyanotic congenital heart disease with decreased pulmonary blood flow*

Tetralogy of Fallot[a]
Trilogy of Fallot
Pulmonary atresia or severe pulmonary stenosis[a]
Isolated hypoplasia of right ventricle
Uhl disease
Tricuspid atresia[a]
Tricuspid stenosis
Ebstein anomaly
Complex cyanotic lesion with obstructed pulmonary blood flow
  Transposition and transposition complexes[a]
  Truncus arteriosus
  Total anomalous pulmonary venous return
  Tricuspid atresia
  Single ventricle
  Double outlet ventricle

[a] More common.

TABLE 6-11. *Cyanotic congenital heart disease with variable or increased pulmonary blood flow*

Variable
Transposition of the great vessels (d-TGV)[a]
Transposition complexes
  Double-outlet right ventricle (DORV type I)
  Taussig-Bing anomaly (DORV type II)
Single ventricle
Tricuspid atresia
  With transposition
  Without transposition
Increased
Truncus arteriosus
Total anomalous pulmonary venous return (TAPVR)
  Supracardiac TAPVR
  Cardiac TAPVR
    Coronary sinus
    Right atrium

[a] More common.

detectable until the arterial oxygen saturation is 85% or less in a patient with a normal hematocrit or when there is a reduced hemoglobin in arterial blood of 3–5 g/dl. With severe anemia (<8 g hemoglobin), cyanosis is not clinically apparent until arterial saturation falls to about 60%. There is obviously an intermediate zone in which the patient is desaturated but not cyanotic.

Cyanosis has causes other than congenital heart disease. These noncardiac causes include primary lung disease, pulmonary arteriovenous malformations, mechanical interference with lung function, primary pulmonary hypertension, poor ventilation because of central nervous system disease, methemoglobinemia, hyperglycemia, hypoglycemia, polycythemia, shock, sepsis, and severe neuromuscular disorders.

TABLE 6-12. *Pulmonary venous hypertension by anatomic level*

Distal to mitral valve—cardiomegaly
  Systemic
    Hypertension
    Fluid overload[a]
    Renal failure[a]
  Aorta
    Coarctation[a]
    Aortic stenosis
    Aortic insufficiency
    Aortic interruption
  Pericardium
    Effusion
    Pericarditis with constriction or tamponade
  Arrhythmia
  Myocardium
    Myocarditis
    Cardiomyopathy
    Endocardial fibroelastosis
    Glycogen storage disease
    Aberrant coronary artery
    Arrhythmia
  Coronary arteries
    Aberrant
    Sclerosis or calcification
    Periarteritis nodosa
    Arteritis
    Kawasaki disease
  Left ventricular tumor
  Hypoplastic left heart syndrome[a]
  Mitral valve
    Mitral stenosis
    Mitral insufficiency
Promixal to mitral valve—normal-size heart
  Left atrium
    Cor triatriatum
    Mitrial ring
    Atrial myxoma
  Pulmonary veins
    Atresia
    Stenosis
  Total anomalous pulmonary venous return with obstruction[a]
  Pulmonary venoocclusive disease

[a] More common.

Cyanosis is a sign of a wide variety of congenital cardiac malformations. However, the basic abnormalities include right-to-left shunts (tricuspid atresia, tetralogy of Fallot), mixing of systemic and pulmonary circulations (truncus arteriosus, single ventricle), right ventricular origin of the aorta (transposition of the great vessels, double-outlet right ventricle), and severe pulmonary edema (cardiomyopathy, hypoplastic left heart syndrome). The first three types allow systemic venous blood to enter the systemic arteries. Severe congestive heart failure with pulmonary edema interferes with normal oxygenation in the pulmonary capillaries so that desaturated blood is returned from the lungs to the left heart and systemic circulation.

The differential diagnosis of congenital heart disease presented is based on the presence or absence of cyanosis and the pulmonary vascularity as shown by chest radiography. Congenital heart disease is categorized as acyanotic with increased pulmonary blood flow (Table 6-8), acyanotic with normal pulmonary blood flow (Table 6-9), cyanotic with decreased pulmonary blood flow (Table 6-10), cyanotic with variable or increased pulmonary blood flow (Table 6-11), and pulmonary venous hypertension (Table 6-12). The pertinent radiologic features of the more common anomalies are discussed below.

SPECIFIC ABNORMALITIES

Acyanotic Congenital Heart Disease with Increased Pulmonary Blood Flow

Ventricular Septal Defect

Incidence

VSD accounts for 25% to 30% of all congenital heart disease and has a frequency of 1.3–3.5 per 1000 births (59). Most centers report VSD as the most common congenital cardiovascular anomaly if one excludes a bicuspid aortic valve from consideration. VSD may be an isolated anomaly, although it is the most common lesion associated with other congenital defects, such as coarctation and patent ductus arteriosus. VSD may also be an integral part of other anomalies such as tetralogy of Fallot, truncus arteriosus, and double-outlet right ventricle. A VSD is the most common congenital heart disease in trisomies 13, 18, and 21 (59).

Anatomy

The ventricular septum is a complex structure curving posteriorly and anteriorly as it extends from the apex of the heart to its base. Defects can occur in any one of the four parts of the ventricular septum (Fig. 6-23): (a) perimembranous; (b) muscular or trabecular; (c) supracristal or outlet; and (d) posterior or inlet. The symptoms, natural history, and

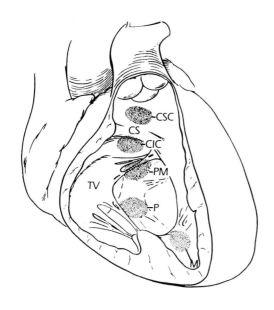

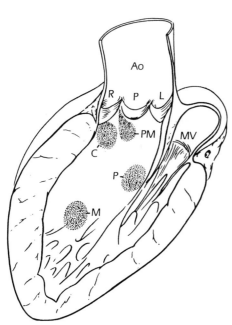

FIG. 6-23. Anatomy of ventricular septal defects. A: Right ventricular view. **B:** Left ventricular view. VSDs may be perimembranous *(PM)*, conal *(C)* opening above the crista supraventricularis *(CSC)*, conal opening below the crista supraventricularis *(CIC)*, muscular *(M)*, or posterior *(P)*. *Ao*, aorta; *CS*, crista supraventricularis; *L*, left aortic cusp; *MV*, mitral valve; *P*, posterior aortic cusp; *R*, right aortic cusp; *TV*, tricuspid valve. Modified from Elliott and Scheibler (2).

surgical approach vary according to the size of the defect, its site, and the pulmonary vascular resistance.

Perimembranous VSD (70% to 80%). These defects (Fig. 6-24C) involve the membranous septum but may extend to involve the inlet, trabecular, or outlet septum; therefore, the term perimembranous is frequently used. The defect is located beneath the anterior aspect of the septal leaflet of the

tricuspid valve and below the crista supraventricularis (see Fig. 6-23).

Muscular VSD (10%). Muscular defects may be single or multiple and small or large. They can occur anywhere in the muscular part of the ventricular septum. They may be hidden within the coarse trabeculations of the right ventricular septum. When multiple VSDs are present, the appearance is that of a "Swiss cheese" septum.

Conal VSD (5%). Conal VSDs are usually supracristal in location. However, because the ventricular septum is concave toward the right ventricle, a VSD that is anterior or conal in location on the left ventricular side may exit either above or below the crista supraventricularis on the right ventricular side (see Fig. 6-23). The upper border of a conal VSD lies beneath the right coronary cusp of the aortic valve; consequent lack of normal septal support may lead to aortic insufficiency. The aortic valve leaflet may prolapse and partially obstruct the ventricular septal defect. The left-to-right shunt is often not significant, but the aortic insufficiency may be progressive, and these patients usually require surgery.

Posterior VSD (5% to 10%). A posterior VSD is an atrioventricular canal defect and involves the posterior ventricular (inlet) septum just in front of the anterior leaflet of the mitral valve (see Fig. 6-23). It is discussed in the section on atrioventricular canal defects.

Physiology

The hemodynamics of VSD are determined by the size of the defect and the pressure difference between the left and right ventricle. In normal children, right ventricular pressure reflects pulmonary vascular resistance. Left ventricular pressure can be elevated when there is left-sided obstruction, e.g., coarctation and aortic stenosis. In patients with VSD's of small or moderate size, there is shunting of blood from the high-pressure left ventricle to the low-pressure right ventricle and low-resistance lungs. In some children, large shunts produce pulmonary arteriolar changes that increase pulmonary vascular resistance. This elevates the right ventricular pressure, which decreases the magnitude of left-to-right shunting. The Eisenmenger physiology, causing cyanosis, is due to a marked increase in pulmonary vascular resistance; pressure in the pulmonary artery becomes equal to or even exceeds aortic pressure, and there is right-to-left shunting at the ventricular level. The Eisenmenger physiology is now rare, as these defects are surgically repaired before pulmonary vascular resistance becomes irreversibly elevated.

Clinical Features

Symptoms and signs vary considerably depending on the size of the shunt and the age of the patient. In neonates there is relatively high pulmonary vascular resistance, and significant left-to-right shunting seldom occurs. When the

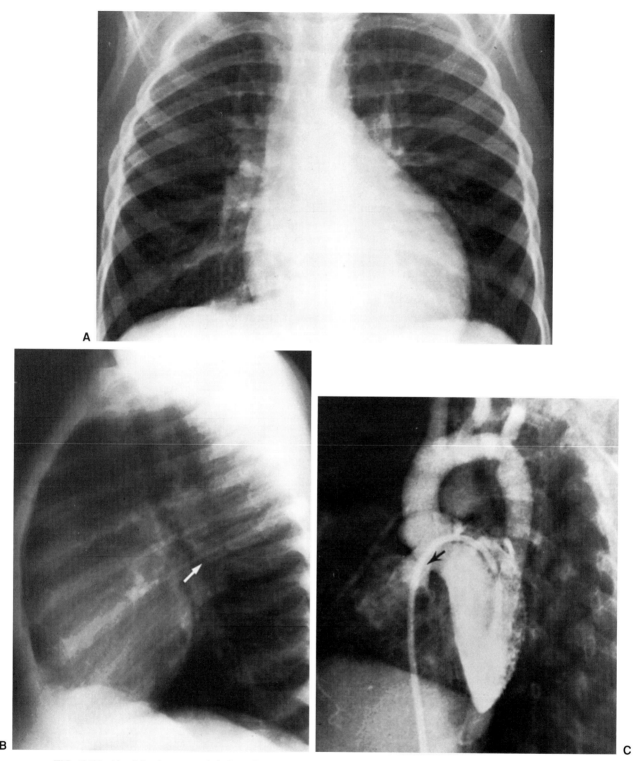

FIG. 6-24. Ventricular septal defect. Three-year-old girl with a heart murmur. **A:** The heart is large, and there is shunt vascularity. The aortic arch is on the left, and the lungs are slightly hyperaerated. **B:** Lateral film confirms hyperaeration and suggests biventricular enlargement. The left main stem bronchus *(arrow)* is displaced posteriorly because of left atrial enlargement. **C:** Selective long axial oblique left ventriculography demonstrates a large perimembranous VSD *(arrow)*.

defect is large, congestive heart failure tends to develop at 1–3 months of age because of the normal decrease in pulmonary vascular resistance. The lower right ventricular pressure allows left-to-right shunting through the VSD. The progressive left ventricular volume overload leads to congestive heart failure, dyspnea, sweating, tachycardia, and poor weight gain. A loud pansystolic murmur is best heard along the left sternal border.

Radiology

The chest radiograph in a child with a small VSD (less than 2:1 Q_p/Q_s ratio or 50% shunt) is normal; a normal chest radiograph does not exclude a small left-to-right shunt. In children with moderate or large VSDs, there is volume overloading resulting in increase in pulmonary blood flow and enlargement of the pulmonary arteries (Fig. 6-24). In infants with large VSDs, the main pulmonary artery dilates and broadens the superior mediastinum; in fact, it is occasionally mistaken for the transverse portion of the aortic arch (see Fig. 6-8). The peripheral pulmonary arterial branches are increased in size and more of them can be seen than usual. Because there is increased venous return to the left atrium, this chamber also enlarges. Enlargement of the left atrium implies that the shunt is distal to the atrial level (Fig. 6-24). However, there are many children with small and moderate-sized VSDs in whom the left atrium appears radiographically normal. Large left-to-right shunts may reduce pulmonary compliance and cause hyperinflation.

In 8% to 10% of children with VSDs, infundibular stenosis slowly develops. Infundibular stenosis increases the right ventricular pressure and therefore decreases the left-to-right shunting. This problem is difficult to diagnose radiographically, as cardiac enlargement diminishes and the pulmonary blood flow looks normal. The radiographic appearance mimics spontaneous closure of the VSD.

If the Eisenmenger physiology develops, there are signs of pulmonary arterial hypertension with prominent central vessels and a decrease in the size of peripheral vessels, producing a "pruned tree" appearance. The main pulmonary artery segment becomes unusually prominent, and there is marked right heart enlargement.

In summary, a small VSD is associated with a normal chest radiograph. Moderate to large VSDs have increased vascularity of the shunt type, an enlarged main pulmonary artery, left atrial enlargement, biventricular hypertrophy or dilatation, and a normal-sized aorta (see Table 6-13).

Echocardiography

Echocardiography and color Doppler sonography accurately assess both anatomic and functional abnormalities and occasionally supplant cardiac catheterization and angiocardiography. Cardiac catheterization is performed to quantify

TABLE 6-13. *Radiologic features of common left-to-right shunts*

Shunt	Aorta	Cardiac enlargement	Left atrium
Secundum atrial septal defect	Small	RV, RA	—
Ventricular septal defect	Normal	RV, LV	↑
Patent ductus arteriosus	Large	LV	↑
Atrioventricular canal	Small	RV, RA, LV	↑ or —

LV, left ventricle; RA, right atrium; RV, right ventricle; ↑, enlarged; —, normal size.

the left to right shunt, measure pulmonary vascular resistance, and characterize the anatomic defect.

Angiocardiography

Left ventriculography in infants and young children can usually be accomplished by passing a catheter across a patent foramen ovale into the left atrium and left ventricle (60). The long axial oblique view images the anterior aspect of the ventricular septum and is ideal for evaluating membranous VSDs. The posterior defect of the atrioventricular canal type is optimally visualized with the four-chamber view. In those patients who have anterior or conal VSDs, aortography assesses dilatation and redundancy or prolapse of the aortic valve cusps and the degree of any associated aortic insufficiency (60).

Treatment and Prognosis

Patients with small VSDs have an excellent prognosis and a normal life expectancy without surgery. At least 30% of all VSDs close spontaneously, and the small defects are the most likely to close (57,61). Closure of membranous defects occurs by adherence of a tricuspid valve leaflet to the septum or by ingrowth of fibrous tissue. During ventricular systole, the site of a closed VSD frequently bulges into the right ventricle. It is called an "aneurysm" or pouch of the ventricular septum and is part of the natural history of closing VSDs (62,63). In most instances, it is not a true aneurysm but represents a spinnaker-like anterior leaflet of the tricuspid valve that is fixed by fibrous tissue in the defect (64). Occasionally, the aneurysm is large and partially obstructs the outflow portion of the right ventricle. Complications of VSDs include recurrent pulmonary infections, bacterial endocarditis, congestive heart failure, and growth failure.

Surgery is indicated in patients who have significant left-to-right shunts, congestive heart failure, or progressive pulmonary hypertension. Many symptomatic children will require surgery during the first year of life. It is unlikely that large defects will close spontaneously; early surgical closure of large VSDs is associated with better long-term results and better left ventricular function (57). For most defects, closure can be accomplished by using a right atrial approach under cardiopulmonary bypass and hypothermia. A Dacron patch is placed on the defect.

Multiple muscular defects present a problem, as they may not be accessible for repair via the right atrium. An apical left ventriculotomy may be necessary. Success has been reported with percutaneous closure using small "umbrella" patches, obviating the need for ventriculotomy (65). Patients who have supracristal ventricular defects associated with aortic insufficiency also present a problem in management. The left-to-right shunt is usually not significant, but they may have progressive aortic insufficiency. When the VSD is repaired, the aortic valve leaflets may need to be plicated and repaired to prevent aortic valve damage requiring subsequent valve replacement.

Atrial Septal Defect

Incidence

ASD accounts for approximately 10% of all congenital heart disease (2,7) and is more common in females. It is often an isolated lesion. ASD is associated with several syndromes, including the Holt-Oram and Ellis-van Creveld syndromes.

Anatomy

Isolated ASDs are subdivided according to their position in the atrial septum (66). The foramen ovale is commonly patent, particularly in the neonate. This disorder, not considered an ASD, is a defect in apposition of the septum secundum to the septum primum. It becomes functionally significant only if elevation of pressure in the right atrium allows a right-to-left shunt through the foramen. An ostium secundum defect, the most common (60%) ASD, is a single opening 1–3 cm in diameter located at the fossa ovalis. Atrial tissue separates the edge of the defect from the atrioventricular valves. The location of the pulmonary venous ostia in the left atrium determines that the right pulmonary veins contribute most of the left-to-right shunt through ostium secundum defects (66,67). A sinus venosus (5%) ASD is located high in the atrial septum at the junction of the superior vena cava with the right atrium. It is almost always associated with anomalous drainage of the right upper pulmonary vein into the superior vena cava (2,66). An ostium primum (35%) defect, due to abnormal formation of the endocardial cushion, produces a large defect in the lower portion of the atrial septum. It is usually part of the complex malformation known as the atrioventricular canal defect, which is discussed later.

Physiology

Due to the defect in the atrial septum, blood passes from the left atrium to the lower pressure right atrium and into the right heart and pulmonary vascular bed. There is an increase in the size of the right atrium, right ventricle, pulmonary artery trunk, pulmonary arteries, and pulmonary veins. The left atrium does not enlarge, as some of the increased blood volume that returns to the left atrium is immediately shunted across the ASD. The size of the ASD has less effect on the flow of blood from the left to the right atrium than do the relative filling resistances in the right and left ventricles.

Clinical Features

Most infants and children with ASD are asymptomatic. The condition usually goes undetected until a heart murmur is heard. The increased flow of blood across the pulmonary valve produces an ejection-type systolic murmur, and the increased volume across the tricuspid valve results in a mid-diastolic murmur. The ECG shows right ventricular enlargement and frequently right atrial enlargement. ASD is the most common congenital heart lesion initially diagnosed in the adult. Among patients with ASD, the incidence of pulmonary vascular disease increases with each decade.

Radiology

In patients with small ASDs, the heart and pulmonary vascularity are normal. However, in the typical ASD of moderate size, the chest radiographs are highly suggestive of the diagnosis. The pulmonary vascularity is increased and of the shunt type. The heart is normal or slightly enlarged, and there may be prominence of the right atrial contour (Fig. 6-25A). The main pulmonary artery is dilated. Because of mediastinal rotation, the superior vena cava may be inapparent (68). In older patients, right ventricular enlargement is manifested by filling in of the retrosternal space. The left atrium is usually normal in size (Fig. 6-25B). In summary, a moderate or large ASD has increased vascularity of the shunt type, right heart enlargement, and no enlargement of the left atrium or aorta (see Table 6-13).

In all patients suspected of having an ASD, the upper lobe pulmonary veins and upper mediastinum should be carefully evaluated. The right upper lobe pulmonary vein is normally oblique. If this vein courses in a more horizontal direction, anomalous right upper lobe pulmonary venous drainage into the cava should be suspected, and the ASD may be of the sinus venosus type (2,67). Partial anomalous pulmonary venous connection may also occur to a vertical vein in the left upper mediastinum; there is an association between this type of partial anomalous venous return and an ostium secundum ASD.

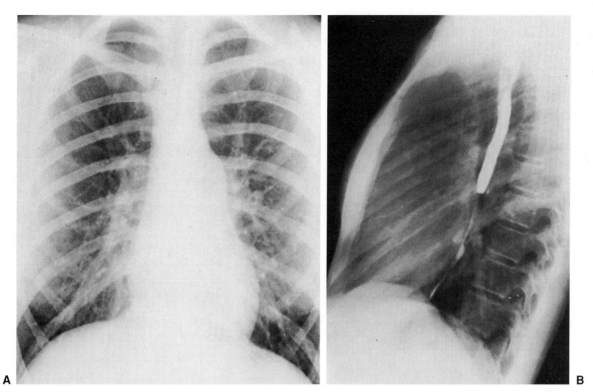

FIG. 6-25. Secundum atrial septal defect. A 14-year-old girl with a heart murmur. **A:** There is shunt vascularity. The heart is not enlarged in its transverse diameter, but there is prominence of the main pulmonary artery segment. The superior vena cava is not visualized. **B:** Retrosternal density is due to right ventricular enlargement. There is no evidence of left atrial enlargement.

Angiocardiography

Cardiac catheterization and angiography are seldom necessary to diagnose ASD, the clinical, radiographic, and echocardiographic features being so typical. Echocardiography has high sensitivity and specificity and furthermore is noninvasive.

However, cardiac catheterization is increasingly used for balloon sizing of the atrial septal defect prior to percutaneous closure. Several devices are available for transcatheter occlusion including the button device and the umbrella and modified umbrella occluders (69–71). Injection into the left atrium in the four-chamber view profiles the atrial septum and the size and position of the ASD. Transesophageal echocardiography is usually used during percutaneous closure; it helps define the site of the ASD and aids in the placement of the occlusion device (70).

In patients with ASDs, injection of contrast into the pulmonary arteries or right ventricle demonstrates mixing of contrast at the atrial level on the levo phase of the study. With the typical secundum ASD there is loss of the normal sharp inferior margin of the left atrial wall because contrast is shunted into the right atrium. Reflux into the inferior vena cava may also be evident. If abnormal pulmonary venous drainage is suspected, catheterization of a right upper pulmonary vein and injection of contrast may be performed. If there is a sinus venosus defect and an anomalous right upper

lobe pulmonary vein, the anomalous ostium into the superior vena cava is just above the defect. The four-chamber view profiles the atrial septum. An ostium secundum defect is in the midseptum; a sinus venosus defect is high; an ostium primum defect involves the lower part of the septum (66).

Treatment and Prognosis

The widespread use of echocardiography has increased the capability for diagnosing small ASDs. The clinical course and spontaneous closure rate of defects thus detected are not yet known. Spontaneous closure rates are related to the size of defects in children diagnosed under 3 months of age by echocardiography; there is 100% closure in defects less than 3 mm in diameter by 18 months of age (72).

Transcatheter occlusion with various devices is feasible, relatively safe, effective, and a viable alternative to surgery (69–72). Devices available for transcatheter occlusion include the button device, the umbrella occluder, and the modified-umbrella occluder (Fig. 6-26). Surgical repair is still the treatment of choice in many institutions. As an ASD is well tolerated in infants, repair is usually deferred until the age of 3–5 years. The repair is through a medium sternotomy and can be accomplished by suture closure or placement of a pericardial or Teflon patch. Postoperative dysrhythmias are common but transient. Major complications of surgery are rare.

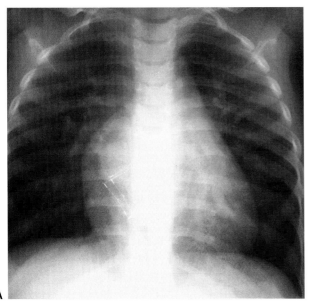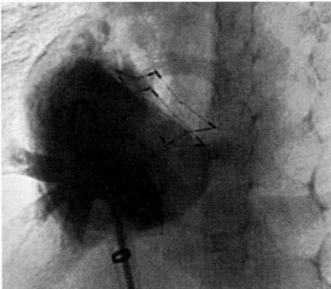

A   B

FIG. 6-26. Transcatheter occlusion of atrial septal defect. A: The chest radiograph was obtained following placement of a percutaneous closure device. **B:** Injection into right atrium shows device straddling atrial septum with no evidence of a shunt.

Despite relatively large left-to-right shunting, pulmonary hypertension rarely develops during childhood. If an ASD is unrecognized or not repaired, pulmonary vascular disease may develop in the adolescent or adult. Pulmonary hypertension and right ventricular hypertrophy result in shunting of blood from the right atrium to the left atrium, and cyanosis ensues. Most of these patients die of complications of pulmonary hypertension during their third or fourth decade. ASD is the most common congenital heart lesion causing pulmonary hypertension in adults.

Patent Ductus Arteriosus

Incidence

The incidence of a persistent PDA in term infants is approximately 1 in 3000. There is a definite female predominance. There is a high incidence of PDA in low birth weight infants (<1000 g) and in newborns with pulmonary disease. Approximately 45% of infants under 1750 g birth weight and 80% of infants under 1200 g birth weight have clinical evidence of a PDA (73). The incidence of PDA in term infants is much higher among those with trisomy 21, trisomy 18, and rubella syndrome. Infants born at high altitude and newborns with birth asphyxia also have a high incidence of PDA.

Anatomy

The ductus arteriosus, a vessel with a musculoelastic wall, extends from the origin of the left pulmonary artery to the descending aorta just beyond the origin of the left subclavian artery (Fig. 6-27). It represents the persistence of a normal embryologic structure, the sixth aortic arch.

Physiology

During fetal life, the ductus arteriosus shunts blood from the main pulmonary artery to the aorta and is about as large as those structures. Although the mechanisms for ductal closure are not fully understood, arterial oxygen saturation and vasoactive substances lead to vasoconstriction. The role of prostaglandins and prostaglandin inhibitors continues to be investigated. Prostaglandins E_1 and E_2 dilate an isolated ductus arteriosus, whereas prostaglandin inhibitors, e.g., indomethacin, constrict the ductus arteriosus and cause closure. Functional closure usually occurs by 24 hours of age. Anatomic closure is normally complete by 2 weeks in 35% of infants, 2 months in 90%, and 1 year in 99%. Autopsy data indicate that anatomic persistence of a PDA is abnormal after the third or fourth month of life (73). Normally, closure of the ductus begins at the pulmonary artery end, and one may see a small ductus diverticulum at the aortic end during infancy. In certain individuals, the normal mechanism for closure of the ductus arteriosus is not activated, and the communication between the aorta and pulmonary artery persists after birth.

In term infants, the systemic pressure rapidly rises above the pulmonary pressure, and blood is shunted from the aorta through the PDA to the pulmonary artery. Shunting occurs during both systole and diastole and is responsible for the continuous machinery murmur. This left-to-right shunt causes an increased volume of blood to pass through the pulmonary arteries, pulmonary veins, left atrium, left ventricle, and aortic arch. The aortic systolic pressure must in-

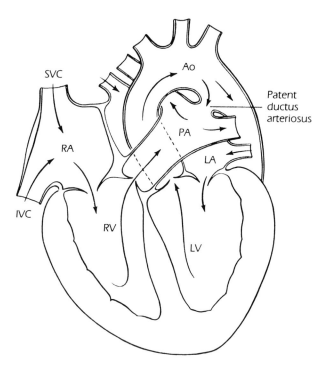

FIG. 6-27. Patent ductus arteriosus. *Ao,* aorta; *IVC,* inferior vena cava; *LA,* left atrium; *LV,* left ventricle; *PA,* pulmonary artery; *RA,* right atrium; *RV,* right ventricle; *SVC,* superior vena cava.

crease to compensate for the diastolic pressure decrease caused by runoff of blood through the ductus arteriosus.

Clinical Features

In newborns and especially in premature infants, a PDA is a common cause of congestive heart failure. During the first week of life, physiologic pulmonary arterial hypertension, worsened by hyaline membrane disease, other pulmonary diseases, and hypoxia, results in bidirectional shunting at the ductal level. As the pulmonary disease improves and pulmonary arterial pressures fall, left-to-right shunting occurs at the ductal level.

Small premature infants with a PDA and left-to-right shunt may not have the classic machinery murmur. In fact, no murmur may be present, or it may be heard intermittently. Evidence of left ventricular failure including tachycardia, tachypnea, and an increased need for ventilatory support may be noted.

Older children with a PDA have a machinery murmur and may present with congestive heart failure or failure to thrive. The increased systolic pressure and decreased diastolic pressure cause a wide pulse pressure and bounding peripheral pulses.

Radiology

Patients with a small PDA have no chest radiographic abnormalities. Moderate to large PDAs show increased vas-

cularity of the shunt type. The vessels and chambers through which blood recirculates are enlarged; there is enlargement of the main pulmonary artery, branch arteries, pulmonary veins, left atrium, left ventricle, and aorta (Fig. 6-28).

A punctate calcification in the ligamentum arteriosum is frequently observed on chest radiographs after spontaneous closure of a ductus arteriosus (74,75). This normal finding, an indication of ductal closure, excludes patency of the ductus. Dystrophic calcification, usually linear with a "railroad track" appearance, is rare in a PDA.

In premature infants, the chest radiographic diagnosis of PDA is subtle and is best assessed by evaluating serial films. A slight increase in cardiac size in a premature infant and hazy, ill-defined pulmonary densities (representing interstitial pulmonary edema) suggest a PDA.

Echocardiography

Color flow Doppler and echocardiography are now essential parts of the screening of high-risk premature infants with a possible PDA. They also quantitate the degree of shunting. One measures left atrial (LA) diameter and compares it to the diameter of the aortic root (AO). The normal LA/AO ratio in infants is between 0.8 and 1.0. A ratio of more than 1.2 suggests left atrial enlargement, which in the absence of left ventricular failure suggests a significant left-to-right shunt distal to the atrial level. Color Doppler analysis of velocity flow profiles in the main pulmonary artery quantify the left-to-right shunting at the ductal level.

Treatment and Prognosis

In premature infants, prostaglandin inhibitors such as indomethacin may be effective in closing a patent ductus arteriosus. When indomethacin is contraindicated, a surgical approach via left thoracotomy is performed. Suture ligation has on occasion been followed by recanalization and, therefore, the duct is usually divided. Video-assisted endoscopic techniques have been increasingly utilized in closing the ductus (76,77). In older children recent advances have been made utilizing a percutaneous arterial or venous approach to place coils in the ductus arteriosus (78,79) (Fig. 6-29). Small residual shunts are common immediately after coil embolization, but most close spontaneously (80).

Role of Ductus Arteriosus in Congenital Cardiac Malformations

Survival in many congenital heart lesions depends on flow through the ductus. Pharmaceutical agents that maintain ductal patency have improved the acute care of critically ill infants, particularly neonates. In some cases of severe tetralogy of Fallot and tricuspid atresia, pulmonary blood flow is dependent on left-to-right shunting through a ductus

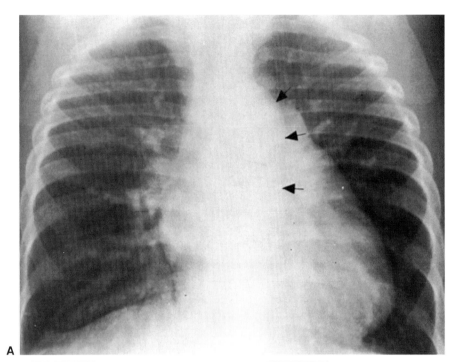

A

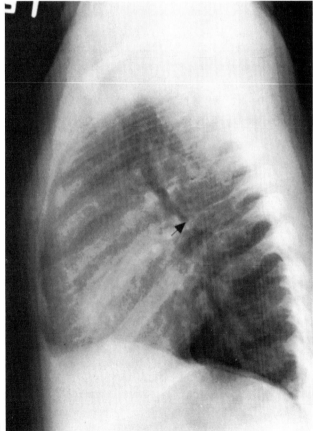

B

FIG. 6-28. Patent ductus arteriosus. A 13-month-old girl with heart murmur and bounding pulses. **A:** There is a left ventricular enlargement and shunt vascularity. The left-sided aortic arch *(top arrow)* and descending thoracic aorta *(lower arrows)* are both prominent. **B:** Lateral film confirms left ventricular enlargement and prominent pulmonary vascularity. The left mainstem bronchus *(arrow)* is displaced posteriorly by left atrial enlargement.

arteriosus. Prostaglandin administration allows vasodilatation of the ductus until a palliative shunt procedure or definitive surgery can be performed. In neonates who have interruption of the aortic arch, hypoplastic left heart syndrome, or severe preductal coarctation, systemic circulation is maintained or augmented by right-to-left shunting through the ductus arteriosus; rapid vasoconstriction of the ductus may result in hypotension and death.

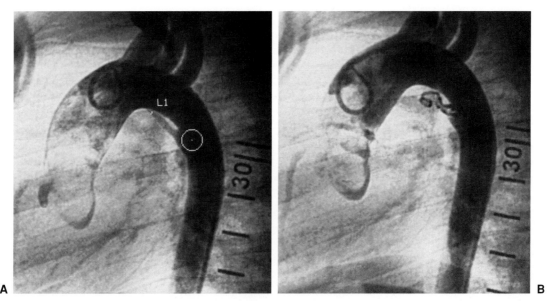

FIG. 6-29. Percutaneous occlusion of patent ductus arteriosus. A: Lateral aortogram showing left-to-right shunt through patent ductus arteriosus. **B:** Percutaneous placement of coil successfully occludes the ductus arteriosus.

Atrioventricular Canal

Incidence

Atrioventricular canal (AVC) defects are sometimes referred to as endocardial cushion defects (ECDs). Abnormalities in the development of the embryologic endocardial cushion tissue cause a spectrum of cardiac anomalies including primum ASD and complete AVC. AVCs represent about 4% of congenital heart lesions (2) (see Table 6-5) and are commonly symptomatic during the first year of life. They are the most common cardiac anomaly in Down syndrome.

Anatomy

The endocardial cushion tissue contributes to the formation of the ventricular septum, the lower part of the atrial septum, and the septal leaflets of the mitral and tricuspid valves (Fig. 6-30A). Abnormalities of growth and fusion of

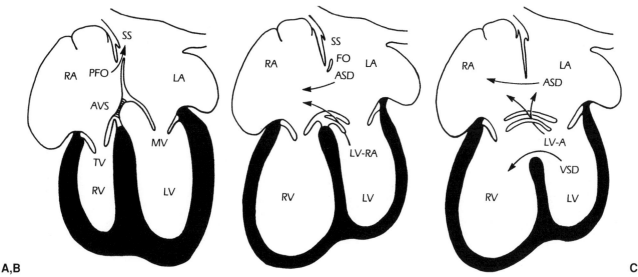

FIG. 6-30. Atrioventricular canal defects. A: Normal cardiac anatomy. Note the relation of the atrioventricular septum *(AVS)* to the mitral and tricuspid valves and to the left ventricle and right atrium. *SS,* septum secundum; *PFO,* patent foramen ovale; *RA,* right atrium; *LA,* left atrium; *TV,* tricuspid valve; *MV,* mitral valve; *RV,* right ventricle; *LV,* left ventricle. **B:** Ostium primum atrial septal defect *(ASD).* Arrows indicate location and direction of intracardiac shunting. *FO,* foramen ovale. **C:** Complete AV canal. Arrows indicate location and direction of intracardiac shunting. From Schwartz (82).

the endocardial cushions produce an absence of the normal atrioventricular septum and various anomalies of the mitral and tricuspid valves: low (ostium primum) ASD, high (posterior) VSD, cleft mitral valve, cleft tricuspid valve, and common atrioventricular valve (81–83). There is usually anomalous insertion of the chordae of the anterior leaflet of the mitral valve on the ventricular septum.

Ostium Primum Defect. An ostium primum defect is located low in the atrial septum just above the AV valve annulus. There is frequently a cleft in the septal leaflet of the mitral valve, and occasionally there is a cleft in the tricuspid valve. There may be left ventricular-right atrial shunting as well as left-to-right shunting at the atrial level (Fig. 6-30B).

Complete Atrioventricular Canal. A complete AVC, the most severe of this family of defects, involves the lower atrial septum, the adjacent part of the ventricular septum, and the septal leaflets of the mitral and tricuspid valves (82,83). The clefts in these leaflets are complete, and the AV valve leaflets are continuous across the ventricular septum. The anomaly may result in the formation of two common AV leaflets that extend from one ventricle to the other (Fig. 6-30C).

Isolated defects of the endocardial cushions may also occur and are considered part of the spectrum of ECD. They include an isolated cleft in the anterior leaflet of the mitral valve or septal leaflet of the tricuspid valve, an isolated posterior VSD, and an isolated ostium primum defect (82,83).

Physiology

The physiology depends on the type of AVC defect present and the extent of the anomaly. Hemodynamic abnormalities include shunting of blood across the ASD (usually present); shunting of blood across the VSD (large in the complete form); shunting of blood from the left ventricle to the right atrium; regurgitation of blood into the atria through incompetent AV valves; and development of pulmonary hypertension with elevated pulmonary vascular resistance. The progression and extent of pulmonary vascular changes in children with Down syndrome and complete canal continues to be debated (84–86). Some studies have shown a relative hypoplasia of the lungs, whereas others have shown no differences in pulmonary vascular changes between Down patients and normal children. In addition to AVC defects, Down children may have chronic nasopharyngeal obstruction, relative hypoventilation, and sleep apnea. Finally, any child with a large left-to-right shunt is at risk for progressive pulmonary hypertension and development of the Eisenmenger physiology.

Clinical Features

The isolated ostium primum type of defect rarely causes major symptoms but is detected because of a murmur. Clinical findings are usually those of a left-to-right atrial shunt,

occasionally associated with mitral insufficiency. The complete type of AV canal defect is characterized by large left-to-right shunting across the ASD and VSD. Symptoms include heart failure, dyspnea, recurrent respiratory infections, and failure to thrive. Patients tend to be small and undernourished with symptoms during the first year of life.

Patients with trisomy 21 (Down syndrome) account for 40% of patients with complete AVC defects. Conversely, 65% of patients with trisomy 21 have congenital heart disease; the most common clinically diagnosed lesion is AVC defect (33%), whereas the most common lesion at autopsy is VSD (40%). The complete type of AV defect is also seen frequently in patients with asplenia and polysplenia.

The most important clue to the diagnosis of AVC defect is the ECG. Left axis deviation occurs in over 95% of cases. First-degree AV heart block is also common (40%).

Radiology

With an ostium primum defect, the heart may be normal or only slightly enlarged. With the complete AV canal type, the heart is moderately to markedly enlarged (Fig. 6-31A, B). Enlargement of the right atrium is suggested by an increased convexity of the right border; the enlargement may be caused by left ventricular-right atrial shunting or left atrial-right atrial shunting. The pulmonary artery is prominent and the pulmonary vascularity increased. The left atrium is normal to markedly enlarged. This atrial enlargement, if present, is secondary to mitral valve incompetence. The aorta is frequently inapparent.

In a young patient with a large left-to-right shunt, one should suspect trisomy 21 and evaluate for other radiographic findings. Twenty percent of patients with trisomy 21 have 11 pairs of ribs; a second manubrial ossification center is present in 90% of Down syndrome children <4 years of age (24).

Echocardiography

The morphologic details including atrial-ventricular communications, valve abnormalities, the relative size of ventricles, and associated lesions are well demonstrated by echocardiography. In most institutions, cardiac catheterization is still performed to determine the size of the shunt and assess the pulmonary vascular resistance.

Angiocardiography

The four-chamber view is ideal for evaluation of the AVC defect. In this view, the anterior and posterior parts of the ventricular septum, the atrial septum, and the status of the AV valve are readily visualized. Left ventriculography allows distinction between an ostium primum defect and a complete AVC defect. Assessment of the degree of mitral

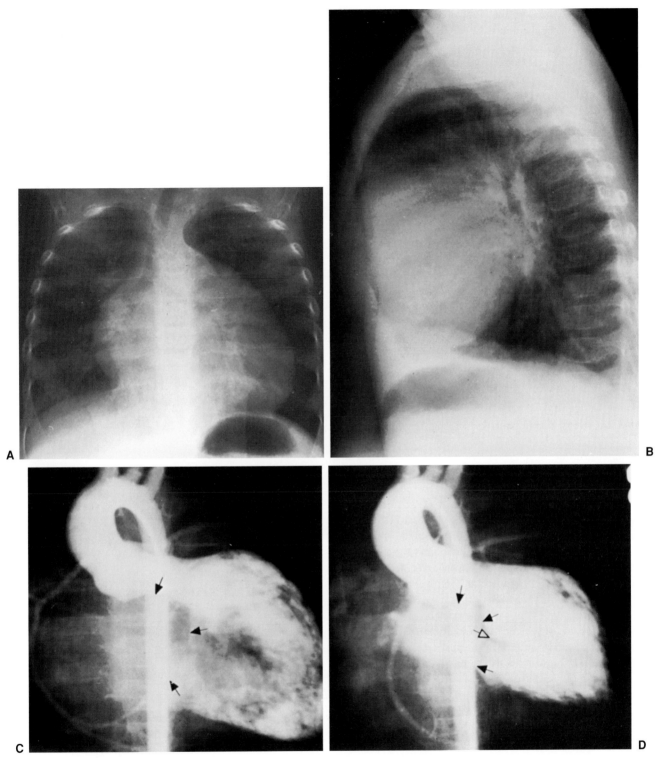

FIG. 6-31. Atrioventricular canal defect. A 20-month-old girl with Down syndrome. **A:** The heart is enlarged, the right atrium is prominent, and there is shunt vascularity. **B:** Lateral chest radiograph demonstrates enlargement of both ventricles and the left atrium. **C, D:** Selective left ventriculography during diastole *(C)* and systole *(D)* shows goose-neck deformity *(solid arrows)* of the left ventricular outflow. There is a cleft in the mitral valve *(open arrow)* and mitral insufficiency.

regurgitation and demonstration of a common atrioventricular valve is of practical importance; they both complicate surgical repair and increase the risk of operation. The 30° right anterior oblique (RAO) view demonstrates the classic "gooseneck" deformity of the left ventricular outflow tract; this deformity is caused by an abnormal attachment of the anterior leaflet of the mitral valve (Fig. 6-31C, D).

Treatment and Prognosis

In symptomatic infants and young children, early complete repair is advocated (87). Early repair may prevent irreversible pulmonary vascular disease and pulmonary hypertension. In asymptomatic children, surgical repair is recommended between 6 months and 1 year of age. For the complete AVC defect, a single patch closes the ASD and VSD; then the left atrioventricular valve is reconstructed. Occasionally, a double-patch technique is used. In patients with an ostium primum defect and a cleft mitral valve, the surgical approach can be from the right atrium. Postoperatively, transient arrhythmias requiring pacing may occur. Mitral insufficiency occurring after repair may necessitate valve replacement.

Cyanotic Congenital Heart Disease with Decreased Pulmonary Blood Flow

Tetralogy of Fallot

Definition and Incidence

The four components of tetralogy of Fallot are (a) right ventricular outflow tract obstruction; (b) large subaortic ventricular septal defect; (c) overriding aorta; and (d) right ventricular hypertrophy. Although the first anatomic description was made by Stenson in 1671, Fallot described the entity in a series of patients in 1888 (88). Tetralogy of Fallot is the most common cyanotic congenital heart lesion of childhood, accounting for 6% of congenital heart disease (Table 6-5). Unparalleled advances in clinical evaluation, angiographic techniques, and surgical repair of this anomaly have occurred over the past 50 years.

Anatomy

The two critical anatomic features of tetralogy of Fallot are obstruction of the right ventricular outflow tract and a large perimembranous VSD in the anterior conal septum immediately below the right aortic cusp (Fig. 6-23). The right ventricular outflow tract obstruction may be at the infundibulum, pulmonary annulus, pulmonary valve, main pulmonary trunk, right or left pulmonary artery, peripheral pulmonary vessels, or entire pulmonary outflow tract. Infundibular stenosis is almost invariably present and relates to anterior displacement or malalignment of the infundibular

septum (89,90). The pulmonary valve is usually bicuspid or unicuspid, and it is stenotic in approximately two thirds of cases. Supravalvular pulmonary arterial narrowing is often seen and is most common at the origin of the right and left pulmonary arteries. The VSD in tetralogy of Fallot is invariably large. The aortic root is anteriorly positioned and lies over the ventricles; however, mitral-aortic continuity is preserved. The overriding aorta permits flow from the right ventricle to cross the VSD and enter the ascending aorta. The ascending aorta is invariably dilated, as it carries the pulmonary venous return and a large part of the systemic venous return (shunted right-to-left through the VSD) (91,92). A right aortic arch is present in 25% of patients with tetralogy of Fallot and in at least 35% of patients with tetralogy of Fallot and pulmonary atresia. Coronary artery anomalies occur with some frequency (93). In 4% of patients the anterior descending division arises from the right coronary artery and crosses the right ventricular outflow tract (93). This configuration is important to recognize, as it may affect the surgical reconstruction of the right ventricular outflow tract.

When an atrial septal defect is associated with tetralogy of Fallot, the entity is referred to as pentalogy of Fallot. The term trilogy of Fallot refers to pulmonary stenosis with an intact ventricular septum and a right-to-left shunt at the atrial level.

Physiology

The severity of obstruction of the right ventricular outflow tract determines the amount of right-to-left shunting. If the obstruction is severe, there is little forward flow into the lungs and severe shunting across the VSD. The natural history of tetralogy of Fallot is that the infundibular stenosis progresses with increasing age and right-to-left shunting increases proportionately.

Clinical Features

The age at which symptoms begin depends on the degree of right ventricular outflow tract obstruction. Severe obstruction leads to presentation shortly after birth with cyanosis and dyspnea. With less severe obstruction, presentation is later. With mild right ventricular outflow obstruction, a left-to-right shunt may predominate (pink or acyanotic tetralogy of Fallot). However, because infundibular stenosis is usually progressive, there is an increase in right ventricular pressure and eventual right-to-left shunting and cyanosis. Polycythemia develops as cyanosis worsens. Tetralogy is frequently associated with other malformations including the VATER complex, trisomy 21, and tracheoesophageal fistula.

The ECG invariably shows right ventricular hypertrophy. Children with tetralogy of Fallot may have hypercyanotic episodes (blue spells) leading to loss of consciousness. Toddlers frequently assume a squatting position; squatting increases systemic resistance and diverts more blood into the pulmonary circulation and thereby an increase in peripheral arterial oxygen saturation. Patients with tetralogy of Fallot have an increased incidence of cerebral infarction, cerebral abscess secondary to right-to-left shunting, and venous thrombosis due to a high hematocrit.

Radiology

The heart is usually not grossly enlarged. However, there is frequently uplifting of the ventricular apex secondary to right ventricular enlargement. There is concavity in the region of the main pulmonary artery segment. The combination of an uplifted apex and a deficient main pulmonary artery segment leads, in middle childhood, to the characteristic boot-shaped or coeur-en-sabot appearance (Fig. 6-32). The pulmonary vascularity is usually decreased. Left pulmonary artery stenosis is common and may cause asymmetric pulmonary blood flow. The ascending aorta, carrying blood from both ventricles, is prominent. A right-sided aortic arch is present in 25% of patients with tetralogy.

Patients occasionally have asymmetric pulmonary artery size because of a palliative shunt into one pulmonary artery. The pulmonary artery may be larger on the side of the thoracotomy, which can be recognized by subtle postoperative rib changes (see Fig. 6-12).

Echocardiography

Angiocardiography and echocardiography are complementary imaging techniques in tetralogy of Fallot. In infants with severe tetralogy, palliative shunts may be performed on the basis of echocardiography alone. Echocardiography demonstrates the ventricular septal defect, the right ventricular outflow tract obstruction, and the degree of aortic overriding. However, angiography demonstrates details of the anatomy of the pulmonary arterial tree, coronary arteries, and collateral blood flow to the lungs.

Angiocardiography

Biplane ventriculography in the four-chamber view demonstrates the sites of outflow tract obstruction and the potential sites of obstruction in the pulmonary arteries (Fig. 6-33A) (94). It also identifies the precise location of the VSD and relation of the aorta to the ventricular septum (Fig. 6-33B). Frequently, a main pulmonary artery injection is performed with cranial angulation to better define the pulmonary artery and its branches. Coronary artery anatomy needs to be defined by echocardiography or coronary angiography so that anomalies will be known prior to surgical repair.

Magnetic Resonance Imaging

In patients with pulmonary atresia and ventricular septal defect and in patients with tetralogy of Fallot, the status of the central pulmonary arteries will affect both palliative treatment and definitive surgical correction (95). Delineation of the main, right, and left pulmonary arteries, and assess-

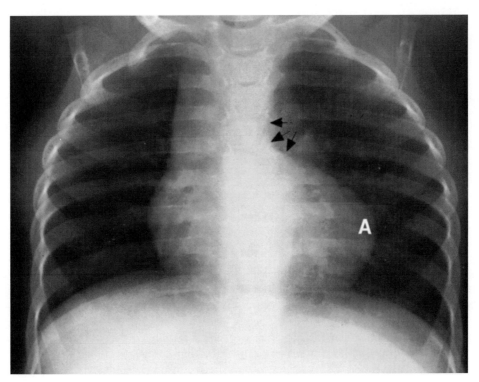

FIG. 6-32. Tetralogy of Fallot. The heart is not enlarged. There is an upturned cardiac apex *(A)*, concave main pulmonary artery segment *(arrows)*, and decreased pulmonary arterial blood flow.

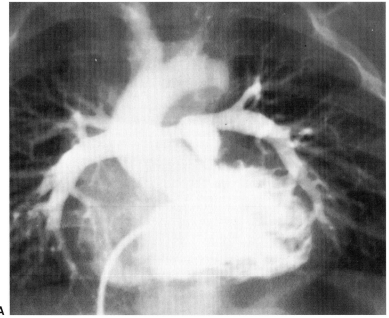

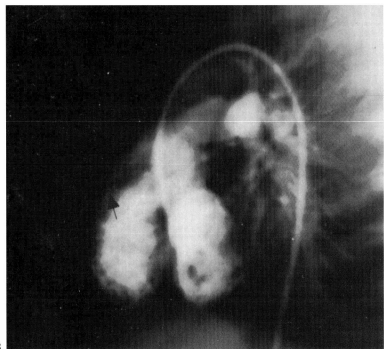

FIG. 6-33. Tetralogy of Fallot. A: Right ventriculography demonstrates multiple sites of right ventricular outflow tract obstruction. There is infundibular stenosis, pulmonary valve stenosis, and stenosis of the origin of the right pulmonary artery. **B:** Left ventriculography shows a high ventricular septal defect and infundibular stenosis *(arrow)*; the ascending aorta overrides the interventricular septum.

ment of aortopulmonary (bronchial) collateral flow is critical information. On occasion, echocardiography and angiography fail to identify a distinct pulmonary arterial confluence (bifurcation), particularly when the proximal right and left branches are extremely hypoplastic. In patients with focal pulmonary artery stenoses central to the hila, MRI may be useful as a map for angioplasty. In the case of dilated pulmonary arteries (absent pulmonary valve), MRI determines the nature and extent of airway compression (28).

Axial planes are usually optimal for evaluating the pulmonary outflow tract (Fig. 6-34). After sagittal, T1-weighted, gated images have been obtained for localization, the plane of the main pulmonary artery is determined. Three- to four-millimeter-thick scans are then obtained through this region. On occasion, two sets of offset (by 1 mm) scans may be useful in confirming the presence of small or atretic pulmonary arteries. Collaterals arising from the descending aorta and surgically created palliative shunts are usually best imaged in a coronal or coronal oblique plane (Fig. 6-35). The large subaortic ventricular septal defect can be visualized with MRI, although this information is readily obtainable by echocardiography and MRI depiction is usually not sig-

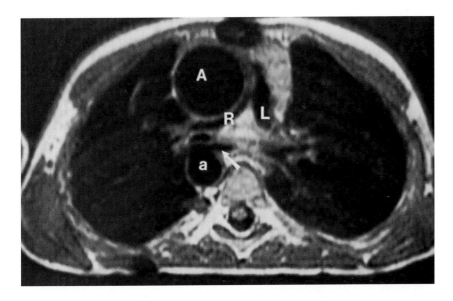

FIG. 6-34. Tetralogy of Fallot. Transaxial MRI through the pulmonary outflow tract. Note the small right pulmonary artery *(R)* and larger but still diminutive left pulmonary artery *(L)*. The asymmetry is due to a previous left Blalock-Taussig shunt. Note also the very large right-sided aortic arch *(A)* and the prominent bronchial collateral vessel *(arrow)* arising from the anterior aspect of the descending aorta *(a)*. From Bisset (28).

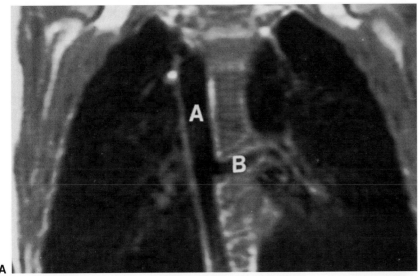

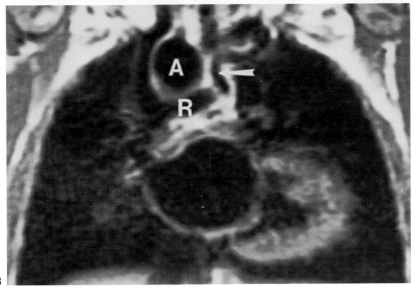

FIG. 6-35 A, B. Tetralogy of Fallot. Sequential, coronal MRI images through the descending aorta and aortic arch. A large bronchial collateral vessel *(B)* supplies blood to the left lung. A Blalock-Taussig shunt *(arrow)* supplies blood to the right pulmonary artery *(R)*. The aortic arch *(A)* is on the right. From Bisset (28).

nificant in the planning of the surgical repair. Additionally, MRI may be used to follow the growth of small pulmonary arteries after a palliative shunt procedure.

Treatment and Prognosis

A landmark in operative palliation occurred at the Johns Hopkins Hospital in 1944 and was based on the technical skills of Dr. Alfred Blalock and the ideas of Dr. Helen Taussig. The Blalock-Taussig shunt is named for their efforts. The innominate artery (later the subclavian artery) was connected to a pulmonary artery, thereby providing additional blood flow to the oligemic lung. Currently, instead of sacrificing a subclavian artery, a synthetic graft is inserted between the subclavian artery and the right or left pulmonary artery. The term *Blalock-Taussig anastomosis* now refers to any surgical connection between the subclavian artery and the pulmonary artery. Palliation is indicated in patients who are symptomatic but are not good candidates for total repair. There is evidence that the pulmonary annulus and pulmonary arteries grow after a Blalock-Taussig shunt, and this makes later definitive repair easier. However, the Blalock-Taussig shunt also may cause stenosis at the anastomotic site; this distorts the pulmonary artery and causes difficulty during the definitive repair.

Although biventricular correction of tetralogy of Fallot has been performed for over four decades, the optimal timing of repair continues to be debated as surgical techniques are progressively refined. Primary repair is increasingly being performed, even in neonates, at the time of diagnosis; this obviates the need for a palliative shunt (96–99). Shunt complications are thus prevented and the incidence of ventricular arrhythmia may be reduced. Risk factors in early surgical repair include small size of the patient, multiple areas of stenosis, small pulmonary arteries, and extracardiac malformations. Definitive surgery includes closing the VSD, removing infundibular muscle causing the obstruction, and inserting either a transannular patch or an external conduit to relieve obstruction between the right ventricle and the main pulmonary artery (100). Late postoperative arrhythmias and right ventricular dysfunction occur after classic repairs, and some advocate the atrial approach or transpulmonary repair rather than ventriculotomy. Closure of any previous palliative shunt must also be performed. Residual right ventricular outflow tract obstruction, pulmonary valve insufficiency, or both may be present after operation. Cardiomegaly following total repair suggests that the patient has right ventricular outflow insufficiency, tricuspid insufficiency, or chronic hypoxic cardiomyopathy leading to right ventricular dysfunction. Reoperation is necessary when there is significant right ventricular outflow obstruction. Most patients have no late complications after surgical repair (101).

Pulmonary Atresia with Ventricular Septal Defect

Definition

Pulmonary atresia with VSD is usually considered a severe form of tetralogy of Fallot. It is also referred to as pseudotruncus and truncus arteriosus type IV. With this entity there is no forward flow from the right ventricle into the main pulmonary artery. Usually there is hypoplasia or atresia of the main pulmonary artery; the atresia may interrupt continuity between the right and left pulmonary arteries. Lack of connection between the right and left pulmonary arteries is termed nonconfluence.

Anatomy

There is absence of luminal continuity between the right ventricle and the pulmonary arteries. Blood supply to the lungs is derived entirely from the systemic arterial circulation. Sources of this collateral supply include the ductus arteriosus, systemic collateral arteries, and networks of bronchial or pleural arteries. The complex patterns of intrapulmonary arterial anatomy have profound surgical implications and are important to define. The most favorable pattern is, beyond the atresia, a large patent ductus arteriosus with pulmonary arteries of nearly normal size. The most difficult patients are those in whom the ductus arteriosus is not patent, the central pulmonary arteries are diminutive or absent, and blood flow to the lungs is by multiple small aortopulmonary collaterals.

Other features of tetralogy of Fallot, such as large outlet VSD, right ventricular hypertrophy, and overriding of the aorta, are present. The ascending aorta is markedly dilated.

Clinical Features

Most affected infants are hypoxic and cyanotic. If the infant does not have adequate systemic collateral vessels, spontaneous closure of the ductus will produce severe hypoxemia and cyanosis. Some patients have such large systemic pulmonary collaterals that they are not cyanotic.

Radiology

The heart is enlarged and often has a prominent upturned apex secondary to right ventricular hypertrophy (Fig. 6-36). There is marked concavity in the region of the main pulmonary artery segment because of underdevelopment of the infundibulum and main pulmonary artery. The dilated aorta is right-sided in approximately 30% of patients (Fig. 6-36). Pulmonary vascular markings have an unusual reticular appearance because of abnormal branching; occasionally these collaterals give the impression, usually false, of increased pulmonary blood flow.

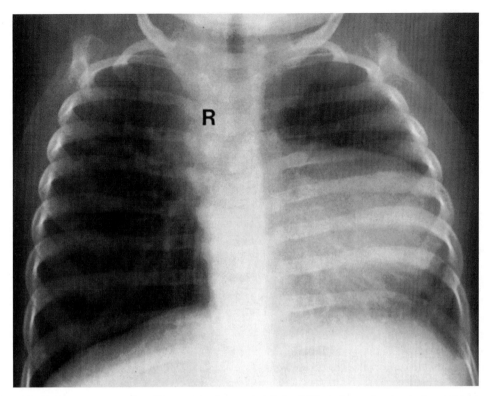

FIG. 6-36. Pulmonary atresia with ventricular septal defect. There is moderate cardiac enlargement, an uplifted apex, a large right aortic arch *(R)*, and a diminutive pulmonary arterial pattern.

MRI has been used to evaluate confluence versus nonconfluence and the size and origin of the pulmonary arteries (see Fig. 6-34).

Angiocardiography

The major purpose of angiography is to define pulmonary blood flow. In severe tetralogy there may be multiple collaterals including branches of the subclavian and internal mammary arteries, bronchial collaterals, and major aorto-pulmonary collaterals. Aortic-pulmonary collaterals can be visualized by selective injection or aortography. In infants, a balloon occlusion aortogram can be performed to define the aortic pulmonary collaterals (Fig. 6-37).

Treatment and Prognosis

Many patients with hypoplastic, nonconfluent pulmonary arteries are not amenable to single-stage repair and will require several surgical procedures. Forward flow from the right ventricle to the pulmonary artery should be established if this is feasible. The ventricular septal defect is left open. If the patient has multiple branch pulmonary artery stenoses, these can be treated by serial percutaneous balloon dilatations (102). When there are several collaterals from the descending aorta, surgical procedures to connect the collaterals to a true pulmonary artery (unifocalization) are attempted.

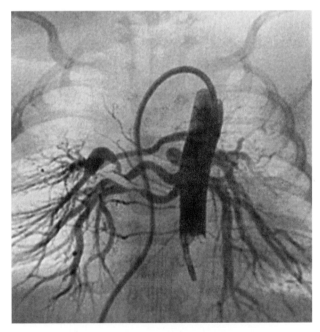

FIG. 6-37. Major aortic pulmonary collaterals. A balloon occlusion aortogram in an infant demonstrates collateral vessels from the descending aorta; they have multiple stenoses and marked tortuosity. The catheter courses through the right atrium, right ventricle, VSD, and ascending aorta to the descending aorta.

The preliminary procedures are then followed by repair of the right ventricular outflow tract obstruction and closure of the VSD.

Tricuspid Atresia

Incidence

Tricuspid atresia accounts for about 1% of all congenital heart disease (2,7,57). It can be an isolated anomaly, but in 30% of the cases there are associated abnormalities, including transposition of the great vessels. Only tricuspid atresia with normally related great vessels will be discussed.

Definition and Anatomy

In tricuspid atresia there is complete agenesis of the tricuspid valve and no direct communication between the right atrium and right ventricle (Fig. 6-38). There is an obligatory right-to-left shunt at the atrial level, usually associated with hypoplasia of the right ventricle and communication between the systemic and pulmonary circulations via a VSD or a PDA.

Physiology

As there is no forward flow from the right atrium to the right ventricle, there must be a right-to-left shunt through a patent foramen ovale (80%), a secundum ASD, or, rarely, a primum ASD. Blood flows from the right atrium to the left atrium and into the left ventricle (Fig. 6-38). Depending on whether there are normally positioned great vessels (70%), complete transposition of the great vessels (d-TGV; 25%), or corrected transposition of the great vessels (l-TGV; 5%), blood enters a great vessel. Frequently a VSD is present, but its left-to-right shunt may progressively diminish and this further reduces pulmonary blood flow.

Clinical Features

More than 50% of patients with tricuspid atresia present with cyanosis on the first day of life. The ECG usually shows left axis deviation, left ventricular hypertrophy, and right atrial enlargement. The presence of left ventricular hypertrophy in a cyanotic neonate suggests tricuspid atresia. Extracardiac anomalies are present in 20% of patients; they particularly involve the gastrointestinal and musculoskeletal systems.

Radiology

The chest radiograph demonstrates a normal or small heart and decreased pulmonary blood flow (Fig. 6-39A). There is convexity of the left cardiac border with an elevated apex

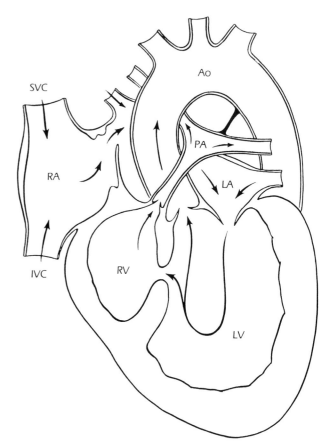

FIG. 6-38. Tricuspid atresia without transposition of the great vessels. *Ao*, aorta; *IVC*, inferior vena cava; *LA*, left atrium; *LV*, left ventricle; *PA*, pulmonary artery; *RA*, right atrium; *RV*, right ventricle; *SVC*, superior vena cava.

and concave main pulmonary artery segment. A right aortic arch is present in 3% to 5% of patients. The right heart border may be straight unless there is right atrial enlargement.

Angiocardiography

The diagnosis of tricuspid atresia and its associated lesions is readily made by echocardiography. Recent developments with the use of biplane transesophageal sonography further improve definition of the anatomy (103). If the atrial septal defect is restrictive, a balloon atrial septostomy may be performed during echocardiography or cardiac catheterization to improve right to left shunting. MRI has been used for anatomic evaluation of tricuspid atresia (104).

Injection of contrast material into the superior vena cava (SVC) demonstrates that there is no forward flow of contrast from the right atrium into the right ventricle. All of the contrast media crosses an ASD into the left atrium or refluxes into the SVC or hepatic sinusoids. There is a nonopaque triangular filling defect to the left of the tricuspid valve in the position normally occupied by the inflow portion of the right ventricle (Fig. 6-39B). Lesions that can mimic the angiocardiographic triangular filling defect of tricuspid atresia

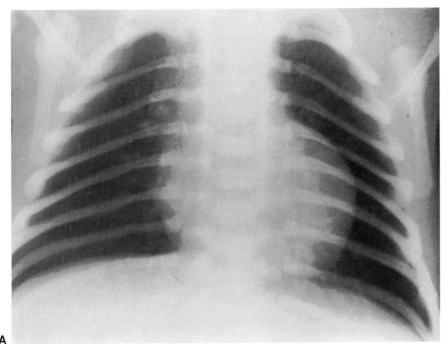

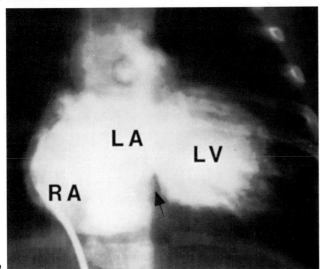

FIG. 6-39. Tricuspid atresia. A: A 2-day-old boy with cyanosis. The heart is not enlarged in its transverse diameter. There is convexity of the lower left cardiac border, an elevated apex, a concave main pulmonary artery segment and decreased pulmonary vascularity. There is slight flattening of the lower right heart border. **B:** A 1-month-old girl with cyanosis. Catheter could not be passed across the tricuspid valve. Injection of contrast material into the right atrium *(RA)* shows opacification of the left atrium *(LA)*, left ventricle *(LV)*, and aorta. There is a triangular lucency *(arrow)* to the left of the tricuspid valve in the position normally occupied by the inflow portion of the right ventricle.

include pulmonary valvular stenosis with patent foramen ovale or ASD, tetralogy of Fallot with ASD, and total anomalous pulmonary venous return; the distinction between these entities and tricuspid atresia is readily made by echocardiography.

Left ventriculography delineates the presence or absence of a VSD, the size of the right ventricle, and any obstruction to pulmonary blood flow. The origin and anatomy of the great vessels are also defined.

Treatment and Prognosis

In newborns with tricuspid atresia and severe cyanosis, pulmonary blood flow may be dependent on a PDA. Vasodil-

atation of the PDA with prostaglandins increases pulmonary blood flow and improves systemic oxygenation. This approach may stabilize the infant for surgical palliation. Palliative surgery (often a modified Blalock-Taussig shunt) is done to increase pulmonary blood flow. In some children, the first surgical procedure will be a Glenn procedure, anastomosis between the SVC and the pulmonary artery. This procedure delivers one third of the total systemic venous return to the pulmonary artery, at a low pressure.

Definitive surgical repair with a Fontan procedure, a right atrial-to-main pulmonary artery direct anastomosis or conduit, is performed in older patients (105,106). Normal pulmonary artery pressure and pulmonary arteriolar resistance have been correlated with favorable outcome after the Fontan procedure (105,107). A more recent approach includes the use of the lateral atrial tunnel technique (cavo-caval baffle) for the Fontan procedure; this may reduce the incidence of atrial arrhythmias and other complications. If the patient's right ventricle is not extremely hypoplastic and is able to generate some forward flow, the pulmonary valve and trunk are used as a conduit between the right atrium and right ventricle (108). Surgical management of children with single functioning ventricles remains challenging. Fontan sounds a cautionary note citing the recent rise in morbidity and mortality (109). Actual changes in morbidity and mortality are not known; surgical techniques continue to be refined, and the postoperative children are not yet adolescents. A potential long-term complication of the Fontan procedure is elevation of systemic venous pressure. The procedure can also be complicated by thrombosis of the pulmonary artery, right atrium, or SVC demonstrable by echocardiography and MRI (46,110).

Glenn and Fontan anastomoses have been associated with the development of pulmonary arteriovenous malformations in as high as 25% of patients (111). The cause of the malformations is unknown; maldistribution of pulmonary blood flow to upper and lower lobes as well as nonpulsatile blood flow have been among the factors suggested. Lack of normal hepatic venous blood flow to the lungs may play a role, and some have implicated hepatic vasoactive agents (112,113).

Ebstein Anomaly

Definition and Anatomy

In Ebstein anomaly, atrialization of part of the right ventricle, there is redundancy of tricuspid valve tissue and adherence of it to the right ventricular wall distal to the tricuspid valve annulus (Fig. 6-40).

Physiology

The right atrium is defined as the chamber proximal to the tricuspid valve. With this anomaly, there is an enlarged chamber projecting into the right ventricle that is described as atrialized, since it is proximal to the tricuspid valve. The degree of impairment of right ventricular function relates to the extent to which the inflow portion is atrialized. When valve tissue adherence occurs, there is loss of normal ventricular contractility. During atrial systole, part of the blood from the right atrium is propelled only into the atrialized portion of the right ventricle. Subsequently, during right ventricular systole, there is forward flow of some blood through the pulmonic valve. Blood within the atrialized portion of the right ventricle is pressed back into the true right atrium. This to-and-fro motion causes additional functional obstruction to the emptying mechanism of the atrium. An interatrial

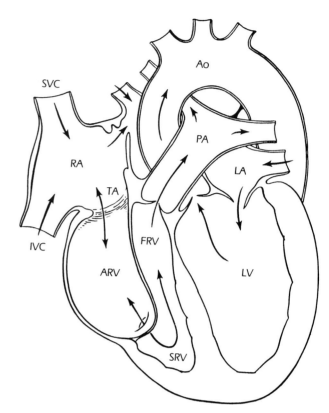

FIG. 6-40. Ebstein anomaly. The tricuspid valve attaches below its normal annulus *(TA)* to divide the right ventricle into a proximal atrialized portion *(ARV)* and a distal, small functional right ventricle *(FRV)*. *Ao*, aorta; *IVC*, inferior vena cava; *LA*, left atrium; *LV*, left ventricle; *PA*, pulmonary artery; *RA*, right atrium; *SVC*, superior vena cava.

communication (either a patent foramen ovale or an ASD) is nearly always present.

Clinical Features

There are a wide variety of clinical manifestations, depending on the degree of tricuspid insufficiency and the status of the atrial septum. During infancy there may be severe obstruction and profound cyanosis. If pulmonary hypertension is present, this elevates right ventricular pressure and makes tricuspid insufficiency worse. Right-to-left shunting occurs at the atrial level. Gradually, as pulmonary artery pressure decreases, there is more forward flow through the pulmonary arteries, and the infant improves. The ECG is always abnormal, demonstrating right bundle branch block, Wolff-Parkinson-White syndrome, or both.

Echocardiography

Echocardiography demonstrates delayed tricuspid valve closure, tricuspid insufficiency, and paradoxical motion of the interventricular septum. The abnormal attachments of

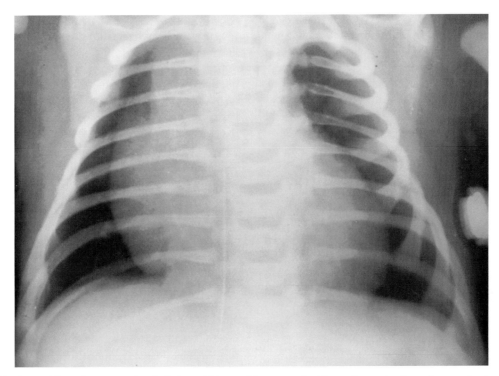

FIG. 6-41. Ebstein anomaly. A 1-day-old boy with cyanosis. There is marked cardiomegaly due to right atrial enlargement. The pulmonary vascularity is decreased.

the tricuspid valve and the reduced size of the right ventricular cavity are well imaged.

Radiology

The appearance on chest radiography depends on the severity of the anomaly. Infants with severe cyanosis may have decreased pulmonary vascularity and massive cardiomegaly due to right atrial enlargement (Fig. 6-41). Older patients, with milder malformations, have adequate right ventricular muscle to propel blood into the pulmonary circulation. The heart may become enlarged and have a ''box-like'' appearance. The right-sided enlargement is due to right atrial enlargement, and the left cardiac contour is abnormal due to displacement of the right ventricular outflow tract. Most patients show some decrease in pulmonary vascularity due to right-to-left shunting at the atrial level.

Angiocardiography

Right ventriculography demonstrates a trilobed appearance. The three lobes are an enlarged right atrium, the smooth-walled atrialized portion of right ventricle, and a trabeculated distal right ventricle. Diagnosis is made by identification of a notch in the right ventricle, which marks the location of the displaced tricuspid valve. The distal portion of the right ventricle is small and empties slowly. There

is to-and-fro movement of contrast between the normal right atrium and the atrialized part of the right ventricle.

Treatment and Prognosis

The prognosis in Ebstein anomaly varies. In infants with severe pulmonary hypertension and profound cyanosis, extracorporeal membrane oxygenation (ECMO) has been used until pulmonary artery pressure decreases; however, these infants have a higher mortality than those not requiring ECMO (114). Palliative surgical procedures have little to offer. When restoration of a competent valve becomes necessary in older children, plastic reconstruction of the tricuspid valve is undertaken; however this may lead to arrhythmias, especially complete heart block (115). Reduction and plication of the redundant right atrial free wall have also been performed with some success. At the other end of the spectrum, some patients with mild degree of the Ebstein anomaly are totally asymptomatic and may need no intervention.

Cyanotic Congenital Heart Disease with Variable Pulmonary Blood Flow

The phrase ''variable flow'' means that the pulmonary blood flow is normal or decreased depending on age and whether pulmonary stenosis is present. Thus, in transposition of the great vessels, pulmonary blood flow may be normal in a neonate. If an arterial switch procedure is not done, pulmonary blood flow increases with age. Children with single ventricles or double-outlet ventricles may have increased flow (no pulmonary stenosis), normal flow (some pulmonary stenosis), or decreased flow (severe pulmonary stenosis).

Transposition of the Great Vessels

Definition and Incidence

Complete transposition of the great vessels (TGV), also called d transposition of the great vessels (d-TGV) or transposition of the great arteries (TGA), is the most common congenital heart disease causing cyanosis during the first 24 hours of life. The incidence varies from 19 to 33 per 100,000 live births. There is a strong male predominance (116). The lesion may be isolated or part of a more complex anomaly. Refinements in diagnosis and surgical management have led to a striking increase in survival over the past 25 years.

Anatomy

With d-TGV, there is an abnormality of arterial relations: the aorta and pulmonary arteries are transposed. The ascending aorta and coronary arteries arise from the right ventricle, and the pulmonary artery arises from the left ventricle. The ascending aorta is usually anterior and to the right of the pulmonary artery, but it may be anterior and to the left, directly anterior, or even posteriorly positioned. The anomaly can also be explained using the terms *concordant* and *discordant*. In normal hearts, the atrial-ventricular-great vessel anatomy is concordant, so that there is a normal relation between the right atrium, right ventricle, and pulmonary artery and a normal relation between the left atrium, left ventricle, and ascending aorta. The term *transposition of the great vessels* indicates discordant ventricular-arterial connections, so the aorta arises entirely or in large part from the right ventricle and the pulmonary artery arises entirely or in large part from the left ventricle. The term *simple transposition* has been used for complete transposition (d-TGV) with an intact ventricular septum or a very small VSD but without other significant associated lesions; in its pure form, the two circulations are completely separate, and the condition is rapidly fatal.

Physiology

In patients who have d transposition of the great vessels, there are two parallel circuits. Desaturated systemic venous blood enters the right atrium, passes into the right ventricle, and is ejected into the aorta. The other circuit involves flow into the pulmonary arteries, pulmonary veins, left atrium, left ventricle, and recirculation into the pulmonary artery. The pulmonary and systemic circulations are in parallel rather than in series, and life is sustained through connections between the two circuits. Communications between the two circulations include a patent foramen ovale, ASD, VSD, PDA, systemic collateral arteries to the lungs, and any combination of the above.

In the normal neonate the right atrial pressure falls as pulmonary vascular resistance decreases and right ventricular pressure decreases. The interatrial pressure gradient in normal patients favors closure of the septum primum flap over the foramen ovale. With d-TGV, however, the right atrium indirectly faces systemic vascular resistance, and the right atrial pressure is persistently elevated. Therefore, there is usually bidirectional shunting at the atrial level or predominant shunting toward the pulmonary circuit. In d-TGV, if shunting is in one direction at one level, it must be in the other direction at some other level; otherwise, one of the parallel circuits would soon accumulate all of the blood.

Clinical Features

With d-TGV the physiology and anatomy are compatible with normal fetal life, and these infants are normal or large for gestational age. Prominent cyanosis is an early and almost universal finding in neonates with TGV. Cyanosis is recognized in the first hour of life in 56% and during the first day of life in 92% of neonates with TGV and intact ventricular septum (116).

Radiology

Historically, d-TGV was grouped among congenital cardiac lesions with increased flow. However, because definitive arterial switch procedures are now performed in the first or second week of life, the classic radiographic appearance (based on findings in older children with transposition) is rarely seen. The appearance of increased pulmonary flow on plain radiographs in neonates with d-TGV may actually represent venous congestion caused by elevation of left atrial pressure, in which case emergent balloon atrial septostomy may be indicated (117).

The ''classic'' radiographic findings of transposition of the great vessels are seen in less than 50% of infants. A normal chest radiograph does not preclude the diagnosis. Radiographic findings include (a) narrowing of the superior mediastinum due to decrease in thymic tissue and abnormal relations of the great vessels; (b) lack of visualization of the malpositioned aortic arch on the left, and lack of the normal shadow of the main pulmonary artery (Fig. 6-42) (118–120); (c) apparent asymmetry of pulmonary arterial flow with the right pulmonary artery being slightly higher and more prominent than the left. The asymmetry is due to left ventricular injection into a main pulmonary artery which is oriented more toward the right pulmonary artery than in normals. In summary, patients with d-TGV can have decreased flow, increased flow, or normal flow, depending on their age and the associated lesions.

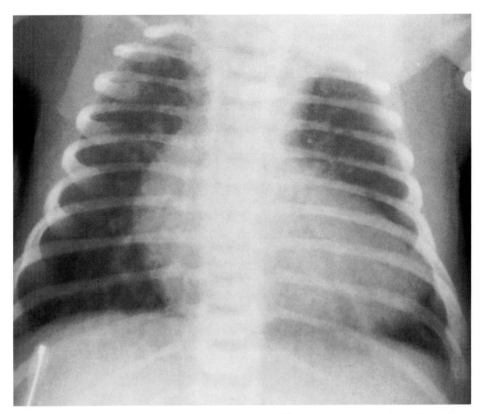

FIG. 6-42. d-TGV. Newborn boy with profound cyanosis. The heart is enlarged and there is a narrow superior mediastinum. The pulmonary vascularity is prominent despite an inapparent main pulmonary artery segment.

Echocardiography

Echocardiography at the bedside plays a dominant role in the diagnosis of patients with TGV. Two-dimensional echocardiography satisfactorily diagnoses d-TGV and any associated lesions and accurately identifies the origins of the coronary arteries. The abnormal position of the aorta and main pulmonary artery is readily identified. Doppler techniques can identify intracardiac shunts and assess flow through a PDA.

Angiocardiography

Two-dimensional echocardiography is so useful that cardiac catheterization is largely restricted to neonates with complex problems. Infants with d-TGV may urgently need a balloon atrial septostomy to improve mixing between the two circuits. This can be performed at the bedside with echocardiographic guidance or in the catheterization laboratory. Left ventriculography shows the left ventricular origin of the pulmonary artery and identifies the subpulmonic infundibulum and the pulmonary bifurcation (Fig. 6-43A, B). During recirculation, left-to-right atrial shunting may be seen if there is an ASD or if the patient has had a balloon atrial septostomy. Right ventriculography shows the right ventricular origin of the aorta, the coronary ostia, the ascending aorta, and the presence or absence of a patent ductus arteriosus (Fig. 6-43C, D). If a VSD is present, the shunt is generally from the systemic right ventricle to the lower pressure left ventricle. The size and position of the VSD, any subvalvular obstruction, and other lesions can be assessed readily.

Postoperative cardiac catheterization is frequently performed to obtain hemodynamic data in many patients with d-TGV. Selective embolization of any residual aortic-pulmonary collaterals may be performed percutaneously.

Treatment and Prognosis

Rashkind Balloon Atrial Septostomy. The Rashkind balloon atrial septostomy is performed to improve mixing at the atrial level. The balloon catheter is placed across the atrial septum, and the balloon is inflated. Once position is verified, the balloon is rapidly withdrawn across the atrial septum, tearing it and enlarging the interatrial communication.

Atrial Correction: Mustard or Senning Procedure. The Mustard and Senning operations correct TGV with an atrial baffle that directs systemic venous return to the left ventricle and pulmonary artery while directing pulmonary venous re-

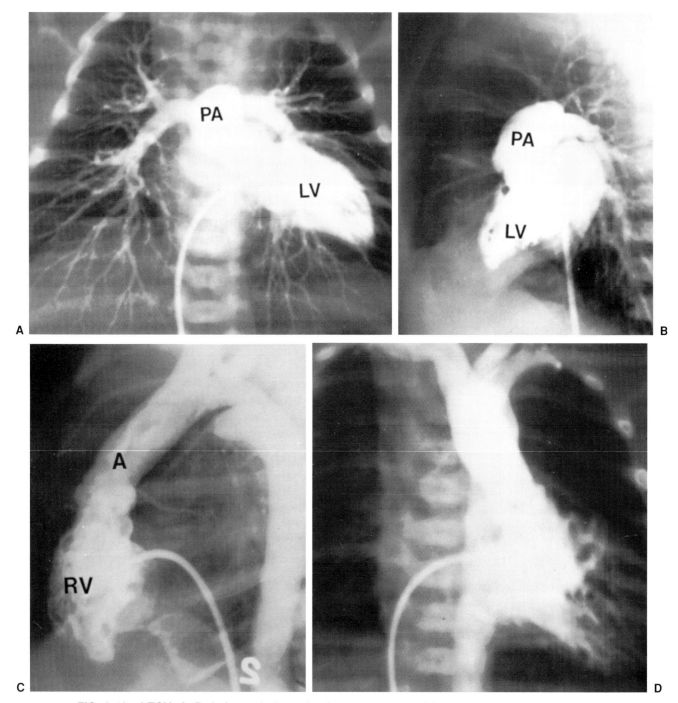

FIG. 6-43. d-TGV. A, B: Left ventriculography demonstrates ventricle-great vessel discordance, the left ventricle *(LV)* giving origin to the pulmonary artery *(PA)*, which is to the right and posteriorly positioned. **C, D:** Right ventriculography shows the right ventricular *(RV)* origin of the aorta *(A)*.

turn to the right ventricle and aorta. Complications of atrial baffle operations include residual interatrial shunt, pulmonary venous or caval obstruction, right ventricular dysfunction, tricuspid insufficiency, and cardiac dysrhythmias. A serious, late complication of both procedures is right ventricular failure. Mustard and Senning operations were the primary surgical techniques during the 1970s and 1980s. Because of late right ventricular dysfunction and failure,

however, alternative surgical approaches have been developed.

Arterial Switch Procedure. The arterial switch (Jatene) procedure has become the procedure of choice for primary surgical repair of d-TGV (121). Jatene and coworkers performed the first arterial switch procedure in 1975 (122). The great arteries are transected above their valves and reanastomosed to the opposite great vessels (Fig. 6-44). The coronary

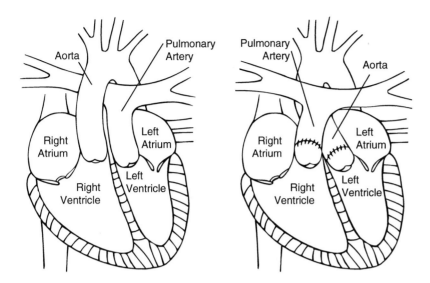

FIG. 6-44. Arterial switch procedure for d-TGV. The great vessels are transected above their valves and cross-anastomosed. The coronaries must be transferred to the systemic vessel.

arteries must also be transferred. With the arterial switch procedure, physiologic correction is accomplished as blood flows from the right atrium to the right ventricle and through the original aortic valve (now attached to the main pulmonary artery) to the lungs. Blood then returns to the left atrium and left ventricle and enters the ascending aorta through the pulmonary valve. A crucial physiologic challenge after repair is the functional adequacy of the left ventricle. Preoperatively the left ventricle is pumping into the lower pressure pulmonary circuit, but postoperatively it must immediately be able to work against systemic resistance. The arterial switch procedure is usually performed during the first week of life when the left ventricle is still prepared by intrauterine physiology to meet the demands of this greater systemic workload.

Without treatment, 30% of infants with d-TGV died during the first week of life, 50% in the first month, and 90% in the first year (116). Aggressive medical and surgical intervention has changed the prognosis dramatically. Among 470 patients who underwent the arterial switch procedure at Children's Hospital, Boston, the survival at 8 years was 91%. Anomalies of the coronary arteries increase risk and are a cause of death (123,124). Complications of the arterial switch procedure are significantly less than those of atrial baffle procedures. The arterial switch procedure allows preservation of ventricular function and is associated with fewer arrhythmias (125,126). Echocardiography and MRI are effective in evaluating postoperative complications of the pulmonary arteries after the arterial switch procedure (127).

Occasionally, older children who develop right ventricular failure years after a Mustard or Senning procedure are referred for two-stage repair. The first stage involves preparation of the left ventricle by banding of the pulmonary artery. This increases the workload of the left ventricle. The tight pulmonary band, however, decreases blood flow to the lung, and so a Blalock-Taussig shunt is also created. When the left ventricle has been strengthened, the arterial switch procedure is performed.

Transposition Complexes

Double-Outlet Right Ventricle

In double-outlet right ventricle, an abnormal relation exists between the aorta and the pulmonary trunk such that both great arteries originate from the morphologic right ventricle (128,129). The only outlet from the left ventricle is a VSD. There may also be an obstruction to pulmonary flow. Classification is based on the site of the VSD in relation to the crista supraventricularis and whether there are normally or abnormally related great vessels.

The radiographic appearance depends on associated lesions. In double-outlet right ventricle without pulmonic stenosis, there is a marked increase in pulmonary blood flow. In double-outlet right ventricle with pulmonic stenosis, the heart is small and the pulmonary blood flow is diminished.

Taussig-Bing Complex

The Taussig-Bing complex (double-outlet right ventricle type II) is considered an incomplete form of transposition. In this entity, the aorta lies anterior and to the right of the pulmonary artery at the level of the semilunar valves. The aorta arises entirely from the right ventricle, and the pulmonary artery overrides the ventricular septum. There is a subpulmonary outlet VSD, which is large. Subaortic stenosis (due to the position of the infundibular septum) and coarctation of the aorta are usually present.

Corrected Transposition of the Great Vessels

Corrected transposition of the great vessels (l-TGV) derives its name from the physiologic correction of the route of blood flow despite major abnormalities in the structure of the heart and great vessels. This type of transposition of the great arteries is synonymous with inversion of the ventricles and AV valves. Systemic venous blood passes into the right atrium and across the mitral valve into the right-sided, morphologic left ventricle. This chamber connects with the pulmonary artery. Oxygenated blood returns from the lungs through the pulmonary veins to the left atrium and crosses a tricuspid valve into a morphologic right ventricle, which is on the left side of the body. This ventricle connects with the transposed aorta which is anterior and to the left of the pulmonary artery. Thus physiologic correction is achieved; systemic venous blood is delivered to the lungs for oxygenation, and oxygenated blood is pumped out to the systemic circulation. In rare cases, there is no additional cardiac anomaly, and cardiac hemodynamics are grossly normal. Described in terms of concordance or discordance by the segmental approach, corrected transposition is atrial-ventricular discordance plus ventricular-arterial discordance.

Because of associated lesions, most patients with corrected transposition develop severe symptoms during the first months of life. The associated lesions include large VSDs, left AV valve insufficiency (tricuspid insufficiency), pulmonary outflow tract obstruction, complete heart block, and polysplenia-asplenia syndromes. The clinical course of children without associated congenital cardiac lesions may include progressive right ventricular enlargement, arrhythmias, and AV valve insufficiency.

The pulmonary vascularity may be normal, increased, or decreased, depending on any associated VSD or pulmonary outflow obstruction. There is frequently an abnormal convexity along the left upper heart border, as the ascending aorta and the right ventricular outflow tract to which it is attached are border forming on the left (2,10,130).

Single Ventricle

Incidence and Anatomy

A single ventricle or univentricular heart is a rare malformation (1% of all congenital heart lesions) in which the interventricular septum is absent. The nomenclature is confusing in this entity. Reference is usually made to the type of inlet (double or single). Inlet refers to the number of AV valves connecting the atria to the single ventricle.

There are three anatomic types of single ventricle. Most commonly, the right ventricle is underdeveloped and the single ventricle has the morphologic configuration of a left ventricle; it is referred to as a single ventricle of the left ventricular type. This type of single ventricle is associated with another, smaller ventricular chamber, termed the infundibulum or rudimentary right ventricle; it is located either on the right side of the single ventricle or in an inverted position on the left side. A VSD is almost always present and connects the single ventricle to the rudimentary chamber. On rare occasions, the single ventricle shows morphologic characteristics of a right ventricle and is termed a single

ventricle of the right ventricular type. An even rarer type of single ventricle is one in which there is only a rudimentary septum in the midportion of the large ventricular cavity; this is referred to as a common ventricle.

Clinical Features

Cyanosis is always present. The degree of cyanosis depends on the amount of pulmonary blood flow. Patients without pulmonary stenosis generally develop congestive heart failure early in infancy because of preferential flow into the low-pressure pulmonary circulation. Clinically, the infants are usually small and have recurrent upper respiratory infections, severe heart failure, sweating, and tachycardia. When pulmonary stenosis is present, the anomaly mimics severe tetralogy of Fallot clinically and radiologically.

Radiology

The chest radiographic appearance of single ventricle depends on the associated lesions. For example, if there is severe pulmonary stenosis or pulmonary atresia, decreased pulmonary flow is seen and the aorta is prominent, as in severe tetralogy of Fallot. In patients without pulmonic stenosis, there is cardiomegaly, a marked increase in the size of the main pulmonary artery, and increased pulmonary blood flow.

The ability of MRI to display anatomy in multiple planes makes it useful in complex anomalies such as these. In single ventricle, MRI shows the atrial anatomy well. It also helps identify the dominant ventricular chamber and accurately depicts coexisting abnormalities such as transposition of the great vessels, VSD, venous anomalies, and the tracheobronchial anatomy of right- or left-sided isomerism.

Treatment and Prognosis

Surgery for single ventricle is still in evolution. A staged repair involves committing the single ventricle to the systemic circuit and then performing a bidirectional Glenn shunt. When the patient is older, a definitive Fontan procedure is performed.

Cyanotic Congenital Heart Disease with Increased Pulmonary Blood Flow

Truncus Arteriosus

Incidence and Definition

An uncommon anomaly (1% of all congenital heart disease), truncus arteriosus is due to failure of division of the primitive truncus arteriosus into aorta and pulmonary artery (57). Therefore, one large vessel—the truncus—originates from the heart to supply the coronary, systemic, and pulmonary circulations. There is always a large, high VSD.

Anatomy

There is no unanimity in classifying the types of truncus arteriosus (131–134). In 1949, Collet and Edwards proposed a classification (Fig. 6-45) that described the origin of the pulmonary arteries from the truncus (133). In the currently used classification of truncus arteriosus described by Van Praagh (33), type I has a short, separate pulmonary trunk. In type II, there is no pulmonary trunk; the pulmonary artery branches arise separately from the truncus. Type III has complete absence of a pulmonary artery; the affected lung is perfused by a patent ductus arteriosus or by collaterals. Type IV has obstruction (usually interruption) of the aorta; the ascending aorta is hypoplastic and the pulmonary trunk is the larger branch of the truncus, giving off a ductus arteriosus that perfuses the descending aorta. Vessels originating from the aorta are referred to as aortopulmonary collaterals. Hemitruncus is another variant; one pulmonary artery arises from the truncus, the opposite lung being supplied by aortic-pulmonary collaterals from the descending aorta.

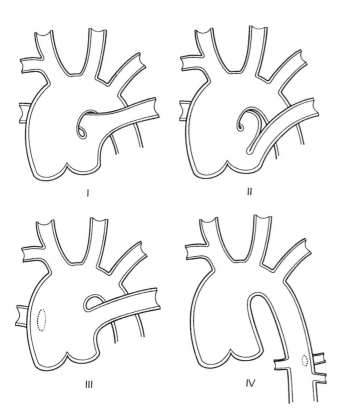

FIG. 6-45. Classification of truncus arteriosus. Type I—origin of main pulmonary artery from the truncus. Type II—separation of the left and right pulmonary arteries at their origin from the truncus. Type III—marked by separate origins of the right and left pulmonary arteries. Type IV (pseudotruncus)—arteries serving the lungs originate from descending aorta. Modified from Collet and Edwards (133).

The VSD in truncus arteriosus results from profound deficiency of the infundibular septum and is generally large. The truncal valve is frequently abnormal and may have two to six cusps, although three cusps are most frequent. The pulmonary artery or arteries most commonly arise from the left posterolateral aspect of the truncus arteriosus a short distance above the truncal valve. The frequent variations in coronary artery origin and distribution may be relevant surgically. A right aortic arch with mirror image branching occurs in approximately 30% of these anomalies.

Physiology

Truncus arteriosus is an admixture lesion at the VSD level. The pressures in the two ventricles are similar. The amount of pulmonary blood flow depends on pulmonary vascular resistance. There is usually a moderate increase in pulmonary flow due to the relatively large pressure gradient between the high-pressure truncus and the low-resistance pulmonary circuit.

Clinical Features

Cyanosis and heart failure often occur early in infancy. Peripheral pulses are bounding, and the pulse pressure is wide because of aortic runoff into the lungs. Truncal valve insufficiency widens the pulse pressure even further.

Radiology

Cardiomegaly is frequently present at birth. As pulmonary vascular resistance decreases (after the second or third day of life), there is a marked increase in pulmonary arterial blood flow (Fig. 6-46A). The left atrium enlarges to accommodate the increased pulmonary venous return. Changes of heart failure may be seen. The truncus or ascending aorta is usually prominent. A right-sided arch is identified in one third of patients and, in conjunction with increased pulmonary vascularity and cardiomegaly, suggests the diagnosis (134). The inferior margin of the left pulmonary artery is occasionally seen at its origin from the truncus.

Angiocardiography

Echocardiography, usually diagnostic, demonstrates the origin and configuration of the pulmonary arteries, the ventricular septal defect, the truncus arteriosus and aortic arch, the status of the truncal valve, and the position of the coronary arteries. Cardiac catheterization is sometimes performed to confirm anatomic details and obtain physiologic data regarding the pulmonary vasculature. In some centers, if echocardiography reveals straightforward anatomy, the

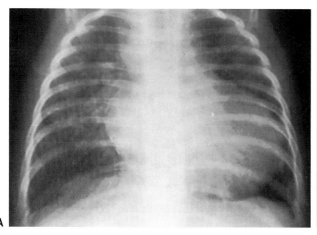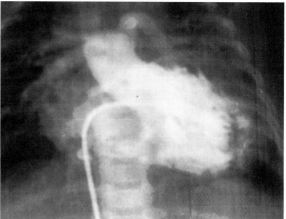

FIG. 6-46. Type II truncus arteriosus. A 3-month-old girl with cyanosis. **A:** The heart is enlarged, the main pulmonary artery segment is concave, the pulmonary vascularity is increased, and there is a right-sided aortic arch. **B:** The pulmonary arteries arise from the posterior aspect of the truncus arteriosus.

patient undergoes repair without catheterization. Infants that present late or have more complex anomalies may require catheterization. During catheterization, because the ventricles have the same pressures, injection can be made into either. The injection will demonstrate a large ventricular septal defect as well as the truncus arteriosus (Fig. 6-46B). Injection of the truncus will demonstrate pulmonary artery anatomy, coronary artery anatomy, and the degree of truncal insufficiency (134). The differential diagnosis of truncus arteriosus in the neonate includes aortopulmonary window and pulmonary atresia with a VSD.

Treatment and Prognosis

Infants previously received pulmonary artery banding to prevent heart failure and decrease the risk of pulmonary vascular changes secondary to high pulmonary flow. Surgical repair of truncus arteriosus is now recommended in the first few days of life (135). The availability of small-valved allografts for the right ventricle-to-pulmonary artery reconstruction avoids the complications of pulmonary hypertension. Patency of the foramen ovale is beneficial postoperatively and may improve outcome, particularly in infants (136).

Total Anomalous Pulmonary Venous Return

Definition

Total anomalous pulmonary venous return (TAPVR) occurs when the common pulmonary vein (a precursor of part of the left atrium) fails to develop fully or is obliterated; the branch pulmonary veins then connect with other venous structures such as the SVC, right atrium, and portal venous system rather than the left atrium.

Anatomy

TAPVR is divided into four types according to the site or sites of connection: supracardiac, cardiac, infracardiac, and mixed (Fig. 6-47). Table 6-14 lists the anomalous sites of connection and their frequency (137). The anomalous venous return may be obstructive or not.

The supracardiac type (type I) is the most common form of TAPVR. All the pulmonary veins converge into the left vertical vein (thought to derive from a primitive anterior cardinal vein rather than the common cardinal vein, as in persistent left SVC), which runs superiorly to drain into the left innominate vein and then into the SVC. In type II TAPVR (cardiac), there is anomalous venous drainage to the coronary sinus or to the right atrium.

In type III TAPVR (infracardiac), the connection is below the diaphragm into the umbilicovitelline system. The pulmo-

TABLE 6-14. *Total anomalous pulmonary venous return*

Anatomy	Frequency (%)
Supracardiac	45
Left vertical vein ("snowman" type)	
Superior vena cava	
Azygos vein	
Right innominate vein	
Cardiac	23
Right atrium	
Coronary sinus	
Persistent sinus venosus	
Infracardiac	21
Portal vein	
Ductus venosus	
Inferior vena cava	
Combined	11
Total	100

Modified from Chen (137).

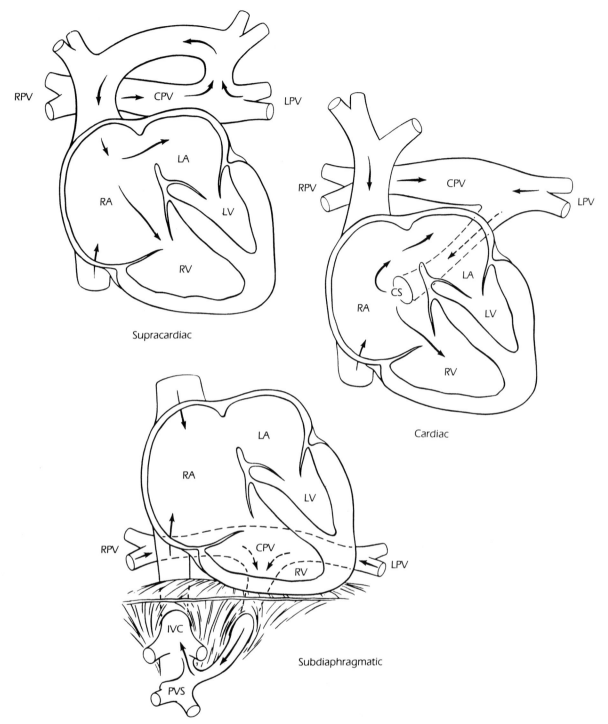

FIG. 6-47. Types of TAPVR. *CPV*, common pulmonary vein; *CS*, coronary sinus; *IVC*, inferior vena cava; *LA*, left atrium; *LPV*, left pulmonary vein; *LV*, left ventricle; *PVS*, portal venous system; *RA*, right atrium; *RPV*, right pulmonary vein; *RV*, right ventricle. Modified from Chen (137).

nary veins from both lungs join to form a confluence immediately behind the left atrium. A common vein from the midportion of this confluence descends immediately anterior to the esophagus and penetrates the diaphragm through the esophageal hiatus. The anomalous vein then joins the portal

vein, ductus venosus, hepatic veins, or inferior vena cava. Obstruction is the result of a combination of factors: length of the common venous channel, obstruction at the diaphragmatic hiatus, closure or restriction of the ductus venosus, and resistance to blood flow through the hepatic sinusoids.

Physiology

Supracardiac TAPVR is seldom associated with pulmonary venous obstruction, although it occasionally occurs at the junction of the common pulmonary vein with the vertical vein. Sometimes the ascending trunk passes between the left pulmonary artery and the left main bronchus and is obstructed there. There is almost always obstruction in type III (infracardiac) TAPVR.

Because both the pulmonary and systemic veins drain to the right atrium, there is increased right atrial blood volume. A widely patent foramen ovale or ASD allows major right-to-left shunting. The right-sided chambers and pulmonary arteries are volume-overloaded and enlarged. When pulmonary venous obstruction exists, the volume overload of the right-sided chambers is replaced by pressure overload, caused by the elevated pulmonary venous pressure, which is transmitted to the capillary bed. Pulmonary edema and pulmonary hypertension develop. Decreased pulmonary blood flow, right ventricular hypertension, and right heart failure ultimately develop.

Clinical Features

Most patients with TAPVR without obstruction develop tachypnea or feeding difficulties during the first month of life. They have large left-to-right shunts, but their cyanosis may be mild and not readily apparent. Patients with obstruction are usually well for the first 12 hours of life and then have progressive hypoxemia and metabolic acidosis.

Radiology

The radiographic appearance of TAPVR varies according to the site of abnormal venous drainage and whether it is obstructed (138). The radiographic appearance of the mediastinum in type I TAPVR has been likened to a snowman (Fig. 6-48); the upper half of the snowman consists of the left vertical vein and dilated SVC (Fig. 6-49A). The body of the snowman is due to the enlarged right atrium. During infancy the snowman shape may not be apparent. On lateral chest radiographs there may be a pretracheal density (Fig. 6-49B), the composite shadow of the left vertical vein and the SVC (Fig. 6-49C) (139). This sign is helpful, particularly in young infants, in distinguishing a normal thymus from the vertical vein of anomalous venous return. Shunt vascularity is present in TAPVR because of increased flow.

In TAPVR at the cardiac level, the pulmonary venous blood flows into the coronary sinus and right atrium. The radiologic findings simulate a large left-to-right shunt at the atrial level. The anomalous vein occasionally indents the barium-filled esophagus (137).

The infracardiac type of TAPVR, which is usually obstructed, demonstrates a normal-sized heart and severe pulmonary edema (Fig. 6-50A). Kerley B lines are often present.

Type IV consists of two or more sites of drainage of the anomalous veins. Occasionally, if there is obstruction of only one side, striking asymmetry of vascularity is present. TAPVR can be isolated or can coexist with other cardiac anomalies.

Echocardiography

Echocardiography is very reliable in establishing the diagnosis of TAPVR. Avoidance of cardiac catheterization in desperately ill neonates with obstructed veins has been an important advance in the preoperative management of these patients (140). In older children, cardiac catheterization measures the degree of pulmonary venous obstruction and provides other important hemodynamic data.

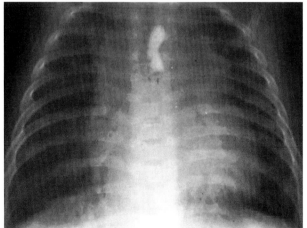
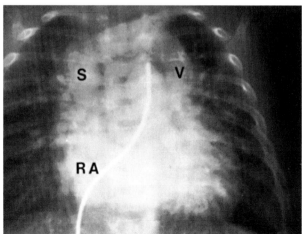

A   B

FIG. 6-48. Supracardiac TAPVR. The snowman configuration on posteroanterior radiographs **(A)** is due to a dilated superior vena cava and vertical vein **(B)**. *RA,* right atrium; *S,* superior vena cava; *V,* vertical vein. Some barium is noted in the esophagus on the chest radiograph.

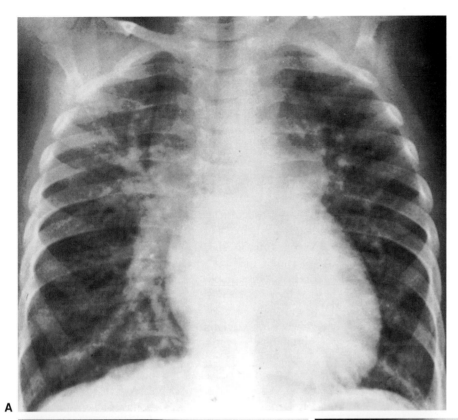

FIG. 6-49. Supracardiac TAPVR.
A: There is a right atrial and right ventricular enlargement. The pulmonary vascularity is prominent. A snowman configuration is present due to dilatation of the vertical vein on the left and the superior vena cava on the right. **B:** A lateral chest radiograph demonstrates a pretracheal soft issue density *(P)*. **C:** The levogram phase of selective right ventricular injection shows that the pretracheal density *(P)* is due to superimposition of the dilated superior vena cava and left vertical vein. (Courtesy of James T. T. Chen, M.D., Durham, North Carolina.)

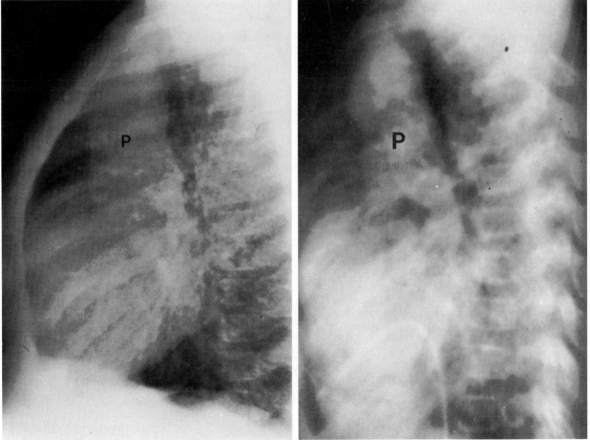

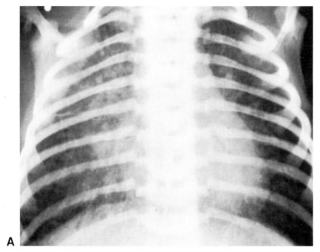

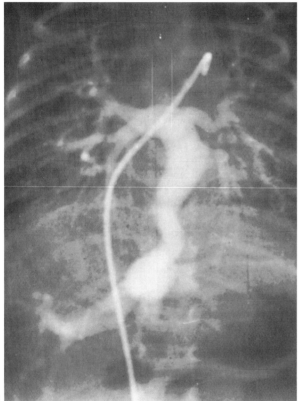

FIG. 6-50. TAPVR below the diaphragm. An 8-day-old infant with marked tachypnea. **A:** There is both interstitial and alveolar pulmonary edema, but the heart is of normal size. **B:** The right and left pulmonary veins join to form a common pulmonary vein. This vein then passes through the esophageal hiatus to drain into the portal venous system.

Angiocardiography

With the supracardiac type of TAPVR, excellent visualization can usually be achieved by direct catheter injection of the anomalous vein. Pulmonary arteriography demonstrates the anomalous pulmonary venous pathway during the levo phase, although significant delay and dilution will occur if obstruction is present (Fig. 6-50B).

Treatment and Prognosis

The combination of earlier diagnosis, aggressive preoperative medical management, and improved surgical techniques has dramatically improved survival in both supracardiac and cardiac types. Prior to 1970, the mortality rate was 50% (141); in the 1970s and 1980s, mortality rates dropped to 10% to 20% (142–144). More recently, mortality rates are 0 to 10% (145). Operative mortality in patients with infracardiac TAPVR or with complex cardiac lesions in association with TAPVR is higher than in other kinds of TAPVR.

Postoperative echocardiography may show pulmonary venous obstruction (146). Some patients develop obstruction at the anastomosis; this may necessitate reoperation if balloon dilatation is not successful. Progressive pulmonary venous occlusive disease due to an obliterative intimal fibrous hyperplasia has been reported in some postoperative patients.

Acyanotic Congenital Heart Disease with Normal Pulmonary Vascularity: Obstructive Lesions

Obstructive lesions may be either left-sided or right-sided. Because pure obstructive lesions produce systolic (pressure) overloading, and because hypertrophy is much more difficult to recognize than dilatation, mild lesions may show little or no radiographic abnormality. A normal chest radiograph in a patient referred for cardiac evaluation does not exclude pathology; normal chest radiographs are fairly common in small left-to-right shunts, and in both right-sided and left-sided obstructive lesions.

Coarctation of the Aorta

Anatomy

Coarctation of the aorta is a congenital narrowing of the aorta. There are localized and diffuse types (Fig. 6-51); the localized type, also termed the adult, postductal, or juxtaductal type, is much more common. In this type, the area of coarctation is located just beyond the left subclavian artery at the level of the ductus arteriosus (Fig. 6-52A). The narrowing is short and discrete, and the external contours of the aorta are correspondingly deformed.

The diffuse type, also known as the infantile, tubular hypoplastic, or preductal type, is characterized by a long segment of aortic narrowing that extends from just distal to the subclavian artery to the ductus arteriosus (Fig. 6-52B). Intracardiac defects (VSD, ASD, deformed mitral valve) are present in half of the patients with the diffuse type of coarctation, and the ductus arteriosus is almost always patent (10).

Clinical Features

The age of development of symptoms and their nature depend on the type of coarctation, its severity, and the pres-

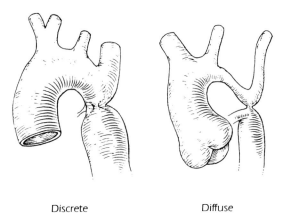

Discrete   *Diffuse*

FIG. 6-51. Coarctation of the aorta. Discrete juxtaductal and diffuse types of coarctation of the aorta. Modified from Elliott and Schiebler (2).

ence or absence of other abnormalities. The diffuse type of coarctation usually presents early in infancy because of the high degree of aortic narrowing and the frequent presence of intracardiac shunts and a PDA. There is congestive heart failure associated with bounding pulses in the upper extremities and nonpalpable leg pulses. The localized type of coarctation is usually diagnosed during late childhood. These patients are frequently asymptomatic but may have upper extremity hypertension.

Radiology

The heart is usually not enlarged in its transverse diameter, but left ventricular enlargement may be detected on the lateral view. There is often dilatation of the ascending aorta. The transverse portion of the thoracic aorta is also dilated when the coarctation is of the localized type. Instead of a smooth, curvilinear contour to the proximal descending thoracic aorta, a notch is present (Fig. 6-53A). The contour of the aorta at this level may resemble the number 3; the upper portion of the 3 is due to the dilated proximal left subclavian artery and aorta proximal to the coarctation; the middle portion of the 3 is due to the coarctation itself; and the lower portion of the 3 is due to poststenotic dilatation of the descending thoracic aorta (Fig. 6-53B, C). Rib notching may

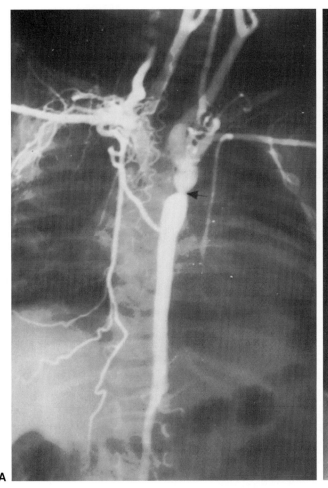

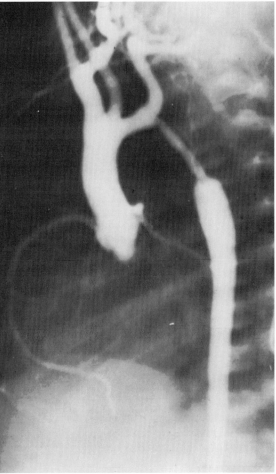

A   B

FIG. 6-52. Coarctation of the aorta. A: Localized or juxtaductal type of coarctation of the aorta *(arrow)*. There are many collaterals from the subclavian arteries. **B:** Diffuse or infantile type of coarctation of the aorta. There is a long segment of narrowed aorta that extends from just distal to the subclavian artery to below the level of the ductus arteriosus.

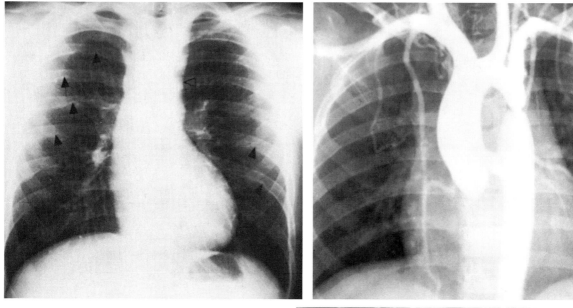

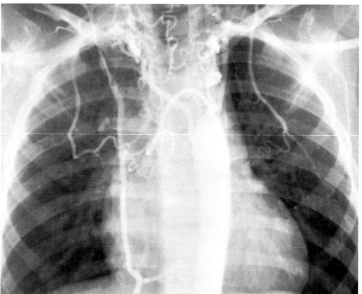

FIG. 6-53. **Localized coarctation of the aorta.** A 13-year-old asymptomatic boy whose hypertension was discovered on routine physical examination. **A:** Posteroanterior chest radiograph. The heart is not enlarged in its transverse diameter, but there is rounding of the left ventricular contour due to hypertrophy. There is slight prominence of the ascending aorta. There is marked bilateral rib notching *(solid arrows)* and discontinuity of the contour of the proximal part of the descending aorta *(open arrow).* **B:** Aortic root injection demonstrates a discrete coarctation just distal to the origin of the left subclavian artery. **C:** Collateral mediastinal vessels fill the descending aorta.

be present and is due to pressure erosion caused by dilated intercostal arteries, which serve as collateral vessels between the internal mammary arteries and the descending aorta. The first, second, and third ribs are not notched, since their intercostal arteries arise from the thyrocervical trunk, which originates from the aorta above the coarctation. On the lateral view, irregular, wavy densities may be seen behind the sternum due to dilatation of the internal mammary arteries, a route of collateral flow. The pulmonary vascularity is normal unless left ventricular failure has developed.

Magnetic Resonance Imaging

Clinical evaluation of the patient suspected of having coarctation of the aorta usually leaves little doubt as to the diagnosis. However, anatomic information that is critical prior to surgical correction are (a) exact site, length, and severity of the coarctation; (b) relationship of the coarctation to the left subclavian artery (which may be used in the operative repair); and (c) anatomy and extent of collateral flow (147). This information is obtained in the neonate with Doppler echocardiography. However, the acoustic window to the thoracic aorta is much more limited in older children because of intervening lung tissue. In the past, the only means of obtaining precise preoperative information was by means of angiocardiography. Currently, MRI is used to acquire detailed anatomic information noninvasively (148–151) (Fig. 6-54). Moreover, velocity-encoded MRI can measure peak pressure gradients (150); cine techniques provide gross assessment of blood flow.

Complications of coarctation repair include restenosis, an-

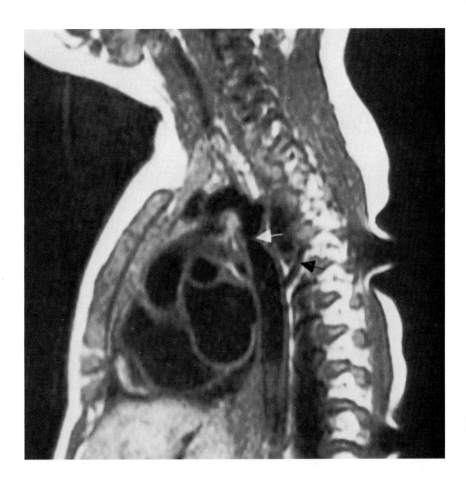

FIG. 6-54. Discrete coarctation of the aorta. Sagittal MRI demonstrates the coarctation *(white arrow)* and a prominent mediastinal collateral vessel *(black arrow)*. From Bisset (28).

eurysm formation, and aortic dissection. MRI is excellent for assessing any of these, but all are rare (151,152).

Treatment and Prognosis

There are currently two approaches to the treatment of coarctation: Primary surgical repair or percutaneous balloon dilatation (153,154). Dilatation of native coarctation in neonates has a 25 to 58% restenosis rate within the first six months (153–156). Many institutions still treat coarctation in infancy surgically. The three methods used for surgery include subclavian flap aortoplasty, resection with reanastomosis, and synthetic patch aortoplasty. Each technique has it advantages and disadvantages, and refinements are continually being made. Surgical complications include phrenic nerve injury, aneurysm formation, residual pressure granient, and restenosis. Balloon angioplasty for recoarctation or restenosis is effective and is associated with accelerated growth of the dilated segment at follow-up in many patients (152, 157). The complication rate is acceptable that includes restenosis and aneurysm development. Large prospective reviews of morbidity and mortality associated with native balloon angioplasty and restenosis coarctation angioplasty will contribute to the knowledge of treatment options. In older patients with native localized coarctation, percutaneous bal-

loon dilation is becoming the treatment of choice in more and more institutions (156).

Valvular Aortic Stenosis

Incidence

It is not widely appreciated that the most common congenital malformation of the heart is a bicuspid aortic valve. This anomaly frequently goes undetected during early life because of lack of symptoms. Bicuspid valves may become stenotic with time and create significant problems during later childhood or adult life. Aortic stenosis is more common in males. In 20% of cases it is associated with other cardiac anomalies, especially coarctation and patent ductus arteriosus (158). In 10%, valvular aortic stenosis presents in early infancy and is referred to as critical aortic stenosis; this will be discussed in the section on neonatal congenital heart disease.

Anatomy

Aortic stenosis occurs in four anatomic types: valvular, supravalvular, and subvalvular (membranous, muscular) (Fig. 6-55). The most common type, valvular aortic stenosis,

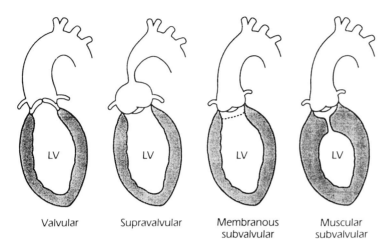

FIG. 6-55. Aortic stenosis. Aortic stenosis may be valvular, supravalvular, or subvalvular. Subvalvular aortic stenosis may be either membranous or muscular. *LV,* left ventricle.

accounts for 60% to 75% of the total. Development of aortic stenosis occurs in a three-cusped valve but is more common in a bicuspid valve. Supravalvular and subvalvular aortic stenosis are discussed separately.

Physiology

Most children and adolescents with aortic stenosis are asymptomatic. With valvular aortic stenosis there is thickening and rigidity of valve tissue. The distortion of blood flow caused by the deformed aortic valve leads to further thickening of the cusps and greater obstruction. This causes systolic overloading and left ventricular hypertrophy. At first the ventricle is able to compensate, and the patient is free of symptoms. At the opposite extreme is heart failure with impaired pump function and reduced contractility. The blood supply to the myocardium may be compromised. Ventricular dysrhythmia and sudden death during physical activity are occasional complications of acute ischemia. Many cases of congenital aortic stenosis are progressive. The commissures are fused and the leaflets are thickened, and bacterial endocarditis eventually may develop.

Radiology

Considerable aortic valvular stenosis may be present despite a normal-appearing radiograph. The lateral film frequently demonstrates a heart contour extending behind the inferior vena cava, indicating left ventricular enlargement (see Fig. 6-11B). There may be dilatation of the ascending aorta on the AP view because of poststenotic dilatation (Fig. 6-56). Dilatation of the ascending aorta is present only in valvular aortic stenosis, not in subvalvular or supravalvular stenosis.

Treatment and Prognosis

Percutaneous balloon dilatation of the aortic valve has been used to treat patients with aortic stenosis. For success

in older patients, two balloons are usually placed, one via each femoral artery.

Aortic valvotomy reduces the pressure gradient across the valve, but some degree of aortic insufficiency usually develops. Management decisions depend on the severity of the obstruction, which is usually estimated from Doppler assessment of gradients. However, pressure gradient estimations depend on flow velocity across the valve and are sometimes unreliable in aortic insufficiency and low cardiac output. Patients with gradients of <25 mm Hg can be followed medically, although 20% of this group will progress. Gradients >50 mm Hg are at risk for arrhythmia and sudden death.

In patients with moderate to severe aortic stenosis, percutaneous balloon aortic valvuloplasty may delay the open valvotomy and/or valve replacement (159–161). However, even after valvuloplasty, progressive stenosis or insufficiency may develop (162–164). Bacterial endocarditis occurs in approximately 4% of patients, and antibiotic prophylaxis is recommended. Prosthetic valve replacement is required in 35% of patients within 15–20 years of surgical valvotomy (165). Surgical options include replacement with a prosthetic aortic valve or an aortic valve or pulmonary valve autograft (166). Recently there has been renewed interest in the Ross procedure, which utilizes the native pulmonary valve to replace the diseased aortic valve. The potential for growth and the proven long-term durability of the native pulmonary valve make it ideal for replacement (167).

Supravalvular Aortic Stenosis

Supravalvular aortic stenosis is a congenital narrowing of the ascending aorta; it can be localized or diffuse but does not involve the aortic valve leaflets or cusps. This lesion is frequently associated with Williams syndrome (idiopathic infantile hypercalcemia) (168). The other components of the syndrome are mild mental retardation, talkativeness and friendly demeanor, elfin facies, and peripheral pulmonic stenosis. They may also have diffuse coarctation of the abdominal aorta and stenosis at the origins of the abdominal vessels. Occasionally, supravalvular stenosis and peripheral pulmo-

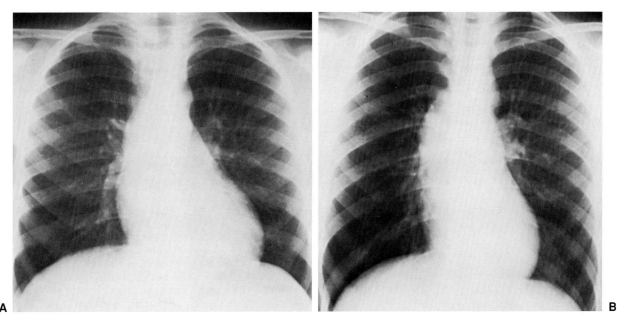

FIG. 6-56. Valvular aortic stenosis. A: An 8-year-old boy. Although not grossly enlarged, the heart has a rounded left ventricular configuration. There is slight prominence of the ascending aorta. **B:** Posteroanterior chest radiograph 5 years later. There is definite left ventricular hypertrophy and a marked increase in prominence of the ascending aorta.

nary stenosis are seen in families without the other features of Williams syndrome. The chest radiographs in supravalvular aortic stenosis are usually negative since dilation of the ascending aorta does not occur.

Patients with supravalvular aortic stenosis have an hourglass deformity of the aortic lumen due to a constricting annular ridge just above the sinuses of Valsalva. The ridge is produced by extreme thickening of the aortic media. The coronary arteries may be dilated and excessively tortuous, the origins of the coronaries being proximal to the obstruction. Surgical repair widens the lumen of the ascending aorta.

Subvalvular Aortic Stenosis

Membranous subvalvular aortic stenosis is caused by a discrete diaphragm that is just below the aortic valve and partially obstructs left ventricular outflow (Fig. 6-57) (169,170). Surgery consists of excising the membrane or fibrous ridge, thereby improving the hemodynamics, and is frequently curative. Distinction between valvular and subvalvular aortic stenosis may be clinically difficult. Echocardiography is useful and can also identify hypertrophic (muscular) subaortic stenosis (171).

Valvular Pulmonary Stenosis

Anatomy

Congenital pulmonary stenosis, a common abnormality, may be isolated or may be combined with other abnormalities. There are two distinct anatomic types of isolated valvular pulmonic stenosis. The classic type—90% of all cases—is caused by severe commissural fusion. The pulmonary valve is conical or dome-shaped, and the fused leaflets impinge on the central orifice. The valve tissue may be slightly thickened but is mobile. The right ventricle develops hypertrophy, particularly noticeable in the infundibular region. The pulmonary artery trunk almost always shows poststenotic dilatation, and the circumference of the trunk frequently exceeds that of the ascending aorta.

In the other 10% of cases, the valve is dysplastic. The commissures are not fused, and stenosis occurs between the valve leaflets, which are thickened and immobile. The annulus of the valve is frequently narrow. Dysplastic pulmonary valves are often familial and may be seen in Noonan syndrome.

Physiology

The right ventricular systolic pressure rises with the degree of stenosis. The right ventricle reacts to obstruction by developing concentric hypertrophy. Most patients with valvular pulmonic stenosis are asymptomatic or only mildly symptomatic. In severe cases, fatigue and dyspnea are present, but right-sided heart failure is rare. Because there is no right-to-left shunting, these patients remain acyanotic, even with severe obstruction.

Radiology

Chest radiographs in mild valvular pulmonic stenosis are normal. With moderate and severe pulmonic stenosis, there

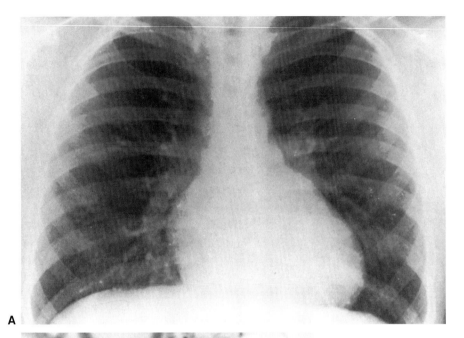

A

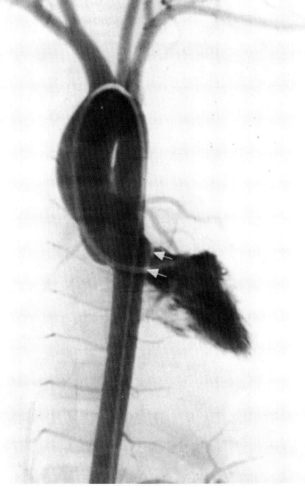

B

FIG. 6-57. Membranous subvalvular aortic stenosis. A 10-year-old boy with fatigue and dyspnea. **A:** Heart is not grossly enlarged in its transverse diameter but has a left ventricular configuration. The ascending aorta is normal. **B:** Selective left ventriculogram in systole. There is a discrete, linear, subvalvular membrane *(arrows)* just below the aortic valve.

is striking dilatation of the main pulmonary artery due to the high-velocity jet of blood ejected through the small valve orifice (Fig. 6-58A, B). The dilatation may extend into the left pulmonary artery (172). The degree of poststenotic dila-

tation is not always proportional to the severity of stenosis. When the stenosis is isolated, right ventricular hypertrophy maintains a normal stroke volume and a normal (not decreased) pulmonary arterial flow. A decrease in pulmonary

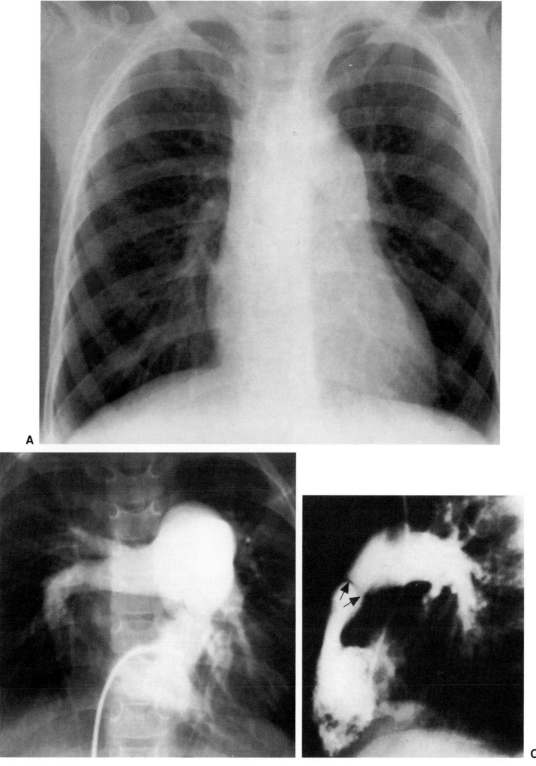

FIG. 6-58. Valvular pulmonary stenosis. A 6-year-old girl with systolic murmur. **A:** The heart is not enlarged in its transverse diameter. There is prominence of the main pulmonary artery segment and increased size of the left pulmonary artery. **B:** Right ventricular injection demonstrates marked dilatation of the main pulmonary artery. **C:** Lateral right ventriculography shows thickening and doming of the pulmonary valve *(arrows)* and poststenotic dilatation of the main pulmonary artery.

blood flow is seen only in some infants with severe pulmonic stenosis, tricuspid insufficiency, and right-to-left shunting at the atrial level.

Angiocardiography

The diagnosis of pulmonary stenosis is made by echocardiography. This technique demonstrates the size of the valve orifice and estimates the pressure gradient. Cardiac catheterization is used as a guide for interventional percutaneous balloon valvuloplasty. Prior to balloon dilatation, biplane angiocardiography with the catheter in the right ventricular chamber demonstrates (in the classic form of pulmonic stenosis) the doming of the thin pulmonary valve leaflets, the size of the orifice, and the jet of opacified blood as it enters the dilated main pulmonary artery (Fig. 6-58B, C). Poststenotic dilatation of the main pulmonary artery and left pulmonary artery are seen.

Angiographic features of the dysplastic valve type of pulmonic stenosis include thickened pulmonary valve leaflets, hypoplasia of the pulmonary valve annulus, and asymmetric doming. There is minimal poststenotic dilatation of the main pulmonary artery, as no systolic jet is present.

Treatment and Prognosis

Percutaneous balloon valvuloplasty is the treatment of choice in patients with classic pulmonary valvular stenosis (173–175). The balloon catheter is advanced over an exchange guidewire positioned in the pulmonary artery. The balloon is inflated across the pulmonary valve, and an indentation ("waist") on the balloon marks the site of the stenotic valve. The success rate of balloon valvuloplasty has been excellent (175). No serious short- or long-term complications have been observed, although mild pulmonary valve insufficiency can occur. Pulmonary balloon valvuloplasty has been used with success in neonates; avoidance of open heart surgery in these patients seems to improve outcome (176).

In children with dysplastic valves and stenosis, narrowing of the valve annulus is almost always present. In these cases, valvuloplasty does not relieve the pressure gradient. Surgical removal of the thickened valve tissue and enlargement of the annulus is usually necessary.

Heart Disease with Pulmonary Venous Prominence

Pulmonary Venous Hypertension

Pulmonary venous hypertension may be due to conditions that cause elevation of left ventricular end-diastolic pressure with subsequent left ventricular failure, primary forms of mitral valve incompetence, or mechanical obstructive lesions located at or proximal to the mitral valve. The differen-

TABLE 6-15. *Causes of pulmonary venous hypertension by anatomic site*

Systemic
  Hypertension
  Renal failure[a]
  Fluid overload[a]
  Arteritis
Aorta
  Coarctation[a]
  Supravalvular aortic stenosis
Aortic valve
  Valvular aortic stenosis
  Aortic insufficiency
Coronary artery disease
Left ventricle
  Subvalvular aortic stenosis
  Myocardial dysfunction[a]
    Pericarditis
      Constriction
      Tamponade
    Myocarditis
    Glycogen storage disease
    Endocardial fibroelastosis
    Anomalous origin of left coronary artery
  Left ventricular tumor
Mitral valve
  Mitral stenosis
    Congenital
    Rheumatic
  Mitral insufficiency
    Congenital
    Acquired
Left atrium
  Supravalvular ring
  Cor triatriatum
  Left atrial myxoma
Pulmonary veins
  TAPVR with obstruction[a]
  Atresia
  Stenosis
  Pulmonary venooclusive disease

TAPVR, total anomalous pulmonary venous return.
[a] More common.

tial diagnosis of pulmonary venous hypertension is based on the anatomic level of the causative lesion or anatomic site of abnormality (Table 6-15; see also Table 6-12).

Many congenital and acquired heart diseases cause pulmonary venous hypertension. They are divided into those with normal-sized hearts and those with cardiomegaly. Lesions beyond the mitral valve usually have cardiomegaly because left ventricular failure or dysfunction is present. Lesions proximal to the mitral valve, such as cor triatriatum, mitral stenosis, left atrial myxoma, and pulmonary venooclusive disease usually have normal-sized hearts (177).

The radiologic signs of pulmonary venous hypertension depend on the age of the patient. Cephalocaudal vascular redistribution does not occur until children assume the erect position (more than 2 years of age) and is difficult to detect until at least age 8. Chest radiographic signs of pulmonary venous hypertension include equalization of blood flow, redistribution of pulmonary blood flow to the upper chest in older children, interstitial edema (Kerley lines, hazy vessel margins), and alveolar pulmonary edema. Pulmonary arteriolar hypertension and right ventricular hypertrophy may occur in chronic pulmonary venous hypertension.

Magnetic Resonance Imaging

In patients with pulmonary venous obstruction without an obvious cause, MRI is useful (178,179). Etiologies, though rare, include total anomalous pulmonary venous return with obstruction, pulmonary vein stenosis, cor triatriatum, supravalvular stenosing mitral ring, and mitral stenosis. All of these abnormalities are characterized by pulmonary venous congestion and right ventricular pressure overload. MRI identifies pulmonary veins better than other modalities (178). MRI should be performed if the cause for pulmonary venous hypertension is in doubt after echocardiography and angiocardiography.

Cor Triatriatum

With cor triatriatum (''heart with three atria''), the pulmonary veins enter a posterior, accessory chamber that drains into the left atrium. This chamber connects with the true left atrium through a membrane with an orifice size of 3 mm to 1 cm. This causes obstruction to pulmonary venous return. Most patients have respiratory symptoms and are misdiagnosed as having primary pulmonary disease. There may be severe pulmonary hypertension.

Cardiac catheterization and injection of contrast material may be fatal, as these patients have severe pulmonary hypertension and may develop pulmonary edema after contrast injection. There may be slow flow in the posterior chamber, obscuring the obstructing membrane (180). MRI can readily demonstrates the membrane, which is always posterior to the left atrial outflow region and mitral valve (179).

Coronary Artery Abnormalities

Anomalous Origin of a Coronary Artery

Definition

Either coronary artery may arise anomalously, but the left coronary artery is much more commonly involved. In this entity, the left coronary artery arises not from the aorta but from the pulmonary artery.

Physiology

During the newborn period there is relative pulmonary hypertension, and blood readily flows from the pulmonary artery into the anomalous coronary artery which then sup-

plies the myocardium. However, as pulmonary vascular resistance decreases, pulmonary pressure falls and antegrade flow through the anomalous artery diminishes. The right coronary artery then enlarges and fills the left coronary artery through collaterals. Rather than perfuse the left ventricular myocardium, the left coronary artery blood takes the lower resistance pathway into the pulmonary artery. Although a left-to-right shunt is then created, the significance of the anomaly lies not in the shunt but in the steal of blood away from the left ventricular myocardium. Myocardial ischemia and infarction may develop.

Clinical Features

The patients are usually asymptomatic until they develop signs and symptoms of myocardial ischemia. Usually the patient's tachypnea, sweating, and irritability are misdiagnosed as an upper respiratory infection. The chest radiograph may show cardiomegaly and the ECG shows changes secondary to ischemia or infarction.

Radiography

Chest radiographs may be entirely normal. However, if the patient has had an infarct, marked cardiomegaly is present (Fig. 6-59A). The enlargement is left ventricular and sometimes left atrial because of mitral insufficiency. Massive cardiomegaly, left bronchial compression, and secondary left lung atelectasis may cause a large opaque hemithorax (181).

Angiography

Selective injection into the right coronary artery demonstrates an enlarged vessel that fills the left coronary artery in a retrograde fashion with subsequent flow into the pulmonary artery (Fig. 6-59B).

Treatment

These children risk death because of myocardial infarction or fatal arrhythmia. Surgical reimplantation of the anomalous coronary artery into the aorta restores the anatomy, but the damaged myocardium may not recover. The diagnosis is ideally made prior to ischemic changes so that repair will be curative.

Coronary Artery Fistula

Definition

A coronary artery fistula, the communication between a dilated main or branch coronary artery and an atrium or

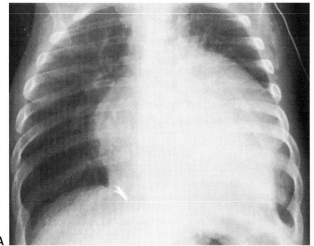

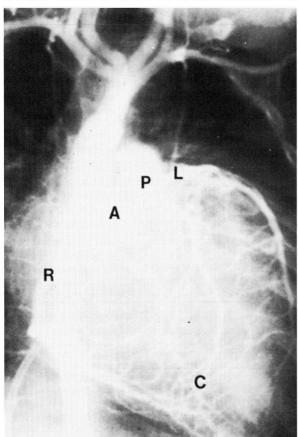

FIG. 6-59. Aberrant left coronary artery. A 3-month-old girl with dyspnea. **A:** There is marked cardiomegaly causing left lower lobe atelectasis. The enlargement is out of proportion to the prominence of the pulmonary vascularity. **B:** The right coronary artery *(R)* arises from the aorta *(A)* and fills the left coronary artery *(L)* in a retrograde manner via collaterals *(C)*. The left coronary artery *(L)* originates from the pulmonary artery *(P)*.

ventricle, probably represents the persistence of a normal fetal vascular communication. Most fistulas, whether from the right or left coronary artery, enter the right side of the heart.

Physiology

Because pressure in the coronary arteries is systemic and pressure in the right-sided heart chambers is much lower, significant left-to-right shunting occurs. Multiple sinusoidal communications may also be present.

Clinical Features

These infants are frequently asymptomatic but may have a murmur suggesting PDA. In other patients, cardiac failure develops in infancy. Echocardiography is diagnostically useful. Doppler sonography demonstrates turbulent flow from a dilated coronary artery into an atrium or a ventricle.

Treatment

Surgical closure of the fistulous connection is successful with low operative morbidity and mortality.

Cardiomyopathy

Despite different etiologies and variable natural histories, cardiomyopathies all adversely affect myocardial function (182). Primary cardiomyopathies have no associated vascular or systemic disease while secondary cardiomyopathies, such as glycogen storage disease, are part of a known systemic disease. Cardiomyopathies may also be classified by their anatomic and functional characteristics as dilated, hypertrophic, and restrictive.

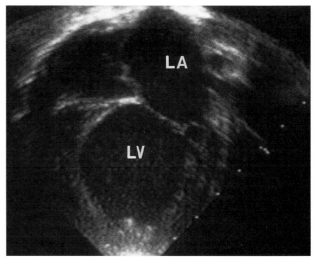

FIG. 6-60. Dilated cardiomyopathy. Four-chambered view echocardiography demonstrates marked dilatation of left atrium *(LA)* and left ventricle *(LV)*.

Dilated Cardiomyopathy

Dilated cardiomyopathy is due to an insult (infection, abnormal immune response, toxin, deposition of abnormal material, nutritional deficiency) that damages the cells of the heart. Most cases are idiopathic. Myocardial cellular dysfunction causes abnormal contraction of the myocardium and heart failure.

Infections frequently damage the myocardium and lead to dilated cardiomyopathy. Myocarditis (inflammation of the myocardium and myocellular necrosis) can be caused by bacterial, viral, rickettsial, fungal, or parasitic organisms. Many believe that in addition to infection, there is an abnormal immunologic response. The most common organisms are viral, particularly the enteroviruses. The diagnosis is suggested by tachypnea, dyspnea, wheezing, and signs of congestive heart failure. ECG and echocardiography document left ventricular dysfunction (Fig. 6-60). Chest radiographs show cardiomegaly, pulmonary edema, and left atrial and left ventricular enlargement (Fig. 6-61A, B). Molecular

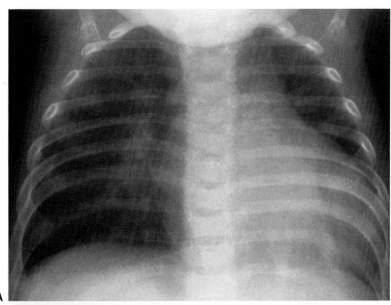

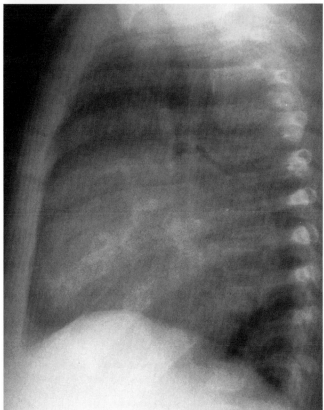

FIG. 6-61. Dilated cardiomyopathy. A: There is marked cardiomegaly and secondary volume loss of the left lower lobe. **B:** The lateral chest radiograph demonstrates marked left atrial and left ventricular enlargement.

biological techniques using DNA probes can detect enteroviral ribonucleuic acid (RNA) in myocardial cells obtained at biopsy (183). Unfortunately, in most cases, the biopsy is not diagnostic (184). Timing of the biopsy so that lymphocytic infiltrate and myocyte damage can be verified is critical (184,185). Biopsy of dilated cardiomyopathy obtained late in the course of disease is nonspecific.

The natural history of children with dilated cardiomyopathy is difficult to predict because of the diverse etiologies (186). The survival rate is 63% to 90% at 1 year and 20% to 80% at 5 years (182,186).

Hypertrophic Cardiomyopathy

Hypertrophic cardiomyopathy is characterized by hypertrophied myocardial cells and a nondilated left ventricle without aortic valvular stenosis. The hypertrophied myocardium creates increased wall thickness, which causes outflow obstruction. The pattern of left ventricular wall thickening varies, but the septum is usually focally involved and contributes to the obstruction. The forward motion of the mitral valve in systole also contributes to the subaortic obstruction. Hypertrophic cardiomyopathy is a hereditary disease; its multiple gene loci account for its heterogeneity.

Chest radiographs usually show cardiomegaly. Serial echocardiograms and ECGs are used to follow progression. Occasionally, ventricular septal myotomy must be performed in patients with high gradients and severe outflow obstruction.

Endocardial Fibroelastosis

Endocardial fibroelastosis may occur as a primary disease or may be secondary to left ventricular obstruction. There is striking deposition of collagen and elastin in the endocardium of the left ventricle. This results in restricted contractility and mitral insufficiency. Chest radiography demonstrates significant enlargement of the left ventricle and left atrium (Fig. 6-62).

Glycogen Storage Disease

Cardiac involvement occurs in glycogen storage disease type II (Pompe disease), which is a deficiency of α_{1-4}-glucosidase, a lysosomal enzyme that hydrolyses glycogen to glucose. There is deposition of glycogen in both skeletal muscles and myocardium. Massive thickening of the ventricular septum and walls causes cardiomyopathy.

Many systems are affected. The ECG shows high voltage, and echocardiography demonstrates thickening of the interventricular septum. Chest radiography shows striking cardiac enlargement, out of proportion to the prominence of the pulmonary vascularity. As the child ages, the increasing left atrial enlargement tends to compress the left lower lobe bronchus and cause collapse. Lateral films show left ventricular enlargement as well as left atrial enlargement.

Acquired Heart Disease

Kawasaki Disease

Kawasaki disease (mucocutaneous lymph node syndrome) is a multisystem illness characterized by fever, rash, conjunctivitis, inflammation and erythema of the lips and oral cavity, cervical adenopathy, and other abnormalities (187,188).

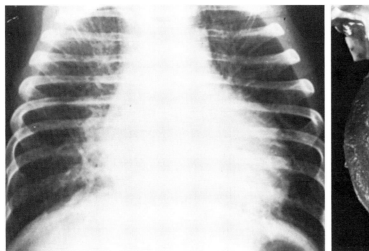
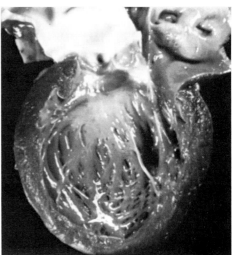

A   B

FIG. 6-62. Endocardial fibroelastosis. A 7-month-old boy with tachypnea and congestive heart failure. **A:** The heart is markedly enlarged. Interstitial pulmonary edema is manifested by hazy vessel margins and Kerley B lines. There are bilateral pleural effusions. **B:** Autopsy specimen. There is marked thickening of the wall of the left ventricle. Whitish material covers the endocardium.

Clinical Features

The acute phase of Kawasaki disease usually starts with the sudden onset of high fever, followed by a rash, nonpurulent conjunctivitis, cervical adenitis, reddening and fissuring of the lips, and erythema of the buccal mucosa. There may be erythema and induration of the hands and feet. There is a generalized vasculitis during the first 10 days of illness. During this acute febrile period, the patients may have acute myocarditis, sinus tachycardia, and a gallop rhythm. During the second to fourth weeks of illness, the patient may show desquamation of the palms and soles. Coronary artery aneurysms tend to arise in the proximal parts of both left and right coronary arteries. During the acute phase, these aneurysms may be fusiform, saccular, cylindrical, or segmental. Low-grade stenosis of the coronary arteries may also occur. Myocardial infarction may be the result; approximately one third of patients are clinically asymptomatic at the time of myocardial infarction.

Radiology

Chest radiographs are usually normal unless myocarditis is severe enough to cause cardiac enlargement. Rarely, cardiac contour abnormalities are caused by aneurysms; occasionally, the coronary aneurysms calcify.

Echocardiography

Echocardiography is the most useful modality for assessing cardiac complications of this disease. Medium and large aneurysms may be found in proximal segments of the major coronary arteries. Intravascular ultrasound used during cardiac catheterization can depict intimal changes and stenoses (40,41).

Angiography

Selective coronary angiography accurately depicts the extent of disease (Fig. 6-63). This study usually follows echocardiographic demonstration of aneurysms. Biplane selective angiography gives a precise delineation of the aneurysms, stenoses, occlusions, and collaterals, which may be important if coronary bypass or thrombolytic therapy is contemplated.

Treatment

Despite intensive research, the etiology of Kawasaki disease remains unknown. Treatment with gamma globulin combined with aspirin decreases the frequency of coronary artery abnormalities (189). Coronary artery bypass procedures have been performed for patients with angina or ECG changes of ischemia.

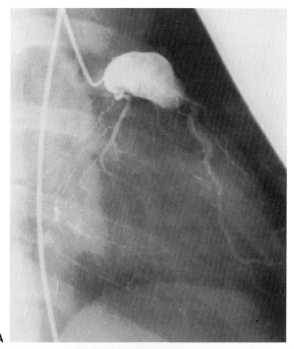

A

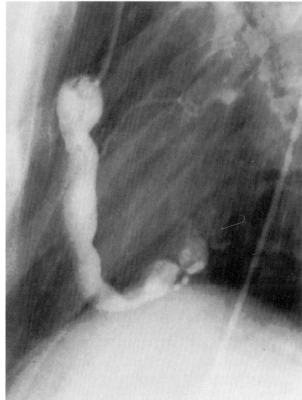

B

FIG. 6-63. Kawasaki disease. A: Selective arteriography shows a large saccular aneurysm of the proximal left coronary artery. **B:** Selective arteriography demonstrates multiple fusiform aneurysms and extensive involvement of the right coronary artery.

Acute Rheumatic Fever

Rheumatic fever is the most common cause, worldwide, of acquired heart disease in children and adults (190). After years of decreasing incidence, there has been a recent moderate resurgence in affluent countries. The prevalence is estimated at 5–15 cases per 1000 children; this translates into a total of several million children per year (191).

Clinical Features

Rheumatic fever is uncommon in children less than 5 years old. Infection by group A *Streptococci* is the precipitating event. However, there are many host factors, including the site of the infection, genetic predisposition, and immune reactivity. Tissue damage is probably related to an immunologic mechanism, either humoral or cellular (190–192).

A multisystem disease, rheumatic fever primarily affects the heart, joints, brain, and skin. Myocarditis, seen in approximately 50% of cases, is the most serious complication of acute rheumatic fever (190). Inflammation of the leaflets of the mitral and aortic valves and of the chordae of the mitral valve is characteristic. The tricuspid and pulmonic valves are rarely involved. Mitral insufficiency is the hallmark of rheumatic carditis. Aortic insufficiency occurs in approximately one fifth of patients, sometimes alone, often associated with mitral insufficiency.

Physiology

As fusion of the valve leaflets and shortening of the chordae tendineae occur, mitral stenosis develops. The left atrium becomes hypertrophied and enlarged. The stenotic

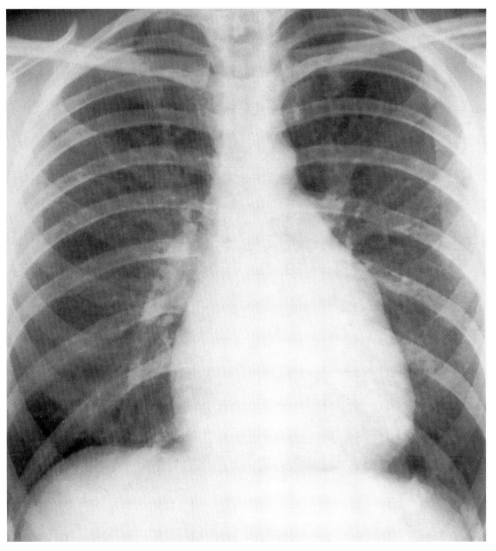

FIG. 6-64. Mitral stenosis. Radiographic findings include an extra bump, or mogul, along the left heart border due to enlargement of the left atrial appendage. Kerley B lines and pulmonary vascular redistribution are present.

valve cannot accommodate the increased flow that accompanies exercise, and the patient develops dyspnea.

Rheumatic aortic valve disease may present with isolated or dominant aortic insufficiency. Mild or moderate stenosis may co-exist. Congenital aortic stenosis is more common than rheumatic stenosis. Although the aortic valve lesion may heal, there is often inadequacy of valve coaptation during diastole and resultant insufficiency. Fusion of the valve leaflets during healing leads to stenosis.

Radiology

With moderate or even severe mitral stenosis, the heart may be normal in size, but there is prominence of the left atrial appendage, creating an extra bump on the left heart border (Fig. 6-64). Kerley B lines may be present, indicating elevated left atrial pressure. With aortic stenosis there may be dilatation of the ascending aorta secondary to the jet through the stenotic valve. In patients with aortic insufficiency, there is both dilatation of the left ventricle and prominence of the ascending aorta.

Echocardiography

Echocardiography demonstrates enlargement of the left atrium, left ventricle, or both. The severity of incompetence can be roughly quantified using spatial mapping and Doppler techniques. Pressure gradients can be assessed and followed serially.

Angiography

Cardiac catheterization and angiography are occasionally useful for precise quantitation of the degree of mitral insufficiency. Catheterization may also be performed if balloon angioplasty of the affected mitral or aortic valve is considered or operative valve replacement is needed.

Treatment

The initial treatment involves eradication of streptococci from the tonsils and other tissues, plus effective prophylaxis. Children with acute carditis are treated with bed rest, aspirin, and occasionally steroids. The valvular disease frequently resolves completely. Acute rheumatic heart disease is seldom fatal.

Congenital Aortic Arch Anomalies

Normal Left Aortic Arch

For understanding normal development and malformations of the aortic arch, the Edwards double-arch system

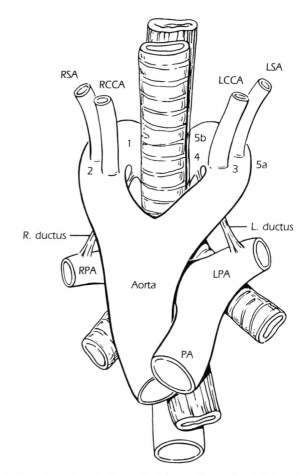

FIG. 6-65. Hypothetical double aortic arch of Edwards. Types of aortic arch depend on the site of interruption (193). The sites of interruptions are numbered. *1*, normal left aortic arch; *2*, left aortic arch with aberrant right subclavian artery; *3*, right aortic arch with aberrant left subclavian artery; *4*, right aortic arch with mirror-image branching; *5a*, *5b*, right aortic arch with isolation of left subclavian artery. *LCCA*, left common carotid artery; *LPA*, left pulmonary artery; *LSA*, left subclavian artery; *PA*, pulmonary artery; *RCCA*, right common carotid artery; *RPA*, right pulmonary artery; *RSA*, right subclavian artery.

(from which both arches are derived) is useful (193). This double arch has a ductus arteriosus on each side. The descending aorta is in the midline (Fig. 6-65). Interruption of this arch system in different locations explains various aortic arch anomalies (Fig. 6-66).

The normal configuration is due to interruption of the dorsal segment of the right arch between the right subclavian artery and descending aorta and involution of the right ductus arteriosus (193). The normal left-sided aortic arch produces a slight extrinsic compression on the trachea and deviates it to the right. It should be stressed that in children with a left-sided aortic arch the trachea is not truly midline but is slightly to the right of midline. In children the trachea bows away from the side of the aortic arch during expiration, deviating the trachea farther to the right in a patient with a normal left-sided aortic arch.

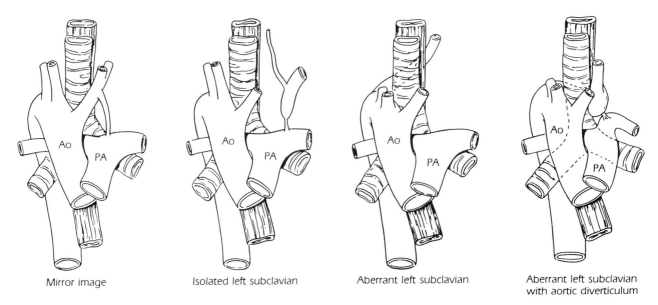

Mirror image   Isolated left subclavian   Aberrant left subclavian   Aberrant left subclavian with aortic diverticulum

FIG. 6-66. Types of right aortic arch. *Ao*, aorta; *PA*, pulmonary artery.

Left Aortic Arch with Aberrant Right Subclavian Artery

The most common congenital arch anomaly is the coexistence of an aberrant right subclavian artery and a left aortic arch. It is a frequent incidental finding during upper gastrointestinal examination. Its incidence in the population is about 1 in 200 (0.5%). The anomaly is due to interruption of the embryonic right arch between the right common carotid and the right subclavian arteries (Fig. 6-65). The right ductus arteriosus almost always disappears, so there is no vascular ring.

Anatomically, the aberrant right subclavian artery arises just distal to the left subclavian artery and passes across the mediastinum posterior to the esophagus to reach the right upper extremity. On esophagography, there is a characteristic oblique posterior indentation on the esophagus, passing from lower left to upper right. A left-sided aortic arch with an aberrant right subclavian artery never or almost never causes tracheal or esophageal compression symptoms. If the aberrant right subclavian artery arises distal to a coarctation, there may be unilateral left-sided rib notching.

Right Aortic Arch with Mirror Image Branching

A right aortic arch with mirror image branching is frequently associated with congenital heart disease. The aortic arch is on the right, and the aorta descends on the right. The first vessel to arise from the aorta is the left innominate artery, followed by the right common carotid artery and the right subclavian artery (Fig. 6-66). This type of arch is due to interruption of the embryonic left arch just distal to the left ductus arteriosus (Fig. 6-65). There is a left ductus arteriosus connecting the left pulmonary artery to the left subclavian

artery. The position of the ductus or ligamentum arteriosum is such that there is no vascular ring.

Plain films show a right-sided aortic arch and right descending aorta. Because there is mirror image branching of the brachiocephalic vessels, there is no posterior indentation on the barium-filled esophagus and no forward displacement of the trachea on the lateral view. If situs inversus is excluded, congenital heart disease is present in 98% of patients with a right aortic arch and mirror-image branching. The anomalies include tetralogy of Fallot (90% of the total), truncus arteriosus (2.5%), transposition of the great vessels (1.5%), atrial or ventricular septal defect (0.5%), and a few other lesions. Approximately 30% of patients with tetralogy of Fallot have a mirror image right aortic arch, as do 35% of patients with truncus arteriosus, a much rarer lesion.

Right Aortic Arch with Aberrant Left Subclavian Artery

A right aortic arch with an aberrant left subclavian artery is the result of interruption of the left arch between the left common carotid and the left subclavian arteries (Fig. 6-65). Except for the ductus or ligamentum, this anomaly is a mirror image of a left arch with an aberrant right subclavian artery discussed (Fig. 6-66). This lesion, in which the left ligamentum or ductus completes the vascular ring, is sometimes symptomatic and sometimes not. The incidence of intracardiac defects (5% to 12%) is higher than in the normal population (<1%) but still considerably less than in patients with mirror-image-branching right aortic arch. Congenital heart lesions occurring in patients with a right-sided aortic arch and aberrant left subclavian artery include tetralogy of Fallot (71%), ASD or VSD (21%), and coarctation of the aorta (7%). Although the ductus or ligamentum completes the ring in all or nearly all of these patients, only 5% develop compression symptoms. In patients with compression of the trachea or esophagus, there is usually a large aortic diverticulum serving the left subclavian artery and a tight left-sided ligamentum arteriosum (Fig. 6-66). This type of right aortic arch is difficult or impossible to differentiate from a double aortic arch by chest radiography or esophagography; MRI clarifies the diagnosis.

Right Aortic Arch with Isolation of Left Subclavian Artery

Right aortic arch with isolation of the left subclavian artery is considerably less common than the previously discussed types of right aortic arch (193). This congenital malformation is explained by interruption of the left arch at two levels: one between the left common carotid and left subclavian arteries, and the other just distal to the left ductus arteriosus (Fig. 6-65). The left subclavian artery is no longer connected to the aorta but is attached to the left pulmonary artery by the left ligamentum or ductus arteriosus (Fig. 6-66). There is a right aortic arch, and the thoracic aorta descends on the right. There is no posterior defect on the barium-filled esophagus.

This anomaly produces a congenital subclavian steal syndrome, as the left subclavian artery is isolated from the aorta and derives its blood supply from the left vertebral artery. The clue is an absent or diminished pulse in the left upper

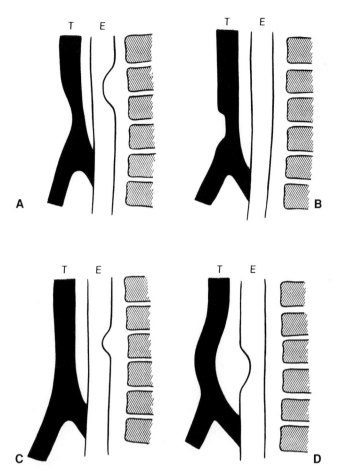

FIG. 6-67. Common vascular rings and other vascular impressions. A: Double aortic arch or right aortic arch with aberrant left subclavian artery, aortic diverticulum, and left ligamentum arteriosum. **B:** Innominate artery or common carotid artery compression. **C:** Left aortic arch with aberrant right subclavian artery. **D:** Pulmonary sling. *E,* esophagus; *T,* trachea. Modified from Berdon and Baker (195).

extremity. Most cases of isolation of the left subclavian artery occur in patients with a right aortic arch and tetralogy of Fallot, although the anomaly has also been described in patients without congenital heart disease (193).

Vascular Rings and Slings

A vascular ring is an anomaly in which there is complete encirclement of the trachea and esophagus by the aortic arch and its vascular derivatives. Vascular anomalies may be divided into those that produce symptoms and those that don't (Table 6-16) (194). If a vascular ring is not complete, there are rarely symptoms. If the ring is complete, symptoms may be due to tracheal compression (respiratory distress, wheezing, tachypnea) or esophageal compression (difficulty swallowing, vomiting, choking, aspiration); tracheal symptoms are more common. Some complete rings, especially right arches with aberrant subclavian arteries, are not tight enough to produce symptoms.

TABLE 6-16. *Congenital aortic anomalies*

Asymptomatic anomalies
  Left aortic arch with aberrant right subclavian artery[a]
  Right aortic arch, aberrant left subclavian artery, loose left ligamentum
  Mirror-image right aortic arch
  Circumflex aorta
    Right aortic arch with left descending aorta
    Left aortic arch with right descending aorta
  Innominate or left common carotid artery compression syndrome[a]
Symptomatic anomalies
  Double aortic arch[a]
    Left descending aorta
    Right descending aorta
  Left aortic arch, aberrant right subclavian artery, right ligamentum
  Right aortic arch, aberrant left subclavian artery, left ligamentum[a]
  Mirror-image right aortic arch—congenital heart disease[a]
  Circumflex aorta
    Right aortic arch, left ligamentum
    Left aortic arch, right ligamentum
  Compression syndrome
    Innominate artery[a]
    Left common carotid artery
  Pulmonary sling: aberrant left pulmonary artery
  Congenital subclavian steal: right aortic arch, isolated left subclavian artery

[a] More common.

Modified from Swischuk and Sapire (10).

The diagnosis and differentiation of vascular rings traditionally has been based on chest radiography and esophagography (Fig. 6-67) (20,194,195). Preoperative angiography is seldom necessary, although occasionally a vascular ring requires repair via a right rather than left thoracotomy (196). However, with the advent of MRI, precise anatomic diagnoses can be made without invasive studies (197). If the chest film demonstrates tracheal compression, probably by a great vessel, the next study should be MRI. T1-weighted, ECG-gaited images are used exclusively. The axial plane provides maximal information concerning the anatomy of the anomaly (197). The coronal plane is also useful in demonstrating the pathology; however, in most cases it is an optional supplement. The inherent natural contrast of intraluminal flowing blood obviates the need for intravenous or intraarterial contrast media. MRI is extremely useful for showing the vascular anomaly and determining the extent of any tracheal compression (Fig. 6-68).

Double Aortic Arch

A double aortic arch, a true vascular ring, encircles the trachea and esophagus (Figs. 6-68 and 6-69). It is the most common symptomatic vascular ring. The anomaly usually exists in isolation but can be associated with congenital heart disease. Symptoms may begin at birth or, if the vascular ring is loose, not until later. Each arch, right and left, gives rise

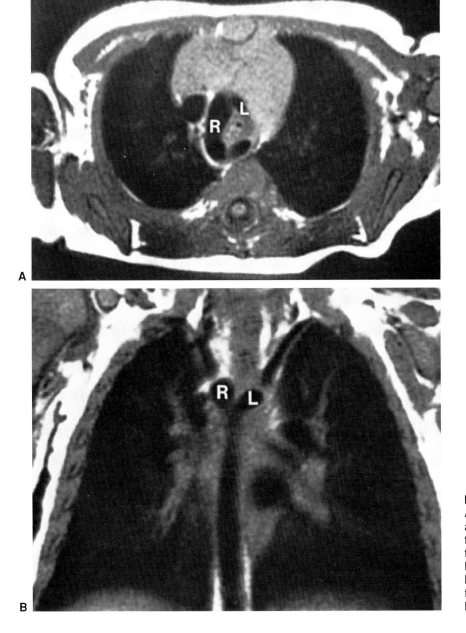

FIG. 6-68. Double aortic arch. A: Axial MRI through the double aortic arch. Both right *(R)* and left *(L)* limbs of the double arch are seen encircling the trachea and esophagus. **B:** Coronal MRI demonstrates that the right *(R)* and left *(L)* limbs of the double arch join posteriorly. The right arch *(R)* is higher and larger. From Bisset et al. (197).

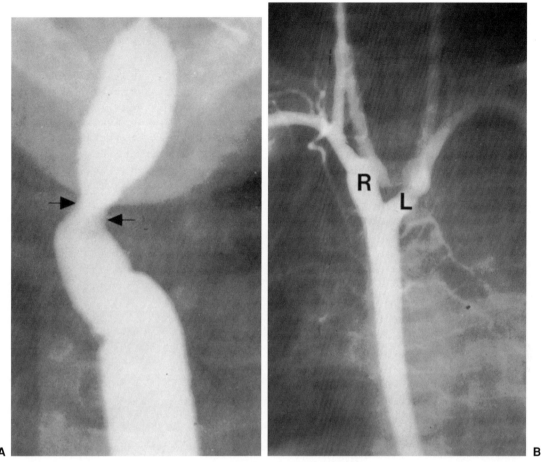

FIG. 6-69. Double aortic arch. A: Anteroposterior esophagogram. There are bilateral extrinsic compressions on the esophagus *(arrows)* to produce a reverse S-shaped appearance. **B:** Thoracic aortogram. A double aortic arch is identified. The right arch *(R)* is larger and higher, and it gives rise to the right subclavian and right common carotid arteries. The left aortic arch *(L)* gives rise to the left subclavian and left common carotid arteries.

to one carotid and one subclavian artery. The ascending aorta arises anterior to the trachea and divides into an anterior (left) and posterior (right) arch; these then join posteriorly to form a common descending aorta. The descending aorta may be on the left or right side. There are many variables, including the relative size of each arch, local areas of nonpatency, the position of the upper descending aorta, and the site of the ductus arteriosus. The right arch is usually larger, more posterior, and higher than the left aortic arch; it passes posterior to the trachea and esophagus to join the left arch.

In infants with a double aortic arch, the aorta may indent the right lateral border of the trachea. The trachea may be malpositioned in the middle of the mediastinum or slightly displaced to the left. The lateral radiograph usually demonstrates anterior bowing of the trachea caused by the retrotracheal aorta. On the AP view of the esophagram, there are bilateral indentations on the esophagus. The higher, larger indentation is caused by the right aortic arch, and the lower indentation is caused by the smaller left aortic arch (Fig.

6-69A). A lateral esophagram shows that the retrotracheal indentation is actually retroesophageal.

Innominate Artery Compression Syndrome

Although not a true vascular ring, the innominate artery and occasionally the common carotid artery origin may produce an isolated anterior tracheal compression (195,198). In young children the normal innominate artery has its aortic origin to the left of the trachea, and it must obliquely cross the trachea as it ascends into the mediastinum and the neck (199). As it crosses the trachea, it sometimes indents the trachea, but usually it does not cause symptoms (198–200). In a small percentage of children (the percentage is controversial), the innominate artery may cause significant persistent compression of the trachea, and the child may have signs and symptoms of airway obstruction. Stridor, cough, dyspnea, and occasionally cyanosis may occur. The term *reflex apnea* is used to describe episodes of reflex respiratory

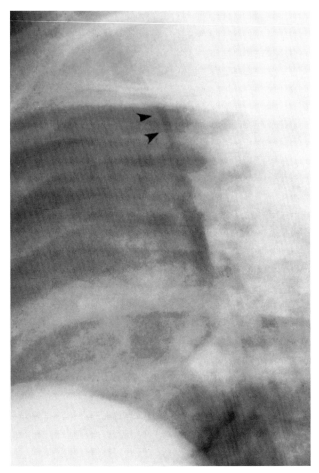

FIG. 6-70. Innominate artery compression syndrome. A lateral chest radiograph demonstrates marked anterior compression of the trachea at the thoracic inlet *(arrowheads)*.

arrest that seem to occur during feeding in patients with severe innominate artery compression syndrome.

Radiographically, the diagnosis can be made by finding persistent anterior narrowing of the trachea at the level of the thoracic inlet on lateral radiographs (Fig. 6-70). In symptomatic patients, fluoroscopy may show persistence of tracheal indentation through the respiratory cycle and collapse during expiration. A barium swallow should be performed to verify that other anomalies are not present and to evaluate for gastroesophageal reflux. There is an increased incidence of innominate artery compression syndrome in patients who have esophageal dilatation secondary to repaired esophageal atresia or severe gastroesophageal reflux. The dilated esophagus compresses the trachea posteriorly and displaces the trachea's anterior wall into the innominate artery. At endoscopy, there is anterior tracheal narrowing by the pulsating innominate artery, and there are frequently abnormal tracheal cartilages. MRI can establish the degree and extent of compression and tracheomalacia. Surgical correction of innominate artery compression is controversial. In the presence of apnea, endoscopic tracheal narrowing, and significant persistent compression as seen by MRI, many surgeons

perform an aortopexy or reimplantation of the innominate artery on the right side of the ascending aorta.

Pulmonary Sling

Anomalous origin of the left pulmonary artery, a sling rather than a ring, may be isolated or part of a more complex anomaly (201). The left pulmonary artery is aberrant and arises from the right pulmonary artery. It crosses over the proximal portion of the right mainstem bronchus or adjacent trachea and then proceeds posteriorly and to the left behind the trachea and in front of the esophagus at or slightly above the level of the carina (Fig. 6-71). The left pulmonary artery then courses to the left, and obliquely downward, in the hilum of the left lung. The distal trachea and carina are often displaced to the left. There may be an impression on the right mainstem bronchus, the trachea, or both by the anomalous vessel. Plain radiographs of the chest usually show hyperinflation or asymmetrical inflation of the lungs, a low position of the left hilum, and anterior bowing of the lower trachea or right mainstem bronchus (Fig. 6-72A) (201). In addition to the posterior indentation on the trachea, there is frequently anterior indentation on the barium-filled esophagus (Fig. 6-72B). This compression is produced by the anomalous vessel as it passes between the esophagus and the trachea. Tracheal stenosis or tracheomalacia may occur at the site of the anomalous vessel. There may be more than one site of tracheal narrowing, and the cartilaginous rings may be complete (202). MRI accurately assesses the vascular anomaly and the degree and extent of the tracheal anomaly (Fig. 6-73).

Cardiac Associations with Types of Situs

Situs Solitus

The cardiac apex, aortic arch, arterial or oxygenated atrium, and spleen are on the left in situs solitus. Although any cardiac anomaly may occur in situs solitus, the overall incidence of congenital heart disease is only 0.6% to 0.8%.

Situs Solitus with Right-Sided Cardiac Apex

In this situation the cardiac apex is on the right, whereas the arterial or oxygenated atrium (left atrium) and spleen are on the left. There is a 95% to 98% incidence of congenital heart disease. Approximately 80% of these patients have l-transposition (corrected transposition). If cyanosis and shunt vascularity are both present, tricuspid atresia is the most likely diagnosis. If cyanosis is present with decreased vascularity, the most likely diagnosis is corrected transposition with VSD and pulmonary atresia. The possibility of asplenia or polysplenia with even more complex congenital heart disease must also be considered.

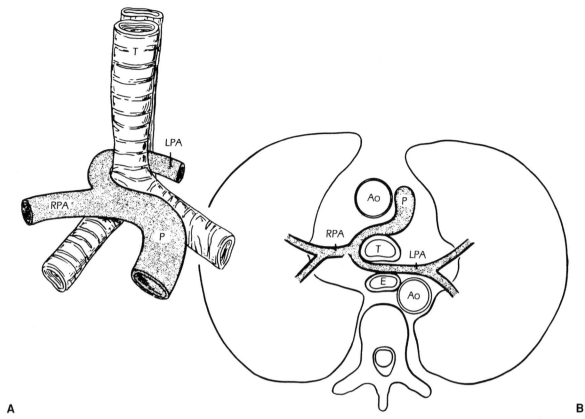

FIG. 6-71. Pulmonary sling. A: Anterior view. **B:** Axial projection. The left pulmonary artery *(LPA)* arises from the right pulmonary artery *(RPA)* and passes between the trachea and esophagus. *Ao,* thoracic aorta; *E,* esophagus; *P,* main pulmonary artery; *T,* trachea.

Situs Inversus

The cardiac apex, aortic arch, arterial atrium (left atrium), and spleen are on the right in situs inversus (Fig. 6-74). This abnormality occurs in 0.01% of the population. The incidence of congenital heart disease in patients with situs inversus, although only 3% to 5%, is still considerably greater than in patients with situs solitus (2). If congenital heart disease is present, the most common malformation is corrected transposition (l-TGV).

Situs Inversus with Left-Sided Cardiac Apex

The cardiac apex is on the left and the aortic arch, arterial atrium (left atrium), and spleen are on the right (Fig. 6-75). This rare abnormality has virtually a 100% association with congenital heart disease, often complex. There is no prevalence of any one cardiac malformation (2).

Situs Solitus with Malposition of Abdominal Viscera

In this abnormality, the cardiac apex, aortic arch, and arterial atrium (left atrium) are on the left and the spleen is on the right (Fig. 6-76). The possibility of asplenia or polysplenia should be considered. Congenital heart disease, usually a left-to-right shunt, is present in most patients. Almost all of these patients have polysplenia with interruption of the infrahepatic segment of the inferior vena cava and azygous continuation (Fig. 6-76B).

Situs Inversus with Malposition of Abdominal Viscera

The cardiac apex, aortic arch, and arterial atrium (left atrium) are on the right and the spleen is on the left. The possibility of asplenia or polysplenia must be considered. Congenital heart disease, usually a left-to-right shunt, is seen in most patients. Most of these patients have polysplenia with azygous continuation of the inferior vena cava.

Asplenia and Polysplenia

The asplenia and polysplenia syndromes are developmental complexes with a striking tendency for the symmetric development of normally asymmetric organs. The abnormalities may include absence of a normal unilateral structure, bilateral development of a normal unilateral organ, or excessive tissue of a normal unilateral organ (Table 6-17).

Radiographically, whenever there is discordance between

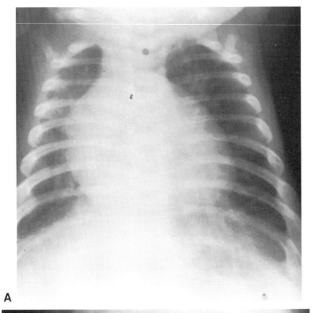

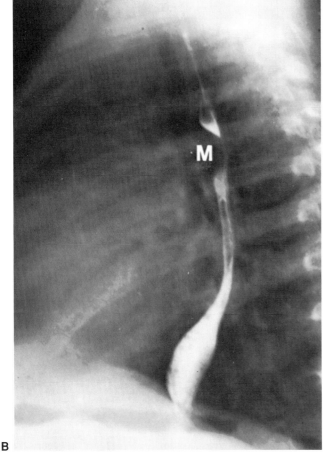

B

FIG. 6-72. **Pulmonary sling.** A 4-year-old girl with VSD and PDA. **A:** The heart is large and there is increased vascularity. The volume and lucency of the left lung are increased compared with the right lung. **B:** Lateral chest with barium in the esophagus shows a soft-tissue mass *(M)* between the anteriorly bowed trachea and the extrinsically compressed esophagus. (Courtesy of Hooshang Taybi, M.D., Oakland, CA.)

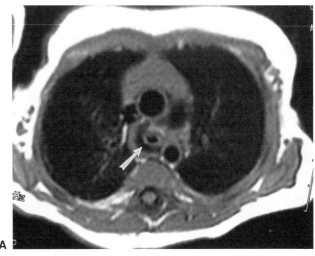

A

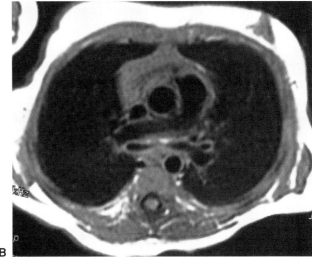

B

FIG. 6-73. **Pulmonary sling. A:** Axial image demonstrates the anomalous left pulmonary artery *(arrow)* passing posterior to the trachea and then entering the left lung. **B:** Axial image shows absence of the normal origin of the left pulmonary artery.

the cardiac apex and situs, one should consider the possibility of polysplenia or asplenia. The best indicator of situs on the chest radiograph is the tracheobronchial anatomy. The longer mainstem bronchus is normally left-sided. The right mainstem bronchus is shorter. In addition to tracheobronchial anatomy, one should also look for venous anomalies. This includes close inspection for the shadow of the inferior vena cava on the lateral film, for a dilated azygous vein in the right superior mediastinum, and for a left SVC.

Asplenia

There is a tendency for bilateral right-sidedness in asplenia. The asplenia syndrome is almost invariably associated with severe, complex congenital heart disease carrying a poor prognosis. The cardiac anomalies, as a group, are

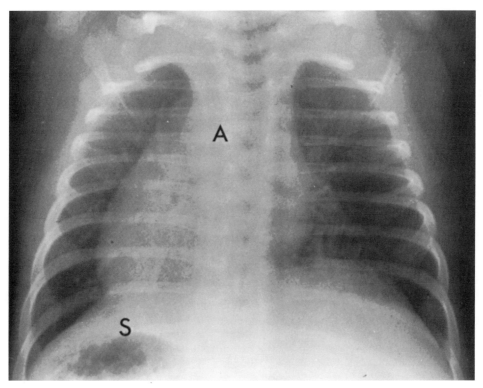

FIG. 6-74. Situs inversus without congenital heart disease. The cardiac apex, aortic arch *(A)*, and stomach *(S)* are on the right. The heart size and pulmonary vascularity are normal.

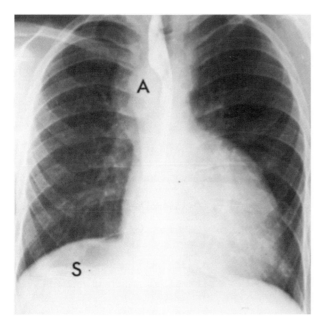

FIG. 6-75. Situs inversus with left-sided cardiac apex. The aortic arch *(A)* and stomach *(S)* are on the right, and the cardiac apex is on the left. Note the decreased pulmonary vascularity. Cardiac catheterization and angiocardiography showed corrected transposition, common ventricle, and pulmonary stenosis.

more complicated than those of polysplenia. Cyanosis is usually present during the neonatal period. Children are at risk for serious infections, such as meningitis and sepsis. Radiologic features include decreased pulmonary vascularity, normal or slightly enlarged heart, cardiac malposition, symmetric liver, midline gastric bubble, midgut malrotation, and bilateral right tracheobronchial pattern (Fig. 6-77) (31,203). There may be mesocardia, levocardia, or dextrocardia. Heinz or Howell-Jolly bodies on peripheral smears confirm the lack of a spleen. Abdominal ultrasonography, CT, and MRI show the tracheobronchial anatomy, the position of intraabdominal structures, and associated vascular anomalies (28,203,204). MRI of the chest and upper abdomen demonstrates the congenital cardiac anomalies and any anomalies of systemic venous return.

Polysplenia

There is a tendency for bilateral left-sidedness or levoisomerism in patients with polysplenia (31). The presentation of patients with polysplenia reflects their underlying congenital heart disease. They are usually acyanotic and have congestive heart failure due to pulmonary overcirculation, either alone or in combination with left-sided obstructive lesions. There is little increased susceptibility to infection. The radiologic features include increased pulmonary vascularity, large heart, absent IVC shadow, dilated azygos vein, cardiac malposition, various hepatic positions, malposition of the stomach, malrotation of the bowel, absence of a minor

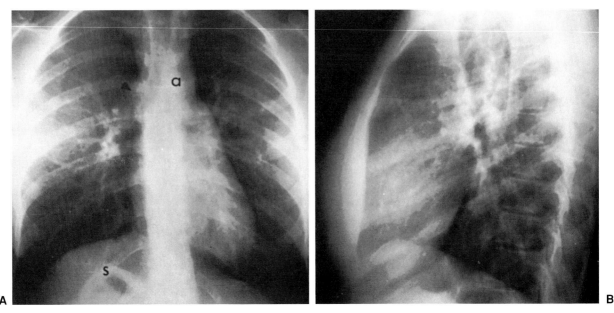

FIG. 6-76. Situs solitus with malposition of abdominal viscera. A: The aortic arch *(a)* and cardiac apex are on the left, and the stomach *(s)* is on the right. There is increased pulmonary vascularity and enlargement of the azygous vein *(arrow)*. **B:** The inferior vena cava is not identified on the lateral chest radiograph. Angiocardiography in this patient with polysplenia demonstrated azygous continuation of the inferior vena cava and a ventricular septal defect.

fissure on either side, and a left tracheobronchial pattern on both sides. Congenital cardiac malformations in the polysplenia syndrome are less severe than those in asplenia and frequently are amenable to surgery.

Operative Procedures for Congenital Heart Disease

A critical step in the evaluation of the chest radiograph of a patient with possible congenital heart disease is careful analysis of the extracardiac structures (see Fig. 6-12). There

may be evidence of previous palliative or corrective surgery for congenital heart disease. Postoperative thoracic wall deformities may be right-sided, left-sided, or midline (i.e., a sternotomy) (Table 6-18). Radiologic signs of thoracotomy include soft-tissue swelling, unevenness (usually insufficient width) of intercostal spaces, pleural fluid or pleural thickening, bony sclerosis, and rib regeneration. Metallic wires in the sternum indicate previous sternotomy. Surgical clips are often noted in the mediastinum. Prosthetic valves are usually radiopaque; they include mitral valve prostheses, aortic valve prostheses, and porcine valves in external conduits.

TABLE 6-17. *Comparison of asplenia and polysplenia*

Organ	Asplenia	Polysplenia
Cardiac	Corrected transposition with VSD or single ventricle	Azygos continuation of IVC
	Pulmonary atresia or stenosis	Anomalous pulmonary venous return
	Common atrium	ASD or common atrium
	Bilateral SVC	VSD
	Total anomalous pulmonary venous return	Bilaterial SVC
	Cardiac malposition	Cardiac malposition
Pulmonary	Trilobed lungs	Bilobed lungs
	Bilateral epiarterial bronchi	Bilateral hyparterial bronchi
	Decreased pulmonary vascularity	Increased pulmonary vascularity
Abdominal	Heterotaxy	Heterotaxy
	Complete: situs inversus	Complete: situs inversus
	Partial	Partial
	Horizontal liver	Horizontal liver
	Malrotation	Malrotation
	Midline gallbladder, gallbladder duplication	Absent gallbladder
	Midline stomach: microgastria	Malposition of stomach

ASD, atrial septal defect; IVC, inferior vena cava; SVC, superior vena cava; VSD, ventricular septal defect.

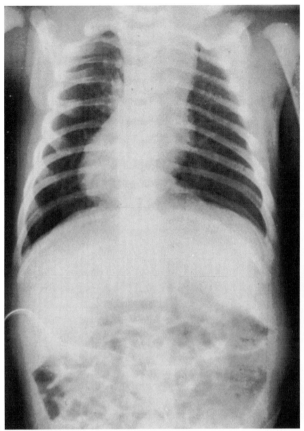
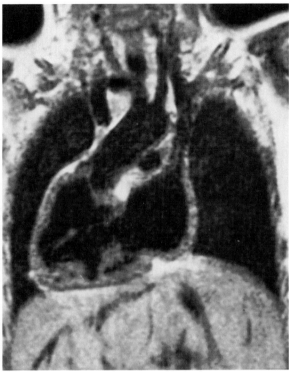

FIG. 6-77. Asplenia. A: A cyanotic newborn who has dextrocardia, midline liver (situs ambiguus), and decreased pulmonary vascularity. **B:** A coronal MRI scan demonstrates midline liver, dextrocardia, left superior vena cava, pulmonary atresia, and corrected transposition.

Embolized coils, often multiple, indicate closure of vessels, usually systemic vessels to the lungs. Clam-shell devices usually indicate closure of an ASD or PDA.

Surgical repairs of ventricular and atrial septal defect, aortic stenosis, pulmonary stenosis, tetralogy of Fallot, and transposition of the great vessels are usually performed through midline sternotomies (Table 6-18). Closure of a patent ductus arteriosus, repair of coarctation of the aorta, pulmonary artery banding, palliative systemic-to-pulmonary anastomosis, and mitral valve commissurotomies are usually performed through a left-sided thoracotomy (Table 6-18).

Blalock-Taussig Shunt

The Blalock-Taussig shunt is an end-to-side anastomosis of a subclavian artery to the ipsilateral pulmonary artery. One modification uses a graft to anastomose a systemic vessel (usually the subclavian artery) to the pulmonary artery (Fig. 6-78). The procedure usually results in asymmetry of the pulmonary arteries, with the side of the shunt having larger arteries. This shunt imposes an extra volume load on the left ventricle. There may also be progressive pulmonary vascular changes due to transmission of arterial pressures through the systemic shunt.

Glenn Shunt

In the classic unidirectional Glenn shunt, the SVC is anastomosed to the right pulmonary artery, which has been di-

TABLE 6-18. *Postoperative thoracic deformity*

Right thoracotomy	Sternotomy	Left thoracotomy
Blalock-Taussig shunt	VSD ASD	Blalock-Taussig shunt PDA
Central conduit shunt	Aortic stenosis Valve replacement	Coarctation
Blalock-Hanlon operation	Pulmonary stenosis Tetralogy repair Conduit Transposition repair Fontan procedure Glenn shunt Cardiac transplantation	PA banding Vascular ring

ASD, atrial septal defect; PA, pulmonary artery; PDA, patent ductus arteriosus; VSD, ventricular septal defect.

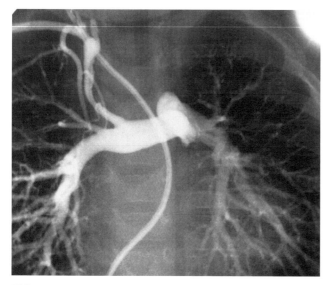

FIG. 6-78. Right Blalock-Taussig shunt. Selective injection of shunt between right subclavian artery and right pulmonary artery. Note the large amount of flow and the retrograde filling of the main and left pulmonary arteries.

vided or separated from the main and left pulmonary artery. A bidirectional Glenn shunt is an end-to-side anastomosis of the SVC to the ipsilateral pulmonary artery, which remains in continuity with the main and left pulmonary arteries; its blood therefore flows in two directions, to the right and to the left (Fig. 6-79). One of the benefits of this type of shunt is that it increases flow of desaturated blood to the pulmonary arteries without volume overload of the left ventricle. A bidirectional Glenn shunt also protects against the development of the pulmonary vascular disease that fol-

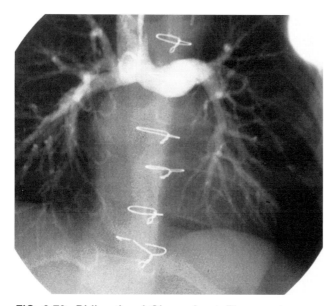

FIG. 6-79. Bidirectional Glenn shunt. The superior vena cava is anastomosed end-to-side to the right pulmonary artery. Both pulmonary arteries fill.

lows many systemic pulmonary shunts. A Glenn shunt is usually ultimately followed by a Fontan repair.

Arterial Switch Procedure

The arterial switch procedure (Jatene procedure) is used in infants for total repair of transposition of the great vessels. With this procedure the great vessels are transected above their respective valves and switched so that the pulmonary artery arises from the right ventricle and the aorta from the left ventricle. The coronary arteries are then moved to the systemic vessel (see Fig. 6-44).

Fontan Procedure

The Fontan procedure is used in patients with single-ventricle, tricuspid atresia, hypoplastic right ventricle, and other complex anomalies. The procedure is a direct anastomosis or placement of a conduit (with or without a valve) from the right atrium to the main pulmonary artery. This diverts systemic venous return to the lungs and bypasses the right ventricle. One modification uses a lateral tunnel or total caval connection: the inferior vena caval return is directed along the right atrial lateral wall using a patch to the inferior aspect of the pulmonary artery or SVC. Another modification incorporates the native pulmonary valve in hopes that the subpulmonary ventricular chamber will be contractile. Complications of the Fontan procedure include elevated systemic venous pressure, elevated right atrial pressure, thrombosis in the right heart chambers, and pulmonary arteriovenous malformations. Some patients have progressive excercise intolerance, effusions, arrhythmias, or protein losing enteropathy. Conversion of other Fontan procedures to the lateral atrial tunnel may afford clinical improvement for some of these patients (205).

A fenestrated Fontan procedure creates a small opening to allow right-to-left interatrial shunting with decompression of the right heart. This small atrial defect can be closed later with occlusive devices.

Mustard or Senning Repair

These surgical procedures are atrial repairs that were formerly used for children with d-TGV. The arterial switch procedure is now the preferred treatment. In the atrial repairs, a pericardial baffle is placed in the common atrium in such a fashion that systemic venous return is directed into the left ventricle and thus to the lungs, and pulmonary venous return is directed to the right ventricle and aorta. Stenosis may develop in the tunnel, which leads to obstruction of the SVC and inferior vena cava and secondary dilatation of the azygous and hemiazygous venous systems. Right heart failure and right ventricular arrhythmias are also late complications of the Mustard and Senning repairs.

Norwood Procedure

The Norwood technique is a two- or three-stage surgical procedure for patients with hypoplastic left heart syndrome (Fig. 6-80A). In stage I, a neo-aorta is constructed using the proximal main pulmonary artery, which is anastomosed with or without a conduit to the descending aorta (Fig. 6-80B). The distal pulmonary artery is oversewn and a Blalock-Taussig shunt or central shunt carries systemic arterial blood to the pulmonary arteries. A large (nonrestrictive) ASD is also created. In stage II, performed approximately 6–12 months later, a bidirectional Glenn shunt is placed and the Blalock-Taussig or central shunt is ligated (Fig. 6-80C). Stage III, performed by 2 years of age, is a conversion of the Glenn shunt to a Fontan procedure (Fig. 6-80D).

Rashkind Balloon Septostomy

The Rashkind procedure is an atrial septostomy performed via a percutaneous technique in patients who have inadequate atrial mixing. The procedure is commonly performed

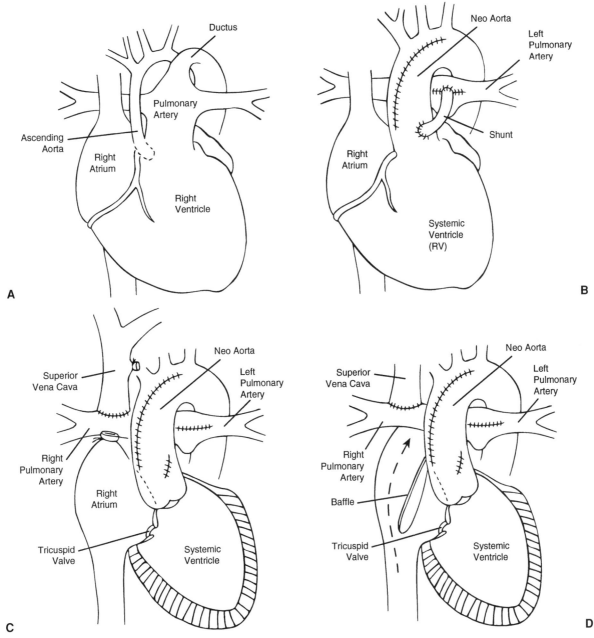

FIG. 6-80. Norwood procedure. A: Hypoplastic left heart. **B:** Stage I. The hypoplastic ascending aorta is incorporated into the main pulmonary artery. The neo-aorta is anastomosed to the descending aorta. The pulmonary arteries are shunted to the lungs. **C:** Stage II. Glenn shunt. **D:** Stage III. Fontan procedure.

in infants with d-TGV and occasionally for tricuspid atresia. A balloon is inflated in the left atrium and rapidly pulled back across the septum. The tear in the atrial septum allows better mixing of blood between the atrial chambers.

Rastelli Procedure

The Rastelli surgical procedure is performed in patients with d-TGV and a large VSD. An external conduit connects the right ventricle to the pulmonary artery. Blood flows from the left ventricle to the ascending aorta through the VSD.

Cardiac Transplantation

Since 1980, several thousand children, ranging in age from newborn to adolescent, have undergone cardiac transplantation. The overall 15-year survival rate is approximately 40% (206). Some indications for cardiac transplantation in infants and children include congenital heart disease with end-stage ventricular dysfunction, hypoplastic left heart syndrome, and cardiomyopathy (206–208). One of the most important considerations prior to transplantation is the match between the size of the donor heart and the chest size of the pediatric recipient. The major causes of death following transplantation include rejection, early graft failure, infection, and sudden death (208,209). Cardiac transplantation evokes an immune response directed to a variety of antigens. Following cardiac transplantation, patients are maintained on immunosuppressive therapy and closely monitored for rejection. Coronary artery disease, caused by an immune response targeted to the vascular endothelium and mediated by T lymphocytes, develops in 30% to 50% of pediatric patients within 5 years of transplantation (210,211). In this complication, angiography demonstrates diffuse concentric narrowing due to intimal proliferation as well as obliteration of distal branches. Cardiac catheterization is performed to monitor patients after cardiac transplantation. Angiography demonstrates ventricular function and coronary artery anatomy; myocardial biopsy tests for rejection (212,213).

Neonatal Congenital Heart Disease

Congenital heart disease is an important cause of infant mortality, and its recognition is a clinical challenge (214,215). Increasingly, diagnosis is made in utero with fetal echocardiography; appropriate management and referral can be accomplished promptly upon delivery.

Color flow Doppler echocardiography has contributed greatly to the diagnosis of heart disease in the newborn. As a result, the chest radiograph has become somewhat less important. It is still used for screening, however, and familiarity with plain film findings of common neonatal congenital lesions has an important role. Furthermore, approximately a third of neonates suspected at first of having congenital heart disease actually have noncardiac illnesses; the chest radiograph is helpful in this distinction.

There are many causes of cardiomegaly in the neonate; they may be congenital cardiovascular anomalies or other causes (Table 6-19) (216). The possibility of correctable causes of cardiomegaly secondary to metabolic abnormalities, arrhythmias, or hematologic abnormalities should always be considered (Fig. 6-81). Although there are a number of abnormalities that may cause heart disease in the neonate, Gyepes and Vincent noted that nine congenital heart lesions account for 75% of the cardiac causes for severe cyanosis or respiratory distress during the neonatal period (Table 6-20) (215).

Physical Examination

All nine lesions causing severe congenital heart disease during the neonatal period may cause cyanosis, respiratory distress, or both during the first few days of life (215). Patients with transposition (d-TGV), pulmonary atresia or severe pulmonary stenosis, and tricuspid atresia usually have marked cyanosis but little or no respiratory distress. Neonates with obstructed TAPVR and hypoplastic left heart syndrome characteristically have marked tachypnea and dyspnea but only slight or questionable cyanosis (215).

Neonates with d-TGV and hypoplastic left heart syndrome may have no murmur, whereas those with coarctation syndrome, Ebstein malformation, and tricuspid atresia have an unimpressive systolic murmur along the left lower sternal margin. Patients with isolated coarctation and hypoplastic left heart syndrome usually have diminished femoral pulses.

Chest Radiography

The first radiologic examination of any neonate suspected of having congenital heart disease is frequently a portable AP chest radiograph, often with no lateral view. Heart size is sometimes difficult to assess because of the thymus (217). Specific chamber enlargement and pulmonary vascularity are more difficult to evaluate in the neonate than in older infants and children. It is common to recognize cardiomegaly but have no idea which chambers are enlarged.

Neonates with decreased pulmonary vascularity usually have one of four lesions in the spectrum of hypoplastic right heart syndrome, in which there is inadequate blood flow from the right heart to the lungs (Table 6-20) and a right-to-left shunt at the atrial or ventricular level. This group includes pulmonary atresia or severe pulmonary stenosis with or without a VSD, tricuspid atresia, and Ebstein malformation. Gross cardiac enlargement, particularly when recognizably of the right atrium, suggests Ebstein malformation (see Fig. 6-41) or pulmonary atresia with an intact septum. If the heart is normal or only slightly enlarged, the infant is more likely to have pulmonary atresia or critical pulmonary stenosis with a ventricular septal defect, or perhaps tricuspid atresia (see Fig. 6-39A).

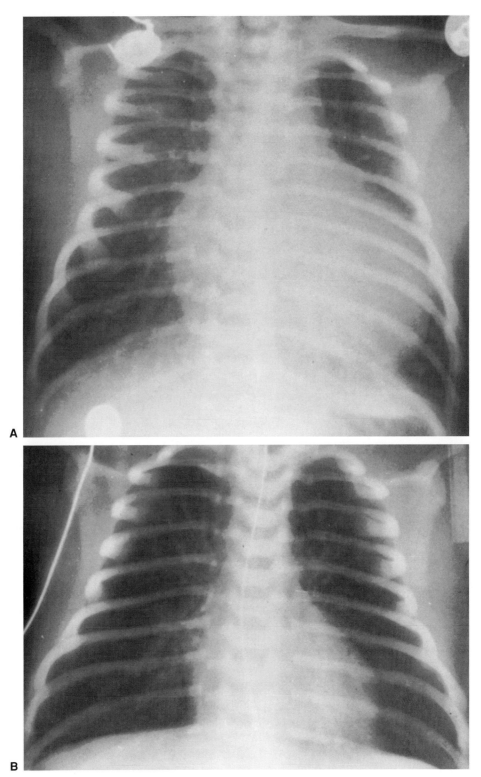

FIG. 6-81. Cardiomegaly secondary to asphyxia. A: Two-day-old boy with severe asphyxia. There is generalized cardiomegaly with pulmonary vascular congestion. **B:** Twenty-four hours after successful therapy of asphyxia. The heart is not enlarged, and pulmonary vascularity is normal.

TABLE 6-19. *Cardiomegaly in the neonate*

Secondary cardiovascular disease	Miscellaneous
Metabolic	Periarteritis
Hypoglycemia	Lupus erythematosus
Potassium	Arteritis
Hyperkalemia	*Congenital cardiovascular anomalies*
Hypokalemia	Acyanotic
Calcium	Left-to-right shunt
Hypercalcemia	Complicated atrial septal defect
Hypocalcemia	Ventricular septal defect[a]
Sodium	Atrioventricular canal defect[a]
Hypernatremia	Patent ductus arteriosus
Hyponatremia	Obstructive lesions
Arrhythmia	Cor triatriatum
Hematologic	Congenital mitral stenosis
Erythrocythemia	Idiopathic obstructive cardiomyopathy
Anemia	Aortic stenosis (valvular, supravalvular)
Erythroblastosis fetalis	Coarctation
Transient tachypnea: wet lung disease[a]	Miscellaneous
Asphyxia: airway obstruction	Endocardial fibroelastosis
Anoxic myocardopathy	Anomalous origin of left coronary artery
Perinatal brain damage	Peripheral arteriovenous fistula
Infant of diabetic mother[a]	Congenital aneurysm
Macrosomia	Cyanotic
Cardiomyopathy	Hypoplastic left heart syndrome[a]
Wet lung disease	Complete transposition (*d*-TGV)[a]
Congenital heart disease	Total anomalous pulmonary venous return—without obstruction
Glycogen storage disease	Truncus arteriosus
Thyroid disease	Pulmonary atresia with intact ventricular septum
Hyperthyroidism	Tricuspid atresia[a]
Hypothyroidism	Hypoplastic right heart complex
Myocarditis	Ebstein malformation[a]
Pericarditis	Persistent fetal circulation[a]
Cardiac tumor	Congenital tricuspid insufficiency
Myocardial infarction	Congenital absence of the pulmonary valve
Coronary sclerosis	
Aberrant coronary artery	
Peripheral arteriovenous malformations	

[a] More common.

TABLE 6-20. *Severe congenital heart disease in the neonate*

Decreased pulmonary vascularity
  Pulmonary atresia or severe pulmonary stenosis
    With intact ventricular septum[a]
    With ventricular septal defect (tetralogy of Fallot)
  Tricuspid atresia
  Ebstein malformation[a]
  Transposition with pulmonary stenosis
Shunt vascularity—active congestion
  Transposition
  Truncus arteriosus
  Total anomalous pulmonary venous return
  Coarctation syndrome[a]
Pulmonary venous hypertension—passive congestion
  Total anomalous pulmonary venous return with obstruction
  Hypoplastic left heart syndrome[a]
  Coarctation of aorta (isolated)[a]

[a] Cardiac enlargement.
Modified from Gyepes and Vincent (215).

If the pulmonary vascularity is increased and of the shunt type, the neonate may well have either d-TGV or coarctation syndrome (Table 6-20). However, neonates with d-TGV may have increased, normal, or even decreased pulmonary vascularity depending on the pulmonary artery pressure (resistance to pulmonary blood flow) and the degree of mixing at the atrial level. With d-TGV, there may be a characteristic egg-shaped cardiac contour due to a narrow cardiac waist (lack of radiographic thymus, malposition of the great vessels), convex left heart border, and prominence of the right atrium (see Fig. 6-42). Patients with d-TGV usually have marked cyanosis. Patients with coarctation syndrome have cardiomegaly, shunt vascularity, and pulmonary venous congestion (Fig. 6-82).

If there is radiologic evidence of pulmonary venous hypertension, the diagnostic considerations include total anomalous pulmonary venous return with obstruction, hypoplastic left heart syndrome, and severe isolated coarctation of the aorta (Table 6-20). The heart of the patient with hypoplastic left heart syndrome is often normal in size during the first

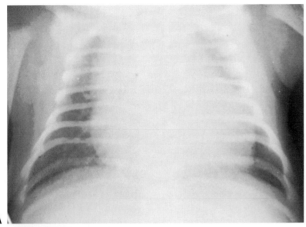

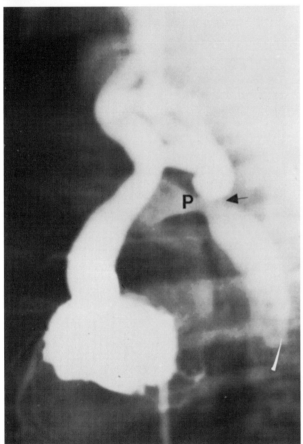

FIG. 6-82. Coarctation syndrome. A 4-day-old boy with congestive heart failure and diminished femoral pulses. **A:** There is cardiomegaly with shunt vascularity and interstitial edema. **B:** Lateral left ventriculogram. There is severe coarctation of the aorta *(arrow)*, and filling of the pulmonary artery through a patent ductus arteriosus *(P)*.

few days of life and then enlarges, whereas it is usually enlarged at birth in patients with severe isolated coarctation of the aorta. If there is severe pulmonary venous hypertension with a normal-sized heart, a likely diagnosis is TAPVR, usually infradiaphragmatic with obstruction (215).

Echocardiography

The development and refinement of pediatric echocardiography has significantly altered the approach to many critically ill newborns. This bedside procedure can usually distinguish neonates with structural congenital heart disease from those with other problems. As many entities mimic congenital heart disease, a normal ECG is of major importance. The availability of ECMO to treat infants with severe pulmonary hypertension and hypoxia mandates that a congenital cardiac anomaly be excluded. Standards have been established for the size of vessels, valves, and cardiac chambers in both premature and term neonates. Thus hypoplastic vessels or ventricles can be diagnosed readily, without more invasive imaging.

Cardiac Catheterization and Angiocardiography

The bedside diagnosis of the ill neonate with congenital heart disease is usually made with echocardiography. Axial angiocardiography further defines anatomy and assesses structure as well as function (218).

Emergency Therapy

Patients with d-TGV may have a balloon atrial septostomy (Rashkind procedure) to allow better mixing of unoxygenated and oxygenated blood at the atrial level. The definitive repair of transposition, the arterial switch or Jatene procedure, is frequently performed during the first weeks of life. Infants with congenital heart lesions and severely decreased flow may be treated with prostaglandins to maintain ductal patency; subsequently, a systemic to pulmonary artery shunt or definitive repair is performed. Infants with critical aortic stenosis or pulmonic stenosis may require emergent percutaneous balloon valvotomy. Isolated coarctation of the aorta is initially treated with intensive medical therapy including prostaglandins to dilate the ductus arteriosus; definitive surgical correction is performed when the infant is stabilized. TAPVR with obstruction requires emergency repair under hypothermia or cardiopulmonary bypass.

Specific Neonatal Cardiovascular Abnormalities

Hypoplastic Left Heart Syndrome

Hypoplastic left heart syndrome (HLHS) is a spectrum of cardiac anomalies including varying degrees of underdevelopment of the aorta, aortic valve, left ventricle, mitral valve, and left atrium. Twenty-eight percent have chromosomal abnormalities (Turner syndrome and trisomies 13, 18 and 21), major extracardiac abnormalities, or both (219).

Anatomy and Physiology

The underdevelopment of the left-sided structures includes varying degrees of hypoplasia, atresia, or stenosis; there is commonly aortic atresia and mitral atresia (1). Survival requires a large interatrial communication with a left-to-right shunt at the atrial level and a widely patent ductus arteriosus with right-to-left shunting. With aortic atresia, there is no forward flow through the aortic valve and the aortic valve ring is small (Fig. 6-83). The left ventricle is usually undersized, the mitral valve is stenotic or atretic, and the mitral valve ring is small. Hypoplasia of the aortic arch is present in varying degrees (Fig. 6-83B); in 80% of patients, there is a shelf-like coarctation at the junction of the ductus arteriosus with the proximal descending aorta.

Clinical Features

The diagnosis of HLHS is increasingly being made by fetal ultrasonography; expeditious transfer can thus be planned in advance. Occasionally, neonates are discharged from the hospital with unsuspected HLHS, become ill, and develop cardiovascular collapse and metabolic acidosis at age 3–5 days. The femoral pulses are generally diminished and the patients usually have severe metabolic acidosis. Hyperkalemia results from decreased systemic perfusion.

Radiography

Usually the heart is in normal position (situs solitus), and its size may be normal to mildly enlarged (Fig. 6-83A). The pulmonary vascular pattern is variable. Sometimes there is pulmonary edema. The near-normal chest radiograph and the clinical severity of the illness are often markedly discrepant.

Echocardiography

Hypoplastic left heart syndrome can be diagnosed at 16–20 weeks of gestation by ultrasonography. In sick neonates, echocardiography provides excellent definition of key features including the size of the ascending aorta, annulus, aortic valve, mitral valve, and left ventricle (Fig. 6-84). There is a greatly enlarged right ventricle and an enlarged pulmonary artery (Fig. 6-85).

Treatment

Hypoplastic left heart syndrome formerly accounted for at least 10% of the deaths in infancy due to structural congenital heart lesions. Infants diagnosed with hypoplastic left heart were considered inoperable and had a 95% fatality rate during the first month of life (1,220). The Norwood procedure was developed in 1983 as a two-stage correction for infants with hypoplastic left heart (221) (see Fig. 6-80).

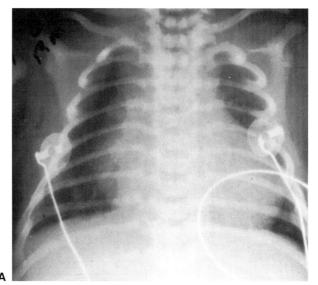

A

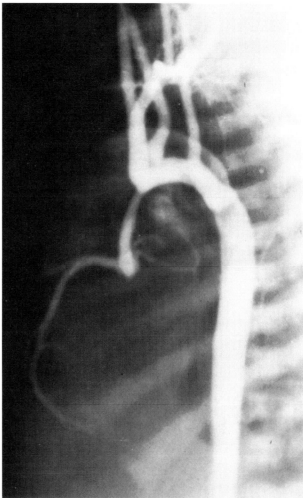

B

FIG. 6-83. Hypoplastic left heart syndrome. A 2-day-old girl with congestive heart failure. **A:** There is generalized cardiomegaly with hazy, indistinct vessel margins because of interstitial edema. **B:** Lateral aortogram. There is severe hypoplasia of the aortic valve and ascending thoracic aorta. Lack of washout of contrast material suggests aortic valve atresia. Autopsy confirmed hypoplasia of the mitral valve, left ventricle, aortic valve, and ascending aorta.

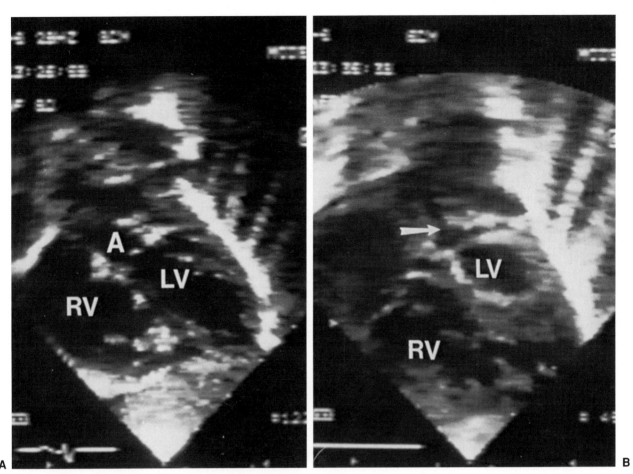

FIG. 6-84. Echocardiography of hypoplastic left heart syndrome. A: Normal inverted apical view for comparison. **B:** Hypoplastic left heart syndrome. Inverted apical view demonstrates a marked decrease in left ventricular size and hypoplasia of the ascending aorta *(arrow)*. The right ventricle is enlarged. LV, left ventricle; RV, right ventricle; A, aorta.

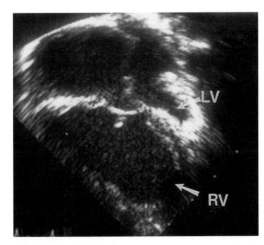

FIG. 6-85. Hypoplastic left heart syndrome. Apical four chambered view shows severe hypoplasia of left ventricle *(LV)* and an enlarged right ventricle *(RV)*.

There have been many advances in management but these patients still present a challenge to the neonatologist, cardiologist, and cardiac surgeon. Early medical management includes infusion of prostaglandins to maintain ductal patency. Oxygen may lower pulmonary artery pressure and therefore be detrimental in certain clinical situations. A delicate balance between the systemic and pulmonary blood flows must be attained. After aggressive medical care and stabilization the first stage of the Norwood procedure is performed (see Fig. 6-80). Modifications of surgery and refinements of management continue to occur for these critically ill infants. In 1991, 50 patients from Philadelphia's Children's Hospital had undergone modified Fontan procedures after the first-stage palliative reconstruction surgery, with an overall mortality rate of 42% (222). Treatment results continue to improve with the continued refinement of surgical techniques and better assessment of risk factors (222–225). Recent advances include earlier caval-pulmonary artery anastomosis and fenestration of the atrium. The late experience with the Mustard and Senning operations suggests that the right ventricle cannot function indefinitely as a systemic ventricle.

An alternative for infants with HLHS is neonatal cardiac transplantation developed by Bailey and coworkers at Loma Linda University (226,227).

Hypoplastic Right Heart Disease

Hypoplastic right heart malformations are characterized by pulmonary atresia and varying degrees of hypoplasia of the right ventricle and tricuspid valve annulus.

Anatomy and Physiology

There is complete obstruction to right heart flow and obligatory right-to-left shunting at the atrial level. The right ventricular pressure may be markedly elevated, and retrograde flow through coronary arteries via myocardial sinusoids occurs. Pulmonary arterial flow may be dependent on left-to-right shunting through a patent ductus arteriosus. As the ductus closes, cyanosis becomes more profound. There is a striking difference in heart size depending on the presence and degree of tricuspid insufficiency; if the tricuspid insufficiency is severe, there is massive enlargement of the right atrium. In patients who have restricted tricuspid flow because of tricuspid stenosis and a small annulus, the right ventricular chamber is small and the heart is not enlarged.

Clinical Features

These infants develop marked cyanosis and hepatomegaly immediately after birth. However, the diagnosis is frequently made by fetal sonography.

Radiology

The chest radiograph shows a heart of normal size except when severe tricuspid insufficiency is present. Pulmonary arterial flow is diminished.

Echocardiography

Echocardiography demonstrates the atretic pulmonary valve, the small pulmonary valve annulus, the size of the right ventricle, and the thickness of the right ventricular wall. Tricuspid valve stenosis and insufficiency are also accurately assessed with this technique.

Angiography

The pressure in the small right ventricle may be systemic. With contrast injection, there is no forward flow into the pulmonary artery (Fig. 6-86). Gross tricuspid insufficiency may be noted. In some cases the tricuspid valve is competent, and there may be filling of the coronary vessels via ventricu-

lar sinusoids due to markedly elevated right ventricular pressure.

Treatment

Prostaglandins are used to maintain patency of the ductus arteriosus. Palliation with a modified Blalock-Taussig shunt maintains adequate pulmonary artery flow. Patients may need a Rashkind balloon atrial septostomy or even a surgical Blalock-Hanlon septectomy to allow significant right-to-left shunting at the atrial level. If the right ventricle is small and severely hypoplastic, the eventual surgical repair is a Fontan procedure.

Persistent Fetal Circulation

In term newborns there are several circumstances in which there is persistence of pulmonary hypertension and the fetal pattern of circulation. The high pulmonary artery pressures lead to right-to-left shunting of blood from the pulmonary artery through the ductus arteriosus into the descending aorta, as is true in fetal life. Persistent fetal circulation (PFC) may be due to diaphragmatic hernia, meconium aspiration, or other lung diseases, or it may be of unknown etiology (primary PFC). When PFC is severe, there is significant right-to-left shunting and the infant is profoundly hypoxemic and acidotic; this situation is often fatal. Chest radiography may show marked decrease in pulmonary vascularity or may be negative (228). ECMO provides oxygen to the blood externally and allows the pulmonary circulation to vasodilate. With further vasodilatation, there is a reduction in pulmonary arterial hypertension and decreased right-to-left shunting. ECMO has had a major impact on the treatment of severe PFC.

Infants of Diabetic Mothers

Infants of diabetic mothers (IDMs) have an increased incidence of congenital cardiac malformations; the most common are VSD and complete d-TGV. IDMs may also have cardiomegaly attributed to asymmetric septal hypertrophy and cardiomyopathy, which is probably secondary to hypoxia or hypoglycemia. Chest radiographs of IDMs often show an increase in subcutaneous fat recognizable along the lateral chest wall. The cardiomegaly may be striking. A specific diagnosis can be made by echocardiography; angiography is usually not performed. The natural history of the disease is regression of septal hypertrophy, clinical improvement, and progression of the chest radiograph to normal.

Arrhythmias

With the increasing use of fetal monitoring, more and more fetal arrhythmias are being recognized in utero. Many

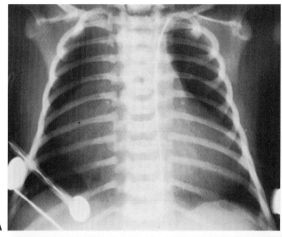

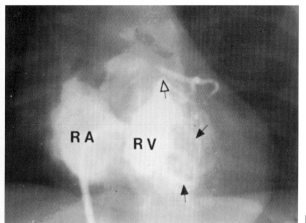

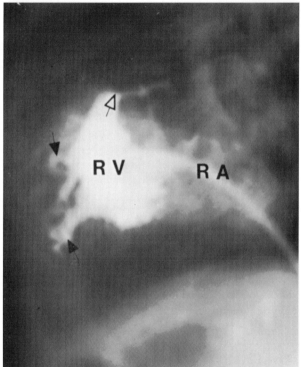

FIG. 6-86. Pulmonary atresia, hypoplastic right ventricle, and intact ventricular septum. Newborn girl with marked cyanosis. **A:** Right-sided cardiac enlargement. The aortic arch is on the left, and the tip of the umbilical arterial catheter is in the left subclavian artery. The pulmonary vascularity is decreased. Anteroposterior **(B)** and lateral **(C)** selective right ventricular angiocardiography. The right ventricle *(RV)* is small, and there is reflux of contrast media across the tricuspid valve into the right atrium *(RA)*. The atresia of the infundibulum *(open arrows)* is apparent. There is filling of numerous myocardial sinusoids *(solid arrows)*.

of the cardiac rhythm disturbances are transitory and benign. Paroxysmal supraventricular tachycardia, however, may cause neonatal hydrops and congestive failure. The initial chest radiograph in these patients may demonstrate cardiomegaly, pulmonary edema, and even anasarca. Complete heart block may be seen in newborns of mothers with systemic lupus erythematosus; it may also occur as an isolated abnormality. There is usually no underlying structural heart disease in neonates with heart block. However, cardiomegaly, with or without mild pulmonary edema, is apparent.

Arteriovenous Malformations

Infants with large arteriovenous malformations (AVMs) or fistulas may develop heart failure during the first few weeks of life. The most common of these causes of failure is an AVM of the vein of Galen. The second most common lesion is a hemangioendothelioma or AVM of the liver. In all of these cases with high flow, chest radiographs demonstrate moderate cardiomegaly and mild changes of heart failure. Echocardiography shows large cardiac chambers and excludes structural heart lesions. Color Doppler sonography may demonstrate increased flow in the intracranial or hepatic AVM.

Vascular Anomalies

The biological classification of vascular anomalies of Mulliken and Glowacki includes two major categories: hemangiomas and vascular malformations (Table 6-21) (229).

TABLE 6-21. *Classification of vascular anomalies*

Hemangioma
Proliferating
Involuting
Involuted
Vascular malformation
High flow
Arteriovenous fistula
Arteriovenous malformation
Low flow
Capillary malformation
Venous malformation
Lymphatic malformation
Macrocystic
Microcystic
Mixed

This classification is supported by clinical, histologic, histochemical, and biochemical differences (229–234) as well as by angiography and imaging (235,236). Hemangiomas are proliferative endothelial cell tumors that typically present in infancy, have a characteristic period of rapid growth during the first year of life, and then slowly involute. Vascular malformations are developmental anomalies that are further classified according to channel abnormalities (arteriovenous, capillary, venous, lymphatic, mixed) and flow characteristics (high-flow, low-flow). The lesions can be readily distinguished by characteristic findings on CT, MRI, and angiography (Table 6-22) (235,236). Interventional radiologic techniques, such as embolization and direct intralesional sclerosant injection, play an important role in the management of pediatric vascular anomalies (234,237–248).

Hemangiomas

Hemangiomas (also discussed in other chapters) are present at birth in 40% of patients; frequently only a faint macular stain is identified (229,230,248). They are more common in females, Caucasians, and premature infants. Hemangiomas usually appear within the first 3 months of life and grow rapidly because of endothelial cell proliferation. This proliferation usually plateaus at about 9 or 10 months of age and is followed by a much slower phase of involution, which may take many years to be complete.

The appearance of a hemangioma depends on its depth and whether the lesion is in its proliferating or involuting phase. Hemangiomas involving the skin surface have a characteristic ``strawberry'' appearance. Deeper lesions may have normal overlying skin or may have a bluish hue, due to draining veins. Hemangiomas are usually warm and may be pulsatile. Some lesions look like arteriovenous malformations, but measurement of urinary levels of fibroblast growth factor, which is produced by hemangiomas and not by vascular malformations, is a reliable means of distinguishing these lesions. During involution, the lesions become softer and

less pulsatile, which reflects cell dropout and fibrofatty replacement.

In the proliferating phase, CT and MRI demonstrate well-circumscribed, lobulated densely and uniformly enhancing lesions with dilated feeding and draining vessels in the center or at the periphery (235). At MRI, the lesions are typically isointense or hypointense to muscle on T1-weighted images, and moderately hyperintense on T2-weighted images (Fig. 6-87). Flow voids are seen within and around the mass on spin-echo images. Gradient imaging demonstrates high flow vessels, usually at the center or along the periphery of the lesion (Fig. 6-87D). The hallmark of the hemangioma is the presence of a high-flow, enhancing parenchymal mass (Fig. 6-88A). Ultrasound, with Doppler interrogation, also demonstrates a parenchymal mass with high-flow vessels (low arterial resistance and increased venous velocity). Angiography, necessary only if endovascular intervention is considered, characteristically demonstrates a hypervascular mass with a dense, prolonged capillary blush and dilated feeding as well as draining vessels (Fig. 6-88) (236,239). During and after involution, the lesions are progressively replaced by fatty tissue, which is most readily demonstrated on CT.

Intracranial hemangiomas are uncommon; they are usually dural or pial in location. Cerebrovascular anomalies, including persistence of embryonic vessels such as the trigeminal artery, carotid and vertebral artery agenesis or hypoplasia, and intracranial aneurysms and obstructive lesions, are occasionally seen in infants with facial hemangiomas (249). Other coexisting anomalies are a cleft sternum, cystic posterior fossa malformations, urogenital anomalies, spinal dysraphism, right aortic arch, and coarctation of the aorta (230,231,249) (Table 6-23).

Because most hemangiomas involute spontaneously, specific treatment is indicated only in certain locations, such as ocular, airway, hepatic, and disseminated hemangiomas. Life-threatening complications also include coagulopathy (Kasabach-Merritt phenomenon), ulceration, and congestive cardiac failure (248,250). Patients with the Kasabach-Merritt phenomenon have a marked decrease in the platelet count (usually <10,000), with or without low levels of fibrinogen and other coagulation factors, because of consumption of clotting factors within the hemangioma. Imaging studies typically demonstrate high flow and diffuse soft-tissue masses with surrounding signal intensity or density of edema. The histology differs from the usual hemangioma; an aggressive (Kaposiform) hemangioendothelioma is the most common pathologic diagnosis. These tumors are notoriously difficult to treat, but the coagulopathy resolves with involution of the lesion.

Specific treatment of hemangiomas includes systemic or intralesional corticosteroids, angiogenesis inhibitors such as interferon, chemotherapy, radiotherapy, and arterial embolization (237,239,245,246,248,251–252). Embolization is indicated only after failure of medical therapy and only in the treatment of complicated life- or organ-endangering heman-

TABLE 6-22. *Imaging findings in pediatric vascular anomalies*

Lesion	Angiography	MRI T1	MRI + Contrast	MRI T2	MRI Gradient	Ultrasound	CT
Hemangioma							
Proliferating	Dilated feeding arts.; cap. stain; dil. draining veins	STM; iso- or hypointense to muscle; flow voids	Uniform intense enhancement	Inc. signal; lobulated STM; flow voids	HFV within and around STM	Discrete STM containing HFV; dec. art. resistance	Uniformly enhancing STM; dil. vessels
Involuting	As above	Variable fat content	As above	Variable fat	As above	As above	Variable fat content
Involuted	Avascular	High signal (fat)	No enhancement	Dec. signal (fat)	No HFV	Echogenic avascular STM	Fat density; no enhancement
Kasabach-Merritt phenomenon	Hypervascular; diffuse cap. stain	Diffuse STM; skin thickening	Diffuse enhancement	Diffuse inc. signal; subcut. stranding	Mildly dil. vessels in and around STM	Diffuse STM with HFV	Diffuse enhancing STM; subcut. stranding
Vascular Malformation							
Arteriovenous malformation	Dil. feeding arts., nidus, early opacification of draining veins	STT; flow voids	Diffuse enhancement	Variable inc. signal; flow voids	HFV throughout abnormal tissue	HFV with low art. resistance; AV shunt; +/− STT	Enhancing vessels and STT; bone sclerosis or destruction
Venous malformation	Contrast puddling on venous phase; sinusoidal spaces and varices on direct injection	Isointense to muscle on T1; +/− high signal thrombi	Diffuse or inhomogeneous enhancement	Septated STM; high signal; signal voids (phleboliths)	No HFV; signal voids (phleboliths)	STM of mixed echogenicity; low-velocity flow; compressible	STM: variable contrast enhancement; lamellated calcifications (phleboliths)
Lymphatic malformation; macrocystic	Avascular STM; Dil. or anom. veins	STM; low signal; septated	Rim or no enhancement	STM; high signal; fluid/fluid levels	No HFV	Cystic STM; +/− vessels in septa	STM; low attenuation; no or rim enhancement
Lymphatic malformation; microcystic	Avascular or capillary staining	STT: hypo- or isointense to muscle	No enhancement	Diffuse increased signal; subcut. stranding	No HFV	STT: echogenic; avascular	Diffuse STT; nonenhancing; subcut. stranding

anom., anomalous; art, arterial; arts., arteries; cap., capillaries; dil., dilated; HFV, high-flow vessels; STM, soft tissue mass; STT, soft tissue thickening; subcut., subcutaneous; dec., decreased; inc., increased.

From Burrows et al. (236).

603

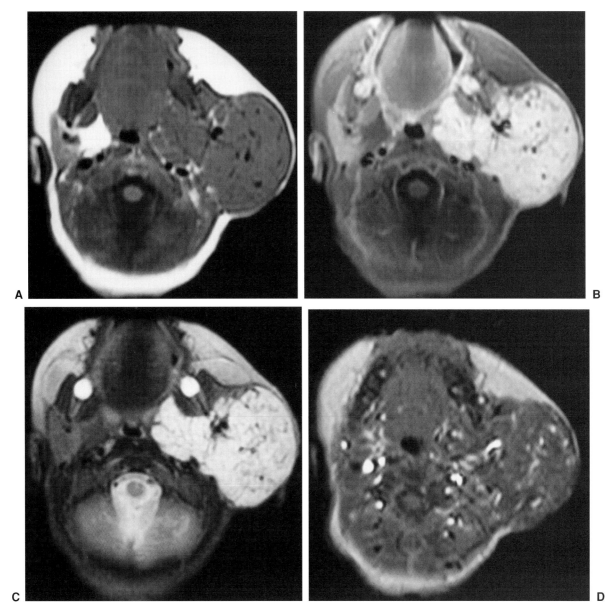

FIG. 6-87. Hemangioma. A 3-month-old infant with rapidly enlarging left facial mass. **A:** Axial T1-weighted MRI demonstrates a discrete soft-tissue mass that is isointense to muscle and contains flow voids. Note the replacement of subcutaneous and parapharyngeal fat as well as displacement of airway and major vessels. **B:** Axial T1-weighted MRI after gadolinium administration. There is uniform contrast enhancement of the mass. **C:** Axial T2-weighted MRI demonstrates homogeneous increased signal with some lobulation and intralesional flow voids. **D:** Gradient-echo image. High flow vessels are identified within and around the hemangioma.

giomas (237–239,245,246,252). Arterial embolization with small particles is usually appropriate, although some lesions with macroscopic arteriovenous shunting (hepatic hemangiomas) require microcoils (245,252). Recurrence after an initial response to embolization is frequent, but the lesions may respond to repeated procedures. Hepatic hemangiomas may have complex vascular anatomy, including systemic collaterals and direct portohepatic or arterioportal shunts, mandating careful angiographic assessment prior to embolization (245,246,252).

Vascular Malformations

Vascular malformations (also discussed in the chapters dealing with the organ involved) are errors of vascular morphogenesis (229,230,234). Although generally considered to be present at birth, they may not become evident or symptomatic until later in life. They tend to grow in proportion to the growth of the child but may enlarge because of hemodynamic changes such as increased blood flow (resulting in vessel elongation and dilatation), obstruction, or thrombosis.

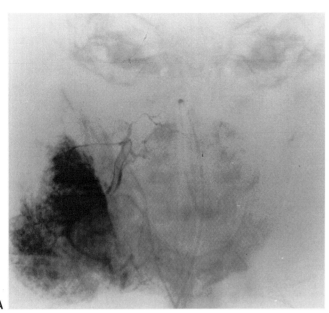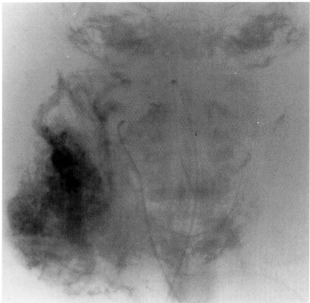

A   B

FIG. 6-88. Hemangioma. A: Late arterial phase of a right facial arteriogram demonstrates enlargement of the facial artery and its branches. There is a diffuse lobular parenchymal blush. **B:** Venous phase demonstrates dilated veins within and around the hemangioma.

The evolution of individual lesions, especially high-flow lesions, may be stimulated by hormonal change (puberty, pregnancy), trauma (surgery, embolization), and infection.

Vascular malformations are classified according to the channel abnormalities present and the flow characteristics (Tables 6-21 and 6-22) (229,230,234). MRI is the most useful imaging modality in their investigation (235,236). The combination of multiplanar spin-echo imaging and flow-sensitive sequences permits accurate characterization of the nature and extent of most lesions. CT is less precise in defining the flow characteristics and extent of the vascular malformation, but it has a role when bony structures are involved. Ultrasound, including Doppler techniques, is valuable for determining tissue and flow characteristics of superficial lesions, but it may fail to demonstrate the extent of the lesion. Plain radiographs are useful in selected patients, mainly to document bony changes. Angiography is generally performed at the time of embolization. In some patients, however, angiography may be necessary to confirm the diagnosis and to demonstrate the extent of soft-tissue arteriovenous malformations and arteriovenous fistulas (236).

High-flow Vascular Malformations

High-flow vascular malformations include arteriovenous fistulas (direct arteriovenous connections without an intervening nidus) and arteriovenous malformations (this is a plexiform nidus of vessels between the feeding arteries and the draining veins). These lesions are characterized, with CT and MRI, by the presence of dilated feeding and draining vessels. In the extracranial soft tissues, the intervening nidus may or may not be detectable, depending on the size of the channels. The lesion should not have an associated parenchymal mass, but some signal abnormalities, possibly related to a fibrofatty matrix or edema, may be evident on MRI. In AVMs of the extracranial soft tissues, CT and MRI frequently show increased thickness of fat, increased thickness and sometimes signal abnormalities of affected muscle, and bony changes. These bony changes include sclerosis, lytic defects, and signal change.

Arteriovenous Fistulas. Congenital arteriovenous fistulas (AVFs) may involve any organ system. Some are symptomatic in the neonatal period because of high output cardiac failure, whereas others are diagnosed by the presence of an audible bruit or palpable pulsation (Fig. 6-89). Congenital AVFs are curable by appropriate endovascular procedures (238,239) and should be treated when diagnosed. Embolization should occlude the fistula itself, not just the feeding artery, to prevent recurrence through collaterals. Effective

TABLE 6-23. *Associations with hemangiomas*

Female gender
Caucasian race
Prematurity
Sternal cleft
Right aortic arch
Coarctation of the aorta
Cervicocranial arterial anomalies (e.g., persistent trigeminal
   artery)
Intracranial arterial occlusions and aneurysms
Cystic malformations of the posterior fossa
Spinal dysraphism
Genitourinary anomalies

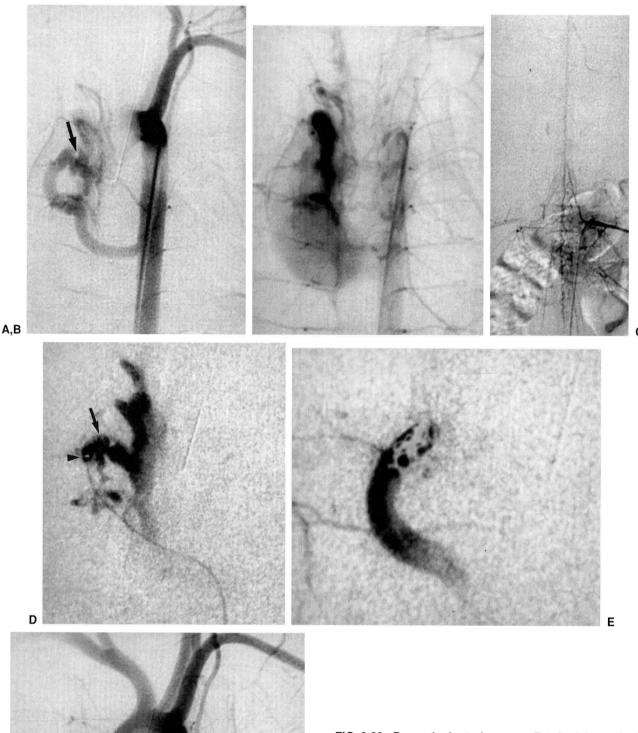

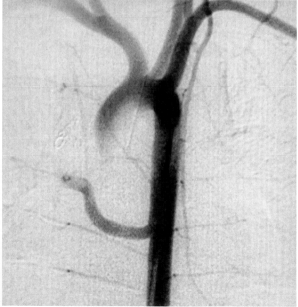

FIG. 6-89. Paraspinal arteriovenous fistula. A 9-month-old boy with a loud bruit over the back. **A, B:** A descending thoracic aortogram demonstrates enlargement of a single right segmental artery. There is a discrete arteriovenous fistula between the right sixth intercostal artery and vein *(arrow)*, which subsequently drains into the azygous and epidural veins **(B)**. **C:** Selective injection of the left 11th segmental artery demonstrates a normal anterior spinal axis. **D:** The tip of the coaxial delivery system with catheter *(arrowhead)* and microcatheter *(arrow)* is placed across the fistula into the draining vein prior to placement of the coils. **E:** Selective injection through the delivery catheter after placement of platinum microcoils across the fistula demonstrates occlusion of fistula and patency of intercostal branches. **F:** An aortogram after embolization confirms occlusion of the fistula and absence of collateral blood supply.

embolization devices include steel wire, platinum fiber coils, detachable balloons, and tissue adhesive (Fig. 6-89).

Arteriovenous Malformations. Arteriovenous malformations consist of a nidus or network of abnormal vascular channels, feeding arteries, and draining veins (Fig. 6-90). Soft-tissue AVMs are not discrete but behave more as field defects, involving large areas and crossing tissue planes. Except for extremely high-flow lesions, which may present with cardiac overload in infancy, most soft-tissue AVMs are asymptomatic in the first decade or two of life. AVMs often have a cutaneous blush with or without underlying soft tissue and osseous hypertrophy. Clinical findings include local hyperthermia, pulsations, thrill, and bruit. The use of continuous-wave Doppler often helps to detect the vascular shunt before it is audible with a stethoscope. Evolution of these lesions often seems to be precipitated by hormonal factors (puberty, pregnancy, hormone therapy), trauma, infection, or surgery (230,234). A combination of arterial steal and venous hypertension results in tissue ischemia, pain, and ulceration, often with severe bleeding. Dental AVMs of the maxilla, mandible, and oral cavity are particularly dangerous, often presenting with life-threatening hemorrhage related to tooth eruption, dental infection, or dental extraction (237,239). Intramuscular AVMs may be associated with pain. Cutaneous AVMs initially demonstrate a superficial blush and warmth; AV shunting can be detected by Doppler sonography. As they evolve, the color intensifies and tortuous, tense veins appear. Dystrophic changes, ulceration, bleeding, and persistent pain follow. Extremity AVMs are usually associated with overgrowth requiring epiphysiodesis; cardiac overload and skin ulcerations are also common and become even more frequent with advancing age.

MRI is useful in confirming the diagnosis of AVM (Fig. 6-90) and in demonstrating its extent, although it is often difficult to distinguish between the actual nidus and the feeding and draining vessels. Intraosseous AVMs typically cause lytic defects that are usually related to dilated draining veins. The affected soft tissues are usually hypertrophied, including skin, subcutaneous fat, and muscle layers. The adjacent bone is often thickened and distorted.

At present, AVMs, except for the smallest lesions, are incurable. Treatment must be planned carefully to avoid stimulating progression and interfering with future management. In particular, proximal ligation and embolization of feeding vessels must be avoided. Superselective arterial embolization is indicated to decrease symptoms, such as pain, bleeding, and ischemic ulceration (234,237–239). Where possible, it should be performed with permanent agents, such as tissue adhesive. Embolization with 100% ethanol has recently been proposed as an ablative procedure (242). However, arterial embolization with ethanol may result in severe tissue ischemia due to capillary penetration. In general, AVMs are impossible to cure by arterial embolization alone. Lesions that are amenable to complete excision are probably best treated by embolization and then excision (234,239). Dental AVMs presenting with bleeding can be managed by

arterial embolization followed by extraction of any loose or involved teeth (237,239,240). Selective arterial embolization followed by direct injection of the intramandibular nidus and draining vein using coils plus sclerosants or tissue adhesive have resulted in apparent obliteration of the nidus with reossification of the affected mandible (240). This approach is preferable to mandibulectomy, especially in the immature facial skeleton. Close follow-up is essential, as AVMs may extend, especially after intervention, into tissue that initially did not appear to be involved. Extremity AVMs presenting with high output cardiac failure in infancy may contain discrete AVFs, and the consequent cardiac failure may respond dramatically to embolization. Overall, however, the prognosis in diffuse extremity AVMs is for progressive worsening and eventual amputation (230,244).

Low-flow Vascular Malformations

Low-flow vascular malformations include capillary malformations, venous malformations, lymphatic malformations, and mixed malformations (see Tables 6-21 and 6-22).

Capillary Malformations. Capillary malformations involving the skin surface include port-wine stains and telangiectasias (230,248). Facial port wine stains are often associated with progressive thickening of the skin and subcutaneous layers as well as overgrowth of the underlying facial skeleton. They often lead to facial asymmetry and dental malocclusion. Although most port wine stains are isolated vascular anomalies, they may signal an underlying deep vascular malformation or a more complex dysmorphogenesis (230,231,248). For example, a port wine stain over the spine may be associated with underlying spinal dysraphism or with a complex high-flow AVM and AVF (e.g., Cobb syndrome) (Table 6-24).

In Sturge-Weber syndrome, a facial port wine stain in the sensory cutaneous area of the first branch of the trigeminal nerve (V1) is associated with underlying ophthalmologic and leptomeningeal vascular anomalies (253). The ocular involvement leads to glaucoma in one third of patients because of the presence of a retinal vascular malformation, probably of a venous type. The intracranial vascular anomalies usually consist of capillary and venous malformations of the brain coverings, associated with progressive cerebral atrophy and cortical calcification, resulting in seizures, focal neurologic deficits, and mental retardation. Intracranial involvement may also include AVMs and AVFs of the calvaria and meninges. The facial malformation may include lymphatic malformations. Approximately 1% to 2% of patients with port wine stains have Sturge-Weber syndrome. The intracranial manifestations are generally not present in patients with port wine stains confined to V2 and V3 distribution, but they may be seen in patients without surface vascular malformations. CT and MRI may be negative in the first 1 or 2 years of life. Typical positive findings include gyral enhancement

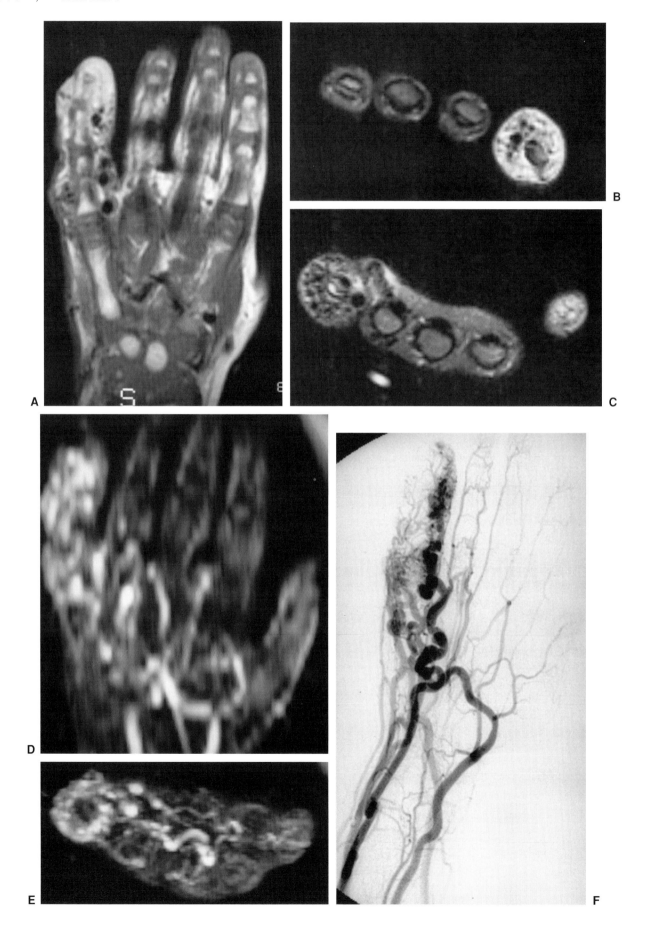

TABLE 6-24. *Examples of syndromes with vascular malformations*

Klippel-Trenaunay, Parkes-Weber
Sturge-Weber
Turner, Noonan
Blue rubber bleb nevus
Maffucci
Bonnet-Dechaume-Blanc
Cobb
Solomon
Riley-Smith
Bannayan
Proteus

and enlargement as well as enhancement of the ipsilateral choroid plexus. Later findings include progressive cortical atrophy and gyral calcification.

Venous Malformations. The signs and symptoms of venous and capillary-venous malformations vary with their depth and extent (230,234). Most of these lesions consist of spongy masses of sinusoidal spaces having variable communications with adjacent veins. Alternately, some venous malformations represent varicosities or dysplasias of small and large venous channels (238,241). The lesions are typically soft and compressible and distend with the Valsalva maneuver or venous compression. They may contain phleboliths. When involved, the overlying skin is blue or purple.

Characteristic MRI findings include focal or diffuse collections of high T2 signal, often containing identifiable spaces of variable size separated by septations (Fig. 6-91) (235,236). Small fluid-fluid levels may be visible. Phleboliths may be evident as areas, most prominent on gradient images, of signal void (Fig. 6-91D). Flow-sensitive images demonstrate no high-flow vessels within or around the lesions but may show an old thrombus. Enhancement may be dense like that of adjacent veins, inhomogeneous, or delayed. CT imaging likewise shows variable contrast enhancement with or without rounded lamellated calcifications.

Angiography is not necessary to make the diagnosis, but it typically shows either no filling of the malformation or delayed opacification of sinusoidal spaces with or without

dysplastic draining veins (236). Direct percutaneous cannulation of the malformation with contrast injection typically shows the interconnecting sinusoidal spaces (241). Communications with adjacent veins may be small or large, and adjacent venous channels may be normal or dysplastic and varicose.

Direct injection of sclerosing agents, most commonly sodium tetradecyl or 100% ethanol, typically results in thrombosis and gradual shrinkage of the malformation and is the preferred treatment at some centers (234,238,239,241–243). This technique involves percutaneous cannulation of the malformation using a needle or Teflon-sheathed needle cannula. After confirming free return of blood, contrast injection is recorded with serial angiographic imaging to document cannula position in the malformation and the presence or absence of venous outflow. In the presence of significant venous outflow, local compression is applied and contrast injections are repeated until the outflow is obstructed. An estimation of the volume of the cannulated part of the malformation is also made from these contrast injections. Contrast medium is then aspirated or expressed from the malformation and an appropriate quantity of sclerosant is injected. The total volume of injected ethanol should not exceed 1 ml/kg. Hemoglobinuria due to hemolysis is a common side effect. The other common complications of ethanol sclerotherapy are skin necrosis and neuropathy. Skin blistering and full-thickness necrosis are most likely to occur when the malformation involves the skin surface. Cardiovascular complications, including bradycardia, arrhythmias, and cardiac arrest, have been reported during embolization and sclerotherapy with 100% ethanol; general anesthesia and close patient monitoring are therefore required. Sclerotherapy is not usually curative but decreases the swelling and pain in most patients (241,243).

Lymphatic Malformations. Lymphatic malformations may be classified as macrocystic, as in cystic hygromas, or microcystic. Those in the head and neck result from maldevelopment of the cervicofacial lymphatic system, which normally arises as paired jugular lymph sacs sprouting from the primitive jugular venous plexus in the 6-week embryo (230). The macrocystic types of lymphatic malformations (cystic

FIG. 6-90. Arteriovenous malformation. A 14-month-old boy with recurrent bleeding from fingertip. **A:** Coronal contrast-enhanced T1-weighted MRI demonstrates diffuse soft-tissue enlargement of the small finger with enhancement and multiple flow voids related to feeding and draining vessels. On this image alone, without the clinical history and arteriogram, it would be difficult to distinguish between AVM and hemangioma. **B, C:** Axial T2-weighted images through the tip **(B)** and base **(C)** of the fingers demonstrate a diffuse increased signal intensity in the ischemic fingertip and nonspecific soft-tissue thickening at the base of the small finger, with flow voids. Some signal abnormality involves the web space between the fourth and fifth rays. **D, E:** An MR angiogram demonstrates dilated feeding and draining vessels throughout the fifth digit. There is circumferential involvement of the fifth digit and adjacent web space. **F:** A brachial arteriogram confirms the diagnosis of a high-flow arteriovenous malformation with arteriovenous shunting that is maximal at the base of the fifth digit. Note the relative avascularity of the finger tip; this indicates that tissue ischemia is the most likely basis for the bleeding and for the signal and enhancement characteristics on MRI.

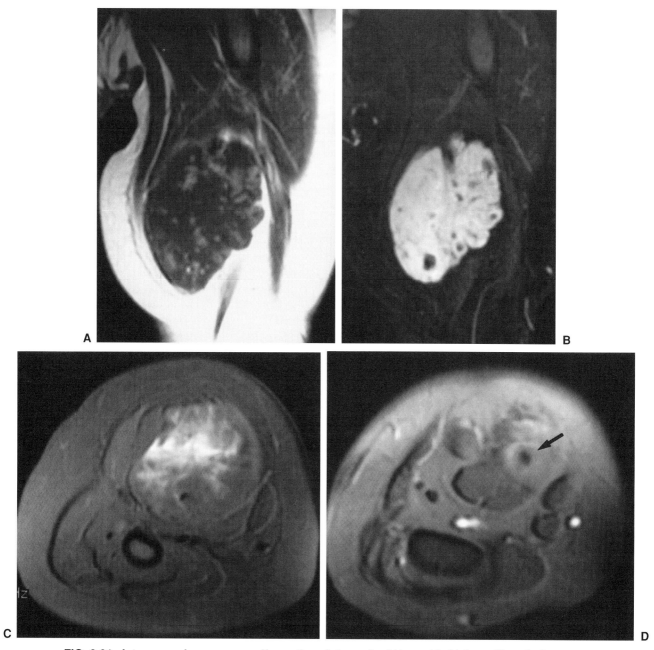

FIG. 6-91. Intramuscular venous malformation. A 1-month-old boy with thigh swelling. **A:** A coronal T1-weighted MRI through the left thigh demonstrates an isointense intramuscular mass with numerous areas of increased signal intensity representing small thrombi or phleboliths. **B:** A T2-weighted coronal MRI at the same level demonstrates a multiseptated mass of high signal intensity containing discrete areas of low signal intensity. These represent phleboliths. **C:** A T1-weighted axial MRI after gadolinium injection. The inhomogeneous contrast enhancement of the mass confirms its venous nature. **D:** Axial gradient image. There are normal arterial and venous channels with no high-flow vessels in the region of the mass. A phlebolith *(arrow)* is accentuated.

hygromas) are believed to result from maldevelopment of the primitive jugular subclavian and axillary sacs, possibly by failure to reestablish venous connections. Interruption or obstruction of the peripheral lymphatic channels presumably results in diffuse or microcystic lymphatic malformations (lymphangiomas).

Lymphatic malformations are usually evident at birth. The macrocystic lesions, most commonly located in the neck, axilla, and chest wall, may be massive and interfere with delivery. Microcystic lesions usually present as diffuse soft-tissue thickening. The lesions typically keep pace with the growth of the child but undergo episodic swelling due to lymphatic obstruction or hemorrhage. Communication is frequently present between the macrocystic lymphatic malformations and adjacent veins.

On physical examination, lymphatic malformations have a rubbery or cystic consistency. Unlike venous malformations, they usually cannot be manually decompressed. The overlying skin may contain capillary malformations, vesicles, or both.

MRI findings in macrocystic lymphatic malformations include cystic fluid collections, often with fluid-fluid levels, associated with lack of contrast enhancement or minimal rim enhancement (Fig. 6-92) (235,236). Evidence of hemorrhage or thrombosis may be present. Enlargement of adjacent veins, including the SVC, has been described in cervicofacial lymphatic malformations (254). Microcystic lymphatic mal-

formations typically appear as diffuse sheets of bright signal on T2-weighted spin-echo MRI and usually have no contrast enhancement. The adjacent subcutaneous fat often shows evidence of lymphedema. CT best demonstrates the bone distortion and shows the soft-tissue component of the malformation to be less dense than surrounding muscle.

The treatment of macrocystic lymphatic malformations is generally early staged surgical excision (230). Residual or recurrent cysts may be treated by injection of sclerosants, including hypertonic glucose, ethanol, deoxycycline, Ethibloc, and OK-432 (238,247).

Mixed Vascular Malformations. Mixed vascular malformations are common. In particular, capillary malformations of the skin are often present in association with deep arteriovenous, lymphatic, or venous malformations.

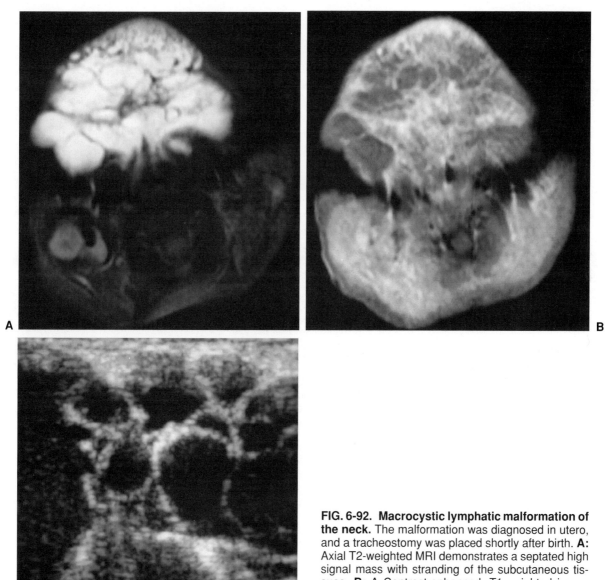

FIG. 6-92. Macrocystic lymphatic malformation of the neck. The malformation was diagnosed in utero, and a tracheostomy was placed shortly after birth. **A:** Axial T2-weighted MRI demonstrates a septated high signal mass with stranding of the subcutaneous tissues. **B:** A Contrast-enhanced, T1-weighted image through the same level demonstrates predominantly rim enhancement of the cystic spaces. **C:** An ultrasound image verifies cysts of varying sizes.

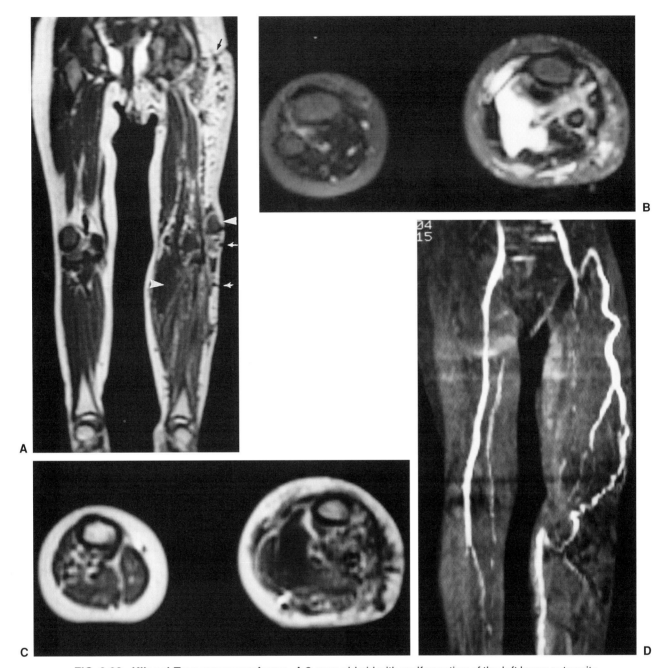

FIG. 6-93. Klippel-Trenaunay syndrome. A 2-year-old girl with malformation of the left lower extremity and pelvis. **A:** Coronal T1-weighted MRI demonstrates increased length and thickness of the left lower extremity, prominent subcutaneous venous channels *(arrows)*, and soft-tissue enlargement due to increased subcutaneous fat and cystic lesions *(arrowheads)* in the subcutaneous and muscular tissues. **B:** An axial T2-weighted image through a cast. There are numerous focal masses of high signal intensity within the intramuscular and subcutaneous layers. **C:** An enhanced T1-weighted image at the same level as **(B)** demonstrates only rim enhancement of the mass lesions, indicating that they are predominantly lymphatic in nature. **D:** An MR venogram of the lower extremities demonstrates normal anatomy on the right side but absence or hypoplasia of the left deep venous system and long saphenous vein. The left-sided venous drainage consists predominantly of a dilated medial superficial vein and a primitive marginal vein (vein of Servelle). These dilated primitive veins account for the visable venous varicosities. Surgery on the varicosities is contraindicated because of absence of a deep venous system.

Syndromes involving vascular malformations are listed in Table 6-24. The most common is Klippel-Trenaunay syndrome, which consists of a spectrum of anomalies involving the extremities, including varicosities of superficial veins, persistence of valveless embryonic channels, deep venous anomalies, lymphatic malformations, and growth disturbance. The affected extremity is usually longer but may be shorter than the normal one. MRI and MR venography are important in defining the underlying venous and soft-tissue abnormalities (Fig. 6-93) (255). Treatment still consists mainly of elastic stockings for compression and epiphysiodesis for extremity length discrepancy.

REFERENCES

General Information

1. Castaneda AR, Jonas RA, Mayer JE Jr, Hanley FL. *Cardiac surgery of the neonate and infant.* Philadelphia: WB Saunders, 1994.
2. Elliott LP, Schiebler GL. *The x-ray diagnosis of congenital heart disease in infants, children, and adults.* Springfield: CC Thomas, 1979.
3. Emmanouilides GC, Riemenschneider TA, Allen HD, Gutgesell HP, eds. *Moss and Adams heart disease in infants, children and adolescents.* Baltimore: Williams and Wilkins, 1995.
4. Garson A Jr, Bricker JT, McNamara DG, eds. *The science and practice of pediatric cardiology.* Philadelphia: Lea and Febiger, 1990.
5. Gedgaudas E, Moller JH, Castaneda-Zuniga WR, Amplatz K. *Cardiovascular radiology.* Philadelphia: WB Saunders, 1985.
6. Keith JD, Rowe RD, Vlad P. *Heart disease in infancy and childhood.* Philadelphia: Macmillan, 1978.
7. Kelley MJ, Jaffe CC, Kleinman CS. *Cardiac imaging in infants and children.* Philadelphia: WB Saunders, 1982.
8. Lefebvre J, Kaufmann HJ. *Clinical practice in pediatric radiology.* New York: Masson, 1979.
9. Silverman FN, Kuhn JP. *Essentials of Caffey's pediatric x-ray diagnosis.* Chicago: Year Book, 1990.
10. Swischuk LE, Sapire DW. *Basic imaging in congenital heart disease.* 3rd ed. Baltimore: Williams and Wilkins, 1986.

Angiocardiography

11. Bargeron LM Jr, Elliott LP, Soto B, et al. Axial cineangiography in congenital heart disease. Section I. Concept, technical and anatomic considerations. *Circulation* 1977;56:1075–1083.
12. Nihill MR. Catheterization and angiography. In: Garson A Jr, Bricker JT, McNamara DG, eds. *The science and practice of pediatric cardiology.* Philadelphia: Lea and Febiger, 1990.
13. Benotti JR. The comparative effects of ionic versus nonionic agents in cardiac catheterization. *Invest Radiol* 1988;23:S366–373.
14. Gertz EW, Wisneski JA, Chiu D, et al. Clinical superiority of a new nonionic contrast agent (iopamidol) for cardiac angiography. *J Am Coll Cardiol* 1985;5:250–258.
15. Arciniegas JG, Soto B, Coghlan HC, Bargeron LM Jr. Congenital heart malformations: sequential angiographic analysis. *AJR* 1981;137:673–681.

Chest Radiography

16. Swischuk LE, Stansberry SD. Pulmonary vascularity in pediatric heart disease. *J Thorac Imaging* 1989;4:1–6.
17. Coussement AM, Gooding CA. Objective radiographic assessment of pulmonary vascularity in children. *Radiology* 1973;109:649–654.
18. Strife JL, Matsumoto J, Bisset GS III, Martin R. The position of the trachea in infants and children with right aortic arch. *Pediatr Radiol* 1989;19:226–229.
19. Stewart JR, Kincaid OW, Titus JL. Right aortic arch: plain film diagnosis and significance. *AJR* 1966;97:377–389.
20. Felson B, Palayew MJ. The two types of right aortic arch. *Radiology* 1963;81:745–759.
21. Rosario-Medina W, Strife JL, Dunbar JS. Normal left atrium: appearance in children on frontal chest radiographs. *Radiology* 1986;161:345–346.
22. Sargent EN, Turner AF, Jacobson G. Superior marginal rib defects. An etiologic classification. *AJR* 1969;106:491–505.
23. Luke MJ, McDonnell EJ. Congenital heart disease and scoliosis. *J Pediatr* 1968;73:725–733.
24. Currarino G, Swanson GE. A developmental variant of ossification of the manubrium sterni in mongolism. *Radiology* 1964;82:916.

Cardiac Malpositions

25. Elliott LP, Jue KL, Amplatz K. A roentgen classification of cardiac malpositions. *Invest Radiol* 1966;1:17–28.
26. Ellis K, Fleming RJ, Griffiths SP, Jameson AG. New concepts in dextrocardia. Angiocardiographic considerations. *AJR* 1966;97:295–313.
27. Van Praagh R. The importance of segmental situs in the diagnosis of congenital heart disease. *Semin Roentgenol* 1985;20:254–271.
28. Bisset GS III. Magnetic resonance imaging of the pediatric cardiovascular system. In: Cohen MD, Edwards MK, eds. *Pediatric magnetic resonance imaging.* BC Decker, Philadelphia, 1990, 541–584.
29. Winer-Muram HT, Tonkin IL. The spectrum of heterotaxic syndromes. *Radiol Clin North Am* 1989;27:1147–1170.
30. Van Mierop LH, Eisen S, Schiebler GL. The radiographic appearance of the tracheobronchial tree as an indicator of visceral situs. *Am J Cardiol* 1970;26:432–435.
31. Landing BH, Lawrence TY, Payne VC Jr, Wells TR. Bronchial anatomy in syndromes with abnormal visceral situs, abnormal spleen and congenital heart disease. *Am J Cardiol* 1971;28:456–462.
32. Soto B, Pacifico AD, Souza AS Jr, et al. Identification of thoracic isomerism from the plain chest radiograph. *AJR* 1978;131:995–1002.
33. Van Praagh R. Terminology of congenital heart disease. Glossary and commentary. *Circulation* 1977;56:139–143.

Echocardiography

34. Meyer RA. Echocardiography. In: Emmanouilides GC, Riemenschneider TA, Allen HD, Gutgesell HP, eds. *Moss and Adams heart disease in infants, children, and adolescents.* Baltimore: Williams and Wilkins, 1995, 241–270.
35. Silverman NH. *Pediatric echocardiography.* Baltimore: Williams and Wilkins, 1993.
36. Snider AR, Bengur AR. Doppler echocardiography. In: Emmanouilides GC, Riemenschneider TA, Allen HD, Gutgesell HP, eds. *Moss and Adams heart disease in infants, children, and adolescents.* Baltimore: Williams and Wilkins, 1995, 270–293.
37. Snider AR, Serwer GA. *Echocardiography in pediatric heart disease.* Chicago: Year Book, 1990.
38. Roberson D, Muhiudeen IA, Silverman NH. Transesophageal echocardiography in pediatrics: techniques and limitations. *Echocardiography* 1990;7:699–712.
39. Latson LA, Tuzcu EM, Nissen S. Coronary intravascular ultrasound in 2 children after cardiac transplantation. *Tex Heart Inst J* 1994;21:310–313.
40. Schratz LM, Schwartz DC, Meyer RA. Pediatric intracoronary ultrasound. *Circulation* 1995;92:II645.
41. Sugimura T, Kato H, Inoue O, et al. Intravascular ultrasound of coronary arteries in children. Assessment of the wall morphology and the lumen after Kawasaki disease. *Circulation* 1994;89:258–265.

Angled Angiocardiography

42. Elliott LP, Bargeron LM Jr, Green CE. Angled angiography. In: Friedman WF, Higgins CB, eds. *Pediatric cardiac imaging.* Philadelphia: WB Saunders, 1984, 1–25.
43. Freedom RM, Culham JAG, Moes CAF. *Angiocardiography of congenital heart disease.* New York: Macmillan, 1984.
44. Elliott LP, Bargeron LM Jr, Soto B, Bream PR. Axial cineangiography in congenital heart disease. *Radiol Clin North Am* 1980;18:515–546.

Magnetic Resonance Imaging

45. Fellows KE, Weinberg PM, Baffa JM, Hoffman EA. Evaluation of congenital heart disease with MR imaging: current and coming attractions. *AJR* 1992;159:925–931.
46. Bisset GS III. Magnetic resonance imaging of congenital heart disease in the pediatric patient. *Radiol Clin North Am* 1991;29:279–291.
47. Higgins CB, Silverman NH, Kersting-Sommerhoff BA, Schmidt K. *Congenital heart disease.* New York: Raven Press, 1990.
48. Kersting-Sommerhoff BA, Diethelm L, Stanger P, et al. Evaluation of complex congenital ventricular anomalies with magnetic resonance imaging. *Am Heart J* 1990;120:133–142.
49. Link KM, Lesko NM. Magnetic resonance imaging in the evaluation of congenital heart disease. *Magn Reson Q* 1991;7:173–190.
50. Mostbeck GH, Caputo GR, Higgins CB. MR measurement of blood flow in the cardiovascular system. *AJR* 1992;159:453–461.
51. Brenner LD, Caputo GR, Mostbeck G, et al. Quantification of left to right atrial shunts with velocity-encoded cine nuclear magnetic resonance imaging. *J Am Coll Cardiol* 1992;20:1246–1250.
52. Akins EW, Martin TD, Alexander JA, et al. MR imaging of double-outlet right ventricle. *AJR* 1989;152:128–130.
53. Donnelly LF, Higgins CB. MR imaging of conotruncal abnormalities. *AJR* 1996;166:925–928.
54. Mayo JR, Roberson D, Sommerhoff B, Higgins CB. MR imaging of double outlet right ventricle. *J Comput Assist Tomogr* 1990;14:336–339.
55. Irsik RD, White RD, Robitaille PM. Cardiac magnetic resonance imaging. In: Emmanouilides GC, Riemenschneider TA, Allen HD, Gutgesell HP, eds. *Moss and Adams heart disease in infants, children, and adolescents.* Baltimore: Williams and Wilkins, 1995, 206–223.
56. Park JH, Han MC, Kim CW. MR imaging of congenitally corrected transposition of the great vessels in adults. *AJR* 1989;153:491–494.

Left-to-Right Shunts

57. Condon VR. The heart and great vessels. In: Silverman FN, Kuhn JP, eds. *Essentials of Caffey's pediatric x-ray diagnosis.* Chicago: Year Book, 1990.
58. Hoffman JIE. Incidence of congenital heart disease: I. Postnatal incidence. *Pediatr Cardiol* 1995;16:103–113.
59. Graham TP Jr, Gutgesell HP. Ventricular septal defects. In: Emmanouilides GC, Riemenschneider TA, Allen HD, Gutgesell HP, eds. *Moss and Adams heart disease in infants, children, and adolescents.* Baltimore: Williams and Wilkins, 1995, 725–746.
60. Santamaria H, Soto B, Ceballos R, et al. Angiographic differentiation of types of ventricular septal defects. *AJR* 1983;141:273–281.
61. Hiraishi S, Agata Y, Nowatari M. Incidence and natural course of trabecular ventricular septal defect: two-dimensional echocardiography and color Doppler flow imaging study. *J Pediatr* 1992;120:409–415.
62. Anderson RH, Lenox CC, Zuberbuhler JR. Mechanisms of closure of perimembranous ventricular septal defect. *Am J Cardiol* 1983;52:341–345.
63. Freedom RM, White RD, Pieroni DR, et al. The natural history of the so-called aneurysm of the membranous ventricular septum in childhood. *Circulation* 1974;49:375–384.
64. Castaneda AR, Jonas RA, Mayer JE Jr, Hanley FL. Ventriculoseptal defects. *Cardiac surgery of the neonate and infant.* Philadelphia: WB Saunders, 1994, 187–201.
65. Lock JE, Block PC, McKay RG, et al. Transcatheter closure of ventricular septal defects. *Circulation* 1988;78:361–368.
66. Carlsson E. Anatomic diagnosis of atrial septal defects. *AJR* 1961; 85:1063–1070.
67. Edwards JE. The pathology of atrial septal defect. *Semin Roentgenol* 1966;1:24.
68. Chait A, Zucker M. The superior vena cava in the evaluation of atrial septal defect. *AJR* 1968;103:104–108.
69. Locke JT, Cockerham JT, Keane JF, et al. Transcatheter umbrella closure of congenital heart defects. *Circulation* 1987;75:593–599.
70. Rao PS, Sideris EB, Hausdorf G, et al. International experience with secundum atrial septal defect occlusion by the buttoned device. *Am Heart J* 1994;128:1022–1035.
71. Reddy SC, Rao PS, Ewenko J, et al. Echocardiographic predictors of success of catheter closure of atrial septal defect with buttoned device. *Am Heart J* 1995;129:76–82.
72. Radzik D, Davignon A, van Doesburg N, et al. Predictive factors for spontaneous closure of atrial septal defects diagnosed in the first 3 months of life. *J Am Coll Cardiol* 1993;22:851–853.
73. Brook MM, Heymann MA. Patent ductus arteriosus. In: Emmanouilides GC, Riemenschneider TA, Allen HD, Gutgesell HP, eds. *Moss and Adams heart disease in infants, children, and adolescents.* Baltimore: Williams and Wilkins, 1995, 746–764.
74. Currarino G, Jackson JH. Calcification of the ductus arteriosus and ligamentum botalli. *Radiology* 1970;94:139–142.
75. Bisceglia M, Donaldson JS. Calcification of the ligamentum arteriosum in children: a normal finding on CT. *AJR* 1991;156:351–352.
76. Burke RP, Wernovsky G, van der Velde M, et al. Video-assisted thoracoscopic surgery for congenital heart disease. *J Thorac Cardiovasc Surg* 1995; 109:499–507.
77. Laborde F, Folliguet T, Batisse A, et al. Video-assisted thoroscopic surgical interruption: the technique of choice for patent ductus arteriosus. Routine experience in 230 pediatric cases. *J Thorac Cardiovasc Surg* 1995;110:1681–1684.
78. Lloyd TR, Fedderly R, Mendelsohn AM, et al. Transcatheter occlusion of patent ductus arteriosus with Gianturco coils. *Circulation* 1993; 88:1412–1420.
79. Hijazi ZM, Lloyd TR, Beekman RH III, Geggel RL. Transcatheter closure with single or multiple Gianturco coils of patent ductus arteriosus in infants weighing < or = 8kg: retrograde versus antegrade approach. *Am Heart J* 1996;132:827–835.
80. Shim D, Fedderly RT, Beekman RH III, et al. Follow-up of coil occlusion of patent ductus arteriosus. *J Am Coll Cardiol* 1996;28:207–211.
81. Baron MG. Endocardial cushion defects. *Radiol Clin North Am* 1968; 6:343–360.
82. Schwartz DC. Atrioventricular septal defects. *Semin Roentgenol* 1985; 20:226–235.
83. Towbin R, Schwartz D. Endocardial cushion defects: embryology, anatomy and angiography. *AJR* 1981;136:157–162.
84. Cooney TP, Thurlbeck WM. Pulmonary hypoplasia in Down's syndrome. *N Engl J Med* 1982;307:1170–1173.
85. Haworth SG. Pulmonary vascular bed in children with complete atrioventricular septal defect: relation between structure and hemodynamic abnormalities. *Am J Cardiol* 1986;57:833–839.
86. Newfeld EA, Sher M, Paul MH, Nikaidoh H. Pulmonary vascular disease in complete atrioventricular canal defect. *Am J Cardiol* 1977; 39:721–726.
87. Hanley FL, Fenton KN, Jonas RA, et al. Surgical repair of complete atrioventricular canal defects in infancy. Twenty year trends. *J Thorac Cardiovasc Surg* 1993;106:387–394.

Cyanotic Congenital Heart Disease

88. Taussig HB. Tetralogy of Fallot: early history and late results. *AJR* 1979;133:423–431.
89. Daves ML. Roentgenology of tetralogy of Fallot. *Semin Roentgenol* 1968;3:377.
90. Kirklin JW. The tetralogy of Fallot. *AJR* 1968;102:253–266.
91. Johnson C. Fallot's tetralogy—a review of the radiological appearances in thirty-three cases. *Clin Radiol* 1965;16:199.
92. Lester RG, Robinson AE, Osteen RT. Tetralogy of Fallot. A detailed angiocardiographic study. *AJR* 1965;94:92–99.
93. Fellows KE, Freed MD, Keane JF, et al. Results of routine preoperative coronary angiography in tetralogy of Fallot. *Circulation* 1975; 51:561–566.
94. Soto B, Pacifico AD, Ceballos R, Bargeron LM Jr. Tetralogy of Fallot: an angiographic-pathologic correlative study. *Circulation* 1981;64: 558–566.
95. Edwards JE, McGoon DC. Absence of anatomic origin from heart of pulmonary arterial supply. *Circulation* 1973;47:393–398.
96. Hennein HA, Mosca RS, Urcelay G, et al. Intermediate results after complete repair of tetralogy of Fallot in neonates. *J Thorac Cardiovasc Surg* 1995;109:332–342.
97. Starnes VA, Luciani GB, Latter DA, Griffin ML. Current surgical management of tetralogy of Fallot. *Ann Thorac Surg* 1994;58: 211–215.
98. Castaneda AR. Classical repair of tetralogy of Fallot: timing, technique, and results. *Semin Thorac Cardiovasc Surg* 1990;2:70–75.

99. Castaneda AR, Mayer JE Jr, Lock JE. Tetralogy of Fallot, pulmonary atresia and diminutive pulmonary arteries. *Prog Pediatr Cardiol* 1992; 1:50.

100. Kirklin JW, Blackstone EH, Kirklin JK, et al. Surgical results and protocols in the spectrum of tetralogy of Fallot. *Ann Surg* 1983;198: 251–265.

101. Katz NM, Blackstone EH, Kirklin JW, et al. Late survival and symptoms after repair of tetralogy of Fallot. *Circulation* 1982;65:403–410.

102. Lock JE, Castaneda-Zuniga WR, Fuhrman BP, Bass JL. Balloon dilation angioplasty of hypoplastic and stenotic pulmonary arteries. *Circulation* 1983;67:962–967.

103. Gentles TL, Rosenfeld HM, Sanders SP, et al. Pediatric biplane transesophageal echocardiography: preliminary experience. *Am Heart J* 1994;128:1225–1233.

104. Fletcher BD, Jacobstein MD, Abramowsky CR, Anderson RH. Right atrioventricular valve atresia: anatomic evaluation with MR imaging. *AJR* 1987;148:671–674.

105. Coles JG, Kielmanowicz S, Freedom RM, et al. Surgical experience with the modified Fontan procedure. *Circulation* 1987;76:III 61–66.

106. Mayer JE Jr, Bridges ND, Lock JE, et al. Factors associated with improved survival after modified Fontan operations. *J Am Coll Cardiol* 1991;17:33A.

107. Knott-Craig CJ, Danielson GK, Schaff HV, et al. The modified Fontan operation. An analysis of risk factors for early postoperative death or takedown in 702 consecutive patients from one institution. *J Thorac Cardiovasc Surg* 1995;109:1237–1243.

108. Gentles TL, Keane JF, Jonas RA, et al. Surgical alternatives to the Fontan procedure incorporating a hypoplastic right ventricle. *Circulation* 1994;90:II 1–6.

109. Fontan F, Kirklin JW, Fernandez G, et al. Outcome after a "perfect" Fontan operation. *Circulation* 1990;81:1520–1536.

110. Jahangiri M, Ross DB, Redington AN, et al. Thromboembolism after the Fontan procedure and its modifications. *Ann Thorac Surg* 1994; 58:1409–1413.

111. Cloutier A, Ash JM, Smallhorn JF, et al. Abnormal distribution of pulmonary blood flow after the Glenn shunt or Fontan procedure: risk of development of arteriovenous fistulae. *Circulation* 1985;72: 471–479.

112. Srivastava D, Preminger T, Lock JE, et al. Hepatic venous blood and the development of pulmonary arteriovenous malformations in congenital heart disease. *Circulation* 1995;92:1217–1222.

113. Berthelot P, Walker JG, Sherlock S, Reid L. Arterial changes in the lungs in cirrhosis of the liver—lung spider nevi. *N Engl J Med* 1966; 274:291–298.

114. Plowden JS, Kimball TR, Bensky A, et al. The use of extracorporeal membrane oxygenation in critically ill neonates with Ebstein's anomaly. *Am Heart J* 1991;121:619–622.

115. Oh JK, Holmes DR Jr, Hayes DL, et al. Cardiac arrhythmias in patients with surgical repair of Ebstein's anomaly. *J Am Coll Cardiol* 1985; 6:1351–1357.

116. Paul MH, Wernovsky G. Transposition of the great arteries. In: Emmanouilides GC, Riemenschneider TA, Allen HD, Gutgesell HP, eds. *Moss and Adams heart disease in infants, children, and adolescents.* Baltimore: Williams and Wilkins, 1995, 1154–1224.

117. Donnelly LF, Hurst DR, Strife JL, Shapiro R. Plain film assessment of the neonate with D-transposition of the great vessels. *Pediatr Radiol* 1995;25:195–197.

118. Barcia A, Kincaid OW, Davis GD, et al. Transposition of the great arteries. An angiocardiographic study. *AJR* 1967;100:249–283.

119. Carey LS, Elliott LP. Complete transposition of the great vessels. Roentgenographic findings. *AJR* 1964;91:529–543.

120. Grainger RG. Transposition of the great arteries and of the pulmonary veins including an account of cardiac embryology and chamber identification. *Clin Radiol* 1970;21:335–354.

121. Kirklin JW, Blackstone EH, Tchervenkov CI, Castaneda AR. Clinical outcomes after the arterial switch operation for transposition. Patient, support, procedural, and institutional risk factors. Congenital Heart Surgeons Society. *Circulation* 1992;86:1501–1515.

122. Jatene AD, Fontes VF, Souza LC, et al. Anatomic correction of transposition of the great arteries. *J Thorac Cardiovasc Surg* 1982;83: 20–26.

123. Wernovsky G, Mayer JE Jr, Jonas RA, et al. Factors influencing early and late outcome of the arterial switch operation for transposition of the great arteries. *J Thorac Cardiovasc Surg* 1995;109:289–301.

124. Bonhoeffer P, Bonnet D, Piechaud JF, et al. Coronary artery obstruction after arterial switch operation for transposition of the great arteries in newborns. *J Am Coll Cardiol* 1997;29:202–206.

125. Rhodes LA, Wernovsky G, Keane JF, et al. Arrhythmias and intracardiac conduction after the arterial switch operation. *J Thorac Cardiovasc Surg* 1995;109:303–310.

126. Colan SD, Boutin C, Castaneda AR, Wernovsky G. Status of the left ventricle after arterial switch operation for transposition of the great arteries. Hemodynamic and echocardiographic evaluation. *J Thorac Cardiovasc Surg* 1995;109:311–321.

127. Blakenberg F, Rhee J, Hardy C, et al. MRI vs. echocardiography in the evaluation of the Jatene procedure. *J Comput Assist Tomogr* 1994; 18:749–754.

128. Hallermann FJ, Kincaid OW, Ritter DG, et al. Angiocardiographic and anatomic findings in origin of both great arteries from the right ventricle. *AJR* 1970;109:51–66.

129. Sridaromont S, Ritter DG, Feldt RH, et al. Double-outlet right ventricle. Anatomic and angiocardiographic correlations. *Mayo Clin Proc* 1978;53:555–577.

130. Bream PR, Elliott LP, Bargeron LM. Plain film findings of anatomically corrected malposition: its association with juxtaposition of the atrial appendages and right aortic arch. *Radiology* 1978;126:589–595.

131. Butto F, Lucas RV Jr, Edwards JE. Persistent truncus arteriosus: pathologic anatomy in 54 cases. *Pediatr Cardiol* 1986;7:95–101.

132. Calder L, Van Praagh R, Van Praagh S, et al. Truncus arteriosus communis. Clinical, angiographic, and pathologic findings in 100 patients. *Am Heart J* 1976;92:23–38.

133. Collet RW, Edwards JE. Persistent truncus arteriosus. A classification according to anatomic subtypes. *Surg Clin North Am* 1949;29:1245.

134. Hallermann FJ, Kincaid OW, Tsakiris AG, et al. Persistent truncus arteriosus: a radiographic and angiocardiographic study. *AJR* 1969; 107:827–834.

135. Hanley FL, Heinemann MK, Jonas RA, et al. Repair of truncus arteriosus in the neonate. *J Thorac Cardiovasc Surg* 1993;105:1047–1056.

136. Truncus arteriosus. In: Castaneda AR, Jonas RA, Mayer JE Jr, Hanley FL, eds. *Cardiac surgery of the neonate and infant.* Philadelphia: WB Saunders, 1994, 281–293.

137. Chen JT. Radiologic demonstration of anomalous pulmonary venous connection and its clinical significance. *CRC Crit Rev Diagn Imaging* 1979;11:383–422.

138. Eisen S, Elliott LP. A plain film sign of total anomalous pulmonary venous connection below the diaphragm. *AJR* 1968;102:372–379.

139. Weaver MD, Chen JTT, Anderson PAW, Lester RG. Total anomalous pulmonary venous connection to the left vertical vein. A plain-film sign useful in early diagnosis. *Radiology* 1976;118:679–683.

140. Sano S, Brawn WJ, Mee RB. Total anomalous pulmonary venous drainage. *J Thorac Cardiovasc Surg* 1989;97:886–892.

141. Behrendt DM, Aberdeen E, Waterson DJ, Bonham-Carter RE. Total anomalous pulmonary venous drainage in infants. Clinical and hemodynamic findings, methods, and results of operation in 37 cases. *Circulation* 1972;46:347–356.

142. Norwood WI, Hougen TJ, Castaneda AR. Total anomalous pulmonary venous connection: surgical considerations. *Cardiovasc Clin* 1981; 11:353–364.

143. Mazzucco A, Rizzoli G, Fracasso A, et al. Experience with operation for total anomalous pulmonary venous connection in infancy. *J Thorac Cardiovasc Surg* 1983;85:686–690.

144. Reardon MJ, et al. Total anomalous pulmonary venous return: report of 201 patients treated surgically. *Tex Heart Inst J* 1985;12:131.

145. Castaneda AR, Jonas AR, Mayer JE Jr, Hanley FL. Anomalies of the pulmonary veins. *Cardiac surgery of the neonate and infant.* Philadelphia: WB Saunders, 1994, 157–166.

146. van der Velde ME, Parness IA, Colan SD, et al. Two-dimensional echocardiography in the pre- and postoperative management of totally anomalous pulmonary venous connection. *J Am Coll Cardiol* 1991; 18:1746–1751.

Obstructive Lesions

147. Kirks DR, Currarino G, Chen JTT. Mediastinal collateral arteries: important vessels in coarctation of the aorta. *AJR* 1986;146:757–762.

148. Gomes AS, Lois JF, George B, et al. Congenital abnormalities of the aortic arch: MR imaging. *Radiology* 1987;165:691–695.

149. Amparo EG, Higgins CB, Shafton EP. Demonstration of coarctation of the aorta by magnetic resonance imaging. *AJR* 1984;143: 1192–1194.

150. Kilner PJ, Firmin DN, Manzara CC, et al. Aortic coarctation assessed by magnetic resonance jet velocity mapping. *Circulation* 1990;82:63.

151. Boxer RA, LaCorte MA, Singh S, et al. Nuclear magnetic resonance imaging in evaluation and follow-up of children treated for coarctation of the aorta. *J Am Coll Cardiol* 1986;7:1095–1098.

152. Anjos R, Qureshi SA, Rosenthal E, et al. Determinants of hemodynamic results of balloon dilation of aortic recoarctation. *Am J Cardiol* 1992;69:665–671.

153. Huggon IC, Qureshi SA, Baker EJ, Tynan M. Effect of introducing balloon dilation of native aortic coarctation on overall outcome in infants and children. *Am J Cardiol* 1994;73:799–807.

154. Johnson MC, Canter CE, Strauss AW, Spray TL. Repair of coarctation of the aorta in infancy: comparison of surgical and balloon angioplasty. *Am Heart J* 1993;125:464–468.

155. Lock JE, Bass JL, Amplatz K, et al. Balloon dilation angioplasty of aortic coarctations in infants and children. *Circulation* 1983;68: 109–116.

156. Morrow WR, Vick GW III, Nihill MR, et al. Balloon dilation of unoperated coarctation of the aorta: short- and intermediate-term results. *J Am Coll Cardiol* 1988;11:133–138.

157. Witsenburg M, The SH, Bogers AJ, Hess J. Balloon angioplasty for aortic recoarctation in children: initial and follow-up results and midterm effect on blood pressure. *Br Heart J* 1993;70:170–174.

158. Braunwald E, Goldblatt A, Aygen MM, et al. Congenital aortic stenosis: clinical and hemodynamic findings in 100 patients. *Circulation* 1963;27:426–562.

159. Kuhn MA, Latson LA, Cheatham JP, et al. Management of pediatric patients with isolated valvar aortic stenosis by balloon aortic valvuloplasty. *Cathet Cardiovasc Diagn* 1996;39:55–61.

160. McKay RG. Balloon valvuloplasty for treating pulmonic, mitral and aortic valve stenosis. *Am J Cardiol* 1988;61:102G–108G.

161. Sholler GF, Keane JF, Perry SB, et al. Balloon dilation of congenital aortic valve stenosis. Results and influence of technical morphological features on outcome. *Circulation* 1988;78:351–360.

162. Moore P, Egito E, Mowrey H, et al. Midterm results of balloon dilation of congenital aortic stenosis: predictors of success. *J Am Coll Cardiol* 1996;27:1257–1263.

163. McCrindle BW. Independent predictors of immediate results of percutaneous balloon aortic valvotomy in children. *Am J Cardiol* 1996;77: 286–293.

164. Mosca RS, Iannettoni MD, Schwartz SM, et al. Critical aortic stenosis in the neonate. A comparison of balloon valvuloplasty and transventricular dilation. *J Thorac Cardiovasc Surg* 1995;109:147–154.

165. Keane JF, Driscoll DJ, Gersony WM, et al. Second natural history study of congenital heart defects. Results of treatment of patients with aortic valvar stenosis. *Circulation* 1993;87:I16–27.

166. Gerosa G, McKay R, Davies J, Ross DN. Comparison of the aortic homograft and the pulmonary autograft for aortic valve or root replacement in children. *J Thorac Cardiovasc Surg* 1991;102:51–61.

167. Reddy VM, Rajasinghe HA, McElhinney DB, et al. Extending the limits of the Ross procedure. *Ann Thorac Surg* 1995;60:S600–603.

168. Antia AU, Wiltse HE, Rowe RD, et al. Pathogenesis of the supravalvular aortic stenosis syndrome. *J Pediatr* 1967;71:431–441.

169. Deutsch V, Shem-Tov A, Yahini JH, Neufeld HN. Subaortic stenosis (discrete form). Classification and angiocardiographic features. *Radiology* 1971;101:275–286.

170. Freedom RM, Culham JAG, Rowe RD. Angiocardiography of subaortic obstruction in infancy. *AJR* 1977;129:813–824.

171. Freundlich IM, McMurray JT, Lehman JS. Idiopathic hypertrophic subaortic stenosis. *AJR* 1967;100:284–289.

172. Chen JT, Robinson AE, Goodrich JK, Lester RG. Uneven distribution of pulmonary blood flow between left and right lungs in isolated valvular pulmonary stenosis. *AJR* 1969;107:343–350.

173. Cheatham JP. Pulmonary stenosis. In: Garson A Jr, Bricker JT, McNamara DG, eds. *The science and practice of pediatric cardiology.* Philadelphia: Lea and Febiger, 1990, 1382.

174. Kan JS, White RI Jr, Mitchell SE, Gardner TJ. Percutaneous balloon valvuloplasty: a new method for treating congenital pulmonary valve stenosis. *N Engl J Med* 1982;307:540–542.

175. Hayes CJ, Gersony WM, Driscoll DJ, et al. Second natural history study of congenital heart defects. Result of treatment of patients with pulmonary valvar stenosis. *Circulation* 1993;87:I28–37.

176. Zeevi B, Keane JF, Fellows KE, Lock JE. Balloon dilation of critical pulmonary stenosis in the first week of life. *J Am Coll Cardiol* 1988; 11:821–824.

177. Shackelford GD, Sacks EJ, Mullins JD, McAlister WH. Pulmonary venoocclusive disease: case report and review of the literature. *AJR* 1977;128:643–648.

178. Masui T, Seelos KC, Kersting-Sommerhoff BA, Higgins CB. Abnormalities of the pulmonary veins: evaluation with MR imaging and comparison with cardiac angiography and echocardiography. *Radiology* 1991;181:645–649.

179. Bisset GS III, Kirks DR, Strife JL, Schwartz DC. Cor triatriatum: diagnosis by MR imaging. *AJR* 1987;149:567–568.

180. Ellis K, Griffiths SP, Jesse MJ, Jameson AG. Cor triatriatium. Angiocardiographic demonstration of the obstructing left atrial membrane. *AJR* 1964;92:669–675.

Cardiomyopathy

181. Wellner LJ, Kirks DR, Merten DF, Armstrong BE. Large opaque hemithorax due to cardiomegaly and atelectasis. *South Med J* 1985; 78:805–809.

182. Chen SC, Nouri S, Balfour I, et al. Clinical profile of congestive cardiomyopathy in children. *J Am Coll Cardiol* 1990;15:189–193.

183. Jin O, Sole MJ, Butany JW, et al. Detection of enterovirus RNA in myocardial biopsies from patients with myocarditis and cardiomyopathy using gene amplification by polymerase chain reaction. *Circulation* 1990;82:8–16.

184. Mason JW. Myocarditis treatment trial investigators: incidence and clinical characteristics of myocarditis (abstract). *Circulation* 1994;84: 2.

185. Billingham ME. The diagnostic criteria of myocarditis by endomyocardial biopsy. *Heart Vessels* 1985;1:133–137.

186. Lewis AB, Chabot M. Outcome of infants and children with dilated cardiomyopathy. *Am J Cardiol* 1991;68:365–369.

Acquired Heart Disease

187. Fukushige J, Nihill MR. Kawasaki disease. In: Garson A Jr, Bricker JT, McNamara DG, eds. *The science and practice of pediatric cardiology.* Philadelphia: Lea and Febiger, 1990, 1542.

188. Melish ME, Hicks RM, Larson EJ. Mucocutaneous lymph node syndrome in the United States. *Am J Dis Child* 1976;130:599–607.

189. Newburger JW, Takahashi M, Burns JC, et al. The treatment of Kawasaki syndrome with intravenous gamma globulin. *N Engl J Med* 1986; 315:341–347.

190. Ayoub EM. Acute rheumatic fever. In: Emmanouilides GC, Riemenschneider TA, Allen HD, Gutgesell HP, eds. *Moss and Adams heart disease in infants, children, and adolescents.* Baltimore: Williams and Wilkins, 1995, 1400–1416.

191. Sanyal SK. Long-term sequelae of the first attack of acute rheumatic fever during childhood. In: Emmanouilides GC, Riemenschneider TA, Allen HD, Gutgesell HP, eds. *Moss and Adams heart disease in infants, children, and adolescents.* Baltimore: Williams and Wilkins, 1995, 1416–1440.

192. El-Said GM, Sorour KA. Acute rheumatic fever. In: Garson A Jr, Bricker JT, McNamara DG, eds. *The science and practice of pediatric cardiology.* Philadelphia: Lea and Febiger, 1990, 1485.

Congenital Aortic Arch Anomalies

193. Shuford WH, Sybers RG, Edwards FK. The three types of right aortic arch. *AJR* 1970;109:67–74.

194. Mandell VS, Braverman RM. Vascular rings and slings. In: Fyler DC, ed. *Nadas' pediatric cardiology.* Philadelphia: Hanley and Belfus, Inc., 1991, 719–726.

195. Berdon WE, Baker DH. Vascular anomalies and the infant lung: rings, slings, and other things. *Semin Roentgenol* 1972;7:39–64.

196. McFaul R, Millard P, Nowicki E. Vascular rings necessitating right thoracotomy. *J Thorac Cardiovasc Surg* 1981;82:306–309.

197. Bisset GS III, Strife JL, Kirks DR, Bailey WW. Vascular rings: MR imaging. *AJR* 1987;149:251–256.
198. Berdon WE, Baker DH, Bordiuk J, Mellins R. Innominate artery compression of the trachea in infants with stridor and apnea. *Radiology* 1969;92:272–278.
199. Strife JL, Baumel AS, Dunbar JS. Tracheal compression by the innominate artery in infancy and childhood. *Radiology* 1981;139:73–75.
200. Swischuk LE. Anterior tracheal indentation in infancy and early childhood: normal or abnormal? *AJR* 1971;112:12–17.
201. Capitanio MA, Ramos R, Kirkpatrick JA. Pulmonary sling. Roentgen observations. *AJR* 1971;112:28–34.
202. Berdon WE, Baker DH, Wung JT, et al. Complete cartilage-ring tracheal stenosis associated with anomalous left pulmonary artery: the ring–sling complex. *Radiology* 1984;152:57–64.

Cardiac Associations with Types of Situs

203. Stanger P, Rudolph AM, Edwards JE. Cardiac malpositions. An overview based on study of sixty-five necropsy specimens. *Circulation* 1977;56:159–172.
204. Tonkin IL, Tonkin AK. Visceroatrial situs abnormalities: sonographic and computed tomographic appearance. *AJR* 1982;138:509–515.

Operative Procedures for Congenital Heart Disease

205. Kreutzer J, Keane JF, Lock JE, et al. Conversion of modified Fontan procedure to lateral atrial tunnel cavopulmonary anastomosis. *J Thorac Cardiovasc Surg* 1996;111:1169–1176.
206. Hosenpud JD, Novick RJ, Breen TJ, Daily OP. The Registry of the International Society for Heart and Lung Transplantation: eleventh official report–1994. *J Heart Lung Transplant* 1994;13:561–570.
207. Fricker JR, Armitage JM. Heart and heart lung transplantation in children and adolescents. In: Emmanouilides GC, Riemenschneider TA, Allen HD, Gutgesell HP, eds. *Moss and Adams heart disease in infants, children, and adolescents.* Baltimore: Williams and Wilkins, 1995, 495–509.
208. Shaddy RE, Naftel DC, Kirklin JK, et al. Outcome of cardiac transplantation in children. Survival in a contemporary multi-institutional experience. Pediatric heart transplant study. *Circulation* 1996;94: II69–73.
209. Chinnock RE, Larsen RL, Emery JR, Bailey LL. Pretransplant risk factors and causes of death or graft loss after heart transplantation during early infancy. Pediatric heart transplant team, Loma Linda. *Circulation* 1995;92(9 Suppl):II206–209.
210. Gao SZ, Schroeder JS, Alderman EL, et al. Prevalence of accelerated coronary artery disease in heart transplant survivors. Comparison of cyclosporine and azathioprine regimens. *Circulation* 1987;80: III100–105.
211. Uretsky BF, Murali S, Reddy PS, et al. Development of coronary disease in cardiac transplant patients receiving immunosuppresive therapy with cyclosporine and prednisone. *Circulation* 1987;76: 827–834.
212. Costanzo-Nordin MR. Cardiac allograft vasculopathy: relationship with acute cellular rejection and histocompatability. *J Heart Lung Transplant* 1992;11:S90–103.
213. Hammond EH, Yowell RL, Price GD, et al. Vascular rejection and its relationship to allograft coronary artery disease. *J Heart Lung Transplant* 1992;11:S111–119.

Neonatal Congenital Heart Disease

214. Castaneda AR, Jonas RA, Mayer JE Jr, Hanley FL. Management of the infant and neonate with congenital heart disease. *Cardiac surgery of the neonate and infant.* Philadelphia: WB Saunders, 1994, 65–87.
215. Gyepes MT, Vincent WR. Severe congenital heart disease in the neonatal period. A functional approach to emergency diagnosis. *AJR* 1972;116:490–500.
216. Taybi H. Roentgen evaluation of cardiomegaly in the newborn period and early infancy. *Pediatr Clin North Am* 1971;18:1031–1058.
217. Edwards DK, Higgins CB, Gilpin EA. The cardiothoracic ratio in newborn infants. *AJR* 1981;136:907–913.
218. Freedom RM. Axial angiocardiography in the critically ill infant. In: Friedman WF, Higgins CB, eds. *Pediatric cardiac imaging.* Philadelphia: WB Saunders, 1984, 26.
219. Natowicz M, Chatten J, Clancy R, et al. Genetic disorders and major extracardiac anomalies associated with the hypoplastic left heart syndrome. *Pediatrics* 1988;82:698–706.
220. Sade RM, Crawford FA Jr, Fyfe DA. Symposium on hypoplastic left heart syndrome (letter to the editor). *J Thorac Cardiovasc Surg* 1986; 91:937–939.
221. Norwood WI, Lang P, Hansen DD. Physiologic repair of aortic atresia-hypoplastic left heart syndrome. *N Engl J Med* 1983;308:23–26.
222. Chang AC, Farrell PE Jr, Murdison KA, et al. Hypoplastic left heart syndrome: hemodynamic and angiographic assessment after initial reconstructive surgery and relevance to modified Fontan procedure. *J Am Coll Cardiol* 1991;17:1143–1149.
223. Bando K, Turrentine MW, Sun K, Sharp TG, Caldwell RL, Darragh RK, Ensing GJ, Cordes TM, Flaspoher T, Brown JW. Surgical management of hypoplastic left heart syndrome. *Ann Thorac Surg* 1996; 62:70–76.
224. Bove EL, Lloyd TR. Staged reconstruction for hypoplastic left heart syndrome. Contemporary results. *Ann Surg* 1996;224:387–394.
225. Forbess JM, Cook N, Roth SJ, et al. Ten-year institutional experience with palliative surgery for hypoplastic left heart syndrome. Risk factors related to stage I mortality. *Circulation* 1995;92:II262–266.
226. Bailey LL, Gundry SR. Hypoplastic left heart syndrome. *Pediatr Clin North Am* 1990;37:137–150.
227. Razzouk AJ, Chinnock RE, Gundry SR, et al. Transplantation as a primary treatment for hypoplastic left heart syndrome: intermediate-term results. *Ann Thorac Surg* 1996;62:1–8
228. Merten DF, Goetzman BW, Wennberg RP. Persistent fetal circulation: an evolving clinical and radiographic concept of pulmonary hypertension of the newborn. *Pediatr Radiol* 1977;6:74–80.

Pediatric Vascular Anomalies

229. Mulliken JB, Glowacki J. Hemangiomas and vascular malformations in infants and children: a classification based on endothelial characteristics. *Plast Reconstr Surg* 1982;69:412–422.
230. Mulliken JB, Young AE. *Vascular birthmarks, hemangiomas and malformations.* Philadelphia: WB Saunders, 1988.
231. Burns AJ, Kaplan LC, Mulliken JB. Is there an association between hemangioma and syndromes with dysmorphic features? *Pediatrics* 1991;88:1257–1267.
232. Takahashi K, Mulliken JB, Kozakewich HP, et al. Cellular markers than distinguish the phases of hemangioma during infancy and childhood. *J Clin Invest* 1994;93:2357–2364.
233. Finn MC, Glowacki J, Mulliken JB. Congenital vascular lesions: clinical application of a new classification. *J Pediatr Surg* 1983;18: 894–900.
234. Jackson IT, Carreno R, Potparic Z, Hussain K. Hemangiomas, vascular malformations, and lymphovenous malformations: classification and methods of treatment. *Plast Reconstr Surg* 1993;91:1216–1230.
235. Meyer JS, Hoffer FA, Barnes PD, Mulliken JB. Biological classification of soft-tissue vascular anomalies: MR correlation. *AJR* 1991;157: 559–564.
236. Burrows PE, Robertson RL, Barnes PD. Angiography and the evaluation of cerebrovascular disease in childhood. *Neuroimaging Clin N Am* 1996;6:561–588.
237. Burrows PE, Lasjaunias PL, Ter Brugge KG, Flodmark O. Urgent and emergent embolization of lesions of the head and neck in children: indications and results. *Pediatrics* 1987;80:386–394.
238. Burrows PE, Fellows KE. Techniques for management of pediatric vascular anomalies. In: Cope C, ed. *Current techniques in interventional radiology.* Philadelphia: Current Medicine, 1995, 12–27.
239. Lasjaunias P, Berenstein A. Craniofacial hemangiomas, vascular malformations and angiomatosis: specific aspects. *Surgical neuroangiography. Endovascular treatment of craniofacial lesions.* Heidelberg: Springer-Verlag, 1987.
240. Chiras J, Hassine D, Goudot P, et al. Treatment of arteriovenous malformations of the mandible by arterial and venous embolization. *AJNR* 1990;11:1191–1194.
241. Dubois JM, Sebag GH, DeProst Y, et al. Soft-tissue venous malformations in children: percutaneous sclerotherapy with Ethibloc. *Radiology* 1991;180:195–198.

242. Yakes WF, Haas DK, Parker SH, et al. Symptomatic vascular malformations: ethanol embolotherapy. *Radiology* 1989;170:1059–1066.

243. de Lorimier AA. Sclerotherapy for venous malformations. *J Pediatr Surg* 1995;30:188–193.

244. Gomes AS. Embolization therapy of congenital arteriovenous malformations: use of alternate approaches. *Radiology* 1994;190:191–198.

245. Fellows KE, Hoffer FA, Markowitz RI, O'Neill JA Jr. Multiple collaterals to hepatic infantile hemangioendotheliomas and arteriovenous malformations: effect on embolization. *Radiology* 1991;181:813–818.

246. McHugh K, Burrows PE. Infantile hepatic hemangioendotheliomas: significance of portal venous and systemic collateral arterial supply. *J Vasc Interv Radiol* 1992;3:337–344.

247. Ogita S, Tsuto T, Deguchi E, et al. OK-432 therapy for unresectable lymphangiomas in children. *J Pediatr Surg* 1991;26:263–268.

248. Enjolras O, Mulliken JB. The current management of vascular birthmarks. *Pediatr Dermatol* 1993;10:311–313.

249. Pascual-Castroviejo I. The association of extracranial and intracranial vascular malformations in children. *Can J Neurol Sci* 1985;12:139–148.

250. Enjolras O, Riche MC, Merland JJ, Escande JP. Management of alarming hemangiomas in infancy: a review of 25 cases. *Pediatrics* 1990;85:491–498.

251. Ezekowitz RAB, Mulliken JB, Folkman J. Interferon alfa-2a therapy for life threatening hemangiomas of infancy. *N Engl J Med* 1992;326:1456–1463.

252. Burrows PE, Fellows KE. Techniques for management of pediatric vascular amomalies. Chapter 2. In: Cope C, ed. *Current techniques in interventional radiology.* 2nd ed. Philadelphia: Current Medicine, 1994, 12–27.

253. Erba G, Cavazzuti V. Sturge-Weber syndrome: natural history and indications for surgery. *J Epilepsy* 1990;3:287–291.

254. Joseph AE, Donaldson JS, Reynolds M. Neck and thorax venous aneurysm: association with cystic hygroma. *Radiology* 1989;170:109–112.

255. Laor T, Burrows PE, Hoffer FA. Magnetic resonance venography of congenital vascular malformations of the extremities. *Pediatr Radiol* 1996;26:371–380.

Practical Pediatric Imaging: Diagnostic Radiology of Infants and Children, Third Edition.
D. R. Kirks, editor and N. T. Griscom, associate editor.
Lippincott–Raven Publishers, Philadelphia © 1998.

CHAPTER 7

Respiratory System

Gary L. Hedlund, N. Thorne Griscom, Robert H. Cleveland, and Donald R. Kirks

Radiology is critical in the diagnostic evaluation of the pediatric respiratory system. Not surprisingly, imaging of the chest and upper airway is extremely common. More than one third of all radiologic examinations performed at children's hospitals each year are chest radiographs, partly because respiratory disorders are so common. Radiologists are repeatedly called upon to choose from an array of imaging tools to investigate acquired and congenital disorders of the pediatric airway and chest. The potential lethality of some obstructive airway lesions and lung diseases makes this topic a priority. One should localize and characterize airway and chest abnormalities so that a practical differential diagnosis facilitates timely patient care. Knowledge of the clinical features of each patient is helpful in distinguishing among the causes of respiratory problems.

Several textbooks and review articles focus on imaging of the respiratory system in general and the radiology of the pediatric respiratory system in particular (1–11). Other review articles, monographs, and textbooks discuss radiology of the newborn chest (7,10,12,13,14), respiratory tract emergencies (8,15,16), and intensive care chest radiology (17).

TECHNIQUES

Evaluation of the Upper Airway

Alterations in pressure across the tracheal wall affect tracheal size (18,19). This change is mainly limited to the cervical trachea. The size of the intrathoracic trachea is controlled by recoil forces of the lungs and chest wall.

During normal inspiration, intrathoracic pressure decreases (becomes more negative), and intrathoracic tracheal lumen diameter increases (Fig. 7-1). Intrathoracic pressure increases during expiration, and intrathoracic tracheal lumen diameter decreases (Fig. 7-1). An increase in pressure in the chest against closed vocal cords or some other obstruction (grunting, straining, shouting, singing loudly, playing a wind instrument) will cause the cervical trachea to bulge outward, sometimes more at the pars membranacea than at the cartilaginous rings. The reverse occurs during vigorous inspiration in children with laryngeal obstruction. A film in a child with croup taken during inspiration, when intrapleural pressure is low and air has difficulty passing through the obstructed

    G. L. Hedlund: Department of Pediatric Imaging, The Children's Hospital, University of Alabama at Birmingham, Birmingham, Alabama 35233.
    N. T. Griscom, R. H. Cleveland, and D. R. Kirks: Department of Radiology, Children's Hospital, Harvard Medical School, Boston, Massachusetts 02115.

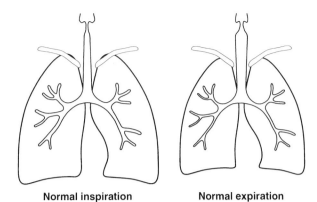

FIG. 7-1. Normal airway caliber. Normal changes in the extrathoracic and intrathoracic airway caliber during inspiration and expiration.

larynx, will show narrowing of the entire upper trachea, not just at the edematous conus elasticus.

The most common indication for radiologic evaluation of the upper airway is stridor. *Stridor* means noisy breathing due to turbulent airflow through a partially obstructed airway. Stridor may be either inspiratory or expiratory and may be associated with voice alteration (8). If stridor is purely inspiratory, the lesion is above the thoracic inlet, usually glottic or supraglottic. If stridor is purely expiratory (wheezing), the lesion is almost always below the thoracic inlet. Obstructive lesions, such as vascular rings, near the thoracic inlet may cause both inspiratory and expiratory stridor (8,20,21). Voice alteration with stridor places the lesion in the glottis or paraglottic region (8).

The radiologic evaluation of a child with inspiratory stridor should include filtered high-kilovoltage anteroposterior (AP) and lateral radiographs of the upper airway (Fig. 7-2) as well as frontal and lateral views of the chest (22). Children suspected of having airway obstruction should never be immobilized in a position that they do not wish to assume. This rule is particularly valid for possible acute epiglottitis, when the child prefers the upright position, and forcing the patient into a supine position is contraindicated (23).

Other indications for radiologic evaluation of the upper airway include nasal obstruction, epistaxis, foreign body, evaluation of nasopharyngeal lymphoid tissue, abnormality of speech, unexplained pulmonary arterial hypertension, hoarseness, trauma, caustic ingestion, abnormal cry, and neck mass (23).

The lateral film of the upper airway is the cornerstone radiograph in children with inspiratory stridor (Fig. 7-3A). This view is excellent for diagnosing epiglottitis, foreign body, and upper airway masses. The AP, high-kilovoltage,

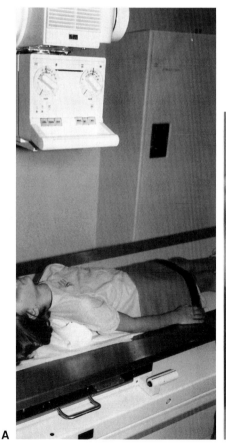
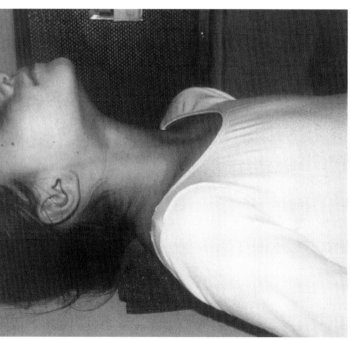

A   B

FIG. 7-2. Positioning for AP and lateral airway radiography. A: The AP airway radiograph is coned to the neck and filtered. **B:** The lateral film is taken in deep inspiration with the neck extended.

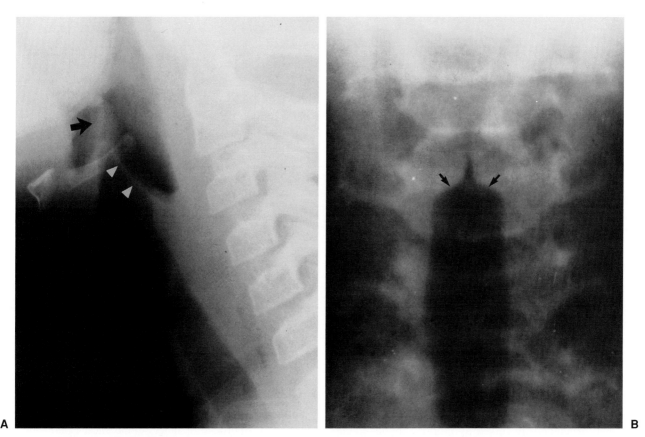

FIG. 7-3. Normal lateral and AP airway radiographs. A: Lateral airway radiography shows normal oropharyngeal distention "small-finger-sized" epiglottis *(arrow)*, and delicate aryepiglottic folds *(arrowheads)*. **B:** Filtered AP airway radiograph shows normal symmetric subglottic "shoulders" *(arrows)*.

tightly coned radiograph with selective filtration removes overlying osseous shadows of the cervical spine and provides the best frontal visualization of the upper airway (Fig. 7-3B) (20). Fluoroscopy is usually not required if epiglottitis or croup is diagnosed by conventional radiography. However, if the cause of inspiratory stridor is not evident from plain films, fluoroscopy should be performed. This technique provides dynamic upper airway evaluation for conditions such as laryngomalacia and small masses like subglottic hemangioma. If both the radiograph and fluoroscopy are normal, a barium esophagogram might well be performed to exclude esophageal foreign body, esophageal inflammatory disease, and vascular ring (24,25).

Ultrasonography is extremely valuable for the evaluation of neck masses in children (26). Computed tomography (CT) exquisitely images trachea and adjacent soft tissues. Normal tracheal cross-sectional areas have been determined for the pediatric population (27–30). A disadvantage of conventional CT is that it only displays axial images and is ineffective in showing dynamic airway changes. Spiral CT technology has the benefit of faster scan times, decreased motion artifact, less need for sedation, and reduced need for intravenous contrast. Although cine CT is not widely available, it depicts tracheal dynamics accurately (31,32). Magnetic resonance imaging (MRI), because of its lack of ionizing

radiation, multiplanar imaging capability, and superior contrast resolution, is an excellent modality for the child with lower (intrathoracic) airway symptoms (33–36). Disadvantages of MRI include expense, length of examination time, difficulty showing the lungs and smaller airways, and frequent need for sedation with monitoring.

Chest Imaging

Conventional Radiography

Indications for radiologic examination of the chest and lower airway include inflammatory disease, deformity of the thoracic cage, palpable mass, heart disease, trauma, chest pain, wheezing, tachypnea, and possible metastatic disease. Chest examinations in children should not be performed routinely on admission to the hospital or for screening purposes. Chest radiography in children is not performed prior to anesthesia unless there are symptoms, signs, or a history of respiratory disease.

Chest Radiography

AP or posteroanterior (PA) and lateral views of the chest are required for accurate evaluation of thoracic abnormalities

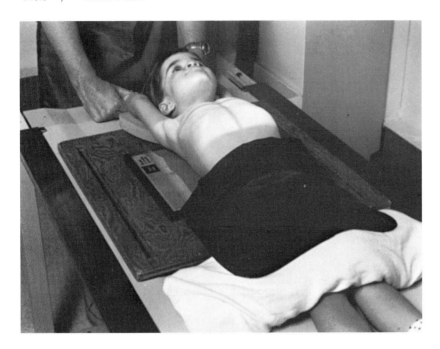

FIG. 7-4. Gonadal shielding during chest radiography. Well-coned AP chest radiograph in a 3-year-old girl. Note the lead drape over the lower abdomen and pelvis.

(8,11,23). Many technologists and radiologists are intimidated by the prospect of radiographing the chest of a crying, wiggling infant (37). The result is frequently a rotated, overexposed, expiratory film that cannot be interpreted. These technical difficulties are solved by properly immobilizing the patient so that the radiograph is obtained near the end of quiet inspiration. Chest radiographs of patients less than 4 years old may be obtained with a variety of immobilization techniques (Fig. 7-4). Use of a pacifier permits exposure during quiet inspiration, not crying. Supine films have the advantage of a more physiologic state, and the radiographs are easier to obtain. In infants, there is little difference in magnification between the supine AP and the erect AP or PA view. It is easier to obtain properly immobilized and exposed films in an uncooperative infant in the supine position (23,37). Cooperative older children (usually over 4 years of age) should have PA and lateral films taken in the erect position. They may be obtained either sitting or standing (Fig. 7-5).

Portable films are obtained in the AP supine (sometimes semierect) position. If needed, a lateral view may be obtained with either a vertical or a horizontal beam. AP supine views of the chest are usually adequate for examinations of neonates; lateral films are required in only a minority of cases (38).

The gonadal dose from a well-collimated chest radiograph is less than 1% of that from a radiograph of the pelvis. The maximum gonadal dosage for AP and lateral views of the chest is less than 10 mrad (39). The use of high-speed films and rare earth screens permits reduction in radiation dosage by at least a futher 75%. Parspeed-equivalent screens and films have usually been used for examinations of the newborn chest in order to decrease quantum mottle in the low kilovoltage that is required. Pediatric rare–earth film-screen systems that have higher speed with less quantum mottle are now being used (see Chapter 1). Even though strict coning to the chest is mandatory, additional protection is achieved by gonadal shielding. A sheet of lead is placed over the gonads for portable or other supine chest examinations of neonates and infants (see Fig. 7-4). A lead shield should be placed between the patient's gonads and the horizontal x-ray beam during erect chest radiography (see Fig. 7-5).

Supplementary Chest Radiography

Abnormalities identified by conventional chest radiographs may require additional plain films for clarification (4). *Oblique views* confirm and evaluate soft tissue, rib, hilar, carinal, and peripheral parenchymal abnormalities. *High-kilovoltage techniques* (130–150 kV) may be useful for mediastinal and airway evaluation. *Inspiration-expiration films* can be used to diagnose air trapping by a mass or foreign body.

The *lateral decubitus view* has classically been used to detect pleural fluid, demonstrate an air-fluid level in a cavity, or confirm and show the size of a pneumothorax. However, when a child is placed in the decubitus position, the dependent hemithorax is also splinted, and its motion restricted (40). This causes the dependent lung to be underaerated and the upper lung to be hyperaerated; it provides an expiration view of the down lung and an inspiration view of the up lung. Therefore, the lateral decubitus view may also be used to demonstrate air trapping in the dependent lung (40) or to clarify a questionable parenchymal opacity in the nondependent lung (41) (Fig. 7-6). One must remember that small amounts of pleural fluid (1.5–2.0 mm thick) may be demonstrated by the lateral decubitus position in normal children (42).

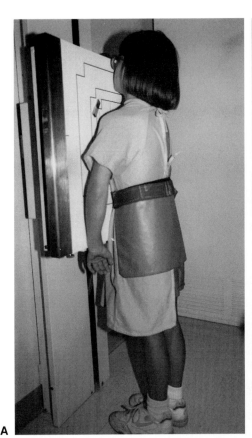
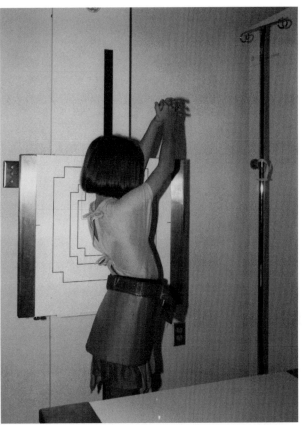

FIG. 7-5. Positioning for upright chest radiography. A: The cooperative older child should be radiographed in an upright PA projection with gonadal shielding in place. **B:** The lateral chest radiograph is taken with the arms elevated.

Fluoroscopy

Fluoroscopy is valuable for dynamic evaluation of pediatric chest abnormalities such as tracheomalacia. Fluoroscopy permits confirmation of a lesion suggested from conventional or supplementary chest radiography, and it allows rotation of the patient during fluoroscopic observation for more accurate localization of a finding. This is particularly important with chest wall lesions. The most informative view may be a fluoroscopic spot film or an overhead radiograph after fluoroscopic positioning. Finally, fluoroscopy permits dynamic observations of any abnormality, such as pulsations, movement with respiration, and movement with positional changes. Dynamic structures such as the heart, airway, and diaphragm can be evaluated. Air trapping and lack of diaphragmatic motion can be detected by fluoroscopy.

Esophagography

Barium studies of the pharynx and esophagus help to define anatomy and rule out vascular rings, extrinsic masses, laryngotracheal clefts, and tracheoesophageal fistulas. The esophagus is located in the posterior part of the middle mediastinum and may be compressed by thoracic masses or adjacent vascular structures. Because of its anatomic position, the barium-filled esophagus is the "road map" of the mediastinum and provides important information about location and extent of adjacent thoracic masses (43); MRI and CT have made this attribute of esophagography less important. Opacification of the esophagus helps to evaluate vascular rings, expiratory stridor (wheezing), and aspiration. Occasionally, the esophagus actually communicates with a bronchopulmonary foregut malformation. Esophagography also demonstrates abnormalities of the esophagus (hiatus hernia, abnormal motility, foreign body) mimicking primary pulmonary or airway disease.

Computed Tomography

CT is now critical in the evaluation of many pediatric chest diseases. Like any other imaging modality, CT must be assessed in terms of diagnostic benefit versus cost and risk to the patient. Chest CT may require sedation in infants and young children less than 5 years of age. There is a skin dose of approximately 2 rad for a CT examination of the chest.

CT demonstrates transaxial anatomy with clarity and in great detail. It frequently clarifies abnormalities that are con-

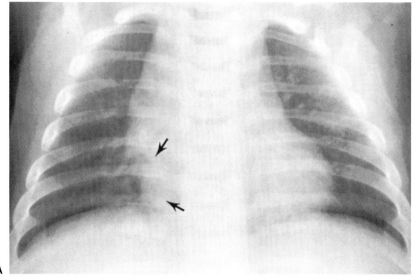

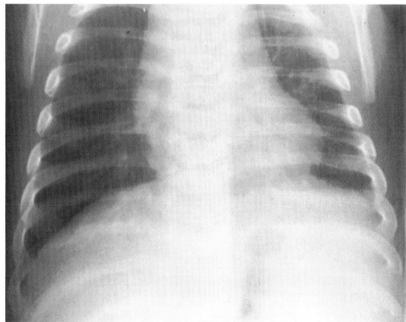

FIG. 7-6. Value of lateral decubitus view.
A: A 3-month-old boy with cough and fever. AP chest radiograph suggests an ill-defined medial right lung opacity *(arrows)* in the "fool's corner." **B:** Left lateral decubitus view hyperinflates the right lung and shows normal branching pulmonary vessels along the right heart border.

fusing or inapparent on conventional chest radiographs. It is able to distinguish density differences with approximately 100 times the sensitivity of conventional radiography. Moreover, the transverse display shows abnormalities of the chest free of overlying mediastinal, diaphragmatic, pulmonary vascular, and bony structures.

CT is ideal for chest wall or pleural lesions, as it shows these abnormalities in cross section. It can detect chest wall extensions of mediastinal masses such as lymphoma. CT accurately demonstrates the trachea and major bronchi, and extrinsic compression and intrinsic masses of the airway are readily diagnosed. CT, especially spiral and high-resolution CT, displays pulmonary parenchymal disease in great detail. It detects many pulmonary nodules that are not demonstrated by conventional chest radiography or chest tomography (44–47). Transverse CT sections demonstrate lesions of the

lung apex, posterior costophrenic sulci, retrosternal area, retrocardiac region, and subpleural areas to particular advantage. CT is the most sensitive and specific method for detecting pulmonary metastatic disease in children (45–48). This is particularly true of high-resolution, thin-section techniques (48,49).

High-resolution CT (HRCT) allows early detection of diffuse pulmonary parenchymal diseases down to the level of the secondary pulmonary lobule. HRCT can characterize opportunistic infections in immunocompromised patients and can direct invasive procedures. A useful technique for examining the lung for diffuse pulmonary disease includes HRCT slices (1.5- to 2-mm thickness) at 1-cm intervals from the lung apices through the bases. A high-resolution algorithm (bone algorithm) is used for edge enhancement. When possible, CT slices are obtained at end-inspiration to diminish vessel crowding and dependent lung edema. The HRCT reconstruction algorithm limits accurate assessment of mediastinal and upper liver lesions, however (48,49).

Although the advantages of conventional chest CT scanning are many, there are challenges unique to imaging the pediatric chest. Voluntary and involuntary (cardiac and respiratory) motion artifacts may degrade the images. The paucity of mediastinal fat in normal children can make it difficult to characterize the shape and extent of a mediastinal abnormality. Spiral CT and ultrafast (cine) CT are particularly suited to investigation of the major intrathoracic airways, cardiovascular structures, and mediastinum. Their advantages include quick scan times, reduced need for sedation, less radiation, and excellent opacification of vascular structures with low contrast volumes (48,50).

Magnetic Resonance Imaging

The multiplanar imaging capabilities of cardiac-gated MRI and magnetic resonance angiography (MRA) make them pivotal methods for investigating cardiac lesions, anomalies of the great vessels, the mediastinal vasculature, mediastinal masses such as bronchopulmonary foregut malformations, chest wall masses, bone marrow abnormalities, and tracheobronchial abnormalities. MRI is being increasingly used to evaluate posterior mediastinal masses. The capability of MRI to characterize tissue allows specific diagnosis of some mediastinal masses (33–36,51,52). Refinements in gating techniques and shortening of scan times will further enhance the role of MRI in evaluating the hila, lung parenchyma, heart, and diaphragm.

Ultrasonography

Ultrasonography is particularly appealing in pediatric diagnosis because it does not use ionizing radiation. Moreover, abnormalities can be evaluated in a number of planes, and without sedation. Unfortunately, air is highly reflective, so that the applications of chest ultrasonography are limited. Sonography is used to evaluate pleural fluid, other pleural lesions, juxtadiaphragmatic masses, neck masses (26), pericardial disease, eventration, diaphragmatic motion, and the thymus (Fig. 7-7) (53). Doppler ultrasound and color flow Doppler aid in the evaluation of vascular catheters, vascular anatomy, and patency of vessels.

Radionuclide Imaging

Nuclear medicine techniques help evaluate cardiac function, right-to-left shunts, pulmonary embolism, inflammatory diseases, neoplasms, and lung ventilation and perfusion.

Bronchography

High-resolution, thin-section CT has almost eliminated the need for bronchography in children (54,55). If per-

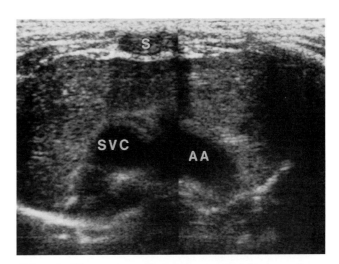

FIG. 7-7. Ultrasonography of the normal thymus. Composite transverse parasternal real time ultrasound image of a 15-month-old boy with a prominent cardiothymic contour on a chest x-ray shows a normal homogeneous thymus located anterior to the great vessels. The gland changed shape during the respiratory cycle. *SVC*, superior vena cava; *AA*, aortic arch; *S*, sternum.

formed, functional bronchography during both inspiration and expiration evaluates not only anatomic but also dynamic abnormalities of the trachea and bronchi (56).

Angiography

Angiography, an invasive procedure, is rarely used to evaluate respiratory disease in children. It can often be replaced by MRI. If performed, the smallest feasible catheter should be used (57). Angiography is essential in the assessment of aneurysms, pulmonary arteriovenous fistulas, sequestrations, and systemic arterial supply to normal lung (2,6,11,23,43).

ORDERED APPROACH

An ordered approach to radiologic examinations of both the upper airway (Table 7-1) and the chest (Table 7-2) is important. This ordered approach should include a systematic analysis of all anatomic regions of the upper airway and chest. One must understand normal anatomy in order to recognize and evaluate abnormalities.

Upper Airway

Anatomic divisions of the airway include the nasal passages, pharynx (nasopharynx, oropharynx, and hypopharynx), larynx, trachea, main bronchi, peripheral bronchi, and bronchioles. The nasopharynx is bounded anteriorly by the posterior nasal choanae and inferiorly by the soft palate. The adenoids often occupy much of this space. The oropharynx

TABLE 7-1. *Ordered approach to upper airway*

Technique
   Inspiration
   Neck extension—moderate
Bony structures
   Base of skull
   Maxilla
   Mandible—tooth buds
   Cervical spine
Soft tissues
   Pretracheal
   Retropharyngeal
Nasopharynx
   Hard palate
   Soft palate
   Uvula
   Adenoidal tissue
Oropharynx
   Tongue
   Uvula
   Palatine tonsils
Hypopharynx—supraglottic larynx
   Base of tongue
   Vallecula
   Epiglottis
   Aryepiglottic folds
   False cords
Glottis—paraglottic larynx
   Laryngeal ventricle
   True cords
   Piriform sinuses
Subglottic larynx
   Trachea
   Cervical esophagus

---

is bounded by the plane of the soft palate superiorly and the tip of the epiglottis inferiorly. The palatine tonsils and tongue are key oropharyngeal structures. The hypopharynx is bounded superiorly by the tip of the epiglottis and inferiorly by the level of the false cords. The larynx consists of three divisions: (a) the supraglottic larynx, including the epiglottis, aryepiglottic folds, and false vocal cords; (b) the glottic portion, extending from the laryngeal ventricle to the lower margin of the true cords; (c) the subglottic larynx, extending down to the lower edge of the cricoid cartilage (Fig. 7-8).

Although AP views of the upper airway are helpful, there is considerably more diagnostic information on lateral views. Normal structures identified on the lateral view include the nasopharynx, adenoids, hard palate, soft palate, uvula, oropharynx, tongue, mandible, base of tongue, vallecula, epiglottis, aryepiglottic folds, pyriform sinuses, laryngeal ventricle, true and false vocal cords, subglottic larynx, and upper trachea (see Table 7-1).

On the lateral film the epiglottis is "rose petal" in shape and "little finger" in size with a concave dorsal surface. The aryepiglottic folds are thin and delicate (Figs. 7-9 and 7-10). The inferior margins of the pyriform sinuses are at the level of the glottis (Fig. 7-9). Although the glottis normally narrows during phonation, narrowing below this level is usu-

ally pathologic (see Figs. 7-39 and 7-40). The aryepiglottic folds and arytenoid cartilages form the lateral and posterior margins of the opening of the glottis, with the epiglottis forming only the anterior margin of this opening (see Figs. 7-9 and 7-35).

There is tremendous variation in the size of normal tonsils and adenoids. The normal newborn has no adenoidal tissue. By 3 months of age, the adenoids are 1–5 mm thick (9,21,58). If adenoidal tissue is not visible by 6 months of age, immunodeficiency should be considered. To be significant, adenoidal enlargement must obliterate or nearly obliter-

TABLE 7-2. *Ordered approach to chest radiograph*

Technique
   Position
      Patient—rotation, lordosis
      Tube—angulation
   Degree of inspiration
   Penetration
   Motion
Systematic approach
   Extrathoracic
      Abdomen
         Liver
         Spleen
         Stomach
         Bowel gas
      Neck
         Soft tissues
         Spine
         Upper airway
   Thorax
      Shape
      Chest wall
         Soft tissues
            Skin
            Subcutaneous fat
            Muscle
         Bony thorax
            Ribs
            Clavicles
            Spine
         Pleura
      Mediastinum
         Airway
            Trachea
            Carina
            Bronchi
         Thymus
         Vessels
            Superior vena cava
            Aorta
         Cardiac
            Heart
            Main pulmonary artery
      Diaphragm
      Pleura
      Parenchyma
         Vessels
         Bronchi
         Lung

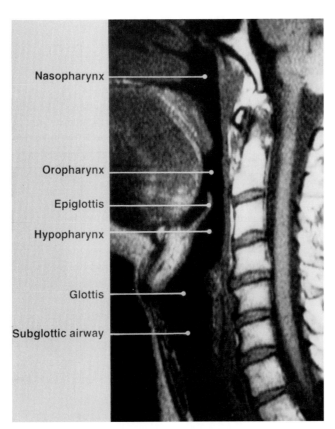

FIG. 7-8. Normal anatomy of the upper airway. T1-weighted sagittal MR image shows normal anatomy. Important structures are labeled.

ate the nasopharynx. Tonsillar enlargement produces a large soft-tissue mass in the oropharynx.

The normal airway buckles anteriorly during expiration, and this may mimic a retropharyngeal abscess (Fig. 7-11). This anterior buckling during expiration is further accentuated by flexion of the neck. For this reason, lateral films of the upper airway should be obtained during inspiration with

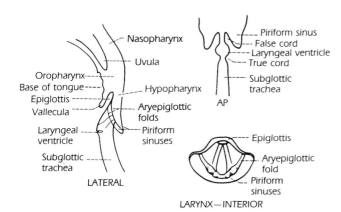

FIG. 7-9. Normal upper airway. Lateral, AP, and cross-sectional views of the upper airway. On the cross-sectional view of the larynx, note that the epiglottis forms only the anterior third of the laryngeal vestibule. From McCook and Kirks (96).

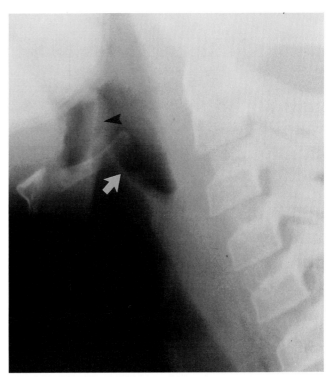

FIG. 7-10. Normal lateral airway. The aryepiglottic folds *(arrow)* are thin. The epiglottis *(arrowhead)* has a "rose petal" configuration with a dorsal concave surface.

the neck extended moderately (see Fig. 7-2B). The prevertebral soft-tissue thickness as seen on the lateral radiograph varies with neck position, degree of inspiration, and age. Rivero and Young reported the normal prevertebral soft-tissue thickness in 586 children (59). Ratios of soft tissue to the sagittal dimension of the vertebral body at C2/C3 were reviewed. Normal infants 1 year and younger had a ratio of 1:1. Children between 1 and 2 years had a ratio of 0.7, 2–4 years 0.6–0.55, and 6–10 years 0.5–0.4 (59). If there is any question about the presence of a retropharyngeal mass, lateral fluoroscopy with or without barium esophagography should be performed.

Chest

Chest radiography is usually performed to evaluate the pulmonary parenchyma. To avoid tunnel vision, all other components of the chest radiograph should be assessed first (Table 7-2). With this type of ordered approach, extrapulmonary abnormalities are less likely to be overlooked.

The chest radiograph should be evaluated first for technique (Table 7-2) (23). If the patient is *rotated*, the distance on the AP view from the center of the vertebral bodies to the medial ends of the clavicles and anterior ribs is not bilaterally symmetric (Fig. 7-12). *Tube angulation* producing a lordotic view of the chest is more common in the neonate than in older children. Such lordotic views are inadvertently obtained either by angling the tube toward the head or by cen-

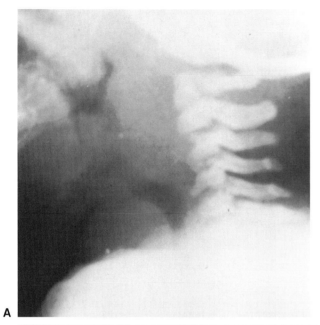

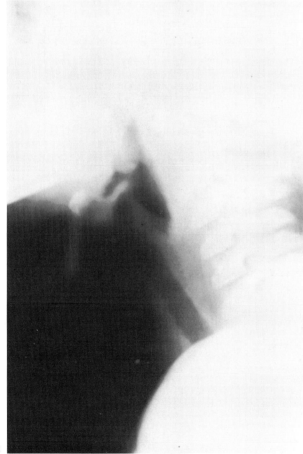

FIG. 7-11. Expiration film of the upper airway. A: A 1-year-old boy referred with the diagnosis of retropharyngeal abscess. The lateral film is taken in expiration with the neck flexed, which causes anterior bowing of the upper airway. **B:** Repeat film during inspiration with the neck extended. The upper airway is normal.

tering the x-ray tube over the upper abdomen so that the beam striking the chest is unduly divergent. The *degree of inspiration* is usually apparent by direct inspection (Fig. 7-13). If one prefers to quantify inspiration by counting ribs, anterior ribs rather than posterior ribs should be used in children, as the dome of the diaphragm is anterior. The diaphragm should be at the level of the sixth anterior rib in adequate inspiration. If the diaphragm is below the eighth rib anteriorly, hyperaeration is likely (Fig. 7-13C). Projection of the hemidiaphragm at or above the fourth anterior rib is seen in hypoaeration. The lateral chest x-ray is often key to the diagnosis of hyperaeration, which causes flattening or eversion of hemidiaphragms and a barrel-shaped thorax. If there is proper *penetration,* intervertebral disk spaces are visible through the heart, and pulmonary vessels are visible in the inner thirds of the lungs without high-intensity illumination. *Motion* is manifested by blurring of the diaphragmatic contours, vessel margins, and other structures.

Next, the abdomen and neck are carefully evaluated. The presence and position of any tubes or catheters are noted. The normal shape of the thorax in the newborn has been likened to a lamp shade; the ribs are horizontal and the thorax, as projected, is trapezoidal (60). As the child grows older, the thorax becomes longer and narrower; the shape assumes the adult rectangular configuration, its greatest length being vertical rather than horizontal (Fig. 7-14). The chest wall, mediastinum, diaphragm, and pleura are then sequentially analyzed (see Table 7-2). A careful survey of the spinal and paraspinal regions is crucial (Fig. 7-15). Finally, the trachea, main bronchi, segmental bronchi, heart, pulmonary vessels, and pulmonary parenchyma are assessed, and any abnormalities are noted.

GENERAL CONSIDERATIONS

Normal Developmental Anatomy of the Respiratory System

Knowledge of the embryologic development of the airway and lungs leads to more accurate recognition of congenital respiratory anomalies on various imaging modalities (61).

The newborn is an obligate nose breather. Obstructions at this level can therefore lead to life-threatening respiratory distress. The nasal cavities begin to develop at about the sixth week of fetal life, as the nasal pits deepen and penetrate the mesenchyme of the frontonasal prominence. The oronasal membrane transiently separates the primitive nasal cavity from the oropharyngeal cavity. Failure of this membrane to perforate leads to membranous or bony choanal obstruction.

Upper airway development is complex. The pharynx, larynx, trachea, bronchi, and alveoli develop from the embryologic foregut (61–64). Between the fourth and sixth fetal weeks, the cranial portion of the foregut changes from a flattened tube into a complicated series of arch-like structures. This branchial apparatus consists of a series of six

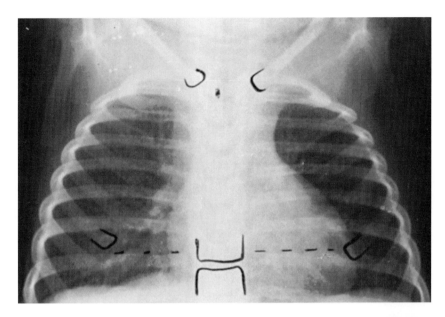

FIG. 7-12. Rotated chest radiograph.
Note the decrease in distance between the center of the vertebral bodies and the medial end of the right clavicle and the anterior right ribs. This is caused by right anterior oblique rotation of the patient.

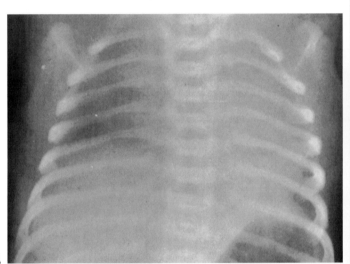

A

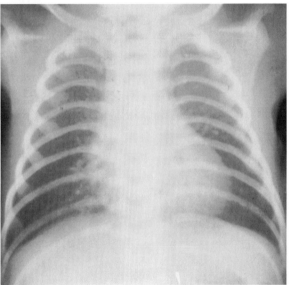

B

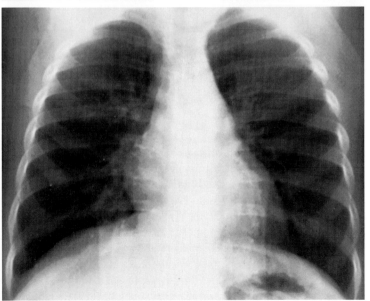

C

FIG. 7-13. Assessing degree of inspiration. A: Hypoaeration: the anterior end of the right fourth rib is at the level of the dome of the diaphragm. **B:** Normal aeration: the diaphragm is at the level of the right sixth anterior rib. **C:** Hyperaeration: hyperlucent lungs in a patient with viral airways disease. The dome of the diaphragm is at the level of the right eighth anterior rib.

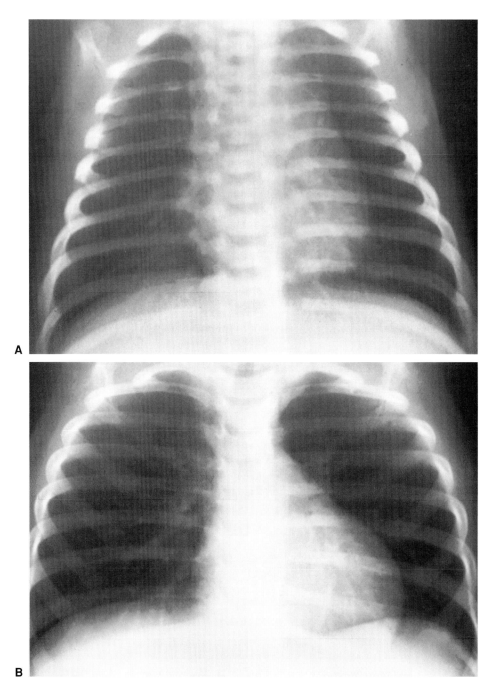

FIG. 7-14. Normal and abnormal shapes of the pediatric thorax. A: Normal newborn chest has a "lamp shade" or trapezoidal shape. **B:** Normal chest at 2 years of age. (*continued*)

mesodermal arches separated from each other externally by branchial clefts or grooves lined by ectoderm. Internally, the arches are separated by endodermally lined pharyngeal pouches. These arches undergo varied regressive and developmental changes. Mesenchyme from the first branchial arch contributes to the body of the tongue, maxilla, and mandible. The Pierre-Robin syndrome is a first-arch malformation characterized by mandibular hypoplasia, cleft palate, and ear and eye anomalies. The third arch contributes to the palatine tonsils and the upper pharyngeal constrictor muscles. The

fourth arch contributes to the lower pharyngeal constrictor musculature, and epiglottic and thyroid cartilage development. The second, third, and fourth arches all contribute to the tongue root. The thyroid gland begins as a cellular proliferation near the tongue root at a site that later becomes the foramen cecum. The larynx undergoes a process of vacuolization and recanalization with development of the laryngeal ventricle, false vocal cords, and true cords (61–63).

As early as the third week of gestation, the primordium of the larynx, trachea, and lungs develops from a ventral

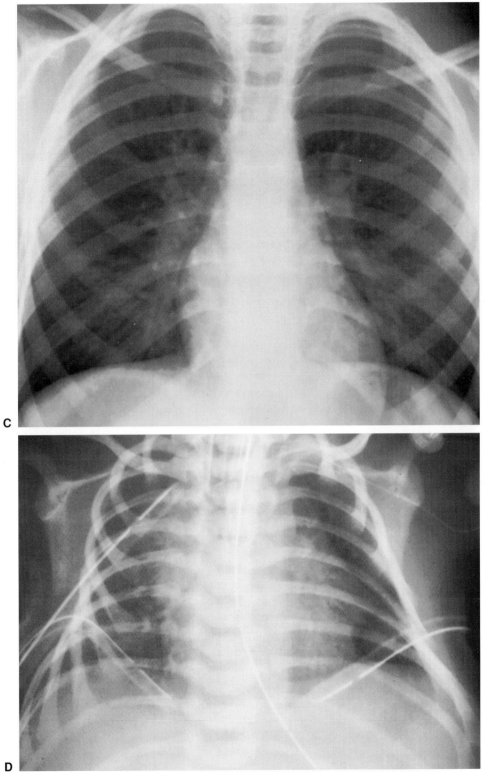

FIG. 7-14. *Continued.* **C:** By 6 years of age the normal pediatric chest is approaching the long, thin shape seen in adults. **D:** This neonate with pulmonary hypoplasia secondary to oligohydramnios has an abnormal, bell-shaped thorax.

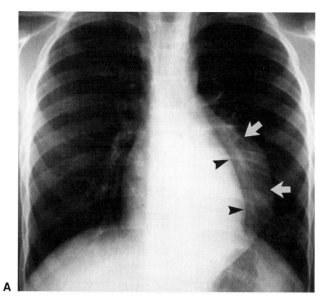

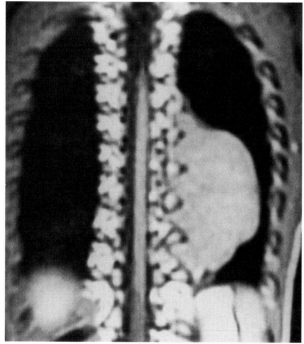

FIG. 7-15. Thoracic paraspinal ganglioneuroma. A: Chest radiograph of a 10-year-old boy with chest pain shows a smooth left paraspinous mass *(arrows)*. Note the normal left cardiac margin *(arrowheads)*. **B:** Coronal T1-weighted MR image shows the large paraspinal and foraminal extent of the tumor, but there is no extradural extension.

diverticulum of the foregut. The esophagotracheal ridges, proceeding from caudal to cranial, ultimately split the dorsal esophagus from the ventral trachea and lung buds. The term "lung bud" is used for the earliest primordium of the tracheobronchial tree. Communication between the respiratory primordium and the foregut is normally maintained only at the larynx. The right lung bud divides into three branches

(lobar bronchi) and the left bud into two (61–63). This is the basis for the development of the lungs into three right and two left lobes. The anomalies associated with this primitive respiratory system budding are referred to as bronchopulmonary foregut abnormalities. These probably include congenital lobar emphysema, bronchogenic cyst, duplication cyst, congenital cystic adenomatoid malformation, and pulmonary sequestration (61–63). With development, the lungs assume a more caudal position; the tracheal bifurcation reaches the level of T4 in the newborn. The development of tracheobronchial tree and the digestive tract explains how anomalies in one system can be related to anomalies in the other, e.g., tracheoesophageal fistula.

Further lung bud development leads to dichotomous bronchial divisions. By the end of the sixth fetal month, approximately 17 generations have been formed (61–63). An additional six divisions occur in postnatal life leading to the respiratory bronchioles. Terminal sacs (primitive alveoli) develop from the terminal bronchioles. During the last two months of prenatal life and for several postnatal years, the number of terminal sacs increases. Growth of the lungs after birth is due mainly to an increase in the number of respiratory bronchioles and alveoli. Approximately one sixth of the adult alveoli are present at birth. The remainder develop in the first decade of postnatal life. Alveolar epithelial cells (types I and II) line these sacs. The type II alveolar cells produce surfactant (61–63). During their development the lung buds penetrate the coelomic cavity and are invested in proliferating mesenchyme. From this mesenchyme the cartilage, muscle, and connective tissue of the lung are formed (65).

Normal development of the anterior chest wall is dependent upon the simultaneous closure of the cranial, caudal, and lateral embryonic folds. Anomalies in closure are reflected in a variety of congenital chest wall and abdominal wall deformities. Chest wall deformities include ectopia cordis, hypoplasia or aplasia of the chest wall, sternal abnormalities, and pectus excavatum and carinatum.

Pectus excavatum (funnel chest) is an inward depression of the sternum and costal cartilages. Although usually an isolated or sporadic anomaly, it may be part of syndromic or nonsyndromic disorders such as Turner syndrome, Marfan syndrome, osteogenesis imperfecta, and muscular dystrophy. Radiographically, the anterior ribs have a steep downward course, the right heart border is partially obscured, and the heart is both rotated and shifted leftward. The lateral radiograph shows sternal depression.

Pectus carinatum (pigeon breast) is abnormal protrusion of the lower sternum. Although often asymptomatic and sporadic, as many as 50% of these children have congenital heart disease, usually acyanotic. This developmental anomaly may also be seen in Noonan syndrome, Morquio syndrome, Marfan syndrome, and Eagle-Barrett (prune belly) syndrome.

The origin of the diaphragm is complex. There are contributions from the septum transversum, which forms the tendinous portion of the diaphragm, and the two pleuroperitoneal membranes, which aide in closure of the connections between the thoracic and abdominal parts of the coelomic cavity. The lateral and dorsal body walls contribute muscular components, and the crura of the diaphragm develop in the mesentery of the esophagus (6,62). A congenital diaphragmatic hernia results from failure of one or both of the pleuroperitoneal membranes to close the pleuroperitoneal canals.

Unique Features of the Pediatric Lung

The small airways of infants are highly susceptible to inflammatory narrowing. Although major bronchial generation is complete by the 16th fetal week, the peripheral airways in children remain relatively and absolutely smaller than in the adult. Conductance of the peripheral airways is at least five times that of the central airways in the adult, but is only equal to that of the central airways in the infant and young child (66,67).

Alveoli develop from terminal air sacs after birth. This saccular proliferation occurs rapidly during the first few years of life, less rapidly thereafter, and slowly after 8 years of age. The size of the lung acinus varies with age, increasing through adolescence. Studies of the human lung show that the acinus (Fig. 7-16) measures 1–2 mm in diameter at birth and then gradually increases to its adult size of 6–10 mm in diameter by adolescence (61,64,68). The lung of a term newborn contains about 20 million alveoli. The lung of the preterm infant has fewer primitive air spaces. By the time a child is 8 years old, there are approximately 300 million alveoli (1,69). Certain developmental anomalies, destructive pulmonary processes, infection, and extrathoracic conditions, such as oligohydramnios, can alter this normal tracheobronchial and alveolar development.

Collateral ventilation in the infant lung is less efficient than in the adult because of relatively underdeveloped pores of Kohn and channels of Lambert as well as thick connective tissue septa and small alveolar size (60,70–72). Near the end of the first decade, the pulmonary architecture is similar to that of an adult; the lungs continue to grow in size until adolescence.

Common Normal Variants

Upper Airway

Accurate interpretation of upper airway radiographs requires knowledge of certain pitfalls that can mimic disease. One of the most common pseudotumors encountered in airway radiography is prominence of the retropharyngeal soft tissues (see Fig. 7-11). An abundance of retropharyngeal tissues is normal in infancy. When technical factors for lat-

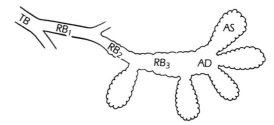

FIG. 7-16. Normal pulmonary acinus. The pulmonary acinus includes all structures distal to a terminal bronchiole. The acinus measures 1–2 mm at birth and grows to adult size of 6–10 mm by approximately 12 years of age (63,68). *AD*, alveolar duct; *AS*, alveolar sacs; *RB*, respiratory bronchiole; *TB*, terminal bronchiole.

eral airway radiography are not optimized, a retropharyngeal pseudotumor may be seen. Swallowing displaces air from the pharynx and can make retropharyngeal tissues look enlarged. Elevation of the hyoid bone and air in the cervical esophagus suggest this sort of swallowing artifact (Fig. 7-17). Neck flexion or a neutral neck position in a young infant can also lead to prominence of the retropharyngeal soft tissues. When the clinical picture suggests retropharyngeal disease and the preliminary radiographs are technically suboptimal or equivocal, fluoroscopy of the airway in the lateral position will soon show whether the retropharyngeal tissues are pathologic or not (23). A lateral barium esophagogram may be a useful supplementary study.

Subglottic membranes seen in bacterial tracheitis (membranous croup) or diphtheria can be mimicked by subglottic mucus. Having the patient cough deeply and repeating the lateral airway radiograph will usually distinguish mobile mucus from adherent inflammatory membranes.

Chest

Evaluation of the chest must always consider the possibility that a supposed abnormality is a normal variant or a pseudotumor. A pseudotumor is a nonneoplastic, nonsurgical mass that simulates a neoplasm (73). Pseudotumors include normal anatomic structures, normal variants, and nonneoplastic masses. Many of the common normal variants and pseudotumors of the thorax (Table 7-3) are individually discussed.

Expiration Chest

An expiration chest is a particularly common cause of confusion in infants and young children. If the findings are bilateral and ill defined, the possibility that the film was taken during limited inspiration (at low lung volumes) should always be considered. Such an expiration chest film may suggest pulmonary edema, bilateral pneumonia, cardiomegaly, and increased pulmonary blood flow (Fig. 7-18A).

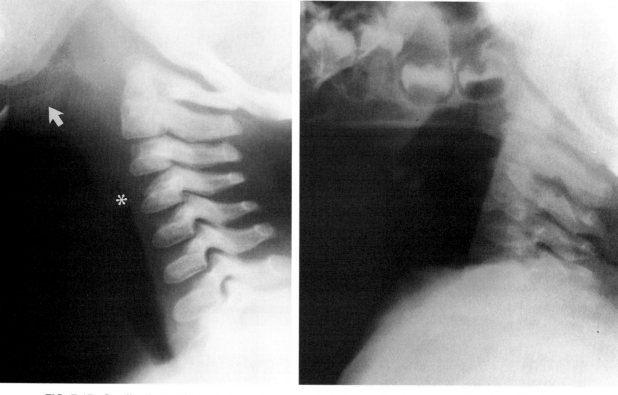

A

B

FIG. 7-17. Swallowing artifact. A: Lateral radiograph during swallowing shows elevation of the hyoid bone *(arrow)* and absence of air in the pharynx. Note air within the cervical esophagus *(*)*. **B:** Repeat radiograph moments later shows normal pharyngeal and precervical anatomy.

TABLE 7-3. *Common normal variants and pseudotumors*

Normal variants	Mediastinum
Expiration chest[a]	Thymus
Prominent thymus[a]	Normal[a]
Vertical fissure line	Thymomegaly
Artifacts	Hemorrhage
Breast tissue	Fat deposition: steroids
Hair braids	Benign adenopathy
Normal pleural fluid in the decubitus position	Immunodeficiency
Chest pseudotumors	Sarcoid
Chest wall	Spine lesion
Rib cartilage[a]	Vertebral osteomyelitis
Rib lesion	Extramedullary hematopoiesis
Fracture	Intrathoracic meningocele
Osteomyelitis	Vascular
Breast tissue	Aneurysm
Lung	Ductus
Pleura	Mycotic
Interlobar effusion	Coarctation or pseudocoarctation
Normal pleural fluid	Prominent normal pulmonary artery[a]
Parenchyma	Absent pulmonary valve
Mucous plug: mucoid impaction	Aberrant left pulmonary artery
Round pneumonia[a]	Aortic nipple
Inflammatory pseudotumor	Dilatation of vena cava (superior, inferior)
Atypical measles	Dilatation of azygos-hemiazygos veins
Atelectasis[a]	Arteriovenous fistula
Pulmonary vessels	Paravertebral
	Intercostal

[a] More common.

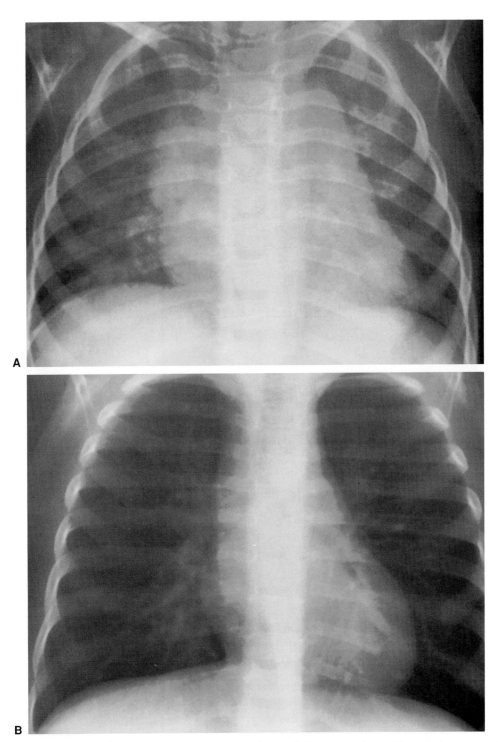

FIG. 7-18. Expiration chest. A: A 2-year-old boy with cough. The central opacities mimic pneumonia and pulmonary edema and the heart looks large. The film was taken during poor inspiration; the diaphragm is at the level of the fourth ribs anteriorly and the trachea is bowed to the right. **B:** Repeat film in inspiration is normal.

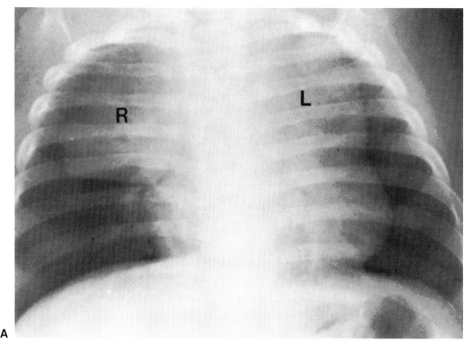

A

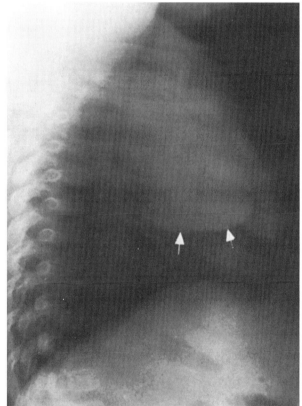

B

FIG. 7-19. Prominent normal thymus. A: Anteroposterior view of the chest in this 6-month-old boy referred for evaluation of mediastinal mass shows large right *(R)* and left *(L)* lobes of the thymus with wavy margins and "sail" configurations. **B:** Lateral view confirms the anterior location of this normal thymus. The sharp, linear inferior margin *(arrows)* is due to extension of the thymus along the minor fissure.

An expiratory film is suggested if both hemidiaphragms are well above the anterior aspects of the sixth ribs and the trachea is bowed away from the side of the aortic arch (74). The limited inspiration causes elevation of both hemidiaphragms and a decrease in vertical height of the thoracic cavity and produces prominence of the heart and central pulmonary vessels. A repeat film taken with an adequate degree of inspi-

ration (Fig. 7-18B) will confirm that these apparent abnormalities are due to expiration.

Normal Thymus

The thymus is usually visible on chest films of infants and young children and is sometimes seen as late as adoles-

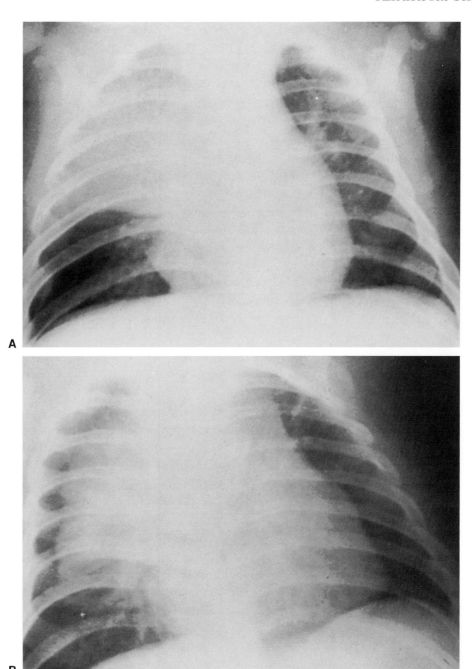

FIG. 7-20. Prominent right lobe of thymus. A: Anteroposterior view of the chest of this 3-month-old boy with cough and suspected right upper lobe pneumonia shows a prominent right upper thoracic opacity. The lack of air bronchograms indicates that the opacity is not in the lung. **B:** Left posterior oblique view confirms that the density is due to a prominent right lobe of the thymus. This view shows the wave sign laterally, indicating that the mass is anterior in location and is indented by the ribs.

cence. A large thymic lobe can mimic a mediastinal mass (Fig. 7-19) or an upper lobe pneumonia (Fig. 7-20). Occasionally, a large but normal thymus in a teenager or an aberrantly positioned thymus in a child cannot be radiographically distinguished from a mediastinal tumor. If the patient is asymptomatic, observation and cross-sectional imaging are recommended, rather than exploratory thoracotomy (52,73,75,76). Although rare, giant idiopathic thymomegaly can simulate a neoplasm and require surgical exploration for definitive diagnosis (77).

The thymus slowly increases in size during childhood and reaches its maximum weight at puberty. However, thymic volume compared to chest volume is greatest during late infancy. For this reason, the normal thymus is frequently

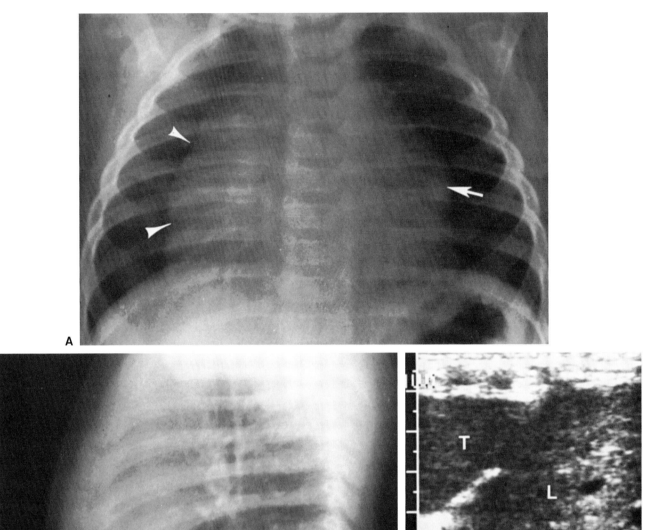

FIG. 7-21. Prominent normal thymus mimicking cardiomegaly. An 8-month-old girl with cough. **A:** Anteroposterior chest radiograph shows a prominent cardiothymic shadow with a "wavy" right margin *(arrowheads)*. A prominent left thymic "notch" is noted *(arrow)*. **B:** Lateral view demonstrates normal heart size. The heart does not extend behind a line drawn down from the trachea. **C:** Longitudinal right parasternal sonography shows a prominent right thymic *(T)* lobe extending inferiorly to abut the hemidiaphragm. *L,* liver.

prominent on chest radiographs between birth and 2 years of age. However, more than 5% of children 5 years of age or older have a recognizable thymus, prominent but normal, on conventional chest radiography. These children sometimes benefit from supplemental imaging (CT or MRI) to characterize their mediastinal "mass" (78,79).

On the AP chest radiograph, the thymus is a smooth, quadrilateral, soft-tissue density that projects from both sides of the superior mediastinum and typically extends from the level of the manubrium down to the fourth costochondral cartilages. Pulmonary vessels and bronchi can be seen through the homogeneous soft-tissue density of the thymus; this finding helps to differentiate the thymus from pneumonia and atelectasis. A lobular thymic contour (except for the wave sign) is abnormal at any age, and displacement of vascular structures or the tracheobronchial tree raises the suspicion of a pathologic mass (80). Other radiographic features of the normal thymus on the frontal view include a notch or cleft at its inferior edge, where it meets the silhouette of the heart, a sail-like extension from the mediastinum, and scalloping of the thymic margin ("wave sign") (Fig. 7-21) (52,78). Sonography can verify that a mediastinal mass is thymus (see Figs. 7-7, 7-21C). The wave sign is most apparent on oblique views and confirms that the structure in question is soft enough to be indented by the anterior costal cartilages and ribs. On lateral chest radiography, the thymus is a homogeneous soft-tissue density located in the anterior and superior mediastinum; a sharp, straight inferior margin is frequently noted on the lateral chest radiograph due to insinuation of thymic tissue along the minor fissure (see Fig. 7-19B). Limited inspiration, recumbency, lordotic positioning, and rotation exaggerate thymic size.

Vertical Fissure Line

The vertical fissure line is a normal variant that should not be confused with a pneumothorax. Initially described by Davis (81), it is sometimes due to reorientation of the plane of the major fissure (Fig. 7-22) (82). The vertical fissure line is seen in patients with cardiomegaly or lower respiratory tract infection and is occasionally seen in a completely normal child. This line in normal children is probably accentuated by a small (normal) amount of pleural fluid. On the AP projection, a vertical line is seen paralleling the lateral chest wall. This line represents the major fissure and extends a variable distance from the diaphragm cephalad (Fig. 7-22) (81,82). Vessels extend beyond this line, which distinguishes the vertical fissure line from a pneumothorax.

Normal Pleural Fluid in Decubitus Position

A small quantity of pleural fluid may be demonstrated in normal children in the decubitus position (42). The lateral decubitus view may be used for confirmation of pathologic quantities of pleural fluid (Fig. 7-23), demonstration of an

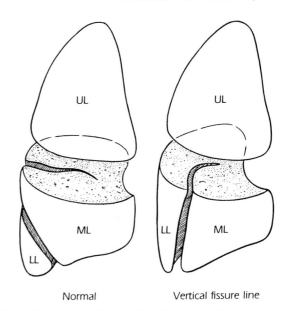

Normal   Vertical fissure line

FIG. 7-22. Vertical fissure line. Normal right lung and vertical fissure line. *LL,* lower lobe; *ML,* middle lobe; *UL,* upper lobe. Modified from Davis (81).

air-fluid level in a cavity, verification of pneumothorax, diagnosis of bronchial foreign body, or clarification of possible pulmonary opacity. When a child is placed in the decubitus position, the dependent lung is underaerated. Conversely, the upper lung on a lateral decubitus chest radiograph is hyperaerated. The decubitus position provides an expiration view of the down lung and an inspiration view of the up lung (40). It should again be stressed that small amounts of pleural fluid (1.5–2.0 mm thick) unassociated with parenchymal or pleural disease may be demonstrated by the lateral decubitus position in normal children (42). This normal pleural fluid is frequently bilateral.

Prominent Rib Cartilage

Not infrequently, a firm lump is noted anteriorly on the chest wall by the child, the child's parents, or an examining physician. This swelling or mass is located just lateral to the sternum. Oblique views of the ribs and sternum with a radiopaque marker over the area of clinical abnormality are normal. There is no bony destruction or discrete mass lesion. This palpable lump is due to focal cartilaginous hypertrophy at one of the costochondral junctions; it is of no clinical importance (73). Sonography can confirm that the mass is cartilage.

Round Pneumonia

Rather than a normal variant, round pneumonia is an unusual disease manifestation peculiar to childhood. Acute pneumonia in children may produce a spherical or rounded density on chest radiographs (Fig. 7-24). These well-circum-

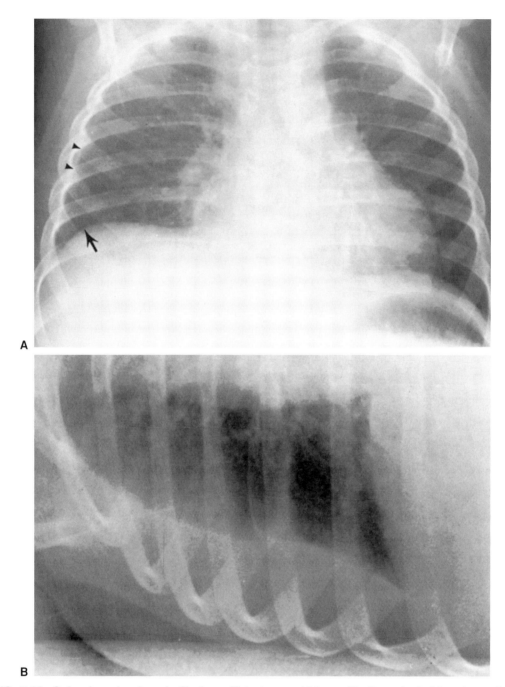

FIG. 7-23. Subpulmonic pleural effusion. This 1-year-old boy with disseminated lymphoma had been referred for right upper quadrant pain. **A:** Erect chest radiograph demonstrates an elevated right diaphragm with lateral position of its dome *(arrow)*. There is increased density of the right upper quadrant and an extraparenchymal soft-tissue stripe *(arrowheads)*. Right pleural fluid was suspected. **B:** Right lateral decubitus view confirms a large pleural effusion.

scribed areas of inflammation may mimic a primary or metastatic lung tumor and launch the unwary on a needless evaluation for neoplasm (67,73,83). The typical clinical presentation is that of a mild respiratory infectious prodrome followed by an acute febrile illness.

Initially, these round lesions are sharply defined. They lose definition and then clear rapidly with antibiotic therapy. Air bronchograms are identified in approximately 20% of round pneumonias. The opacities are almost always posterior and are usually in a lower lobe. This posterior location is

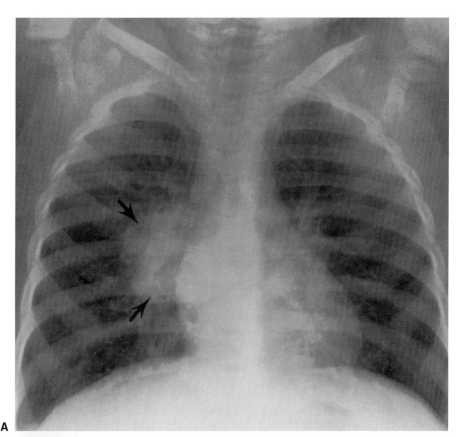

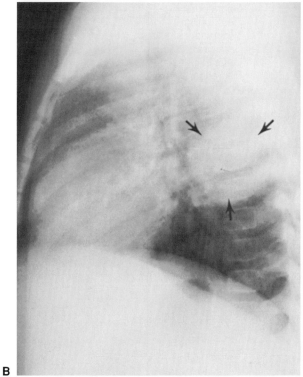

FIG. 7-24. Round pneumonia. This 14-month-old girl had a respiratory prodrome, cough, fever, and leukocytosis. Anteroposterior **(A)** and lateral **(B)** chest radiographs demonstrate a pseudotumor of the superior segment of the right lower lobe actually representing round pneumonia *(arrows)*.

possibly due to gravitational effect on bacteria-laden fluid in children, who usually sleep in the supine position (83).

Round pneumonias are almost always bacterial; most are pneumococcal in origin. After 8 years of age, round pneumonia is uncommon, perhaps because of the greater development of the pathways of collateral ventilation (pores of Kohn, channels of Lambert). A round pneumonia in the older child or adult suggests inadequate host response (immunodeficiency) or an atypical pathogen (e.g., fungus). Round pneumonias are not rare, and their recognition should prompt appropriate treatment rather than unnecessary diagnostic procedures (73,83). A ''round pneumonia'' in a posteromedial location with erosion of adjacent bony structures usually turns out to be a neuroblastoma, however.

Aortic Nipple

The aortic nipple is a common normal variant of the chest. It is due to the course of the supreme intercostal vein (84). A small rounded density is seen adjacent to the aortic knob (84).

SPECIFIC ABNORMALITIES

Upper Airway Obstruction

Patients with upper airway obstruction usually have inspiratory stridor. Diagnostic considerations include congenital disorders (choanal atresia, encephalocele, laryngomalacia), infectious disease (croup, epiglottitis), foreign body (airway, esophageal), and upper airway masses (Table 7-4) (21,58,85).

Choanal Atresia

Choanal atresia is a threat to life in the neonatal period. It is a congenital obstruction of the posterior nasopharynx that can be bony (90%) or membranous, bilateral (33%) or unilateral, complete or incomplete (86). Choanal atresia is the most common congenital anomaly of the nasal cavity (87). Unilateral choanal atresia is frequently asymptomatic and may remain undiagnosed until older childhood. Because the newborn is an obligate nasal breather, bilateral choanal atresia causes severe respiratory distress, especially during

TABLE 7-4. *Causes of upper airway obstruction*

Congenital causes	Trauma
Choanal atresia	Foreign body[a]
Micrognathia or macroglossia	Airway
Ectopic thyroid and thyroglossal duct cyst	Esophageal
Laryngomalacia[a]	Hematoma
Congenital laryngeal stenosis	Hemophilia
Congenital subglottic tracheal stenosis	Laceration
Nasal encephalocele	Secondary tracheal stenosis
Inflammatory causes	Caustic ingestion[a]
Enlarged tonsils and adenoids[a]	Radiation
Retropharyngeal abscess	Thermal injury
Infectious mononucleosis	Miscellaneous causes
Croup[a]	Vocal cord paralysis
Epiglottitis	Tracheomalacia[a]
Esophageal inflammatory disease	Vascular ring[a]
Stevens-Johnson syndrome	Hemophilia
Mass	Angioneurotic edema
Pharyngeal mass	Stevens-Johnson syndrome
Laryngeal cyst	Laryngeal web
Aryepiglottic cyst	Extrinsic compression
Retention cyst	Dilated esophagus after
Lymphangioma	repair of atresia
Cystic hygroma	
Epiglottic cyst	
Retention	
Lymphangioma	
Cystic hygroma	
Papilloma	
Hemangioma	
Fibroma	
Soft tissue sarcoma	
Rhabdomyosarcoma	
Dermoid-teratoma	

[a] More common.

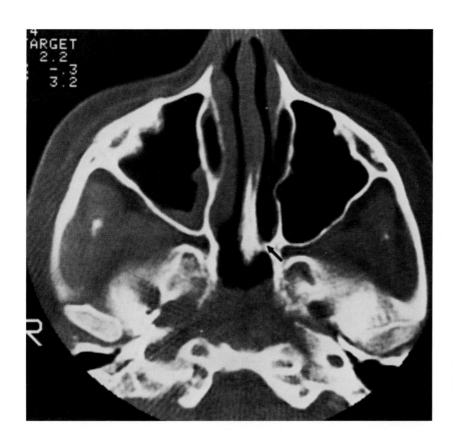

FIG. 7-25. Unilateral choanal atresia. A 7-year-old boy with nasal congestion. Axial CT section demonstrates obstructing bony plate *(arrow)*. *R*, right. (Courtesy of Janet L. Strife, M.D., Cincinnati, Ohio.)

feeding. Plain radiographs of the nasopharynx usually show no abnormality. The diagnosis is suspected clinically by failure to pass an enteric tube through one or both nostrils into the nasopharynx. Diagnosis is confirmed by CT (Fig. 7-25) (87). In bony atresia, which is more common, the lateral wall of the nasal cavity is thickened and medially bowed. The vomer is usually enlarged and fused with the bony wall of the nasal cavity (Fig. 7-25). In the membranous type, obstruction is at the level of the pterygoid plates. Congenital maxillary hypoplasia, nasal turbinate hyperplasia, and anterior nasal aperture (bony inlet) stenosis can also lead to nasal obstruction (21,88). Administration of topical decongestants and nasal suctioning prior to CT avoids the pitfall of thickened tissues in the nasal cavity and accumulated secretions that may mimic choanal atresia.

Nasal Encephalocele

Meningoceles and encephaloceles may involve the nasal cavity. Meninges alone (meningocele) or meninges and brain (encephalocele) herniate into the nasal cavity. This herniation occurs through a defect in the cribriform plate or through an open suture. The patient usually presents with nasal obstruction, rhinorrhea, or epistaxis. Radiographically, a soft-tissue mass in the nose or paranasal sinuses is seen in association with a bony defect (89). MRI is the examination of choice for determining the precise extent of the soft-tissue mass and nature of the bony defect prior to surgical treatment (Fig. 7-26).

Juvenile Nasal Angiofibroma

Juvenile nasal angiofibroma is a highly vascular, benign tumor of the posterior nasal cavity. It typically originates in the nasopharynx and pterygopalatine fossa. Although histologically benign, it can be locally invasive. Symptoms are caused by tumor extension into the nose, orbit, or skull base (90). The tumor occurs almost exclusively in adolescent boys, who typically develop epistaxis and nasal obstruction. Lateral radiographs show a soft-tissue mass in the nasal cavity and pterygopalatine fossa causing anterior bowing of the posterior wall of the maxillary sinus (antral sign) (Fig. 7-27). In addition to the clinical exam and sinus radiographs, MRI is the best imaging test to define extent of disease; at least 5% have orbital or intracranial extension (Fig. 7-28). MRI can also differentiate fluid within an obstructed sinus from actual tumor extension. Although not necessary for diagnosis, preoperative angiography with embolization will improve surgical outcome (91).

Other nasal cavity and nasopharyngeal masses include antrochoanal polyp, teratoma, osteoma, hemangioma, lymphoepithelioma, rhabdomyosarcoma, nasopharyngeal carcinoma, and lymphoma. Pterygoid bone destruction on the lateral airway film indicates an aggressive process.

Macroglossia

Tongue enlargement may cause upper airway obstruction. Hypothyroidism, Down syndrome, Pompe disease, and

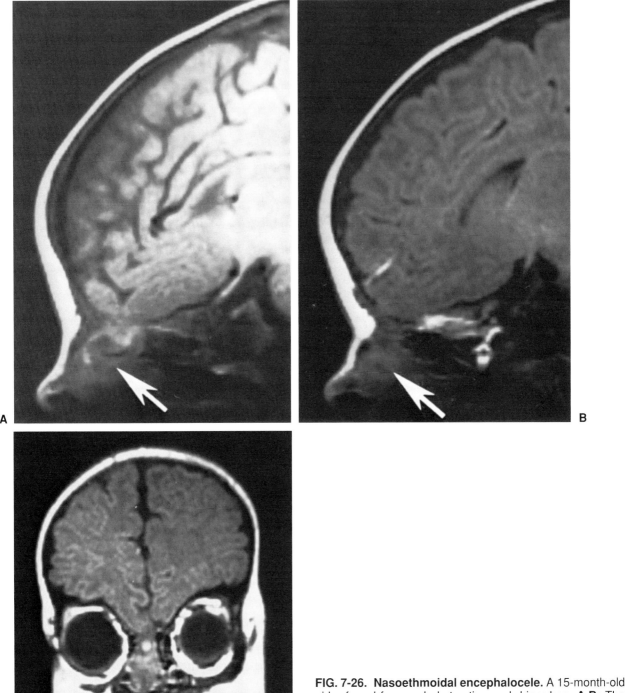

FIG. 7-26. Nasoethmoidal encephalocele. A 15-month-old girl referred for nasal obstruction and rhinorrhea. **A,B:** The parasagittal MR T1 images show a soft-tissue mass isointense to brain in the anterior right ethmoid sinus and nasal cavity *(arrows)*. The mass is contiguous with the inferior medial right frontal lobe through a defect in the cribriform plate. **C:** The coronal T1 image confirms contiguity of the nasoethmoidal encephalocele with the frontal lobe and precisely demonstrates the extent of the mass. (Courtesy of William S. Ball, Jr., M.D., Cincinnati, Ohio.)

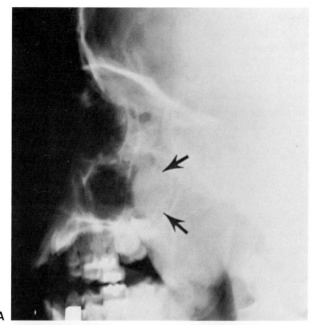

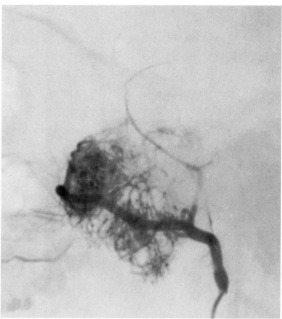

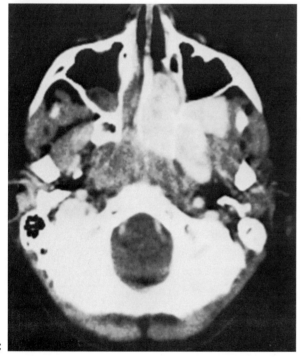

FIG. 7-27. Juvenile nasal angiofibroma. A 14-year-old boy with epistaxis and nasal obstruction. **A:** Lateral view of the paranasal sinuses shows an ovoid soft-tissue mass arising in and expanding the pterygopalatine fossa *(arrows)*. **B:** Lateral arteriogram from a selective maxillary artery injection shows a densely staining hypervascular mass. **C:** Contrast-enhanced axial CT at the level of the skull base demonstrates a vascular mass that extends into the nasal cavity and infratemporal fossa. (Courtesy of Janet L. Strife, M.D., Cincinnati, Ohio.)

Beckwith-Wiedemann syndrome (Fig. 7-29) may be associated with macroglossia. Conditions causing micrognathia (Pierre Robin syndrome and cerebrocostomandibular syndrome) have relative macroglossia because of micrognathia and a small oral cavity.

Tongue Lesions

Focal lesions of the tongue can lead to oral and oropharyngeal airway obstruction. Base of tongue lesions include enlargement of lingual tonsils, lingual thyroid, dermoid, ranula, and thyroglossal duct cyst (25% are suprahyoid) (92). Lingual tonsils and a lingual thyroid rarely cause airway obstruction. Other focal tongue masses include hemangioma, lymphangioma, rhabdomyosarcoma, and fibrous lesions.

Tonsillar Enlargement

Adenoids are normal collections of lymphoid tissue located in the posterior nasopharynx. Palatine tonsils are similar normal lymphoid aggregates in the oropharynx. Enlargement of these lymphoid collections represents the most

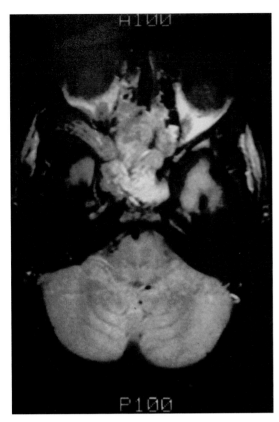

FIG. 7-28. Juvenile nasal angiofibroma. Axial proton density MR image in a 14-year-old boy with nasal congestion and epistaxis shows a lobulated nasopharyngeal mass with sphenoid, ethmoid, and right pterygopalatine fossa extension. (Courtesy of Brian Wiatrak, M.D., Birmingham, Alabama.)

common cause of sleep-associated upper airway obstruction in children. Certain patients (e.g., Down syndrome) are particularly susceptible to this complication. Chronic upper airway obstruction due to tonsillar enlargement may lead to chronic hypoxemia, hypercapnia, respiratory acidosis, pulmonary hypertension, and, eventually, cor pulmonale. The lateral radiograph with mouth closed during deep inspiration optimizes visualization of the adenoids and nasopharynx. Large tonsils and adenoids can occur in healthy asymptomatic children; a radiograph for tonsillar enlargement rarely provides information that is not already clinically apparent (Fig. 7-30). However, radiography will sometimes prevent tonsillectomy in a child whose adenoids are normal in size or only slightly enlarged. After 3 months of life, the adenoids become progressively more prominent. It is not unusual to see adenoid tissue greater than 2 cm in thickness in a normal older child. Absence of adenoidal tissue after 3–6 months of age warrants evaluation for immune deficiency. Radiographic clues to an adenoidal tumor rather than mere physiologic enlargement include mass effect on the uvula and pterygoid plate erosion or destruction.

Adenoidal and tonsillar enlargement can occur with acute infection. Infectious mononucleosis, typically caused by Epstein-Barr virus (less often by cytomegalovirus), may be associated with marked tonsillar and adenoidal enlargement (93). This disease is rare in children under 3 years of age. The mean age of infectious mononucleosis is 14 years; this is older than patients with physiologic lymphoid tissue enlargement. Malaise, sore throat, splenomegaly, liver dysfunction, and atypical lymphocytes are usually also present in patients with infectious mononucleosis (93).

Lingual Thyroid Tissue

A mass at the base of the tongue may be lingual thyroid tissue, a thyroglossal duct cyst, or a neoplasm of the tongue such as a hemangioma (Table 7-5). The possibility that such a mass represents ectopic thyroid tissue necessitates thyroid imaging prior to surgical intervention (Fig. 7-31) (94). If the thyroid gland is in normal position, a mass at the base of the tongue may be surgically excised or, if cystic, marsupialized (95).

Hypopharyngeal Cysts

Tumors that involve the epiglottis and aryepiglottic folds are infrequent and are usually benign. These masses may be

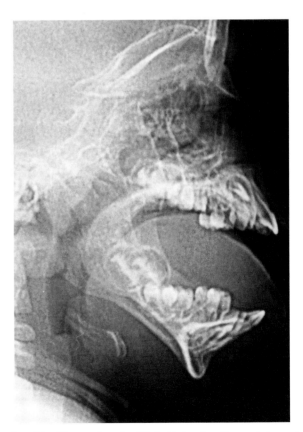

FIG. 7-29. Macroglossia. Digital lateral radiograph in an infant with Beckwith-Wiedemann syndrome shows marked enlargement of the tongue. (Courtesy of Sam T. Auringer, M.D., Winston Salem, N.C.)

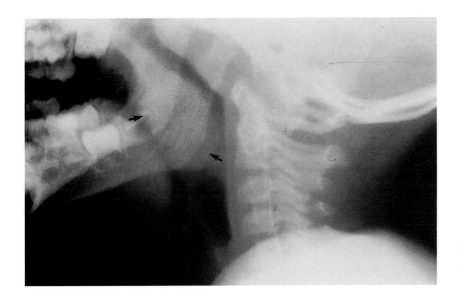

FIG. 7-30. Tonsillar enlargement. Lateral soft-tissue neck radiograph in a 5-year-old boy with sleep-associated, upper airway obstruction shows marked enlargement of the palatine tonsils *(arrows).*

retention cysts or lymphatic tumors such as lymphangioma or cystic hygroma. The histology may be nonspecific. Signs and symptoms are usually those of inspiratory stridor or choking during feeding. Lateral films of the upper airway show a soft-tissue mass that involves the epiglottis or aryepiglottic folds (Fig. 7-32). It may be impossible to determine if the mass arises from the epiglottis itself or if the epiglottis is secondarily involved by extension of a mass of the aryepiglottic folds (96).

Laryngomalacia

Laryngomalacia is the most common cause of inspiratory stridor in the first year of life. The cause is a lax epiglottis

TABLE 7-5. *Upper airway masses*

Nasal cavity and nasopharynx	Dermoid, teratoma
Polyp[a]	Fibrous tumor
Teratoma	Duplication
Nasal glioma	Rhabdomyosarcoma
Encephalocele	Thyroid
Angiofibroma	Lingual thyroid
Papilloma	Thyroglossal duct cyst
Histiocytoma	Hypopharynx and larynx
Neurofibroma	Epiglottic cyst
Hemangioma	Aryepiglottic cyst
Carcinoma	Papillomas[a]
Rhabdomyosarcoma[a]	Laryngeal cyst
Lymphoma[a]	Trachea
Neuroblastoma[a]	Hemangioma[a]
Chordoma	Chordoma
Esthesioneuroblastoma	Papillomas[a]
Oral cavity and oropharynx	Histiocytosis
Tongue	Neurofibroma
Hemangioma[a]	Carcinoma
Lymphangioma	Rhabdomyosarcoma
Cretinism	Cylindroma
Beckwith-Wiedemann syndrome	Adenoma
Glycogen storage disease	Fibroma
Mucopolysaccharidosis	Hamartoma
Neurofibromatosis	Lymphoma
Myotonia congenita	

[a] More common.

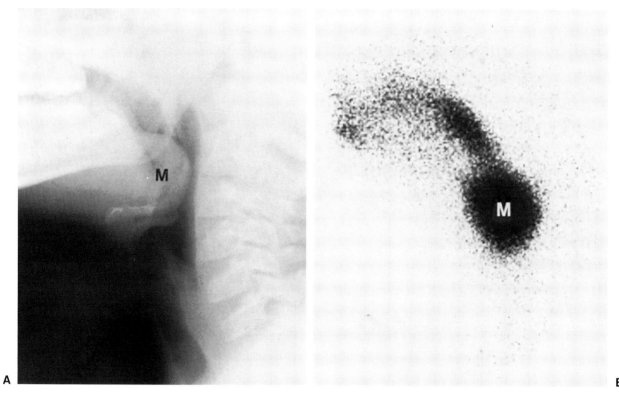

FIG. 7-31. Lingual thyroid. A 5-year-old girl with mild respiratory difficulty. **A:** Lateral radiograph of the upper airway shows a large mass *(M)* of the tongue base. **B:** Thyroid scintigraphy confirms that this mass *(M)* is ectopic thyroid tissue. There is no thyroid tissue present in the neck.

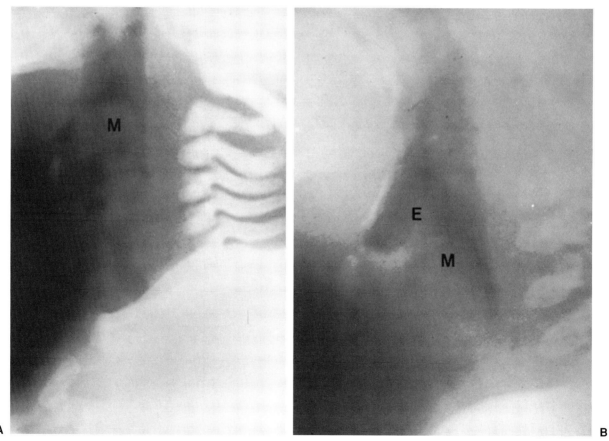

FIG. 7-32. Supraglottic tumors. A: Aryepiglottic cyst. A large mass *(M)* arises from the aryepiglottic fold and involves the epiglottis. **B:** Aryepiglottic cyst. Lobular mass *(M)* involves the aryepiglottic fold. There is also epiglottic enlargement *(E). (continued)*

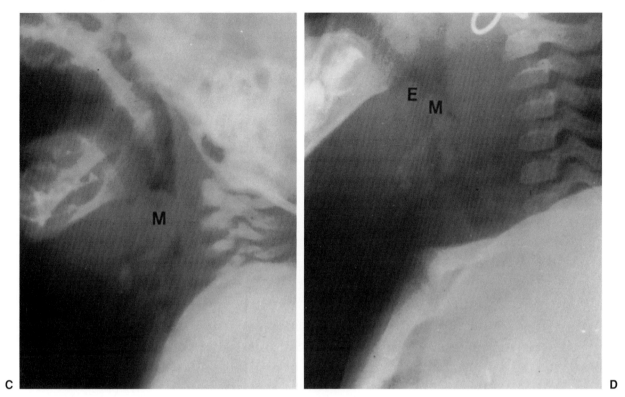

C   D

FIG. 7-32. *Continued.* **C:** Epiglottic cyst. A large mass *(M)* involves the region of the epiglottis and aryepiglottic folds. **D:** Epiglottic lymphangioma. A lobular mass *(M)* arises from the region of the base of the epiglottis *(E)* and aryepiglottic folds. From McCook and Kirks (96).

and redundant aryepiglottic folds that are drawn into the glottic region during inspiration creating airway obstruction (97). The larynx of an infant is relatively flaccid. The stridor lessens with crying or excitement. In 90% of patients with laryngomalacia, symptoms resolve by age 2. During the fluoroscopic evaluation of the symptomatic patient there is ante-

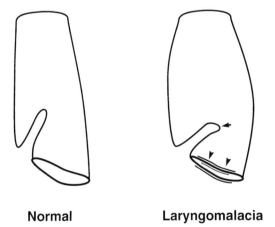

Normal   **Laryngomalacia**

FIG. 7-33. Laryngomalacia. Line diagrams of normal lateral supraglottic anatomy and characteristic features of laryngomalacia: horizontal orientation of the epiglottis *(arrow)*, redundancy in aryepiglottic folds *(arrowheads)*, and inspiratory ballooning of the oropharynx.

rior buckling of the aryepiglottic folds, horizontal orientation of the epiglottis, and ballooning of the pyriform recesses (Fig. 7-33). The stridor is loudest during quiet breathing and disappears with crying. In many clinical practices, fiberoptic endoscopy has supplanted fluoroscopy for confirmation of this diagnosis.

Epiglottitis

Epiglottitis, now largely preventable by immunization, is less common but much more dangerous than croup. It usually affects older children than croup; the peak incidence is at about 3-1/2 years of age (58,98). There is an abrupt onset of inspiratory stridor, fever, restlessness, and severe dysphagia. The usual pathogen is *Hemophilus influenzae*. Cases of epiglottitis have also been caused by group A *Streptococcus*, usually in older (mean age 6 years) children. A patient with acute epiglottitis is in mortal danger. No physical or radiologic examination that makes it more difficult for the patient to breathe should be performed. The minimum that is necessary to establish the diagnosis is done. If an enlarged epiglottis is not identified by careful physical examination, a single lateral radiograph of the neck, with the patient erect in a position of comfort, will confirm the diagnosis. The clinician must accompany the patient to the radiology department, and equipment for endotracheal intubation or tracheostomy must be immediately available. The diagnosis is often estab-

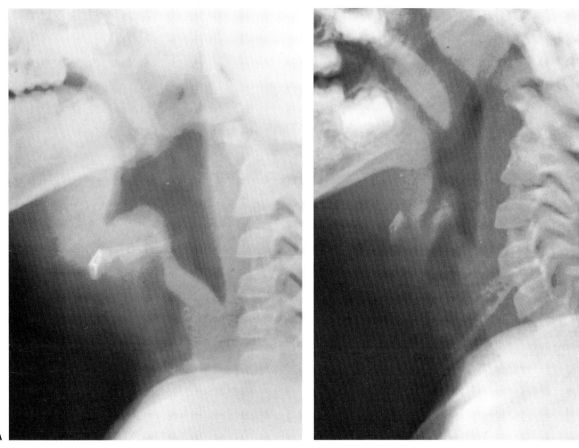

A

B

FIG. 7-34. Epiglottitis. A 2-year-old girl with inspiratory stridor. **A:** Epiglottic enlargement and marked thickening of aryepiglottic folds. **B:** Normal upper airway after 2 weeks of antibiotic therapy.

lished by physical examination or endoscopy; this makes a radiograph superfluous.

The lateral radiograph shows marked enlargement of the epiglottis and thickening of the aryepiglottic folds (Fig. 7-34) (98). Although the epiglottis is enlarged, the airway obstruction is mostly due to marked thickening of the aryepiglottic folds (Fig. 7-35) (99). For this reason, some have advocated the term *supraglottitis* rather than *epiglottitis*. However, at least 25% of children with proved acute bacterial epiglottitis also have subglottic edema (Fig. 7-36); the appearance on an AP radiograph is indistinguishable from that seen with croup (85,96,100). Occasionally, hypoaeration of the lungs is the clue to upper airway obstruction (Fig. 7-36A) (101).

Although bacterial infection is the most common cause, other entities may cause radiographic enlargement of the epiglottis. These include omega-shaped epiglottis, prominent normal epiglottis, hemophilia with local bleeding, angioneurotic edema, chronic epiglottitis, Stevens-Johnson syndrome, aryepiglottic cyst, epiglottic cyst, foreign body, trauma, caustic or chemical ingestion, leukemia, and thermal and irradiative injury (96); these are all rare. Acute epiglottic swelling has also been described with brown recluse spider bites, bee stings, and poisoning (96,97).

Papilloma and Papillomatosis

Papillomas are the most common tumors of the larynx in children. These lesions are usually small and asymptomatic. The site of involvement is usually the anterior larynx, often the anterior one third of the vocal cords.

Chronic laryngeal papillomatosis is an uncommon condition in the preadolescent child (95). There is progressive hoarseness, and typical papillomas will be shown at laryngoscopy. Occasionally, radiologic examination shows enlargement and deformity of the vocal cords by irregular nodular masses (Fig. 7-37). The pharynx and esophagus are occasionally involved. Laryngeal papillomatosis is probably due to viral infection. Human papilloma virus is implicated. As many as 50% of cases have a maternal history of *condyloma accuminatum.*

Transbronchial spread of laryngeal papillomas (papillomatosis) is rare (102). This unusual complication (less than 5% of all cases) occurs in patients with large masses requiring repeated surgical procedures (95). It is thought that there is spread of the causative agent down the tracheobronchial tree during surgery and development of pulmonary nodules that then cavitate (Fig. 7-38) (102). The posterior location of these lesions supports the concept of transbronchial spread

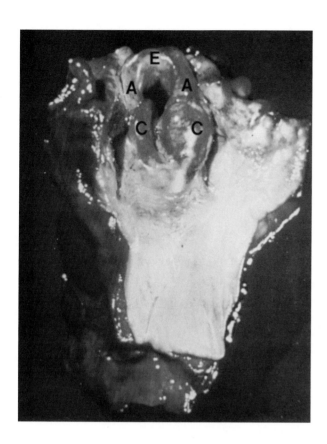

FIG. 7-35. Gross specimen of acute epiglottitis. The esophagus is opened and the upper airway is viewed from behind. There is mild enlargement of the epiglottis *(E)*. Note the marked thickening of the aryepiglottic folds *(A)* and in the arytenoid cartilage region *(C)*. The epiglottis forms only the anterior third of the laryngeal vestibule. The critical airway obstruction is due largely to thickening of the aryepiglottic folds and arytenoid regions.

with aspiration while the patient is supine. Severe morbidity and even mortality due to hemorrhage, lung destruction, and restrictive lung disease sometimes develop (102).

Other rare tumors of the larynx include chondroma, hamartoma, granular cell myoblastoma, fibroma, and neurofibroma.

Vocal Cord Paralysis

Paralysis of the vocal cords can produce signs and symptoms of upper airway obstruction. Bilateral vocal cord paralysis is life threatening. A weak or absent voice and inspiratory stridor are observed. Paralysis of the vocal cords may be secondary to Chiari II or III malformations, severe neonatal hydrocephalus, intracranial hemorrhage, birth asphyxia, postviral neuropathy, central nervous system (CNS) tumor, or trauma to the recurrent laryngeal nerve. Normally, the true vocal cords move symmetrically toward midline during phonation and retract laterally during rest and respiration. Paralyzed cords fail to retract. Fluoroscopy and high-resolution ultrasonography can confirm the vocal cord paralysis. In most cases, endoscopy has supplanted fluoroscopy for diagnosis.

Croup

Croup is the most common cause of acute obstructive airway disease in infants and young children (21,58). This infection is the most common cause of stridor in childhood (85). Most cases are viral (parainfluenza type 1, influenza A). Although the entire airway is inflamed (the term "laryngotracheobronchitis" may be used), the critical narrowing is located just 1 cm below the vocal cords, at the "conus elasticus." There is loose attachment of the mucosa at this level, so edema readily elevates it and narrows the airway. This subglottic tracheal narrowing is accentuated by the lack of compliance of the cricoid cartilage and the fact that it is a complete ring. Croup is a disease of infants and young children, the peak incidence being between 6 months and 3 years (mean age of 12 months) (95,98). The child presents with a mild barky cough and intermittent inspiratory stridor. Frequently, there is a history of antecedent or simultaneous lower respiratory tract infection.

Anteroposterior radiographs show loss of the normal lateral convexities ("shoulders") of the subglottic trachea. There is narrowing of the subglottic lumen to produce an inverted V or "church steeple" (Fig. 7-39). This subglottic narrowing extends well below a line drawn through the lower margins of the pyriform sinuses. Lateral radiographs demonstrate hypopharyngeal overdistention during inspiration, normality of the epiglottis and aryepiglottic folds, loss of definition of the laryngotracheal lumen just below the vocal cords, and narrowing of the subglottic part of the larynx and trachea. This subglottic narrowing is somewhat variable (Fig. 7-40). The change in caliber between normal trachea below and narrowed airway above is accentuated in expiration (Fig. 7-40B) (103). The hypopharyngeal overdistention

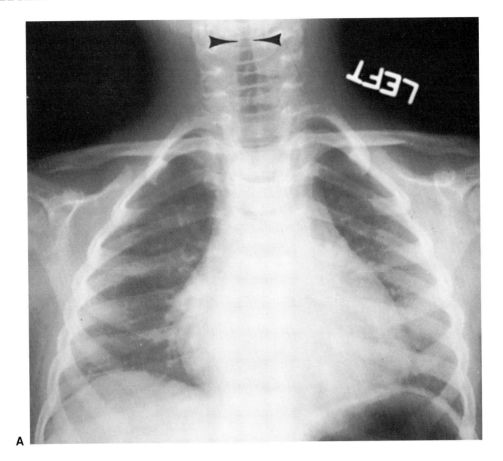

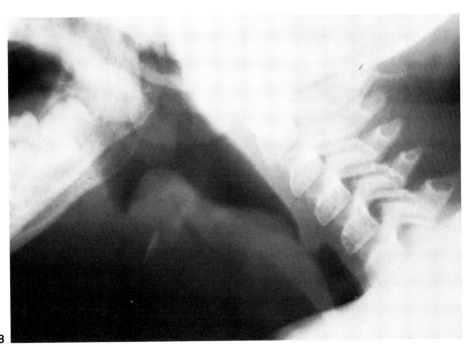

FIG. 7-36. Hypoaeration of lungs secondary to epiglottitis. A: Chest radiograph of a 2-year-old boy with fever, restlessness, and air hunger shows hypoaeration of lungs. Symmetric subglottic airway narrowing is noted *(arrowheads)*. **B:** Lateral view of the upper airway demonstrates the typical findings of epiglottitis.

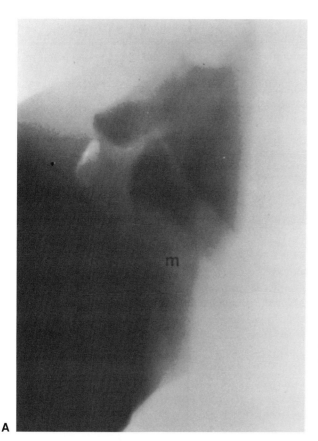

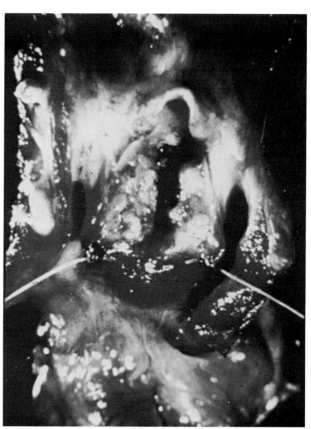

A

B

FIG. 7-37. Laryngeal papillomatosis. A 2-year-old boy with inspiratory stridor, cough, and hoarseness. **A:** Lobular soft-tissue mass *(m)* in the larynx. **B:** Gross appearance of laryngeal papillomatosis. Suture material is seen in the dorsal margins of the vocal cords. There are many soft-tissue excrescences arising from the entire length of both vocal cords.

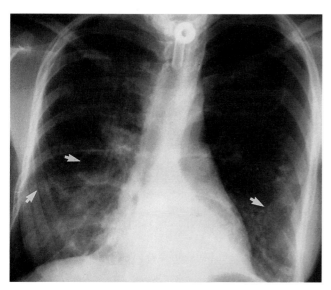

FIG. 7-38. Transbronchial spread of laryngeal papillomas. An 18-year-old girl with history of chronic laryngeal papillomatosis. Note the numerous cavitary lung lesions *(arrows)* due to transbronchial spread.

is a physiologic response and acts to diminish upper airway resistance (104).

The child suspected of having croup should have AP and lateral views of the upper airway as well as frontal and lateral views of the chest. If these findings are equivocal or normal, a complete radiologic evaluation for stridor, including fluoroscopy and esophagography, should be considered (21,24,25,58). Although the features of croup are characteristic, the real purpose of the radiologic examination is not to diagnose croup but to exclude other causes of inspiratory stridor that mimic croup such as congenital or acquired subglottic stenosis, subglottic hemangioma, airway foreign body, esophageal foreign body, and epiglottitis. As a rule, croup lasts only a few days; persistence of symptoms lasting more than 7 days warrants further evaluation.

Membranous Croup

Several bacteria cause this uncommon bacterial inflammation of the larynx, trachea, and bronchi. *Staphylococcus aureus* is the most common organism. Membranous croup probably represents a primary bacterial infection rather than a bacterial infection superimposed on severe viral croup.

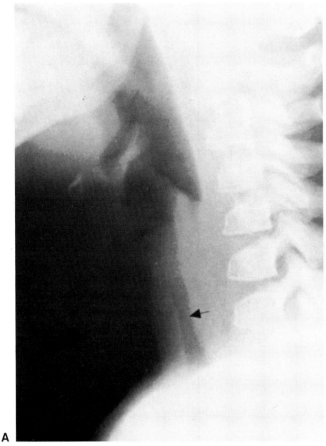

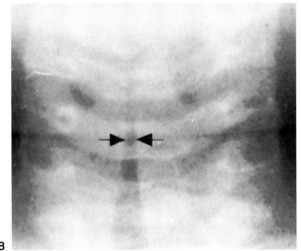

FIG. 7-39. Croup. A 2-year-old girl with inspiratory stridor. **A:** Lateral view of the upper airway shows pharyngeal disten-tion and subglottic tracheal narrowing *(arrow).* **B:** Anteropos-terior view of the upper airway shows subglottic narrowing well below the level of the pyriform sinuses, producing a "church steeple" or inverted "V" appearance *(arrows).*

Generally, patients with membranous croup are older than children with viral croup; they have more severe respiratory symptoms and are more systemically affected. In addition to the usual radiographic signs of croup, there is irregularity

of the tracheal walls due to membranes in the subglottic airway (Fig. 7-41) (105). Nonadherent mucus can mimic membranous croup, but mucous debris should clear or shift with coughing (73,105). Pneumomediastinum may occa-sionally be an associated abnormality. The differential diag-nosis includes subglottic tracheal foreign body and diph-theria; fortunately, the latter is readily prevented by immuni-zation.

Subglottic Hemangioma

Hemangioma of the trachea is the most common subglot-tic soft-tissue mass causing upper respiratory tract obstruc-tion in infants and young children (21,95,106). The hemangi-omas usually occur along the lateral or posterior wall of the subglottic trachea. The patient with a subglottic hemangioma usually develops cough (Fig. 7-42A) and inspiratory stridor during the neonatal period. The stridor is frequently intermit-tent. Approximately 50% of patients also have cutaneous hemangiomas. Spontaneous involution of the subglottic hemangioma by 18 months is common. Some small heman-giomas are identified only at endoscopy. The classic radio-logic appearance of the larger subglottic hemangiomas is an eccentric mass, sometimes lumpy (Fig. 7-42B), deforming the subglottic trachea (21,58,106). The eccentricity of the mass or airway deformity differentiates this lesion from croup and congenital subglottic stenosis. Plain radiographs cannot distinguish subglottic hemangiomas from subglottic cysts, eccentric subglottic stenoses, subglottic mucoceles, ectopic thyroid tissue, and granulation tissue; laryngoscopy is required for definitive diagnosis (107).

Retropharyngeal Cellulitis and Abscess

Infants and young children with retropharyngeal cellulitis, adenitis, or abscess typically have a history of an upper respi-ratory tract infection followed by the sudden onset of neck pain and stiffness, dysphagia, and a higher fever. Rarely, retropharyngeal abscess is the result of pharyngeal or esoph-ageal perforation. Stridor is usually a minor symptom. Cervi-cal adenopathy is common. The many lymph nodes and lym-phatic chains in the retropharyngeal space between the posterior pharyngeal wall and prevertebral fascia, drain the posterior nasal passage, nasopharynx, middle ear, and ton-sils. Pyogenic infection may spread through this lymphatic system to the retropharyngeal area. At the onset of symp-toms, the retropharyngeal swelling is due to edema and lym-phangitis; retropharyngeal cellulitis is much more common than retropharyngeal abscess. Fifty percent of retropharyn-geal abscesses occur between 6 and 12 months of age. Com-plications include dissection of the abscess into the mediasti-num and jugular vein thrombosis.

The lateral radiograph of the neck shows thickening of the retropharyngeal soft tissues with forward bulging and

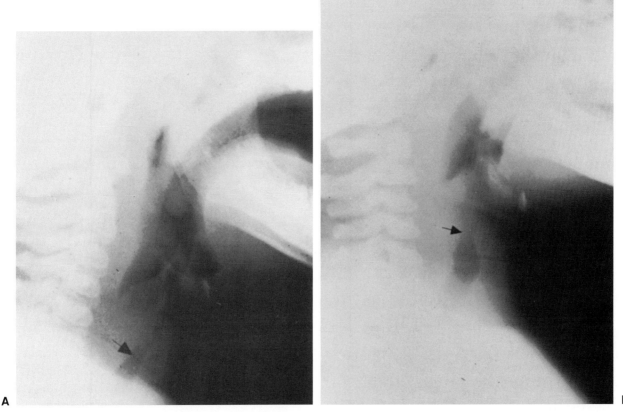

A

B

FIG. 7-40. Croup. A 1-year-old boy with inspiratory stridor. Inspiration **(A)** and expiration **(B)** views of the upper airway demonstrate subglottic tracheal narrowing *(arrows).* There is some widening of the narrowed segment during expiration. The discrepancy in caliber between the segment of subglottic narrowing *(arrow)* and the normal trachea below it is more apparent in expiration.

displacement of the airway (Figs. 7-43, 7-44, 7-45). The most reliable radiographic sign of retropharyngeal pathology is a curved anterior displacement of the posterior pharyngeal airway with loss of the normal step off at the level of the larynx (Fig. 7-45A) (108). There is often straightening of the normal cervical lordosis because of muscle spasm. The thickness of the tissue between the pharyngeal lumen and the vertebrae should normally be three fourths of the antero-posterior diameter of the body of the adjacent vertebra or less (108). However, patient age has some effect on these criteria for precervical soft-tissue thickness (59). If gas is present within the retropharyngeal soft-tissue mass, this confirms the diagnosis (Fig. 7-43B). If there is no gas, plain radiography cannot distinguish between retropharyngeal cellulitis and abscess. If the radiographic findings are minimal or equivocal, a barium swallow might be helpful; this shows anterior displacement of the pharynx and esophagus, and confirms the presence of soft-tissue swelling of the retropharyngeal space (Fig. 7-44B). CT, which has largely supplanted esophagography, cannot confidently distinguish adenitis from abscess unless a collection of pus is shown (Fig. 7-45B); however, it can accurately assess extent of disease and identify complications. Ultrasound, which can distin-

guish adenitis from abscess, is frequently useful (26,109). Retropharyngeal abscess is the most common acute cause of a retropharyngeal mass.

Other retropharyngeal mass lesions in infants and young children include cystic hygroma, hemangioma, neuroblastoma, neurofibroma, ectopic goitrous thyroid tissue, the myxedema of hypothyroidism, foreign body, traumatic instrumentation, and edema or hematoma from cervical spine injury. Enlarged lymph nodes due to lymphoma, leukemia, histiocytosis, infectious mononucleosis, and tuberculosis (scrofula) must also be considered (108). Edema from superior vena cava (SVC) obstruction and augmented venous return in a vascular anomaly, such as malformation of the vein of Galen, may also thicken the retropharyngeal space.

Esophageal Foreign Body and Esophageal Inflammatory Disease

Complete radiologic evaluation of problematic cases of stridor includes AP and lateral chest radiographs including the laryngeal region, fluoroscopy and radiographs of the upper airway, and esophagography (24,25). The esophagogram is particularly important if conventional radiographs

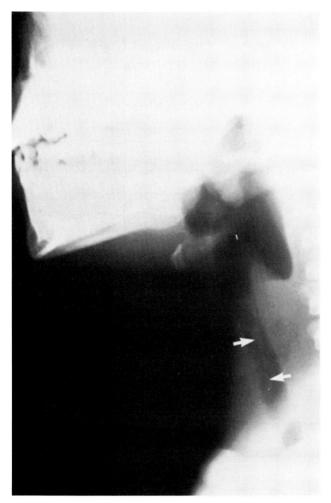

FIG. 7-41. Membranous croup. This 9-year-old boy had severe respiratory distress and high fever. This lateral airway radiograph shows subglottic narrowing and linear membranes *(arrows)*. The membranes were removed endoscopically; culture of the trachea grew *Staphylococcus aureus*.

and fluoroscopy of the upper airway are normal or only questionably abnormal. Esophageal inflammatory disease is an unusual cause of stridor in infants and children. Esophageal foreign bodies may cause respiratory symptoms (cough, stridor, pneumonia) before esophageal symptoms (dysphagia, drooling, pain) are evident. The most common locations for retained esophageal foreign bodies are the thoracic inlet just below the cricopharyngeus, the level of the left main bronchus, and just above the esophagogastric junction. Stridor in infants due to esophageal foreign bodies may occur because of direct mechanical compression, periesophageal inflammation, abscess formation, or direct extension of the inflammatory process into the trachea by ulceration and fistula formation (21,25). Stridor may also be caused by esophageal inflammation (Figs. 7-46, 7-47) (25,110). Smooth esophageal foreign bodies such as metallic coins may be removed in children using a Foley catheter with fluoroscopic guidance. However, this type of interventional radiologic technique is contraindicated when there is evidence of parae-

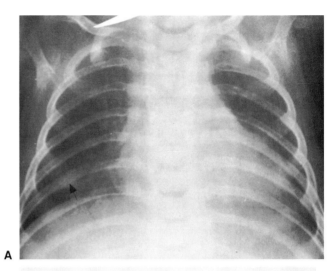

A

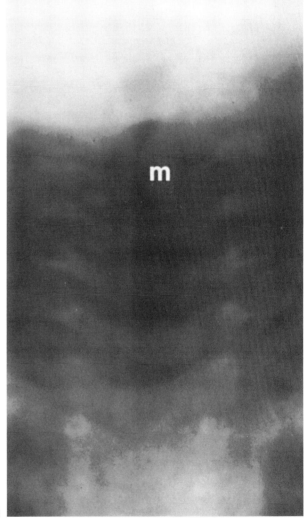

B

FIG. 7-42. Subglottic hemangioma. A: Anteroposterior chest radiograph of a 3-month-old boy who had had intermittent cough and inspiratory stridor since birth. There is generalized underaeration and a cough fracture *(arrow)* involving the posterior aspect of the right seventh rib. **B:** Anteroposterior view of the upper airway. Note the asymmetric subglottic mass *(m)* on the left.

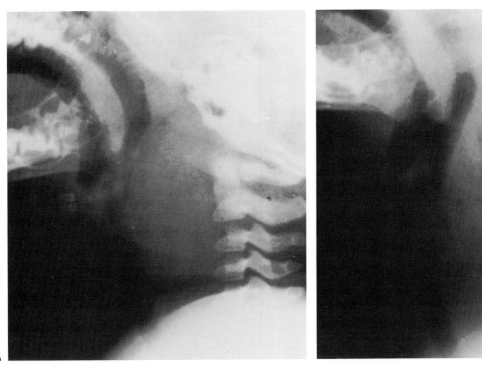

FIG. 7-43. Retropharyngeal cellulitis progressing to abscess. A 6-month-old boy with dysphagia. **A:** There is a large retropharyngeal soft-tissue mass. **B:** A lateral film obtained 4 days later shows a linear collection of air in the mass *(arrow)*. This is due to spontaneous communication between the retropharyngeal abscess and the hypopharynx.

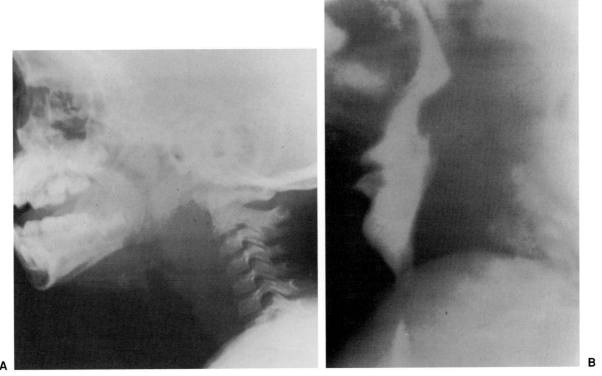

FIG. 7-44. Retropharyngeal abscess or cellulitis. A 2-year-old girl with fever and difficulty swallowing. **A:** A lateral film of the upper airway shows a large retropharyngeal soft-tissue mass. **B:** An esophagogram confirms that both the esophagus and the trachea are displaced anteriorly.

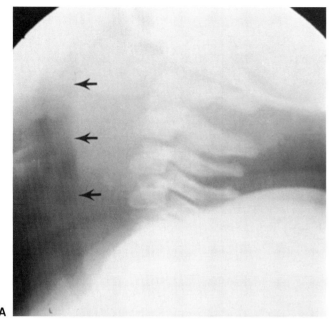

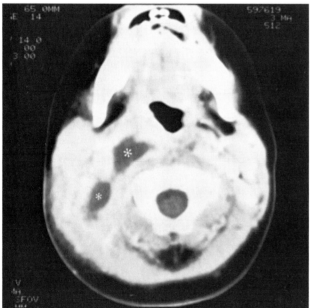

FIG. 7-45. Retropharyngeal abscess. A 14-month-old boy with fever and drooling. **A:** There is a large retropharyngeal mass that displaces the airway anteriorly *(arrows)*. **B:** CT shows both right parapharyngeal and posterior cervical low attenuation masses *(*)*. The abscesses were surgically drained.

sophageal inflammatory reaction (Fig. 7-46) or stridor, or the coin has been present for more than a few hours. Radiologic evaluation of the esophagus is mandatory in a child with unexplained inspiratory stridor or pneumomediastinum (21, 25,58,110).

Cystic Hygroma

Cystic hygromas are congenital malformations of the cervical lymph sacs, most commonly involving the posterior triangle of the neck and supraclavicular fossa. The cause of these tumors is not known. Although these lesions are histologically benign, they often infiltrate into surrounding tissues. Large cystic hygromas may extend into the mediastinum or invade the retropharyngeal space. At least 50% of these tumors appear at birth as soft-tissue masses. Growth of the tumor is commonly proportional to the infant's growth. The appearance of these lesions on plain film depends on the size of the tumor, its location, and the extent

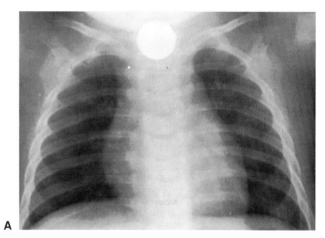

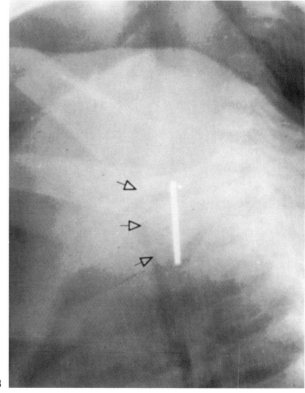

FIG. 7-46. Stridor due to esophageal foreign body. The anteroposterior chest radiograph **(A)** and the lateral radiograph of the upper airway **(B)** demonstrate a metallic coin in the esophagus at the level of the thoracic inlet. There is soft-tissue swelling around the esophagus. The trachea is bowed forward and narrowed *(arrows)* by the paraesophageal inflammatory reaction. The foreign body was difficult to remove endoscopically. From Kirks and Merten (25).

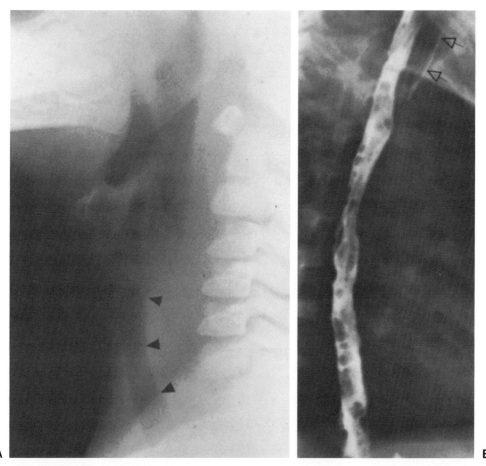

FIG. 7-47. Stridor due to esophageal moniliasis. A 21-month-old boy with acute lymphocytic leukemia in remission, inspiratory stridor, and hoarseness. **A:** Lateral radiograph of the upper airway shows minimal extrinsic compression of the subglottic trachea *(arrowheads)*. The remainder of the upper airway is normal. **B:** Esophagogram. Note the cobblestone appearance of the atonic esophagus due to submucosal inflammation. There is some aspiration of barium *(arrows)*. From Kirks and Merten (25).

of involvement (Fig. 7-48A). Sonography typically shows a multilocular cystic mass (Fig. 7-48B). CT and MRI demonstrate the extent of these tumors most precisely (111).

Chest Radiography in Upper Airway Obstruction

Because the history and physical examination are frequently confusing in infants with upper airway obstruction, a chest radiograph may be the initial examination. The radiologist must be aware of the chest film findings in children with upper airway obstruction. These findings alert one to evaluate the upper airway more carefully and to obtain detailed conventional films or perform fluoroscopy (see Fig. 7-36A).

With obstruction above the thoracic inlet, sufficient air cannot enter the chest during inspiration; the chest radiograph may consequently show underaeration (see Figs. 7-36A and 7-42A). Moreover, there is frequently a paradoxical increase in heart size during inspiration (101). Normally, the heart becomes smaller during inspiration; with glottic or supraglottic obstruction, the inspiratory intrathoracic pres-

sures become deeply negative, causing increased venous return to the heart, which becomes larger (101). Underaeration of the lungs with paradoxical increase in heart size during inspiration and decrease in heart size during expiration suggest upper airway obstruction (101).

Congenital Abnormalities

Tracheobronchial Abnormalities

The airways have only one major function: to carry air to the pulmonary periphery, where oxygen and carbon dioxide can be exchanged, and to return the modified air back to the outside. They are also the only major anatomic system with a back-and-forth, ebb-and-flow motion. Most diseases of the airways come to attention because they interfere with this tidal flow of air.

The trachea buds from the embryonic foregut and then sequentially bifurcates into about 24 generations of branches, ending with the alveoli. The total cross-sectional area of the airway changes slowly, from the larynx to the

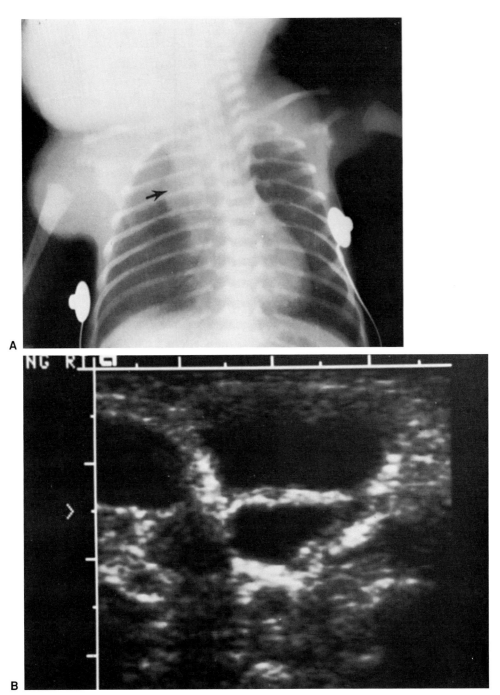

FIG. 7-48. Cystic hygroma. A: Portable chest radiograph. There is a large soft-tissue mass of the right neck and axilla that extends into the mediastinum *(arrow).* **B:** Longitudinal sonography of the neck shows a multilocular cystic mass.

bronchioles (generations 5–16) (112,113). Then it rapidly expands as the number of airways increases phenomenally. The major resistance to the flow of gas is in the smaller bronchi and largest bronchioles. Though very small, the peripheral airways are so numerous that they contribute much less total resistance than the central airways. In healthy adults, less than 20% of airway resistance is attributable to

airways less than 2 mm in diameter; the situation is quite different in bronchiolitic infants. In the trachea, gas flow is mostly turbulent, especially during rapid, deep respirations. It becomes fully laminar only in the very small airways. Velocity falls off steeply in the periphery because the total cross sectional area through which the air is moving is so very large (114).

Before birth, the airways and lungs are filled not with gas but with liquid, which is slowly passed up into the pharynx and is either swallowed or escapes into the amniotic fluid. Obstruction of the fetal airway therefore leads to fluid-filled enlargement of the obstructed pulmonary segments, not to the air trapping and atelectasis seen at all other times of life (115).

The important points in the anatomy of the trachea are its C-shaped cartilaginous rings and the fact that the rings are completed posteriorly by fibrous tissue and smooth muscle, the pars membranacea. In the bronchi, the rings are much less regular; the smallest bronchi have none. Particularly in childhood, these rings are elastic. The bronchi and trachea are lined by ciliated columnar mucosa and are bathed in mucus, formed by the mucosa and by the mucus glands in the wall of the trachea. The mucus is propelled toward the vocal cords by ciliary action at the rate of 1–3 cm/min (19).

CT readily shows tracheal size and shape. Conventional or spiral CT shows static anatomy more precisely; ultrafast (electron beam) CT is more sensitive to changes during the respiratory cycle (31). In middle childhood and in adolescence, the trachea is almost round in cross section at the end of a deep inspiration. Its shape is less circular in the elderly, at low lung volumes, and in various tracheal abnormalities. The length, diameters, cross-sectional area, and volume of the pediatric trachea have been measured and plotted against body height, gender, and age (30). There is a disproportionate increase in tracheal dimensions in boys at adolescence.

Those who see only static images of the trachea often think of it as an unchanging rigid organ. However, tracheal dimensions in the chest are sensitive to the phase of respiration and the intrapleural pressure. The retracting forces of the chest wall and lungs cause the intrathoracic trachea to be large at high lung volumes, when intrapleural pressure is most deeply negative. Fluoroscopy readily confirms that the trachea and bronchi get larger during inspiration and smaller during expiration.

Alterations in pressure across the wall also govern tracheal size (18,19). This pressure-governed change is limited to the cervical trachea because the size of the intrathoracic trachea is controlled by the recoil forces of the lungs and chest wall. If the vocal cords are closed, a rise in pressure within the chest (grunting, straining, shouting, singing loudly, playing a wind instrument) will cause the cervical trachea to bulge outward, sometimes more at the pars membranacea than at the cartilaginous rings. The reverse occurs during vigorous inspiration in children with laryngeal obstruction. A film in a child with croup taken during inspiration, when intrapleural pressure is low and air has difficulty passing through the obstructed larynx, will show narrowing of the entire upper trachea, not merely at the conus elasticus.

Tracheal Agenesis

This rare tracheal abnormality is commonly associated with maternal polyhydramnios and almost always with tra-

cheo- or bronchoesophageal fistula. The basic clinical features are immediate, severe respiratory distress, absence of cry, and inability to intubate the airway below the larynx (116). Three forms of tracheal agenesis occur. In type 1, the upper trachea is absent and the lower trachea connects to the esophagus. Type 2 has a common bronchus connecting right and left main bronchi to the esophagus while the trachea is absent (Fig. 7-49). In type 3 the right and left main bronchi arise independently from the esophagus. Congenital heart disease, radial ray anomalies, and duodenal atresia are common. Adequate ventilation of the lungs from esophageal intubation may suggest the diagnosis and permit survival long enough for surgical repair to be attempted. Chest films may show absence of the tracheal air shadow, abnormal carinal position, and placement of the "endotracheal" catheter within the esophagus (Fig. 7-49) (113,116,117). Injection of contrast material into the esophagus confirms the diagnosis (Fig. 7-49C).

Tracheal Stenosis

While acquired stenosis of the trachea occurs as a consequence of intubation or traumatic tracheobronchial suctioning, congenital stenosis of the trachea due to complete cartilaginous rings is rare. Approximately 50% of congenital tracheal stenoses are focal, 30% generalized, and 20% funnel-shaped (118). The latter type is commonly seen with pulmonary artery sling. The diagnosis of congenital tracheal stenosis should prompt a search for associated anomalies (tracheoesophageal fistula [TEF], lung agenesis or hypoplasia, pulmonary artery sling, and bronchial stenosis). Most children (90%) present during the first year of life, often with biphasic stridor. Determining the cause of fixed intrinsic tracheal narrowing in a symptomatic child is crucial. Bronchoscopy may not adequately evaluate the extent of the narrowing and its causes. Fluoroscopy provides a rapid, inexpensive means of distinguishing tracheal stenosis from tracheomalacia. CT is useful in showing the presence and extent of tracheal narrowing (Fig. 7-50). CT is superior in this regard compared to chest ragiography and high kV airway films (118). When combined with bolus enhancement, CT will show extrinsic mass lesions and vascular anomalies.

MRI is as accurate as bronchoscopy in evaluating the anatomy of the airway (36,58). Moreover, MRI can identify mediastinal masses and blood vessels as well as their relationship to the trachea. The limitations of MRI in airway evaluation are its inability to demonstrate dynamic changes and its inability to show aerated lungs well.

Symptoms similar to those of tracheal stenosis can be caused by foreign body, croup, epiglottitis, granulation tissue after intubation, tracheomalacia, and neoplasms (papilloma, fibroma, hemangioma, adenoma, cylindroma, granular cell myoblastoma, schwannoma).

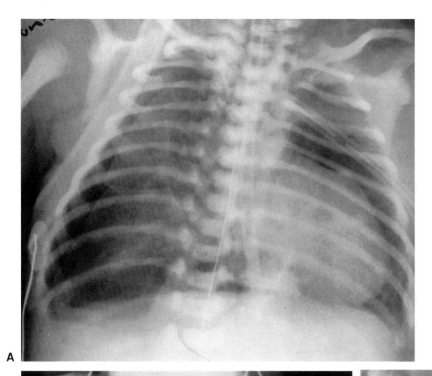

A

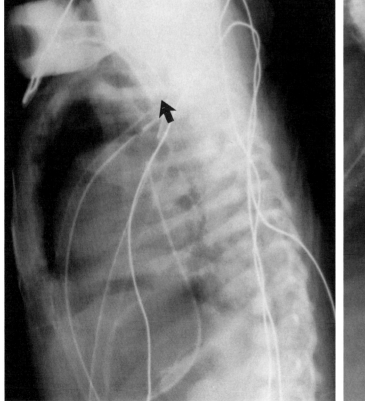

B

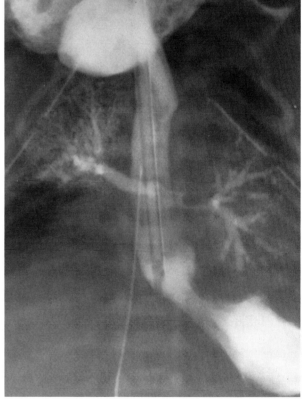

C

FIG. 7-49. Tracheal agenesis (type 2).
A: Anteroposterior chest radiograph of a term newborn with severe respiratory distress shows bilateral pneumothoraces. Note the absence of the tracheal air shadow. **B:** Lateral chest radiograph shows anterior pneumothoraces (retrosternal lucency). Note the esophageal position *(arrow)* of the tracheostomy tube. **C:** Postmortem AP esophagogram shows a common bronchus arising from the esophagus and branching into right and left main bronchi.

Tracheomalacia

Tracheomalacia is defined as tracheal wall softening; this softening is supposedly due to an abnormality of the cartilaginous ring. Congenital or primary tracheomalacia, an exceedingly rare condition, may be seen sporadically or in association with chondrodystrophies, such as the Ellis-van Creveld syndrome and Larsen syndrome. Prematurity is associated with tracheomalacia, perhaps because of the repeated trauma of intubation. Tracheomalacia may be secondary to tracheostomy, esophageal atresia/TEF, chronic inflammation (cystic fibrosis, recurrent aspiration, immuno-

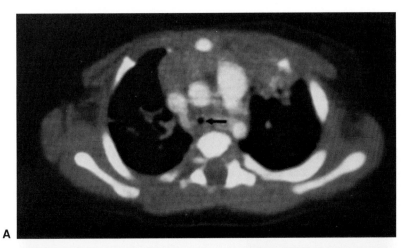

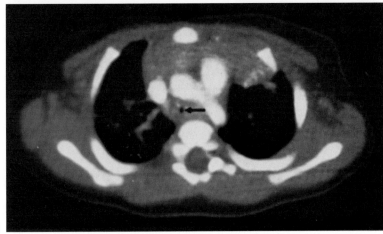

FIG. 7-50. Congenital tracheal stenosis. A, B: Axial, contrast-enhanced CT sections demonstrate severe narrowing of the tracheal lumen. The narrowed lumen *(arrows)* is a "perfect circle" rather than oval. (Courtesy of Janet L. Strife, M.D., Cincinnati, Ohio.)

deficiency), extrinsic compression (vascular ring, sling, or aberrancy) and neoplasm. Tracheomalacia causes expiratory stridor (wheezing) that is most severe with crying and may disappear at rest. Infants so affected may experience "dying spells" (reflex apnea). Cyanosis and bradycardia may occur, particularly after feeding.

Lateral fluoroscopy and esophagography can be diagnostic (21,58,119). Fluoroscopy shows an exaggerated decrease in the caliber of the trachea during expiration. Wheezing is loudest during crying or forced expiration. Although limited in its availability, cine CT allows dynamic cross-sectional evaluation of tracheal compliance and regional anatomy. MRI, although comprehensive in showing the relationship of vascular and nonvascular structures to the abnormal trachea (Fig. 7-51), lacks the capability to evaluate the airway dynamically.

Tracheoesophageal Fistula

TEF may present with choking, cyanosis, coughing at the time of feeding, or severe chronic recurrent pulmonary problems (5,120). If esophageal atresia co-exists, the presentation may include maternal polyhydramnios and excessive neonatal oral secretions. This topic is further discussed in Chapter 8.

Bronchial Atresia

Occasionally, lobar or segmental bronchi are congenitally atretic. The upper lobe bronchi are more frequently affected. In the newborn period, bronchial atresia presents as a water density "mass," usually occupying part or all of an upper lobe. The "mass" is fetal lung liquid, trapped behind the atresia (112,113,115). Later in childhood, the fetal lung liquid having escaped (perhaps through the pores of Kohn and channels of Lambert), bronchial atresia is found because of local air trapping. There is frequently a round opacity at the site of the atresia, central to the air trapping; this represents accumulated mucus just distal to the atresia (113). CT shows these relationships well. Bronchial atresia may be associated with other anomalies such as bronchogenic cyst, intralobar sequestration, and cystic adenomatoid malformation.

Tracheal Bronchus

The incidence of tracheal bronchus (right upper lobe bronchus arising directly from the trachea) is approximately 1% in the general population. Bronchial ectopia is much more common on the right (2.5–7 times more frequent). The tracheal bronchus supplies the entire right upper lobe or its

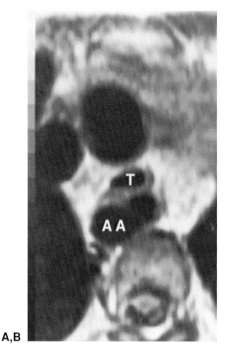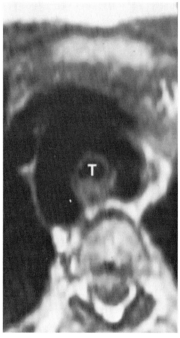

FIG. 7-51. Double aortic arch. A, B: Two axial MR images demonstrate a double aortic arch and narrowing of the trachea *(T)*; the larger arch is right and posterior *(AA)*. (Courtesy of Janet L. Strife, M.D., Cincinnati, Ohio.)

apical segment (Fig. 7-52). The bronchus may also lead to a supernumerary segment. The diagnosis of tracheal bronchus should be considered in cases of persistent or recurrent upper lobe pneumonia, atelectasis, or air trapping (112).

Other Bronchial Branching Anomalies

Isomerism syndromes are associated with unique bronchial branching patterns. Asplenia or Ivemark syndrome includes bilateral right lung (trilobed) bronchial pattern, absence of spleen, single ventricle, functionally single atrium, anomalous pulmonary venous return, pulmonic stenosis or atresia, and transposition of the great vessels. Polysplenia is a left lung isomerism syndrome. It includes bilateral left lung bronchial pattern, intestinal malrotation, multiple small spleens, interrupted inferior vena cava (IVC), and atrial or ventricular septal defects (Fig. 7-53) (112). These conditions are discussed in greater detail in Chapter 6.

Bronchial Stenosis

Bronchial stenosis, like tracheal stenosis, is usually acquired. Prematurity with intubation and repeated tracheo-

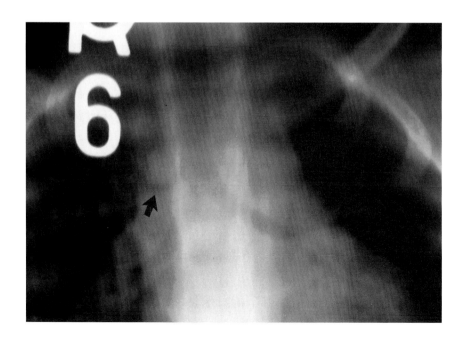

FIG. 7-52. Tracheal bronchus. Anteroposterior chest tomography of a 4-year-old boy with recurrent pneumonia shows a tracheal bronchus *(arrow)* supplying the entire right upper lobe.

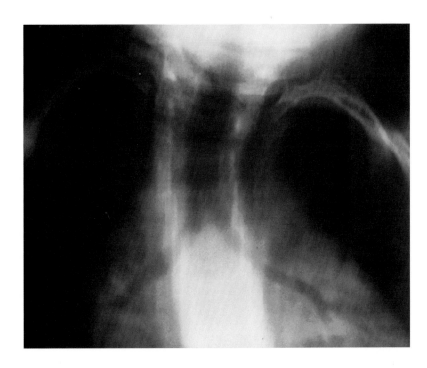

FIG. 7-53. Polysplenia. Anteroposterior spinal tomography for the evaluation of scoliosis in this 5-year-old boy fortuitously showed bilateral left (long) mainstem bronchi.

bronchial suctioning is followed by stenosis and secondary chronic or recurrent segmental or lobar pneumonia, atelectasis, or air trapping. The right upper lobe is often affected (112,113). In pulmonary tuberculosis, the bronchi may be extrinsically compressed by lymph nodes or intrinsically narrowed by granuloma formation. The diagnosis of childhood tuberculosis should be considered when the asymptomatic or mildly symptomatic child with segmental atelectasis or air trapping is noted to have mediastinal or hilar adenopathy.

Bronchial Fistulas

Bronchial communication with the esophagus (communicating bronchopulmonary foregut malformation) is often associated with esophageal atresia. These communications are usually on the right. Recurrent pneumonias may plague the patient. Chest radiography typically shows a segmental area of air space opacity, collapse, or bronchiectasis. The esophagogram is diagnostic. Congenital bronchobiliary fistula (connection between airway and biliary tree) is a rare anomaly.

Pulmonary Underdevelopment

Pulmonary underdevelopment, including congenital absence of a lung, is fairly common. Patients are asymptomatic unless there is an associated cardiovascular abnormality or a superimposed illness. The three forms of pulmonary underdevelopment are agenesis, aplasia, and hypoplasia (112,113,117). *Agenesis* is complete absence of a lung or lobe and its bronchi. *Aplasia* is absence of lung tissue but presence of a rudimentary bronchus. *Hypoplasia* is the presence of both bronchi and alveoli in an underdeveloped lobe (112,117,121).

Lung Agenesis

Complete agenesis of a lung is easily recognized, as there is a small completely opaque hemithorax with displacement of the mediastinal structures, diaphragm, and normal lung toward that side (Fig. 7-54). This entity may be detected at birth or may become manifest later when a superimposed infection, such as bronchiolitis, accentuates the limited pulmonary reserve. Either lung may be absent (117,122). Right lung agenesis is associated with a higher mortality rate, possibly because of the higher incidence of cardiovascular anomalies. Bronchography or bronchoscopy verifies that the mainstem bronchus is completely missing, and angiography demonstrates that there are no pulmonary or bronchial arteries on the side of the absent lung (Fig. 7-54B). Other frequently associated anomalies include TEF, imperforate anus, renal dysgenesis or agenesis, and hemivertebrae. If the aortic arch is located on the side opposite the agenetic lung, the trachea may be narrowed extrinsically by the aortic arch as it courses from the displaced heart (117,122).

Lobar Underdevelopment

Pulmonary hypoplasia is caused by factors directly or indirectly compromising the thoracic space available for lung growth (121). These causes may be intrathoracic (diaphragmatic hernia, extralobar sequestration [ELS]) or extrathoracic (oligohydramnios, arthrogryposis). Lobar underdevelopment (agenesis, aplasia, hypoplasia) classically involves

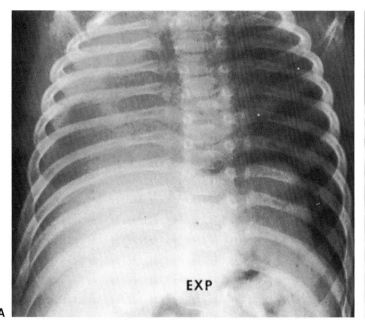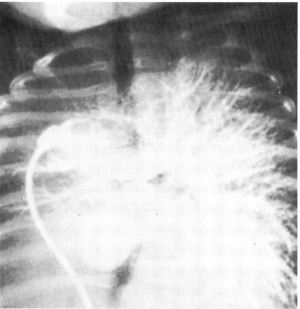

FIG. 7-54. Pulmonary agenesis. A: Expiration view of the chest. Complete opacity of right hemithorax with displacement of heart and mediastinum from left to right. There is also a left diaphragmatic eventration. **B:** Pulmonary arteriogram. Normal left pulmonary artery and branches; complete absence of right pulmonary artery.

the right lung. The association of pulmonary hypoplasia with right-sided obstructive congenital heart defects suggests that pulmonary blood flow is an important factor in normal lung development. In right lung hypoplasia, there is a decrease in the volume of the right hemithorax, normal or increased density on that side, and displacement of the heart and mediastinum toward the right. This mediastinal shift is accentuated during inspiration because there is increased compensatory ventilation of the left lung. There is obscuration of the right heart border and ascending aorta due to extrapleural areolar tissue, best seen on the lateral film (Fig. 7-55) (123). This extrapleural areolar tissue on the lateral film is sharply outlined posteriorly by the parietal pleura of the small but otherwise normal right lung. This anterior pleural line and opacity have been mistakenly referred to as an accessory hemidiaphragm. Extrapleural areolar tissue has a shape different from that of right upper lobe collapse, which does not extend to the diaphragm and has a hilar connection with a wedge appearance (112, 121,122,124). Significant anomalies associated with pulmonary hypoplasia are usually diaphragmatic (diaphragmatic hernia) or renal (dysgenesis, agenesis) (125,126).

Scimitar Syndrome

The scimitar syndrome, or congenital pulmonary venolobar syndrome, is a unique form of lobar agenesis or aplasia associated with other anomalies of the pulmonary vessels and thorax (112,121,122,124). The common feature in all cases of pulmonary venolobar syndrome is hypoplasia or aplasia of one or more lobes of the right lung (127–129). The variable components include partial anomalous pulmonary venous return from the abnormal lung (frequently seen as a scimitar-shaped vein); absent or small pulmonary artery perfusing the abnormal lung; arterial supply to the abnormal segment of lung partly or wholly from the thoracic aorta, abdominal aorta, or celiac axis; anomalies of the hemidiaphragm on the affected side, including accessory diaphragm, phrenic cyst, or diaphragmatic hernia; absence of the IVC and anomalies of the bony thorax or thoracic soft tissues with excessive extrapleural areolar tissue (112,124,127,128).

The syndrome may be dominantly inherited, but has variable expression (112,124). The term *congenital pulmonary venolobar syndrome* emphasizes that the anomaly may be part of an embryologic spectrum that includes systemic segmental or subsegmental arterial supply to normal pulmonary tissue, unilateral pulmonary or lobar hypoplasia, intralobular or extralobular segmental dysplasia, cystic adenomatoid hamartomatous malformation, bronchogenic cyst, bronchopulmonary foregut malformation, and sequestration (129).

Radiologically, one sees a small right hemithorax, obscuration of the right heart border, and a retrosternal soft-tissue density (Figs. 7-55 and 7-56). On the AP chest radiograph, the anomalous vein has the appearance of a Turkish scimitar (Fig. 7-56A). This anomalous vessel usually drains to the IVC but may also end in the portal vein, a hepatic vein, or right atrium (112,121,124,127,128). There may be an atrial septal defect. The right pulmonary artery may be completely or partly absent, and there is frequently a systemic vessel arising from the lower thoracic or upper abdominal aorta to supply the involved right lower lobe (Fig. 7-56D). There may be a mass of abnormal tissue in this right lower lobe (pulmonary sequestration).

Other Pulmonary Developmental Anomalies

The most common clinically significant pulmonary developmental anomalies span a continuum of maldevelopment. These abnormalities include congenital lobar emphysema (CLE), intrathoracic foregut cysts (bronchogenic, enteric, neurenteric), congenital cystic adenomatoid malformation (CCAM), sequestrations of the lung, hypogenetic lung syndrome (scimitar syndrome), and pulmonary arteriovenous malformation. At one end of the spectrum, normal pulmonary vessels connect to abnormal parenchyma (CLE). At the other end of the spectrum, abnormal pulmonary vessels course through normal pulmonary tissue (pulmonary arteriovenous malformation). Between these two extremes are anomalies with varied combinations of pulmonary and vascular maldevelopment. This continuum has been referred to as the sequestration spectrum (130).

Congenital Lobar Emphysema

CLE is a condition characterized by progressive overdistention of a lobe or, occasionally, two lobes. The term *emphysema* is really a misnomer, as there is no destruction of alveolar walls. The etiology of congenital lobar emphysema remains unknown in more than 50% of cases even after pathologic examination of the emphysematous lobe. Many cases seem to be due to obstruction of a bronchus by a ball valve mechanism. Postulated causes of this obstruction include bronchial cartilage deficiency, dysplasia, or immaturity; inflammatory exudate; inspissated mucus; mucosal fold or web; bronchial stenosis; extrinsic vascular compression; and extrinsic mass compression (131). Some cases of unknown etiology co-exist with an actual increase in alveolar number. The emphysematous lobe remains expanded after sectioning. Microscopic examination may show distended alveoli with thinned septa or normal alveolar size with an increase in alveolar number (polyalveolar type).

Most patients with congenital lobar emphysema become symptomatic during the neonatal period. There is a male/female incidence of 3:1 (7,10,12). Associated anomalies have been reported in 14% to 50% of children. These anomalies frequently involve the cardiovascular system (70%). Patent ductus arteriosus, ventricular septal defect (VSD), and tetralogy of Fallot are most common.

Congenital lobar emphysema usually involves one of the upper lobes or the right middle lobe. The distribution of lobar involvement is as follows: left upper lobe 43%; right

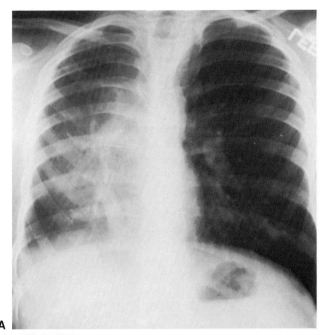

A

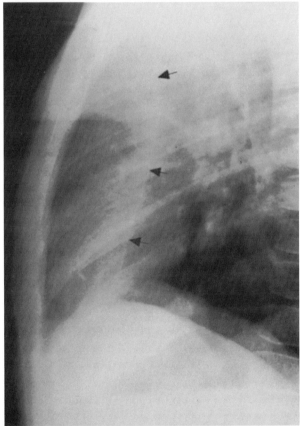

B

FIG. 7-55. Pulmonary hypoplasia in scimitar syndrome. **A:** Decreased aeration of the right hemithorax with displacement of the heart and mediastinum from left to right. There is loss of the right heart border. A large anomalous vein drains the right lung, producing a scimitar appearance. **B:** Lateral chest radiograph. The retrosternal opacity is due to extrapleural areolar tissue anterior to the right lung *(arrows)*.

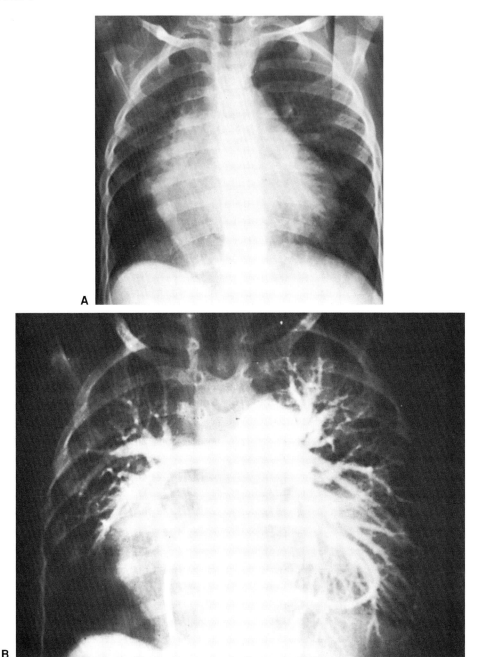

FIG. 7-56. Scimitar syndrome. A: Hypoplasia of right lung and anomalous vein in right lower lobe. **B:** Pulmonary arteriogram, arterial phase. Absence of branches to right lower lobe. (*continued*)

middle lobe 32%; right upper lobe 20%; and the lower lobes 5% (10,131). During the first few days of life, lung fluid may be trapped in the involved lobe, producing an opaque, enlarged hemithorax (Fig. 7-57A). This opacity is due to impaired clearance of lung fluid from alveoli through the bronchi (132). As vascular and lymphatic resorption progresses, the involved lobe may develop a reticular appearance. Subsequently, the classic radiologic appearance of an emphysematous lobe with generalized radiolucency develops (Fig. 7-57B). Pulmonary vessels are markedly attenuated but can usually be seen extending into the periphery of the

hyperlucent lobe. Compression of adjacent lobes provides a useful radiologic clue to the diagnosis. Nuclear scintigraphy shows decreased ventilation, matching decreased perfusion, and delayed tracer washout in the emphysematous lobe (Fig. 7-58). In summary, the radiographic appearance is that of an overdistended lobe that progresses from alveolar opacification to interstitial reticulation to general hyperlucency (Figs. 7-57 and 7-58) (7,10,12).

On the basis of early radiographic findings, fluid-filled lobar emphysema may be confused with other intrathoracic masses such as cystic adenomatoid malformation, pulmo-

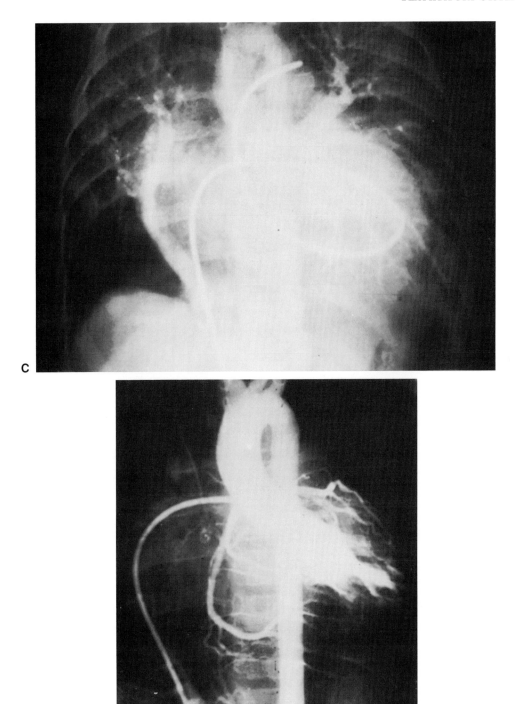

FIG. 7-56 *Continued.* **C:** Pulmonary arteriogram, venous phase. An anomalous vein drains the right lower lobe into the inferior vena cava. **D:** Aortogram. Systemic vessel from the aorta below the diaphragm supplies the right lower lobe. (Courtesy of Edward B. Singleton, M.D., Houston, Texas.)

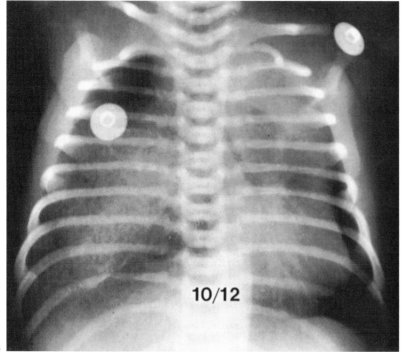

10/12

A

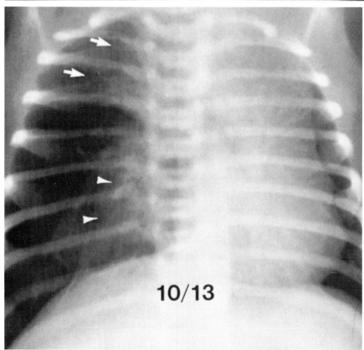

10/13

B

FIG. 7-57. Congenital lobar emphysema. A:
Film at 2 hours of age shows a large opacity in the
right chest displacing the heart and mediastinum
to the left. B: Fluid has started to clear from the
emphysematous right middle lobe by 24 hours to
produce a lucent mass with reticular densities.
Note the compressive atelectasis of the right upper
lobe *(arrows)* and right lower lobe *(arrowheads).*

nary sling, neurogenic tumor, neurenteric cyst, enterogenous
cyst, bronchogenic cyst, teratoma, cystic hygroma, diaphragmatic hernia, hamartoma, fibrosarcoma, and sequestration
(7). If it appears that there is emphysema of an entire lung,
barium esophagography should be performed to exclude a
mediastinal bronchogenic cyst or pulmonary sling. Congenital lobar emphysema may rarely be confused with pneumothorax and solitary lung cyst. In difficult cases, CT may be

helpful. As previously noted, pulmonary vessels do extend
to the periphery of the hyperexpanded lobe of congenital
lobar emphysema, and there is no visualization of a pleural
line as in tension pneumothorax. Decubitus and cross-table
lateral views help to distinguish congenital lobar emphysema
from tension pneumothorax. Bronchoscopy should be performed prior to surgery to rule out the possibility of an endobronchial lesion. Definitive treatment for congenital lobar

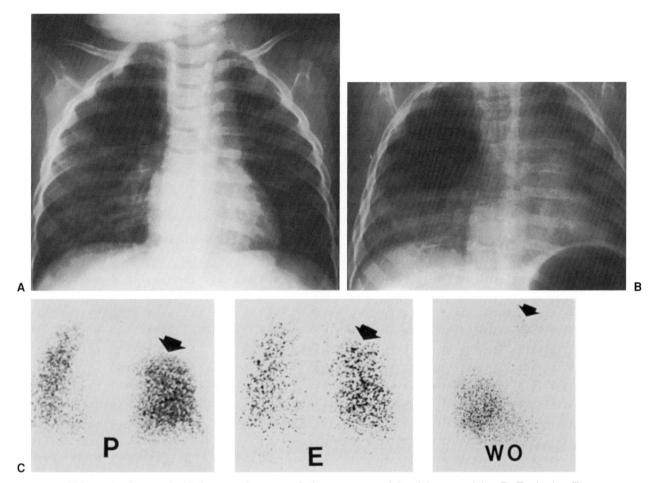

FIG. 7-58. Congenital lobar emphysema. A: Lucent mass of the right upper lobe. **B:** Expiration film. Air trapping is evident in the emphysematous right upper lobe. **C:** Ventilation-perfusion scintigraphy (posterior images). *Left:* absence of activity in right upper lobe *(arrow)* on the perfusion scan *(P). Center:* lack of ventilation in the same region *(arrow)* on an equilibrium ventilation scan *(E). Right:* trapping of tracer in right upper lobe *(arrow)* on washout phase *(WO)* of ventilation scan.

emphysema is surgical resection of the involved lobe; the prognosis is excellent (7,10,12,131).

Bronchopulmonary Foregut Malformations

This term refers to a subset of pulmonary developmental anomalies that result from abnormal budding of the embryonic foregut and tracheobronchial tree. Bronchopulmonary foregut malformations include foregut cysts, bronchogenic cysts, enteric cysts, and neurenteric cysts (133,134). CCAM and pulmonary sequestration are often included in this spectrum (130).

Foregut Cysts. Intrathoracic foregut cysts (enteric, bronchogenic, and neurenteric cysts) are derived from the primitive foregut and represent an abnormality of either foregut or tracheobronchial budding. Most authors rely on a combination of embryology, histology, and the relationship of the cyst to normal structures to classify intrathoracic foregut cysts.

Bronchogenic cysts account for approximately half of all congenital intrathoracic cysts and may be mediastinal or intrapulmonary. The much more common mediastinal bronchogenic cyst represents an earlier budding abnormality; intrapulmonary bronchogenic cysts result from later budding defects. These cysts are lined by ciliated epithelium. Their walls contain smooth muscle and often cartilage. Mediastinal bronchogenic cysts can be paratracheal (usually right-sided), carinal, or hilar. The carinal location is common (135). The intrapulmonary cysts are rounded, sharply marginated, and typically within the medial third of the lung. Bronchogenic cysts do not initially communicate with the tracheobronchial tree. Instrumentation of the cyst or infection may lead to an air-filled cyst or an air-fluid level (130,136,137). The benign-appearing aerated intrapulmonary cyst must be differentiated from an acquired cyst and the rare but potentially malignant cystic mesenchymal hamartoma (138).

Enteric cysts form earlier in embryogenesis than bronchogenic cysts and are generally in the posterior mediasti-

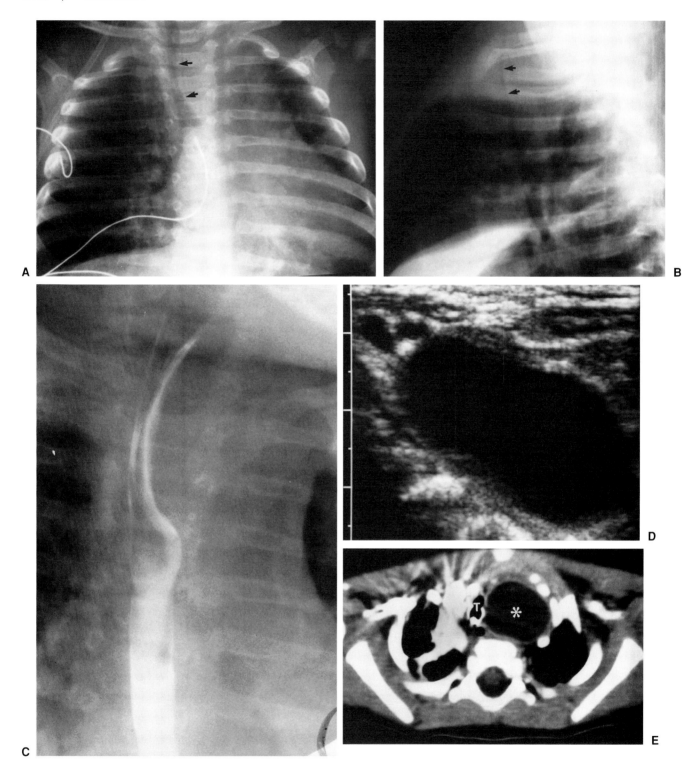

FIG. 7-59. Mediastinal enteric cyst. A: Anteroposterior chest radiograph in a 6-month-old boy with a history of stridor since birth. There is a left paratracheal mass effect *(arrows)*. **B:** Lateral chest x-ray shows marked tracheal narrowing and anterior displacement *(arrows)*. **C:** Anterior spot film from an esophagogram shows a left upper esophageal impression. **D:** Suprasternal sagittal sonogram. The ovoid cervicothoracic mass is sonolucent. **E:** Contrast-enhanced CT image at the level of the thoracic inlet. A superior mediastinal, paraesophageal, low-density mass *(*)* displaces the trachea to the right. *T*, trachea. (Courtesy of Chris Guion, M.D., Birmingham, Alabama.)

num. They may contain gastric mucosa. Those that are found in the esophageal wall are referred to as esophageal cysts or duplications. These cysts usually appear early in life, as acid and pepsin secretions in the cyst may rupture into the tracheobronchial tree and cause hemoptysis. A large posterior or middle mediastinal mass, usually on the right side, is noted radiologically (Fig. 7-59). Pleural effusion and parenchymal opacity due to aspiration of the caustic cyst contents may occur. There may be associated spinal anomalies. The mediastinal uptake of technetium (^{99m}Tc) pertechnetate is strong confirmatory evidence that the enteric cyst contains gastric mucosa. Intrathoracic gastrogenic cysts are potentially life threatening and should be resected (139).

Neurenteric cysts (see also Chapter 4) present as posterior mediastinal masses associated with vertebral anomalies (130,136). MRI is the method of choice for evaluating both thoracic and spinal components of neurenteric cysts.

Clinical symptoms in patients with intrathoracic foregut cysts are variable. Symptoms are due to the size and position of the cyst (Fig. 7-59). Because of the frequent central location of these cysts, compression of the airway can lead to obstructive overinflation, often involving an entire lung. The clinical presentation may mimic asthma, vascular ring, viral lower airways disease, or airway foreign body. Some patients are completely asymptomatic. In older children, adolescents, and adults, bronchogenic cysts may be diagnosed incidentally or when the cyst becomes infected.

Most bronchogenic, enteric, and neurenteric cysts are filled with serous or mucoid fluid. Therefore, they appear as water density mass lesions on chest x-ray (Fig. 7-60). They are typically solitary and unilocular. Mediastinal bron-

chogenic cysts are often infracarinal or paratracheal. An esophagogram commonly shows anterior esophageal indentation and a posterior mass effect upon the carina or trachea. Intrapulmonary bronchogenic cysts are fluid-filled masses that may become air containing (Fig. 7-61) as a result of infection or instrumentation.

Cross-sectional imaging plays an important role in the evaluation of intrathoracic foregut cysts. CT has the capability of localizing an intrathoracic cyst, defining the extent and relation to key structures, and characterizing the intrinsic density. The cyst contents may be watery or viscous. Therefore, attenuation values are variable; the density of mucus-containing cysts is often surprisingly high (140). Regardless of the CT density, a lack of enhancement is expected (Fig. 7-61). Cysts complicated by infection may show wall enhancement. In the neonatal chest, sonography may accurately characterize the cystic nature of the mass. T1-weighted MRI images show intrinsic signal intensities ranging from low to high depending on cyst contents (serous, mucinous, proteinaceous, milk of calcium). T2-weighted images are typically high in signal intensity (141,142). Both MRI and contrast-enhanced CT can confidently exclude vascular lesions such as a pulmonary artery sling.

Congenital Cystic Adenomatoid Malformation

Congenital cystic adenomatoid malformation of the lung consists of a hamartomatous proliferation of terminal bronchioles at the expense of alveolar development. The lesion is composed of both cystic and solid tissue. The cysts are lined by respiratory epithelium and usually communicate

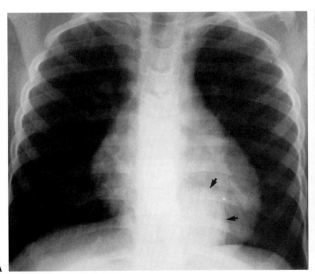
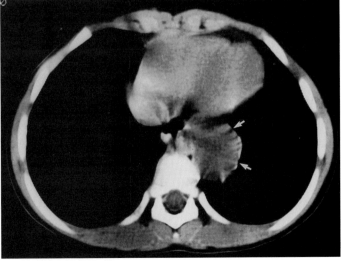

FIG. 7-60. Mediastinal bronchogenic cyst. A: A 2-year-old girl evaluated for cough and fever. The chest radiograph shows a rounded left retrocardiac opacity *(arrows).* **B:** Contrast-enhanced CT shows a nonenhancing water–density middle mediastinal mass *(arrows).*

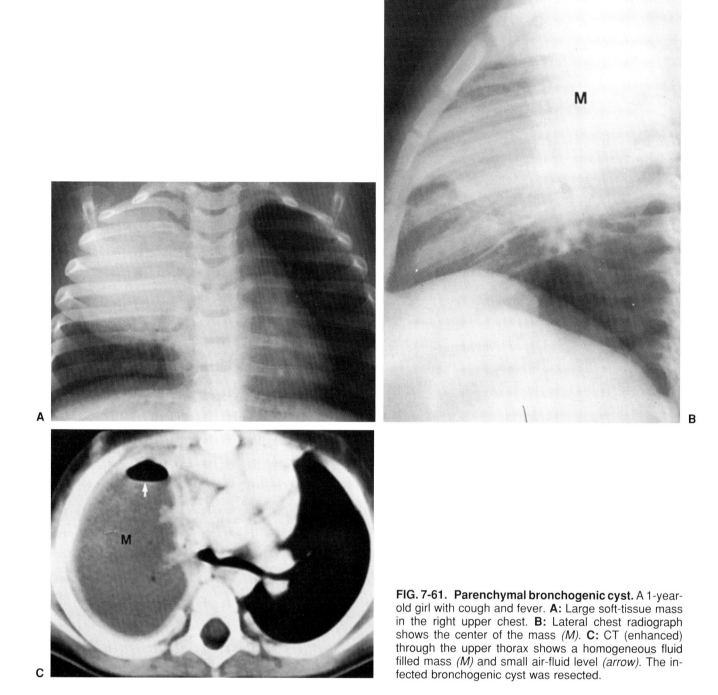

FIG. 7-61. **Parenchymal bronchogenic cyst.** A 1-year-old girl with cough and fever. **A:** Large soft-tissue mass in the right upper chest. **B:** Lateral chest radiograph shows the center of the mass *(M)*. **C:** CT (enhanced) through the upper thorax shows a homogeneous fluid filled mass *(M)* and small air-fluid level *(arrow)*. The infected bronchogenic cyst was resected.

with the tracheobronchial tree. There is a slight predilection for the upper lobes. This malformation can be classified on the basis of clinical, radiographic, and histologic features (65,143). Type I, composed of variable-sized cysts with at least one dominant cyst (>2 cm in diameter), is most common (50%). The prognosis is excellent; other congenital malformations are infrequent (5%). Type II (41%) is composed of smaller more uniform cysts up to 2cm in diameter

(1–10 mm); congenital malformations (renal, intestinal, cardiac, skeletal) are common (50%). Type III CCAM is the least common (9%). These lesions are composed of microcysts and appear solid to visual inspection. Fetal hydrops and maternal polyhydramnios are common with type III CCAM; because of associated abnormalities and respiratory compromise, the prognosis is poor. All types of CCAM have normal vascular supply and drainage (65,130,137,143).

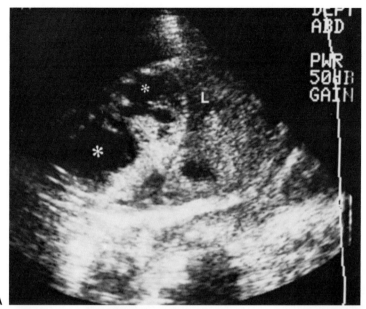

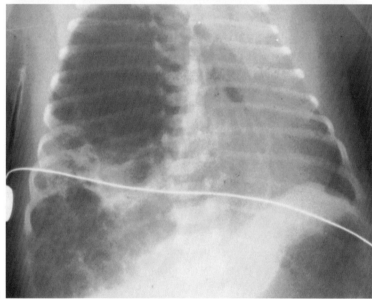

FIG. 7-62. Cystic adenomatoid malformation.
A: Antenatal longitudinal ultrasonography shows a multilocular cystic mass in the right thorax *(*)* that everts the right hemidiaphragm. *L*, liver. **B:** At 4 hours of age, an irregular cystic mass occupies the right thorax, displacing mediastinal structures to the left. (Courtesy of Randy Osborne, M.D., Colorado Springs, Colorado.) (*continued*)

The radiographic appearance of CCAM depends on the type, age of the patient, and presence of complications such as infection. Immediately after birth CCAM appears as a water density mass with mediastinal shift toward the other side. In a short time and with egress of fluid, a reticulated or bubbly appearance is seen (Fig. 7-62) (65,143).

Radiographically, type I lesions have one or more dominant cysts with adjacent smaller cysts and solid tissue elements (Fig. 7-63). Type II lesions display smaller, more evenly sized and spaced cysts (Fig. 7-64). Type III CCAM images as a solid mass and may be associated with fetal hydrops. In time, type I and II CCAM may show progressive enlargement of air-filled cysts and sometimes mimic congenital diaphragmatic hernia. Unlike diaphragmatic hernia, the distribution of abdominal bowel gas will be normal. The distended dominant cysts of CCAM may also mimic congenital lobar emphysema. Pneumonia with pneumatoceles, lung abscess, complicated bronchogenic cyst, and the rare cystic mesenchymal hamartoma are other differential diagnostic considerations. CT can be useful in characterizing CCAM by showing location and extent (65,144). On CT, a variably sized cystic mass with associated soft-tissue elements is typically seen (types I and II) (Figs. 7-63 and 7-64). Air-fluid levels may be seen with or without superimposed infection (65,144).

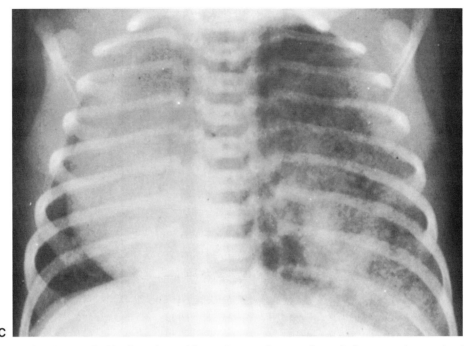

C

FIG. 7-62. *Continued.* **C:** Newborn boy with respiratory distress. Irregularly aerated mass in the left chest displaces the mediastinal structures to the right. There was a normal bowel gas pattern. (Courtesy of Gary D. Shackelford, M.D., St. Louis, Missouri.)

Pulmonary Sequestration

Sequestered lung is defined as "a congenital mass of aberrant pulmonary tissue that has no normal connection with the bronchial tree or with the pulmonary arteries" (124). It is usually supplied by an anomalous artery arising from the aorta, and its venous drainage is via the azygous system, the pulmonary veins, or the IVC (124,145). Although frequently asymptomatic, children with sequestered lung are usually seen because of superimposed infection. The sequestration is usually located in one of the basilar segments of a lower lobe (Fig. 7-65). If bronchography is performed, normal bronchi drape around the sequestration (Fig. 7-66B). Aortography demonstrates one or more systemic vessels entering the mass, often arising from the aorta just at or slightly below the level of the diaphragm (Fig. 7-66). The systemic vessel

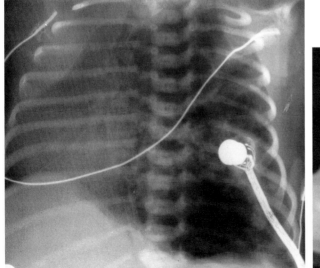

A

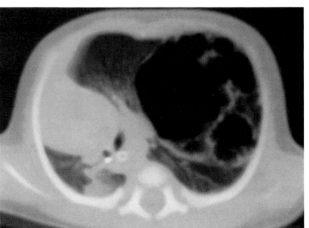

B

FIG. 7-63. **Type I congenital cystic adenomatoid malformation. A:** Chest radiograph at 4 hours of age shows a large cystic left lung mass with rightward mediastinal shift. **B:** Contrast enhanced chest CT shows a complex mass of the LUL containing cysts of various size and interposed soft-tissue elements.

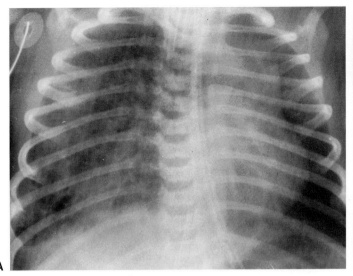
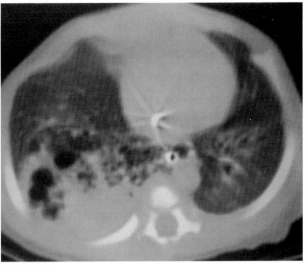

FIG. 7-64. **Type II congenital cystic adenomatoid malformation. A:** Newborn chest radiograph obtained for tachypnea shows a heterogeneous bubbly mass of the mid and lower right lung with mediastinal shift to the left. **B:** Contrast-enhanced CT shows a complex cystic RLL mass. There is more uniformity in the smaller cysts than seen in type I CCAM. Note the solid components. (Courtesy of Kenneth Hawkins, M.D., Birmingham, Alabama.)

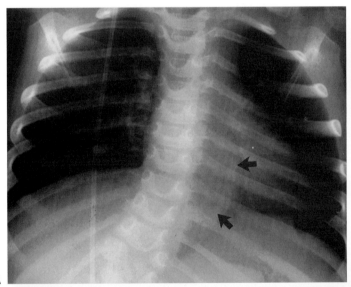
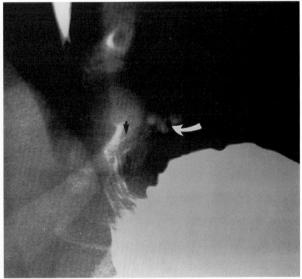
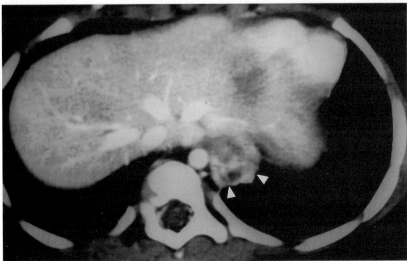

FIG. 7-65. **Sequestration. A:** Chest radiograph in a 5-year-old boy with cough, spina bifida, and congenital scoliosis. A vague medial LLL opacity *(arrows)* is noted; this failed to clear on follow-up radiographs. **B:** Contrast-enhanced chest CT shows a complex mass *(arrowheads)* of the medial basilar segment of the LLL. **C:** Esophagogram shows a fistulous connection *(arrows)* between the distal esophagus and the LLL sequestration *(curved arrow).*

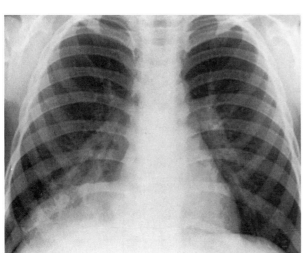

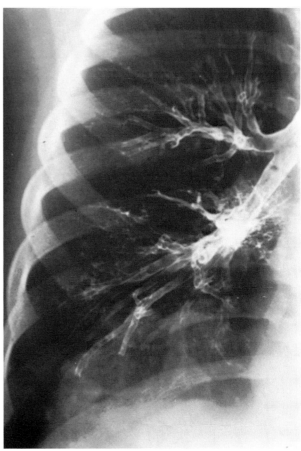

FIG. 7-66. Sequestration. A 7-year-old boy with recurrent pneumonia in posterior basilar segment of right lower lobe. **A:** Chest radiograph shows mass in right lower lobe. **B:** Anteroposterior bronchogram. The bronchi to the posterior basilar segment of the right lower lobe drape around but do not enter the mass. (*continued*)

runs in the inferior pulmonary ligament to reach the sequestered tissue.

Intralobar sequestration (ILS) is contained within the lung, has no separate pleural covering, and is intimately connected to adjacent lung (124,130,145). Venous drainage is usually by pulmonary veins (145). ILS is confined to a lower lobe in 98% of cases. The medial part of the left lower lobe is most often involved (Fig. 7-65). Although common in extralobar sequestration (ELS) (65%), CLE (42%), and type II CCAM (26%), anomalies elsewhere are present in only 12% of patients with ILS. Twenty-five percent of these associated anomalies are esophagobronchial fistulas (see Fig. 7-65).

ELS is located between the lower lobe and the diaphragm and has its own pleural covering (146). Ninety percent of ELS lesions are left-sided. They are usually drained by the azygous venous system (124,130,145,146). However, the venous drainage is not always clear-cut, and this is one reason many authorities consider the two types of sequestration to be embryologically related. Accessory lung bud development prior to pleural development leads, in theory, to intralobar sequestration whereas ELS occurs when the accessory lung budding occurs after pleural investments have formed, but this distinction may not be valid.

The modes of presentations of ILS and ELS are different. Most cases of intralobar sequestration are diagnosed after adolescence. Symptoms are often those of pneumonia, recurrent or refractory to therapy. It is uncommon to see symptomatic ILS in neonates and infants. ELS, on the other hand, presents most frequently during the first 6 months of life. Dyspnea, cyanosis, and feeding difficulties are common. Other associated anomalies are common (65%) with ELS; they include pulmonary hypoplasia, horseshoe lung, CCAM, bronchogenic cyst, diaphragmatic hernia, and cardiovascular anomalies such as truncus arteriosus and total anomalous pulmonary vessel return.

The imaging of suspected pulmonary sequestration is directed to identification of sequestered or dysplastic lung tissue; identification of aberrant arterial and venous connections; evaluation of possible bronchial or gastrointestinal connections; finding of associated lung anomalies such as horseshoe lung or hypoplasia; and assessment for diaphragmatic defects (146,147).

The radiographic appearance of ILS depends on the degree of aeration and the presence or absence of infection in the sequestered tissue. An airless opacity in the lung base (usually left) is a common early finding (Figs. 7-65

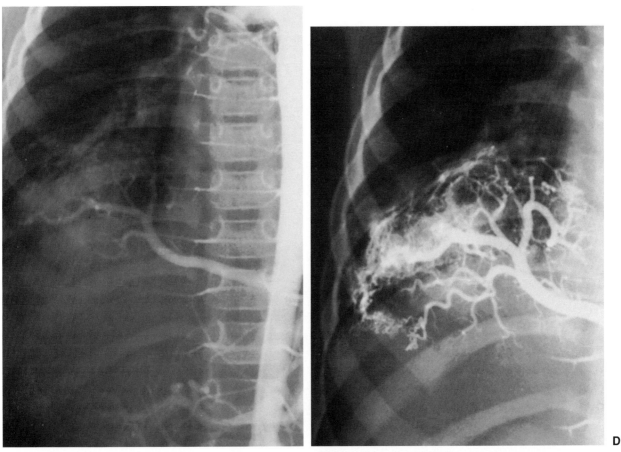

C   **D**

FIG. 7-66. *Continued.* **C, D:** Thoracic aortography **(C)** and selective arteriography **(D)** demonstrate a large systemic vessel arising from the aorta below the diaphragm and supplying the sequestration. Several hypertrophied bronchial arteries **(C)** also supply the sequestration because of recurrent infection.

and 7-66). With recurrent or chronic infection, a mixed cystic and water-density opacity is identified (Fig. 7-65). The newborn or infant with ELS typically shows a persistent water-density mass in the posteromedial thorax, usually on the left (Fig. 7-67). Barium studies may be used to rule out communication with the stomach or esophagus (Fig. 7-65C) (147). Pulmonary sequestrations may be demonstrated with sonography (Fig. 7-67B). This modality is particularly useful in the newborn or infant with a mass near the liver or diaphragm. Antenatal sonography depicting hydramnios and a fetal chest mass strongly suggests the diagnosis of ELS. Real-time, duplex, and color Doppler may demonstrate vascular connections to the sequestration (147).

CT in ILS localizes and shows the extent of abnormality; it may demonstrate arterial and venous connections (147). If infection has complicated the sequestration, then CT demonstrates a multicystic mass in the lung base (Fig. 7-65B). An ELS is a solid soft-tissue mass with variable enhancement next to the diaphragm (Fig. 7-67C).

MRI of pulmonary sequestration can characterize the pulmonary abnormalities and vascular connections in multiple imaging planes. In most cases, MRI with MR angiography (MRA) makes catheter angiography unnecessary (141,147).

However, selective angiography (particularly digital subtraction) may be necessary to characterize systemic arterial feeders and show venous anatomy preoperatively. Surgical treatment of sequestration requires complete removal of the involved parenchyma to prevent recurrent infection.

Not all pulmonary lesions with systemic arterial supply are sequestrations (148–150). Other congenital causes of systemic arterial supply include arteriovenous fistula, pulmonary artery aplasia or atresia, and systemic arterial supply to normal lung. Systemic arterial supply to an otherwise normal part of the lung is a rare congenital abnormality with characteristic radiologic features (Fig. 7-68). The opacity is usually in the basilar segment of the left lower lobe, but there is no mass effect or cystic change in the pulmonary parenchyma. The heart may be enlarged because of the left-to-left shunt. Bronchoscopy and bronchography demonstrate a normal bronchial supply to the involved segment of lung. Aortography and pulmonary angiography show a large systemic artery arising from the aorta just above the diaphragm providing part or all of the arterial supply to the involved segment (Fig. 7-68) (150). Acquired causes of systemic arterial supply to the lung include destructive bronchopulmonary disease, severe pulmonary infection, pleurectomy, and iatrogenic anastomosis, such as Blalock-Taussis shunt (148,150).

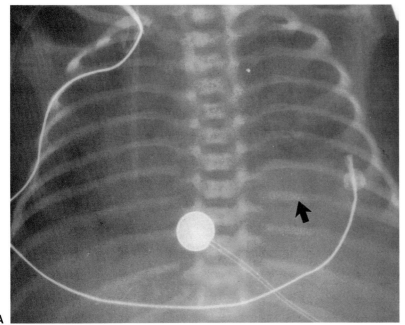

A

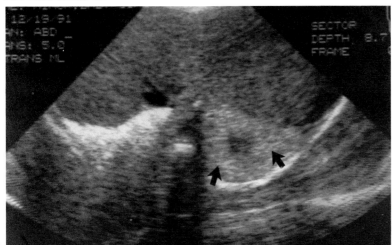

B

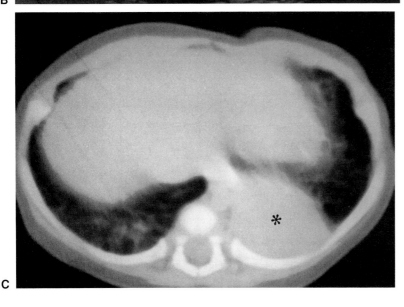

C

FIG. 7-67. Pulmonary sequestration. A: At 22 hours of age, chest radiography in this tachypneic newborn shows a left basilar water density mass *(arrow).* **B:** Transverse transabdominal ultrasonography shows a well-delineated, slightly hyperechoic oval mass in the left lower thorax *(arrows).* **C:** CT confirms a homogeneous soft-tissue mass in the left lower thorax *(*).*

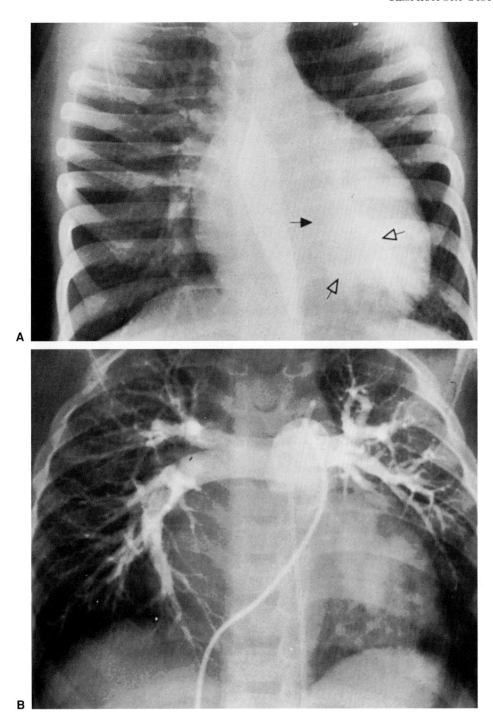

FIG. 7-68. Systemic arterial supply to normal lung. A: Chest radiograph of a 6-month-old boy with a continuous heart murmur heard best below the left clavicle. The heart is enlarged, and there is a density in the left lower lobe *(open arrows)* that obscures a portion of the descending aorta *(closed arrow).* **B:** Pulmonary angiogram. There are no vessels supplying the basilar segments of the left lower lobe. (*continued*)

Pulmonary Arteriovenous Malformation

Abnormal communications between blood vessels in the lung are acquired or congenital (151). Acquired connections are called *pulmonary fistulas* and are associated with liver disease, cyanotic heart disease, chronic pulmonary infection, and emphysema. Congenital arteriovenous malformations (AVMs) are abnormal communications between pulmonary arteries and veins without an intervening capillary bed. These lesions are usually clinically silent in infancy and childhood. However, cyanosis, polycythemia, dyspnea, and digital clubbing sometimes develop. Multiple lesions are

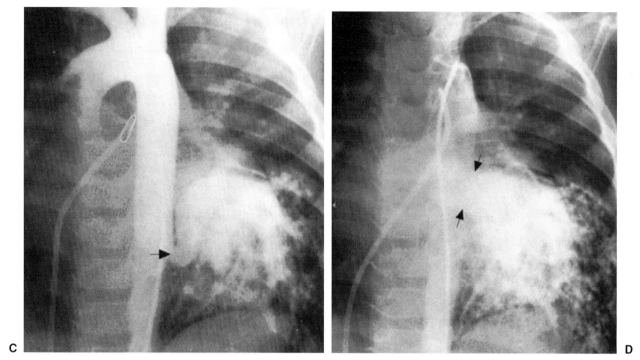

C

D

FIG. 7-68. *Continued.* **C:** Thoracic aortogram, arterial phase. A large artery off the descending aorta *(arrow)* supplies the basilar segments of the left lower lobe. **D:** Thoracic aortogram, venous phase. There is drainage of the basilar segments into the left atrium by a large inferior pulmonary vein *(arrows)*. From Kirks et al. (150).

common (33% to 50%) as is bilaterality (8% to 20%) (130). About 60% are in the lower lobes, and 60% occur in patients with the autosomal dominant disorder Osler-Weber-Rendu disease (hereditary hemorrhagic telangiectasia) (130).

The typical radiographic finding is a round or oval, well-defined pulmonary mass that often is lobulated (Fig. 7-69). Feeding or draining vessels are pathognomonic (Fig. 7-69D). The Valsalva and Mueller maneuvers alter lesion size. Contrast-enhanced CT or MRI can show the vascular nature of the lesion and characterize it further. Pulmonary angiography is used to identify other lesions, evaluate the contralateral lung, and guide occlusive therapy (Fig. 7-69D) (130, 151,152).

Horseshoe Lung

Horseshoe lung is a very rare congenital anomaly of pulmonary development in which the bases of the left and right lungs are joined by a parenchymal isthmus posterior to the heart (127,153). It is associated with anomalies of bronchopulmonary and cardiovascular development. The isthmus may be demonstrated by CT, MRI, or autopsy.

Diagnosis of horseshoe lung is based on the demonstration of lung fusion without intervening pleura. Accessory bronchi and pulmonary vessels pass through this isthmus. The pulmonary arteries, veins, bronchi, and esophagus should be carefully evaluated prior to surgery (127,153).

Diaphragmatic Abnormalities

Anomalies such as diaphragmatic hernia, eventration, and agenesis may be associated with malformations of the lung and may cause severe respiratory symptoms.

Congenital Diaphragmatic Hernia

Bochdalek hernia (hernia through the posterior pleuroperitoneal foramen) usually causes severe respiratory distress in the neonate. It is one of the most common congenital anomalies of the thorax. The diagnosis is frequently made by prenatal sonography. The left pleuroperitoneal foramen is usually involved (75%). The neonatal radiographic appearance may be that of a large intrathoracic mass of soft-tissue density (Fig 7-70A). The more characteristic pattern of many intrathoracic air-filled loops of bowel is found after several hours (Fig. 7-70B). There is an absence of normal amounts of gas-containing bowel in the abdomen, and the abdomen is scaphoid on physical examination. The prognosis in neonates with congenital diaphragmatic hernia correlates with the degree of underlying lung hypoplasia (125). Other causes of cystic or cystic-appearing intrathoracic masses in the newborn include lobar emphysema, cystic adenomatoid malformation, sequestration, bronchogenic cyst, and other developmental lesions of the lung (130).

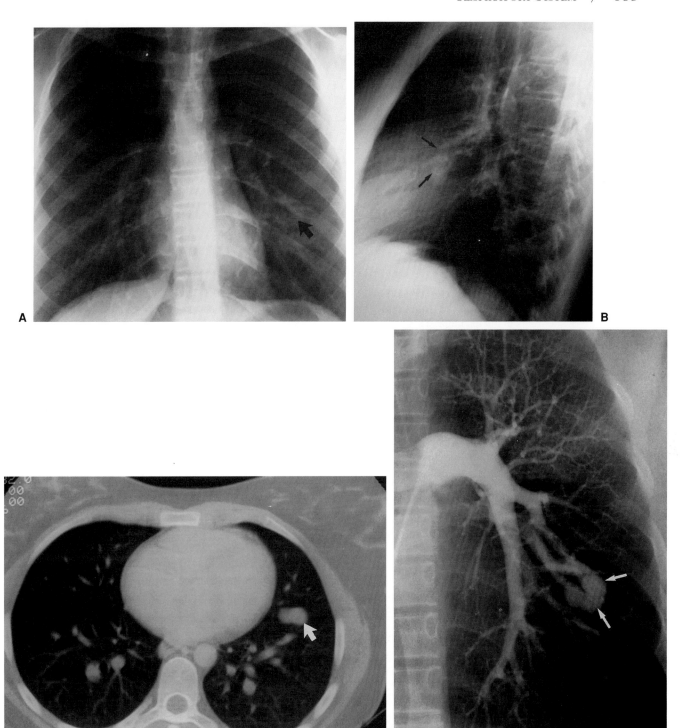

FIG. 7-69. Congenital pulmonary arteriovenous malformation (AVM). A: This 15-year-old girl had fever and cough. The PA chest radiograph shows a lobular lingular mass *(arrow)*. **B:** The comet-tail appearance on the lateral chest radiograph *(arrows)* suggests a vascular lesion. **C:** Contrast-enhanced CT shows an enhancing lobular varicose lingular mass *(arrow)*. **D:** Pulmonary angiography demonstrates a lingular arteriovenous malformation *(arrows)*. (Courtesy of Yoginder Vaid, M.D., Birmingham, Alabama.)

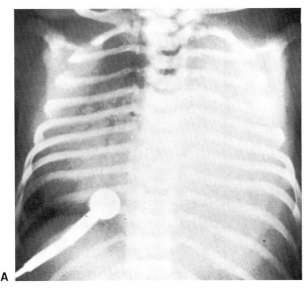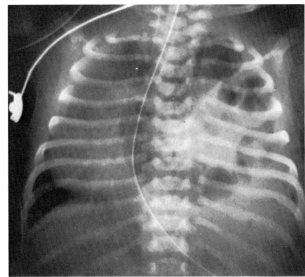

A

B

FIG. 7-70. Diaphragmatic (Bochdalek) hernia. A: Newborn male with respiratory distress. Large soft-tissue mass of the left chest displaces the heart and trachea to the right. **B:** By 6 hours of age, air-filled loops of bowel are identified in the left thorax.

Congenital Eventration of the Diaphragm

Congenital diaphragmatic eventration is either partial or complete and is usually right-sided. Hypoplasia of the diaphragmatic muscle is supposedly the cause (154–156). Patients who have pulmonary symptoms may require surgical plication (Fig. 7-71). When severe, the condition causes severe neonatal respiratory distress; plain films may mimic those of diaphragmatic hernia. However, most eventrations are minor, transitory, local diaphragmatic elevations found incidentally on chest films in the first few years of life. They disappear with age.

Diaphragmatic Paresis and Paralysis

Serial chest radiographs and knowledge of a central neurologic or phrenic nerve insult aid in making this diagnosis (Fig. 7-72). In some cases, bedside sonography or fluoroscopy will be required to distinguish a weak (paretic) from a paralyzed hemidiaphragm (157,158). Imaging assessment should be performed with the patient temporarily off of ventilatory support. It may be impossible to distinguish a severe congenital eventration from a paralyzed hemidiaphragm (159).

Vascular Rings

The infant or child who presents with apneic episodes, choking, stridulous breathing, wheezing, or dysphagia warrants a prompt and comprehensive workup. The possibility of a vascular ring must be considered when these symptoms develop. A well-positioned, properly penetrated chest radio-graph is an excellent screening study for symptomatic vascular ring; the major aortic shadow will be found on the right. A normal esophagogram almost always rules out the diagnosis. MRI has become the imaging procedure of choice to define anatomy (33,141). This topic is further discussed in Chapter 6.

General Abnormalities

Abnormalities of Aeration

Abnormalities of lung aeration may be localized or generalized. Localized abnormalities of aeration are often due to intrinsic or extrinsic narrowing of the airway to a localized segment of lung. Common causes of localized abnormalities of aeration include foreign body and mucous plugging.

Abnormalities of aeration of the lung include hypoaeration and hyperaeration (Table 7-6). Normal aeration of the lung depends on integrated function of the CNS, neuromuscular system, thoracic cage, and pulmonary parenchyma. Generalized abnormalities of aeration may be congenital, inflammatory, neoplastic, or miscellaneous (Table 7-6).

Hypoaeration is manifested radiologically by elevation of the diaphragm and loss of the normal cylindrical shape of the thorax. In the newborn, hypoaeration produces a bell-shaped thorax (see Fig. 7-14D). Hypoaeration leads to an increase in the transverse diameter of the heart and prominence of the central pulmonary vascularity. Hypoaeration is most frequently due to chest radiographs being obtained near or at expiration (see Fig. 7-13). It may also be due to CNS abnormalities, interruption of the normal neural and muscular activity of the diaphragm or other thoracic muscles, intrinsic or extrinsic abnormalities of the skeletal components

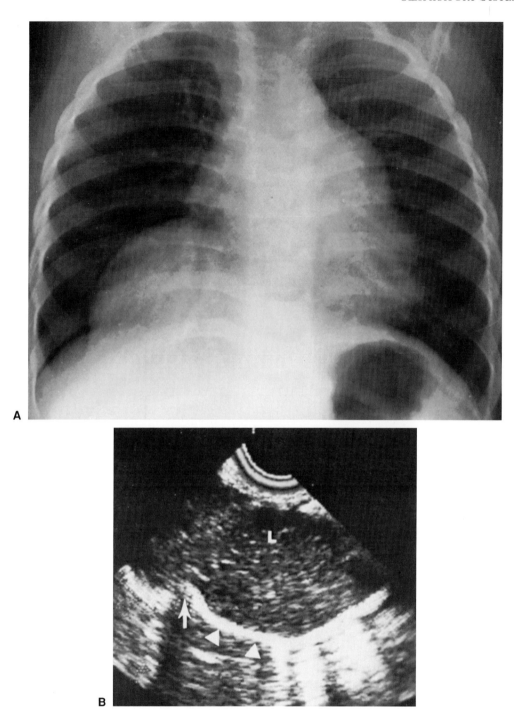

FIG. 7-71. Anteromedial diaphragmatic defect. A: Chest radiograph of an 18-month-old boy with recurrent respiratory tract infection shows focal anteromedial elevation of the right hemidiaphragm. **B:** Longitudinal right parasagittal sonography demonstrates diaphragm *(arrowheads)*, diaphragmatic discontinuity *(arrow)*, and liver *(L)*. Ultrasonography confirmed cephalad movement of the herniated liver as the diaphragm moved inferiorly. (*continued*)

of the thorax, or primary pulmonary abnormalities (Table 7-6) (101).

Hyperaeration is manifested radiologically by an increased lung volume. The diaphragms are flattened on both AP and lateral projections. There is an increase in the retrosternal lucency and anterior convexity of the sternum. In the AP projection, the diaphragms are below the level of the eighth ribs anteriorly or the tenth ribs posteriorly (see Fig. 7-13C). The pulmonary parenchyma is lucent; however, lucency is also caused by overpenetration. Generalized hyperaeration may be due to increased central respiratory drive, increased air flow to the lungs, partial obstruction of bronchi

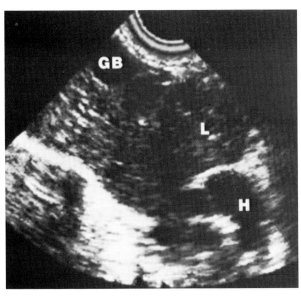
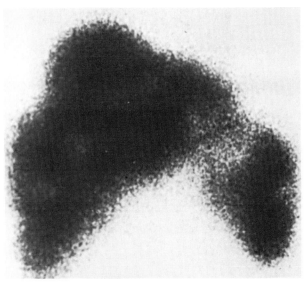

FIG. 7-71. *Continued.* **C:** Subcostal oblique view extending from the gallbladder *(GB)* to the heart *(H)*. The relation of the herniated liver *(L)* and the heart is noted. **D:** ^{99m}Tc sulfur colloid scan shows focal hepatic herniation. From Merten et al. (154).

TABLE 7-6. *Abnormalities of aeration*

Hypoaeration	Hyperaeration
Normal	Congenital
Expiration[a]	Cystic fibrosis[a]
Rapid eye movement (REM) sleep	α_1-Antitrypsin deficiency
Neuromuscular	Inflammatory
Central nervous system (CNS) depression	Viral airways disease[a]
Coma	Bronchiolitis
Drugs	Bronchitis, laryngotracheobronchitis
CNS tumor	Bronchopneumonia
Ondine's curse	Asthma[a]
Postoperative complications[a]	Tumor
Muscular	Endotracheal
Trauma	Compression
Amyotonia	Miscellaneous
Myasthenia	Asthma[a]
Myotonic dystrophy	Congenital heart disease[a]
Thoracic	Failure
Bone dysplasia	Shunt
Asphyxiating thoracic dystrophy	Emphysema
Osteogenesis imperfecta	Airway obstruction or compression
Lethal dwarfism	Foreign body[a]
Flail chest	Vascular ring
Abdominal distention[a]	Tumor
Ascites	Tracheomalacia
Mass	Tracheal stenosis
Intestinal obstruction	Hyperventilation
Pulmonary	Acidosis
Airway	Dehydration
Mucous plug[a]	Sepsis
Malpositioned endotracheal tube[a]	Respirator therapy[a]
Foreign body	Adult respiratory distress syndrome (ARDS)
Trauma	Tracheoesophageal fistula
Parenchyma	
Pneumonia	
Irradiation	
Hyaline membrane disease[a]	
Hypoplasia	

[a] More common.

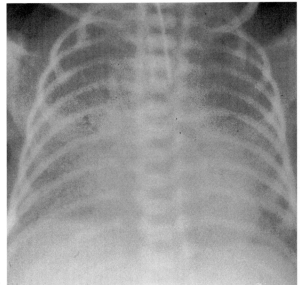

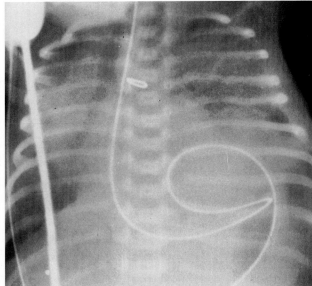

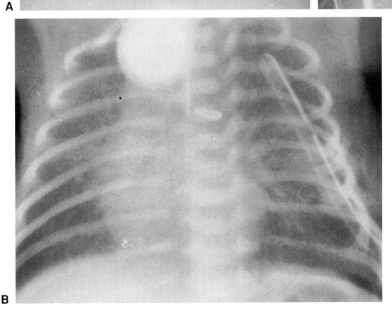

FIG. 7-72. Left hemidiaphragmatic paralysis. A: Chest radiograph at 72 hours of age in this premature newborn with respiratory distress shows diffuse pulmonary granularity consistent with respiratory distress syndrome and superimposed interstitial edema due to a patent ductus arteriosus (PDA). **B:** Chest radiograph immediately after PDA ligation. There are postoperative changes and symmetric hemidiaphragm positions. **C:** Chest x-ray 10 days after surgery. Left hemidiaphragm is elevated, presumably because of iatrogenic left phrenic nerve injury and diaphragmatic paralysis. Note the position of the stomach, marked by the enteric tube.

and bronchioles, or pulmonary parenchymal destruction (Table 7-6).

Abnormal aeration may be manifest as asymmetric lung aeration. Determining which side is abnormal may be a challenge (Table 7-7). The physiologic interrelation between lung size, aeration, and pulmonary blood flow yields clues to the diagnosis (160,161). On an inspiratory frontal chest radiograph, the hemithorax with normal or increased vascularity is usually normal. The hemithorax (large or small) with diminished vascularity is usually the abnormal side. The hemithorax, which changes least on an inspiratory-expiratory film, is abnormal (121,160). A large opaque hemithorax is most commonly caused by infection (empyema). Large pleural effusion from tumor (lymphoma or primitive neurectodermal tumor), a primary pulmonary mass, and trauma (hemothorax) must also be considered (Fig. 7-73) (162). Pulmonary agenesis gives rise to a small opaque hemi-

thorax (see Fig. 7-54). Pulmonary atelectasis may show a small opaque or semiopaque hemithorax. The normally sized partially opaque hemithorax is commonly due to posterior layering of an effusion. The large hyperlucent hemithorax is usually due to obstructive or compensatory emphysema (Fig. 7-74); Inspiratory-expiratory and decubitus views can help to make the distinction (8,9,163). Finally, a small hyperlucent lung may be secondary to pulmonary artery or lung hypoplasia or the Swyer-James syndrome; the latter shows air trapping on an expiratory film (Table 7-7).

Pleura and Pleural Effusion

The lungs are surrounded by two layers of pleura, a membrane that covers the lung (visceral pleura) and the inner lining of the thorax (parietal pleura). Between the two is a

TABLE 7-7. *Unilateral hyperlucent lung*

Extrapulmonary causes	Large hilus
Technical problems	External bronchial obstruction
Rotation[a]	Nodes
Poor positioning	Tumor
Scoliosis[a]	Asymmetric chronic pulmonary disease
Grid cutoff	Cystic fibrosis[a]
Lateral decentering	Chronic obstructive pulmonary disease
Decubitus film	Congenital bronchial atresia
Soft tissues	Pulmonary sling (aberrant left pulmonary
Breast	artery)
Asymmetry	Congenital absence of pulmonary value
Mastectomy	No air trapping
Absent pectoralis muscles	Small hilus
Congenital (Poland syndrome)	Pulmonary underdevelopment
Surgical	Agenesis
Hemiatrophy	Aplasia
Skeletal disorders	Hypoplasia
Scoliosis[a]	Proximal interruption of pulmonary artery
Pectus excavatum or carinatum	Postlobectomy
Hemiatrophy	Normal hilus
Pulmonary causes	Compensatory hyperinflation
Air trapping	Congenital heart disease
Small hilus	Tetralogy of Fallot[a]
Swyer-James syndrome	Pulmonary stenosis
Congenital lobar emphysema	Patent ductus arteriosus
Normal hilus	Contralateral disease
Endobronchial obstruction	Chest wall
Inflammation	Pleural
Foreign body[a]	Parenchymal[a]
Tumor	Pneumothorax[a]
Parenchymal disease	Pulmonary artery branch stenosis
Bulla	Large hilus
Cysts	Pulmonary artery occlusion
Bronchiectasis	Embolus
	Thrombus
	Tumor
	Scimitar syndrome

[a] More common.

Modified from Cumming et al. (160), Kirkpatrick (72), and MacPherson et al. (161).

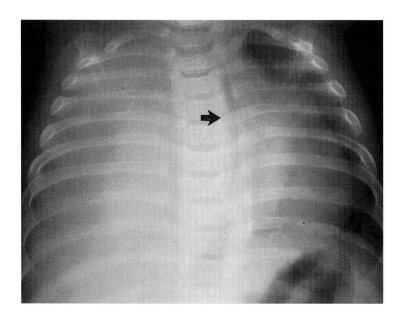

FIG. 7-73. Large opaque hemithorax. Newborn with tachypnea. The AP chest radiograph shows a large opaque right hemithorax. Note the tracheal displacement *(arrow)*, depression of right main bronchus, and cardiomediastinal shift. A large, infected, parenchymal bronchogenic cyst was surgically resected.

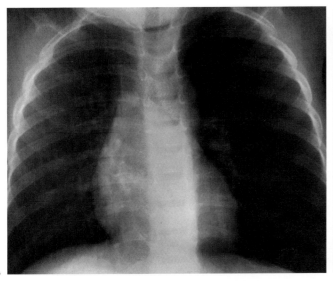

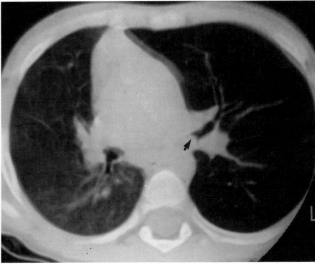

A

B

FIG. 7-74. **Asymmetric lung aeration.** A 3-year-old boy with chronic cough. **A:** Chest x-ray shows a large, hyperlucent left lung with diminished vascularity and shift of the mediastinum from left to right. **B:** CT section through the level of the left mainstem bronchus. A peanut *(arrow)* is obstructing the bronchus and causing hyperinflation of the left lung.

potential space. The pleural membranes are lined by mesothelial cells. Pulmonary artery branches supply the visceral pleural; intercostal artery branches supply the parietal pleura. Subepithelial lymphatics of the parietal pleura drain into the internal mammary, intercostal, and mediastinal nodes. The visceral pleura drains into mediastinal nodes (1).

Pleural fluid is usually evident on PA and lateral views of the chest. However, a minimum of 400 ml of pleural liquid is required for radiographic visualization on an upright adult chest x-ray. Expiratory views optimize visibility of small collections. Fluid fills the lateral and posterior costophrenic sulci and then tracks along the lateral and posterior chest walls in a meniscus configuration (1,8). Occasionally, pleural fluid is purely subpulmonic in location. The diaphragm appears elevated and what seems to be its dome on the AP film is more lateral in location than normal (see Fig. 7-23). Pleural fluid also may be seen in the medial pleural space as a triangular density to the left, and sometimes to the right, of the lower thoracic spine. Many children are radiographed supine; in this position, pleural fluid tends to accumulate posteriorly and causes a general increase in the density of the hemithorax. In the supine patient, fluid may also cap the lung apex. Decubitus films are sensitive to small amounts of pleural fluid (as little as 50 ml), which usually layers in the dependent part of the pleural space (see Fig. 7-23B). It must be stressed that the decubitus technique may show a small amount of pleural fluid (a layer 1.5–2.0 mm thick) in normal children (42). Sonography is valuable for confirming pleural effusion. It can also localize loculated collections and guide pleural drainage.

The pleural space is kept nearly empty of liquid through equilibrium between filtration and absorption. When filtration exceeds absorption, pleural effusions form. Starling forces may be altered when capillary permeability is increased, as in infection and systemic lupus erythematosus, when capillary hydrostatic pressure is increased (overhydration), plasma oncotic pressure is decreased (hypoalbuminemia), or parenchymal oncotic pressure is increased (pulmonary infarction). Altered lymphatic flow due to nephrosis, hepatic cirrhosis, adenopathy, tumor, or lymphatic disruption may also lead to pleural effusions (Fig. 7-75).

The differential diagnosis of pleural effusion in infants

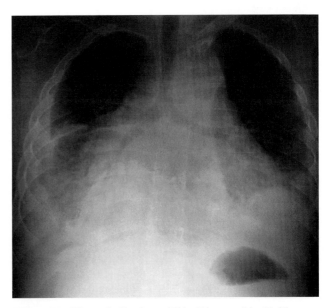

FIG. 7-75. **Pleural effusions.** This 15-year-old with Noonan syndrome, hypertrophic cardiomyopathy, and pulmonary valvular stenosis shows interlobular septal lines (Kerley lines) and large, bilateral pleural effusions.

TABLE 7-8. *Differential diagnosis of pleural effusion*

Idiopathic	Trauma
Congenital	Hemorrhage
Chylothorax[a]	Chylothorax
Erythroblastosis fetalis	Hydrocarbon pneumonitis
Lymphangiectasia	Esophageal rupture
Primary	Irradiation
Secondary	Iatrogenic
Generalized	Postoperative:
Congenital nephrosis	postpneumonectomy[a]
Infection	Miscellaneous
Bacterial	Wet lung disease[a]
Pneumococcal[a]	Congestive heart failure[a]
Staphylococcal	Hypoproteinemia
Hemophilus	Renal disease[a]
Tuberculosis	Nephrotic syndrome
Empyema	Glomerulonephritis
Fungal	Cirrhosis
Viral (unusual)	Collagen vascular
Neoplasm	disease
Generalized	Lupus erythematosus
Lymphoma-leukemia	Rheumatoid disease
Neuroblastoma	Abdominal inflammatory
Skeletal	disease
Askin tumor	Appendicitis
Ewing sarcoma	Abscess
Osteogenic sarcoma	Pancreatitis
Metastatic disease	Lymphatic obstruction
Pleural	Tumor
Sarcoma	Parasite
Metastatic disease	Mediterranean fever
Mesothelioma	Niemann-Pick disease
Parenchymal	Ruptured aneurysm
Lymphoma-leukemia[a]	Mycotic
Sarcoma	Coarctation
Mesenchymoma	Sarcoidosis
Lymphangioma	Venous obstruction
Hemangioma	
Dermoid cyst	

[a] More common.

and children is extensive (Table 7-8) (2,6,8,9,164). Density in the pleural space, as in any other cavity, may be blood, pus, water, or cells. A small pleural effusion in the newborn is usually due to wet lung disease and delayed clearance of lung fluid. Larger amounts of pleural fluid in the newborn suggest chylothorax.

Pleural fluid in association with lobar consolidation is usually an exudate caused by bacterial infection. The most common cause of pulmonary consolidation and pleural effusion in children in the United States is still pneumococcal (*Streptococcus pneumoniae*) pneumonia. However, the possibilities of primary tuberculosis, *Staphylococcus aureus* pneumonia, or *Hemophilus influenzae* pneumonia should also be considered. A pleural tap with stain, culture, and cytology is useful for diagnosis. Pleural fluid in association with bacterial infection may be due to parenchymal edema, lymphatic congestion, or actual extension of infection into the pleural space (empyema). Pleural effusion in viral pneumonia is unusual (2,6,8,9,164). Pulmonary infection may also be

complicated by other pleural problems, such as pneumothorax and bronchopleural fistulas.

Pleural effusion due to pulmonary neoplasm is less common in the child than in the adult. It may be seen with tumors of the chest wall, pleura, pulmonary parenchyma, or mediastinum. Pleural effusion in association with thymic enlargement suggests T-cell leukemia or T-cell non-Hodgkin's lymphoma (NHL). Pleural effusion may be the presenting radiologic sign of Ewing sarcoma of the bony thorax and of metastatic neuroblastoma (Table 7-8).

Another cause of pleural effusion is an abnormality of oncotic forces which allows fluid (transudate) to pass into the pleural space. Common examples are congestive heart failure, renal disease, and hypoproteinemia. Other causes of pleural effusion in infants and children include trauma, abdominal inflammatory disease, collagen vascular disease, and SVC occlusion causing chylothorax (Table 7-8) (9,164).

Newborn Chest Radiology

General Abnormalities

Profound physiologic changes occur during conversion from placental dependence for respiratory function to pulmonary dependence (113). Substantially complete aeration of the lungs occurs within two to three breaths in the normal newborn. Respiratory distress is the most common abnormality of the newborn (7,10,60). Lung disorders are responsible for approximately half of all deaths in newborn infants and for significant morbidity in those who survive (7,60).

Many disorders cause dyspnea during the first days of life (Table 7-9) (165). Radiology plays a critical role in its evaluation. The history and physical examination in the neonate are of much less value than in the older child and adult; thus radiologic examination becomes very important. All newborns with respiratory distress should have AP views of the chest, and the films should be interpreted immediately (60). Lateral films may be obtained if needed.

There are extrathoracic and intrathoracic causes of respiratory distress (Table 7-9). Intrathoracic causes may be of the chest wall, pleural, cardiac, or pulmonary. Pulmonary causes of respiratory distress in the newborn may be surgical or medical (Table 7-9) (7,10,60). Surgical disease, in contrast to medical disease, is usually asymmetric (166); there is almost always evidence of mass effect in abnormalities requiring surgical intervention (7,12).

Normal Newborn Chest

One must have an ordered approach to the newborn chest radiograph (see Table 7-2). General technique should be assessed by analyzing positioning, degree of inspiration, penetration, and motion. The chest film is then systematically analyzed beginning with extrathoracic structures and progressing to the thorax, heart, and lungs (60).

TABLE 7-9. *Respiratory distress in the newborn*

Extrathoracic causes
  Intracranial
    Hemorrhage[a]
    Tumor
  Neuromuscular
    Depression (low Apgar score)[a]
    Narcotized[a]
    Myasthenia
    Muscular dystrophy
    Cord laceration
  Abdominal
    Mass
    Perforation
    Obstruction
    Ascites
  Systemic
    Sepsis[a]
    Anemia
Intrathoracic causes
  Cardiac[a]
  Pulmonary
    Surgical
      Bochdalek hernia[a]
      Esophageal atresia/TEF[a]
      Diaphragm
        Paresis
        Paralysis
        Eventration
      Cephalic fold defect
      Lobar emphysema[a]
      Mass
        Neurenteric cyst
        Cystic adenomatoid malformation
        Sequestration
        Bronchogenic cyst
        Mesenchymoma
        Pulmonary sling with airway obstruction
        Neurogenic tumor
        Mediastinal mass
      Pleural effusion
        Chyle
        Blood
        Pus
      Pneumomediastinum[a]
      Pneumothorax[a]
    Medical
      Wet lung disease[a]
      Immature lung
      Hyaline membrane disease (respiratory distress syndrome)[a]
      Chronic pulmonary disease
        Wilson-Mikity syndrome
        Bronchopulmonary dysplasia[a]
      Atelectasis[a]
      Meconium aspiration[a]
      Aspiration
      Neonatal pneumonia[a]
      Pulmonary hemorrhage
      Pulmonary lymphangiectasia
      Erythrocythemia
      Chest wall
        Muscular disease
        Bony thorax abnormality

[a] More common
TEF, tracheoesophageal fistula

In the normal newborn thorax, the anteroposterior and transverse diameters are nearly equal. For this reason, there is an increase of only 2–4 kilovoltage peak (kVp) from the AP view to the lateral view. The normal newborn thorax has a trapezoidal or lamp shade shape on AP radiographs, with the ribs being fairly horizontal (60). The lateral margins of the thorax diverge slightly in a caudal direction (see Fig. 7-14A). The thorax is abnormally bell-shaped with CNS damage, neuromuscular abnormality, an abnormal thoracic cage, or severe pulmonary parenchymal disease (see Fig. 7-14D) (7,9,10). In these conditions, the narrowing of the upper thorax and flaring of the lower ribs are associated with a more vertical position of the ribs, to produce a sagging appearance of the chest and a bell-shaped configuration (see Fig. 7-14D).

The thymus is usually identified in term newborns and may be quite prominent, particularly in patients with hyaline membrane disease. This organ consists of right and left lobes and occupies the anterior part of the superior mediastinum. There is usually a notch where the inferior margin of the thymus meets the silhouette of the heart. Occasionally, the lateral margin of the thymus has a wavy contour, which is due to anterior costal cartilages indenting the soft thymus at several levels. This "wave sign" is more apparent on oblique views. The thymus frequently extends into the minor fissure or pushes the right upper lobe out over the fissure on both AP and lateral views. The sharp inferior margin on the AP view produces a "sail sign." The thymus looks even more prominent on an expiration film.

The heart is more globular in shape in the newborn infant than in the older child (7,60). This is due to normal prominence of the right-sided cardiac structures, but it makes individual cardiac chambers even more difficult to identify. The aortic arch may be hidden behind the overlying thymus. The trachea just above its bifurcation deviates away from the side of the aortic arch; this is exaggerated during expiration, but neonatal chest films often fail to show the side of the aorta clearly. There is a wide range of normal for the cardiothorax index of newborns; the upper limit is about 65% (60). However, when the newborn heart enlarges, it usually does so in all directions; therefore the distance between the posterior margin of the heart and the spine is decreased on the lateral view. The posterior border of the normal heart should not extend behind the trachea on the lateral film. The heart should be considered enlarged if the cardiothoracic index is greater than 65% or the posterior margin of the heart projects behind a line drawn as a continuation of the trachea in a patient with a normal thoracic configuration (60).

The hemidiaphragms are smooth and dome-like on both frontal and lateral views. Their domes are anterior and medial to their midportion (7,10,60). At quiet inspiration, the hemidiaphragms on an AP view are at the levels of the sixth ribs anteriorly and the eighth or ninth ribs posteriorly.

The lungs of the normal newborn are more radiolucent than those of older children. Air bronchograms may be seen normally in the medial thirds of the lung parenchyma.

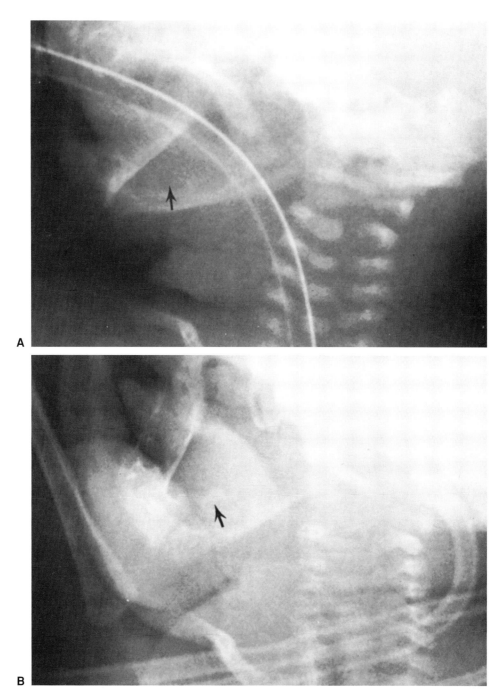

FIG. 7-76. Tooth maturation for determining gestational age. A: Premature infant, less than 33 weeks gestation. No enamel is seen in the first molar cusp *(arrow)*. **B:** A 33-week-gestation premature infant. Oblique view of the mandible from a chest radiograph shows some enamel in the first molar cusp *(arrow)*. (*continued*)

Knowledge of the gestational age and skeletal maturation in the newborn is important for the diagnosis of many abnormalities. For example, pulmonary disease in a newborn of 30 weeks gestation is much more likely to be immature lung or respiratory distress syndrome (RDS) than in a 40-week, small-for-date baby (7,23). The presence of the proximal humeral ossification center indicates a term newborn; ossification here never occurs before 36 weeks gestation but is seen in 40% of patients between 40 and 41 weeks gestation and in 82% at 42 weeks gestation (23). The presence of the proximal humeral ossification center in a neonate with cyanosis suggests complete transposition of the great vessels (23). Skeletal maturation is delayed by many intrauterine disorders.

Tooth maturation is the most useful guide for determining gestational age from chest radiographs (23). Enamel is seen

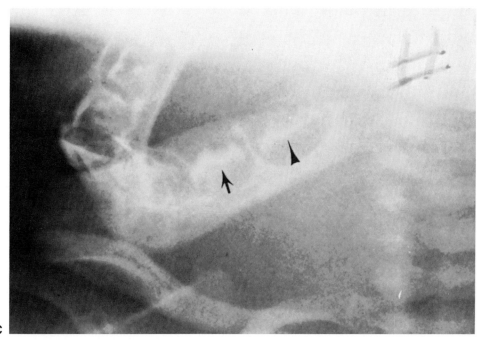

FIG. 7-76. *Continued.* **C:** Well-formed enamel is seen in the cusps of the first *(arrow)* and second *(arrowhead)* molar cusps of a term newborn (>36 weeks gestation).

in the cusps of the first deciduous molars at 33 weeks gestation and in the second deciduous molars at 36 weeks gestation (Fig. 7-76) (23).

Immature Lung Disease

Immature lung is a condition of small premature infants whose clinical, radiologic, and prognostic features are different from those of patients with RDS (167,168). These small, premature infants have birth weights of less than 1500 g; the average is approximately 1000 g (167). Unlike RDS, there is usually absence of clinical signs of respiratory distress until 4–7 days of life. Surfactant phospholipid components are present probably because of accelerated production of surfactant from intrauterine stress (167). However, there is typically insufficient surfactant to maintain alveolar ventilation.

Patients with immature lung disease have diffuse granularity of the lungs, which may be confused with RDS. However, there is a relative absence of air bronchograms and little or no lung underaeration (167,169). The radiologic granularity of the lungs is probably due to summation of densities of the thickened interstitium (167,169). The initial radiographs may be normal in immature lung disease.

Complications of immature lung disease include apnea with bradycardia and persistent patency of the ductus arteriosus (167). These complications may require ventilation, but the incidence of air block phenomena is much lower than with respiratory distress syndrome because only low ventilator pressures and rates are required for support. Intraventricular hemorrhage, bronchopulmonary dysplasia, necrotizing enterocolitis, and death are fairly common in those patients

born at <1000 g. This entity should be distinguished from RDS, as the overall survival (82%) for immature lung disease is considerably better than that for RDS (167,168).

Respiratory Distress Syndrome

Etiology

Respiratory distress syndrome, also known as hyaline membrane disease (HMD), is a disease of hypoventilation and a manifestation of pulmonary immaturity. It is seen predominantly in newborns under 36–38 weeks of gestational age who weigh less than 2.5 kg. RDS remains the leading cause of death in liveborn infants. Clinical symptoms have their onset shortly after birth and are characterized by abnormal retraction of the chest wall, cyanosis, increased respiratory rate, and expiratory grunting. At autopsy, the lungs are noncompliant and atelectatic; the interstitium of the lung is thickened, and the dilated terminal airways are usually lined with hyaline membranes (7,13,14). RDS, a distinct pathologic entity, is due to a deficiency of pulmonary surfactant (170). Surfactant is a phospholipid complex synthesized by the type II pneumocyte, which coats the alveolar lining cells and prevents atelectasis by lowering surface tension in alveoli. This effect increases pulmonary compliance and decreases breathing effort (13,14). Hyaline membranes not only may be seen with other disease processes but also are frequently absent in patients with RDS who die at less than 4 hours of age. These facts support the use of the term *respiratory distress syndrome* (RDS) rather than the classic term *hyaline membrane disease* (HMD).

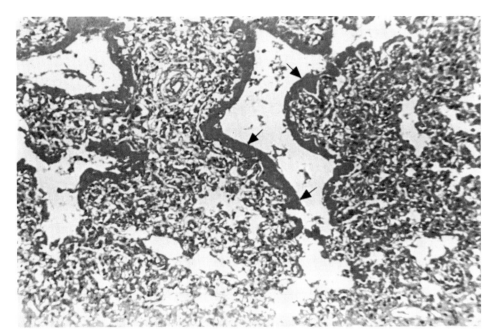

FIG. 7-77. Histology of respiratory distress syndrome (hyaline membrane disease). There are many atelectatic alveoli and hyaline membranes *(arrows).*

Pathology

The hallmark pathologic finding in RDS is acinar atelectasis (Fig. 7-77). The diffuse collapse of alveoli is associated with interstitial edema and damage to alveolar epithelium (168). There is overdistention of the terminal bronchioles and terminal air sacs in association with the acinar atelectasis, which can lead to rupture of the terminal air sacs with air block complications (pneumothorax, pneumomediastinum, and pulmonary interstitial emphysema). Exposure to air rapidly leads to the development of hyaline membranes containing fibrin and cellular debris (Fig. 7-77). Hyaline membranes are formed by proteinaceous exudate; there is frequently epithelial necrosis beneath the hyaline membranes (7). The lungs in RDS are almost impossible to inflate and look grossly like liver. Alveolar atelectasis and dilatation of terminal airways, rather than the presence of hyaline membranes, are the important pathologic characteristics of RDS (170).

Clinical Features

The primary factors predisposing to RDS are prematurity and perinatal asphyxia. Surfactant production begins at approximately 24 weeks gestation and increases with gestational age. For this reason, the incidence of RDS decreases with increasing maturity as follows: less than 1000 g, 66%; 1000 g (27 weeks gestation), 50%; 1500 g (31 weeks gestation), 16%; 2000 g (34 weeks gestation), 5%; 2500 g (36 weeks gestation), 1% (7,59). Males are affected almost twice

as often as females. RDS is more common at any given gestational age in whites than in blacks. The onset of clinical symptoms is usually at birth and always within the first 2 hours of life. The findings include dyspnea, inspiratory retractions, tachypnea, nasal flaring, expiratory grunting, and progressive cyanosis. Laboratory findings correlate with the severity of the RDS and include hypoxemia, hypercapnia, respiratory acidosis, and hypoglycemia.

Radiology

The spectrum of radiologic abnormalities in RDS, from mild to severe, correlates fairly well with clinical severity. The radiologic hallmark of RDS is reticulogranularity of the lungs. This reticulogranularity is due to superimposition of multiple acinar nodules caused by atelectatic alveoli and diffuse microscopic underaeration (Fig. 7-77). Generalized hypoaeration of the lungs and air bronchograms are common. Due to severe retraction, air may be seen in the suprasternal fossa (171). This occasionally mimics air in the dilated proximal pouch of esophageal atresia on the AP chest radiograph (171). Because RDS is characterized by microscopic underaeration, the best radiologic criterion for diagnosis remains reticulogranular densities within the pulmonary parenchyma (Fig. 7-78). General aeration may remain normal if the child is large or on a respirator. The development of air bronchograms is dependent on the coalescence of areas of acinar atelectasis around dilated terminal bronchioles. Rupture of alveoli and air sacs can lead to pulmonary interstitial emphysema.

A

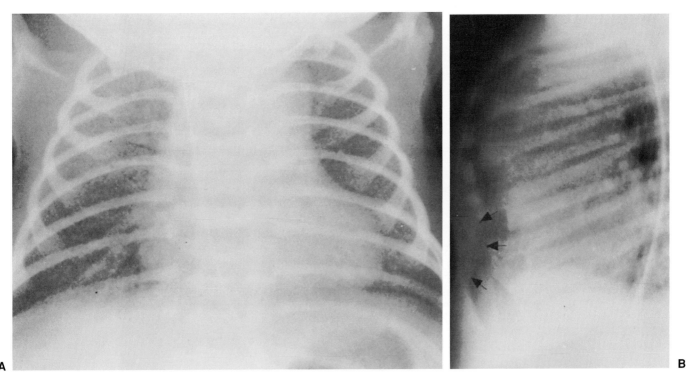

B

FIG. 7-78. **Classic respiratory distress syndrome. A:** Anteroposterior chest radiograph. The bell-shaped thorax is due to generalized underaeration. Reticulogranular densities caused by acinar atelectasis indicate microscopic underaeration. Air bronchograms are present. **B:** A lateral film confirms underaeration as well as lower chest retraction *(arrows)*.

The same factors (prematurity, perinatal asphyxia, cesarean section) that predispose to RDS also predispose to wet lung disease. The initial chest radiograph may show extensive acinar and interstitial opacities in both of these disease processes. As fluid is cleared from the lungs through the bronchi, lymphatics, and capillaries, the associated wet lung syndrome disappears, and one is left with the classic radiologic appearance of RDS.

A normal chest film at 6 hours of age virtually rules out RDS (13,60). Other causes (cardiac, abdominal, CNS, sepsis) of respiratory distress should be considered. The granular densities and hypoaeration persist for 3–5 days in patients with mild to moderate RDS. Clearing, which extends from peripheral to central and from upper lobe to lower lobe (172), begins at the end of the first week of life.

Severe RDS is characterized by progressive hypoaeration of the lungs and diffuse bilateral opacities. The opacity is due to coalescence of the basic acinar atelectasis complicated by interstitial and alveolar edema. There may be superimposed parenchymal hemorrhage. This type of severe and progressive RDS often leads to death, usually within 72 hours (7,13).

If one sees reticulogranular densities, a diagnosis of RDS can be made with a 90% confidence level. Other entities that may produce similar densities include immature lung, wet lung disease, neonatal pneumonia (particularly β-hemolytic streptococcal pneumonia), idiopathic hypoglycemia,

congestive heart failure, maternal diabeties, and early pulmonary hemorrhage (7,60).

Treatment

Therapy is aimed at preventing severe acidosis and hypoxemia by maintaining normal temperature, oxygen concentration, and electrolytes, usually in a neonatal intensive care unit. Intravenous fluids, electrolytes, and calories are administered to correct metabolic acidosis, hypoglycemia, hypocalcemia, and hyperkalemia. Patients with RDS are given prophylactic antibiotics. Mechanical ventilation with positive end-expiratory pressure is performed to maintain patency of the terminal air sacs and maintain adequate oxygenation (7,10,13,60). In children successfully managed with short courses of assisted ventilation at an FiO_2 below 0.4–0.6, the radiographs usually evolve from classic RDS to hazy diffuse opacification of the lungs to normal over a period of several days to 3 weeks.

Since glucocorticoids accelerate lung maturation, the incidence of RDS in babies born at <32 weeks gestation can be significantly reduced by administering betamethasone to the mother for several days before delivery. Two postnatal treatments (artificial surfactant and high-frequency ventilation) have significantly improved the clinical course of RDS and altered the radiologic appearance. In addition to improv-

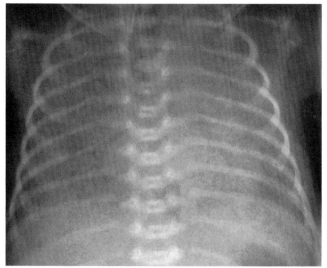
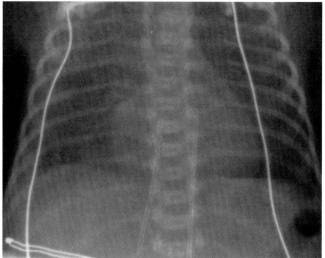

FIG. 7-79. Respiratory distress syndrome. A: Chest radiograph performed at 5 hours of age on a 1900-g boy demonstrates underaeration and the reticulogranularity of hyaline membrane disease. **B:** At 19 hours of age (3 hours after treatment with artificial surfactant) there is marked improvement in lung aeration. The O_2 saturation also markedly improved.

ing the prognosis of patients with RDS, artificial surfactant has reduced the frequency of pneumothorax, formerly seen in up to 10% of ventilated babies (7,13,60). Artificial surfactant is given soon after birth; some babies receive four additional doses in the first 48 hours of life (173,174). This regimen has significantly improved the early survival and course of these children, although long-term consequences of their disease, such as bronchopulmonary dysplasia (BPD), may not have changed (173–177). Artificial surfactant, given as liquid boluses via an endotracheal tube, has also produced changes in the radiographic appearance. Since the surfactant is not evenly distributed throughout the lungs, it is common to see areas of improved lung alternating with areas of unchanged RDS (Fig. 7-79) (175,178,179). This uneven distribution of surfactant leads to a radiographic appearance which simulates other entities such as neonatal pneumonia and meconium aspiration syndrome. In addition, the surfactant may cause sudden distention of multiple acinar units and produce a radiographic appearance quite suggestive of pulmonary interstitial emphysema (PIE) (173–176,178). Babies with uneven surfactant effect generally improve quickly whereas those with PIE tend to deteriorate.

High-frequency ventilation (HiFi) is also used to treat RDS; air block complications from barotrauma are significantly less with HiFi than with conventional respirator therapy (180). The effect on long-term prognosis of HiFi, just as for surfactant therapy, has not yet been determined. The radiographic appearance of babies receiving HiFi is similar to that seen with conventional ventilator therapy. However, the degree of pulmonary inflation is used to adjust mean airway pressure (MAP). Ideally, the dome of the diaphragm should project over the sixth to eighth anterior ribs if MAP is appropriately adjusted.

Complications of Respiratory Distress Syndrome

There are many acute and chronic complications that may occur during the course of RDS (Table 7-10) (181–183). These complications may be iatrogenic or be caused by the disease process itself.

Air Block Complications and Spontaneous Air Block Phenomena

The lungs of the premature infant are immature and are vulnerable to damage. Alveolar rupture may lead to various air block complications. These include parenchymal pseudocyst, pulmonary interstitial emphysema, pneumomediastinum, pneumothorax, pneumopericardium, intravascular air, and air in the extrathoracic soft tissues. Macklin and Macklin during the late 1930s demonstrated experimentally that an increase in transalveolar pressure led to alveolar rupture, dissection of air along peribronchial and perivascular spaces of the interstitium to reach the mediastinum, and subsequent decompression of this pneumomediastinum into the pleural space as a pneumothorax. In addition to this mechanism, Wood has shown that interstitial air (primarily within lymphatics) may directly rupture through the visceral pleura to produce pneumothorax (184).

Mild forms of air block phenomena occur in 1% to 2% of all neonates (7,10,60,185). This incidence increases to as much as 10% with mechanical ventilation (Fig. 7-80). When alveolar rupture occurs, air may localize and coalesce in the parenchyma to produce a pulmonary pseudocyst (Fig. 7-80C) (186). More frequently, particularly in the poorly compliant lung, air accumulates in the peribronchial and perivascular spaces to produce PIE. PIE is almost always preceded

TABLE 7-10. *Complications of respiratory distress syndrome*

Acute complications	Aspiration
Malposition of ancillary equipment	Pulmonary hemorrhage
Endotracheal tube[a]	Congestive heart failure
Catheters[a]	Fluid overload
Arterial	Patent ductus arteriosus[a]
Venous	Hemorrhage
Enteric	Pulmonary
Air block complications	Intracranial[a]
Parenchymal pseudocyst	Subependymal germinal matrix
Pulmonary interstitial emphysema[a]	Intraventricular
Pneumomediastinum[a]	Parenchymal
Pneumothorax[a]	Subarachnoid
Pneumopericardium	Periventricular leukomalacia[a]
Subcutaneous emphysema	Necrotizing enterocolitis[a]
Retroperitoneal air	*Chronic complications*
Pneumoperitoneum	Parenchymal pseudocyst
Gas embolism: pulmonary venous air embolism	Lobar emphysema
Intravascular air	Localized pulmonary interstitial emphysema
Diffuse opacity—"white out"	Delayed onset of diaphragmatic hernia
Apnea: breathing high oxygen content	Bronchopulmonary dysplasia[a]
Atelectasis[a]	Hyperinflation[a]
Mucus plugging[a]	Recurrent respiratory tract infection[a]
Breathing high oxygen content	Upper
Post–extubation	Lower
Coalescence and progression of respiratory distress syndrome	Tracheomalacia
Superimposed pneumonia	Tracheal stenosis
	Retrolental fibroplasia

[a] More common.

by some form of positive pressure assisted ventilation. PIE is manifested as tortuous linear lucencies, relatively uniform in size, radiating outward from the hilar regions throughout the lung (Figs. 7-80B and 7-81). These linear lucencies do not empty on expiration and extend to the periphery of the lung (183,187). Another common pattern is that of small round lucencies in the lung. Peripheral PIE can produce subpleural blebs and ultimately rupture into the pleural space to produce a pneumothorax (168) or extend centrally to produce pneumomediastinum or pneumopericardium (Fig. 7-82A). PIE may be localized in the pulmonary parenchyma, often in the lung, to produce a mass effect (188); this has been treated by decubitus positioning, selective bronchial intubation, and surgical resection (189). Air in the mediastinum may subsequently dissect and lead to pneumothorax, subcutaneous emphysema, retroperitoneal or anterior body wall air, and pneumoperitoneum. In addition to parenchymal pseudocysts and PIE, alveolar rupture may allow entry of air into the pulmonary venous system. This leads to systemic air embolism and intravascular air (Fig. 7-82B), which, when severe enough to be radiologically visible, is almost always fatal.

Pneumomediastinum. Spontaneous pneumomediastinum is not uncommon in the newborn (185). Most cases are clinically insignificant. Rarely, a pneumomediastinum becomes large enough to produce tamponade. Approximately half of all cases of pneumomediastinum cannot be detected without a lateral film (60).

A pneumomediastinum of moderate size frequently has the radiographic appearance of an air mass. This mass may displace the heart to the right (190). The mass effect is due to persistence of the sternopericardial ligament and a fibrofatty mediastinal meshwork, which restricts air to the anterior mediastinum, prevents dissection of air into the neck, and causes air to displace adjacent structures (190). On the AP film, radiolucency outlines the heart, often on both sides. There may be a continuous diaphragm sign (191) caused by air in the mediastinum beneath the heart (Fig. 7-83A). The thymus is frequently elevated by the air in the anterior mediastinum (Fig. 7-83B). The lateral view is confirmatory (Fig. 7-83C).

It may be difficult to distinguish pneumomediastinum from pneumopericardium or a medially located pneumothorax. With pneumopericardium, air completely outlines the heart on both AP and lateral views. Moreover, air limited to the pericardium cannot extend beyond the origins of the aorta and pulmonary artery (Fig. 7-82A). Pneumopericardium and medial pneumothorax do not elevate or outline the thymus on either AP or cross-table lateral views. In the decubitus position, a medial pneumothorax usually shifts to the less dependent part of the pleural space, whereas a pneumomediastinum remains central.

Pneumothorax. Essentially, every pneumothorax in the newborn is a tension pneumothorax. The radiologic findings of pneumothorax in the neonate are an increase in volume of the hemithorax, contralateral shift of the heart

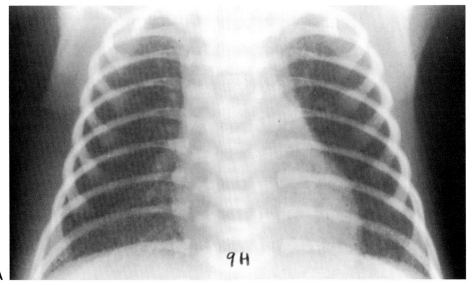

A

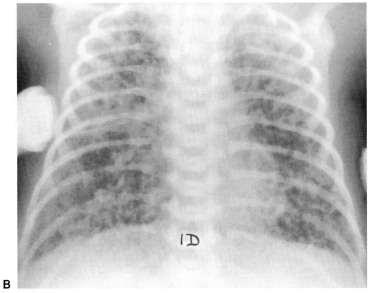

B

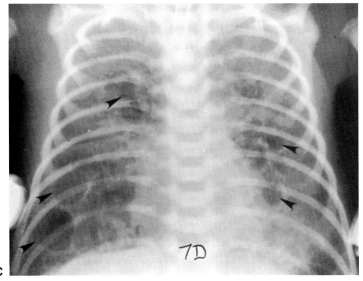

C

FIG. 7-80. Air block complications. A: At 9 hours of age, there are diffuse reticulogranular densities consistent with respiratory distress syndrome. **B:** Bilateral pulmonary interstitial emphysema at 1 day of age. **C:** Bilateral interstitial pseudocysts *(arrowheads)* at 1 week of age.

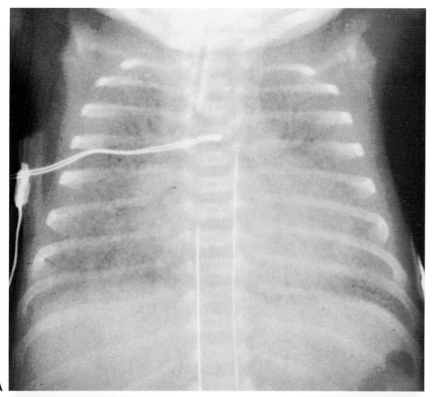

A

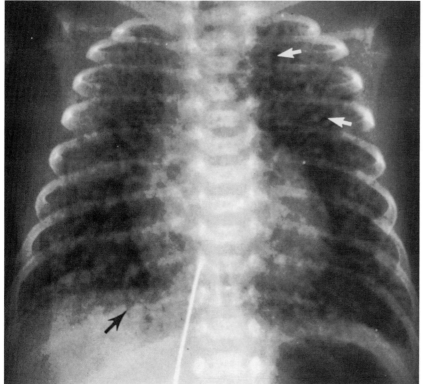

B

FIG. 7-81. Complication of respiratory distress syndrome. A: Classic pattern of diffuse reticulogranular densities and generalized underaeration in RDS. **B:** After ventilatory therapy, this premature infant developed bilateral pulmonary interstitial emphysema with discrete linear gas collections *(arrows)* within the interlobular septa.

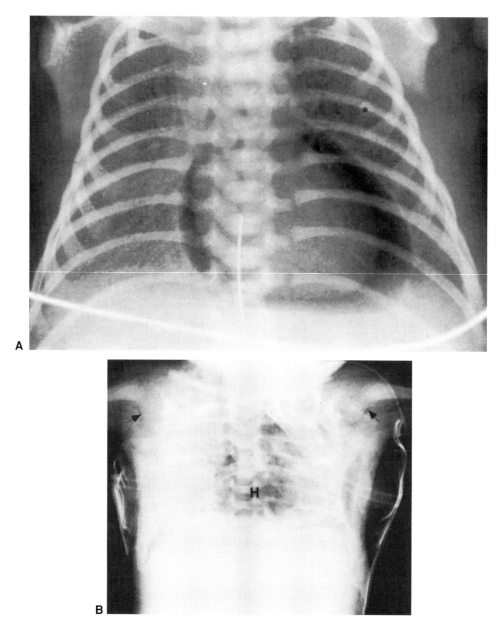

FIG. 7-82. Air block complications. A: Pneumopericardium. **B:** Systemic air embolism with intravascular air. Air is seen in the heart *(H)* and axillary vessels *(arrows)*.

and mediastinum, depression of the diaphragm, and separation of the intercostal spaces. In the supine position, pleural air tends to accumulate anteriorly and medially. The AP film may show nothing but increased radiolucency of the involved hemithorax, as the lung itself falls posteriorly behind the anterior pleural air collection (192,193). Medial herniation of the air-containing pleural spaces in front of the heart is a common sign of pneumothorax on the supine AP chest radiograph (194). The lack of medial displacement of the lung may prevent air from outlining the lateral lung border on the AP supine film. The anterior junction line is well visualized in neonates with bilateral pneumothorax (195).

Usually, a small amount of air is seen lateral and superior to the lung (Fig. 7-84). The cross-table lateral view is excellent for determining the size and extent of a tension pneumothorax (Fig. 7-84B) (196). Lucency is seen anterior to a smooth nearly-straight line that represents the ventral surface of the displaced lung (Fig. 7-84B). Massive pneumothorax is readily apparent and is frequently associated with pulmonary interstitial emphysema (Fig. 7-85). A chest tube should be inserted anteriorly for optimal decompres-

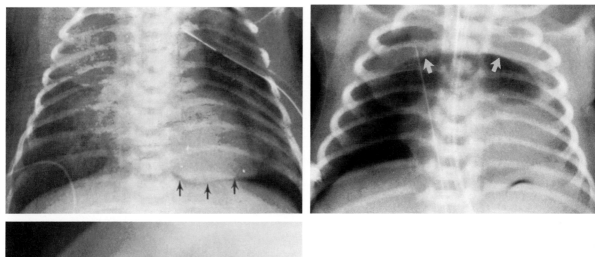

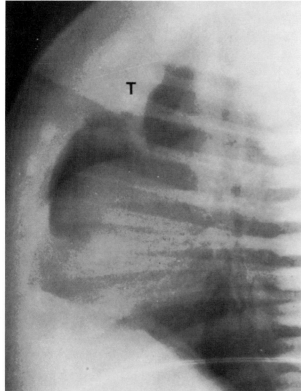

FIG. 7-83. Pneumomediastinum. A: The continuous diaphragm sign *(arrows)* is due to air in the mediastinum beneath the heart. **B:** Elevation of the thymus due to pneumomediastinum *(arrows).* **C:** A lateral film confirms air in the mediastinum outlining the thymus *(T).*

sion of a tension pneumothorax if the child is to be kept supine, as is usual.

Endotracheal Tube Malposition

There are several complications of intubation (181,197). The endotracheal tube (ET) may be placed in the esophagus, not the trachea (Fig. 7-86B), may become occluded by blood or mucus (181), and most commonly may be positioned in a mainstem bronchus or at in incorrect level of the trachea (Fig. 7-86A). Chest radiography remains the only certain way of demonstrating the position of the ET tip. The ideal position in a term newborn is at least 1.2 cm below the vocal

cords and 2.0 cm above the carina with the neonate's head in neutral position (197); the tip of the ET in this position is just below the medial ends of the clavicles on the AP chest radiograph.

There may be marked changes in ET position with head movement. Donn and Kuhns (198) conceptualized the upper end of the ET as being attached to a lever arm that runs from the anterior margin of the maxilla to the first cervical vertebra, moving about a fulcrum at the upper cervical spine (197). If the neck is flexed, the lever arm is angled inferiorly and the tip of the ET is pushed distally (199). When the neck is extended, the functional lever arm is elevated and pulls the tip cephalad. Rotatory motion directs the lever arm away from the carina; the tip of the ET is pulled cephalad

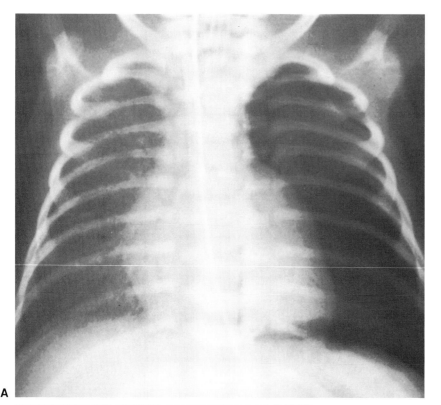

A

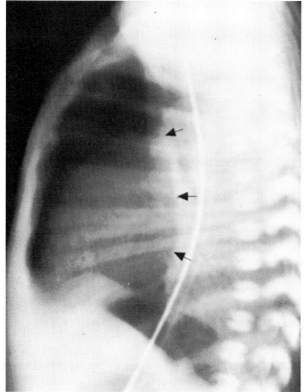

B

FIG. 7-84. Tension pneumothorax. A: Anteroposterior supine chest radiograph. Lucency of left hemithorax with small amount of air beneath the base and above the apex of the left lung. **B:** Cross-table lateral view. Note the large anterior tension pneumothorax. The ventral surface of the left lung (arrows) is displaced posteriorly.

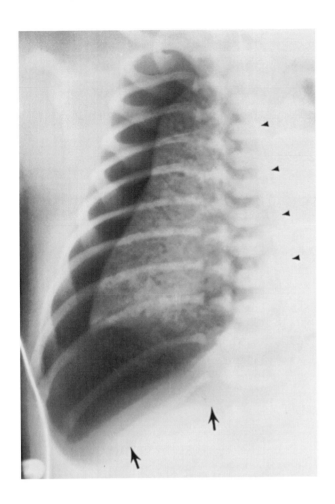

FIG. 7-85. Tension pneumothorax. Tension pneumothorax and interstitial emphysema of right lung. There is eversion of the right hemidiaphragm *(arrows)* and marked leftward mediastinal shift with bowing of the nasogastric tube *(arrowheads)* and displacement of the heart.

with lateral head movement (197). This concept of lever arms and their fulcrum provides an explanation for ET movement: caudad with flexion, cephalad with extension, and cephalad with lateral rotation of the head and neck (197). The mandible, therefore, should be included on chest radiographs obtained for evaluation of ET placement. If the neck is in flexion during AP radiographs of the chest, the tip of the ET may falsely appear to be too low. If the radiograph is obtained with the neck in extension or the head rotated to the side, the ET may falsely appear to be too high (197,200).

Umbilical Catheter Malposition

Umbilical arterial catheters are used for both monitoring and treating sick neonates. The umbilical arteries dip into the pelvis before joining the internal iliac arteries. The umbilical arterial catheter passes through the umbilicus, umbilical artery, internal iliac artery, and common iliac artery and then into the aorta (Fig. 7-87A) (7). The tip of the catheter should be kept away from the vessels to abdominal and retroperitoneal viscera. A good location is below the renal arteries at approximately L3 or L4; others prefer a T_8–T_{10} location.

Umbilical venous catheters are also frequently used. The umbilical vein runs cephalad to join the left portal vein. The tip of an umbilical venous catheter should ideally be at the

junction of the IVC and right atrium. To reach this position, the catheter passes through the umbilicus, umbilical vein, medial part of left portal vein, ductus venosus, IVC, and right atrium. On the AP view, there is a gentle convexity of the catheter to the right in the liver (Fig. 7-87A). Straightening of this intrahepatic course of the catheter is an indirect sign of hepatomegaly. On the lateral view, the normal umbilical venous catheter describes a gentle S-shaped curve prior to reaching the heart (Fig. 7-87B). An umbilical venous catheter may be malpositioned in the umbilical vein, left portal vein or branch, common portal vein, right portal vein or branch, splenic vein, mesenteric vein, IVC, SVC, coronary sinus, right atrium, right ventricle, pulmonary artery, left atrium, or pulmonary vein (38).

Enteric Catheter Malposition

Polyethylene enteric catheters are frequently used for gastrointestinal decompression or tube feedings. These enteric tubes are usually placed in the stomach for bowel decompression. Duodenal tubes are frequently used for feedings. Because duodenal perforations secondary to enteric tubes usually occur at the superior flexure (junction of duodenal bulb and descending duodenum) or inferior flexure (junction of descending duodenum and horizontal duodenum), the tip of a feeding enteric tube should be in the third

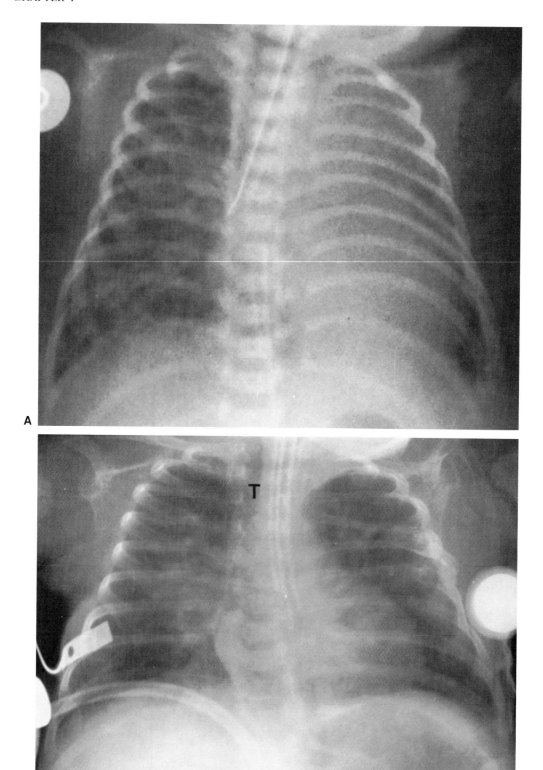

FIG. 7-86. Endotracheal tube malposition. A: The tip of the endotracheal tube is in the right mainstem bronchus. There is partial atelectasis of the left lung. **B:** Endotracheal tube in esophagus. Note the position of the trachea *(T)*.

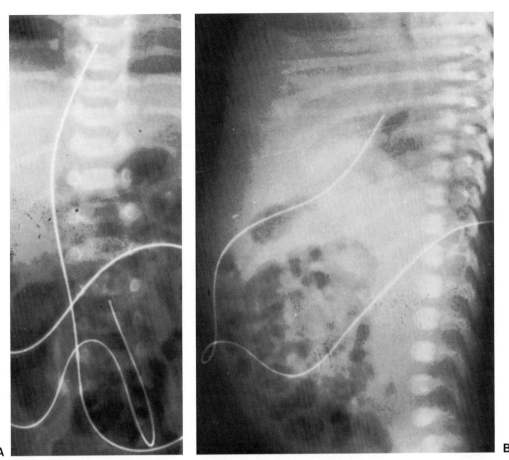

FIG. 7-87. Normal umbilical catheter positions. A: Anteroposterior view of the abdomen. The umbilical arterial catheter tip is at the level of L3–4. The umbilical venous catheter tip is in the right atrium. **B:** Lateral view of the abdomen. The normal S-shaped curve of umbilical venous catheter as it passes from the umbilicus to the right atrium. Note that the postero-inferior part of the catheter is outside the patient.

(transverse) or fourth (ascending) part of the duodenum. The ideal location is approximately 1 cm proximal to the duodenojejunal junction (ligament of Treitz) (7). Polyethylene tubes become stiff and hard when exposed to enteric secretions. The neonatal duodenum is redundant, and the ligament of Treitz is not always fixed; consequently, enteric tubes may have a broad C-shaped curve that falsely suggests perforation (7).

Pneumoperitoneum

Patients with RDS who are being ventilated at high pressures may develop pneumomediastinum, retroperitoneal air, and pneumoperitoneum. Patients with pneumoperitoneum secondary to respirator therapy usually have other air block phenomena, such as PIE, pneumomediastinum, or pneumothorax. It may still be difficult, however, to decide whether a pneumoperitoneum is due to extension of air from the chest or to perforation of the gastrointestinal tract. A long air-fluid level in the peritoneum is common following gastrointestinal perforation but may also occasionally be seen with pneumoperitoneum due to air block (7). Nonionic contrast agents administered through a feeding tube provide a safe and reliable method for determining the presence or absence of gastrointestinal perforation in the neonate (Fig. 7-88).

Lung White-out

Diffuse parenchymal opacity, even apparent airlessness, may develop during the treatment and course of RDS. If apnea or atelectasis develops in a patient who is being ventilated on high PO_2 concentrations, rapid resorption of oxygen from alveoli may produce generalized areas of opacity (201). Decreasing ventilatory settings may also cause parenchymal opacification. Other, more severe causes of a "white-out" in patients with RDS include progression and coalescence of RDS, superimposed pneumonia, aspiration, pulmonary hemorrhage (Fig. 7-89) (202), and congestive heart failure (Table 7-10).

Patent Ductus Arteriosus

The normal ductus arteriosus functionally closes, in response to high oxygen concentrations, within a day or two

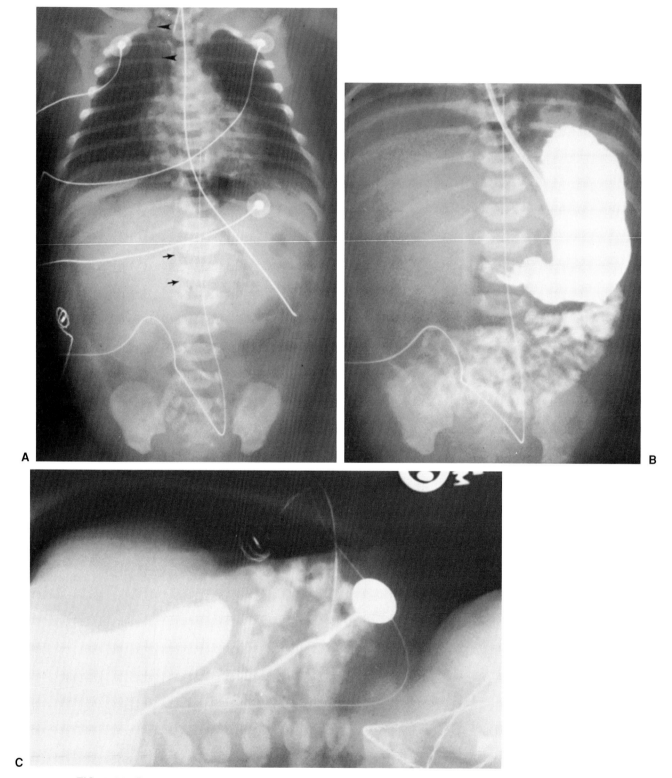

FIG. 7-88. Pneumoperitoneum secondary to air block complications. A: Anteroposterior supine film of the chest and abdomen of a newborn with neonatal pneumonia requiring respirator therapy. There is a pneumomediastinum *(arrowheads)*. Free intraperitoneal air outlines the falciform ligament *(arrows)*. **B:** Nonionic contrast study is normal without any leaks from the stomach, duodenum, or proximal small bowel. **C:** Cross-table supine lateral abdomen radiograph shows a large amount of free intraperitoneal gas. Note the contrast in the upper gastrointestinal tract.

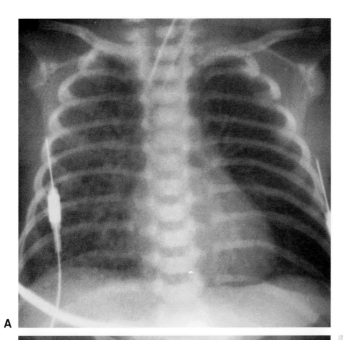

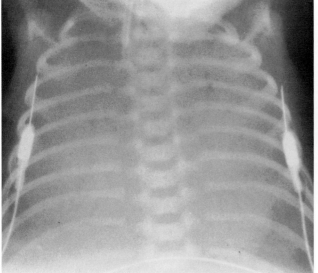

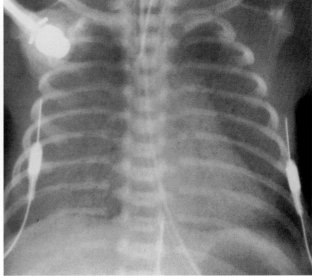

FIG. 7-89. Pulmonary hemorrhage. A: The diffuse reticulogranular lung densities of hyaline membrane disease and the discrete right lung rounded and linear lucencies of pulmonary interstitial emphysema. **B:** After sudden deterioration, the chest radiograph shows opacity of the whole lung. Blood was suctioned from the trachea. **C:** By 12 hours there was notable clearing. This appearance is compatible with resolving pulmonary hemorrhage.

of birth. Because patients with RDS are usually severely hypoxic, the ductus arteriosus may remain patent. During the first few days of life, pulmonary arterial pressure is elevated; the poorly compliant lungs of RDS and the associated hypoxia and acidosis accentuate this pulmonary hypertension. Shunting across the patent ductus arteriosus (PDA) is bidirectional or right to left. By the end of the first week, as pulmonary artery pressure decreases because of the increased compliance of the healing lungs of RDS, shunting becomes left to right (7). There may be no appreciable change in the chest radiograph, although usually there is a slight increase in heart size. More importantly, the central pulmonary vascularity may become prominent and the vessel margins ill defined; the last finding indicates interstitial pulmonary edema (Fig. 7-90) (203). These radiologic changes may be apparent several hours before clinical symptoms or signs. Confirmation of the diagnosis is by Doppler echocardiography.

The stimuli for closure of the ductus arteriosus are normal oxygen levels, normal pH, and normal levels of prostaglandin. Treatment with indomethacin often results in ductal closure by inhibiting prostaglandin; gastrointestinal perforation and osteoarthropathy are known complications of this therapy. Transcatheter occlusion or surgery may be necessary for closure of a persistent PDA. Treatment of PDA is critical in extremely sick neonates and in patients with associated malformations or syndromes (38,200,203). Patent ductus arteriosus is discussed further in Chapter 6.

Lobar Distention

RDS is sometimes followed by acquired lobar emphysema or by pulmonary interstitial emphysema localized to one lobe

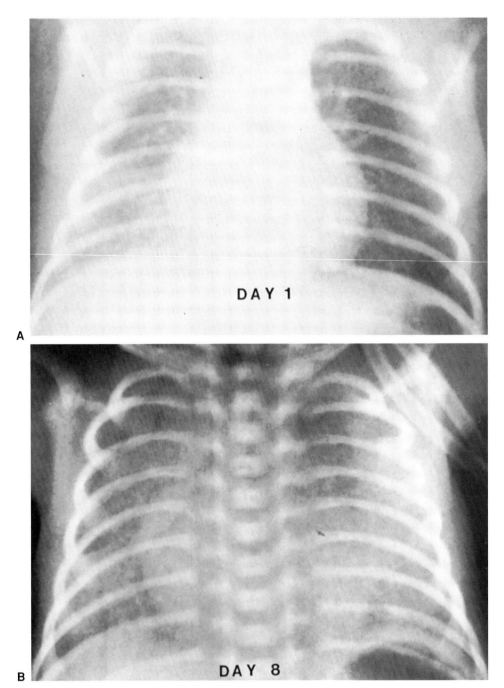

FIG. 7-90. Patent ductus arteriosus. A 1500-g infant with respiratory distress. **A:** *Day 1*. Diffuse granular parenchymal densities typical of the respiratory distress syndrome. **B:** *Day 8*. Cardiomegaly and prominent central vessels with indistinct margins presumably representing congestive heart failure. A PDA was confirmed by Doppler echocardiography.

(7,189). Infants with the acquired form of lobar emphysema frequently have radiologic evidence of bronchopulmonary dysplasia. The distention is presumably related to a bronchial abnormality, such as mucosal proliferation, granulation tissue, chronic mucous plugging, or a mucosal web. Lobectomy may rarely be required. Ventilation-perfusion scanning will characterize the altered lung physiology.

Bronchopulmonary Dysplasia

BPD (chronic lung disease of prematurity) is a common, significant complication in newborns who require ventilatory therapy. The clinical, radiologic, and pathologic features of BPD were originally described by Northway and Rosan in 1967 (204) and 1968 (205). BPD has been the subject of

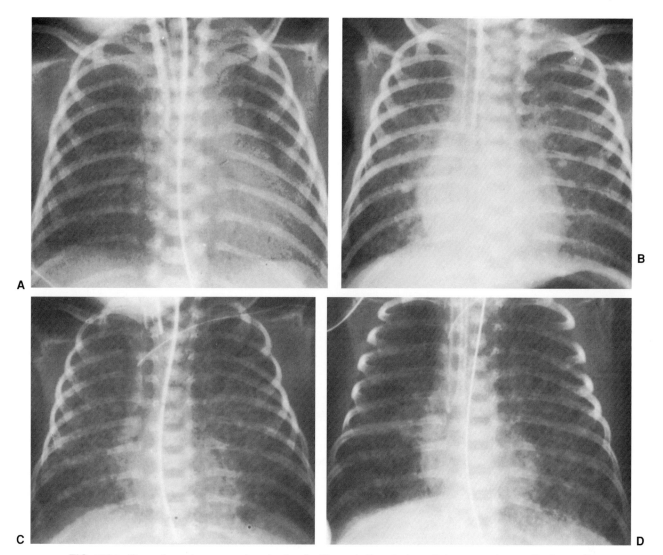

FIG. 7-91. Bronchopulmonary dysplasia. A: Stage I. Respiratory distress syndrome. **B:** Stage II. Bilateral pulmonary opacities. There is a patent ductus arteriosus; densities are presumably partly due to congestive heart failure. **C:** Stage III. 21 days of age. Note the bilateral parenchymal densities, producing bubbly lungs. **D:** Stage IV. 5 weeks of age. Note the persistence of circular lucencies and curvilinear densities, producing a honeycomb appearance of the lungs.

many publications since its recognition (206–210). BPD is a distinct pulmonary disease affecting all of the tissues of the developing lung after prolonged oxygen or respirator therapy of RDS. It was initially thought to represent oxygen toxicity.

Northway and Rosan identified four stages of BPD (205). Stage I BPD is identical with RDS clinically and radiologically (Fig. 7-91A). Pathologically, mucosal necrosis is present. Stage II BPD develops between 4 and 10 days of age. Radiologically there is marked opacity of the lungs, producing a "white-out" (Fig. 7-91B). Pathologically, there is exudative necrosis and repair of alveolar epithelium, with persistent hyaline membranes, patchy bronchiolar necrosis, eosinophilic exudate within alveoli and airways, squamous

metaplasia, and interstitial edema (205). Congestive heart failure from a patent ductus arteriosus may complicate this stage (Fig. 7-91B). Stage III BPD develops between 10 and 20 days of age and is characterized by a bubbly radiologic appearance of the lungs (Fig. 7-91C). This honeycomb appearance has poorly defined, variable sized, rounded lucencies surrounded by linear densities. The bubbly lucencies are due to overdistention of alveoli and acini within scarred lungs. Pathologically, there is persistent injury to alveolar epithelium but superimposed widespread bronchial and bronchiolar mucosal metaplasia and hyperplasia with mucous secretion and exudation of alveolar macrophages as well as histiocytes into the airways (205). Stage IV BPD develops after 1 month of age. There is again a honeycomb

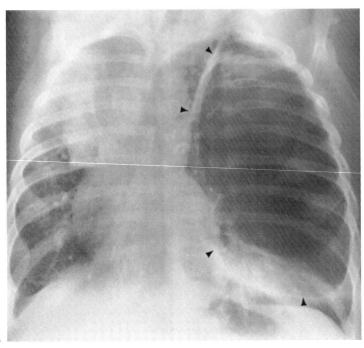
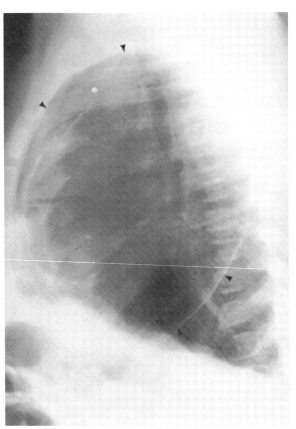

A   B

FIG. 7-92. **Complication of bronchopulmonary dysplasia.** Anteroposterior **(A)** and lateral **(B)** chest radiographs of a 5-month-old boy with known bronchopulmonary dysplasia show a large "cyst" of the left upper lobe *(arrowheads)*. It is either acquired left upper lobe emphysema or an interstitial cyst. Note the mass effect on the mediastinum and the secondary right upper lobe compressive atelectasis.

or bubbly appearance of the lungs, with alternating cyst-like lucencies surrounded by curvilinear strands of soft-tissue density (Fig. 7-91D). There is also hyperaeration, which may be much more marked at the bases, and frequently cardiomegaly is present.

Occasionally, a large interstitial cyst or acquired emphysema develops (Fig. 7-92). Histologically, there are focal groups of distended alveoli, with deposition of collagen and elastin fibers in the interstitium and septal walls and with associated tortuosity and dilatation of lymphatics.

The radiologic appearances of stage III and stage IV BPD are identical. These stages are distinguished by the temporal setting: BPD in a patient over 1 month of age is considered to be stage IV. BPD is probably due to both oxygen toxicity and barotrauma. Indolent pulmonary infection may lead to a longer course of O$_2$ and ventilator support.

The radiologic appearance and course of BPD have changed since the initial descriptions (210). An orderly progression through the four stages as first described is rarely seen (170). Frequently, a patient with RDS requires prolonged respirator and oxygen therapy. By the end of the first or second week of life, there is a persistent haziness of vessel margins progressing to linear densities that persist into the third or fourth week of life. At this point, there is the gradual

development of a bubbly appearance of the lungs associated with hyperaeration, frequently more pronounced at the bases. This picture persists beyond 1 month of age and represents a modified form of stage IV BPD. Radiologic changes of stage II BPD are now rarely identified. Perhaps many of the patients who were thought to have had stage II BPD actually had persistent patency of the ductus arteriosus.

The prognosis of patients with BPD has improved. Stage IV BPD is now associated with a mortality of <40% (210). More than one third of patients with stage IV BPD are clinically normal by 3 years of age, and 29% have only minor handicaps (209). Sequential chest radiographs in patients with BPD frequently show persistent hyperaeration during infancy with gradual clearing of the circular lucencies and linear densities (207,208). Further radiologic improvement occurs, although a majority still have minor radiologic abnormalities at age 8 (207). Pulmonary function studies are frequently abnormal, and lower respiratory tract infection is common (209,210).

Precocious dysplastic pulmonary changes (severe BPD seen at the end of the second postnatal week) have been described in low birth weight (<1000 g) infants with *Ureaplasma urealyticum* lower respiratory tract infection (211).

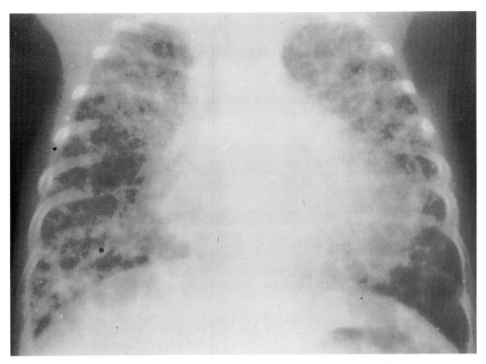

FIG. 7-93. Wilson-Mikity syndrome. A 2-month-old boy with no history of respirator or oxygen therapy. The strands of density and the bubbly appearance of the lungs are indistinguishable from stage IV bronchopulmonary dysplasia. The heart is large because of cor pulmonale.

Wilson-Mikity Syndrome

The Wilson-Mikity syndrome is also referred to as pulmonary dysmaturity (7,13,212). The similarity of the clinical, radiologic, and pathologic features of Wilson-Mikity syndrome and BPD is marked; some authorities consider them to be the same disease. The two disorders presumably represent the effects of exogenous insults on the developing lung. The insult is oxygen or respirator therapy or both in patients who develop BPD; it may be nothing but room air for the smaller group of patients who develop Wilson-Mikity syndrome.

Patients with Wilson-Mikity syndrome are premature and may be asymptomatic or have only mild respiratory distress during the immediate newborn period. The mild or absent clinical symptoms makes oxygen or respirator therapy unnecessary. By 10–14 days of age, there is the gradual onset of respiratory distress. Chest radiography at this time shows findings similar to stage III or IV BPD (Fig. 7-93) (7,13,212).

Persistent Fetal Circulation Syndrome

The high pulmonary vascular resistance present in fetal life decreases in the newborn period in response to pulmonary expansion and oxygenation. Failure of this normal physiologic transition and the continuation of high pulmonary vascular resistance is termed the persistent fetal circulation syndrome (PFC) or persistent pulmonary hypertension of the neonate (7,10,13). Neonates with this condition may have right-to-left shunting at the foramen ovale or ductus arteriosus if pulmonary artery pressure is in excess of systemic arterial pressure. Persistent fetal circulation syndrome may occur as a primary form of pulmonary hypertension. The etiology of the disorder, which usually occurs in full-term babies, is unknown. Pathology shows pulmonary arteriolar narrowing and thickening. The secondary form of PFC is due to hypoxemia and is seen in neonatal pneumonia, severe pulmonary hypoplasia accompanying congenital diaphragmatic hernia, and meconium aspiration syndrome. The pulmonary arteriolar vasoconstriction, pulmonary artery hypertension, and systemic arterial desaturation may be profound.

Radiography in neonates with primary PFC may be negative or may show diminished pulmonary vascularity, mild cardiomegaly, and hepatomegaly (Fig. 7-94) (7). Neonates with secondary PFC have a radiographic picture reflecting the primary underlying pulmonary abnormality.

Wet Lung Disease

Etiology

Wet lung disease, due to delayed resorption and clearance of fluid from the lung, is one of the most common causes of respiratory distress in the newborn. It has characteristic radiologic and clinical features. It is synonymous with transient tachypnea of the newborn and transient respiratory dis-

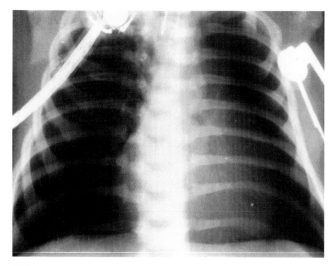

FIG. 7-94. Persistent fetal circulation. Chest x-ray in a term newborn with PFC due to sepsis shows markedly decreased pulmonary vascularity and hyperinflation.

tress of the newborn. Because the radiologic appearance represents delayed clearance of normal lung fluid and because this is the cause of the symptoms, the term wet lung disease is preferred (213).

Pathophysiology

Normal lung fluid is cleared through bronchi by the thoracic squeeze during vaginal delivery (30%), and through lymphatics (30%) and capillaries (40%). Conditions that predispose to wet lung disease include cesarean section, a minor or moderate degree of prematurity, maternal diabetes, and precipitous delivery (213,214). Most of these conditions have a decrease in the thoracic squeeze, which normally clears approximately one third of the fetal lung fluid through the tracheobronchial tree. Other factors in the pathogenesis include hypoproteinemia, hypervolemia, erythrocythemia, and decreased pulmonary lymph flow.

Aspiration of clear amniotic fluid is an entity clinically and radiologically indistinguishable from wet lung disease (213). Conditions predisposing to aspiration of clear amniotic fluid include mild fetal distress and breech delivery. Distinction between wet lung disease and aspiration of clear amniotic fluid is purely academic, as both are benign conditions and both are treated conservatively (213).

Clinical Features

Sex distribution among patients with wet lung disease is equal. There is often a history of cesarean section, prematurity, or maternal sedation. Tachypnea develops during the first 6 hours of life, with the respiratory rate being fairly normal during the first hour and then gradually increasing over the next 4–6 hours (215). The respiratory rate peaks at

1 day of age and returns to normal by 2–3 days of age. There may be mild cyanosis, substernal retraction, and expiratory grunting in association with mild hypercarbia, hypoxia, and acidosis (215). Patients with wet lung disease are almost always hyperoxygenated on 100% (FiO$_2$ of 1.0) inspired oxygen.

Radiologic Features

Chest films obtained at 2–6 hours of age show fluid within the lungs and sometimes mild cardiomegaly. There may be prominence of vascular markings with hazy margins, fluid within fissures, and a small amount of pleural fluid. More severe cases may show alveolar edema with patchy rounded areas of opacity (Fig. 7-95A) (213,214). The lungs begin to clear within 10–12 hours. During this clearing phase, there may be reticulogranular densities that mimic RDS. This temporary finding is associated with normal aeration or hyperaeration, not hypoaeration. The alveolar edema clears with interval development of pulmonary vascular congestion, interstitial edema, and engorged lymphatics. Clearing continues from peripheral to central and from upper to lower lung. The heart is never significantly enlarged in wet lung disease. On cross-table lateral films, the acinar and interstitial opacities of wet lung disease are most prominent at the posterior, dependent portions of the lungs. The chest film is usually normal by 48–72 hours of age (Fig. 7-95B). It the infant actually had aspiration of clear amniotic fluid, hyperaeration may persist for 4–5 days (7).

Differential diagnostic considerations include RDS, neonatal pneumonia, congestive heart failure, erythroblastosis fetalis, maternal diabetes, idiopathic hypoglycemia, neonatal polycythemia, erythrocythemia, and idiopathic hypervolemia. Persistent prominence of or an increase in the pulmonary vascularity with a normal-sized heart suggests total anomalous pulmonary venous return below the diaphragm in a term neonate and PDA in a premature infant.

Treatment

Because wet lung disease is a benign condition, treatment is conservative and supportive. The prognosis for both wet lung disease and aspiration of clear amniotic fluid is excellent.

Meconium Aspiration Syndrome

The meconium aspiration syndrome (MAS) is caused by the intrauterine or intrapartum aspiration of meconium-stained amniotic fluid (13,216,217). Aspiration of meconium into the tracheobronchial tree produces characteristic radiologic findings. Meconium staining of amniotic fluid is present in approximately 10% to 15% of live births, but only 1% to 1.5% of newborns have MAS with meconium in the

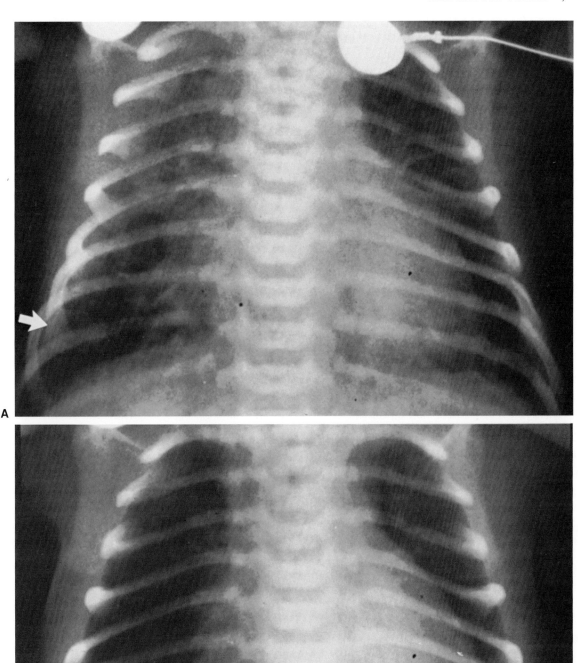

FIG. 7-95. Wet lung disease. Term boy neonate with moderate respiratory distress. **A:** The heart is at the upper limits of normal in transverse diameter. There is a slight increase in vascularity with hazy margins and diffuse patchy interstitial and acinar opacities. There is a small, right pleural effusion *(arrow)*. **B:** Normal chest radiograph at 24 hours of age.

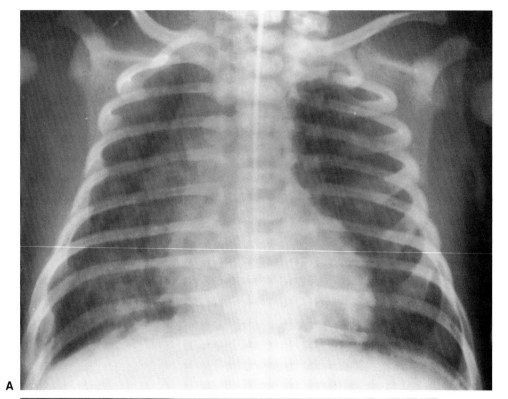

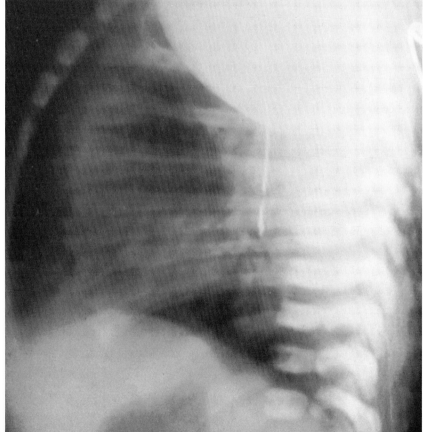

FIG. 7-96. Meconium aspiration. A: Patchy pulmonary parenchymal opacities. **B:** Hyperaeration manifested by flattening of the diaphragm and anterior bowing of the sternum.

airway below the vocal cords. Meconium is a tenacious, viscous, greenish black material that contains mucus, epithelial cells, fatty acids, swallowed material, debris, and bile. Severe in utero hypoxemia causes fetal defecation and gasping, which leads to aspiration of meconium-containing amniotic fluid into the tracheobronchial tree. This aspired meconium produces bronchial obstruction and chemical pneumonitis.

Clinical

The sex distribution in patients with MAS is equal. This syndrome most commonly occurs in babies who are postmature (mean of 10 days past expected delivery date), are small for gestational age, or have had intrauterine stress causing hypoxia. The diagnosis is confirmed by visualization of meconium in the airway below the vocal cords. The respiratory distress may be severe, with cyanosis, wheezing, and hyperaeration and profound hypercarbia, hypoxia, and acidosis (7,13).

Pathology

Aspiration of meconium produces partial or complete bronchial obstruction. There are patchy areas of subsegmental atelectasis that occur peripheral to obstructed bronchi and compensatory areas of hyperinflation. Because of the marked hyperinflation, there is a propensity for alveolar rupture, leading to air block complications such as pneumomediastinum and pneumothorax. Chemical pneumonitis is often present, and there may be superimposed bronchopneumonia.

Radiologic Features

The radiographic findings of MAS vary, partly with the severity of the aspiration. There are patchy, bilateral, asymmetric areas of opacity. These opacities are usually acinar and may appear rounded (Figs. 7-96 and 7-97A). There is marked hyperaeration of the lungs with flattening of the domes of the diaphragm on both the AP and lateral views (Fig. 7-96) (7,13). Air block complications such as pneumomediastinum or pneumothorax are seen in approximately 25% of patients with proven MAS (216,217). The asymmetric, coarse, patchy infiltrates are due to subsegmental atelectasis, which is usually present at birth and is associated with hyperaeration of the lungs; areas of atelectasis alternating with areas of hyperinflation are characteristic. Because the meconium produces a chemical pneumonitis, clearing of the radiologic opacities may take several weeks, despite rapid clinical improvement; radiologic clearing lags well behind clinical improvement. Other causes of such acinar opacities include severe wet lung disease, neonatal pneumonia, and pulmonary hemorrhage (7,9).

Treatment

In the past, treatment was primarily supportive, with oxygen given as required and antibiotics administered routinely. Due to a mortality rate of up to 25% in babies with MAS, extracorporeal membrane oxygenation (ECMO) is increasing used to treat severe meconium aspiration (Fig. 7-97) as well as other causes of intractable respiratory failure (218,219). Liquid ventilation has also been used for treating respiratory failure (220). ECMO provides a circulatory bypass of the lungs; pulmonary inflation is at a minimum, whereas oxygen tension and oxygen saturation are maintained at physiologic levels (219). On ECMO therapy, the lungs are almost airless (Fig. 7-97B) (221). Ultrasonography may be extremely helpful in evaluating the CNS, chest, and abdomen of infants undergoing ECMO therapy (222).

Neonatal Pneumonia

Neonatal pneumonia may be acquired in utero as an ascending infection or transplacental infection, during delivery, or after birth (7,10,13). Etiologic organisms include viruses, bacteria, protozoa, and fungi. Symptomatology is variable but usually includes nonspecific respiratory distress. The chest radiograph may be the first suggestion of infection.

Ascending infection is associated with premature rupture of membranes and prolonged labor. Organisms causing neonatal pneumonia acquired through the ascending route or during delivery are normal inhabitants of the vagina: Staphylococcus aureus, streptococci, diphtheroids, anaerobic organisms, Escherichia coli, Proteus, and Listeria (7,10). Neonatal pneumonia may also be due to Pseudomonas aeruginosa and other gram-negative organisms.

Group B streptococcal pneumonia is common in the newborn. At least 25% of women in labor are colonized with this organism. The radiologic appearance may be identical to that of RDS: reticulogranular densities, often with pleural fluid (Fig. 7-98) (223,224). Pleural effusions are common (up to 67% of cases) in neonatal pneumonia but are rare in uncomplicated RDS. Lower ventilatory pressure requirements than those for RDS suggest the pressure of β-hemolytic streptococcal pneumonia. Confirmation of the diagnosis and institution of appropriate antibiotic therapy are critical in decreasing the high mortality of streptococcal neonatal pneumonia.

Unlike β-hemolytic streptococcal pneumonia, most neonatal pneumonias are characterized by patchy, asymmetric pulmonary opacities and hyperaeration (Fig. 7-99) (225). Empyema associated with neonatal pneumonia suggests staphylococcal or Klebsiella pneumonia. During the healing stages of staphylococcal pneumonia, pneumatoceles may develop. If the nephrotic syndrome, ascites, hepatosplenomegaly, or osteomyelitis predominantly involving long bones is present, one must consider the possibility of syphilitic pneumonia (pneumonia alba) (226). Small nodular or mili-

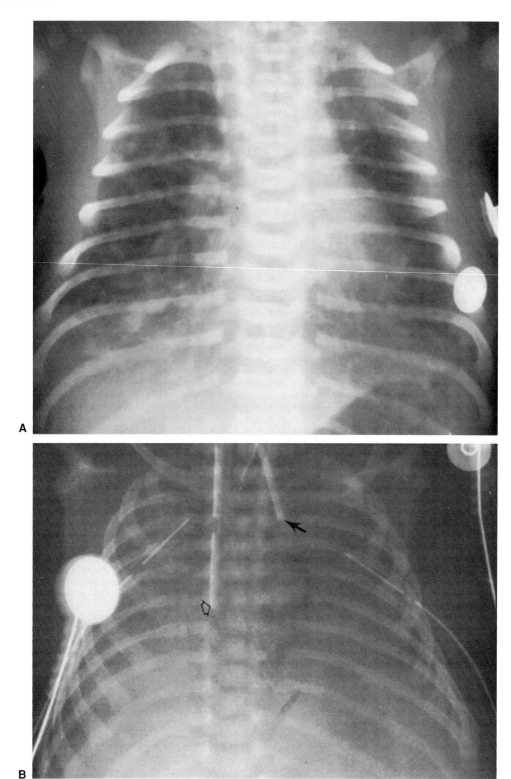

FIG. 7-97. Meconium aspiration and extracorporeal membrane oxygenation (ECMO) therapy. A: A chest radiograph prior to ECMO shows patchy bilateral lung opacities. **B:** Day 3 on ECMO. There is marked pulmonary opacification and volume loss. Note the position of the bypass cannulas in the right atrium (*open arrow*) and the brachiocephalic artery *(solid arrow)*.

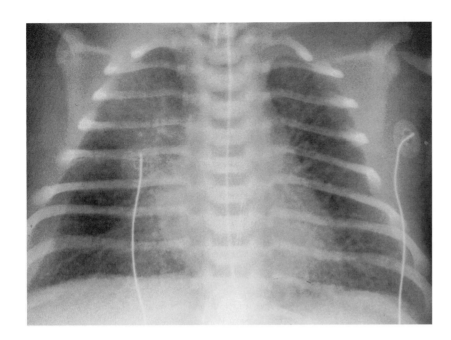

FIG. 7-98. Group B streptococcal pneumonia. Newborn boy with respiratory distress and sepsis shows diffuse reticulonodular densities mimicking RDS. There is a right pleural effusion.

ary opacities may be due to transplacentally acquired tuberculosis, listeriosis, or fungal disease (10).

Several infants have been reported with the late onset of a right-sided diaphragmatic hernia in association with neonatal pneumonia (227,228). Presumably the diaphragmatic defect was preexisting. Respiratory distress and hyperaeration associated with the pneumonia may prevent herniation of abdominal viscera, or the pneumonia may simply be a chance association.

Chylothorax

Chylothorax is the most common cause of a large pleural effusion in the newborn. There is an accumulation of lymph

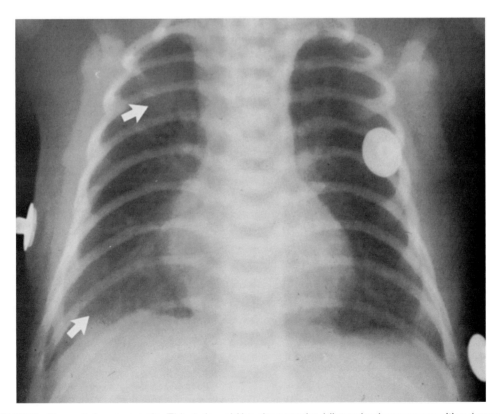

FIG. 7-99. Neonatal pneumonia. This 4-day-old boy has patchy, bilateral pulmonary opacities *(arrows)*.

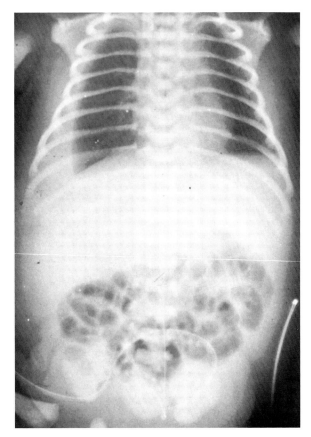

FIG. 7-100. Chylothorax. Newborn boy with large right pleural effusion due to chylothorax. Chylous ascites is also present. (Courtesy of Bruce Mewborne, M.D., San Antonio, Texas.)

it necessary to explore the thoracic duct. The prognosis is excellent except when the chylothorax is bilateral (10).

Other causes of pleural effusion in the newborn include erythroblastosis fetalis, congestive heart failure, infantile polycystic kidneys, polycythemia, congenital cystic adenomatoid malformation, ELS, idiopathic or iatrogenic hypervolemia, obstruction of pulmonary venous return, esophageal rupture, erosion by a gastroenteric cyst, wet lung disease, and Turner syndrome and its associated pulmonary lymphangiectasia (7,9,10).

Congenital Pulmonary Lymphangiectasia

Babies with congenital pulmonary lymphangiectasia often have symptoms similar to those of hyaline membrane disease (13). Most patients diagnosed at birth do not survive. Radiographs often reveal a coarse interstitial infiltrate secondary to the distended and abnormally draining lymphatics (Fig. 7-101) (7,10). Kerley B lines are common (see Fig. 7-104). Pleural fluid, sometimes chylous, is common. The diagnosis is confirmed by lung biopsy; there is marked hyperplasia of lymph channels in the pulmonary interstitium.

Congenital Heart Disease Mimicking Lung Disease

Congenital heart disease may mimic several of these neonatal pulmonary diseases (229). Congestive pulmonary interstitial edema may be difficult to distinguish from neonatal

in the pleural space, but it does not become truly chylous until milk or formula has been ingested. Neonates with spontaneous chylothorax are usually born at term after a normal labor and delivery. Half of the patients develop symptoms within the first day of life, and 70% have symptoms by the end of the first week (10). Males are affected twice as frequently as females. The majority occur on the right. Occasionally they are bilateral or are associated with chylous ascites (Fig. 7-100). The etiology of chylothorax usually remains unknown. It is postulated that there is rupture of the thoracic duct or transient central venous hypertension during delivery. Lymph accumulates in the mediastinum and extends into the pleural space (10). Congenital anomalies of the lymphatic system occasionally cause neonatal chylothorax (7).

Decubitus films verify the amount of effusion. In severe cases, there is complete opacification of the involved hemithorax, shift of the heart and mediastinum to the opposite side, and widening of the ipsilateral ribs.

Most patients respond to single or repeated thoracenteses. A large chylothorax may require chest tube drainage. Treatment with medium chain triglycerides is helpful. Rarely is

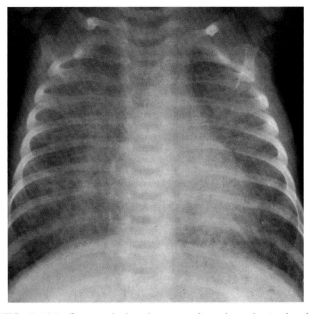

FIG. 7-101. Congenital pulmonary lymphangiectasia. A 3-week-old infant with persistent oxygen requirement. There is a diffuse increase in interstitial markings. Echocardiography excluded pulmonary venous obstruction. Lung biopsy showed pulmonary lymphangiectasia.

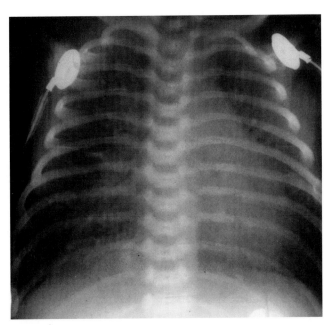

FIG. 7-102. Total anomalous pulmonary venous return (TAPVR) below the diaphragm. A 5-day-old boy with tachypnea. There is interstitial and alveolar pulmonary edema but a normal-sized heart. The common pulmonary vein passed through the esophageal hiatus to drain into the portal venous system.

pneumonia and wet lung disease. Congenital heart lesions producing obstruction to pulmonary venous return but no cardiac enlargement are particularly confusing. These lesions include valvular and supravalvular mitral stenosis, cor triatriatum, stenosis of a common pulmonary vein, and total anomalous pulmonary venous return (TAPVR) with obstruction (7). If the obstruction is marked, cyanosis (in severe cases) or signs of pulmonary edema, dyspnea, and feeding difficulties (in less severe cases) develop in the first week of life. A chest radiograph will show pulmonary venous hypertension but not an enlarged heart (Fig. 7-102). Most patients with TAPVR below the diaphragm have pulmonary venous obstruction (230).

Significant cardiac enlargement suggests congestive heart failure. During the first week of life, before the pulmonary vascular resistance drops enough to allow left-to-right shunting, congestive failure is usually secondary to pressure overload, obligatory volume overload, or myocardial dysfunction. The lesions most commonly producing these phenomena are critical aortic stenosis, hypoplastic left heart syndrome, coarctation of the aorta, interruption of the aortic arch, myocarditis, dysrhythmias, myocardial ischemia, and vascular malformations. By the second week of life, after pulmonary resistance has dropped, volume overload lesions are the usual causes of congestive failure. These include ventricular septal defect, endocardial cushion defect, patent ductus arteriosus, and aorticopulmonary window. Congeni-

tal heart disease in newborns is discussed in greater detail in Chapter 6.

Pulmonary Infection

Respiratory tract infection is the most common human illness. Viruses are the major cause of pulmonary infection in children, especially below age 5 years. Bacteria become an increasingly important cause of pneumonia in older children and in the hospitalized child (66,71,72,231–234). Many bacterial pneumonias in infants and children are superimposed on a viral lower respiratory tract infection. Pneumonias due to fungal, protozoan, and chemical agents are much less common than bacterial infection (232,234).

Pulmonary infection may involve the peripheral air spaces, interstitium, or conducting airways. Infections can be located in the peripheral gas-exchanging lung (consolidative pneumonia), the conducting airways and adjacent air spaces (bronchopneumonia), or the conducting airways alone (airways infection) (8,235,236). If infection involves the peripheral air spaces, inflammatory exudate may spread through collateral pathways (the pores of Kohn and channels of Lambert) to fill adjacent air spaces. The bronchi and perihilar lung parenchyma are usually spared at first in this type of *consolidative pneumonia*. The inflammatory exudate of *bronchopneumonia* involves the bronchi, bronchioles, and adjacent air spaces, frequently in multiple, scattered foci. The inflammatory reaction is initially limited to bronchi or bronchioles in *airways infection* (70,233,236).

The patterns of pulmonary inflammatory disease, its sequelae, and its radiologic appearances are determined by both anatomic and functional factors unique to the child (66,234).

Pediatric peripheral airways are smaller and more collapsible than those of an adult, and collateral pathways of air drift are less effective. There is a higher concentration of mucous glands lining the pediatric airway. The small size and decreased conductance of the peripheral airways are further compromised in airways infection by superimposed edema, mucous secretions, and inflammatory debris; this causes partial or complete occlusion of bronchi or bronchioles and consequent air trapping or atelectasis (66,233,234). Therefore, the radiographic patterns of pulmonary inflammatory disease are determined by both anatomic and functional factors that are unique in the child (66,67).

Collateral ventilation in the infant lung is less efficient than in the adult due to relative underdevelopment of the accessory ventilatory channels (the pores of Kohn and channels of Lambert) and the thickness of the connective tissue septa. These anatomic limitations on collateral ventilation influence the pathophysiology and radiologic patterns

TABLE 7-11. *Etiologies of pediatric pulmonary infection*

Infection	Common cause	Less common cause
Virus	Respiratory syncytial virus	Cytomegalovirus
	Adenovirus	Rubeola
	Parainfluenzae viruses (types 1, 2, 3)	Varicella
Bacteria	*Streptococcus pneumoniae* (pneumococcal)	*Klebsiella*
	Staphylococcus aureus	*Pseudomonas*
	Streptococcus pyogenes	*Escherichia coli*
	Hemophilus influenzae	Mixed flora
	Tuberculosis	
Mycoplasma	*Mycoplasma pneumoniae*	
Protozoa	*Pneumocystis carinii*	Toxoplasmosis
Mycoses		Histoplasmosis
		Blastomycosis
		Coccidioidomycosis
		Cryptococcosis
		Aspergillosis
Nocardia		*Nocardia asteroides*
Rickettsia and *Chlamydia*	*Chlamydia trachomatis*	Ornithosis
		Psittacosis

Modified from Osborne et al. (234).

of pneumonia in children (8,66,67,70,233,236). After 8 years of age, pulmonary architecture is similar to that in the adult.

The defense mechanisms of the respiratory system are categorized as mechanical (e.g., ciliary action), phagocytic, and immune. All three are fully functional and working in concert in the normal child.

Etiology

Pediatric pulmonary infections are caused by a variety of organisms (Table 7-11). Viral organisms tend to cause bronchiolitis, bronchitis, or bronchopneumonia. Bacterial organisms usually cause bronchopneumonia or consolidative (lobar, segmental, subsegmental) pneumonia (234,235).

The role of imaging is to confirm or exclude a clinically suspected pneumonia, to localize it anatomically, to characterize it, and to evaluate progress or complications. Imaging methods demonstrate gross, not microscopic, pathology. One airspace disease tends to look like another, regardless of the pathogen, and the same is true of airway disease. These factors severely limit etiologic diagnosis, and any radiologic evaluation must give great weight to the clinical setting (8,70,233,234,237,238).

Pulmonary parenchymal opacities, patchy parenchymal collapse, and pulmonary overinflation occurring in neonatal pneumonia are nonspecific. However, airspace disease is the characteristic finding of neonatal pneumonia and is most frequently due to nonhemolytic *Streptococcus, Staphylococcus, Escherichia coli,* or *Hemophilus influenzae* (71,234).

Viral pneumonia tends to affect ambulatory children under the age of 5 years (71,239). The most frequent of-fender is the respiratory syncytial virus (RSV), which produces yearly epidemics, but parainfluenza virus, adenovirus, and influenza virus infections may also cause pneumonia in the preschool child (Table 7-12) (234).

Bacterial infection in children <5 years old is usually due to *Streptococcus pneumoniae* (pneumococcal pneumonia). *Mycoplasma pneumoniae* plays an increasingly important role in school-age children, causing 30% of all childhood pneumonias (71,239,240). Gram-negative aerobic or anaerobic infections as well as pneumococcal and staphylococcal organisms should be considered in hospitalized patients. These etiologies are particularly likely when cavitation or pleural effusion is present.

Chronically ill and immunologically compromised children often develop pneumonia caused by less common pathogens. *Pneumocystis* pneumonia is important in this latter group, as are cytomegalovirus (CMV), fungal, and *Nocardia* infections (241,242). Pulmonary opacities in children with acquired immunodeficiency syndrome (AIDS) may be due to infection or to lymphoid hyperplasia in the lungs (241,242).

Race, geography, social status, and unusual exposures also affect the etiology of pulmonary infection. The radiologic features, patient age, and clinical factors must be integrated before an etiologic diagnosis is suggested (8,234,237,238).

Radiologic Manifestations

Acute pulmonary infection during childhood causes abnormal pulmonary densities on the chest radiograph. The radiologic features reflect the pulmonary pathology as fol-

TABLE 7-12. *Patient age and etiologic agents in infectious pneumonia*

Agent	Most likely organisms, by age		
	0–3 months	4 months to 5 years	6–16 years
Nonbacterial			
Common	*Chlamydia trachomatis,* RSV, CMV	RSV, parainfluenza 3, influenza A	*Mycoplasma,* influenza A
Less common	Influenza viruses, parainfluenza viruses	Varicella (chickenpox), adenovirus, paramyxovirus (measles)	Adenovirus, paramyxovirus
Bacterial			
Common	Streptococcus B and D, enteric bacilli, *Streptococcus pneumoniae*	*S. pneumoniae, Hemophilus influenzae*	*S. pneumoniae*
Less common	*Staphylococcus aureus, H. influenzae*	Streptococcus A, *S. aureus*	*H. influenzae,* streptococcus A, *S. aureus*

RSV, respiratory syncytial virus; CMV, cytomegalovirus.
Modified from Schweich (240).

lows: (a) infections that primarily involve peripheral air spaces; (b) infections that primarily involve airways; (c) infections that involve both airways and airspaces (bronchopneumonia). If infection involves the airways, atelectasis and altered aeration are often present.

Certain patterns suggest specific organisms and disease processes. In general, respiratory infection in the infant primarily involves small airways. The respiratory distress that results from peripheral airways obstruction is radiographically manifest as regions of subsegmental atelectasis, air trapping, and linear or discoid regions of perihilar opacity. Viral organisms are most commonly implicated. In older children and adolescents, pulmonary infections may involve either the interstitium or airspaces, and bacterial infections are more common (8,68,236).

Streptococcus pneumoniae (pneumococcal) pneumonia commonly causes a rounded infiltrate; staphylococcal pneumonia leads to segmental patchy airspace infiltrates, pneumatoceles, emphyema, and pneumothorax. Tuberculosis causes paratracheal and mediastinal adenopathy, unchanging airspace disease, and consolidation with collapse. *Mycoplasma pneumoniae* may present with localized lobar, segmental, or subsegmental consolidation in the child with respiratory symptoms or a more diffuse pattern of peribronchial thickening and interstitial opacities in patients with systemic symptoms. Septic pulmonary emboli create multiple cavitary pulmonary nodules, typically with ill-defined margins. Although these radiologic patterns may be helpful, they lack specificity and require correlation with clinical and laboratory information.

Parenchymal Opacities

Widespread pulmonary disease produces radiologic opacities. Basic patterns of this type of disseminated pulmonary disease include vascular, acinar, interstitial, and mixed (234). Volume loss, partial or complete, may be associated with any of these basic patterns. Because opacities are frequently mixed, basing the differential diagnosis purely on the radiologic appearance can be misleading. Pulmonary edema, a classic example of an acinar pattern, graphically demonstrates this point, as both alveoli and the interstitium are involved. Conversely, viral pneumonias in children, which classically present as peribronchial interstitial disease, may also involve contiguous acini. It is particularly difficult to distinguish acinar from interstitial disease in neonates and young infants because of the anatomic size of the acinus. If one understands these limitations, it is frequently helpful to base a differential diagnosis on the radiologic appearance of either acinar disease (Table 7-13) (243) or interstitial disease (Table 7-14) (244).

Acinar Disease

A pulmonary acinus is that portion of lung distal to a terminal bronchiole. It consists of respiratory bronchioles, alveolar ducts, alveolar sacs, and alveoli (see Fig. 7-16). The terminal bronchiole is the last purely conducting structure in the lung and serves the basic functional respiratory unit of the lung (64,68,245). It divides into two or more respiratory bronchioles, which serve alveolar ducts, alveolar sacs, and alveoli (see Fig. 7-16). The acinus increases in diameter from 1 to 2 mm at birth to 3 to 4 mm by 6 months of age to the normal adult size of 6 to 10 mm by 16 years of age (64,68). Fluid filling the acini may be inflammatory (exudate or frank pus), transudate, blood, edema, cellular infiltrate, or extension of cellular material from the interstitium (Table 7-13). At the periphery of the lesion there is usually a mixture of normal acini and partially filled acini. There may be contiguous spread of the acinar filling process to involve adjacent alveoli and produce peribronchiolar nodules (64,68,243).

TABLE 7-13. *Acinar disease in infants and children*

Acute disease
  Pneumonia[a]
    Bacterial[a]
    Mycoplasma[a]
    Viral[a]
  Primary tuberculosis
  Atelectasis[a]
  Pulmonary edema[a]
  Hyaline membrane disease[a]
  Aspiration[a]
  Hemorrhage
    Trauma
    Hemosiderosis
  Wet lung disease[a]
  Hypersensitivity
    Drug
    Inhalation
Chronic disease
  Pneumonia[a]
    Chronic
    Recurrent
  Aspiration[a]
    Chronic
    Recurrent
  Lymphoma-leukemia
  Sarcoidosis
  Pulmonary alveolar proteinosis
  Fungus infection
  Tuberculosis
  Alveolar microlithiasis
  "Interstitial" pneumonitis
    Desquamative
    Lymphocytic
    Others

[a] More common.
Modified from Felson (243).

(243). The size of these acinar nodules depends on the age of the patient. Acinar disease tends to have a more rapid course and is more radiopaque than interstitial disease. Acinar disease is classified as acute or chronic (Table 7-13).

Interstitial Disease

The pulmonary interstitium is the fibrous and structural framework of the lung (244,245). It includes alveolar walls and interstitial septa. There are vascular (arteries, capillaries, veins, lymphatics) and supporting structures in the interstitium (245).

The basic pathologic process in interstitial disease is thickening of the interstitial tissues. The thickening may involve individual alveolar walls and extend into large septa. Because of this interstitial thickening, there is frequently a jux-

TABLE 7-14. *Interstitial disease in infants and children*

Acute disease
  Pneumonia
    Viral[a]
    Mycoplasma
    Bacterial
  Interstitial edema[a]
  Tuberculosis
  Fungus infection
  Hypersensitivity
    Drug
    Inhalation
  Glomerulonephritis
  Hemorrhage
  Wet lung disease[a]
  Hypoproteinemia
Chronic disease
  Cystic fibrosis[a]
  Bronchopulmonary dysplasia[a]
  Wilson-Mikity syndrome
  Histiocytosis
  Metastatic disease
  Sarcoidosis
  Collagen vascular disease
  Irradiation
  Gaucher disease
  Niemann-Pick disease
  Rheumatoid arthritis
  Tuberous sclerosis
  Interstitial pneumonitis
    Usual
    Desquamative
    Lymphocytic
    Others—AIDS
  Drug therapy
  Lymphangiectasia
    Primary
    Secondary
  Neurofibromatosis

[a] More common.
Modified from Felson (244).

This spread of airspace disease typically occurs centrifugally via the pores of Kohn and channels of Lambert.

Other terms used to describe the acinar pattern include airspace disease, alveolar pattern, alveolar opacification, and parenchymal consolidation. The acinar radiologic pattern is characterized by fluffy, ill-defined margins. There is frequently coalescence of disease as intervening acini become involved (243). Pneumonia with an acinar pattern of lobar, segmental, or subsegmental distribution is usually bacterial (8,234,235). However, viral inflammatory disease, *Mycoplasma* pneumonia, and noninfectious inflammatory reactions can also cause this radiologic appearance.

Widespread acinar disease is usually segmental or lobar in distribution. The so-called butterfly or bat-wing pattern is due to coalescent opacity, more prominent centrally and fading toward the periphery of the lung (Fig. 7-103) (243). Air-filled bronchi surrounded by acinar density produce air bronchograms, whereas air-filled acini surrounded by acinar opacities produce air acinograms. Individual acinar nodules may be seen as small, ill-defined, rosette-like opacities

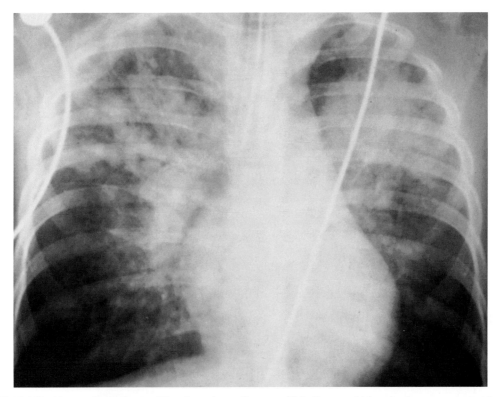

FIG. 7-103. Parenchymal opacities in acinar disease. This 5-year-old boy had severe closed head injury and neurogenic pulmonary edema. Portable chest radiograph shows a central "bat-wing" pattern of fluffy coalescent parenchymal acinar opacities.

taposition of adjacent air containing cystic structures. Moreover, local thickening of the interstitium may contrast with adjacent air-filled acini to produce a nodular appearance.

The radiologic hallmark of interstitial disease is sharp outlines and margins of a diffuse process (Fig. 7-104). Coalescence occurs late if at all (244). The radiologic appearance may include linear densities, fine and irregular nodules, large and variable nodules, and honeycombing (244). Pneumothorax is a potential complication of interstitial disease. There are both acute and chronic causes of interstitial disease in infants and children (Table 7-14). Viral pneumonia is a common cause of acute interstitial lung disease (8).

Mixed Pulmonary Opacities

Many pulmonary infections produce a mixture of these patterns and have characteristics of both airspace and airway disease. Radiographs may show bilateral patchy parenchymal and interstitial opacities plus hyperinflation or irregularity of inflation. This radiographic appearance is most frequently due to viral agents but can also be seen with *Mycoplasma* infection and bacterial pneumonia (231, 233–235,246). Bronchopneumonia of whatever cause spreads peripherally through the bronchial system to produce a segmental pattern of mixed airspace and interstitial opacities.

Atelectasis

Subsegmental atelectasis is common among infants and young children with pulmonary infections and particularly with viral lower airways disease. Lobar and segmental collapse is a less likely result of infection. Pathologically, atelectasis is a loss of air, complete or incomplete, from the pulmonary parenchyma. Radiographically, there are discoid and band-like opacities, often radiating from the hila. Definitive radiographic diagnosis is based on direct or indirect signs of volume loss. Direct signs include displaced fissures bounding the affected region, radiopacity (loss of aeration), and crowding of bronchovascular structures. Indirect signs of collapse include elevation of a hemidiaphragm, shift of mediastinal structures toward the side of the affected lobe, rib crowding on that side, hilar displacement, and compensatory hyperaeration of adjacent uninvolved lobes.

Round atelectasis may mimic a paravertebral tumor but is uncommon in children (47). Atypical peripheral upper lobe atelectasis may simulate an apical mass. This unusual appearance is due to the outer surface of the upper lobe remaining adjacent to the parietal pleura of the chest, while the lower and middle lobes expand both anterior and posterior to the collapsed lobe (247,248). Total atelectasis of the left lung secondary to massive cardiomegaly may simulate a left chest mass (Fig. 7-105). Despite the total atelectasis of the left lung, the left hemithorax is both large and opaque

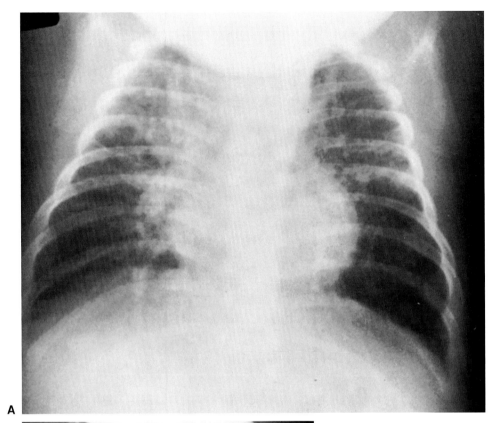

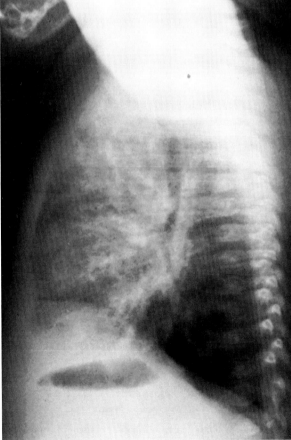

FIG. 7-104. Parenchymal opacities in interstitial disease. A 4-week-old boy was referred for respiratory distress and later proved to have pulmonary lymphangiectasia. AP **(A)** and lateral **(B)** chest radiographs show bilateral reticulolinear densities scattered throughout both lungs; Kerley B lines are present. Biopsy confirmed hyperplasia of lymph channels in the lung interstitium. (Courtesy of Dr. David Boldt, Melbourne, Australia.)

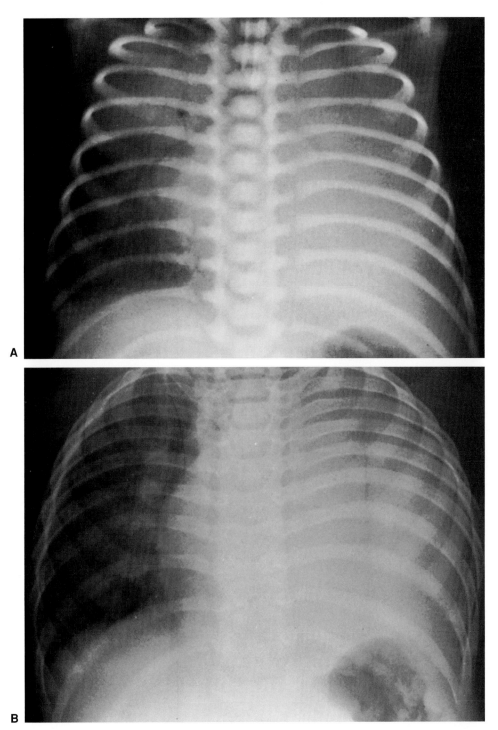

FIG. 7-105. Total atelectasis due to cardiomegaly. A: Newborn with severe subaortic stenosis. There is complete atelectasis of the left lung. The opaque left hemithorax remains large due to the combination of atelectasis and cardiomegaly. **B:** A 9-month-old girl with endocardial fibroelastosis. Large opaque left hemithorax due to atelectasis and cardiomegaly.

because of the massive cardiomegaly. Noninvasive procedures such as high-kilovoltage chest radiography, esophagography, computed tomography, electrocardiography, and echocardiography should lead to the correct diagnosis (73).

Viral Pneumonia and Airway Infection

Viruses are common causes of pneumonia, especially in children under 5 years of age. Viral pneumonia is usually preceded by cough and rhinitis. Viral pneumonia causes less systemic toxicity than bacterial pneumonia, although fever is common. The common viral etiologies of pulmonary infection include respiratory syncytial virus (RSV), parainfluenza viruses (types I, II, and III), the adenoviruses, enterovi-

rus, and influenza virus (see Tables 7-11 and 7-12) (234). Other less common viral causes of pediatric pneumonia include herpes simplex virus, rhinovirus, and, in the immunocompromised patient, CMV.

These viruses produce a surface infection of the respiratory mucous membranes and multiplication of viruses in the mucosa. There is necrosis of ciliated epithelial cells, goblet cells, and bronchial mucous glands. The bronchial and bronchiolar walls become edematous and infiltrated with inflammatory cells. There is frequently involvement of peribronchial tissues and interlobular septa, with extension of necrosis and edema into the terminal air passages and alveoli. The inflammatory process tends to affect only the airways, sparing adjacent airspaces (Fig. 7-106). Resolution is characterized by epithelial regeneration and proliferation

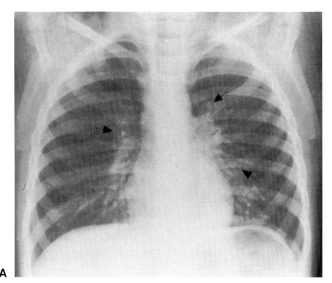

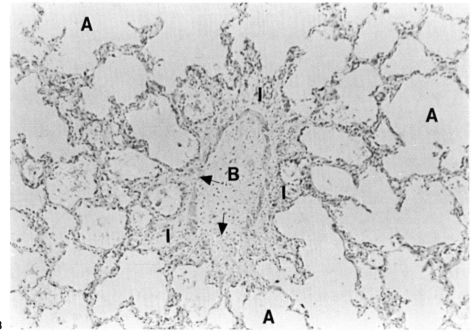

FIG. 7-106. **Viral airways disease. A:** A 2-year-old boy with viral bronchitis. The lungs are mildly hyperaerated, and there is a diffuse increase in linear markings in the parahilar regions with associated peribronchial cuffing *(arrows)*. **B:** Microscopic lung section of a patient who died of adenovirus pneumonia. The alveoli *(A)* are normally aerated and contain no inflammatory exudate. There is a marked inflammatory exudate within a bronchiole *(B)* with associated bronchiolar necrosis *(arrows)* and peribronchial interstitial extension of the inflammatory process *(I)*. (Courtesy of Dennis Osborne, M.D., Brisbane, Australia.)

(231,246). The radiographic appearance of viral pneumonia reflects the airway distribution of disease. Disease is usually bilateral, and is often associated with hyperaeration and air trapping. There are areas of bronchial wall thickening and peribronchial opacification to produce peribronchial cuffing; bronchial wall thickening produces parahilar linear densities. Some patchy areas of opacification are present in approximately half the cases (234). Segmental or lobar consolidation, hilar adenopathy, and pleural effusion are rare (8,66,231,234,235,246).

Bronchiolitis is a clinical syndrome, viral in etiology, which occurs in patients <1 year of age. These infants have tachypnea, wheezing, fever of lower grade than that caused by bacterial pneumonia, chest retractions, and pulmonary overaeration. RSV is the most common cause of bronchiolitis; epidemics tend to occur during the winter months. Recurrent attacks of "bronchiolitis" should suggest some other process such as asthma or cystic fibrosis. Radiographically, bronchiolitis is characterized by marked hyperaeration, moderate peribronchial cuffing, and minimal parahilar linear opacities (Fig. 7-107) (66,234).

Bronchitis usually occurs in older infants or young children and is characterized by hyperaeration, moderate to marked peribronchial cuffing, and parahilar linear opacities (see Fig. 7-106) (8,234,246). Bronchitis with bronchial wall thickening and peribronchial opacification has been referred to as a "dirty chest."

Bronchopneumonia is characterized by patchy areas of parenchymal opacification (Fig. 7-108). These opacities are due to peribronchial extension of infection as well as atelectasis associated with airway disease. Much of the opacity seen in viral airways disease is actually due to atelectasis caused by bronchial and bronchiolar mucus plugging (234).

One tends to think of viral airway disease as a benign process. However, there may be a 2- to 3-week lag in radiologic resolution despite marked clinical improvement much earlier. Although resolution usually occurs without sequelae, viral airway infection sometimes causes bronchiectasis (234). Epidemics of adenovirus type 21 pneumonia producing severe bronchiectasis (Fig. 7-109) in susceptible races have been reported (234). Adenovirus infections may occasionally cause bronchiolitis obliterans and the unilateral hyperlucent lung syndrome (Swyer-James syndrome).

Incompletely immunized children may develop atypical measles after exposure to natural measles virus. The illness is characterized by fever, headache, cough, abdominal pain, muscle cramps, and a maculopapular rash that initially appears on the hands and feet and progresses centrally (249). Pulmonary involvement with acute atypical measles usually causes bilateral acinar opacities with or without pleural effusion and hilar adenopathy. The parenchymal opacities may be nodular. Failure of immunization causes hypersensitivity to natural measles virus rather than immunity. The response is one of immune complex (viral antigen-host-antibody-complement) formation in the lungs with resultant pulmonary tissue injury (249). Wood and Bernstein (249) believed

that acute atypical measles pneumonia is due to a more rapid and better contained formation of pulmonary immune complexes with resultant nodular tissue injury. Nodular residuals following atypical measles pneumonia are common (249). These nodules are usually peripheral, may contain calcification, and may persist for years (250).

Bacterial Pneumonia

Bacterial pneumonia is a major cause of morbidity among infants and children in the United States. Factors that predispose to bacterial pneumonia include urban living, poor socioeconomic status, increased number of siblings, parental smoking, and preterm delivery (240). Other conditions, such as tracheoesophageal fistula, other causes of aspiration, developmental pulmonary anomalies, acquired or congenital immune defects, congenital heart disease, and cystic fibrosis, increase a patient's susceptibility to pneumonia (233,234).

Normally, the respiratory system from the sublaryngeal region to the alveoli is sterile. The lungs are protected from bacterial infection by several mechanisms: (a) intact swallowing and gag reflex (prevents aspiration); (b) cough reflex (to expel material, sometimes containing bacteria); (c) normal mucosal mucus blanket and ciliated epithelium (to entrap and expel organisms); and (d) intact host immune system.

Bacterial pneumonia in children is often due to *Streptococcus pneumoniae* (pneumococcal), *Streptococcus,* or *Staphylococcus.* Less common etiologies include *Hemophilus influenzae, Klebsiella,* and *Pseudomonas* (see Tables 7-11 and 7-12) (8,233,234,236). There is typically a peripheral airspace exudate that is centrifugally progressive from a small nidus to involve a bronchopulmonary segment or an entire lobe (Fig. 7-110) (231,235). Pathologically, exudate fills alveoli (Fig. 7-110C).

Bacterial pneumonia is often preceded by an upper respiratory tract viral infection. Cough, fever, chest pain, and headache are common symptoms. It is not unusual for the child with bacterial pneumonia to present with abdominal pain and fever (Fig. 7-111). Most children with bacterial pneumonia rapidly respond to antibiotics. Radiographic resolution is influenced by patient age, host immune response, and extent of parenchymal and pleural disease. Typically, there is resolution with 2–4 weeks. When the pneumonia fails to clear in a timely fashion, an underlying pathologic process must be considered; possibilities include an endobronchial foreign body, adenopathy due to tuberculosis or granulomatous disease causing airway compression, and congenital anomalies, such as sequestration or bronchopulmonary foregut cyst.

Radiologic consolidation is usually lobar or segmental and frequently contains air bronchograms (Fig. 7-110). A central lucency may represent normal aerated lung, cavitation, or a pneumatocele. A round pneumonia, typically

Text continues on p. 733.

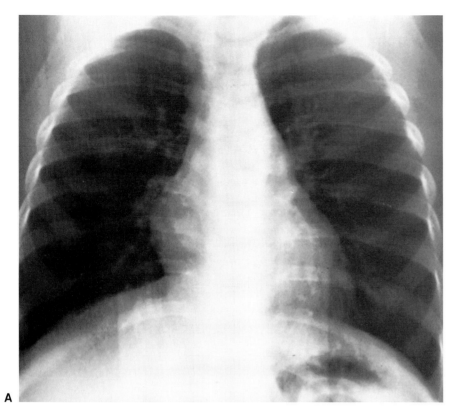

A

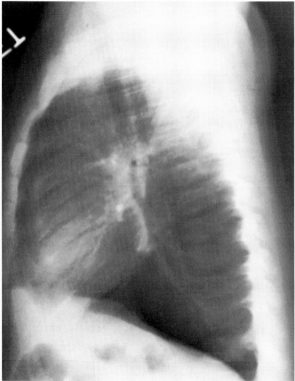

B

FIG. 7-107. Hyperaeration in bronchiolitis. An 11-month-old girl with cough and fever. **A:** Anteroposterior chest radiograph shows markedly hyperaerated lungs. Domes of hemidiaphragms are at the level of the eighth ribs anteriorly. There is minimal increase in parahilar markings. **B:** The lateral radiograph shows an increase in retrosternal lucency and marked flattening of the hemidiaphragms.

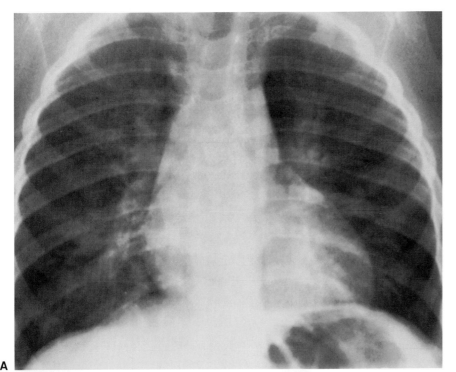

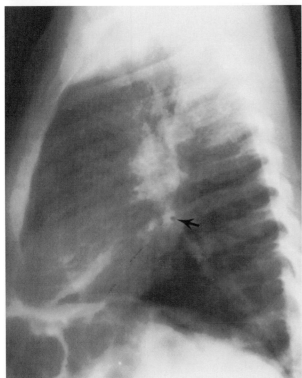

FIG. 7-108. Viral bronchopneumonia. Anteroposterior **(A)** and lateral **(B)** chest radiographs of a 12-month-old girl demonstrate hyperaeration, peribronchial cuffing *(arrow)*, increased linear parahilar markings, and patchy bilateral parenchymal opacities.

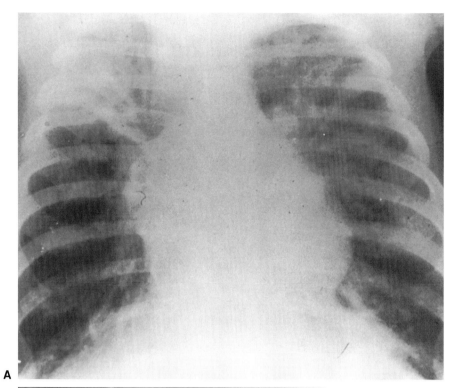

A

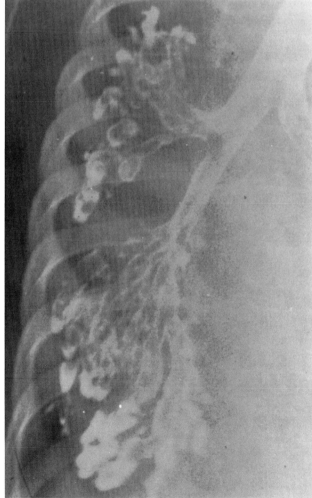

B

FIG. 7-109. Bronchiectasis complicating viral pneumonia. **A:** A 6-month-old infant with proven adenovirus 21 infection. **B:** Bronchogram 6 months later shows severe bronchiectasis. (Courtesy of Dennis Osborne, M.D., Brisbane, Australia.)

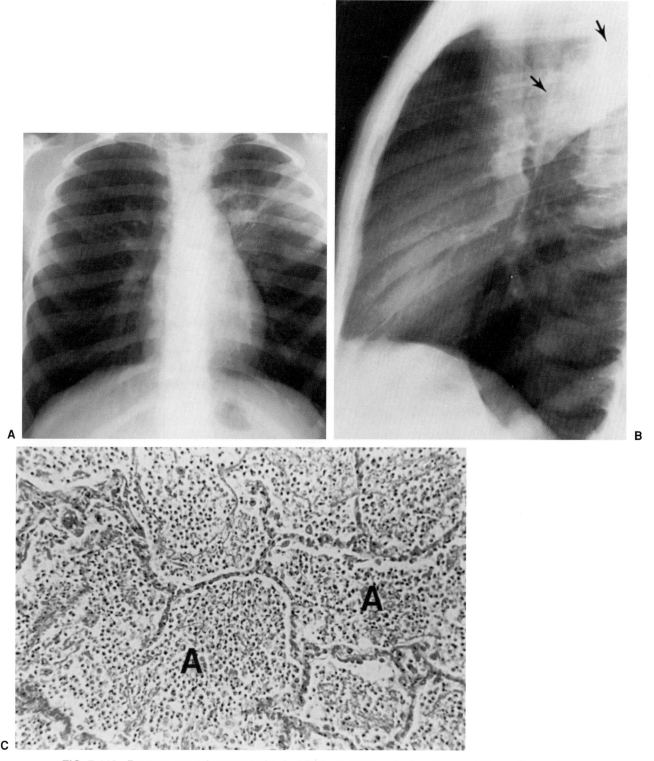

FIG. 7-110. Pneumococcal pneumonia. A: AP chest radiograph of an 8-year-old boy with cough and fever shows segmental consolidation in the left upper lobe. **B:** Lateral view confirms left upper lobe consolidation *(arrows).* **C:** Histologic section of a patient with pneumococcal pneumonia. Alveoli *(A)* are completely filled with organisms and inflammatory exudate.

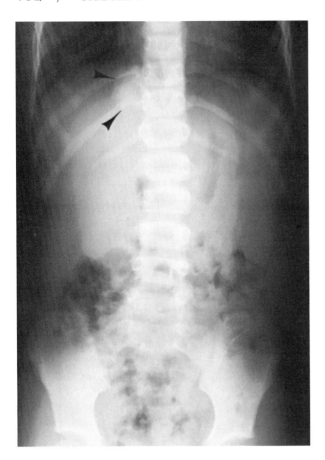

FIG. 7-111. Round pneumonia presenting as an acute abdomen. An 8-year-old girl with right lower quadrant pain, abdominal tenderness, and fever. The supine anteroposterior abdominal radiograph shows a rounded infiltrate in the right lung base *(arrowhead)*.

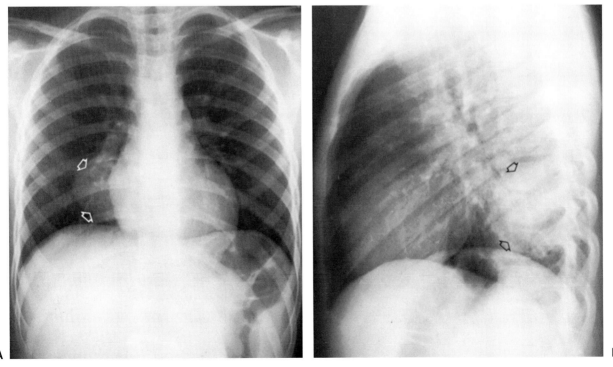

A   B

FIG. 7-112. Round pneumonia. A, B: An 11-year-old boy with fever, abdominal pain, and cough. The AP **(A)** and lateral **(B)** chest radiographs show a rounded opacity in the right lower lobe *(arrows)*.

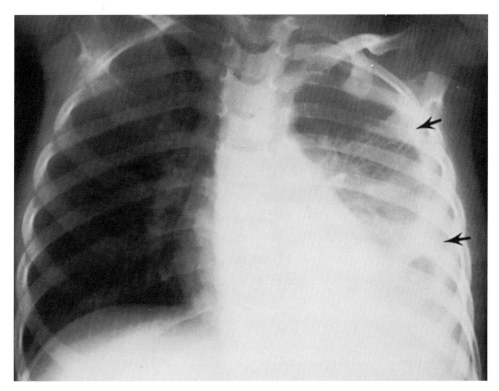

FIG. 7-113. Pneumonia and pleural effusion or empyema. Anteroposterior chest radiograph of a 2-year-old boy with proved pneumococcal pneumonia shows consolidation of the left lower lobe and pleural effusion or empyema *(arrows).*

seen in children <8 years of age (Fig. 7-112), is usually pneumococcal in origin. Pleural effusion suggests pneumococcal, staphylococcal, tuberculous, or *Hemophilus* pneumonia (Fig. 7-113). When pleural fluid is seen, with or without parenchymal infiltrate or hilar adenopathy, primary tuberculosis must be considered (234). Distinguishing sterile pleural fluid from empyema is impossible radiographically. The appearance of pleural fluid in the setting of pneumonia suggests empyema. Thoracentesis confirms the diagnosis (Fig. 7-114) (240). Pneumatoceles suggest staphylococcal (Fig. 7-115) or gram-negative pneumonia. Pneumatocele formation may also occur after hydrocarbon aspiration or pulmonary trauma. A pneumatocele is distinguished from a pulmonary abscess by the radiographic appearance and time of occurrence. A pneumatocele is thin-walled and occurs 10–14 days after the onset of infection, when the patient is clinically improving.

Although rare, lung abscesses represent a significant complication of bacterial pneumonia; *Staphylococcus* and *H. influenzae* are the most common organisms. Abscesses tend to occur early in the course of disease, when the patient is clinically ill. Multiple scattered abscesses suggest bacterial endocarditis. Pathologically, lung consolidation progresses to lung necrosis and central cavitation with bronchial communication. Radiographically, a lung abscess has a thick irregular wall, and there are variable amounts of fluid and air within the cavity. It may be difficult to differentiate be-

tween lung abscess, infected pneumatocele, and loculated empyema with a bronchopleural fistula. CT can ususally distinguish a lung abscess from empyema (Fig. 7-116) (1,234,251).

In general, follow-up chest radiography during convalescence is not necessary unless complications such as abscess, pneumatocele, pneumothorax, or bronchopleural fistula are suspected. Follow-up radiographs are suggested if there is a strong suspicion that the consolidation represents an infected developmental abnormality, such as sequestration, if the patient has a compromised immune system, or if the patient has sickle cell disease. When follow-up radiographs are obtained, the usual tendency is to get them too early. Ideally, all symptoms should have resolved and 14 to 21 days should have passed before the follow-up examination is obtained.

Mycoplasma Pneumonia

Mycoplasma pneumoniae causes up to 30% of pneumonia in older childhood. The organism is neither a bacterium nor a virus. The course can range from an indolent illness , consisting of malaise, lethargy, and dyspnea, to an acute pneumonia with cough, fever, and myalgias.

The radiologic changes in *M. pneumoniae* pneumonia can mimic other pulmonary diseases (252). The most frequent pattern is one of bronchopneumonic infiltrates, especially of

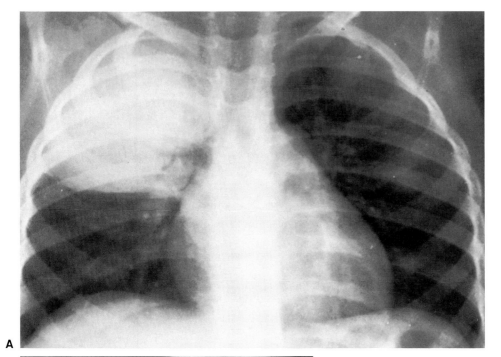

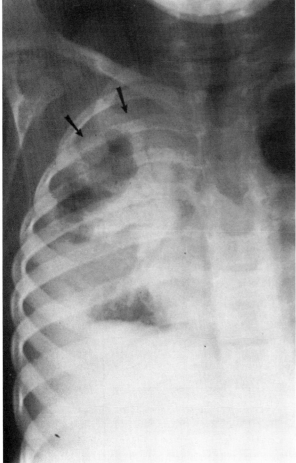

FIG. 7-114. Empyema. A 2-year-old boy with known pneumo-coccal pneumonia. **A:** The initial anteroposterior chest radio-graph shows consolidation of the entire right upper lobe. **B:** After 1 week of antibiotic therapy, the patient remained ill with cough and fever. The chest radiograph shows right upper lobe and right lower lobe consolidation with an area of extraparenchymal soft-tissue density in the right upper thorax *(arrows)*. Thoracentesis confirmed empyema.

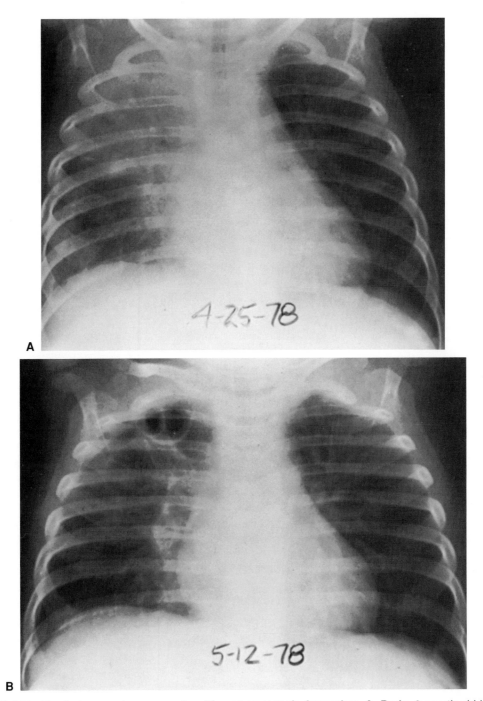

FIG. 7-115. Staphylococcal pneumonia with pneumatocele formation. A, B: An 8-month-old boy with cough and fever. Admission chest radiograph **(A)** shows right upper lobe consolidation and pleural thickening. Chest radiograph after 2 weeks of antibiotic therapy **(B)** shows that pneumatoceles have developed in the right upper lobe. (*continued*)

the lower lobes. Bilateral, reticulonodular interstitial infiltrates and discoid shadows of segmental and subsegmental atelectasis are common; these patients, whose radiographic findings suggest viral airway disease, tend to have an indolent course (253). Less common is consolidation in a segmental or subsegmental distribution; the latter pattern is seen in acutely ill, toxic children with respiratory symptoms (Fig.

7-117) (253). Pleural effusions are not uncommon but tend to be small and transient. Other radiographic manifestations of this disease include diffuse nodular interstitial densities which may mimic miliary tuberculosis and hilar lymph node enlargement with parenchymal infiltrates resembling pulmonary sarcoidosis (252,253).

Text continues on p. 739.

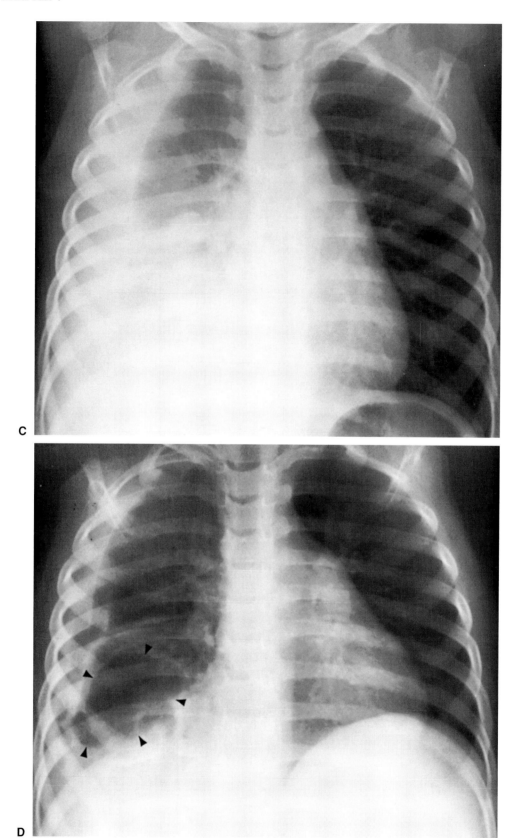

FIG. 7-115. *Continued.* **C, D:** A 2-year-old girl with cough and fever. Admission chest radiograph **(C)** shows right lower lobe consolidation with a large pleural effusion. Chest radiograph after 10 days of antibiotic therapy **(D)**. The patient was asymptomatic, but a pneumatocele has developed in the right lower lobe *(arrowheads)*.

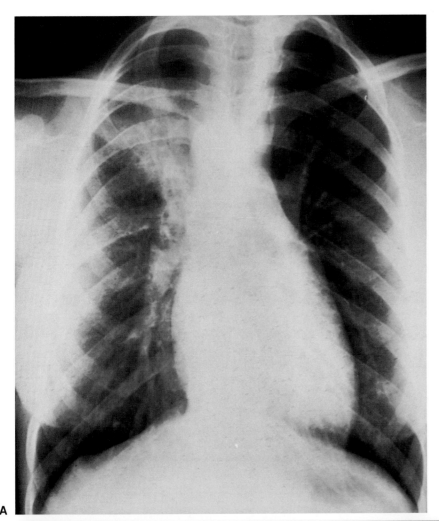

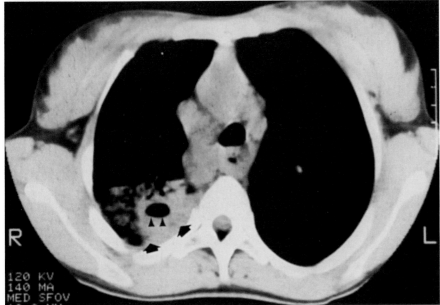

FIG. 7-116. Lung abscess. A 16-year-old girl with immunodeficiency. Cough and fever persisted despite antibiotics to cover "community-acquired" pneumonia. **A:** Chest radiograph shows right upper lobe consolidation. **B:** Chest CT demonstrates right upper lobe consolidation with a central cavity and an air-fluid level *(arrowheads)*. Note the adjacent pleural reaction *(arrows)*.

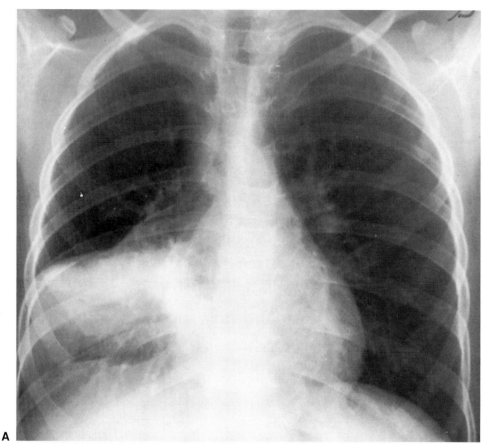

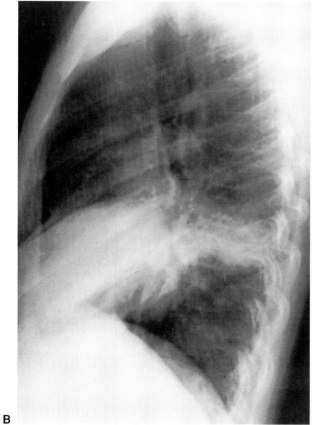

FIG. 7-117. *Mycoplasma* **pneumonia.** A 9-year-old boy with myalgias, cough, and a palpable spleen. The patient had a positive cold agglutinin test for *Mycoplasma pneumoniae.* Anteroposterior **(A)** and lateral **(B)** chest radiographs show right middle lobe and right lower lobe consolidations.

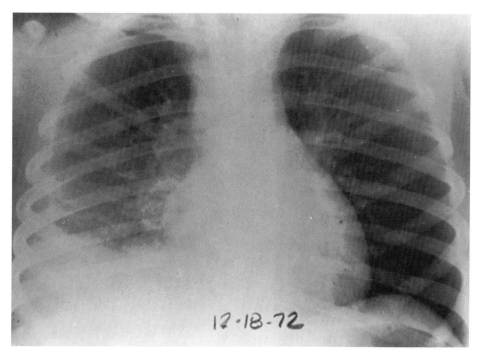

FIG. 7-118. Primary tuberculosis. There is a right lower lobe opacity, a right pleural effusion, and right hilar adenopathy.

Tuberculosis

A high index of suspicion is required for an early diagnosis of tuberculosis, which has been increasing in frequency in the United States, particularly in regions inhabited by large populations of immigrants and refugees (254–256). Other factors contributing to its continuing recurrence are poverty, homelessness, and the epidemic of human immunodeficiency virus (HIV) (257).

The initial pulmonary inflammatory exudate of tuberculosis (primary tuberculosis) produces localized airspace disease in any pulmonary segment or lobe (258,259). There may be regional lymph node enlargement and pleural effusion (Fig. 7-118). The infection spreads from the peripheral airspace focus to central lymph nodes by lymphatic channels (Fig. 7-119). After several weeks, hypersensitivity develops and there is regional lymph node enlargement and sometimes caseation necrosis in the inflammatory foci (Fig. 7-120) (258,259). With the development of resistance, the inflammatory reactions in the parenchyma and lymph nodes involute and may calcify. These calcifications may produce a peripheral Ghon focus or a Ranke complex (calcification in parenchyma and central lymph nodes). If host resistance is poor or there is overwhelming infection, the primary parenchymal process extends to involve large segments of lung, and this is usually associated with a pleural effusion (260). There may also be spread of organisms from the lymphatic system into the venous system through the thoracic duct (see Fig. 7-119). Subsequent seeding of organisms to the lungs leads to miliary or secondary tuberculosis (Fig. 7-121) (254,261).

Radiologic examination is critical in the early diagnosis of tuberculosis (260). The chest radiograph may be sufficiently characteristic to suggest the correct diagnosis. If airspace disease is present in association with hilar adenopathy or pleural effusion, particularly if the child is not acutely ill, tuberculosis is likely (see Fig. 7-118). The radiologic appearance of miliary tuberculosis is fairly characteristic: multiple, small nodular opacities of a relatively uniform size (2–3 mm) scattered throughout both lungs (Fig. 7-121). HRCT demonstrates the interstitial thickening and nodularity of miliary tuberculosis (254,261). Unlike adolescents and adults, infants with miliary tuberculosis may have few symptoms. Certain pulmonary mycotic infections such as histoplasmosis (midwestern United States) and coccidioidomycosis (southwestern United States) and viral pneumonia may mimic the radiologic pattern of pulmonary tuberculosis (256,257).

Chlamydia Pneumonia

Pneumonia due to chlamydial infection is increasingly recognized (262–265). The agent responsible for this infection is *Chlamydia trachomatis,* an obligate intracelluar parasite with features of both a bacterium and a virus. The organism can produce a pneumonia characterized by both alveolar and interstitial lymphocytic and phagocytic infiltration. There may be pulmonary hemorrhage. Infection with this organism is acquired from the mother during vaginal delivery. There is frequently a history of previous conjunctivitis or rhinitis. Approximately 50% will have peripheral eosino-

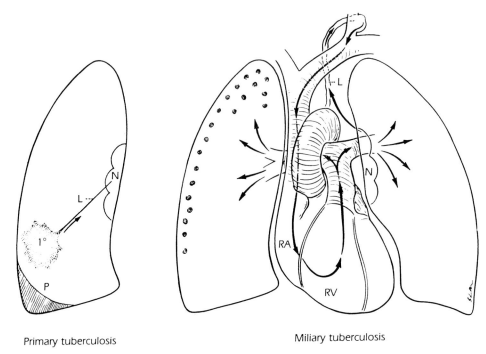

Primary tuberculosis

Miliary tuberculosis

FIG. 7-119. Pathophysiology of tuberculosis. Primary tuberculosis produces pulmonary consolidation (1°) and there may be a pleural effusion (P). Organisms tend to spread through lymphatics (L) to central lymph nodes (N). If immunity is inadequate or infection is overwhelming, organisms spread from central lymph nodes to the thoracic duct and the systemic venous circulation. Subsequent seeding of the lungs produces miliary tuberculosis. *RA,* right atrium; *RV,* right ventricle.

philia. The average age at onset of symptoms is 6 weeks with a range of 4–12 weeks. There is frequently a staccato cough with minimal fever or leukocytosis.

The radiologic appearance, frequently much more impressive than would be predicted by the history and physical examination, is similar to that of viral airway disease (265). There is generalized hyperaeration plus areas of atelectasis. Numerous linear and reticulonodular interstitial densities are scattered symmetrically throughout the lungs (Fig. 7-122). Radiologic resolution requires weeks to months and lags well behind clinical improvement (8,234,235,262,265).

Mycoses

Mycotic (fungal) diseases that involve the lung include histoplasmosis, aspergillosis, blastomycosis, mucormycosis, coccidioidomycosis, and candidiasis. Nocardiosis and actinomycosis have some fungal attributes (234). Although these infections are uncommon in children, they must be considered when the clinical or radiographic features are those of a chronic or otherwise unusual pneumonia (235). Radiography is not sufficiently specific to differentiate among them.

Histoplasmosis occurs endemically in the Ohio, Mississippi, and Missouri river valleys. The disease is due to inhalation of spores of *Histoplasma capsulatum.* The primary disease is often asymptomatic and is detected by a positive

histoplasmin skin test. Patients with acute primary pulmonary histoplasmosis may have a normal chest radiograph. Other radiographic manifestations of the disease include subsegmental patchy infiltrates, fleeting alveolar opacities, variable hilar adenopathy, and eventually small residual parenchymal opacities. Hilar, mediastinal, and intrapulmonary lymph node enlargement is common (Fig. 7-123). Acute, massive histoplasmosis infection occurs after exposure to a heavy inoculum of spores; this carries a high morbidity and mortality. The chest radiograph typically shows a pattern of interstitial pneumonia, often with a nodular component. Fibrosing mediastinitis, which entraps and obstructs mediastinal structures, is a rare complication of histoplasmosis.

Pulmonary aspergillosis occurs in three clinical forms (266): (a) *Allergic bronchopulmonary* aspergillosis complicates chronic asthma or cystic fibrosis (266). Radiography during the acute stage shows patchy consolidation mixed with atelectasis. An upper lung predominance is common. Finger-like opacities due to mucoid impaction in dilated bronchi are characteristic (Fig. 7-124) (267). In the later stages of disease, bronchiectasis and pulmonary fibrosis may be seen. (b) *Aspergilloma* (intracavitary fungus ball), like allergic aspergillosis, is a noninvasive form of the disease (266). The antecedent pulmonary cavitation may be caused by pulmonary tuberculosis, fungal infection, bronchiectasis, developmental lung cyst, sarcoidosis, pneumatocele, or a chronic abscess cavity. (c) *Invasive aspergillosis* is a life-

Text continues on p. 744.

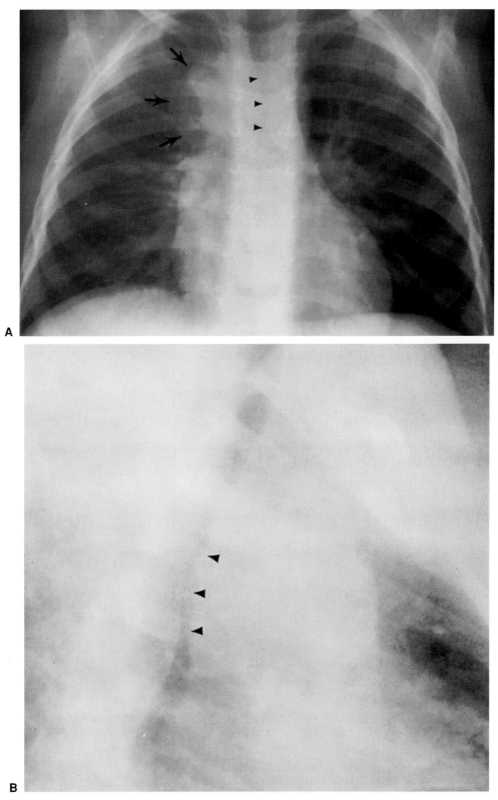

FIG. 7-120. Primary tuberculosis. A: Anteroposterior chest radiograph of a 2-year-old boy with expiratory stridor (wheezing) and positive PPD shows bulky right paratracheal adenopathy *(arrows)* compressing the trachea *(arrowheads)*. **B:** Lateral chest radiograph shows posterior bowing and narrowing of the trachea *(arrowheads)* due to mediastinal adenopathy.

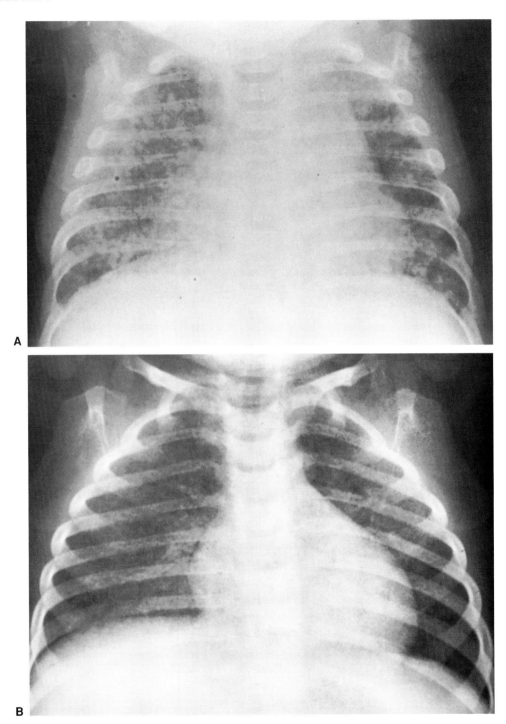

FIG. 7-121. Miliary tuberculosis. A: A 3-month-old mildly symptomatic boy. Note the multiple miliary lung nodules. **B:** A 9-month-old boy. There are multiple small miliary nodules scattered throughout the lungs in this patient, who only had mild pulmonary symptoms.

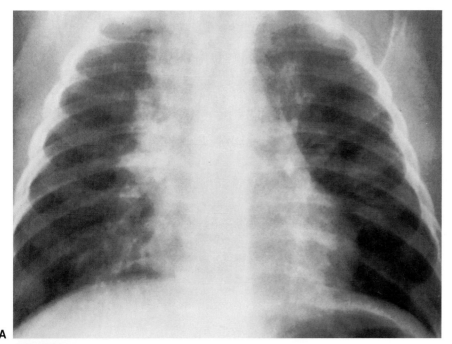

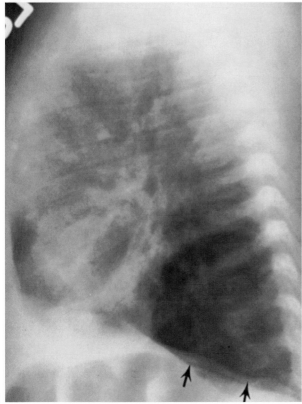

FIG. 7-122. *Chlamydia* **pneumonia.** A 2-month-old boy with staccato cough, previous rhinitis, and conjunctivitis. **A:** There is hyperaeration, an increase in linear parahilar markings, peribronchial cuffing, and patchy acinar opacities. **B:** The lateral chest radiograph confirms peribronchial cuffing and hyperaeration *(arrows).*

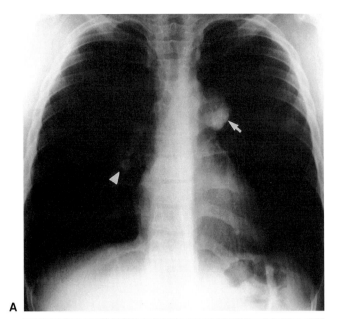

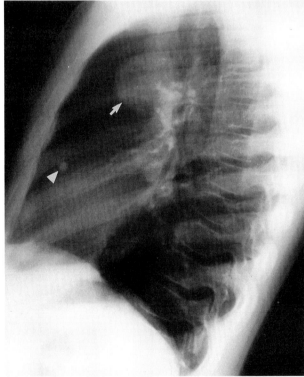

FIG. 7-123. Histoplasmosis. AP **(A)** and lateral **(B)** chest radiographs of a 14-year-old boy show left paraaortic and middle mediastinal adenopathy *(arrows)*. Note the calcified granuloma in the right middle lobe *(arrowhead)*.

threatening infection of immunocompromised patients manifested radiographically by nonspecific multifocal parenchymal opacities (Fig. 7-125) (266). The wedge-shaped opacity of pulmonary infarction may be an early finding.

Radiographic differentiation among the various pulmonary mycoses is often impossible; each may have pulmonary opacification with or without cavitation, calcification, and adenopathy (2,6).

Opportunistic Infection

Children with altered immune status are at risk for pulmonary infection caused by opportunistic agents. Leukemia, lymphoma, congenital and acquired immunodeficiency

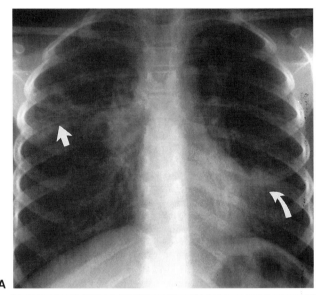

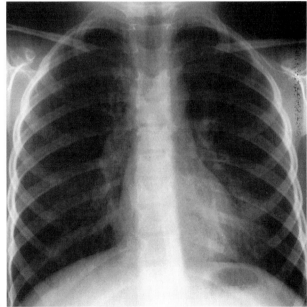

FIG. 7-124. Allergic bronchopulmonary aspergillosis. This 8-year-old girl with known asthma developed cough and eosinophilia in her blood and sputum. **A:** At presentation, the chest radiograph shows homogeneous tubular opacities in the right upper lobe due to bronchi filled with secretions *(arrow)*. A patchy area of lingular atelectasis is also noted *(curved arrow)*. **B:** Follow-up at 3 months shows resolution of right upper lobe opacities but persistent lingular atelectasis.

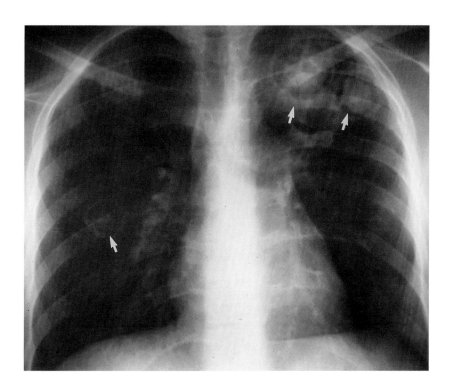

FIG. 7-125. Invasive pulmonary aspergillosis. This 13-year-old neutropenic boy with acute lymphocytic leukemia had cough and fever. The chest radiograph shows multiple cavitating pulmonary nodules *(arrows)*.

states, corticosteroid treatment, and cytotoxic drug therapy predispose to infection with *Pneumocystis carinii,* measles, chickenpox, CMV, and fungal organisms.

Pneumocystis carinii frequently causes pneumonia in the immunosuppressed child, especially with AIDS. Early symptoms, though mild (often only cough and malaise), may rapidly progress to respiratory failure. Like most pulmonary infections in the immunocompromised host, a *P. carinii* pneumonia has no specific features. The early, subtle radiographic changes of interstitial disease may suggest early pulmonary edema or viral infection (Fig. 7-126A). Progression to diffuse airspace disease is common (Fig. 7-126B). Bronchoscopy and lavage or open lung biopsy may be necessary to confirm the diagnosis (241,242).

Complications of Pneumonia

Pleural Inflammation

In the pediatric patient, inflammation of the pleural membranes often accompanies pneumonia. In fact, thickening of the pleural shadows may be an even earlier radiographic sign of bacterial pneumonia than pulmonary infiltrate. Other causes of pleural thickening include trauma, neoplasm, granulomatous inflammatory disease, generalized inflammatory disease affecting serous membranes, lymphatic abnormalities, and pulmonary vascular obstruction (2,6,8,9). Infections in the adjacent lung associated with pleurisy and empyema in infants and children are generally caused by bacteria (*Hemophilus influenzae, Streptococcus pneumoniae,* and

Staphylococcus aureus), tuberculosis, fungal infection, *Mycoplasma* pneumonia, and viral disease (1). Chest radiographs are sensitive to pleural disease. A pleural effusion usually fills and obliterates the costophrenic sulcus even when small. Uncomplicated pleural effusions shift with change in patient position. Empyema on the other hand, because of its thick fibrinopurulent nature, typically shows little movement with radiographs obtained in different patient positions. An accumulation of pleural fluid on a decubitus radiograph of 10 mm or more in thickness is significant (see Fig. 7-115), and thoracentesis should be considered.

Ultrasonography can help to distinguish pleural thickening from pleural effusion, characterize the fluid collection, and determine the best location for thoracentesis or chest tube insertion. It may be difficult to distinguish a pyopneumothorax from a peripheral lung abscess; CT is extremely helpful. In the former (empyema), an obtuse angle is created where the empyema meets the chest wall. Pulmonary abscess typically forms an acute angle with the inner chest wall (see Fig. 7-116B) (46). In the setting of pleurisy and large pleural effusion, a careful search should be made for radiologic signs of extrapleural disease (bone erosion, rib splaying, pedicle destruction), since tumors may mimic thoracopulmonary infection.

Lung Abscess

A lung abscess is pulmonary parenchymal suppuration and necrosis. The abscess is typically circumscribed and thick-walled. With more sophisticated antibiotics and more

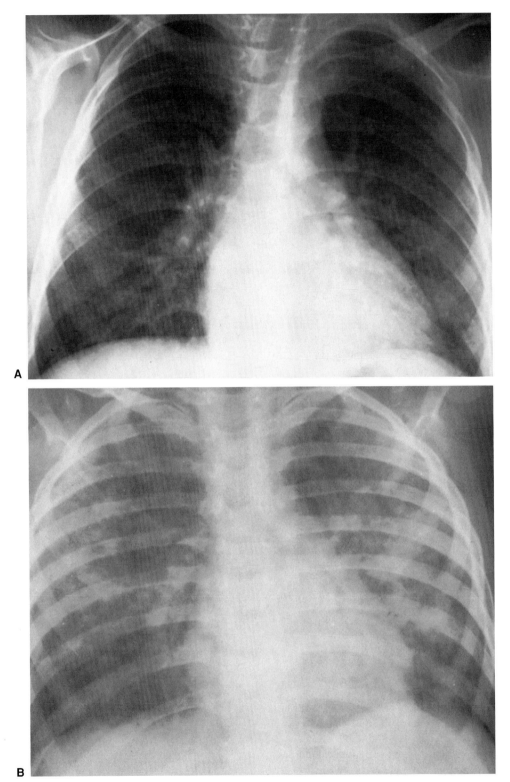

FIG. 7-126. *Pneumocystis carinii* pneumonia. **A:** An 11-year-old boy with acute lymphocytic leukemia. The chest radiograph shows an indistinctness of central pulmonary vessels due to interstitial disease. **B:** A 3-year-old boy with acute lymphocytic leukemia and cough. Airspace and interstitial disease are present.

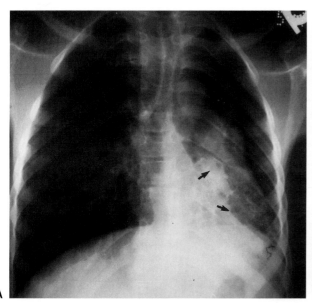
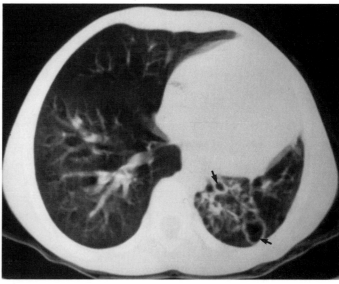

FIG. 7-127. Bronchiectasis. A 10-year-old boy with IGA deficiency and severe bronchiectasis secondary to recurrent bacterial infection. **A:** Chest radiograph shows LLL cystic spaces and tram lines consistent with bronchiectasis *(arrows)*. There is also volume loss. **B:** CT confirms LLL saccular bronchiectasis *(arrows)*.

modern management of infected tonsils, the incidence of pulmonary abscess has declined dramatically. The interplay between host immune status and virulence of causative organism governs which patients are at risk for abscess. Primary pulmonary abscesses occur in an otherwise healthy child. Secondary abscesses are seen in an infant or child who is compromised. This compromise may be a congenital or acquired immune disorder, a predisposition to chronic or recurrent aspiration, or an extensive and severe bronchopneumonia due to staphylococcal or gram-negative organisms. Primary abscesses are typically solitary. Prior to communication with the airway, the pulmonary abscess is an oval or rounded water density mass. CT with intravenous contrast can differentiate an early lung abscess without an air-containing cavity from consolidated lung. Most pulmonary abscesses will communicate with the airway and eventually develop into thick-walled cavities with air-fluid levels. CT can characterize the intrinsic nature of the abscess, assess proximity to the pleura, and plan percutaneous drainage (see Fig. 7-116B) (268).

Pneumatocele

A pneumatocele, quite different from a pulmonary abscess, is an interstitial air accumulation that sometimes follows acute or chronic pneumonia (269). Other causes include trauma, hydrocarbon aspiration (270), and barotrauma. A pneumatocele (rounded, thin-walled lucency) develops when the patient is clinically improving; these usually develop 10–14 days into the course of pulmonary infection (16). Pulmonary abscess, on the other hand, develops early

in the course of disease when the patient is still quite ill (16). The wall of a pneumatocele is thinner than a pulmonary abscess (see Figs. 7-115 and 7-116); abscesses frequently contain an air-fluid level. Most pneumatoceles will, in time, resolve without sequelae. An air-fluid level in a pneumatocele suggests complicating infection.

Bronchiectasis

Bronchiectasis is defined as localized bronchial dilatation (4,271). The usual cause is infection. Reversible bronchiectasis may occur during an acute pneumonia. Childhood bronchiectasis may be due to adenovirus infection (see Fig. 7-109) or bacterial pneumonia (Fig. 7-127). Bronchiectasis is classified as cylindrical (tubular dilatation with a smooth outline), varicose (dilatation and distortion by constrictions), and saccular or cystic (dilatation, with ballooned terminations) (4). Varicose and saccular bronchiectasis are irreversible.

CT has markedly decreased the indications for bronchography in children (54,55,271). High-resolution CT confirms the presence and extent of bronchiectasis (Fig. 7-127). However, bronchography sometimes shows the site and extent of bronchiectasis to better advantage (see Fig. 7-109B). Evaluation of other segments of lung is particularly important if surgical resection is contemplated. If indicated, functional bronchography (films taken during both inspiration and expiration) should be performed (56). Fluoroscopy as well as overhead films in AP, oblique, and lateral projections are obtained to visualize the bronchial anatomy (Fig. 7-128).

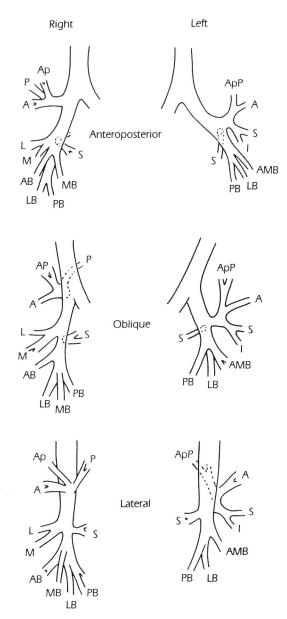

Right   Left

Anteroposterior

Oblique

Lateral

FIG. 7-128. Normal bronchial anatomy. The normal segmental bronchial anatomy of the right and left lungs is shown in AP, oblique, and lateral projections. *A*, anterior; *AB*, anterior basal; *AMB*, anteromedial basal; *Ap*, apical; *ApP*, apical posterior; *I*, inferior; *L*, lateral; *LB*, lateral basal; *M*, medial; *MB*, medial basal; *P*, posterior; *PB*, posterior basal; *S*, superior.

Swyer-James Syndrome

The Swyer-James syndrome (MacLeod syndrome, idiopathic unilateral hyperlucent lung) is a clinical, radiologic, and pathologic syndrome characterized by unilateral hyperlucency of a lung associated with a decrease in the size and number of pulmonary vessels as well as absence of peripheral filling at bronchography (160,161). The majority of cases in the literature have had repeated childhood respiratory infections. It is thought that viral (often adenovirus) pneumonia leads to a necrotizing bronchiolitis, which heals

by fibrosis to produce an obliterative bronchiolitis and unilateral lung hyperlucency (160,161).

Chest radiography shows a hyperlucent, but enlarged, lung or lobe. The increased lucency is easier to recognize when it involves the entire lung but is often lobar or subsegmental (Fig. 7-129A). There is a decrease in the number and size of pulmonary vessels. *Review of chest radiographs* usually shows previous pneumonia. The interval between the initial chest films showing pneumonia and subsequent unilateral or local hyperlucency varies from 7 to 30 months (160,161). *Expiration views* obtained by radiography, fluoroscopy, or decubitus positioning demonstrate lack of ventilation and air trapping in the hyperlucent region. *Bronchography* shows mild cylindrical bronchiectasis in the affected lung with an abrupt cutoff of peripheral filling at the fourth or fifth bronchial generation producing a pruned tree appearance (Fig. 7-129). This appearance is due to bronchiolitis obliterans (160,161). *Pulmonary angiography,* if performed, shows diminished vascularity to the affected region, lobe, or lung (Fig. 7-129D). *Lung scintigraphy* shows decreased perfusion to the hyperlucent lung as well as abnormal ventilation, with delayed wash-in and wash-out due to air trapping (Fig. 7-130).

There are a variety of other causes of unilateral hyperlucency lung (see Table 7-7) (9). In children, unilateral hyperlucency is most frequently due to an endobronchial foreign body, pneumothorax, congenital lobar emphysema, pulmonary artery hypoplasia or occlusion, or compensatory hyperinflation (see Fig. 7-74). Radiologic evidence of diminished vascularity and perfusion accompanied by normal or reduced size of the affected lung or region suggests that hypovascularity rather than overinflation is the major cause of the hyperlucency. Expiration views will confirm any air trapping.

Aspiration Pneumonia and Gastroesophageal Reflux

Aspiration pneumonia may be either acute or chronic. Aspiration may occur at rest, during sleep, during feeding, or with vomiting. Underlying pathologic conditions such as gastroesophageal reflux (GER), neurologic impairment, or tracheoesophageal fistula are often implicated (120). Dysfunctional swallowing, cleft lip, cleft palate, and choanal atresia also predispose to aspiration. The patient's position at the time of the aspiration determines the radiographic pattern. Supine aspiration leads to right upper lobe and perihilar opacities (Fig. 7-131). The toddler or ambulatory child who aspirates while erect develops right lower lobe or bilateral basal opacities. Massive aspiration may mimic pulmonary edema. Chronic aspiration and recurrent pneumonia sometimes lead to bronchiectasis (120,272,273). The pathophysiologic relationship between GER and reactive airway disease is less clearly understood. Some patients with GER may have an asthma-like syndrome secondary to GER. Silent aspiration of small quantities of gastric contents may incite severe bronchospasm. GER may also precipitate reactive air-

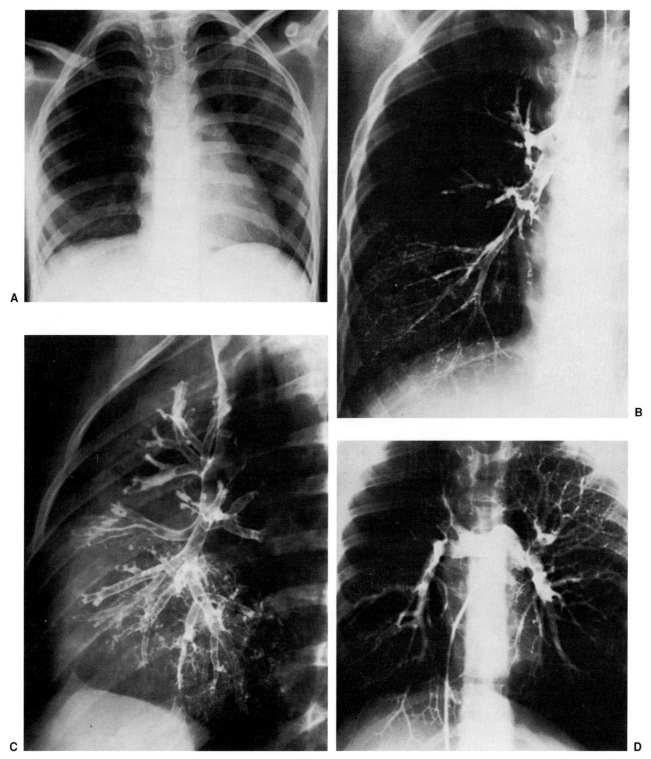

FIG. 7-129. Swyer-James syndrome. A 9-year-old boy with previous pneumonia. **A:** An expiration posteroanterior chest radiograph shows lucency due to air trapping in the right upper and middle lobes. **B:** An anteroposterior bronchogram shows a "pruned tree" appearance of the right upper and middle lobe bronchi. **C:** An oblique dynamic bronchogram demonstrates inability to alveolarize contrast into the parenchyma of the right upper and middle lobes. **D:** Pulmonary angiogram. There is decreased vascularity on the right with some stretching of vessels.

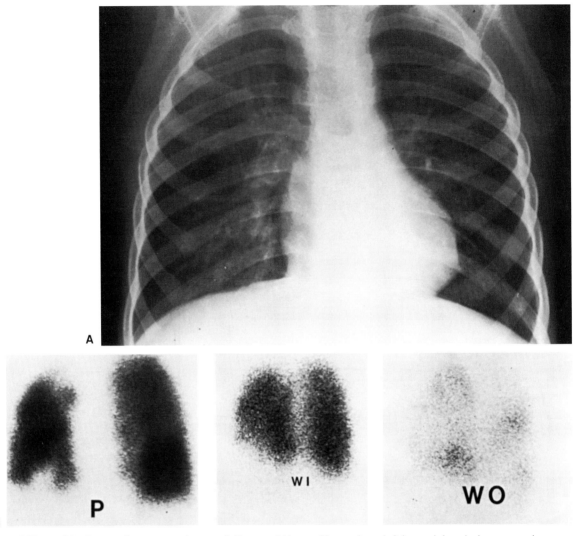

FIG. 7-130. Swyer-James syndrome. A 5-year-old boy with previous left lower lobe viral pneumonia. **A:** There is lucency of the left lung, particularly at the base. **B:** Posterior nuclear scintigraphy. *Left:* Patchy decreased perfusion of the left lower lobe. *Center:* Decreased wash-in *(WI)* of tracer. *Right:* Air trapping during wash-out *(WO)* in the left lower lobe.

way disease by activating esophageal stretch, pH, or thermal mucosal receptors. Nighttime cough, wheezing, recurrent pneumonia, and recurrent otitis media suggest underlying GER and/or aspiration.

Acute Chest Syndrome in Sickle Cell Disease

Children with sickle cell anemia frequently develop chest pain, fever, hypoxia, and pulmonary opacities. The condition is termed the acute chest syndrome; the term reflects the uncertainty about whether the etiology is infection or infarction (274). The opacities are unsharp, often irregular in shape, and frequently bilateral (Fig. 7-132). They seldom involve an entire lobe or segment. The syndrome is usually treated empirically with antibiotics. Chest radiographs help

follow the course of disease. Thin section CT may show a paucity of small vessels near opacities, which suggests an occlusive rather than an infectious etiology (274).

Chronic or Recurrent Pulmonary Disease

Myriad abnormalities cause chronic or recurrent pulmonary disease in infants and children (Table 7-15) (5,272,273). An extensive differential diagnosis is of little help when confronted with an individual case. The radiologist should be aware that there are many etiologic possibilities and have some concept of those in which radiologic evaluation may lead to a definitive diagnosis or narrow the differential diagnostic possibilities (273). The etiology of chronic or recurrent pulmonary disease is based on the corre-

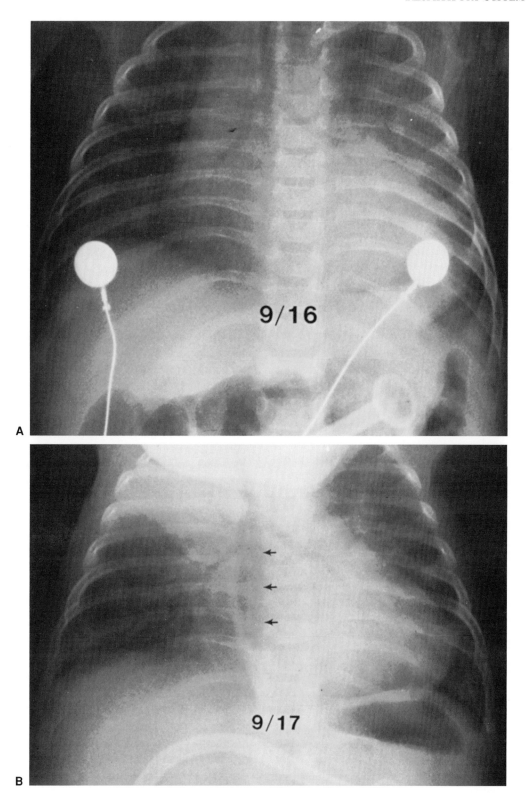

FIG. 7-131. Aspiration pneumonia. A: The baseline anteroposterior chest radiograph of a 3-year-old boy with neurologic impairment and known severe gastroesophageal reflux is normal. **B:** After an acute episode of respiratory distress, the chest radiograph shows consolidation and volume loss in the right upper lobe. Note the air-filled esophagus *(arrows).*

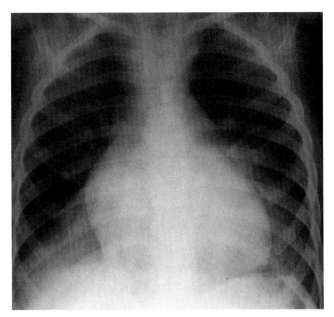

FIG. 7-132. Acute chest syndrome. A 6-year-old boy with sickle cell disease and the clinical presentation of sickle crisis. This chest radiograph shows mild cardiomegaly and bilateral lower lobe airspace disease.

lation of clinical, laboratory, and radiologic data. Some diseases require lung biopsy for diagnosis.

The primary radiologic tools are chest radiography, review of previous chest radiographs, and esophagography. Chest radiography demonstrates the gross pathology in the lungs (273). Important features include the distribution and pattern of the opacities, the presence or absence of lymphadenopathy, the presence or absence of pleural involvement, cardiac size, the appearance of the pulmonary vascularity, and the appearance of the soft tissues and bony structures of the thorax (5,272,273). The basic evaluation includes frontal and lateral views of the chest. Supplementary techniques, such as oblique films, fluoroscopy, an inspiration-expiration pair, high-kilovoltage films, and decubitus films, may be required. *Review of previous* films is critical. If the area of opacity is always in the same location and is segmental or lobar, an anatomic cause (such as foreign body, bronchial stricture, or sequestration) of the chronic or recurrent parenchymal disease should be considered. Persistent or recurrent right upper lobe opacity suggests aspiration. Patchy areas of opacity in varying locations decrease the likelihood of a localized endobronchial or anatomic lesion.

Esophagography is used to evaluate swallowing function, esophageal peristalsis, and the anatomy of the esophagus. To evaluate the swallowing mechanism, barium should be administered orally. One may demonstrate nasal reflux (which suggests poor neuromuscular control of swallowing), aspiration, abnormal esophageal peristalsis, extrinsic compression of the esophagus by a mass, a tracheoesophageal fistula, a hiatus hernia, or GER.

Immunodeficiency Diseases

General Concepts

Primary immunodeficiency diseases are rare. They usually require complex diagnostic evaluations of the immune system and treatment at tertiary medical centers (275–277). The incidence of agammaglobulinemia and/or hypoglobulinemia is estimated, for example, at 1 in 50,000 (276). Secondary immunodeficiency states occur with AIDS and after irradiation, bone marrow transplantation, or chemotherapy.

The immune system consists of antibody production, cellular immunity, the complement system, and phagocytic function (Table 7-16). Bone marrow stem cells differentiate into two divergent, immunologically active populations. B lymphocytes (named for the bursa of Fabricius in chickens) are linked to humoral antibody production. B cells, which are restricted to lymph nodes, differentiate into plasma cells which produce immunoglobulin antibodies. T lymphocytes, which are thymus-dependent, are responsible for cellular immunity. T cells are associated with delayed hypersensitivity, immunologic memory, killer cells in graft reactions, immunosurveillance for malignancy, and release of cytotoxic, chemotactic, and macrophage reactive factors (276). T-cell function is damaged by the AIDS virus (278).

Phagocytosis, the engulfing of microorganisms by leukocytes, occurs later in the immune response. Disorders of the phagocytic response are considered separately. The complement system is the primary humoral mediator of antigen-antibody reactions. An activated complement system lyses organisms and mediates the inflammatory response (276). Moreover, complement is capable of recruiting the participation of other humoral and cellular systems, induces histamine release, directs the migration of leukocytes, and releases lysozymes.

The 1970 World Health Organization (WHO) classification for immunodeficiency disorders presented a possible cellular deficit (T cell, B cell, or stem cell) for each broad category of immunodeficiency. However, cells having surface markers characteristic of T or B lymphocytes are rarely completely lacking in any of these conditions (276).

Antibody deficiency disorders may be congenital or acquired. Deficiencies may be found in all immunoglobulin classes (agammaglobulinemia, hypogammaglobulinemia) or in one or more classes (dysgammaglobulinemia). Clinical characteristics of antibody deficiency disorders include recurrent infections with high-grade extracellular encapsulated pathogens (pneumococci, streptococci, and *Hemophilus*), fungal and viral infections, chronic sinopulmonary disease, antibody deficiency in serum and secretions, and presence or lack of B lymphocytes with surface immunoglobulins or complement receptors. There may be a paucity of palpable lymphoid and visible nasopharyngeal tissue in X-linked agammaglobulinemia (Bruton hypogammaglobulinemia),

TABLE 7-15. *Chronic and recurrent pulmonary disease*

Aspiration	Immunodeficiency[a]
Central nervous system[a]	Prematurity
Malformation	Immunoglobulin
Trauma	Acquired immunodeficiency syndrome (AIDS)
Tumor	Ataxia-telangiectasia
Prematurity	Neutropenia
Dysfunction[a]	Wiskott-Aldrich syndrome
Riley-Day syndrome	Physical agents
Central nervous system	Foreign body[a]
Postoperative	Hydrocarbon aspiration
Prematurity	Drugs
Foregut	Methotrexate
Dysfunction	Bleomycin
Esophageal atresia	Others
Tracheoesophageal fistula	Radiation[a]
Vascular ring	Noxious gases
Hiatus hernia	Bronchopulmonary dysplasia[a]
Chalasia	Wilson-Mikity syndrome
Reflux	Lipoid pneumonia
Achalasia	Cardiovascular[a]
Cleft palate	Left-to-right shunt[a]
Anomaly	Pulmonary artery stenosis
Underdevelopment of lung	Vascular ring
Agenesis	Congestive heart failure
Aplasia	Neoplastic disorders
Hypoplasia	Histiocytosis
Vascular	Leukemia-lymphoma
Anomalies of tracheobronchial tree	Infection[a]
Congenital lobar emphysema: other cystic disease	Tuberculosis
Pulmonary sling	Fungus
Bronchopulmonary foregut malformation	*Mycoplasma*[a]
Sequestration	Viruses[a]
Duplication	*Pneumocystis*
Bronchogenic cyst	Giant cell pneumonia
Skeletal	Bronchiectasis[a]
Asphyxiating thoracic dystrophy	Worm infestation
Osteogenesis imperfecta	Miscellaneous disorders
Kartagener syndrome	Sarcoid
Allergy	Hemosiderosis
Asthma[a]	Pulmonary alveolar proteinosis
Loeffler pneumonia	Collagen vascular disease
Allergic alveolitis	Hamman-Rich syndrome
Milk allergy	Interstitial pneumonia
Antigens	Desquamative interstitial pneumonitis (DIP)
Bacteria	Lymphoid associated diseases
Mycobacteria	Lymphocytic interstitial pneumonitis (LIP)
Fungi	Bronchiolar-associated lymphoid tissue (BALT)
Viral	Chronic interstitial pneumonitis (CIP)
Systemic disease	Trauma
Cystic fibrosis[a]	Other
Riley-Day syndrome	
Amyotonia congenita	
Ectodermal dysplasia	

[a] More common.

Modified from Kirkpatrick (273) and Silverman (5).

common variable agammaglobulinemia, selective IgA deficiency, and transient hypogammaglobulinemia of infancy (Table 7-16).

Aside from AIDS, defects in T cells are rare (Table 7-16). Cellular immunodeficiency disorders are often referred to as examples of isolated defects of the T-cell system, as serum immunoglobulin concentrations are usually normal or elevated. However, B-cell function is also compromised due to a deficiency of T-helper cells (276). Clinical characteristics of cellular immunodeficiency disorders include recur-

TABLE 7-16. *Classification of immunodeficiency disease*

Antibody deficiency disorders
    X-linked agammaglobulinemia or hypogammaglobulinemia
      (Bruton type)
    Common-variable immunodeficiency (acquired)[a]
    Transient hypogammaglobulinemia of infancy
    Selective IgA deficiency[a]
    Immunodeficiency with elevated IgM
    X-lined lymphoproliferative disease
    Others
Cellular immunodeficiency disorders
    Acquired immunodeficiency syndrome (AIDS)[a]
    Thymic hypoplasia (DiGeorge syndrome)
    Cartilage hair hypoplasia
    Cellular immunodeficiency with immunoglobulins (Nezelof
      syndrome)
    Others
Severe combined immunodeficiency disorders (SCID)
    Autosomal recessive SCID with adenosine deaminase defi-
      ciency
    X-linked recessive SCID
    SCID with leukopenia (reticular dysgenesis)
    Others
Partial combined immunodeficiency disorders
    Wiskott-Aldrich syndrome
    Ataxia-telangiectasia
    Immunodeficiency
      With short-limbed dwarfism
      With thymoma
    Hyper-IgE (Job or Buckley syndrome)
    Chronic mucocutaneous candidiasis
    Others
Complement component deficiencies
Phagocytic dysfunction
    Disorders of production
      Hereditary neutropenia
      Cyclic neutropenia
      Neutropenia with immunodeficiency
      Acquired[a]
    Disorders of function
      Chemotaxis
      Opsonic
      Ingestion
      Killing: chronic granulomatous disease
    Others

[a] More common.

Modified from Buckley (276).

rent infections with low-grade or opportunistic infectious agents (fungi, viruses, *Pneumocystis*), delayed cutaneous anergy, growth retardation and diarrhea, susceptibility to graft-versus-host disease, high incidence of malignancy, and short life span (276). *Pneumocystis carinii* pneumonia is common and may be life threatening (278). It is rare that patients with primary cellular immunodeficiency disorders survive childhood. Cellular immunodeficiency disorders include AIDS, thymic hypoplasia (DiGeorge syndrome), and cellular immunodeficiency with immunoglobulins (Nezelof syndrome) (275–279).

Antibody Immunodeficiency Disorders

Selective Immunoglobulin A Deficiency

Selective immunoglobulin A (IgA) deficiency is the most common primary immunodeficiency disorder, with an incidence of approximately 1 in 800. The absence of IgA predisposes the patient to chronic sinopulmonary infections (viral and bacterial), allergies, celiac disease, ulcerative colitis, regional enteritis (Crohn disease), systemic lupus erythematosus, rheumatoid arthritis, and malignancy. There is frequently lymphoid hyperplasia of the gastrointestinal tract.

Congenital X-linked Hypogammaglobulinemia

Congenital X-linked hypogammaglobulinemia (Bruton type), an isolated defect in humoral immunity, is a recessive disorder occurring only in males. Serum immunoglobulin levels are very low. There are usually inflammatory changes in the lungs, including consolidation, interstitial opacities, or bronchiectasis. Opacification of paranasal sinuses due to infection is common. There may be absence of lymphoid tissue on the lateral view of the nasopharynx. Lymphoma and leukemia are the only malignancies that have been reported with this disorder, the risk of malignancy being approximately 6% (280).

Cellular Immunodeficiency Disorders

DiGeorge Syndrome

DiGeorge syndrome is a primary defect in cellular immunity caused by absence or hypoplasia of the thymus. The parathyroid glands, also derived from the third and fourth pharyngeal pouches, are frequently absent; this may cause neonatal tetany. There may be abnormalities of other structures related to or developing at the same time as the pharyngeal pouches, causing micrognathia, low-set ears, hypertelorism, and congenital heart disease (especially interrupted aortic arch and truncus arteriosus). The diagnosis should be suggested in the newborn if one sees a narrow superior mediastinum and retrosternal lucency due to absence of the thymus (Fig. 7-133). There is no known association of malignancy with DiGeorge syndrome. Fungal (particularly moniliasis) and viral infections may be fatal in these patients.

Cartilage-Hair Hypoplasia

This autosomal recessive short-limbed bone dysplasia is more common among the Amish than in the general population. The hair is fine and sparse. The immune defect is an almost complete absence of T-cell function. Viruses, such as varicella, are the most common cause of infection. Neutropenia and lymphopenia are seen in about one fourth of cases.

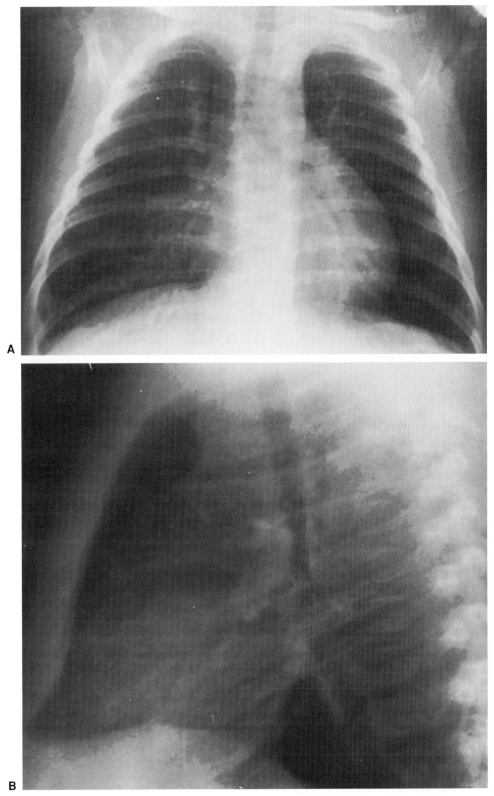

FIG. 7-133. DiGeorge syndrome. A 2-day old boy with hypocalcemic tetany. Anteroposterior **(A)** and lateral **(B)** chest radiographs show a slight increase in parahilar linear markings. The retrosternal lucency on the lateral radiograph is due to absence of the thymus.

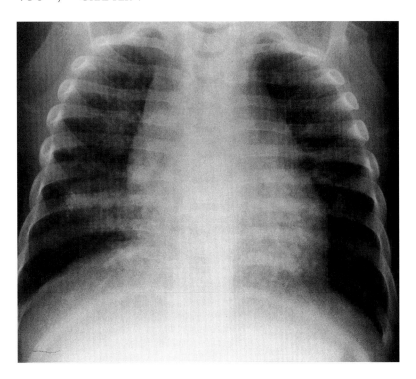

FIG. 7-134. Lymphocytic interstitial pneumonitis in acquired immunodeficiency syndrom (AIDS). A 2-year-old boy whose mother was a drug addict. The anteroposterior chest radiograph shows diffuse reticulonodular densities. Open lung biopsy showed lymphocytic interstitial pneumonitis.

Acquired Immunodeficiency Syndrome

AIDS is a growing problem in children and an increasing cause of secondary immunodeficiency disease (241,242,278,281–284). The disease is caused by a lymphotropic retrovirus. Approximately 2% of all AIDS cases occur in children. As in the adult, the AIDS virus (HIV) impairs T-cell function (241,278). The signs and symptoms include failure to thrive, chronic diarrhea, generalized lymphadenopathy, pulmonary infections, and hepatosplenomegaly. Chronic parotid gland swelling is common. Causes of secondary immunodeficiency (chemotherapy, irradiation, bone marrow transplantation) and primary immunodeficiency states must be excluded (241,242,278). Maternal transmission and blood transfusions represent the major risk factors for children. The former is much more common (over 80% and increasing).

The pulmonary disease in pediatric AIDS is of two major types: acute pulmonary infections (*Pneumocystis carinii* pneumonia, CMV pneumonia) and noninfectious interstitial pneumonitis (chronic lymphocytic infiltration) (Fig. 7-134) (281,283,284). Pyogenic infections are also common. Patients with *P. carinii* or CMV pneumonia are usually clinically ill. The early radiographic findings are central interstitial infiltrates; this pattern may rapidly evolve into confluent airspace disease (278,281).

Noninfectious interstitial pneumonitis (chronic lymphocytic infiltration) in children with AIDS includes lymphocytic interstitial pneumonitis (LIP), desquamative interstitial pneumonitis (DIP), and chronic interstitial pneumonitis. The pulmonary lymphoid proliferation seen in LIP is probably a pulmonary response to injury. At least half of pulmonary

disease in children with AIDS is due to lymphoid-associated diseases including pulmonary lymphoid hyperplasia (PLH), bronchiolar-associated lymphoid tissue (BALT), and polymorphic polyclonal B-cell lymphoproliferative disorder (PBLD). Radiographically, BALT causes central peribronchial nodular interstitial densities. LIP usually has an insidious clinical onset with only mild cough and dyspnea; radiographically, there are diffuse reticulonodular densities (Fig. 7-134). It is impossible to distinguish the various types of chronic lymphocytic infiltration on chest radiography with any certainty. Histologic examination of lung tissue is required for confirmation of diagnosis and classification of the disease process. The development of pulmonary lymphoid hyperplasia indicates the persistence of some, although a diminished, immune response. Pediatric AIDS patients with pulmonary lymphoid hyperplasia are, therefore, at less risk of pulmonary infection than those with no immune response (281).

Combined Immunodeficiency Disorders

Severe Combined Immunodeficiency Disease

Severe combined immunodeficiency disease is characterized by complete absence of both T-cell and B-cell immunity. The child has susceptibility to infection (lack of T-cell function: recurrent viral and fungal infections; lack of B-cell function: recurrent pyogenic infections). Patients rarely survive beyond a year of age without bone marrow transplantation. Findings include failure to thrive, chronic diarrhea, persistent oral thrush, pneumonia, and sepsis. Thymic tissue is frequently radiologically absent. Treatment is bone marrow transplantation, followed by an approximate 2% risk of a lymphoproliferative neoplasm (280).

Common Variable Immunodeficiency

Patients with common variable immunodeficiency are usually not symptomatic until later childhood or early adulthood. This acquired condition affects boys and girls equally, and there is no known genetic transmission. Cell-mediated immunity is intact early but usually becomes deficient late in the course of the disease. There is radiologic evidence of both acute and chronic sinopulmonary infection. There may be marked lymphadenopathy due to lymphoid hyperplasia. There is an 8% risk of malignancy; lymphoreticular tumors predominate, although gastric carcinoma and thymoma have also been reported (280).

Wiskott-Aldrich Syndrome

Wiskott-Aldrich syndrome includes the triad of eczema, recurrent pyogenic infections, and thrombocytopenia. Serum levels of IgM are low, but other immunoglobulins may be elevated or normal. Initially, T-cell functions are normal, but they decrease with increasing age. The syndrome is inherited as an X-linked recessive trait. Pyogenic infections usually start before 1 year of age and may include meningitis, otitis media, pneumonia, and sepsis. Lymphoid tissue may be absent in the nasopharynx on lateral airway films. There is an increased risk (8%) of lymphoreticular malignancies (280).

Ataxia Telangiectasia

The complete syndrome of ataxia telangiectasia includes cerebellar ataxia, telangiectasia of the conjunctiva and skin, and recurrent sinopulmonary infections. The disease is inherited as an autosomal recessive trait, and there is selective IgA deficiency in approximately 40% of patients. There are variable degrees of T-cell deficiencies, which become more severe with increasing age. These patients are susceptible to both viral and bacterial infections. Recurrent pneumonia and recurrent severe sinusitis in a child with truncal ataxia strongly suggests the diagnosis. The thymus and lymph tissues are radiologically absent. There is a 10% estimated risk for the development of lymphoreticular malignancies, leukemia, or nonlymphoid tumors (280). This is the only disease known to raise the risk of radiation-induced malignancy; radiologists must be especially careful with the use of diagnostic x-rays. The cause of death is usually overwhelming infection or lymphoreticular malignancy.

Phagocytic Dysfunction

Chronic Granulomatous Disease

Chronic granulomatous disease is usually inherited as an X-linked recessive disorder. Clinical manifestations usually occur before 3 years of age. Patients are particularly susceptible to infection with catalase-positive bacteria, such as *Staphylococcus aureus* and various gram-negative bacteria and fungi (276).

Clinical manifestations include granulomatous lesions of the skin, thyroiditis, lymphadenopathy, hepatosplenomegaly, pneumonia, osteomyelitis of unusual bones, diarrhea, intermittent abdominal pain, perianal abscesses, cystitis, and esophageal strictures. Enzymatic defects in polymorphonuclear leukocytes lead to an inability to kill certain bacteria and fungi after cellular infection. Both antibody function and cell-mediated immunity are normal. Calcification may occur in granulomas in the lungs, liver, and lymph nodes; this provides a helpful radiologic clue to the diagnosis (285). Pulmonary infiltrates may persist for several weeks despite "appropriate therapy." Gastric antral narrowing may be the initial presentation (279,285).

Other Syndromes

Other conditions may be associated with defective phagocytic cell chemotaxis and serious chronic or recurrent infections. *Chediak-Higashi syndrome* is an autosomal recessive disorder associated with pneumonias, abscesses of solid organs, and osteomyelitis. Neurologic abnormalities (retardation, cerebellar and long tract signs), partial oculocutaneous albinism, and abnormal neutrophils are also characteristic of this disorder. *Job syndrome* (hyper-IgE syndrome, Buckley syndrome) carries a susceptibility to recurrent infections of the skin, lungs, joints, and muscles. In addition to defective phagocytic cell chemotaxis, these patients have elevated serum IgE. *Schwachman-Diamond syndrome* is a syndrome of recurrent infections, neutropenia, pancreatic insufficiency, and sometimes metaphyseal dysplasia. Although 100 times less common than cystic fibrosis, this disorder is the second most common pancreatic cause of malabsorption in children; it probably is inherited as an autosomal recessive trait.

Malignancy Associated with Immunodeficiency Disorders

In addition to preventing infection, the immune system plays an important role in preventing malignancy, apparently being able to recognize and destroy neoplastic cells. There is a dramatic increase in the incidence of malignancies in both primary and secondary immunodeficiencies. The incidence of malignancy in children with immunodeficiency is 100–10,000 times that of age-matched controls (276,280).

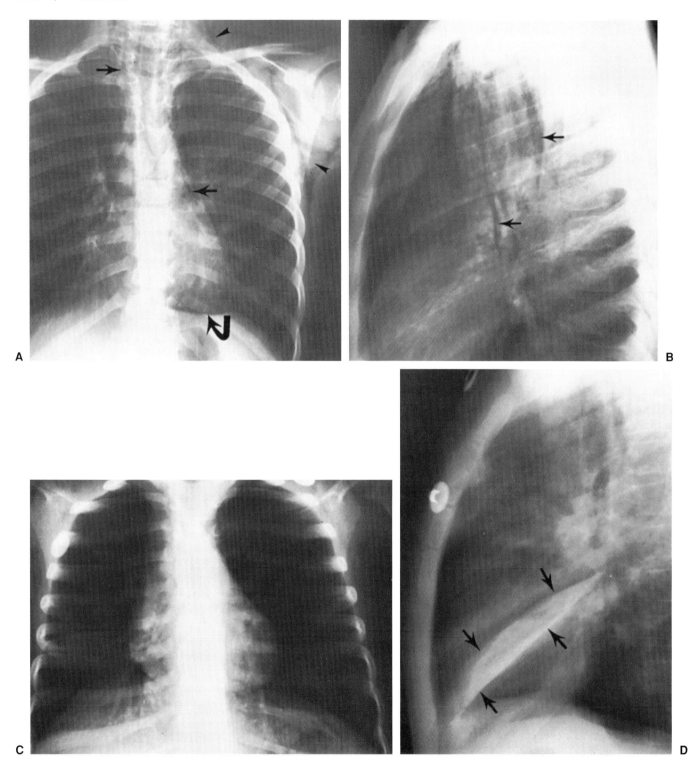

FIG. 7-135. Complications of asthma. A, B: Posteroanterior **(A)** and lateral **(B)** chest radiographs of a 9-year-old girl with asthma show pneumomediastinum *(arrows)* and subcutaneous emphysema *(arrowheads)*. Note the "continuous diaphragm sign" *(curved arrow)*. **C, D:** Posteroanterior **(C)** and lateral **(D)** radiographs of a 5-year-old boy with asthma. There is atelectasis of the right middle lobe *(arrows)*. *(continued)*

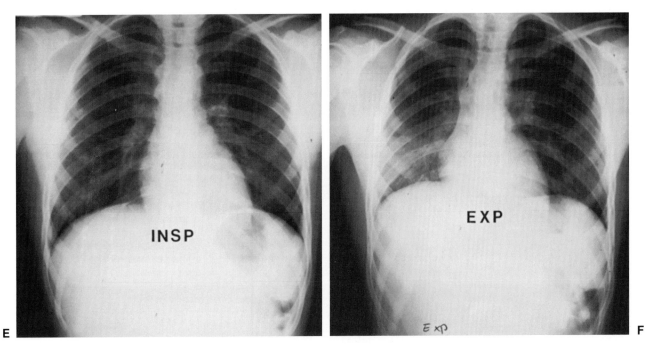

7-135. *Continued.* **E, F:** Inspiration **(E)** and expiration **(F)** radiographs of an 11-year-old girl asthmatic with severe shortness of breath and hypoxemia. There is marked air trapping in both upper lungs, demonstrated only in expiration.

The immunodeficiency disorders that have a particularly high risk of malignancy are AIDS and ataxia telangiectasia. Also at risk are children with X-linked agammaglobulinemia, severe combined immunodeficiency, common variable immunodeficiency, Wiskott-Aldrich syndrome, and selective IgA immunodeficiency (275–277,279). Lymphoproliferative tumors and leukemia are the most common neoplasms; immunodeficiency patients may also develop carcinomas and sarcomas, particularly of the gastrointestinal tract and soft tissues.

Other Chronic Pulmonary Disorders

Asthma

Asthma is a disorder of the tracheobronchial tree characterized by varying degrees of obstruction to air flow. The clinical hallmark of this illness is wheezing, caused by partial obstruction of the larger intrathoracic airways. An antibody-antigen reaction on the tracheobronchial mucosal surface releases mediators to produce bronchospasm. Most cases of childhood asthma come to attention before age 8. There is often a family history of asthma, allergic rhinitis, and atopic dermatitis. Asthma co-exists with other allergic disorders. Precipitating and aggravating factors include allergens, infections (particularly RSV), irritants, weather changes, emotional factors, GER, and certain drugs, for example, aspirin and nonsteroidal antiinflammatory agents. The typical baseline chest radiograph of a patient with asthma shows normal to mildly increased aeration, mild prominence of the parahilar linear markings, and minor peribronchial cuffing (286).

Chest radiographs are obtained more to exclude a complication than to demonstrate the presence of asthma (287). Complications include atelectasis, pneumonia, obstructive emphysema, and air block phenomena (pneumomediastinum, pneumothorax, subcutaneous emphysema) (Fig. 7-135) (286–288). The major concern in asthma, the one prompting most of the chest films, is the possibility of pneumonia. A good working rule is that nearly all of the pulmonary opacities found in asthmatic children represent atelectasis rather than pneumonia. If atelectasis persists for several days, infection may be superimposed. Although there are features (the shadows are linear, multiple, changeable, and fleeting) that suggest atelectasis, one is certain of the diagnosis only when the opacity clears without antibiotic therapy.

Atelectasis and obstructive emphysema are related to mucous plugging, which is made worse by acute bronchospasm and superimposed lower respiratory tract infection. Significant localized air trapping is well demonstrated by fluoroscopy or by chest radiographs in expiration. Air block complications are due to profound air trapping during acute episodes of bronchospasm (286,288,289). However, pneumothorax is so rare in asthma that its presence should raise the possibility that the wheezing is caused by foreign body aspiration. Chest radiographic abnormalities in children admitted to the hospital for acute asthma include marked hyperinflation (67%), opacity (21%), definite atelectasis (30%), and pneumomediastinum (2%) (Fig. 7-135) (286). Pneumomediastinum is manifested by the continuous diaphragm

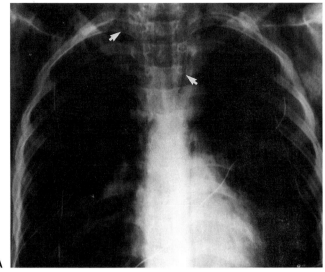

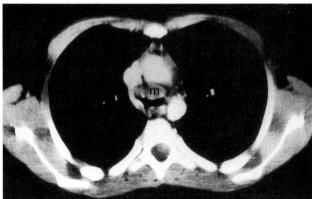

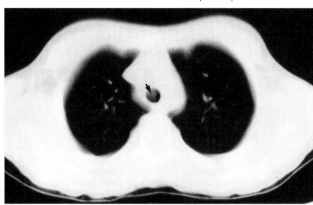

FIG. 7-136. Tracheal cylindroma presenting as asthma. A 9-year-old boy presenting with the recent onset of wheezing. **A:** An AP chest x-ray shows hyperinflation and pneumomediastinum *(arrows)*. Note the sharp outline of the descending aorta and main pulmonary artery, due to air in the mediastinum. **B:** Enhanced CT at the level of the carina shows a precarinal mass *(m)* and extrinsic compression of the anterior trachea at that level. **C:** CT scan just above the carina shows an intratracheal mass *(arrow)*.

sign, elevation and outlining of the thymus, and outlining of other mediastinal structures (aorta, central pulmonary arteries) by air. There may also be subcutaneous emphysema (Fig. 7-135A). Asthma is the most common cause of pneumomediastinum in older children (289).

The conditions to be differentiated from asthma depends on the age. Important considerations include laryngotracheobronchomalacia, cystic fibrosis, chronic viral infection, airway foreign body, croup, congenital anomalies, and extrinsic or intrinsic tracheobronchial tumors (Fig. 7-136). Airway foreign body must be considered when there is the sudden onset of wheezing, particularly if the patient is <3 years of age and the respiratory symptoms persist.

Allergic Lung Disease

The exposure of the lung to various stimuli in infancy, childhood, or adolescence can produce an allergic response. The clinical and radiologic presentation of patients with nonasthmatic allergic pulmonary disease is based on the characteristics of the offending agent, the intensity and duration of the exposure, and the host response. Differentiating asthma from nonasthmatic allergic pulmonary disease is a difficult

clinical challenge; the diagnosis of allergic lung disease is usually suggested only when other causes of airway disease and recurrent infectious pneumonia have been excluded.

Many substances have been implicated in allergic lung disease, including medications such as aspirin, penicillin, and nitrofurantoin, and organic dusts. These agents are capable of inducing non-IgE-mediated allergic pneumonitis. Nonasthmatic allergic lung disease can be broken into three groups: hypersensitivity pneumonitis, allergic bronchopulmonary disease, and pulmonary hypersensitivity reactions. *Hypersensitivity pneumonitis* is an allergic pulmonary disease resulting from inhalation of dust particles (proteins of animal origin and molds), chemicals, or drugs. *Allergic bronchopulmonary disease* has characteristics of both IgE-mediated allergy and hypersensitivity pneumonitis. Allergic bronchopulmonary aspergillosis (ABPA) is included in this category of nonasthmatic allergic lung disease and represents an immune bronchial disease to aspergilli that occurs in atopic children, often after many years of asthma. ABPA may also develop as a late complication of cystic fibrosis. *Pulmonary hypersensitivity reactions* are reactions of the lung to a variety of other allergic substances.

The radiographic manifestations of allergic lung disease in the infant may suggest bronchiolitis or recurrent pneumo-

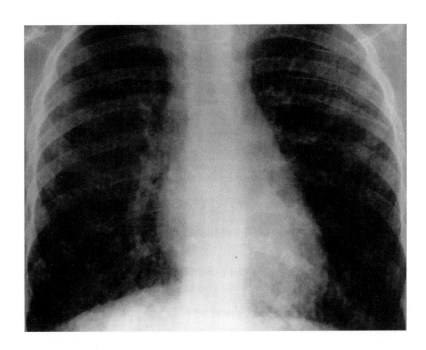

FIG. 7-137. Hypersensitivity pneumonitis. This 14-year-old boy raised pigeons as a hobby. He presented with cough and wheezing. The chest x-ray shows diffuse reticulonodular interstitial opacities.

nia. In the older child and adolescent, the chest radiograph may mimic asthma (Fig. 7-137). Radiographic manifestations of allergic pulmonary disease include diffuse pulmonary interstitial opacities, small nodular interstitial densities, and patchy subsegmental atelectasis (Fig. 7-137). Chronic changes include bronchial wall thickening and interstitial fibrosis (1).

Cystic Fibrosis

Among children, adolescents, and young adults of Caucasian descent, cystic fibrosis is the most important chronic respiratory illness, with the exception of asthma (290). Cystic fibrosis is an autosomal recessive illness. The cystic fibrosis gene resides on chromosome 7; if both alleles are abnormal, cystic fibrosis is present. The most common of the many mutations that occur is deletion of three base pairs, leading to the absence of phenylalanine; this deletion accounts for about 70% of the mutant genes in the United States (291). Over 400 other mutations make up the remaining 30%; many are very rare. These other mutations apparently lead to somewhat different expressions of the illness, but these differences are still being worked out (291).

The cystic fibrosis gene expresses itself through abnormalities in the cystic fibrosis transmembrane conductance regulator. This regulating protein controls the passage of chloride and, secondarily, water out of epithelial cells to the epithelial surface. It consequently determines the hydration of respiratory mucus. Inadequate hydration at the cell surface leads to inspissated secretions and impaired ciliary clearance; this in turn promotes bacterial infection. This pathophysiology is the rationale of treatment with amiloride, which blocks sodium resorption and retains water on the epithelial surface.

About 1 in 25 individuals of northern European extraction carries one abnormal cystic fibrosis gene, but these heterozygotes are free of symptoms. In 1 of approximately 625 marriages, both partners are carriers. One in four of their children (i.e., 1 in roughly 2500 births) will be homozygous and affected. Cystic fibrosis genes are rare in Asian populations and are uncommon in African-Americans.

Clinical Features

The diagnosis of cystic fibrosis is suggested by respiratory systems, gastrointestinal symptoms, or a positive family history. In a small group (approximately 5%) of patients with cystic fibrosis, the earliest and most debilitating symptoms are gastrointestinal. These manifestations include meconium ileus, meconium ileus equivalent, steatorrhea, malabsorption, failure to thrive, fatty liver, and cirrhosis. Pulmonary manifestations usually have their onset during later infancy or middle childhood but sometimes in adolescence or adult life. Chest symptoms and signs are chronic cough, recurrent pulmonary infection, atelectasis, and obstructive pulmonary disease. Focal disease is more common in an upper lobe than elsewhere. As respiratory disease progresses, systemic symptoms (fatigue, weight loss, and productive cough) supervene. Respiratory insufficiency and progressive pulmonary arterial hypertension develop in later stages of the disease. Nasal polyps are common, and by adolescence sinus opacity due to sinonasal polyps or sinusitis is almost always present (292).

Pathology

The pulmonary pathology of cystic fibrosis is limited at first to the airways. Even at autopsy, it is striking how se-

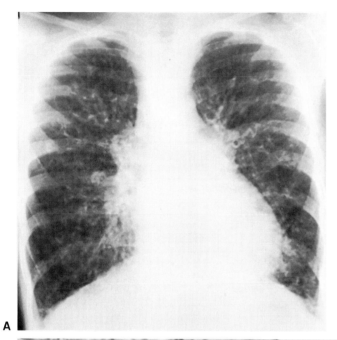

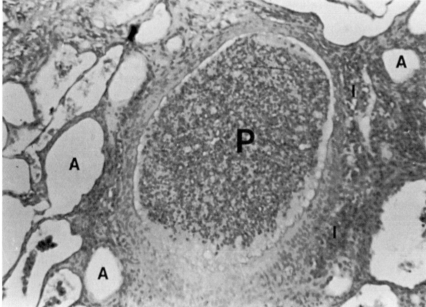

FIG. 7-138. Cystic fibrosis. A: A 7-year-old girl with severe cystic fibrosis. Note the hyperaeration, increase in linear markings particularly in the parahilar regions, peribronchial cuffing, prominent hilar structures, and bronchial mucous plugging. **B:** Histologic section of the resected lung of a patient with cystic fibrosis. The alveoli *(A)* are normally aerated, but a large mucous plug *(P)* occupies a bronchus surrounded by inflammatory reaction *(I)*. This histologic section emphasizes that cystic fibrosis is primarily an airways disease.

verely the airways are affected despite fairly normal appearing airspaces (Fig. 7-138B). The viscous mucus accumulates within small airways, producing obstruction and harboring bacteria that lead to infection, bronchitis, and bronchiectasis (291). The most commonly cultured organisms from patients with cystic fibrosis are *Staphylococcus aureus* and *Pseudomonas aeruginosa* (291). Breakdown of cells, especially the polymorphonuclear leukocytes in pus, liberates deoxyribonucleic acid (DNA), which forms sticky, obstructing complexes with respiratory mucus. This is the basis for treatment with DNase, which liquefies these complexes and allows the infected mucus to be brought up by ciliary action or coughing (293).

Bronchitis, bronchial plugging, and bronchopneumonia are present in patients with cystic fibrosis. The pathologic changes of bronchiectasis can be found in all patients over 6 months of age (291). True emphysema (alveolar destruction) is encountered only in older patients and is rarely severe. Late in the course of the disease, patients may develop pneumothorax and pleural thickening of a mild degree.

Radiologic Findings

Chest radiography is almost always the initial imaging modality in patients with cystic fibrosis. In the infant and

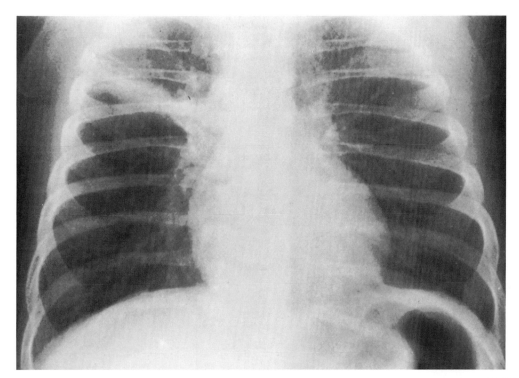

FIG. 7-139. Early manifestation of cystic fibrosis. A 2-month-old girl thought to have bronchiolitis. The lungs are hyperaerated, and there is subsegmental atelectasis of the right upper lobe. A sweat test confirmed the diagnosis of cystic fibrosis.

young child, cystic fibrosis is sometimes diagnosed when chest films are still normal. Infants with cystic fibrosis are particularly prone to develop atelectasis and focal or generalized hyperaeration (Fig. 7-139). Mucous plugging partially obstructs airways and produces secondary hyperaeration or atelectasis. In older children, chest radiographs show hyperaeration, increased linear parahilar markings, peribronchial cuffing, bronchial mucous plugging, and bronchiectasis (see Fig. 7-138) (290,292).

Progressive mucous plugging and superimposed infection cause chronic airway disease. This condition produces bronchial wall thickening, which is manifested radiologically as peribronchial cuffing and parahilar linear densities that radiate from the hilar regions (290,292). These changes rarely completely clear. Mucoid impaction commonly occurs in dilated bronchi and bronchioles; it is manifested as rounded soft-tissue densities or finger-like linear densities in a bronchial distribution. Bronchiectatic cavities may be filled with fluid or air, or may contain air-fluid levels. Prominence of the hilar regions is a common finding in patients with cystic fibrosis; it is due to hilar adenopathy or large pulmonary arteries associated with pulmonary arterial hypertension, usually the former (290,292).

A number of scoring methods are used for the evaluation of chest radiographs in patients with cystic fibrosis (294). The method of Brasfield is simple, has a high degree of interobserver reproducibility, and is recommended (290). This radiographic scoring system (based on air trapping, lin-

ear markings, nodular cystic lesions, large pulmonary opacities, general severity, and presence of complications) correlates with pulmonary function testing, the Shwachman clinical scoring system, and morbidity (290).

CT demonstrates the pulmonary and bronchial changes of cystic fibrosis very well (Fig. 7-140). Plain films show far less bronchiectasis than will be revealed by CT. However, it is not yet clear that this exquisite demonstration of pathologic anatomy actually leads to an improved outcome for the patient. If lobectomy is being considered because of unusually localized disease, CT of the entire chest should be performed to show the extent and severity of disease elsewhere.

Scintigraphic ventilation-perfusion studies in patients with cystic fibrosis will provide additional information about regional lung function (Fig. 7-141). Patchy areas of decreased ventilation or perfusion, which are usually matched, are commonly present; there is only a fair match between these functional abnormalities and the gross anatomic abnormalities shown by radiographs (290). The ventilation-perfusion study may demonstrate disease before radiographs become abnormal. In mildly affected patients, hypoventilation and hypoperfusion are frequently noted in the lower lung zones, and occasionally profound perfusion defects not suggested by the chest radiograph are demonstrated (Fig. 7-141). Ventilation-perfusion studies are not necessary in most patients with cystic fibrosis but help assess regional abnormalities in minimally affected patients, patients being con-

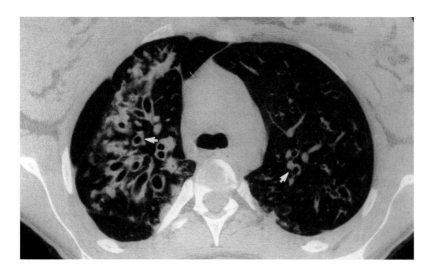

FIG. 7-140. Cystic fibrosis. High-resolution CT scan (1.5 mm collimation, high-resolution algorithm) in a 15-year-old boy with cystic fibrosis shows severe right upper lobe bronchiectasis. Note the signet ring signs *(arrows)*.

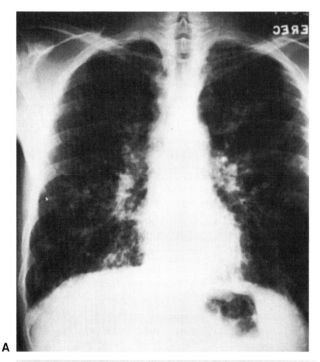

A

FIG. 7-141. Cystic fibrosis. A: Posteroanterior chest radiograph shows moderate radiographic changes of cystic fibrosis. **B:** Posterior perfusion *(P)* and ventilation *(V)* scintigraphy demonstrates matching areas of decreased activity.

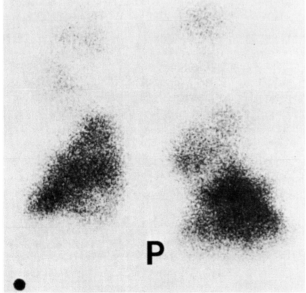

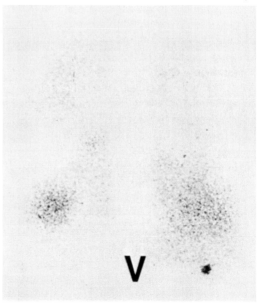

B

sidered for lobe resection, prior to lung transplantation, and to assess therapy (290).

Complications

As cystic fibrosis progresses, patients are increasingly at risk for complications. Pneumothorax occurs most frequently in the adolescent or young adult with significant lung disease and is usually secondary to rupture of bullae or blebs (290). This complication leads to severe dyspnea and, rarely, to sudden death. There is frequently radiologic evidence of tension pneumothorax; because of abnormal compliance, the diseased lung collapses only partly (Fig. 7-142). These pneumothoraces are usually spontaneous but occasionally are secondary to positive pressure ventilation or trauma. Patients who have had a previous pneumothorax may be able to diagnose its recurrence. A small pneumothorax may require decubitus positioning and expiration views for confirmation. Chest tube evacuation of pneumothorax is effective in approximately 65% of patients (290). Recurrent pneumothorax may require percutaneous injection of sclerosing agents into the pleural space or, rarely, open thoracotomy with pleurectomy.

Hemoptysis is an uncommon but serious complication in patients with long-standing cystic fibrosis. The bleeding site may be demonstrated by selective bronchial arteriography (Fig. 7-143B). Bronchial artery embolization sometimes controls hemoptysis in patients with cystic fibrosis (Fig. 7-143C) (295). A considerable amount of the upper lobe opacity seen in cystic fibrosis (Fig. 7-143) actually represents dilated bronchial arteries.

Lobar atelectasis is a common complication of cystic fibrosis, usually involving the right upper lobe. Prolonged collapse with superimposed localized infection is the most common indication for pulmonary resection (290).

Pulmonary hypertension and cor pulmonale frequently develop in severe cystic fibrosis. In such patients, hilar prominence is usually due to both adenopathy and enlarged pulmonary arteries. Progressive heart enlargement is evident on serial films in patients who are developing cor pulmonale. The heart usually looks very small in patients with cystic fibrosis because of hyperaeration (296); therefore, a seemingly normal heart may actually represent cardiomegaly due to cor pulmonale. Echocardiographic evaluation of right ventricular size and septal wall motion can detect cor pulmonale prior to electrocardiographic changes (290).

Hypertrophic pulmonary osteoarthropathy is a rare extrapulmonary complication of cystic fibrosis. The leg and forearm are most frequently affected. Clinically, there is pain and swelling, which may be associated with clubbing. Radiographically, there is periosteal new bone formation, particularly along the shafts of the long bones.

The paranasal sinuses in patients with cystic fibrosis are usually completely opacified from early childhood. Although the sinuses are opaque, they may be large and well

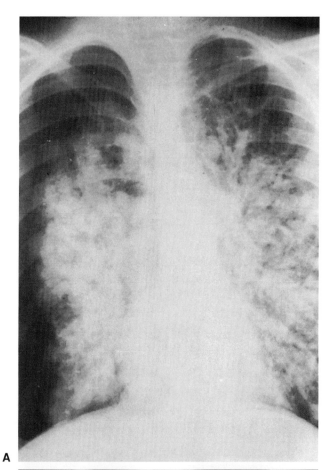

A

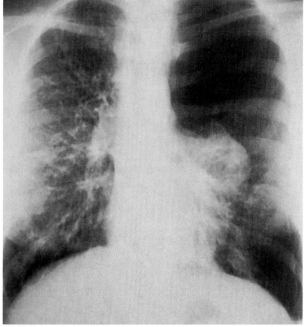

B

FIG. 7-142. Pneumothorax complicating cystic fibrosis.
A: A 13-year-old boy with severe cystic fibrosis and a large right tension pneumothorax. **B:** A 16-year-old girl with cystic fibrosis and sudden onset of shortness of breath. There is a large left tension pneumothorax. In both examples, the incomplete lung collapse, despite a tension pneumothorax, is due to decreased lung compliance.

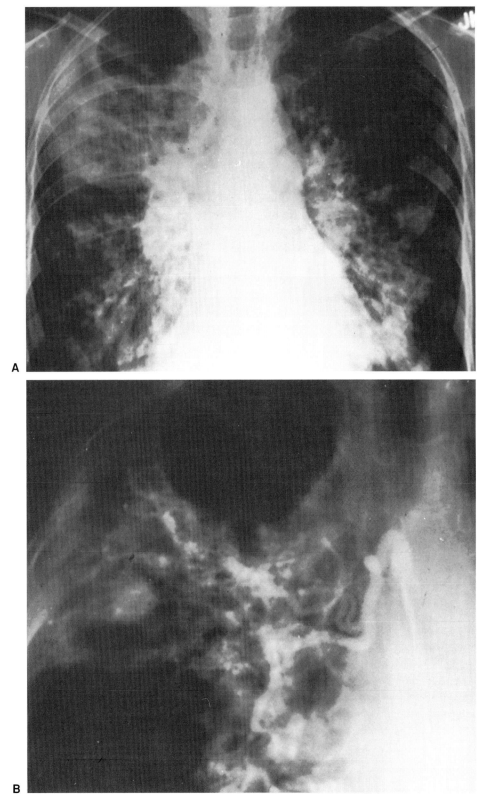

FIG. 7-143. Bronchial embolization in cystic fibrosis. A 14-year-old boy with severe hemoptysis. **A:** Severe cystic fibrosis. There are opacities and blebs in the right upper lobe. **B:** Large tortuous and dilated bronchial arteries to the right upper lobe. (*continued*)

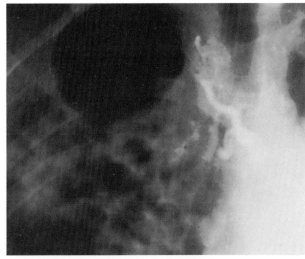

C

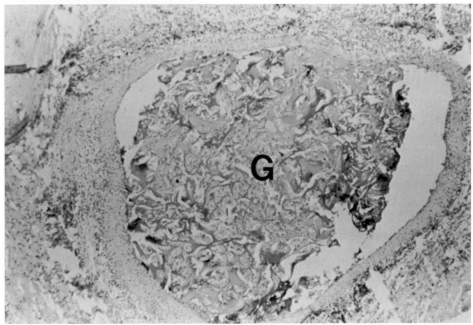

D

FIG. 7-143. *Continued.* **C:** Bronchial arterial occlusion following gelfoam particulate embolization. The massive hemoptysis stopped within 2 hours of embolization, but the patient died 12 hours later because of respiratory failure. **D:** Histologic section shows gelfoam embolus *(G)* in a bronchial arteriole.

developed. There is seldom evidence of bone destruction or loss of the mucoperiosteal line. The frontal sinuses are usually hypoplastic. Nasal polyps are frequently present.

Kartagener Syndrome

Kartagener described a syndrome of situs inversus, sinusitis, and bronchiectasis. It has been shown that Kartagener syndrome (immotile or dysmotile cilia syndrome) is due to deficiency of the dynein arms of cilia (Fig. 7-144). This deficiency is responsible for immotility of respiratory, auditory, and spermatocyte cilia, which causes bronchiectasis, sinusitis, deafness, and male infertility. Impaired ciliary action in developing cells may be responsible for the equal distribution of situs solitus and situs inversus (290). The term *dysmotile cilia syndrome* has been used as a broader entity that includes, in addition to classical Kartagener syndrome, patients with normal situs or situs ambiguus, and problems due to ineffective cilia. Thus, previously confusing cases of bronchiectasis in normal-situs siblings of patients with Kartagener syndrome can now be included in the dysmotile cilia syndrome (297).

The radiologist frequently suggests the diagnosis of Kartagener syndrome or the dysmotile cilia syndrome by observing two or more of the classic components or by observing one component in a patient with a history suggestive of infertility or deafness (290,297). Electron microscopy (Fig. 7-144C) and ciliary motility studies are confirmatory (290).

Rheumatic Disorders

The rheumatic disorders that may involve the lungs include collagen vascular diseases, connective tissue diseases, and rheumatic diseases (1). The common denominator is

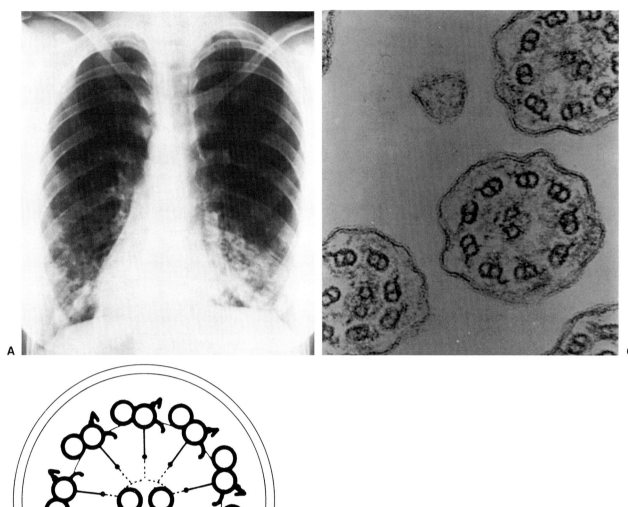

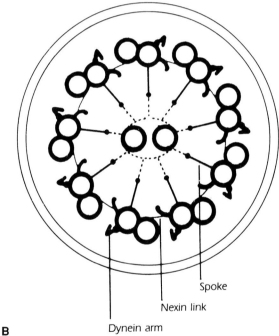

Spoke

Nexin link

Dynein arm

B

FIG. 7-144. Kartagener syndrome. A: A 14-year-old girl with situs inversus and lower lobe bronchiectasis. Films of the sinuses showed marked mucosal thickening in both maxillary antra. **B:** Line drawing of electron microscopy of normal cilia for comparison. **C:** Electron microscopy in this patient. Note the absence of inner arms (nexin links, inner dynein arms, and spokes).

chronic or recurrent tissue inflammation of unknown etiology. Although an infectious cause for rheumatic disorders has not been revealed, there are serologic abnormalities, and antigenic stimulation is likely. The rheumatic disorders that may have pulmonary involvement are systemic lupus erythematosus (SLE) (298), juvenile rheumatoid arthritis, Henoch-Schönlein purpura, dermatomyositis, scleroderma, mixed connective tissue disease, Wegener granulomatosis (299,300), Behçet syndrome, and acute rheumatic fever (1).

Pulmonary inflammation and injury in these rheumatic diseases is due to pulmonary antigen exposure, immune complex deposition, and inflammatory system amplification. The richly vascularized lung tissue is a prime target for injury. Pulmonary hemorrhage, particularly in SLE, can occur as the first manifestation of illness (298).

The radiographic patterns encountered in patients with rheumatic disease are varied. Acute or subacute disease may show bilateral patchy parenchymal infiltrates representing alveolar hemorrhage or edema, pleural effusion, and pericardial effusion. Later findings are reticular or reticulonodular

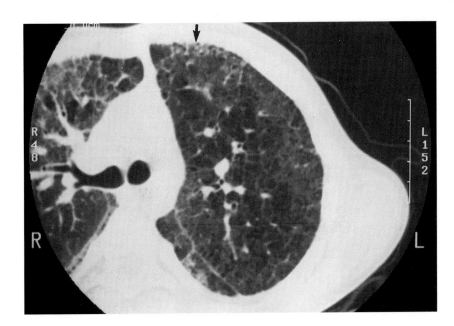

FIG. 7-145. Mixed connective tissue disease. High-resolution CT demonstrates patchy areas of peripheral interstitial fibrosis *(arrow)* and "ground glass" densities. Ground glass density may be due to ongoing inflammation and is potentially reversible. (Courtesy of Thomas C. Hay, D.O., Denver, Colorado.)

interstitial changes consistent with pulmonary fibrosis (Fig. 7-145). Airspace infiltrates and pleural effusions are usually not present. A honeycomb pattern, due to chronic interstitial lung disease and fibrosis, develops in some patients.

Chronic Interstitial Lung Disease

Chronic inflammation of the lung can lead to either a granulomatous or nongranulomatous response, and subsequent end-stage interstitial lung disease (1). A granulomatous response is seen in sarcoid and sarcoid-like illnesses. A nongranulomatous response occurs in the usual form of interstitial pneumonia and in bronchiolitis with or without organizing pneumonia. Neoplastic processes such as Langerhans cell histiocytosis, lymphangiomyomatosis, and lymphoproliferative disorders may also cause a desmoplastic interstitial response and result in chronic interstitial lung disease (301).

When chronic lung inflammation disrupts the epithelial surface of the alveolar wall, the usual form of interstitial pneumonia (UIP) may cause thickened interstitial tissues. A variant of UIP occurs when organization of inflammatory exudate occurs within the distal airways; hence, bronchiolitis obliterans (BO) is characterized by endobronchiolar and peribronchiolar inflammation (302). When inflammatory exudate occludes the distal airways, bronchiolitis obliterans with organizing pneumonia (BOOP) develops (303). BO and BOOP may be caused by infections such as mycoplasma, drugs, toxic exposures, and rheumatic disorders of the lung; they may also be idiopathic. Chest radiographs in both BO and BOOP tend to show bilateral ground glass opacities (302–305).

CT or HRCT can help in the early detection and quantification of disease and analysis of the therapeutic response of patients with chronic interstitial lung disease. Certain pat-

terns suggest a specific diagnosis. The interface sign of interstitial disease refers to the irregular interfaces of the lung parenchyma with pleura, mediastinum, and pulmonary vessels. Subpleural zone lung densities in the periphery may indicate irreversible damage (pulmonary fibrosis). Peribronchial and perivascular distribution may be seen in granulomatous causes of interstitial lung disease (sarcoidosis). Peripheral lung nodules or "mass-like" opacities have been described in BOOP (303–305).

Pulmonary Sarcoidosis

Sarcoidosis is a systemic granulomatous disease of unknown etiology (306). Although sarcoidosis is considered rare in children, there is some evidence to suggest that the overall incidence of childhood sarcoidosis, both symptomatic and asymptomatic, may be similar to that of the adult population (307). The disease can occur as early as 2 1/2 years of age (307). Over 80% of patients are black. There is no gender predominance. The initial symptoms may be constitutional, respiratory, visual, cutaneous, musculoskeletal, cardiac, or salivary glandular (307). The most sensitive clinical indicator of pulmonary sarcoidosis is pulmonary function testing. Lung impairment, which is predominantly restrictive, is usually most pronounced during the acute phase of the disease. There is little correlation between the degree of pulmonary function impairment and the severity of radiologic abnormalities (307).

The patterns of pulmonary sarcoidosis during childhood differ from those seen in adults. Thoracic lymphadenopathy is more frequent at diagnosis (100%) than in adults (84%) (306,307). Bilateral hilar lymphadenopathy, found in all patients in a series of 26 children (Fig. 7-146) and seen only slightly less frequently in adults (90% to 98%), is the radiographic hallmark of sarcoidosis at all ages; however, the

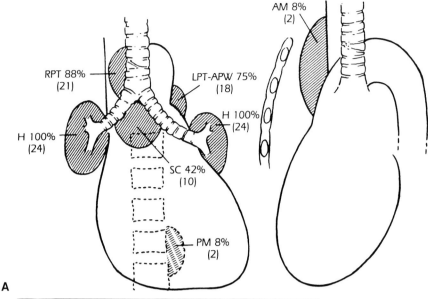

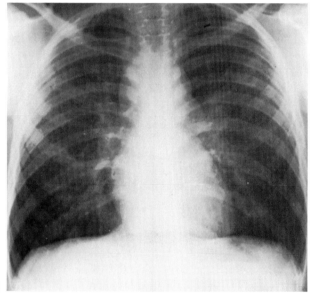

FIG. 7-146. Pulmonary sarcoidosis. A: Representation of lymph node involvement in 24 pediatric cases of pulmonary sarcoidosis: hilar *(H)*, right paratracheal *(RPT)*, left paratracheal aorticopulmonary window *(LPT APW)*, subcarinal *(SC)*, anterior mediastinum *(AM)*, posterior mediastinum *(PM)*. Percentages represent the number of patients in whom specific lymphadenopathy was present, in a total of 26 patients. **B:** Typical bilateral hilar and paratracheal lymphadenopathy with a generalized pattern of small, irregular pulmonary parenchymal involvement. From Merten et al. (307).

pattern of bilateral paratracheal lymphadenopathy with hilar adenopathy is even more common in childhood sarcoidosis (88%) than the 31% to 37% incidence observed in adults (306,307). Unilateral right paratracheal disease associated with bilateral hilar adenopathy (the 1–2–3 sign) is unusual during childhood (13%). Involvement of other mediastinal lymph nodes (subcarinal, anterior mediastinal, posterior mediastinal) along with hilar and paratracheal nodes is sometimes seen (307). Pulmonary parenchymal involvement during childhood is similar in frequency (63%) to that observed in adults (307). The pattern of pulmonary parenchymal involvement can be reticulonodular, miliary, acinar, or fibrotic (306). A small, irregular reticulonodular interstitial pattern is the most common (73%) radiologic pattern in childhood sarcoidosis (307).

Langerhans Cell Histiocytosis

Langerhans cell histiocytosis, the new term for histiocytosis X, includes the spectrum of Letterer-Siwe disease, Hand-Schuller-Christian disease, and eosinophilic granuloma. Its cause remains unknown. It frequently involves the spine and ribs, causing vertebra plana or rib destruction. In the mediastinum, it occasionally causes punctate thymic calcification and thymic cysts, a few of which may contain gas (308). There may be diffuse interstitial lung disease (Fig. 7-147). The interstitial shadows, reticulonodular at first, may become cystic and lead to a honeycombed appearance. Pneumothorax is an occasional complication. Though Langerhans cell histiocytosis occasionally is limited to the lungs in adults, isolated pulmonary involvement is rare in children (309).

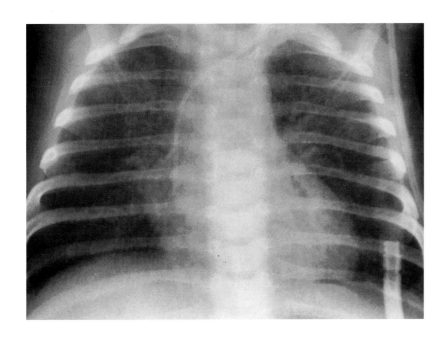

FIG. 7-147. Langerhans cell histiocytosis. The chest film of this 8-month-old boy with known histiocytosis shows diffuse reticulonodular densities.

Lymphoproliferative Disorders

Lymphoid hyperplasia in the lung can occur in either a nodular or diffuse pattern. When diffuse, it is referred to as lymphocytic interstitial pneumonitis. This disorder has been associated with several systemic diseases: chronic active hepatitis, Sjögren syndrome, myasthenia gravis, and especially AIDS. Radiographs show peribronchial and perivascular opacities.

Lymphangiomyomatosis

This is thought by some to be a variant of tuberous sclerosis. It is most common in women of reproductive age. A proliferation of spindle-shaped cells resembling smooth muscle occurs in the interstitium and along lymphatics. Hyperinflation, reticulonodular opacities, and pleural effusion may be present (Fig. 7-148). Like Langerhans histiocytosis, this disorder leads to honeycomb lung with hyperaeration rather than lung contraction.

α_1-Antitrypsin Deficiency

α_1-Antitrypsin is normally secreted by the liver into the circulation. Deficiency of α_1-antitrypsin leads to intrahepatic obstructive cholestasis and ultimately to cirrhosis. In childhood, liver disease is a much more common manifestation of the illness than pulmonary disease. However, a few patients with this deficiency develop respiratory problems as children. α_1-Antitrypsin inhibits neutrophil elastase, an enzyme that destroys the connective tissues of the alveolar walls. Deficiency of it leads to connective tissue destruction which, in many adults and a few older children, leads to emphysema. Exposure to cigarette smoke apparently hastens and worsens the lung damage (310).

Dyspnea, wheezing, cough, air trapping, and biopsy proven panacinar emphysema are signs and symptoms. Radiographs show hyperinflation, often difficult to distinguish from the hyperinflation of ordinary asthma. In adult life, the emphysema has a predilection for the lung bases.

Idiopathic Pulmonary Hemosiderosis

Pulmonary hemosiderosis is a disease of unknown etiology characterized by intraalveolar hemorrhage. It is thought to be an autoimmune disease. Some cases are related to sensitivity to proteins in cow's milk.

The symptoms depend on the temporal course and severity of the pulmonary hemorrhages. They include cough, fever, severe respiratory distress, failure to thrive, fatigue, and pallor. Severe bleeding leads to hemoptysis and hematemesis. The dyspnea, tachycardia, and fever may be marked. Hypochromic, microcytic anemia due to chronic blood loss, reticulocytosis, and eosinophilia are often present (8,311).

Following an acute hemorrhage, there are bilateral, hazy opacities that may simulate pulmonary edema (8,311). As blood is cleared from the alveoli and hemosiderin is deposited in the lung septa, the acinar pattern evolves into a reticulonodular interstitial pattern (Fig. 7-149) (8,311).

The diagnosis is made by identifying hemosiderin-laden macrophages in the sputum or in gastric washings (311). MRI may verify that the parenchymal opacities contain blood, hemosiderin, or other blood products. Frequently, needle lung aspiration or open lung biopsy is required for

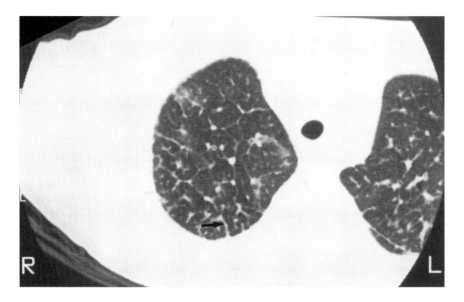

FIG. 7-148. Pulmonary lymphangiomatosis. High-resolution CT shows septal thickening *(arrow)* with mild irregularity of the pleural surface. Septal thickening bordering the secondary pulmonary lobules is characteristic of both lymphangiomatous and hemangiomatous lesions of the lung. (Courtesy of Thomas C. Hay, D.O., Denver, Colorado.)

definitive diagnosis. Steroid therapy has been successful in some cases. Death may be due to massive pulmonary hemorrhage, progressive respiratory insufficiency, or cor pulmonale (311).

Pulmonary Alveolar Proteinosis

Pulmonary alveolar proteinosis (PAP) is an uncommon disease of unknown etiology characterized by deposition within the alveolar spaces of a flocculent, granular material high in protein and lipid content. There is a 2 : 1 male/female ratio; most patients are aged 20–50 at the time of diagnosis. Approximately 40 cases of PAP have been reported in children (312). Almost 30% of these patients have had thymic alymphoplasia, and it has been speculated that immunologic incompetency is a causative factor, particularly in children under 1 year (312). Similar pathologic and radiologic abnormalities are seen in patients with surfactant protein B deficiency (313).

The clinical symptoms are is highly variable. There is frequently diarrhea and vomiting. Other symptoms include failure to thrive, exertional dyspnea, and cyanosis. If there is no superimposed infection, laboratory studies are normal.

The radiologic findings are frequently much more severe than the clinical abnormalities. The chest radiograph frequently shows small acinar nodules that may assume a miliary pattern (Fig. 7-150). These nodules may coalesce to form larger nodular densities or small areas of consolidation, as is commonly seen in adults (312). Pleural effusions and adenopathy are absent unless there is superimposed infection. CT of the chest shows scattered airspace densities, greater in the bases and decreasing gradually toward the apices. These opacities presumably represent acini filled with periodic acid– Schiff–positive eosinophilic material (312). Lung biopsy confirms the diagnosis (Fig. 7-150B). Bronchopul-

monary lavage, the therapy of choice for childhood PAP, has decreased the mortality of this disease, previously uniformly fatal in childhood (312).

Thoracic Tumors

Chest Wall Masses

Tumors of the chest wall are the rarest of all chest masses in infants and children (Table 7-17). A limited number of

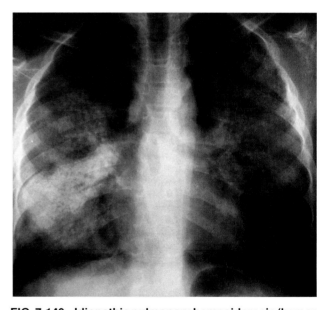

FIG. 7-149. Idiopathic pulmonary hemosiderosis (hemorrhage). An 8-year-old girl with cough, dyspnea, hemoptysis, and iron deficiency anemia. There are bilateral acinar opacities due to hemorrhages superimposed upon diffuse nodular interstitial lung disease representing hemosiderin deposition in the interstitium.

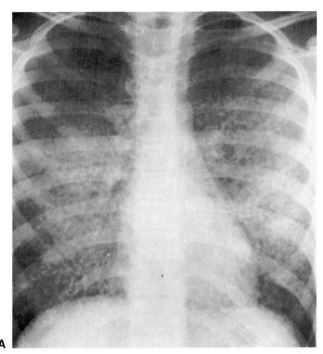

A

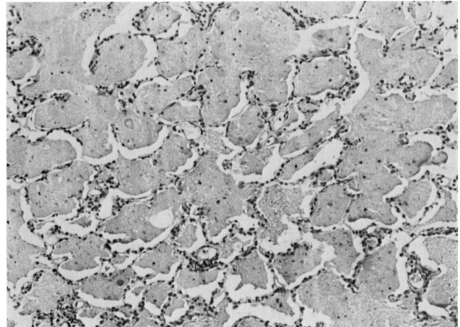

B

FIG. 7-150. Pulmonary alveolar proteinosis. A: A 7-year-old girl with bilateral acinar nodules mimicking miliary disease. **B:** Lung biopsy. The alveoli are filled with periodic acid–Schiff (PAS)–positive material. From McCook et al. (312).

pediatric cases have been separately reported and discussed in the literature (43,314).

With conventional chest radiography, it may be difficult to confirm that a mass arises from the chest wall (Table 7-18) rather than from the pulmonary parenchyma or mediastinum (Table 7-17). Bone destruction, not just bone erosion or rib splaying, indicates that the mass arises from the chest wall. If there is a pleural effusion, the extrapleural nature of the mass may not be radiographically apparent until after thoracentesis (314). CT and MRI are helpful for determining whether a chest wall mass is soft-tissue, bony, or extrapleural-intrathoracic in location (Table 7-17) (46,47,141).

Skeletal scintigraphy complements cross-sectional imaging, showing extent of bony involvement and multiplicity of involved sites in metastatic disease.

Soft-Tissue Masses

Soft-tissue masses of the thorax may arise from cutaneous or subcutaneous tissues. Breast masses are much less common in children than adults (315); these tumors are not included in this discussion. Benign tumors (Table 7-18) are more common than malignant neoplasms. Physical examina-

TABLE 7-17. *Diagnostic approach to pediatric chest masses*

Location
    Chest wall
        Soft tissues
        Bony thorax
        Extrapleural space
    Lung
        Pleura
        Parenchyma
    Mediastinum
Density
    Air
    Fat
    Soft tissue
    Calcification
    Ossification
Contrast enhancement
Borders
Size
Shape
Associated abnormalities
    Direct
        Displacement
        Erosion
        Destruction
    Indirect
        Organomegaly
        Anomalies

Modified from Kirks et al. (43).

tion helps characterize the lesion and its extent. Tangential radiography or fluoroscopy confirms the soft-tissue mass and the absence of rib or lung abnormalities. A radiopaque marker may be placed over the mass for localization. Radiologic examination occasionally demonstrates calcification in a mesenchymoma or fat in a lipoma. CT and MRI both show the internal features and extent of the mass. MRI provides better tissue characterization than CT and demonstrates vascular compression or encasement better.

Skeletal Tumors

Generalized bone diseases causing bony thoracic (spine, clavicle, rib, scapula) lesions include Langerhans cell histiocytosis, multiple hereditary exostoses, and neurofibromatosis (Table 7-18). Langerhans cell histiocytosis of a rib may be associated with bony lesions elsewhere. Multiple hereditary exostoses may involve the ribs, clavicles, or scapulas. The irregular, wavy ribs and the notched ribs of neurofibromatosis are thought to be a part of a generalized mesenchymal maldevelopment; occasionally, true intercostal neurofibromas tumors develop.

Most other thoracic skeletal tumors (Table 7-18) in children are malignant (Fig. 7-151). Metastatic disease is more common than primary neoplasm (314). Multiple extrapleural masses and areas of rib destruction suggest metastatic disease; neuroblastoma and leukemia are the usual causes.

Ewing sarcoma is the most common primary skeletal

tumor of the thoracic cage (314). It usually causes rib expansion, destruction of the cortex and medulla, periosteal bone formation, and a soft-tissue mass (Fig. 7-152). The radiologic appearance may be that of a pleural effusion hiding the underlying rib destruction. MRI is the examination of choice for characterization of the tumor's internal matrix, its extent, and its relationship to adjacent structures of the chest wall (Fig. 7-152).

An Askin tumor (primitive neuroectodermal tumor [PNET]) is a malignant, small cell neuroepithelioma that originates in the chest wall or lung (316,317). PNETs simulate Ewing sarcomas clinically, radiographically (Fig. 7-153), and histologically. Special immunocytochemical and electron microscopic features distinguish this tumor from Ewing sarcoma and other malignant, small, round cell neoplasms (2,318,319).

Extrapleural Intrathoracic Tumors

Extrapleural intrathoracic tumors are rare in children but are usually malignant even if there is no associated rib destruction. Rhabdomyosarcoma is the most common nonskeletal extrapleural chest wall tumor in children (Table 7-18). The radiologic features are those of an extrapleural mass, sometimes difficult to distinguish from a Ewing sarcoma or PNET (43,317).

TABLE 7-18. *Chest wall masses*

Soft-tissue tumors	Bony thorax tumors
Benign[a]	Generalized bone disease
Lymphangioma[a]	Neurofibromatosis
Cystic hygroma[a]	Multiple hereditary
Lipoma[a]	exostoses
Hemangioma	Primary skeletal tumors
Neurofibroma	Benign
Hamartoma	Fibrous dysplasia[a]
Desmoid	Osteochondroma
Malignant	(exostosis)
Askin tumor (PNET)	Eosinophilic
Rhabdomyosarcoma	granuloma[a]
Large cell lymphoma	Enchondroma
Undifferentiated	Aneurysmal bone cyst
sarcoma	Osteoblastoma
Malignant	Chondroblastoma
mesenchymoma	Unicameral bone cyst
Fibrosarcoma	Malignant tumors[a]
Synovioma	Metastatic[a]
Extrapleural-intrathoracic	Neuroblastoma[a]
tumors	Leukemia[a]
Benign	Ewing sarcoma
Mesenchymoma	Chloroma
Lipoma	Primary
Malignant[a]	Ewing sarcoma[a]
Rhabdomyosarcoma[a]	Askin tumor (PNET)[a]
Mesenchymoma	Chondrosarcoma
	Osteogenic sarcoma

[a] More common.
PNET, primitive neuroectodermal tumor
Modified from Franken et al. (314) and Kirks et al. (43).

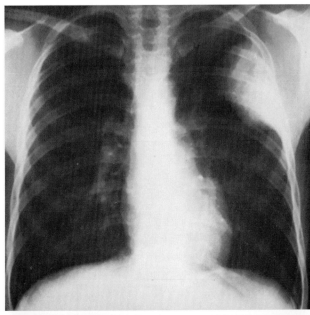

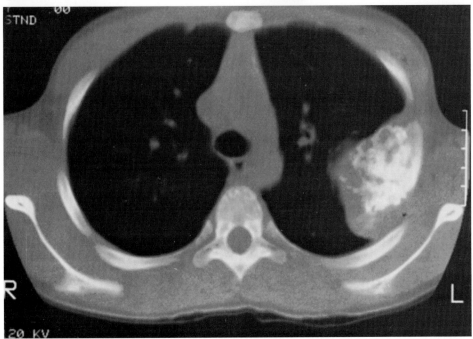

FIG. 7-151. Chondrosarcoma of bony thorax. A 14-year-old boy with chronic left chest pain. **A:** Posteroanterior chest radiograph shows a smoothly marginated left chest wall mass that appears to be extrapleural. **B:** Transaxial CT shows a large rib mass with a prominent chondroid matrix. The precise extent of the lesion is demonstrated.

Mediastinal Masses

The radiologic approach to pediatric mediastinal masses is complex, intellectually challenging, and diagnostically critical (43,47,320). The signs and symptoms depend on the age, the size and the location of the mass, and its relation to other intrathoracic structures. Approximately 75% of children found to have mediastinal masses are at least mildly symptomatic. Esophageal compression leads to dysphagia, cough may indicate airway involvement, and venous distention reflects SVC obstruction. Imaging evaluation of the mediastinum demands a thorough knowledge of normal anatomy and normal variants. Initial evaluation is made by chest radiography. Anterior and middle mediastinal masses are often further evaluated with CT. Posterior mediastinal masses may involve the extradural space and thus are best imaged with MRI (141). As technology continues to improve, MRI will become the definitive imaging method for all mediastinal masses in infants and children.

The mediastinum is the central anatomic space between the two lungs and their parietal pleurae. It extends from the thoracic inlet cranially to the diaphragm caudally and from the sternum ventrally to the vertebral column dorsally. It contains all of the thoracic viscera with the exception of the lungs and their pleurae.

The mediastinum is the most common location of primary

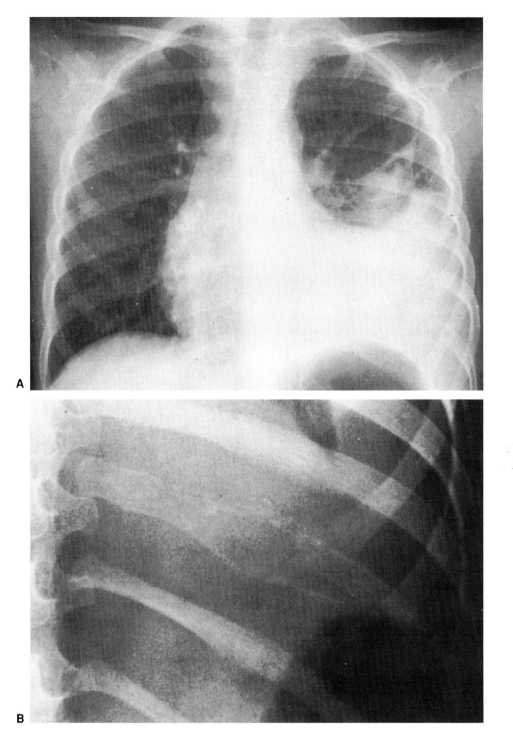

FIG. 7-152. Ewing sarcoma. A: A 5-year-old girl with a large left pleural effusion. **B:** Collimated high-kilovoltage film shows an expansile, destructive lesion of the posterior part of the left tenth rib. From Kirks et al. (43).

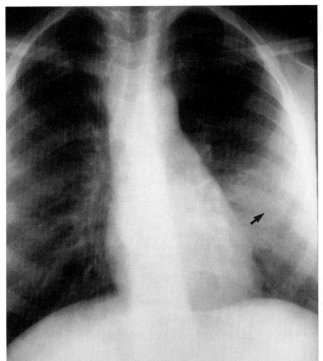

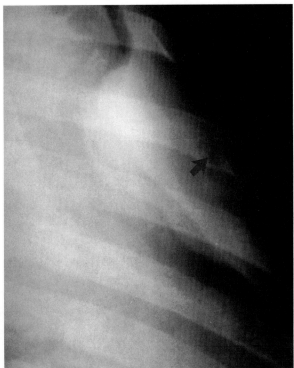

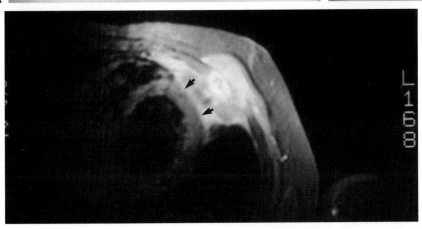

FIG. 7-153. Askin tumor (primitive neuroectodermal tumor [PNET]) of chest wall. A 7-year-old girl with cough and chest pain. **A:** AP chest x-ray shows a left thoracic opacity, vague and poorly marginated in this projection. Note the indistinct appearance of the left anterior fourth rib *(arrow)*. **B:** Oblique radiography shows a large extrapleural mass and permeative fourth rib destruction *(arrow)*. **C:** Axial T1-weighted MR image. The extent of the chest wall tumor and the obliteration of the fibrous pericardium *(arrows)* are exquisitely demonstrated. Pericardial invasion was confirmed at thoracotomy.

thoracic masses in children. Moreover, at least one third of all mediastinal masses occur in patients <15 years of age (43,320,321).

Radiographic Compartments

Classically, the mediastinum has been divided into upper and lower portions by a line drawn from the sternal angle (angle of Louis) to the fourth thoracic intervertebral disk space (T4–T5). The upper compartment is referred to as the superior mediastinum. The lower part is divided into the anterior mediastinum in front of the heart, the middle mediastinum containing the pericardium and heart, and the posterior mediastinum behind the heart. These classic anatomic divisions of the mediastinum are not practical for pediatric imaging analysis and differential diagnosis (43,321,322).

Modification of the radiologic compartments of Hope et al. (321) and Felson (322) for the analysis of mediastinal masses in infants and children has proven to be practical (Fig. 7-154) (43).

By this modified approach, the posterior mediastinum lies behind a line drawn tangential to the ventral margins of the vertebral bodies. Most posterior mediastinal masses actually arise in a paravertebral gutter, so that their posterior surfaces are not outlined by air on the lateral chest radiograph. The anterior mediastinum is in front of a line drawn parallel to the previously described posterior line and extending from the most cephalic portion of the manubrium to the diaphragm. The middle mediastinum is between the anterior and posterior mediastinal compartments (Fig. 7-154). These compartments may be extrapolated from the lateral chest radiograph (Fig. 7-154A) to axial CT (Fig. 7-154B) as well as axial, sagittal, and coronal MR images.

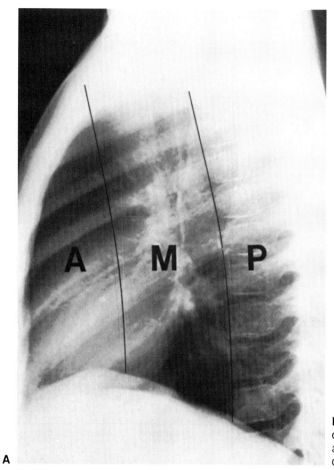

A

FIG. 7-154. Mediastinal compartments. **A:** Lateral chest radiograph. **B:** Axial CT section at the level of the carina. *A*, anterior mediastinum; *M*, middle mediastinum; *P*, posterior mediastinum. From Kirks and Korobkin (47).

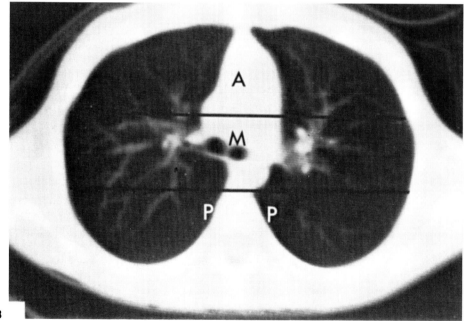

B

Radiologic Analysis of Mediastinal Masses

The various compartments of the mediastinum are superimposed on the frontal chest radiograph. The hilum overlay sign and cervicothoracic sign aid in the localization of mediastinal masses on the PA or AP radiograph (322). However, the lateral view is critical for placement of the mass in one of the three mediastinal compartments (Fig. 7-154A).

Because the mediastinum is enclosed by pleura, tumors within the mediastinum have the radiologic features of an extrapleural mass. The mediastinal mass, like a marble under a rug, is convex toward the lung parenchyma, with a sharp, well-defined lateral margin and an obtuse angle at the upper and lower junctions of the mass with the normal mediastinal pleural reflections. Air bronchograms are not present in a mediastinal mass. Any spine, rib, or sternal abnormalities confirm the extrapleural mediastinal location of the mass.

The lateral radiograph permits localization of a mass to the anterior, middle, or posterior mediastinum. These compartments are not separated by anatomic tissue planes. Because mediastinal masses may involve more than one compartment, the center of a mass should be considered as the anatomic site of origin for differential diagnostic purposes (Table 7-19). A posterior mediastinal mass is located in the paravertebral gutter on cross-sectional images (43), and its posterior surface is not outlined by air on the lateral chest radiograph (322).

Anterior Mediastinum

The anterior mediastinum contains thymus, lymph nodes, the anterior part of the heart, part of the main pulmonary artery, the proximal ascending aorta, the phrenic nerves, and sometimes a substernal extension of the thyroid (43). Approximately 30% of pediatric mediastinal tumors arise in the anterior compartment (43,323,324). They usually arise from either thymus or lymph nodes. The radiologic differential diagnosis (Table 7-19) includes the four "T's": teratoma (germ cell tumor), thymic tumor, "terrible" lymphoma or leukemia, and thyroid tumor. A prominent, but normal, thymus is the most common pseudotumor of the anterior mediastinum. Because tumors of the thymus and thyroid are very unusual in infants and children, the primary differential diagnostic considerations of a pediatric anterior mediastinal mass are lymphoma and teratoma.

Thymus. The thymus is a common pseudotumor and uncommon pathologic mass of the anterior mediastinum. Un-

TABLE 7-19. *Mediastinal masses*

Etiology	Anterior mediastinum (30%)	Middle mediastinum (30%)	Posterior mediastinum (40%)
Congenital	Normal thymus[a]	Foregut cyst:[a] enteric, respiratory	Foregut cyst: enteric, respiratory, neurenteric
	Thymic cyst	Esophagus:[a] hiatus hernia, achalasia, reflux, chalasia	Lateral meningocele
			Bochdalek hernia
	Thymomegaly	Extension of normal thymus	Ectopic thymus
	Morgagni hernia		
Inflammatory	Mediastinitis	Mediastinitis	Mediastinitis
	Lymphadenopathy	Lymphadenopathy[a]	Lymphadenopathy
	Sternal inflammatory disease		Spinal inflammatory disease
Neoplasm	Lymphoma-leukemia[a]	Lymphoma-leukemia[a]	Neurogenic tumor
	Teratoma[a]	Lymphadenopathy[a]: primary, metastatic	Neural crest tumor[a]
	Other germ cell tumors		Peripheral nerve tumor
			Lymphoma-leukemia
	Seminoma		Teratoma
	Thymoma		
	Thyroid or parathyroid tumor	Thyroid or parathyroid tumor	
	Hamartoma	Hamartoma	Hamartoma
	Mesenchymal tumor	Mesenchymal tumor	Mesenchymal tumor
	Lymphangioma-hemangioma	Lymphangioma-hemangioma	Lymphangioma-hemangioma
	Lipoma	Lymphoid hamartoma	Pheochromocytoma
	Phrenic nerve tumor	Vagus nerve tumor	Melanoma
	Pericardial cyst or tumor	Pericardial cyst or tumor	Thoracic duct cyst
	Cardiac tumor or aneurysm	Cardiac tumor or aneurysm	Osteocartilaginous tumor
Traumatic	Hematoma	Hematoma	Hematoma
	Sternal fracture	Diaphragmatic rupture	Spinal fracture
	Thymic hemorrhage		
Vascular	Aneurysm of sinus of Valsalva	Aneurysm: aorta; ductus	Aneurysm of descending aorta
	Anomalous vessel	Dilated superior or inferior vena cava	Dilated azygous or hemiazygous veins
		Anomalies of great vessels	
		Pulmonary varix	
Miscellaneous	Histiocystosis	Pancreatic pseudocyst	Histiocytosis
	Sarcoidosis	Sarcoidosis	Extramedullary hematopoiesis
		Histiocytosis	Sarcoidosis

(%) Percentage of mediastinal masses in each compartment.
[a] More common lesions.
Modified from Kirks et al. (43).

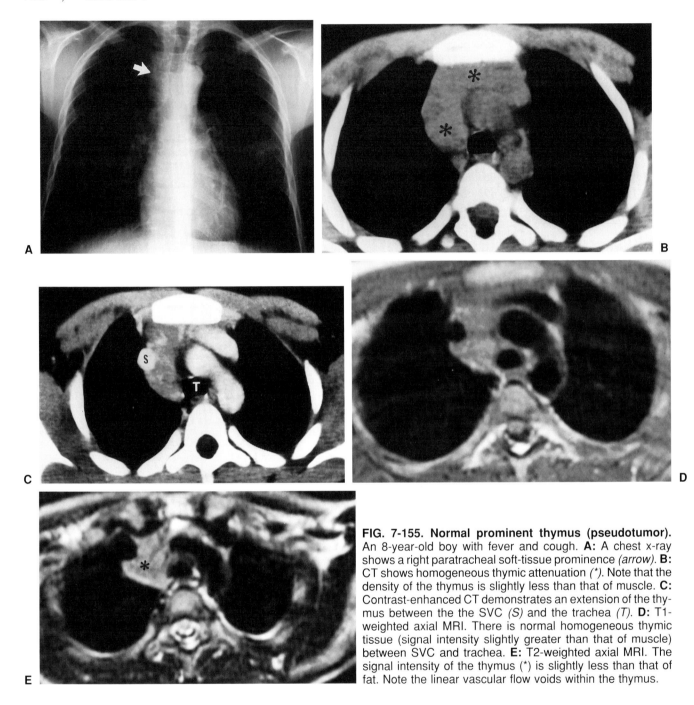

FIG. 7-155. Normal prominent thymus (pseudotumor).
An 8-year-old boy with fever and cough. **A:** A chest x-ray shows a right paratracheal soft-tissue prominence *(arrow)*. **B:** CT shows homogeneous thymic attenuation *(*)*. Note that the density of the thymus is slightly less than that of muscle. **C:** Contrast-enhanced CT demonstrates an extension of the thymus between the the SVC *(S)* and the trachea *(T)*. **D:** T1-weighted axial MRI. There is normal homogeneous thymic tissue (signal intensity slightly greater than that of muscle) between SVC and trachea. **E:** T2-weighted axial MRI. The signal intensity of the thymus (*) is slightly less than that of fat. Note the linear vascular flow voids within the thymus.

derstanding the variable appearance of the normal thymus is important. Infants and young children may show a variety of typical thymic shapes (sail sign, wave sign, and notch sign). In the first 5 years of life, the thymus is usually prominent on the chest radiograph and is often quadrilateral. Toward the end of the first decade, the thymus becomes relatively inconspicuous. Questions often arise as to whether the thymus is normal but prominent, or pathologically enlarged. Knowledge of the expected location, shape, size, and internal features of the normal thymus allows the radiologist to recognize an abnormality and plan an integrated imaging strat-

egy. On chest radiography, the thymus should be considered to be pathologically enlarged when its borders have an unusual shape. Marked lobularity of the thymus is never normal, at any age. The displacement of vessels or the airway is strongly suggestive of pathology. Posterior extension of the thymus between the trachea and SVC is an exception to this rule. In this circumstance, a mild tracheal mass effect may be seen (Fig. 7-155A).

CT evaluation of the thymus offers better spatial resolution and contrast sensitivity than chest radiography; it can precisely evaluate thymic size, shape, and density. By CT,

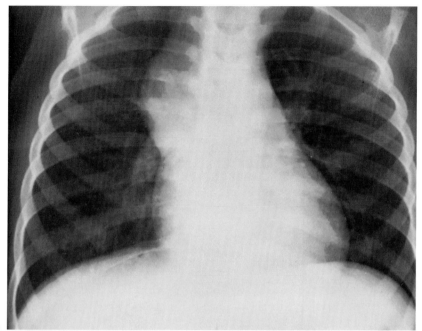

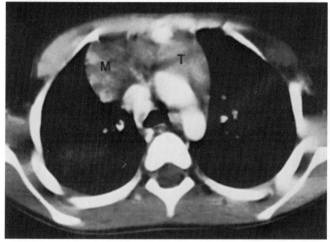

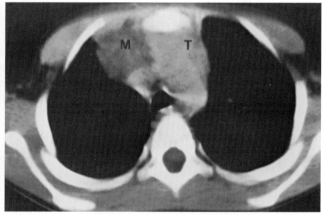

FIG. 7-156. Primary thymic lymphangioma/hemangioma. A 5-year-old boy with cough and fever. **A:** A chest radiograph shows a smooth right upper mediastinal mass. **B:** Enhanced CT at the level of the carina demonstrates an inhomogeneous right anterior mediastinal mass *(M)*. This mass is inseparable from homogeneous, normal thymic tissue *(T)*. **C:** A delayed CT image accentuates the difference between abnormal tissue *(M)* and the normal left thymic lobe *(T)*.

the normal childhood thymus is a quadrilateral gland with homogeneous density similar to that of skeletal muscle (Fig. 7-155B, C). The lateral margins are slightly convex outward. After puberty, the thymus is more triangular. Normal age-related measurements for thymic lobe thickness have been determined (79). For neonates and infants, parasternal sonography can be a useful adjunct to the chest radiograph. Thymic tissue is homogeneous and similar to liver in echo texture (53). MRI has been helpful in the characterization of normal and abnormal thymic tissue; it is ideal for conditions causing thymic infiltration (lymphoma, leukemia). Normally, the T1-weighted appearance of the thymus is slightly hyperintense relative to muscle (Fig. 7-155D) (52). On T2-weighted images, it is slightly less bright than fat (Fig. 7-155E). The thymic signal should be homogeneous.

Apart from the prominent normal thymus (pseudotumor), true masses of the thymus during childhood are unusual. Hy-perplasia, teratoma, thymic cyst (325), hemorrhage, thymolipoma, thymoma, lymphoma, and lymphangioma/hemangioma (Fig. 7-156) may cause pathologic thymic enlargement.

Thymoma. Thymoma is most common between the fourth and sixth decades. In childhood it is rare. Derived from thymic epithelium, this encapsulated lesion sometimes contains areas of necrosis, hemorrhage, cyst formation, and calcification. Approximately 30% of these lesions are malignant. Parathymic syndromes (myasthenia gravis, hypogammaglobulinemia, and red cell aplasia) may be part of the clinical picture. Forty percent of patients with thymona have one of the paraneoplastic syndromes; approximately 35% of patients with thymoma have myasthenia gravis (MG), whereas only 15% of patients with MG have a thymoma (326). Thymic follicular hyperplasia is common (65%) in MG (326).

Germ Cell Tumor. Germ cell tumors occur most commonly in the anterior mediastinum in close proximity to or

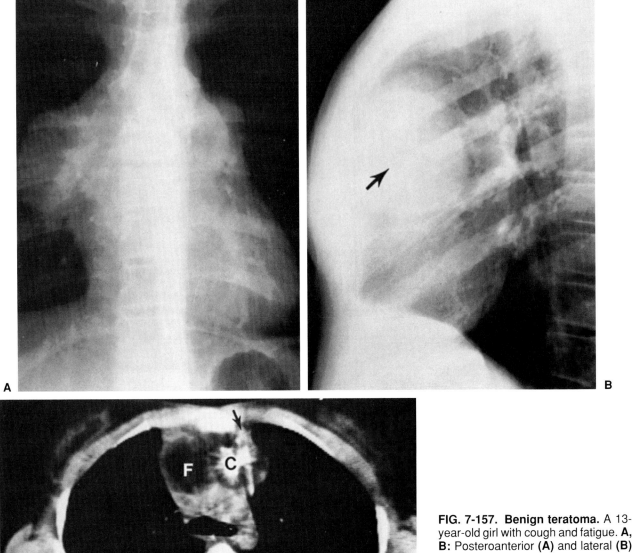

FIG. 7-157. Benign teratoma. A 13-year-old girl with cough and fatigue. **A, B:** Posteroanterior **(A)** and lateral **(B)** chest radiographs show a large lobular mediastinal mass. The center of the mass is in the anterior mediastinum *(arrow)*. **C:** A CT section at the level of the carina demonstrates an anterior mediastinal mass that contains fat *(F)*, calcification *(C)*, and soft tissue *(arrow)*. From Kirks and Korobkin (47).

within the thymus. Germ cell tumors of the mediastinum include teratoma, teratocarcinoma, choriocarcinoma, seminoma, endodermal sinus (yolk sac) tumor, and mixed germ cell tumor (327–329). Teratomas of the anterior mediastinum can be distinguished from other germ cell tumors if they contain soft tissue, fat, and calcification (Fig. 7-157). Although histologically benign, mature teratomas can cause significant compression effects (Fig. 7-158).

Homogeneous tumors with very low attenuation coefficients in the mass should be considered to be benign fatty teratomas. A mediastinal tumor with more variable attenua-

tion may be benign or malignant germ cell tumor, a mixed tumor, or a liposarcoma (327–329). Malignant germ cell tumors of the mediastinum are most common in adolescents and young male adults. Seminoma (germinoma) is the most common primary malignant mediastinal germ cell tumor. Nonseminomatous malignant germ cell tumors include endodermal sinus tumors (α-fetoprotein marker), choriocarcinoma (human chorionic gonadotropin marker), and mixed germ cell tumors. In such cases, a large mass may expand the mediastinum to fill a hemithorax. Radiographic hints that the chest opacity is due to a tumor include ipsilateral hilar

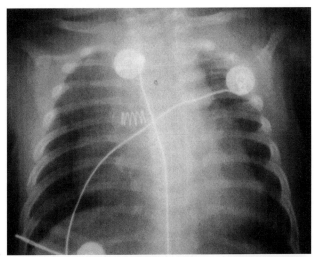

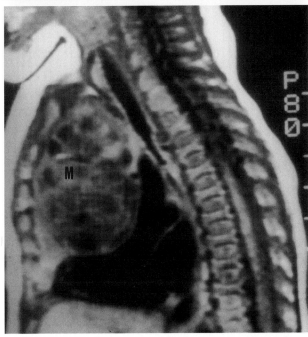

FIG. 7-158. Benign teratoma. Newborn with severe respiratory distress. **A:** AP chest radiograph shows widening of the upper mediastinum and loss of the tracheal air shadow. **B:** Sagittal T1-weighted MRI demonstrates a large heterogeneous mass *(M)* and marked tracheal and cardiac compression. Courtesy of Sam T. Auringer, M.D., Winston-Salem, North Carolina.

and main bronchus compression, mediastinal adenopathy, and metastases to the contralateral lung.

Lymphoma. After leukemia and tumors of the CNS, lymphoma is the third most common neoplasm in children less than 16 years old (319). At least 60% of pediatric lymphomas are NHL, and 40% are Hodgkin's disease. NHL of childhood is usually a disseminated disease. It has marked similarities to acute lymphocytic leukemia (ALL) (319, 330), and differentiation between them may be difficult or arbitrary. This has led to the frequent use of the term "lymphoma-leukemia" in pediatric imaging (319,330). Although there are some similarities in childhood between NHL and Hodgkin's disease, they are far outweighed by the many differences in clinical features, imaging appearance, histologic features, biological behavior, and response to therapy. For this reason, it is important to discuss these two malignancies separately (319,331).

Non-Hodgkin's lymphoma. NHL of childhood differs dramatically from both pediatric Hodgkin's disease and adult NHL (332). NHL accounts for about 60% of pediatric lymphomas and 6% of all childhood cancers. The peak age of presentation is between 7 and 11 years (mean 9 years). The male to female ratio is 3:1 (319).

The histopathologic classification of NHL is based on cell type, degree of differentiation, and cell markers (333). The broadest classification separates NHL into lymphoblastic and nonlymphoblastic types. Nonlymphoblastic NHL is further subdivided into histiocytic (large cell) and undifferentiated. Undifferentiated, nonlymphoblastic NHL includes Burkitt and non-Burkitt types. The criteria for separation into various groups are based on not only histopathologic findings but also cytomorphologic features, chemical markers, and immunologic markers. There are four major types of childhood NHL: lymphoblastic (30% to 35%), undifferentiated non-Burkitt (25% to 30%), undifferentiated Burkitt (20% to 25%), and histiocytic or large cell (15% to 20%) (330,333,334).

There is excellent correlation between the type of NHL and the site of involvement. Lymphoblastic NHL is usually supradiaphragmatic and presents as a mediastinal mass, often with cervical lymphadenopathy. Undifferentiated (small noncleaved cell) NHL (non-Burkitt and Burkitt types) usually occurs in the abdomen, the ileocecal region being the most common site of involvement. Large cell (histiocytic) NHL occurs in various anatomic regions but is seldom mediastinal. Abdominal NHL usually arises from B cells; mediastinal NHL is derived from T cells; and peripheral nodal NHL may arise from B cells, T cells, or non-B, non-T-cell types (319,330,333). More than 70% of NHL in children is disseminated at the time of diagnosis. Most childhood NHL is extranodal, in contrast both with adult NHL and with Hodgkin's disease at any age. The most frequent primary site of childhood NHL is the abdomen, particularly the ileocecal region; the second most common site is the mediastinum (approximately 25%) (319,330,333).

Mediastinal lymphoma, when large and bulky, produces the SVC syndrome and extrinsic airway compression. Mediastinal CT or MRI demonstrates a small number of large discrete lymph nodes or a more conglomerate mass in which individual nodes are no longer identifiable (Fig. 7-159) (334). Extranodal disease involving the spleen, liver, kidneys, and gastrointestinal tract causes single or multiple low-attenuation areas in the parenchyma or a diffuse infiltrating pattern on CT. The similarity between NHL and ALL of childhood is particularly evident in mediastinal disease (Fig. 7-160) (335). With this type of involvement, the percentage of malignant cells in the bone marrow is used to decide whether to call the disease ALL or NHL (330,331).

Because more than 70% of pediatric NHL is widely disseminated when diagnosed, microscopic metastases are assumed and chemotherapy is given to all patients. Staging is not as detailed or meticulous as with Hodgkin's disease. In addition to the size and extent of primary mediastinal disease, other regional or systemic areas of potential involvement may be evaluated. Therapy and prognosis are influenced by the presence or absence of bone marrow and CNS involvement.

Hodgkin's disease. Hodgkin's disease is less frequent in children than NHL, accounting for approximately 5% of all malignancies in infants and children (319). Pediatric Hodgkin's disease, usually appearing during adolescence, accounts for only 10% of all cases of Hodgkin's disease. The clinical features, imaging appearance, histologic features, treatment, and prognosis of pediatric Hodgkin's disease are almost identical to those of adult Hodgkin's disease. However, the male predominance is more marked during childhood and is strongest during the first decade of life (319).

The relative frequencies of the histologic types of Hodgkin's disease in children are as follows: nodular sclerosis, 60% to 70%; mixed cellularity, 15% to 25%; lymphocytic predominance, 10% to 15%; and lymphocytic depletion, 1% to 5% (319,336). It is difficult to make a definitive diagnosis of Hodgkin's disease without an open biopsy. The Reed-Sternberg cell has a classic appearance in fixed sections stained with hematoxylin and eosin (Fig. 7-161). It is typically binucleate and has a prominent, centrally located nucleolus in each nucleus, a well-demarcated nuclear membrane, and eosinophilic cytoplasm with a perinuclear halo. This cell, with its "owl-eye" appearance, is believed to represent the neoplastic cell of the disease. However, the surrounding cells, which presumably represent a reactive or stromal cell component, actually compose a much larger part of the tumor (336).

Hodgkin's disease almost always arises in lymph nodes. Cervical lymphadenopathy is the most likely symptom at presentation. Involvement of the thorax (85%), paraaortic lymph nodes (35%), and spleen (35%) is also common. The disease usually progresses via lymphatic pathways to contiguous lymph node groups and the spleen. The frequent involvement of certain abdominal lymph nodes groups is another difference between Hodgkin's disease and NHL. In Hodgkin's disease, mesenteric lymph nodes are rarely involved, whereas paraaortic and celiac nodes are common sites of disease.

Intrathoracic lymph node involvement is seen in about 85% of patients at the time of presentation. In almost all such patients, the superior prevascular and paratracheal lymph node groups are involved (Fig. 7-162), either alone or with other intrathoracic manifestations of disease. Hilar nodes are involved in more than 25% of patients with Hodgkin's disease. Involvement of the subcarinal (22%), posterior mediastinal (5%), and cardiophrenic angle (8%) lymph node groups can affect radiation therapy planning. Pulmonary parenchymal involvement is seen in approximately 10% of patients at presentation. Lung involvement occurs only with radiographically demonstrable mediastinal (usually ipsilateral hilar) lymph node enlargement. Pleural effusions, occurring in approximately 15% of patients with Hodgkin's disease, are assumed to be due to lymphatic venous obstruction rather than involvement of the pleural surfaces by tumor, unless pleural masses are also identified (319).

Staging of the disease at diagnosis governs the therapy and determines the prognosis. According to the Ann Arbor classification, there are four major stages. Imaging studies are a critical part of staging. CT and MRI are invaluable for assessing the extent of the disease at diagnosis and the subsequent response to therapy (337,338); treatment planning is altered by these studies in at least 10% of cases (51).

Tracheobronchial compression occurs in up to 55% of children with newly diagnosed Hodgkin's lymphoma. CT not only is more sensitive than chest radiography for the detection of intrathoracic tracheal narrowing but also can be used to quantitate this decrease in cross-sectional area (Fig. 7-162C) (27,339,340). Patients with mediastinal masses producing significant respiratory symptoms usually have tracheal cross-sectional areas below the lower range of normal (339,340).

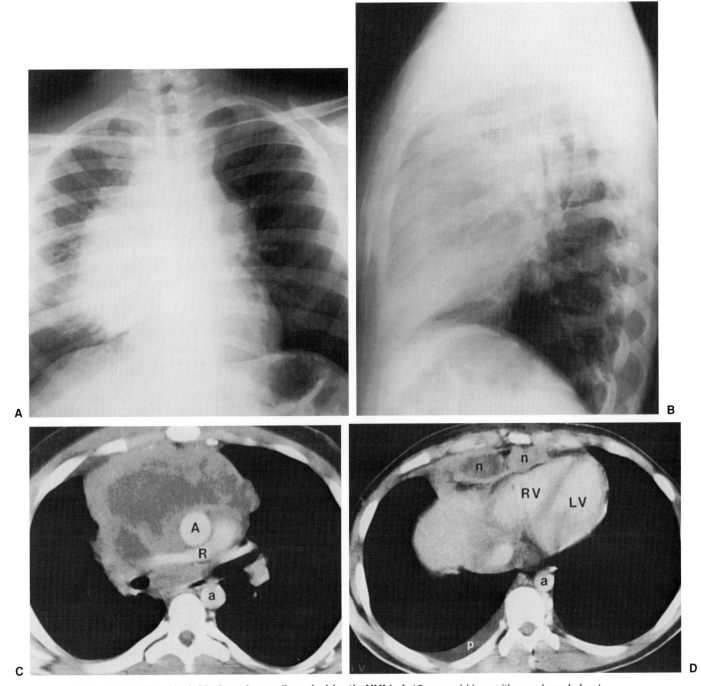

FIG. 7-159. Non-Hodgkin lymphoma (lymphoblastic NHL). A 16-year-old boy with cough and chest pain. **A, B:** Posteroanterior **(A)** and lateral **(B)** chest radiographs demonstrate a bulky anterior mediastinal mass. Note the "filling in" of the retrosternal space on the lateral view. **C:** Enhanced transaxial CT at the level of the ascending aorta *(A)* shows the bulky, conglomerate, anterior mediastinal mass with decreased central attenuation due to necrosis. *R,* right pulmonary artery; *a,* descending thoracic aorta. **D:** CT section at the level of the cardiac apex. Note the enlarged, discrete cardiophrenic lymph nodes *(n)* and the small right pleural effusion *(p)*. *RV,* right ventricle; *LV,* left ventricle.

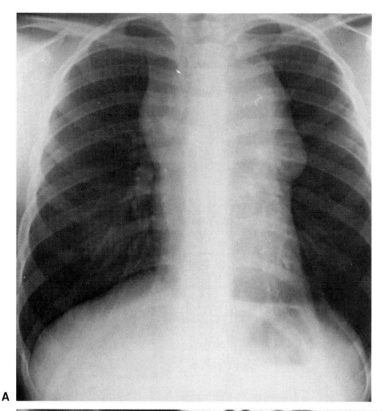

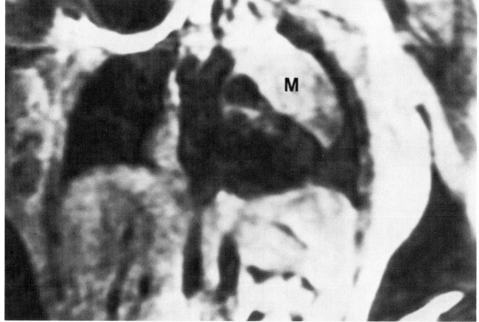

FIG. 7-160. T cell-leukemia. A 13-year-old boy with a palpable left neck mass. **A:** A posteroanterior chest radiograph shows a lobular anterior mediastinal mass. **B:** Coronal, T1-weighted MRI demonstrates a high-signal-intensity mass *(M)* involving the thymus. The signal intensity of normal thymus on T1-weighted images should be slightly greater than skeletal muscle. Note the similarity in imaging between this case and childhood non-Hodgkin's lymphoma (see Fig. 7-159).

Middle Mediastinum

The middle mediastinum contains the posterior part of the heart, the aortic arch and origins of the brachiocephalic vessels, the pulmonary arteries, the trachea, the major bronchi, lymph nodes, the right and left vagus nerves, the venae cavae, the azygos vein, and the esophagus (43). Approximately 30% of pediatric mediastinal tumors arise in this

compartment (43,320). Although the diagnostic considerations are extensive (Table 7-19), the primary differential diagnosis is remembered by the letters AB. Masses usually arise from lymph nodes (A, adenopathy) or primitive foregut (B, bronchopulmonary foregut malformation). Common abnormalities include infectious adenopathy (bacterial or granulomatous), neoplastic adenopathy (lymphoma/leukemia, metastatic), and bronchopulmonary foregut malformations

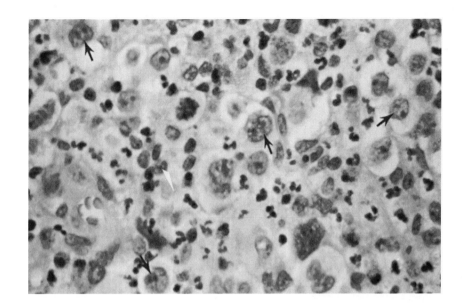

FIG. 7-161. Histologic appearance of Hodgkin's disease. Numerous Reed-Sternberg cells *(arrows)* are surrounded by reactive stromal cells.

(bronchogenic cyst, neurenteric cyst, enteric duplication cyst, sequestration) (43,320). Other mediastinal cystic lesions include pericardial cysts (usually located near a cardiophrenic angle), hiatal hernias, cystic degenerations of a hematoma or neoplasm, and parasitic infection; the last is rare.

The esophagus is the "road map" of the middle mediastinum and is an important anatomic landmark. Occasionally, a mediastinal mass is esophageal in origin (e.g., hiatus hernia) and the esophagogram is diagnostic (Fig. 7-163).

Adenopathy. Adenopathy may be paratracheal, tracheobronchial, or bronchopulmonary and may compress an adjacent airway. Node enlargement is usually due to malignant or inflammatory disease. Middle mediastinal lymph nodes are frequently involved by lymphoma; however, the center of the adenopathy is usually more anterior. Wilms tumor and osteogenic sarcoma may metastasize to lymph nodes and produce a middle mediastinal mass.

Inflammatory adenopathy is usually bacterial or granulomatous. Parenchymal consolidation and secondary adenopathy may occur in bacterial pneumonia (especially pneumococcal, staphylococcal, and *Hemophilus* pneumonia) and in primary tuberculosis. Occasionally, tuberculosis causes a unilateral nodal mass without detectable parenchymal disease. Histoplasmosis is a frequent cause of granulomatous middle mediastinal adenopathy (Fig. 7-164).

The CT features of mediastinal adenopathy may lead to the diagnosis. Low-attenuation nodes are typically seen with necrosis in the setting of aggressive neoplasia. Tuberculosis (TB), fungal disease, and lymphoma should also be considered. Markedly enhancing nodes may be seen with metastases (for example, from thyroid carcinoma, neurofibrosarcoma, melanoma, or leiomyosarcoma), Castleman disease, angioimmunoblastic lymphadenopathy, and sarcoidosis. Calcified nodes may be seen with TB, fungal infection and sarcoidosis. Metastatic mucinous adenocarcinoma, osteosarcoma, and chondrosarcoma may calcify.

Bronchopulmonary Foregut Malformations. Bronchopulmonary foregut malformations include intralobar and extralobar sequestrations, pulmonary sequestrations with partial or complete enteric communications, congenital esophageal or gastric diverticula, communicating and noncommunicating esophageal duplication, enteric cysts, neurenteric cysts, and bronchogenic (respiratory) cysts (134). Malformations during the critical period of foregut embryogenesis may cause either enteric or bronchogenic malformations. This etiologic hypothesis allows a number of congenital thoracic anomalies all to be considered bronchopulmonary foregut malformations (134). Sequestrations have been discussed earlier in this chapter.

Bronchogenic cysts. Foregut cysts (enteric, bronchogenic) are sharply marginated, homogeneous, water density masses. They rarely contain air but occasionally have peripheral linear calcifications. These foregut cysts are usually single and are round or oval. Bronchogenic cysts may be in the middle mediastinum (see Figs. 7-60 and 7-165) or pulmonary parenchyma; they tend to be less than three posterior rib interspaces in diameter (341). Depending on the content of the fluid in the mass, bronchogenic cysts are hypo-, iso-, or hyperdense on CT (140). However, contrast-enhanced CT shows a wall that enhances more than the cyst content. MRI confirms not only the location of the mass in the middle mediastinum but also its fluid content (Fig. 7-165). Enteric cysts tend to be larger than bronchogenic cysts and are located in the middle or posterior mediastinum. Both bronchogenic and enteric cysts are more common on the right than on the left.

Neurenteric cysts. Neurenteric cysts (see also Chapter 4) cause posterior mediastinal masses in association with vertebral anomalies (130). They cannot be histologically distinguished from other enteric cysts. Neurenteric cysts are due to incomplete or delayed obliteration of the primitive neurenteric canal, a connection from the yolk sac to the amniotic

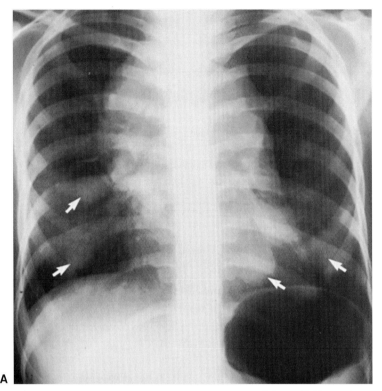

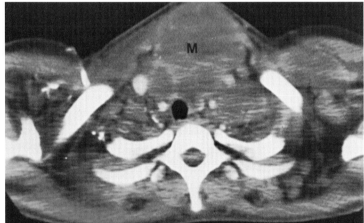

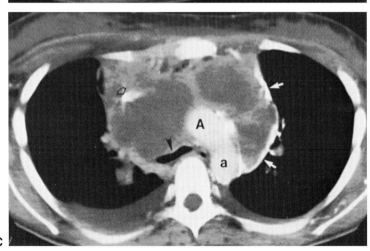

FIG. 7-162. Nodular sclerosing Hodgkin's disease. A 16-year-old girl with shortness of breath and superior vena cava syndrome. **A:** A posteroanterior chest radiograph shows a large, lobulated mediastinal mass (*arrows*) that extends above the thoracic inlet (cervicothoracic sign). Note the many patchy parenchymal opacities, presumably representing parenchymal Hodgkin's disease. **B:** Enhanced CT at the level of the thoracic inlet demonstrates a bulky prevascular cervicothoracic mass *(M)* that displaces the trachea posteriorly. **C:** A CT section at the level of the transverse aorta shows a large lobular mediastinal mass and bilateral pleural effusions. A catheter *(open arrow)* is in the partially occluded superior vena cava. Numerous pericardial venous collaterals are apparent *(arrows)*. There is marked extrinsic compression of the trachea *(arrowhead)*. *A*, ascending aorta; *a*, descending aorta.

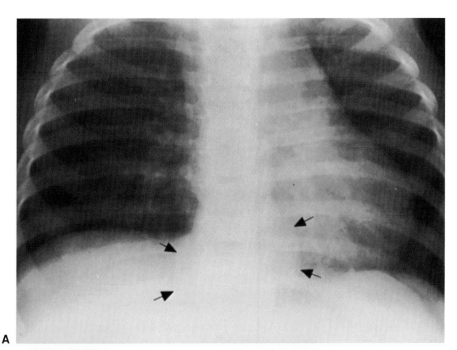

A

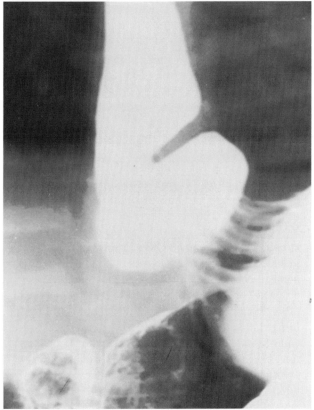

B

FIG. 7-163. Hiatus hernia. A: Bilateral paraspinal masses *(arrows).* **B:** Esophagogram demonstrates large, sliding hiatus hernia. From Kirks et al. (43).

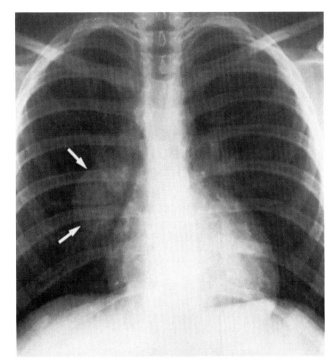

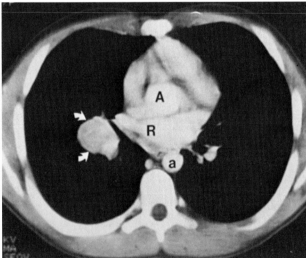

FIG. 7-164. Mediastinal histoplasmosis. This 14-year-old girl was referred because of an abnormality on a routine chest radiograph. **A:** A posteroanterior chest radiograph shows a right hilar mass *(arrows)*. The lateral view confirmed the mass. **B:** Enhanced CT at the level of the right pulmonary artery demonstrates an avascular mass *(curved arrows)* due to enlarged right bronchopulmonary lymph nodes. *A*, ascending aorta; *a*, descending aorta; *R*, right pulmonary artery.

cavity. There may also be cord anomalies, including syringohydromyelia, tethering of the cord, a patent fistulous tract to the cyst, or an intradural cyst containing enteric mucosa. The vertebral anomalies vary from scoliosis, anterior spina bifida, hemivertebra, posterior spina bifida, and fusion of vertebrae to an actual bony cleft through a vertebra. The vertebral anomalies may be at the same level as the cyst or,

more commonly, cranial to the cyst in the cervical or upper thoracic spine. MRI is the method of choice for evaluating the thoracic and spinal contents of neurenteric cysts.

Enteric cysts. Enteric cysts may contain gastric mucosa. These gastrogenic cysts usually appear early in life, as acid and pepsin secretions of the cyst may rupture into the tracheobronchial tree causing hemoptysis. A large posterior or middle mediastinal mass, usually on the right side, is noted radiologically. There may be associated pleural effusions and parenchymal opacity due to aspiration of acid contents of the cyst. There may be associated spinal anomalies. The mediastinal uptake of technetium (^{99m}Tc) pertechnetate is strong confirmatory evidence that the enteric cyst contains gastric mucosa (139). These intrathoracic gastrogenic cysts are potentially life threatening and should be resected.

Posterior Mediastinum

The posterior mediastinum contains the thoracic duct, the descending thoracic aorta, the azygos and hemiazygos veins (but not the azygous arch), the anterior and lateral surface of the spinal column, nerve roots, and the paravertebral sympathetic chain (43). Approximately 40% of pediatric mediastinal tumors arise in this compartment (43,320,321); neurogenic tumors account for 95% of them. The primary differential diagnostic considerations are all tumors of sympathetic ganglion origin: neuroblastoma, ganglioneuroblastoma, and ganglioneuroma (Table 7-19).

Neurogenic tumors are the most common mediastinal masses of childhood. Neuroblastoma is much more frequent than ganglioneuroblastoma or ganglioneuroma and usually occurs in children <2 years of age (318,342). Ten percent to 15% of neuroblastomas occur in the thorax. Although neuroblastoma is highly malignant, it generally has a favorable prognosis when diagnosed before 1 year of age, particularly in the mediastinum. Other factors that affect prognosis include stage of disease, DNA index, and N-myc gene copy number. N-myc amplification and diploidy are unfavorable prognostic indicators. Ganglioneuroblastoma is more highly differentiated and has histologic features of both ganglioneuroma and neuroblastoma. It has a good prognosis even in children older than 1 year (318). Ganglioneuroma is a mature, benign tumor that occurs in older children and has an excellent prognosis. Much rarer than these ganglion series tumors are tumors of nerve sheath origin (schwannoma and neurofibroma) and paragangliomas (342).

Neuroblastoma and its more highly differentiated forms, ganglioneuroblastoma and ganglioneuroma, arise from primitive sympathetic neuroblasts of the embryonic neural crest. The small, round cells of neuroblastoma may be difficult to differentiate from those of Ewing sarcoma, rhabdomyosarcoma, leukemia, and lymphoma; however, neuroblastoma is the only one that commonly forms tumor rosettes in bone marrow (318). Neuroblastomas are composed entirely of undifferentiated sympathoblasts. The tumor is usually well

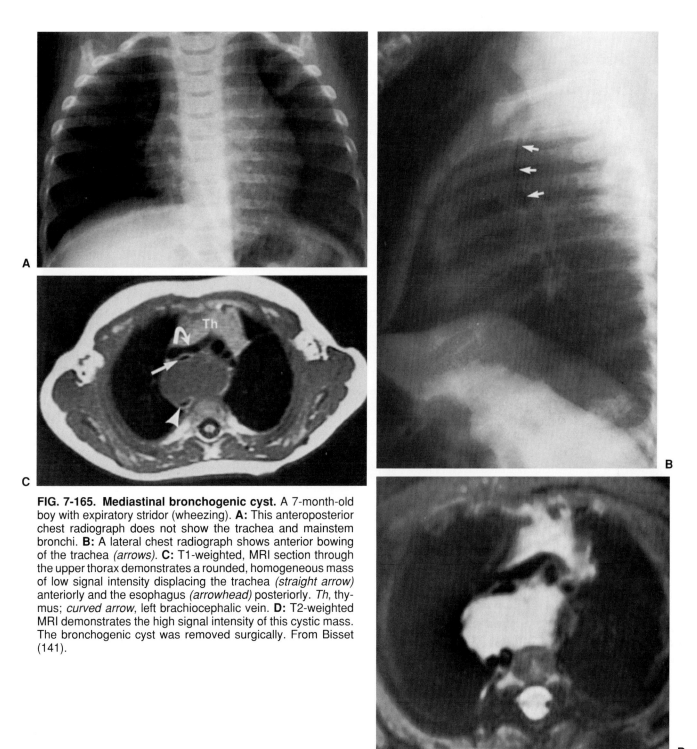

FIG. 7-165. Mediastinal bronchogenic cyst. A 7-month-old boy with expiratory stridor (wheezing). **A:** This anteroposterior chest radiograph does not show the trachea and mainstem bronchi. **B:** A lateral chest radiograph shows anterior bowing of the trachea *(arrows)*. **C:** T1-weighted, MRI section through the upper thorax demonstrates a rounded, homogeneous mass of low signal intensity displacing the trachea *(straight arrow)* anteriorly and the esophagus *(arrowhead)* posteriorly. *Th*, thymus; *curved arrow*, left brachiocephalic vein. **D:** T2-weighted MRI demonstrates the high signal intensity of this cystic mass. The bronchogenic cyst was removed surgically. From Bisset (141).

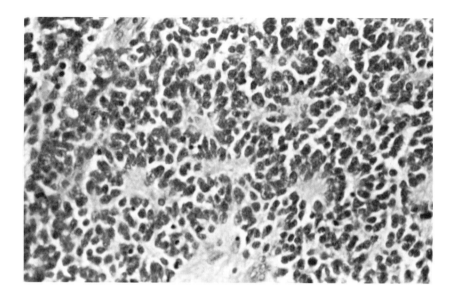

FIG. 7-166. Histologic appearance of neuroblastoma. The neoplasm consists of small, round, dark-staining cells that form tumor rosettes. From Bousvaros et al. (318).

demarcated and may contain gross or microscopic calcification, but it lacks capsular structures. At histologic examination, there are nests of primitive round cells with dark-staining nuclei and scanty cytoplasm that form tumor rosettes (Fig. 7-166). Ganglioneuroblastoma is a less malignant tumor containing undifferentiated neuroblasts and mature ganglion cells. The tumor may be partially or totally encapsulated and frequently contains granular calcification. Ganglioneuroma is a benign tumor, is well circumscribed and encapsulated, and often contains gross flecks of calcium (Fig. 7-167).. The tumor is composed of mature ganglion cells, abundant cytoplasm, and axonal structures. Ganglioneuroblastoma and ganglioneuroma tend to occur in older children rather than infants. Neuroblastoma occasionally modifies itself spontaneously into one of the more mature tumors.

Neuroblastoma is usually silent until it invades or compresses adjacent structures, metastasizes to distant sites, or produces unusual paraneoplastic syndromes. Its nonspecific symptoms and signs include fever, irritability, weight loss, and anemia. Ten percent to 15% of neuroblastomas and 43% of ganglioneuromas are thoracic, arising in the sympathetic ganglia of the posterior mediastinum.

Neuroblastoma, particularly when thoracic in location, is notorious for dumbbell extradural tumor extension, causing spinal cord compression, paraplegia, extremity weakness, alteration in bowel or bladder function, or radicular pain (Fig. 7-168). In a small child, Horner syndrome and heterochromia of the iris are highly suggestive of cervical or apical thoracic neuroblastoma (318,343). In approximately half of children with myoclonic encephalopathy of infancy (opsoclonus-myoclonus syndrome) due to neuroblastoma, the tumors are in the posterior mediastinum (318). Chest radiographs show nearly all thoracic neuroblastomas. These tumors are almost always located in the posterior mediastinum; about a quarter contain radiographically visible calcification. There may be erosion of ribs or enlargement of intervertebral foramina, particularly the former. Subtle calcifications may

be identified with CT, confirming the neurogenic nature of the tumor (Fig. 7-168) Additionally, pulmonary parenchymal metastases, although rare, are accurately shown by CT.

CT and MRI have become the imaging modalities of choice for evaluating pediatric neuroblastoma (318). Cross-sectional imaging (CT or MRI) is critical for the confirmation, localization, and staging of neuroblastoma, whether the tumor is thoracic, abdominal, pelvic, cervical, or intracranial.

The frequency of extradural extension in neuroblastoma makes MRI particularly helpful (Fig. 7-169). MRI enables assessment of intraspinal involvement without intrathecal contrast (141,344). Multiplanar imaging allows the longitudinal extent along the spine to be shown. The high lipid and water content of these tumors tend to create high signal on T1- and T2-weighted images. Any patient with suspected or confirmed neuroblastoma should undergo CT or MRI and bone scintigraphy for staging. These modalities in conjunction with clinical data and the results of bone marrow aspiration permit accurate staging of at least 95% of patients by the Evans system (51,318).

Children with extensive extradural extension of neurogenic tumors often undergo irradiation, chemotherapy, or decompressive laminectomy before definitive removal of the posterior mediastinal mass. This prevents neurologic morbidity due to cord compression by hemorrage during removal of the mediastinal mass (43,141).

Overall survival for all stages of neuroblastoma is 72% if the patient is less than 1 year of age; 28% for patients aged 1–2 years; and 12% for patients older than 2 years (318). Patients with thoracic neuroblastomas have an overall 61% survival rate, compared with a 20% survival for patients with abdominal tumors. The better prognosis for patients with thoracic lesions may be due to discovery of the tumor at an earlier stage (318). In summary, the prognosis in patients with neuroblastoma is related to age, stage, and location: younger age at diagnosis, better prognosis; higher stage of disease, worse prognosis; thoracic location of neuroblastoma, better prognosis.

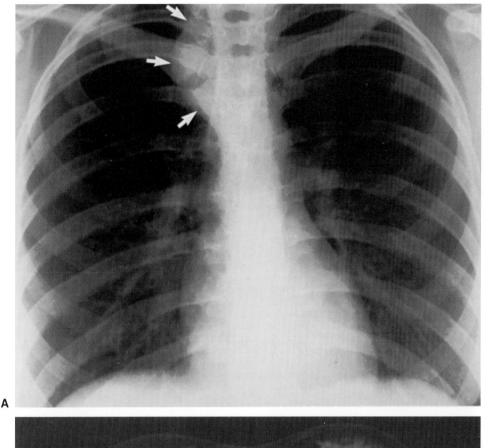

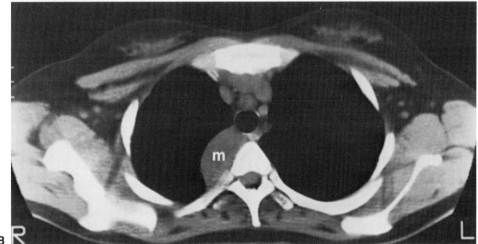

FIG. 7-167. Ganglioneuroma. A: Chest radiograph of this 16-year-old girl obtained after mild chest trauma shows a smooth right paraspinous mass *(arrows)*. The superior extent of the mass extends above the thoracic inlet and has sharply defined margins. **B:** Enhanced CT at the level of the lung apices demonstrates a nonvascular, oval, posterior mediastinal mass *(m)*.

Vascular Mediastinal Masses

Aneurysms, though rare in children, must be considered in the differential diagnosis of a mediastinal mass, particularly when it cannot be separated from the aorta, main pulmonary artery, or right or left pulmonary artery. Aneurysms can present in any of the three mediastinal compartments (43,320).

Lung Tumors

Lung tumors in infants and children may involve the pleura or parenchyma (Table 7-20). Metastatic lesions are, by far, the most common lung tumors in children. In contrast to the adult, primary malignant pulmonary tumors are rare in children (43,46).

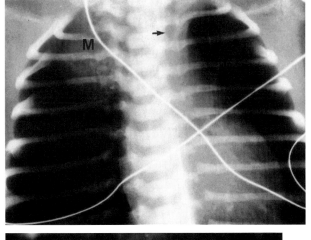

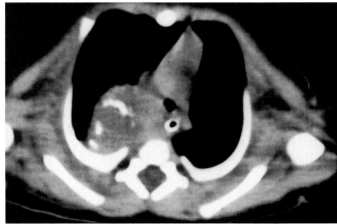

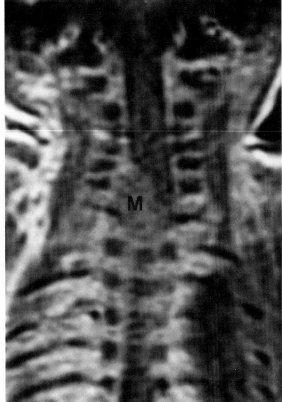

FIG. 7-168. Apical neuroblastoma. Term newborn with respiratory distress. **A:** An AP chest radiograph shows a right upper thoracic apical mediastinal mass *(M)* with leftward tracheal deviation *(arrow)*. **B:** CT shows a partially calcified posterior mediastinal mass. Note the tracheal and esophageal displacement. **C:** A coronal T1-weighted MR image shows a mass *(M)* with extradural extension. The spinal cord is displaced to the left.

Most primary parenchymal tumors in children are benign. In fact, the most common primary lung tumor in the child is not a neoplasm but an inflammatory pseudotumor (345–348). Approximately two thirds of pediatric pulmonary tumors are either inflammatory pseudotumors or bronchial adenomas (349,350). Primary pediatric pulmonary neoplasms include epithelial tumors (bronchial carcinoid, cylindroma, mucoepidermoid, bronchogenic carcinoma), pleuropulmonary blastoma, Askin tumor (PNET), teratoma, rhabdomyosarcoma, fibrous lesions (fibroma, fibromatosis, fibrosarcoma), neurogenic tumors, chondroid tumors, and vascular lesions. Primary sarcomas of the lung, though rare, are 10 times as frequent as bronchogenic carcinoma (Table 7-20) (137).

Parenchymal Bronchogenic Cyst

Bronchogenic cysts are congenital lesions formed by abnormal budding of the tracheobronchial primordium. It is assumed that intrapulmonary bronchogenic cysts are due to abnormal branching late in lung development, in contrast to mediastinal bronchogenic cysts, which are due to an earlier branching abnormality. These lesions are often asymptomatic but become clinically apparent when there is respiratory distress or superimposed infection. The hilar or subcarinal location of many mediastinal bronchogenic cysts has been stressed (135). However, parenchymal bronchogenic cysts are as common as mediastinal lesions (351). They appear as well-defined masses, without calcification. They are round

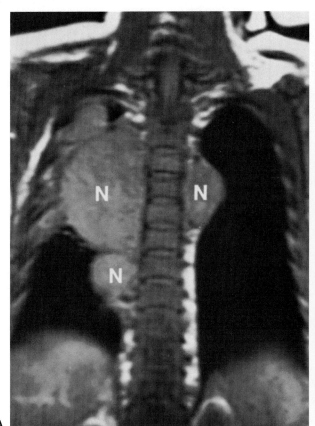 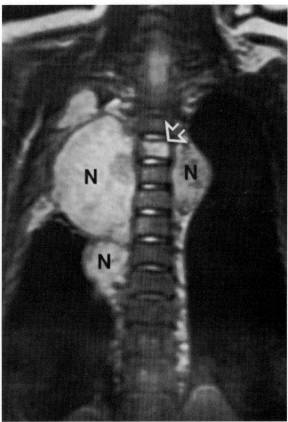

FIG. 7-169. Recurrent thoracic neuroblastoma. A, B: Coronal, proton density–weighted **(A)** and T2-weighted **(B)** MR sections through the thoracic spine of a 6-month-old girl who had previously undergone resection of stage I thoracic neuroblastoma. There are bilateral lobular paravertebral masses representing recurrent neuroblastoma *(N)*. Moreover, high signal intensity within one of the midthoracic vertebral bodies *(arrow)* indicates vertebral metastatic disease. Bone marrow aspirate confirmed stage IV disease. *(continued)*

or oval and may be large (see Fig. 7-61) (351). If communication with the airway develops because of instrumentation or superimposed infection, an air-fluid level may develop in the cyst (see Fig. 7-61C).

Cystic Mesenchymal Hamartoma

Cystic lung lesions are relatively common in children. Every attempt should be made to determine if a pediatric lung cyst developed prenatally or was acquired after birth, usually as a consequence of some other illness. Cysts that arise prenatally are defined in terms of position, histologic characteristics, and associated lesions. These include parenchymal bronchogenic cyst, congenital cystic adenomatoid malformations, complicated bronchopulmonary sequestrations, and cystic mesenchymal hamartomas. The last is radiographically benign but has neoplastic potential (Fig. 7-170) (138,352). A lung cyst may antedate the appearance of an aggressive lung tumor, such as a sarcoma. Therefore, the lung cyst that cannot be defined as acquired (pneumatoceles, posttraumatic cysts, post-BPD cysts) should be assumed to be developmental and elective resection should be planned (138,352).

Inflammatory Pulmonary Pseudotumor

Other terms such as plasma cell granuloma, xanthogranuloma, and fibrous xanthoma have been used to describe this reactive myofibroblastic inflammatory process seen in children (346). It accounts for about half of the benign lung tumors of childhood. This lesion is usually clinically silent. Radiographs typically show a variably sized rounded or lobulated pulmonary parenchymal mass. Many of these lesions are >4 cm in diameter when detected (346,347). Calcification is common; unlike the central calcification in a large granuloma or the popcorn calcification of a pulmonary hamartoma, the calcification of inflammatory pulmonary pseudotumor is often amorphous and scattered (Fig. 7-171) (345,348). At times, although histologically benign, this lesion may grow aggressively.

Bronchial Adenoma

Bronchial adenomas arise from the duct epithelium of bronchial mucous glands. The carcinoid type is far more common than the salivary gland type and is the most

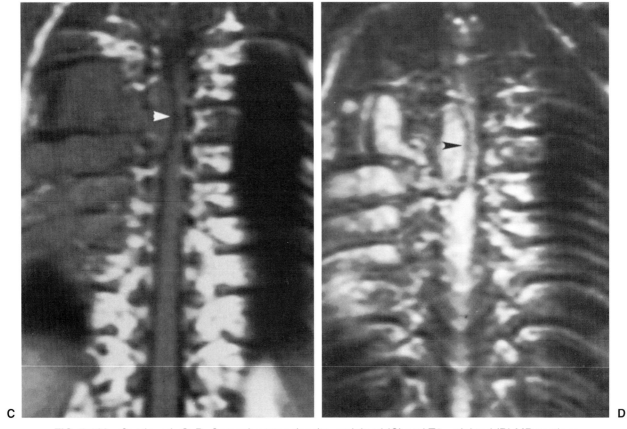

FIG. 7-169. *Continued.* **C, D:** Coronal, proton density–weighted **(C)** and T2-weighted **(D)** MR sections through the spinal canal demonstrate an extradural tumor extension *(arrowheads)* that obliterates the subarachnoid space and displaces the spinal cord to the left. From Bisset (141).

common bronchial tumor in children (353). Approximately 80% of bronchial adenomas are located in major bronchi (43). Affected children usually have cough, fever, wheezing, recurrent pneumonia, hemoptysis, or chest pain. Peripheral adenomas are usually asymptomatic. The radiologic features depend on the location of the mass. Peripheral adenomas are not associated with bronchial obstruction and have the appearance of a pulmonary nodule. Centrally located adenomas mimic foreign bodies and may cause air trapping, air leak, atelectasis, recurrent infection, abscess, or bronchiectasis. CT will suggest an intramural or intraluminal bronchial mass. Diagnosis is confirmed by bronchoscopy and biopsy. With prompt surgery, the prognosis is excellent.

Tracheal Tumors

Tracheobronchial tumors are rare in children. Tracheal papillomas, fibromas, angiomas, and cylindromas (adenoid cystic carcinomas) have been reported. These tumors often cause asthma-like wheezing and dyspnea on exertion. Radiographs may show absence of a portion of the tracheal air column (the missing segment sign), air trapping, atelec-

tasis, pneumomediastinum, or pneumothorax (see Fig. 7-136).

Pleuropulmonary Blastoma

This lesion differs in many respects from the classic pulmonary blastoma seen in adults. It has blastematous, primordial features like many of the other more familiar and more common dysontogenic neoplasms of childhood, such as Wilms tumor, hepatoblastoma, and embryonal rhabdomyosarcoma. The median age at diagnosis is 32 months (354). Chest pain, cough, and, occasionally, fever are seen. A large solid pulmonary, or less commonly pleural, mass is found on chest radiography (355,356). The mixed solid and cystic features of the lesion can be demonstrated by CT or MRI (Fig. 7-172) (354–356).

Metastatic Lung Tumors

Metastatic tumors, usually hematogenously spread, are far more common in children than primary lung tumors (137). Less commonly, metastatic neoplasms may spread to the lung through lymphatics, bronchi, or the pleural space, or

TABLE 7-20. *Lung tumors*

Pleural masses
    Metastatic[a]
    Mesothelioma
    Lymphoma—leukemia
    Askin tumor (PNET)
Parenchymal masses
    Primary
        Benign[a]
            Parenchymal bronchogenic cyst[a]
            Sequestration[a]
            Bronchial adenoma
            Round pneumonia[a]
            Inflammatory pseudo-tumor
            Hamartoma
            Hemangioma
            Cystic mesenchymal hamartoma
        Malignant
            Sarcoma[a]
            Pulmonary blastoma
            Bronchogenic carcinoma
    Secondary[a]
        Benign: papillomatosis
        Malignant[a]
            Wilms tumor[a]
            Osteogenic sarcoma[a]
            Soft-tissue sarcoma
            Rhabdomyosarcoma
            Neuroblastoma
            Teratoma
            Angiosarcoma
            Other

[a] More common lesions.
PNET, primitive neuroectodermal tumor.
Modified from Kirks et al. (43) and Sane and Girdany (137).

by direct invasion. Wilms tumor, the most common metastatic lung tumor of childhood, spreads through systemic veins with embolic seeding of the pulmonary parenchyma. Other tumors with a propensity to metastasize to the lungs include primary malignant skeletal tumors (osteosarcoma, Ewing sarcoma), soft-tissue sarcomas (rhabdomyosarcoma, fibrosarcoma), and reticulum cell sarcoma.

Metastatic disease usually causes many rounded or oval pulmonary nodules (Fig. 7-173). These variably sized nodules are usually peripheral, often subpleural. Occasionally there is a pleural effusion. A pneumothorax may develop because of metastases from a Wilms tumor or with metastatic sarcoma, such as osteogenic sarcoma, rhabdomyosarcoma, or Ewing sarcoma. CT is particularly useful in the diagnosis and follow-up of metastatic disease in children. CT may show a decrease in both size and attenuation coefficient of pulmonary metastases after chemotherapy.

Primary Malignant Lung Tumors

Unlike adults, children rarely have primary malignant lung tumors (43,46,137). A pulmonary sarcoma is usually a large, round, homogeneous mass on the chest radiograph without calcification or adenopathy. Definitive diagnosis is made by tissue biopsy.

Integrated Imaging of Pediatric Chest Masses

The chest radiograph remains the fundamental examination for evaluation of a pediatric chest mass (43). PA and lateral chest radiographs permit localization of a chest mass to the lung parenchyma, mediastinum, or chest wall. Oblique views may be necessary, especially for chest wall masses (43). However, further characterization, precise localization and demonstration of the extent of the mass, require CT or MRI (Fig. 7-174) (51).

MRI provides superior information about chest wall masses and mediastinal abnormalities (Fig. 7-174). Two limitations of MRI for mediastinal masses are its failure to detect small calcifications in a tumor and the potential for mistaking a cluster of normal-sized lymph nodes for a pathologic mass because of inferior spatial resolution. Tracheal and bronchial abnormalities are better seen with CT because of its superior spatial resolution. MRI is better for determining the relationship of a mass to vessels. MRI provides excellent visualization of flowing blood and cardiac chambers without intravenous contrast material (141). MRI has excellent soft-tissue contrast; it is particularly valuable in determining the relationship of neurogenic lesions to the vertebral canal, extradural space, and spinal cord (344).

MRI of the pediatric thorax should be performed with the use of cardiac gating. Children under 5 years of age are almost always sedated. T1-weighted images are obtained in axial, sagittal, and, frequently, coronal planes for anatomic information. Proton density and T2-weighted axial images assess the signal intensity of the mass, extent of disease, and any mass effect on contiguous structures.

Because of the long examination time, need for sedation, and expense of MRI, CT currently remains the modality of choice for evaluating anterior and middle mediastinal masses. MRI is the method of choice for evaluating posterior mediastinal masses because of their propensity for extradural extension (see Figs. 7-168 and 7-169). However, MRI is increasingly used to evaluate pediatric mediastinal masses in all compartments (141).

Pulmonary Critical Care, Chest Trauma, and Miscellaneous Pulmonary Insults

Radiography in the Critical Care Environment

The radiologist providing service to intensive care units (ICUs) must be skilled in the accurate and timely interpretation of portable chest radiographs (17,357–359). These examinations assess cardiopulmonary alterations and therapeutic effects. The ICU patient is typically on mechanical ventilation, is invasively monitored, and has indwelling cath-

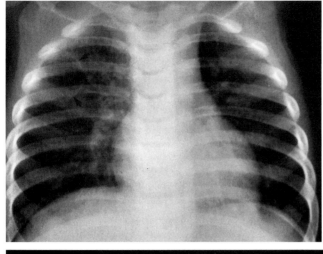

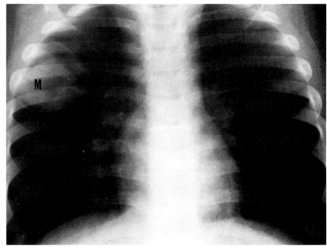

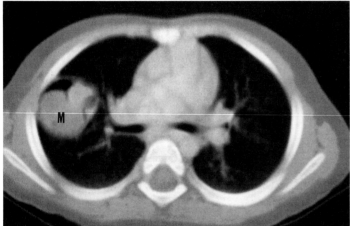

FIG. 7-170. Pulmonary rhabdomyosarcoma arising in cystic mesenchymal hamartoma. A: A chest x-ray in an 18-month-old boy with cough and fever shows a "benign" appearing right upper lobe lung cyst *(arrows)* and features of viral airways disease. **B:** A chest x-ray at 24 months of age shows a water-density mass *(M)* within the cavity. **C:** CT demonstrates a variably enhancing lobular mass *(M)* within the cystic lung lesion. Histologic examination showed a rhabdomyosarcoma within a cystic mesenchymal hamartoma. From Hedlund et al. (138).

eters. The presence of these support measures often mandates daily radiographs. The portable ICU chest radiograph leads to the decision to change vascular catheter position in as many as 20% of patients (360). The ideal position for the ET tip is just below the level of the inferomedial ends of the clavicles. If the chin is seen at the top of the chest radiograph, the neck is in flexion; this moves the ET toward the carina (198,199). Complications of ET position include selective main bronchial intubation with consequent atelectasis or pneumothorax, esophageal intubation, and tracheal rupture.

The subclavian and jugular veins are commonly used for monitoring venous pressure, medication administration, and parenteral nutrition. A clear understanding of normal vascular anatomy allows early detection of potentially life-threatening catheter complications (361). Two important radiographic signs of impending catheter perforation are (a) catheter tip position against the wall of a vessel or heart chamber; and (b) curved tip sign (change in SVC catheter shape from straight to curved), suggesting that the tip is lodged in a mural thrombus or the vessel wall (361). The tip should be placed in the SVC just above the azygous vein (361); this is the level of the pericardial reflection over the SVC.

Bedside ICU chest radiographs allow a rapid assessment of abnormal extra alveolar air collections (pneumothorax, pneumomediastinum, and pulmonary interstitial emphysema) often associated with rapid clinical deterioration (17,357,358,360). Hydrostatic (fluid overload) and increased permeability (adult respiratory distress syndrome) forms of pulmonary edema can also be assessed on ICU chest radiographs (359).

Adult Respiratory Distress Syndrome

Adult respiratory distress syndrome (ARDS) refers to acute respiratory failure after an insult that may or may not have injured the lungs directly. The syndrome is well described in adults (362,363). The same pathophysiology of increased capillary permeability, pulmonary edema, and hemorrhage leading to respiratory failure occurs in children (364,365). Some of the insults that lead to ARDS include infection, inhalation injury, aspiration, near-drowning, trauma, sepsis, and certain drugs, including salicylates and barbiturates. ARDS causes dyspnea, tachypnea, cyanosis refractory to O_2 therapy, decrease in lung compliance, and

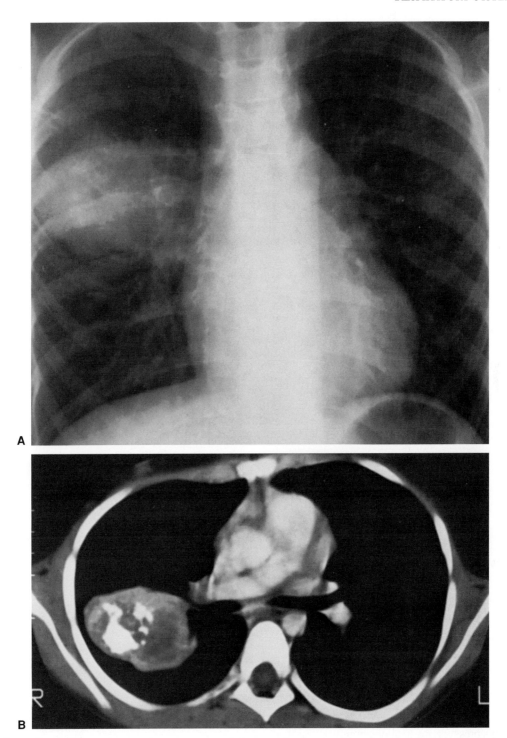

FIG. 7-171. Inflammatory pulmonary pseudotumor. An 8-year-old asymptomatic boy. **A:** A chest radiograph shows a large, well-demarcated, calcium-containing mass in the right lung. **B:** Enhanced chest CT shows a mixed-density, calcium-containing mass in the superior segment of the right lower lobe. The tumor contained many histiocytes and plasma cells.

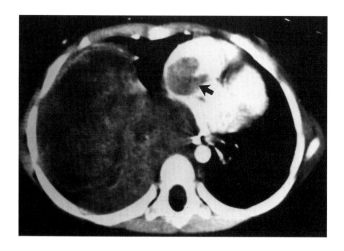

FIG. 7-172. Pleuropulmonary blastoma. This 2-year-old girl presented with respiratory distress and superior vena cava obstruction. Contrast-enhanced CT shows a bulky heterogeneous right pulmonary mass that extends into the right atrium *(arrow)*.

diffuse alveolar infiltrates. No matter what the insult, the course typically follows four stages (362). In stage I, or *acute injury,* there are no specific signs and the chest x-ray is normal, except for hyperventilation. Stage II, or the *latent period,* lasts from 6 to 48 hours after the insult. Although this represents a time of relative cardiovascular and clinical stability, there are physiologic alterations in the arterial oxy-

gen content and pulmonary vascular resistance. The chest x-ray during this phase often shows fine reticular interstitial opacities. Stage III, *acute respiratory failure,* is the stage at which the diagnosis is made. Mixed interstitial and airspace opacities are seen on chest x-rays (Fig. 7-175A). Stage IV, *severe physiologic abnormality,* indicates severe disease (which may be reversible) characterized clinically by hyper-

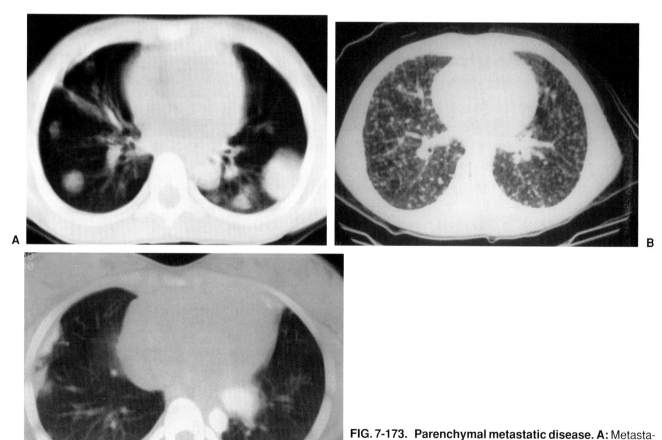

FIG. 7-173. Parenchymal metastatic disease. A: Metastases from Wilms tumor. **B:** Miliary metastases from follicular thyroid carcinoma. **C:** Multiple high density (partially calcified) metastases from osteogenic sarcoma.

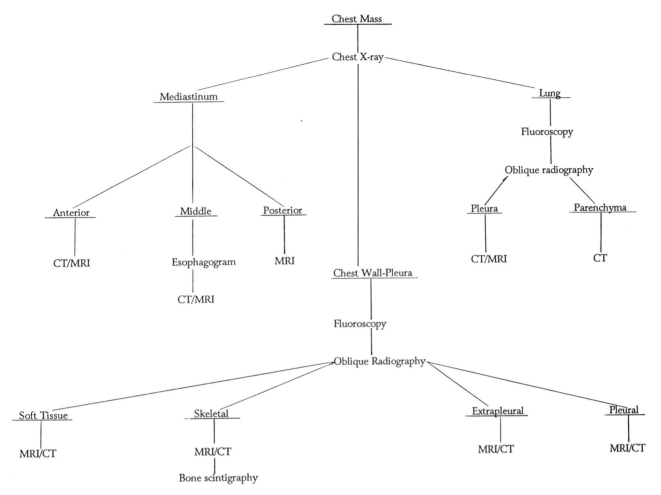

FIG. 7-174. An algorithm for imaging pediatric chest masses. *CT*, computed tomography; *MRI*, magnetic resonance imaging.

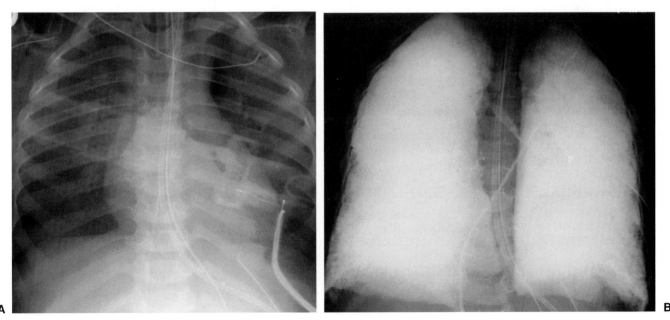

FIG. 7-175. Treatment of adult respiratory distress syndrome. This 3-year-old boy developed respiratory failure after surgery and general anesthesia. **A:** Anteroposterior chest radiography shows pulmonary edema. **B:** After failing maximal medical and ventilator support, the patient was placed on liquid ventilation (perflubron). The chest x-ray shows high-density opacity of both lungs.

capnia and radiographically by large flocculent areas of consolidation. Respiratory support may be necessary for weeks to months (365). In neonates, infants, and some young children, liquid ventilation with perflubron (Fig. 7-175B) may allow salvage when other forms of therapy have failed (366).

Chest Trauma

Radiologic findings in children after chest trauma, penetrating or blunt, are similar to those in adults. The initial clinical, laboratory, and radiologic findings may greatly underestimate the true severity of the injury. Rib fractures, sternal fractures, pulmonary lacerations, pulmonary contusions, pulmonary hematomas, traumatic pneumatoceles, bronchial fractures, tracheal tears, pericardial effusions, myocardial contusions, aortic disruptions, and traumatic pseudoaneurysms all occur (15,367–373). The first chest radiograph should be carefully assessed for spine fractures and for clues to other injuries; a rib fracture suggests splenic or hepatic injury, while hemidiaphragm indistinctness suggests diaphragmatic rupture. Pulmonary *contusions* produce homogeneous or nodular parenchymal opacities, often unsharp, which usually become larger and denser during the first 24–48 hours after injury (Fig. 7-176). A pulmonary contusion may eventually contract into a mass-like lesion (15). Pulmonary *hematomas* produce round or oval opacities on the initial chest radiograph. These opacities are slow to resolve and may cavitate during their resolution. *Traumatic pneumatoceles* after blunt chest trauma may be pulmonary or mediastinal (368,372). They usually occur with other manifestations of pulmonary injury and develop within minutes or hours of the injury. They are thin-walled and may enlarge rapidly. When mediastinal, the air collections are usually elongated and paraspinal or paracardiac in location, often lying in or beneath an inferior pulmonary ligament (368,374,375). Traumatic pneumatoceles slowly become smaller and disappear after 2–3 weeks (368). *Bronchial and tracheal fractures* may cause massive persistent atelectasis or air leak following blunt chest trauma (Fig. 7-177) (373,376,377). *Aortic laceration* causes superior mediastinal widening, rightward tracheal or esophageal displacement, caudal displacement of the left main bronchus, widening of the soft-tissue shadows along the spine and aorta, a left hemothorax, and pleural fluid (blood) over the apex of the left lung (Fig. 7-178) (370). Any of these signs suggests mediastinal hematoma; immediate aortography should be considered. CT has been used to evaluate blunt chest trauma in children (369); thoracic aortography is indicated if CT shows an abnormality of the aorta or evidence of a mediastinal hematoma.

Penetrating injuries to the chest, heart, and great vessels produce findings similar to those seen with blunt chest trauma. In addition, there may be air within the pleural space, heart, mediastinum, or great vessels. A metallic foreign body may be seen in the heart, mediastinum, lungs, or spine. De-

layed complications such as tears of the heart or a great vessel, and hemopericardium are infrequent.

Lower Airway Foreign Bodies

Airway foreign bodies are a common, serious clinical problem in children. Small infants may ingest almost anything, and foreign body aspiration occurs commonly (8,16,378). An airway foreign body is suspected clinically if there is a history of possible aspiration followed by cough, wheezing, respiratory distress or decreased breath sounds. However, these symptoms may quickly subside. There may be no available history of aspiration, the patients presenting with "cough and fever—rule out pneumonia" or wheezing. If wheezing develops in the absence of a known pulmonary disease such as asthma, foreign body or some other obstructive lesion such as a vascular ring should be strongly considered (378). An airway foreign body is always a lurking possiblilty in a child <3 years of age with clinically or radiologically suspected pneumonia (16); expiration radiographs are critical for diagnosis (Fig. 7-179). If a pneumonia fails to clear within the usual time (10–14 days), further investigation for possible foreign body aspiration should be considered.

The age range of children with airway foreign bodies is 9 months to 16 years; the peak age is 1–2 years (378). Airway foreign bodies are more common on the right (55%) than the left (33%). Fortunately, only 7% are bilateral, and 5% are in the trachea (Fig. 7-180) (378). No more than 10% of foreign bodies are radiopaque (Fig. 7-181) (378). Most foreign bodies are vegetable material (84%). Peanuts are the most common offenders (16). Other common foreign bodies include sunflower seeds, meat, eggshells, metal pins, and plastic toys. Because metallic foriegn bodies cause little reaction, radiologic evaluation and diagnosis may be delayed for several months.

The radiologic findings of tracheal or bronchial foreign bodies include hyperinflation, air trapping, regional oligemia, atelectasis, consolidation, pleural fluid, pneumomediastinum, pneumothorax, and bronchiectasis. The cross-sectional area of the bronchi increases with inspiration and decreases with expiration (see Fig. 7-179). A small foreign body (e.g., a sunflower seed) may cause no obstruction to air flow during either inspiration or expiration. Fortunately, a foreign body of this type is found in fewer than 1% of cases (378). If a bronchus is completely obstructed, there is distal consolidation or atelectasis (Fig. 7-181); this occurs with approximately 20% of all lower airway foreign bodies (16). Usually, there is a medium-sized foreign body (for example, a peanut) with mild bronchial mucosal reaction; the airway is unobstructed or partially obstructed during inspiration but completely obstructed during expiration due to the normal expiratory decrease in bronchial diameter (see Fig. 7-179). Inspiratory chest radiographs are normal in approximately 20%–30% of patients with bronchial foreign

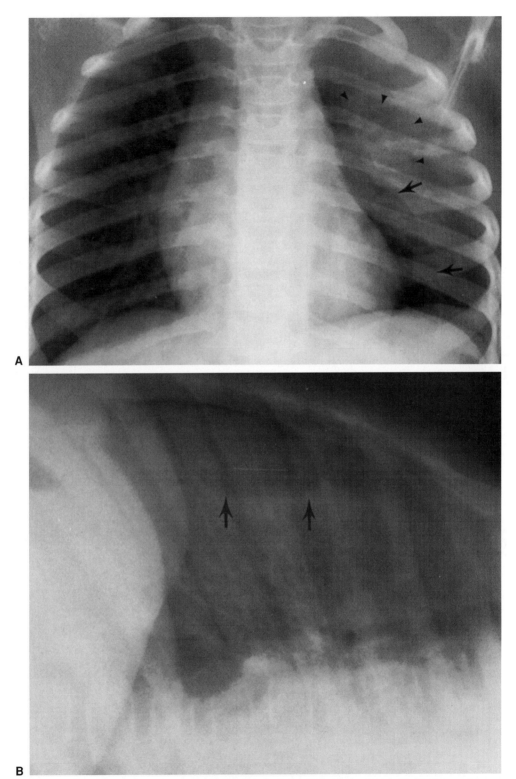

FIG. 7-176. Lung contusion and anteromedial pneumothorax. A 2-year-old boy after blunt chest trauma. **A:** An anteroposterior chest radiograph suggests a left medial pneumothorax *(arrows)*. Note the patchy opacity in the left upper lobe presumed to be a contusion *(arrowheads)*. **B:** A supine cross table lateral view confirms retrosternal intrapleural air *(arrows)*. From Hedlund and Kirks (16).

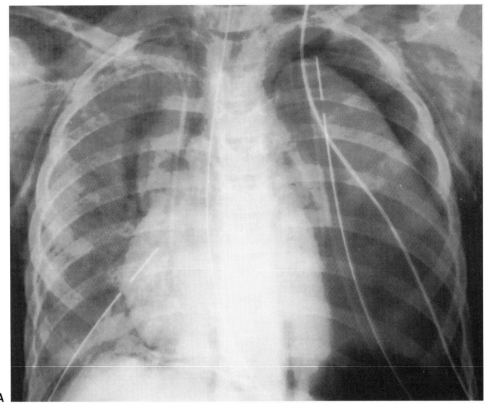

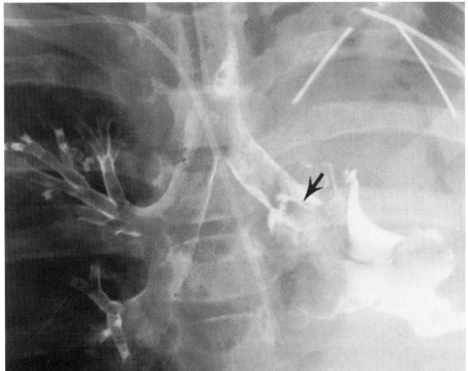

FIG. 7-177. Bronchial fracture. A 10-year-old boy who sustained severe blunt chest trauma. **A:** A chest radiograph shows a large, persistent left pneumothorax despite 24 hours of chest tube drainage. Note the pneumomediastinum, massive subcutaneous air, and pulmonary contusion. **B:** A bronchogram confirmed a fracture of the left mainstem bronchus *(arrow)*. From Hedlund and Kirks (16).

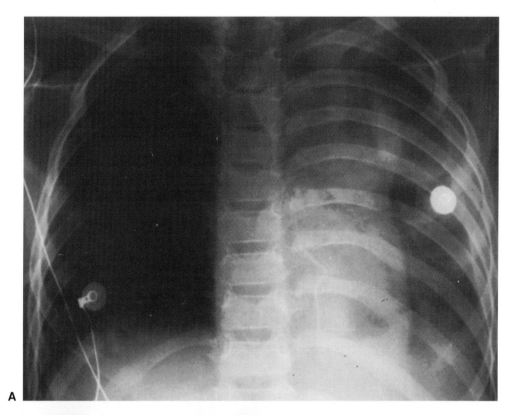

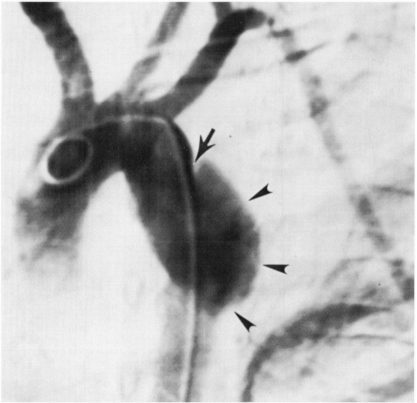

FIG. 7-178. Mediastinal hematoma secondary to aortic transection. An 8-year-old boy with blunt chest trauma. **A:** A chest radiograph shows a widened superior mediastinum, an indistinct transverse aorta, left pleural fluid, and patchy left lung opacities due to lung contusion. **B:** An aortogram confirms the aortic transection *(arrow)* and a pseudoaneurysm *(arrowheads)*. From Hedlund and Kirks (16).

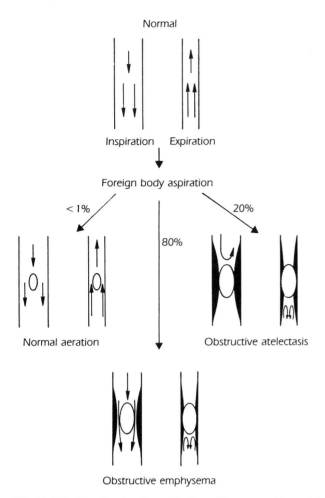

FIG. 7-179. Foreign body aspiration. The normal bronchi increase in diameter during inspiration and decrease in diameter during expiration. Foreign body aspiration may be associated with normal aeration (<1%), obstructive atelectasis (20%), or obstructive emphysema (80%).

bodies (Fig. 7-182) (16); thus, standard inspiratory chest radiographs are not sensitive to airway foreign bodies (379). Unilateral air trapping can be demonstrated by an expiration film, fluoroscopy, or decubitus views.

Because a normal inspiration chest radiograph may be seen in a child with an airway foreign body, at least one supplementary diagnostic maneuver (expiration film, fluoroscopy, decubitus films) should always be performed if the diagnosis is suspected (Fig. 7-183). If the child is cooperative, inspiration and expiration views of the chest are recommended (16). Uncooperative children require fluoroscopy or decubitus views (Fig. 7-183). Accentuation of expiration by manual compression of the upper abdomen during fluoroscopy helps to demonstrate air trapping (Fig. 7-183D) (380). The radiologist must always be alert for direct or indirect signs of air trapping. The aeration problems caused by foreign bodies can lead to pneumomediastinum (381) and pneumothorax (Fig. 7-184) (382). An air block complication in a

child <3 years of age with or without a parenchymal opacity suggests the presence of an airway foreign body (381,382).

Bronchoscopy and removal of the foreign body should be performed immediately after diagnosis. If there is a convincing history of foreign body aspiration, bronchoscopy is mandatory regardless of the radiologic findings. Standard (inspiratory) PA and lateral chest radiography may be completely normal in as many as 30% of patients with endoscopically proven lower airway foreign bodies (379). CT is occasionally helpful in confirming the presence and location of a foreign body (see Fig. 7-74).

Hydrocarbon Pneumonitis

Among the substances that children ingest are hydrocarbons such as furniture polish, gasoline, kerosene, and char-

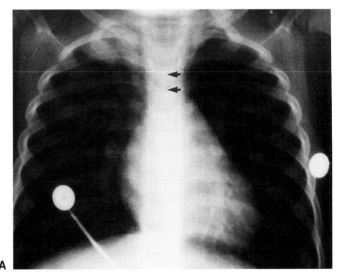

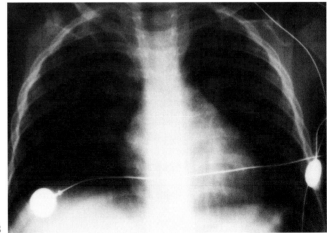

FIG. 7-180. Tracheal foreign body. A: An anteroposterior chest radiograph in an acutely symptomatic 18-month-old boy shows bilateral hyperaeration and a missing segment of the tracheal air shadow *(arrows).* **B:** Following the bronchoscopic removal of three peanuts, the entire trachea is well visualized.

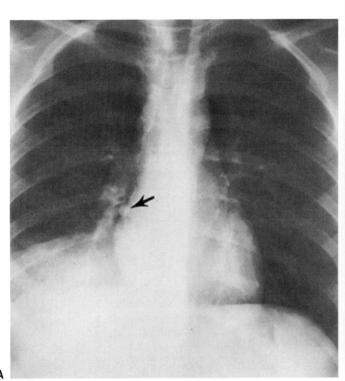
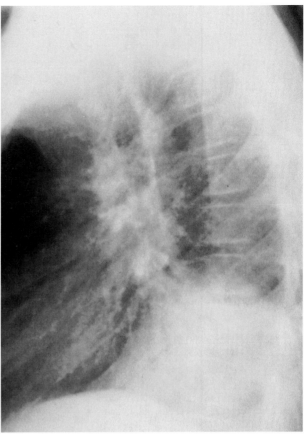

FIG. 7-181. Obstructive atelectasis secondary to an airway foreign body. A 10-year-old boy with cough and fever after surgery under general anesthesia. **A:** An anteroposterior chest radiograph shows elevation of the right hemidiaphragm and atelectasis of the right lower lobe. Note the rounded radiodensity along the right heart border *(arrow)*. **B:** A lateral view confirms marked atelectasis of the right lower lobe. At bronchoscopy, a tooth was removed from the right lower lobe bronchus. From Hedlund and Kirks (16).

coal lighter fluid. Because of the low viscosity and surface tension of these hydrocarbons, they are readily aspirated into the tracheobronchial tree. A chemical pneumonitis caused by this aspiration may develop within several hours. There is no evidence that hydrocarbon absorption from the gastrointestinal tract plays any role in the development of hydrocarbon pneumonitis (383). Hydrocarbons produce a profound chemical pneumonitis with surfactant destruction, atelectasis of alveoli, and difficulties in gas exchange. The chemical pneumonitis also produces hyperemia, bronchial and bronchiolar necrosis, peribronchial edema, small vessel thromboses, and destructive bronchopneumonia (120,384).

Radiologic changes of hydrocarbon pneumonitis may not be seen for 6–12 hours after ingestion and aspiration. If the chest radiograph is normal 24 hours after ingestion, there has not been significant hydrocarbon aspiration (16,384,385). The opacities are usually fluffy and confluent and have nodular acinar components (Fig. 7-185A). Bronchial and bronchiolar necrosis with complicating air trap-

ping may lead to pneumatocele (Fig. 7-185B) (270). Because the pneumonitis is chemical, radiologic improvement lags well behind clinical improvement. The chest radiographs may remain abnormal for several weeks or months.

Near-drowning

Near-drowning is a form of aspiration. The extent and severity of radiographic findings are related to the amount, not the type, of water ingested (386–388). The patchy parahilar acinar densities resemble pulmonary edema, but the heart is not enlarged (Fig. 7-186) (389).

If pulmonary edema is cardiac in origin, the heart is almost always large. In noncardiac pulmonary edema, the heart size is usually normal (389). Near-drowning is one of many conditions that can cause noncardiac pulmonary edema. Other causes and types of noncardiac pulmonary edema during childhood include acute glomerulonephritis, fluid overload, aspiration states (massive aspiration, hydrocarbon pneumo-

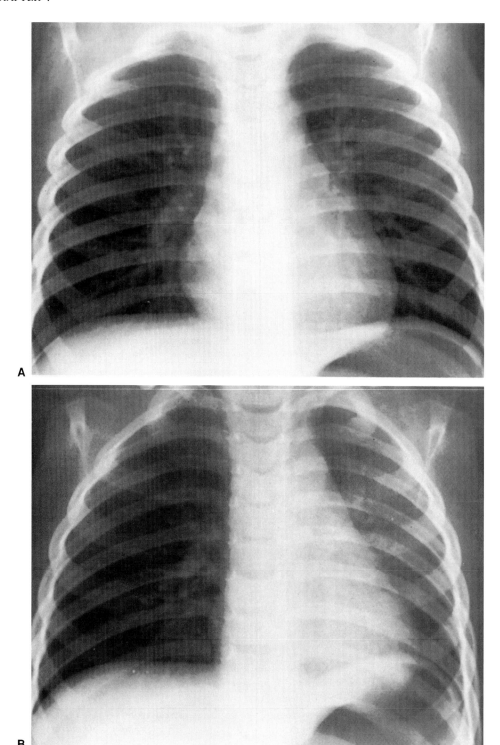

FIG. 7-182. Airway foreign body. A 2-year-old boy with cough and fever. **A:** An anteroposterior chest radiograph demonstrates symmetric lung aeration. **B:** Expiration view shows air trapping on the right. At bronchoscopy, a peanut was removed from the right main bronchus.

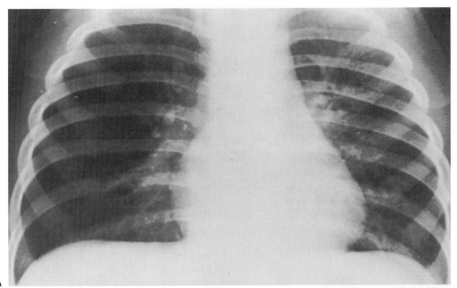

A

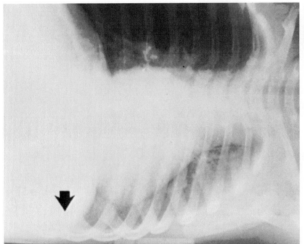

B

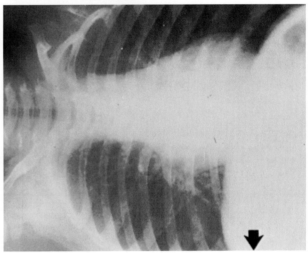

C

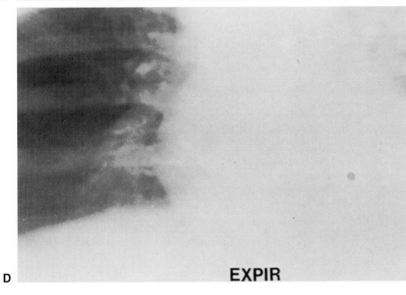

D

EXPIR

FIG. 7-183. Foreign body aspiration. A 2-year-old girl with cough and fever. **A:** An anteroposterior chest radiograph in inspiration demonstrates hyperaeration of the right lung. **B:** A left lateral decubitus view shows normal deaeration of the dependent left lung. **C:** A right lateral decubitus view demonstrates air trapping in the dependent right lung. The *arrows* in **B** and **C** indicate the dependent hemithorax. **D:** Expiration fluoroscopic spot film. Expiration was accentuated by manual abdominal compression while the child was crying (380). The air trapping in the right lung was due to the tip of a yellow crayon in the right main bronchus.

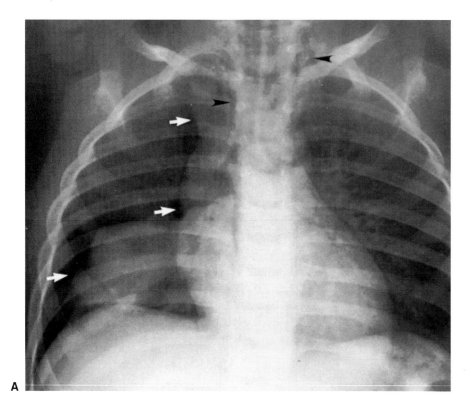

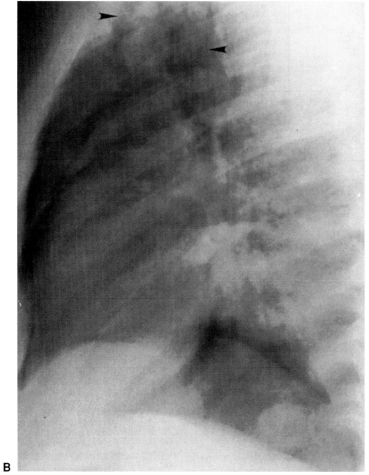

FIG. 7-184. Air block complication due to airway foreign body. A 2-year-old boy developed cough while eating candy. Anteroposterior **(A)** and lateral **(B)** chest radiographs demonstrate a pneumomediastinum *(arrowheads)* and a right pneumothorax *(arrows)*. A candy fragment was removed from the right main bronchus at bronchoscopy. From Hedlund and Kirks (16).

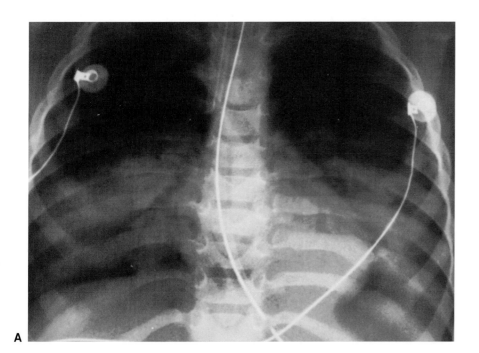

A

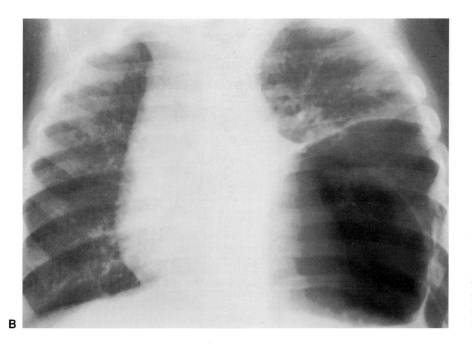

B

FIG. 7-185. Hydrocarbon aspiration. An 18-month-old girl with severe respiratory distress after aspirating furniture polish. **A:** A chest radiograph 12 hours after ingestion and aspiration shows extensive bibasilar consolidations. **B:** Two weeks later, there is a large pneumatocele in the left lower lobe. From Hedlund and Kirks (16).

nitis), inhalation injuries, neurogenic pulmonary edema, rheumatic pneumonitis, collagen vascular disease, allergic pneumonitis, and adult respiratory distress syndrome (8,9,16). With severe forms of near-drowning, neurogenic pulmonary edema accentuates the central opacities of aspiration. Moreover, the radiologic findings of "dry" near-drowning (that is, without aspiration) are identical to aspiration near-drowning but are due to hypoxia and neurogenic pulmonary edema, rather than aspiration of water into the tracheobronchial tree (16).

The chest film may remain normal in patients with severe clinical deterioration from near-drowning. Clinical assessment and serial blood gas determinations are much more important than chest radiography for following the course of the illness; there is a poor correlation between the severity of the chest radiographic abnormalities and the outcome (387). The radiologic opacities persist despite marked clinical improvement (388). The severity of the CNS hypoxia governs the outcome much more than the degree of lung damage.

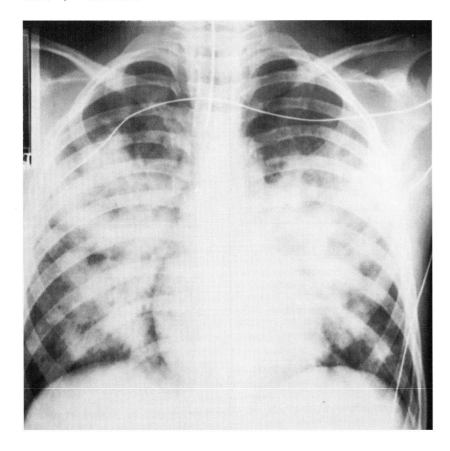

FIG. 7-186. Near-drowning. The heart of this 8-year-old boy is not enlarged. There are confluent bilateral central opacities in a "bat-wing" or "butterfly" distribution.

REFERENCES

General Information

1. Chernick V, ed. *Kendig's disorders of the respiratory tract in children.* 5th ed. Philadelphia: W.B. Saunders, 1990.
2. Felman AH. *Radiology of the pediatric chest: clinical and pathological correlations.* New York: McGraw-Hill, 1987.
3. Lefebvre J. *Clinical practice in pediatric radiology, vol. 2: The respiratory system.* New York: Masson, 1979.
4. Putman CE, ed. *Pulmonary diagnosis: imaging and other techniques.* New York: Appleton-Century-Crofts, 1981.
5. Silverman FN. Chronic lung disorders in childhood. In: Eklof O, ed. *Current concepts in pediatric radiology.* Vol. 1. New York: Springer, 1977, 13–27.
6. Singleton EB, Wagner ML, Dutton RV. *Radiologic atlas of pulmonary abnormalities in children,* 2nd ed. Philadelphia: W.B. Saunders, 1988.
7. Swischuk LE. *Imaging of the newborn, infant, and young child.* 3rd ed. Baltimore: Williams & Wilkins, 1989.
8. Swischuk LE. *Emergency imaging of the acutely ill or injured child.* 3rd ed. Baltimore: Williams & Wilkins, 1994.
9. Swischuk LE, John SD. *Differential diagnosis in pediatric radiology,* 2nd ed. Baltimore: Williams & Wilkins, 1995.
10. Wesenberg RL. *The newborn chest.* Hagerstown, MD: Harper & Row, 1973.
11. Sty JR, Wells RG, Starshak RJ, Gregg DC. *Diagnostic imaging of infants and children,* Vol 3. Gaithersburg, MD: Aspen, 1992.
12. Alford BA. Neonatal chest: conditions requiring intervention or surgery. In: Kirks DR, ed. *Emergency pediatric radiology. A problem-oriented approach.* Reston, VA: American Roentgen Ray Society, 1995, 205–209.
13. Cleveland RH. Imaging of the newborn chest: medical disease. In: Kirks DR, ed. *Emergency pediatric radiology. A problem-oriented approach.* Reston, VA: American Roentgen Ray Society, 1995, 197–203.
14. Cleveland RH. A radiologic update on medical diseases of the newborn chest. *Pediatr Radiol* 1995;25:631–637.
15. Wagner RB, Crawford WO Jr, Schimpf PP. Classification of parenchymal injuries of the lung. *Radiology* 1988;167:77–82.
16. Hedlund GL, Kirks DR. Emergency radiology of the pediatric chest. *Curr Probl Diagn Radiol* 1990;19:133–164.
17. Markowitz RI. Chest radiology in the pediatric intensive care unit. In: Kirks DR, ed. *Emergency pediatric radiology. A problem-oriented approach.* Reston, VA: American Roentgen Ray Society, 1995, 217–223.

Techniques

18. Griscom NT, Wohl MEB. Tracheal size and shape: effects of change in intraluminal pressure. *Radiology* 1983;149:27–30.
19. West JB. Respiration. In: West JB, ed. *Best and Taylor's physiological basis of medical practice.* Baltimore: Williams & Wilkins, 1990, 518–604.
20. Berdon WE, Baker DH, Bordiuk J, Mellins R. Innominate artery compression of the trachea in infants with stridor and apnea. *Radiology* 1969;92:272–278.
21. Swischuk LE, Smith PC, Fagan CJ. Abnormalities of the pharynx and larynx in childhood. *Semin Roentgenol* 1974;9:283–300.
22. Joseph PM, Berdon WE, Baker DH, et al. Upper airway obstruction in infants and small children. Improved radiographic diagnosis by combining filtration, high kilovoltage, and magnification. *Radiology* 1976;121:143–148.
23. Poznanski AK. *Practical approaches to pediatric radiology.* Chicago: Year Book, 1976.
24. Grunebaum M. Respiratory stridor—a challenge for the paediatric radiologist. *Clin Radiol* 1973;24:485–490.
25. Kirks DR, Merten DF. Stridor in infants and children due to esophageal inflammatory disease. *Gastrointest Radiol* 1980;5:321–323.
26. Kraus R, Han BK, Babcock DS, Oestreich AE. Sonography of neck masses in children. *AJR* 1986;146:609–613.

27. Effmann EL, Fram EK, Vock P, Kirks DR. Tracheal cross-sectional area in children: CT determination. *Radiology* 1983;149:137–140.

28. Griscom NT. Computed tomographic determination of tracheal dimensions in children and adolescents. *Radiology* 1982;145:361–364.

29. Griscom NT, Wohl MEB. Dimensions of the growing trachea related to age and gender. *AJR* 1986;146:233–237.

30. Griscom NT. CT measurement of the tracheal lumen in children and adolescents. *AJR* 1991;156:371–372.

31. Frey EE, Sato Y, Smith WL, Franken EA Jr. Cine CT of the mediastinum in pediatric patients. *Radiology* 1987;165:19–23.

32. Peschmann RK, Napel S, Couch JL, et al. High speed computed tomography: systems and performance. *Appl Opt* 1985;24:4052–4060.

33. Bisset GS III, Strife JL, Kirks DR, Bailey WW. Vascular rings: MR imaging. *AJR* 1987;149:251–256.

34. Fletcher BD, Dearborn DG, Mulopulos GP. MR imaging in infants with airway obstruction: preliminary observations. *Radiology* 1986;160:245–249.

35. Hedlund GL, Bisset GS III. Esophageal duplication cyst and aberrant right subclavian artery mimicking a symptomatic vascular ring. *Pediatr Radiol* 1989;19:543–544.

36. Simoneaux SF, Bank ER, Webber JB, Parks WJ. MR imaging of the pediatric airway. *RadioGraphics* 1995;15:287–298.

37. Davis LA, Davis LT. Radiographic technique and the normal infant chest. *Semin Roentgenol* 1972;7:31–38.

38. Singleton EB. Radiologic considerations of intensive care in the premature infant. *Radiology* 1981;140:291–300.

39. Aspin N. The gonadal x-ray dose to children from diagnostic radiographic technics. *Radiology* 1965;85:944–951.

40. Capitanio MA, Kirkpatrick JA. The lateral decubitus film. An aid in determining air–trapping in children. *Radiology* 1972;103:460–462.

41. Kaufman AS, Kuhns LR. The lateral decubitus view: an aid in evaluating poorly defined pulmonary densities in children. *AJR* 1977;129:885–888.

42. Eklof O, Torngren A. Pleural fluid in healthy children. *Acta Radiol* 1971;11:346–349.

43. Kirks DR, Effmann EL, Osborne D. Chest masses in infants and children: a selective overview. In: Putman CE, ed. *Pulmonary diagnosis: imaging and other techniques*. New York: Appleton-Century-Crofts, 1981, 263–287.

44. Muhm JR, Brown LR, Crowe JK, et al. Comparison of whole lung tomography and computed tomography for detecting pulmonary nodules. *AJR* 1978;131:981–984.

45. Kirks DR, Korobkin M. Chest computed tomography in infants and children. An analysis of 50 patients. *Pediatr Radiol* 1980;10:75–82.

46. Kirks DR, Korobkin M. Computed tomography of the chest wall, pleura, and pulmonary parenchyma in infants and children. *Radiol Clin North Am* 1981;19:421–429.

47. Kirks DR, Korobkin M. Computed tomography of the chest in infants and children: techniques and mediastinal evaluation. *Radiol Clin North Am* 1981;19:409–419.

48. Lynch DA, Brasch RC, Hardy KA, Webb WR. Pediatric pulmonary disease: assessment with high-resolution ultrafast CT. *Radiology* 1990;176:243–248.

49. Mayo JR, Webb WR, Gould R, et al. High-resolution CT of the lungs: an optimal approach. *Radiology* 1987;163:507–510.

50. Kao SC, Smith WL, Sato Y, et al. Ultrafast CT of laryngeal and tracheobronchial obstruction in symptomatic postoperative infants with esophageal atresia and tracheoesophageal fistula. *AJR* 1990;154:345–350.

51. Siegel MJ, Nadel SN, Glazer HS, Sagel SS. Mediastinal lesions in children: comparison of CT and MR. *Radiology* 1986;160:241–244.

52. Siegel MJ, Glazer HS, Wiener JI, Molina PL. Normal and abnormal thymus in childhood: MR imaging. *Radiology* 1989;172:367–371.

53. Han BK, Babcock DS, Oestreich AE. Normal thymus in infancy: sonographic characteristics. *Radiology* 1989;170:471–474.

54. Herman M, Michalkova K, Kopriva F. High-resolution CT in the assessment of bronchiectasis in children. *Pediatr Radiol* 1993;23:376–379.

55. Kornreich L, Horev G, Ziv N, Grunebaum M. Bronchiectasis in children: assessment by CT. *Pediatr Radiol* 1993;23:120–123.

56. Meradji M, Kerrebijn KF. Functional bronchography in children. *Ann Radiol* 1976;19:67–75.

57. Kirks DR, Fitz CR, Harwood-Nash DC. Pediatric abdominal angiography: practical guide to catheter selection, flow rates, and contrast dosage. *Pediatr Radiol* 1976;5:19–23.

58. Strife JL. Pediatric airway obstruction: imaging in the 1990's. In: Kirks DR, ed. *Emergency pediatric radiology. A problem-oriented approach*. Reston, VA: American Roentgen Ray Society, 1995, 225–232.

59. Silverman FN, Kuhn JP, eds. *Caffey's pediatric x-ray diagnosis*. 9th ed. St. Louis: Mosby, 1993.

60. Ablow RC. Radiologic diagnosis of the newborn chest. *Curr Probl Pediatr* 1971;1:1–55.

61. Reid L. The lung: its growth and remodeling in health and disease. *AJR* 1977;129:777–788.

General Considerations

62. Skandalakis JE, Gray SW, eds. *Embryology for surgeons: the embryological basis for the treatment of congenital anomalies*. 2nd ed. Baltimore: Williams & Wilkins, 1994.

63. Inselman LS, Mellins RB. Growth and development of the lung. *J Pediatr* 1981;98:1–15.

64. Lui YM, Taylor JR, Zylak CJ. Roentgen–anatomical correlation of the individual human pulmonary acinus. *Radiology* 1973;109:1–5.

65. Rosado-de-Christenson ML, Stocker JT. Congenital cystic adenomatoid malformation. *RadioGraphics* 1991;11:865–886.

66. Griscom NT, Wohl MEB, Kirkpatrick JA Jr. Lower respiratory infections: how infants differ from adults. *Radiol Clin North Am* 1978;16:367–387.

67. Burko H. Considerations in the roentgen diagnosis of pneumonia in children. *AJR* 1962;88:555–565.

68. Osborne DRS, Effmann EL, Hedlund LW. Postnatal growth and size of the pulmonary acinus and secondary lobule in man. *AJR* 1983;140:449–454.

69. Langston C, Kida K, Reed M, Thurlbeck WM. Human lung growth in late gestation and in the neonate. *Am Rev Respir Dis* 1984;129:607–613.

70. Condon VR. Pneumonia in children. *J Thorac Imag* 1991;6:31–44.

71. Glezen P, Denny FW. Epidemiology of acute lower respiratory disease in children. *N Engl J Med* 1973;288:498–505.

72. Kirkpatrick JA. Pneumonia in children as it differs from adult pneumonia. *Semin Roentgenol* 1980;15:96–103.

Common Normal Variants

73. Taybi H. Pseudoneoplastic masses (pseudotumors) in children. Part two: pseudotumors of abdomen, skeleton, and soft tissue. *Med Radiogr Photogr* 1978;54:41–71.

74. Chang LWM, Lee FA, Gwinn JL. Normal lateral deviation of the trachea in infants and children. *AJR* 1970;109:247–251.

75. de Geer G, Webb WR, Gamsu G. Normal thymus: assessment with MR and CT. *Radiology* 1986;158:313–317.

76. Molina PL, Siegel MJ, Glazer HS. Thymic masses on MR imaging. *AJR* 1990;155:495–500.

77. Barth K, Schnauffer L, Kaufmann HJ. Giant idiopathic thymomegaly. *Pediatr Radiol* 1976;4:117–119.

78. Francis IR, Glazer GM, Bookstein FL, Gross BH. The thymus: reexamination of age-related changes in size and shape. *AJR* 1985;145:249–254.

79. St. Amour TE, Siegel MJ, Glazer HS, Nadel SN. CT appearances of the normal and abnormal thymus in childhood. *J Comput Assist Tomogr* 1987;11:645–650.

80. Shackelford GD, McAlister WH. The aberrantly positioned thymus: a cause of mediastinal or neck masses in children. *AJR* 1974;120:291–296.

81. Davis LA. The vertical fissure line. *AJR* 1960;84:451-453.

82. Proto AV, Ball JB Jr. The superolateral major fissures. *AJR* 1983;140:431–437.

83. Rose RW, Ward BH. Spherical pneumonias in children simulating pulmonary and mediastinal masses. *Radiology* 1973;106:179–182.

84. McDonald CJ, Castellino RA, Blank N. The aortic ''nipple.'' The left superior intercostal vein. *Radiology* 1970;96:533–536.

Upper Airway Obstruction

85. John SD, Swischuk LE. Stridor and upper airway obstruction in infants and children. *RadioGraphics* 1992;12:625–643.

86. Williams HJ. Posterior choanal atresia. *AJR* 1971;112:1–11.

87. Slovis TL, Renfro B, Watts FB, et al. Choanal atresia: precise CT evaluation. *Radiology* 1985;155:345–348.

88. Ey EH, Han BK, Towbin RB, Jaun WK. Bony inlet stenosis as a cause of nasal airway obstruction. *Radiology* 1988;168:477–479.

89. Zizmor J, Noyek AM. Cysts, benign tumors, and malignant tumors of the paranasal sinuses. *Otolaryngol Clin North Am* 1973;6:487–508.

90. Sinha PP, Aziz HI. Juvenile nasopharyngeal angiofibroma. A report of seven cases. *Radiology* 1978;127:501–505.

91. Davis KR. Embolization of epistaxis and juvenile nasopharyngeal angiofibromas. *AJNR* 1986;7:953–962.

92. Wadsworth DT, Siegel MJ. Thyroglossal duct cysts: variability of sonographic findings. *AJR* 1994;163:1475–1477.

93. Sato Y, Dunbar JS. Abnormalities of the pharynx and prevertebral soft tissues in infectious mononucleosis. *AJR* 1980;134:149–152.

94. Mahboubi S, Tenore A, Kirkpatrick JA. Diagnosis of ectopic thyroid: value of pretracheal soft-tissue measurements. *AJR* 1981;137: 717–719.

95. Dunbar JS. Upper respiratory tract obstruction in infants and children. *AJR* 1970;109:227–246.

96. McCook TA, Kirks DR. Epiglottic enlargement in infants and children: another radiologic look. *Pediatr Radiol* 1982;12:227–234.

97. Capitanio MA, Kirkpatrick JA. Upper respiratory tract obstruction in infants and children. *Radiol Clin North Am* 1968;6:265–277.

98. Dunbar JS. Epiglottitis and croup. *J Can Assoc Radiol* 1961;12:86–95.

99. John SD, Swischuk LE, Hayden CK Jr, Freeman DH Jr. Aryepiglottic fold width in patients with epiglottitis: where should measurements be obtained? *Radiology* 1994;190:123–125.

100. Shackelford GD, Siegel MJ, McAlister WH. Subglottic edema in acute epiglottitis in children. *AJR* 1978;131:603–605.

101. Capitanio MA, Kirkpatrick JA. Obstructions of the upper airway in children as reflected on the chest radiograph. *Radiology* 1973;107: 159–161.

102. Kramer SS, Wehunt WD, Stocker JT, Kashima H. Pulmonary manifestations of juvenile laryngotracheal papillomatosis. *AJR* 1985;144: 687–694.

103. Currarino G, Williams B. Lateral inspiration and expiration radiographs of the neck in children with laryngotracheitis.(croup). *Radiology* 1982;145:365–366.

104. Meine FJ, Lorenzo RL, Lynch PF, et al. Pharyngeal distension associated with upper airway obstruction. Experimental observations in dogs. *Radiology* 1974;111:395–398.

105. Han BK, Dunbar JS, Striker TW. Membranous laryngotracheobronchitis (membranous croup). *AJR* 1979;133:53–58.

106. Sutton TJ, Nogrady MB. Radiologic diagnosis of subglottic hemangioma in infants. *Pediatr Radiol* 1973;1:211–216.

107. Cooper M, Slovis TL, Madgy DN, Levitsky D. Congenital subglottic hemangioma: frequency of symmetric subglottic narrowing on frontal radiographs of the neck. *AJR* 1992;159:1269–1271.

108. McCook TA, Felman AH. Retropharyngeal masses in infants and young children. *Am J Dis Child* 1979;133:41–43.

109. Ben-Ami T, Yousefzadeh DK, Aramburo MJ. Pre-suppurative phase of retropharyngeal infection: contribution of ultrasonography in the diagnosis and treatment. *Pediatr Radiol* 1990;21:23–26.

110. Woodruff WW III, Merten DF, Kirks DR. Pneumomediastinum: an unusual complication of acute gastrointestinal disease. *Pediatr Radiol* 1985;15:196–198.

111. Miller EM, Norman D. The role of computed tomography in the evaluation of neck masses. *Radiology* 1979;133:145–149.

Congenital Abnormalities

112. Landing BH, Wells TR. *Tracheobronchial anomalies in children.* In: Rosenberg HS, Bolande RP. *Perspectives in pediatric pathology.* Vol 1. Chicago: Year Book, 1973, 1–32.

113. Landing BH. Congenital malformations of the larynx and trachea. In: Saldana MJ, ed. *Pathology of pulmonary disease.* Philadelphia: JB Lippincott, 1994.

114. Griscom NT. Diseases of the trachea, bronchi, and smaller airways. *Radiol Clin North Am* 1993;31:605–615.

115. Griscom NT, Harris GBC, Wohl MEB, et al. Fluid-filled lung due to airway obstruction in the newborn. *Pediatrics* 1969;43:383–390.

116. Effmann EL, Spackman TJ, Berdon WE, et al. Tracheal agenesis. *AJR* 1975;125:767–781.

117. Felson B. Pulmonary agenesis and related anomalies. *Semin Roentgenol* 1972;7:17–30.

118. Hernandez RJ, Tucker GF. Congenital tracheal stenosis: role of CT and high kV films. *Pediatr Radiol* 1987;17:192–196.

119. Wittenborg MH, Gyepes MT, Crocker D. Tracheal dynamics in infants with respiratory distress, stridor, and collapsing trachea. *Radiology* 1967;88:653–662.

120. Neuhauser EBD, Griscom NT. Aspiration pneumonitis in children. *Progr Pediatr Radiol* 1967;1:265–293.

121. Currarino G, Williams B. Causes of congenital unilateral pulmonary hypoplasia: a study of 33 cases. *Pediatr Radiol* 1985;15:15–24.

122. Maltz DL, Nadas AS. Agenesis of the lung. Presentation of eight new cases and review of the literature. *Pediatrics* 1968;42:175–188.

123. Cremin BJ, Bass EM. Retrosternal density: a sign of pulmonary hypoplasia. *Pediatr Radiol* 1975;3:145–147.

124. Felson B. The many faces of pulmonary sequestration. *Semin Roentgenol* 1972;7:3–16.

125. Boyden EA. The structure of compressed lungs in congenital diaphragmatic hernia. *Am J Anat* 1972;134:497–507.

126. Kitagawa M, Hislop A, Boyden EA, Reid L. Lung hypoplasia in congenital diaphragmatic hernia. A quantitative study of airway, artery, and alveolar development. *Br J Surg* 1971;58:342–346.

127. Freedom RM, Burrows PE, Moes CAF. ''Horseshoe'' lung: report of five new cases. *AJR* 1986;146:211–215.

128. Gao YA, Burrows PE, Benson LN, et al. Scimitar syndrome in infancy. *J Am Coll Cardiol* 1993;22:873–882.

129. Tomsick TA, Moesner SE, Smith WL. The congenital pulmonary venolobar syndrome in three successive generations. *J Can Assoc Radiol* 1976;27:196–199.

130. Panicek DM, Heitzman ER, Randall PA, et al. The continuum of pulmonary developmental anomalies. *RadioGraphics* 1987;7: 747–772.

131. Cremin BJ, Movsowitz H. Lobar emphysema in infants. *Br J Radiol* 1971;44:692–696.

132. Fagan CJ, Swischuk LE. The opaque lung in lobar emphysema. *AJR* 1972;114:300–304.

133. Fowler CL, Pokorny WJ, Wagner ML, Kessler MS. Review of bronchopulmonary foregut malformations. *J Pediatr Surg* 1988;23: 793–797.

134. Gerle RD, Jaretzki A III, Ashley CA, Berne AS. Congenital bronchopulmonary–foregut malformation. Pulmonary sequestration communicating with the gastrointestinal tract. *N Engl J Med* 1968;278: 1413–1419.

135. Eraklis AJ, Griscom NT, McGovern JB. Bronchogenic cysts of the mediastinum in infancy. *N Engl J Med* 1969;281:1150–1155.

136. Stocker JT, Drake RM, Madewell JE. Cystic and congenital lung disease in the newborn. *Perspect Pediatr Pathol* 1978;4:93–154.

137. Sane SM, Girdany BR. Cysts and neoplasms in the infant lung. *Semin Roentgenol* 1972;7:122–148.

138. Hedlund GL, Bisset GS III, Bove KE. Malignant neoplasms arising in cystic hamartomas of the lung in childhood. *Radiology* 1989;173: 77–79.

139. Macpherson RI, Reed MH, Ferguson CC. Intrathoracic gastrogenic cysts: a cause of lethal pulmonary hemorrhage in infants. *J Can Assoc Radiol* 1973;24:362–369.

140. Mendelson DS, Rose JS, Efremidis SC, et al. Bronchogenic cysts with high CT numbers. *AJR* 1983;140:463–465.

141. Bisset GS III. Pediatric thoracic applications of magnetic resonance imaging. *J Thorac Imaging* 1989;4:51–57.

142. von Schulthess GK, McMurdo K, Tscholakoff D, et al. Mediastinal masses: MR imaging. *Radiology* 1986;158:289–296.

143. Madewell JE, Stocker JT, Korsower JM. Cystic adenomatoid malformation of the lung. Morphologic analysis. *AJR* 1975;124:436–448.

144. Shackelford GD, Siegel MJ. CT appearance of cystic adenomatoid malformations. *J Comput Assist Tomogr* 1989;13:612–616.

145. Stocker JT. Sequestrations of the lung. *Semin Diagn Pathol* 1986;3: 106–121.

146. Rosado-de-Christenson ML, Frazier AA, Stocker JT, Templeton PA.

From the archives of the AFIP. Extralobar sequestration: radiologic-pathologic correlation. *RadioGraphics* 1993;13:425–441.

147. Felker RE, Tonkin IL. Imaging of pulmonary sequestration. *AJR* 1990; 154:241–249.

148. Currarino G, Willis K, Miller W. Congenital fistula between an aberrant systemic artery and a pulmonary vein without sequestration. A report of three cases. *J Pediatr* 1975;554–557.

149. Currarino G, Willis KW, Johnson AF Jr, Miller WW. Pulmonary telangiectasia. *AJR* 1976;127:775–779.

150. Kirks DR, Kane PE, Free EA, Taybi H. Systemic arterial supply to normal basilar segments of the left lower lobe. *AJR* 1976;126: 817–821.

151. Higgins CB, Wexler L. Clinical and angiographic features of pulmonary arteriovenous fistulas in children. *Radiology* 1976;119:171–175.

152. White RI, Mitchell SE, Barth KH, et al. Angioarchitecture of pulmonary arteriovenous malformations: an important consideration before embolotherapy. *AJR* 1983;140:681–686.

153. Frank JL, Poole CA, Rosas G. Horseshoe lung: clinical, pathologic, and radiologic features and a new plain film finding. *AJR* 1986;146: 217–226.

154. Merten DF, Bowie JD, Kirks DR, Grossman H. Anteromedial diaphragmatic defects in infancy: current approaches to diagnostic imaging. *Radiology* 1982;142:361–365.

155. Robinson AE, Gooneratne NS, Blackburn WR, Brogdon BG. Bilateral anteromedial defect of the diaphragm in children. *AJR* 1980;135: 301–306.

156. Wayne ER, Campbell JB, Burrington JD, Davis WS. Eventration of the diaphragm. *J Pediatr Surg* 1974;9:643–651.

157. Diament MJ, Boechat MI, Kangarloo H. Real-time sector ultrasound in the evaluation of suspected abnormalities of diaphragmatic motion. *J Clin Ultrasound* 1985;13:539–543.

158. McCauley RGK, Labib KB. Diaphragmatic paralysis evaluated by phrenic nerve stimulation during fluoroscopy or real–time ultrasound. *Radiology* 1984;153:33–36.

159. Wexler HA, Poole CA. Neonatal diaphragmatic dysfunction. *AJR* 1976;127:617–622.

General Abnormalities

160. Cumming GR, MacPherson RI, Chernick V. Unilateral hyperlucent lung syndrome in children. *J Pediatr* 1971;78:250–260.

161. Macpherson RI, Cumming GR, Chernick V. Unilateral hyperlucent lung: a complication of viral pneumonia. *J Can Assoc Radiol* 1969; 20:225–231.

162. Seibert RW, Seibert JJ, Williamson SL. The opaque chest: when to suspect a bronchial foreign body. *Pediatr Radiol* 1986;16:193–196.

163. Capitanio MA, Ramos R, Kirkpatrick JA. Pulmonary sling. Roentgen observations. *AJR* 1971;112:28–34.

164. Wolfe WG, Spock A, Bradford WD. Pleural fluid in infants and children. *Am Rev Respir Dis* 1968;98:1027–1032.

Newborn Chest Radiology

165. Giedion A. Radiology of respiratory distress in the newborn. *Curr Concepts Pediatr Radiol* 1977;1:1–12.

166. Alford BA, McIlhenny J, Jones JE, et al. Asymmetric radiographic findings in the pediatric chest: approach to early diagnosis. *RadioGraphics* 1993;13:77–93.

167. Edwards DK, Jacob J, Gluck L. The immature lung: radiographic appearance, course and complications. *AJR* 1980;135:659–666.

168. Wood BP, Davitt MA, Metlay LA. Lung disease in the very immature neonate: radiographic and microscopic correlation. *Pediatr Radiol* 1989;20:33–40.

169. Fletcher BD, Fanaroff AA. The "immature lung" and RDS. *AJR* 1981;136:840.

170. Swischuk LE, John SD. Immature lung problems: can our nomenclature be more specific? *AJR* 1996;166:917–918.

171. Hernandez R, Kuhns LR, Holt JF. The suprasternal fossa on chest radiographs in newborns. *AJR* 1978;130:745–746.

172. Ablow RC, Orzalesi MM. Localized roentgenographic pattern of hyaline membrane disease. Evidence that the upper lobes of human lung mature earlier than the lower lobes. *AJR* 1971;112:23–27.

173. Couser RJ, Ferrara TB, Ebert J, et al. Effects of exogenous surfactant therapy on dynamic compliance during mechanical breathing in preterm infants with hyaline membrane disease. *J Pediatr* 1990;116: 119–124.

174. Merenstein GB, Cassady G, Erenberg A, et al. Surfactant replacement therapy for respiratory distress syndrome. *Pediatrics* 1991;87: 946–947.

175. Edwards DK, Hilton SVW, Merritt TA, et al. Respiratory distress syndrome treated with human surfactant: radiographic findings. *Radiology* 1985;157:329–334.

176. Liechty EA, Donovan E, Purohit D, et al. Reduction of neonatal mortality after multiple doses of bovine surfactant in low birth weight neonates with respiratory distress syndrome. *Pediatr* 1991;88:19–28.

177. Hallman M, Merritt TA, Jarvenpaa AL. Exogenous human surfactant for treatment of severe respiratory distress syndrome: a randomized prospective clinical trial. *J Pediatr* 1985;106:963–969.

178. Levine D, Edwards DK III, Merritt TA. Synthetic vs. human surfactants in the treatment of respiratory distress syndrome: radiographic findings. *AJR* 1991;157:371–374.

179. Wood BP, Sinkin RA, Kendig JW, et al. Exogenous lung surfactant: effect on radiographic appearance in premature infants. *Radiology* 1987;165:11–13.

180. Jackson JC, Truog WE, Standaert TA, et al. Effect of high-frequency ventilation on the development of alveolar edema in premature monkeys at risk for hyaline membrane disease. *Am Rev Respir Dis* 1991; 143:865–871.

181. Macpherson RI, Chernick V, Reed M. The complications of respirator therapy in the newborn. *J Can Assoc Radiol* 1972;23:91–102.

182. Strife JL, Smith P, Dunbar JS, Steven JM. Chest tube perforation of the lung in premature infants: radiographic recognition. *AJR* 1983; 141:73–75.

183. Weller MH. The roentgenographic course and complications of hyaline membrane disease. *Pediatr Clin North Am* 1973;20:381–406.

184. Wood BP, Anderson VM, Mauk JE, Merritt TA. Pulmonary lymphatic air: locating "pulmonary interstitial emphysema" of the premature infant. *AJR* 1982;138:809–814.

185. Steele RW, Metz JR, Bass JW, DuBois JJ. Pneumothorax and pneumomediastinum in the newborn. *Radiology* 1971;98:629–632.

186. Williams DW, Merten DF, Effmann EL, Scatliff JH. Ventilator-induced pulmonary pseudocysts in preterm neonates. *AJR* 1988;150: 885–887.

187. Swischuk LE. Bubbles in hyaline membrane disease. Differentiation of three types. *Radiology* 1977;122:417–426.

188. Magilner AD, Capitanio MA, Wertheimer I, Burko H. Persistent localized intrapulmonary interstitial emphysema: an observation in three infants. *Radiology* 1974;111:379–384.

189. Schwartz AN, Graham CB. Neonatal tension pulmonary interstitial emphysema in bronchopulmonary dysplasia: treatment with lateral decubitus positioning. *Radiology* 1986;161:351–354.

190. Franken EA Jr. Pneumomediastinum in newborn with associated dextroposition of the heart. *AJR* 1970;109:252–260.

191. Levin B. The continuous diaphragm sign. A newly-recognized sign of pneumomediastinum. *Clin Radiol* 1973;24:337–338.

192. Moskowitz PS, Griscom NT. The medial pneumothorax. *Radiology* 1976;120:143–147.

193. Swischuk LE. Two lesser known but useful signs of neonatal pneumothorax. *AJR* 1976;127:623–627.

194. Fletcher BD. Medial herniation of the parietal pleura: a useful sign of pneumothorax in supine neonates. *AJR* 1978;130:469–472.

195. Markowitz RI. The anterior junction line: a radiographic sign of bilateral pneumothorax in neonates. *Radiology* 1988;167:717–719.

196. Hoffer FA, Ablow RC. The cross-table lateral view in neonatal pneumothorax. *AJR* 1984;142:1283–1286.

197. Kuhns LR, Poznanski AK. Endotracheal tube position in the infant. *J Pediatr* 1971;78:991–996.

198. Donn SM, Kuhns LR. Mechanism of endotracheal tube movement with change of head position in the neonate. *Pediatr Radiol* 1980;9: 37–40.

199. Conrardy PA, Goodman LR, Lainge F, Singer MM. Alternation of endotracheal tube position. Flexion and extension of the neck. *Crit Care Med* 1976;4:7–12.

200. McSweeney WJ. Radiologic evaluation of the newborn with respiratory distress. *Semin Roentgenol* 1972;7:65–83.

201. Fletcher BD, Avery ME. The effects of airway occlusion after oxygen breathing on the lungs of newborn infants. Radiologic demonstration in the experimental animal. *Radiology* 1973;109:655–657.

202. Bomsel F, Couchard M, Larroche JC, Magder L. Radiologic diagnosis of massive pulmonary haemorrhage of the newborn. *Ann Radiol* 1975; 18:419-430.

203. Slovis TL, Shankaran S. Patent ductus arteriosus in hyaline membrane disease: chest radiography. *AJR* 1980;135:307–309.

204. Northway WH Jr, Rosan RC, Porter DY. Pulmonary disease following respirator therapy of hyaline-membrane disease. Bronchopulmonary dysplasia. *N Engl J Med* 1967;276:357–368.

205. Northway WH Jr, Rosan RC. Radiographic features of pulmonary oxygen toxicity in the newborn: bronchopulmonary dysplasia. *Radiology* 1968;91:49–58.

206. Edwards DK, Colby TV, Northway WH Jr. Radiographic-pathologic correlation in bronchopulmonary dysplasia. *J Pediatr* 1979;95: 834–836.

207. Griscom NT, Wheeler WB, Sweezey NB, et al. Bronchopulmonary dysplasia: radiographic appearance in middle childhood. *Radiology* 1989;171:811–814.

208. Griscom NT. Respiratory problems of early life now allowing survival into adulthood: concepts for radiologists. *AJR* 1992;158:1–8.

209. Northway WH Jr. Observations on bronchopulmonary dysplasia. *J Pediatr* 1979;95:815–818.

210. Northway WH Jr. Bronchopulmonary dysplasia and research in diagnostic radiology. *AJR* 1991;156:681–687.

211. Crouse DT, Odrezin GT, Cutter GR, et al. Radiographic changes associated with tracheal isolation of ureaplasma urealyticum from neonates. *Clin Infect Dis* 1993;17:S122–130.

212. Grossman H, Berdon WE, Mizrahi A, Baker DH. Neonatal focal hyperaeration of the lungs (Wilson-Mikity syndrome). *Radiology* 1965; 85:409–417.

213. Wesenberg RL, Graven SN, McCabe EB. Radiological findings in wet-lung disease. *Radiology* 1971;98:69–74.

214. Swischuk LE. Transient respiratory distress of the newborn (TRDN). A temporary disturbance of a normal phenomenon. *AJR* 1970;108: 557–563.

215. Steele RW, Copeland GA. Delayed resorption of pulmonary alveolar fluid in the neonate. *Radiology* 1972;103:637–639.

216. Gooding CA, Gregory GA. Roentgenographic analysis of meconium aspiration of the newborn. *Radiology* 1971;100:131–140.

217. Gregory GA, Gooding CA, Phibbs RH, Tooley WH. Meconium aspiration in infants: a prospective study. *J Pediatr* 1974;85:848–852.

218. Bartlett RH, Gazzaniga AB, Toomasian J, et al. Extracorporeal membrane oxygenation (ECMO) in neonatal respiratory failure. 100 cases. *Ann Surg* 1986;204:236–245.

219. Brudno DS, Boedy RF, Kanto WP Jr. Compliance, alveolar-arterial oxygen difference, and oxygenation index changes in patients managed with extracorporeal membrane oxygenation. *Pediatr Pulmonol* 1990;9:19–23.

220. Gross GW, Greenspan JS, Fox WW, et al. Use of liquid ventilation with Perflubron during extracorporeal membrane oxygenation: chest radiographic appearances. *Radiology* 1995;194:717–720.

221. Taylor GA, Lotze A, Kapur S, Short BL. Diffuse pulmonary opacification in infants undergoing extracorporeal membrane oxygenation: clinical and pathologic correlation. *Radiology* 1986;161:347–350.

222. Slovis TL, Sell LL, Bedard MP, Klein MD. Ultrasonographic findings (CNS, thorax, abdomen) in infants undergoing extracorporeal oxygenation therapy. *Pediatr Radiol* 1988;18:112–117.

223. Ablow RC, Driscoll SG, Effmann EL, et al. A comparison of early–onset group B streptococcal neonatal infection and the respiratory–distress syndrome of the newborn. *N Engl J Med* 1976;294: 65–70.

224. Ablow RC, Gross I, Effmann EL, et al. The radiographic features of early onset group B streptococcal neonatal sepsis. *Radiology* 1977; 124:771–777.

225. Haney PJ, Bohlman M, Sun CC. Radiographic findings in neonatal pneumonia. *AJR* 1984;143:23–26.

226. Austin R, Melhem RE. Pulmonary changes in congenital syphilis. *Pediatr Radiol* 1991;21:404–405.

227. Leonidas JC, Hall RT, Beatty EC, Fellows RA. Radiographic findings in early onset neonatal group B streptococcal septicemia. *Pediatrics* 1977;59 Suppl:1006–1011.

228. McCarten KM, Rosenberg HK, Borden S IV, Mandell GA. Delayed

appearance of right diaphragmatic hernia associated with group B streptococcal infection in newborns. *Radiology* 1981;139:385–389.

229. Freed MD. Congenital cardiac malformations. In: Taeusch HW, Ballard RA, Avery ME, eds. *Schaffer and Avery's diseases of the newborn.* Philadelphia: WB Saunders, 1991, 591–633.

230. Cleveland R. Total anomalous pulmonary venous connection: case 10. In: Siegel MJ, Bisset GS, Cleveland RH, et al, eds. *ACR pediatric disease test and syllabus.* Reston: American College of Radiology, 1993, 272–302.

Pulmonary Infection

231. Bettenay FAL, de Campo JF, McCrossin DB. Differentiating bacterial from viral pneumonias in children. *Pediatr Radiol* 1988;18:453–454.

232. Denny FW, Clyde WA Jr. Acute lower respiratory tract infections in nonhospitalized children. *J Pediatr* 1986;108:635–646.

233. Griscom NT. Pneumonia in children and some of its variants. *Radiology* 1988;167:297–302.

234. Osborne D, Kirks DR, Effmann EL. Pneumonia in the child. In: Putman CE, ed. *Pulmonary diagnosis: imaging and other techniques.* New York: Appleton-Century-Crofts, 1981, 219–245.

235. Swischuk LE, Hayden CK Jr. Viral vs. bacterial pulmonary infections in children. (Is roentgenographic differentiation possible?) *Pediatr Radiol* 1986;16:278–284.

236. Swischuk LE. Chest disease in infants and children. In: Kirks DR, ed. *Emergency pediatric radiology. A problem-oriented approach.* Reston, VA: American Roentgen Ray Society, 1995, 211–216.

237. Heulitt MJ, Ablow RC, Santos CC, et al. Febrile infants less than 3 months old: value of chest radiography. *Radiology* 1988;167: 135–137.

238. Patterson RJ, Bisset GS III, Kirks DR, Vanness A. Chest radiographs in the evaluation of the febrile infant. *AJR* 1990;155:833–835.

239. Smith CB, Overall JC Jr. Clinical and epidemiologic clues to the diagnosis of respiratory infections. *Radiol Clin North Am* 1973;11: 261–278.

240. Schweich P. Lower respiratory tract infections. In: Schwartz MW, ed. *Principles and practice of clinical pediatrics.* Chicago: Year Book, 1987, 441–448.

241. Singleton EB, Orson LW. Pulmonary complication of acquired immune deficiency syndrome in infants and children. *Int Pediatr* 1988; 3:312–317.

242. Zimmerman BL, Haller JO, Price AP, et al. Children with AIDS—Is pathologic diagnosis possible based on chest radiographs? *Pediatr Radiol* 1987;17:303–307.

243. Felson B. The roentgen diagnosis of disseminated pulmonary alveolar diseases. *Semin Roentgenol* 1967;2:3–22.

244. Felson B. Disseminated interstitial diseases of the lung. *Ann Radiol* 1966;9:325–345.

245. Weibel ER. Looking into the lung: what can it tell us? *AJR* 1979; 133:1021–1031.

246. Osborne D. Radiologic appearance of viral disease of the lower respiratory tract in infants and children. *AJR* 1978;130:29–33.

247. Franken EA Jr, Klatte EC. Atypical (peripheral) upper lobe collapse. *Ann Radiol* 1977;20:87–93.

248. Tamaki Y, Pandit R, Gooding CA. Neonatal atypical peripheral atelectasis. *Pediatr Radiol* 1994;24:589–591.

249. Wood BP, Bernstein RM. Pulmonary nodular "pneumonia" during the acute atypical measles illness. *Ann Radiol* 1978;21:193–198.

250. Young LW, Smith DI, Glasgow LA. Pneumonia of atypical measles. Residual nodular lesions. *AJR* 1970;110:439–448.

251. Stark DD, Federle MP, Goodman PC, et al. Differentiating lung abscess and empyema: radiography and computed tomography. *AJR* 1983;141:163–167.

252. Guckel C, Benz-Bohm G, Widemann B. Mycoplasmal pneumonias in childhood. Roentgen features, differential diagnosis and review of literature. *Pediatr Radiol* 1989;19:499–503.

253. Putman CE, Curtis AM, Simeone JF, Jensen P. Mycoplasma pneumonia. Clinical and roentgenographic patterns. *AJR* 1975;124:417–422.

254. Cremin BJ. Tuberculosis: the resurgence of our most lethal infectious disease—a review. *Pediatr Radiol* 1995;25:620–626.

255. Buckner CB, Leithiser RE, Walker CW, Allison JW. The changing epidemiology of tuberculosis and other mycobacterial infections in the United States: implications for the radiologist. *AJR* 1991;156: 255–264.

256. Rieder HL, Cauthen GM, Kelly GD, et al. Tuberculosis in the United States. *JAMA* 1989;262:385–389.

257. Snider DE Jr, Rieder HL, Combs D, et al. Tuberculosis in children. *Pediatr Infect Dis J* 1988;7:271–278.

258. Lamont AC, Cremin BJ, Pelteret RM. Radiological patterns of pulmonary tuberculosis in the paediatric age group. *Pediatr Radiol* 1986; 16:2–7.

259. Stansberry SD. Tuberculosis in infants and children. *J Thorac Imaging* 1990;5:17–27.

260. Leung AN, Muller NL, Pineda PR, Fitzgerald JM. Primary tuberculosis in childhood: radiographic manifestations. *Radiology* 1992;182: 87–91.

261. Jamieson DH, Cremin BJ. High resolution CT of the lungs in acute disseminated tuberculosis and a pediatric radiology perspective of the term ''miliary''. *Pediatr Radiol* 1993;23:380–383.

262. Radkowski MA, Kranzler JK, Beem MO, Tipple MA. Chlamydia pneumonia in infants: radiography in 125 cases. *AJR* 1981;137: 703–706.

263. Schachter J. Chlamydial infections. *N Engl J Med* 1978;298:490–495.

264. Wood BP. Infantile chlamydia trachomatis pneumonia: radiographic features. *Ann Radiol* 1979;22:213–216.

265. Stickney RH, Bjelland JC, Capp MP, et al. Chlamydia trachomatis: a cause of an infantile pneumonia syndrome. *AJR* 1978;131:914–915.

266. Greene R. The pulmonary aspergilloses: three distinct entities or a spectrum of disease. *Radiology* 1981;140:527–530.

267. Klein DL, Gamsu G. Thoracic manifestations of aspergillosis. *AJR* 1980;134:543–552.

268. Ball WS Jr, Bisset GS III, Towbin RB. Percutaneous drainage of chest abscesses in children. *Radiology* 1989;171:431–434.

269. Quigley MJ, Fraser RS. Pulmonary pneumatocele: pathology and pathogenesis. *AJR* 1988;150:1275–1277.

270. Harris VJ, Brown R. Pneumatoceles as a complication of chemical pneumonia after hydrocarbon ingestion. *AJR* 1975;125:531–537.

271. Coleman LT, Kramer SS, Markowitz RI, Kravitz RM. Bronchiectasis in children. *J Thorac Imaging* 1995;10:268–279.

272. Baker DH. Chronic pulmonary disease in infants and children. *Radiol Clin North Am* 1963;1:519–537.

273. Kirkpatrick JA. The problem of chronic and recurrent pulmonary disease. *Prog Pediatr Radiol* 1967;1:294–325.

274. Bhalla M, Abboud MR, McLoud TC, et al. Acute chest syndrome in sickle cell disease: CT evidence of microvascular occlusion. *Radiology* 1993;187:45–49.

Immunodeficiency Diseases

275. Brasch RC. *The child with immunodeficiency: what the radiologist should know. Syllabus for diagnostic radiology*. San Francisco: University of California, 1978.

276. Buckley RH. Primary immunodeficiency diseases. In: Bennett JC, Plum FC. *Cecil textbook of medicine*. 20th ed. Philadelphia: WB Saunders, 1996, 1401–1408.

277. Kirkpatrick JA, Capitanio MA, Marcondes Pereira RM. Immunologic abnormalities: roentgen observations. *Radiol Clin North Am* 1972;10: 245–259.

278. Amodio JB, Abramson S, Berdon WE, Levy J. Pediatric AIDS. *Semin Roentgenol* 1987;22:66–76.

279. Stiehm ER, ed. *Immunologic disorders in infants and children*. Philadelphia: WB Saunders, 1989.

280. Shackelford GD, McAlister WH. Primary immunodeficiency diseases and malignancy. *AJR* 1975;123:144–153.

281. Haller JO, Cohen HL. Pediatric HIV infection: an imaging update. *Pediatr Radiol* 1994;24:224–230.

282. Haney PJ, Yale-Loehr AJ, Nussbaum AR, Gellad FE. Imaging of infants and children with AIDS. *AJR* 1989;153:1033–1041.

283. Marquis JR, Berman CZ, DiCarlo F, Oleske JM. Radiographic patterns of PLH/LIP in HIV positive children. *Pediatr Radiol* 1993;23: 328–330.

284. Wood BP. Children with acquired immune deficiency syndrome. Radiographic features. *Invest Radiol* 1992;27:964–970.

285. Wolfson JJ, Quie PG, Laxdal SD, Good RA. Roentgenologic manifestations in children with a genetic defect of polymorphonuclear leukocyte function. Chronic granulomatous disease of childhood. *Radiology* 1968;91:37–48.

Chronic Pulmonary Disorders

286. Eggleston PA, Ward BH, Pierson WE, Bierman CW. Radiographic abnormalities in acute asthma in children. *Pediatrics* 1974;54: 442–449.

287. Zieverink SE, Harper AP, Holden RW, et al. Emergency room radiography of asthma: an efficacy study. *Radiology* 1982;145:27–29.

288. Gillies JD, Reed MH, Simons FE. Radiologic findings in acute childhood asthma. *J Can Assoc Radiol* 1978;29:28–33.

289. McSweeney WJ, Stempel DA. Noniatrogenic pneumomediastinum in infancy and childhood. *Pediatr Radiol* 1973;1:139–144.

290. Effmann EF, Osborne D, Kirks DR. Cystic fibrosis and other genetic diseases affecting the tracheobronchial tree. In: Putman CE, ed. *Pulmonary diagnosis: imaging and other techniques*. New York: Appleton-Century-Crofts, 1981, 247–262.

291. Colin AA, Wohl ME. Cystic fibrosis. *Pediatr Rev* 1994;15:192–200.

292. Amodio JB, Berdon WE, Abramson S, Baker D. Cystic fibrosis in childhood: pulmonary, paranasal sinus, and skeletal manifestations. *Semin Roentgenol* 1987;22:125–135.

293. Hubbard RC, McElvaney NG, Birrer P, et al. A preliminary study of aerosolized recombinant human deoxyribonuclease I in the treatment of cystic fibrosis. *N Engl J Med* 1992;326:812–815.

294. te Meerman GJ, Dankert-Roelse J, Martijn A, van Woerden HH. A comparison of the Shwachman, Chrispin-Norman and Brasfield methods for scoring of chest radiographs of patients with cystic fibrosis. *Pediatr Radiol* 1985;15:98–101.

295. Fellows KE, Stigol L, Shuster S, et al. Selective bronchial arteriography in patients with cystic fibrosis and massive hemoptysis. *Radiology* 1975;114:551–556.

296. Swischuk LE. Microcardia: an uncommon diagnostic problem. *AJR* 1968;103:115–118.

297. Nadel HR, Stringer DA, Levinson H, et al. The immotile cilia syndrome: radiological manifestations. *Radiology* 1985;154:651–655.

298. Ramirez RE, Glasier C, Kirks D, et al. Pulmonary hemorrhage associated with systemic lupus erythematosus in children. *Radiology* 1984; 152:409–412.

299. McHugh K, Manson D, Eberhard BA, et al. Wegener's granulomatosis in childhood. *Pediatr Radiol* 1991;21:552–555.

300. Wadsworth DT, Siegel MJ, Day DL. Wegener's granulomatosis in children: chest radiographic manifestations. *AJR* 1994;163:901–904.

301. Hogg JC. Chronic interstitial lung disease of unknown cause: a new classification based on pathogenesis. *AJR* 1991;156:225–233.

302. McLoud TC, Epler GR, Colby TV, et al. Bronchiolitis obliterans. *Radiology* 1986;159:1–8.

303. Epler GR, Colby TV, McLoud TC, et al. Bronchiolitis obliterans organizing pneumonia. *N Engl J Med* 1985;312:152–158.

304. Bouchardy LM, Kuhlman JE, Ball WC Jr, et al. CT findings in bronchiolitis obliterans organizing pneumonia. (BOOP) with radiographic, clinical, and histologic correlation. *J Comput Assist Tomogr* 1993;17: 352–357.

305. Helton KJ, Kuhn JP, Fletcher BD, et al. Bronchiolitis obliterans-organizing pneumonia (BOOP) in children with malignant disease. *Pediatr Radiol* 1992;22:270–274.

306. Kirks DR, McCormick VD, Greenspan RH. Pulmonary sarcoidosis. Roentgenologic analysis of 150 patients. *AJR* 1973;117:777–786.

307. Merten DF, Kirks DR, Grossman H. Pulmonary sarcoidosis in childhood. *AJR* 1980;135:673–679.

308. Sumner TE, Auringer ST, Preston AA. Thymic calcification in histiocytosis X. *Pediatr Radiol* 1993;23:204–205.

309. Ha SY, Helms P, Fletcher M, et al. Lung involvement in Langerhans' cell histiocytosis: prevalence, clinical features, and outcome. *Pediatrics* 1992;89:466–469.

310. Burdelski M. Diagnostic, preventive, medical, and surgical management of alpha 1-antitrypsin deficiency in childhood. *Acta Pediatr Suppl* 1994;393:33–36.

311. Anonymous. Care records of the Massachusetts General Hospital. Weekly clinicopathological exercises. Case 30-1979. Idiopathic pulmonary hemosiderosis. *N Engl J Med* 1979;301:201–208.

312. McCook TA, Kirks DR, Merten DF, et al. Pulmonary alveolar proteinosis in children. *AJR* 1981;137:1023–1027.

313. Herman TE, Nogee LM, McAlister WH, Dehner LP. Surfactant protein B deficiency: radiographic manifestations. *Pediatr Radiol* 1993; 23:373–375.

Thoracic Tumors

314. Franken EA Jr, Smith JA, Smith WL. Tumors of the chest wall in infants and children. *Pediatr Radiol* 1977;6:13–18.
315. Boothroyd A, Carty H. Breast masses in childhood and adolescence. A presentation of 17 cases and a review of the literature. *Pediatr Radiol* 1994;24:81–84.
316. Fink IJ, Kurtz DW, Cazenave L, et al. Malignant thoracopulmonary small-cell ("Askin") tumor. *AJR* 1985;145:517–520.
317. Winer-Muram HT, Kauffman WM, Gronemeyer SA, Jennings SG. Primitive neuroectodermal tumors of the chest wall (Askin tumors): CT and MR findings. *AJR* 1993;161:265–268.
318. Bousvaros A, Kirks DR, Grossman H. Imaging of neuroblastoma: an overview. *Pediatr Radiol* 1986;16:89–106.
319. Miller JH, ed. *Imaging in pediatric oncology.* Baltimore: Williams and Wilkins, 1985.
320. Merten DF. Diagnostic imaging of mediastinal masses in children. *AJR* 1992;158:825–832.
321. Hope JW, Borns PF, Koop CE. Radiologic diagnosis of mediastinal masses in infants and children. *Radiol Clin North Am* 1963;1:17–50.
322. Felson B. The mediastinum. *Semin Roentgenol* 1969;4:41–58.
323. Bower RJ, Kiesewetter WB. Mediastinal masses in infants and children. *Arch Surg* 1977;112:1003–1009.
324. King RM, Telander RL, Smithson WA, et al. Primary mediastinal tumors in children. *J Pediatr Surg* 1982;17:512–520.
325. Jaramillo D, Perez-Atayde A, Griscom NT. Apparent association between thymic cysts and prior thoracotomy. *Radiology* 1989;172:207–209.
326. Rosado-de-Christenson ML, Galobardes J, Moran CA. Thymoma: radiologic-pathologic correlation. *RadioGraphics* 1992;12:151–168.
327. Brown LR, Muhm JR, Aughenbaugh GL, et al. Computed tomography of benign mature teratomas of the mediastinum. *J Thorac Imaging* 1987;2:66–71.
328. Levitt RG, Husband JE, Glazer HS. CT of primary germ-cell tumors of the mediastinum. *AJR* 1984;142:73–78.
329. Rosado-de-Christenson ML, Templeton PA, Moran CA. Mediastinal germ cell tumors: radiologic and pathologic correlation. *Radio-Graphics* 1992;12:1013–1030.
330. Kjeldsberg CR, Wilson JF, Berard CW. Non-Hodgkin's lymphoma in children. *Hum Pathol* 1983;14:612–627.
331. Cohen MD, Siddiqui A, Weetman R, et al. Hodgkin disease and non-Hodgkin lymphomas in children: utilization of radiological modalities. *Radiology* 1986;158:499–505.
332. Bragg DG, Colby TV, Ward JH. New concepts in non-Hodgkin lymphomas: radiologic implications. *Radiology* 1986;159:289–304.
333. Wang Y. Classification of non-Hodgkin's lymphoma. *AJR* 1986;147:205–208.
334. Hamrick-Turner JE, Saif MF, Powers CI, et al. Imaging of childhood non-Hodgkin lymphoma: assessment by histologic subtype. *Radio-Graphics* 1994;14:11–28.
335. Castellino RA, Bellani FF, Gasparini M, Musumeci R. Radiographic findings in previously untreated children with non-Hodgkin's lymphoma. *Radiology* 1975;117:657–663.
336. Urba WJ, Longo DL. Hodgkin's disease. *N Engl J Med* 1992;326:678–687.
337. Elkowitz SS, Leonidas JC, Lopez M, et al. Comparison of CT and MRI in the evaluation of therapeutic response in thoracic Hodgkin disease. *Pediatr Radiol* 1993;23:301–304.
338. Luker GD, Siegel MJ. Mediastinal Hodgkin disease in children: response to therapy. *Radiology* 1993;189:737–740.
339. Kirks DR, Fram EK, Vock P, Effmann EL. Tracheal compression by mediastinal masses in children: CT evaluation. *AJR* 1983;141:647–651.
340. Shamberger RC, Holzman RS, Griscom NT, et al. CT quantitation of tracheal cross-sectional area as a guide to the surgical and anesthetic management of children with anterior mediastinal masses. *J Pediatr Surg* 1991;26:138–142.
341. Reed JC, Sobonya RE. Morphologic analysis of foregut cysts in the thorax. *AJR* 1974;120:851–860.
342. Reed JC, Hallet KK, Feigin DS. Neural tumors of the thorax: subject review from the AFIP. *Radiology* 1978;126:9–17.
343. Riggs W Jr, Benton C, Wood B. Cervical neurogenic tumors presenting as thoracic apical masses in infants and children. *Pediatr Radiol* 1977;5:201–203.
344. Siegel MJ, Jamroz GA, Glazer HS, Abramson CL. MR imaging of intraspinal extension of neuroblastoma. *J Comput Assist Tomogr* 1986;10:593–595.
345. Kaufman RA. Calcified postinflammatory pseudotumor of the lung: CT features. *J Comput Assist Tomogr* 1988;12:653–655.
346. Laufer L, Cohen Z, Mares AJ, et al. Pulmonary plasma cell granuloma. *Pediatr Radiol* 1990;20:289–290.
347. Pearl M. Postinflammatory pseudotumor of the lung in children. *Radiology* 1972;105:391–395.
348. Schwartz EE, Katz SM, Mandell GA. Postinflammatory pseudotumors of the lung: fibrous histiocytoma and related lesions. *Radiology* 1980;136:609–613.
349. Hartman GE, Shochat SJ. Primary pulmonary neoplasms of childhood: a review. *Ann Thorac Surg* 1983;36:108–119.
350. Shady K, Siegel MJ, Glazer HS. CT of focal pulmonary masses in childhood. *RadioGraphics* 1992;12:505–514.
351. Rogers LF, Osmer JC. Bronchogenic cyst. A review of 46 cases. *AJR* 1964;91:273–283.
352. Weinberg AG, Currarino G, Moore GC, Votteler TP. Mesenchymal neoplasia and congenital pulmonary cysts. *Pediatr Radiol* 1980;9:179–182.
353. Bellah RD, Mahboubi S, Berdon WE. Malignant endobronchial lesions of adolescence. *Pediatr Radiol* 1992;22:563–567.
354. Manivel JC, Priest JR, Watterson J, et al. Pleuropulmonary blastoma. The so-called pulmonary blastoma of childhood. *Cancer* 1988;62:1516–1526.
355. Ohtomo K, Araki T, Yashiro N, Iio M. Pulmonary blastoma in children. Two case reports and a review of the literature. *Radiology* 1983;147:101–104.
356. Senac MO Jr, Wood BP, Isaacs H, Weller M. Pulmonary blastoma: a rare childhood malignancy. *Radiology* 1991;179:743–746.

Pulmonary Critical Care and Trauma

357. Markowitz RI. Radiologic assessment in the pediatric intensive care unit. *Yale J Biol Med* 1984;57:49–82.
358. Sivit CJ, Taylor GA, Hauser GJ, et al. Efficacy of chest radiography in pediatric intensive care. *AJR* 1989;152:575–577.
359. Milne EN. A physiological approach to reading critical care unit films. *J Thorac Imaging* 1986;1:60–90.
360. Greenbaum DM, Marschall KE. The value of routine daily chest x-rays in intubated patients in the medical intensive care unit. *Crit Care Med* 1982;10:29–30.
361. Tocino IM, Watanabe A. Impending catheter perforation of superior vena cava: radiographic recognition. *AJR* 1986;146:487–490.
362. Greene R. Adult respiratory distress syndrome: acute alveolar damage. *Radiology* 1987;163:57–66.
363. Putman CE, Minagi H, Blaisdell FW. The roentgen appearance of disseminated intravascular coagulation (DIC). *Radiology* 1973;109:13–18.
364. Effmann EL, Merten DF, Kirks DR, et al. Adult respiratory distress syndrome in children. *Radiology* 1985;157:69–74.
365. Royall JA, Levin DL. Adult respiratory distress syndrome in pediatric patients. I. Clinical aspects, pathophysiology, pathology and mechanisms of lung injury. *J Pediatr* 1988;112:169–180.
366. Hirschl RB, Parent A, Tooley R, et al. Liquid ventilation improves pulmonary function, gas exchange, and lung injury in a model of respiratory failure. *Ann Surg* 1995;221:79–88.
367. Crawford WO Jr. Pulmonary injury in thoracic and non-thoracic trauma. *Radiol Clin North Am* 1973;11:527–541.
368. Fagan CJ, Swischuk LE. Traumatic lung and paramediastinal pneumatoceles. *Radiology* 1976;120:11–18.
369. Manson D, Babyn PS, Palder S, Bergman K. CT of blunt chest trauma in children. *Pediatr Radiol* 1993;23:1–5.
370. Simeone JF, Minagi H, Putman CE. Traumatic disruption of the thoracic aorta: significance of the left apical extrapleural cap. *Radiology* 1975;117:265–268.
371. Sivit CJ, Taylor GA, Eichelberger MR. Chest injury in children with blunt abdominal trauma: evaluation with CT. *Radiology* 1989;171:815–818.
372. Sorsdahl OA, Powell JW. Cavitary pulmonary lesions following nonpenetrating chest trauma in children. *AJR* 1965;95:118–124.
373. Wiener Y, Simansky D, Yellin A. Main bronchial rupture from blunt trauma in a 2-year-old child. *J Pediatr Surg* 1993;28:1530–1531.

374. Bowen A III, Quattromani FL. Infraazygous pneumomediastinum in the newborn. *AJR* 1980;135:1017–1021.

375. Volberg FM Jr, Everett CJ, Brill PW. Radiologic features of inferior pulmonary ligament air collections in neonates with respiratory distress. *Radiology* 1979;130:357–360.

376. Mahboubi S, O'Hara AE. Bronchial rupture in children following blunt chest trauma. Report of five cases with emphasis on radiologic findings. *Pediatr Radiol* 1981;10:133–138.

377. Oh KS, Fleischner FG, Wyman SM. Characteristic pulmonary finding in traumatic complete transection of a main-stem bronchus. *Radiology* 1969;92:371–372.

378. Reed MH. Radiology of airway foreign bodies in children. *J Can Assoc Radiol* 1977;28:111–118.

379. Svedstrom E, Puhakka H, Kero P. How accurate is chest radiography in the diagnosis of tracheobronchial foreign bodies in children? *Pediatr Radiol* 1989;19:520–522.

380. Wesenberg RL, Blumhagen JD. Assisted expiratory chest radiography. An effective technique for the diagnosis of foreign body aspiration. *Radiology* 1979;130:538–539.

381. Burton EM, Riggs W Jr, Kaufman RA, Houston CS. Pneumomediastinum caused by foreign body aspiration in children. *Pediatr Radiol* 1989;20:45–47.

382. Berdon WE, Dee GJ, Abramson SJ, et al. Localized pneumnothorax adjacent to a collapsed lobe: a sign of bronchial obstruction. *Radiology* 1984;150:691–694.

383. Wolfe BM, Brodeur AE, Shields JB. The role of gastrointestinal absorption of kerosene in producing pneumonitis in dogs. *J Pediatr* 1970;76:867–873.

384. Daeschner CW, Blattner RJ, Collins VP. Hydrocarbon pneumonitis: respiratory disorders. *Pediatr Clin North Am* 1957;4:243–253.

385. Eade NR, Taussig LM, Marks MI. Hydrocarbon pneumonitis. *Pediatrics* 1974;54:351–357.

386. Modell JH. Drowning. *N Engl J Med* 1993;328:253–256.

387. Putman CE, Tummillo AM, Myerson DA, Myerson PJ. Drowning: another plunge. *AJR* 1975;125:543–548.

388. Wintemute GJ. Childhood drowning and near-drowning in the United States. *Am J Dis Child* 1990;144:663–669.

389. Harle TS, Kountoupis JT, Boone ML, Fred HL. Pulmonary edema without cardiomegaly. *AJR* 1968;103:555–560.

Practical Pediatric Imaging: Diagnostic Radiology of Infants and Children, Third Edition.
D. R. Kirks, editor and N. T. Griscom, associate editor.
Lippincott–Raven Publishers, Philadelphia © 1998.

CHAPTER 8

Gastrointestinal Tract

Carlo Buonomo, George A. Taylor, Jane C. Share, and Donald R. Kirks

C. Buonomo, G. A. Taylor, J. C. Share, and D. R. Kirks: Department of Radiology, Children's Hospital, Harvard Medical School, Boston, Massachusetts 02115.

Gastrointestinal (GI) radiology in children has little in common with GI radiology in adults. The diseases that are of greatest interest to the pediatric radiologist, such as malrotation and intussusception, are usually the least familiar to general radiologists, and the fluoroscopic techniques used by the pediatric radiologist are often quite different from those used for adults. There is of course some common ground between pediatric and adult GI imaging. The basic principles of fluoroscopic, ultrasonographic, and computed tomographic (CT) diagnosis are the same in children and adults, and certain conditions, such as inflammatory bowel disease, are important in both pediatrics and adult medicine. This chapter, however, will concentrate on those conditions that occur exclusively or almost exclusively in children and on the radiologic techniques used to evaluate them. When a disease is common in both children and adults, the manifestations unique to childhood will be emphasized. Diseases that are of great importance in adult GI imaging but occur only rarely in children, such as carcinoma, will be mentioned in passing or not at all.

The aim is to help the reader develop a practical, informed approach to the imaging of the more common pediatric GI diseases. The chapter is comprehensive but not exhaustive, covering those topics with which any radiologist who cares for children should be familiar. For a more detailed discussion, the reader is referred to the excellent textbooks of Franken and Smith (1) and Stringer (2).

The chapter has seven sections. In the first, the radiologic techniques used in pediatric GI imaging are discussed. The second section is devoted to the radiologic approach to a few general pediatric abnormalities, such as abdominal masses and GI bleeding. The third and largest section describes diseases of the bowel and is organized by patient age. The fourth, fifth, and sixth sections cover the liver, spleen, and pancreas. The final section is devoted to imaging of blunt abdominal trauma.

TECHNIQUES

This section provides a general description of the most important techniques used in pediatric GI radiology. Detailed discussions of techniques for specific clinical situations, e.g., ultrasonography in pyloric stenosis, are found in the sections devoted to those conditions.

Radiography

Abdominal Radiography

Plain films of the abdomen are the foundation of GI imaging and should be obtained before contrast examinations and other special studies. Pediatric GI radiology is above all plain film radiology. In many situations, including vague or chronic abdominal pain and constipation, an anteroposterior (AP) supine radiograph of the abdomen is the only film required. One of the most common, and most important, indications for abdominal radiography is evaluation of the acute abdomen. The primary objective of abdominal films in this setting is to distinguish surgical from nonsurgical disease: a horizontal beam radiograph is thus necessary in addition to the supine film in order to demonstrate free intraperitoneal air or air-fluid levels in obstructed bowel. The horizontal beam film may be obtained by erect, supine cross-table lateral, or decubitus positioning.

Berdon and colleagues have emphasized the advantages of prone abdominal films (3). Plain films of the abdomen should be considered contrast studies of the intestine using air as the contrast medium. In the supine position, air fills ventral portions of the alimentary tract, namely, the gastric antrum, anteriorly located small bowel loops, and the transverse and sigmoid colon. In the prone position, air moves into the gastric fundus, the duodenal bulb, more posteriorly located small bowel loops, ascending and descending colon, and the rectum. The prone film may thus be very helpful in distinguishing large from small bowel and for excluding small bowel obstruction (Fig. 8-1). A supine AP film and a horizontal beam film make up the basic acute abdominal series. The usefulness of the prone film should be stressed but the decision to obtain one left to the individual radiologist.

Upper Gastrointestinal Series

Techniques for examination of the upper gastrointestinal (UGI) tract depend on the indication, patient age, and differential diagnostic considerations. To perform a thorough evaluation with a minimum of radiation, the examination must be tailored to the child's problem. The most common indications in a newborn or infant are vomiting, especially bilious vomiting, and respiratory problems such as apnea, stridor, or pneumonia, possibly caused by aspiration, gastroesophageal reflux, or a tracheoesophageal fistula. In older children, the study is usually performed for vomiting, abdominal pain, or failure to thrive.

Very little preparation of the patient is necessary (see Appendix 1). As a general rule, feeding is withheld for the usual interval between feedings. A child who is not hungry will not drink barium; a child, however, who has fasted for too long is usually irritable and is even less likely to drink barium. Premature infants and newborns should thus fast for no more than 2 or 3 hours before the study; older infants and young children for 3 or 4 hours. In older children, a 6-hour fast is adequate. Preparation of older children for a double-contrast UGI is the same as for adults.

Parents are encouraged and almost always agree to stay with the child during the exam. We do not use any devices to immobilize infants for a UGI series or for a contrast enema. Those devices are not necessary, and their use causes unnecessary anxiety for the patient and family. The technologist and parent(s) sit at the head of the fluoroscopy table, hold the upper body, and feed the baby; the radiologist helps

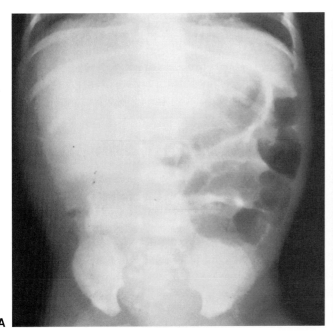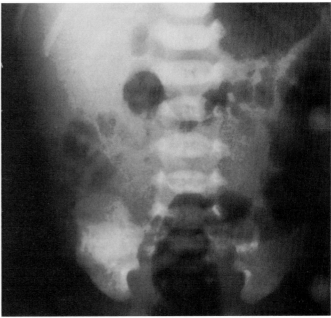

A B

FIG. 8-1. Value of prone abdominal radiograph to exclude small bowel obstruction. A: Supine abdominal radiograph demonstrates distended bowel in the left abdomen and a paucity of bowel gas distally, suggesting obstruction. **B:** Prone abdominal radiograph clearly distinguishes large and small bowel. Air has moved to the rectosigmoid and descending colon. There is no evidence of mechanical obstruction. (From Johnson JF, Robinson L. Localized bowel distention in the newborn: a review of plain film analysis and differential diagnosis. *Pediatrics* 1984;73:206–215.)

immobilize and comfort the baby (Fig. 8-2). Radiation exposure is minimized by use of digital low-dose fluoroscopy, small field size, and gonadal shielding.

Barium is the best contrast agent for UGI examinations. It is inexpensive and safe and provides the best images. The primary use of water-soluble contrast agents is when perforation or postoperative anastomotic leakage is suspected. High-osmolality, water-soluble contrast agents such as meglumine diatrizoate (Gastrografin, ER Squibb and Co., New Brunswick, NJ) and intravenous contrast agents have no place in UGI studies in children because their hyperosmolal-ity may lead to significant fluid shifts and, if aspirated, to severe pulmonary edema. Cystographic agents such as iotha-lamate meglumine (Cystoconray II, Mallinckrodt Inc., St. Louis, MO) are not markedly hypertonic, but their low iodine concentration makes them unsatisfactory for use in the UGI tract. However, low-osmolality nonionic water-soluble contrast media such as metrizamide, iopamidol, iohexol, and ioxaglate have become very important in pediatric GI radiology (4). These compounds contain enough iodine for acceptable images at only slightly hyperosmolar concentrations (see Appendix 5). Because they are nearly iso-osmolar, there

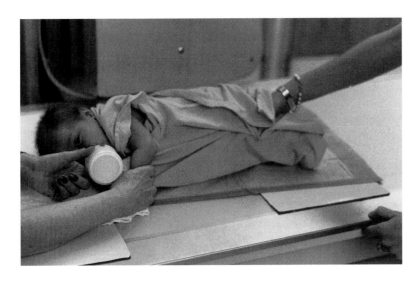

FIG. 8-2. Upper gastrointestinal series. Adequate immobilization for a UGI series is provided by the radiologist and technologist or parent(s).

is little risk of fluid shifts; as a consequence, they not only are safer but also do not become diluted and thus allow high-quality images for prolonged periods. These are also the least harmful agents if aspirated (4,5). Because these agents are much more expensive than barium and do not opacify the bowel as well (6), they should be used in only a few situations. They are the agents of choice to show the proximal pouch in esophageal atresia, to show an esophageal perforation or leak after repair of esophageal atresia, when there is very high risk of aspiration as in neurologically impaired children, and when a UGI must be performed in a small child with massive gastroesophageal reflux and lessened ability to protect the airway. They are also the best agents in premature infants in whom there are nonspecific abdominal signs. They allow prolonged imaging in babies who may have unsuspected necrotizing enterocolitis, perforation, or obstruction, and who, even in the absence of specific abnormalities, often have very slow intestinal transit (7).

In a young child, the administration of barium may be difficult. Infants will usually take barium readily from a bottle. Older children can drink from a cup, directly or with a straw. The infant or young child who is unwilling to drink and whose examination requires only a small amount of barium can usually be fed from a catheter-tipped syringe, with care taken to not overfill the mouth. In uncooperative children for whom larger amounts of barium are needed, a nasogastric tube, usually an 8-French feeding tube, may be used. After the tip of the tube is fluoroscopically shown to be in the stomach, barium is injected; after this, barium can be injected into the esophagus as the tube is withdrawn. Most children tolerate tube placement quite well, and an expeditious study via a nasogastric tube is more acceptable than a prolonged struggle with a child who is unwilling or unable to drink. Barium should be administered through a nasogastric tube in newborns suspected of having upper intestinal obstruction; in this setting, the tube is needed to empty the stomach before the study and to drain it of barium after the study. The tube also allows more precise control of the amount of barium given and prevents overfilling.

At first, barium is administered in the lateral position, with the left side down. In this position, the barium collects in the gastric fundus. The stomach must not empty until the radiologist has evaluated the esophagus; premature filling of the duodenum may make it impossible to locate the duodenojejunal junction. In the left lateral position swallowing function, esophageal peristalsis and esophageal contour are evaluated. Special attention is given to any extrinsic impressions on the esophagus (Fig. 8-3A). The child is then turned supine, and the contour of the esophagus evaluated again (Fig. 8-3B). The child is then rotated into a prone right anterior oblique (RAO) position, which allows barium to flow into the gastric antrum (Fig. 8-3C). Barium then passes into the duodenum. In the neonate or young infant, a nearly lateral position may be required for demonstration of the pylorus and duodenum. After barium has filled the duodenum, the infant is quickly turned to the supine position to locate the duodenojejunal junction (ligament of Treitz) (Fig. 8-3D).

The patient may then be returned to the prone RAO position for additional evaluation of the pylorus and duodenal bulb. In most cases, a single AP overhead film of the abdomen is then obtained to evaluate the proximal small bowel. No other routine films are obtained. This standard exam thus includes a scout film of the abdomen, spot films of the esophagus in lateral and frontal projections, the stomach and duodenal sweep in the RAO projection, and, most importantly, the stomach and duodenum in the supine position to demonstrate the duodenojejunal junction. No UGI series is complete without a frontal film showing the duodenojejunal junction, which should be to the left of the spine at the level of the duodenal bulb, approximately halfway between the greater and lesser curvatures of the stomach (Fig. 8-3D).

In older children who can cooperate and in whom there is an appropriate indication such as the suspicion of ulcer, a double-contrast exam may be performed, as in the adult.

Small Bowel Series

Common indications for small bowel examination in children include chronic or recurrent abdominal pain, unexplained GI blood loss, malabsorption, suspicion of inflammatory bowel disease, chronic small intestinal obstruction, and protein-losing enteropathy.

The small bowel is usually examined by antegrade examination after evaluation of the esophagus, stomach, and duodenum. The use of greater amounts of barium reduces the number of radiographs needed to show all parts of the small bowel: additional barium must therefore be given after the completion of the UGI series. Films are taken at 30- to 60-minute intervals until barium can be seen in the cecum. Each film is immediately reviewed after processing. Fluoroscopy and compression spot films are used if any pathology is identified on overhead films and always to show the terminal ileum. The anatomy and peristaltic activity of the terminal ileum are evaluated at fluoroscopy with manual compression. When inflammatory bowel disease is suspected the barium is frequently followed into the colon. There is good correlation between findings on so-called antegrade colonography and colonoscopy. Antegrade colonography requires no more than an additional film or two, provides information about areas of the colon that may not be seen by endoscopy, and occasionally reveals unexpected pathology (8).

The terminal ileum can also be examined by refluxing barium into the ileum during an enema. Enteroclysis (small bowel enema) is rarely indicated in children, and the diagnostic yield is low in a child who has had a negative, good-quality small bowel follow-through (9,10). Enteroclysis is sometimes used to evaluate a small bowel mass seen on a small bowel series or an area of possibly abnormal small bowel seen on a small bowel series in a child with the question of inflammatory bowel disease. Good results are obtained with the method of enteroclysis used by Stringer and colleagues (2,9).

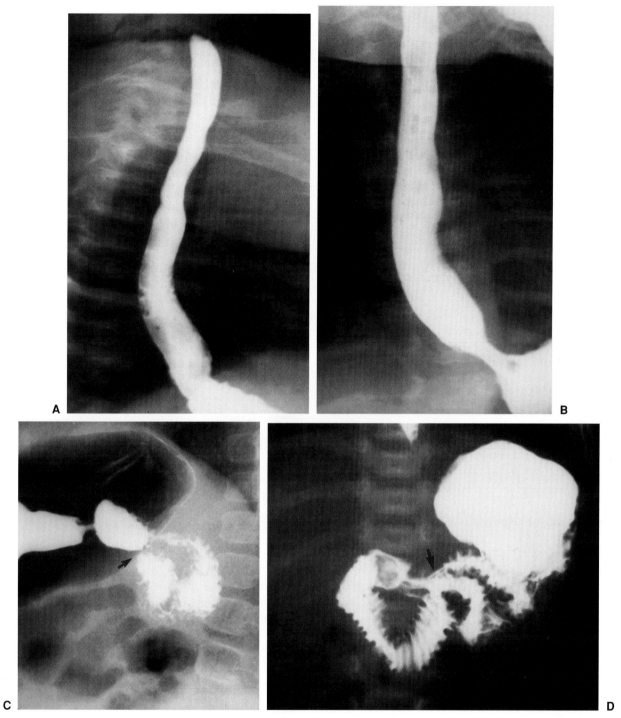

FIG. 8-3. Normal UGI Series. A: Lateral view of esophagus. **B:** AP view of esophagus. **C:** Steep RAO view demonstrating the pylorus, duodenal bulb, and duodenojejunal junction *(arrow)*. **D:** AP view demonstrating normal duodenojejunal junction *(arrow)*.

Contrast Enema

The main indication for contrast enemas in newborns is the possiblity of low intestinal obstruction. In older infants and children, the usual indications are obscure abdominal pain, constipation, and lower GI bleeding.

For enemas in newborns with low intestinal obstruction, a dilute water-soluble agent such as Cystoconray II is used. Details about this extremely important subject are given in the discussion of intestinal obstruction in the newborn. In older infants and children, water-soluble contrast is used only when perforation is suspected. Undiluted hypertonic agents such as Gastrografin have no role in diagnostic studies in infants and children, for reasons already given. The expensive low-osmolar nonionic agents are also not used for enemas. Air is used for the diagnosis and treatment of intussusception. In all other situations, barium is the agent of choice.

Rigorous cleansing of the colon is seldom required in children (see Appendix 1). One is usually not searching for small intraluminal or mucosal lesions unless there is lower GI bleeding. If the study is for chronic constipation (''rule out Hirschsprung disease''), no bowel preparation is given. Patients with acute inflammatory bowel disease or other acute abdominal conditions also require no preparation; in fact, they rarely need a contrast enema at all. In the child with rectal bleeding thought to be due to polyps or inflammatory bowel disease, a double-contrast enema is performed after thorough cleansing of the colon. In inflammatory bowel disease, cleansing is accomplished with a liquid diet and enemas. If polyps are suspected, adequate cleansing requires a liquid diet, laxatives, and enemas (see Appendix 1).

The use of a balloon-type enema tip is not advised in infants and young children, as it may perforate the rectum or misleadingly distend the narrowed rectum of Hirschsprung disease. In neonates and infants, a blunt red rubber catheter of appropriate size (usually 14–24 French) is used. The catheter may be modified by the addition of a metal washer placed an appropriate distance from its tip (11). The metal washer serves three functions: it marks the anus, it prevents pushing the tube too far into the rectum, and it helps keep the tube taped in place. In older children, standard disposable enema tips may be used (11) (Fig. 8-4).

The patient is immobilized by the technologist and parent with the arms above the head, as for a UGI series. No restraining devices are employed. The enema tip is introduced an appropriate distance into the rectum, and the buttocks are taped shut around the tubing and metal washer. Contrast should be administered by gravity whenever possible; a syringe may be used for the fluoroscopically monitored injection of contrast in the neonate.

Fluoroscopic examination must begin with the patient in the lateral position to allow visualization of the caliber and contour of the rectum during filling. Spot films of the rectum in the lateral position must be obtained. The patient is then turned into various positions as barium fills each segment of the colon. The examination is ended when there is definite

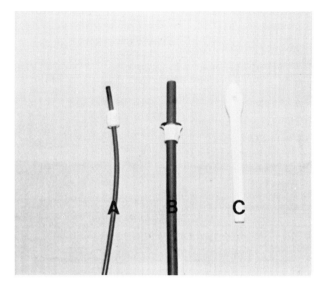

FIG. 8-4. Pediatric enema tips. A: A 14-French red Robinson catheter with metal washer, for newborns and infants less than 6 months of age. **B:** A 24-French red Robinson catheter with metal washer, for older infants and young children. **C:** Plastic enema tip, for children over 5 years of age. From Kirks et al. (11).

filling of the cecum, confirmed by complete filling of the appendix or reflux of contrast into the terminal ileum. In studies performed on constipated children in whom Hirschsprung disease is the only consideration, filling to the splenic flexure is usually sufficient.

The number and type of overhead films depend on the indications for the examination and the pathology demonstrated at fluoroscopy. Preevacuation and postevacuation overhead AP radiographs of the abdomen often suffice. Double-contrast exams, as in adults, require many overhead films.

Modified Barium Swallow

Evaluation of swallowing should be a part of all UGI series, especially in newborns and infants. The complexity and speed of swallowing, however, make thorough evaluation difficult on the routine UGI series. Patients with swallowing problems are better evaluated with a modified barium swallow (video swallowing study), which differs from a standard UGI in several respects. The child eats or is fed in the position in which he would eat at home, usually sitting. This is facilitated by special chairs adapted for fluoroscopy (see Fig. 1-20). Children are fed different types and textures of food to exclude aspiration and assess the ease with which they are consumed. The study is videotaped so that the complex process of swallowing can be viewed repeatedly and in slow motion. The study is preferably done with experienced speech pathologists and therapists, who can formulate a feeding plan based on the findings. The modified barium swallow is most useful in children with cerebral palsy or other types of neurologic impairment.

Ultrasonography

Ultrasonography has many applications in pediatric GI imaging. Structures and abnormalities that may be imaged include masses and inflammation of the solid organs (liver, spleen, pancreas), the gallbladder and biliary tree, the GI tract (pyloric stenosis, appendicitis, GI inflammation), and ascites.

Ultrasonography should be guided in part by the history and by abnormalities shown by conventional radiography. Ultrasonography is less rewarding when performed because of vague symptoms without clinical or radiologic localization of an abnormality.

Pediatric abdominal sonographic examinations should include systematic evaluation of all abdominal and pelvic organs. One should develop a thorough, ordered routine. A good method is to begin with transverse views of the liver and its vessels, particularly including the hepatic veins and left, main, and right portal veins, keeping in mind that the left lobe of a baby's liver can be quite prominent. Transverse views of the pancreas, gallbladder, and right kidney are obtained. The relationship between the superior mesenteric artery (SMA) and vein (SMV) is evaluated; an abnormal orientation of these two vessels suggests malrotation. Transverse views are followed by longitudinal views of the liver, pancreas, gallbladder, aorta, inferior vena cava (IVC), and right kidney. The left upper quadrant is saved for next-to-last because children are often ticklish there. Longitudinal and transverse views of the spleen and left kidney are obtained. Before placing the child prone, views of the urinary bladder and the space behind it (to check for ascites) are obtained. The child is then placed prone for additional images of the kidneys, unless the likelihood of renal pathology is low.

A transducer of the highest frequency that allows penetration should be used. In infants, a 5-MHz linear array or sector transducer is used. A 7.5-MHz transducer can be used in the premature infant. In toddlers and small school-aged children, a 5-MHz transducer is appropriate. For older or chubby children, transducers appropriate for adults are used. A complete study is performed on most patients referred for any abdominal examination in order to search for unsuspected abnormalities and to provide a baseline for future comparisons.

Computed Tomography

CT is most commonly used to detect and delineate neoplasms, trauma, adenopathy, abscesses, complex fluid collections, and the complications of inflammatory bowel disease. Each examination should be tailored to the specific questions being asked to minimize radiation exposure, shorten the examination time, and ensure the child's cooperation. Except after blunt trauma, abdominal CT is never the first imaging study in newborns and young infants but is reserved for specific problems not solved with ultrasound (US).

With few exceptions, oral and intravenous (IV) contrast should be used routinely when scanning children. Two such exceptions are the immunocompromised child in whom microabscesses of the liver or spleen are suspected and the child with blunt abdominal trauma: these children do not usually need oral contrast. For specific information regarding slice thickness and oral and IV contrast, please refer to Chapter 1.

Magnetic Resonance Imaging

Magnetic resonance imaging (MRI), with its superb ability to distinguish among soft tissues, multiplanar imaging capability, lack of ionizing radiation, and ability to image vascular structures without intravenous contrast agents, is often used in the evaluation of neoplastic, inflammatory, and metabolic lesions of the liver (e.g., hemochromatosis) and, to a lesser extent, of the spleen and pancreas. Because of motion from intestinal peristalsis and limited spatial resolution, MRI is seldom used to study the GI tract itself.

The radiologist needs to tailor each MRI examination to its indications, combining different pulse sequences to detect and accentuate abnormalities. Because even minimal motion can create artifacts rendering the MR images nondiagnostic, children <6 years of age will usually need sedation. MRI is therefore not risk-free in infants and young children and should almost never be used as a first-line imaging modality. Specific scanning techniques, protocols, and sedation methods are given in Chapter 1.

Angiography

The utility of angiography in the evaluation of the GI tract is limited. The increasing availability of noninvasive imaging modalities such as US with duplex and color Doppler, helical CT, and magnetic resonance angiography have eliminated many of the previous indications for abdominal angiography. Much of pediatric GI angiography is now therapeutic rather than diagnostic. Indications for angiography include ischemia after organ transplantation, GI bleeding, vascular malformations, and, rarely, preoperative tumor evaluation with possible embolization prior to resection and chemotherapy infusion.

Although angiography is invasive and requires deep sedation or general anesthesia, the use of techniques and devices tailored to pediatric patients keeps risks and complications low. A more detailed discussion of pediatric angiographic techniques is given in Chapter 1.

Nuclear Medicine

Nuclear medicine provides physiologic information about the GI tract and solid abdominal organs. Esophageal and gastric motility, gastroesophageal reflux, and aspiration can be studied after the ingestion of a small dose of radiotracer, typically ^{99m}Tc-sulfur colloid. GI bleeding may be evaluated by searching for ectopic gastric mucosa in a Meckel diverticulum after administration of ^{99m}Tc-pertechnetate. Acute GI bleeding may be assessed after administration of ^{99m}Tc-labeled red blood cells (RBCs) or ^{99m}Tc-sulfur colloid. Leukocytes labeled with either ^{99m}Tc or ^{111}In have been used to evaluate children with inflammatory bowel disease and in the diagnostic workup of appendicitis. Imaging with ^{99m}Tc-labeled iminodiacetic acid (IDA) analogs is important in hepatic and biliary abnormalities, particularly neonatal jaundice and choledochal cyst, and in assessing the results of hepatic resection, liver transplantation, and portoenterostomy (Kasai procedure). Radionuclide imaging of the spleen after administration of heat-denatured ^{99m}Tc-RBCs or ^{99m}Tc-sulfur colloid can demonstrate the presence or absence of functioning splenic tissue and evaluate the possibility of polysplenia in cases of heterotaxy. Scintigraphy is also used to evaluate abnormalities of splenic position, splenosis after trauma or splenectomy, and splenic perfusion and function in children with sickle cell disease. Scintigraphy is rarely performed to evaluate solid hepatic masses in children.

GENERAL ABNORMALITIES

Common Abdominal Emergencies

Acute abdominal disease in children is caused by many pathologic processes. Many of these abnormalities are peculiar to childhood and have unique radiologic manifestations. Imaging is frequently critical for accurate diagnosis and proper treatment of acute pediatric abdominal disease. This is particularly true in infants and young children in whom the history may be unhelpful, abnormalities in one anatomic region may be referred to another, and the physical examination may be nonspecific.

Some of the more common general abdominal emergencies of childhood are discussed below. The diagnostic approach, imaging techniques, and radiologic features of specific abdominal emergencies of infants and children are presented in subsequent sections. The emphasis is on practical approaches to common pediatric abnormalities.

Pneumoperitoneum

Pneumoperitoneum is the presence of free air in the peritoneal cavity. It is due to an abnormal communication between an air-containing space and the peritoneal cavity. Entry of air into the peritoneal cavity is usually due to a perforation of the GI tract, air block with dissection of air from the chest into the abdomen, or recent abdominal surgery. In the absence of a history of recent surgery and air block, pneumoperitoneum strongly suggests a bowel perforation and is a surgical emergency.

The etiology of pneumoperitoneum is different at different ages (Table 8-1). By far the most common cause of neonatal

TABLE 8-1. *Causes of pneumoperitoneum*

Neonate
  Perforation of gastrointestinal tract
    Necrotizing enterocolitis (NEC)[a]
    Idiopathic gastric perforation
    Distal intestinal obstruction[a]
    Isolated perforation not associated with NEC
    Ruptured Meckel diverticulum
    Stress ulcer or peptic ulcer
  Iatrogenic
    Air-block: dissection from penumomediastinum[a]
    Gastric performation[a]
      Nasogastric tube
      Mechanical ventilation
      Indomethacin
    Small bowel perforation due to indomethacin
    Colon perforation
      Thermometer
      Enema
    Laparotomy
    Paracentesis
    Resuscitation
Older infant and child
  Perforation of gastrointestinal tract
    Peptic ulcer or stress ulcer[a]
    Ruptured Meckel diverticulum
    Blunt trauma
    Perforated appendix
  Iatrogenic
    Air-block: dissection from pneumomediastinum[a]
    Laparotomy[a]
    Paracentesis
    Percutaneous biopsy
    Resuscitation
  Perforation of other viscus
    Uterus
    Vagina
    Air-filled bladder
  Traumatic passage of air from vagina through Fallopian tubes

[a] More common.

pneumoperitoneum is perforation due to necrotizing enterocolitis (NEC). Other causes include idiopathic gastric perforation, isolated perforation not associated with NEC, dissection of air from a pneumomediastinum, distal bowel obstruction, and iatrogenic causes such as perforation of the stomach by nasogastric tubes or mechanical ventilation (12,13), perforation due to indomethacin therapy (14), and perforation of the rectum caused by an enema or a thermometer (15). Common causes of pneumoperitoneum in the older infant and child include perforated ulcer and dissection from a pneumomediastinum.

Pneumoperitoneum may be caused by the dissection of air from the chest into the peritoneal cavity (Fig. 8-5) (16). It usually occurs in neonates with hyaline membrane disease who develop pulmonary interstitial emphysema, pneumomediastinum, and pneumothorax while receiving positive pressure ventilation. As initially described by Macklin and Macklin, air may dissect directly from the mediastinum through the diaphragmatic hiatus into the retroperitoneum

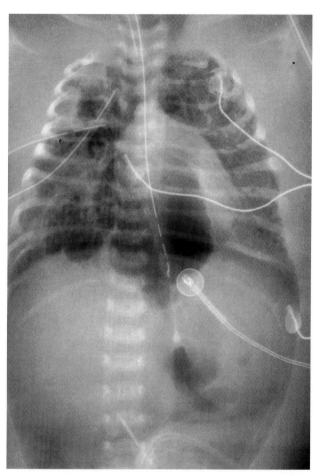

FIG. 8-5. Pneumoperitoneum secondary to air block. Massive pneumoperitoneum in an infant with severe viral pneumonia and pneumomediastinum; air in the left retrocardiac region is probably in or beneath the pulmonary ligament.

cavity after surgery usually indicates perforation or anastomotic breakdown.

The radiologist must be familiar with the subtle signs of pneumoperitoneum on supine abdominal radiographs. Diagnosis can be confirmed by a horizontal beam radiograph. This may be an erect, left lateral decubitus, or supine cross-table lateral view; the latter two are more usual in an ill child. A detailed discussion of the plain film findings of pneumoperitoneum is given in the section on NEC.

GI Bleeding

A number of entities can cause GI bleeding in infants and children; these entities are, in general, quite different from those that cause GI bleeding in the adult (Table 8-2) (20, 21). The list of causes varies with the child's age and the severity and character of the bleeding. Bright red or coffee-ground emesis or aspirated gastric fluid and melena indicate a site of hemorrhage proximal to the ligament of Treitz. Passage of red blood via the rectum usually implies a colonic source of hemorrhage. Lower GI bleeding is much more

TABLE 8-2. *Causes of gastrointestinal bleeding*

Newborn
    Swallowed maternal blood[a]
    Anal fissure[a]
    Gastritis
    Necrotizing enterocolitis[a]
    Allergic colitis[a]
    Infectious colitis
    Midgut volvulus
    Systemic hypoperfusion, shock
Infants and young children
    Esophagitis[a]
    Gastritis[a]
    Stress ulcer
    Peptic ulcer
    Meckel diverticulum
    Intussusception[a]
    Anal fissure[a]
    Allergic colitis[a]
    Infectious colitis
    Colonic polyp
    Henoch-Schönlein purpura
    Foreign body
Older children
    Esophagitis[a]
    Esophageal varices
    Gastritis[a]
    Peptic ulcer[a]
    Meckel diverticulum[a]
    Colonic polyp[a]
    Anal fissure[a]
    Foreign body
    Infectious colitis[a]
    Inflammatory bowel disease[a]
    Henoch-Schönlein purpura
    Hemolytic-uremic syndrome

[a] More common

with subsequent rupture of air into the peritoneal cavity (17). Air may also dissect from the mediastinum through the sternocostal attachments of the diaphragm into the anterior extraperitoneal space (18). The development of pneumoperitoneum in a patient who is on a respirator without other evidence of air block phenomena can be a diagnostic problem. Has this air dissected from the chest, or does the patient have a GI perforation? The presence of air-fluid levels in the peritoneal cavity by a horizontal beam film makes a perforation more likely. A small amount of fluid, however, may be seen in the peritoneal cavity in patients with dissection of air from the chest, and the absence of air-fluid levels does not exclude a ruptured viscus. Paracentesis and fluid analysis may indicate a GI perforation. Examination of the GI tract with water-soluble contrast material may be indicated to exclude or confirm the presence of GI perforation (see Fig. 8-98) (19).

The amount of persistent intraperitoneal air following laparotomy correlates with the size of the patient; postoperative air disappears more quickly in children than in adults. Postoperative intraperitoneal air in children usually disappears in 3 or 4 days. An increasing amount of air within the peritoneal

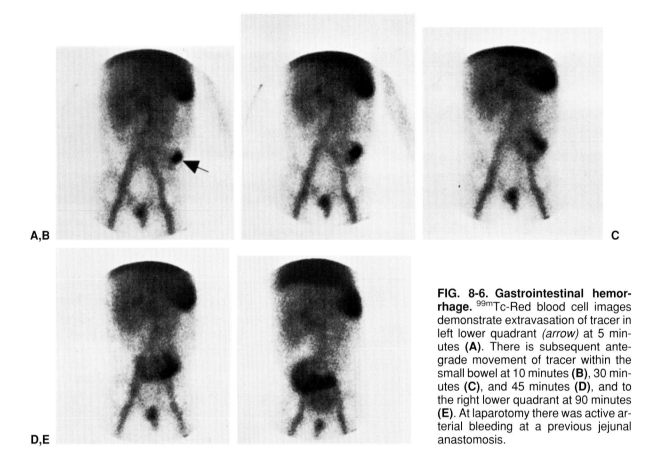

A,B

C

D,E

FIG. 8-6. Gastrointestinal hemorrhage. ^{99m}Tc-Red blood cell images demonstrate extravasation of tracer in left lower quadrant *(arrow)* at 5 minutes **(A)**. There is subsequent antegrade movement of tracer within the small bowel at 10 minutes **(B)**, 30 minutes **(C)**, and 45 minutes **(D)**, and to the right lower quadrant at 90 minutes **(E)**. At laparotomy there was active arterial bleeding at a previous jejunal anastomosis.

common in childhood than upper GI bleeding. Massive hemorrhage is unusual in children, unless there is a hemorrhagic diathesis, portal hypertension, or a vascular malformation of the GI tract. Less common causes of massive hemorrhage are gastritis, ulcer disease, and Meckel diverticulum.

GI bleeding is usually not an isolated symptom in newborns. When it is isolated, it usually ceases spontaneously and rarely has a surgical cause (22). Blood may be present in the stool in such very important conditions as malrotation with volvulus and the colitis associated with Hirschsprung disease, but other symptoms usually dominate. In premature infants, bloody stool often indicates necrotizing enterocolitis, but again it is part of a larger symptom complex. In asymptomatic newborns, hematemesis or "heme-positive stool" is frequently due to swallowed maternal blood. Blood staining of the diaper is usually due to an anal fissure. Babies with milk-protein allergy may have blood loss without other symptoms. In infants and young children without other symptoms, bleeding is likely to be due to a Meckel diverticulum or a juvenile polyp. Bloody stool in infants and children is also common in intussusception, infectious colitis, Henoch-Schönlein purpura, hemolytic uremic syndrome, and inflammatory bowel disease; again, there are usually other symptoms.

The diagnostic approach to isolated GI bleeding must be

tailored to the age and the suspected site of bleeding. Endoscopy is the procedure of choice for infants and children with isolated upper GI bleeding (23). The upper GI series is not useful in acute bleeding and should be reserved for children in whom there is chronic or intermittent blood loss. The small bowel series is the best study when Crohn's disease is suspected. In acute lower GI bleeding, sigmoidoscopy is the procedure of choice; the barium enema is reserved for patients with chronic blood loss.

When the site of bleeding remains obscure despite the history and physical examination, scintigraphy performed with ^{99m}Tc-labeled red blood cells can accurately localize sites of active bleeding (Fig. 8-6). Rates of bleeding as slow as 0.1–0.4 ml/min can be detected with this method (24). If the lesion is a Meckel diverticulum, it can be localized with scintigraphy employing ^{99m}Tc-pertechnetate, which is taken up by ectopic gastric mucosa in the diverticulum. Angiography is usually reserved for patients in whom therapeutic angiographic intervention is anticipated.

In summary, GI bleeding is a much less common problem in pediatrics than in adult medicine, and its causes are very different. Most GI bleeding is accompanied by other signs and symptoms that suggest the correct diagnosis; when this is not true, radiologic techniques are useful as adjuncts to endoscopy.

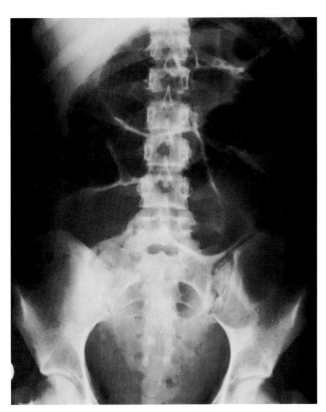

FIG. 8-7. Mechanical small bowel obstruction. Supine film demonstrates many dilated loops of small bowel but no air in the colon or rectum. The soft-tissue mass in the pelvis is a cul-de-sac abscess following an appendiceal perforation.

Acquired Intestinal Obstruction

Obstruction is defined as failure of passage of intestinal contents (including air) through the alimentary tract. It may be congenital or acquired. The approach to intestinal obstruction in the newborn is very different from the approach to acquired intestinal obstruction, which is the subject here. It is important to distinguish mechanical obstruction from paralytic ileus. *Mechanical obstruction* is an impeded intestinal passage of contents due to any mechanical hindrance. *Paralytic ileus* (adynamic ileus) is impedance, usually temporary, of the passage of intestinal contents due to lack of peristalsis (25).

The radiologic hallmark of mechanical small bowel obstruction is disproportionate dilatation of a portion of small bowel compared to the more distal small bowel or colon (Fig. 8-7). The number of dilated small bowel loops depends on the anatomic level of obstruction. This dilatation is at first local, immediately above the obstruction. Eventually, distention affects loop after loop of bowel to produce the classic "step-ladder" appearance. Air-fluid levels are usually present; air-fluid levels in the same loop of bowel may be at different heights. The diagnosis of mechanical small bowel obstruction may be difficult if there are many fluid-filled loops of bowel or if there is displacement of bowel by a mass.

In older children the small bowel can usually be readily distinguished from the colon by both appearance and location. Distended small bowel is usually centrally located, and valvulae conniventes can be seen extending completely across its lumen. Distended colon lies peripherally in the abdomen, and its haustra do not extend completely across the lumen. Unfortunately, in newborns and infants the distinction between small bowel and colon may be difficult or impossible. Well-defined haustra are not present early in life; moreover, distended small bowel frequently displaces the colon and may thus be much more lateral than normal (see Fig. 8-59). Prone views may help make the distinction (see Fig. 8-1), but contrast studies are often necessary.

One of the aims of this chapter is to remind the reader of the differential diagnosis of acquired small bowel obstruction in children (Table 8-3). This aim is spelled AAIIMM, with the letters standing for the common causes of acquired small bowel obstruction in children: adhesions from previous surgery; appendicitis, frequently with abscess formation; incarcerated inguinal hernia; intussusception; malrotation with volvulus; and miscellaneous (e.g., Meckel diverticulum, duplication, ingested foreign body). Malrotation, Meckel diverticulum, and duplication are not, of course, truly acquired anomalies. They are included in this mnemonic, however, to stress that unlike most other causes of congenital intestinal obstruction they may and frequently do present well into childhood. Even if one includes congenital causes, intussusception is the most common cause of mechanical obstruction of infants and children.

Adynamic (paralytic) ileus frequently occurs after major abdominal, retroperitoneal, and spinal surgery. It is also common with inflammatory diseases such as sepsis, pneumonia, peritonitis, pancreatitis, and urinary tract infection (Table 8-3). Functional intestinal disturbances are also seen with electrolyte disturbances, dehydration, autonomic nervous system dysfunction, various drugs, hypothyroidism, and idiopathic intestinal pseudoobstruction.

Paralytic ileus is characterized by accumulation of both gas and fluid in all parts of the GI tract. The distal bowel seldom empties itself, which distinguishes paralytic ileus from mechanical obstruction. Pain is not an important clinical feature until abdominal distention becomes marked. There is no visible peristalsis, and no bowel sounds are audible by auscultation. There may be numerous, short air-fluid levels on upright films in patients with paralytic ileus. In confusing cases a prone film and even a contrast enema may be necessary to clarify the location and caliber of the colon and exclude mechanical obstruction.

Intraperitoneal Fluid

There are many causes of intraperitoneal fluid in infants and children. These causes may be classified by the age of the patient (neonates versus infants and older children) and

TABLE 8-3. *Acquired gastrointestinal obstruction*

Mechanical obstruction
  Esophagus
    Foreign body[a]
    Stricture
    Achalasia
    Prior surgery[a]
  Stomach
    Hypertrophic pyloric stenosis[a]
    Peptic ulcer
    Hematoma
    Bezoar
    Gastric volvulus
  Duodenum and small bowel
    Peptic ulcer
    Superior mesenteric artery syndrome
    Adhesions[a]
    Meckel diverticulum
    Appendicitis[a]
    Inguinal hernia[a]
    Intussusception[a]
    Neoplasm
    Bezoar
    Malrotation[a], volvulus[a]
    Henoch-Schönlein purpura
  Colon
    Post-necrotizing enterocolitis stricture[a]
    Inflammatory stricture
    Stricture associated with cystic fibrosis
    Ischemic stricture
    Posttraumatic stricture
    Volvulus: cecal; sigmoid
    Adhesions
    Inguinal hernia[a]
    Intussusception
    Neoplasm
    Duplication
    Hemolytic uremic syndrome
Paralytic ileus
  Inflammatory[a]
    Sepsis
    Gastroenteritis
    Peritonitis
    Pancreatitis
    Urinary tract infection
  Trauma[a]
    Major surgery
    Blunt trauma
  Metabolic
    Hypokalemia
    Hypoglycemia
    Disordered calcium metabolism
    Dehydration
  Miscellaneous
    Vasculitis
    Henoch-Schönlein purpura
    Hemolytic uremic syndrome
    Autonomic nervous system dysfunction
    Anemia
    Hypothyroidism

[a] More common

TABLE 8-4. *Causes of intraperitoneal fluid*

Newborn
  Hydrops, immune and non-immune[a]
  Sepsis
  Fluid overload
  Congestive heart failure[a]
  Liver disease
  Portal vein thrombosis
  Perforation of the common bile duct
  Idiopathic gastric perforation
  Necrotizing enterocolitis[a]
  Bowel obstruction with perforation[a]
  Urinary tract obstruction with forniceal rupture[a]
  Congenital nephrosis
  Renal vein thrombosis
  Chylous ascites
  Hemoperitoneum after birth trauma
  Other trauma
Infants and older children
  Sepsis
  Fluid overload
  Congestive heart failure[a]
  Liver disease[a]
  Portal vein thrombosis
  Pancreatitis[a]
  Peritonitis
  Serositis (collagen vascular disease)
  Malignant ascites
  Bowel perforation[a]
  Inflammatory or infectious enteritis[a]
  Protein-losing enteropathy
  Appendicitis[a]
  Renal disease[a]
  Bladder rupture after augmentation
  Pelvic inflammatory disease
  Ruptured ovarian cyst[a]
  Trauma, including child abuse[a]

[a] More common

type of fluid (transudate, exudate, blood, chyle, urine, bile, intestinal contents) (Table 8-4).

Intraperitoneal fluid is best demonstrated by conventional radiography when it is located close to structures (properitoneal fat, bowel) that have a different density. Small amounts of intraperitoneal fluid accumulate first in the pelvis when the patient is erect or supine. Fluid then extends up the paracolic gutters into Morison's pouch. By this time, there is some fluid between loops of small bowel. Large amounts of intraperitoneal fluid may be interposed between the diaphragm and the liver even in the erect position. Common radiologic findings of intraperitoneal fluid in children include blurring of the tip of the liver or spleen, opacity lateral to the colon in the paracolic gutters, soft-tissue density in the pelvis, and central location of bowel loops (26). Ascertaining the cause of intraperitoneal fluid may require conventional radiography, ultrasonography, voiding cystourethrography, excretory urography, GI contrast studies, nuclear scintigraphy, CT, or MRI. Intraperitoneal fluid is easily demonstrated by US, which is the method of choice for confirming the diagnosis of intraperitoneal fluid, as it does not use

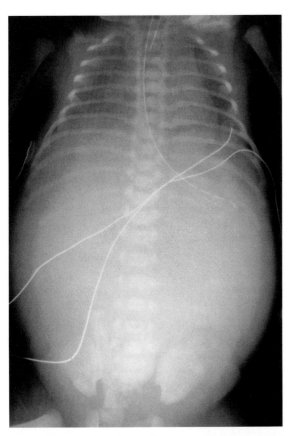

FIG. 8-8. Neonatal ascites. Supine radiograph reveals a gasless abdomen in a newborn boy with meconium peritonitis and ascites due to ileal perforation. The baby had cystic fibrosis. The opacities overlying the pelvis are the umbilical cord and its clip.

radiation, is simple, and detects small amounts of fluid. US is especially useful when the abdomen is gasless (27).

There are many causes of neonatal ascites; prompt diagnosis and appropriate therapy are necessary. In the newborn, the amount of intraperitoneal fluid is frequently large, causing centrally located and separated floating bowel loops, or even a gasless abdomen (Fig. 8-8). In newborns, ascites can sometimes be seen as a distinct lucency lateral to the denser liver (28). If there is vomiting or if bowel loops are abnormal on conventional films, a GI cause such as obstruction with perforation and peritonitis is likely. If there is peripheral or body wall edema, one should consider infection, heart disease, liver disease, or one of the causes of hydrops fetalis. If hepatomegaly is present, infectious, cardiac, and hepatic causes of ascites are likely. Urinary ascites accounts for at least 25% of cases and is the most common cause of ascites in male newborns (28). Urinary ascites is due to distal obstruction with back-pressure causing rupture of a calyceal fornix. This forniceal rupture results in passage of urine into the perirenal space and then the peritoneal cavity. In boys with urinary ascites, posterior urethral valves must be excluded.

Chylous ascites, an uncommon form of ascites, may occur at any age and may be congenital or acquired. Chylous ascites may be due to obstruction or trauma or may be idiopathic. Chyle has a high fat content after feeding has begun; before that, it is serous. The clinical and radiologic features of chylous ascites are those of any other cause of intraperitoneal fluid. Chylous ascites may be associated with chylothorax. There may be spontaneous recovery from chylous ascites. Treatment, if necessary, is usually drainage and institution of a diet of medium-chain triglycerides. These triglycerides are apparently absorbed directly into the portal system and bypass the lymphatic circulation.

Hemoperitoneum secondary to abdominal trauma may occur at any age. In the newborn, hemoperitoneum is related to birth trauma and is most frequently caused by a ruptured subcapsular hematoma of the liver. Laceration of an umbilical vessel occurs occasionally (29).

Abdominal Calcifications

Calcifications are uncommon on abdominal radiographs in children and should be assumed to be pathologic until proven otherwise (Table 8-5). As always in pediatrics, the most important diagnostic consideration is the patient's age. Another critical consideration is the precise anatomic location of the calcification.

In newborns calcification often occurs in the peritoneal cavity and is evidence of in utero intestinal perforation and subsequent meconium peritonitis. These calcifications are found anywhere in the peritoneum and may be punctate or in clumps (Fig. 8-9) but are often linear and peripheral, and as such can be easily identified as conforming to the peritoneum. Peritoneal calcifications may also be associated with a mass, the so-called meconium pseudocyst (see Fig. 8-74). In newborns calcification may occur in neoplasms, especially neuroblastoma; the calcifications may be found in the region, of the adrenal or in the pelvis. Adrenal hemorrhage occurs in children in whom there has been perinatal stress of many types; the hemorrhagic adrenal may calcify rapidly. Teratomas, either in the retroperitoneum or sacrococcygeal region may also calcify or ossify. Intrahepatic calcifications are found more and more frequently on prenatal US; although these calcifications can be associated with infection, an etiology is rarely found; if the calcifications are not associated with a mass, they appear to have little clinical importance (30). Neonatal liver tumors are usually not calcified. Meconium calcifies when it comes into contact with urine, as occurs in boys with anorectal malformations (Fig. 8-10) (31), in girls with the cloacal malformation, and when there is severe stasis of the intestinal contents, as may occur in intestinal atresias or total colonic Hirschsprung disease; newborns with these conditions may thus have intraluminal calcifications in the small or large intestine. In girls an ovary may become necrotic and calcify after torsion of an ovarian cyst; the calcified ovary may be amputated and then wander about the abdomen.

TABLE 8-5. *Abdominal calcification in children*

Peritoneal	Kidney
Meconium pseudocyst[a]	Nephrocalcinosis[a]
Meconium peritonitis[a]	Nephrolithiasis[a]
Mesenteric cyst	Tumor
Implants from ovarian teratoma	Wilms
Liver	Renal cell carcinoma
Inflammation	Metastatic
TORCHS	Urinoma
Abscess	Renal vein thrombosis
Granuloma	Necrosis
Tumor	Cortical
Hemangioendothelioma	Papillary
Hepatoblastoma[a]	Tubular
Hepatocellular carcinoma	Glomerulonephritis
Metastatic disease: neuroblastoma	Hematoma
Hepatic necrois	Focal ischemia
Post traumatic	Adrenal
Vascular	Adrenal hemorrhage[a]
Portal vein thromboemboli	Infarct
After umbilical vein catheterization	Tumor
Idiopathic[a]	Neuroblastoma[a]
Spleen	Carcinoma
Infection	Metastatic
TORCHS	Wolman disease
Histoplasmosis	Retroperitoneal teratoma
Tuberculosis	Scrotum
Hematoma	Meconium peritonitis
Tumor	Teratoma
Epidermoid	Gallbladder (Gallstones)
Dermoid	Idiopathic[a]
Sickle cell disease[a]	Hemolytic anemia[a]
Splenic cyst	Sickle cell anemia[a]
Bowel	Cystic fibrosis
Bowel stenosis or atresia	Interruption of enterohepatic circulation
Hirschsprung disease	Prolonged fasting, total parenteral nutrition[a]
Imperforate anus with rectourinary communication	Diuretics
Foreign body	Transfusions[a]
Appendicolith[a]	Anatomic malformation of biliary tract
Stone in Meckel diverticulum	Postoperative[a]
Pancreas	Sepsis
Pancreatitis[a]	Vascular system
Pseudocyst	Renal disease[a]
Chronic malnutrition	Catheter induced
Diabetes mellitus	Tumor thrombus
Cystic fibrosis	Inferior vena cava calcification
Granulomatous infection	Obliterated structures
	Umbilical veins
	Umbilical arteries
	Ductus venosus
	Genital
	Teratoma[a]
	Infarcted ovary

[a] More common

Source: Modified from Taybi H. Thoracic and abdominal calcifications in children. In: Margulis AR, Gooding, CA, eds. *Diagnostic radiology.* San Francisco: University of California, 1988.

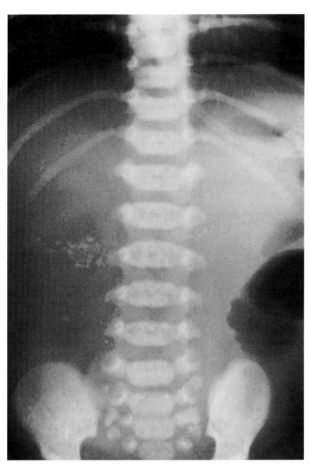

FIG. 8-9. Meconium peritonitis. Newborn male with jejunal atresia and meconium peritonitis. There are many punctate calcifications in the right midabdomen and several loops of distended jejunum in the left abdomen. From Kirks (96).

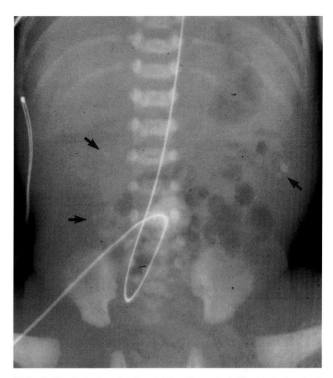

FIG. 8-10. Intraluminal calcification. Calcified intraluminal meconium *(arrows)* in a newborn boy with a high imperforate anus and a rectourethral fistula.

In infants and older children with calcifications one must think of tumors of the adrenal, liver, and ovary; calculi in the kidney and gallbladder; and appendicoliths. The exact location of the calcification is usually not difficult to ascertain in older children. When the etiology is unclear, US and CT are very useful.

Abdominal Masses

The diagnostic evaluation of an abdominal mass in an infant or child is a challenging problem. The role of diagnostic imaging is to identify the precise anatomic location, the organ of origin, and the extent of the pathologic process with a minimal number of imaging procedures.

This overview presents the differential diagnosis of abdominal masses in the neonate and then in the older child. The modern imaging modalities (US, nuclear scintigraphy, CT, and MRI) have dramatically changed the traditional approach to an abdominal mass in a child. The more common pediatric abdominal masses are discussed later in this chapter and in Chapter 9.

Imaging Modalities

Imaging modalities frequently used for the evaluation of pediatric abdominal masses include radiography, US, CT, MRI, and nuclear scintigraphy. Abdominal radiography is limited by its ability to distinguish only four densities: bone or mineral, soft tissue, fat, and air. The general location of a mass may be shown by radiography and the presence of calcification noted. Contrast studies of the GI tract are performed if the mass is thought to be intestinal in origin or intimately related to the GI tract.

US is the favored initial imaging modality, after preliminary radiography, for pediatric abdominal masses. It is readily available, does not utilize radiation, and is diagnostically accurate. US is particularly important in the newborn.

CT and MRI are superior in anatomic detail to other imaging modalities. CT and MRI are excellent for evaluating retroperitoneal masses, such as Wilms tumor and neuroblastoma. They provide anatomic and physiologic information about organs and vascular structures despite overlying gas and bone. MRI demonstrates beautifully the extent of disease, its effect on vascular and neural structures, and bone marrow involvement.

Nuclear scintigraphy has only a limited role in the evaluation of pediatric abdominal masses. Renal scintigraphy is superior to excretory urography for imaging and quantifying renal function, particularly during the first week of life. Angiography is currently indicated for abdominal masses only if a precise knowledge of segmental vascular anatomy is required (as for hepatoblastoma prior to resection) or if interventional techniques (e.g., embolization) are contemplated.

Excretory urography, once the cornerstone of the radiologic evaluation of abdominal masses in children, is now seldom used (32). However, a plain film or digital radiograph of the abdomen may be obtained after contrast-enhanced CT to obtain a "poor man's" excretory urogram.

Neonatal Abdominal Masses

The discovery of an abdominal mass in the first month of life is frightening to both parent and clinician. However, most neonatal abdominal masses are benign and have an excellent prognosis (Table 8-6) (33).

Ultrasonography provides detailed anatomic information about the abdominal contents during the neonatal period. Sonography should be the second study in a neonate thought to have an abdominal mass, after a plain film is obtained to look for calcifications and evaluate the bowel gas pattern. If the US study is completely normal, no further evaluation is required.

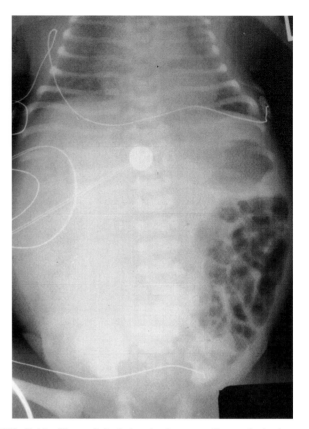

FIG. 8-11. Neonatal abdominal mass. Severely hydronephrotic right kidney presenting as an abdominal mass in a newborn boy.

TABLE 8-6. *Neonatal abdominal masses*

Lesion	Incidence (%)
Renal	55
Hydronephrosis[a]	(25)
Multicystic dysplastic kidney[a]	(15)
Polycystic kidney disease	
Mesoblastic nephroma	
Renal ectopia	
Renal vein thrombosis	
Nephroblastomatosis	
Wilms tumor	
Nonrenal retroperitoneal masses	10
Adrenal hemorrhage[a]	
Neuroblastoma[a]	
Teratoma	
Genital masses	15
Hydrometrocolpos	
Ovarian cyst[a]	
Gastrointestinal masses	15
Duplication[a]	
Complicated meconium ileus[a]	
Mesenteric or omental cyst	
Dilated bowel proximal to atresia	
Hepatosplenobiliary masses	5
Hemangioendothelioma[a], hemangioma	
Hepatoblastoma	
Hepatic cyst	
Splenic hematoma	
Splenic cyst	
Choledochal cyst	
Hydrops of gallbladder	
TOTAL	100

[a] More common

Source: Modified from Griscom (33) and Kirks et al (32).

Neonatal Renal Masses

Approximately half of neonatal abdominal masses arise from the kidney (Table 8-6). Hydronephrosis is the most common abdominal mass in the neonate, but the diagnosis may not be clinically suspected during the first 24 hours of life (Fig. 8-11). More and more cases of hydronephrosis are detected by in utero sonography, and this expedites neonatal evaluation and therapy. As a further consequence, milder cases are identified in the newborn period, and fewer cases turn up later in childhood. Specific causes of neonatal hydronephrosis include ureteropelvic junction obstruction, posterior urethral valves, duplex kidney with ectopic ureterocele, vesicoureteral reflux, prune-belly syndrome, and ureteral or ureterovesical obstruction (32). If the hydronephrosis is not recognized during the first week of life, the presenting symptom may be recurrent fever or failure to thrive secondary to superimposed infection rather than the mass itself.

A multicystic dysplastic kidney is the second most common abdominal mass occurring in the neonate. As with hydronephrosis, many cases are now diagnosed in utero by sonography and verified by imaging during the newborn period. Other less common neonatal renal masses include infantile polycystic kidney disease, adult polycystic kidney disease, mesoblastic nephroma (fetal renal hamartoma), renal ectopia, renal vein thrombosis, and nephroblastomatosis. Wilms tumor is very unusual in neonates, but the rare rhabdoid tumor of the kidney may occur in the newborn period.

Ultrasonography will reveal the renal origin of masses and often provides a definitive diagnosis. Excretory urography is of limited value during the first few days of life because of the decreased glomerular filtration rate and concentrating ability of the kidney. The neonate has a large extracellular volume, low renal plasma flow, and poor tubular concentration. In addition to these physiologic considerations, the high osmolarity of excretory urographic contrast agents very occasionally causes congestive heart failure or dehydration in a sick neonate. Renal scintigraphy shows physiology and function well.

Neonatal Genital Masses

Hydrometrocolpos and ovarian cyst are the two genital mass lesions found in newborn girls. Hydrometrocolpos is a fluid-filled, dilated vagina and uterus (34). Clinically, there is usually a firm, fixed, midline pelvic or abdominopelvic mass. There are often other congenital anomalies such as imperforate anus. Plain films demonstrate a midline mass that may contain air, from a rectal fistula. Sonography confirms echolucent or echogenic fluid in the dilated uterus or vagina. Cystography, genitography, and barium enema may be required to demonstrate the anatomy of complex lesions.

Ovarian cysts are very common in newborn girls. They are probably the result of an exaggeration of normal follicular development stimulated by maternal hormones. Ovarian cysts are usually of germinal or Graafian epithelial origin. They are usually lateral to the midline and mobile. When the cyst is uncomplicated, US confirms the presence of an anechoic mass, which may be primarily abdominal rather than pelvic. A cyst that has undergone hemorrhage or torsion may appear solid sonographically or may contain echogenic material or a fluid-debris level (35). Unless particularly large (more than 6 cm), ovarian cysts may be treated conservatively; many undergo spontaneous involution.

Neonatal GI Masses

If plain films demonstrate an abdominal mass associated with intestinal obstruction, a GI origin is most likely (36). Duplication is the most common GI tract mass in the neonate (33). These duplications are usually discrete and round or oval. Sonography may be diagnostic of enteric duplication by demonstrating a characteristic wall consisting of an inner echogenic layer (mucosa) and outer hypoechoic layer (muscle) (37). Meconium pseudocyst, mesenteric cyst, and dilatation of bowel proximal to atresia are other GI causes of a neonatal abdominal mass. All of these GI masses are usually associated with plain film evidence of intestinal obstruction.

Neonatal Nonrenal Retroperitoneal Masses

Nonrenal retroperitoneal masses in the neonate include adrenal hemorrhage, neuroblastoma, and teratoma. Sonography can often distinguish between neuroblastoma (usually echogenic) and neonatal adrenal hemorrhage (usually hypoechoic). However, some cases of congenital neuroblastoma are cystic, and the differentiation between hemorrhage and tumor cannot always be made on a single examination (38). Because congenital adrenal neuroblastoma has an excellent prognosis, serial sonography is an acceptable way to diagnose the unusual case in which the history, physical examination, and initial sonography are not diagnostic; adrenal hemorrhage becomes smaller and often calcifies whereas neuroblastoma either does not change or becomes larger.

Neonatal Hepatobiliary and Splenic Masses

The hepatobiliary system and the spleen are the least common anatomic sites of neonatal abdominal masses. Neonatal masses in the liver, spleen, or biliary system include hemangioendothelioma/hemangioma, hepatoblastoma, hepatic cyst, splenic hematoma, splenic cyst, choledochal cyst, and hydrops of the gallbladder. Sonography is usually diagnostic. Nuclear scintigraphy is of supplemental value for diagnosing choledochal cyst. There is an association between choledochal cyst and biliary atresia. A combination of US and hepatobiliary scintigraphy can show the associated atresia when a choledochal cyst is found in a neonate (39).

Abdominal Masses in Older Infants and Children

Pediatric abdominal masses found after the neonatal period are still predominantly retroperitoneal; however, there is a significant increase in malignant tumors, and there are important differences in the incidences of specific masses (Table 8-7) (32). Renal masses account for about the same fraction of the total, but many of them are Wilms tumors. Other retroperitoneal tumors are also encountered more frequently, especially neuroblastoma. There is thus a considerably higher percentage of malignant neoplasms in the older infant and child than in the neonate. Because of these important differences, CT and MRI play a much more important diagnostic role in older children than in neonates. They are capable not only of demonstrating the anatomic features of a mass but also of determining the local and metastatic extent of malignant lesions.

Abdominal masses of genital origin are less common in older children than in neonates. Almost all of these masses are ovarian; most are cystic. They usually present clinically as asymptomatic pelvic masses but can cause acute abdominal pain secondary to torsion. Calcifications are frequently demonstrated; dermoids may contain well-defined teeth, bone, or fat. Ultrasonography confirms the cystic nature of the mass and the pelvic location of the tumor.

TABLE 8-7. *Abdominal masses in older infants and children*

Lesion	Incidence (%)
Renal masses	55
Wilms tumor[a]	(22)
Hydronephrosis[a]	(20)
Cyst	
Congenital malformations	
Nonrenal retroperitoneal masses	23
Neuroblastoma[a]	(21)
Teratoma	
Other neoplasms	
Genital masses	4
Ovarian cyst	
Teratoma	
Hydrometrocolpos	
Other	
Gastrointestinal masses	12
Appendiceal abscess[a]	(10)
Other neoplasms	
Congenital malformations	
Hepatosplenobiliary masses	6
TOTAL	100

[a] More common

Source: Modified from Kirks et al (32).

Abdominal abscess is the most common GI mass in older infants and children. Extension of appendiceal abscesses into the cul-de-sac occurs frequently, forming a mass between bladder and rectum. Ultrasonography confirms the mixed echo pattern of the abscess as well as its location.

Hepatobiliary masses represent approximately 6% of all abdominal tumors in pediatric patients after the neonatal period. Most of these masses arise in the liver and are malignant. Specific hepatobiliary masses are discussed later in this chapter.

Integrated Imaging of Pediatric Abdominal Masses

Many diagnostic modalities can be used to image pediatric abdominal masses. The ultimate goal of imaging, better patient care, depends on the coordinated efforts of the radiologist, pediatrician, and surgeon. The age of the patient and the physical examination guide the initial imaging technique. Precise diagnostic evaluation allows selection of the proper surgical or medical therapy.

The role of radiology is to confirm, characterize, and determine the extent of an abdominal mass. The initial imaging shows whether a mass is truly present. Sonography may demonstrate that the ''mass'' is merely a normal neonatal organ, in which case no further evaluation is indicated. Second, the location of the mass is clarified. The abdominal mass may be retroperitoneal or intraperitoneal. Finally, local extent and distant spread of a malignant lesion are determined. Cystic and anechoic abdominal masses are almost always benign; solid, echogenic, and vascular masses are frequently malignant.

The development of CT, MRI, and US has led to the formulation of algorithmic approaches for imaging an abdominal mass in the neonate and older child (Fig. 8-12). The purpose of these decision trees is not to dictate a diagnostic approach but to suggest imaging modalities that may allow expeditious preoperative diagnosis and definition. These approaches to pediatric abdominal masses are continually being modified by clinical trials of imaging protocols.

The maximal amount of diagnostic information should be obtained with minimal cost, trauma, and radiation to the patient. This type of expedient, selective integration of imaging modalities with clinical data is critical for improved medical care. This integrated approach demands complete review of clinical and imaging findings at each step and frequently requires repeated revision of the diagnostic plan. The approach avoids inflexible choices and requires that expected diagnostic yields as well as risks and costs be determined for each modality. One can no longer assume that all imaging modalities are ''complementary.''

SPECIFIC ABNORMALITIES OF THE ABDOMEN

Newborn

Anomalies of the Abdominal Wall

Closure of the anterior abdominal wall in the fetus is a complex process requiring infolding of four mesenchymal ''folds'' (cephalic, caudal, and two lateral) (40). These folds meet at the umbilicus, and their fusion closes the ventral surface of the fetus except for the attachment of the umbilical cord. Although the precise pathogenesis of abdominal wall defects is uncertain, these defects may be thought of as resulting from maldevelopment of one or more of these mesenchymal folds.

Cephalic Fold Defect

Failure of closure of the cephalic fold results in a group of defects described as thoracoabdominal ectopia cordis (pentalogy of Cantrell) (41). These include a supraumbilical ventral hernia; defects in the sternum, anterior portion of the diaphragm, and pericardium; and congenital heart disease. If the lateral folds also fail to fuse there will be an omphalocele as well. The diagnosis is obvious, and survival depends on the severity of the congenital heart disease.

Omphalocele

Omphalocele is a midline abdominal wall defect thought to result from maldevelopment of the lateral folds. Any abdominal organ or organs may herniate into the defect. The herniated viscera are covered by a sac of peritoneum and amnion, into the apex of which the umbilical cord inserts.

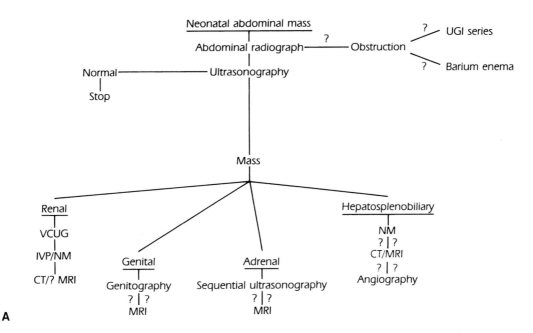

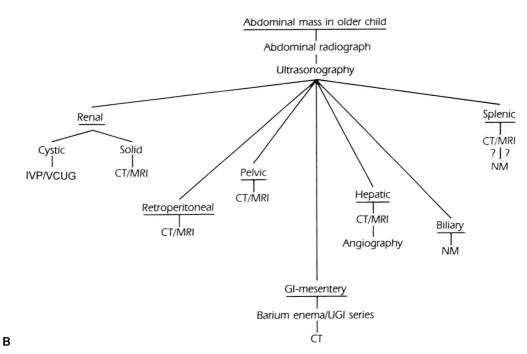

FIG. 8-12. Possible algorithms for pediatric abdominal masses. A: Neonatal abdominal mass. **B:** Abdominal mass in older child. *CT*, computed tomography; *IVP*, intravenous pyelogram; *MRI*, magnetic resonance imaging; *NM*, nuclear medicine imaging; *UGI*, upper gastrointestinal series; *VCUG*, voiding cystourethrogram.

The size and contents of the omphalocele are variable: small sacs may contain only a loop of bowel, large ones the entire intestine and liver.

About two thirds of babies with omphalocele have associated anomalies, most frequently of the cardiovascular system (42). Chromosomal abnormalities (trisomies 13, 18, and 21) often coexist with omphalocele. Omphalocele is also a part of the Beckwith-Wiedemann syndrome (43). Malrotation of

the intestine is an almost inevitable consequence of omphalocele, although few of these patients develop volvulus. Survival is excellent and quality of life generally good in patients with omphalocele if there are no other serious anomalies (44). Preoperative imaging of newborns with omphalocele is usually not indicated. If a plain abdominal radiograph is obtained it will show a protruding soft-tissue mass. Individual bowel loops will be surrounded by air only if the

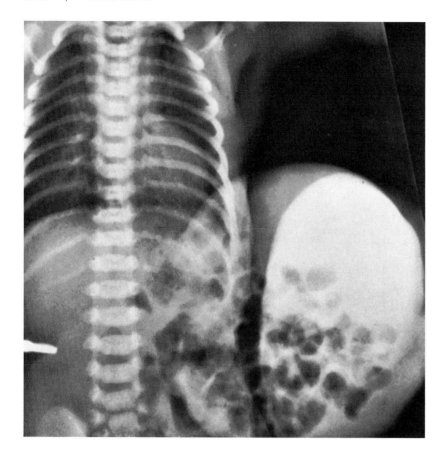

FIG. 8-13. Omphalocele. There is herniation of bowel into a smooth (membrane-covered) mass that originates at the umbilicus.

sac has ruptured (Fig. 8-13). Postoperative imaging may be confusing if the history of omphalocele is not available, as the abdominal organs are usually malpositioned. The kidneys, for example, may be immediately subdiaphragmatic in location; presumably the ascent of the kidneys from the pelvis, normally arrested by the liver, continues in fetuses with omphalocele until the diaphragm is reached (45) (Fig. 8-14).

Gastroschisis

Gastroschisis is a defect in the abdominal wall located lateral to and usually to the right of the midline, next to a normally positioned umbilicus. It may be due to a vascular accident leading to the loss of the medial part of the right lateral fold (46). The theory that gastroschisis is caused by a local vascular abnormality rather than a more general abnormality of differentiation is supported by the infrequent association of gastroschisis with other congenital anomalies.

In gastroschisis it is usually only bowel that herniates through the abdominal wall defect. Unlike the bowel in omphalocele, which is covered by a membrane, the bowel in gastroschisis is exposed to amniotic fluid. Contact with amniotic fluid somehow injures the bowel; this injury is grossly manifested as shortening of bowel, frequently associated with stenosis or atresia, and as an inflammatory "peel" that

covers the bowel (47). The bowel in gastroschisis always has disordered motility, which may have serious clinical effects (48). Most of the morbidity of gastroschisis is due to these abnormalities.

A plain film of the abdomen in a newborn with gastroschisis shows herniated bowel loops individually outlined by air and a normally positioned umbilicus (Fig. 8-15). Upper GI studies obtained in the postoperative period will frequently demonstrate gastroesophageal reflux, dilated bowel, and very slow transit time, mimicking obstruction (48–51). There is also a relatively high incidence of necrotizing enterocolitis in babies with repaired gastroschisis (49).

Cloacal Exstrophy

Cloacal exstrophy is a rare, severe anomaly in which there is maldevelopment of the caudal portion of the fetal abdominal wall and cloacal membrane (52). This results in omphalocele, epispadias, and bladder exstrophy. The exstrophied bladder is bisected in the midline by an area of exposed intestinal mucosa; this exposed mucosal plate is the ileum and cecum. The externalized intestine usually has two openings: the superior one is the orifice of the proximal bowel, and the inferior one is the hindgut, which is hypoplastic and ends blindly. No anus is present.

All patients with classic cloacal exstrophy have widely

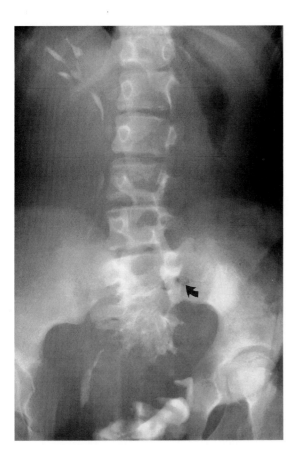

FIG. 8-14. Cloacal exstrophy with omphalocele. An IVP demonstrates a right kidney that is subdiaphragmatic. The left kidney *(curved arrow)* is pelvic in location. Many vertebral anomalies and a widened pubic symphysis are present.

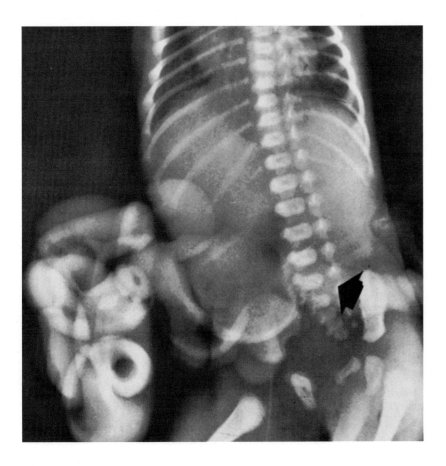

FIG. 8-15. Gastroschisis. The bowel is herniated through an abdominal wall defect. The umbilicus *(arrow)* is in normal position. Some of the bowel loops are surrounded by air.

diastatic pubic bones and spinal dysraphism (53) (see Fig. 8-14). Limb anomalies and renal anomalies are very common. Malrotation is present in at least half; duplication of the large bowel also occurs. The small bowel may be short. The first step in the repair of the GI malformation is usually tubularizing the exposed ileocecal "plate" and blind-ending hindgut, anastomosing it to the ileum and bringing it out as an end-colostomy. Postoperative contrast studies are used to estimate the length of bowel; MRI is able to show the musculature of the pelvic floor.

Cloacal exstrophy should not be confused with the cloacal malformation (54). This very different entity is discussed in Chapter 9.

Anomalies of the Diaphragm

Bochdalek Hernia and Eventration of the Diaphragm

The most important congenital abnormality of the diaphragm is the posterolateral or Bochdalek hernia, the result of incomplete closure of the pleuroperitoneal canal. This common and often severe anomaly is also discussed in Chapter 7 ("Respiratory System") because it almost always causes respiratory symptoms. Newborns with a large Bochdalek hernia have severe respiratory distress. At first the herniated liver and bowel produce a large, opaque hemithorax. After air is swallowed, the bowel in the hernia becomes gas-filled (Fig. 8-16). Bochdalek hernias are five times as common on the left side as on the right. Because bowel dilatation in the hernia can cause cardiorespiratory compromise and arrest, the stomach should be decompressed by tube as soon as the condition is diagnosed.

The morbidity of Bochdalek hernia is caused by pulmonary hypoplasia, contralateral and especially ipsilateral to the hernia. Patients with Bochdalek hernia always have malrotation and abnormal fixation of bowel; they seem, however, to be at surprisingly low risk for midgut volvulus (55). Gastroesophageal reflux is common in survivors of congenital diaphragmatic hernia and may be severe (56).

The presentation of a Bochdalek hernia is occasionally delayed. These delayed hernias are much more common on the right than on the left; it is postulated that the liver may somehow temporarily plug the diaphragmatic defect. Poor lung compliance and assisted ventilation may also delay the appearance of a Bochdalek hernia (57). There is also an increased incidence of delayed, right-sided Bochdalek hernia in patients with neonatal streptococcal pneumonia (58). The reason for this peculiar association is not known.

Eventration of the diaphragm is defined as a usually focal but sometimes generalized attenuation or absence of the muscle of the diaphragm, without a frank communication between the pleural and peritoneal cavities (59). Small areas of eventration are usually transitory and asymptomatic and are found only when a chest radiograph is obtained for other reasons. Eventrations may, however, present in infancy with

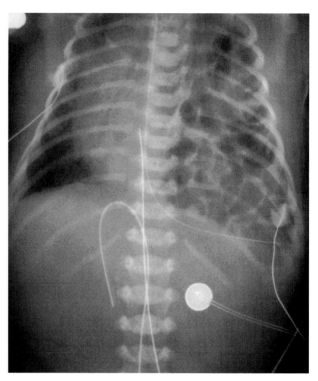

FIG. 8-16. Congenital diaphragmatic hernia (Bochdalek). The air-filled herniated intestine has a mass effect and shifts the heart, mediastinum, and aorta (marked by the straight catheter) to the right. The abdomen is gasless.

severe respiratory distress and mimic a Bochdalek hernia both clinically and radiographically. The distinction between hernia and severe eventration is very difficult by any radiographic method, and in the newborn with respiratory distress the distinction is not important because both conditions require surgical repair.

Morgagni Hernia

A much less common type of diaphragmatic hernia is the Morgagni hernia, caused by an anteromedial defect in the diaphragm extending from the sternum laterally to the ribs. Patients with Morgagni hernias usually present in adult life, the hernia being found incidentally on a chest x-ray. Rare patients present in infancy with respiratory distress (60,61). Many newborns with Morgagni hernias have other congenital anomalies. On AP chest radiographs there is an opacity in the cardiophrenic angle, usually on the right side, which may displace the heart to the left; on the lateral view, Morgagni hernias are anterior (Fig. 8-17). The defects may be bilateral; these hernias, however, are more common on the right because a defect on the left is reinforced by heart and pericardium. When bowel is present in the hernia the diagnosis is usually straightforward. If the hernia contains liver, as it may in infants with respiratory distress, the diagnosis is more difficult. Ultrasonography may allow localization of the diaphragmatic defect and identification of the herniated

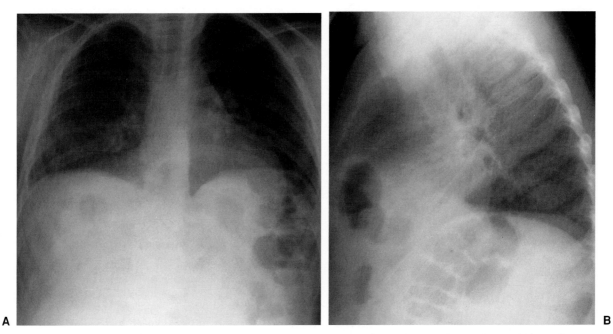

FIG. 8-17. Morgagni hernia. A: An AP chest radiograph reveals an ill-defined mass in the right cardi-ophrenic angle and air collections behind the sternum and over the liver. **B:** A lateral chest radiograph clearly shows that the mass is anterior and contains bowel.

viscera (62). Differentiation of a Morgagni hernia from an eventration may be difficult. In hernias the most cephalic portion usually abuts the anterior chest wall; most eventrations are more posterior.

Esophageal Atresia and Tracheoesophageal Fistula

Definition and Classification

The trachea and esophagus begin fetal life as a single structure. Errors in the differentiation of the trachea from the esophagus result in a spectrum of congenital anomalies. The most important of these is segmental atresia of the esophagus, with or without a persistent communication between the trachea and esophagus, a tracheoesophageal fistula (TEF). Esophageal atresia usually occurs at the junction of the upper and middle thirds of the esophagus. The length of the gap between the upper and lower esophageal segments varies and is generally longest when there is no fistula. In the most common form of esophageal atresia, the upper segment of the esophagus ends blindly, and the proximal end of the lower part of the esophagus communicates with the trachea, usually just above the carina (Fig. 8-18). In much less common forms of esophageal atresia the proximal end of the lower portion of the esophagus may be blind with the upper portion of the esophagus communicating with the trachea, or both upper and lower esophageal segments may communicate with the trachea (Fig. 8-18). Esophageal atresia may be present without a TEF, and there may be a TEF without esophageal atresia, the so-called H-type fistula (Fig. 8-18).

There are several classifications of esophageal atresia. For the radiologist, however, it suffices to remember that one may have pure esophageal atresia without a TEF; esophageal atresia with a fistula that may be proximal, distal, or both; or an isolated TEF without esophageal atresia. All types other than atresia with a distal fistula are uncommon. For effective communication with clinicians, these simple descriptive terms are better than numbers or letters.

Clinical Features and Associated Anomalies

The presence of esophageal atresia may be suspected prenatally because of polyhydramnios, due to obstruction of fetal swallowing. Fetuses without a fistula are more likely to have polyhydramnios; in these cases a definitive prenatal diagnosis is possible due to the nonvisualization of the fetal stomach on US. Many children with esophageal atresia are born prematurely.

Almost all children with esophageal atresia will present soon after birth with drooling, coughing, choking, and sometimes cyanosis. All symptoms become more dramatic if the infant is fed. Attempts to pass a tube into the stomach will fail. Children with TEF without esophageal atresia are usually diagnosed somewhat later in life: symptoms of coughing and choking during feeding, recurrent pneumonias, and gaseous distention of the abdomen, however, often begin at birth (63,64).

About half of all children with esophageal atresia have other congenital anomalies (65,66). This association of anomalies has been described by the acronym VATER, for

Esophageal atresia

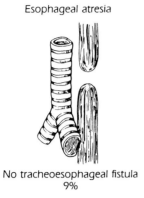

No tracheoesophageal fistula
9%

Esophageal atresia and tracheoesophageal fistula

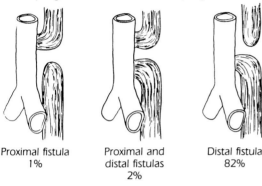

Proximal fistula
1%

Proximal and
distal fistulas
2%

Distal fistula
82%

Tracheoesophageal fistula

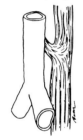

No esophageal atresia
6%

FIG. 8-18. Esophageal atresia and tracheoesophageal fistula. There may be esophageal atresia alone *(top)*, esophageal atresia and tracheoesophageal fistula *(middle)*, or tracheoesophageal fistula alone *(bottom)*. The approximate frequency of each type is shown.

*v*ertebral defects, *a*nal atresia, *t*racheo*e*sophageal fistula, and *r*adial and *r*enal dysplasia (67,68). The acronym has been expanded to VACTERL to include cardiac and limb anomalies (69). Those who coined the term VATER stress that these anomalies do not represent a single syndrome with a defined etiology. They are rather a nonrandom association of abnormalities that result from an unknown error or errors in embryogenesis occurring by the fifth week of gestation. Thus, while many babies with esophageal atresia have one or more of the anomalies of the VATER or VACTERL association, very few will have all of them. Overall, the most

commonly found anomalies in babies with esophageal atresia are of the cardiovascular and GI systems (66). The most commonly found cardiac anomalies are ventricular septal defect, patent ductus arteriosus, and tetralogy of Fallot. Of the associated GI anomalies, other atresias, especially of the anus and duodenum, are most common (65,66). With advances in neonatology and surgical technique most of the mortality in esophageal atresia is due to associated anomalies, not the esophageal atresia itself. The cardiac abnormalities are the most likely to be lethal (66).

Radiology

The radiologist will usually first see the newborn with esophageal atresia after an unsuccessful attempt to place a nasogastric tube. The initial films of the chest and abdomen will typically show the nasogastric tube curled in the upper chest, in the proximal esophageal pouch (Fig. 8-19). The presence of air in the stomach and intestines implies that there is a distal fistula or possibly both proximal and distal fistulas (70). The absence of GI air implies that there is esophageal atresia but no fistula (Fig. 8-20) or, very rarely, atresia with only a proximal fistula (Fig. 8-21) (71). The films should also be carefully inspected for associated anomalies, particularly of the heart and spine (Fig. 8-20).

After this initial examination the radiologist's involvement in the care of these babies varies from hospital to hospital. For many surgeons, the plain film alone provides sufficient preoperative information; they feel that the rare proximal fistula will be discovered at surgery during mobilization of the proximal esophageal segment. However, some surgeons prefer that the diagnosis of esophageal atresia be further proven, that traumatic pharyngeal perforation be excluded, and that pouch anatomy be further defined. This is readily accomplished by the injection, under fluoroscopic control, of air into the proximal esophageal pouch via a nasal or oral tube (Fig. 8-22). As a contrast agent, air is cheap, readily available, and nontoxic to the lungs. The pouch usually distends easily. Liquid contrast is rarely placed in the pouch. This fluoroscopically monitored injection is reserved for two situations: first, when the pouch cannot be distended with air, suggesting that it is decompressing via a proximal fistula (Fig. 8-21); and second, when there is a suspicion that the baby has a perforation of the pharynx or esophagus (pseudodiverticulum) rather than esophageal atresia.

Although a traumatic perinatal or postnatal abnormality rather than a congenital anomaly, pharyngeal perforation is discussed here because of its resemblance to esophageal atresia. Injury to the pharynx may occur during delivery but is more likely to result from the attempt to pass either an endotracheal tube or a nasogastric tube that perforates the posterior wall of the pharynx (72). This perforation causes a pharyngeal pseudodiverticulum that may track from the retropharyngeal space into the mediastinum or pleural space (73). If a nasogastric tube is subsequently passed it may

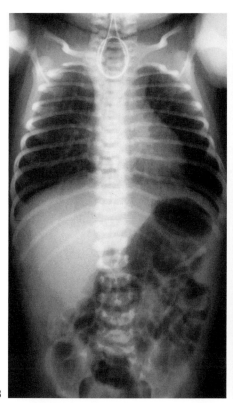
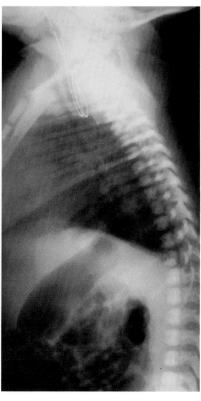

FIG. 8-19. Esophageal atresia with distal tracheoesophageal fistula. AP **(A)** and lateral **(B)** radiographs of the chest and abdomen demonstrate an enteric tube coiled in the upper esophageal pouch. The air in the bowel indicates a distal tracheoesophageal communication.

A,B

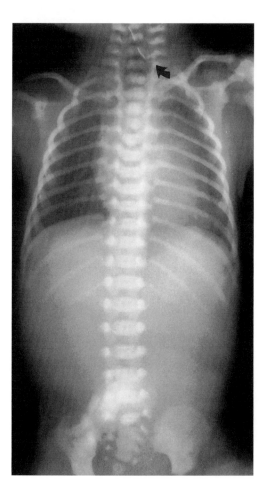

FIG. 8-20. Esophageal atresia without tracheoesophageal fistula. An enteric tube is in the upper esophageal pouch *(arrow)*. There is no gas in the abdomen. A minor sacral anomaly is also present.

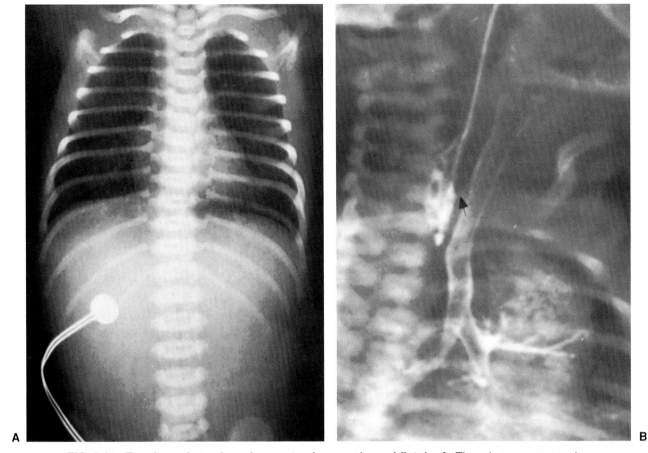

FIG. 8-21. **Esophageal atresia and upper tracheoesophageal fistula. A:** There is an upper esophageal pouch but no air within the abdomen. **B:** Small amount of contrast injected into the upper pouch through an enteric tube. A tracheoesophageal fistula *(arrow)* is identified proximal to the atresia.

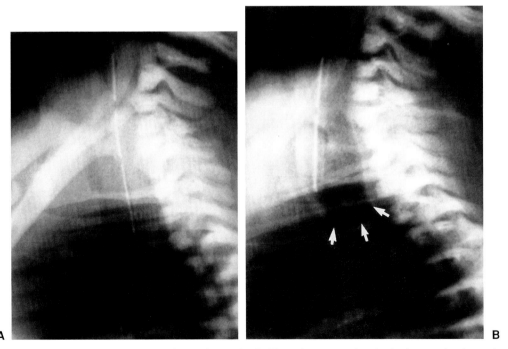

FIG. 8-22. **Proximal pouch of esophageal atresia. A:** There is an enteric tube in the proximal esophageal pouch. **B:** The pouch *(arrows)* is more clearly defined after injection of air.

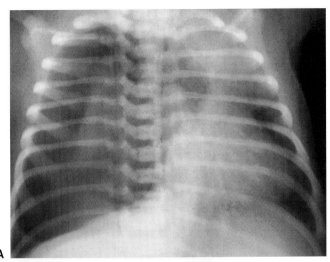

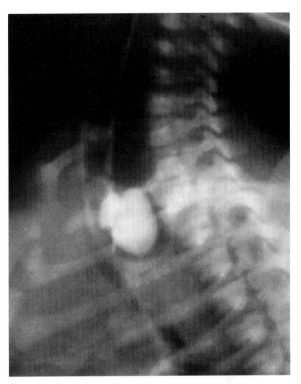

FIG. 8-24. Esophageal atresia. Proximal esophageal pouch distended with air and a small amount of contrast. The margins of the pouch are smooth.

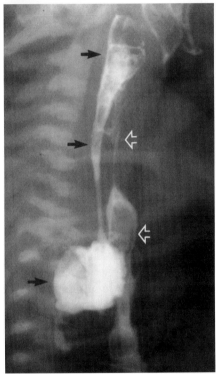

FIG. 8-23. Pharyngeal pseudodiverticulum. A: A large right pneumothorax in a newborn with a history of traumatic intubation. **B:** Contrast fills a pharyngeal pseudodiverticulum, which tracks into the mediastinum *(arrows)* behind the normal esophagus *(open arrows).*

enter the false passage, fail to descend further, and mimic esophageal atresia. A pneumomediastinum or pneumothorax in a patient with clinically suspected esophageal atresia or with a history of traumatic tube placement suggests pharyngeal perforation (Fig. 8-23). If one injects contrast it is usually not difficult to distinguish a pharyngeal pseudodiverticulum from the pouch of esophageal atresia. The pseudodiverticulum is more posterior than an esophageal pouch and, unlike the esophageal pouch, it is usually irregular in contour (Figs. 8-23 and 8-24). Contrast injected into

a pseudodiverticulum frequently passes into the mediastinum or pleural cavity (Fig. 8-23) and is difficult to remove from the false passage.

If indicated for one of the above reasons, one should use a low osmolar, nonionic, water-soluble contrast agent. A small amount is injected under fluoroscopic control, in the lateral projection, with the head slightly elevated. A proximal fistula is carefully looked for, as are signs of pharyngeal perforation. The contrast is then completely removed via the enteric tube.

Because the surgical approach to esophageal atresia is a posterolateral thoracotomy on the side opposite the aortic arch, most surgeons will, if the situs of the arch is not evident from the plain film, ask for another study. Cardiac US, is fast and easy to perform and also screens for cardiac anomalies.

The evaluation of TEF without associated atresia, the "H-type" TEF, is different from the routine described above. Most affected children present somewhat later in life with coughing and choking during feeding and recurrent pneumonia. Plain radiographs of the chest sometimes show chronic lung disease but may be normal. Occasionally, there is gaseous distention of the esophagus or intestine, reflecting the open tracheoesophageal communication (74). Most children referred for radiologic evaluation to "rule out H-type TEF" do not have it; aspiration and gastroesophageal reflux cause coughing and choking during feeding and are much more frequent causes of recurrent pneumonia. The evaluation begins with a routine barium swallow with the patient drinking from a bottle or cup; careful attention is paid to the swallowing mechanism, possible aspiration (best detected in the lateral position), esophageal motility and anatomy, and the presence or absence of reflux. Many H-type fistulas are readily diagnosed on routine studies, but others are very difficult to find (75). Careful fluoroscopy and adequate esophageal distention are critical. Repeated studies may be necessary. Though some authors recommend routine performance of esophagography via an esophageal tube, sometimes with the patient prone, this is seldom necessary to show an H-type fistula. Tubes are used when adequate esophageal distention cannot be obtained via nipple or cup and when there is a high suspicion of fistula but previous studies have been negative. If a tube is used it should be positioned in the distal esophagus and withdrawn to the proximal esophagus with injections of contrast every centimeter or two. The entire trachea and larynx should be included in the field of view, as aspiration is common with this technique.

The appearance of an H-type TEF is the same with oral or tube administration. The fistulas may be at any level but are most frequently found near the thoracic inlet (63). The fistulas are generally quite small and may open only intermittently. They extend in a cephalad direction from the esophagus to the trachea (Fig. 8-25). Some prefer to describe the

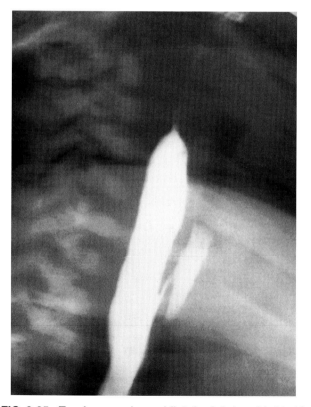

FIG. 8-25. Tracheoesophageal fistula. A 6-day-old girl with coughing and cyanosis during feeding. The fistula is identified at the level of C6–7 passing obliquely upward from the esophagus to the trachea.

isolated TEF as an ''N fistula'' rather than an ''H fistula'' because the morphology of the letter N is more anatomically correct (63).

The diagnosis of esophageal atresia and tracheoesophageal fistula is usually straightforward. The role of the radiologist should be to provide the surgeon with as much information as he or she feels is necessary before operating. Positive contrast injection of a proximal esophageal pouch is rarely necessary but can be done safely. In the case of H-type fistula, the routine use of a tube esophagram is not necessary; whatever method one uses, however, adequate esophageal distention, careful fluoroscopy, and persistence are necessary (75).

Postoperative Radiology

The immediate postoperative complications of repair of esophageal atresia and tracheoesophageal fistula are anastomotic leak and recurrent TEF. Recurrent TEFs, which occur in as many as 10% of cases, can be extremely difficult to find and, as is the case with isolated TEF, may require several examinations (76). The combination of radiography and endoscopy is usually successful, however.

Though most children with repaired esophageal atresia do reasonably well, many experience recurrent GI and respiratory problems such as coughing and choking, dysphagia, failure to thrive, apnea, cyanosis, and stridor. These symptoms are a challenge to the radiologist and clinician (77,78). Probably the most common cause of dysphagia is an anastomotic stricture. Food impaction proximal to a narrowed anastomosis is quite common (Fig. 8-26). Virtually all children with esophageal atresia have disordered esophageal peristalsis (79,80). Gastroesophageal reflux also occurs in most children after repair of atresia and may cause esophagitis and stricture (81). Though most strictures after repair of esophageal atresia are peptic, a small number are congenital. Some of these congenital strictures are associated with tracheobronchial rests (82,83).

Respiratory difficulties after repair of esophageal atresia may be due to recurrent aspiration secondary to obstruction or reflux or to tracheomalacia, which leads to intermittent tracheal narrowing (Fig. 8-27) (78). Though tracheomalacia is present to some extent in almost all patients with repaired atresia (84,85) and may cause few or no symptoms, in some it is severe enough to cause life-threatening apnea requiring aortopexy (86).

Severe, progressive scoliosis, with concavity toward the thoracotomy site, may become apparent years after repair of esophageal atresia (87). This complication is most common after postoperative anastomotic leaks.

High Intestinal Obstruction

Intestinal obstruction is the most common abdominal emergency in the newborn period. Neonatal obstructions

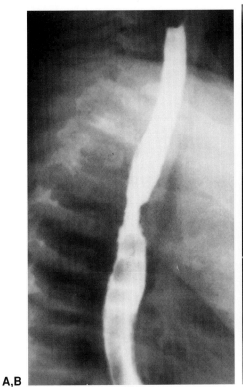
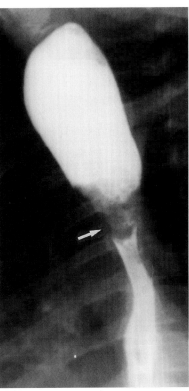

A,B

FIG. 8-26. Anastomotic stricture after repair of esophageal atresia. A: Routine postoperative esophagram in a child with repaired esophageal atresia shows mild anastomotic narrowing. **B:** Same child several months later. A foreign body (piece of bread) is impacted at the anastomosis *(arrow).*

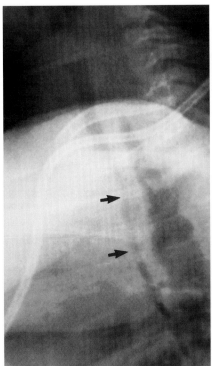
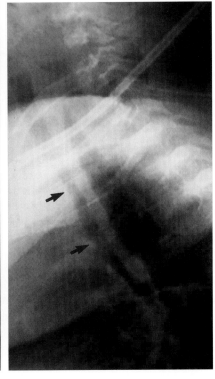

A,B

FIG. 8-27. Tracheomalacia. Fluoroscopic images of the trachea *(arrows)* in a child with repaired esophageal atresia show marked tracheal narrowing in expiration **(A)** compared to inspiration **(B)**.

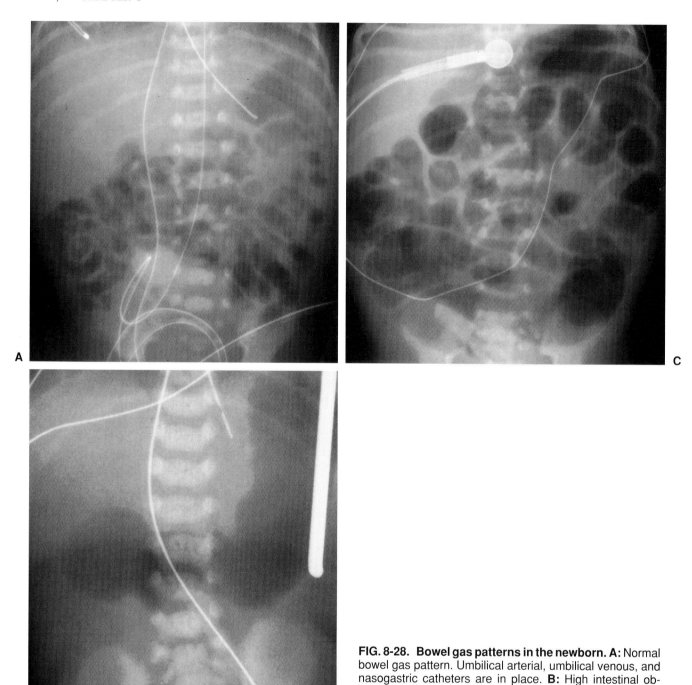

FIG. 8-28. Bowel gas patterns in the newborn. A: Normal bowel gas pattern. Umbilical arterial, umbilical venous, and nasogastric catheters are in place. **B:** High intestinal obstruction. The stomach and duodenal bulb are dilated (double bubble) in a newborn with duodenal atresia. **C:** Low intestinal obstruction. Many dilated bowel loops in a newborn with Hirschsprung disease. From Buonomo (88).

may be classified as high or low. Obstructions that occur proximal to the midileum, i.e., obstructions involving the stomach, duodenum, jejunum, or proximal ileum, are called high or upper intestinal obstructions. Obstructions that involve the distal ileum or colon are called low intestinal obstructions. The presentation of the two types of obstruction may be identical. Either type may present with poor feeding, vomiting (often bilious), abdominal distention, and failure to pass meconium within 24 hours or very sluggish passage

of meconium. The distinction between high and low obstructions can almost always be made on the basis of plain films. Air proceeds distally in the GI tract until stopped at the obstruction; plain films in babies with high obstruction thus will reveal one, two, or a few dilated air-filled bowel loops; films in low obstructions will show many dilated air-filled loops (Fig. 8-28) (88). The distinction is critical: children with high obstructions usually need little or no radiologic evaluation after the plain film; the specific diagnosis will be

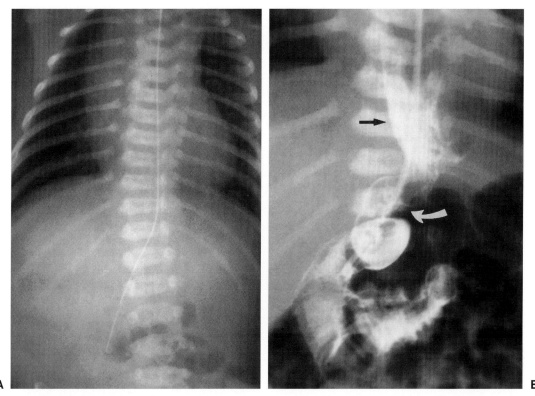

A

B

FIG. 8-29. Microgastria. A: Plain film of the abdomen in a newborn with nonbilious emesis. The course of the enteric tube is abnormal. **B:** UGI demonstrates a small tubular midline stomach *(curved arrow)* and a dilated distal esophagus *(arrow).*

made in the operating room. Newborns with low obstructions need a contrast enema, which usually provides a specific diagnosis and may be therapeutic (89).

Obstruction of the Stomach

Congenital obstruction of the stomach is very uncommon. Complete absence of the stomach virtually never occurs. Hypoplasia of the stomach, or microgastria, is rare and may exist as an isolated malformation or with other anomalies, especially asplenia. The radiologic appearance is characteristic: a small tubular midline stomach and a dilated distal esophagus (Fig. 8-29) (90).

Atresia of the stomach occurs at the antrum or pylorus. Although a complete gap between segments of the stomach may occur, gastric obstruction is more frequently produced by a mucosal web or diaphragm. If the web is perforated, as it often is, symptoms, most commonly nonbilious vomiting, may arise only later in childhood (91), although a web occasionally presents in the newborn period (92). Plain films of the abdomen in a newborn with complete gastric atresia will show a distended stomach and no distal air (Fig. 8-30). A newborn with a distended stomach on an abdominal film is much more likely to have an obstruction of the duodenum than of the stomach (Fig. 8-31).

Duodenal Atresia, Stenosis, and Web

Definition and Clinical Features. Intestinal atresia is the most common cause of high obstruction in the newborn, and the duodenum is the most common site of atresia. In atresia there is complete obliteration of the intestinal lumen; in stenosis, partial occlusion. Atresia is much more common than stenosis (93), but the etiology is the same. There are several types (Fig. 8-32) including complete or partial obstruction by a diaphragm or web. Atresia and stenosis occur when the duodenum, which is a solid tube from about 3–6 weeks gestation, fails to recanalize or to recanalize completely. Atresia and stenosis almost always occur in the region of the ampulla of Vater (about 80% are just distal to the ampulla); thus it is not surprising that they are frequently accompanied by abnormalities of the bile duct and pancreas. If membranous atresia or stenosis is present, the ampulla may actually insert into the obstructing diaphragm. Annular pancreas, in which the persistent ventral anlage of the pancreas surrounds the second portion of the duodenum, occurs in as many as 20% of patients with duodenal atresia or stenosis (93). The annular pancreas may contribute to the duodenal obstruction but is seldom or never found without intrinsic obstruction of the duodenum itself (93). Preduodenal portal vein is an unusual malformation which may occur with duodenal obstruction; as is the case with annular pan-

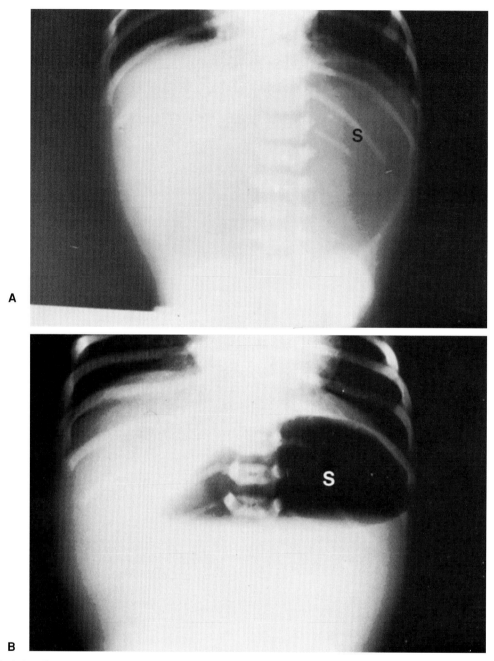

FIG. 8-30. Antral atresia. Newborn with vomiting. Anteroposterior **(A)** and erect **(B)** films demonstrate a markedly dilated stomach *(S)* with an air-fluid level. (Courtesy of James H. Scatliff, M.D., Chapel Hill, N.C.)

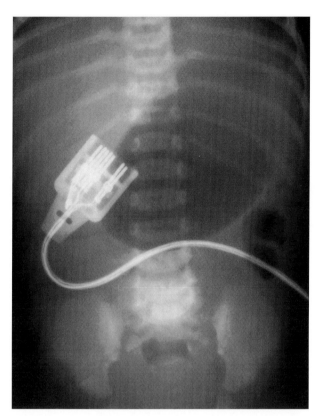

FIG. 8-31. Duodenal obstruction causing gastric outlet obstruction. Marked gastric distention with little distal gas in a newborn with a midgut volvulus.

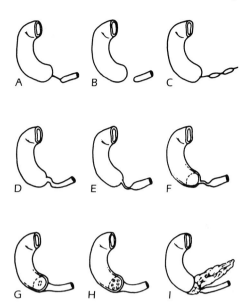

FIG. 8-32. Congenital intrinsic duodenal obstruction. A: Atresia with string-like connection. **B:** Atresia with two blind ends. **C:** Multiple duodenal atresias. **D:** Short duodenal stenosis. **E:** Long duodenal stenosis. **F:** Complete duodenal diaphragm. **G:** Incomplete duodenal diaphragm with single opening. **H:** Incomplete duodenal diaphragm with multiple openings. **I:** Annular pancreas with duodenal stenosis. (Modified from Salonen I. Congenital duodenal obstruction: a review of the literature and a clinical study of 66 patients, including a histopathologic study of annular pancreas and a follow-up study of 36 survivors. *Acta Paediatr Scan* 1978; 272:1–87.)

creas, the preduodenal portal vein is rarely the sole cause of obstruction (94).

Duodenal atresia and stenosis may be associated with other congenital anomalies. These include other intestinal atresias and congenital heart disease. About 30% of patients with duodenal atresia or stenosis have Down syndrome, and in these babies the coexistence of heart disease is particularly high (93). Duodenal atresia and stenosis may also be part of the VATER association.

Duodenal atresia and stenosis occur with equal frequency in boys and girls. Prematurity is common, as is maternal polyhydramnios. Bilious emesis in the first hours of life is the cardinal symptom, as it is with most cases of intestinal obstruction in the newborn. The 20% of atresias that are preampullary have nonbilious emesis.

Radiology. In duodenal atresia the abdominal radiograph is usually diagnostic. Air is present in the stomach and usually in the proximal duodenum, but there is no distal air. When both the stomach and duodenal bulb are dilated, as is usual, the film shows the classic "double bubble" of duodenal atresia (Fig. 8-33). Occasionally, only the stomach will appear to be distended. In the very uncommon type of duodenal atresia in which a bifid common bile duct inserts both above and below the atresia, air may be present in distal bowel (95).

In duodenal stenosis, whether due to segmental narrowing or an incomplete web or diaphragm, the stomach and duodenal bulb will usually be distended, but air will be present in the distal bowel. Atresia due to a complete web will of course be indistinguishable from other types of atresia.

Gastric perforation, gastric emphysema, and air in the biliary tree occur only rarely in babies with duodenal obstruction (96). In babies with duodenal atresia and esophageal atresia but no tracheoesophageal fistula, there is a distended gasless abdomen, due to the enormously dilated, fluid-filled stomach (97). Sonography shows a fluid-filled and distended stomach and duodenal bulb.

In newborns with evidence of complete duodenal obstruction on an abdominal radiograph, there is almost never an indication for further radiologic investigation (98). Air is an excellent contrast medium. Positive contrast media provide no more information; duodenal atresia, on film, looks the same in black (air) as it does in white (barium). Sometimes in babies with duodenal obstruction the stomach and or duodenum will have been partially decompressed by vomiting or by a nasogastric tube. In these cases injection of a small amount of air via a nasogastric tube will confirm the diagnosis (Fig. 8-34). Most newborns with evidence of complete duodenal obstruction on plain film are taken directly to surgery.

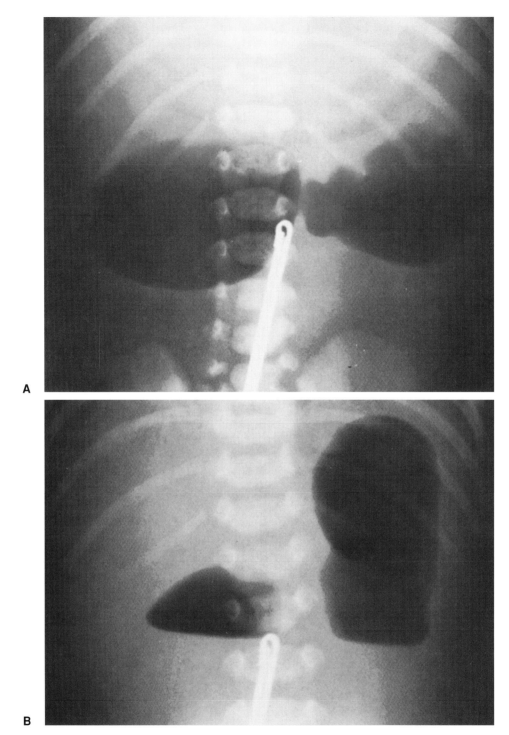

FIG. 8-33. Duodenal atresia. A: Supine radiograph demonstrates gas in the stomach and markedly dilated duodenal bulb. **B:** Double bubble with air-fluid levels in both stomach and duodenum on erect film. From Kirks (96).

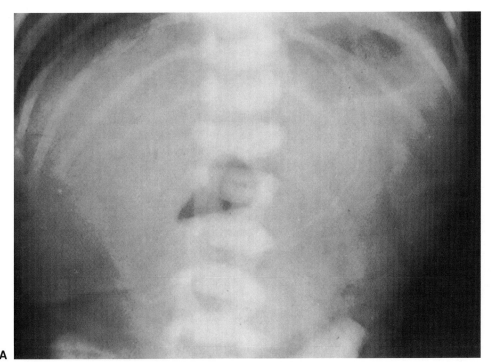

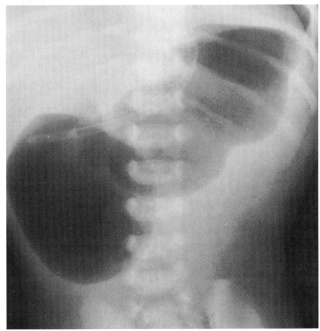

FIG. 8-34. Duodenal atresia. A: Small collections of gas in the stomach and duodenum. **B:** Complete duodenal obstruction demonstrated after injection of 10 cc of air. From Kirks (96).

Some surgeons will ask for a contrast enema in patients with complete duodenal obstruction. In babies with a single proximal intestinal atresia the colon should be of normal or nearly normal caliber; as will be discussed below, a microcolon implies that there are one or more distal atresias (see Fig. 8-60).

Like the newborn with complete duodenal obstruction, the newborn with partial duodenal obstruction will frequently be taken to surgery without any radiologic investigation after the plain films. This is because there is no cause of congenital

duodenal obstruction, complete or partial, which does not require surgery; the surgeon is content to make a specific diagnosis in the operating room. Sometimes, however, the surgeon will ask for radiologic help in distinguishing a type of partial obstruction for which operation may be delayed, such as duodenal stenosis, from midgut volvulus, which requires immediate surgery. In these cases, an upper GI may be very useful, but only if the child is clinically stable. Duodenal stenosis will appear as a narrowed area in the second portion of the duodenum (Fig. 8-35). The findings on UGI

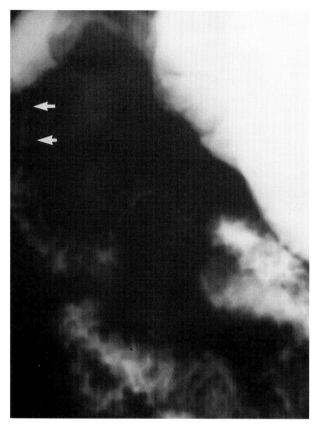

FIG. 8-35. Duodenal stenosis. Marked narrowing of the second portion of the duodenum *(arrows)* in a neonate.

in patients with duodenal webs vary from narrowing to complete obstruction (98). The most diagnostic appearance of a web is that of a thin, curvilinear defect extending a variable distance across the lumen of the duodenum (Fig. 8-36). The wind-sock appearance that a duodenal web may have in an adult or older child, the so-called intraluminal duodenal diverticulum, is not seen in newborns and is probably due to stretching and redundancy of the web caused by years of peristalsis against an incomplete obstruction (Fig. 8-37) (99) .

The duodenal bulb is usually more distended in duodenal atresia or stenosis than in midgut volvulus, but this is not invariably true (see Fig. 8-45). In a baby with a very distended bulb and partial duodenal obstruction, a UGI should be performed to exclude malrotation if surgery is to be delayed (98). Furthermore, some babies with malrotation have complete duodenal obstruction, with no distal air: not every child with complete duodenal obstruction has duodenal atresia (see Fig. 8-44) (100).

Treatment. Duodenoduodenostomy and duodenojejunostomy are the usual surgical procedures for duodenal atresia and stenosis. Care must be taken to identify the ampulla of Vater, which may enter the site of stenosis or web. Survival is excellent; mortality is due to associated anomalies. Postoperative imaging is straightforward. The duodenal bulb may remain distended for many years after repair of duodenal obstruction.

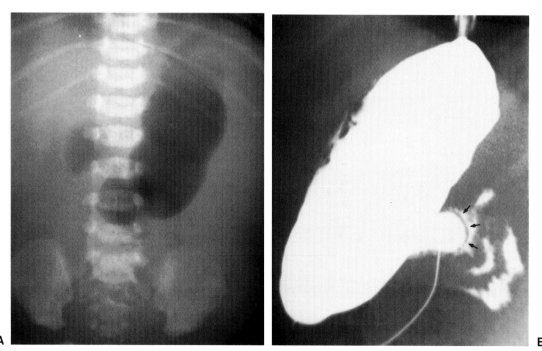

A   B

FIG. 8-36. Duodenal web. A: Supine abdominal radiograph in a newborn with bilious emesis demonstrates a dilated stomach and duodenal bulb. There is little distal gas. B: UGI series shows a duodenal web *(arrows)*. The baby also had trisomy 21 (Down syndrome). From Buonomo (88).

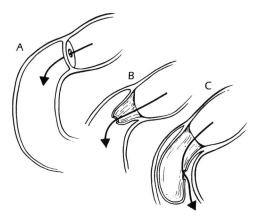

FIG. 8-37. Development of an intraluminal duodenal diverticulum. A: Duodenal diaphragm with central opening. **B:** Stretching of diaphragm secondary to pressure from above. **C:** Typical wind-sock appearance of intraluminal diverticulum in an older child or adult with an eccentric opening in the diverticulum. From Kirks (96); modified from Pratt (99).

Malrotation

Knowledge of the embryology of intestinal development leads to an understanding of malrotation, one of the most important topics in pediatric radiology. The GI tract begins in fetal life as a straight, short tube. The process by which this tube elongates and assumes an orderly, stable arrangement in the peritoneal cavity is very complicated. In the classic

description of Snyder and Chaffin (101), the straight, midline tube of the primitive midgut is divided into two parts by the axis of the SMA. The proximal, prearterial, or duodenojejunal loop lies above and anterior to the SMA. The distal, postarterial, or cecocolic loop (comprising what will be the distal ileum, right colon, and proximal two thirds of the transverse colon) lies below and behind the SMA (Fig. 8-38). As the intestine elongates the two loops rotate independently in a counterclockwise direction around the axis of the SMA. Thus the duodenojejunal loop rotates to the right 90°, then another 90° to a position posterior to the SMA, and finally another 90° to lie left of the artery. This 270° counterclockwise rotation results in the second portion of the duodenum lying to the right of the SMA, the third portion posterior to the SMA, and the duodenojejunal junction to the left and posterior to the SMA. The cecocolic loop also rotates 270° counterclockwise, with the cecum coming to lie finally in the right lower quadrant and the transverse colon anterior to the SMA (Fig. 8-38). As the process of rotation is completed, the bowel becomes fixed and stabilized in its final position by the mesentery. The normal mesentery thus has a broad base which extends from the left upper quadrant at the duodenojejunal junction (ligament of Treitz) to the cecum in the right lower quadrant (Fig. 8-39).

Snyder and Chaffin used the analogy of a rope on a board (Fig. 8-40) to explain the complicated process of normal rotation and to emphasize that rotation is a continuum, not a series of discrete 90° turns. The process can be arrested at

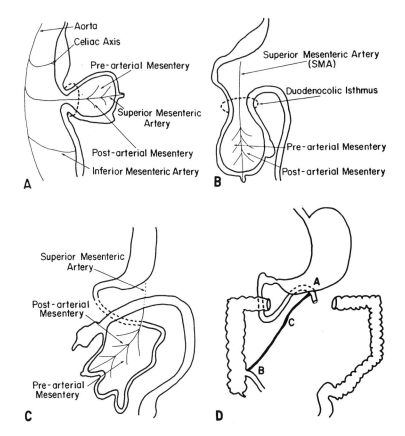

FIG. 8-38. Normal intestinal rotation. A: Lateral view of the gut at fifth to sixth fetal week. **B:** AP view of the gut at eighth fetal week. **C:** AP view of the gut at the eleventh fetal week. **D:** AP view at birth. *A,* ligament of Treitz; *B,* ileocecal junction; *C,* root of mesentery. See text for details. From Houston and Wittenborg (100).

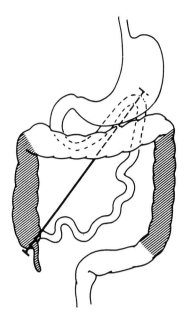

FIG. 8-39. Normal small bowel mesenteric attachment. Normal broad base of the mesenteric attachment extends from the ligament of Treitz (duodenojejunal junction) in the left upper quadrant to the ileocecal valve in the right lower quadrant. The ascending and descending colon *(hatched)* are fixed in the retroperitoneum. From Kirks (96).

any point, in either loop or in both. Thus, in theory at least, an enormous number of variations of rotation are possible (102). ''Malrotation'' is the general term for any abnormal variation in intestinal rotation. Classification of malrotation into subtypes is of little use. Any variety of malrotation seen on an x-ray study in a child with abdominal symptoms should be assumed to be the cause of the symptoms unless there are very strong reasons to believe otherwise.

Malposition of the intestines in itself does not generally cause problems. Malposition of the intestines, however, is usually accompanied by malfixation, which may have catastrophic consequences. When the duodenojejunal junction and the ileocecal junction, the normal points of fixation of the mesentery, are not in their usual location, the mesentery is likely to have only a narrow base (Fig. 8-41). Since the entire jejunum and ileum are attached to this narrow pedicle there is a tendency for the intestines to twist around it: this leads to extrinsic compression of the bowel, obstruction at the base of the pedicle, and, if the twist persists, to occlusion of the mesenteric vessels (Fig. 8-41). The twist of malfixed intestines around their short mesentery is called midgut volvulus. Patients with malfixation of the bowel also frequently have abnormal peritoneal fibrous bands (103). These so-called Ladd bands extend from the malpositioned cecum across the duodenum and attach to the liver, posterior peritoneum, or abdominal wall and may contribute to duodenal obstruction (Fig. 8-42).

The symptoms of malrotation are usually those of proximal bowel obstruction. They may be accompanied by symptoms of vascular occlusion, depending on whether a volvulus is present and on the degree and duration of the twist. The bowel obstruction may be caused by the volvulus, by Ladd bands, or both. In most children with malrotation at any age, obstruction is caused by the volvulus, the bands playing a lesser role or no role at all (104–106).

The incidence of malrotation is unknown; people with malrotation may be asymptomatic for their whole lives. Symptoms may occur at any age, but most patients with symptomatic malrotation present in the first month of life, especially in the first week (104–107). Emesis is nearly always present and is usually bilious. Bilious emesis in a new-

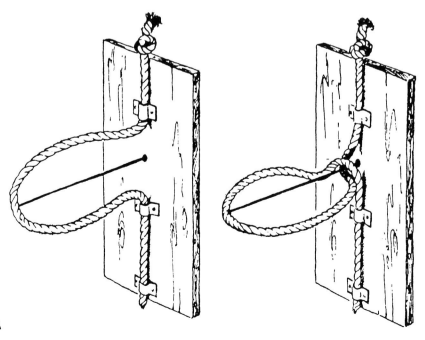

A **B**

FIG. 8-40. Normal intestinal rotation. A: The top limb of the loop corresponds to the duodenojejunum, the wire to the SMA, and the bottom limb to the distal ileum, cecum, and right colon. **B:** The loops have been rotated through an arc of 270° about the wire as an axis in a counterclockwise direction. Thus, the top limb has become the bottom one and the bottom one the top. From Snyder and Chaffin (101).

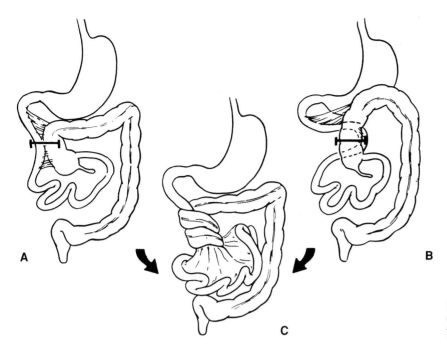

A

B

C

FIG. 8-41. Midgut volvulus. Narrow mesenteric attachment as in **A** or **B** may lead to midgut volvulus **(C)**. From Kirks (96).

born who has been normal for the first few days should be considered to be due to midgut volvulus until proven otherwise; however, in only a minority of newborns with bilious emesis can any organic cause for their vomiting be identified (108). The clinical condition of the child with midgut volvulus ranges from normal to moribund, depending on the degree of vascular compromise. Bloody stool is occasionally present. The physical examination may be negative.

The older the child, the more atypical the symptoms of malrotation can be. Chronic or recurrent abdominal pain, intermittent vomiting, failure to thrive, diarrhea, and malabsorption may be presenting symptoms (105,109–111). The malabsorptive state may result from chronic venous and lymphatic obstruction (112). Though midgut volvulus is less likely in older children with malrotation than in infants, volvulus can occur at any age (113,114).

Malrotation is an integral component of congenital anom-

alies such as omphalocele, gastroschisis, and diaphragmatic hernia. Midgut volvulus rarely develops after surgical correction of these anomalies (55,107). Malrotation is also common in babies with congenital heart disease and heterotaxy (115). In the absence of one of these clinically obvious conditions, malrotation is usually an isolated abnormality (105). Up to 5% of babies with malrotation, however, have an intrinsic obstructing duodenal lesion, often stenosis, in addition to duodenal obstruction due to Ladd bands or volvulus (105,107).

A special situation is that of prenatal midgut volvulus. This may lead to extensive necrosis of bowel and atresia or atresias (100,116).

Radiology. The child with malrotation and midgut volvulus may present with an acute abdomen; time should not be wasted performing radiologic studies, apart from plain films, on such sick patients. A child with bilious emesis on the first day of life and a film showing complete duodenal obstruction needs surgery, not more imaging. All other children with bilious emesis or other symptoms that suggest malrotation need radiologic evaluation.

The first step is a plain film of the abdomen (104). The findings on the plain film are due to obstruction of the duodenum and bowel ischemia. Thus an abdominal film may be negative between episodes of volvulus; it may be negative even if volvulus is present, if the constriction is not tight enough to cause findings. Because the stomach is so much larger and more distensible than the duodenum, plain films may suggest a gastric outlet obstruction when the obstruction is actually duodenal (see Fig. 8-31). The classic finding on a plain film is partial obstruction of the duodenum (Fig. 8-43) (100,104,117), although in other patients the obstruction

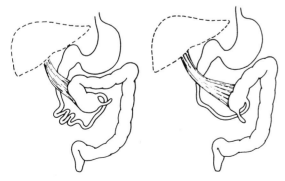

FIG. 8-42. Ladd bands. Peritoneal bands may extend from the malpositioned cecum, across the duodenum, to the posterolateral abdomen and porta hepatis. From Kirks (96).

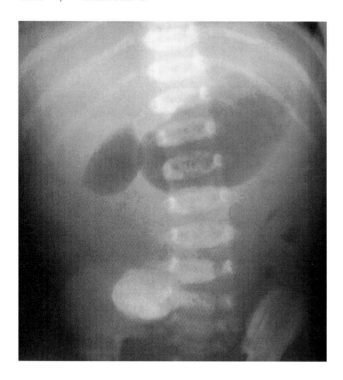

FIG. 8-43. Malrotation with midgut volvulus: partial duodenal obstruction. Supine abdominal radiograph in a neonate with bilious emesis shows a dilated stomach and duodenum with a small amount of distal bowel gas.

is complete (Fig. 8-44) (98). The child who vomits bile at birth and whose film demonstrates a double bubble with no distal intestinal air probably has duodenal atresia; the abdominal film of a baby with midgut volvulus, however, may also demonstrate complete duodenal obstruction (Fig. 8-44) or marked gastric and duodenal distention (Fig. 8-45). Close communication with the surgical staff is mandatory in these difficult cases. After the immediate postnatal period,

any duodenal obstruction should be assumed to be midgut volvulus until proven otherwise.

The plain films of babies with midgut volvulus may also show a pattern of ileus or distal small bowel obstruction with multiple dilated loops and air-fluid levels (Fig. 8-46) (100,104). This is an ominous sign, sometimes reflecting a closed loop obstruction and nonabsorption of gas from the necrotic intestine (118,119). Finally, the abdomen in midgut

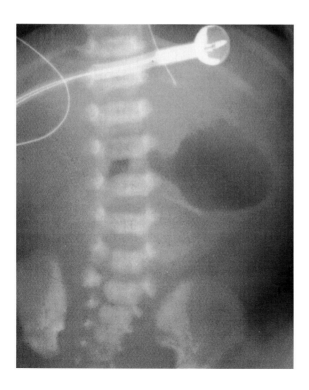

FIG. 8-44. Midgut volvulus with complete duodenal obstruction. AP film of a newborn with bilious vomiting shows air in the stomach and probably in the first part of the duodenum. No air is present distally. A midgut volvulus was present at surgery.

definite distal bowel obstruction in which case a contrastenema should be performed. This particularly includes infants and children who have previously been well and newborns who have bilious emesis but normal films. Of all the anomalies that cause bilious emesis, only malrotation is likely to produce a normal abdominal film.

The truly important abnormality in malrotation is malfixation of the intestines. Malfixation is inferred from malposition of the duodenojejunal junction and of the cecum (see Figs. 8-38 and 8-41). The barium enema was formerly employed to diagnose malrotation. The entire colon may be abnormally positioned; more frequently, however, the colon is normal in position except for the cecum and ascending colon. The ascending colon appears shortened and the cecum ends above the iliac fossa. This high cecum is often directed transversely, back to the midline (100,104) (Fig. 8-46). The high cecum of malrotation, usually fixed in position by Ladd bands and at or directed to the midline, needs to be distinguished from the high, normally oriented but mobile cecum frequently found as a normal variant. Over the years the barium enema has fallen out of favor as the initial study for malrotation (100,120). This is partly because of confusion caused by a normal but high cecum, but especially because the cecum may be normally positioned in up to 20% of children with malrotation (121–125).

The location of the duodenojejunal junction is a more accurate indication of malrotation. The normal duodenojejunal junction is to the left of the left pedicles of the spine and is at the level of the duodenal bulb (125). Virtually all patients with malrotation will have a duodenojejunal junction lying to the right of or below the normal position (Fig. 8-47). In a child with malrotation but no obstruction, the abnormally located duodenojejunal junction may be the only finding. In addition, in malrotation the jejunum will usually be on the right. The obstruction may be complete or partial (Figs. 8-47 to 8-49). One occasionally sees the pathognomonic ''corkscrew'' pattern of the twisted duodenum and jejunum (Figs. 8-46 and 8-50). Only very rare cases of malrotation have none of these findings (124,125,126). When the location of the duodenojejunal junction is uncertain, following the barium to show the location of the jejunum, ileum, and cecum often helps. Abnormal position of the cecum facilitates the diagnosis. Ultimately, however, in the absence of duodenal obstruction or a corkscrew duodenum and jejunum, the most specific sign of malrotation is the abnormally positioned duodenojejunal junction (126). The radiologist, however, should be aware that the duodenojejunal junction is mobile in children and may be displaced down and to the right by distended bowel, by masses, and by enlarged organs such as the spleen (Fig. 8-51) (125–127).

Ultrasonography is also useful in malrotation. The actual duodenal obstruction or volvulus may be visualized (128–132). The majority of patients with malrotation will have inversion of the normal relationship of the SMA and SMV; in malrotation the SMV lies to the left of the SMA

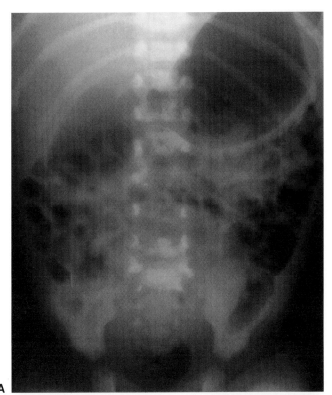

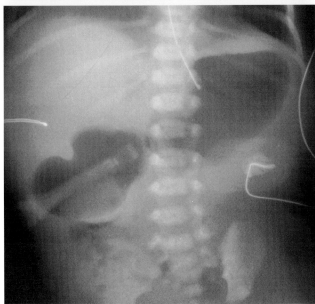

FIG. 8-45. Incomplete duodenal obstruction. Abdominal films of two newborns with partial duodenal obstructions. The baby in **(A)** had a duodenal web; the baby in **(B)** a midgut volvulus. From Buonomo (88).

volvulus may be gasless because of either proximal obstruction or diffuse bowel necrosis (119).

With the exceptions described above (the neonate with complete duodenal obstruction and the critically ill infant with bilious emesis), all newborns with bilious emesis need a UGI series, unless their abdominal film demonstrates a

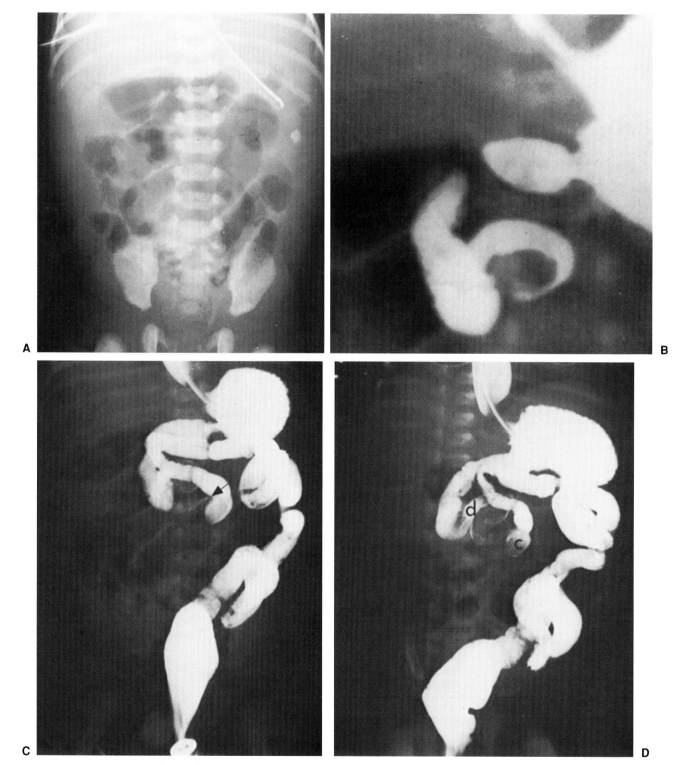

FIG. 8-46. Midgut volvulus with apparent distal small bowel obstruction. A: Supine radiograph. There are many dilated loops of small bowel mimicking mechanical distal small bowel obstruction. **B:** UGI series. Note the spiral or corkscrew appearance of the duodenum. **C:** Anteroposterior film after opacification of the colon. The cecum is high and midline. The ileocecal valve *(arrow)* opens to the right. **D:** Left posterior oblique film. The narrow mesenteric attachment between the duodenum *(d)* and the cecum *(c)* is apparent. From Kirks (96).

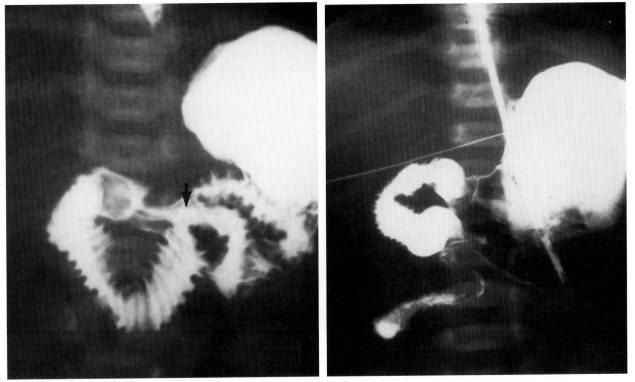

FIG. 8-47. Upper gastrointestinal series in malrotation. A: Normal duodenojejunal junction *(arrow)*. **B:** Malrotation. The duodenum does not reach to the left of the spine or the level of the duodenal bulb. There is a "corkscrew" appearance of the distal duodenum.

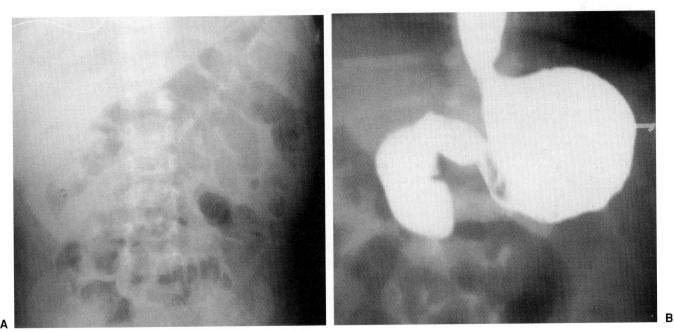

FIG. 8-48. Midgut volvulus with complete duodenal obstruction. A: AP film demonstrates air throughout bowel. **B:** UGI series demonstrates complete obstruction of the third portion of the duodenum.

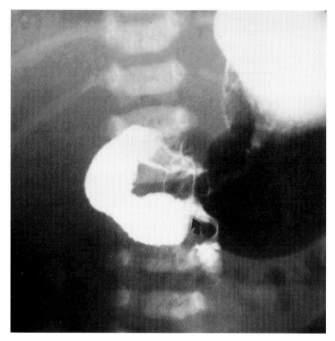

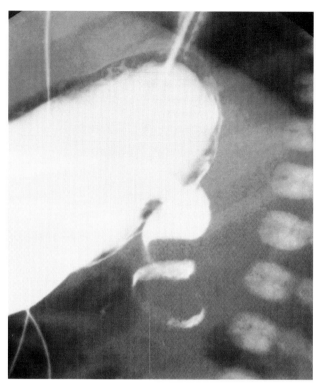

FIG. 8-49. Midgut volvulus with partial duodenal obstruction. The duodenum is partially obstructed *(curved arrow)*. The duodenojejunal junction is inferior and medial to its normal location.

FIG. 8-50. Midgut volvulus. Classic "corkscrew" appearance of duodenum and proximal jejunum.

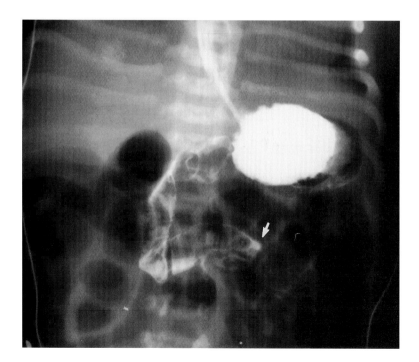

FIG. 8-51. Displacement of duodenojejunal junction due to distended bowel. Marked bowel distention in a newborn due to Hirschsprung disease. The duodenojejunal junction *(arrow)* is displaced inferiorly by the distended bowel. At surgery there was normal intestinal rotation.

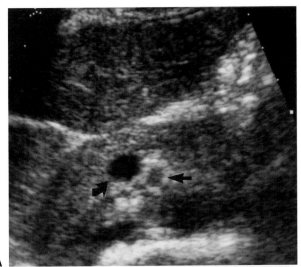

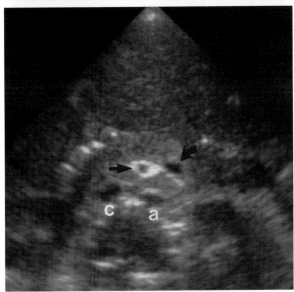

FIG. 8-52. Abnormal position of the superior mesenteric artery and vein (SMA, SMV) by US in malrotation. A: Normal relationship of the SMA *(arrow)* which lies to the left of the SMV *(curved arrow)*. **B:** Malrotation. The SMA *(arrow)* lies to the right of the SMV *(curved arrow)*. There was malrotation at surgery. *a,* aorta, *c,* inferior vena cava. From Buonomo (89).

(Fig. 8-52) (133–135). However, about a third of patients with surgically proven malrotation have a normal relationship of these vessels, and some patients with an abnormal position of the SMA and SMV do not have malrotation (136). Thus, US is neither sensitive nor specific enough, and the UGI remains the best diagnostic method. Abnormal position of the mesenteric vessels may also be shown by CT or MRI (137,138).

Treatment. Malrotation is a surgical emergency because of the high frequency of midgut volvulus and its sequel, ischemic necrosis. The accepted surgical procedure (Ladd operation) includes reduction of the volvulus (untwisting the volvulus), resection of nonviable bowel, transection of ab-

normal peritoneal bands, exclusion of an associated duodenal stenosis or web, and placement of the small bowel in the right abdomen and the colon on the left. The mesentery of the small bowel is thus spread smoothly from right to left with a broad attachment. Recurrent volvulus after a Ladd procedure is very unusual, perhaps because of the formation of adhesions.

Although all surgeons agree asymptomatic malrotation in an infant or young child should be operated on, there is disagreement about surgical repair of a malrotation found incidentally in older children and adults (139). It is clear, however, that the possibility of midgut volvulus exists at any age. There is also disagreement about performing a Ladd procedure for children with malrotation associated with cardiac disease (140); some of these children will develop volvulus (141,142).

Jejunal Atresia and Stenosis

Definition and Clinical Features. Atresia or stenosis of the jejunum or proximal ileum presents as a high intestinal obstruction, distal ileal atresia or stenosis as low obstruction. The clinical and radiologic features of distal ileal atresia and stenosis will be discussed in the section on low obstruction. The embryology of all these conditions is the same and will be discussed here.

Atresia and stenosis are slightly more common in the proximal jejunum and distal ileum than in the intervening small intestine (143). As is the case in the duodenum, atresia is much more common than stenosis (Fig. 8-53). Unlike duodenal atresia, however, jejunoileal atresia is caused not by a failure of recanalization but by ischemic injury. The ischemia may be due to a primary vascular accident or to a mechanical obstruction as with in utero volvulus. Babies with jejunoileal atresia have fewer associated anomalies than those with duodenal atresia.

Two unusual forms of atresia may be inherited. In apple-peel (Christmas tree) atresia (Figs. 8-53 and 8-54) there is distal duodenal or proximal jejunal atresia associated with absence of the distal SMA, shortening of the small bowel distal to the atresia, and absence of part of the mesentery (144). This type of atresia is probably caused by prenatal occlusion of the SMA distal to the origin of the midcolic artery. The bowel distal to the atresia is supplied by collaterals from the middle, right, and ileocolic arteries. The distal small intestine spirals around this vascular supply and gives this type of atresia its name (Fig. 8-54).

The syndrome of multiple intestinal atresias with intraluminal calcification is found most frequently in infants of French-Canadian ancestry and is transmitted in an autosomal recessive pattern. There are multiple atresias from stomach to rectum. The radiologic hallmark of this syndrome is extensive calcification of intraluminal contents between the atresias (145). Nonhereditary bowel atresias occasionally also cause intraluminal calcification.

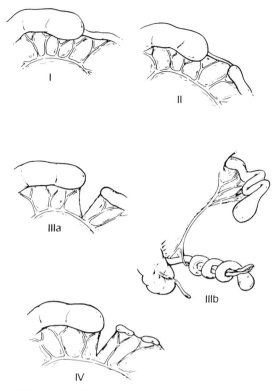

FIG. 8-53. Classification of intestinal atresia. *Type I*, membranous atresia; *type II*, blind ends separated by fibrous cord; *type IIIa*, blind ends separated with an associated V-shaped mesenteric gap; *type IIIb*, apple-peel small bowel atresia; *type IV*, multiple atresias. From Kirks (96).

Newborns with jejunoileal atresia will usually present with bilious emesis. The abdomen is likely to be distended, especially when the atresia is fairly distal.

Radiology. The abdominal radiograph of a child with jejunal atresia will usually show a few dilated bowel loops, more than duodenal atresia but fewer than ileal atresia or other types of low bowel obstruction (Fig. 8-55). The loop just proximal to the atresia is frequently disproportionately dilated and has a bulbous end (Fig. 8-56) (146). Occasionally, this bulbous segment is completely filled with fluid and produces, on plain films, a mass of soft-tissue density. If the ischemic event that produced the atresia also caused a perforation, there may be peritoneal calcification and meconium peritonitis. Intraluminal calcification is rarely present. The apple peel type of atresia does not have distinctive plain film findings.

As is the case with duodenal atresia or stenosis, the child with jejunal atresia or stenosis usually needs no further radiologic investigation. A UGI is rarely indicated. Some surgeons will request an enema to confirm or exclude additional sites of atresia. In isolated proximal atresia of the jejunum, the colon will be normal or nearly normal in size; in more distal atresias, the colon will be smaller (Fig. 8-57). An enema in a child with apple-peel atresia may demonstrate the typical spiral configuration of the distal small bowel (Fig. 8-58) (147).

Treatment. Surgical treatment consists of primary anastomosis with resection of nonviable bowel and tapering of very

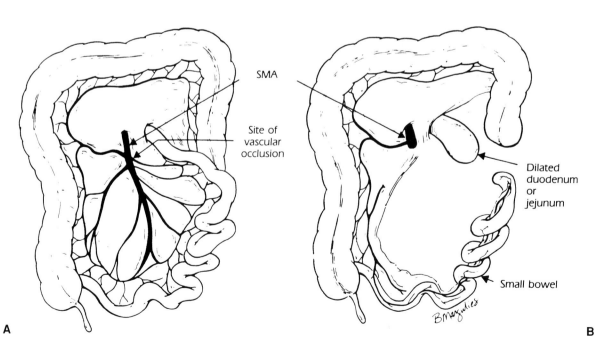

FIG. 8-54. Apple-peel small bowel atresia. A: Normal distribution of the superior mesenteric artery (SMA). **B:** In utero occlusion of the SMA produces apple-peel atresia. From Kirks (96).

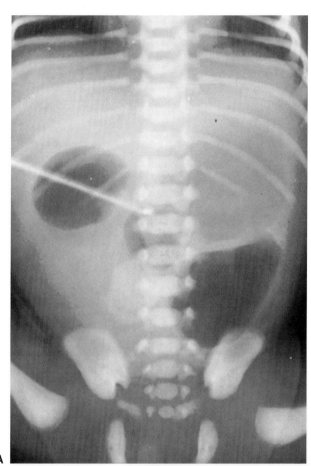

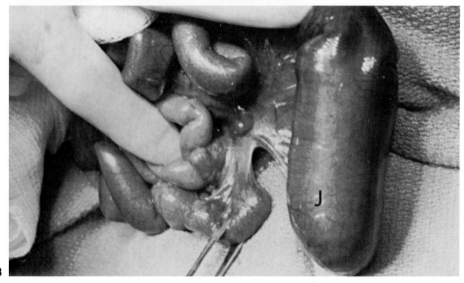

FIG. 8-55. Jejunal atresia. A: Triple bubble due to gas in dilated stomach, duodenum, and proximal jejunum. **B:** Type IIIa atresia with dilated jejunum *(J)* proximal to the atresia; the forceps are on the collapsed jejunum distal to the atresia; a V-shaped mesenteric gap lies between the separated blind ends. (Courtesy of Howard C. Filston, M.D., Knoxville, TN.)

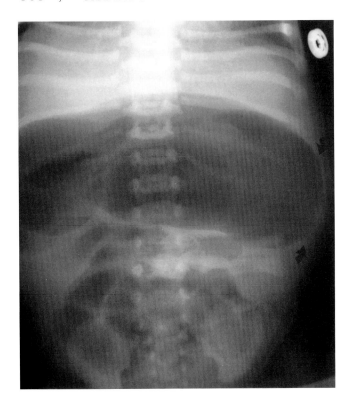

FIG. 8-56. Jejunal atresia. Supine radiograph in a newborn with abdominal distention and bilious emesis. Jejunal atresia was present at surgery. Note that the loop just proximal to the atresia is disproportionately dilated and has a "bulbous" end *(curved arrows)*.

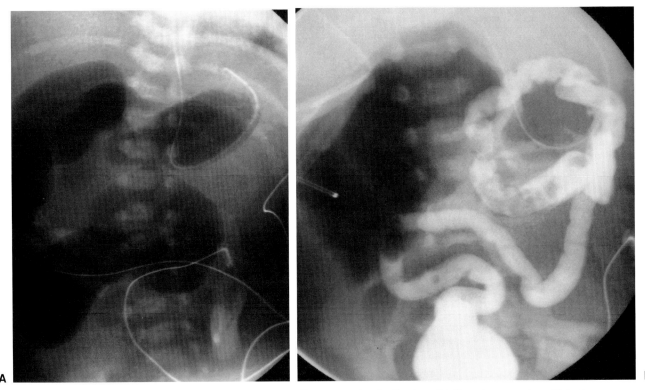

A

B

FIG. 8-57. Multiple atresias. Newborn with bilious emesis. A: Supine AP film shows a few dilated loops consistent with proximal jejunal atresia. B: Contrast enema demonstrates a small colon. Five additional small bowel atresias, including a distal ileal atresia, were found at surgery. The colon is displaced to the left by the dilated small bowel; this is not malrotation.

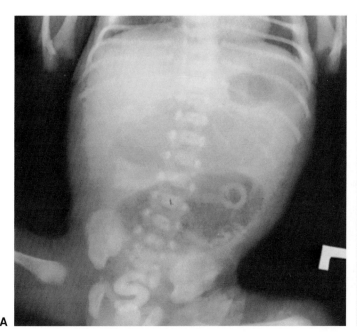
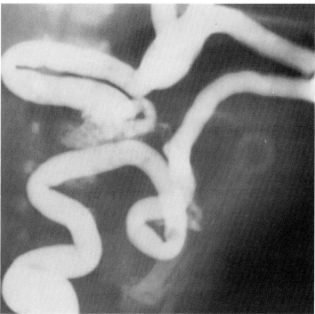

A

B

FIG. 8-58. Apple-peel small bowel atresia. A: Triple bubble on supine radiograph due to distention of stomach and two loops of proximal small bowel. Contrast in the rectum from previous enema. **B:** Contrast enema. The colon is unused. The spiral course of the distal small bowel is consistent with apple-peel small bowel atresia.

dilated segments. The bulbous bowel just proximal to the atresia is frequently poorly functioning. On postoperative examination there is often very delayed passage of contrast through this loop even when the anastomosis is widely patent.

Survival in babies with intestinal atresia is very good; the major morbidity is the short gut syndrome in babies who have had extensive loss of bowel leaving insufficient absorbing surface. Short gut syndrome is especially likely to occur in apple-peel atresia. The familial form of multiple intestinal atresias is usually fatal.

Low Intestinal Obstruction

Low intestinal obstruction may be defined as one occurring in the distal ileum or colon. The differential diagnosis of low intestinal obstruction in the neonate, for practical purposes, consists of only four conditions. Two involve the colon, i.e., Hirschsprung disease and "functional immaturity of the colon" (also known as meconium plug syndrome and small left colon syndrome). Two involve the distal ileum, i.e., meconium ileus and ileal atresia. These four conditions comprise nearly all neonatal low obstructions. Other causes include anorectal malformations (common, but seldom a diagnostic problem), colon atresia, megacystis–microcolon-intestinal hypoperistalsis syndrome, and neonatal intussusception.

That an obstruction is low is usually obvious from the plain film. However, whether a low obstruction is at the level of the distal ileum or at the level of the colon, and in the latter case in what part of the colon, is difficult or impossible to determine from the plain film. When confronted with a plain film showing many distended loops, we can only rarely state with any confidence whether the distention involves only small bowel (i.e., the obstruction is in the distal ileum) or small bowel and colon (i.e., the point of obstruction is in the colon). This distinction can be readily made with a contrast enema (Fig. 8-59).

Virtually all newborns with plain film evidence of low obstruction need a contrast enema. For diagnostic enemas in newborns a relatively dilute, ionic, water-soluble contrast, such as is used for cystography should be employed (see Appendix 5); the osmolality of these agents is not high, so that large fluid shifts into bowel do not occur, and the iodine concentration is high enough to provide satisfactory images. It is not necessary to use the high-cost, low-osmolar, non-ionic, water-soluble agents. In neonates, water-soluble agents are preferable to barium for several reasons. First, though it is rare, perforation due to the obstruction may not be detected on the plain film, and contrast may spill into the peritoneal cavity. Second, babies with either functional immaturity of the colon or meconium ileus (especially the latter) benefit from enemas with water-soluble contrast; therapy thus begins immediately, with the diagnostic study. Moreover, there has been greater success in reducing meconium ileus using water-soluble contrast for the initial diagnostic enema rather than barium. Finally, in this setting, barium offers no particular advantages over water-soluble contrast. Depiction of fine mucosal detail is not usually im-

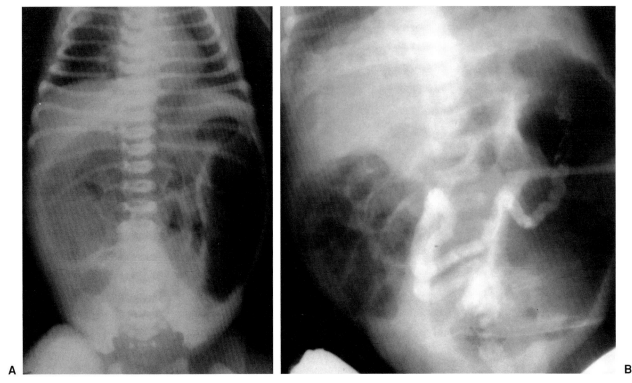

FIG. 8-59. Low intestinal obstruction. A: A supine radiograph of newborn with abdominal distention demonstrates a very dilated bowel loop in the left flank. This could be mistaken for colon. **B:** A contrast enema demonstrates a microcolon. The dilated loop in the left flank is shown to be small bowel. The baby had meconium ileus.

portant in newborns, and poor evacuation of barium on delayed films, though a finding in Hirschsprung disease, is neither sensitive nor specific enough in itself to make a diagnosis; delayed films are only rarely obtained when Hirschsprung disease is suspected.

The critical differential diagnostic finding on the contrast enema of a newborn with low bowel obstruction is the presence or absence of a microcolon (148). A microcolon is a colon of very small caliber, generally less than 1 cm in diameter (Fig. 8-60). The entire colon must be involved, not just a portion, as in the small left colon syndrome. The diagnosis is usually obvious, though the judgment is necessarily subjective. A microcolon is an unused colon: the caliber of the colon depends on the amount of succus entericus which reaches it. If little or no succus entericus reaches the colon, it will be tiny. Therefore, with the exceptions of the microcolon of prematurity and the microcolon of total colonic Hirschsprung disease (both discussed below), the presence of a microcolon means that the baby has a high-grade, distal small bowel obstruction, i.e., for all practical purposes, meconium ileus or ileal atresia. Isolated atresias of the more proximal small bowel will not lead to a microcolon since the remaining small bowel distal to the atresia will produce enough succus entericus to give a colon of normal caliber (see Fig. 8-57) (148). Proximal ileal atresia, which is unusual, leads to a colon of variable size.

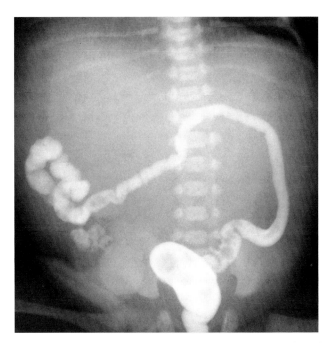

FIG. 8-60. Microcolon. Unused colon in a newborn with multiple intestinal atresias. From Buonomo (88).

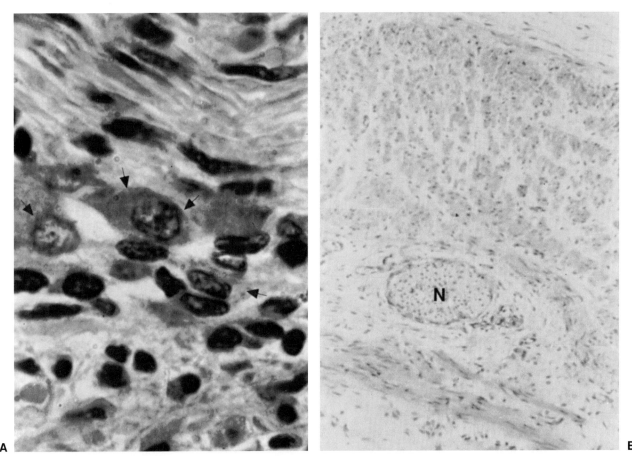

FIG. 8-61. Myenteric plexus. A: Normal. High-power view of myenteric plexus with normal ganglion cells *(arrows)*. **B:** Hirschsprung disease. Low-power view of the myenteric plexus containing a hypertrophied nerve *(N)*, frequently seen in Hirschsprung disease. No ganglion cells are identified. (Courtesy of Howard C. Filston, M.D., Knoxville, TN.)

Hirschsprung Disease

Hirschsprung disease is caused by the absence of intramural ganglion cells in the distal bowel. The ganglion cells of the intestine migrate in a craniocaudad direction and reach the distal colon by about the twelfth week of gestation (149). Hirschsprung disease results when there is an arrest in this migration of neural cells; the area of aganglionosis extends distally from the point of neuronal arrest to the anus (Fig. 8-61). The region of aganglionosis is continuous; the existence of ''skip areas'' is extraordinarily rare (150). The aganglionic region may involve only the rectum and a portion of the sigmoid colon (short segment disease; this accounts for about three fourths of the cases) may extend a variable distance proximal to the sigmoid (long segment disease), or may affect the entire colon and a variable amount of small intestine (total colonic disease). Ultrashort segment disease with aganglionosis limited to the region of the internal sphincter is very rare, as is aganglionosis involving the entire alimentary tract (151).

Hirschsprung disease is three or four times as common in boys as in girls (151) and, for obscure reasons, is very uncommon in premature infants. In the unusual total colonic variant, the incidence in boys and girls is more nearly equal, and there is a strong hereditary tendency (151). Serious associated anomalies are uncommon in children with Hirschsprung disease (152), although approximately 5% have Down syndrome. An interesting and unusual association of Hirschsprung disease is with congenital hypoventilation syndrome (Ondine curse) and congenital neuroblastoma (153); all three disorders are due to the maldevelopment of cells derived from the neural crest.

The absence of ganglion cells in Hirschsprung disease results in the failure of the distal intestine to relax normally. Peristaltic waves do not pass through the aganglionic segment, and defecation is abnormal, which leads to functional obstruction. Most children with Hirschsprung disease present in the newborn period with intestinal obstruction. A few patients are found later in infancy or childhood, usually with chronic, severe constipation. Up to a third of patients with Hirschsprung disease develop enterocolitis, either at presentation or after surgery (154). The pathogenesis of the enterocolitis is unclear; its manifestations range from diarrhea to fulminant colitis with sepsis and shock. Any newborn with

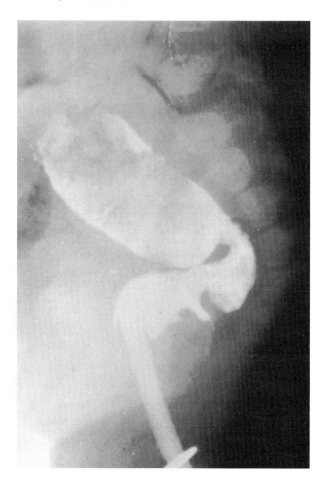

FIG. 8-62. Hirschsprung disease. A 4-month-old boy with constipation since birth. The metallic washer marks the external anus. There is a transition zone in the rectum and irregularity of the distal aganglionic bowel. Surgical exploration confirmed aganglionosis.

symptoms of obstruction and colitis should be suspected of having Hirschsprung disease.

Radiology. Plain films of the abdomen in the newborn with Hirschsprung disease will demonstrate low bowel obstruction. About 5% present with pneumoperitoneum secondary to perforation (155). Most of those babies have total colonic disease, although enterocolitis is not usually present. The perforation may be in the appendix. As in all causes of low obstruction, definitive diagnosis requires a contrast enema. Balloon catheters should never be used; they may obscure the diagnosis, or perforate the stiff, aganglionic rectum. The catheter should barely be in the rectum, to avoid obscuring a transition zone. The critical view is the lateral view of the rectum, obtained during slow filling (156). The most specific sign of Hirschsprung disease is the transition zone from the normal or slightly small aganglionic bowel to dilated normally innervated proximal bowel (Fig. 8-62) (157, 158). Unfortunately, a discrete zone of transition is infrequent in newborns; in these cases, the "rectosigmoid index" is helpful (159). In normal children and in children with other causes of low obstruction, any barium enema film should show the widest rectal diameter to be greater than the maximal diameter of the sigmoid colon; the ratio of rectal to sigmoid diameter, or rectosigmoid index, is normally ≥1. In newborns with Hirschsprung disease this ratio is <1 (Fig.

8-63). Another finding on contrast enema in children with Hirschsprung disease is irregular contractions, once called anorectal dyskinesia (157), in the aganglionic segment (Fig. 8-62); though quite specific, these contractions are infrequently seen (158). If barium has been used as the contrast agent, films obtained after 24 hours may show an unusual degree of retention of barium. However, the finding is not specific, and good evacuation does not rule out Hirschsprung disease (158). This lack of specificity and sensitivity limits the usefulness of delayed films. In any case, in many newborns with obstruction, delay in therapy is inappropriate. If the enema suggests Hirschsprung disease, a rectal biopsy should be obtained promptly. Lastly, and importantly, the contrast enema in newborns with Hirschsprung disease may be normal.

In children with Hirschsprung disease and colitis, the enema may show mucosal edema and ulceration (160) (Fig. 8-64). Clearly, enemas should not be performed in newborns who are critically ill with colitis.

The radiologic diagnosis of total colonic Hirschsprung disease is very difficult (Fig. 8-65) (161–163). Findings include a normal barium enema, a short colon of normal caliber, a microcolon, and a transition zone in the ileum. Additional findings include easy, extensive reflux far back into small bowel (164), a pseudo-transition zone in the

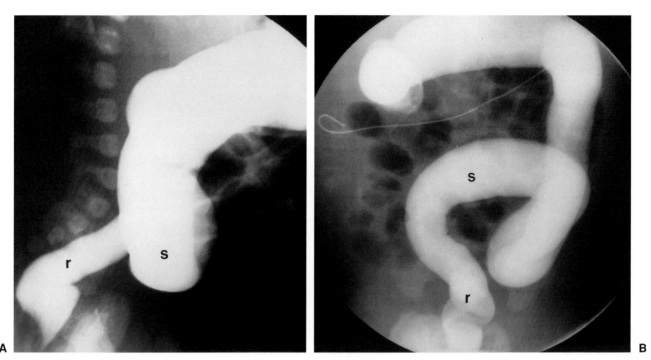

FIG. 8-63. Hirschsprung disease. Abnormal rectosigmoid index. The diameter of the sigmoid colon *(s)* is greater than that of the rectum *(r)* on lateral **(A)** and anteroposterior **(B)** views.

colon (165), and intraluminal small bowel calcification (166).

Treatment. Definitive diagnosis of Hirschsprung disease is made by rectal biopsy, to demonstrate the lack of normal ganglion cells (see Fig. 8-61). Care must be taken to obtain the biopsy at least 1.5 cm above the pectinate line because hypoganglionosis is normal in the rectum below this level. The presence of ganglion cells on a suction biopsy, obtainable at the bedside, excludes the diagnosis. If ganglion cells are not present, a full-thickness biopsy is necessary because false positives may occur with the suction technique. Surgical correction is usually accomplished in two steps; the first is a colostomy just proximal to the pathologic transition zone; the later step is definitive repair, usually by the Soave endorectal pull-through. Most patients with short-segment disease do quite well; those with long segment and total colonic disease often have chronic bowel dysfunction.

Functional Immaturity of the Colon

In 1956, Clatworthy and colleagues described a form of low intestinal obstruction that they felt was the consequence of "the inability of the colon to rid itself of the meconium residue of 9 months of fetal life" (167). Barium enemas revealed a strikingly narrow rectosigmoid and descending colon and transition to a dilated colon at the splenic flexure. Clatworthy labeled this the "meconium plug syndrome," reflecting the belief that the obstruction was probably due to an "alteration in the character of the most distal portion

of the meconium mass" (167). In 1974, Davis et al. (168) described the "small left colon syndrome" in 20 neonates with clinical and radiographic features very similar to those reported by Clatworthy. These authors felt that the syndrome was distinct from the meconium plug syndrome and their name for the syndrome emphasized their belief that it was the smallness of the colon and not abnormalities of the meconium that was the cause of obstruction. In 1975, LeQuesne and Reilly emphasized in a review article that a small left colon and evidence of bowel obstruction could be seen with or without meconium plugs (169). Finally, in 1977 Berdon and coworkers, reviewing their own and published experience, postulated that meconium plug syndrome and small left colon syndrome were overlapping entities in the spectrum of functional neonatal intestinal obstruction (170). Their view is now widely accepted. Most pediatric radiologists now use "meconium plug syndrome" and "small left colon" synonymously, or simply use the generic term "functional immaturity of the colon."

Functional immaturity of the colon is a common cause of neonatal obstruction. Many feel that it is a result of abnormalities in intestinal motility (171). The babies are frequently infants of diabetic mothers (172) or mothers who have received magnesium sulfate for eclampsia (173), though sometimes no risk factors are present. There is no association with cystic fibrosis. Affected newborns present with signs of intestinal obstruction. Babies with functional immaturity of the colon tend not to be as sick as babies with other types of obstruction. Plain films reveal evidence of low

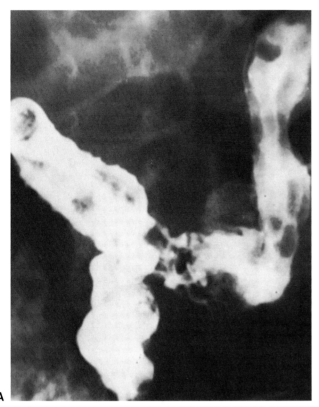

A

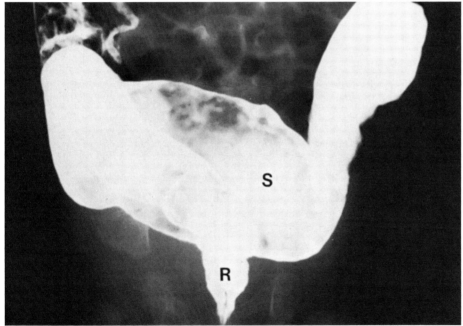

B

FIG. 8-64. Hirschsprung disease with colitis. A: There are mucosal irregularities and submucosal edema of the colon. B: A radiograph at 72 hours demonstrates a marked discrepancy in caliber between the maximal diameter of the rectum *(R)* and the maximal diameter of the sigmoid colon *(S)*. There has been improvement of the colitis proximal to the transition zone.

obstruction. A contrast enema will demonstrate distention of the right and transverse colon and a transition near the splenic flexure to a descending and rectosigmoid colon of narrow diameter. The rectum is usually quite distensible (Fig. 8-66). The amount of meconium in the colon is variable, and discrete "plugs" of meconium at the point of transition may or may not be seen. During or after the enema meconium may be passed; the classic finding is passage of a discrete "plug" (Fig. 8-67). However, this is infrequent; in fact, large amounts of meconium are often passed during enemas by newborns with any type of low obstruction. After the enema there is usually clinical improvement, and over the course of hours or days radiographic and clinical signs of obstruction resolve. Although babies with this form of functional obstruction usually do quite well, a benign course is not invariable, and perforation may occur (174).

The important differential diagnostic alternative in babies with the findings described above is Hirschsprung disease (170,175). Careful analysis of the enema findings is often helpful (170). Only the unusual case of Hirschsprung disease has a transition zone at the splenic flexure. In addition, the apparent transition zone of functional immaturity tends to be quite abrupt whereas the transition zone in Hirschsprung disease is usually cone-shaped and gradual. In Hirschsprung disease the aganglionic colon is usually of nearly normal caliber; in functional immaturity the left colon is usually small. In most newborns with functional immaturity the rectum is quite distensible, whereas in Hirschsprung disease

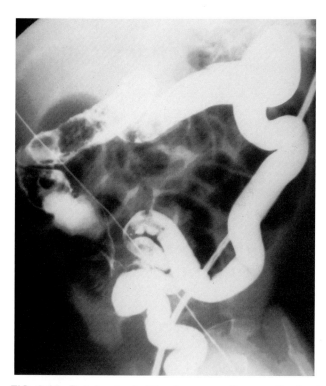

FIG. 8-65. Total colonic Hirschsprung disease. Contrast enema. The entire colon is somewhat small in caliber. The histologic transition zone was in the distal ileum.

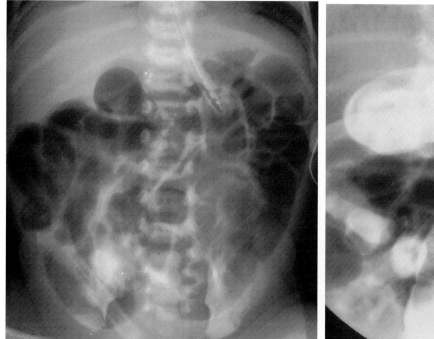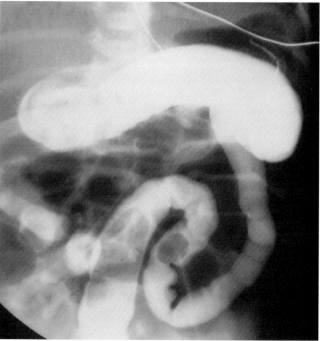

A B

FIG. 8-66. Functional immaturity of the colon (small left colon syndrome). Plain film **(A)** and contrast enema **(B)** in a newborn with abdominal distention and failure to pass meconium. The left colon is small with a transition to dilated colon at the splenic flexure. There is little meconium in the colon.

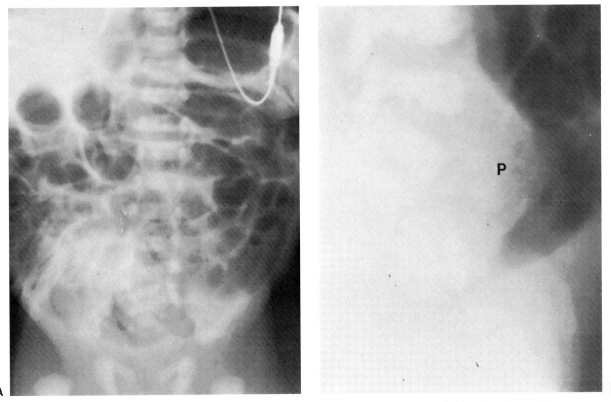

FIG. 8-67. Functional immaturity of the colon (meconium plug syndrome). Newborn boy with obstruction. **A:** There is dilatation of many loops of bowel, suggesting distal obstruction. **B:** Lateral film shows a presacral pseudotumor *(P)* due to the meconium within the rectosigmoid colon. *(Continued)*

the aganglionic colon is usually little larger than the anus. However, a distinction between the two entities is not always possible. In children whose symptoms do not resolve, a biopsy should be performed (Fig. 8-68).

Functional obstruction is frequently present in premature infants (176). In very premature infants the functional obstruction, presumably the result of immaturity of the neuronal apparatus (177), may be so severe as to prevent feeding. The natural history of this disorder is unknown. The contrast enema may be normal or may show a microcolon (178).

Colon Atresia

Colon atresia is much rarer than atresia of the small bowel. As in small bowel atresia, the atresia may have the form of a diaphragm (web) or there may be a fibrous cord or complete gap between the blind segments (see Fig. 8-53). Atresias are evenly distributed in the colon, which supports an intrauterine vascular etiology.

Plain films demonstrate low bowel obstruction, occasionally with a disproportionately dilated loop of proximal colon. Contrast enemas show a microcolon distal to the atresia (Fig. 8-69) (179). If the atresia is due to a web or diaphragm,

the enema may show a club-shaped microcolon next to or ballooning into the air-filled proximal colon (wind-sock deformity) (Fig. 8-70) (179,180). Atresias of the colon may coexist with other intestinal atresias. Stenosis of the colon is very rare.

Anorectal Malformations

The terms "imperforate anus" and "anorectal malformation" are used synonymously. The former term is more frequently employed but is a misleading simplification of the complexity which actually exists. The etiology is unknown but involves abnormal separation of the genitourinary system from the hindgut. The malformations are best thought of as anal or anorectal atresia in which the atretic anorectum most often terminates in the genitourinary tract. Though it is customary to describe the communication between the rectum and genitourinary tract as a "fistula," this communication is in fact the actual termination of the hindgut.

Anorectal malformations are classified as high or low, depending on whether or not the rectum ends above or below the puborectalis sling; the lesions are then subclassified according to the anatomy of the termination. In low lesions there is usually a visible perineal orifice, which may be ste-

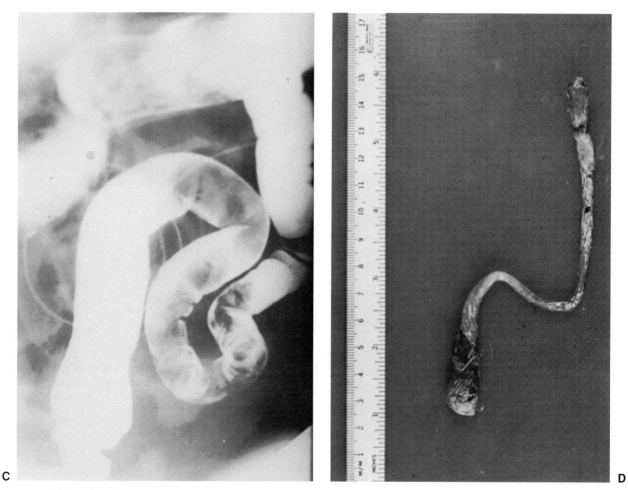

C

D

FIG. 8-67. *(continued)* **C:** Contrast enema demonstrates many filling defects due to meconium in the rectosigmoid colon. The rectum is distensible. **D:** A long meconium plug passed after contrast enema.

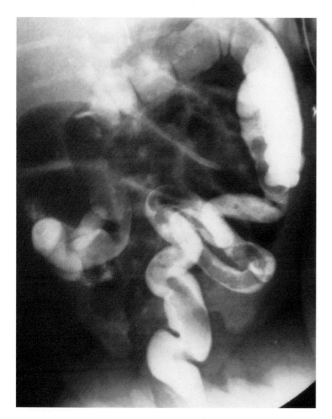

FIG. 8-68. Hirschsprung disease mimicking small left colon syndrome. Apparent transition zone at the splenic flexure. Biopsy showed no ganglion cells distal to the distal ileum. Note that the rectum is not distensible and that there are ''meconium plugs'' in the left colon.

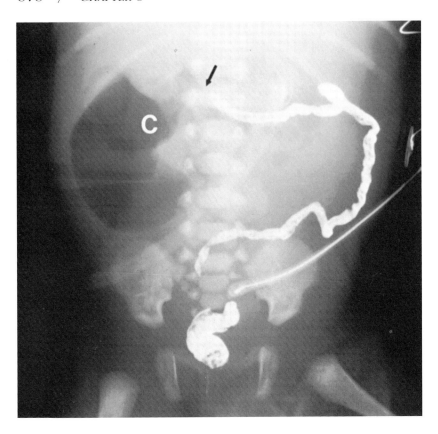

FIG. 8-69. Colon atresia. A water-soluble contrast enema demonstrates an unused distal colon that tapers toward the right transverse colon *(C)*. Note that the gas-filled transverse colon also has a beak-like distal end *(arrow)* at the site of atresia.

notic or completely covered; there is no communication with the genitourinary tract. In boys with high lesions, the rectum almost always terminates in the posterior urethra; much less frequently the rectum terminates in the bladder or anterior urethra (181) or ends blindly. In girls with high lesions, the rectum terminates in the vagina or vestibule or, rarely, ends blindly.

The classification of anorectal malformations as high or low has prognostic and therapeutic significance. The international classification of anorectal malformations also recognizes an intermediate category, but most surgeons treat these lesions as high lesions (182). Low lesions can be managed at birth by anoplasty or dilatation; high lesions require a colostomy, with later definitive repair by posterior sagittal anoplasty.

The distinction between high and low lesions can usually be made on clinical grounds, based on the presence or absence of a visible perineal opening or passage of meconium via the vagina or urethra (183). The radiologic distinction between high and low lesions is unreliable and is seldom used (184). In the few cases in which the level is not clear from clinical examination, most surgeons will perform a diverting colostomy; approaching a high lesion as if it were low invites disaster.

What is the role of the radiologist in the evaluation of imperforate anus? The initial abdominal film may suggest the level of the lesion: meconium may calcify when it comes in contact in utero with urine (see Fig. 8-10) (31). Calcified intraluminal meconium in a boy with imperforate anus is evidence of a rectourethral communication and a high lesion. Air may also be present in the bladder in boys with high lesions. In girls with high malformations, the rectum communicates with the vagina, so these findings will not be present.

Babies with imperforate anus, especially high lesions, frequently have associated anomalies, especially of the lumbosacral spine and urinary tract (185,186). About a third of children with high imperforate anus, and a few with low lesions, will have spinal dysraphism; this has important implications for future bowel function. Special mention should be made of the Currarino triad of anorectal malformation, sacral deformity, and presacral mass (187,188).

Half to two thirds of babies with imperforate anus have associated urinary tract anomalies, again with a much higher incidence in patients with high lesions (185). The abnormalities include horseshoe kidney, renal agenesis and hypoplasia, hydronephrosis, and vesicoureteral reflux.

Babies with low lesions usually need only renal US preoperatively. Babies with high lesions generally need only renal US and a plain film of the abdomen preoperatively. Before definitive repair, the rectourethral communication may also be demonstrated by injection of the distal

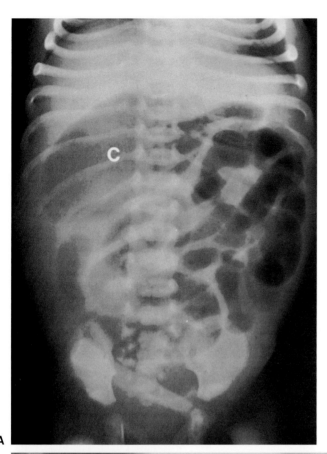

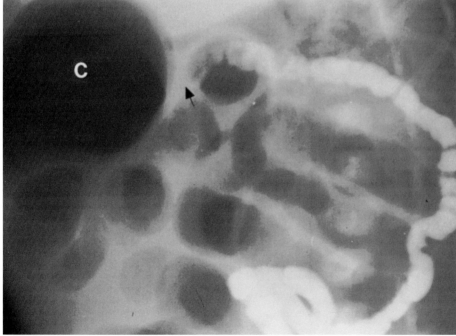

FIG. 8-70. Colon atresia. Male newborn with vomiting and abdominal distention. **A:** There is a markedly dilated loop of bowel in the right upper quadrant *(C)*, with moderate diffuse dilatation of bowel. **B:** Water-soluble contrast enema demonstrates an unused distal colon, which has a club-shaped termination *(arrow)* distal to the markedly dilated right transverse colon *(C)*. (Courtesy of Guido Currarino, M.D., Dallas, TX.)

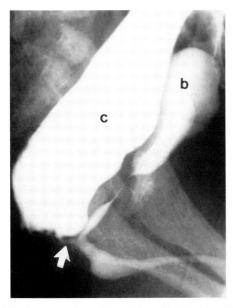

FIG. 8-71. Anorectal malformation. This baby with a high imperforate anus has had a colostomy. Injection of the distal limb of the colostomy with water-soluble contrast demonstrates a fistula *(arrows)* from the rectum to the posterior urethra. *c,* colon; *b,* bladder.

limb of the colostomy (Fig. 8-71). All patients should also have an MRI of the spine. In children with postoperative incontinence, MRI may be helpful in evaluating the anatomy of the pelvic musculature and the position of the neorectum (Fig. 8-72) (189).

Megacystis-Microcolon-Intestinal Hypoperistalsis Syndrome

Megacystis-microcolon-intestinal hypoperistalsis syndrome, described by Berdon and colleagues in 1973 (190), is a rare cause of intestinal obstruction in the newborn. Almost all of the reported cases have involved girls (190,191). Affected newborns present with intestinal obstruction. Their abdominal distention is due to a distended bladder as well as dilated bowel loops. A contrast enema will show a microcolon; this, however, is a transient finding, as follow-up studies will demonstrate a colon of normal size. The initial microcolon is probably due to very poor small intestinal motility, which results in an unused colon. An upper GI series will demonstrate markedly decreased intestinal peristalsis; the intestinal length may be decreased, and malrotation is common. Evaluation of the urinary tract will show a markedly distended bladder and usually dilated pelvicalyceal systems and ureters. The upper tract dilatation may not be permanent. Affected infants usually require parenteral nutrition, and long-term survival is rare.

Meconium Ileus

Meconium ileus is low intestinal obstruction caused by the inspissation of abnormal meconium in the distal ileum and colon. It almost always occurs in babies with cystic fibrosis (CF) and is the presenting feature in about 5% to 10% of patients. Babies with CF who develop meconium ileus produce a tenacious and viscous meconium that in utero occludes the small intestinal lumen and results in a high-grade distal small bowel obstruction. Meconium ileus is often complicated by volvulus of a distal intestinal loop, atresia, perforation, or peritonitis. Presumably these are the result of twisting of a heavy, meconium-laden loop and consequent ischemia.

Babies with meconium ileus have signs and symptoms of low intestinal obstruction. Obstruction is sometimes suggested prenatally by the presence of dilated bowel on US (192).

Plain films in babies with uncomplicated meconium ileus show low obstruction (193). The classic findings of meconium ileus—namely, a bubbly appearance in the right lower quadrant due to air mixed with meconium (Fig. 8-73), marked variation in the caliber of the distended bowel loops, and a paucity of air fluid levels on horizontal beam radiography—are neither sensitive nor specific (193). In complicated meconium ileus, there may be peritoneal gas, fluid, or calcification (see Fig. 8-9) or a mass effect. The mass effect is usually due to a so-called meconium pseudocyst, a mass of necrotic loops of intestine and fluid with a fibrous cyst wall that may be calcified (Fig. 8-74). Unfortunately, in many cases of complicated meconium ileus, the plain film may demonstrate only low obstruction and thus fail to distinguish complicated from uncomplicated cases (193).

The findings on contrast enema are diagnostic. There is a microcolon; the smallest of all colons occurs in meconium ileus. The colon is empty except for occasional pellets of meconium. The distal 10–30 cm of ileum are relatively small, yet larger than the colon, and contain many round or oval filling defects representing inspissated meconium. Further filling refluxes contrast into proximal, distended loops of ileum (Fig. 8-75).

In 1968 Noblett introduced the nonoperative treatment of meconium ileus by meglumine diatrizoate (Gastrografin) enema (194). This very hyperosmolar agent thins the abnormal meconium by drawing water into the bowel lumen. Thirty years later, there is still no consensus about the best way to perform the enema, what contrast to use, how many enemas can and should be performed, and what the success rate is. Most pediatric radiologists now agree that full-strength meglumine diatrizoate is not necessary for therapeutic effect and can be dangerous (195). Serial enemas may be performed safely, as long as there is progressive clinical improvement and the baby's electrolyte status is monitored. The overall success rate in uncomplicated meconium ileus is 50% to 60%. The perforation rate is 2% or 3%; higher

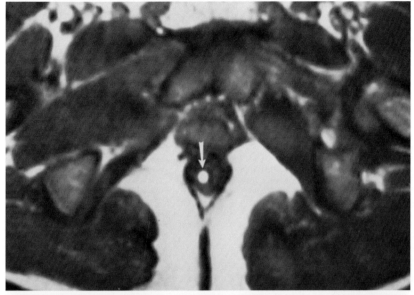

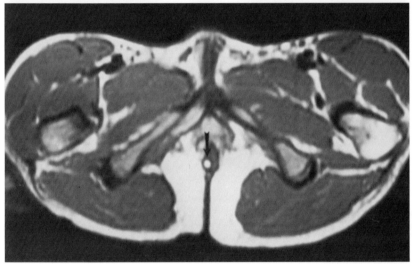

FIG. 8-72. MRI evaluation of postoperative anorectal malformation. A: Normal sphincter and neorectum. The ring-shaped anal sphincter surrounds the centrally located anus *(arrow)*. High signal intensity in anus is due to chloral hydrate marker. **B:** Hypoplastic sphincter and eccentric neorectum. The anal sphincter is underdeveloped on the right. The chloral hydrate anal marker *(arrow)* is eccentrically positioned in the sphincter.

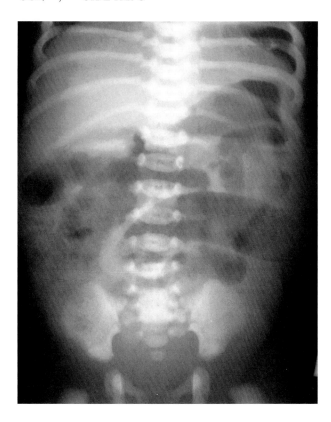

FIG. 8-73. Meconium ileus. This supine radiograph of a newborn with meconium ileus demonstrates low intestinal obstruction; the mottled gas pattern in the right lower quadrant is a mixture of air and meconium.

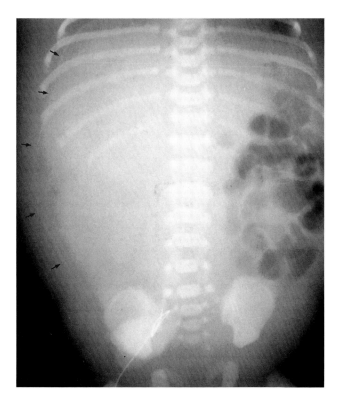

FIG. 8-74. Complicated meconium ileus with meconium pseudocyst. This supine radiograph of a newborn demonstrates a large right-sided mass. The mass is associated with calcification *(arrows)* along the peritoneal surface over the dome of the liver. At surgery, meconium ileus, ileal perforation, and a meconium pseudocyst were found. The baby had cystic fibrosis.

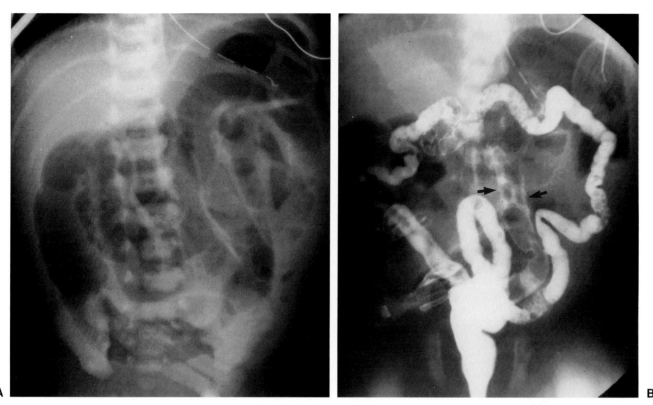

A **B**

FIG. 8-75. Meconium ileus. A: An abdominal film in a newborn with abdominal distention shows many dilated bowel loops containing gas mixed with solid material. **B:** A contrast enema demonstrates a microcolon. The distal ileum *(arrows)* is impacted with meconium.

perforation rates date from early experience with the hydrostatic technique (195).

The following approach seems reasonable. As with all cases of low obstruction, the initial (diagnostic) enema is performed with water-soluble contrast. An initial enema with barium seems to decrease the chance of later success. In a few cases, the initial water-soluble enema may relieve the obstruction completely. Usually, additional enemas using half-strength meglumine diatrizoate are required. Effort must be taken to reflux contrast into the ileum, and if possible back into dilated bowel (Fig. 8-76). One or two enemas can be performed daily until the obstruction is relieved. There must be clinical evidence that the obstruction is improving. Unfortunately, because of the nonspecificity of plain film findings, it is common that the diagnosis of complicated meconium ileus (by definition not medically treatable) is made only in the operating room after a series of therapeutic enemas have failed. However, this approach leads to reasonable success with few significant complications. If hydrostatic therapy fails, surgery is necessary to relieve the obstruction.

Ileal Atresia

The embryology of ileal atresia is described in the section on jejunal atresia and stenosis, where proximal ileal atresia

is also discussed. Babies with distal ileal atresia have low obstruction, and plain films will so indicate (Fig. 8-77). The enema will reveal a microcolon except in the rare instance in which the atresia is due to ischemia late in pregnancy, after the colon has accumulated enough meconium to be normal or nearly normal in size (Fig. 8-77). Some cases of ileal atresia are secondary to meconium ileus.

Necrotizing Enterocolitis

Definition and Clinical Features

Necrotizing enterocolitis (NEC) refers to the idiopathic, often severe enterocolitis seen in premature infants in neonatal intensive care units (196). Its precise etiology remains unknown, but hypoxia and infection are both important. Unfed babies seldom develop NEC; milk or formula probably serves as a substrate for the growth of microorganisms. NEC does occur, however, in infants in whom none of these predisposing factors are present (197). Occasionally there are epidemic outbreaks of NEC in newborn nurseries, which suggests an infectious etiology.

In NEC the inflammation of the intestine begins in the mucosa and submucosa and may extend through the full thickness of the bowel wall. Involvement may be diffuse but is usually patchy. The distal ileum and right colon are

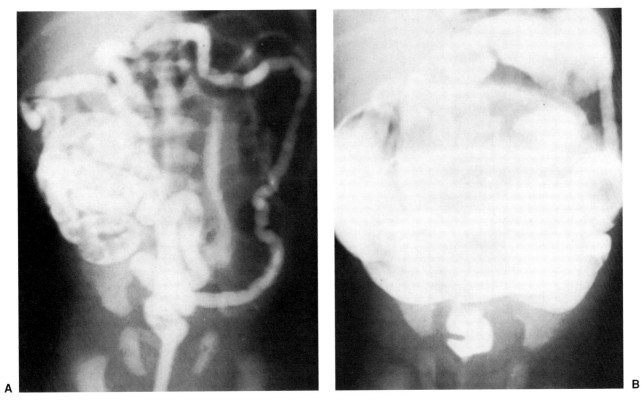

A   B

FIG. 8-76. Meconium ileus. A: Microcolon in newborn with meconium ileus. **B:** A therapeutic enema fills markedly dilated ileum proximal to the obstruction.

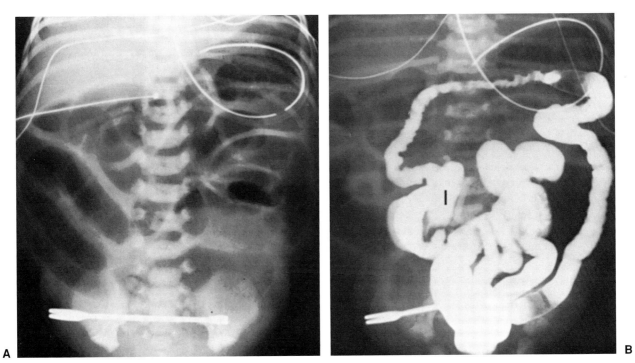

A   B

FIG. 8-77. Ileal atresia. A: A supine radiograph shows many loops of dilated bowel. **B:** Contrast flows freely through the unused microcolon without reflux beyond the terminal 2 cm of the ileum *(I)*. From Kirks (96).

involved far more frequently than other sites, though any part of the intestine may be affected.

The majority of cases occur in children who weigh less than 2000 g at birth. Symptoms usually develop in the first week of life, often in the first few days. Extremely low birth weight infants (those weighing less than 1000 g) may develop the disease somewhat later, often after 2 weeks (198).

The signs of NEC include abdominal distention, feeding intolerance, vomiting, blood in the stool, and diarrhea. Lethargy, instability of temperature and blood pressure, and apnea are also seen. Severe disease may present as shock. In advanced disease, the signs may include erythema of the body wall and palpable, distended bowel loops. The mortality of NEC is about 30% but is higher in very low birth weight infants.

Radiology

When NEC is suspected, routine abdominal films are obtained, usually supine films of the abdomen every 12–24 hours depending on the infant's status. If the child is more severely ill, the supine film is accompanied by one using a horizontal beam to detect free air. Either a supine cross-table lateral view or a left-side-down decubitus view may be used.

Both are extremely sensitive to free air, but the cross-table lateral disturbs the baby less. Small amounts of free air may be more visible to the inexperienced on a decubitus view (see Fig. 8-91). The choice will also depend on the condition of the baby and the skill and experience of the technologists. The duration of the so-called NEC watch depends on the status of the baby. Because most perforations occur within 2 days of diagnosis (199), routine horizontal beam films are often discontinued after 2 or 3 days.

The diagnosis of NEC must be based on both clinical signs and symptoms and radiographic findings. The radiographic findings are quite nonspecific, however, especially in the very early and very advanced stages of NEC. The most widely used system of staging NEC, that of Bell and colleagues, recognizes three stages: stage I, early or suspected NEC; stage II, definite NEC; and stage III, advanced disease (200). Most radiologists will thus attempt to characterize the radiographic findings as suspicious for NEC or compatible with early NEC, as specific for NEC, or as diagnostic of advanced disease.

In early NEC the goal should be to make a diagnosis when the systemic or GI signs are nonspecific. Unfortunately, the radiographic signs of early NEC are just as nonspecific.

The most commonly detected abnormality is diffuse gaseous distention of the intestine (Fig. 8-78) (201). Many pre-

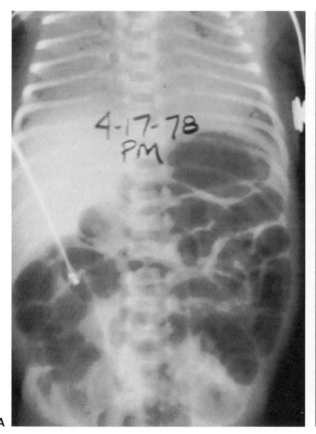

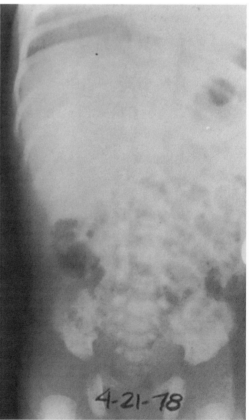

FIG. 8-78. Necrotizing enterocolitis. A 3-day-old girl with abdominal distention, vomiting, and bloody stool. **A:** An anteroposterior supine abdominal radiograph demonstrates diffuse bowel distention. **B:** The patient was treated for NEC for 3 days. The bowel gas pattern is now normal.

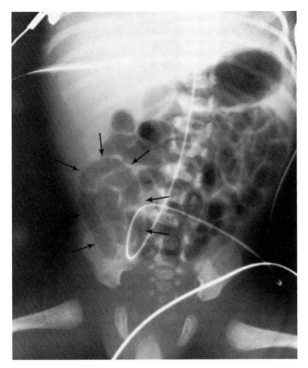

FIG. 8-79. Necrotizing enterocolitis. There is focal distention of bowel in the right lower quadrant *(arrows)* an early sign of NEC. The focally distended bowel has straight margins and is unwound into a tubular configuration.

mature babies who do not turn out to have NEC, however, also have mildly distended intestines. The most severely premature seem to suffer from intestinal inertia, a vague term that reflects lack of understanding of intestinal function in very low birth weight babies, who are frequently distended and intolerant of feeding in the absence of any detectable anatomic abnormality. Babies who are treated with nasal continuous positive airway pressure (CPAP) also often have distended abdomens (202); these children are usually otherwise well.

A slightly more useful sign of early NEC is the loss of the normal symmetric distribution of bowel gas (201,203). There may be a paucity of gas in one part of the abdomen and dilatation in another (Fig. 8-79). This uneven distribution presumably reflects focality of disease. This finding is also nonspecific.

Because of the nonspecificity of the findings of early NEC, some radiologists have advocated contrast enemas to exclude the diagnosis and thus spare the baby unnecessary treatment (204). Enemas in babies with NEC demonstrate mucosal irregularity and edema (Fig. 8-80). Enemas can decrease the number of false-positive diagnoses of NEC, at the cost of a few false negatives but without complications from the procedure (204). Despite these data, contrast enemas are not widely used for the diagnosis of NEC. This is partly because of what some authorities feel is the risk of perfora-

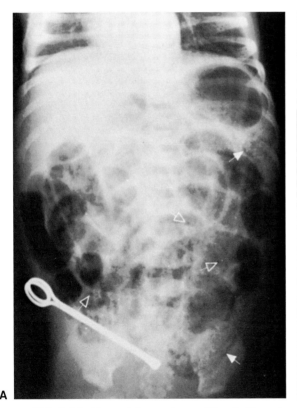

A

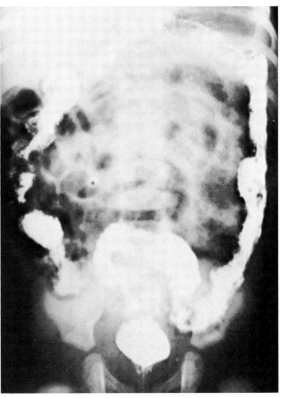

B

FIG. 8-80. Necrotizing enterocolitis. A: There is extensive subserosal *(solid arrows)* and submucosal *(open arrows)* air in the bowel wall. **B:** A postevacuation film after a water-soluble contrast enema. Mucosal irregularity and pneumatosis intestinalis are best appreciated in the descending and rectosigmoid colon.

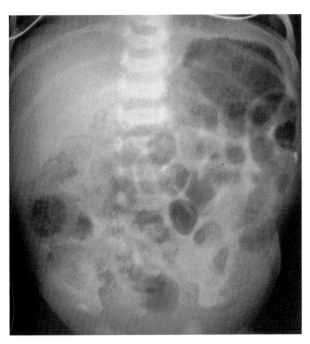

FIG. 8-81. Necrotizing enterocolitis. A supine radiograph demonstrates pneumatosis intestinalis involving much of the colon.

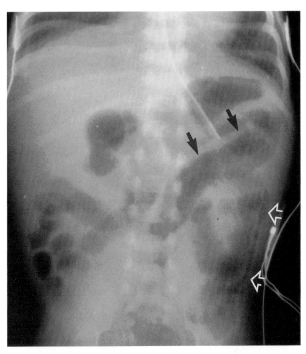

FIG. 8-82. Necrotizing enterocolitis. Bubbly pattern of pneumatosis due to submucosal air in transverse colon *(arrows)*. Linear lucency in descending colon is due to subserosal air *(open arrows)*. The bowel gas distention is asymmetric, as is typical of NEC.

tion (2) and partly because many neonatologists are comfortable with short courses of medical therapy in suspected NEC.

Interpretation of abdominal films is more straightforward in cases of definite NEC. In the neonatal intensive care unit the presence of intramural gas (pneumatosis intestinalis) is virtually pathognomonic of NEC. The reported incidence of pneumatosis in NEC varies widely, depending largely on how NEC is defined; perhaps it occurs in about three quarters of patients (201,205–207). The pneumatosis may be diffuse or localized but most frequently involves the distal small bowel and the colon (Fig. 8-81). The intramural gas may be submucosal, where it has a bubbly or cystic appearance, or subserosal, where it is more linear (Figs. 8-82 and 8-83). The bubbly morphology of pneumatosis is easily confused with stool or meconium in a normal colon. In practice, however, abdominal films of normal premature infants, especially those less than 2 weeks old, seldom demonstrate this pattern (208). Thus, a bubbly area on the film of a premature baby in the appropriate clinical setting should be assumed to be pneumatosis. In difficult cases follow-up films are helpful, as stool will usually move whereas pneumatosis may not (Fig. 8-84). Different views, including prone views, may also be helpful in distinguishing pneumatosis from stool (209).

Pneumatosis may be an early finding in NEC, i.e., in babies without clinically severe disease (201,206,210). Conversely, some children with severe or fatal NEC never develop pneumatosis (201,206). Although in most cases resolution of pneumatosis heralds clinical improvement, in some babies its disappearance coincides with clinical wors-

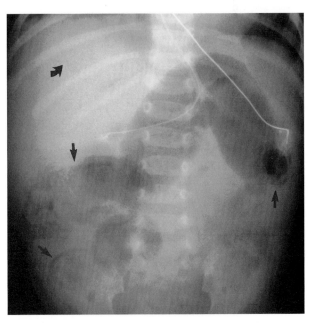

FIG. 8-83. Necrotizing enterocolitis. Extensive submucosal and subserosal air *(arrows)* in an infant with NEC secondary to ischemia due to severe coarctation of the aorta. Air can be faintly seen in the portal venous system *(curved arrow)*.

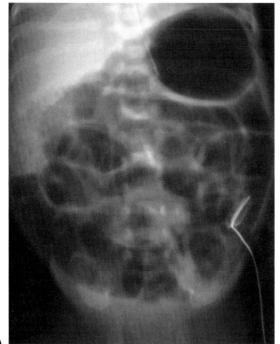

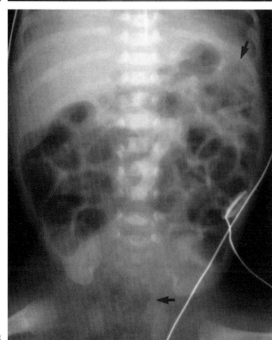

FIG. 8-84. Stool mimicking pneumatosis. A: Mottled or bubbly area in right upper quadrant in a newborn with blood in the stool. **B:** A film 12 hours later demonstrates that the "bubbles" have moved to the left upper quadrant and rectum *(arrows)* which confirms that the appearance was due to stool in the colon. The child was clinically well.

ening. Generalized pneumatosis suggests serious disease (210).

Along with pneumatosis, the other virtually pathognomonic sign of NEC is gas in the portal venous system. The reported incidence of portal venous gas (PVG) in NEC varies widely, but it probably occurs in between 10% and 30% of patients (201,205–207). Although gas in the portal veins does not always indicate a fatal outcome, it is almost always associated with severe disease (211,212). Some authors have suggested that PVG is an indication for operation (212,213).

PVG gas appears as fine branching lucencies projected over the liver (Figs. 8-83 and 8-85). PVG may be better seen on a cross-table lateral view than on an AP film (Fig. 8-86) (214). PVG may also be ultrasonographically visible as moving foci of echogenicity in the portal veins (Fig. 8-87) (215). Clinical improvement does not always accompany the radiographic disappearance of PVG.

In NEC, death is caused by intestinal necrosis with perforation, peritonitis, sepsis, and shock. The goal of the radiologist is to identify those patients in whom perforation is imminent or has just occurred and in whom an operation may prevent or minimize peritonitis. Unfortunately, just as the early radiographic findings of NEC are nonspecific, so are some of the advanced findings. No radiographic signs are completely sensitive or specific for identifying the babies at maximum risk of perforation. Some feel that PVG is an indication for surgery (212,213). Another sign that marks advanced disease is the persistent loop sign, a dilated loop of intestine that remains unchanged over 24–36 hours (Fig. 8-88) (201,216). Another ominous sign is the shift from generalized to unevenly distributed bowel dilatation (Fig. 8-89) (201).

Ascites is another sign of perforation or impending perforation (210,217). Small amounts of ascites are difficult to

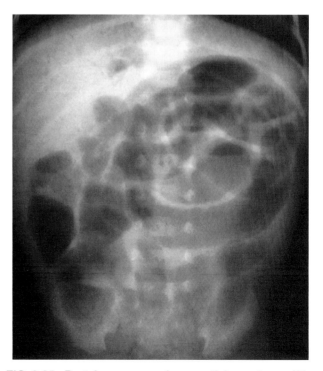

FIG. 8-85. Portal venous gas in necrotizing enterocolitis. The branching lucencies in the liver are due to air in the portal venous system.

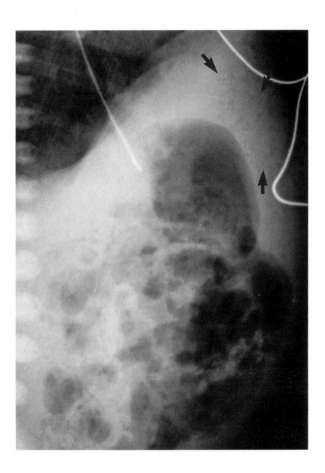

FIG. 8-86. Portal venous gas in necrotizing enterocolitis. (Same patient as Fig. 8-81.) A supine cross-table lateral film demonstrates portal venous gas *(arrows)* not visible on an AP radiograph taken at the same time. Extensive pneumatosis is also apparent.

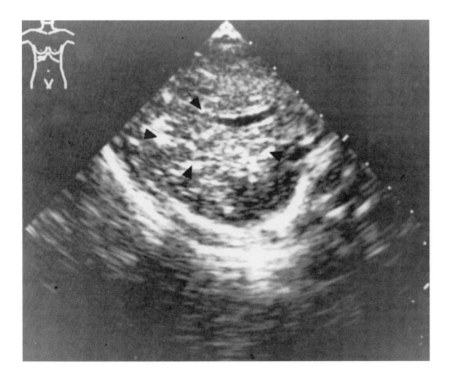

FIG. 8-87. Sonography of portal venous gas. Right upper quadrant sonography in a neonate with NEC. The foci of increased echogenicity *(arrows)* are due to gas in the portal venous system. Movement of air within portal veins was demonstrated during real-time sonographic examination.

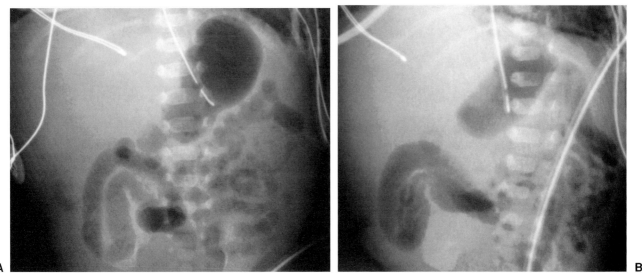

A   B

FIG. 8-88. Persistent loop sign of necrotizing enterocolitis. A: Abdominal film in a premature infant with NEC demonstrates a dilated loop of bowel in the right lower quadrant. **B:** A film obtained 24 hours later shows that the loop is fixed and more dilated. Perforation occurred shortly after this radiograph.

detect on abdominal films and US may thus be useful (218,219). The presence of intraperitoneal fluid in a child with NEC and clinical deterioration may be an indication for surgery.

The only absolute indication for surgical intervention in NEC is pneumoperitoneum. Unfortunately, only one half

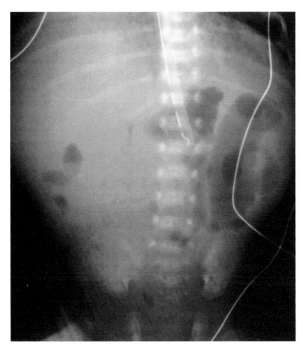

FIG. 8-89. Necrotizing enterocolitis. Markedly asymmetrical bowel gas pattern with dilated loops in the left upper quadrant and a paucity of gas in the right lower quadrant. The baby was operated on after this film and was found to have multiple ileal and colonic perforations.

to three quarters of patients with perforation have free air detectable even on horizontal beam films (199,201); in addition, pneumoperitoneum identifies only those patients who have already had a perforation. Small amounts of free air may be identified on supine cross-table lateral films, where it may be seen as triangular lucencies (''tell-tale triangle'') between loops of bowel below the anterior abdomen wall (Fig. 8-90) (220). Free air is also seen on the left decubitus film over the liver (Fig. 8-91). The most important task of the radiologist, however, is to identify a pneumoperitoneum on a supine film, which may be the only film obtained. Massive pneumoperitoneum is not difficult to detect; free air gives an overall lucency to the abdomen, and the air outlines intraperitoneal structures such as the falciform ligament, the umbilical arteries (221), and the urachus (Figs. 8-92, 8-97, and 8-98). These signs are all due to an abnormal interface between air and soft tissue. Small amounts of air collecting in the posterior hepatorenal space (pouch of Morison) may be seen on supine films as a triangular lucency projected over the liver (Fig. 8-93) (222). Air in the Morison's pouch may not rise over the liver on decubitus films. Air may be seen on both sides of the bowel wall (Rigler sign) (Fig. 8-94); one must be cautious, however, about using this sign in neonates with marked diffuse gaseous distention since multiple air-bowel interfaces and the thinness of the bowel wall may give the appearance of air on both sides of it.

In summary, the signs on abdominal films of early NEC are nonspecific. Of the classic signs of NEC, pneumatosis is most frequently seen. Its presence, unless extensive, is not necessarily an indication of severe disease, and its disappearance does not always imply improvement. Portal venous gas is a sign of advanced disease, and some support its use as an indication for surgery. No sign is specific for impending

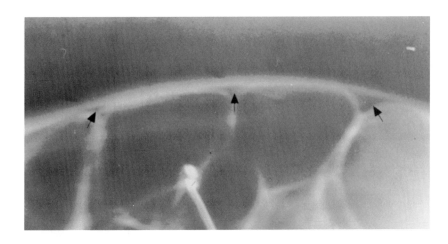

FIG. 8-90. Pneumoperitoneum: "Tell-tale triangle." A 19-day-old male with necrotizing enterocolitis. The triangular lucencies *(arrows)* are due to small anterior collections of free intraperitoneal air bordered by the peritoneal surface and adjacent bowel loops.

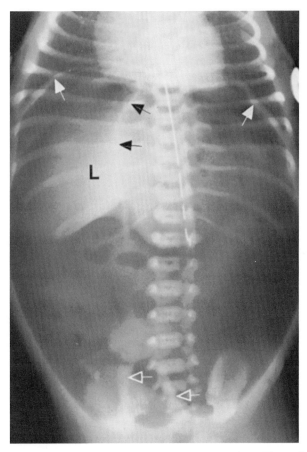

FIG. 8-92. Pneumoperitoneum: football sign. There is overall lucency of the abdomen with an abnormal interface between free air and the peritoneum producing the "football" sign. The abnormal air–soft-tissue interfaces demonstrate liver *(L)*, diaphragm *(white arrows)*, falciform ligament *(black arrows)*, and umbilical arteries *(open arrows)*.

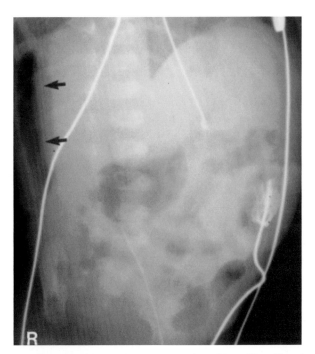

FIG. 8-91. Pneumoperitoneum on decubitus film. Free intraperitoneal air collects over the liver *(arrows)* on this decubitus film in a child with NEC.

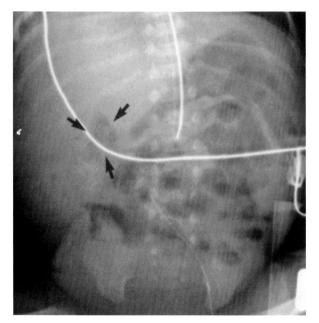

FIG. 8-93. Pneumoperitoneum: air in Morison's pouch. Supine abdominal film. The triangular air collection in the right upper quadrant *(arrows)* is air in the hepatorenal space. A perforation of the ileum was found at surgery.

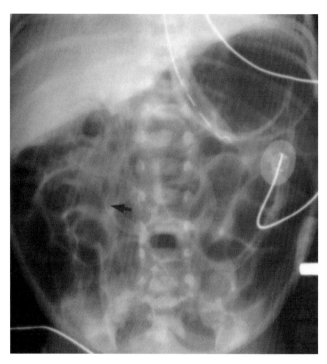

FIG. 8-94. Pneumoperitoneum: Rigler sign. Supine film in a neonate with NEC. Air outlines both sides of the bowel wall *(arrow)*.

perforation, and all the signs of advanced disease are insensitive. Pneumoperitoneum is an indication for surgery but is not present in all babies with perforations. Obviously, proper diagnosis and management of NEC require close cooperation between radiologist, neonatologist, and surgeon.

Complications

Intestinal strictures may follow either medical or surgical treatment of NEC and occur in 10% to 20% of survivors. The strictures may be asymptomatic, but most cause bowel obstruction weeks or months after the episode of NEC. Even a child whose NEC was not severe may develop a stricture; thus any survivor of NEC with symptoms of obstruction should undergo a contrast enema.

NEC strictures may be single or multiple. Although NEC mostly affects the distal ileum and right colon, most strictures occur in the left colon (Figs. 8-95 and 8-96) (223). Spontaneous resolution of NEC strictures rarely occurs, and asymptomatic patients with strictures may be watched (224). Routine barium enemas after NEC are probably not worthwhile. In children who have had diversion by either ileostomy or colostomy, it is important to evaluate the distal defunctionalized bowel before reestablishment of continuity because a stricture may be concealed there.

Infants who have had extensive bowel resection may develop short gut syndrome with its attendant complications. Unusual complications of NEC include enteroenteric fistulas (225) and, in children with multiple strictures, enterocysts (226).

NEC in the Full-Term Infant

NEC may occur in full-term infants. Specific risk factors can frequently be identified; these include polycythemia and hypoxia. Children who have had major cardiac surgery may

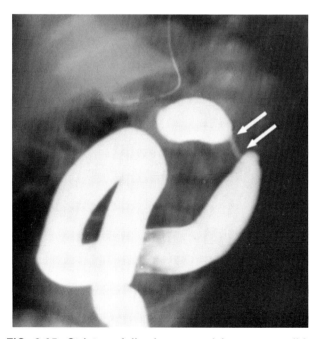

FIG. 8-95. Stricture following necrotizing enterocolitis. The splenic flexure is the most common site of stricture *(arrows)* after NEC.

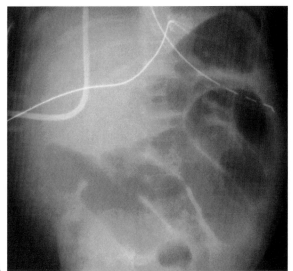

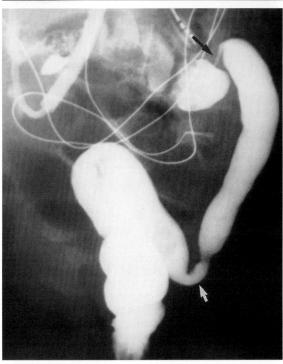

FIG. 8-96. Stricture following necrotizing enterocolitis.
A: An abdominal film demonstrates a distal bowel obstruction in a baby 6 weeks after medically treated NEC. **B:** An AP view from a contrast enema reveals strictures at the junction of the sigmoid and descending colon *(white arrow)* and near the splenic flexure *(black arrow)*.

develop NEC, apparently because of poor bowel perfusion (see Fig. 8-83) (227). Abdominal surgery, particularly repair of gastroschisis and repair of intestinal atresia, is also sometimes followed by NEC (49,228). These babies tend to develop symptoms relatively late, several weeks after surgery; their clinical course is often severe. The precise etiology of this type of NEC is not clear. Babies born to mothers who abuse cocaine probably also have a higher incidence of NEC (229).

Idiopathic Gastric Perforation

Spontaneous or idiopathic perforation of the stomach is an uncommon event but is one of the more common causes of pneumoperitoneum in the term neonate. The perforation usually occurs in the anterior or posterior wall of the greater curvature of the stomach. The cause is unknown, although perforation can be produced experimentally with acute gastric distention. Ischemia may play a role in some cases (230).

Idiopathic gastric perforation usually occurs in the first 2–5 days of life in a previously healthy term newborn. The first sign may be abdominal distention during a well-baby physical examination. The illness can also be catastrophic. Symptoms include poor feeding, vomiting, respiratory distress, abdominal distention, and shock (231). Plain films of the abdomen show pneumoperitoneum, usually large (Fig. 8-97). In neonatal gastric perforation an air-fluid level can seldom be found in the stomach, whereas a gastric air-fluid level is frequently present when the perforation is elsewhere (232). Neonatal gastric perforation may also be secondary to distention due to mechanical ventilation, especially in association with prematurity (12), indomethacin therapy (14), NEC, nasogastric intubation (12), or ischemia (Fig. 8-98).

Infant and Young Child

Esophageal Foreign Body

Infants and young children swallow many foreign objects. Most foreign bodies pass through the GI tract without complication. Occasionally, however, a foreign body lodges in the esophagus and must be removed. Esophageal foreign bodies in children include coins, pieces of plastic, buttons, bone fragments, pins, fruit pits, poorly chewed food, toys, and small batteries (233). It is not understood why foreign bodies lodge in the esophagus of some children but not in others, as the esophagus is intrinsically normal in almost all instances. If a foreign body lodges in the esophagus, it usually does so at the thoracic inlet (the most common site of impaction), the level of the aortic arch or left mainstem bronchus, and (least frequently) the gastroesophageal junction. A foreign body at other sites in the esophagus suggests that there is an underlying abnormality, most commonly an anastomotic stricture after repair of esophageal atresia (see Fig. 8-26).

Most infants and children with esophageal foreign bodies are acutely symptomatic. There may be chest pain, worsened by swallowing. Salivation, increased secretions, drooling, and gagging are common. Young infants may refuse to eat or be irritable. Occasionally the child with an esophageal foreign body simply has symptoms of upper airway obstruction suggesting croup (234). This presentation is more common in young children, especially when the foreign body has been impacted for a long time. In

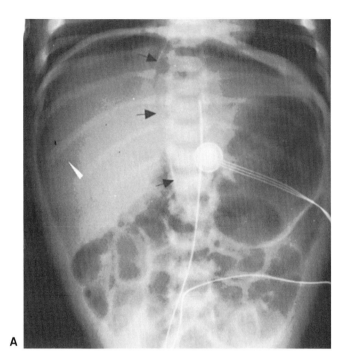

A

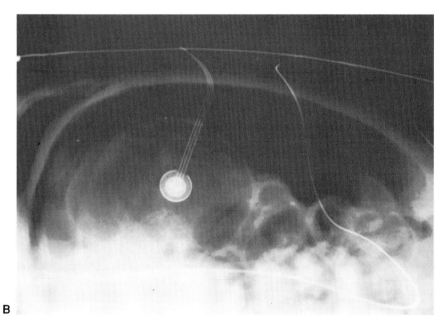

B

FIG. 8-97. Pneumoperitoneum due to idiopathic gastric perforation. A: An anteroposterior supine radiograph shows lucency of the upper abdomen with air contacting the diaphragm and right abdominal wall. The falciform ligament *(arrows)* is identified. **B:** Right lateral decubitus radiograph. Free intraperitoneal air is confirmed. Both the outer and inner walls of bowel are visible. An air-fluid level is not identified in the stomach.

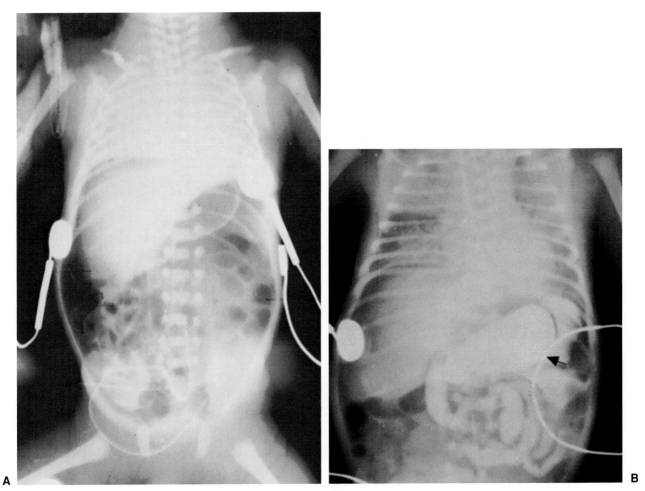

FIG. 8-98. Pneumoperitoneum due to gastric rupture. 1-day-old female with severe lung disease. **A:** Massive pneumoperitoneum. **B:** A water-soluble contrast study demonstrates perforation *(arrow)* of the greater curvature of the stomach.

addition, the longer a foreign body has been impacted, the more likely are complications. The most common complication is perforation and subsequent mediastinitis. Rarer complications include tracheoesophageal fistula and aortoesophageal fistula. Complications are more likely to occur with sharp objects such as pins and bones. Aluminum can ''pop-tops'' are difficult to see radiologically and are likely to cause perforations (235).

Plain films for a suspected foreign body should include the entire GI tract, nasopharynx to anus. This prevents overlooking a foreign body in an unsuspected location and may detect multiple foreign bodies. This survey usually requires two films, a lateral view of the neck and upper thorax, and an AP view of the chest and abdomen. Most foreign bodies are opaque and will be seen on one of these views.

Coins, which are the most frequently swallowed foreign bodies, have a typical appearance in the esophagus. On the AP view the flat surface of the coin is seen; on the lateral view the coin is on edge (Fig. 8-99). The opposite

occurs when a coin is present in the trachea—a very rare event. Special note should be made of the radiographic appearance of disk batteries of the type used in cameras and hearing aids. These batteries may be mistaken for coins but careful attention will reveal a different and characteristic appearance (236). On an AP view a double density is present because of the bilaminar structure of the battery, whereas on a lateral view a step-off is visible between the anode and cathode. Identification of batteries is important because they may cause chemical injury to the esophagus.

Particular attention should be paid to signs of inflammation, such as an abnormally increased distance between the trachea and esophagus (Fig. 8-99), tracheal narrowing (Fig. 8-100), or a mediastinal mass. Occult esophageal foreign bodies may mimic airway disease, chronic pneumonia, or a mediastinal tumor. If plain films are negative and an esophageal foreign body is still suspected, a contrast examination using nonionic, low-osmolar, water-soluble contrast is per-

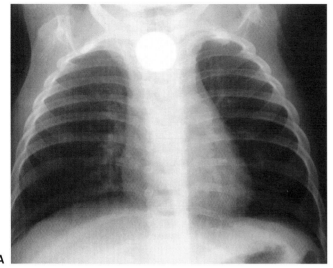

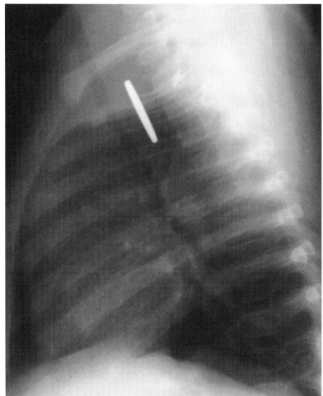

FIG. 8-99. Esophageal foreign body. A swallowed coin is lodged in the esophagus at the level of the aortic arch. On an AP view **(A)** the flat surface of the coin is visible; on the lateral view **(B)** the coin is seen on edge. Note also on the lateral view the abnormally increased distance, due to inflammatory reaction, between the trachea and esophagus at the level of impaction. The coin was removed endoscopically.

formed (Fig. 8-100). Water-soluble contrast is used because of the possibility of occult perforation.

Esophageal foreign bodies should be promptly removed to prevent complications. Some foreign bodies must be removed endoscopically, under general anesthesia. Many opaque foreign bodies, particularly coins, can be removed

using a nonoperative Foley catheter technique (237,238). Contraindications to catheter removal include symptoms or signs of airway obstruction, radiologic evidence of narrowing of the airway, mediastinal inflammation (Fig. 8-99), or the fact that the esophageal foreign body is sharp (239). If the foreign body is blunt, is not associated with inflammatory changes, and has been in the esophagus for less than 8–12 hours, it can almost always be removed with a catheter under fluoroscopic control.

A Foley catheter (12 or 14 French) is passed through the nose or mouth to a point just beyond the foreign body and the balloon of the catheter is inflated with contrast material. The patient is positioned for balloon extraction of a foreign body in a prone-oblique or lateral position with the head down. The catheter is then withdrawn from the esophagus with gentle, steady traction, and the balloon pulls the foreign body. As the foreign body emerges from the esophagus, gravity allows it to fall out of the mouth onto the table (Fig. 8-101). The balloon must be deflated before the catheter is withdrawn through the nose. After successful removal of a foreign body, an esophagram should be performed, initially with water-soluble contrast, if there is any suspicion of a complication.

The published experience with thousands of Foley catheter extractions has proved that the method is quick, easy, and safe (240,241). It avoids the slight risks inherent in esophagoscopy and general anesthesia. It is certainly cost-effective (242). The technique, however, remains controversial because of the possibility of aspiration of the foreign body into the airway (243). All agree that the criteria for removal outlined above must be strictly adhered to and that the procedure must be done only by physicians with experience. (241,242).

Chemical Injury to the Esophagus

Young children, in addition to swallowing any small object that they get their hands on, may also drink anything they find including, unfortunately, caustic agents. A number of household chemical agents produce esophageal injury; the most common are alkaline caustics, acids, and ammonium chloride. The type and location of caustic damage to the GI tract depends on the chemical nature of the agent. Acid produces maximal effect on the prepyloric region of the stomach (Fig. 8-102B). Common alkali caustic injury produces a penetrating burn of the mouth, pharynx, and esophagus (Fig. 8-102A). There is usually inadequate ingestion to produce damage to the stomach and small bowel. Bleach usually produces only superficial mucosal damage to the esophagus.

The type and concentration of alkali also influence the degree and location of injury. Crystals are usually expectorated after ingestion, and the maximum damage is to the mouth and pharynx. Liquid agents are usually swallowed and produce caustic damage on the esophagus.

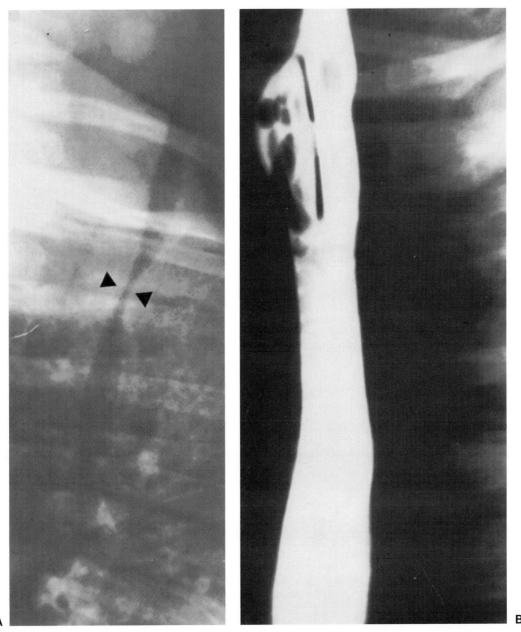

FIG. 8-100. Occult esophageal foreign body. Infant referred for evaluation of a mediastinal mass. **A:** There is circumferential narrowing *(arrowheads)* of the upper thoracic airway just below the thoracic inlet and adjacent mediastinal fullness. **B:** Esophagogram. The intraluminal foreign body is a piece of plastic material. (Courtesy of William J. McSweeney, M.D., Washington, DC.)

The diagnosis of caustic ingestion is usually obvious from the history. Clinical detection of oral and pharyngeal burns in a child with lye ingestion indicates probable esophageal damage, but their absence does not rule out significant esophageal injury (244).

Chest radiography after acute caustic ingestion may show mediastinal widening, pneumomediastinum, or pleural effusion, all of which suggest esophageal perforation. Inflammation of the periesophageal tissues with resultant mass effect on the trachea may, however, occur without perforation.

Evaluation of the esophagus after acute caustic ingestion is difficult. Esophagogastroscopy allows direct inspection of the mucosa but may be dangerous. Contrast esophagography frequently underestimates the severity of damage (244). Patterns of acute injury include esophageal atony, rigidity of the esophagus, irritability of the esophagus due to mucosal injury or damage to the Auerbach plexus, and aspiration. Hypopharyngeal burns may cause enlargement of the epiglottis.

Perforation is the most common acute complication of chemical esophagitis. Esophageal strictures develop in up to a third of children with alkali esophageal burns. Location of

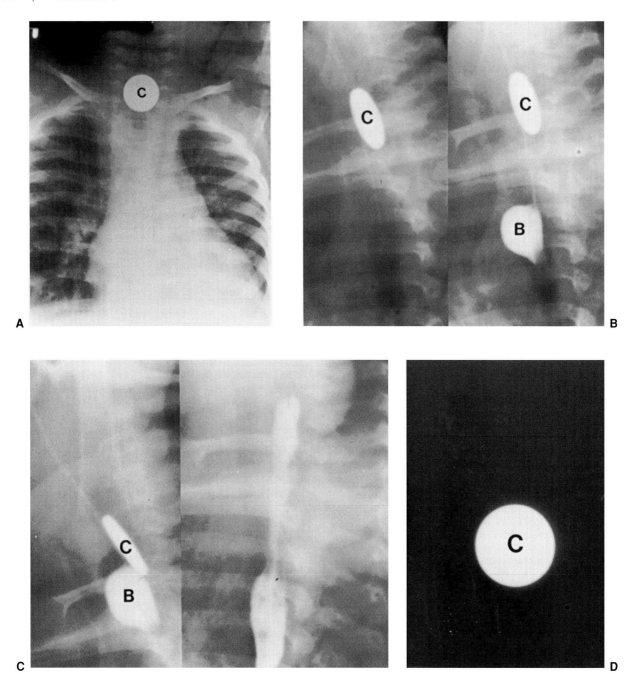

FIG. 8-101. Fluoroscopic catheter removal of esophageal foreign body. A 1-year-old boy who was playing with a coin bank. **A:** The coin *(C)* in the upper esophagus. **B:** A Foley catheter is passed beyond the coin *(left)*, and its balloon *(B)* is inflated with water-soluble contrast material *(right)*. **C:** The coin falls against the balloon as the catheter is withdrawn *(left)*. Esophagography after coin removal with water-soluble contrast *(right)* is normal. **D:** Radiograph of dime *(C)* removed from the esophagus.

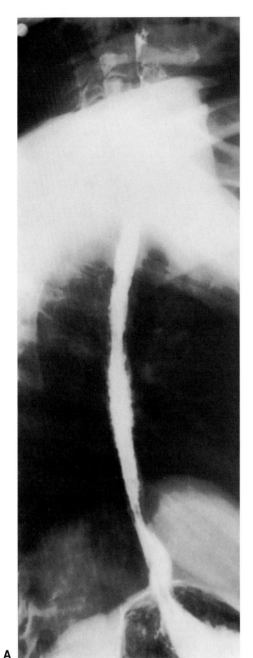

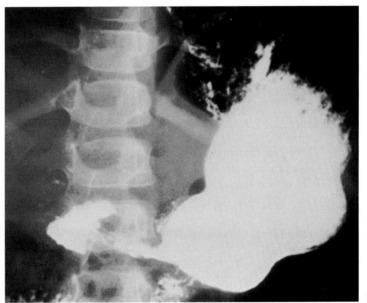

FIG. 8-102. Corrosive ingestion. A: Lye ingestion. A lateral esophagram 3 weeks after lye ingestion demonstrates extensive ulceration and multiple strictures. **B:** Acid ingestion. UGI series several months after ingestion of hydrochloric acid shows a severe antral stricture.

A

B

these strictures is random, depending on the site and severity of the spasm at the time of the ingestion. The length of the strictures is variable, and they may be multiple (Fig. 8-102A). The most typical appearance is of a smooth, tapered stricture.

Hypertrophic Pyloric Stenosis

Definition and Clinical Features

Hypertrophic pyloric stenosis (HPS) is a very common cause of vomiting in young infants. Its diagnosis is straight-

forward and its treatment safe and effective. The disease itself, however, is somewhat mysterious. In HPS hypertrophy and hyperplasia of the circular muscle layer of the pylorus lead to lengthening and thickening of the pylorus. The thickened muscle encroaches on the lumen of the pylorus, gradually producing gastric outlet obstruction (Fig. 8-103). Hirschsprung, who coined the term "pyloric stenosis" in 1888, believed that the pyloric narrowing was congenital. HPS, however, is not found in utero or at birth. The cause of the muscular hypertrophy remains unknown, though there is evidence that it is due to abnormal innervation of the circular muscle (245). Genetic factors are also important

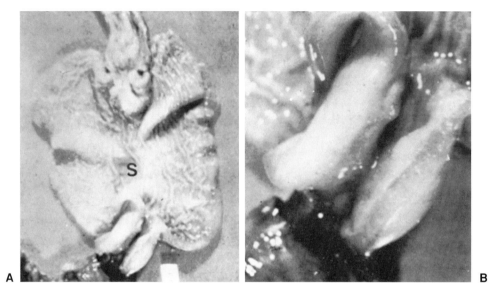

FIG. 8-103. Hypertrophic pyloric stenosis. Gross pathologic specimen of hypertrophic pyloric stenosis in a patient who died of other causes. **A:** The dilated stomach *(S)* is opened. **B:** A close-up view demonstrates marked thickening of the circular musculature of the pylorus. (Courtesy of Gary D. Shackelford, M.D., St. Louis, MO.)

since it is more common in babies with an affected parent or sibling. Babies with HPS do not usually have other problems, except that there is an unexplained association with esophageal atresia (246). There is no evidence of an increased incidence of renal anomalies in infants with HPS (247).

Hirschsprung's belief that HPS is a congenital anomaly is easy to understand because most cases are found in the second to sixth week of life. HPS is rare in children who are less than l week old or greater than 3 months old. Preterm infants may develop HPS before what would have been their due date. HPS is more common in boys than in girls (4:1) and in white than in black or Oriental children. The often-quoted increased incidence of HPS in first-born babies is probably not correct.

Babies with HPS have usually been well, though many have been spitting up since birth. Actual vomiting begins in the second or third week of life and progresses from what may appear to be simple regurgitation to projectile vomiting after every feeding. The vomitus is not bilious, though it may be blood-tinged because of associated gastritis. The vomiting is occasionally severe enough to cause dehydration and alkalosis. The presentation of HPS may be atypical in sick or premature infants (248).

Radiology

The current debate about whether US is necessary for the diagnosis of HPS echoes the controversy of an earlier era about the utility of the UGI series (249). The diagnosis of HPS can certainly be made on purely clinical grounds, by palpation of the hypertrophied pyloric mass (olive) in a baby

with an appropriate history. Although some studies suggest that the mass can be felt in up to 80% of cases of HPS, the increasing reliance on radiology has resulted in fewer physicians being able to palpate the mass, the only pathognomonic clinical sign of HPS (250,251). Since a false-positive diagnosis of HPS leads to unnecessary surgery, most surgeons today choose to obtain an imaging study, especially because US, the current study of choice, is safe, painless, and in experienced hands has a sensitivity and specificity approaching 100%.

What study should be done in a child under 3 months of age with nonbilious vomiting is controversial. US is often used as the first imaging modality; gastroesophageal reflux, inflammatory disease of the stomach, and duodenal abnormalities are searched for as well as HPS. However, most pediatric radiologists, pediatricians, and pediatric surgeons, feel uncomfortable with US for the diagnosis of causes of vomiting other than HPS and perform a UGI if the US examination is negative (252,253). Thus, in order to avoid a second study, it is important to select patients for US appropriately. A reasonable policy is to perform US as the initial study in babies with nonbilious vomiting only when by age and history HPS is clearly the most likely diagnosis. In other babies a UGI, which will diagnose HPS as well as other causes of vomiting, is performed. This approach leads to very few second studies.

Ultrasound

No preparation is required for the US examination of HPS (254). With the baby in the supine right posterior oblique position, aided by a rolled towel under the baby's left side,

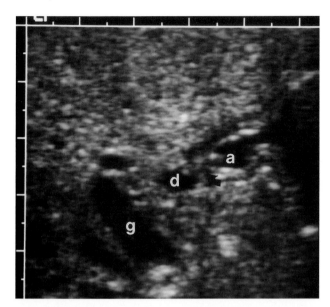

FIG. 8-104. Normal pylorus by sonography. The normal pyloric channel *(curved arrow)* is short and often difficult to find. *a*, antrum; *d*, duodenal bulb; *g*, gallbladder.

a high-frequency linear array transducer (5 MHz or greater) is used. The transducer is held in a transverse or oblique (angled toward the right shoulder) orientation over the right upper quadrant and then moved slowly along the abdominal wall until the antrum and pylorus are found. The gallbladder is a good landmark for the antropyloric region (Fig. 8-104). Most babies with HPS will have quite a bit of gastric fluid, which facilitates visualization of the pylorus. If the stomach is empty, a small amount of sugar water from a bottle sometimes helps. Massive overdistention of the stomach pushes the pylorus posteriorly and makes it difficult to visualize; a nasogastric tube must then drain the stomach.

When the pyloric channel is located, the transducer is angled until it is aligned with its long axis. In babies without HPS, identification of the normal pylorus can be difficult (Fig. 8-104). The hypertrophied muscle is usually less echogenic than the liver, though at certain angles it may appear nearly as echogenic as the liver (255). The muscle is always less echoic than the highly echogenic mucosa, which appears as parallel echogenic lines between the hypertrophied muscle (Fig. 8-105). The hypertrophied muscle mass indents the duodenal bulb and bulges into the gastric antrum (''cervix sign'') (256). Redundant pyloric mucosa may also protrude into the antrum (''mucosal nipple'' sign) (Fig. 8-105). Another important sign of HPS is hyperperistalsis of the stomach; the hyperperistasis stops at the pylorus, gastric contents failing to pass into the duodenum.

The ultrasonographic diagnosis of HPS is usually obvious and measurements merely support the visual impression. Most pediatric radiologists will measure only the thickness of the pyloric muscle and the length of the pyloric channel. The thickness of the muscle, measured from the outer edge of the echogenic mucosal complex to the outer edge of the

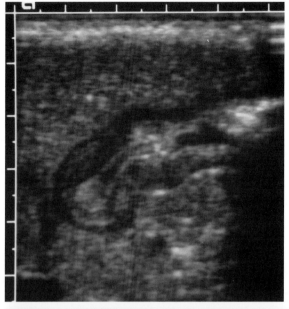

A

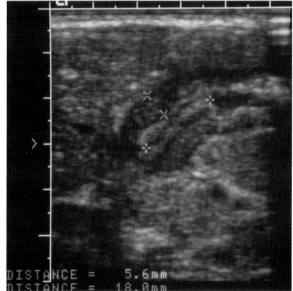

B

FIG. 8-105. Ultrasonography of hypertrophic pyloric stenosis. A: Hypertrophic pyloric stenosis. **B:** Measurements of abnormal muscle thickness (5.6 mm) between *X*'s and elongated (18 mm) pyloric channel between + 's. See text for the details of measurements.

muscle, is the most sensitive and specific sign of HPS (257–259). Recent work has shown that a muscle thickness of 3 mm or greater is virtually 100% specific for HPS (259). A more conservative criterion is 3.5 mm or greater; the extra half a millimeter assures that no false-positive diagnoses are made. In fact, most babies with HPS will have muscle thickness of 4 mm or greater (257–259). The muscle thickness increases with the age at diagnosis. No adjustment needs to be made for the patient's gestational age (258). Measurements should be made on a midline longitudinal view, at the midportion of the pylorus (Fig. 8-105B).

Normal pyloric muscle is usually <2.0 mm thick (258). Muscle thickness between 2 and 3 mm may be seen in pylorospasm (antral spasm), an ill-defined condition sometimes associated with inflammatory disease of the stomach (258). In pylorospasm the pylorus may open during scanning, unlike the pylorus in HPS. Muscle thickness between 2 and 3 mm also occurs in early pyloric stenosis (258,259).

Channel length is a more variable parameter than muscle thickness and should also be measured on midline longitudinal views of the pylorus (Fig. 8-105B). Most babies with HPS will have pyloric channel lengths of >16 mm, but some patients without HPS will also have lengths >16 mm (257). Thus, the diagnosis should not be made on channel length alone.

The technique takes some time to master, but once mastered there is usually little difficulty in distinguishing normal from abnormal. There are only two common pitfalls (260). A greatly overdistended stomach may make identification of the pylorus difficult, but this can be overcome by careful scanning and positioning and by decompressing the stomach when necessary. A false-positive diagnosis of HPS may be made when the contracted antrum is scanned in tangent: this makes the muscle look abnormally thick. This pitfall is easily avoided by making measurements only in the longitudinal plane because the lumen of the pylorus is always a straight line in HPS.

Pyloric stenosis is not a surgical emergency, and there is no need to make the diagnosis in the middle of the night. False-positive diagnoses must be avoided; a child with borderline measurements may be reexamined in a day or two. No child should have an unnecessary operation because of mismeasurement by a fraction of a millimeter.

Upper GI

Some vomiting babies examined by UGI turn out to have HPS; knowledge of the features of HPS on UGI therefore remains important. A scout film of the abdomen is the first step. Though there are no pathognomonic signs of HPS on plain film, massive distention of the stomach, little small bowel or colonic air, and visible waves of gastric peristalsis (the caterpillar sign) are very suggestive, especially in combination (261) (Fig. 8-106).

In HPS, the upper GI series is diagnostically very reliable (249). The stomach may be so distended in HPS that it is necessary to drain it via a nasogastric tube. All babies with HPS will have delayed gastric emptying and hyperperistaltic waves that stop at the pylorus. In most cases of HPS enough barium will pass into the pyloric channel to visualize the pyloric hypertrophy (Fig. 8-107). The canal will be elongated and narrowed (string sign) (Fig. 8-108B). The pylorus usually turns upward to the patient's left (Figs. 8-108B and 8-109). The elongated and narrowed channel may appear as a double track of barium if the hypertrophied muscle squeezes the lumen into separate compartments (Fig. 8-109).

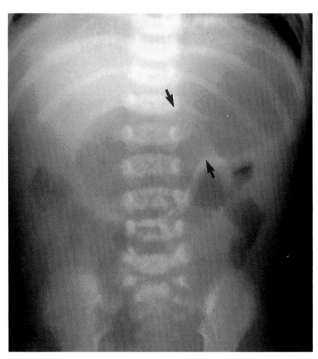

FIG. 8-106. Plain film findings in hypertrophic pyloric stenosis. A supine radiograph demonstrates a dilated stomach with little distal bowel gas. A deep peristaltic wave *(arrows)* gives the stomach a "caterpillar" appearance.

The hypertrophied muscle indents the antrum (Fig. 8-108) and the duodenal bulb (the "mushroom sign") (Fig. 8-109). The "pyloric tit" deformity on the lesser curve adjacent to the pylorus is due to a peristaltic wave arrested at that point (249).

The UGI may be difficult to interpret when gastric emptying is so delayed that barium fails to reach the duodenal bulb. In these cases it may be helpful to perform the Currarino

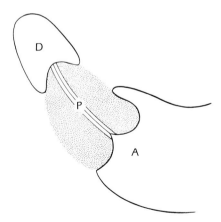

FIG. 8-107. Hypertrophic pyloric stenosis. Radiologic and imaging findings of hypertrophic pyloric stenosis. The soft-tissue mass of hypertrophied muscle *(stippled)* surrounds the pylorus *(P)*. This mass indents the gastric antrum *(A)* and duodenal bulb *(D)*, and narrows and elongates the pyloric canal *(P)*.

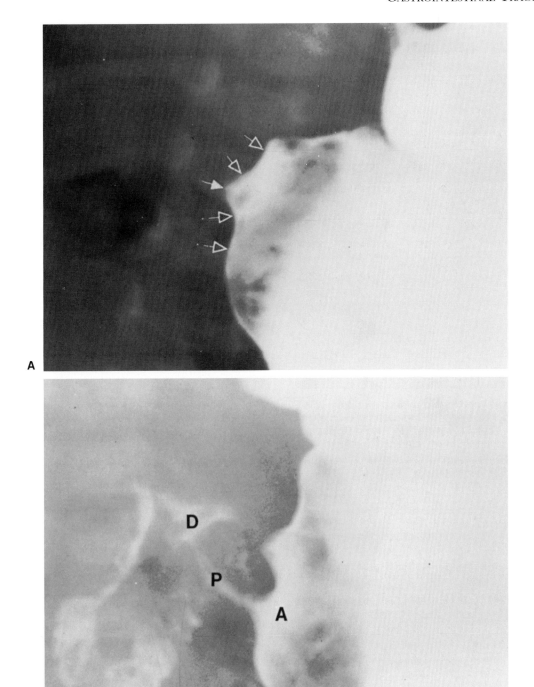

FIG. 8-108. UGI of hypertrophic pyloric stenosis. A 5-week-old boy with vomiting. **A:** Air-contrast view of the gastric antrum with manual compression (Currarino maneuver [262]) demonstrates mass effect on the gastric antrum *(open arrows)* and narrowing of the proximal pyloric canal *(solid arrow)*. **B:** Delayed film confirms classic mass effects of hypertrophic pyloric muscle on gastric antrum *(A)* and duodenal bulb *(D)*; there is elongation and narrowing of the pylorus *(P)*, the string sign.

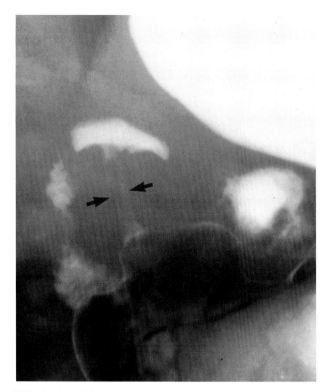

FIG. 8-109. UGI of hypertrophic pyloric stenosis. "Double-track" sign of pyloric stenosis. The hypertrophied pyloric muscle may intrude centrally into the pyloric lumen to produce a double track of barium *(arrows)*. Also note the abnormally cephalad course of the pylorus and the mass effect of the pyloric muscle on the duodenal bulb ("mushroom" sign).

maneuver (262). An air-contrast view of the antrum and pylorus is obtained by placing the patient supine with the right side elevated and manually compressing the antrum toward the pylorus. Frequently the ''shoulder sign'' of the antrum will become visible (Fig. 8-108). The diagnosis of HPS cannot be made by delayed emptying alone, because this can be caused by gastritis and pylorospasm.

After the study, if positive for HPS and if the stomach is still full, the stomach should be emptied by nasogastric tube. Though very uncommon, barium aspiration after a UGI can be fatal (263).

In summary, US is the most sensitive and specific test for HPS; it is painless, does not expose the child to radiation, and is very easy in experienced hands. The UGI, also very sensitive and specific, should be reserved for those cases in which HPS is not considered the most likely cause of vomiting. HPS is not an emergency, and if one is uncomfortable with the diagnosis made by either UGI or US, there is little harm in waiting and repeating the study. Nearly all false positives can be avoided.

Treatment

The treatment for HPS is the Ramstedt pyloromyotomy, which incises and spreads the hypertrophied muscle without violating the mucosa. The procedure has virtually no morbidity or mortality and is nearly always effective. After successful pyloromyotomy, the pyloric muscle thickness and pyloric channel length may remain abnormal on US for up to 6 weeks (264). Deformity may also be present on UGI series for months after surgery. The most important finding in the immediate postoperative period is persistently delayed gastric emptying. After incomplete or inadequate myotomy, the pylorus looks the same as on the preoperative studies by both US and UGI (265). UGI is the better examination in the unusual child with vomiting after pyloromyotomy because gastric emptying is easier to assess than with US, and other, unrelated abnormalities may be found.

Differential Diagnosis

The major differential diagnostic concern is pylorospasm, as described above. Children with the findings of pylorospasm on US or UGI may progress to HPS (266).

Delayed emptying may be due to antral gastritis, seen on both US or GI as thickened folds or on US as thickened mucosa. Gastritis due to hyperplasia of the antral mucosa is sometimes caused by administration of prostaglandin E, a drug used to maintain patency of the ductus arteriosus in newborns with cyanotic heart disease (267). The mucosal hyperplasia may cause gastric outlet obstruction. In these babies the UGI shows elongation of the pyloric channel, but US shows that the narrowing is due not to muscle hypertrophy but to mucosal hyperplasia (Fig. 8-110) (267,268). The obstruction disappears after therapy is discontinued.

Antral webs or diaphragms, incomplete forms of gastric atresia, are uncommon lesions that may cause symptoms at any age. These children usually present before 6 months of age (91,269) with symptoms of recurrent nonbilious emesis. The webs may be difficult to find on UGI but are usually visualized as thin (1–4 mm), often mobile filling defects stretching across the antrum about 1–2 cm proximal to the pylorus (Fig. 8-111) (91). Gastric emptying may be delayed. The treatment of obstructing webs is surgical.

Gastroesophageal Reflux

Gastroesophageal reflux (GER) is the retrograde passage of gastric contents into the esophagus. GER is described as regurgitant when the refluxed material reaches the mouth and nonregurgitant when gastric contents reach only the esophagus. Regurgitation may be of small or large volume. In infancy it may be difficult to distinguish regurgitation from vomiting, which is the forceful expulsion of gastric contents. Vomiting is never normal, whereas some degree of regurgitation, the ''spitting up'' with which all parents are familiar, is normal and common in infancy. When does spitting up become pathologic GER? No tables give normal values for the frequency of regurgitation in infancy. In effect, GER is deemed pathologic when it has pathologic conse-

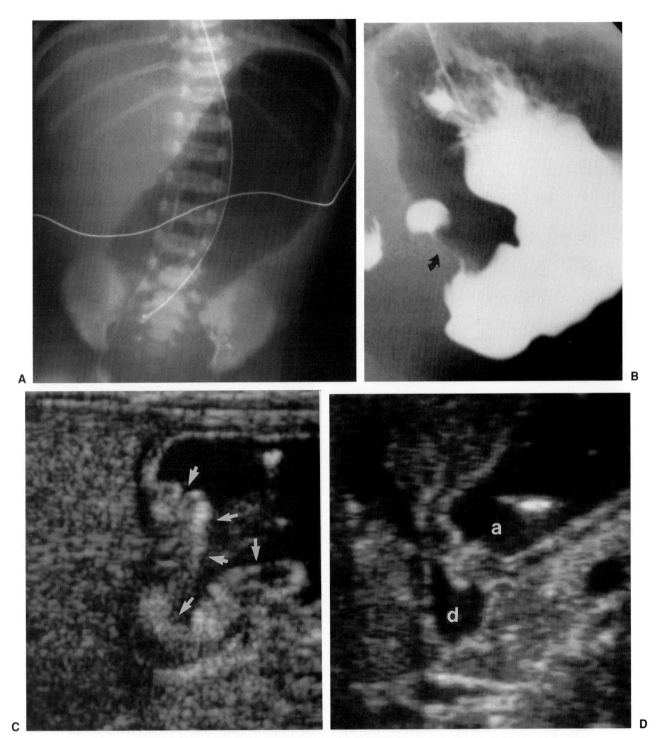

FIG. 8-110. Prostaglandin-induced antral mucosal hyperplasia. A: Supine abdominal radiograph of a 10-day-old boy with cyanotic heart disease on prostaglandin since birth. The stomach is markedly distended, and there is no distal gas. The baby had been vomiting persistently. **B:** UGI series demonstrates an elongated, upwardly directed, narrow pylorus *(curved arrows)* mimicking pyloric stenosis. **C:** US performed shortly after UGI demonstrates grossly thickened antral mucosa *(arrows)*. There is no significant thickening of the muscular layer. **D:** Normal antral mucosa for comparison. *a*, antrum; *d*, duodenum.

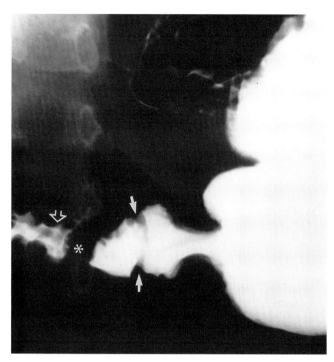

FIG. 8-111. Antral web. UGI series. The web appears as a filling defect *(arrows)* extending across the antrum (*, pylorus; *open arrow,* duodenal bulb).

quences. The questions therefore are: What are the pathologic consequences and clinical manifestations of reflux in infancy and childhood? How can the diagnosis of pathologic reflux be made, and can inconsequential physiologic reflux be reliably distinguished from pathologic reflux? Finally, what is the role of the radiologist?

Older children with reflux usually have symptoms like those of adults, namely, heartburn and dysphagia. The symptoms, if any, of infants and young children are very different. They fall into two groups, the results of reflux esophagitis and the effects of GER on the respiratory tract. Infants who regurgitate large volumes of feeding may become malnourished and fail to thrive. However, failure to thrive is more frequently a consequence of esophagitis and its accompanying irritability and poor feeding. Infants and children with esophagitis may be asymptomatic or only have occult blood in the stool. The late consequences of esophagitis include peptic strictures and Barrett's esophagus, which are described below.

The respiratory consequences of GER are less familiar, more confusing, and more controversial (270). GER may result in the aspiration of refluxed gastric contents, causing pneumonitis and perhaps apnea. The other, less well understood connection of GER with respiratory disease is through laryngospastic and bronchospastic reflexes, triggered by GER and mediated by afferent nerves from the esophagus. These reflexes may be responsible for apnea and some cases of sudden infant death syndrome (271) and may exacerbate asthma.

Most pediatricians will undertake a diagnostic evaluation of babies with clinical reflux (regurgitation) with these pathologic consequences and babies without regurgitation who have symptoms, either GI or respiratory, suggestive of GER. The evaluation of GER varies widely from institution to institution. Endoscopy is frequently used in children with symptoms of esophagitis. Endoscopy with biopsy may unequivocally establish the diagnosis of reflux esophagitis. Endoscopy, however is not a perfect test; not all significant reflux causes esophagitis, and the presence of esophagitis does not necessarily confirm that other symptoms are also caused by reflux. Endoscopy is also invasive. Twenty-four-hour pH probe monitoring is considered the gold standard for detection of reflux and allows correlation of symptoms with episodes of reflux. However, it is also invasive and generally requires at least an overnight admission to the hospital. The pH probe compares the number and duration of episodes of GER with normal standards for the age; this method inevitably leads to some false-positive and false-negative determinations of pathologic GER.

Scintigraphy is becoming more widely used for the evaluation of GER. Tc-sulfur colloid, which is not absorbed from the GI tract, is mixed with the child's food (usually milk or formula). The child is imaged continuously for at least an hour and esophageal activity is measured (Fig. 8-112). Imaging of the lungs, looking for aspiration, is also performed.

The sensitivity of scintigraphy to GER is similar to that of the pH probe (272); the specificity of scintigraphy for determination of pathologic GER, however, is uncertain (273).

The utility of the UGI series for the evaluation of reflux has been a topic of debate ever since the first description of the fluoroscopic appearance of GER in 1947 (274). The authors of that paper came to have great misgivings about the concepts presented therein. A UGI series tailored for the evaluation of GER with administration of amounts of barium equal to a normal feeding, and intermittent fluoroscopy for several minutes after a routine UGI will show GER in the majority of infants and in up to 80% of newborns (275–277), many or most of whom have no symptoms attributable to reflux. Therefore, the role of UGI series is not to diagnose reflux but to rule out structural lesions causing the patient's symptoms (276,277). Most patients with regurgitation or vomiting have no anatomic abnormalities (278). A small number, however, will have a hiatal hernia, esophageal stricture, gastric outlet obstruction, malrotation, or some other abnormality. The seriousness of these lesions makes the UGI indispensable in the work-up in any child with enough emesis to worry the pediatrician.

In children who are referred for "rule out reflux," a standard UGI series should be performed, paying careful attention to swallowing, esophageal motility and anatomy, gastric emptying, and the position of the duodenojejunal junction. No special maneuvers are used to elicit reflux. Reflux and the level reached are noted, but no attempt is made to grade reflux based on this level; higher reflux does not always correlate with symptoms and significance (276,279).

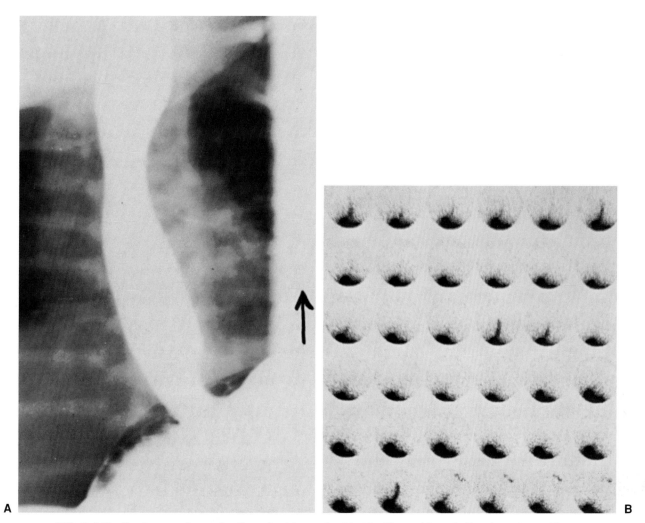

FIG. 8-112. Gastroesophageal reflux. An 11-month old girl with vomiting. **A:** Esophagogram. There is gross gastroesophageal reflux. At fluoroscopy the gastroesophageal junction remained open, and there was absence of peristalsis in the distal esophagus. **B:** Nuclear scintigraphy. Multiple posterior images, each of 30 seconds duration, were obtained after feeding of Tc-sulfur colloid and formula. There are several episodes of gastroesophageal reflux. Refluxed material reaches the oropharynx, as shown on the bottom row of images. The stomach is at the bottom of each image. There is no evidence of aspiration.

The single-contrast barium study (all that can be performed in infants) is insensitive to all but the most severe esophagitis (279). Peptic strictures, a common consequence of reflux even in infants and small children, are well seen. Children with strictures typically present with dysphagia or gradual refusal to eat solid foods. Babies taking only liquids may not develops symptoms from their strictures until they begin to take solids; the reflux causing the stricture may have been silent. Peptic strictures may be long or short and smooth or ulcerated and are usually in the mid and distal esophagus (Fig. 8-113).

Barrett's esophagus, or columnar metaplasia of the squamous esophageal epithelium, is a serious consequence of reflux esophagitis. It is especially common in those with conditions predisposing to severe reflux, such as repaired esophageal atresia and neurologic impairment (280). The most serious complication of Barrett's esophagus is the later development of adenocarcinoma of the esophagus; this consideration is especially important in children, who have many years of risk. Children with Barrett's esophagus usually have no symptoms other than those of esophagitis and perhaps stricture. There are no pathognomonic radiologic signs of Barrett's esophagus. Most patients will have reflux; one third to one half will have strictures, sometimes ulcerated (280,281). The strictures are typically in the mid- and distal esophagus. Because the radiologic findings of Barrett esophagus are nonspecific, endoscopy and biopsy are recommended in all children with esophageal strictures.

In summary, GER is a common problem in infancy and childhood, producing symptoms, especially respiratory symptoms, that are unique to childhood. There is no perfect test for GER. The mere detection of GER does not mean that it is pathologic. The available tests measure and detect different aspects of GER and are best used as complements

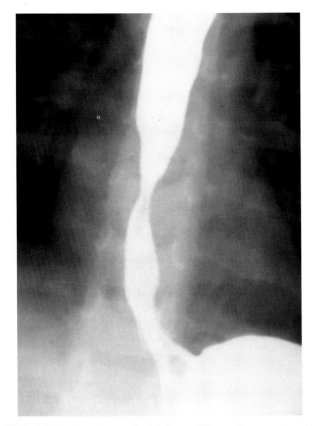

FIG. 8-113. Esophageal stricture. AP esophagram in a 4-year-old boy with gradual refusal to take solid foods. There is a short smooth stricture of the distal esophagus. Endoscopy and biopsy revealed severe reflux esophagitis. He had never had symptoms of reflux even as an infant.

to one another and in conjunction with clinical data (282, 283). The role of the UGI is a crucial, if limited, one: to exclude anatomic lesions that may lead to, exacerbate, or result from reflux.

Hiatal Hernia

Small sliding hiatal hernias of the type commonly seen in adults with GER are uncommon in childhood. Because of differences in the definition of hiatal hernia and in UGI series techniques, however, the incidence of hiatal hernia reported in childhood varies widely (284). Large hiatal hernias do occur in childhood, many in the neurologically impaired; they may be asymptomatic but are often associated with severe reflux (285). When the hernia is large it is visible on plain radiographs of the chest as a large posterior retrocardiac mass, sometimes extending toward the right lateral chest wall (Fig. 8-114) (285). Contrast studies will demonstrate that the hernia is of the sliding type, the gastroesophageal junction lying above the diaphragm. The esophagus appears short and may be kinked. The stomach is usually twisted to some degree, and complete organoaxial volvulus may be present. The antrum and fundus are frequently at the

same level, and the pylorus and duodenum may be directed inferiorly and to the left (Fig. 8-114). There may be delayed gastric emptying because of pyloric obstruction. Because the stomach lies next to the esophagus these hernias are frequently mislabeled paraesophageal. However, since the G-E junction is in the chest, they are true hiatal hernias. Paraesophageal hernias are unusual in childhood. The symptoms of hiatal hernia are usually those of reflux; ischemic symptoms are rare despite the fact that some degree of gastric volvulus is usually present. The treatment is surgical.

Gastric Volvulus

The stomach is normally fixed by the gastrohepatic, gastrophrenic, gastrosplenic, and gastrocolic ligaments. Volvulus of the stomach is uncommon and in childhood usually occurs only when there is deficient fixation of the stomach, as occurs with asplenia, diaphragmatic hernia or eventration, hiatus hernia, and malrotation (286,287).

Gastric volvulus is usually described as either mesenteroaxial or organoaxial (Fig. 8-115). Mesenteroaxial volvulus is rotation of the stomach about a mesenteric axis perpendicular to the long axis of the stomach. The gastric antrum passes superiorly and anteriorly and from right to left, so that the gastroesophageal junction is lower than normal and the antrum is near the expected location of the gastroesophageal junction (Fig. 8-115B). Obstruction may occur at the gastroesophageal junction or the pylorus. Organoaxial volvulus is rotation of the stomach about its long axis, which places the greater curvature of the stomach superiorly and the lesser curvature of the stomach inferiorly (Fig. 8-115A).

Mesenteroaxial volvulus is more common in newborns and infants, and is usually acute (287–289). The classic presentation is abdominal pain and retching without vomiting, but symptoms may be atypical in the newborn (287). Supine abdominal films will usually show marked gastric distention; erect films will show an air-fluid level, or levels, with a "beak" at the displaced antrum (Fig. 8-116) (287). Contrast studies are usually not necessary but will demonstrate the anatomy and any obstruction better.

Organoaxial volvulus is rare in children and is usually associated with a large hiatus hernia. Plain films will show a distended stomach, which is usually intrathoracic. There may be gastric outlet obstruction. The volvulus may be chronic or intermittent and lead to chronic pain and failure to thrive (290). Treatment of both types of volvulus is surgery.

Bezoar

A bezoar is a mass of ingested foreign material in the stomach. Types include trichobezoar (hair), phytobezoar (vegetable fiber), lactobezoar (milk precipitates), and gastrolith (concretion of various materials). Lactobezoars, seen in newborns, presumably are caused by mixing of the formula with an insufficient amount of water. A trichobezoar, the

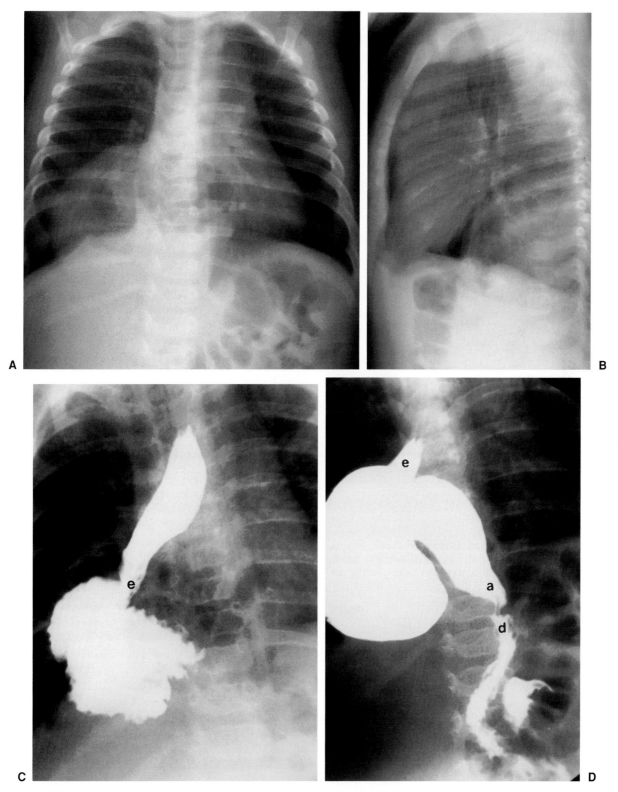

FIG. 8-114. Hiatal hernia. AP **(A)** and lateral **(B)** chest radiographs in a 9-month-old with vomiting since birth. There is a large air-containing mass projected over the right cardiophrenic angle; it is posterior on lateral view. Early **(C)** and later **(D)** views from a UGI series show that the GE junction *(e)* is in the chest. The stomach is twisted with the antrum *(a)* lying to the left. The pylorus and duodenum *(d)* are directed to the left and inferiorly.

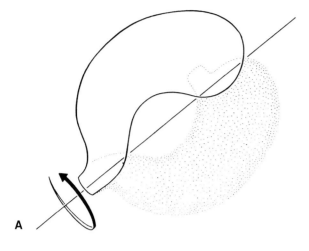

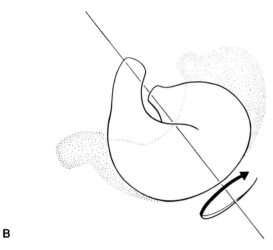

FIG. 8-115. Gastric volvulus. A: Organoaxial volvulus; rotation is around the long axis of the stomach. **B:** Mesenteroaxial volvulus; rotation is around the mesentery along a line perpendicular to the long axis of the stomach. Modified from Franken and Smith (1).

most common bezoar in older children, is usually due to chronic hair swallowing by emotionally disturbed children (Fig. 8-117) (291).

Abdominal radiographs show an intraluminal gastric mass with a mottled appearance resembling ingested food. Trichobezoars are often large and may fill the entire stomach. A barium UGI series confirms that the mass is intraluminal and not attached to the wall. The bezoar is frequently best delineated on delayed radiographs, which may show extension of the bezoar into the duodenum and jejunum.

Lactobezoars usually disappear after formula adjustment and increased water intake (292). Trichobezoars and phytobezoars usually require surgical removal, to prevent ulceration, perforation, hemorrhage, intestinal obstruction, and protein-losing enteropathy.

Intussusception

Definition and Clinical Features

Intussusception is the invagination of a segment of intestine (the "intussusceptum") into the contiguous distal segment of bowel (the "intussuscipiens"). The mechanical consequences of intussusception are obstruction and ischemia. The latter occurs because the mesentery intussuscepts along with the bowel; the resulting mesenteric vascular obstruction may lead to frank intestinal necrosis. About 90% of intussusceptions are ileocolic, the remainder are ileoileocolic, ileoileal, and colocolic; the last is very rare (Fig. 8-118).

Intussusception in childhood is usually idiopathic, i.e., no specific pathologic lesion can be identified as a lead point. At surgery hypertrophied lymphoid tissue is very frequently found in the distal small bowel, and it has long been assumed that this acts as a lead point in idiopathic intussusception. In less than 10% of childhood intussusceptions does some other pathologic lesion serve as a lead point (293–296). Lead points can occur at any age but are found most frequently in children of less than 1 month or more than 4 years; at those ages as many as half of intussusceptions may be caused by lead points (295–298). The most common lead point is a Meckel diverticulum; others include enteric duplication cysts, polyps of the ileum or colon, an inflamed appendix, bowel wall hemorrhage (as in Henoch-Schönlein purpura), and lymphoma or lymphosarcoma. Malignant lead points are more common in older children. One disease in which intussusception may also occur, although rarely, is cystic fibrosis, with abnormal stool seeming to serve as the lead point.

Though intussusception may occur at any age, idiopathic intussusception is most common in infants under 2 years old; the majority occur in infants between 3 months and 1 year of age. Boys are affected about twice as frequently as girls. Intussusception is more common in the winter and spring, when viral infections are common; this seasonal variation suggests that viral infection leads to lymphoid hypertrophy in the bowel which in turn leads to intussusception. Only a minority of patients with intussusception, however, have an identifiable viral prodrome and, in some hospitals, intussusception is common throughout the year.

The child with intussusception has usually been well. Most develop abdominal pain, typically intermittent. The attacks may be accompanied by drawing of the legs up on the abdomen. Vomiting is frequently present and may be bilious. Bowel movements may be normal at first, but the stool usually begins to contain blood, which may be occult or be mixed with mucus to produce the classic currant jelly stool of intussusception. Frank rectal bleeding may occur, usually in children with prolonged symptoms. Diarrhea may also be present. Most children with intussusception are seen within 24 hours of the onset of symptoms, but there is sometimes a delay of several days. Children with intussusception are often lethargic; lethargy may be the sole or most striking

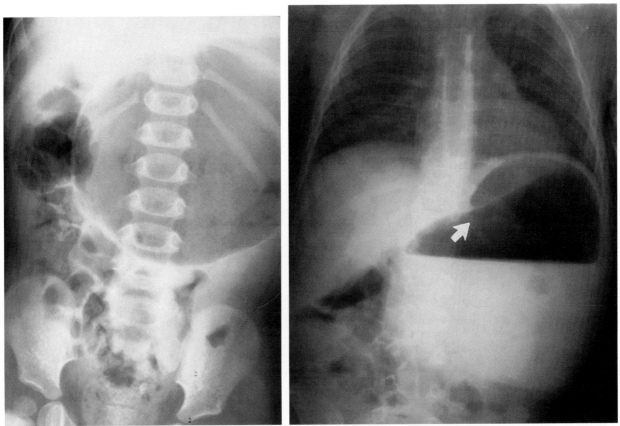

FIG. 8-116. Mesenteroaxial gastric volvulus. A: A supine film in an infant with retching without vomiting demonstrates marked gastric distention. The stomach is unusually round. **B:** An erect film demonstrates mesenteroaxial gastric volvulus with "beak" *(arrow)* at the malpositioned gastric antrum. (Courtesy of J. G. Blickman, M.D., Boston, MA.)

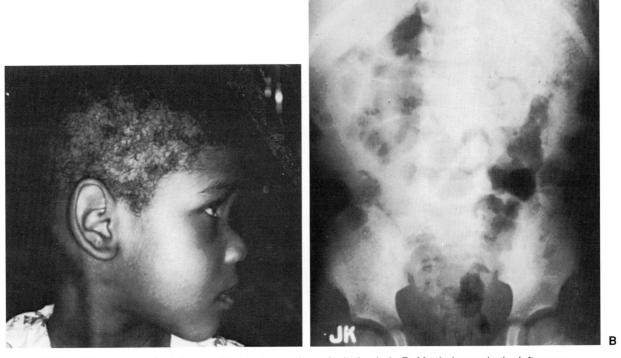

FIG. 8-117. Bezoar. A: A 3-year-old girl with patches of missing hair. **B:** Mottled mass in the left upper quadrant. *(Continued)*

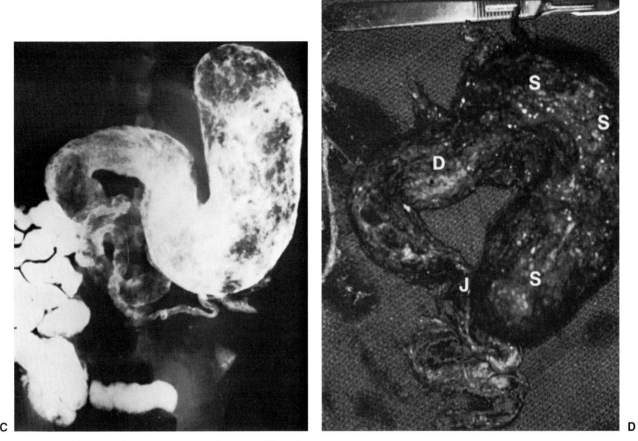

C   D

FIG. 8-117. *(continued)* **C:** The irregular filling defects in the stomach are due to the trichobezoar. Note that the bezoar extends into the duodenum and proximal small bowel. **D:** Large trichobezoar of the stomach *(S)*, duodenum *(D)*, and jejunum *(J)* removed surgically. (Courtesy of T. P. Votteler, M.D., Dallas TX.)

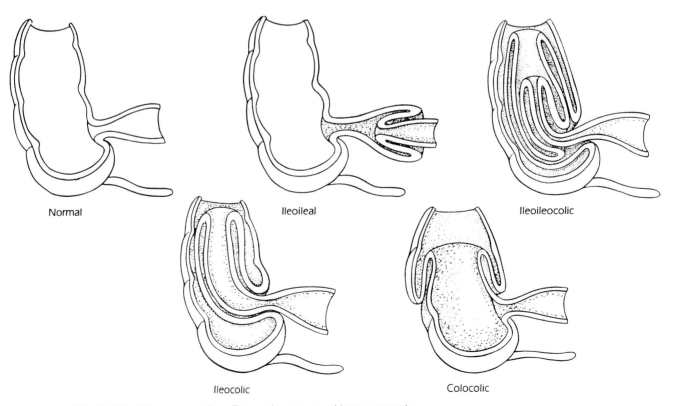

FIG. 8-118. Intussusception. The various types of intussusception.

symptom of intussusception. Without treatment, tachycardia and eventually hypotension may occur. Fever may be present. Abdominal palpation may reveal an abdominal mass, typically described as sausage-shaped, often in the right lower quadrant.

Suspected intussusception is an emergency. Surgical consultation is imperative, not only for physical diagnosis but because it is ultimately the surgeon who must decide whether the child should undergo an attempt at enema reduction or proceed directly to the operating room. Children with suspected intussusception should have radiologic evaluation only when they are hemodynamically stable. They should be accompanied by personnel trained to care for them if decompensation occurs.

Radiology

Evaluation of the child with suspected intussusception begins with plain films of the abdomen. There is no agreement about the utility of plain films in intussusception (299–304). Most children with intussusception will have abnormal plain films, and in many cases the abnormalities correctly suggest the diagnosis. The findings on plain films can be explained by the pathologic anatomy: the distal small bowel in most intussusceptions invaginates the colon, the leading edge of

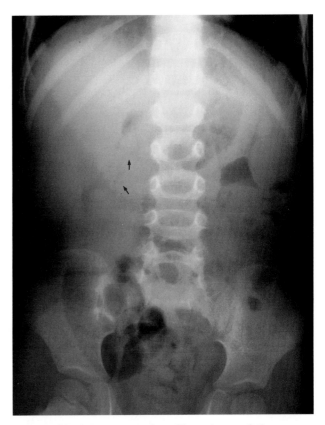

FIG. 8-120. Intussusception. There is a soft-tissue mass in the right upper quadrant. Lucencies *(arrows)* in the mass represent intussuscepted mesenteric fat. Note also the lateralization of ileum, overall paucity of gas, and loss of the subhepatic angle.

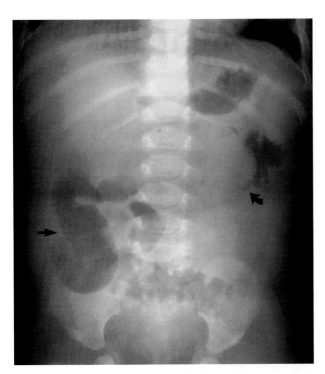

FIG. 8-119. Intussusception. Supine abdominal radiograph. There is a paucity of air in the proximal small bowel. The ileum *(arrow)* is dilated and is more lateral than normal. The intussusception is outlined by air near the splenic flexure *(curved arrow)*.

the intussusceptum usually reaching the hepatic flexure or transverse colon. Thus, in most patients one will not be able to identify the cecum and right colon. Especially if vomiting and diarrhea are present, there may be a paucity of gas in the proximal small bowel, and of gas and feces in the colon distal to the intussusception. The combination of paucity of air in the proximal small bowel, the presence of air in normal or dilated distal small bowel, and the lateral location (in the expected position of the right colon) of that small bowel is very suggestive of intussusception and is due to the distal small bowel being carried distally with the intussusceptum (Fig. 8-119). In about half of cases, the actual mass of the intussusceptum is shown (Figs. 8-120, 8-121; see also Figs. 8-124, 8-125A, and 8-130A). The specificity of this finding is increased by the presence of characteristic lucencies within the mass (see Figs. 8-120 and 8-130A). These lucencies, which are occasionally seen as two concentric rings inside a soft-tissue density, usually to the right of the spine ("target sign") (305) probably represent mesenteric fat trapped in the intussusception (Fig. 8-120) (306). The presence of air outlining the leading edge of the mass ("crescent sign") is virtually pathognomonic of intussusception (Figs.

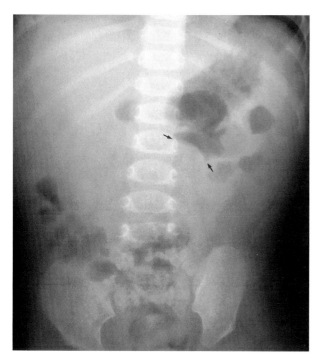

FIG. 8-121. Intussusception. Air outlines the leading edge of the intussusception *(arrows)* seen as a soft-tissue mass in the transverse colon. No air is present in the right upper quadrant.

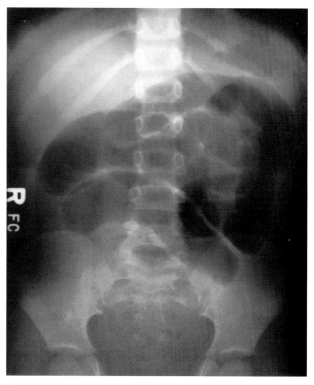

FIG. 8-122. Intussusception. Small bowel obstruction in an infant with intussusception. The intussusception was successfully reduced with air.

8-119 and 8-121). In 10% to 25% of cases, frank small bowel obstruction is present (Fig. 8-122) (307). Small bowel obstruction is not specific for intussusception but is very suggestive in a child of the appropriate age.

The sensitivity and specificity of the plain film for the diagnosis of intussusception is enhanced by multiple views. In addition to the supine view, a film with a horizontal beam, either a supine cross-table lateral, an upright, or a left side down decubitus view, is useful. The horizontal beam film is used not only to exclude pneumoperitoneum, which though rarely present would lead to immediate surgery, but also because the intussusception itself may be more readily visible on this view (308,309). If the supine and horizontal beam films are nondiagnostic, a prone film may be obtained. Prone positioning drives air from the transverse colon into the right colon and cecum (Fig. 8-123). Definite visualization of the cecum with air virtually excludes intussusception; failure to identify the cecum on a prone film should raise the suspicion of intussusception.

Most pediatric radiologists find abdominal plain films very helpful in intussusception. Children with intussusception will seldom have normal films. However, when a radiologist is asked to rule out intussusception, a rigorous definition of normal must be applied: the entire cecal pole must be visualized to exclude intussusception. Care must be taken not to mistake dilated small bowel in the right lower quadrant

for the cecum. Furthermore, when the clinical suspicion is very high and no abnormality can be found on plain films, some other means, usually a contrast enema, must be used to exclude an intussusception.

Children with clearly normal films are usually observed without further testing. If the films are not definitively normal or are clearly abnormal, an intussusception is excluded by air enema. In some centers, if the plain film in a child with suspected intussusception is normal or equivocal, abdominal US is performed. Several studies have shown that in the proper hands, US is nearly 100% sensitive for intussusception (310–312). At some centers, in fact, US is the initial test, either before or without plain films (313). The appearance of intussusception on US is characteristic but not completely specific (314). On transverse section, it appears as a hypoechoic ring surrounding an echogenic center, the so-called target or donut sign (Fig. 8-124) (315). On longitudinal scans, the appearance has been described as the sandwich or pseudokidney sign (316). The echogenic center is probably the mucosa of the intussusceptum and the outer hypoechoic rim the edematous wall of the intussusceptum (316,317). In some cases a series of concentric rings can be observed (318,319). These rings represent additional layers of bowel wall and mesentery; their visualization may be dependent on the amount of edema present.

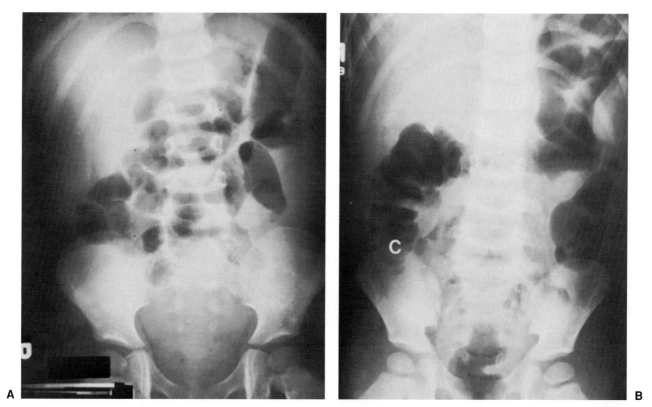

FIG. 8-123. Value of prone radiograph to exclude intussusception. A: Supine abdominal radiograph. There is distended bowel in the upper abdomen but it is impossible to distinguish between large and small bowel. **B:** Prone abdominal radiograph. Gas has distended the ascending colon, descending colon, and rectum; there is no evidence of bowel obstruction. There is gaseous distention of the terminal ileum and cecal pole *(C)* and no evidence of the soft-tissue mass of intussusception.

Management

By the mid-nineteenth century reduction of intussusception by water or saline enemas, or by rectal insufflation of air to literally "blow the intussuscepting bowel back into its original position," were well-established techniques, safer and more effective than surgery (320). As surgical techniques improved, enema reduction gradually fell out of favor, especially in North America. Even in the 1930s and 1940s, however, operative mortality remained high, which led a surgeon, Mark Ravitch, to reevaluate enema reduction. His careful clinical and experimental work, using barium enemas and fluoroscopy, finally led to the acceptance of hydrostatic reduction as the treatment of choice for intussusception (321). The barium enema became the most widely used method of reduction in Europe and North America in the 1970s and 1980s. In China and some other places physicians used air as the agent (322,323). Air reduction was introduced to North America in the 1980s and is now widely used (324).

Contraindications to Enema Reduction and Factors Influencing Success. The only absolute contraindications to attempted pneumatic or hydrostatic reduction of intussusception are pneumoperitoneum and the clinical evidence of peritonitis. Small or moderate amounts of peritoneal fluid may be seen on abdominal US in about half of patients with intussusception and in the absence of other findings should not be taken as evidence of peritonitis (325,326). Large amounts of free fluid should lead one to question the diagnosis of uncomplicated intussusception. Recent work suggests that lack of flow on color Doppler US predicts greater difficulty in reduction (327,328), but reduction should still probably be attempted.

Small bowel obstruction (SBO) is not a contraindication to reduction (307). However, the rate of successful reduction is lower in children with SBO (329,330). Children with symptoms for more than 24 hours or rectal bleeding may also have a lower rate of reduction (329, 330). In general, the more distal intussusceptions are harder to reduce, but even intussusceptions that have prolapsed through the anus can be completely reduced. Ileo-ileal and ileo-ileocolic intussusceptions are very difficult to reduce. None of these conditions are contraindications to enema reduction; their presence may, however, influence how aggressively reduction is attempted. Nearly every child, unless there are signs of peritonitis, should undergo enema reduction, provided adequate medical assistance is present during the attempt.

Patient Preparation. Some children with intussusception

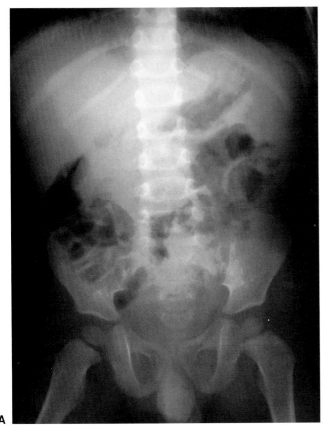

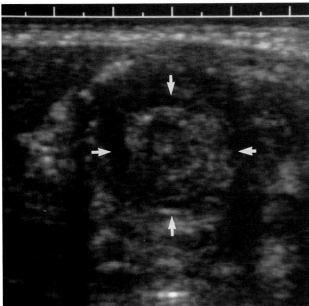

FIG. 8-124. Ultrasound of intussusception. A: A supine radiograph of an infant with abdominal pain and vomiting demonstrates a soft-tissue mass in the right upper quadrant. The appearance strongly suggests intussusception. **B:** A transverse sonographic image of the right upper quadrant reveals intussusception *(arrows)*.

are very ill and have dehydration, tachycardia, and hypotension. These children need to be stabilized before fluoroscopy and must have adequate intravenous access. A surgeon should be present during the reduction, though this will not be possible in every hospital. At the least, surgical consultation *must* be obtained *before* any attempt at enema reduction.

Children with suspected intussusception sometimes receive antibiotics before attempted reduction; there are few data to support or dispute this practice. Glucagon has not been shown to be effective and is rarely used (331). Sedation during enema reduction is more controversial (332–335). Clinical and experimental work has shown that at least during air enemas, the Valsalva maneuver, probably eliminated or attenuated by sedation, protects against bowel perforation and increases the reducing pressure during the enema (336); this has led many radiologists not to use sedation.

The procedure should be thoroughly explained to the parents, who should be informed of the small risk of perforation. The parents should also be warned that if an intussusception is present, reduction probably will be painful. If no sedation is employed, the rationale for this choice should be explained.

Technique of Reduction

Hydrostatic Reduction. Barium is still, according to the most recent surveys, the most widely used medium for intussusception reduction (334,335). Because of the risk of perforation, some radiologists prefer water-soluble agents, such as iothalamate meglumine (Cystoconray) or dilute meglumine diatrizoate. In a few centers water or saline enemas are used for reduction, with monitoring by US (337). The technique is reportedly very safe and effective.

The largest bore catheter that the anus can safely admit is inserted and secured with tape. Balloon catheters are usually not employed though their use is advocated by some radiologists. The enema tubing is connected to the bag of contrast, which by custom, mostly based on the data of Ravitch (321), is placed about 1 m or 3 feet above the table top.

If an intussusception is not encountered and there is free flow of contrast into the small bowel, the exam is terminated. If present, the intussusception is usually encountered in the transverse colon, though it may be seen anywhere from the anus to the cecum. The intussusception will appear as a convex intraluminal filling defect (Fig. 8-125). As contrast insinuates itself between the intussusceptum and the intussuscipiens the filling defect may take on the classic coiled spring appearance (Fig. 8-126). Although extensive tracking of barium between the intussusceptum and intussuscipiens ("dissection sign") (338) without movement of the intussusception was once thought to indicate nonreducibility, these intussusceptions are often reducible with a second or third attempt (329,339). Nearly all intussusceptions are at least partly reducible, but completion of reduction into the ileum may be difficult. If 3 minutes pass without further progress,

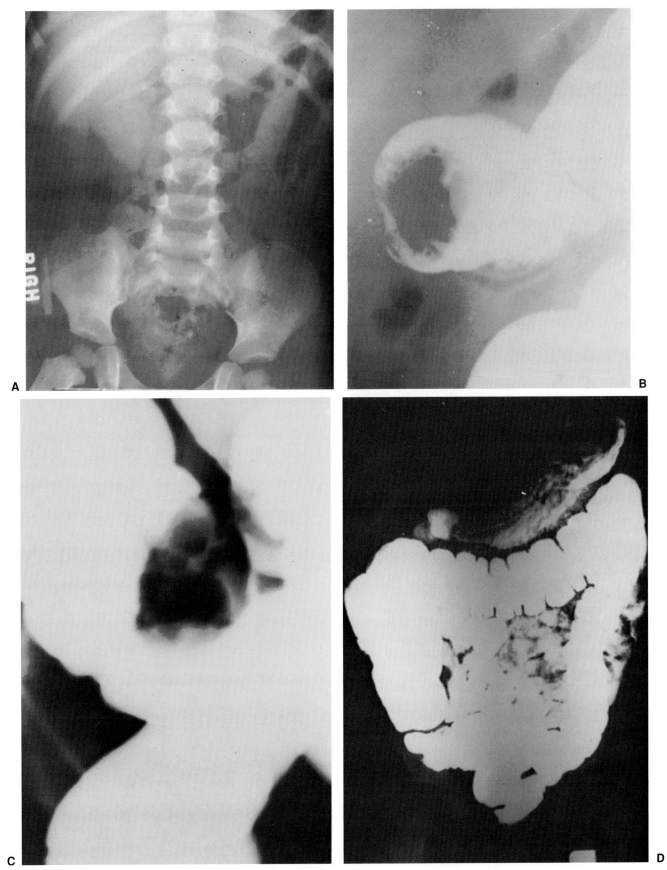

FIG. 8-125. Hydrostatic reduction of intussusception. A 2-year-old boy with acute abdominal pain.
A: There is a paucity of gas in the right upper quadrant and loss of the subhepatic angle. **B:** Intussusception in right transverse colon. **C:** Reduction of intussusception to the level of ileocecal valve. **D:** Free
flow of contrast material into distal small bowel with further retrograde flow to duodenum and stomach.

917

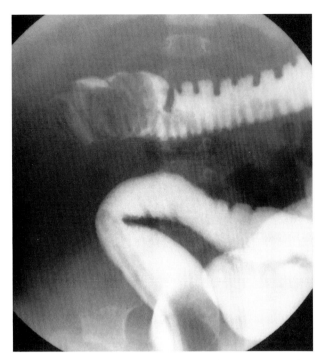

FIG. 8-126. Hydrostatic reduction of intussusception. Spot film during barium enema demonstrates intussusceptum in proximal transverse colon with the appearance of a coiled spring.

the barium is siphoned out by lowering the reservoir to the floor and the infant is allowed to evacuate. The enema is begun again. Attempts at reduction are terminated if the barium column remains obstructed after three attempts of 3–5 minutes of constant hydrostatic pressure, with intervening evacuation. This method has been referred to as the rule of 3's: 3 attempts of 3 minutes duration each, with the barium column rising 3 feet above the table. Many experienced pediatric radiologists will raise the enema bag higher than 1 m and try for longer than 9–15 minutes. In most departments the rule of 3's is used as a guide, not an absolute prescription. The hydrostatic pressures generated by different contrast media are quite different. A barium solution diluted to approximately 25% weight/volume generates a pressure of about 85 mm Hg, at a height 1 m; dilute water-soluble preparations generate less (340,341).

Successful reduction is indicated by free flow of contrast material into the terminal ileum (Fig. 8-125). One should attempt to reflux contrast as far back into the ileum as is possible to assure that reduction is complete. Filling of the appendix frequently occurs; this should not be mistaken for successful reduction. Contrast sometimes refluxes into the ileum before reduction; care must be taken that there is no persistent mass in the cecum. The edematous ileocecal valve is often visible but should be distinguishable from a residual intussusception by its mural rather than intraluminal location on the medial wall of the cecum.

Occasionally, complete colonic reduction appears to have occurred but there is no reflux into the ileum. When there

is no residual mass in the cecum, the postevacuation films are normal, and pain and other signs and symptoms disappear, it is safe merely to observe the child. In the great majority of cases clinical and radiologic evidence of successful reduction will be clear (342,343). This approach is probably valid for reductions with both air and liquid contrast. Some radiologists will use US to document successful reduction, but care must be taken not to confuse edematous bowel with residual intussusception because both may have a donut appearance. The edematous donut seen after reduction is usually smaller (344).

After reduction, a postevacuation film should be obtained. As documented by Eklof and Hugosson (345), the postevacuation film of a successfully treated intussusception should demonstrate free reflux into the small bowel, often more than on the preevacuation film, and no dilatation of small bowel above the contrast medium; dilatation implies more proximal obstruction. Colonic contrast is evacuated poorly in children with successful reduction but nearly completely in children with unreduced or recurrent intussusception (Figs. 8-125D and 8-127).

Occasionally, a smooth filling defect at the cecal wall, not in the location of the ileocecal valve, can be seen after successful reduction. This probably represents edema or hemorrhage into the cecal wall (346). It should be carefully distinguished from the intraluminal defect of a residual intussusception. There should be no filling defects in the colon or

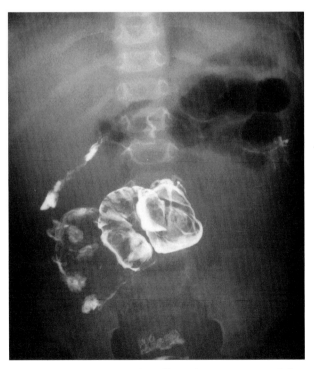

FIG. 8-127. Postevacuation film after unsuccessful reduction of intussusception. An AP radiograph after a barium enema demonstrates a persistent ileal filling defect that at surgery was a Meckel diverticulum. The patient has evacuated the colon nearly completely.

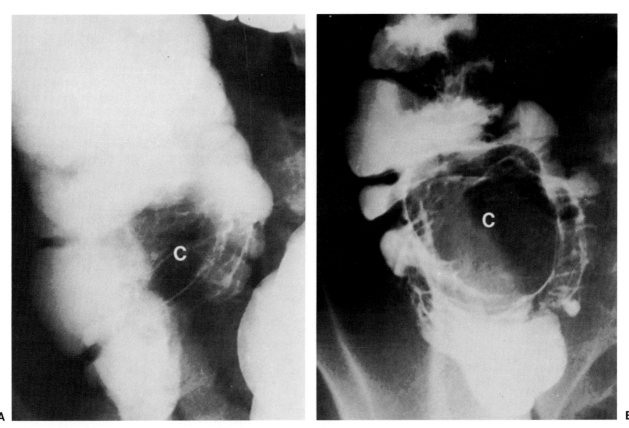

FIG. 8-128. Intussusception due to non-Hodgkin lymphoma. A 14-year-old boy with intermittent abdominal pain and a right lower quadrant mass. **A:** A soft-tissue mass in the cecum *(C)* with a coiled-spring appearance due to intussusception. **B:** Postevacuation radiograph. The cecal mass *(C)* is again demonstrated well. This intussusception could not be hydrostatically reduced.

small bowel, except for lymphoid hyperplasia in the terminal ileum and edema of the ileocecal valve. A persistent filling defect in the small bowel after an apparently successful reduction should suggest a lead point (Fig. 8-127). Hydrostatic (but not pneumatic) reduction of lead points is unusual (347). The limited experience with successful reduction of lead points suggests that they are often easy to see at fluoroscopy (Figs. 8-127 and 8-128).

The reported success rate of hydrostatic reduction varies greatly. It depends on the experience and persistence of the radiologist and the patient referral pattern. Most centers report success rates between 60% and 80%. After failed reduction, children are usually operated on immediately. If the child is stable, additional delayed attempts at reduction are sometimes performed (348). This approach has been used after attempted reduction with both liquid and air.

Pneumatic Reduction. The commercially available Shiels intussusception air reduction system (Custom Medical Products, Maineville, OH) works well for pneumatic reduction (349). This device consists of two parts: a reusable aneroid gauge and insufflator, similar to that of a sphygmomanometer, and a disposable tubing set with an enema tip, a filter, and a three-way stopcock (Fig. 8-129A). The stopcock attaches to the gauge and allows for easy, rapid decompression of the colon during the examination. For effective reduction

it is essential that an air-tight system be used. This is facilitated by creating an occlusive seal using a plug made of wrapped 1/2-in. tape and a 1.5-in. centrally perforated disk that is pulled down to the tape plug (Fig. 8-129B). The tube is taped to the buttocks securely. The patient may be supine or prone. Air insufflation then proceeds. When an intussusception is encountered it is usually easily seen as an intraluminal filling defect, and insufflation pressure usually rises (Fig. 8-130). If no intussusception is encountered air flows freely filling the colon and, often after a short delay, refluxes into the ileum. Reflux of contrast into the ileum before complete reduction is achieved occurs more frequently with air than with barium, and care must be taken that no residual filling defects are present in the cecum (350). A postevacuation film is always obtained. Films after air enemas are useful in the same way as films after opaque enemas, namely, to show absence of filling defects and obstruction and the completeness of evacuation.

Exclusion of intussusception by air enema usually requires less than a minute of fluoroscopy time. Pressures average approximately 60 mm Hg but are frequently lower (351). The insufflation pressure, with the child at rest (i.e., not straining or screaming), should be no more than 120 mm Hg. Pressures may rise substantially higher when the patient strains (performs a Valsalva maneuver). Experimental work

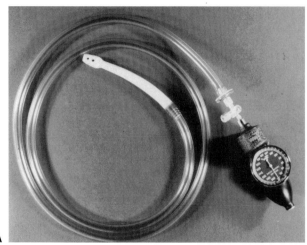

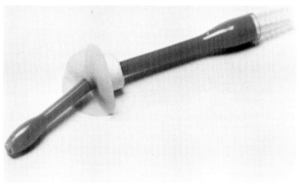

FIG. 8-129. Shiels air insufflation device and enema tip.
A: Reusable, hand-held insufflator/gauge (Tycos Life Science, Arden, NC) is connected with filter to disposable tubing set by a three-way stopcock for immediate colonic decompression. **B:** Preparation of catheter tip for air enema. Flex-tip catheter wrapped with 0.5-in. tape. A 1.5-in. centrally perforated latex rubber disk is pulled down to the tape plug to occlude the anus and reduce leakage of air. This enema tip may be used for air, barium, water-soluble, or double-contrast enemas. Modified from Shiels et al. (349).

sure is exerted on the intussusception during hydrostatic reduction, reduction with air is an intermittent process with widely fluctuating pressures. Time limits for reduction attempts are therefore difficult to state, but complications are rare as long as the maximum pressure of 120 mm Hg at rest is not exceeded. When a child is very ill, has some of the predictors of a lower rate of reduction, or has what have been identified as risk factors for perforation (see following) *and* in whom no progress in reduction is being made, the study should be terminated earlier than usual.

Success rates reported with air reduction have varied. As experience with the technique has increased, so has the success rate, and rates of 80% to 90% are now common (351–353). Because air reduction is faster and cleaner for both the patient and the radiologist and because in experienced hands rates of reduction are often higher with air than with barium, air reduction has replaced barium reduction at many pediatric centers (353). However, concerns about air enemas have been voiced (354,355). The most important concern has been safety, as will be discussed later. Concerns about visualization of the intussusception have proved unfounded; even in cases of small bowel obstruction it is rare not to see the intussusception easily. A more valid concern has been the ability of air to detect lead points. The available data suggest that in many cases lead points will not be seen on air enemas (356) and, moreover, that the lead points may be reduced all too easily with air (356,357). Ultrasonography may be useful when suspicious filling defects persist after air enemas and in those patients old enough to make a lead point likely (358).

Complications

There is a 5% to 10% recurrence rate after successful hydrostatic or pneumatic reduction of intussusception (293,294,359,360). The recurrence rate after surgical reduction is <5% (359,360). Most recurrences occur within 72 hours of the reduction, but occasionally occur more than a year later. Recurrences may be multiple. There are no significant differences in age or symptoms between children who go on to have recurrent intussusception and those who have only one episode (360). Children with recurrent intussusception appear to be no more likely to have a lead point than those with single episodes (359,360). Children who present with recurrence should thus undergo enema reduction; as many as five intussusceptions have been reduced in one child. In older children with recurrence, however, one should fluoroscope with extra care and then, if necessary, use US or barium studies to exclude a lead point.

has demonstrated, and this seems to be true in clinical practice, that the Valsalva maneuver protects against perforation by preventing large pressure gradients across the bowel wall; it thus allows higher intracolonic pressures and more effective reduction (336). Sedation is not used during air reduction to allow the child to perform the Valsalva maneuver at will. The average pressure required for enema reduction is about 100 mm Hg. There is no easy guideline for air reduction analogous to the rule of 3's for hydrostatic reduction. This is mainly because while more or less continuous pres-

FIG. 8-130. Air reduction of intussusception. A 2-year-old girl with crampy, intermittent abdominal pain. A supine abdominal radiograph demonstrates a soft-tissue mass in the right upper quadrant with obliteration of the subhepatic angle **(A)**. There is dilatation of a loop of small bowel in the right mid-abdomen. The images show successful reduction of the intussusception *(I)* from the right transverse colon **(B)** to the ascending colon **(C)** to the cecum **(D)** into the small bowel **(E)**. A postreduction film **(F)** shows free flow of air into the ileum and disappearance of the soft-tissue mass. *(Continued)*

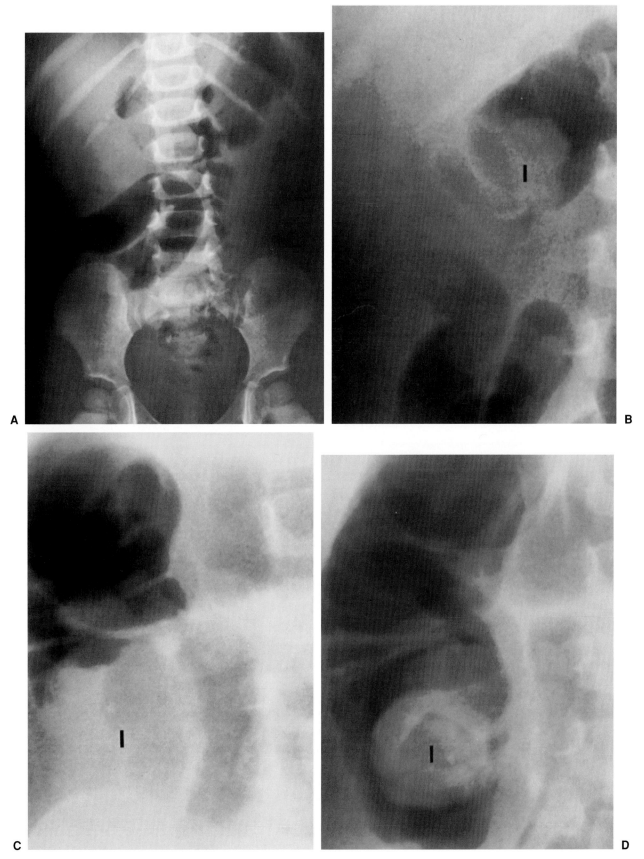

FIG. 8-130. *(Continued)*

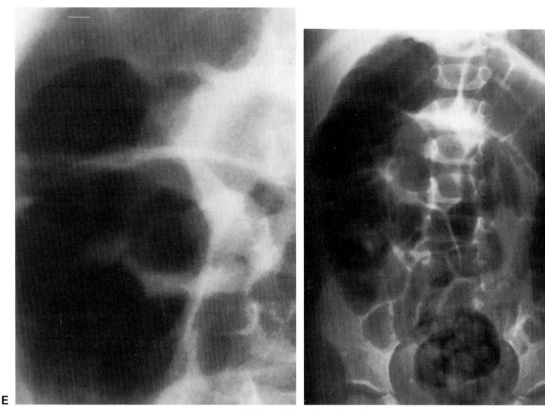

E

F

FIG. 8-130. (Continued)

Perforation of the intestine is a rare complication of enema reduction. The historical perforation rate with hydrostatic reduction is <0.5% (361). Initial reports of air reduction reported rates as high as 2.8% (352). Some of these perforations occurred with pressures of greater than 120 mm Hg. As awareness of the dangers of high pressures has increased, the perforation rates with air have declined and now are similar to those with barium (351,355,362). The perforation rate in the enormous Chinese experience with air is comparable to the historical barium rate (363).

A rare sequel of perforation during air reduction is tension pneumoperitoneum. Though this is very unusual, an 18-gauge needle should always be available for immediate decompression. Leak of either air or barium is usually seen at fluoroscopy (362).

Perforation due to intussusception usually occurs in the intussuscipiens at or proximal to the intussusception (362). The perforating bowel wall is usually necrotic: this has led to the theory that the perforation is not caused by but is merely uncovered by the enema during reduction (364). This theory does not explain all perforations, as some occur through normal bowel wall (362). Rarely, perforation occurs distal to the intussusception (365). Perforation seems to be more common in babies <6 months of age with a longer duration of symptoms (362,366), though this is not true in some series (367). Caution should therefore be exercised in very sick babies who have been symptomatic for a long time.

Perforations during air enemas are smaller than perforations during hydrostatic reduction, there is less fecal soiling, and obviously there is no barium to cause barium peritonitis (336,362). Most children with perforation with either medium do well; as Eklof has said, perforation should be regarded as ''less a failure of method than an unfortunate but rare complication of the examination'' (25).

Inguinal Hernia

In fetal life the parietal peritoneal membrane extends through the internal inguinal ring to form the processus vaginalis. During the normal descent of the testis from the abdomen into the scrotum late in gestation the processus vaginalis becomes attached to the testis, which carries it into the scrotum. The portion of the processus that covers the testis becomes the tunica vaginalis; the remainder of the processus vaginalis involutes, thus eliminating the communication between the scrotum and the peritoneal cavity. The processus vaginalis may remain patent and cause no symptoms throughout life but in most people closes during infancy. The patent processus vaginalis becomes a hernia (indirect inguinal hernia) when abdominal contents enter it. In boys it is usually bowel which enters the sac; in girls it may be bowel, ovary, or fallopian tube.

Indirect inguinal hernias are much more common in boys than in girls and much more common in premature than in

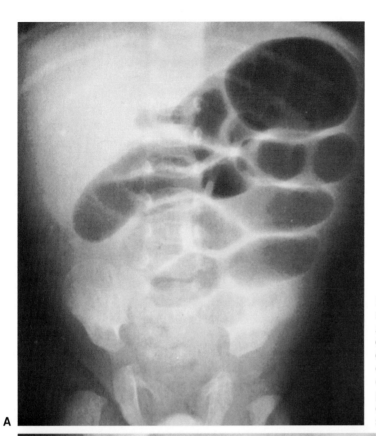

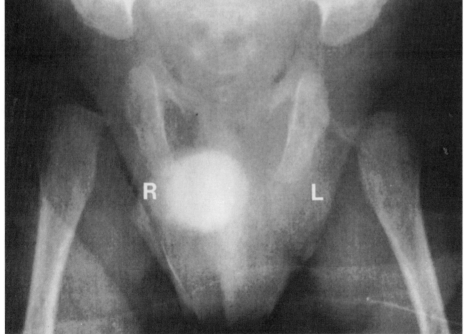

FIG. 8-131. Incarcerated inguinal hernia. A 5-week-old boy with bilious vomiting. **A:** Anteroposterior supine abdominal radiograph. The disproportionate gaseous distention of small bowel compared to colon indicates mechanical small bowel obstruction. **B:** Coned-down AP view of the pelvis. There is thickening of the left *(L)* compared to the normal right *(R)* inguinoscrotal fold.

full-term infants. They are frequently bilateral. The major complication of an indirect inguinal hernia is incarceration, which may lead to intestinal obstruction. Incarcerated hernia is one of the most common causes of bowel obstruction during infancy. Incarceration is most common in young infants. The incarceration sometimes leads to strangulation.

The diagnosis of incarcerated hernia is usually straightfor-

ward. Occasionally, when the presentation is less obvious, a plain film may be obtained. The film may show mechanical obstruction. An air-containing loop of bowel may be identified in the inguinal canal or scrotum; usually, however, the incarcerated loops are airless. The diagnosis also may be suggested by a thickened inguinoscrotal fold (Fig. 8-131) (368). Normally, the two inguinoscrotal folds are symmetric.

A swollen inguinoscrotal fold may also be seen with a hydrocele, an undescended testis, and adenitis. When it is not clear as to what causes the swollen fold or large scrotum, US may identify the fluid, bowel, or mass.

Most incarcerated hernias can be reduced nonoperatively and repaired later. If there is evidence of strangulation or the hernia is nonreducible, immediate surgery is necessary.

Anomalies of the Omphalomesenteric Duct

The omphalomesenteric (vitelline) duct is a tubular structure which in fetal life runs in the umbilical cord connecting the midgut, at the level of what will become the ileum, with the extraembryonic yolk sac. The duct normally involutes by about the ninth week of fetal life. Persistence of all or part of the duct results in a variety of postnatal anomalies (Fig. 8-132) (369). When the entire duct persists there is communication of the ileum with the umbilicus and fecal umbilical discharge; injection of contrast into this draining

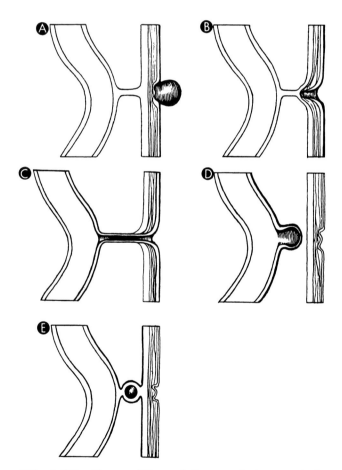

FIG. 8-132. Abnormalities of the omphalomesenteric duct. A: Mucosal polyp at umbilicus, with a band from the bowel to the umbilicus. **B:** Omphalomesenteric band or cord and umbilical sinus. **C:** Omphalomesenteric fistula. **D:** Meckel diverticulum. **E:** Omphalomesenteric cyst. (From Shaw A. Disorders of the umbilicus. In: Welch K, Randolph JG, Ravitch MM, eds. *Pediatric surgery.* Chicago: Year Book, 1986, 731–739.)

omphalomesenteric fistula will opacify small bowel. An umbilical sinus occurs when only the distal portion of the duct persists. If the proximal (juxta-ileal) part of the duct remains patent, a Meckel diverticulum is the result. Meckel diverticula are by far the most common and important of the omphalomesenteric remnants. They are located on the antimesenteric border of the ileum, usually within 60 cm of the ileocecal valve. The diverticula contain all layers of intestinal wall and frequently have ectopic mucosa within them, especially gastric mucosa; the ectopic mucosa may produce symptoms. When both ends of the embryonic duct involute, leaving only the central portion patent, an omphalomesenteric cyst results; these cysts often produce no symptoms but may present as a mass or cause bowel obstruction. Finally, the entire duct may involute except for a fibrous band connecting the umbilicus and the ileum.

Omphalomesenteric remnants cause symptoms in two ways. One way is bowel obstruction, which is most common in young infants (370). In these babies the obstruction is usually due to a volvulus of the small intestine around a fibrous duct remnant. High-grade distal small bowel obstruction will then develop; bowel necrosis is common (371). An enema may show beaking of the cecum or ileum and thus suggest volvulus. Obstruction in older infants and young children is usually due to an intussusception with a Meckel diverticulum as a lead point.

The other common presentation of an omphalomesenteric remnant, usual in older infants and young children, is GI bleeding due to ectopic gastric mucosa in a Meckel diverticulum (370). The bleeding is usually painless and self-limited but occasionally is massive, requiring emergency operation. The rectal blood is usually maroon or bright red.

The best imaging modality for detecting Meckel diverticula is nuclear scintigraphy with ^{99m}Tc pertechnetate, which accumulates in gastric mucosa. Ectopic gastric mucosa is present in only about 25% of Meckel diverticula but is almost always present in those that bleed. Patients are usually premedicated with pentagastrin to increase pertechnetate uptake by gastric mucosa. A Meckel diverticulum will be seen as a well-defined area of increased uptake, usually in the right lower quadrant (Fig. 8-133). The activity in ectopic mucosa generally appears at about the same time as activity in the stomach and gradually increases. The overall accuracy of scintigraphy for detection of Meckel diverticula is about 90%.

Meckel diverticula are notoriously difficult to demonstrate on barium studies; the studies are frequently negative, or may demonstrate evidence a mass effect on bowel near the diverticulum (Fig. 8-133). Occasionally, the diverticulum fills with contrast and can be recognized.

Less common complications of a Meckel diverticulum include nonhemorrhagic inflammation due to ulceration from ectopic mucosa, perforation, and formation of a giant diverticulum. The treatment for all symptomatic diverticula is surgery.

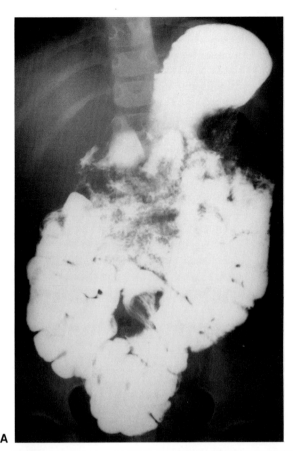

A

FIG. 8-133. Meckel diverticulum. A: A film from a small bowel series on a child with several episodes of painless rectal bleeding. There is mass effect on distal small bowel loops near the midline. **B:** A spot film confirms the mass. **C:** A delayed anterior scintigraphic image of the abdomen at 1 hour shows a round focal accumulation of ^{99m}Tc-pertechnetate in the midabdomen *(arrow)*, corresponding to the mass seen on barium studies. *S,* stomach; *b,* bladder.

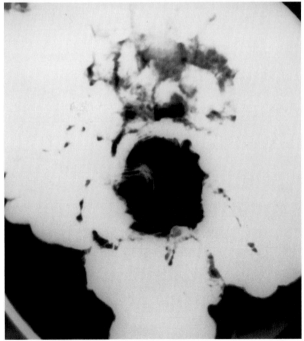

B

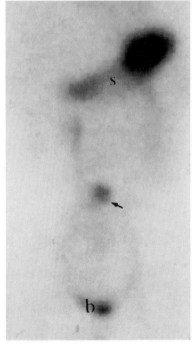

C

Gastrointestinal Duplication

A gastrointestinal (GI) duplication (enteric cyst) is a spherical or tubular cystic structure that is lined with alimentary tract epithelium, has smooth muscle in its wall, and is usually attached to the GI tract. Duplications generally share a common muscular wall and blood supply with adjacent bowel. The lining may not be identical to the mucosa of the adjacent intestine. The most frequently found ectopic tissues are gastric mucosa and pancreatic tissue. Enteric duplications are named for the adjacent part of the GI tract, not for the type of mucosa present. Spherical duplications do not usually communicate with the GI tract; the much less common tubular types frequently do. Although duplications may occur anywhere from the tongue to the anus, most occur in the distal ileum; the esophagus is the next most common site (Fig. 8-134) (372).

The signs and symptoms and the radiologic findings depend on the location of the duplication. Most duplications present during the first year of life (373).

Duplications of the esophagus are most common in the distal third. They frequently produce no symptoms and are detected as posterior mediastinal masses on chest x-rays obtained for unrelated reasons. Duplications of the upper two thirds of the esophagus may cause compression of the airway. Esophageal duplications may be associated with other congenital anomalies. They frequently contain gastric mucosa, which may lead to ulceration and rarely to perforation and hemorrhage.

On plain films, esophageal duplications usually appear as mediastinal masses. Air may be seen within them. Esophagrams will show displacement of the esophagus and an extraluminal mass (Fig. 8-135). The duplications rarely communicate with the esophagus. US is useful only if the mass extends into the neck. CT and MRI are helpful but are often nonspecific, demonstrating a rounded, fluid-filled mass near the esophagus (Fig. 8-136). The mass is sometimes paraspinal rather than directly adjacent to the esophagus.

Infants with duplications of the stomach and small bowel are most likely to present with abdominal pain, distention, and symptoms of obstruction or an abdominal mass. Obstruction may be caused by compression or, in the distal small bowel, by intussusception. Contrast studies will show compression of adjacent bowel (Figs. 8-137 and 8-138). The diagnosis of a gastric or small bowel duplication is usually established by US. Duplications have a typical appearance on US, wherever their location: a cystic mass, the wall of which has an inner echogenic layer corresponding to mucosa and an outer hypoechoic layer corresponding to muscle (Figs. 8-137 and 8-138). This gut signature is virtually pathognomonic of a duplication (37).

Duplications of the colon may be spherical, in which case their presenting features and radiologic findings are similar to those of small bowel duplications. Nearly half of colonic duplications, however, are tubular. The frequently involve the entire colon, the duplicated colon lying side by side with the normal colon and communicating with it. The duplicated colon may end blindly, at a second perineal orifice, or in the genitourinary system. Other anomalies are frequently present.

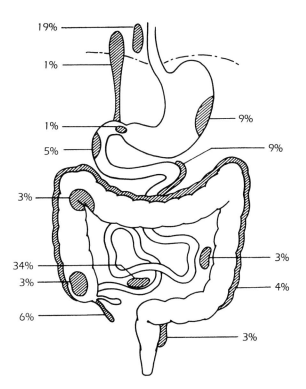

FIG. 8-134. Frequency of anatomic locations of gastrointestinal duplications. The most common sites of duplication are the terminal ileum, distal esophagus, stomach, and jejunum. From Kirks (96).

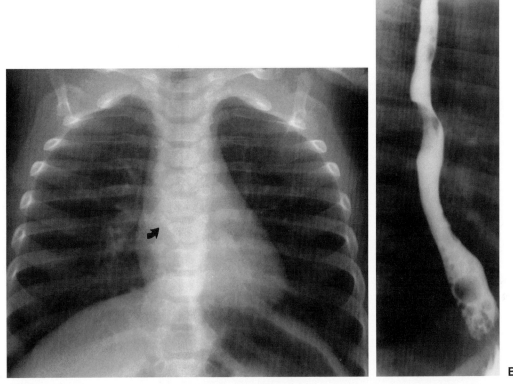

FIG. 8-135. Esophageal duplication. A: AP radiograph of the chest demonstrates a contour abnormality *(curved arrow)* in the azygoesophageal recess. **B:** Oblique esophagram demonstrates external compression of the mid esophagus by a mass. An esophageal duplication was removed.

Mesenteric Cyst (Lymphangioma)

Mesenteric cyst is a nonspecific term used to describe a number of benign cystic abdominal masses. In children, what are called mesenteric cysts are invariably cystic lymphangiomas (374). These uncommon lesions are probably developmental anomalies in which the lymphatic vessels of the mesentery fail to establish communications with the central lymphatic system, resulting in the formation of a large mass of dilated, fluid-filled lymphatic spaces. The mass is usually confined to the small bowel mesentery or, less often, the omentum. Although lymphangiomas may adhere to adjacent organs, they do not invade them. Intraabdominal lymphangiomas are rarely associated with lymphatic malformations elsewhere.

Children with intraabdominal lymphangiomas usually present in the first few years of life but only rarely in the newborn period. The most common symptoms are abdominal pain and distention. Plain radiographs will show a large noncalcified mass. US will usually show a multiloculated, cystic mass, usually with thin septations (Fig. 8-139) (375). The fluid is usually anechoic but may contain echoes if bloody, chylous, or purulent. CT and MRI are generally not as helpful as US. The attenuation and signal intensity of the fluid will vary with its composition (Fig. 8-139) (376). The treatment is resection.

Polyps and Polyposis Syndromes

Because the term polyp is so nonspecific, and because different types of polyps may have drastically different clinical significance, the radiologist must have a clear understanding of the different types of GI tract polyps in children. Polyps and polyposis syndromes are usually classified into four groups: isolated juvenile polyps; inherited hamartomatous polyposis syndromes (juvenile polyposis, Peutz-Jeghers syndrome, and Cowden syndrome); inherited adenomatous polyposis syndromes (familial polyposis, Gardner syndrome, and Turcot syndrome); and noninherited polyposes, the prime example of which is the Cronkhite-Canada syndrome. Most radiologists are familiar with the adenomatous polyposes, which will not be discussed further here. The most important syndromes that occur in children are isolated juvenile polyps, juvenile polyposis, and Peutz-Jeghers syndrome.

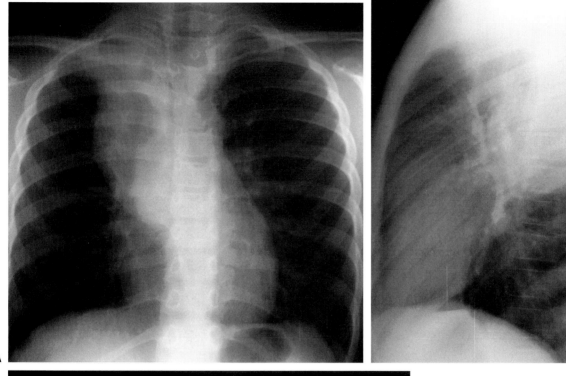

A

B

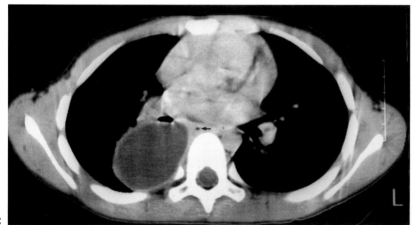

C

FIG. 8-136. Esophageal duplication. AP **(A)** and lateral **(B)** chest radiographs in a 7-year-old boy with cough and fever show a large posterior mediastinal mass. **C:** CT scan with intravenous contrast demonstrates a fluid-filled, thin-walled mass adjacent to esophagus *(arrow).*

Isolated Juvenile Polyps

The most common tumor of the colon in childhood is the juvenile polyp. Some consider juvenile polyps to be inflammatory; others to be hamartomas (377). They are not true neoplasms, unlike adenomatous polyps in the adult. Histologically, juvenile polyps consist of large, cystically dilated glands and an inflamed lamina propria; little smooth muscle is present. Juvenile polyps may be single or multiple. A child with five or fewer juvenile polyps in the colon is considered to have "isolated juvenile polyps" (377). The polyps are most frequently found in the rectum and sigmoid but may occur elsewhere in the colon.

Children with juvenile polyps almost always present between the ages of 2 and 10 years with painless rectal bleeding. The bleeding is usually intermittent and is rarely pro-

fuse, but anemia may develop. Rectal prolapse of a juvenile polyp is unusual, and colocolic intussusception due to a polyp even more uncommon.

Most children with rectal bleeding are referred for endoscopy. When imaging is decided on, painless rectal bleeding is one of the few indications for a double-contrast barium enema. The polyps are easily visible because they are usually quite large (1–5 cm) and pedunculated (Figs. 8-140 and 8-141). The entire colon should be carefully examined, looking for multiple lesions. If the diagnosis is established by enema, the child must undergo endoscopy; the polyp may be removed endoscopically to be examined pathologically and to prevent further symptoms. Though isolated juvenile polyps are not true neoplasms, there have been a few reports of adenomas or carcinomas in juvenile polyps, and of adenomas occurring simultaneously with juvenile polyps (377).

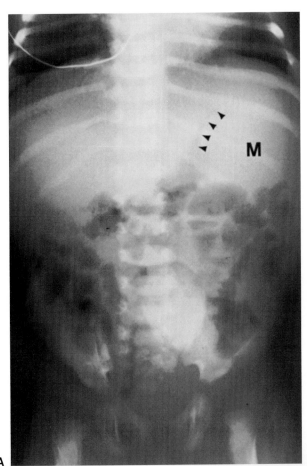

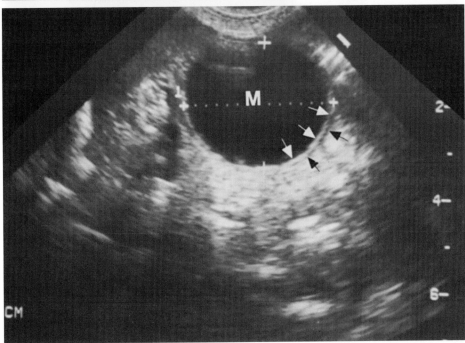

FIG. 8-137. Gastric duplication cyst. A: A left upper quadrant mass *(M)* extrinsically compresses the stomach *(arrowheads)*. **B:** Longitudinal sonography confirms that the mass *(M)* is cystic (anechoic, sharp posterior wall, increased through-transmission). The mucosa is echogenic *(white arrows)* and the adjacent muscle sonolucent *(black arrows)*.

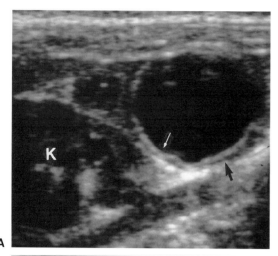

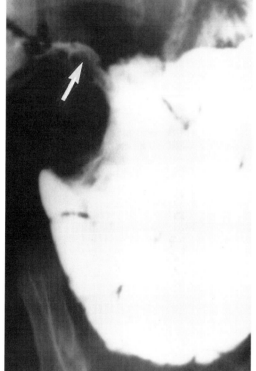

FIG. 8-138. Ileal duplication cyst. **A:** A sonogram of the right flank in a newborn with an abdominal mass demonstrates a cystic mass inferior to the right kidney *(K)*. The inner wall *(white arrow)* of the cyst is echogenic, the outer wall *(black arrow)* sonolucent. **B:** A spot film from a UGI/SBFT demonstrates a mass effect on the terminal ileum *(arrow)*. **C:** The resected surgical specimen, a spherical noncommunicating duplication cyst *(d)* of the terminal ileum. *a,* appendix; *c,* cecum; *i,* ileum.

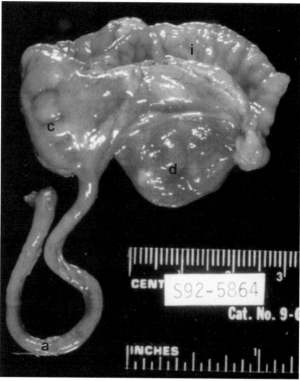

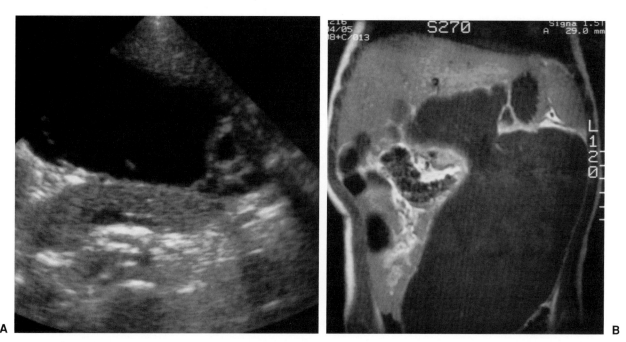

FIG. 8-139. Omental cyst (cystic abdominal lymphangioma). A: Transverse sonogram at level of pancreas in a 3-½-year-old boy with a history of a protuberant abdomen and intermittent abdominal pain. There is a sonolucent mass with septations. **B:** Coronal T1-weighted (600/15) MR image demonstrates a fluid-filled intraperitoneal mass extending from the lesser sac. A lymphangioma arising from the lesser omentum and adherent to the lesser curvature of the stomach was resected. (From Buonomo C, Griscom NT. Cystic lymphangioma (omental cyst). *RadioGraphics* 1991;11:1146–1148.)

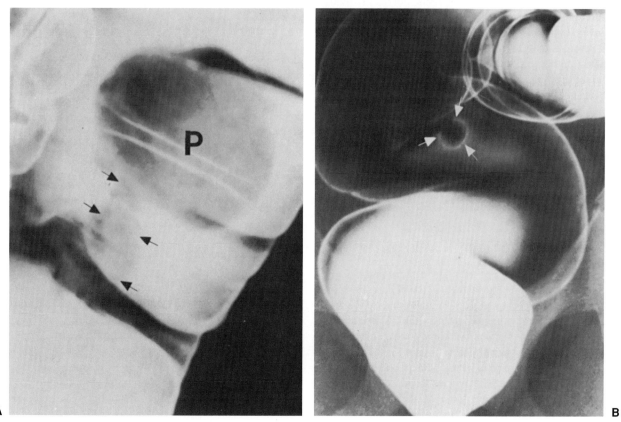

FIG. 8-140. Juvenile polyps. A: Large polyp *(P)* of the descending colon with a long stalk *(arrows)*. **B:** Round, broad-based juvenile polyp of the rectum *(arrows)*.

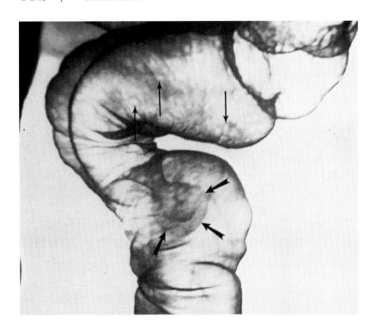

FIG. 8-141. Juvenile polyp. There is a pedunculated polyp *(large arrows)* of the descending colon. Note the lymphoid follicular pattern *(small arrows)* of the colonic mucosa; these lymphoid follicles are seen normally in children on air-contrast enemas with good mucosal coating.

Even though malignancy in juvenile polyps is very rare, the risk of malignancy and of further bleeding warrants removal of all colonic polyps in children.

Juvenile Polyposis

Children who have six or more juvenile polyps involving the colon or who have juvenile polyps in other parts of the alimentary tract are considered to have juvenile polyposis (377). About half of these children have a family history of polyposis, and autosomal dominant transmission is identified in some cases. Any child with a juvenile polyp and a family history of juvenile polyposis is considered to have juvenile polyposis. These children are at risk for GI neoplasms, especially carcinoma of the colon.

A severe form of juvenile polyposis, so-called juvenile polyposis of infancy, presents in the first year or two of life with bloody diarrhea, intussusception, and malabsorption. A family history is usually not present. Most such children die in the first few years of life.

Peutz-Jeghers Syndrome

Peutz-Jeghers syndrome is an autosomal dominant disorder characterized by mucocutaneous pigmentation (most commonly of the buccal mucosa), GI hamartomas, and an increased risk of GI and other neoplasms (378). The hamartomatous polyp of Peutz-Jeghers syndrome has a characteristic smooth muscle core and is specific for that syndrome. The polyps occur from stomach to rectum and are most common in the jejunum and ileum. The major clinical manifestations of Peutz-Jeghers syndrome are due to small bowel intussusceptions (Fig. 8-142). The intussusceptions frequently resolve spontaneously but may lead to obstruction and intestinal necrosis. Patients with Peutz-Jeghers syndrome have an in-

creased risk of adenocarcinoma of the alimentary tract, especially of the stomach, duodenum, and colon. Whether these lesions arise from malignant transformation of the Peutz-Jeghers polyp or independently is unclear. Patients with this syndrome also develop extraintestinal malignancies, especially of the pancreas, breast, and reproductive organs (379).

The polyps of Peutz-Jeghers syndrome are best evaluated by the small bowel series. They may be multiple and may be sessile or pedunculated (Fig. 8-142). They tend to occur in clusters; a cluster of polyps may resemble a single lobulated carcinoma. Transient intussusceptions are frequently seen. Current treatment of the Peutz-Jeghers syndrome is endoscopic removal of as many polyps as is feasible, plus careful clinical and radiologic screening for neoplasms.

Henoch-Schönlein Purpura

Henoch-Schönlein purpura (HSP) is a disorder of unknown cause characterized by a purpuric rash, usually involving the lower extremities and buttocks, abdominal pain, arthritis, and sometimes nephritis. The signs and symptoms of HSP are due to small vessel vasculitis. The etiology of the vasculitis is unknown, but some cases of HSP follow upper respiratory infection or use of drugs such as penicillin.

HSP usually affects children between the ages of 3 and 7 (380). Boys are affected more frequently than girls. GI symptoms occur in most patients. Children with HSP typically have colicky abdominal pain. Occult or gross blood is usually present in the vomitus or stool. The clinical diagnosis of HSP in the child with abdominal pain is usually clear but may be confusing if abdominal symptoms precede the characteristic rash or if the abdominal symptoms are very severe; it is these children who will come to radiologic attention. The radiologic findings in children with HSP reflect the pathophysiology of the disorder, edema and hemorrhage

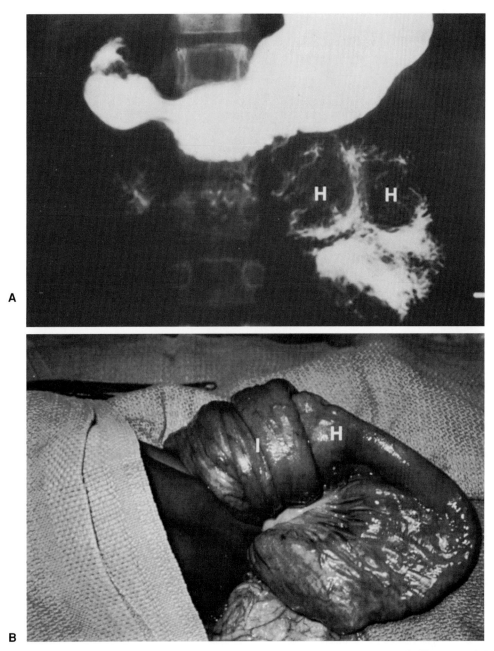

FIG. 8-142. Peutz-Jeghers syndrome. A 14-year-old girl with abdominal pain. **A:** There are lobular masses *(H)* in the proximal jejunum. **B:** A small bowel hamartoma *(H)* intussuscepting into the distal bowel *(I)*.

of the bowel wall. A small bowel series may show fold thickening, ranging from subtle to frank thumbprinting (Fig. 8-143) (380,381). The involvement may be diffuse or localized; the jejunum is probably the area most frequently involved (381); colonic disease is unusual. Areas of hemorrhage may serve as lead points for intussusception; these are usually transient but may result in bowel obstruction. Usually of small bowel into small bowel, the intussusceptions are rarely amenable to air or hydrostatic reduction. Bowel wall thickening may also be seen on US or CT (Fig. 8-

143). HSP usually resolves spontaneously. The prognosis is excellent unless catastrophic central nervous system (CNS), renal, or GI complications occur.

Older Child

Achalasia

In achalasia, there is failure of normal relaxation of the lower esophageal sphincter during swallowing and absence

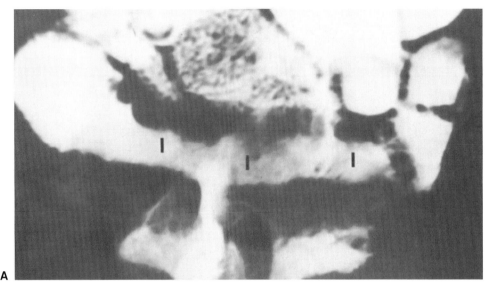

A

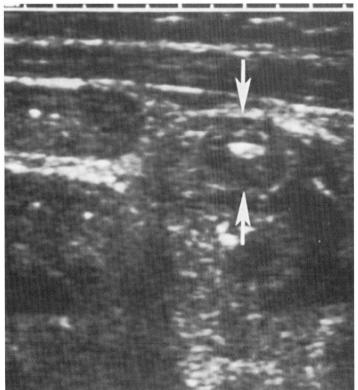

B

FIG. 8-143. Henoch-Schönlein purpura. A 3-year-old girl with purpuric skin rash and abdominal pain. **A:** Spot film from a small bowel series. There is ulceration and thickening of the wall of several loops of ileum *(I)*. **B:** Sonography. Hemorrhage into the bowel wall produces the "target" sign *(arrows)*. The central echogenicity is due to compressed mucosa and submucosa; the surrounding hypoechoic area is due to edema and hemorrhage of deeper layers of the bowel wall.

of normal propulsive contractions in the body of the esophagus. These abnormalities result in functional obstruction of the distal esophagus. The esophagus empties only with increased hydrostatic pressure. Esophagitis may develop because of stasis of food. The cause is unknown.

Fewer than 5% of cases of achalasia occur in children (382). As is true in adults, most cases of achalasia in childhood are sporadic, although occasionally a child with achalasia will have a family history of the disorder. The diagnosis of achalasia is difficult to make in young children who may have minimal esophageal symptoms and present with failure

to thrive or pulmonary disease (recurrent pneumonia, asthma, chronic cough) (383). Older children usually have weight loss, chest pain, dysphagia, and regurgitation (382).

A dilated esophagus may be visible on chest radiographs, often with an air-fluid level. On esophagrams the esophagus is dilated and has no normal peristaltic activity. Occasionally there are nonpropulsive contractions. The distal esophagus is tapered (beak appearance) and slowly empties into the stomach (Fig. 8-144) (384,385). The findings may be subtle in infancy. The radiologic differential diagnosis includes esophageal stricture (rare at the gastroesophageal junction),

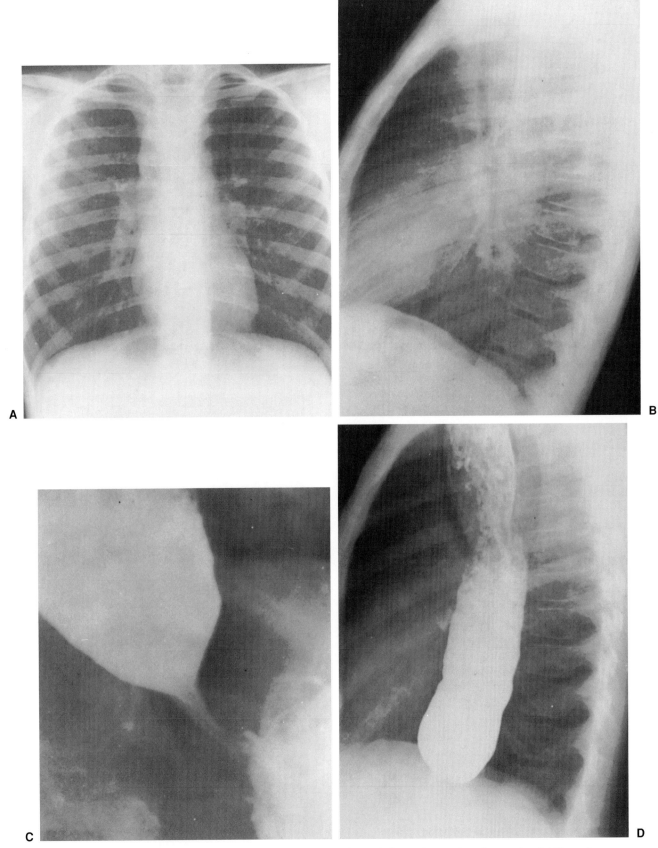

FIG. 8-144. Achalasia. A 9-year-old boy with nocturnal cough, intermittent wheezing, and weight loss. **A:** There is slight widening of the superior mediastinum. **B:** The trachea is bowed anteriorly and narrowed. There is a soft-tissue density behind the heart. **C:** The lower esophagus is dilated, with V-shaped narrowing of the gastroesophageal junction. **D:** The dilated esophagus contains both barium and undigested food. The trachea is displaced and narrowed by the dilated upper esophagus. From Maravilla et al. (385).

and carcinoma and leiomyoma of the esophagus (both very rare in children).

The esophagram is almost always diagnostic in achalasia and is usually followed by manometry and endoscopy. Manometric findings include failure of lower esophageal sphincter relaxation and lack of normal propulsive peristalsis.

Achalasia is treated by relieving the functional obstruction of the distal esophagus, by repeated dilatations or surgical myotomy.

Ulcer Disease and Gastritis

Gastritis, duodenitis, and peptic ulcer disease, though much less common in children than in adults, are nonetheless important problems in pediatrics. All three probably arise from similar pathogenetic processes; they are in some way related to an imbalance between production of hydrochloric acid by the stomach and the mechanisms that protect the stomach and duodenum from the acid. The most important advance in understanding peptic disease has been the recognition of the role of infection by *Helicobacter pylori*.

Gastritis and ulcers are usefully classified as primary or secondary. The most important causes of secondary disease are stress and medications. Factors that lead to stress-induced gastritis or stress ulceration include trauma, burns, sepsis, major surgery, and diseases of the CNS. Nonsteroidal antiinflammatory drugs are the medications most frequently associated with gastritis. Ingestion of acid may cause gastritis, which is also sometimes seen after alkali ingestion (see Fig. 8-102B).

The symptoms of ulcer disease vary with the cause of the ulcers and the age of the child. In newborns and young infants, in whom gastritis and ulcers are usually stress-induced, feeding difficulties, vomiting, and GI bleeding are common. Perforation, though rare, may be the presenting manifestation. Ulcers in the pyloric channel may cause obstruction and mimic pyloric stenosis (Fig. 8-145A). In young children, gastric ulcers are probably more common than duodenal ulcers (386,387) and cause feeding difficulties, nausea and vomiting, chronic abdominal pain, and GI bleeding (sometimes occult). In older children duodenal ulcers are more common and present with the typical adult pattern of epigastric pain relieved by food (386,387).

Endoscopy is the best diagnostic procedure in children with acute GI bleeding. Children with other signs and symptoms of ulcer disease may be referred for radiologic evaluation. In small children, in whom only single contrast examinations can be performed, the well-established insensitivity of the exam to small ulcers limits its usefulness. Patient, persistent fluoroscopy, the use of compression, and varying the position of the child often yield rewards. Sonography, though not the primary modality for visualizing the stomach, may demonstrate thickened gastric folds and even discrete ulcers (388,389). In older children double-contrast examinations can be performed; the criteria for diagnosis of gastric

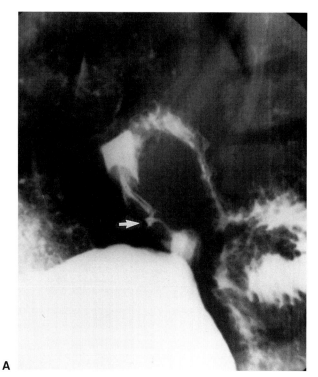

A

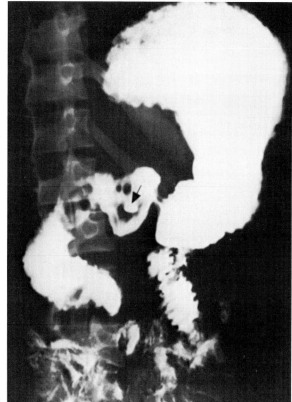

B

FIG. 8-145. Peptic ulcer disease. A: Antral ulcer *(arrow)* causing partial gastric outlet obstruction in an infant. Note also the diffuse narrowing of the antrum and pylorus. **B:** Duodenal ulcer *(arrow)* with surrounding edema.

and duodenal ulcers are identical to those for adults. *H. pylori* infection, in addition to producing typical ulcers, may also produce markedly enlarged gastric folds (390).

Several unusual pediatric gastropathies are worth mentioning. The antral gastritis produced by prostaglandins was previously discussed (see Fig. 8-110). Menetrier disease, or hypertrophic gastropathy, is rare in childhood and is probably a different disease from the one seen in adults (391). In children it is usually an acute but transient and self-limited disease and may be due to allergy or infection, perhaps by cytomegalovirus (392,393). Affected children present with nausea and vomiting and signs of protein-losing enteropathy such as anemia and edema. The upper GI series will show marked thickening of gastric folds; fold thickening may be present throughout the stomach, without the classic antral sparing described in adults (Fig. 8-146) (394).

Idiopathic eosinophilic gastroenteritis (as opposed to eosinophilic enteritis with a known cause, such as allergy to milk or soy proteins) is an uncommon disorder in which there is peripheral eosinophilia and variable eosinophilic infiltration of the intestinal wall. The eosinophilic involvement may occur anywhere in the intestine but is most common in the stomach and proximal intestine (395). The symptoms are usually those of protein-losing enteropathy. Systemic atopic symptoms are usually present. Esophageal stricture (396) and gastric outlet obstruction may occur. The radiographic appearance—nodularity and thickening of gastric and jejunal folds—is nonspecific (395).

Other systemic conditions that may involve the stomach in children are Crohn's disease and chronic granulomatous disease (397).

Superior Mesenteric Artery Syndrome

A rare form of bowel obstruction, the SMA syndrome, is caused by compression of the third part of the duodenum by the SMA as it crosses in front of the duodenum. The primary syndrome is quite rare. A much more frequently seen mid-duodenal obstruction, perhaps erroneously labeled the SMA syndrome, occurs in malnourished children, especially those with neurologic disease, and in children in body casts or who have had spinal fusion for scoliosis. In these children, who have an abnormal or unaccustomed posture or have lost a great deal of weight, the spine is very close to the anterior abdominal wall, and it is probably the spine rather than the SMA which compresses the duodenum. Plain films demonstrate a dilated stomach and duodenum (Fig. 8-147). A UGI will show a dilated hyperperistaltic proximal duodenum with an abrupt caliber change and obstruction as it crosses the spine. Treatment is usually supportive with either parenteral nutrition or nasojejunal tube feeding. This allows the patient to gain weight and afford the duodenum sufficient space between the spine and the anterior abdominal wall.

Inflammatory Bowel Disease

The term "inflammatory bowel disease" (IBD) usually refers to both Crohn's disease and ulcerative colitis (UC), the two most common and important idiopathic diseases of bowel. In pediatrics, the use of the less specific term IBD is often appropriate because it is often difficult to distinguish between Crohn's disease and UC on clinical, radiologic, endoscopic, and pathologic criteria (398). A child carrying the clinical and endoscopic diagnosis of UC often has a small bowel series demonstrating terminal ileal disease and a consequent change of diagnosis to Crohn's disease.

Crohn's Disease

Crohn's disease is a transmural granulomatous inflammatory disease that may affect any part of the GI tract, from mouth to anus (399). The etiology is unknown; infection and altered immunity have been suggested. Up to 10% of patients with Crohn's disease have a family history of IBD (399). The peak incidence of Crohn's disease is between 20 and 40 years of age, but many cases begin in childhood, especially in the early teenage years. Crohn's disease is very uncommon in infants and young children.

The presentation is quite variable. Abdominal pain and diarrhea are common, but GI symptoms may be mild or absent. Weight loss, growth failure, delayed puberty, or fever of unknown origin may be the only complaint. Extraintestinal manifestations such as arthritis and sclerosing cholangitis seem less common than in adults. Crohn's disease occasionally mimics an acute process such as appendicitis, with severe right lower quadrant pain.

The terminal ileum is involved in the majority of cases. Most children will have involvement of the distal ileum and right colon. Children also may have isolated small bowel disease, with a normal terminal ileum, or isolated colonic disease (Fig. 8-148) (400). Involvement of the esophagus, stomach, or duodenum is unusual.

The role of radiology in suspected Crohn's disease depends on the presenting complaints. In patients with symptoms (such as bloody diarrhea) suggesting colonic disease, endoscopy will usually be the first study employed, and the nature and extent of colonic disease will be determined. Because the distinction between Crohn's disease and UC is often difficult by colonoscopy and biopsy, a small bowel examination is usually performed to evaluate the small intestine. Enemas are seldom used to evaluate IBD. If performed, double-contrast exams are better than single-contrast exams (401). The findings are aphthous ulcerations and deep mucosal ulcers in an asymmetric and discontinuous distribution, the right colon being most frequently involved. Crohn's disease is occasionally indistinguishable from UC on barium enema when there is diffuse superficial involvement.

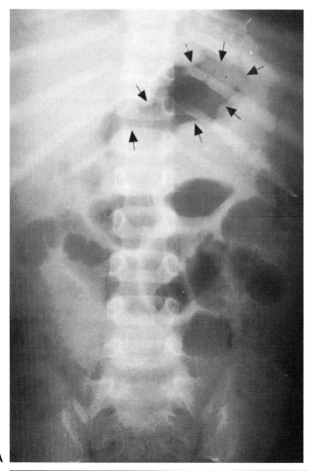

A

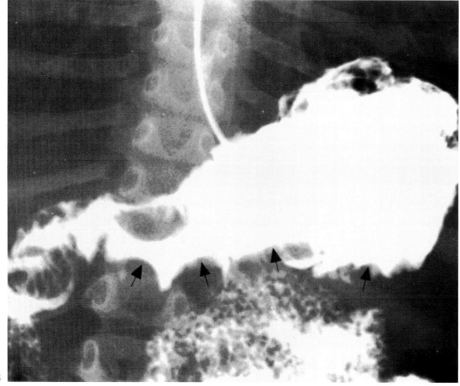

B

FIG. 8-146. **Menetrier disease.** A 3-year-old boy with peripheral edema and anemia. **A:** A supine abdominal radiography shows thumbprinting of the wall of the stomach *(arrows).* **B:** UGI examination shows submucosal edema of the entire stomach, most pronounced along the greater curvature of the antrum and body *(arrows) (Continued).*

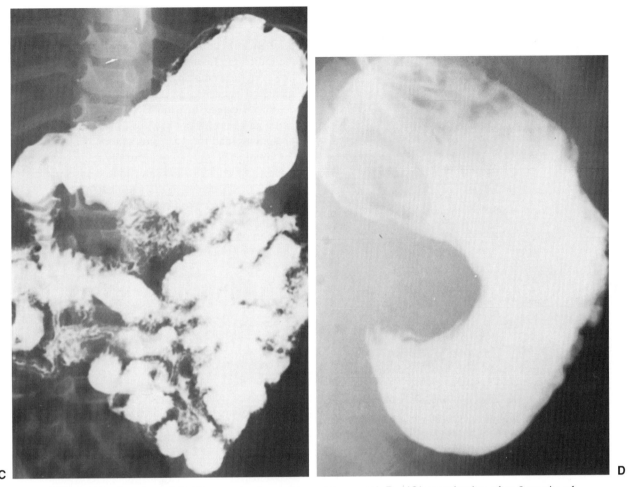

C

D

FIG. 8-146. *(continued)* C: The proximal small bowel is normal. D: UGI examination after 2 weeks of conservative therapy, the anemia and peripheral edema having resolved, is negative.

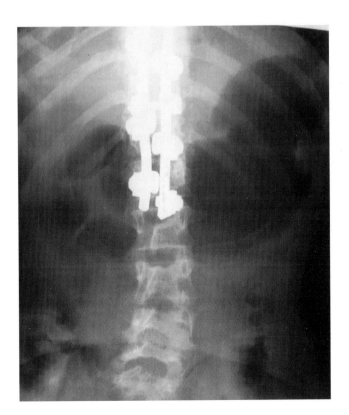

FIG. 8-147. **Superior mesenteric artery syndrome.** Supine radiograph in a boy with persistent vomiting after spinal fusion for scoliosis. The stomach and duodenum are dilated, the latter to the point where it crosses the spine. The patient is in a body cast.

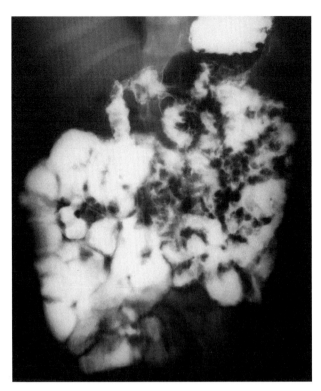

FIG. 8-148. Crohn's disease. UGI series in a 7-year-old girl with diarrhea, abdominal pain, and weight loss. The abnormalities are limited to the duodenum and jejunum, which have nodular, thickened folds. The terminal ileum is normal.

Most children who present with nonspecific abdominal signs and symptoms or with systemic signs and who are suspected of having Crohn's disease will undergo UGI-small bowel follow-through (SBFT). Scout films may demonstrate an abnormal bowel gas pattern and a lack of formed stool in the colon (402). Since the disease seldom involves the esophagus, stomach, or duodenum, a double-contrast examination of the UGI tract is worthwhile only when there are signs or symptoms referable to the esophagus, stomach, or duodenum. Otherwise, a careful single-contrast exam is performed because better demonstration of the most relevant area, the distal small bowel, is obtained with lower density barium. Frequent overhead films and intermittent fluoroscopy are employed. Enteroclysis is rarely necessary. Prolonging the small bowel exam into the colon may help the gastroenterologist stage the disease and obviate colonoscopy to the right colon (8).

On small bowel follow-through the findings are similar to those seen in adults. The bowel is rigid with a thickened wall and irregular mucosa (Figs. 8-149 and 8-150). The classic cobblestone appearance is usually due to deep transverse and linear ulcers between areas of edematous mucosa. The cecum is frequently spastic and irregular in contour (Fig. 8-149). When Crohn's disease is limited to the proximal small bowel, thickened folds may be the only finding (Fig. 8-148).

When the diagnosis of Crohn's disease has been established, there is little role for routine follow-up studies. There

is often little correlation between the clinical course and the radiologic findings. The radiologist's role is important, however, in evaluating complications. There is a slightly increased incidence of carcinoma of the small bowel and colorectal cancer in patients with Crohn's disease. CT is particularly useful in showing sinuses, fistulas, abscesses, phlegmons, and focal fat proliferation (Fig. 8-151) (403).

Crohn's disease may occasionally mimic acute processes such as appendicitis and infectious ileitis due to *Yersinia.* Barium or CT studies usually separate these entities. Lymphoma may also involve the ileum and mimic Crohn's disease. The most important diagnostic consideration, however, is not to mistake the quite nodular normal terminal ileum of childhood for disease (Fig. 8-152).

Ulcerative Colitis

The epidemiology of UC is similar to that of Crohn's disease. UC is most common in young adults but occurs in adolescents and children and rarely in infants. It is more common in children with a family history of disease and in whites. The cause is unknown.

The presentation of children with UC is less variable than that of children with Crohn's disease. They are less likely to have only growth failure. The vast majority present with bloody diarrhea and abdominal pain. Symptoms may arise insidiously or acutely. In a few children, especially in infants, the onset may be fulminant, with profuse bloody diarrhea and signs of toxicity such as fever, hypotension, and leukocytosis. Some may have toxic megacolon. The fulminant variety of UC in infants may be fatal and can often be controlled only with colectomy.

There are many extraintestinal manifestations of UC. The most notable is arthritis, which is of two types: an arthritis mainly involving the large joints of the lower extremities that flares with active IBD, and a spondylitis the course of which is independent of the colonic disease. Hepatobiliary disease (hepatitis, cirrhosis, pericholangitis or sclerosing cholangitis) occurs in a small number of UC patients. The last is the most classic lesion, may predate the development of IBD, and may be unresponsive to therapy, including colectomy.

The inflammatory lesions of UC are limited to the mucosa. There is only secondary involvement of the submucosa, except in cases of fulminant colitis, when the inflammation may be transmural. UC involves the rectum and extends proximally a variable distance without skip areas. Rectal sparing is unusual.

Children suspected of having colitis usually proceed to endoscopy and come to radiology later for a UGI-SBFT to exclude involvement of the small intestine and help the gastroenterologist distinguish between UC and the colitis of Crohn's disease. Thus, enemas are seldom performed in children with colitis. If an enema is performed and if the child is not seriously ill, a double-contrast exam is preferable. In

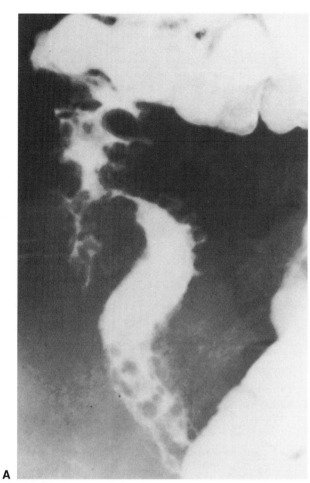

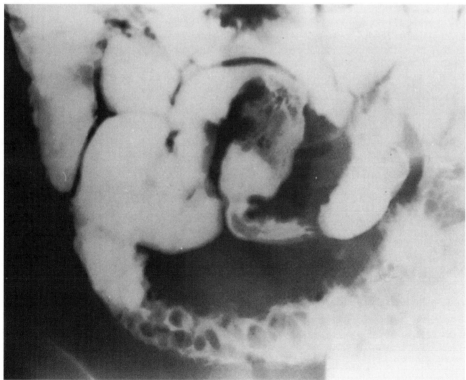

FIG. 8-149. Crohn's disease. A: Ileocolic disease. There is submucosal edema, ulceration, and narrowing of the terminal ileum and spasm, narrowing, and edema of the cecum. **B:** Small bowel involvement with normal terminal ileum. The cobblestone appearance of the distal small bowel is due to mucosal and submucosal components of transmural disease. Fluoroscopically, both the anatomy and peristalsis of the terminal ileum were normal.

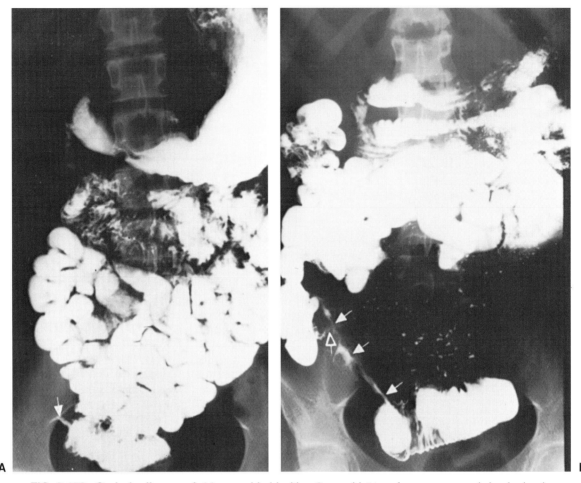

FIG. 8-150. Crohn's disease. A 14-year-old girl with a 2-year history of vague upper abdominal pain, weight loss, and recurrent diarrhea. Three previous UGI series at other hospitals were normal; the distal small bowel was never evaluated. **A:** Small bowel series. A film at 45 minutes shows a normal stomach, duodenal bulb, duodenal sweep, and proximal small bowel. There is a questionable area of narrowing *(arrow)* of the distal small bowel. **B:** A 90-minute film shows that contrast material has passed through the markedly narrowed terminal ileum *(solid arrows)* into the colon. An ileocecal fistula *(open arrow)* is also present.

the early stages of UC a fine granular mucosal pattern may be detected (Fig. 8-153). There may also be fine mucosal stippling due to superficial ulcers. With more advanced disease the ulcers become deep enough to be seen on single-contrast examinations. Regenerating mucosa may produce so-called pseudopolyps. As the disease becomes chronic, extensive fibrosis develops, and there is shortening of the colon with loss of haustration.

The most serious long-term complication of UC is adenocarcinoma of the colon. The risk of cancer begins only after about 10 years of disease, but the subsequent risk is about 20% per decade (404). The extent and duration of disease are important risk factors, as may be the age at diagnosis (405). There is no consensus about the optimal approach to screening for cancer or timing of colectomy (406).

The differential diagnosis of UC in older children is mainly infectious colitis, especially that caused by *Campylobacter* and *Clostridium difficile,* but also that of *E. coli, Shi-*

gella, Salmonella, and *Yersinia.* The colitis of hemolytic-uremic syndrome may also be bloody. In the fulminant variant of UC (which usually occurs in infants), NEC, Hirschsprung colitis, and allergic colitis must also be considered.

The Immunocompromised Child

Immune deficiency may be congenital or acquired. Congenital syndromes of immune deficiency are quite varied in their manifestations, and no general statements can be made about GI problems in children with these unusual disorders. Specific mention may be made of chronic granulomatous disease of childhood, a rare, inherited disease of phagocyte dysfunction in which marked thickening of the wall of the gastric antrum may lead to gastric outlet obstruction (397).

The radiologist is, however, frequently involved in the care of children with acquired immune deficiency due to

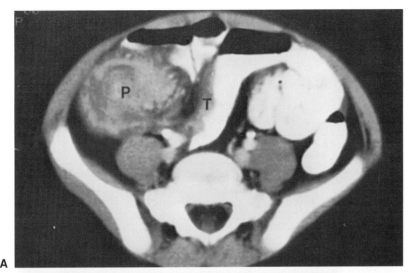

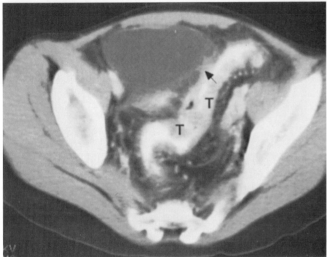

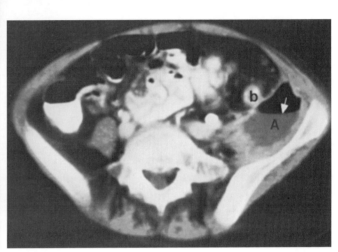

FIG. 8-151. Complications of Crohn's disease. A: Phlegmon. CT demonstrates a right lower quadrant inflammatory mass or phlegmon *(P)*, separation of bowel loops, and adjacent, eccentric bowel wall thickening *(T)*. **B:** Extensive bowel wall thickening. CT demonstrates marked bowel wall thickening *(T)* of the sigmoid colon with mesenteric spiculations indicating transmural disease. Eccentric thickening of the left bladder wall *(arrow)* suggests the development of an enterovesical fistula. **C:** Iliopsoas abscess. CT demonstrates replacement of the left iliopsoas muscle by a large fluid collection *(A)* with an air-fluid level *(arrow)*. There is presumably a fistula from the adjacent thick-walled loop of bowel *(b)*. (From Auringer ST, Bisset GS, III, Kirks DR. Pediatric gastrointestinal imaging: an update. In: Balistreri WF, Vanderhoff JA, eds. *Pediatric gastroenterology and nutrition.* London: Chapman and Hall, 1990, 244–257.)

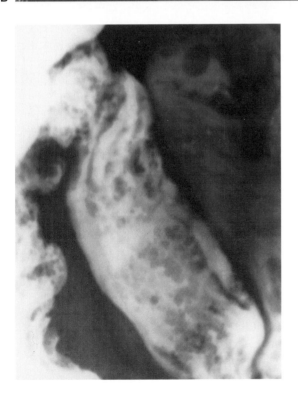

FIG. 8-152. Normal terminal ileum. The terminal ileum in children is quite nodular because of lymphoid tissue. Fluoroscopy of the terminal ileum must include evaluation of peristalsis.

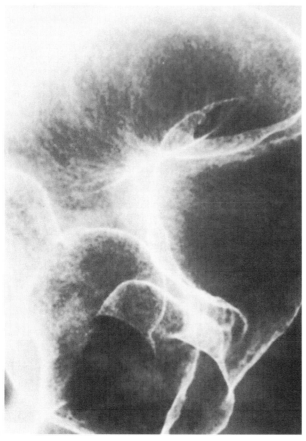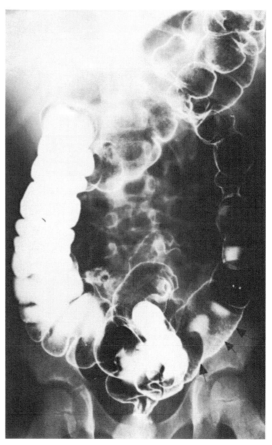

A
B

FIG. 8-153. Ulcerative colitis. An 8-year-old boy with a 2-year history of intermittent bloody diarrhea. **A:** A double-contrast barium enema. This coned-down view of splenic flexure shows a granular appearance due to diffuse, fine mucosal ulcerations and mucosal edema. **B:** The postevacuation film. There is a granular appearance of the entire colon. Marginal irregularities due to ulcerations *(arrows)* are noted in the descending colon and rectosigmoid colon.

infection with the human immunodeficiency virus (acquired immune deficiency syndrome, or AIDS), or chemotherapy or radiation therapy for cancer. In children with AIDS, the GI symptoms are due primarily to acute and chronic enteric infections and much less often to GI neoplasms. As many as a one fourth of children with AIDS suffer from malnutrition and failure to thrive (407). Imaging findings in the GI tract in children with AIDS are, for the most part, similar to those found in adults. Esophagitis due to *Candida,* cytomegalovirus (CMV), and herpes simplex virus (HSV) is common. CMV infection may also involve the stomach, typically causing deep ulceration. Thickened gastric folds are frequently found in children with AIDS and may be caused by *H. pylori, Cryptosporidium,* or the lymphoproliferative disorder known as gut-associated lymphoid tissue (GALT) (407). Chronic diarrhea is one of the most disabling manifestations of AIDS, and may be due to opportunistic organisms such as *Cryptosporidium* and *Isospora belli* or to more common pathogens like *Salmonella, Shigella, Campylobacter,* and *Giardia. Cryptosporidium* typically causes thickened folds in the proximal small intestine; findings on

SBFT, however, in children with enteritis are nonspecific and biopsy is usually necessary for definitive diagnosis.

Diarrhea in children with AIDS may also be due to colitis, most notably due to CMV. CMV colitis is often quite severe and may result in pneumatosis, stricture, toxic megacolon, and perforation (407). The findings on barium enema include thickened folds, superficial and deep ulcerations, and strictures.

Intraabdominal lymphadenopathy, common in children with AIDS, is often due to lymphoma or infection with *Mycobacterium avium intracellulare* (MAI). The lymphadenopathy is frequently massive, and the nodes in both infection and lymphoma may have low-density necrotic centers. MAI and lymphoma may also cause lesions in the liver and spleen.

Children whose immune systems have been suppressed by chemotherapy or radiation therapy are also subject to GI problems. Children who have undergone bone marrow transplantation are at risk of graft versus host disease (GVHD), which may be acute or chronic. In the acute form, one of the major target organs is the small intestine, in which small bowel fold thickening or small bowel fold effacement (''ribbon bowel'') may occur (408). Intestinal involvement by GVHD is most common in the jejunum but may occur anywhere in the intestine, including the colon. Other conditions, most notably viral infection and ischemia, may mimic GVHD. In the chronic form of GVHD, the major target organ in the GI tract is the esophagus, where mid- and upper esophageal strictures and webs develop (409).

Typhlitis (neutropenic colitis) is a necrotizing inflammation of the colon and ileum in neutropenic patients (410). The cecum (*typhlon* in Greek) is the region most frequently involved. Typhlitis most commonly occurs in leukemia but may also develop in lymphoma, aplastic anemia, cyclic neutropenia, AIDS, and after organ transplantation (411). The precise pathogenesis is unknown, but it is probably bacterial invasion of a colonic wall compromised by chemotherapy. The most common symptoms of typhlitis are fever, abdominal pain, and distention; vomiting, diarrhea, and bloody stool are also seen (411). The right lower quadrant pain it causes may suggest appendicitis. Plain films may show an absence of gas in the right lower quadrant, bowel wall thickening, pneumatosis intestinalis, and small bowel obstruction or ileus (412,413). These findings are vividly shown by US and CT (Fig. 8-154) (414,415). Contrast studies are usually contraindicated.

Treatment of typhlitis is supportive, plus antibiotics. Surgery is usually reserved for secondary perforation and peritonitis.

Appendicitis

Definition and Clinical Features

Acute appendicitis is the most common condition requiring abdominal surgery in children. The disease is rare in infants but becomes more common during each year of childhood. It may be difficult to diagnose; appendicitis should always be considered in infants and children with confusing abdominal symptoms.

The etiology of appendicitis is probably obstruction of the appendiceal lumen: this leads to retention of secretions, superimposed bacterial inflammation, and vascular compromise. It may progress to perforation and abscess formation.

In older children with nonperforated appendicitis, the clinical findings usually suggest the correct diagnosis. Their pain shifts from the periumbilical region to the right lower quadrant. The pain may be associated with anorexia, nausea, vomiting, and diarrhea; the symptoms may suggest gastroenteritis. The periumbilical pain usually precedes vomiting. Direct tenderness over the inflamed appendix (McBurney sign) is the most important physical finding. In young children with appendicitis there is an increased incidence of perforation and a decrease in the specificity of the physical findings (416). Delay in diagnosis can cause increased morbidity; this has led to the increased use of radiographs and

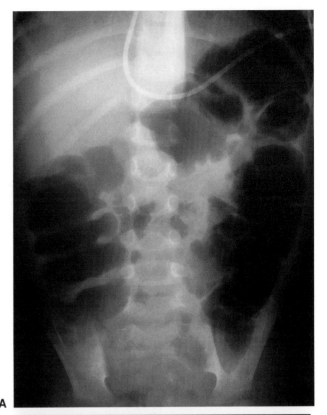

A

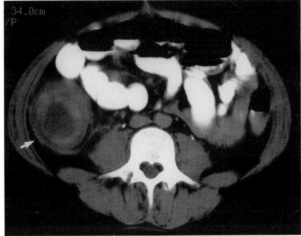

B

FIG. 8-154. Typhlitis. A: Abdominal radiograph in a young child with acute lymphocytic leukemia (ALL) and abdominal pain shows distention of the cecum and thickening of the haustral folds. **B:** CT scan of a 15-year-old boy with ALL demonstrates a markedly thickened wall of the cecum and ascending colon *(arrow)*.

other imaging to differentiate appendicitis from other conditions, particularly in younger children.

Radiology

Radiologic evaluation is performed only if the clinical presentation is confusing. Up to a third of children with

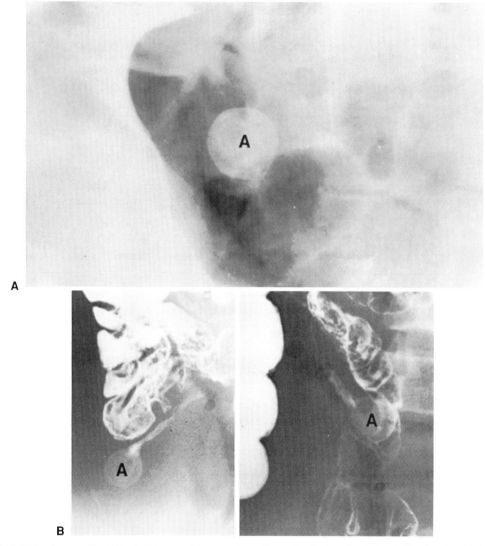

FIG. 8-155. Appendicolith. A 15-year-old asymptomatic male. **A:** Laminated calcific density *(A)* in the right lower quadrant. **B:** The density *(A)* is at the tip of the appendix and can be freely moved laterally *(left)* and medially *(right)*. *(Continued)*

appendicitis, however, have atypical signs and symptoms. The goal of imaging is to make a diagnosis before perforation and to reduce the rate of "negative laparotomy," which in most hospitals is approximately 20%.

Radiography. Plain films of the abdomen may be completely normal in patients with acute appendicitis. An appendicolith can be seen in 5% to 10% of cases. It may be laminated and is usually in the right lower quadrant (Fig. 8-155). A right posterior oblique view of the pelvis is frequently helpful confirming in questionable cases. Identification of an appendicolith in a child with acute abdominal pain is virtually diagnostic of appendicitis; at least half of these patients have perforation, abscess, or both. Prophylactic appendectomy should be performed on an asymptomatic, healthy child with an appendicolith because of the high frequency of later appendicitis with perforation.

Radiographs frequently contain signs of right lower quadrant inflammatory disease. These inflammatory changes include air-fluid levels in the terminal ileum and cecum, thickening of the cecal wall, a soft-tissue mass effect on the cecum, loss of the obturator internus fat plane, fluid between the cecum and properitoneal fat line, and scoliosis (splinting) convex to the left (417).

The clinical diagnosis of appendicitis becomes more difficult after perforation; fortunately, the plain film findings become more distinctive (418,419). Free intraperitoneal air is uncommon after appendiceal perforation. Extraluminal gas does occur in some patients but is rarely the only radiographic finding of appendiceal perforation (419). Extraluminal gas collections may be located between the colon and the properitoneal fat line and may be bubbly, oval, or triangular.

The colon cutoff sign occurs in some children with ap-

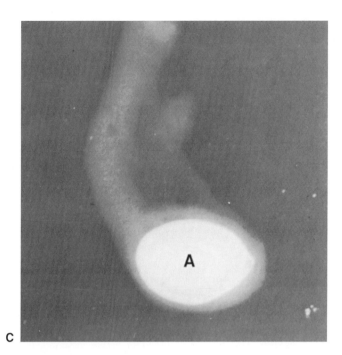

C

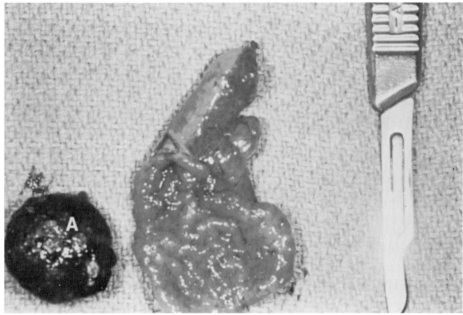

D

FIG. 8-155. *(continued)* **C:** Radiograph of resected appendix. The laminated appendicolith *(A)* is located at the tip of the appendix. **D:** The large appendicolith *(A)* is compared with the removed appendix *(center)*, its mesentery, and the end of a surgical scalpel.

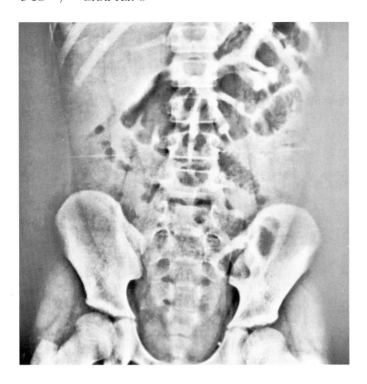

FIG. 8-156. Appendicitis with perforation. Anteroposterior supine radiograph demonstrates all three components of the colon cutoff sign: absence of gas and feces in the cecum and right colon; reflex dilatation of the transverse colon; and amputation of colonic gas at the hepatic flexure. The distention of small bowel indicates early small bowel obstruction. From Johnson et al. (418).

pendiceal perforation (419). This sign is absence of gas and feces in the right lower quadrant, dilatation of the transverse colon, and a sharp cut-off of gas at the hepatic flexure (Fig. 8-156). A prone radiograph distinguishes inflammatory spasm due to appendicitis from mere collapse of the ascending colon particularly well.

Small bowel obstruction is a common manifestation of perforated appendicitis. Obstruction is caused by fibrinous adhesions and inflammatory reaction around the perforated appendix (Fig. 8-157). In children with a perforated appendix and small bowel obstruction, there may be disproportionate jejunal dilatation and the suggestion of high small bowel obstruction (420). If peritonitis complicates appendicitis, paralytic ileus develops. Other plain film findings of perforated appendicitis include a mass in the right lower quadrant and obliteration of pelvic fat planes.

The barium enema, widely used before the advent of US and CT, is not sensitive to the illness, nor is it specific enough to exclude appendicitis. It is now rarely used (421).

Ultrasonography. Since Puylaert's 1986 report (422) of the ultrasonographic diagnosis of appendicitis using graded compression, there have been many studies documenting its utility in both adults and children. The sensitivity and specificity of US for the diagnosis of appendicitis are both between about 85% and 95% (423–427).

Sonography is performed using a 5.0- or 7.5-MHz linear transducer. With the patient supine, transverse sonography is performed with slowly and gradually applied compression of the right lower quadrant. The appendix is usually identi-

fied just medial and inferior to the tip of the cecum and anterior and lateral to the iliac vessels and psoas muscle. The identification of a normal appendix depends on the persistence of the sonographer (427). The normal appendix is a tubular structure traceable to the cecum at one end, blind at the other. It has an echogenic inner layer and a hypoechoic outer layer. Acute appendicitis is diagnosed when a noncompressible appendix with a cross-sectional diameter of 6 mm or greater is seen (Fig. 8-158). Other findings include an appendiceal wall thickness of 2 mm or greater, disruption of the echogenic mucosal line, and an appendicolith (Fig. 8-159). Inflammation may be limited to the tip of the appendix. After perforation, it may be more difficult to demonstrate the appendix. A periappendiceal mass may be seen, as well as interloop fluid, a phlegmon, or a frank abscess. Localized pericecal fluid is a much more specific sign of appendicitis than free fluid. Color Doppler demonstration of increased appendiceal blood flow may help in equivocal cases (428).

The ultrasonographic diagnosis of appendicitis is not always straightforward. With any radiologic technique, especially one as operator-dependent as US, there will inevitably be false positives and false negatives. Both the radiologist and the referring surgeon must be aware of pitfalls. A retrocecal appendix may be very difficult to see, as may inflammation confined to the tip of the appendix. A recently perforated appendix may be difficult to visualize if the appendix is no longer distended and there is no organized accumulation of pus. Other diseases, including typhlitis, Crohn's disease, and the constipation of cystic fibrosis (without appendi-

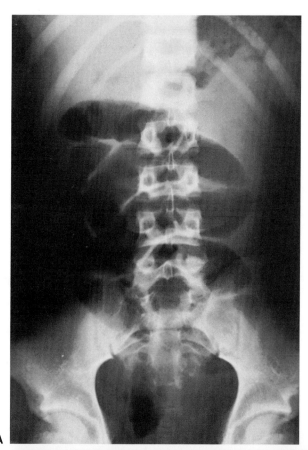

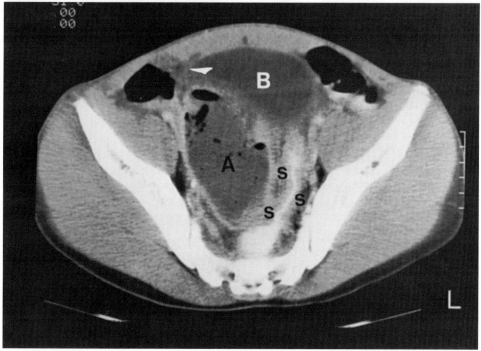

FIG. 8-157. Appendiceal abscess with small bowel obstruction. A 15-year-old boy with abdominal pain and fever. **A:** An anteroposterior supine abdominal radiograph shows disproportionate dilatation of the proximal small bowel compared to distal bowel. There is a suggestion of a soft-tissue pelvic mass. **B:** A CT section shows a large cul-de-sac abscess *(A)* containing fluid and air and pressing on the bladder *(B)*. Note the thickening of the wall of the sigmoid colon *(s)* next to the abscess.

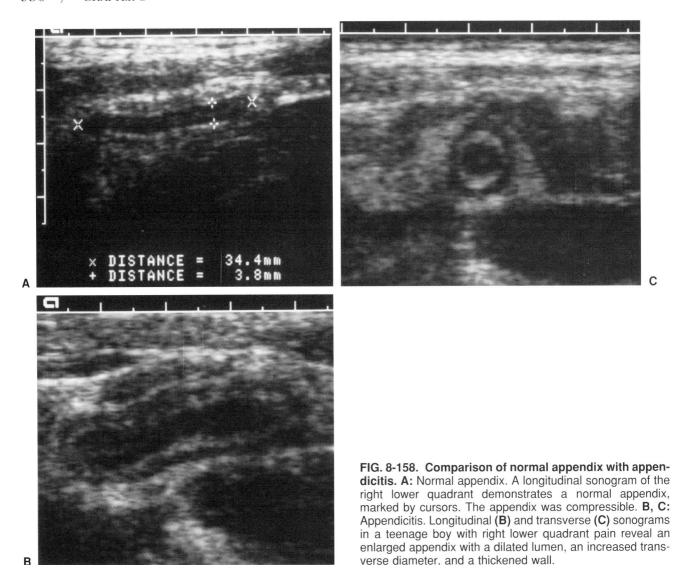

FIG. 8-158. Comparison of normal appendix with appendicitis. A: Normal appendix. A longitudinal sonogram of the right lower quadrant demonstrates a normal appendix, marked by cursors. The appendix was compressible. **B, C:** Appendicitis. Longitudinal **(B)** and transverse **(C)** sonograms in a teenage boy with right lower quadrant pain reveal an enlarged appendix with a dilated lumen, an increased transverse diameter, and a thickened wall.

citis), may resemble acute appendicitis. Appendicitis remains primarily a clinical diagnosis. US is most useful in patients with atypical or ambiguous signs; it is in that group that unexpected findings may turn up (427,429–432). Mesenteric adenitis, the most common mimic of appendicitis, can be diagnosed when enlarged mesenteric nodes and sometimes thickening of the terminal ileum are seen but the appendix is normal. The most serious condition that mimics appendicitis is torsion of the right ovary; thus, the US evaluation of a girl of any age with right lower quadrant pain and a sonographically normal appendix must include visualization of the ovaries.

Computed Tomography. CT is the best modality for evaluating patients with complicated appendicitis and possible abscess. CT not only detects periappendiceal and pelvic abscesses but shows their effects on adjacent structures and any abdominal extensions (Figs. 8-157 and 8-160) (433). CT is invaluable in the management of periappendiceal and pelvic inflammatory masses.

Complications of Cystic Fibrosis

Chronic pulmonary disease is the most common and important manifestation of cystic fibrosis (CF). CF, however, is a multisystem disease, and its GI complications are a significant cause of morbidity (434,435). Radiologists must be familiar with the GI manifestations of CF, not to establish the diagnosis, but because many of the most typical findings are of little clinical importance and must be kept in perspective.

As previously discussed, the most characteristic GI manifestation of CF is meconium ileus. Older children and adults

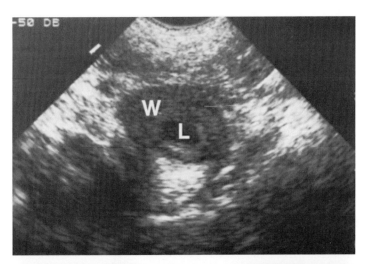

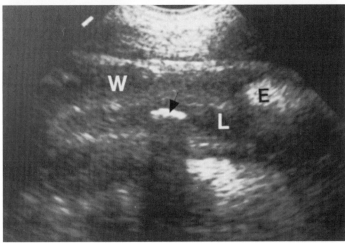

FIG. 8-159. Appendicitis. Sonography of appendicitis in a 16-year-old boy with right lower quadrant and pelvic pain. Transverse *(above)* and longitudinal *(below)* sonographic sections demonstrate a dilated appendiceal lumen *(L)*, a thickened appendiceal wall *(W)*, and an appendicolith *(arrow)* with acoustic shadowing. Note the increased echogenicity *(E)* within the thickened wall of the tip of the appendix due to hemorrhage and necrosis. Acute appendicitis, an appendicolith, and a periappendiceal abscess were found at surgery.

may develop intestinal obstruction due to inspissation of their abnormally viscid intestinal contents in the distal small bowel. This syndrome is currently termed the distal intestinal obstruction syndrome (DIOS), though many pediatricians and radiologists refer to it by its traditional name, meconium ileus equivalent. Patients with DIOS may have chronic recurrent abdominal pain but usually come to the radiologist's attention only when there are symptoms of acute obstruction. Plain films of the abdomen demonstrate large amounts of formed feces in the distal small bowel, cecum, and right colon and evidence of mechanical obstruction (Fig. 8-161) (434). DIOS can usually be successfully treated with nasogastric suction, oral *N*-acetylcysteine, and oral lavage solutions such as Golytely. When these methods fail, enemas with gastrografin (meglumine diatrizoate) under fluoroscopic control, are very effective. As with meconium ileus, the radiologist should make every effort to reflux contrast into the terminal ileum.

There are other less common causes of mechanical

bowel obstruction in patients with CF, notably appendicitis and intussusception (434). Another cause of bowel obstruction in children with CF, colonic stricture, has recently been described (436–438). That these strictures are caused by high-strength pancreatic enzyme supplements is suspected but not yet proven. The disease may begin as an inflammatory disease, of which the end result is stricture (439). The strictures are typically found in the right colon but may involve the entire colon (437). In general, children with strictures are younger (usually <10 years) than children with DIOS.

Other important GI problems in patients with CF include biliary cirrhosis, gallstones, malabsorption and consequent malnourishment, rectal prolapse, constipation, and gastroesophageal reflux. Radiologists should be aware of the typical findings of CF on UGI and SBFT: thickened duodenal and small bowel folds, nodular filling defects, and dilated bowel (440,441). The findings are especially striking in the duodenum (Fig. 8-162). The cause of these abnormalities is uncertain, but they have little or no clinical significance.

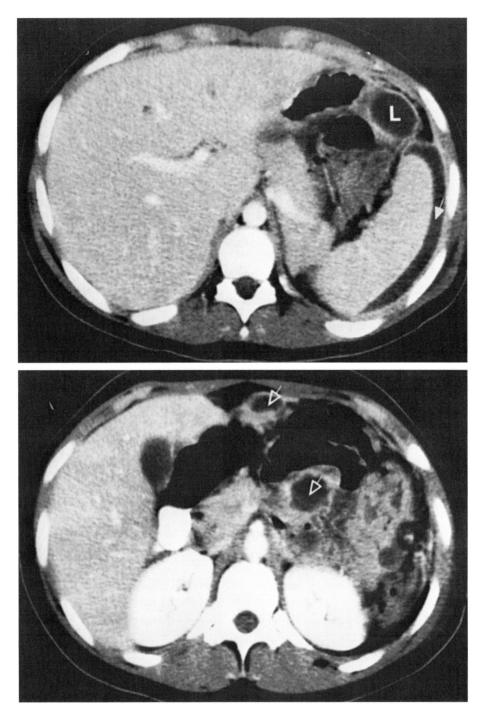

FIG. 8-160. Appendicitis with perforation. Appendiceal perforation with peritoneal spread producing lesser sac *(L)*, perisplenic *(arrow)*, interloop *(open arrows)*, and pelvic *(not shown)* abscesses. These abscesses are shown as areas of decreased density (fluid) with enhancing margins.

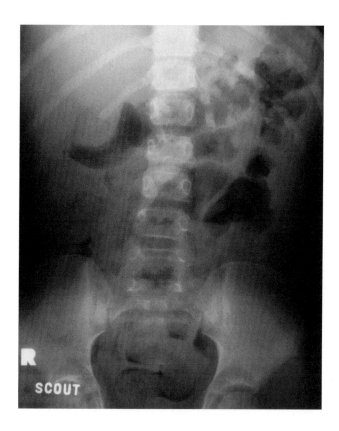

FIG. 8-161. Distal intestinal obstruction syndrome (meconium ileus equivalent). A supine abdominal film in a 10-year-old girl with cystic fibrosis shows large amounts of stool in the colon and small bowel distention.

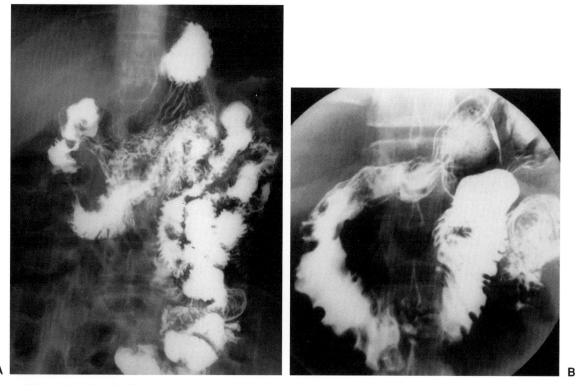

A

B

FIG. 8-162. Cystic fibrosis. An overhead film **(A)** from an UGI series and a spot film of the duodenum **(B)** in a girl with cystic fibrosis demonstrate the characteristic thickened folds, most evident in the duodenum ("smudged" duodenum).

ABNORMALITIES OF THE HEPATOBILIARY SYSTEM

Imaging Techniques

Radiography

Plain radiographs occasionally help by identifying abnormal parenchymal calcifications, biliary calculi, or enlargement of the liver.

Ultrasonography

Ultrasonography is particularly valuable. It should be the first imaging study in newborns and infants with suspected hepato biliary disease and in older children with biliary colic, jaundice, or portal hypertension. Imaging of the newborn and young infant is best performed using 7-MHz linear and sector transducers. Older infants and young children can be imaged with 5-MHz transducers. Older or obese children generally require 3.5-MHz transducers for adequate penetration. Duplex and color Doppler evaluation of the hepatic vasculature should be a routine part of the liver examination. The hepatic veins, portal vein, hepatic artery, and IVC should be evaluated for presence, direction, pulsatility, and turbulence of flow. The abdomen should also be inspected for periumbilical and periportal varices.

Computed Tomography

CT is usually reserved for evaluation of hepatic masses, metastatic disease, abscesses, and surgical complications of transplantation, especially if US is not definitive. Other indications for CT of the liver include evaluation of diffuse parenchymal disease such as cirrhosis, fatty infiltration, and hemochromatosis. Evaluation of the liver is best performed using bolus injection of intravenous contrast and either dynamic or helical scanning. Extensive noncontrast scanning of the liver is usually not necessary.

Magnetic Resonance Imaging

As with CT, MRI is most useful in the evaluation of complex anatomy and diffuse parenchymal disease. Its multiplanar capabilities and its sensitivity to minute differences in tissue composition make it a superb tool to determine the resectability of hepatic masses and show the extent of extrahepatic disease. Use of appropriately sized surface coils is essential for maximizing the signal-to-noise ratio and resolution. Evaluation of the liver should include both T1- and T2-weighted sequences. Gradient-recalled-echo and inversion recovery sequences are also helpful for evaluation of the hepatic vasculature and biliary system, respectively.

Nuclear Medicine

Nuclear medicine techniques used in children include hepatobiliary and reticuloendothelial system (RES) scintigraphy. Hepatobiliary imaging uses ^{99m}Tc-labeled iminodiacetic acid derivatives that are rapidly taken up by hepatocytes and excreted into the biliary system. Its most common use is in neonatal jaundice, to distinguish between neonatal hepatitis and biliary atresia. Other indications include the evaluation of choledochal cyst, arteriohepatic dysplasia, Caroli disease, and biliary leak. High-resolution, parallel hole collimation is essential for maximal spatial resolution. RES scintigraphy employs ^{99m}Tc-labeled sulfur colloid, which permits imaging of functioning hepatic parenchyma by its localization in cells of the RES. Less frequently used than hepatobiliary scintigraphy, it evaluates the size, position, displacement, and replacement of functional hepatic tissue.

Angiography

With the advent of the cross-sectional methods, angiography is used less frequently. Recent advances in interventional techniques, however, have led to renewed interest in angiography. Current indications include preoperative vascular roadmapping of hepatic malignancies and vascular malformations, especially when embolotherapy is considered, and the evaluation of portal hypertension.

Congenital and Neonatal Abnormalities

Biliary Atresia and Neonatal Hepatitis

Neonatal jaundice, a common clinical problem, is caused by a variety of diseases. The causes include infectious hepatitis, biliary atresia, intravascular hemolysis, extravascular hemolysis, resorption of local hemorrhage, metabolic abnormalities such as α_1-antitrypsin deficiency, various enzymatic deficiencies, and bile duct obstruction (442). Jaundice that persists beyond 4 weeks of age is due to biliary atresia or neonatal hepatitis in 90% of cases (443). These two entities have similar clinical, biochemical, and histologic manifestations. Diagnostic imaging therefore has an important role in identifying patients with biliary atresia for prompt surgery while avoiding laparotomy in patients with neonatal hepatitis (442).

Pathologic features of neonatal hepatitis include multinucleated giant cells, parenchymal disruption, and bile duct canaliculi that are relatively free of bile. Cirrhosis may develop. Neonatal hepatitis may be due to cytomegalovirus, hepatitis A or B, rubella, toxoplasma, or spirochetes. Metabolic causes of neonatal hepatitis include α_1-antitrypsin deficiency, familial recurrent cholestasis, and other inborn errors of metabolism. In patients with biliary atresia, the liver characteristically shows periportal fibrosis, intrahepatic small bile duct proliferation, absence of multinucleated giant cells, and focal or total absence of extrahepatic ducts. Cirrhosis ultimately develops unless there is spontaneous healing or corrective surgery.

The clinical features of biliary atresia and neonatal hepatitis are nearly identical. Both cause obstructive jaundice between 1 and 4 weeks of age in an otherwise healthy neonate. The liver and spleen may be enlarged in both conditions. Laboratory tests of liver function and bilirubin metabolism are similar. Biliary atresia and neonatal hepatitis may in fact be variations of the same infectious process, with biliary ''atresia'' resulting from sclerosing cholangitis of extrahepatic or intrahepatic bile ducts (444). In any case, biliary atresia is a dynamic, postnatally progressive, obstructive process. Surgical results are significantly better when surgery is performed before 10 weeks of age, presumably because of loss of microscopic ductal patency at the porta hepatis by 3 months of age.

The distinction of biliary atresia from neonatal hepatitis depends on the demonstration of the morphology and function of the biliary ductal system. The intrahepatic and extrahepatic bile duct system is patent but small in neonatal hepatitis (Fig. 8-163). Some or all of the major hepatic ducts are absent in biliary atresia; despite this mechanical obstruction, however, in biliary atresia the proximal intrahepatic ducts are usually small.

The initial imaging procedure in patients with neonatal jaundice is usually US to exclude choledochal cyst and dilatation of the extrahepatic biliary system. Sonography of the hepatic parenchyma and intrahepatic bile ducts is usually normal in both hepatitis and biliary atresia in the neonate. Only about 20% of patients with biliary atresia have an identifiable gallbladder (442), and thus, though the finding of a normal gallbladder supports the diagnosis of hepatitis, sonography cannot wholly distinguish between biliary atresia and neonatal hepatitis.

Hepatobiliary scintigraphy with ^{99m}Tc-labeled iminodiacetic acid (IDA) derivatives usually permits accurate differentiation of biliary atresia from other causes of neonatal jaundice (445). The patient is treated with oral phenobarbital (5 mg/kg/day) for at least 5 days prior to the examination (446). After intravenous injection of an IDA compound in a dose of 0.05 mCi/kg (minimum 0.25 mCi), sequential images of the abdomen are obtained every 30 seconds for an hour. Additional images at 2, 4, 6, 12, and 24 hours may be obtained if needed. Normally, the ^{99m}Tc-labeled IDA derivatives are rapidly extracted from the blood by the hepatocytes and excreted into the biliary system and intestinal tract. The tracer begins to accumulate in the liver within 5 minutes of injection, and the gallbladder is usually visualized within 15 minutes. The tracer appears in the proximal small bowel by

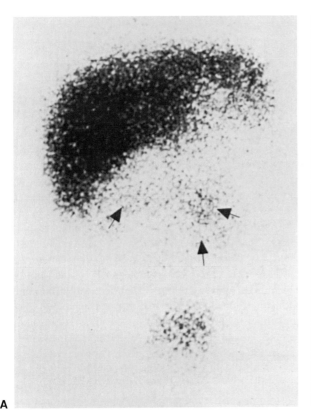
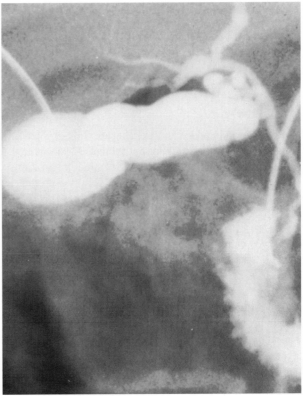

A
B

FIG. 8-163. Neonatal hepatitis. A 6-week-old boy with jaundice. **A:** Hepatobiliary scintigraphy. Tracer activity has reached the gastrointestinal tract *(arrows)*. **B:** Operative cholangiogram. The gallbladder and cystic duct are of normal size. The hepatic ducts and common bile duct are small but patent. Contrast medium readily flows into the duodenum.

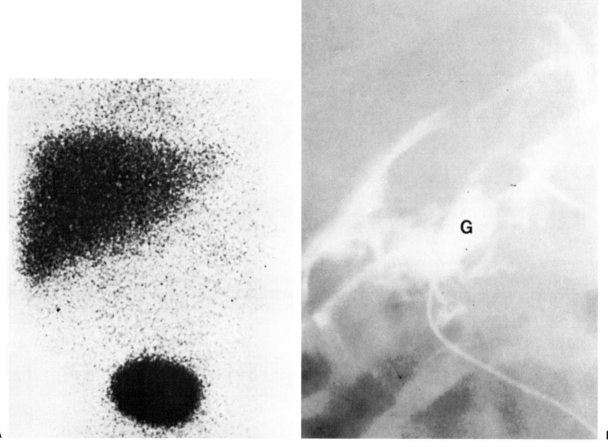

FIG. 8-164. Biliary atresia. A 2-month-old boy with jaundice. **A:** Hepatobiliary scintigraphy. There is good uptake of tracer within the liver at 4 hours but no activity in the gastrointestinal tract. Note the increased genitourinary tract excretion of tracer. **B:** Operative cholangiogram. Contrast material was injected into the small gallbladder *(G)*. There is extravasation of contrast medium; no extrahepatic bile ducts are identified.

30 minutes. The gallbladder and extrahepatic biliary ducts are frequently not identified in normal infants. Most of the tracer is in the colon by 6 hours, with little remaining in the liver. Five to fifteen percent of the tracer is normally excreted by the kidneys, but renal excretion is significantly increased in hepatobiliary disease.

In infants less than 3 months of age with biliary atresia, the hepatic extraction of tracer is good and the definition of liver boundaries persists throughout the examination (Fig. 8-164). In infants with severe neonatal hepatitis there is poor hepatic extraction, so that tracer accumulation in the liver is due to blood pool activity rather than hepatocyte uptake. It may be impossible to distinguish biliary atresia with severe cirrhosis from severe neonatal hepatitis in infants over 3 months of age.

Hepatobiliary scintigraphy in the neonate with jaundice thus demonstrates one of three patterns: (a) normal hepatic extraction of tracer and excretion into the GI tract (normal, neonatal hepatitis, some other cause of jaundice); (b) normal hepatic extraction of tracer but no excretion into the GI tract (biliary atresia); and (c) poor hepatic extraction and poor or no excretion into the GI tract (severe neonatal hepatitis, he-

patic necrosis, biliary atresia, advanced cirrhosis). Scintigraphic visualization of tracer in the GI tract indicates patency of the extrahepatic biliary ducts and excludes biliary atresia (Fig. 8-163). Lateral images help distinguish renal from bowel radioactivity.

If hepatobiliary scintigraphy does not demonstrate ductal patency, exploratory laparotomy is performed. If the gallbladder is identified, a cholangiogram is performed via the gallbladder. In severe neonatal hepatitis, a small but otherwise normal biliary system is demonstrated. The common bile duct, duodenum, and right and left hepatic ducts must be well visualized (Fig. 8-163). The liver is biopsied, but no other surgery is performed. With biliary atresia, the pattern of the operative cholangiogram varies according to the type of atresia (Fig. 8-165). The liver hilus must frequently be explored to determine if the lesion is correctable by an anastomotic procedure (Fig. 8-165). An occasional case of neonatal hepatitis will be confused with biliary atresia when operative cholangiography fails to fill part of the biliary tree.

Only 12% of infants with biliary atresia have a type that is correctable by surgical anastomosis of intact bile ducts (Fig. 8-165) (447). If surgical drainage is possible in biliary

Correctable
12%

"Not correctable"
88%

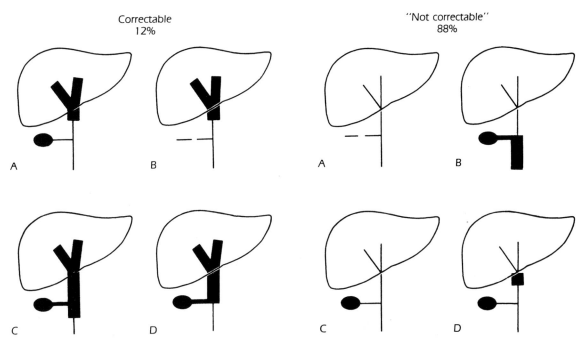

A   B

C   D

A   B

C   D

FIG. 8-165. Types of biliary atresia. Only 12% of cases are correctable by direct anastomotic procedures. The remainder are usually treated by a Kasai hepatic portoenterostomy. Modified from Franken and Smith (1).

atresia by anastomotic bypassing of atretic segments or a Kasai hepatic portoenterostomy, recovery may occur. The Kasai procedure is anastomosis of an intestinal loop to the raw surface of the dissected porta hepatis and may be used in those cases that are not otherwise correctable. Results of the Kasai procedure depend on the age at which it is attempted. Hepatobiliary scintigraphy may help evaluate the integrity and function of the portoenterostomy (Fig. 8-166) as well as detect complications such as bile cyst or bile leakage. The prognosis in biliary atresia depends on the presence or absence of cirrhosis (448). Liver transplantation may be life saving in surgically noncorrectable cases, failed Kasai procedures, and cirrhosis progressing to hepatic failure.

Choledochal Cyst and Caroli disease

A choledochal cyst is a localized dilatation of the biliary ductal system. Five types (Fig. 8-167) have been described: type 1A, localized dilatation of the common bile duct below the cystic duct; type 1B, dilatation of the common bile and hepatic ducts; type 2, a localized, eccentric, cystic diverticulum off the common duct; type 3, dilatation of the distal intramural portion of the common bile duct (choledochocele); and type 4, multiple cystic dilatations involving intrahepatic and extrahepatic biliary radicles (Caroli disease) (449,450). Caroli disease is also defined as saccular dilatation of major intrahepatic bile ducts without other evidence of obstruction (451). Although its cause is unknown and despite the classification given above, it is probably an entity distinct from choledochal cyst. Caroli disease may be complicated by cholangitis, stone formation, or biliary cirrhosis (449,450).

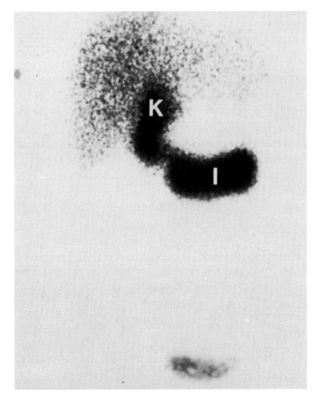

FIG. 8-166. Successful Kasai procedure for biliary atresia. Hepatobiliary scintigraphy (DISIDA scan) obtained 2 months after a Kasai procedure. There is fair extraction of tracer by the liver. Tracer passes through the hepatic portoenterostomy *(K)* into the proximal gastrointestinal tract *(I)*.

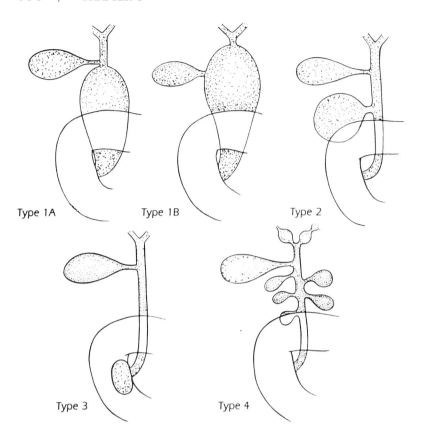

Type 1A   Type 1B   Type 2

Type 3   Type 4

FIG. 8-167. Types of choledochal cyst. Please see text for discussion.

Although the precise etiology of choledochal cyst is unknown, there appear to be two broad groups. The first group is seen in neonates with jaundice and is caused by stenosis or atresia of part of the biliary tree. The association of neonatal choledochal cyst with biliary atresia is important to remember. A second group is diagnosed later in life, often accompanied by pancreatitis and common duct stones; it is less frequently complicated by cirrhosis. Babbitt noted a local anomaly of the orifices of the common bile duct and pancreatic duct in patients with the latter type of choledochal cyst allowing reflux of pancreatic secretions into the biliary tree (452). He proposed that this type is caused by bile duct inflammation due to pancreatic secretions. It thus appears that there are two groups of choledochal cysts: congenital cysts and acquired cysts, the latter perhaps caused by pancreatic-biliary reflux.

Choledochal cysts are uncommon; the incidence is increased in females and Orientals. The cysts may be found at any age, but half of the patients are between 1 and 10 years of age at diagnosis. Another 20% of patients are diagnosed

between 10 and 16 years of age. One third of patients have jaundice during the first year of life. The triad of intermittent jaundice, pain, and abdominal mass is characteristic in the older child but is present in only a minority of younger children with choledochal cysts. Other less specific findings include recurrent pancreatitis and biliary cirrhosis with portal hypertension (449). Five percent of cases of obstructive jaundice during infancy are due to choledochal cysts.

Plain films may show a right upper quadrant mass displacing bowel gas. Calcification of the wall of a choledochal cyst is rare (453). GI contrast studies show displacement of the gastric antrum anteriorly, inferiorly, and to the left. The duodenal bulb is usually compressed, and the descending part of the duodenum is displaced laterally. A choledochocele produces a rounded filling defect in the duodenum near the ampulla of Vater.

Ultrasonography and hepatobiliary scintigraphy often allow a specific diagnosis. Ultrasonography shows the cystic mass in the porta hepatis, fluid-filled and separate from the gallbladder (Fig. 8-168). Demonstration of the distended common bile duct, cystic duct, or hepatic duct emptying

FIG. 8-168. Choledochal cyst. A 7-year-old girl with a right upper quadrant mass, jaundice, and intermittent abdominal pain. **A:** Transverse ultrasonography. A large, cystic mass *(C)* connects with a bile duct medially *(arrow)* and is located anterior to the right kidney *(K)*. The mass is separate from the gallbladder *(g)*. **B:** Longitudinal ultrasonography. The large choledochal cyst *(C)* communicates with bile ducts *(arrows)* and extrinsically compresses the inferior vena cava *(I)*. **C:** Anterior view of DISIDA scan at 5 hours. No tracer is identified in the gastrointestinal tract. The irregular accumulation below the liver *(arrows)* is in the choledochal cyst. **D:** An operative cholangiogram demonstrates a type 1B choledochal cyst.

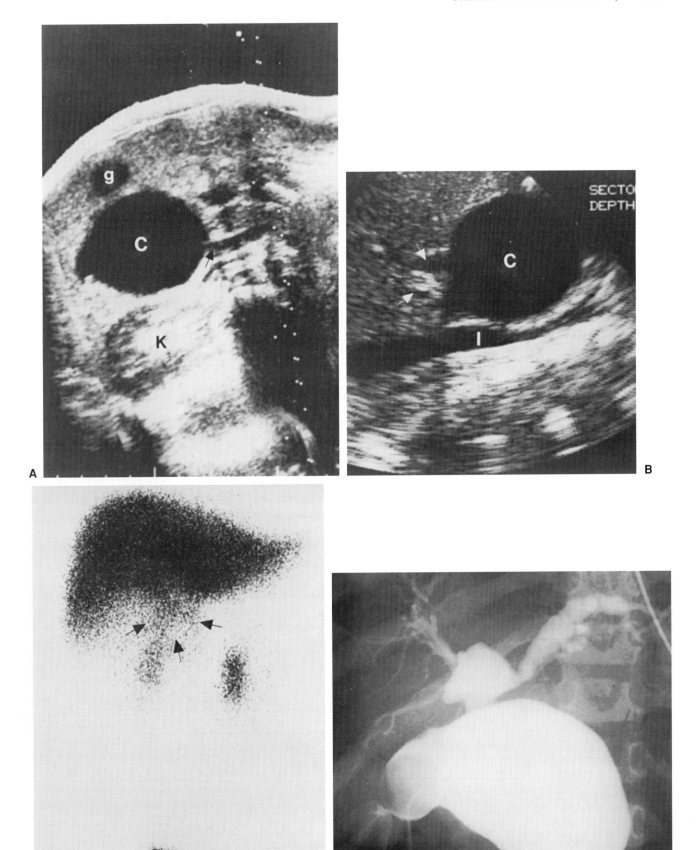

directly into the cystic mass confirms the diagnosis (Fig. 8-168). Hepatobiliary scintigraphy demonstrates normal uptake by the liver and accumulation and stasis of tracer in the choledochal cyst (Fig. 8-168). There is frequently biliary obstruction with no drainage of IDA derivatives into the GI tract (Fig. 8-168). Cholangiography is performed at the time of resection (Fig. 8-168) and is essential for operative planning. Choledochal cysts may also be identified by CT, percutaneous transhepatic cholangiography, and endoscopic retrograde cholangiopancreatography (ERCP).

The differential diagnosis of choledochal cyst includes other fluid-filled masses, e.g., hepatic cyst, pancreatic pseudocyst, ovarian cyst, omental cyst, mesenteric cyst, enteric duplication, hepatic artery aneurysm, and spontaneous perforation of an extrahepatic bile duct. The combination of ultrasonography and hepatobiliary scintigraphy usually allows a specific preoperative diagnosis. The preferred treatment for choledochal cyst is total excision with enteric loop drainage. This treatment prevents recurrent jaundice, ascending cholangitis, and bile duct cancer in any residual cyst wall.

Cholelithiasis and Cholecystitis

Gallstones in childhood are not uncommon and with the widespread use of US are more and more frequently found in asymptomatic children. In newborns and infants cholelithiasis may be idiopathic but is often seen in association with total parenteral nutrition, diuretics, sepsis, and small bowel disease. In older children hemolytic anemia, scoliosis surgery, cystic fibrosis, and abnormal enterohepatic circulation of bile salts due to ileal disease may lead to gallstones (454). In adolescents, in addition to the causes listed above, pregnancy and oral contraceptive use may be implicated.

Approximately 50% of gallstones in children are opaque and can be seen on plain films (Fig. 8-169). Pigmented stones associated with hemolytic disorders are more commonly calcified (50%) than cholesterol stones (15%) (455). Sonography is the diagnostic modality of choice for evaluation of the gallbladder. By US gallstones are echogenic opacities in the gallbladder with acoustic shadowing (Fig. 8-170) or echogenic opacities that shift position with gravity. The distinction between small nonshadowing gallstones and biliary sludge may be difficult.

Neonatal gallstones may be asymptomatic or, rarely, cause biliary obstruction; they may spontaneously resolve (456). Cholecystitis due to cholelithiasis is relatively rare in young children but becomes more common with increasing age. Gallbladder wall thickening and pericholecystic fluid associated with gallstones suggest cholecystitis. The gallbladder will not be visualized on hepatobiliary scintigraphy in the vast majority of children with cholecystitis. False-negative ultrasonography and scintigraphy, however, do occur.

Children may also develop cholecystitis in the absence of gallstones (acalculous cholecystitis). This occurs usually in very ill children who have had trauma, surgery, or burns or are septic. On ultrasonography, the gallbladder is usually enlarged and tender with a thickened wall; on scintigraphy, the gallbladder is usually not visualized.

Acalculous cholecystitis should be distinguished from gallbladder hydrops, which is distention of the gallbladder without inflammation. Hydrops tends to develop in patients who are not as ill as those with acalculous cholecystitis; the most common cause is Kawasaki disease (457). US will show a distended gallbladder without wall thickening. The clinical and radiologic differentiation of hydrops from acalculous cholecystitis may be difficult. Isolated gallbladder wall thickening may be seen in patients with hepatitis, ascites, and AIDS-related cholangitis (Fig. 8-171) (458,459).

Hepatobiliary Tumors

The liver is the third most common site (after the kidney and adrenal glands) of origin of abdominal malignancies in infants and children. Liver tumors represent approximately 6% of abdominal tumors in pediatric patients. Hepatic masses may be primary or metastatic in origin. Approximately one third of primary liver tumors in children are benign. They can be further classified according to their cell of origin as epithelial or mesenchymal (Table 8-8) (460).

The main roles of imaging in primary hepatic tumors are to (a) distinguish benign from malignant tumors; (b) define the extent of the lesion and therefore its resectability; (c) assess the response to treatment (461). When the tumor shows a characteristic imaging appearance (e.g., hemangioma or cystic mesenchymal hamartoma), a definitive diagnosis can be made. However, in most cases diagnostic certainty is not possible with imaging alone. Clinical presentation, age, and serum level of α-fetoprotein (AFP) aid in the differential diagnosis. In patients less than 5 years of age, hepatoblastoma, mesenchymal hamartoma, and hemangioma are the most commonly encountered lesions. In patients over 5, hepatocellular carcinoma (especially in children over 10) and mesenchymal sarcoma (especially in children between 5 and 10) are more likely.

TABLE 8-8. *Pediatric hepatic tumors*

Cell of Origin	Tumor
Benign	
Epithelial	Focal nodular hyperplasia (3%)
	Adenoma (1%)
Mesenchymal	Hemangioma/hemangiodenothelioma (18%)
Other	(4%)
Malignant	
Epithelial	Hepatoblastoma (36%)
	Hepatocellular carcinoma (20%)
Mesenchymal	Mesenchymal sarcoma (7%)
Other	(11%)

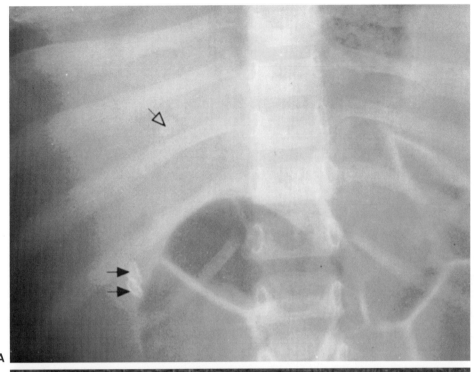

A

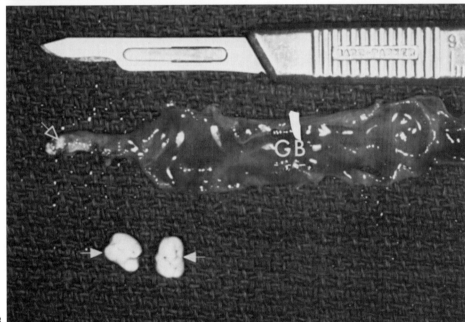

B

FIG. 8-169. Cholelithiasis due to interruption of the enterohepatic circulation of bile salts. A 4-year-old girl with right upper quadrant pain and previous small bowel resection for midgut volvulus. **A:** Stones in the gallbladder *(solid arrows)* and cystic duct *(open arrows)*. **B:** Cholecystectomy specimen. Pale, faceted cholesterol stones *(solid arrows)* were removed from the open gallbladder *(GB)*. A third cholesterol stone *(open arrows)* was impacted in the cystic duct. From Kirks (454).

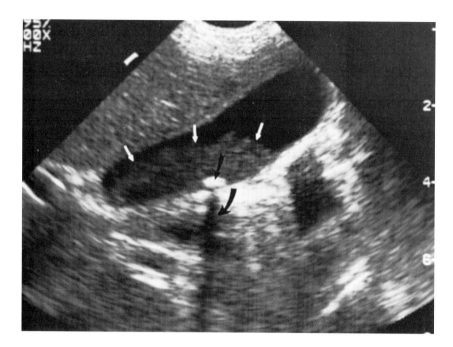

FIG. 8-170. Ultrasonography of cholelithiasis. Longitudinal sonography demonstrates a single echogenic focus *(black arrow)* within sludge *(white arrows)*. The gallstone produces distal shadowing *(curved black arrow)*.

Although the liver is classically divided into right and left lobes, there are three important surgical divisions of the liver. As seen by imaging modalities, the right and left lobes of the liver are separated by a plane that connects the IVC and gallbladder (Fig. 8-172). It is critical to identify the medial and lateral segments of the left lobe of the liver, which are separated by the intersegmental fissure (Fig. 8-172). A tumor of the right lobe of the liver that involves the medial segment of the left lobe is still resectable by means of an extended right hepatectomy. However, a lesion of both segments of the left lobe that also involves the right lobe is usually unresectable (462).

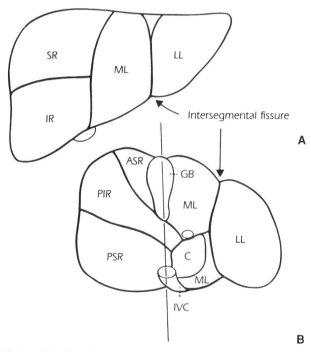

FIG. 8-172. Divisions of the liver. Anterior **(A)** and inferior **(B)** schematic views of the liver. The right lobe of the liver is separated from the left lobe of the liver by a line connecting the inferior vena cava *(IVC)* and the gallbladder fossa *(GB)*. The intersegmental fissure *(arrows)* separates the medial *(ML)* and lateral *(LL)* segments of the left lobe of the liver. *ASR*, anterior segment of right lobe; *C*, caudate lobe; *IR*, inferior segment of right lobe; *PIR*, posterior inferior segment of right lobe; *PSR*, posterior superior segment of right lobe; *SR*, superior segment of right lobe.

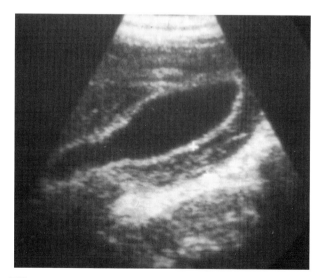

FIG. 8-171. Gallbladder wall thickening due to hepatitis. An 11-year-old boy with hemophilia and transfusion-related hepatitis. The gallbladder wall is 1 cm thick.

Imaging-guided percutaneous biopsy often allows benign lesions to be observed nonoperatively and malignant lesions to be treated with the appropriate chemotherapeutic regimen if they are not resectable. Chemoembolization of unresectable or progressive malignant liver tumors may also be performed.

Abdominal radiography may show hepatic enlargement, diaphragmatic elevation, and displacement of bowel gas. Although nonspecific, hepatic calcifications or the presence of pulmonary metastases may be diagnostically helpful. Although sonography shows the cystic or solid nature of the mass lesion, the echotexture of solid hepatic masses is a poor indicator of histology. Color flow Doppler examination is useful for assessing the vascularity of neoplasms (463,464); sonography may also be used to guide fluid aspiration or tissue biopsy. MRI and CT are excellent for the preoperative evaluation of hepatic masses and are equal in their ability to determine resectability (465). MRI, however, appears to detect postoperative recurrences better (466,467). Angiography accurately assesses hepatic artery and portal venous anatomy, but it is usually reserved for those cases that require detailed preoperative vascular mapping or interventional embolotherapy.

Benign Tumors

Mesenchymal Hamartoma

This uncommon, benign lesion is considered a failure of normal development rather than a true neoplasm (468). Most patients are less than 2 years old, and there is a slight male predominance. The lesion is usually very large (12–15 cm on average). Up to 75% are situated in the right lobe where they may form a pedunculated mass attached to the inferior hepatic surface. The lesion is usually cystic, fluid having accumulated in mesenchyma or in spaces lined by biliary epithelium (469). Mesenchymal hamartomas have variable amounts of stroma. Congestive failure may develop because of a large vascular component and arteriovenous (AV) shunting (470). However, patients usually present with only an asymptomatic enlarging abdominal mass. Surgical resection is the definitive treatment. The prognosis is excellent (471).

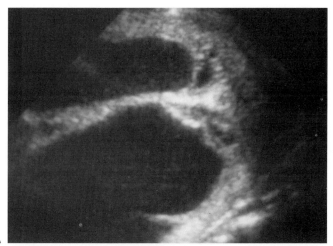

A

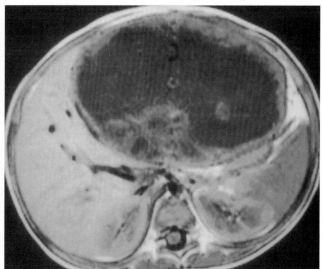

FIG. 8-173. Mesenchymal hamartoma of the liver. A: Transverse ultrasound image. **B:** Contrast-enhanced CT. **C:** T1-weighted MRI. A large cystic mass is shown in the liver. There is a solid component posteriorly.

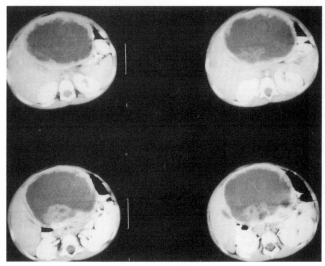

B

C

The imaging appearance depends on the amount of stroma in the hamartoma. Large cystic areas can be seen clearly by US, CT, or MRI (Fig. 8-173). The septa and the solid components enhance. Calcification has not been reported (469). On angiography, the appearance ranges from predominantly hypovascular (mostly cystic) to hypervascular (mostly solid). At times, the outline of individual arteries is irregular and suggests malignant neovascularity. When the typical appearance of a large hepatic mass with many large cystic spaces is seen on imaging, the diagnosis of mesenchymal hamartoma can be made. However, when the hamartoma is mostly solid, differentiation from hepatoblastoma is difficult and biopsy is needed (469).

Hemangioma (Hemangioendothelioma)

The nomenclature used for these lesions is confusing. Here the term hemangioma will be used to refer to what has been known as infantile hemangioendothelioma and infantile "cavernous" hemangioma. The most widely used classification (472) divides this benign vascular tumor of the liver into hemangioendotheliomas (types 1 and 2) and cavernous hemangiomas. Work by Mulliken and Glowacki (473) and Mulliken and Young (474) suggests that hemangioendotheliomas and infantile cavernous hemangiomas are probably the same entity in different phases of evolution. The "cavernous hemangiomas" that do not involute and the "hemangiomas" found in adult livers are probably venous malformations.

So defined (473,474), hemangioma is a true neoplasm characterized by hypercellularity and endothelial cell proliferation in its early phase, usually in the first 18 months of life. The formation of new feeding and draining vessels both within and around the hemangioma accompanies cellular proliferation. The sinusoidal spaces in the hemangioma have low vascular resistance, and the lesion can cause significant AV shunting. This proliferative phase is followed by a long involutional phase that lasts for 5–8 years. As the hemangioma involutes, the endothelial hyperplasia decreases and fibrous and fatty tissues begin to separate the vascular spaces. Some of the vascular spaces dilate and the endothelium begins to flatten, and a cavernous appearance develops (472). Although hemangiomas are typically multicentric, scattered in the liver parenchyma, large solitary lesions may be seen.

The nomenclature difficulties make the true incidence unclear. It is reported that 85% or more of hepatic hemangiomas present at 6 months of age or younger. They are twice as common in girls, and 40% to 50% of affected infants also have cutaneous hemangiomas. The patients may present with asymptomatic hepatomegaly, congestive failure, anemia, jaundice, or the Kasabach-Merritt syndrome (platelet trapping by the hemangioma leading to thrombocytopenic coagulopathy) (474).

The diagnosis can be made by imaging, especially when the presentation is typical. US shows many hypoechoic, well-circumscribed hepatic lesions and abnormally large vessels with high flow (Fig. 8-174) (475). Abrupt tapering of the abdominal aorta distal to the celiac axis and SMA is seen when the amount of blood flowing through the hemangioma is large. On CT, these lesions are of low density on unenhanced scans and show early peripheral enhancement and later filling-in of the lesions. On MRI, hemangiomas have low signal intensity on T1-weighted images and very high signal intensity on T2-weighted images, especially with fat suppression. There are large flow voids on T1-weighted images and high intensity on gradient-recalled-echo sequences, which indicates high flow. Enhancement with gadolinium indicates the presence of solid tissue in this true neoplasm. On angiography in the symptomatic high-flow hemangioma, the hepatic arteries are dilated and tortuous and the hepatic veins fill early. Opacification of multiple discrete homogeneous nodules and collections of contrast in sinusoidal spaces can be seen in the parenchymal phase. When a hemangioma presents as a solitary hepatic mass, especially if there is little AV shunting, the differentiation from hepatoblastoma can be difficult with imaging alone.

If the patient is not significantly compromised by the AV shunting, the prognosis is excellent; all hemangiomas eventually involute. Therapy for symptomatic hemangioma includes medications to treat congestive heart failure, high-dose steroids, and interferon-α2a (antiangiogenesis factor) therapy (476). If there is life-threatening failure or hemorrhage secondary to the Kasabach-Merritt syndrome, embolization of the feeding hepatic arterial branches and systemic collaterals can decrease the degree of AV shunting to the point where medical therapy can control the symptoms until the hemangioma involutes (477). Aggressive embolization can cause significant hepatic necrosis, especially when there is a portal venous supply to the hemangioma.

Focal Nodular Hyperplasia

Focal nodular hyperplasia (FNH) is a nonneoplastic lesion of the liver typically seen in young women with a history of oral contraceptive use. FNH accounts for 2% to 6% of hepatic tumors in childhood, and approximately 15% of cases are reported in children (460). Hemihypertrophy, familial glioblastoma, and sickle cell disease are conditions reported to be associated with FNH. The lesion consists of nodules of normal-appearing hepatocytes arranged in cords and surrounded by fibrous septa. Imaging findings are similar to those in adults: a well-defined mass with one or more stellate fibrous scars in the center of the lesion. Although there is no known association between FNH and hepatocellular carcinoma, surgical resection remains the recommended form of therapy (478).

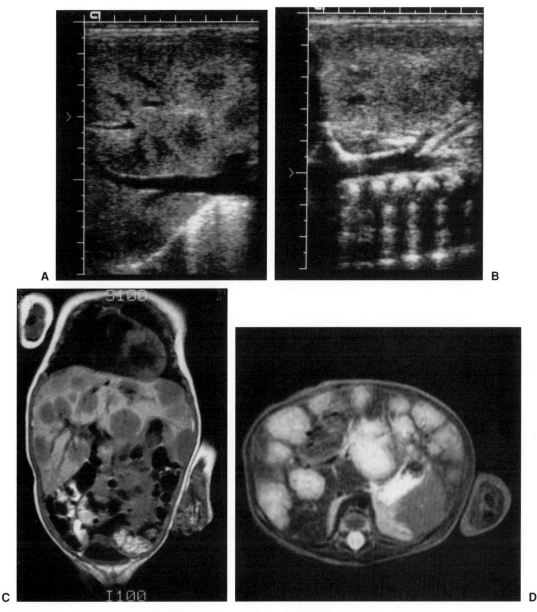

FIG. 8-174. Hemangioendothelioma (hemangioma). Newborn with a palpable liver and congestive heart failure. **A:** Transverse ultrasound image. There are many hypoechoic nodules in the liver. **B:** Sagittal ultrasound image. The prominent celiac axis and abrupt tapering of the aorta at and below the superior mesenteric artery are due to increased blood flow to the liver. **C:** A T1-weighted coronal MR image shows many low intensity foci of tumor. **D:** T2-weighted fast spin-echo transverse MR image. Note the vascular flow voids associated with the nodules.

Malignant Neoplasms

Hepatoblastoma

Hepatoblastoma is the most common primary hepatic tumor of childhood. It is usually found in children less than 5 years old. Approximately two thirds of the patients are less than 2 years old (479). The tumor can be present at birth. There is an increased incidence in boys. Risk factors for the tumor include siblings with hepatoblastoma, trisomy 18, hemihypertrophy, Beckwith-Wiedemann syndrome, fa-

milial adenomatous polyposis, fetal alcohol syndrome, maternal use of gonadotropins, and maternal exposure to metals or petroleum products. Cirrhosis is not a risk factor. Over 60% arise in the right lobe. The tumor is usually large (10–12 cm), solitary, and well delineated with a pseudocapsule. The tumor is most commonly made up solely of epithelial cells, either of the fetal type (the most favorable histology), embryonal type, or mixed fetal-embryonal type. Less commonly the tumor is made up of mixed epithelial-mesenchymal (anaplastic) cells (the least favorable histology); this subtype can have differentiated mesenchymal tissues such as osteoid and cartilage.

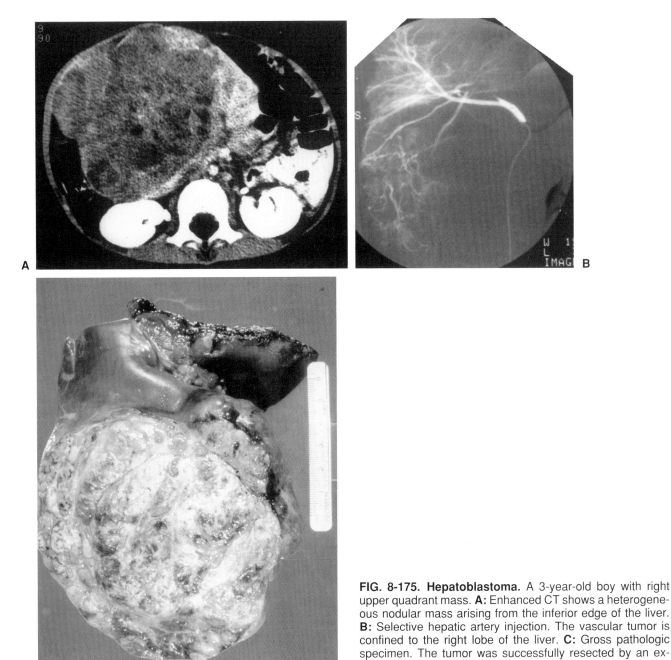

FIG. 8-175. Hepatoblastoma. A 3-year-old boy with right upper quadrant mass. **A:** Enhanced CT shows a heterogeneous nodular mass arising from the inferior edge of the liver. **B:** Selective hepatic artery injection. The vascular tumor is confined to the right lobe of the liver. **C:** Gross pathologic specimen. The tumor was successfully resected by an extended right hepatectomy.

Early symptoms and signs are uncommon, and the tumor is often large when discovered. The serum AFP is elevated in 90% of cases. Elevated levels of human chorionic gonadotropin have been reported in children with precocious puberty and hepatoblastoma.

Abdominal radiographs show hepatic calcifications in up to half of cases. On US, the mass is hypervascular. Its typical mixed echogenicity reflects areas of hemorrhage and necrosis. Evaluation with duplex or color Doppler US demonstrates hypervascularity. The margins of the tumor are better defined by MRI or CT (Figs. 8-175 and 8-176) (480). The tumor is usually of lower density on unenhanced CT images

than the surrounding normal parenchyma and enhances less. On MRI, the tumor is hypointense on T1-weighted images and hyperintense on T2-weighted images. With gradient–recalled-echo sequences, the patency of blood vessels compressed or invaded by tumor can be assessed without any contrast agent. Purely epithelial tumors have more homogeneous density and signal intensity on CT and MR and more homogenous enhancement of the tumor. On angiography, hepatoblastomas are hypervascular and have areas of neovascularization and encasement of vessels. Sometimes a typical spoke wheel arrangement of the arteries is present. Arteriovenous shunting is occasionally demonstrated.

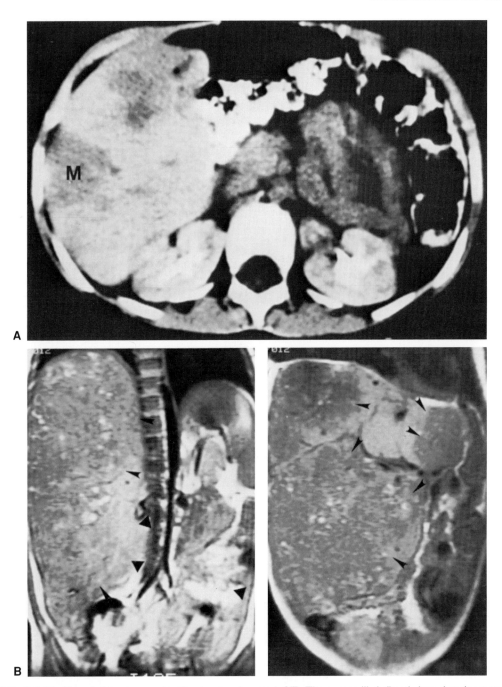

FIG. 8-176. Hepatoblastoma. A: Contrast-enhanced CT. There are ill-defined, low-density masses *(M)* in the right lobe of the liver. **B:** Coronal T1-weighted MRI. There is extensive involvement of both lobes of the liver *(arrowheads)*, making the tumor unresectable.

Long-term survival is impossible without complete resection. Fortunately, between 50% and 70% of these tumors are resectable when diagnosed.

Hepatocellular Carcinoma

Hepatocellular carcinoma (HCC) is the second most common primary hepatic tumor in children. It is usually found in children older than 5 years of age (mean age at presentation 12–14 years). There is a slight male predominance. Slightly more than half of the patients have elevated serum AFP levels. Except for age, the signs and symptoms are quite similar to those of hepatoblastoma. Several chronic liver diseases increase the risk of subsequent HCC. These include cirrhosis, glycogen storage disease, tyrosinemia, biliary atresia, and hepatitis. The association of childhood HCC with hepatitis B virus infection is well documented in Africa and Asia.

HCC may present as a focal mass or as a diffusely infiltrating process. It involves the right lobe more commonly, but both lobes may be involved with multifocal disease. The prognosis is worse than that of hepatoblastoma. Only 15% to 30% of these tumors are resectable at presentation (Fig. 8-177). Hemorrhage, necrosis, and cystic areas are common (480). With imaging alone, HCC cannot be distinguished from hepatoblastoma.

A variant, the fibrolamellar type, constitutes approximately 3% of HCC. It is usually a tumor of the young adult (mean age of 20 years). There is an equal sex distribution. There is no association with chronic liver disease. Although it has a better prognosis than typical HCC, cure of the fibrolamellar variant is not possible without complete resection. Approximately half are resectable at presentation. The hallmark of this variant is the presence of a central scar that is sometimes calcified. This tumor is found more commonly in the left lobe.

Mesenchymal Sarcoma

This is a rare primary malignant tumor affecting children between the ages of 5 and 10 years. It is also called malignant mesenchymoma and undifferentiated (embryonal) sarcoma. Boys and girls are equally affected. The right lobe is more commonly involved (481). It is usually a large, hypovascular mass with well-defined borders lined by a fibrous pseudocapsule. Necrosis and hemorrhage are common. The cut surface has a mucoid and partially cystic appearance. Histologically, the tumor cells are undifferentiated sarcomatous (spindle) cells.

The imaging appearance of the tumor depends on the amount of cyst formation in the mass. No calcifications are seen (482). The septa between the cystic areas, the solid portion of the tumor, and the pseudocapsule often enhance after contrast administration (483). There is a propensity for local recurrence and for direct spread into the diaphragm, the lung, and other contiguous structures.

Although the prognosis is very poor (<10% cure), survival has been reported after complete resection.

Hepatic Metastases

The most common secondary hepatic malignancies of childhood are metastases from neuroblastoma, Wilms tumor,

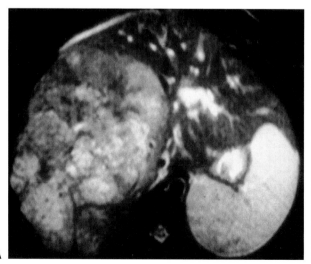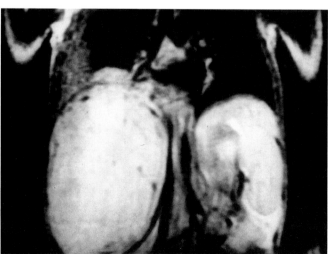

A   B

FIG. 8-177. Hepatocellular carcinoma. A: A T2-weighted axial MRI image shows a well-defined nodular tumor involving the right lobe of the liver. **B:** A coronal T1-weighted image after gadolinium enhancement shows tumor eroding through the right hemidiaphragm and causing a pleural effusion. The tumor is clearly unresectable.

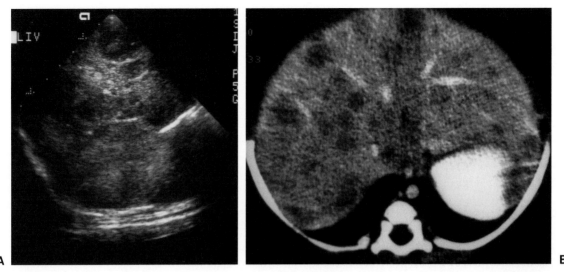

FIG. 8-178. Neuroblastoma metastases to liver. A: A sagittal ultrasound image shows several hypo-echoic nodules in the liver. **B:** A contrast-enhanced CT shows hypodense nodules with peripheral contrast enhancement.

leukemia, and lymphoma. Metastases generally are detected as one or more nodules in the parenchyma of the liver. Cystic metastases are rare in childhood. On sonography, metastases are seen as focal or ill-defined areas of abnormal echogenicity and may be associated with neovascularity detectable by color Doppler. Contrast-enhanced CT will often show nodules with poor central enhancement but increased enhancement at the periphery of the nodule (Fig. 8-178). Metastases vary in appearance on MRI. On T2-weighted images most metastases are hyperintense relative to normal liver. With T1-weighted sequences the intensity varies and can be less than, equal to, or greater than adjacent liver parenchyma.

Rhabdomyosarcoma of the Biliary Tree

Although rhabdomyosarcoma of the biliary tract is rare, it is the most common neoplasm of the biliary tree in children. Histologically this tumor is classified as an embryonal rhabdomyosarcoma. The age at diagnosis varies widely. There is no gender predilection. Imaging findings include dilatation of the common and intrahepatic biliary ducts and a lobulated intraluminal mass.

Diffuse Hepatic Parenchymal Disease

Hepatitis

Except in newborns, viral hepatitis is the most common cause of hepatic inflammation. The liver usually appears normal on CT and US; these imaging studies are therefore seldom requested. Gallbladder wall thickening is sometimes seen on right upper quadrant sonography in patients with hepatitis (see Fig. 8-171).

Fatty Replacement

The normal child's liver has a fat content of less than 5%. Diseases causing increased fat deposition in the liver may make the organ appear lucent by conventional radiography (484). The radiologic signs of fatty liver include lucency of the liver, sharp outline of the right kidney margin due to the fat–soft-tissue interface, fat-muscle interface between the liver and abdominal musculature, fat-fluid interface between the fatty liver and ascites, hollow viscus wall sign due to fatty liver adjacent to air-filled bowel, and blurring of the medial margin of the right properitoneal fat stripe (484,485).

Fatty infiltration of the liver is detected much earlier by cross-sectional imaging than by conventional radiography. Sonography shows focal or diffuse increased echogenicity of the liver (Fig. 8-179A). CT shows markedly decreased attenuation of the hepatic parenchyma due to generalized fatty replacement (Fig. 8-179B). MRI demonstrates fatty replacement as high signal intensity on T1-weighted images (Fig. 8-180) and variable signal intensity on T2-weighted images. CT and MRI demonstrate that most patients with malnutrition or long-term hyperalimentation develop fatty replacement in the liver, either generalized or focal.

Other causes of a radiologically visible fatty liver in children include cystic fibrosis, Reye syndrome, acute starvation, kwashiorkor, malabsorption, high-dose steroid therapy, glycogen storage disease, acute hepatitis, liver toxins, cirrhosis, and previous severe liver damage (484,485).

Cirrhosis

Cirrhosis is characterized by irreversible widespread hepatic fibrosis and nodular parenchymal regeneration. Although the precise etiology of cirrhosis is often not

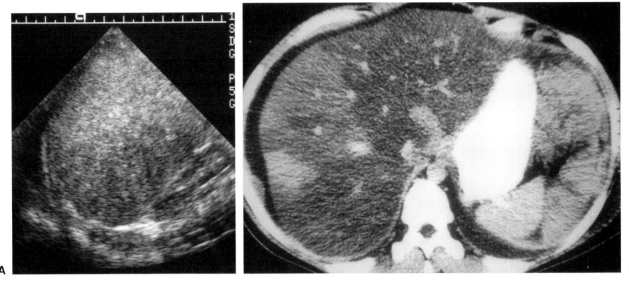

FIG. 8-179. Diffuse fatty replacement due to cystic fibrosis. A 3-year-old boy with cystic fibrosis. **A:** Sagittal ultrasonography shows a diffusely echogenic liver. **B:** Contrast-enhanced CT. The enlarged liver has diffusely decreased attenuation because of fatty replacement.

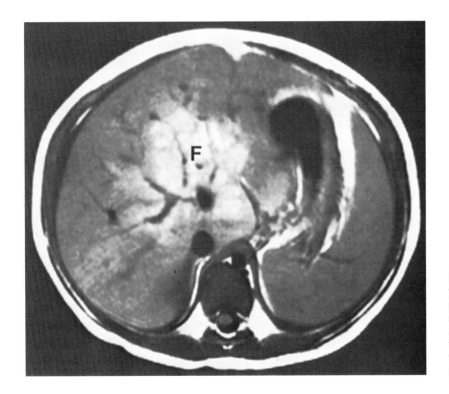

FIG. 8-180. Focal fatty replacement. A 4-year-old boy with chronic liver failure due to paucity of intrahepatic bile ducts (Alagille syndrome). T1-weighted MRI demonstrates a poorly marginated area of high signal intensity *(F)*; this signal intensity is similar to that of subcutaneous fat. Intrahepatic vessels are neither displaced nor invaded.

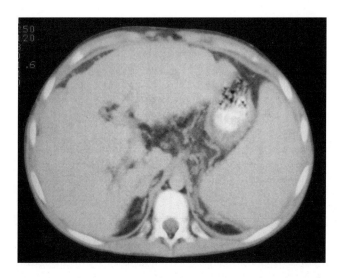

FIG. 8-181. Cirrhosis. A 14-year-old girl with cystic fibrosis and biliary cirrhosis. Contrast-enhanced CT shows nodular hepatomegaly, splenomegaly, and multiple retrogastric varices.

elucidated in children, common causes include chronic cholestasis (cystic fibrosis, biliary atresia); genetically transmitted disorders such as tyrosinemia, galactosemia, and α_1-antitrypsin deficiency, and diseases associated with acquired cholestasis (viral or chronic active hepatitis). On pathologic examination the liver is firm and nodular and is traversed throughout by narrow bands of connective tissue. Common clinical symptoms include failure to thrive, anorexia, jaundice, and a bleeding diathesis.

Morphologic features of cirrhosis (enlargement of the left hepatic and caudate lobes, nodularity, and compression of intrahepatic vessels) and varices can be demonstrated by US, CT, and MRI (Figs. 8-181 and 8-182). Increased echogenicity in a diffuse or patchy distribution is an additional sonographic characteristic of cirrhosis. Regenerating liver nodules usually have MRI signal characteristics similar to those of normal liver. Fatty degeneration within these nodules may cause increased signal intensity on T1-weighted images. For a discussion of the hemodynamic changes of cirrhosis, please see the following section.

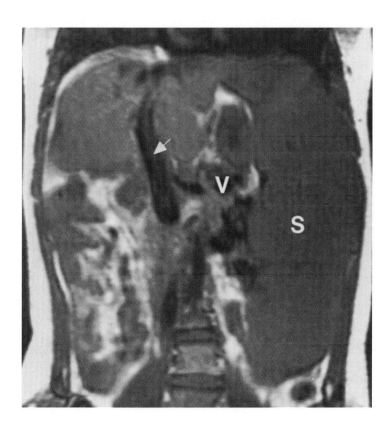

FIG. 8-182. MRI of end-stage liver disease. T1-weighted (SE 600/20) MRI. Note the massive splenomegaly *(S)*, numerous varices *(V)*, and small liver. The increased signal intensity *(arrows)* verifies abnormal blood flow in the portal vein.

Vascular Abnormalities

Portal Hypertension

Portal hypertension is caused by increased resistance to portal venous blood flow (486). It may be due to extrahepatic obstruction, intrahepatic obstruction, or hepatic venous hypertension (Table 8-9). Extrahepatic portal obstruction is considerably more common in children than in adults; more-

TABLE 8-9. *Portal hypertension in children*

Extrahepatic obstruction
    Portal vein occlusion: thrombus
        Idiopathic[a]
        Omphalitis
        Umbilical vein catheterization
    Extrinsic portal vein compression
Intrahepatic obstruction: cirrhosis, chronic liver disease
    Posthepatitis
        Postinfectious hepatitis[a]
        Postneonatal hepatitis[a]
    Chronic active hepatitis
    Childhood cirrhosis
    Genetic and metabolic disorders
        Wilson disease
        Histiocytosis
        α_1-Antitrypsin deficiency[a]
        Gaucher diseae
        Porphyria
        Hemoglobinopathies
        Gycogen storage disease
        Mucopolysaccharidoses
        Galactosemia
        Tyrosinemia
    Kwashiorkor
    Toxins
        Drugs
        Poisons
        Others
    Inflammatory bowel disease
    Biliary cirrhosis
        Biliary atresia[a]
        Choledochal cyst
        Cystic fibrosis[a]
        Alagille syndrome
        Familial intrahepatic cholestasis
    Hepatic venous hypertension
    Hepatic vein thrombosis: Budd-Chiari syndrome
    Passive venous congestion
        Pericarditis
        Congenital heart disease
Hyperkinetic hypertension: increased flow
    Arteriovenous malformation
        Spleen
        Bowel
Blood dyscrasias
    Leukemia
    Others

[a] More common.

Modified from Berger PE, Afshani E. Angiography. In: Franken EA Jr., Smith WL, eds. *Gastrointestinal imaging in pediatrics*. Philadelphia: Harper & Row, 1982:473–489.

over, in children extrahepatic obstruction due to portal vein occlusion (Fig. 8-183A) is a more common cause of portal hypertension than intrahepatic obstruction due to cirrhosis (Fig. 8-183B). Because of the increased resistance to portal venous blood flow, collaterals develop for hepatopetal flow (flow toward the liver by portal-portal collaterals) or hepatofugal flow (flow away from the liver through portosystemic collaterals).

Portal vein thrombosis (followed by cavernous transformation of the portal vein or cavernoma) leading to portal hypertension is the most common cause of massive GI bleeding during childhood (487). Thrombosis of the portal vein usually presents between the ages of 3 and 10 years with massive GI bleeding and splenomegaly (486). Liver function tests and liver biopsy are usually normal. The bleeding is spontaneous and is due to esophageal varices. Most cases of portal vein occlusion are idiopathic (Table 8-9). A few cases can be directly related to ascending omphalitis or are complications of umbilical venous catheterization.

Patients with cirrhosis often progress to obstruction at the sinusoidal level and then to portal hypertension. These children usually develop signs of liver disease prior to variceal bleeding. Unlike in extrahepatic portal vein obstruction, liver function tests and liver biopsy are abnormal because of hepatic parenchymal disease.

In the past, the evaluation of portal hypertension was a common indication for abdominal angiography. Duplex and color Doppler sonography have now replaced arteriography in most cases. However, angiography can still be useful in determining the location of portal venous obstruction and of active GI hemorrhage, in the evaluation of vascular hemodynamics prior to shunting, and in detecting thromboses in portosystemic shunts. Arterial portography evaluates hepatic and celiac axis arterial anatomy as well as the superior mesenteric, splenic, and portal veins (Fig. 8-184). It usually requires the prolonged injection of large volumes of contrast material into the splenic artery and SMA with tolazoline (Priscoline) enhancement. If the spleen is markedly enlarged, there may be poor visualization of the splenic vein and portosystemic collaterals.

Sonographic evaluation of patients suspected of having portal hypertension should include a determination of the size of the portal vein and the direction of portal venous flow as well as a search for portosystemic collateral circulation (488). Normal portal venous flow is toward the liver (hepatopetal) and varies with respiration (Fig. 8-185A). The earliest sign of portal hypertension is loss of this respiratory variation; flow subsequently reverses altogether (488). Portal vein pulsatility (with arterial systole) is commonly seen in children with end-stage liver disease and portal hypertension (Fig. 8-185B) (489). It is postulated that loss of compliance of the liver parenchyma due to progressive fibrosis results in impedance of portal venous flow during arterial systole. Portal vein pulsatility can also be present in congestive heart failure and tricuspid regurgitation (490,491). Severe portal hypertension causes thickening of the lesser omentum due

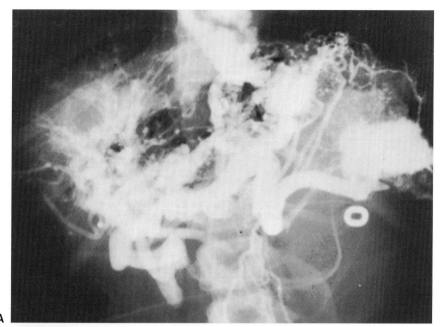

A

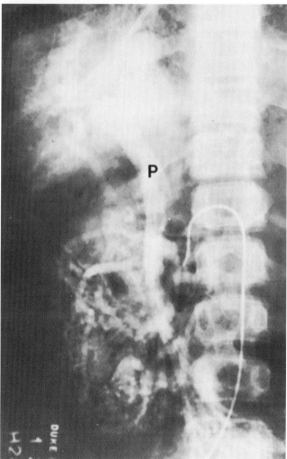

B

FIG. 8-183. Common pediatric causes of portal hypertension. A: A 9-year-old girl with cavernous transformation of the portal vein. This splenoportogram demonstrates a patent splenic vein, occlusion of the portal vein, collaterals in the region of the porta hepatis (cavernous transformation, cavernoma), and many esophageal varices. **B:** A 15-year-old boy with cystic fibrosis and biliary cirrhosis. Arterial portography after superior mesenteric artery injection demonstrates a patent portal vein *(P)*.

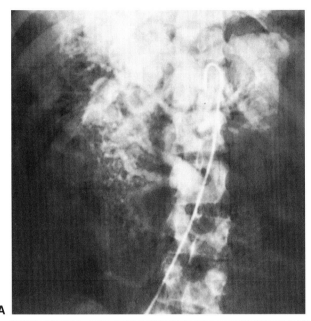

A

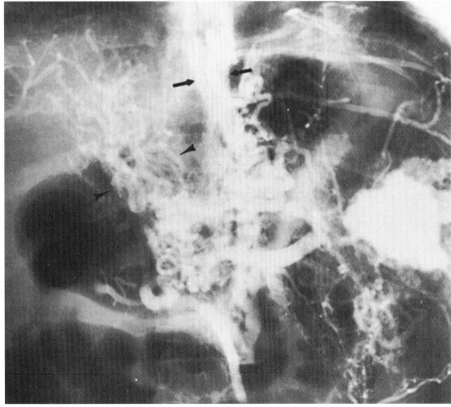

B

FIG. 8-184. Cavernous transformation of the portal vein.
A: Arterial portography in a 12-year-old girl demonstrates many collateral portal venous vessels. **B:** A splenoportogram in a 7-year-old girl shows cavernous transformation of the portal vein *(arrowheads)* and many porto-systemic collateral pathways including esophageal varices *(arrows)*. The splenic pulp pressure was 40 cm of water (normal 13.5 cm water). (From Moore AV, Kirks DR, Mills SR, et al. Pediatric abdominal angiography: panacea or passe. *AJR* 1982;138:433–443.)

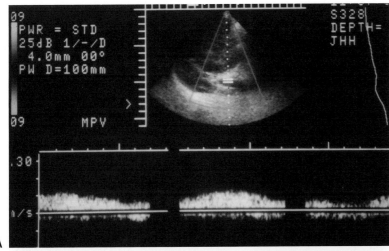

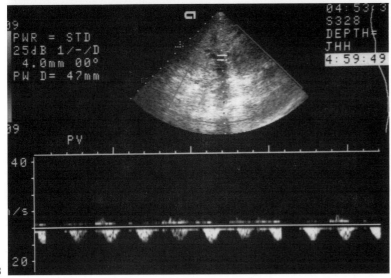

FIG. 8-185. Doppler demonstration of portal vein hemodynamics. A: Normal portal vein. Flow is toward the liver (hepatopetal), and there is respiratory variation. **B:** Portal hypertension. Flow is away from the liver (hepatofugal) and pulsatile with the heart beat.

to varices (Fig. 8-186) (492). Portal vein thrombosis (Fig. 8-187) and secondary cavernous transformation of the portal vein (portal-portal collaterals) are readily demonstrated by sonography, CT, and MRI (Fig. 8-188). Portal vein branch occlusions are difficult to define by sonography; angiography is more sensitive to such occlusions. Sonography with color and duplex Doppler is useful for follow-up of patients with portosystemic shunts (493,494). Continuous hepatofugal flow in the portal vein is expected after a portosystemic shunt (Fig. 8-189).

Budd-Chiari Syndrome

Hepatic venous obstruction (Budd-Chiari syndrome) is uncommon during childhood. Most patients present with abdominal distention of rapid onset, ascites, hepatomegaly, and abdominal pain. The causes include leukemia, sickle cell disease, and inflammatory bowel disease; in the majority of patients, however, no cause can be identified. Doppler sonography can be used for rapid, noninvasive diagnosis.

Typical findings include diminution in caliber of and absence of flow in hepatic veins and prominence of the veins draining the caudate lobe into the IVC (Fig. 8-190).

Liver Transplantation

Preoperative Evaluation

Liver transplantation is now an accepted and successful treatment for end-stage liver disease in children. The most common indications for liver transplantation are biliary atresia, fulminant hepatic failure, α_1-antitrypsin deficiency, cryptogenic cirrhosis, and chronic active hepatitis (495). Other causes of liver failure requiring liver transplantation include severe neonatal hepatitis, Wilson disease, chronic cholestasis, tyrosinemia, and (rarely) an inoperable hepatic neoplasm. Imaging is critical for both planning and follow-up of liver transplantation. Goals of preoperative imaging evaluation include (a) assessment of portal vein size and hemodynamics, (b) detection and mapping of varices, (c)

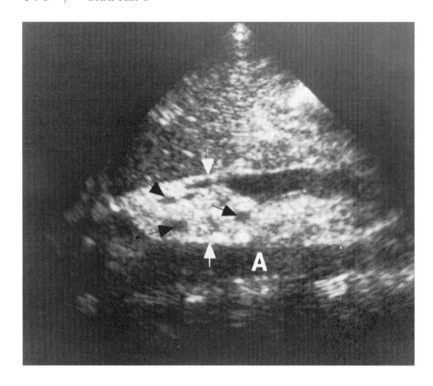

FIG. 8-186. Lesser omental varices in portal hypertension. A 10-year-old girl with portal hypertension accompanying cavernous transformation of the portal vein. In this left paramedian sagittal sonogram, the lesser omentum *(white arrows)* is approximately twice as thick as the abdominal aorta *(A)*. The many hypoechoic areas *(black arrows)* in the omentum are varices.

detection of unsuspected tumors, and (d) identification of anatomic abnormalities that might make transplantation difficult or impossible (496). Although sonography is most commonly used for preoperative imaging, MRI and CT can also play a role, especially in children who are difficult to examine by US and in those with complex anatomy.

Postoperative Imaging

Two types of transplantations are performed in children: whole-liver cadaveric transplants, and reduced-size transplants from a living related donor. Because the postoperative

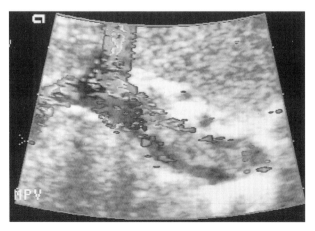

FIG. 8-187. Portal vein thrombosis. A 2-year-old boy with a hypercoagulable state. A color Doppler image shows a partially occluding portal vein thrombus.

appearance is very different, it is essential to know which procedure was performed before examining these patients (495).

In whole-liver transplantation, the hepatic vascular structures are in their expected anatomic location at the hilum. Hepatic artery anastomoses are usually performed end to end, donor to recipient, or the donor celiac axis with part of the aorta is anastomosed to the recipient aorta. The portal vein anastomosis is usually end to end or by means of an interposed graft. The recipient hepatic portion of the IVC is usually resected, and the donor segment of the IVC is interposed. Biliary anastomoses vary; choledochojejunostomy with internal or external stenting and choledocho-choledochostomy with stent are employed most often.

The scarcity of matched donor livers of a size suitable for children has made reduced-size liver transplantation (RSLT) an increasingly common alternative (497). Although several variations have been described, the most commonly performed RSLT utilizes either the entire left hepatic lobe or its lateral segment. Because of size constraints, previous surgery, or abnormalities in abdominal situs, the transplanted segment is not placed in its normal anatomic orientation. Consultation with the surgeon is essential if the locations of donor vessels and ducts and their anastomoses are to be understood.

Common postoperative complications after both types of transplantation include hepatic artery thrombosis, biliary anastomotic leaks (Fig. 8-191) and strictures, perihepatic fluid collections, and hepatic infarction (495). Periportal edema is seen in about 20% of all transplants and is an expected early finding (Fig. 8-192). Doppler sonography is

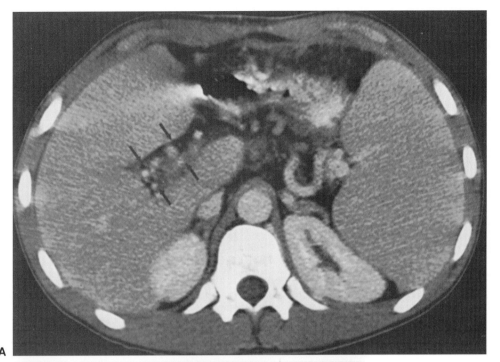

A

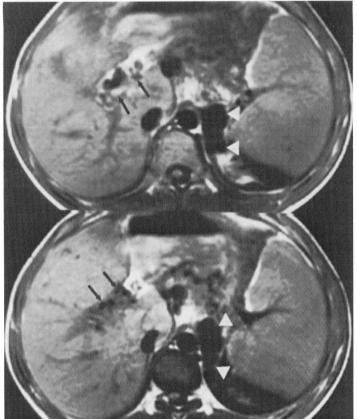

B

FIG. 8-188. Cavernous transformation of the portal vein. A 14-year-old girl with omphalitis as an infant and subsequent portal vein thrombosis. **A:** Contrast-enhanced CT. Note the many collateral vessels *(arrows)* in the porta hepatis. The liver parenchyma appears normal, but there is moderate splenomegaly. **B:** T1-weighted MRI. The cavernous transformation *(arrows)*, splenomegaly, and perisplenic collateral vessels *(arrowheads)* are well demonstrated.

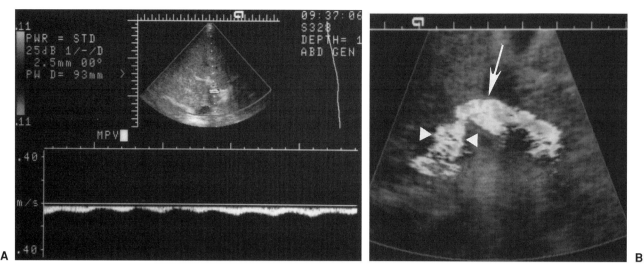

FIG. 8-189. Doppler evaluation of a surgically created portosystemic shunt. A 14-year-old girl with idiopathic portal hypertension after a surgical splenocaval shunt. **A:** A Duplex Doppler tracing of the main portal vein shows hepatofugal flow. **B:** A transverse color Doppler image shows that the splenic vein *(arrow)* drains directly into the inferior vena cava *(arrowheads)*.

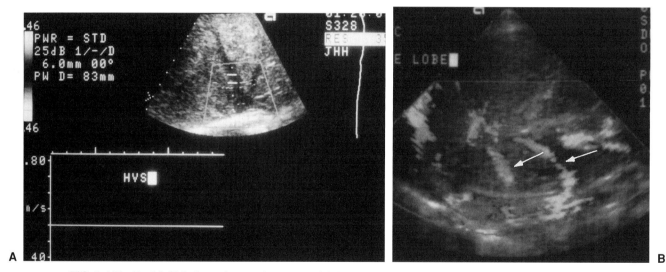

FIG. 8-190. Budd-Chiari syndrome. An 8-year-old girl with hepatic vein occlusion. **A:** A Duplex Doppler tracing shows no flow in the middle hepatic vein. **B:** A sagittal color Doppler image shows enlarged caudate lobe veins *(arrows)* draining directly into the inferior vena cava.

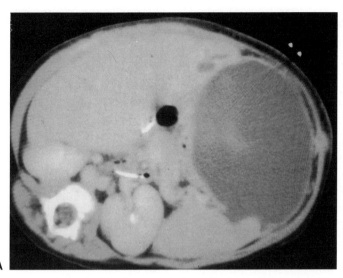
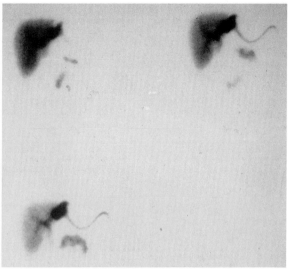

A

B

FIG. 8-191. Postoperative bile leak after reduced-size liver transplant. A: Contrast-enhanced CT shows a large fluid collection adjacent to the cut surface of the transplanted liver. The collection was drained percutaneously. B: Hepatobiliary scintigraphy shows accumulation of tracer outside the liver and drainage into the percutaneous catheter.

routinely performed in the immediate postoperative period and during periods of acute hepatic dysfunction to assess the patency of and hemodynamics in the portal vein and hepatic artery. MRI cholangiography using heavily T2-weighted, fast spin-echo sequences with fat saturation can be helpful in identifying biliary complications (Fig. 8-193).

SPLENIC ABNORMALITIES

Normal Spleen

Although standards for normal splenic size in children have been developed for CT and nuclear medicine, US is the modality most commonly used to evaluate splenic size and texture in the child. Reproducible splenic measurements can be obtained by imaging the spleen in its coronal plane, to include the splenic dome, hilum, and tip. Values for normal splenic size, as a function of age, have been developed (Table 8-10) (498). The normal spleen as seen by US is homogeneous in its echogenicity, has a tapered lower margin, and does not extend below the lower border of the left kidney (Fig. 8-194).

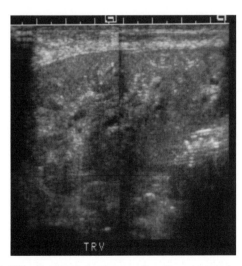

FIG. 8-192. Periportal edema after liver transplantation. A composite transverse ultrasound image shows branching echogenic structures, consistent with periportal edema, coursing along the portal vessels.

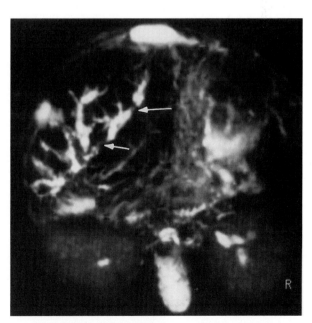

FIG. 8-193. MR cholangiography. A MR cholangiogram in a 1-year-old boy with a reduced-size liver transplant shows a dilated biliary tree with several stenoses (arrows). (Courtesy of Tal Laor, M.D., Boston, MA.)

TABLE 8-10. *Normal splenic size on ultrasonography*

Age (Number of patients)	Length of Spleen (cm)			
	10th %ile	Median	90th %ile	Suggested upper limit
0–3 months (n = 28)	3.3	4.5	5.8	6.0
3–6 months (n = 13)	4.9	5.3	6.4	6.5
6–12 months (n = 17)	5.2	6.2	6.8	7.0
1–2 years (n = 12)	5.4	6.9	7.5	8.0
2–4 years (n = 24)	6.4	7.4	8.6	9.0
4–6 years (n = 39)	6.9	7.8	8.8	9.5
6–8 years (n = 21)	7.0	8.2	9.6	10.0
8–10 years (n = 16)	7.9	9.2	10.5	11.0
10–12 years (n = 17)	8.6	9.9	10.9	11.5
12–15 years (n = 26)	8.7	10.1	11.4	12.0
15–20 years (n = 17)				
Female	9.0	10.0	11.7	12.0
Male	10.1	11.2	12.6	13.0

Source: Rosenberg HK et al (498).

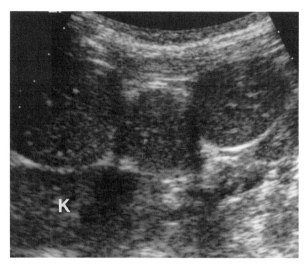

FIG. 8-195. Polysplenia. Three well-defined splenic nodules were noted in the left upper quadrant in this 9-year-old boy. He was born with biliary atresia and had undergone a Kasai procedure at one month of life. *K*, kidney.

Congenital Anomalies

Asplenia and polysplenia are part of the heterotaxy syndromes. In asplenia, complex and severe cardiac anomalies are usually present. Radionuclide scanning, US, and MRI can be used to document the absence of the spleen (499).

In polysplenia, the cardiac anomalies are usually less severe. Multiple splenules may be present along the greater curvature of the stomach. Interruption of the intrahepatic IVC with azygous continuation and preduodenal portal vein are associated anomalies and should be searched for whenever polysplenia is identified. Biliary atresia is also associated with the polysplenia syndrome (Fig. 8-195) (500).

Accessory splenic tissue should not be confused with polysplenia. An accessory spleen is a small, round, soft-tissue structure adjacent to the splenic hilum or along the lower border of an otherwise normal spleen (Fig. 8-196). An accessory spleen is almost always an incidental finding and seldom causes symptoms. Torsion of an accessory spleen is a rare cause of acute abdominal pain (501).

Wandering or ectopic spleen is a condition in which the supporting ligaments of the spleen are lax or do not develop. The spleen lies in an abnormal location. Wandering spleen may cause few or no symptoms, or it may cause acute abdominal pain if complicated by torsion (502). Abdominal US of wandering spleen shows lack of splenic tissue in the left upper quadrant and a soft-tissue mass, the malpositioned spleen, elsewhere in the abdomen. If the echogenicity of the spleen is altered and no vascular signals are demonstrated within it, torsion and infarction should be considered (503). The CT findings of wandering spleen with torsion include abnormal splenic location, inhomogeneous enhancement, and vascular thrombosis (502,503). A whorled appearance of the tissues at the splenic hilum, if seen, represents the twisted splenic pedicle intermixed with fat (504).

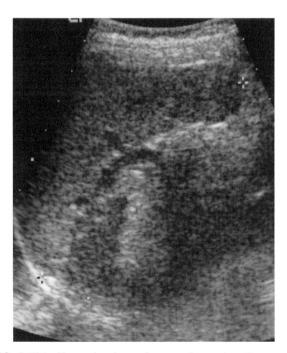

FIG. 8-194. Normal spleen. A coronal scan in a 9-year-old girl demonstrates a normal spleen, measuring 9 cm in length.

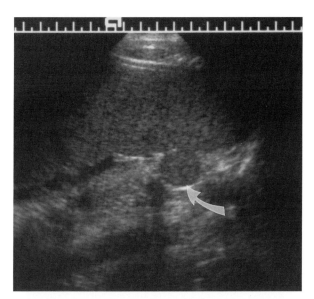

FIG. 8-196. Accessory spleen. Accessory splenic tissue *(arrow)* was an incidental finding in this asymptomatic child. This should not be confused with polysplenia.

Splenomegaly

Chronic liver disease with portal hypertension is one of the most common causes of splenomegaly in children. Although most cases of portal hypertension are clinically evident, an occasional patient will present with splenomegaly as the only sign of the disorder. Whenever an enlarged spleen is seen on a screening abdominal ultrasonogram, the examination should be extended to include Doppler evaluation of the splenic and portal vessels.

Marked enlargement of the spleen can occur with leukemia and lymphoma; there may also be associated distortion of the splenic echotexture (505). Other diseases associated with splenic enlargement in children include viral illness, collagen vascular disease, the hemolytic anemias, and Langerhans cell histiocytosis. Splenic enlargement has been noted in neonates during treatment with extracorporeal membrane oxygenation (ECMO); the cause is felt to be accumulation of damaged blood products in the spleen (506).

Some metabolic disorders cause splenomegaly (Fig. 8-197). Splenic enlargement is almost universal in Gaucher disease, a storage disease caused by a deficiency in glucocerebrosidase, which leads to abnormal accumulations of glucocerebroside. Focal splenic lesions representing clumps of Gaucher cells, infarction, or fibrosis can be seen in the enlarged spleen (507). The splenic lesions of Gaucher disease are also visible on MRI (508).

Splenic enlargement can be seen in both the homozygous and heterozygous forms of sickle cell anemia. In the young child with homozygous sickle cell disease, marked pooling of blood in the spleen, known as splenic sequestration, can lead to splenomegaly (509). Splenomegaly associated with hemorrhage, infarction, or rupture can occur in the heterozy-

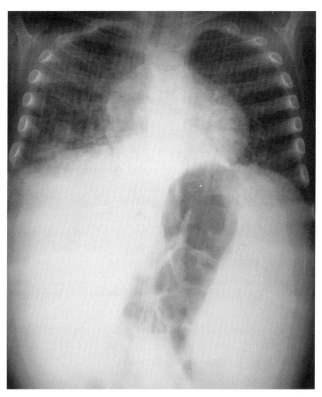

FIG. 8-197. Splenomegaly. A child with Niemann-Pick disease and marked hepatosplenomegaly. This disorder is characterized by accumulation of sphingomyelin in various organs including the spleen, liver, and lung. Note the diffuse interstitial lung disease.

gous forms of sickle cell disease. The classic appearance of recent splenic infarction is that of wedge-shaped defect(s) in the periphery of the spleen, of low density on CT, and hypo- or anechoic on US (Fig. 8-198). A healed infarct is hyperechoic on US (510). Repeated splenic infarctions lead

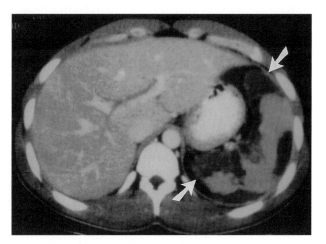

FIG. 8-198. Splenic infarct. Many low-density infarcts are seen in the spleen *(between arrows)* in this patient heterozygous for sickle cell disease. The patient presented with left upper quadrant pain. (Courtesy of Stephen O'Connor, M.D., Boston, MA.)

to shrinkage of the spleen and autosplenectomy, usually by the age of 5 years. A spleen that has undergone autosplenectomy may be small and densely calcified on radiography or CT (511), and it may be impossible to see with US.

Focal Lesions

A splenic cyst can be congenital (primary) or secondary to trauma, infarction, or hydatid disease. Although hydatid disease is the most common cause of splenic cyst worldwide, congenital or epidermoid cysts are more common in North America (512). A congenital splenic cyst may be an incidental finding at US or it may present as a left upper quadrant mass or as local discomfort. Splenic cysts often occur in a readily recognized pattern, i.e., in a healthy adolescent girl with minor abdominal symptoms and an enormous left upper quadrant mass (513).

On imaging studies, congenital splenic cysts are usually solitary, but "daughter" cysts may be present. A congenital splenic cyst can become infected and may rupture or bleed after trauma to the abdomen (514). The cyst is surrounded by a rim of normal splenic tissue (Fig. 8-199). It may be echogenic on US or of high density on CT if the cyst contains fat or cholesterol or has been complicated by hemorrhage or infection (Fig. 8-200) (512). Congenital splenic cysts are lined by epithelium, which distinguishes them from splenic pseudocysts (secondary cysts), which do not have an epithelial lining and are felt to be secondary to trauma or infarction.

Conditions predisposing to splenic abscess include bacterial endocarditis, sickle cell disease, trauma, and pyogenic infection elsewhere. A splenic abscess usually appears on

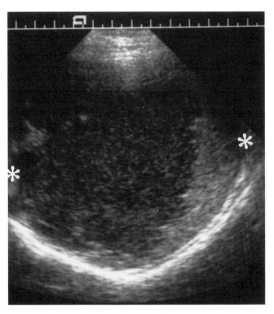

FIG. 8-200. Epidermoid cyst. A 13-year-old boy with a 1-month history of left upper quadrant pain. A transverse view of the spleen *(between asterisks)* shows a unilocular lesion containing debris. It contained "greasy yellow fluid" and was an epidermoid cyst.

US as a sonolucent mass. There may be septations within the mass or internal echogenicity caused by debris. Highly echogenic material within the abscess may represent gas (515). Multiple small sonolucent lesions are characteristic US findings of splenic involvement with candidiasis. On CT, the most common pattern is one of numerous round lesions of low attenuation (516).

Cat-scratch disease is an infection thought to be caused by a gram-negative organism. Although most cases are confined to regional lymph nodes, splenic and hepatic involvement have been described. On CT, the lesions are of low attenuation and become more apparent with the administration of contrast material (517). US shows round hypoechoic lesions (Fig. 8-201). The lesions of cat-scratch disease may calcify over time (518). Other causes of splenic calcification are tuberculosis, histoplasmosis, and chronic granulomatous disease of childhood (Fig. 8-202).

Splenic tumors, except for leukemia and lymphoma, are exceedingly rare. Arteriovenous and lymphatic malformations can occur in the spleen; the lymphatic lesions can be unilocular or contain numerous cystic spaces. Lymphatic malformations of other parts of the body, such as the mediastinum, axilla, neck, and abdominal viscera, are seen in some patients with lymphatic malformations of the spleen (Fig. 8-203) (519).

Abdominal trauma and its effects on the spleen are discussed later in this chapter. Nontraumatic rupture of the spleen can occur in the setting of infectious mononucleosis (520). The imaging findings are similar to those seen in traumatic rupture.

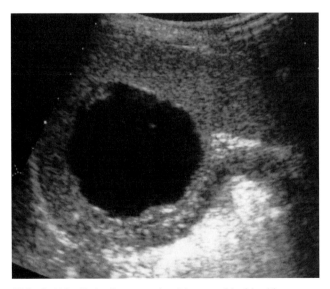

FIG. 8-199. Splenic cyst. An 11-year-old girl with severe abdominal pain with no history of trauma. A solitary unilocular cyst was noted in the upper pole of the spleen. Presumed to be congenital, the cyst has been followed for 3 years and has not changed.

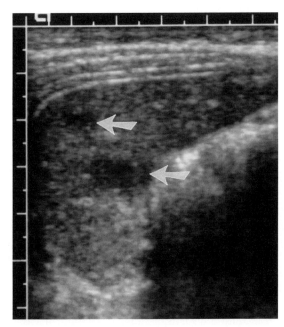

FIG. 8-201. Splenic granulomata. A 7-year old girl presented with 2 weeks of high fever. Abdominal sonography shows numerous low-density lesions in the spleen *(arrows)*. Liver lesions were also noted. Biopsy of one of the splenic lesions showed granulomatous inflammation, but an organism was never found. The patient was presumed to have cat-scratch disease.

PANCREATIC ABNORMALITIES

Normal Pancreas

US is usually the first imaging modality for pancreatic disease in children. The normal pancreas has an echogenicity equal to or slightly greater than that of liver. Siegel and

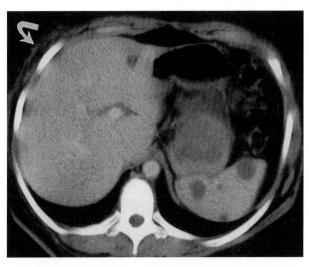

FIG. 8-203. Lymphatic malformations. Many well-defined low-attenuation lesions were noted in the spleen in this 16-year-old girl with a lymphatic malformation of the right upper extremity and chest wall. Although never biopsied, the splenic lesions are apparently also lymphatic malformations. Note the involvement of the right chest wall *(curved arrow)*.

colleagues have shown that pancreatic dimensions correlate with age (521). The head and tail of the pancreas are usually of similar size and are wider than the pancreatic body (Fig. 8-204). The pancreatic duct, if visible, is an echogenic line usually less than 1 mm wide (521).

Developmental Abnormalities

In fetal life the pancreas consists of a dorsal and a ventral bud. Both buds have ducts, which drain separately into the

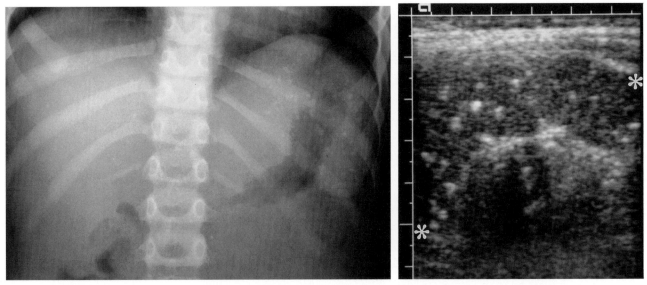

FIG. 8-202. Splenic calcification. A: A radiograph of the upper abdomen shows many calcifications in the liver and spleen in this 4-year-old girl, who had been treated for pulmonary tuberculosis. B: The splenic calcifications are well seen on ultrasound as echogenic foci *(asterisks mark the spleen)*.

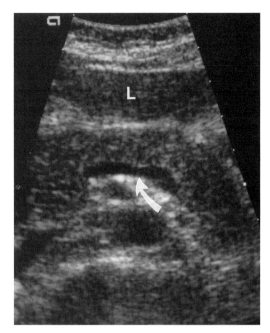

FIG. 8-204. Normal pancreas. Transverse view of the pancreas in this 10-year-old girl shows normal anatomy. The pancreas sits on the splenic vein *(curved arrow). L,* liver.

duodenum. The two buds usually fuse before birth. The dorsal bud forms the tail, body, and part of the head of the pancreas; the ventral bud evolves into the uncinate process of the head. After fusion, the ventral duct joins the part of the dorsal duct in the pancreatic head to form the main pancreatic duct (duct of Wirsung), which drains most of the pancreas. The remainder of the dorsal duct may regress or persist as the accessory pancreatic duct (duct of Santorini).

In pancreas divisum, the ventral and dorsal buds do not fuse. Thus the pancreas derived from the dorsal bud, the larger part, must drain through the accessory duct. The main duct drains the smaller (ventral) pancreas. Pancreas divisum has been implicated as a cause of acute pancreatitis. The small size of the accessory duct, required to carry most of the pancreatic secretions, is thought to impede their flow (522). US is typically unable to diagnose pancreas divisum. Thin-section CT may show the separate dorsal and ventral moieties (523), and ERCP can convincingly show the ductal anatomy.

Annular pancreas usually coexists with intrinsic duodenal stenosis or atresia. While most cases of annular pancreas are diagnosed in infancy during repair of duodenal atresia or stenosis, some cases are discovered later in life because of intermittent nausea and vomiting. Annular pancreas appears on cross-sectional imaging as a soft-tissue mass contiguous with the pancreas and encircling the duodenum (523,524).

A duplication cyst of the foregut communicating with the pancreatic duct is an unusual cause of intermittent abdominal pain, nausea, and vomiting. Laboratory values may be normal. This rare anomaly is suggested by an irregular cyst, with a thickened wall, in the pancreas. Debris may be present in the cyst. ERCP is diagnostic if there is free communication (Fig. 8-205).

Hereditary Disorders

Cystic fibrosis (CF) was named for the pathologic changes in the pancreas. The pathologic changes range from mild (accumulation of mucus in the ducts) to severe (total obstruction of the ducts and ductules by mucus, leading to atrophy,

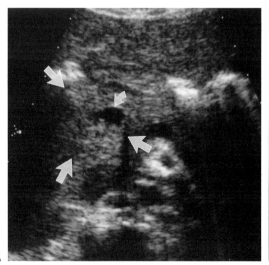

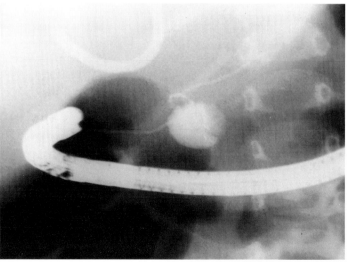

FIG. 8-205. Duplication cyst. This 18-month-old boy was referred for ultrasonography because of recurrent pancreatitis. A transverse view of the pancreatic head **(A)** showed it to be enlarged *(straight arrows)* and to contain a small cyst *(curved arrow).* A subsequent ERCP **(B)** showed a well-defined collection of contrast, the duplication, communicating with the pancreatic duct. The diagnosis of duplication cyst was confirmed at surgery.

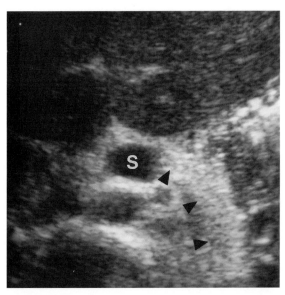

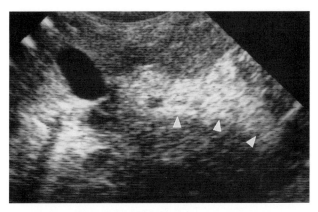

FIG. 8-208. Schwachman-Diamond syndrome. An 18-month-old with Schwachman-Diamond syndrome, failure to thrive, neutropenia, and relapsing fevers. The pancreas *(arrowheads)* is extremely echogenic.

FIG. 8-206. Cystic fibrosis. The pancreas *(arrowheads)* is small and densely echogenic. *S,* superior mesenteric vein.

fibrosis, and cyst formation. Severe pancreatic dysfunction is seen in many patients with CF.

On US, the pancreas of a patient with CF is usually small and echogenic because of replacement with fat and fibrous tissue (Figs. 8-206 and 8-207) (525,526); it is an example of the white pancreas described by Schneider (527). Other causes of white (i.e., hyperechoic) pancreas include the Shwachman-Diamond syndrome (exocrine pancreatic insufficiency and bone marrow dysfunction), hemosiderosis, and chronic pancreatitis (Fig. 8-208). On CT, the pancreas of CF is typically small and has the attenuation value of fat (523,526). Calcifications and small cysts may be seen by either US or CT. If the calcification is severe enough, it will be visible by plain film. Total replacement of the pancreas

with macroscopic cysts, termed pancreatic cystosis, can occur in CF and should not be mistaken for a cystic tumor (528).

Von Hippel-Lindau disease (VHLD) is an autosomal dominant condition characterized by CNS hemangioblastomas, retinal angiomas, and visceral lesions, including renal cysts and carcinomas, pheochromocytomas, and cysts of the adrenal glands, liver, spleen, mesentery, and epididymis. The pancreatic lesions seen in this disease include cysts and (very rarely in children) microcystic adenomas and islet cell tumors (529). The cysts, the most common lesions (Fig. 8-209), may be numerous or few and vary in size. Cystic replacement of the pancreas can occur. Pancreatic lesions may be the first or only manifestation of VHLD, which may be important when there is a family history of the disorder. The disease is also discussed in Chapter 2.

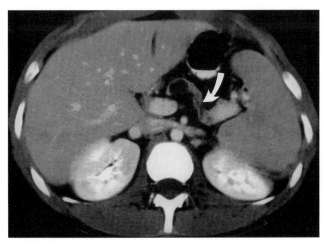

FIG. 8-207. Atrophic pancreas in cystic fibrosis. Young woman with cystic fibrosis. The pancreas *(arrow)* is small and contains many small cysts.

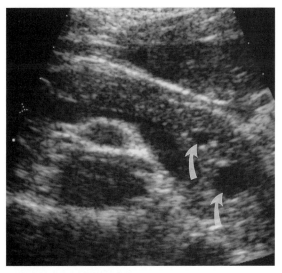

FIG. 8-209. Von Hippel-Lindau disease. There are two cysts *(curved arrows)* in the pancreas of this young man with Von Hippel-Lindau disease. He also had bilateral renal cysts. A cerebellar hemangioblastoma had been resected.

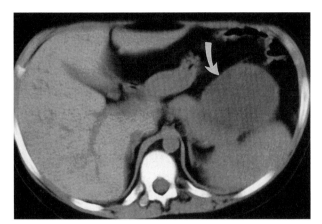

FIG. 8-210. Pseudocyst. This 13-year-old boy with a transplanted kidney developed two pancreatic pseudocysts after pancreatitis secondary to valproic acid therapy. One of them, shown here, is anterior to the distal pancreas *(curved arrow).*

Autosomal dominant polycystic kidney disease is sometimes associated with cysts in the pancreas.

Pseudocysts and Congenital Cysts

A pseudocyst secondary to trauma or inflammation is the most commonly encountered cystic lesion of the pancreas. A pseudocyst is usually a well-defined fluid collection with a thick wall. The fluid is hypoechoic on US and of water attenuation on CT unless there has been hemorrhage or infection. A history of trauma or pancreatitis is often obtained (Fig. 8-210). In early childhood, an unexplained pseudocyst suggests child abuse.

True congenital pancreatic cysts are extremely rare (530). A true cyst of the pancreas is lined by epithelium, as opposed to a pseudocyst, which has only a fibrous wall. Characteristics which distinguish a congenital cyst from a pseudocyst are its thinner wall, loculations or septations within the cyst, and normal-appearing adjacent pancreatic tissue.

Pancreatic Tumors

Pancreatic tumors are rare in children. Grosfeld et al. reported only 13 neoplasms at two institutions over a 20-year period (531). Six were malignant (rhabdomyosarcoma 2, carcinoma 4); seven were benign (insulinoma 5, mucinous cystadenoma 2). Other tumors of the pancreas include nonfunctioning islet cell tumors and secondary lesions (neuroblastoma, Burkitt lymphoma). Burkitt lymphoma causes the pancreas to appear diffusely and irregularly enlarged (Fig. 8-211) (532).

Mucinous cystadenoma deserves special mention. Although usually described as a benign tumor, it is considered premalignant. It is seen most commonly in females, in the body and tail of the pancreas. It can become quite large.

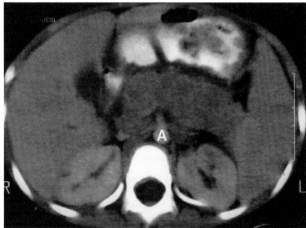

A

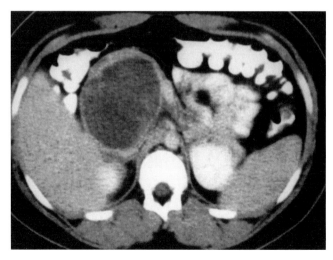

B

FIG. 8-211. Burkitt lymphoma. Ultrasonography **(A)** and computed tomography **(B)** show nodular tumorous enlargement of the pancreas in this 4-year-old boy with stage IV Burkitt lymphoma. *A,* aorta; *L,* liver.

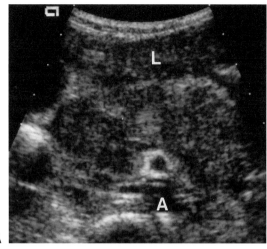

FIG. 8-212. Mucinous cystadenoma. This 14-year-old girl presented with right upper quadrant pain, nausea, and vomiting. CT shows a cystic mass in the head of the pancreas. Although the cyst wall is well defined, its thickness varies.

While it is often multilocular, when unilocular it can be confused with a pancreatic pseudocyst (Fig. 8-212) (533).

Pancreatitis

Causes of acute pancreatitis in childhood include infection (especially viral), drug toxicity (L-asparaginase, valproic acid, steroids, acetaminophen), peptic disease, gallstones, cystic fibrosis, structural anomalies (pancreas divisum, pancreatic intestinal duplication cyst), Kawasaki disease, and accidental and nonaccidental trauma (534). Trauma, a common cause of pancreatitis in childhood, is discussed later in this chapter. Some cases of pancreatitis are idiopathic.

The diagnosis of acute pancreatitis is based on the history, physical examination, and laboratory data. The classic symptoms are nausea, vomiting, and abdominal pain. Elevated levels of amylase and lipase in the serum and amylase in the urine are evidence of pancreatitis. Imaging, especially US, is often employed. While the examination may be negative, pancreatic enlargement, dilatation of the duct, and abnormal echogenicity are signs of acute pancreatitis (Fig. 8-213) (521).

CT may show a normal-sized or enlarged pancreas. Fluid collections may be demonstrated in the pancreas. Extrapancreatic fluid collections can be seen in children with acute pancreatitis; they often diminish or resolve altogether without intervention (535).

While cross-sectional imaging helps confirm the diagnosis of acute pancreatitis in confusing or difficult cases, it probably plays a greater role in searching for structural causes of pancreatitis and for consequences of the process such as pseudocyst. Pancreatic pseudocyst occurs after about 10% of cases of pancreatitis (see Fig. 8-210) (534).

Recurrent pancreatitis is seen in children with CF, after chemotherapy, and with hereditary pancreatitis. However, it is often idiopathic. ERCP is used to evaluate the patient with recurrent pancreatitis with no demonstrable cause. The goal of ERCP is to outline the anatomy of the biliary and pancreatic ductal systems and uncover a structural cause (536).

Chronic fibrosing pancreatitis, a rare entity of unknown cause, is histologically characterized by bands of collagenous tissue surround normal-appearing acini. Pancreatic autodigestion, often present in acute pancreatitis, is not seen in chronic fibrosing pancreatitis. Diffuse enlargement of the entire pancreas may be seen, or there may be focal enlargement of the pancreatic head simulating a mass. Compression of the common bile duct by the enlarged pancreas can cause obstructive jaundice (537).

Hereditary pancreatitis is an autosomal dominant condition characterized by recurrent episodes of abdominal pain beginning in childhood. Marked ductal dilatation and large round ductal calcifications are hallmarks of this disorder (Figs. 8-214 and 8-215). Pancreatic carcinoma can be a late complication (538).

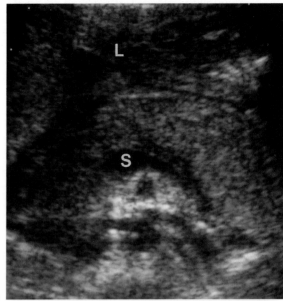

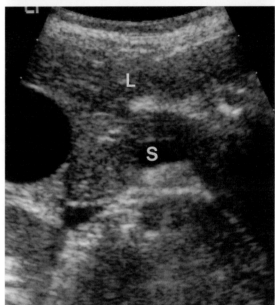

FIG. 8-213. Acute pancreatitis. This 4-year-old girl presented with abdominal pain, vomiting, and jaundice. Laboratory studies suggested hepatitis and pancreatitis. Ultrasonography **(A)** shows generalized enlargement of the pancreas. **B:** Follow-up examination. The pancreas is now normal. A distended gallbladder is next to the pancreatic head. *L,* liver; *S,* splenic vein.

IMAGING OF BLUNT ABDOMINAL TRAUMA

Injuries are the most common cause of death in children between their first and twentieth birthdays. In 1986, over 22,000 children died from trauma in the United States, 600,000 were hospitalized, and 16 million received treatment in emergency departments. Blunt abdominal injury accounts for approximately 5% of pediatric trauma admissions

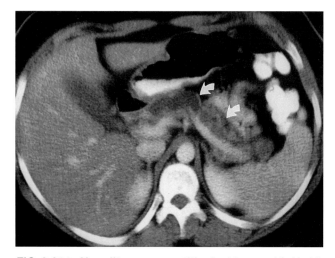

FIG. 8-214. Hereditary pancreatitis. An 18-year-old girl with epigastric pain, elevated serum amylase and lipase, and a family history of pancreatitis. CT shows an atrophic pancreas *(arrows)* and a dilated pancreatic duct due to chronic pancreatitis.

and is most commonly caused by motor vehicle accidents, falls, blows to the abdomen, and child abuse (539).

CT has become the primary imaging tool in blunt abdominal trauma. It has almost entirely replaced peritoneal lavage and scintigraphy in hemodynamically stable patients, and it has contributed to a continuing reduction in exploratory laparotomy (540). Although sonography has been suggested as a rapid, readily available alternative, the current literature suggests that US cannot match the accuracy of CT in detecting and depicting pediatric abdominal injuries (541). This section will review the identification of children at high and low risk of abdominal injury, CT technique, patterns of injury unique to children, and the clinical implications and outcomes of CT appearances after blunt trauma.

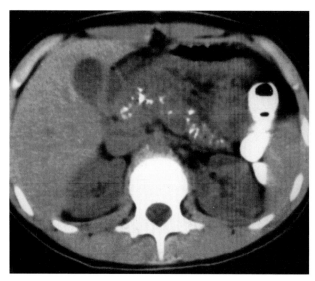

FIG. 8-215. Pancreatic calcifications. Irregular calcifications throughout the pancreas of this patient with hereditary pancreatitis.

Radiographic Evaluation

After the initial physical examination, a supine radiograph of the abdomen and pelvis should be obtained to identify pelvic fractures, peritoneal air or fluid, and displacement of normal structures by hematoma. A supine film is of course much less sensitive to a small pneumoperitoneum than an upright film. Diagnostic peritoneal lavage is indicated, although only rarely, in the unstable patient with suspected abdominal bleeding or intestinal perforation, or if CT is not available.

Computed Tomography

Indications

Because children are often unable to report their symptoms and localization of pain can be difficult, many centers use the CT scan to screen for significant occult intraabdominal injury. Although there is still debate about specific indications for CT, a group of variables associated with a significantly higher risk of abdominal injury has been identified (Table 8-11) (540,542).

One of the most important clinical findings is the presence of a lap-belt ecchymosis (Fig. 8-216). It is a high-risk indicator of intraabdominal injury and should prompt a careful search for lumbar spine, bowel, and bladder injuries. Although lap-belt injuries are present in only a minority of children examined with CT after blunt trauma, they account for up to 68% of all identified bowel and thoracolumbar spine injuries (543,544). Shearing forces due to rapid deceleration are distributed against the small area of the lap belt resulting in compression of a bowel loop or some other viscus between the seat belt and the spine. Migration of the

TABLE 8-11. *Variables associated with increased risk for significant abdominal injury by logistic regression*

Variable	Odds ratio[a]	p Value
Mechanism of injury		
Lap belt ecchymosis	7.17	.0001
Fall or bicycle injury	2.80	.0001
Abuse or assault	2.09	.0001
Gross hematuria	4.20	.0001
Abdominal tenderness	3.29	.0001
Trauma score ≤12	2.75	.0005
Fractured pelvis	2.62	.008
Hematocrit <30%	2.34	.0005
Chest trauma[b]	2.06	.047
Abdominal distension	1.99	.006
Absent bowel sounds	1.72	.028

[a] Compared to patients without the individual variable.

[b] Chest trauma is defined as the presence of thoracic abrasions or contusions on physical examination, rib or thoracic spine fracture, hemothorax, pneumothorax, parenchymal opacification, or hematoma on the initial plain radiograph of the chest.

Table modified from Taylor et al (540).

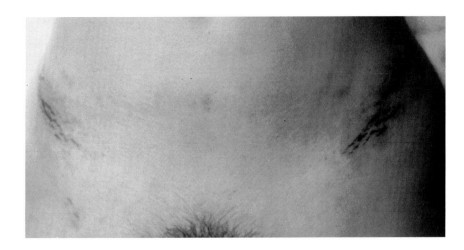

FIG. 8-216. Lap-belt ecchymosis. Photograph of a girl injured as a passenger in a motor vehicle accident shows typical linear, oblique lap-belt ecchymoses across the anterior abdominal wall. (Courtesy of Steven Fishman, M.D., Boston, MA.)

belt up the abdominal wall, the relative lack of abdominal wall protective thickness, and their higher center of gravity make children especially vulnerable to acute hyperflexion injury of the upper lumbar spine during sudden deceleration.

Gross hematuria also appears to be a strong indicator of underlying abdominal injuries. The most commonly injured organ in children with hematuria is not the kidney (26%) but rather the spleen (37%) or liver (33%) (545). The high risk of nonurinary injuries in children with gross hematuria suggests CT rather than excretory urography for initial evaluation. However, the association between microscopic hematuria and abdominal injury is high only in children with other abdominal signs of trauma. Asymptomatic hematuria is a low-yield indication of underlying injury (545,546).

Neurologic impairment is another common reason for requesting abdominal CT examination after trauma. Comatose children (Glasgow Coma Scale <8) who have signs referable to the abdomen are at risk for significant abdominal injury. However, neurologic impairment in the absence of abdominal signs or symptoms is only a low-yield indication for abdominal CT (547). Abdominal injuries in this group are rare and typically minor.

Abdominal CT is generally contraindicated in the presence of shock or extraabdominal life-threatening injury. Because CT is not free or infinitely available, the decision to obtain an emergency abdominal CT after blunt trauma must be based on the likelihood of underlying injury. The Abdominal Injury Score (AIS) has been developed as a triage tool for determining the risk of abdominal injury after blunt trauma in children (542). It is derived from clinical features at presentation that, based on a logistic regression model, predict the presence of abdominal injury. The probability of abdominal injury can be estimated by adding the individual partial scores (Table 8-12) and applying the sum to the nomogram (Fig. 8-217). For example, a child with a lap belt injury (partial score = 24), gross hematuria (partial score = 14), abdominal tenderness (partial score = 12), and a

Trauma Score of 15 (partial score = 0) would have a total AIS of 50 and a predicted probability of significant abdominal injury of approximately 65% (Fig. 8-217). Low scores predict a low risk of abdominal injury; higher scores, a progressively higher risk. Using the AIS, there is a good correlation between the observed and predicted frequencies of abdominal injury (542).

Technique

To obtain a rapid and diagnostically accurate computed tomogram, careful attention to technique is essential. Most injured children can be examined without sedation. A preliminary anteroposterior scout image of the abdomen and lower chest is obtained in all cases. A lateral scout image

TABLE 8-12. *Abdominal injury score*

Features of presentation	Score
Mechanism of injury	4
MVA, pasenger	8
MVA, pedestrian	15
Fall	15
Bicycle	12
Abuse or assault	24
Lap belt	0
Other	
Trauma score ≤12	10
Abdominal tenderness	12
Abdominal distension	7
Absent bowel sounds	5
Fracture of pelvis	10
Gross hematuria	14
Chest trauma	7
Hematocrit <30%	9

MVA, motor vehicle accident.
From Taylor et al (542)

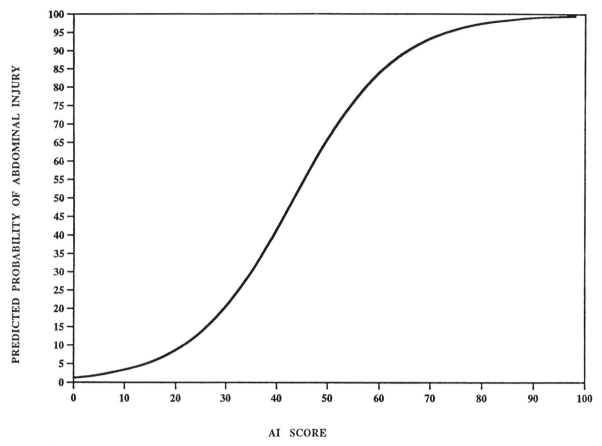

FIG. 8-217. Abdominal Injury Score. Nomogram for predicting the risk of abdominal injury in children after blunt trauma. See text for details. Modified from Taylor et al. (542).

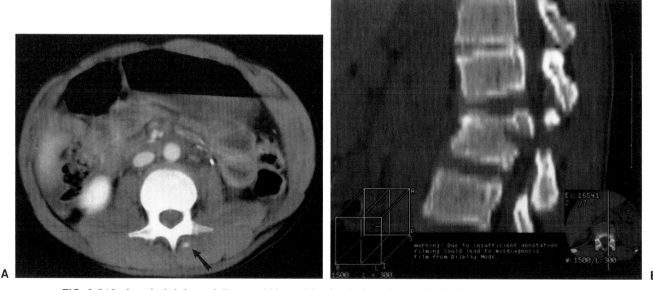

FIG. 8-218. Lap-belt injury. A 7-year-old boy with a lap-belt ecchymosis. **A:** Abdominal CT at the level of the L1 vertebral body shows only small radiodensities posterior to the left lamina *(arrow).* **B:** Sagittal reconstruction of spiral CT of the lumbar spine shows a Chance-type fracture of L1.

TABLE 8-13. *Location of intra-abdominal injury in 326 injured children*

Organ	Number (%)
Liver	118 (36)
Spleen	112 (34)
Kidney	73 (22)
Pancreas	20 (6)
Adrenal	36 (11)
Bowel	26 (8)
Bladder	8 (2)
Shock Bowel	34 (10)
Total	427[a]

[a] 70 patients (21%) had injury to two or more intraabdominal organs.

Table modified from Taylor and Sivit (548).

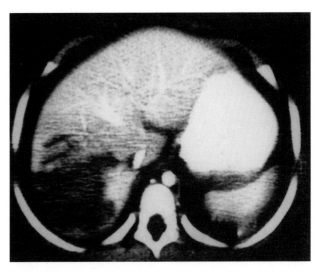

FIG. 8-220. Liver hematoma. A 4-year-old girl in a motor vehicle accident. CT shows a large hematoma of the posterior segment of the right lobe of the liver with extension to the lateral border of the inferior vena cava.

is recommended for children with lap-belt marks across the abdomen. Significant lumbar spine injuries can be missed on CT when lateral preliminary images are not obtained (Fig. 8-218). The abdomen should be examined using spiral technique or a dynamic sequence of incremental 8- to 10-mm sections through the entire abdomen, starting a few centimeters above the diaphragm and extending through the bony pelvis. Enhancement given by rapid intravenous injection is imperative for the identification of visceral injury. Extensive imaging without intravenous contrast is not indicated in the acute trauma situation.

Although this is controversial, many pediatric radiologists do not use oral contrast routinely when scanning injured children. It often remains in the stomach, with only poor opacification of the small bowel, and has not been helpful in identifying bowel injury. However, oral contrast may be useful in pancreatic injury. Please refer to Chapter 1 for additional information on CT techniques in children.

Specific Injuries

Solid Organ Injury

Table 8-13 shows the distribution of abdominal injuries in a large series of children scanned after blunt trauma. Up to 21% of children with abdominal injury have injury to more than one organ (548). In children, injury to the liver is common. Up to 83% of injuries occur in the larger, more exposed right lobe (Fig. 8-219), the posterior segment of the right lobe being injured most often (Fig. 8-220) (549). Periportal lucency in the setting of trauma may represent either hemorrhage or edema secondary to vigorous hydration (Fig. 8-221) (550). It is seen in up to 79% of children with

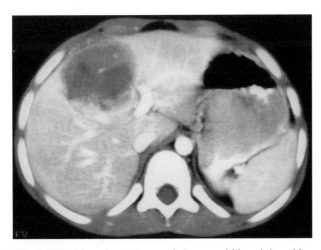

FIG. 8-219. Liver hematoma. A 6-year-old boy injured in a fall. CT through the upper abdomen shows a large hematoma in the anterior segment of the right lobe of the liver. The patient was treated conservatively.

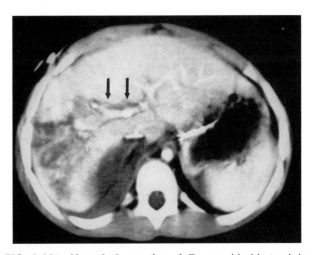

FIG. 8-221. Hepatic laceration. A 7-year-old girl struck by a car. CT shows irregular laceration of the right lobe of the liver and periportal lucencies medial to the injury *(arrows)*. Note the associated right adrenal hematoma and the collapsed inferior vena cava.

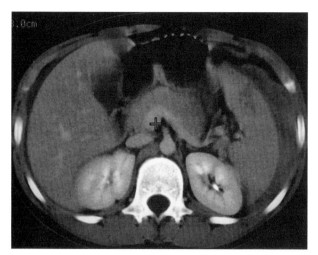

FIG. 8-222. Splenic laceration. A 13-year-old boy injured while roller-skating. CT shows a small laceration in the anterior part of the spleen and a perisplenic sentinel clot.

hepatic injury and is associated with physiologic instability and a higher (approximately 13%) mortality rate (551).

Splenic injuries are also quite common in children. The majority of splenic injuries are associated with a perisplenic sentinel clot or a hemoperitoneum (Fig 8-222) (552). It is important to recognize streak artifacts from overlying ribs and inhomogeneous enhancement of the splenic parenchyma due to the rapidity of the bolus contrast enhancement; these are common causes of the heterogeneous appearance of normal splenic parenchyma. The compliant nature of the chest wall in children often allows upper abdominal and lung injury; the liver and spleen may sustain extensive injury despite the absence of rib fractures.

Although grading systems have been developed for the CT categorization of hepatic and splenic injuries, their accuracy in predicting clinical outcome has not been encouraging (553,554). In children, the size and extent of injury on CT do not correlate well with the need for operative management (555). Even large parenchymal hematomas or lacerations usually heal without surgery (Fig. 8-223).

The kidney is the most commonly injured organ in the retroperitoneum (Fig. 8-224). Parenchymal contusions and incomplete lacerations account for the majority of renal injuries (40% to 60%), followed by complete lacerations (20% to 47%) and multifragment shattered kidney (4% to 14%). Arterial injury is the least common pattern of injury (5% to 9%) (556,557). The presence of perirenal or periureteric fluid is not a good predictor of the extent of renal injury. However, fluid collections in the anterior pararenal space, psoas, and interfascial spaces are often associated with significant renal injury (557). Fortunately, complete healing and preservation of significant renal function are possible in most cases without surgery (Fig. 8-225). Large, persistent urinomas often become infected and may require surgical drainage. In addition, renovascular injury with incomplete

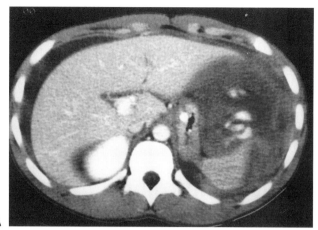

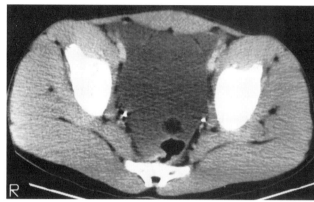

FIG. 8-223. Splenic fracture. A 15-year-old boy hit by car. CT of the upper abdomen **(A)** shows a splenic fracture with a large perisplenic hematoma. Despite a large amount of blood in the pelvis **(B)**, this patient was successfully treated without surgical intervention.

occlusion of a renal artery may cause hypertension and require a revascularization procedure.

Injury to the pancreas, unlike other solid viscera, can be difficult to identify with CT (Fig. 8-226) (558). There may be little change in parenchymal density and minimal separa-

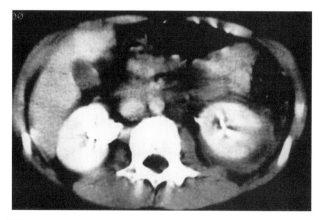

FIG. 8-224. Renal laceration. An 8-year-old boy injured after bicycle accident. CT shows a laceration of the left kidney extending to the lateral renal margin. There is a perinephric hematoma.

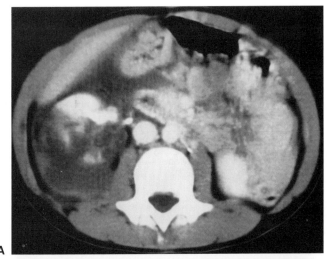

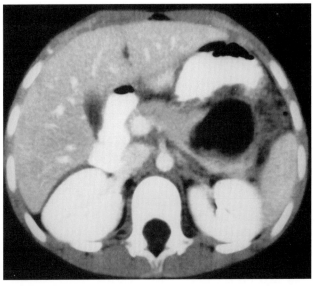

FIG. 8-227. Traumatic pancreatic pseudocyst. An 8-year-old boy fell on his bicycle handlebars 2 weeks previously. CT shows a pseudocyst arising from the pancreatic tail. Note the irregular margins of the cyst and the adjacent inflammatory reaction.

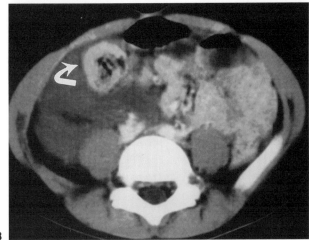

FIG. 8-225. Renal fracture. A 6-year-old boy struck by a car. CT shows a shattered lower pole of the right kidney **(A)**, and a perinephric hematoma that extends inferiorly **(B)** and displaces the right colon medially *(arrow)*. No surgical treatment was necessary.

tion of pancreatic fragments during the acute phase. The presence of fluid in the lesser sac is a useful marker. It is present in up to 72% of children with pancreatic injury and is rare (<1%) in children without this injury (558). Surgical exploration is necessary in over half of children with pancreatic injury for repair of ductal disruption or drainage of a pseudocyst (Fig. 8-227).

Hematoma or laceration of the adrenal gland occurs in approximately 3% of children with abdominal trauma and is usually associated with injury to other intraabdominal organs (Fig. 8-228). These injuries are typically unilateral and are

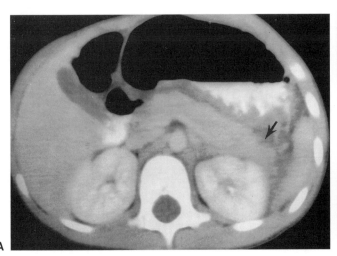

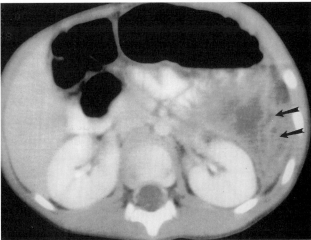

FIG. 8-226. Pancreatic Injury. A 4-year-old boy with abdominal pain and elevated serum amylase after a car accident. CT images through the upper abdomen **(A** and **B)** show a fracture of the pancreatic tail *(arrow)* and fluid in the peripancreatic and left anterior pararenal spaces *(arrows)*.

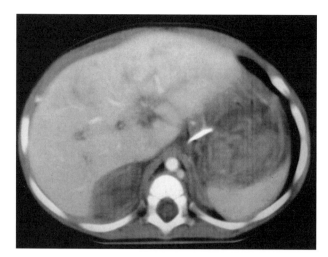

FIG. 8-228. Adrenal hematoma. A 2-year-old girl injured by her caretaker. CT shows a right adrenal hematoma.

more common on the right. Adrenal hematomas rarely or never require surgical treatment and do not result in clinically evident adrenal insufficiency (559).

Peritoneal Fluid

Peritoneal fluid occurs in over 60% of children with significant abdominal injuries. Commonly associated injuries include hepatic and splenic injury (74%), retroperitoneal hematoma (5%), isolated pelvic fracture (5%), and bowel or bladder injury (5%). Children with hemoperitoneum tend to have more severe splenic injuries, and many of them have injuries to more than one abdominal organ (548). The amount of hemoperitoneum indicates the cumulative amount of bleeding since injury. Larger peritoneal fluid collections are associated with an increased frequency of systemic hypotension, greater need for surgical intervention, and higher mortality (560). However, a large hemoperitoneum does not necessarily indicate either continuing hemorrhage or the need for surgical exploration. In a large series of patients, only 23% of children with solid organ injury and a large hemoperitoneum required laparotomy (548).

Peritoneal fluid collections may represent blood, intestinal contents, extravasated unopacified urine, or fluid instilled during diagnostic peritoneal lavage. Because the density of hemoperitoneum is variable (15–75 HU), it is difficult to determine the composition of peritoneal fluid on CT imaging (561). Although small amounts of peritoneal fluid may be found in the cul-de-sac without any clear cause, these unexplained fluid collections are uncommon (2%) in the setting of blunt trauma (548). The finding of focal peritoneal fluid collections or collections of moderate size in the absence of demonstrable solid organ injury or pelvic fracture should suggest bowel or bladder perforation (560).

On occasion, active peritoneal hemorrhage can be demonstrated with CT by identifying a dense collection of extrava-

sated intravascular contrast associated with either a large hematoma or hemoperitoneum. The CT attenuation of the hemoperitoneum may be inhomogeneous because of incomplete mixing of opacified and unopacified blood (Fig. 8-229) (562). Showing active hemorrhage by CT appears to be more common in children with solid organ injury than in adults. Although many of these children are hemodynamically unstable and require urgent surgical intervention, most of them survive (563).

Hollow Organ Injury

Injury to the GI tract or mesentery is present in less than 10% of children after blunt trauma (564). CT findings can

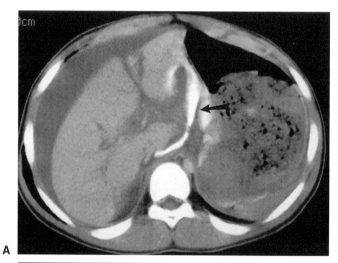

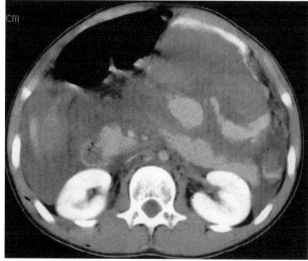

FIG. 8-229. Active arterial bleeding. A 13-year-old boy injured as a passenger in a motor vehicle accident. CT through the upper abdomen **(A)** shows a dense jet of contrast-enhanced blood along the medial surface of the liver *(arrow)*. A lower CT section **(B)** shows a large soft-tissue clot with extravasated dense blood layering beneath the anterior abdominal wall. At laparotomy, several tears of the hepatic artery were repaired. From Taylor et al. (563).

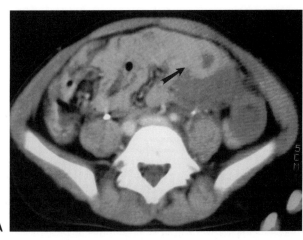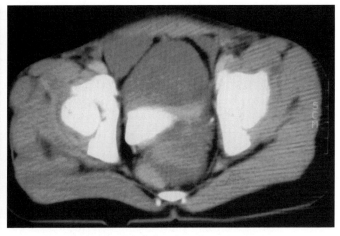

FIG. 8-230. Bowel injury. An 8-year-old girl run over by a car. **(A)** CT through lower abdomen shows focal thickening of a single loop of bowel *(arrow)*, surrounded by peritoneal fluid. CT through the pelvis **(B)** shows a moderate peritoneal fluid collection in the pouch of Douglas. No solid organ injuries were identified by CT. A tear of the jejunum was repaired at laparotomy.

be subtle and nonspecific (Figs. 8-230 and 8-231) (565). Despite these limitations, the CT diagnosis of bowel injury can be made by detecting any one of the following: pneumoperitoneum, bowel wall thickening, or unexplained peritoneal fluid (fluid present without associated pelvic fracture or solid organ injury). Pneumoperitoneum is detected in as few as 30% to 40% of patients with intestinal injury and is not a sensitive test for bowel disruption (564). Similarly, the size of the pneumoperitoneum does not correlate with the degree of bowel injury. Even large tears may seal quickly, with little or no air escaping into the peritoneum. Bowel injury may result in nonperforating, ischemic injury and present later as small bowel obstruction due to a stricture or adhesions (566).

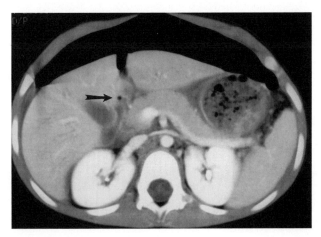

FIG. 8-231. Gastric perforation. A 4-year-old boy with a lap-belt ecchymosis. CT through upper abdomen shows a large hydropneumoperitoneum, with a small bubble of gas in the subhepatic space *(arrow)*. A perforation of the gastric antrum was repaired at laparotomy.

Rupture of the urinary bladder is also uncommon in children after blunt abdominal trauma (<1%). However, prompt diagnosis is essential because of the increased mortality associated with delayed repair. The most common findings include extravasation of urinary contrast and thickening of the bladder wall (567). Determination of the site of bladder rupture is important because extraperitoneal rupture is typically managed nonoperatively, whereas intraperitoneal rupture requires immediate surgical repair. The two types of rupture can be distinguished on the basis of the location of extravasated urinary contrast; extraperitoneal fluid will accumulate in the perivesical spaces surrounding the bladder, perhaps extending up to the umbilicus and posteriorly behind the rectum (Fig. 8-232), whereas intraperitoneal rupture will result in fluid in the pouch of Douglas and the paravesical peritoneal recesses and between bowel loops.

Hypoperfusion Syndrome

The hypoperfusion or shock bowel syndrome is a complex of CT findings consisting of diffuse dilatation of the intestine with fluid; abnormally intense contrast enhancement of the bowel wall, mesentery, kidneys, and pancreas; moderate to large amounts of fluid in the greater and lesser peritoneal sacs, and diminished caliber of the abdominal aorta, IVC, and mesenteric vessels, all occurring in children with a history of shock (Fig. 8-233) (568). These patients typically respond to initial resuscitative measures and appear to be hemodynamically stable prior to CT. Clinically occult hypovolemia, with resultant vasoconstriction, replacement of a depleted vascular volume with iodinated contrast, and large third space fluid losses into the GI tract and peritoneum are probably responsible for this CT appearance. The hypoperfu-

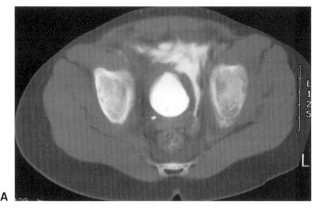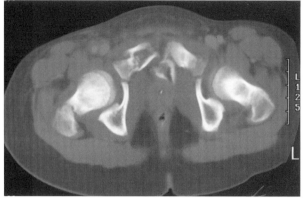

FIG. 8-232. Bladder rupture. A 7-year-old girl injured in car accident. CT through the pelvis **(A)** shows extraperitoneal extravasation of contrast-containing urine into the perivesical spaces anterior to the bladder. Note the bladder wall thickening and the absence of contrast in the pouch of Douglas. A lower scan **(B)** shows extravasated urine anterior to the urethra and a fracture of the right pubic bone.

sion complex is associated with a poor clinical outcome; the reported mortality is up to 85% within a week of injury (569).

CT is a highly effective tool for the diagnosis of abdominal injury in children. With the increasing use of nonoperative therapy for solid organ injury, the clinical impact of abdominal CT in children is changing. CT information now primarily influences decisions regarding the level of monitoring while in the hospital, the length of restriction from certain physical activities, and the need and time for clinical follow-up. There is still no consensus regarding the necessity, type, and frequency of imaging for follow-up of solid organ injuries treated nonoperatively.

REFERENCES

General Information

1. Franken EA Jr, Smith WL, eds. *Gastrointestinal imaging in pediatrics.* New York: Harper and Row, 1982.
2. Stringer DA. *Pediatric gastrointestinal imaging.* Toronto: Brian Decker, 1989.

Techniques

3. Berdon WE, Baker DH, Leonidas J. Advantages of prone positioning in gastrointestinal and genitourinary roentgenologic studies in infants and children. *AJR* 1968;103:444–455.

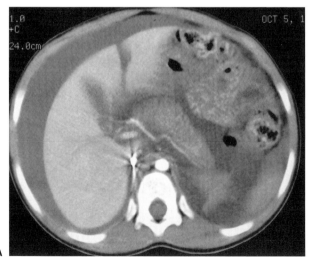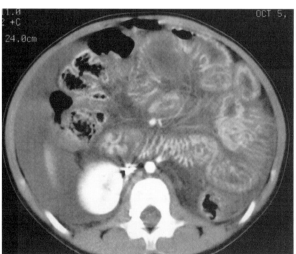

FIG. 8-233. Hypoperfusion complex. A 7-year-old girl hit by car. **A:** CT through the upper abdomen shows large peritoneal fluid collections in the greater and lesser peritoneal sacs, and decreased caliber of the portal vein, aorta, and inferior vena cava (IVC). There is a catheter in the small IVC. **B:** CT image through the lower abdomen shows abnormally dense enhancement of the right kidney and bowel wall, a large peritoneal fluid collection, fluid-filled and distended bowel loops, and decreased caliber of the mesenteric vessels. (Courtesy of Robert A. Kaufman, M.D., Memphis, TN.)

4. Cohen MD. Choosing contrast media for the evaluation of the gastrointestinal tract of neonates and infants. *Radiology* 1987;162:447–456.
5. Ratcliffe JF. The use of low osmolality water soluble (LOWS) contrast media in the pediatric gastrointestinal tract. A report of 115 examinations. *Pediatr Radiol* 1986;16:47–52.
6. Cohen MD, Towbin R, Baker S, et al. Comparison of Iohexol with barium in gastrointestinal studies of infants and children. *AJR* 1991; 156:345–350.
7. Cohen MD, Weber TR, Grosfeld JL. Bowel perforation in the newborn: diagnosis with metrizamide. *Radiology* 1984;150:65–69.
8. Dangman BC, Leichtner AM, Teele RL. The antegrade colonogram: extending the small bowel follow through for children suspected of having colonic disease. *Pediatr Radiol* 1992;22:573–576.
9. Stringer DA, Cloutier S, Daneman A, Durie P. The value of the small bowel enema in children. *J Can Assoc Radiol* 1986;37:13–16.
10. Baath L, Ekberg O, Borulf S, et al. Small bowel barium examination in children. Diagnostic accuracy and clinical value as evaluated from 331 enteroclysis and follow-through examinations. *Acta Radiol* 1989; 30:621–626.
11. Kirks DR, Kane PE, Taybi H. Pediatric enema tips. *Radiology* 1976; 118:232.

Common Abdominal Emergencies

12. Tan CE, Kiely EM, Agrawal M, et al. Neonatal gastrointestinal perforation. *J Pediatr Surg* 1989;24:888–892.
13. Uceda JE, Laos CA, Kolni HW, Klein AM. Intestinal perforations in infants with a very low birth weight: a disease of increasing survival? *J Pediatr Surg* 1995;30:1314–1316.
14. Nagaraj HS, Sandhu AS, Cook LN, et al. Gastrointestinal perforation following indomethacin therapy in very low birth weight infants. *J Pediatr Surg* 1981;16:1003–1007.
15. Fonkalsrud EW, Clatworthy HW Jr. Accidental perforation of colon and rectum in newborn infants. *N Engl J Med* 1965;272:1097–1100.
16. Campbell RE, Boggs TR Jr, Kirkpatrick JA Jr. Early neonatal pneumoperitoneum from progressive massive tension pneumomediastinum. *Radiology* 1975;114:121–126.
17. Macklin M, Macklin C. Malignant interstitial emphysema of the lung and mediastinum as an important occult complication in many respiratory diseases and other conditions. *Medicine* 1944;23:281–358.
18. Kleinman PK, Brill PW, Whalen JP. Anterior pathway for transdiaphragmatic extension of pneumomediastinum. *AJR* 1978;131: 271–275.
19. Cohen MD, Schreiner R, Lemons J. Neonatal pneumoperitoneum without significant adventitial pulmonary air: use of metrizamide to rule out perforation of the bowel. *Pediatrics* 1982;69:587–589.
20. Spencer R. Gastrointestinal hemorrhage in infancy and childhood: 476 cases. *Surgery* 1964;55:718–734.
21. Vinton NE. Gastrointestinal bleeding in infancy and childhood. *Gastroenterol Clin North Am* 1994;23:93–122.
22. Sherman NJ, Clatworthy HW Jr. Gastrointestinal bleeding in neonates: a study of 94 cases. *Surgery* 1967;62:614–619.
23. Treem WR. Gastrointestinal bleeding in children. *Gastrointest Endosc Clin North Am* 1994;4:75–97.
24. Treves ST, Grand R. Gastrointestinal bleeding. In: Treves ST, ed. *Pediatric nuclear medicine.* 2nd ed. New York: Springer-Verlag, 1995, 453–465.
25. Eklof O. Acquired small bowel obstruction. In: Franken EA Jr, Smith WL, eds. *Gastrointestinal imaging in pediatrics.* 2nd ed. New York: Harper and Row, 1982, 244–261.

Intraperitoneal Fluid

26. Franken EA Jr. Ascites in infants and children. Roentgen diagnosis. *Radiology* 1972;102:393–398.
27. Seibert JJ, Williamson SL, Golladay ES, et al. The distended gasless abdomen: a fertile field for ultrasound. *J Ultrasound Med* 1986;5: 301–308.
28. Griscom NT, Colodny AH, Rosenberg HK, et al. Diagnostic aspects of neonatal ascites: report of 27 cases. *AJR* 1977;128:961–969.
29. Cywes S, Cremin BJ. The roentgenologic features of hemoperitoneum in the newborn. *AJR* 1969;106:193–199.

Abdominal Calcifications

30. Stein B, Bromley B, Michlewitz H, et al. Fetal liver calcifications: sonographic appearance and postnatal outcome. *Radiology* 1995;197: 489–492.
31. Berdon WE, Baker DH, Wigger HJ, et al. Calcified intraluminal meconium in newborn males with imperforate anus. Enterolithiasis in the newborn. *AJR* 1975;125:449–455.

Abdominal Masses

32. Kirks DR, Merten DF, Grossman H, Bowie JD. Diagnostic imaging of pediatric abdominal masses: an overview. *Radiol Clin North Am* 1981;19:527–545.
33. Griscom NT. The roentgenology of neonatal abdominal masses. *AJR* 1965;93:447–463.
34. Reed MH, Griscom NT. Hydrometrocolpos in infancy. *AJR* 1973; 118:1–13.
35. Nussbaum AR, Sanders RC, Hartman DS, et al. Neonatal ovarian cysts: sonographic-pathologic correlation. *Radiology* 1988;168: 817–821.
36. Effmann EL, Griscom NT, Colodny AH, Vawter GF. Neonatal gastrointestinal masses arising late in gestation. *AJR* 1980;135:681–686.
37. Barr LL, Hayden CK Jr, Stansberry SD, Swischuk LE. Enteric duplication cysts in children: are their ultrasonographic wall characteristics diagnostic? *Pediatr Radiol* 1990;20:326–328.
38. Forman HP, Leonidas JC, Berdon WE, et al. Congenital neuroblastoma: evaluation with multimodality imaging. *Radiology* 1990;175: 365–368.
39. Torrisi JM, Haller JO, Velcek FT. Choledochal cyst and biliary atresia in the neonate: imaging findings in five cases. *AJR* 1990;155: 1273–1276.

Anomalies of the Abdominal Wall

40. Franken EA Jr. Anomalies of the anterior abdominal wall: classification and roentgenology. *AJR* 1971;112:58–67.
41. Cantrell J, Haller J, Ravitch M. A syndrome of congenital defects involving the abdominal wall, sternum, diaphragm, pericardium and heart. *Surg Gynecol Obstet* 1958;107:602–614.
42. Mayer T, Black R, Matlak ME, Johnson DG. Gastroschisis and omphalocele. *Ann Surg* 1980;192:783–787.
43. Hughes MD, Nyberg DA, Mack LA, Pretorius DH. Fetal omphalocele: prenatal US detection of concurrent anomalies and other predictors of outcome. *Radiology* 1989;173:371–376.
44. Tunell WP, Puffinbarger NK, Tuggle DW, et al. Abdominal wall defects in infants. Survival and implications for adult life. *Ann Surg* 1995;221:525–528.
45. Pinckney LE, Moskowitz PS, Lebowitz RL, Fritsche P. Renal malposition associated with omphalocele. *Radiology* 1978;129:677–682.
46. Hoyme HE, Higginbottom MC, Jones KL. The vascular pathogenesis of gastroschisis: intrauterine interruption of the omphalomesenteric artery. *J Pediatr* 1981;98:228–231.
47. Touloukian RJ, Spackman TJ. Gastrointestinal function and radiographic appearance following gastroschisis repair. *J Pediatr Surg* 1971;6:427–434.
48. Oh KS, Dorst JP, Dominguez R, Girdany BR. Abnormal intestinal motility in gastroschisis. *Radiology* 1978;127:457–460.
49. Blane CE, Wesley JR, DiPietro MA, et al. Gastrointestinal complications of gastroschisis. *AJR* 1985;144:589–591.
50. Soboleski D, Daneman A, Manson D, Ein S. Tailoring the small-bowel follow-through examination postoperatively in gastroschisis patients. *Pediatr Radiol* 1995;25:267–268.
51. Ramsden WH, Arthur RJ, Martinez D. Gastroschisis: a radiological and clinical review. *Pediatr Radiol* 1997;27:166–169.
52. Wood BP. Cloacal malformations and exstrophy syndromes. *Radiology* 1990;177:326–327.
53. Meglin AJ, Balotin RJ, Jelinek JS, et al. Cloacal exstrophy: radiologic findings in 13 patients. *AJR* 1990;155:1267–1272.
54. Jaramillo D, Lebowitz RL, Hendren WH. The cloacal malformation: radiologic findings and imaging recommendations. *Radiology* 1990; 177:441–448.

Anomalies of the Diaphragm

55. Levin TL, Liebling MS, Ruzal-Shapiro C, et al. Midgut malfixation in patients with congenital diaphragmatic hernia: what is the risk of midgut volvulus? *Pediatr Radiol* 1995;25:259–261.
56. Stolar CJ, Levy JP, Dillon PW, et al. Anatomic and functional abnormalities of the esophagus in infants surviving congenital diaphragmatic hernia. *Am J Surg* 1990;159:204–207.
57. Kirchner SG, Burko H, O'Neill JA, Stahlman M. Delayed radiographic presentation of congenital right diaphragmatic hernia. *Radiology* 1975;115:155–156.
58. McCarten KM, Rosenberg HK, Borden S IV, Mandell GA. Delayed appearance of right diaphragmatic hernia associated with group B streptococcal infection in newborns. *Radiology* 1981;139:385–389.
59. Moccia W, Kaude JV, Felman AH. Congenital eventration of the diaphragm. Diagnosis by ultrasound. *Pediatr Radiol* 1981;10:197–200.
60. Baran EM, Houston HE, Lynn HB, O'Connell EJ. Foramen of Morgagni hernias in children. *Surgery* 1967;62:1076–1081.
61. Pokorny WJ, McGill CW, Harberg FJ. Morgagni hernias during infancy: presentation and associated anomalies. *J Pediatr Surg* 1984;19:394–397.
62. Merten DF, Bowie JD, Kirks DR, Grossman H. Anteromedial diaphragmatic defects in infancy: current approaches to diagnostic imaging. *Radiology* 1982;142:361–365.

Esophageal Atresia and Tracheoesophageal Fistula

63. Kappelman MM, Dorst J, Haller JA, Stambler A. H-type tracheoesophageal fistula. *Am J Dis Child* 1969;118:568–575.
64. Thomas PS, Chrispin AR. Congenital tracheo-oesophageal fistula without oesophageal atresia. *Clin Radiol* 1969;20:371–374.
65. Holder TM, Cloud DT, Lewis JE, Pilling GP IV. Esophageal atresia and tracheoesophageal fistula. A survey of its members by the Surgical Section of the American Academy of Pediatrics. *Pediatrics* 1964;34:542–549.
66. Chittmittrapap S, Spitz L, Kiely E, Brereton RJ. Oesophageal atresia and associated anomalies. *Arch Dis Child* 1989;64:364–368.
67. Kirkpatrick JA, Wagner ML, Pilling GP IV. A complex of anomalies associated with tracheoesophageal fistula and esophaeal atresia. *AJR* 1965;95:208–211.
68. Quan L, Smith DW. The VATER association. Vertebral defects, Anal atresia, T-E fistula with esophageal atresia, Radial and Renal dysplasia: a spectrum of associated defects. *J Pediatr* 1973;82:104–107.
69. Temtamy SA, Miller JD. Extending the scope of the VATER association: definition of the VATER syndrome. *J Pediatr* 1974;85:345–349.
70. Goodwin CD, Ashcraft KW, Holder TM, et al. Esophageal atresia with double tracheoesophageal fistula. *J Pediatr Surg* 1978;13:269–273.
71. Berdon WE, Baker DH. Radiographic findings in esophageal atresia with proximal pouch fistula (type B). *Pediatr Radiol* 1975;3:70–74.
72. Osman MZ, Girdany BR. Traumatic pseudodiverticulums of the pharynx in infants and children. *Ann Radiol* 1973;16:143–147.
73. Kassner EG, Baumstark A, Balsam D, Haller JO. Passage of feeding catheters into the pleural space: a radiographic sign of trauma to the pharynx and esophagus in the newborn. *AJR* 1977;128:19–22.
74. Smith WL, Franken EA Jr, Smith JA. Pneumoesophagus as a sign of H type tracheoesophageal fistula. *Pediatrics* 1976;58:907–909.
75. Benjamin B, Pham T. Diagnosis of H-type tracheoesophageal fistula. *J Pediatr Surg* 1991;26:667–671.
76. Stringer DA, Ein SH. Recurrent tracheo-esophageal fistula: a protocol for investigation. *Radiology* 1984;151:637–641.
77. Biller JA, Allen JL, Schuster SR, et al. Long-term evaluation of esophageal and pulmonary function in patients with repaired esophageal atresia and tracheoesophageal fistula. *Dig Dis Sci* 1987;32:985–990.
78. Griscom NT. Respiratory problems of early life now allowing survival into adulthood: concepts for radiologists. *AJR* 1992;158:1–8.
79. Kirkpatrick JA, Cresson SL, Pilling GP IV. The motor activity of the esophagus in association with esophageal atresia and tracheoesophageal fistula. *AJR* 1961;86:884–887.
80. Werlin SL, Dodds WJ, Hogan WJ, et al. Esophageal function in esophageal atresia. *Dig Dis Sci* 1981;26:796–800.
81. Jolley SG, Johnson DG, Roberts CC, et al. Patterns of gastroesophageal reflux in children following repair of esophageal atresia and distal tracheoesophageal fistula. *J Pediatr Surg* 1980;15:857–862.

82. Thomason MA, Gay BB. Esophageal stenosis with esophageal atresia. *Pediatr Radiol* 1987;17:197–201.
83. Neilson IR, Croitoru DP, Guttman FM, et al. Distal congenital esophageal stenosis associated with esophageal atresia. *J Pediatr Surg* 1991;26:478–481.
84. Rideout DT, Hayashi AH, Gillis DA, et al. The absence of clinically significant tracheomalacia in patients having esophageal atresia without tracheoesophageal fistula. *J Pediatr Surg* 1991;26:1303–1305.
85. Wailoo MP, Emery JL. The trachea in children with tracheo-esophageal fistula. *Histopathology* 1979;3:329–338.
86. Blair GK, Cohen R, Filler RM. Treatment of tracheomalacia: eight years' experience. *J Pediatr Surg* 1986;21:781–785.
87. Gilsanz V, Boechat IM, Birnberg FA, King JD. Scoliosis after thoracotomy for esophageal atresia. *AJR* 1983;141:457–460.

High Intestinal Obstruction

88. Buonomo C. Neonatal gastrointestinal disease: surgical emergencies. In: Kirks DR, ed. *Emergency pediatric radiology. A problem-oriented approach.* Reston, VA: American Roentgen Ray Society, 1995, 123–128.
89. Buonomo C. Neonatal gastrointestinal emergencies. *Radiol Clin North Am* 1997;35:845–864.
90. Shackelford GD, McAlister WH, Brodeur AE, Ragsdale EF. Congenital microgastria. *AJR* 1973;118:72–76.
91. Bell MJ, Ternberg JL, McAlister W, et al. Antral diaphragm—a cause of gastric outlet obstruction in infants and children. *J Pediatr* 1977;90:196–202.
92. Cremin BJ. Congenital pyloric antral membranes in infancy. *Radiology* 1969;92:509–512.
93. Fonkalsrud EW, de Lorimier AA, Hays DM. Congenital atresia and stenosis of the duodenum. A review compiled from the members of the Surgical Section of the American Academy of Pediatrics. *Pediatrics* 1969;43:79–83.
94. McCarten KM, Teele RL. Preduodenal portal vein: venography, ultrasonography, and review of the literature. *Ann Radiol* 1978;21:155–160.
95. Kassner EG, Sutton AL, De Groot TJ. Bile duct anomalies associated with duodenal atresia: paradoxical presence of small bowel gas. *AJR* 1972;116:577–583.
96. Kirks DR. Anomalies of the small bowel. In: Franken EA Jr, Smith WL, eds. *Gastrointestinal imaging in pediatrics.* 2nd ed. New York: Harper and Row, 1982, 151–188.
97. Crowe JE, Sumner TE. Combined esophageal and duodenal atresia without tracheoesophageal fistula: characteristic radiographic changes. *AJR* 1978;130:167–168.
98. Lee FA, Mahour GH, Gwinn JL. Roentgenographic aspects of intrinsic duodenal obstruction. *Ann Radiol* 1978;21:133–142.
99. Pratt AD Jr. Current concepts of the obstructing duodenal diaphragm. *Radiology* 1971;100:637–643.
100. Houston CS, Wittenborg MH. Roentgen evaluation of anomalies of rotation and fixation of the bowel in children. *Radiology* 1965;84:1–17.
101. Snyder WH, Chaffin L. Embryology and pathology of the intestinal tract: presentation of 40 cases of malrotation. *Ann Surg* 1954;140:368–380.
102. Balthazar EJ. Intestinal malrotation in adults. Roentgenographic assessment with emphasis on isolated complete and partial nonrotations. *AJR* 1976;126:358–367.
103. Ladd W. Surgical diseases of the alimentary tract in infants. *N Engl J Med* 1936;205:705–708.
104. Berdon WE, Baker DH, Bull S, Santulli TV. Midgut malrotation and volvulus. Which films are most helpful? *Radiology* 1970;96:375–384.
105. Stewart DR, Colodny AL, Daggett WC. Malrotation of the bowel in infants and children: a 15 year review. *Surgery* 1976;79:716–720.
106. Torres AM, Ziegler MM. Malrotation of the intestine. *World J Surg* 1993;17:326–331.
107. Ford EG, Senac MO Jr, Srikanth MS, Weitzman JJ. Malrotation of the intestine in children. *Ann Surg* 1992;215:172–178.
108. Lilien LD, Srinivasan G, Pyati SP, et al. Green vomiting in the first 72 hours in normal infants. *Am J Dis Child* 1986;140:662–664.
109. Steiner GM. The misplaced caecum and the root of the mesentery. *Br J Radiol* 1978;51:406–413.
110. Yanez R, Spitz L. Intestinal malrotation presenting outside the neonatal period. *Arch Dis Child* 1986;61:682–685.

111. Powell DM, Othersen HB, Smith CD. Malrotation of the intestines in children: the effect of age on presentation and therapy. *J Pediatr Surg* 1989;24:777–780.

112. Mori H, Hayashi K, Futagawa S, et al. Vascular compromise in chronic volvulus with midgut malrotation. *Pediatr Radiol* 1987;17: 277–281.

113. Firor HV, Steiger E. Morbidity of rotational abnormalities of the gut beyond infancy. *Cleve Clin Q* 1983;50:303–309.

114. Spigland N, Brandt ML, Yazbeck S. Malrotation presenting beyond the neonatal period. *J Pediatr Surg* 1990;25:1139–1142.

115. Moller JH, Amplatz K, Wolfson J. Malrotation of the bowel in patients with congenital heart disease associated with splenic anomalies. *Radiology* 1971;99:393–398.

116. Mercado MG, Bulas DI, Chandra R. Prenatal diagnosis and management of congenital volvulus. *Pediatr Radiol* 1993;23:601–602.

117. Potts SR, Thomas PS, Garstin WI, McGoldrick J. The duodenal triangle: a plain film sign of midgut malrotation and volvulus in the neonate. *Clin Radiol* 1985;36:47–49.

118. Frye TR, Mah CL, Schiller M. Roentgenographic evidence of gangrenous bowel in midgut volvulus with observations in experimental volvulus. *AJR* 1972;114:394–401.

119. Kassner EG, Kottmeier PK. Absence and retention of small bowel gas in infants with midgut volvulus: mechanisms and significance. *Pediatr Radiol* 1975;4:28–30.

120. Simpson AJ, Leonidas JC, Krasna IH, et al. Roentgen diagnosis of midgut malrotation: value of upper gastrointestinal radiographic study. *J Pediatr Surg* 1972;7:243–252.

121. Humphry A. Intestinal obstruction due to abnormal duodenal fixation in infants. *J Can Assoc Radiol* 1970;21:251–256.

122. Firor HV, Harris VJ. Rotational abnormalities of the gut. Re-emphasis of a neglected facet, isolated incomplete rotation of the duodenum. *AJR* 1974;120:315–321.

123. Slovis TL, Klein MD, Watts FB Jr. Incomplete rotation of the intestine with a normal cecal position. *Surgery* 1980;87:325–330.

124. Beasley SW, de Campo JF. Pitfalls in the radiological diagnosis of malrotation. *Australas Radiol* 1987;31:376–383.

125. Katz ME, Siegel MJ, Shackelford GD, McAlister WH. The position and mobility of the duodenum in children. *AJR* 1987;148:947–951.

126. Long FR, Kramer SS, Markowitz RI, et al. Intestinal malrotation in children: tutorial on radiographic diagnosis in difficult cases. *Radiology* 1996;198:775–780.

127. Taylor GA, Teele RL. Chronic intestinal obstruction mimicking malrotation in children. *Pediatr Radiol* 1985;15:392–394.

128. Hayden CK Jr, Boulden TF, Swischuk LE, Lobe TE. Sonographic demonstration of duodenal obstruction with midgut volvulus. *AJR* 1984;143:9–10.

129. Cohen HL, Haller JO, Mestel AL, et al. Neonatal duodenum: fluid-aided US examination. *Radiology* 1987;164:805–809.

130. Leonidas JC, Magid N, Soberman N, Glass TS. Midgut volvulus in infants: diagnosis with US. Work in progress. *Radiology* 1991;179: 491–493.

131. Pracros JP, Sann L, Genin G, et al. Ultrasound diagnosis of midgut volvulus: the "whirlpool" sign. *Pediatr Radiol* 1992;22:18–20.

132. Shimanuki Y, Aihara T, Takano H, et al. Clockwise whirlpool sign at color Doppler US: an objective and definite sign of midgut volvulus. *Radiology* 1996;199:261–264.

133. Gaines PA, Saunders AJ, Drake D. Midgut malrotation diagnosed by US. *Clin Radiol* 1987;38:51–53.

134. Loyer E, Eggli KD. Sonographic evaluation of superior mesenteric vascular relationship in malrotation. *Pediatr Radiol* 1989;19: 173–175.

135. Weinberger E, Winters WD, Liddell RM, et al. Sonographic diagnosis of intestinal malrotation in infants: importance of the relative positions of the superior mesenteric vein and artery. *AJR* 1992;159:825–828.

136. Zerin JM, DiPietro MA. Superior mesenteric vascular anatomy at US in patients with surgically proved malrotation of the midgut. *Radiology* 1992;183:693–694.

137. Nichols DM, Li DK. Superior mesenteric vein rotation: a CT sign of midgut malrotation. *AJR* 1983;141:707–708.

138. Shatzkes D, Gordon DH, Haller JO, et al. Malrotation of the bowel: malalignment of the superior mesenteric artery—vein complex shown by CT and MR. *J Comput Assist Tomogr* 1990;14:93–95.

139. Filston HC, Kirks DR. Malrotation—the ubiquitous anomaly. *J Pediatr Surg* 1981;16:614–620.

140. Chang J, Brueckner M, Touloukian RJ. Intestinal rotation and fixation in heterotaxia: early detection and management. *J Pediatr Surg* 1993; 28:1281–1285.

141. Ruben GD, Templeton JM Jr, Ziegler MM. Situs inversus: the complex inducing neonatal intestinal obstruction. *J Pediatr Surg* 1983; 18:751–756.

142. Sharland MR, Chowcat NL, Qureshi A, Drake DP. Intestinal obstruction caused by malrotation of the gut in atrial isomerism. *Arch Dis Child* 1989;64:1623–1624.

143. de Lorimier AA, Fonkalsrud EW, Hays DM. Congenital atresia and stenosis of the jejunum and ileum. *Surgery* 1969;65:819–827.

144. Leonidas JC, Amoury RA, Ashcraft KW, Fellows RA. Duodenojejunal atresia with "apple peel" small bowel. A distinct form of intestinal atresia. *Radiology* 1976;118:661–665.

145. Daneman A, Martin DJ. A syndrome of multiple intestinal atresias with intraluminal calcification. A report of a case and a review of the literature. *Pediatr Radiol* 1979;8:227–231.

146. Gaisie G, Odagiri K, Oh KS, Young LW. The bulbous bowel segment: a sign of congenital small bowel obstruction. *Radiology* 1980;135: 331–334.

147. Schiavetti E, Massotti G, Torricelli M, Perfetti L. "Apple peel" syndrome. A radiological study. *Pediatr Radiol* 1984;14:380–383.

Low Intestinal Obstruction

148. Berdon WE, Baker DH, Santulli TV, et al. Microcolon in newborn infants with intestinal obstruction. Its correlation with the level and time of onset of obstruction. *Radiology* 1968;90:878–885.

149. Ohamoto E, Veda T. Embryogenesis of intramural ganglia of the gut and its relationship to Hirschsprung's disease. *J Pediatr Surg* 1967; 2:437–442.

150. Haney PJ, Hill JL, Sun CC. Zonal colonic aganglionosis. *Pediatr Radiol* 1982;12:258–261.

151. Kleinhaus S, Boley SJ, Sheran M, Sieber WK. Hirschsprung's disease—a survey of the members of the Surgical Section of the American Academy of Pediatrics. *J Pediatr Surg* 1979;14:588–597.

152. Berdon WE, Baker DH. The roentgenographic diagnosis of Hirschsprung's disease in infancy. *AJR* 1965;93:432–446.

153. Roshkow JE, Haller JO, Berdon WE, Sane SM. Hirschsprung's disease, Ondine's curse and neuroblastoma—manifestations of neurocristopathy. *Pediatr Radiol* 1988;19:45–49.

154. Elhalaby EA, Coran AG, Blane CE, et al. Enterocolitis associated with Hirschsprung's disease: a clinical-radiological characterization based on 168 patients. *J Pediatr Surg* 1995;30:76-83.

155. Newman B, Nussbaum A, Kirkpatrick JA Jr. Bowel perforation in Hirschsprung's disease. *AJR* 1987;148:1195–1197.

156. Cremin BJ. The early diagnosis of Hirschsprung's disease. *Pediatr Radiol* 1974;2:23–28.

157. Swenson O, Neuhauser EBD, Pickett LK. New concepts of etiology, diagnosis and treatment of congenital megacolon (Hirschsprung's disease). *Pediatrics* 1949;4:201–209.

158. Rosenfield NS, Ablow RC, Markowitz RI, et al. Hirschsprung disease: accuracy of the barium enema examination. *Radiology* 1984;150: 393–400.

159. Pochaczevsky R, Leonidas JC. The "recto-sigmoid index". A measurement for the early diagnosis of Hirschsprung's disease. *AJR* 1975; 123:770–777.

160. Blane CE, Elhalaby E, Coran AG. Enterocolitis following endorectal pull-through procedure in children with Hirschsprung's disease. *Pediatr Radiol* 1994;24:164–166.

161. De Campo JF, Mayne V, Boldt DW, De Campo M. Radiological findings in total aganglionosis coli. *Pediatr Radiol* 1984;14:205–209.

162. Berdon WE, Koontz P, Baker DH. The diagnosis of colonic and terminal ileal aganglionosis. *AJR* 1964;91:680–689.

163. Sane SM, Girdany BR. Total aganglionosis coli. Clinical and roentgenographic manifestations. *Radiology* 1973;107:397–404.

164. Chandler NW, Zwiren GT. Complete reflux of the small bowel in total colon Hirschsprung's disease. *Radiology* 1970;94:335–339.

165. Johnson JF, Cronk RL. The pseudotransition zone in long segment Hirschsprung's disease. *Pediatr Radiol* 1980;10:87–89.

166. Fletcher BD, Yulish BS. Intraluminal calcifications in the small bowel of newborn infants with total colonic aganglionosis. *Radiology* 1978;126:451–455.

167. Clatworthy H, Howard W, Lloyd J. The meconium plug syndrome. *Surgery* 1956;39:131–141.

168. Davis WS, Allen RP, Favara BE, Slovis TL. Neonatal small left colon syndrome. *AJR* 1974;120:322–329.

169. Le Quesne GW, Reilly BJ. Functional immaturity of the large bowel in the newborn infant. *Radiol Clin North Am* 1975;13:331–342.

170. Berdon WE, Slovis TL, Campbell JB, et al. Neonatal small left colon syndrome: its relationship to aganglionosis and meconium plug syndrome. *Radiology* 1977;125:457–462.

171. Philippart AI, Reed JO, Georgeson KE. Neonatal small left colon syndrome: intramural not intraluminal obstruction. *J Pediatr Surg* 1975;10:733–740.

172. Davis WS, Campbell JB. Neonatal small left colon syndrome. Occurrence in asymptomatic infants of diabetic mothers. *Am J Dis Child* 1975;129:1024–1027.

173. Sokal MM, Koenigsberger MR, Rose JS, et al. Neonatal hypermagnesemia and the meconium plug syndrome. *N Engl J Med* 1972;286:823–825.

174. Nixon GW, Condon VR, Stewart DR. Intestinal perforation as a complication of the neonatal small left colon syndrome. *AJR* 1975;125:75–80.

175. Ellis DG, Clatworthy HW Jr. The meconium plug syndrome revisited. *J Pediatr Surg* 1966;1:54–61.

176. Cremin BJ. Functional intestinal obstruction in premature infants. *Pediatr Radiol* 1973;1:109–112.

177. Vanhoutte JJ, Katzman D. Roentgenographic manifestations of immaturity of the intestinal neural plexus in premature infants. *Radiology* 1973;106:363–367.

178. Amodio J, Berdon W, Abramson SJ, Stolar C. Microcolon of prematurity: a form of functional obstruction. *AJR* 1986;146:239–244.

179. Bley WR, Franken EA Jr. Roentgenology of colon atresia. *Pediatr Radiol* 1973;1:105–108.

180. Winters WD, Weinberger E, Hatch EI. Atresia of the colon in neonates: radiographic findings. *AJR* 1992;159:1273–1276.

181. Currarino G, Votteler TP, Kirks DR. Anal agenesis with rectobulbar fistula. *Radiology* 1978;126:457–461.

182. Pena A. *Atlas of surgical management of anorectal malformations.* New York: Springer-Verlag, 1990.

183. Seibert JJ, Golladay ES. Clinical evaluation of imperforate anus: clue to type of anal-rectal anomaly. *AJR* 1979;133:289–292.

184. Berdon WE, Baker DH, Santulli TV, Amoury R. The radiologic evaluation of imperforate anus. An approach correlated with current surgical concepts. *Radiology* 1968;90:466–471.

185. Berdon WE, Hochberg B, Baker DH, et al. The association of lumbosacral spine and genitourinary anomalies with imperforate anus. *AJR* 1966;98:181–191.

186. Appignani BA, Jaramillo D, Barnes PD, Poussaint TY. Dysraphic myelodysplasias associated with urogenital and anorectal anomalies: prevalence and types seen with MR imaging. *AJR* 1994;163:1199–1203.

187. Currarino G, Coln D, Votteler T. Triad of anorectal, sacral and presacral anomalies. *AJR* 1981;137:395–398.

188. Kirks DR, Merten DF, Filston HC, Oakes WJ. The Currarino triad: complex of anorectal malformation, sacral bony abnormality, and presacral mass. *Pediatr Radiol* 1984;14:220–225.

189. Sato Y, Pringle KC, Bergman RA, et al. Congenital anorectal anomalies: MR imaging. *Radiology* 1988;168:157–162.

190. Berdon WE, Baker DH, Blanc WA, et al. Megacystis-microcolon-intestinal hypoperistalsis syndrome: a new cause of intestinal obstruction in the newborn. Report of radiologic findings in five newborn girls. *AJR* 1976;126:957–964.

191. Young LW, Yunis EJ, Girdany BR, Sieber WK. Megacystis-microcolon-intestinal hypoperistalsis syndrome: additional clinical, radiologic, surgical and histopathologic aspects. *AJR* 1981;137:749–755.

192. Estroff JA, Parad RB, Benacerraf BR. Prevalence of cystic fibrosis in fetuses with dilated bowel. *Radiology* 1992;183:677–680.

193. Leonidas JC, Berdon WE, Baker DH, Santulli TV. Meconium ileus and its complications. A reappraisal of plain film roentgen diagnostic criteria. *AJR* 1970;108:598–609.

194. Noblett HR. Treatment of uncomplicated meconium ileus by Gastrografin enema: a preliminary report. *J Pediatr Surg* 1969;4:190–197.

195. Kao SCS, Franken EA Jr. Nonoperative treatment of simple meconium ileus: a survey of the Society for Pediatric Radiology. *Pediatr Radiol* 1995;25:97–100.

Necrotizing Enterocolitis

196. Berdon WE, Grossman H, Baker DH. Necrotizing enterocolitis in the premature infant. *Ann Radiol* 1965;8:85–89.

197. Kliegman RM, Fanaroff AA. Necrotizing enterocolitis. *N Engl J Med* 1984;310:1093–1103.

198. Rowe MI, Reblock KK, Kurkchubasche AG. Healy PJ. Necrotizing enterocolitis in the extremely low birth weight infant. *J Pediatr Surg* 1994;29:987–990.

199. Frey EE, Smith W, Franken EA Jr, Wintermeyer KA. Analysis of bowel perforation in necrotizing enterocolitis. *Pediatr Radiol* 1987;17:380–382.

200. Bell MJ, Ternberg JL, Feigin RD, et al. Neonatal necrotizing enterocolitis. Therapeutic decisions based upon clinical staging. *Ann Surg* 1978;187:1–7.

201. Daneman A, Woodward S, de Silva M. The radiology of neonatal necrotizing enterocolitis (NEC). A review of 47 cases and the literature. *Pediatr Radiol* 1978;7:70–77.

202. Jaile JC, Levin T, Wung JT, et al. Benign gaseous distension of the bowel in premature infants treated with nasal continuous airway pressure: a study of contributing factors. *AJR* 1992;158:125–127.

203. Kogutt MS. Necrotizing enterocolitis of infancy. Early roentgen patterns as a guide to prompt diagnosis. *Radiology* 1979;130:367–370.

204. Kao SCS, Smith WL, Franken EA Jr, et al. Contrast enema diagnosis of necrotizing enterocolitis. *Pediatr Radiol* 1992;22:115–117.

205. Santulli TV, Schullinger JN, Heird WC, et al. Acute necrotizing enterocolitis in infancy: a review of 64 cases. *Pediatrics* 1975;55:376–387.

206. Rabinowitz JG, Siegle RL. Changing clinical and roentgenographic patterns of necrotizing enterocolitis. *AJR* 1976;126:560–566.

207. Virjee J, Somers S, DeSa D, Stevenson G. Changing patterns of neonatal necrotizing enterocolitis. *Gastrointest Radiol* 1979;4:169–175.

208. Patriquin HB, Fisch C, Bureau M, Black R. Radiologically visible fecal gas patterns in "normal" newborns and young infants. *Pediatr Radiol* 1984;14:87–90.

209. Johnson JF. Pneumatosis in the descending colon: preliminary observations on the value of prone positioning. *Pediatr Radiol* 1988;19:25–27.

210. Leonidas JC, Hall RT, Amoury RA. Critical evaluation of the roentgen signs of neonatal necrotizing enterocolitis. *Ann Radiol* 1976;19:123–132.

211. Kosloske AM, Musemeche CA, Ball WS Jr, et al. Necrotizing enterocolitis: value of radiographic findings to predict outcome. *AJR* 1988;151:771–774.

212. Cikrit D, Mastandrea J, Grosfeld JL, et al. Significance of portal vein air in necrotizing enterocolitis: analysis of 53 cases. *J Pediatr Surg* 1985;20:425–430.

213. Kosloske AM. Indications for operation in necrotizing enterocolitis revisited. *J Pediatr Surg* 1994;29:663–666.

214. Kirks DR, O'Byrne SA. The value of the lateral abdominal roentgenogram in the diagnosis of neonatal hepatic portal venous gas (HPVG). *AJR* 1974;122:153–158.

215. Merritt CR, Goldsmith JP, Sharp MJ. Sonographic detection of portal venous gas in infants with necrotizing enterocolitis. *AJR* 1984;143:1059–1062.

216. Wexler HA. The persistent loop sign in neonatal necrotizing enterocolitis: a new indication for surgical intervention? *Radiology* 1978;126:201–204.

217. Leonidas JC, Krasna IH, Fox HA, Broder MS. Peritoneal fluid in necrotizing enterocolitis: a radiologic sign of clinical deterioration. *J Pediatr* 1973;82:672–675.

218. Kodroff MB, Hartenberg MA, Goldschmidt RA. Ultrasonographic diagnosis of gangrenous bowel in neonatal necrotizing enterocolitis. *Pediatr Radiol* 1984;14:168–170.

219. Miller SF, Seibert JJ, Kinder DL, Wilson AR. Use of ultrasound in the detection of occult bowel perforation in neonates. *J Ultrasound Med* 1993;12:531–535.

220. Seibert JJ, Parvey LS. The telltale triangle: use of the supine cross-table lateral radiograph of the abdomen in early detection of pneumoperitoneum. *Pediatr Radiol* 1977;5:209–210.

221. Coussement AM, Gooding CA, Taybi H, Faure CC. Roentgenographic visualization of the umbilical arteries in pneumoperitoneum in the newborn. *AJR* 1973;118:46–48.

222. Brill PW, Olson SR, Winchester P. Neonatal necrotizing enterocolitis: air in Morison pouch. *Radiology* 1990;174:469–471.

223. Costin BS, Singleton EB. Bowel stenosis as a late complication of acute necrotizing enterocolitis. *Radiology* 1978;128:435–438.

224. Tonkin IL, Bjelland JC, Hunter TB, et al. Spontaneous resolution of colonic strictures caused by necrotizing enterocolitis: therapeutic implications. *AJR* 1978;130:1077–1081.

225. Levin TL, Brill PW, Winchester P. Enteric fistula formation secondary to necrotizing enterocolitis. *Pediatr Radiol* 1991;21:309–311.

226. Ball TI, Wyly JB. Enterocyst formation: a late complication of neonatal necrotizing enterocolitis. *AJR* 1986;147:806–808.

227. Kleinman PK, Winchester P, Brill PW. Necrotizing enterocolitis after open heart surgery employing hypothermia and cardiopulmonary bypass. *AJR* 1976;127:757–760.

228. Amoury RA, Goodwin CD, McGill CW, et al. Necrotizing enterocolitis following operation in the neonatal period. *J Pediatr Surg* 1980; 15:1–8.

229. Czyrko C, Del Pin CA, O'Neill JA Jr, Maternal cocaine abuse and necrotizing enterocolitis: outcome and survival. *J Pediatr Surg* 1991; 26:414–418.

Idiopathic Gastric Perforation

230. Lloyd JR. The etiology of gastrointestinal perforations in the newborn. *J Pediatr Surg* 1969;4:77–84.

231. Rosser SB, Clark CH, Elechi EN. Spontaneous neonatal gastric perforation. *J Pediatr Surg* 1982;17:390–394.

232. Pochaczevsky R, Bryk D. New roentgenographic signs of neonatal gastric perforation. *Radiology* 1972;102:145–147.

Esophageal Foreign Body

233. Nandi P, Ong GB. Foreign body in the oesophagus: review of 2394 cases. *Br J Surg* 1978;65:5–9.

234. Newman DE. The radiolucent esophageal foreign body: an often-forgotten cause of respiratory symptoms. *J Pediatr* 1978;92:60–63.

235. Eggli KD, Potter BM, Garcia V, et al. Delayed diagnosis of esophageal perforation by aluminum foreign bodies. *Pediatr Radiol* 1986;16:511–513.

236. Maves MD, Lloyd TV, Carithers JS. Radiographic identification of ingested disc batteries. *Pediatr Radiol* 1986;16:154–156.

237. Shackelford GD, McAlister WH, Robertson CL. The use of a Foley catheter for removal of blunt esophageal foreign bodies from children. *Radiology* 1972;105:455–456.

238. Campbell JB, Davis WS. Catheter technique for extraction of blunt esophageal foreign bodies. *Radiology* 1973;108:438–440.

239. Towbin R, Lederman HM, Dunbar JS, et al. Esophageal edema as a predictor of unsuccessful balloon extraction of esophageal foreign body. *Pediatr Radiol* 1989;19:359–360.

240. Campbell JB, Condon VR. Catheter removal of blunt esophageal foreign bodies in children. Survey of the Society for Pediatric Radiology. *Pediatr Radiol* 1989;19:361–365.

241. Harned RK II, Strain JD, Hay TC, Douglas MR. Esophageal foreign bodies: safety and efficacy of Foley catheter extraction of coins. *AJR* 1997;168:443–446.

242. Kirks DR. Fluoroscopic catheter removal of blunt esophageal foreign bodies. A pediatric radiologist's perspective. *Pediatr Radiol* 1992;22:64–65.

243. Myer CM III. Potential hazards of esophageal foreign body extraction. *Pediatr Radiol* 1991;21:97–98.

Chemical Injury to the Esophagus

244. Franken EA Jr. Caustic damage of the gastrointestinal tract: roentgen features. *AJR* 1973;118:77–85.

Hypertrophic Pyloric Stenosis

245. Vanderwinden JM, Mailleux P, Schiffmann SN, et al. Nitric oxide synthase activity in infantile hypertrophic pyloric stenosis. *N Engl J Med* 1992;327:511–515.

246. Franken EA Jr, Saldino RM. Hypertrophic pyloric stenosis complicating esophageal atresia with tracheoesophageal fistula. *Am J Surg* 1969; 117:647–649.

247. Fernbach SK, Morello FP. Renal abnormalities in children with hypertrophic pyloric stenosis—fact or fallacy? *Pediatr Radiol* 1993;23:286–288.

248. Tach ED, Perlman JM, Bower RJ, McAlister WH. Pyloric stenosis in the sick premature infant. Clinical and radiological findings. *Am J Dis Child* 1988;142:68–70.

249. Shopfner CE, Kalmon EH Jr, Coin CG. The diagnosis of hypertrophic pyloric stenosis. *AJR* 1964;91:796–800.

250. Breaux CW Jr, Georgeson KE, Royal SE, Curnow AJ. Changing patterns in the diagnosis of hypertrophic pyloric stenosis. *Pediatrics* 1988;81:213–217.

251. Anonymous. Is ultrasound really necessary for the diagnosis of pyloric stenosis? *Lancet* 1988;1:1146.

252. Foley LC, Slovis TL, Campbell JB, et al. Evaluation of the vomiting infant. *Am J Dis Child* 1989;143:660–661.

253. Forman HP, Leonidas JC, Kronfeld GD. A rational approach to the diagnosis of hypertrophic pyloric stenosis: do the results match the claims? *J Pediatr Surg* 1990;25:262–266.

254. Teele RL, Smith EH. Ultrasound in the diagnosis of idiopathic hypertrophic pyloric stenosis. *N Engl J Med* 1977;296:1149–1150.

255. Spevak MR, Ahmadjian JM, Kleinman PK, et al. Sonography of hypertrophic pyloric stenosis: frequency and cause of nonuniform echogenicity of the thickened pyloric muscle. *AJR* 1992;158:129–132.

256. Ball TI, Atkinson GO Jr, Gay BB Jr. Ultrasound diagnosis of hypertrophic pyloric stenosis: real-time application and the demonstration of a new sonographic sign. *Radiology* 1983;147:499–502.

257. Blumhagen JD, Maclin L, Krauter D, et al. Sonographic diagnosis of hypertrophic pyloric stenosis. *AJR* 1988;150:1367–1370.

258. O'Keeffe FN, Stansberry SD, Swischuk LE, Hayden CK Jr. Antropyloric muscle thickness at US in infants: what is normal? *Radiology* 1991;178:827–830.

259. Hernanz-Schulman M, Sells LL, Ambrosino MM, et al. Hypertrophic pyloric stenosis in the infant without a palpable olive: accuracy of sonographic diagnosis. *Radiology* 1994;193:771–776.

260. Swischuk LE, Hayden CK Jr, Stansberry SD. Sonographic pitfalls in imaging of the antropyloric region in infants. *RadioGraphics* 1989; 9:437–447.

261. Riggs W, Long W Jr. The value of the plain film roentgenogram in pyloric stenosis. *AJR* 1971;112:77–82.

262. Currarino G. The value of double-contrast examination of the stomach with pressure ''spots'' in the diagnosis of infantile hypertrophic pyloric stenosis. *Radiology* 1964;83:873–878.

263. McAlister WH, Siegel MJ. Fatal aspirations in infancy during gastrointestinal series. *Pediatr Radiol* 1984;14:81–83.

264. Sauerbrei EE, Paloschi GG. The ultrasonic features of hypertrophic pyloric stenosis with emphasis on the postoperative appearance. *Radiology* 1983;147:503–506.

265. Jamroz GA, Blocker SH, McAlister WH. Radiographic findings after incomplete pyloromyotomy. *Gastrointest Radiol* 1986;11:139–141.

266. Geer LL, Gaisie G, Mandell VS, et al. Evolution of pyloric stenosis in the first week of life. *Pediatr Radiol* 1985;15:205–206.

267. Peled N, Dagan O, Babyn P, et al. Gastric-outlet obstruction induced by prostaglandin therapy in neonates. *N Engl J Med* 1992;327:505–510.

268. Mercado-Deane MG, Burton EM, Brawley AV, Hatley R. Prostaglandin-induced foveolar hyperplasia simulating pyloric stenosis in an infant with cyanotic heart disease. *Pediatr Radiol* 1994;24:45–46.

269. Campbell DP, Vanhoutte JJ, Smith EI. Partially obstructing antral web—a distinct clinical entity. *J Pediatr Surg* 1973;8:723–728.

Gastroesophageal Reflux

270. Orenstein SR, Orenstein DM. Gastroesophageal reflux and respiratory disease in children. *J Pediatr* 1988;112:847–858.

271. See CC, Newman LJ, Berezin S, et al. Gastroesophageal reflux-induced hypoxemia in infants with apparent life-threatening event(s). *Am J Dis Child* 1989;143:951–954.

272. Seibert JJ, Byrne WJ, Euler AR, et al. Gastroesophageal reflux—the acid test: scintigraphy or the pH probe? *AJR* 1983;140:1087–1090.

273. Tolia V, Calhoun JA, Kuhns LR, Kauffman RE. Lack of correlation between extended pH monitoring and scintigraphy in the evaluation of infants with gastroesophageal reflux. *J Lab Clin Med* 1990;115:559–563.

274. Neuhauser EBD, Berenberg W. Cardio-esophageal relaxation as a cause of vomiting in infants. *Radiology* 1947;48:480–483.

275. McCauley RGK, Darling DB, Leonidas JC, Schwartz AM. Gastro-esophageal reflux in infants and children: a useful classification and reliable physiologic technique for its demonstration. *AJR* 1978;130: 47–50.

276. Cleveland RH, Kushner DC, Schwartz AN. Gastroesophageal reflux in children: results of a standardized fluoroscopic approach. *AJR* 1983; 141:53–56.

277. Leonidas JC. Gastroesophageal reflux in infants: role of the upper gastrointestinal series. *AJR* 1984;143:1350–1351.

278. Arthur RJ, Ziervogel MA, Azmy AF. Barium meal examination of infants under 4 months of age presenting with vomiting. A review of 100 cases. *Pediatr Radiol* 1984;14:84–86.

279. Darling DB, McCauley RGK, Leape LL, et al. The child with peptic esophagitis: a correlation of radiologic signs with esophageal pathology. *Radiology* 1982;145:673–676.

280. Yulish BS, Rothstein FC, Halpin TC Jr. Radiographic findings in children and young adults with Barrett's esophagus. *AJR* 1987;148: 353–357.

281. Hassall E, Weinstein WM, Ament ME. Barrett's esophagus in childhood. *Gastroenterology* 1985;84:1331–1337.

282. Meyers WF, Roberts CC, Johnson DG, Herbst JJ. Value of tests for evaluation of gastroesophageal reflux in children. *J Pediatr Surg* 1985; 20:515–520.

283. Blane CE, Klein MD, Drongowski RA, et al. Gastroesophageal reflux in children: is there a place for the upper gastrointestinal study? *Gastrointest Radiol* 1986;11:346–348.

Hiatal Hernia

284. Darling DB. Hiatal hernia and gastroesophageal reflux in infancy and childhood. Analysis of the radiologic findings. *AJR* 1975;123: 724–736.

285. Daneman A, Kozlowski K. Large hiatus hernias in infancy and childhood. *Australas Radiol* 1977;21:133–139.

Gastric Volvulus

286. Ziprkowski MN, Teele RL. Gastric volvulus in childhood. *AJR* 1979; 132:921–925.

287. Campbell JB. Neonatal gastric volvulus. *AJR* 1979;132:723–725.

288. Cole BC, Dickinson SJ. Acute volvulus of the stomach in infants and children. *Surgery* 1971;70:707–717.

289. Campbell JB, Rappaport LN, Skerker LB. Acute mesentero-axial volvulus of the stomach. *Radiology* 1972;103:153–156.

290. De Giacomo C, Maggiore G, Fiori P, et al. Chronic gastric torsion in infancy: a revisited diagnosis. *Australas Radiol* 1989;33:252–254.

Bezoar

291. DeBakey M, Ochsner A. Bezoars and concretions: a comprehensive review of the literature with an analysis of 303 collected cases and a presentation of 8 additional cases. *Surgery* 1938;4:934–963.

292. Cremin BJ, Fisher RM, Stokes NJ, Rabkin J. Four cases of lactobezoar in neonates. *Pediatr Radiol* 1974;2:107–110.

Intussusception

293. Ein SH, Stephens CA. Intussusception: 354 cases in 10 years. *J Pediatr Surg* 1971;6:16–27.

294. Wayne ER, Campbell JB, Burrington JD, Davis WS. Management of 344 children with intussusception. *Radiology* 1973;107:597–601.

295. Ein SH. Leading points in childhood intussusception. *J Pediatr Surg* 1976;11:209–211.

296. Ong NT, Beasley SW. The leadpoint in intussusception. *J Pediatr Surg* 1990;25:640–643.

297. Patriquin HB, Afshani E, Effmann E, et al. Neonatal intussusception. Report of 12 cases. *Radiology* 1977;125:463–466.

298. Eklof OA, Johanson L, Lohr G. Childhood intussusception: hydrostatic reducibility and incidence of leading points in different age groups. *Pediatr Radiol* 1980;10:83–86.

299. Levine M, Schwartz S, Katz J, et al. Plain film findings in intussusception. *Br J Radiol* 1967;37:678–681.

300. Eklof O, Hartelius H. Reliability of the abdominal plain film diagnosis in pediatric patients with suspected intussusception. *Pediatr Radiol* 1980;9:199–206.

301. Eklof O, Thonell S. Conventional abdominal radiography as a means to rule out ileo-caecal intussusception. *Acta Radiol (Diagn)* 1984;25: 265–267.

302. Ratcliffe JF, Fong S, Cheong I, O'Connell P. The plain abdominal film in intussusception: the accuracy and incidence of radiographic findings. *Pediatr Radiol* 1992;22:110–111.

303. Meradji M, Hussain SM, Robben SGF, Hop WCJ. Plain film diagnosis in intussusception. *Br J Radiol* 1994;67:147–149.

304. Sargent MA, Babyn P, Alton DJ. Plain abdominal radiography in suspected intussusception: a reassessment. *Pediatr Radiol* 1994;24: 17–20.

305. Ratcliffe JF, Fong S, Cheong I, O'Connell P. Plain film diagnosis of intussusception: prevalence of the target sign. *AJR* 1992;158: 619–621.

306. Lee JM, Kim H, Byun JY, et al. Intussusception: characteristic radiolucencies of the abdominal radiograph. *Pediatr Radiol* 1994;24: 293–295.

307. Leonidas JC. Treatment of intussusception with small bowel obstruction: application of decision analysis. *AJR* 1985;145:665–669.

308. White SJ, Blane CE. Intussusception: additional observations on the plain radiograph. *AJR* 1982;139:511–513.

309. Johnson JF, Woisard KK. Ileocolic intussusception: new sign on the supine cross-table lateral radiograph. *Radiology* 1989;170:483–486.

310. Pracros JP, Tran-Minh VA, Morin de Finfe CH, et al. Acute intestinal intussusception in children. Contribution of ultrasonography (145 cases). *Ann Radiol* 1987;30:525–530.

311. Verschelden P, Filiatrault D, Garel L, et al. Intussusception in children: reliability of US in diagnosis—a prospective study. *Radiology* 1992;184:741–744.

312. Shanbhogue RLK, Hussain SM, Meradji M, et al. Ultrasonography is accurate enough for the diagnosis of intussusception. *J Pediatr Surg* 1994;29:324–327.

313. Bhisitkul DM, Listernick R, Shkolnik A, et al. Clinical application of ultrasonography in the diagnosis of intussusception. *J Pediatr* 1992; 121:182–186.

314. Weinberger E, Winters WD. Intussusception in children: the role of sonography. *Radiology* 1992;184:601–602.

315. Bowerman RA, Silver TM, Jaffe MH. Real-time ultrasound diagnosis of intussusception in children. *Radiology* 1982;143:527–529.

316. Swischuk LE, Hayden CK, Boulden T. Intussusception: indications for ultrasonography and an explanation of the doughnut and pseudokidney signs. *Pediatr Radiol* 1985;15:388–391.

317. del-Pozo G, Albillos JC, Tejedor D. Intussusception: US findings with pathologic correlation—the crescent-in-doughnut sign. *Radiology* 1996;199:688–692.

318. Holt S, Samuel E. Multiple concentric ring sign in the ultrasonographic ultrasonographic diagnosis of intussusception. *Gastrointest Radiol* 1978;3:307–309.

319. Montali G, Croce F, De Pra L, Solbiati L. Intussusception of the bowel: a new sonographic pattern. *Br J Radiol* 1983;56:621–623.

320. McDermott VG. Childhood intussusception and approaches to treatment: a historical review. *Pediatr Radiol* 1994;24:153–155.

321. Ravitch MM, McCune RM. Reduction of intussusception by barium enema: a clinical and experimental study. *Ann Surg* 1948;128: 904–913.

322. Guo JZ, Ma XY, Zhou QH. Results of air pressure enema reduction of intussusception: 6,396 cases in 13 years. *J Pediatr Surg* 1986;21: 1201–1203.

323. Fiorito ES, Recalde Cuestas LA. Diagnosis and treatment of acute intestinal intussusception with controlled insufflation of air. *Pediatrics* 1959;24:241–244.

324. Gu L, Alton DJ, Daneman A, et al. Intussusception reduction in children by rectal insufflation of air. *AJR* 1988;150:1345–1348.

325. Swischuk LE, Stansberry SD. Ultrasonographic detection of free peritoneal fluid in uncomplicated intussusception. *Pediatr Radiol* 1991; 21:350–351.

326. Feinstein KA, Myers M, Fernbach SK, Bhisitkul DM. Peritoneal fluid in children with intussusception: its sonographic detection and relationship to successful reduction. *Abdom Imaging* 1993;18:277–279.

327. Lam AH, Firman K. Value of sonography including color Doppler in the diagnosis and management of long standing intussusception. *Pediatr Radiol* 1992;22:112–114.

328. Lim HK, Bae SH, Lee KH, et al. Assessment of reducibility of ileocolic intussusception in children: usefulness of color Doppler sonography. *Radiology* 1994;191:781–785.

329. Stephenson CA, Seibert JJ, Strain JD, et al. Intussusception: clinical and radiographic factors influencing reducibility. *Pediatr Radiol* 1984;20:57–60.

330. Katz M, Phelan E, Carlin JB, Beasley SW. Gas enema for the reduction of intussusception: relationship between clinical signs and symptoms and outcome. *AJR* 1993;160:363–366.

331. Franken EA Jr, Smith WL, Chernish SM, et al. The use of glucagon in hydrostatic reduction of intussusception: a double-blind study of 30 patients. *Radiology* 1983;146:687–689.

332. Touloukian RJ, O'Connell JB, Markowitz RI, et al. Analgesic premedication in the management of ileocolic intussusception. *Pediatrics* 1987;79:432–434.

333. Markowitz RI, Meyer JS. Pneumatic versus hydrostatic reduction of intussusception. *Radiology* 1992;183:623–624.

334. Katz ME, Kolm P. Intussusception reduction 1991: an international survey of pediatric radiologists. *Pediatr Radiol* 1992;22:318–322.

335. Meyer JS. The current radiologic management of intussusception: a survey and review. *Pediatr Radiol* 1992;22:323–325.

336. Shiels WE II, Kirks DR, Keller GL, et al. Colonic perforation by air and liquid enemas: comparison study in young pigs. *AJR* 1993;160:931–935.

337. Woo SK, Kim JS, Suh SJ, et al. Childhood intussusception: US-guided hydrostatic reduction. *Radiology* 1992;182:77–80.

338. Fishman MC, Borden S, Cooper A. The dissection sign of nonreducible ileocolic intussusception. *AJR* 1984;143:5–8.

339. Johnson JF, Shiels WE II. Ileocolic intussusception: hydrostatic reduction in the presence of the dissection sign. *Pediatr Radiol* 1986;16:514–515.

340. Kuta AJ, Benator RM. Intussusception: hydrostatic pressure equivalents for barium and meglumine sodium diatrizoate. *Radiology* 1990;175:125–126.

341. Sargent MA, Wilson BPM. Are hydrostatic and pneumatic methods of intussusception reduction comparable? *Pediatr Radiol* 1991;21:346–349.

342. Pierro A, Donnell SC, Paraskevopoulou C, et al. Indications for laparotomy after hydrostatic reduction for intussusception. *J Pediatr Surg* 1993;28:1154–1157.

343. Ein SH, Palder SB, Alton DJ, Daneman A. Intussusception: toward less surgery? *J Pediatr Surg* 1994;29:433–435.

344. Rohrschneider W, Troger J, Betsch B. The post-reduction donut sign. *Pediatr Radiol* 1994;24:156–160.

345. Eklof O, Hugosson C. Post-evacuation findings in barium enema treated intussusceptions. *Ann Radiol* 1976;19:133–139.

346. Devred P, Faure F, Padovani J. Pseudotumoral cecum after hydrostatic reduction of intussusception. *Pediatr Radiol* 1984;14:295–298.

347. Ein SH, Shandling B, Reilly BJ, Stringer DA. Hydrostatic reduction of intussusceptions caused by lead points. *J Pediatr Surg* 1986;21:883–886.

348. Connolly B, Alton DJ, Ein SH, Daneman A. Partially reduced intussusception: when are repeated delayed reduction attempts appropriate? *Pediatr Radiol* 1995;25:104–107.

349. Shiels WE II, Bisset GS III, Kirks DR. Simple device for air reduction of intussusception. *Pediatr Radiol* 1990;20:472–474.

350. Hedlund GL, Johnson JF, Strife JL. Ileocolic intussusception: extensive reflux of air preceding pneumatic reduction. *Radiology* 1990;174:187–189.

351. Shiels WE II, Maves CK, Hedlund GL, Kirks DR. Air enema for diagnosis and reduction of intussusception: clinical experience and pressure correlates. *Radiology* 1991;181:169–172.

352. Stein M, Alton DJ, Daneman A. Pneumatic reduction of intussusception: 5-year experience. *Radiology* 1992;183:681–684.

353. Kirks DR. Air intussusception reduction: "the winds of change." *Pediatr Radiol* 1995;25:89–91.

354. Poznanski AK. Why I still use barium for intussusception. *Pediatr Radiol* 1995;25:92–93.

355. Daneman A, Alton DJ. Intussusception. Issues and controversies related to diagnosis and reduction. *Radiol Clin North Am* 1996;34:743–756.

356. Miller SF, Landes AB, Dautenhahn LW, et al. Intussusception: ability of fluoroscopic images obtained during air enemas to depict lead points and other abnormalities. *Radiology* 1995;197:493–496.

357. Don S, Cohen MD, Wells LJ, Rescorla FJ. Air reduction of an intussusception caused by a pathologic lead point in an infant. *Pediatr Radiol* 1992;22:326–327.

358. Lam AH, Firman K. Ultrasound of intussusception with lead points. *Australas Radiol* 1991;35:343–345.

359. Ein SH. Recurrent intussusception in children. *J Pediatr Surg* 1975;10:751–755.

360. Champoux AN, Del Beccaro MA, Nazar-Stewart V. Recurrent intussusception. Risks and features. *Arch Pediatr Adolesc Med* 1994;148:474–478.

361. Campbell JB. Contrast media in intussusception. *Pediatr Radiol* 1989;19:293–296.

362. Daneman A, Alton DJ, Ein S, et al. Perforation during attempted intussusception reduction in children—a comparison of perforation with barium and air. *Pediatr Radiol* 1995;25:81–88.

363. Gu L, Wong S, Gu A. Perforations during attempted intussusception reduction: 14 patients from 9,028 examinations over a 20 year period. *J Interv Radiol* 1993;2:36–38.

364. Bramson RT, Blickman JG. Perforation during hydrostatic reduction of intussusception: proposed mechanism and review of the literature. *J Pediatr Surg* 1992;27:589–591.

365. Armstrong EA, Dunbar JS, Graviss ER, et al. Intussusception complicated by distal perforation of the colon. *Radiology* 1980;136:77–81.

366. Humphry A, Ein SH, Mok PM. Perforation of the intussuscepted colon. *AJR* 1981;137:1135–1138.

367. Blane CE, DiPietro ME, White SJ, et al. An analysis of bowel perforation in patients with intussusception. *J Can Assoc Radiol* 1984;35:113–115.

Inguinal Hernia

368. Currarino G. Incarcerated inguinal hernia in infants: plain films and barium enema. *Pediatr Radiol* 1974;2:247–250.

Anomalies of the Omphalomesenteric Duct

369. DiSantis DJ, Siegel MJ, Katz ME. Simplified approach to umbilical remnant abnormalities. *RadioGraphics* 1991;11:59–66.

370. Vane DW, West KW, Grosfeld JL. Vitelline duct anomalies. Experience with 217 childhood cases. *Arch Surg* 1987;122:542–547.

371. Gaisie G, Curnes JT, Scatliff JH, et al. Neonatal intestinal obstruction from omphalomesenteric duct remnants. *AJR* 1985;144:109–112.

Gastrointestinal Duplication

372. Macpherson RI. Gastrointestinal tract duplications: clinical, pathologic, etiologic, and radiologic considerations. *RadioGraphics* 1993;13:1063–1080.

373. Bower RJ, Sieber WK, Kiesewetter WB. Alimentary tract duplications in children. *Ann Surg* 1978;188:669–674.

Mesenteric Cyst (Lymphangioma)

374. Ros PR, Olmsted WW, Moser RP Jr, et al. Mesenteric and omental cysts: histologic classification with imaging correlation. *Radiology* 1987;164:327–332.

375. Blumhagen JD, Wood BJ, Rosenbaum DM. Sonographic evaluation of abdominal lymphangiomas in children. *J Ultrasound Med* 1987;6:487–495.

376. Siegel MJ, Glazer HS, St. Amour TE, Rosenthal DD. Lymphangiomas in children: MR imaging. *Radiology* 1989;170:467–470.

Juvenile Polyps and Polyposis Syndromes

377. Harned RK, Buck JL, Sobin LH. The hamartomatous polyposis syndromes: clinical and radiologic features. *AJR* 1995;164:565–571.

378. Buck JL, Harned RK, Lichtenstein JE, Sobin LH. Peutz-Jeghers syndrome. *RadioGraphics* 1992;12:365–378.

379. Giardiello FM, Welsh SB, Hamilton SR, et al. Increased risk of cancer in the Peutz-Jeghers syndrome. *N Engl J Med* 1987;316:1511–1514.

Henoch-Schönlein Purpura

380. Grossman H, Berdon WE, Baker DH. Abdominal pain in Schonlein-Henoch syndrome. Its correlation with small bowel barium roentgen study. *Am J Dis Child* 1964;108:67–72.
381. Glasier CM, Siegel MJ, McAlister WH, Shackelford GD. Henoch-Schonlein syndrome in children: gastrointestinal manifestations. *AJR* 1981;136:1081–1085.

Achalasia

382. Azizkhan RG, Tapper D, Eraklis A. Achalasia in childhood: a 20-year experience. *J Pediatr Surg* 1980;15:452–456.
383. Vaughn WH, Williams JL. Familial achalasia with pulmonary complications in children. *Radiology* 1973;107:407–409.
384. Sorsdahl OA, Gay BB Jr. Achalasia of the esophagus in childhood. *Am J Dis Child* 1965;109:141–146.
385. Maravilla AM, Barnes JC, Kirks DR. Achalasia: radiological case of the month. *Am J Dis Child* 1979;133:855–856.

Gastritis and Ulcer Disease

386. Nord KS. Peptic ulcer disease in the pediatric population. *Pediatr Clin North Am* 1988;35:117–140.
387. Gryboski JD. Peptic ulcer disease in children. *Pediatr Rev* 1990;12:15–21.
388. Stringer DA, Daneman A, Brunelle F, et al. Sonography of the normal and abnormal stomach (excluding hypertrophic pyloric stenosis) in children. *J Ultrasound Med* 1986;5:183–188.
389. Hayden CK Jr, Swischuk LE, Rytting JE. Gastric ulcer disease in infants: US findings. *Radiology* 1987;164:131–134.
390. Morrison S, Dahms BB, Hoffenberg E, Czinn SJ. Enlarged gastric folds in association with *Campylobacter pylori* gastritis. *Radiology* 1989;171:819–821.
391. Baker A, Volberg F, Sumner T, Moran R. Childhood Menetrier's disease: four new cases and discussion of the literature. *Gastrointest Radiol* 1986;11:131–134.
392. Marks MP, Lanza MV, Kahlstrom EJ, et al. Pediatric hypertrophic gastropathy. *AJR* 1986;147:1031–1034.
393. Coad NAG, Shah KJ. Menetrier's disease in childhood associated with cytomegalovirus infection: a case report and review of the literature. *Br J Radiol* 1986;59:615–620.
394. Burns B, Gay BB Jr. Menetrier's disease of the stomach in children. *AJR* 1968;103:300–306.
395. Teele RL, Katz AJ, Goldman H, Kettell RM. Radiographic features of eosinophilic gastroenteritis (allergic gastroenteropathy) of childhood. *AJR* 1979;132:575–580.
396. Matzinger MA, Daneman A. Esophageal involvement in eosinophilic gastroenteritis. *Pediatr Radiol* 1983;13:35–38.
397. Griscom NT, Kirkpatrick JA Jr, Girdany BR, et al. Gastric antral narrowing in chronic granulomatous disease of childhood. *Pediatrics* 1974;54:456–460.

Inflammatory Bowel Disease

398. Stringer DA. Imaging inflammatory bowel disease in the pediatric patient. *Radiol Clin North Am* 1987;25:93–113.
399. Wills JS, Lobis IF, Denstman FJ. Crohn disease: state of the art. *Radiology* 1997;202:597–610.
400. Kirks DR, Currarino G. Regional enteritis in children: small bowel disease with normal terminal ileum. *Pediatr Radiol* 1978;7:10–14.
401. Winthrop JD, Balfe DM, Shackelford GD, et al. Ulcerative and granulomatous colitis in children. Comparison of double- and single-contrast studies. *Radiology* 1985;154:657–660.
402. Taylor GA, Nancarrow PA, Hernanz-Schulman M, Teele RL. Plain abdominal radiographs in children with inflammatory bowel disease. *Pediatr Radiol* 1986;16:206–209.
403. Jabra AA, Fishman EK, Taylor GA. CT findings in inflammatory bowel disease in children. *AJR* 1994;162:975–979.
404. Devroede GJ, Taylor WF, Sauer WG, et al. Cancer risk and life expectancy of children with ulcerative colitis. *N Engl J Med* 1971;285:17–21.
405. Ekbom A, Helmick C, Zack M, Adami HO. Ulcerative colitis and colorectal cancer. A population-based study. *N Engl J Med* 1990;323:1228–1233.

406. Korelitz BI. Considerations of surveillance, dysplasia, and carcinoma of the colon in the management of ulcerative colitis and Crohn's disease. *Med Clin North Am* 1990;74:189–199.

The Immunocompromised Child

407. Haller JO, Cohen HL. Gastrointestinal manifestations of AIDS in children. *AJR* 1994;162:387–393.
408. Fisk JD, Shulman HM, Greening RR, et al. Gastrointestinal radiographic features of human graft-vs.-host disease. *AJR* 1981;136:329–336.
409. McDonald GB, Sullivan KM, Plumley TF. Radiographic features of esophageal involvement in chronic graft-vs.-host disease. *AJR* 1984;142:501–506.
410. Wagner ML, Rosenberg HS, Fernbach DJ, Singleton EB. Typhlitis: a complication of leukemia in childhood. *AJR* 1970;109:341–350.
411. Katz JA, Wagner ML, Gresik MV, et al. Typhlitis. An 18-year experience and postmortem review. *Cancer* 1990;65:1041–1047.
412. Abramson SJ, Berdon WE, Baker DH. Childhood typhlitis: its increasing association with acute myelogenous leukemia. Report of five cases. *Radiology* 1983;146:61–64.
413. McNamara MJ, Chalmers AG, Morgan M, Smith SE. Typhlitis in acute childhood leukaemia: radiological features. *Clin Radiol* 1986;37:83–86.
414. Frick MP, Maile CW, Crass JR, et al. Computed tomography of neutropenic colitis. *AJR* 1984;143:763–765.
415. Alexander JE, Williamson SL, Seibert JJ, et al. The ultrasonographic diagnosis of typhlitis (neutropenic colitis). *Pediatr Radiol* 1988;18:200–204.

Appendicitis

416. Wilkinson RH, Bartlett RH, Eraklis AJ. Diagnosis of appendicitis in infancy. The value of abdominal radiographs. *Am J Dis Child* 1969;118:687–690.
417. Joffe N. Radiology of acute appendicitis and its complications. *Crit Rev Clin Radiol Nucl Med* 1975;7:97–160.
418. Johnson JF, Coughlin WF, Stark P. The sensitivity of plain films for detecting perforation in children with appendicitis. *Fortschr Geb Rontgenstr Nuklearmed* 1988;149:619–623.
419. Johnson JF, Coughlin WF. Plain film diagnosis of appendiceal perforation in children. *Semin Ultrasound CT MR* 1989;10:306–313.
420. Riggs W Jr, Parvey LS. Perforated appendix presenting with disproportionate jejunal distention. *Pediatr Radiol* 1976;5:47–49.
421. Fedyshin P, Kelvin FM, Rice RP. Nonspecificity of barium enema findings in acute appendicitis. *AJR* 1984;143:99–102.
422. Puylaert JBCM. Acute appendicitis: US evaluation using graded compression. *Radiology* 1986;158:355–360.
423. Abu-Yousef MM, Bleicher JJ, Maher JW, et al. High-resolution sonography of acute appendicitis. *AJR* 1987;149:53–58.
424. Jeffrey RB Jr, Laing FC, Townsend RR. Acute appendicitis: sonographic criteria based on 250 cases. *Radiology* 1988;167:327–329.
425. Kao SCS, Smith WL, Abu-Yousef MM, et al. Acute appendicitis in children: sonographic findings. *AJR* 1989;153:375–379.
426. Vignault F, Filiatrault D, Brandt ML, et al. Acute appendicitis in children: evaluation with US. *Radiology* 1990;176:501–504.
427. Sivit CJ, Newman KD, Boenning DA, et al. Appendicitis: usefulness of US in diagnosis in a pediatric population. *Radiology* 1992;185:549–552.
428. Quillin SP, Siegel MJ. Appendicitis: efficacy of color Doppler sonography. *Radiology* 1994;191:557–560.
429. Siegel MJ, Carel C, Surratt S. Ultrasonography of acute abdominal pain in children. *JAMA* 1991;266:1987–1989.
430. Gaensler EHL, Jeffrey RB Jr, Laing FC, Townsend RR. Sonography in patients with suspected acute appendicitis: value in establishing alternative diagnoses. *AJR* 1989;152:49–51.
431. Larson JM, Peirce JC, Ellinger DM, et al. The validity and utility of sonography in the diagnosis of appendicitis in the community setting. *AJR* 1989;153:687–691.
432. Siegel MJ. Acute appendicitis in childhood: the role of US. *Radiology* 1992;185:341–342.
433. Friedland JA, Siegel MJ. CT appearance of acute appendicitis in childhood. *AJR* 1997;168:439–442.

Complications of Cystic Fibrosis

434. Abramson SJ, Baker DH, Amodio JB, Berdon WE. Gastrointestinal manifestations of cystic fibrosis. *Semin Roentgenol* 1987;22:97–113.
435. Agrons GA, Corse WR, Markowitz RI, et al. Gastrointestinal manifestations of cystic fibrosis: radiologic-pathologic correlation. *RadioGraphics* 1996;16:871–893.
436. Smyth RL, van Velzen D, Smyth AR, et al. Strictures of the ascending colon in cystic fibrosis and high-strength pancreatic enzymes. *Lancet* 1994;343:85–86.
437. Zerin JM, Kuhn-Fulton J, White SJ, et al. Colonic strictures in children with cystic fibrosis. *Radiology* 1995;194:223–226.
438. Pettei MJ, Leonidas JC, Levine JJ, Gorvoy JD. Pancolonic disease in cystic fibrosis and high-dose pancreatic enzyme therapy. *J Pediatr* 1994;125:587–589.
439. Ablin DS, Ziegler M. Ulcerative type of colitis associated with the use of high strength pancreatic enzyme supplements in cystic fibrosis. *Pediatr Radiol* 1995;25:113–116.
440. Berk RN, Lee FA. The late gastrointestinal manifestations of cystic fibrosis of the pancreas. *Radiology* 1973;106:377–381.
441. Taussig LM, Saldino RM, Di Sant'Agnese PA. Radiographic abnormalities of the duodenum and small bowel in cystic fibrosis of the pancreas (mucoviscidosis). *Radiology* 1973;106:369–376.

Biliary Atresia and Neonatal Hepatitis

442. Kirks DR, Coleman RE, Filston HC, et al. An imaging approach to persistent neonatal jaundice. *AJR* 1984;142:461–465.
443. Hirsig J, Rickham PP. Early differential diagnosis between neonatal hepatitis and biliary atresia. *J Pediatr Surg* 1980;15:13–15.
444. Landing BH. Considerations of the pathogenesis of neonatal hepatitis, biliary atresia and choledochal cyst: the concept of infantile obstructive cholangiopathy. *Prog Pediatr Surg* 1974;6:113–139.
445. Majd M, Reba RC, Altman RP. Hepatobiliary scintigraphy with ^{99m}TC-IDA scintigraphy in the evaluation of neonatal jaundice. *Pediatrics* 1981;67:140–145.
446. Majd M, Reba RC, Altman RP. Effect of phenobarbital on ^{99m}Tc-IDA scintigraphy in the evaluation of neonatal jaundice. *Semin Nucl Med* 1981;11:194–204.
447. Izant RJ Jr, et al. *Biliary atresia survey.* Washington, DC: American Academy of Pediatrics, 1964.
448. Kasai M, Watanabe I, Ohi R. Follow-up studies of long-term survivors after hepatic portoenterostomy for "noncorrectable" biliary atresia. *J Pediatr Surg* 1975;10:173–182.

Choledochal Cyst and Caroli Disease

449. O'Neill JA Jr. Choledochal cyst. *Curr Probl Surg* 1992;29:361–410.
450. Altman RP. Choledochal cyst. *Semin Pediatr Surg* 1992;1:130–133.
451. Caroli J. Diseases of intrahepatic bile ducts. *Isr J Med* Sci 1968;4:21–35.
452. Babbitt DP, Starshak RJ, Clemett AR. Choledochal cyst: a concept of etiology. *AJR* 1973;119:57–62.
453. Rosenfield N, Griscom NT. Choledochal cysts: roentgenographic techniques. *Radiology* 1975;114:113–119.

Cholelithiasis and Cholecystitis

454. Kirks DR. Lithiasis due to interruption of the enterohepatic circulation of bile salts. *AJR* 1979;133:383–388.
455. Reif S, Sloven DG, Lebenthal E. Gallstones in children. Characterization by age, etiology, and outcome. *Am J Dis Child* 1991;145:105–108.
456. Keller MS, Markle BM, Laffey PA, et al. Spontaneous resolution of cholelithiasis in infants. *Radiology* 1985;157:345–348.
457. Slovis TL, Hight DW, Philippart AI, Dubois RS. Sonography in the diagnosis and management of hydrops of the gallbladder in children with mucocutaneous lymph node syndrome. *Pediatrics* 1980;65:789–794.
458. Patriquin HB, DiPietro M, Barber FE, Teele RL. Sonography of thickened gallbladder wall: causes in children. *AJR* 1983;141:57–60.
459. Chung CJ, Sivit CJ, Rakusan TA, et al. Hepatobiliary abnormalities on sonography in children with HIV infection. *J Ultrasound Med* 1994;13:205–210.

Hepatobiliary Tumors

460. Dehner LP. Liver, gallbladder, and extrahepatic biliary tract. In: Dehner LP. *Pediatric surgical pathology.* Baltimore: Williams and Wilkins, 1987, 433–523.
461. Cohen MD. Gastrointestinal tumors. In: *Imaging of Children with Cancer.* St. Louis: Mosby–Year Book, 1992, 20–42.
462. Mukai JK, Stack CM, Turner DA, et al. Imaging of surgically relevant hepatic vascular and segmental anatomy. Part 2. Extent and resectability of hepatic neoplasms. *AJR* 1987;149:293–297.
463. VanCampenhout I, Patriquin H. Malignant microvasculature in abdominal tumors in children: detection with Doppler US. *Radiology* 1992;183:445–448.
464. Taylor GA, Perlman EJ, Scherer LR, et al. Vascularity of tumors in children: evaluation with color Doppler imaging. *AJR* 1991;157:1267–1271.
465. Boechat MI, Kangarloo H, Ortega J, et al. Primary liver tumors in children: comparison of CT and MR imaging. *Radiology* 1988;169:727–732.
466. Boechat MI, Kangarloo H, Gilsanz V. Hepatic masses in children. *Semin Roentgenol* 1988;23:185–193.
467. Weinreb JC, Cohen JM, Armstrong E, Smith T. Imaging of the pediatric liver: MRI and CT. *AJR* 1986;147:785–790.
468. Stocker JT, Ishak KG. Mesenchymal hamartoma of the liver: report of 30 cases and review of the literature. *Pediatr Pathol* 1983;1:245–267.
469. Ros PR, Goodman ZD, Ishak KG, et al. Mesenchymal hamartoma of the liver: radiologic-pathologic correlation. *Radiology* 1986;158:619–624.
470. Smith WL, Ballantine TVN, Gonzalez-Crussi F. Hepatic mesenchymal hamartoma causing heart failure in the neonate. *J Pediatr Surg* 1978;13:183–185.
471. DeMaioribus CA, Lally KP, Sim K, et al. Mesenchymal hamartoma of the liver. A 35-year review. *Arch Surg* 1990;125:598–600.
472. Dehner LP, Ishak KG. Vascular tumors of the liver in infants and children. A study of 30 cases and review of the literature. *Arch Pathol* 1971;92:101–111.
473. Mulliken JB, Glowacki J. Hemangiomas and vascular malformations in infants and children: a classification based on endothelial characteristics. *Plast Reconstr Surg* 1982;69:412–422.
474. Mulliken JB, Young AE. *Vascular birthmarks: hemangiomas and malformations.* Philadelphia: WB Saunders, 1988.
475. Paltiel HJ, Patriquin HB, Keller MS, et al. Infantile hepatic hemangioma: doppler US. *Radiology* 1992;182:735–742.
476. Ezekowitz RAB, Mulliken JB, Folkman J. Interferon alfa-2a therapy for life-threatening hemangiomas of infancy. *N Engl J Med* 1992;326:1456–1463.
477. Fellows KE, Hoffer FA, Markowitz RI, O'Neill JA Jr. Multiple collaterals to hepatic infantile hemangioendotheliomas and arteriovenous malformations: effect of embolization. *Radiology* 1991;181:813–818.
478. Reymond D, Plaschkes J, Luthy AR. Focal nodular hyperplasia of the liver in children: review of follow-up and outcome. *J Pediatr Surg* 1995;30:1590–1593.
479. Dachman AH, Pakter RL, Ros PR, et al. Hepatoblastoma: radiologic-pathologic correlation in 50 cases. *Radiology* 1987;164:15–19.
480. Powers C, Ros PR, Stoupis C, et al. Primary liver neoplasms: MR imaging with pathologic correlation. *RadioGraphics* 1994;14:459–482.
481. Newman KD, Schisgall R, Reaman G, Guzzetta PC. Malignant mesenchymoma of the liver in children. *J Pediatr Surg* 1989;24:781–783.
482. Ros PR, Olmsted WW, Dachman AH, et al. Undifferentiated (embryonal) sarcoma of the liver: radiologic-pathologic correlation. *Radiology* 1986;161:141–145.
483. Marti-Bonmati L, Ferrer D, Menor F, Galant J. Hepatic mesenchymal sarcoma: MRI findings. *Abdom Imaging* 1993;18:176–179.

Diffuse Hepatic Parenchymal Disease

484. Griscom NT, Capitanio MA, Wagoner ML, et al. The visibly fatty liver. *Radiology* 1975;117:385–389.
485. Yousefzadeh DK, Lupetin AR, Jackson JH Jr. The radiographic signs of fatty liver. *Radiology* 1979;131:351–355.

Vascular Abnormalities

486. Karrer FM. Portal hypertension. *Semin Pediatr Surg* 1992;1:134–144.
487. Rosch J, Dotter CT. Extrahepatic portal obstruction in childhood and its angiographic diagnosis. *AJR* 1971;112:143–149.
488. Patriquin H, Lafortune M, Burns PN, Dauzat M. Duplex Doppler examination in portal hypertension: technique and anatomy. *AJR* 1987;149:71–76.
489. Westra SJ, Zaninovic AC, Vargas J, et al. The value of portal vein pulsatility on duplex sonograms as a sign of portal hypertension in children with liver disease. *AJR* 1995;165:167–172.
490. Abu-Yousef MM. Duplex Doppler sonography of the hepatic vein in tricuspid regurgitation. *AJR* 1991;156:79–83.
491. Cressman JB, Strife JL, Meyer RA, Iwamoto H. *Duplex Doppler sonography of the portal vein: evaluation of waveform pulsatility with changes in right atrial pressure.* Colorado Springs, CO: The Society for Pediatric Radiology, 1994, 102.
492. Patriquin H, Tessier G, Grignon A, Boisvert J. Lesser omental thickness in normal children: baseline for detection of portal hypertension. *AJR* 1985;145:693–696.
493. Lafortune M, Patriquin H, Pomier G, et al. Hemodynamic changes in portal circulation after portosystemic shunts: use of duplex sonography in 43 patients. *AJR* 1987;149:701–706.
494. Patriquin H, Lafortune M, Weber A, et al. Surgical portosystemic shunts in children: assessment with duplex Doppler US. Work in progress. *Radiology* 1987;165:25–28.

Liver Transplantation

495. Westra SJ, Zaninovic AC, Hall TR, et al. Imaging in pediatric liver transplantation. *RadioGraphics* 1993;13:1081–1099.
496. Bisset GS III, Strife JL, Balistreri WF. Evaluation of children for liver transplantation: value of MR imaging and sonography. *AJR* 1990;155:351–356.
497. Ben-Ami TE, Martich V, Yousefzadeh DK, et al. Anatomic features of reduced-size liver transplant: postsurgical imaging characteristics. *Radiology* 1993;187:165–170.

Splenic Abnormalities

498. Rosenberg HK, Markowitz RI, Kolberg H, et al. Normal splenic size in infants and children: sonographic measurements. *AJR* 1991;157:119–121.
499. Hernanz-Schulman M, Ambrosino MM, Genieser NB. Current evaluation of the patient with abnormal visceroatrial situs. *AJR* 1990;154:797–802.
500. Abramson SJ, Berdon WE, Altman RP, et al. Biliary atresia and noncardiac polysplenic syndrome: US and surgical considerations. *Radiology* 1987;163:377–379.
501. Seo T, Ito T, Watanabe Y, Umeda T. Torsion of an accessory spleen presenting as an acute abdomen with an inflammatory mass. US, CT, and MRI findings. *Pediatr Radiol* 1994;24:532–534.
502. Herman TE, Siegel MJ. CT of acute splenic torsion in children with wandering spleen. *AJR* 1991;156:151–153.
503. Nemcek AA Jr, Miller FH, Fitzgerald SW. Acute torsion of a wandering spleen: diagnosis by CT and duplex Doppler and color flow sonography. *AJR* 1991;157:307–309.
504. Swischuk LE, Williams JB, John SD. Torsion of wandering spleen: the whorled appearance of the splenic pedicle on CT. *Pediatr Radiol* 1993;23:476–477.
505. Gore RM, Shkolnik A. Abdominal manifestations of pediatric leukemias: sonographic assessment. *Radiology* 1982;143:207–210.
506. Klippenstein DL, Zerin JM, Hirschl RB, Donn SM. Splenic enlargement in neonates during ECMO. *Radiology* 1994;190:411–412.
507. Hill SC, Reinig JW, Barranger JA, et al. Gaucher disease: sonographic appearance of the spleen. *Radiology* 1986;160:631–634.
508. Hill SC, Damaska BM, Ling A, et al. Gaucher disease: abdominal MR imaging findings in 46 patients. *Radiology* 1992;184:561–566.
509. Topley JM, Rogers DW, Stevens MCG, Serjeant GR. Acute splenic sequestration and hypersplenism in the first five years in homozygous sickle cell disease. *Arch Dis Child* 1981;56:765–769.
510. Weingarten MJ, Fakhry J, McCarthy J, et al. Sonography after splenic embolization: the wedge-shaped acute infarct. *AJR* 1984;141:957–959.

511. Magid D, Fishman EK, Siegelman SS. Computed tomography of the spleen and liver in sickle cell disease. *AJR* 1984;143:245–249.
512. Daneman A, Martin DJ. Congenital epithelial splenic cysts in children. Emphasis on sonographic appearances and some unusual features. *Pediatr Radiol* 1982;12:119–125.
513. Griscom NT, Hargreaves HK, Schwartz MZ, et al. Huge splenic cyst in a newborn: comparison with 10 cases in later childhood and adolescence. *AJR* 1977;129:889–891.
514. Musy P-A, Roche B, Belli D, et al. Splenic cysts in pediatric patients—a report on 8 cases and review of the literature. *Eur J Pediatr Surg* 1992;2:137–140.
515. Rudick MG, Wood BP, Lerner RM. Splenic abscess diagnosed by ultrasound in the pediatric patient. Report of three cases. *Pediatr Radiol* 1983;13:269–271.
516. Freeman JL, Jafri SZH, Roberts JL, et al. CT of congenital and acquired abnormalities of the spleen. *RadioGraphics* 1993;13:597–610.
517. Rappaport DC, Cumming WA, Ros PR. Disseminated hepatic and splenic lesions in cat-scratch disease: imaging features. *AJR* 1991;156:1227–1228.
518. Talenti E, Cesaro S, Scapinello A, et al. Disseminated hepatic and splenic calcifications following cat-scratch disease. *Pediatr Radiol* 1994;24:342–343.
519. Morgenstern L, Bello JM, Fisher BL, Verham RP. The clinical spectrum of lymphangiomas and lymphangiomatosis of the spleen. *Ann Surg* 1992;58:599–603.
520. Johnson MA, Cooperberg PL, Boisvert J, et al. Spontaneous splenic rupture in infectious mononucleosis: sonographic diagnosis and follow-up. *AJR* 1981;136:111–114.

Pancreatic Abnormalities

521. Siegel MJ, Martin KW, Worthington JL. Normal and abnormal pancreas in children: US studies. *Radiology* 1987;165:15–18.
522. Yedlin ST, Dubois RS, Philippart AI. Pancreas divisum: a cause of acute pancreatitis in childhood. *J Pediatr Surg* 1984;19:793–794.
523. Herman TE, Siegel MJ. CT of the pancreas in children. *AJR* 1991;157:375–379.
524. Orr LA, Powell RW, Melhem RE. Sonographic demonstration of annular pancreas in the newborn. *J Ultrasound Med* 1992;11:373–375.
525. Willi UV, Reddish JM, Teele RL. Cystic fibrosis: its characteristic appearance on abdominal sonography. *AJR* 1980;134:1005–1010.
526. Daneman A, Gaskin K, Martin DJ, Cutz E. Pancreatic changes in cystic fibrosis: CT and sonographic appearances. *AJR* 1983;141:653–655.
527. Schneider K, Harms K, Fendel H. The increased echogenicity of the pancreas in infants and children: the white pancreas. *Eur J Pediatr* 1987;146:508–511.
528. Hernanz-Schulman M, Teele RL, Perez-Atayde A, et al. Pancreatic cystosis in cystic fibrosis. *Radiology* 1986;158:629–631.
529. Hough DM, Stephens DH, Johnson CD, Binkovitz LA. Pancreatic lesions in von Hippel-Lindau disease: prevalence, clinical significance, and CT findings. *AJR* 1994;162:1091–1094.
530. Baker LL, Hartman GE, Northway WH. Sonographic detection of congenital pancreatic cysts in the newborn: report of a case and review of the literature. *Pediatr Radiol* 1990;20:488–490.
531. Grosfeld JL, Vane DW, Rescorla FJ, et al. Pancreatic tumors in childhood: analysis of 13 cases. *J Pediatr Surg* 1990;25:1057–1062.
532. Vade A, Blane CE. Imaging of Burkitt lymphoma in pediatric patients. *Pediatr Radiol* 1985;15:123–126.
533. Poustchi-Amin M, Leonidas JC, Valderrama E, et al. Papillary-cystic neoplasm of the pancreas. *Pediatr Radiol* 1995;25:509–511.
534. Weizman Z, Durie PR. Acute pancreatitis in childhood. *J Pediatr* 1988;113:24–29.
535. King LR, Siegel MJ, Balfe DM. Acute pancreatitis in children: CT findings of intra- and extrapancreatic fluid collections. *Radiology* 1995;195:196–200.
536. Brown CW, Werlin SL, Geenan JE, Schmalz M. The diagnostic and therapeutic role of endoscopic retrograde cholangiopancreatography in children. *J Pediatr Gastroenterol Nutr* 1993;17:19–23.
537. Atkinson GO Jr, Wyly JB, Gay BB Jr, et al. Idiopathic fibrosing pancreatitis: a cause of obstructive jaundice in childhood. *Pediatr Radiol* 1988;18:28–31.
538. Spencer JA, Lindsell DRM, Isaacs D. Hereditary pancreatitis: early ultrasound appearances. *Pediatr Radiol* 1990;20:293–295.

Imaging of Blunt Abdominal Trauma

539. Division of Injury Control—Center for Environmental Health and Injury Control—Centers for Disease Control. Childhood injuries in the United States. *Am J Dis Child* 1990;144:627–646.

540. Taylor GA, Eichelberger MR, O'Donnell R, Bowman L. Indications for computed tomography in children with blunt abdominal trauma. *Ann Surg* 1991;213:212–218.

541. Taylor GA, Kaufman RA. Emergency department sonography in the initial evaluation of blunt abdominal injury in children. *Pediatr Radiol* 1993;23:161–163.

542. Taylor GA, O'Donnell R, Sivit CJ, Eichelberger MR. Abdominal injury score: a clinical score for the assignment of risk in children after blunt trauma. *Radiology* 1994;190:689–694.

543. Newman KD, Bowman LM, Eichelberger MR, et al. The lap belt complex: intestinal and lumbar spine injury in children. *J Trauma* 1990;30:1133–1138.

544. Sivit CJ, Taylor GA, Newman KD, et al. Safety belt injuries in children with lap-belt ecchymosis: CT findings in 61 patients. *AJR* 1991; 157:111–114.

545. Taylor GA, Eichelberger MR, Potter BM. Hematuria. A marker of abdominal injury in children after blunt trauma. *Ann Surg* 1988;208: 688–693.

546. Stalker HP, Kaufman RA, Stedje K. The significance of hematuria in children after blunt abdominal trauma. *AJR* 1990;154:569–571.

547. Taylor GA, Eichelberger MR. Abdominal CT in children with neurologic impairment following blunt trauma. Abdominal CT in comatose children. *Ann Surg* 1989;210:229–233.

548. Taylor GA, Sivit CJ. Post-traumatic peritoneal fluid: is it a reliable indicator of intraabdominal injury in children? *J Pediatr Surg* 1995; 30:1644–1648.

549. Stalker HP, Kaufman RA, Towbin R. Patterns of liver injury in childhood: CT analysis. *AJR* 1986;147:1199–1205.

550. Patrick LE, Ball TI, Atkinson GO, Winn KJ. Pediatric blunt abdominal trauma: periportal tracking at CT. *Radiology* 1992;183:689–691.

551. Sivit CJ, Taylor GA, Eichelberger MR, et al. Significance of periportal low-attenuation zones following blunt trauma in children. *Pediatr Radiol* 1993;23:388–390.

552. Federle MP, Griffiths B, Minagi H, Jeffrey RB Jr. Splenic trauma: evaluation with CT. *Radiology* 1987;162:69–71.

553. Mirvis SE, Whitley NO, Gens DR. Blunt splenic trauma in adults: CT-based classification and correlation with prognosis and treatment. *Radiology* 1989;171:33–39.

554. Umlas SL, Cronan JJ. Splenic trauma: can CT grading systems enable prediction of successful nonsurgical treatment? *Radiology* 1991;178: 481–487.

555. Brick SH, Taylor GA, Potter BM, Eichelberger MR. Hepatic and splenic injury in children: role of CT in the decision for laparotomy. *Radiology* 1987;165:643–646.

556. Yale-Loehr AJ, Kramer SS, Quinlan DM, et al. CT of severe renal trauma in children: evaluation and course of healing with conservative therapy. *AJR* 1989;152:109–113.

557. Siegel MJ, Balfe DM. Blunt renal and ureteral trauma in childhood: CT patterns of fluid collections. *AJR* 1989;152:1043–1047.

558. Sivit CJ, Eichelberger MR, Taylor GA, et al. Blunt pancreatic trauma in children: CT diagnosis. *AJR* 1992;158:1097–1100.

559. Sivit CJ, Ingram JD, Taylor GA, et al. Posttraumatic adrenal hemorrhage in children: CT findings in 34 patients. *AJR* 1992;158: 1299–1302.

560. Sivit CJ, Taylor GA, Bulas DI, et al. Blunt trauma in children: significance of peritoneal fluid. *Radiology* 1991;178:185–188.

561. Federle MP, Jeffrey RB Jr. Hemoperitoneum studied by computed tomography. *Radiology* 1983;148:187–192.

562. Sivit CJ, Peclet MH, Taylor GA. Life-threatening intraperitoneal bleeding: demonstration with CT. *Radiology* 1989;171:430.

563. Taylor GA, Kaufman RA, Sivit CJ. Active hemorrhage in children after thoracoabdominal trauma: clinical and CT features. *AJR* 1994; 162:401–404.

564. Bulas DI, Taylor GA, Eichelberger MR. The value of CT in detecting bowel perforation in children after blunt abdominal trauma. *AJR* 1989; 153:561–564.

565. Rizzo MJ, Federle MP, Griffiths BG. Bowel and mesenteric injury following blunt abdominal trauma: evaluation with CT. *Radiology* 1989;173:143–148.

566. Shalaby-Rana E, Eichelberger M, Kerzner B, Kapur S. Intestinal stricture due to lap-belt injury. *AJR* 1992;158:63–64.

567. Sivit CJ, Cutting JP, Eichelberger MR. CT diagnosis and localization of rupture of the bladder in children with blunt abdominal trauma: significance of contrast material extravasation in the pelvis. *AJR* 1995; 164:1243–1246.

568. Taylor GA, Fallat ME, Eichelberger MR. Hypovolemic shock in children: abdominal CT manifestations. *Radiology* 1987;164:479–481.

569. Sivit CJ, Taylor GA, Bulas DI, et al. Post traumatic shock in children: CT findings associated with hemodynamic instability. *Radiology* 1992;182:723–726.

Practical Pediatric Imaging: Diagnostic Radiology of Infants and Children, Third Edition.
D. R. Kirks, editor and N. T. Griscom, associate editor.
Lippincott–Raven Publishers, Philadelphia © 1998.

CHAPTER 9

Genitourinary Tract

Carol E. Barnewolt, Harriet J. Paltiel, Robert L. Lebowitz, and Donald R. Kirks

Radiology plays a critical role in the evaluation of abnormalities of the genitourinary tract in infants and children. A variety of modalities, including both noninvasive and interventional techniques, are used to assess abnormalities of the kidneys, ureters, bladder, urethra, adrenal glands, and genitalia (1–15).

Until the 1980s, intravenous urography (IVU) and voiding cystourethrography (VCUG) were central to the evaluation of the urinary tract in infants and children. However, modern diagnostic imaging modalities (ultrasonography [US], nuclear medicine, computed tomography [CT], magnetic resonance imaging [MRI]) have assumed an increasingly important role. Interventional techniques now sometimes provide additional diagnostic information and definitive treatment. The indications and techniques for evaluating the genitourinary tract in children by conventional radiologic methods and other imaging modalities are presented in this chapter.

Common clinical problems that prompt radiologic evaluation of the genitourinary tract include urinary tract infection, abnormal prenatal sonography, and palpable abdominal mass. Hydronephrosis and multicystic dysplastic kidney now almost never present as flank masses but are discovered during prenatal sonographic screening. Prenatal sonography has given us a much more accurate estimation of the incidence of congenital genitourinary abnormalities, allowed an understanding of their natural history with and without intervention, and provided insight into previously unquestioned therapy.

The general topic of abdominal masses in the neonate and older child is presented in Chapter 8. Specific tumors of the kidneys, adrenals, and genital tract are discussed in detail in this chapter. Other abnormalities discussed and illustrated in this chapter include congenital genitourinary anomalies, trauma, hypertension, intersex problems, hematuria, voiding problems, flank or pelvic pain, renal failure, precocious puberty, scrotal pain, and congenital lesions of bone or viscera likely to be associated with renal abnormalities.

Both the patient's age and the presenting problem guide the imaging evaluation. This chapter is organized by disease, not by mode of presentation. General abnormalities and differential diagnostic considerations are discussed first, followed by specific congenital and acquired abnormalities. Several tables of differential diagnostic considerations are included; these are as important as the text itself. Sometimes the distinction between congenital and acquired disease is difficult, either because causation is not well understood or because of overlap, but the division between the two has been kept as logical as possible.

TECHNIQUES

Imaging of the genitourinary tract of children is significantly different from that of adults. Because many diagnostic modalities may be used, the ultimate medical goal—better patient care—requires the coordinated effort of radiologist and referring physician. The age of the patient, the findings on physical examination, and the clinical problem dictate the initial imaging technique. US is frequently the first and sometimes the only examination that is necessary.

Diagnostic imaging should be performed only for precise indications. Complete, accurate clinical information is essential for proper selection and performance of diagnostic imaging. A team approach among the various pediatric subspecialties with frequent, welcome, and constructive interdisciplinary dialogue inevitably improves patient care.

The gonads are frequently in the area of interest, and radiation exposure must be kept to a minimum. Uncooperative patients require adequate immobilization and sometimes even sedation. The maximum diagnostic information should be obtained with a minimum of cost, patient discomfort, delay, and radiation exposure. An expeditious, selective integration of imaging modalities with nonradiologic data and disease incidence is critical for patient care. After precise diagnostic evaluation, the appropriate surgical, medical, or radiologic therapy is selected.

Radiography and Fluoroscopy

Voiding Cystourethrography

VCUG demonstrates both the anatomy of the bladder and urethra and the presence or absence of vesicoureteral reflux. It also provides information about the function and coordination of the bladder and the urethral sphincter. Indications for VCUG include urinary tract infection; hydronephrosis or hydroureter on sonography (prenatal or postnatal) or intravenous urography; hematuria; voiding abnormalities; neonatal ascites; day and night wetting in a previously continent boy; and, in some children, congenital anomalies such as anorectal malformation, myelodysplasia, and prune-belly syndrome (10,16,17).

Preparation

No physical preparation is necessary. However, the fact that this examination uses radiation and requires urethral catheterization can cause great anxiety in parents. Children have a fear of both pain and the unknown. For these reasons, psychological preparation of both the parents and the child is mandatory. An explanatory pamphlet for parents and children provided ahead of time describing the technique and explaining efforts to assure comfort and safety in nonmedical terms can be very useful. The pamphlet should include ways that the parent can explain the procedure to the child before entering the medical environment. Just before the actual examination, the procedure should be explained again to both the parents and the child using words and pictures. Questions are encouraged. The child should be told repeatedly that

C. E. Barnewolt, H. J. Paltiel, R. L. Lebowitz, and D. R. Kirks: Department of Radiology, Children's Hospital, Harvard Medical School, Boston, Massachusetts 02115.

there will be no surprises. As radiologists and clinicians, we must be true to our word. These efforts are extremely helpful to the child, parent(s), and radiologist (18).

Supplies

The supplies for VCUG include a catheterization tray, polyethylene catheters (5 Fr, 8 Fr), warmed 2% Hibiclens (chlorhexidine gluconate) cleaning solution, contrast medium and intravenous drip bottles, plastic tubing, needles, plastic syringes (10–50 ml), a sterile specimen cup, 2% xylocaine (lidocaine) jelly, tape, and urine culture bottles (10).

Contrast Media

The contrast medium for VCUG is usually 17% Cystoconray II, 18% Cystografin–dilute, or 25% Hypaque (Hypaque 25). Depending on the predicted bladder capacity, a small (250 cm^3) or large (500 cm^3) glass bottle is suspended approximately 1 m above the level of the urinary bladder and is connected to the bladder catheter by plastic extension tubing.

Technique

VCUG should always be performed under fluoroscopic guidance with the child awake (19). The duration of fluoroscopy should be kept to a minimum, and low-dose techniques should be used whenever possible (20). If the child is able to cooperate, the bladder should be emptied just before the study. Adult companions (typically parents) should probably stay with the child throughout the procedure unless pregnant. If pregnant, the parent stays with the child during the catheterization but must leave before fluoroscopy begins.

The patient is catheterized on the fluoroscopy table. After cleaning of the interlabial area or penile tip, the area is draped. Once cleaning has begun, the labia must be kept separated to avoid contamination. In an uncircumcised boy, the foreskin is carefully retracted before cleaning. In uncircumcised infants, sterility is maintained by retracting the foreskin only partially, aligning its opening with the urethral meatus, and cleaning the area before catheterization.

Occasionally, labial adhesions (synechiae vulvae) are discovered in girls when attempts are made to separate the labia for cleaning (Fig. 9-1) (21). If exposure of the urethra is adequate without undue patient discomfort, the examination can proceed. If not, the labial adhesions are treated medically or surgically, and the need for VCUG is reassessed.

An 8-Fr catheter is used in all children except small premature infants, when a 5-Fr tube is substituted. After the penile tip is cleaned, the urethra of older boys is anesthetized. Lidocaine jelly is placed on the urethral meatus, and the entire urethra is then filled with lidocaine jelly by injecting 6–10 cm^3 in a retrograde manner using a syringe and fistula tip. In both boys and girls, the catheter should be inserted

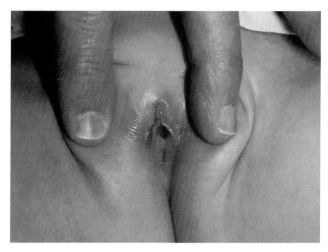

FIG. 9-1. Labial adhesions. Labial adhesions (synechiae vulvae) between the labia minora.

until it loops once in the urinary bladder. In girls, the catheter is secured by taping it to the upper inner thigh. In boys, the catheter is secured to the low anterior abdominal wall and penis. The urine obtained by catheter from the bladder is placed in a sterile container for culture.

The position of the catheter should be confirmed before the bladder is filled. A scout fluoroscopic spot film of the bladder region is obtained; any unusual catheter position is noted (Figs. 9-2 and 9-3). Contrast is then instilled by gravity drip through intravenous tubing. With the patient supine, the bladder is evaluated periodically during low-volume filling and then until complete filling. During early filling, the bladder is carefully observed for a ureterocele. Any abnormalities of bladder contour are noted. The patient is turned in both oblique projections to visualize the regions of the ureterovesical junctions (UVJs) for reflux or other abnormality (Fig. 9-4). During voiding the male urethra is seen best in the oblique projection, whereas the female urethra is seen well in the anteroposterior (AP) projection. The bladder should again be observed in the supine position at the end of voiding. The absence of vesicoureteral reflux should be documented with spot films of the kidneys at the end of the study (Table 9-1). If reflux is present, the level and amount of distention should be documented. The UVJs should again be evaluated for the course and insertion of the distal ureters (Fig. 9-4) and the presence or absence of bladder diverticula (Table 9-1).

If the child is calm, cessation of flow of contrast medium into the system is the endpoint for filling. Older children are able to state when the bladder is full. Signs of a full bladder in infants include crying and plantar flexion of the toes. For infants under 1 year of age, bladder capacity in milliliters is predicted by multiplying the weight in kilograms by 7. The predicted bladder capacity in milliliters of children more than 1 year old is the age in years plus 2 multiplied by 30 (22,23). An attempt should always be made to fill the bladder at least to predicted capacity; reflux can be missed with un-

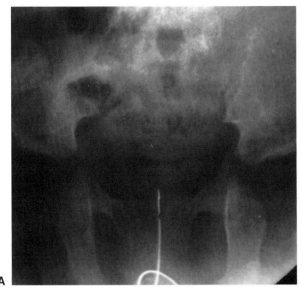

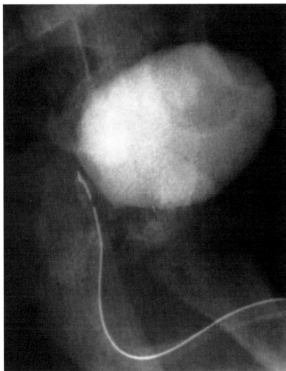

FIG. 9-2. Catheter in posterior urethra. A: An AP spot film shows an unusually low position of the tip of the catheter. **B:** A lateral film after filling the bladder. The tip of the catheter is in the posterior urethra.

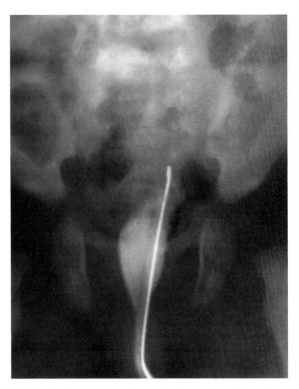

FIG. 9-3. Inadvertent catheterization of vagina. Contrast fills the vagina, the long axis of which is vertical. No bladder neck is identified, and contrast material immediately drains out along the catheter. Note that the vagina extends well below the pelvic floor.

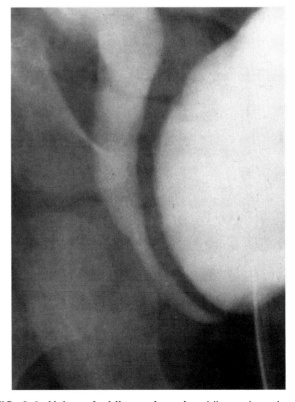

FIG. 9-4. Value of oblique view. An oblique view shows ectopic insertion of the refluxing ureter into the bladder neck.

derfilling. If filling to predicted capacity is not possible, this should be noted (24).

Younger children and infants void spontaneously. Initiation of voiding may be a problem in older children, particularly in adolescent girls. Helpful maneuvers include complete filling of the urinary bladder, encouragement, erect positioning, dimming of room lights, the sound of running water, and dripping warm water on the toes or perineum. Everyone involved must remain patient and calm.

TABLE 9-1. *Sequence for voiding cystourethrography*

Confirm catheter position[a]
Bladder, low-volume filling: supine[a]
Ureterovesical junctions, bladder filled: obliques
Urethra, voiding
    Male: oblique[a]
    Female: supine[a]
Bladder, end of voiding: supine[a]
Reflux
    Absent: kidneys[a]
    Present
        Document level and distention[a]
        Ureterovesical junctions
        Ureters
        Kidneys
        Rate and completeness of drainage

[a] Spot films.

The cyclic VCUG is a variation of standard VCUG technique. Several cycles of filling and voiding with the catheter remaining in place are observed. This procedure enhances the demonstration of reflux, especially in infants and in those patients who have ureteral ectopia or massive hydronephrosis (Fig. 9-5) (25,26).

Fluoroscopy should be brief and intermittent during bladder filling. One should continue filling the bladder until the patient voids around the catheter. The catheter is then removed during voiding, and spot films of the urethra are obtained. Infants are able to void in the horizontal position on the fluoroscopic table, but older children, especially boys, may void more readily upright.

Intravenous Urography

Indications and Contraindications

Before US and other cross-sectional methods became available, intravenous urography (IVU) was the mainstay of genitourinary imaging. It still provides morphologic information about the urinary tract and semiquantitative assessment of renal function. Current indications for IVU are (a) assessment of function and obstruction of both single and duplicated collecting systems; (b) evaluation of girls with continuous day and night wetting to confirm and characterize an ectopic ureter; (c) postoperative evaluation of the urinary tract. IVU may also be indicated to clarify an abnormal ultrasound examination of the kidneys and verify possible urinary tract calculi. The need for IVU must be determined on a case-by-case basis. An abdominal radiograph after contrast-enhanced CT or angiocardiography often shows the urinary tract fairly well.

The radiologist must be totally familiar with the history, physical examination, laboratory data, previous radiologic studies, and clinical considerations before an IVU is performed. The status of fluid and electrolyte balance and renal function must be known. The radiologist should question the patient, parent, and referring physician about allergies or previous contrast reactions.

Severe dehydration and shock are among the few contraindications to IVU in children (10). Pregnancy is another contraindication, and this possibility should always be considered in teenage girls.

The glomerular filtration rate during the immediate newborn period is 20% of that in the adult. This figure increases to 30% of the adult rate by the third day and then to 50% at 10 days of age. Because opacification by IVU depends on the glomerular filtration rate and plasma concentration, the concentration of contrast medium in the kidneys with IVU is usually poor during the first 7–10 days of life (1,26a). US and nuclear scintigraphy are more frequently used to evaluate the genitourinary tract during this period (27).

Preparation

No preparation is required for IVU. Because some ionic contrast media used for IVU are hyperosmolar, fluid should not be withheld from infants for more than 3–4 hours when those agents are used. Moreover, any dehydration should be corrected prior to the examination. In infants, bottle feeding is withheld immediately before the study. With nonionic contrast media, nausea and vomiting are rarely encountered so that fluid deprivation is not necessary. Ionic agents sometimes cause vomiting. Older, cooperative patients are asked to empty the bladder prior to injection; a full bladder may cause upper urinary tract dilatation mimicking hydronephrosis.

Contrast Media

Commonly used contrast media for excretory urography previously included meglumine diatrizoate (Reno-M-60; Bracco Diagnostics, Inc., Princeton, NJ) and sodium diatrizoate (Hypaque-50; NYCOMED Inc., New York, NY) (10).

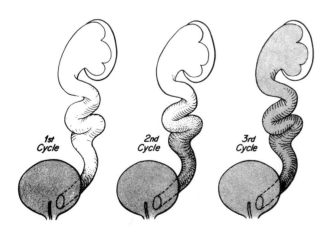

FIG. 9-5. Cyclic VCUG in refluxing hydronephrosis. Diagrammatic representation of massive reflux. With each cycle of filling and voiding, the dilated, poorly draining ureter fills with more contrast material.

Both have iodine concentrations in the range of 280–300 mg/ml. Their osmolalities are in the range of 1500–1600 mOsm/L; they are markedly hyperosmolar. Higher concentrations of contrast media should not be used for excretory urography in infants; they may cause severe dehydration and seizures.

Attempts to improve the safety of intravascular contrast media led to the development of nonionic agents. Iopamidol (Isovue; Bracco Diagnostics Inc., Princeton, NJ) and iohexol (Omnipaque; NYCOMED, Inc., New York, NY) are nonionic contrast media commonly used for IVU. The benefits of nonionic agents include a decrease in minor side effects and adverse reactions (28). Additional benefits in children include decreased osmotic load (600–700 mOsm/L), less irritation with intravenous injection, and fewer harmful effects if extravasation occurs (28). The trend has been to use nonionic contrast agents more and more frequently in children.

The recommended dose of ionic contrast is 2 ml/kg; the maximum dose is 4 ml/kg. Nonionic contrast media are used in a dose of 1–3 ml/kg. This dosage schedule results in total doses of 300–600 mg/kg of iodine, a concentration that produces diagnostically satisfactory IVUs.

Injection of Contrast Medium

The contrast medium should be injected intravenously by a physician or by some other skilled person with a physi-cian in the immediate area. The contrast should be drawn up immediately before administration.

The container from which the contrast medium has been drawn should be checked before injection to confirm the correctness of the preparation. The dosage should be checked before each study. The preferred injection sites are the veins of the hand, wrist, and antecubital fossa. The contrast medium is injected as rapidly as the needle allows. Any reaction to contrast medium should be noted on the patient's x-ray jacket, radiologic report, and chart, and the patient and parent should be fully informed.

Filming

Because of the K-absorption edge of iodine, the kilovoltage should be kept as close to 70 kVp as possible. Techniques vary from approximately 60–70 kVp for small infants to 90 kVp for large children.

Every effort should be made to minimize radiation exposure to the gonads. The male gonads are excluded from direct exposure by both beam collimation and gonadal shielding for all films. The female gonads are externally shielded for films collimated to the kidneys. The number of films is minimized.

If an infant is known to have vesicoureteral reflux, a catheter should be placed in the bladder to keep the bladder empty so that reflux does not mimic renal function (Fig. 9-6). A preliminary film is always obtained, for several reasons: (a)

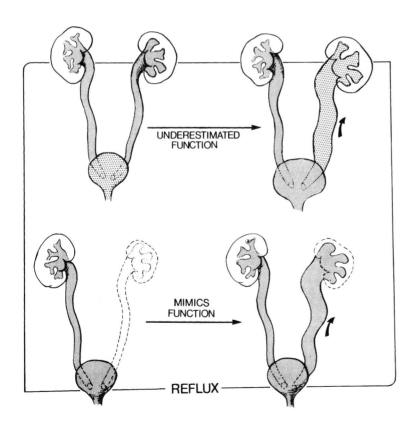

FIG. 9-6. Importance of catheter drainage in patients with severe reflux. Reflux of nonopaque urine into a ureter and collecting system of a normal kidney can lead to underestimation of renal function *(above)*. Reflux of contrast material excreted by one kidney can mimic function by the other *(below)*. Catheter drainage of the bladder during intravenous urography (IVU) and renal scintigraphy prevents these errors.

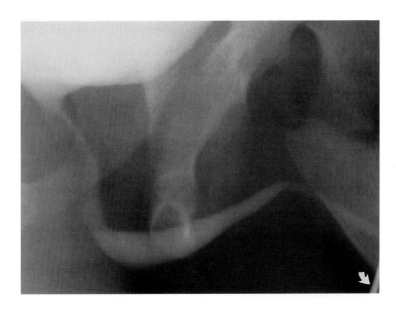

FIG. 9-7. Antegrade urethrography. A Zipser clamp *(curved arrow)* partially obstructs urethral flow. The contrast material excreted during IVU opacifies both the posterior and anterior urethra.

to verify proper radiographic technique; (b) to detect urinary tract calcification; (c) to evaluate anomalies of the spine; and (d) to show the effects of previous urinary tract surgery or radiation therapy. The preliminary film extends from the base of the lungs to the pubis. On an initial IVU, at least two postcontrast films are essential. A coned-down AP film of the kidneys is obtained approximately 3 minutes after injection. This view is particularly helpful for showing renal contours and nephrographic density. The next and often final film is taken 15 minutes after injection. If these films are normal or if it is a follow-up study, the IVU is usually complete. In other circumstances an AP or PA film may be obtained at 30 minutes. If obstructive uropathy is suspected, delayed films are necessary to clarify the site of obstruction. Prone and upright views help distinguish between ureteropelvic and ureterovesical obstruction. Voiding against partial obstruction (Zipser antegrade urethrography) opacifies both the posterior and anterior (male) urethra (Fig. 9-7).

Retrograde Urethrography

Retrograde urethrography (RUG) is used in males to assess anterior urethral strictures, the postoperative status of urethral reconstructions, infrasphincteric rectourethral fistulas in patients with anorectal malformations, and anterior urethral injuries. Water-soluble contrast media are used in the same concentrations as for VCUG. The tip of a Foley catheter is placed in the distal urethra. The balloon is then gently inflated in the fossa navicularis (Fig. 9-8A). Contrast medium is injected from a syringe. The patient is positioned in a steep oblique or lateral projection.

The technique is performed only in boys and accurately evaluates only the anterior urethra. Because of inadequate filling, the urethra proximal to the external sphincter cannot be evaluated (Fig 9-8B).

Nephrostography

A nephrostogram is usually performed to exclude obstruction or extravasation after a surgical or percutaneous nephrostomy. Contrast is infused by gravity during continuous fluoroscopic monitoring. In the normal patient, there should be free flow of contrast medium through the anastomosis, down the ureter, and into the bladder. If leakage or obstruction is identified, the infusion should be discontinued and additional views should be obtained to characterize the site and extent of the abnormality. Delayed films are helpful for determining the severity of obstruction.

Conduit Opacification

Urinary conduits may be created from portions of small or large bowel. These conduits are designed not as reservoirs but as channels for urine flow. The conduit is occluded by inflating a Foley catheter just inside the external stoma. The balloon is then gently pulled against the fascia to form a seal. After a scout film, contrast (17% concentration, as in VCUG) is instilled by gravity.

Rectal Opacification

Rectal opacification is often necessary to determine the site and nature of rectogenitourinary connections in patients with a high imperforate anus or a cloacal malformation. A Foley catheter is placed in the distal limb of the colostomy created in the newborn period, and 17% iodinated contrast material is instilled by gravity or injected by syringe to opacify the rectum and its connection with the genitourinary tract. These connections are best demonstrated in the true lateral position.

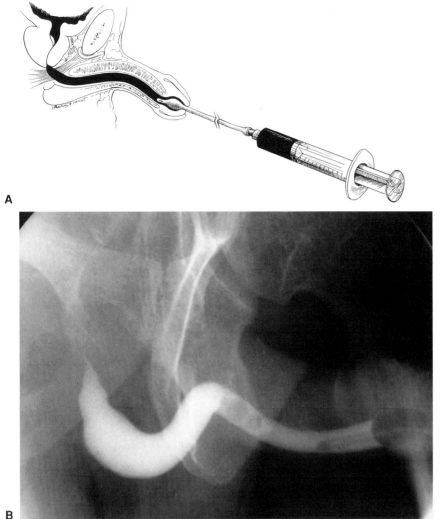

A

B

FIG. 9-8. Retrograde urethrography. A: The balloon of a Foley catheter is inflated in the fossa navicularis. Contrast material distends the anterior urethra to the level of the external sphincter. A small amount of contrast material usually opacifies a collapsed posterior urethra and the base of the urinary bladder. **B:** The inflated balloon of the Foley catheter is in the fossa navicularis. A few air bubbles are seen in the distended anterior urethra. The normal bulbous urethra has a tapered narrowing at the level of the closed external sphincter.

Genitography

Genitography and vaginography are still performed for evaluating selected genital abnormalities, ambiguous genitalia, a urogenital sinus, and the cloacal malformation (10,29). The examination is performed under fluoroscopic control.

The technique varies with the anatomy and age of the patient. If the perineal opening is a penis-like structure, a polyethylene feeding tube is used. If the anatomy is more female or if a urogenital sinus is being evaluated, a polyethylene feeding tube passed through a single-hole nipple (10) or an inflated Foley balloon catheter placed against the perineum is used for injection. AP and lateral fluoroscopy with videotaping and films are required; opacification is usually transitory.

Ultrasonography

US is particularly useful in children as it does not utilize ionizing radiation, is relatively inexpensive, and is diagnosti-

cally accurate (12,27,30–34). Current indications for genitourinary sonography include postnatal evaluation of abnormalities seen on prenatal sonograms, a palpable abdominal mass, urinary tract infection, conditions associated with renal anomalies or tumors, possible obstructive uropathy, ambiguous genitalia, neonatal ascites and anasarca, suspected renal agenesis or ectopia, localization for renal biopsy, evaluation of a transplanted kidney, suspected urachal remnants, scrotal pain and scrotal masses, pelvic masses, pelvic pain in girls, and pregnancy (31–34).

The child is evaluated in both the supine and prone positions. Transverse and longitudinal scans of the kidneys, ureters, bladder, and pelvis are performed. Renal length is best assessed in the prone position. Transducer choice depends on the size of the patient. In very small premature infants, the kidneys are best imaged with a 7-MHz linear array transducer. The kidneys of larger infants and children are usually best imaged with a 5- or 3-MHz phased- or curved-array transducer.

Color and pulsed Doppler imaging is utilized to assess renal vascularity (30,35). However, Doppler sonography is of only questionable usefulness in patients with possible renovascular hypertension. Color Doppler energy (CDE) and ultrasound contrast agents improve the assessment of renal blood flow and perfusion; this is important in renal trauma, infarction, and ischemia (36,37).

The superficial location of transplanted kidneys makes them accessible to ultrasound imaging with high-frequency transducers. Accurate serial dimensions are particularly helpful in identifying edema, a sign of rejection. Both color and pulsed Doppler sonography should always be used to evaluate renal transplants for patency of arterial and venous blood flow. The resistive index should be calculated; an elevated resistive index suggests rejection (38).

A full bladder is mandatory as an acoustic window for sonographic evaluation of the pelvis. Older boys and girls are instructed to arrive for evaluation with a full urinary bladder. If the bladder is not full, the child and parents must be told of the need to wait for it to fill. In an emergency situation, the bladder is filled with saline by catheterization.

In many institutions, US has become the examination of choice for testicular torsion. The testes are best imaged with either a 5- or 7-MHz linear array transducer. Demonstration of both normal color Doppler and normal pulsed Doppler waveforms of testicular arterial flow is necessary to exclude torsion. Demonstration of blood flow is usually easiest in the transverse plane at the level of the testicular hilum. Ultrasound is also the best examination to show whether a palpable scrotal mass is intratesticular or extratesticular.

Nuclear Medicine

Technetium-99m (^{99m}Tc) is an ideal radioisotope for pediatric studies when used with a gamma camera. Many compounds permitting study of specific organ anatomy and function can be labeled with this isotope. Radiation dosage to the whole body and to the specific organ is low with ^{99m}Tc; it is a gamma emitter with a half-life of only 6 hours.

Mercaptoacetyltriglycine (MAG 3) is rapidly cleared by tubular secretion and is not retained in the parenchyma of normal kidneys. It affords excellent delineation of the renal pelves and ureters and good assessment of drainage. ^{99m}Tc-MAG 3 is now the most widely used agent for renal scintigraphy.

The clearance of diethylenetriaminepentaacetic acid (DTPA) is almost purely dependent on glomerular filtration; there is little tubular absorption or excretion. Therefore, ^{99m}Tc-DTPA may be used to assess many physiologic parameters: differential renal function, renal plasma flow, glomerular filtration, and renal clearance (1,3,14). Morphologic information regarding kidney size, amount of functioning parenchyma, and drainage from the kidneys into the ureters and bladder can be obtained from sequential scans (1,3,14).

Radionuclide Cystography

Many imaging studies are prompted by urinary tract infection and vesicoureteral reflux. Because of its low radiation dosage, radionuclide cystography (RNC) has become increasingly important for the latter and is a very common nuclear medicine study.

The preparation and catheterization of the patient is identical to that for VCUG. The catheter is connected to a bottle of normal saline that is dripped into the urinary bladder by gravity. Tc-^{99m} pertechnetate (1-2 mCi) is injected into the flowing saline. The abdomen and pelvis are continuously monitored on the persistence scope of the gamma camera during the filling and voiding phases. The urinary bladder is filled to predicted capacity. There are three grades of reflux on RNC (see Fig. 9-78).

In its estimate of the presence and degree of vesicoureteral reflux, isotope cystography, particularly catheter isotope cystography, correlates well with conventional VCUG (1). Its low radiation dose makes it ideal for older children with urinary tract infection who are unlikely to have reflux or bladder abnormalities, for follow-up of patients with known vesicoureteral reflux, for siblings or offspring of patients with a history of reflux, and for evaluation after antireflux surgery. Conventional VCUG is still preferred as the initial imaging procedure in all boys and in girls suspected of having an anatomic abnormality such as a bladder diverticulum or ectopic ureter. If RNC is not available, alternatives using a tailored, low-dose fluoroscopic technique may be used (39,40).

Cortical Scintigraphy

The scintigraphic agents, ^{99m}Tc-labeled dimercaptosuccinic acid (DMSA) and ^{99m}Tc-labled glucoheptonate, have a high affinity for the renal cortex because of their concentration by tubular cells. These agents, which produce a fairly high level of renal detail, are particularly appropriate for studying renal morphology. DMSA is currently the best cortical agent; 60% of the administered dose is concentrated by the cells of the proximal tubules.

Indications for cortical scintigraphy include the question of acute pyelonephritis, assessment of renal cortical scarring, localization of small amounts of renal parenchyma, identification of malpositioned kidneys, and confirmation of a pseudotumor due to a column of Bertin (1). The use of single-photon emission computed tomography (SPECT) increases the sensitivity of DMSA to changes of acute pyelonephritis and renal scarring (41).

Diuretic Renography

Diuretic (furosemide) renography with ^{99m}Tc-MAG 3 or ^{99m}Tc-DTPA is particularly useful in determining whether a dilated ureter or pelvicalyceal system is obstructed. The

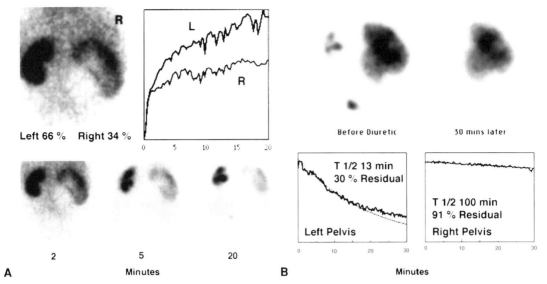

FIG. 9-9. Renal scintigraphy of severe obstruction. A: Dynamic ^{99m}Tc-MAG 3 study shows a large right kidney with delayed transit time and significant retention of tracer. Note that the normal left kidney provides 66% of total renal function. **B:** Diuretic renography. The right renal collecting system is markedly dilated, and the drainage of the tracer is abnormal.

absence of a well-defined transition point by US, VCUG, or IVU suggests nonobstructive dilatation rather than obstruction.

Radiotracer is administered intravenously (0.1 mCi/kg of MAG 3, using a minimum of 1 mCi), and filling of the collecting system is continuously monitored. When the dilated collecting system is filled with tracer, intravenous furosemide (1 mg/kg, up to a maximum dose of 40 mg) is administered. Digital images are then collected over a 30-minute period, a renogram curve (activity versus time) is generated, and the half-time for tracer clearance is calculated. The anatomic images, washout curve, and clearance half-time are analyzed to determine whether obstruction is present (Fig. 9-9) or absent (Fig. 9-10). There is a good correlation between diuretic venography and the Whitaker test in the determination of obstruction (42).

Captopril Renography

Captopril renography is used to screen for renal artery stenosis in children with hypertension. Intrarenal perfusion pressure is decreased by renal artery stenosis, and glomerular filtration rate (GFR) consequently decreases. This stimulates angiotensin-converting enzyme (ACE) to form angiotensin II, which constricts the efferent arteriole of the glomerulus; this autoregulatory effect maintains GFR despite decreased perfusion pressures. Captopril is an ACE inhibitor and decreases the effectiveness of autoregulation. Renography is performed both before and after the administration of captopril; decreased function of a kidney after captopril is highly suggestive of unilateral renal artery stenosis, and angiography should probably be performed (42). Captopril renography may be falsely negative if the stenosis is bilateral.

Computed Tomography

CT accurately assesses many pediatric renal abnormalities (15,43–45). It provides a cross-sectional display of anatomy less dependent on renal function than IVU. It is also able to discriminate small density differences after intravenous contrast material administration, and it thus provides a more precise assessment of limited function. Calcifications are

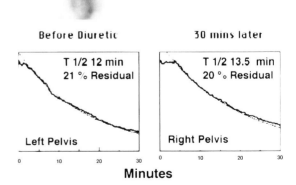

FIG. 9-10. Renal scintigraphy of dilated collecting systems without obstruction. Posterior renal scintigraphy shows dilation of the renal collecting structures, more marked on the right. Diuretic renography shows washout of tracer from both kidneys.

readily apparent, and the nature of renal masses may be ascertained (44). CT shows anatomic detail much better than scintigraphy. Unlike IVU, it shows the kidneys even if renal function is compromised. Unlike US, CT is not adversely affected by overlying gas or bone and is capable of evaluating renal function. It also displays anatomy more precisely.

Computed tomography is usually preceded by US. It may clarify sonographic findings or, as with tumors, it may provide new information. In patients with a malignancy, CT (along with MRI) delineates the involvement of adjacent anatomic structures and forms the basis for tumor staging. CT is the diagnostic modality of choice in patients with renal trauma (44).

CT with thin sections is also excellent for identifying and localizing poorly functioning, dysplastic renal tissue. This can be particularly helpful in children with an ectopically inserting ureter draining a kidney that does not visualize by IVU (see Fig. 9-98). Spiral CT is particularly helpful in evaluating urinary tract calcifications and stones.

Meticulous attention to technique improves CT information. To decrease the risk of vomiting, movement during injection, stimulation of a sedated patient, and contrast reactions, many pediatric radiologists use only nonionic contrast for CT. Injection is usually performed in an upper extremity vein in order to visualize the renal arteries and veins without high-density caval artifacts caused by lower extremity injection. Delayed scans may be necessary to visualize the ureters or to document delayed excretion in hydronephrosis (44). An abdominal radiograph after contrast-enhanced CT may be obtained, particularly in trauma patients, to further assess the urinary tract.

Magnetic Resonance Imaging

MRI of the genitourinary tract is used almost exclusively for characterizing and staging malignancies. The advantages of MRI include lack of ionizing radiation, absence of the hazards of iodinated contrast material, and multiplanar imaging capabilities. The latter is particularly helpful in determining the organ of origin of very large abdominal masses. The disadvantages of MRI include greater expense, less availability, and more frequent need for sedation because of longer examination times. Currently, many or most pediatric genitourinary neoplasms are evaluated with MRI.

Coils should be selected to optimize the signal-to-noise ratio while including the entire area of interest. Both T1-weighted sequences (delineation of anatomy) and fast spin-echo T2-weighted sequences (definition of pathology) are performed. A postgadolinium T1 sequence is almost always obtained to assess the perfusion of the neoplasm. Assessment of tumor vascularity may be helpful in diagnosis as well as showing the effects of therapy.

Renal Angiography

With the emergence of less invasive modalities, there has been a dramatic decline in the use of pediatric angiography.

Evaluation of renovascular hypertension remains the most common indication for renal angiography (46). Arteriography is still indicated in children with suspected main renal artery or segmental renal artery stenosis. The advent of transluminal angioplasty has made nonsurgical therapy possible for some of these lesions. Segmental and main renal vein sampling for renin is also frequently performed.

Other indications for renal angiography include assessment of a donor kidney prior to transplantation, characterization of a vasculopathy such as polyarteritis nodosa, and diagnosis and transcatheter embolization of acute bleeding after renal vascular trauma. The techniques of pediatric angiography are discussed in detail in Chapter 1.

Percutaneous Procedures

Percutaneous interventional procedures of the genitourinary tract include needle biopsy, abscess drainage, and nephrostomy. Percutaneous procedures may be guided by fluoroscopy, US, or CT.

The Whitaker test may help to determine whether or not a collecting system is obstructed when other studies are equivocal. Pressures in the pelvicalyceal system and the bladder are compared during perfusion of the nephrostomy catheter with saline at a rate of 10 cc/minute. If the renal pelvic pressure is 15 cm of water greater than the bladder pressure, obstruction is present (47). A false-positive occurs when the rate of perfusion is greater than the maximum rate of urine production by the kidney. Interpretation of pressure differences in infants is controversial.

NORMAL GENITOURINARY TRACT

Renal Position and Size

The kidneys are retroperitoneal, the upper poles being more posterior and closer to the spine than the lower poles. The right kidney is lower than the left in approximately 60% of normal patients, the kidneys are at the same level in one third, and the left kidney is lower in 6% (48). The pelvis of the right kidney is usually at the level of the L2 vertebral body, and the left renal pelvis is usually at the L1−2 interspace (48). If the two kidneys are not at the same level, the difference is usually less than one vertebral body height. Renal position is not influenced by the age or sex of the child (48,49).

Renal size is important in the evaluation of several abnormalities of the pediatric genitourinary tract. Renal length is measured to determine renal growth and to compare with the opposite kidney. Length and apparent length are affected by changes in the opposite kidney (compensatory hypertrophy), by dilatation of the collecting system, and by rotation of the kidney (10). Renal size is measured by ultrasound examination in the supine and prone positions (50). The longest diameter, usually measured in the prone position, is compared to standard nomograms (Fig. 9-11). These renal

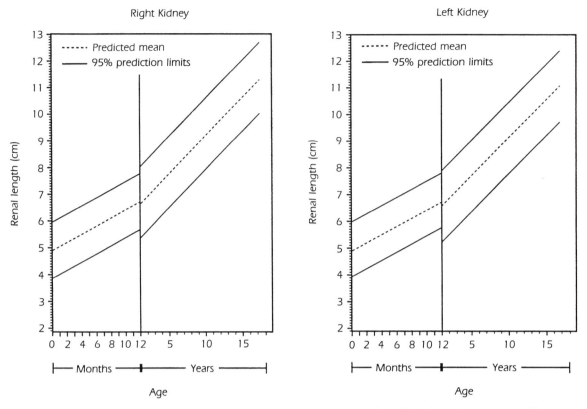

FIG. 9-11. Normal renal length by sonography. Maximal renal length is plotted versus age. From Han and Babcock (53).

lengths are slightly greater than those obtained with IVU, in which foreshortening of the kidneys may be present because of their tilt. By IVU, children over 18 months of age have an average kidney length corresponding to the height of the first four lumbar vertebral bodies including three intervertebral disks (48); the length of the kidney normally equals the distance from the superior endplate of the vertebral body of L1 to the inferior endplate of L4. In younger children the kidney is relatively large; renal length may be as great as the height of five or even six vertebral bodies (10,48).

More precise length standards for IVU are available from the data of Eklöf and Ringertz (Fig. 9-12A) (49). The greatest length of the kidney by IVU is compared to the distance from the upper margin of the vertebral body of L1 to the lower margin of the vertebral body of L3 (49). A nomogram similar to that for ultrasound examinations allows determination of the number of standard deviations that a kidney deviates from the normal (Fig. 9-12).

Parenchymal Thickness and Character

Careful measurements of parenchymal thickness should always be made in order to detect subtle changes of atrophy and scarring (10,51). By sonography, the relatively hypoechoic cortical margins should be of equal thickness (mea-

suring from the outer margin of the central echo complex to the renal capsule) in each of the two polar regions and in the middle third of the kidney. Focal thinning suggests scar formation. With IVU, the thickness of the renal parenchyma is assessed by drawing the Hodson intercalyceal line (51). This line connects the outermost papillae (Fig. 9-13). The thickness of the renal parenchyma is then determined as the distance between this line and the renal outline. The renal parenchyma or renal substance thickness is measured for the two polar regions and the middle third for each kidney (Fig. 9-13). The polar measurements should be approximately equal (51). The sum of the parenchymal thicknesses in the two polar regions of the kidney accounts for up to 60% of the length of the kidney during childhood but only 50% in the adult. The relatively larger size of the kidney in children is due to this increase in renal substance thickness, particularly at the poles (51). The earliest sign of an atrophic pyelonephritic scar is a slight reduction in renal substance thickness at one of the poles.

Ultrasonographic characterization of the echogenicity of the renal parenchyma is important. In general, renal echogenicity should be compared with that of the adjacent hepatic or splenic parenchyma. In premature infants, the renal parenchyma is more echogenic than liver, probably because the total volume of the glomeruli is relatively larger. There is

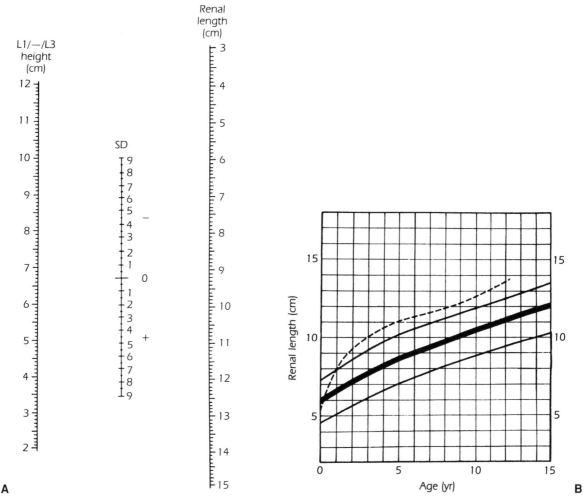

FIG. 9-12. Normal renal lengths by excretory urography. A: Nomogram for renal length. The distance from the top of L1 to the bottom of L3 is measured in centimeters and plotted on the line to the left. The greatest renal length is measured in centimeters and plotted on the line to the right. A *straight line* connecting these two points intersects the standard deviation line in the center. The normal range for renal length is ±2 SD. From Eklöf and Ringertz (49). **B:** Graph for renal length. The *solid lines* plot normal renal length ±2 SD by age. The *dotted line* plots compensatory hypertrophy of a single functioning kidney by age. From Lebowitz and Colodny (61).

also then a greater proportion of cellular components in the glomerular tuft and a larger number of cortical loops of Henle. Term infants demonstrate cortical echogenicity equal to or slightly greater than hepatic parenchymal echogenicity. After 5–6 months of age, the renal parenchymal echogenicity is similar to that of the adult, i.e., less than that of adjacent liver. The corticomedullary junction is well delineated. The renal sinus is echogenic in older children because of the fat and blood vessels there.

Particularly during fetal life and early infancy, normal kidneys have an undulating contour on IVU and renal sonography (Fig. 9-14). This normal appearance is due to fetal lobation (52). The small indentations between the lobes should not be confused with renal scars, as there is no local loss of renal cortical tissue. As the infant grows, the cortical surface grows smoother and individual lobes can no longer

be seen. The medullary pyramids are strikingly more hypoechoic than the cortex in normal infants (Fig. 9-14); this appearance should not be mistaken for calyceal dilation and hydronephrosis (53,54).

Bladder

The dome and base of the bladder have different embryologic developments and separate functions. In the neonate and young child, the dome and body of the bladder are located primarily in the abdomen. Structures that can usually be identified at VCUG include the interureteric ridge, trigonal canal, and baseplate of the bladder. Complete filling occasionally shows a remnant of the urachus at the dome of the bladder. The sonographic thickness of the bladder wall

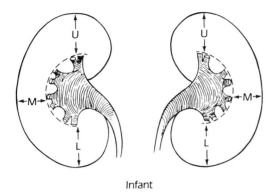

Infant

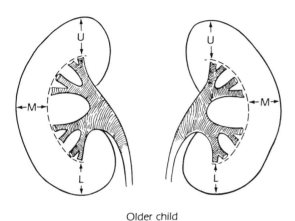

Older child

FIG. 9-13. Measurement of renal parenchymal thickness or IVU. The Hodson intercalyceal line is drawn by connecting the outermost papillae. The renal parenchymal thickness is the distance between this intercalyceal line and the renal outline. The renal parenchymal thickness of the upper poles *(U)* and lower poles *(L)* should be bilaterally symmetric. The renal parenchymal thickness of the midportion *(M)* of the right and left kidneys should be equal. Modified from Hodson (51).

should be no more than 3 mm when distended and 5 mm when collapsed.

Urethra

The female urethra corresponds anatomically to the posterior urethra of the male (Fig. 9-15). Anatomic features that can usually be identified in the girl include the urethrovesical junction, intermuscular incisura, urethral sphincter, and distal urethral segment (16,17). There is reflux of contrast material during voiding from the perineum into the vagina in up to 60% of normal girls; this occurs in all positions.

The components of the male urethra include the prostatic or posterior urethra, membranous urethra, bulbous urethra, and penile urethra (Fig. 9-15). There are obvious similarities between the male prostatic and membranous urethra and the entire female urethra (Fig. 9-15) (16). Anatomic structures that can usually be identified in the boy include the urethrovesical junction, intermuscular incisura, veru-

montanum, membranous urethra at the level of the urogenital diaphragm, bulbous urethra, suspensory ligament of the penis, penile urethra, and fossa navicularis (Figs. 9-15 and 9-16).

Gonads

Ovaries

The ovaries are located in the pelvis, within the mesovarium of the broad ligament. Their long axes are usually parallel to the iliac vessels. The size and appearance of the ovaries change with age and, after puberty, with the stage of the menstrual cycle.

US is the initial and usually the only imaging modality required in evaluation of female infants, children, and adolescents who present with pelvic pain, abnormal sexual development, or a pelvic mass. CT and MRI are occasionally useful if the origin of a pelvic mass cannot be determined with sonography or when precise delineation of extent is required.

Neonatal ovaries are readily shown by US. They measure, on average, about 1 cm³ in volume. They frequently contain 1 or more small cysts, usually <1 cm in diameter (55). Ovarian volume decreases slightly after infancy, presumably because of a decline in gonadotropin levels, but then increases at puberty (55,56). From approximately 2 years of age until puberty, the ovaries are usually solid and homogeneous in echotexture. Some ovaries contain small cysts, probably follicular in nature (Fig. 9-17). The normal postpubertal ovary has a mean volume of 7.8 cm³ with a normal range of 1.7–18.5 cm³ (57). In addition to being larger than prepuber-

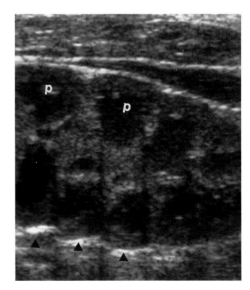

FIG. 9-14. Normal newborn renal sonography. The contour of the normal newborn kidney has an undulating appearance. Each mound *(arrowheads)* corresponds to an individual renal lobe. The renal pyramids *(p)* of young infants are less echoic than surrounding cortex; this normal appearance should not be mistaken for hydronephrosis.

Indications for scrotal imaging include cryptorchidism, a painless scrotal mass, painful scrotal swelling, trauma, and precocious puberty. US, often with duplex and color Doppler imaging, is the best modality for scrotal imaging. Supplementary evaluation with nuclear scintigraphy or MRI will sometimes be required. Sonography provides high-resolution images of the scrotum and its contents; Doppler imaging assesses blood flow. Scintigraphy provides further information about blood flow to the scrotum, testes, and epididymes (58).

The normal testicle is oval and has smooth contours with homogeneous, medium-level echotexture. The testes should be symmetric in size and shape and have equal echogenicity. Testicular size depends on age and stage of sexual development. Prior to age 12, the volume of one testis is 1 to 2 cm^3 (Fig. 9-19). Volumes range from 2 to 5 cm^3 at 12 years, 5 to 10 cm^3 at 13 years, and 12 to 14 cm^3 at 15 years (Fig. 9-20) (59).

Since blood flow to the scrotum and its contents is relatively low in normals, radionuclide angiography rarely demonstrates tracer activity in the scrotum. Tracer is detected in the femoral and iliac vessels as well as diffusely in the thighs and pelvis (Fig. 9-21A). Testicular uptake usually is as intense as that in the soft tissues of the adjacent thighs during the static or tissue phase (Fig. 9-21B). Pinhole images should demonstrate activity in the scrotum with little or no background activity (Fig. 9-21C). Tracer uptake in the scrotum is usually uniform and bilaterally symmetric.

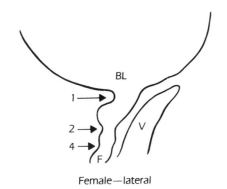
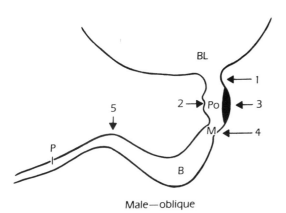

FIG. 9-15. Normal female and male urethra. The structures commonly visualized during voiding cystourethrography (VCUG) in the normal female include the bladder *(BL)*, bladder neck or urethrovesical junction *(1)*, intermuscular incisura *(2)*, membranous urethra at the level of the urogenital diaphragm or urethral sphincter *(4)*, fossa navicularis *(F)*, and vagina *(V)*. Anatomic structures commonly identified during VCUG in the normal male include the bladder *(BL)*, bladder neck or urethrovesical junction *(1)*, intermuscular incisura *(2)*, verumontanum *(3)*, membranous urethra at the level of the urogenital diaphragm or urethral sphincter *(4)*, and suspensory ligament of the penis *(5)*. The female urethra corresponds to the male posterior urethra. Components of the male urethra include prostatic or posterior urethra *(Po)*, membranous urethra *(M)*, bulbous urethra *(B)*, and penile urethra *(P)*.

tal ovaries, postpubertal ovaries frequently have larger and more asymmetric follicular cysts (Fig. 9-18).

Scrotum and Contents

Normal scrotal contents include the testis, epididymis, a small amount of fluid between the layers of the tunica vaginalis, spermatic artery, pampiniform venous plexus, and vas deferens. The appendix testis, a müllerian duct remnant, is located at the upper pole of the testicle. The appendix epididymis and the paradidymis, mesonephric remnants, are situated respectively on the head of the epididymis and in the anterior portion of the spermatic cord.

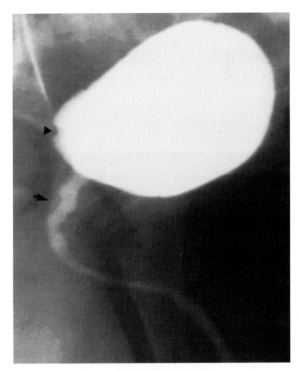

FIG. 9-16. Normal VCUG. A 3-month-old boy with urinary tract infection. The crescentic impression at the base of the bladder *(arrowhead)* is the interureteric ridge. The normal verumontanum *(arrow)* is seen in the posterior urethra.

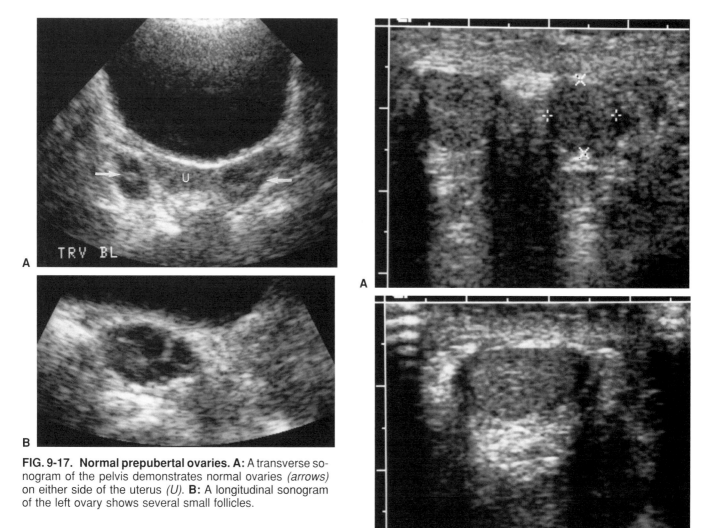

FIG. 9-17. Normal prepubertal ovaries. A: A transverse sonogram of the pelvis demonstrates normal ovaries *(arrows)* on either side of the uterus *(U)*. B: A longitudinal sonogram of the left ovary shows several small follicles.

FIG. 9-19. Normal prepubertal testes. A: A transverse sonogram demonstrates normal right and left testes. The left testis is marked by *cursors*. B: Longitudinal sonography shows smooth contours and a homogeneous parenchyma.

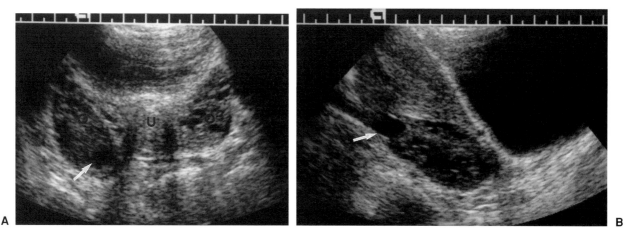

FIG. 9-18. Normal postpubertal ovaries. A: A transverse sonogram demonstrates a normal uterus *(U)* and ovaries *(O)*. There are several follicles in each ovary, including a large follicle in the right ovary *(arrow)*. B: Longitudinal sonography of the right ovary. Several follicles, including a dominant follicle *(arrow)*, are well visualized.

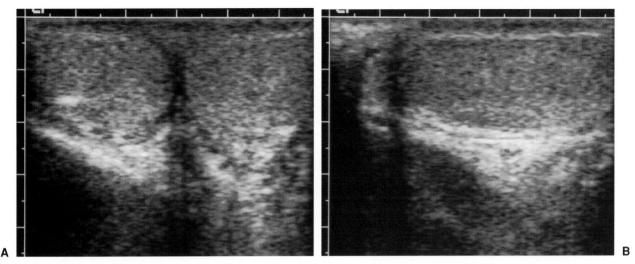

FIG. 9-20. Normal postpubertal testes. Transverse **(A)** and longitudinal **(B)** sonography shows symmetric size and shape. Postpubertal testes are both larger and more echogenic than prepubertal testes.

GENERAL ABNORMALITIES

Normal Variants

Kidney

Fetal lobations represent persistence of the normal fetal state. The kidney is a multilobed organ during fetal life, with seven anterior and seven posterior lobes separated by a fibrous longitudinal groove. The sites of fusion of these lobes with one another are often represented by surface depressions or grooves (see Fig. 9-14).

On occasion, the fibrous band separating the anterior and posterior parts of the kidney remains visible on US as the *interrenicular septum* (Fig. 9-22); it may also be confused with scarring if sectioned in a medial parasagittal plane. The interrenicular septum is distinguished from cortical scarring by the absence of loss of cortical tissue and the presence of an ultrasonographic connection between the junction of the two reniculi and the central sinus echoes (60).

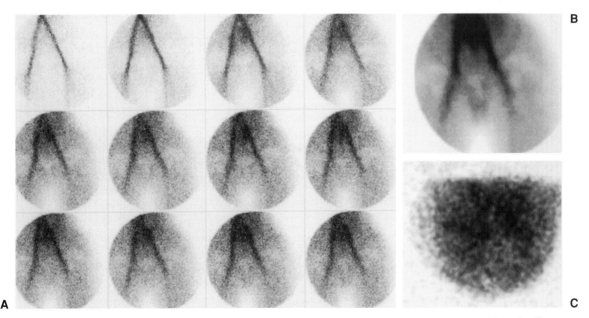

FIG. 9-21. Normal scrotal scintigraphy. A: Radionuclide angiography shows tracer within the iliac and femoral vessels. Perfusion of the scrotum and testicles is usually not perceptible. **B:** Immediate static image. Tracer is noted within the soft tissues as well as the iliac, femoral, scrotal, and testicular vessels. **C:** Pinhole magnification image with lead shielding. There is a homogeneous distribution of tracer in the scrotum. Normally the testicles are not identified.

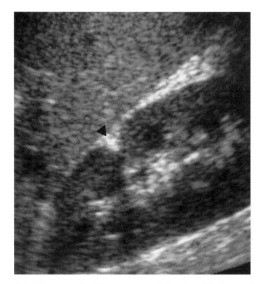

FIG. 9-22. Interrenicular septum. The focal indentation *(arrowhead)* is the cleft or septum at the junction of the two reniculi. This normal variant should not be mistaken for a parenchymal scar caused by chronic pyelonephritis. The renal length and cortical volume are normal.

Grooves between fetal lobations and between the anterior and posterior reniculi should not be confused with chronic atrophic pyelonephritic scarring. In contrast to the pyelonephritic scar, a persistent fetal groove is located between calyceal groups rather than opposite a calyx (Fig. 9-23). Moreover, patients with fetal lobations and fetal grooves have no calyceal distortion (61).

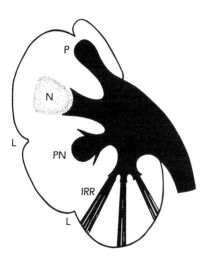

FIG. 9-23. Normal and abnormal renal anatomy. The normal papilla *(N)* of a medullary pyramid fits into a cupped calyx. Fetal lobations *(L)* are located between calyceal groups. A pyelonephritic scar *(P)* is opposite a clubbed calyx, and there is loss of adjacent renal parenchymal thickness. Papillary necrosis *(PN)* may be difficult to distinguish from an everted calyx. Intrarenal reflux *(IRR)* usually occurs at the upper or lower pole of the kidney. Modified from Lebowitz and Colodny (61).

An *aberrant papilla* may project directly into the lumen of the calyceal infundibulum or renal pelvis without distorting or obstructing an adjacent collecting system. This otherwise normal papilla appears as a conical projection into the lumen or as a round or oval structure (62). It is a radiolucent defect at IVU that should not be confused with a tumor, calculus, blood clot, air bubble, papillary necrosis, or pyelitis cystica.

Ureter

Transverse folds may produce a corkscrew appearance of the upper segment of the ureter at intravenous urography (Fig. 9-24). This tortuous appearance is due to transverse folds, which are full-thickness inward projections of the ureteral wall (63). They represent persistence of normal fetal tortuosity of the ureter. Externally, the ureters are smooth. Retrograde injection and longitudinal sections show that the tortuosity is due to intraluminal projections of the ureteral wall. Microscopically, these folds contain mucosa, muscularis, and extensions of the adventitia. The frequency of these transverse folds in the proximal ureter is highest in the neonate (75%) and decreases in frequency to an 11% incidence at 2 years of age. These upper ureteral folds have no postnatal clinical significance (63).

Vascular impressions are broad, band-like filling defects in the infundibulum or ureter. These defects often have a notch-like configuration. Vascular impressions are usually broader than transverse folds (62).

Bladder

The dome of the bladder in the infant and small child is intraabdominal and anterior, whereas the base is intrapelvic and posterior (64). This positioning produces a bichambered configuration. *Bowel impressions* are common. They extrinsically compress the intraabdominal (superior) compartment of the bladder when it is filled with contrast material. This appearance should not be confused with an intravesical mass or extrinsic compression of the bladder by a pelvic mass.

The ureter normally inserts into the full urinary bladder approximately one quarter of the way from the bladder base to the bladder dome. Insertion at any lower point along the bladder base or into the urethra or vagina is abnormal or ectopic. *Fake ureteral ectopia* (Fig. 9-25) is produced in three ways: (a) a refluxing ureter is observed only in the late phase of voiding; (b) the site of ureteral insertion is determined from a prone (not a supine) IVU radiograph (Fig. 9-25B); (c) reflux into the ureter overlies contrast that has refluxed into the vagina (Fig. 9-25C). The normal bladder has a superior compartment that is anterior and an inferior compartment that is posterior (Fig. 9-25A) (64). When the child is prone, contrast material fills the dome of the bladder, but the base of the bladder may be filled with nonopaque urine. The ureter then appears to insert infravesically (64).

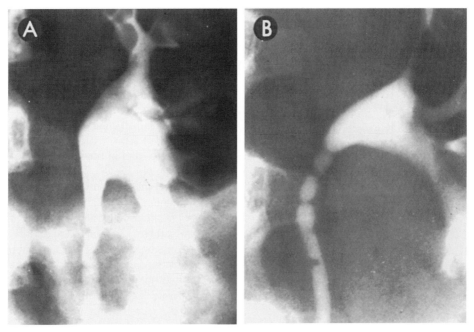

FIG. 9-24. Transverse upper ureteral folds at excretory urography. A: A 16-month-old boy. **B:** 2-year-old girl. From Kirks et al. (63).

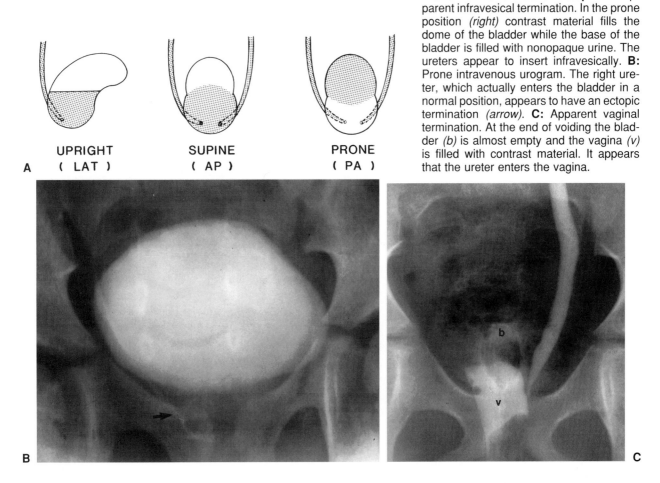

UPRIGHT
(LAT)

SUPINE
(AP)

PRONE
(PA)

FIG. 9-25. Fake ureteral ectopia. A: Apparent infravesical termination. In the prone position *(right)* contrast material fills the dome of the bladder while the base of the bladder is filled with nonopaque urine. The ureters appear to insert infravesically. **B:** Prone intravenous urogram. The right ureter, which actually enters the bladder in a normal position, appears to have an ectopic termination *(arrow).* **C:** Apparent vaginal termination. At the end of voiding the bladder *(b)* is almost empty and the vagina *(v)* is filled with contrast material. It appears that the ureter enters the vagina.

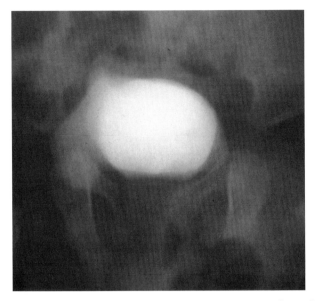

FIG. 9-26. Bladder ears. In this child, the extraperitoneal herniation of bladder (bladder ears) is larger on the right than the left. This normal appearance should not be mistaken for a bladder diverticulum.

A supine radiograph shows the true position of the ureterovesical junction.

Bladder ears are normal lateral protrusions of the urinary bladder commonly seen in infants less than 6 months of age (Fig. 9-26). These transitory protrusions are most apparent when the bladder is partially filled. Bladder ears represent extraperitoneal herniations of the bladder through the internal inguinal ring into the inguinal canal. Approximately 20% of infants with bladder ears also have inguinal hernias (65). This association may reflect the presence of a patent or partially patent processus vaginalis that allows both bowel and bladder to herniate into the inguinal canal (65). Rarely one can see lateral protrusions of the rectum in this same location, producing a normal variant termed ''rectal ears.''

Urethra

The *spinning top female urethra* is a transitory, dynamic phenomenon. At one time, this appearance was believed to be secondary to meatal stenosis or a urethral ring. This misconception led to many unnecessary urethral dilatations (66). Currently, most believe that the spinning top urethra is a normal variant; because the distal urethral segment is less distensible, there may be intermittent and variable dilatation of the more proximal urethra during voiding. Others (67) have performed video urodynamic studies in some of these patients and demonstrated bladder detrusor instability (dyssynergy), a congenitally wide bladder neck anomaly, or both.

Normal anatomic folds are frequently visualized in the posterior urethra of the male. They should not be confused with obstructing valves. Unlike posterior urethral valves, these folds do not produce dilatation of the more proximal

posterior urethra or decrease the urinary stream. The *intermuscular incisura* produces an indentation in the midportion of the posterior urethra (Fig. 9-27) (see Fig. 9-15). It is located at the level of the middle of the verumontanum. This incisura is due to an abundance of collagenous tissue at the point where smooth muscle reflected from the bladder around the upper half of the urethra meets the paraurethral striated muscle, which is reflected upward around the lower urethra (16,17). This incisura is more prominent anteriorly (see Fig. 9-15) and in boys (16,17). Occasionally, a prominent *insertion of the plicae colliculae* is present. Plicae are normal folds that extend distally from the distal end of the verumontanum (Fig. 9-27). There may be a circumferential fold where these plicae insert into the distal portion of the posterior urethra just above the membranous urethra (Fig. 9-27). They form a continuum from a normal variant through minor posterior urethral valves to obstructing valves.

The urethral (external) sphincter or urogenital diaphragm extends from the midportion of the verumontanum to just beyond the membranous urethra. During voiding, incomplete relaxation of the sphincter can produce narrowings or partial obstructions of the urethra (Fig. 9-28A). Fluoroscopy during VCUG will verify that the urethra is normal (Fig. 9-28B).

Cowper glands are paired pea-sized glands situated behind and on each side of the membranous urethra between the two fascial layers of the urogenital membrane (68). Each of these glands is drained by a large main duct that empties into the floor of the bulbous urethra. Occasionally, these *Cowper gland ducts* are filled during voiding cystography or retrograde urethrography. A tubular structure, which originates from the floor of the bulbous urethra, is noted (see Figs. 9-107 and 9-108). These ducts course posteriorly, close to the undersurface of the urethra on each side and terminate near the external sphincter. Filling of Cowper gland ducts may result from an incompetent ostium of the duct or from rupture of a previous Cowper gland duct cyst. Filling of this structure should not be confused with a urethral diverticulum, partial duplication, stricture, false passage, extravasation, or fistula.

A *urinal artifact* may be produced in the male during voiding. The urethral stream is compressed at the level of the penoscrotal junction by the plastic urinal. This artifact should not be confused with a stricture of the penile urethra (Fig. 9-29A). A film during voiding without compression by the urinal confirms normal urethral caliber (Fig. 9-29B).

The *foreskin artifact* is due to retraction of a tight foreskin and consequent narrowing of the distal urethra (Fig. 9-30). This can mimic a distal urethral stricture. Reduction of the foreskin makes the appearance normal.

Pseudotumors

Renal Pseudotumors

Hypertrophy of a column of Bertin is a well-known simulator of a renal neoplasm (62). A normal column (septum)

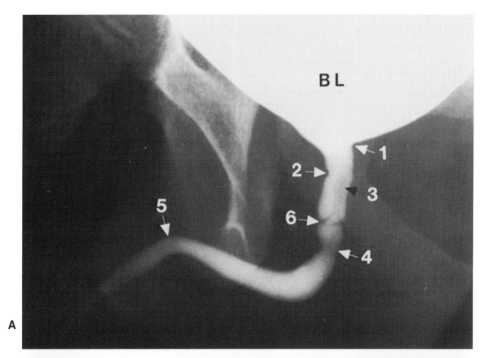

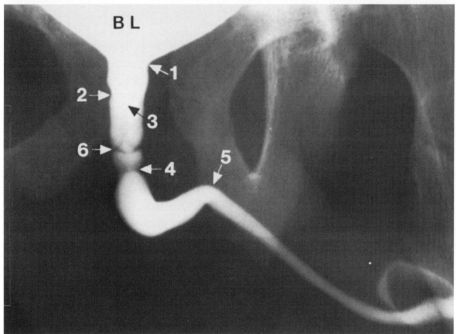

FIG. 9-27. Normal urethral folds. A 9-year-old boy with urinary tract infection. VCUG in right posterior oblique **(A)** and left posterior oblique **(B)** positions. The bladder *(BL)*, bladder neck or urethrovesical junction *(1)*, intermuscular incisura *(2)*, verumontanum *(3)*, membranous urethra passing through the external or urethral sphincter *(4)*, and suspensory ligament of the penis *(5)* are readily apparent. Prominent plicae colliculae extend from the verumontanum distally. There is a circumferential fold *(6)* where these plicae insert into the posterior urethra just above the membranous urethra.

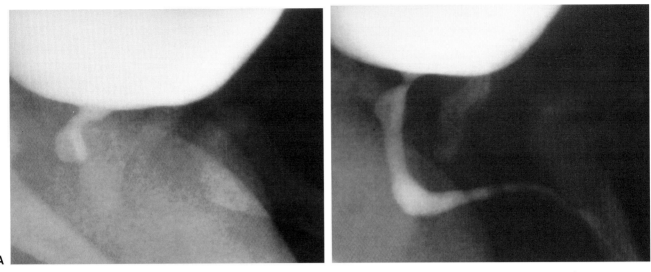

FIG. 9-28. Normal VCUG. A: The bladder neck (urethrovesical junction) is open but the sphincter is contracted. The upper portion of the verumontanum is seen as a filling defect in the posterior part of the urethra. **B:** The sphincter is now relaxed and urethra is well visualized. The entire verumontanum is now seen. Dynamic studies, such as this, verify that the urethral (external) sphincter begins at the level of the middle of the verumontanum.

of Bertin is cortical renal tissue inserted between adjacent renal pyramids. If it becomes focally hypertrophied, it may cause splaying of the renal calyces and infundibula. This hypertrophy and infolding of cortical tissue usually occurs between the calyces of the upper and middle poles. The density of this column of Bertin during the nephrographic phase of excretory urography is greater than that of the adjacent medulla and equal to or greater than the density of the adjacent renal cortex. If there is a centrally placed medulla within this column of Bertin, there may be an area of radiolucency surrounded by a dense cortical blush. Sonography demonstrates a mass with echogenicity similar to that of normal renal cortex. Doppler sonography, or renal angiography if performed, shows that the intralobar arteries are displaced in a curvilinear manner around the pseudotumor, but neovascularity and arteriovenous shunting are not present.

Renal scintigraphy with ^{99m}Tc-DMSA shows increased uptake in this infolded cortical tissue. Compared with surrounding normal tissue, the column of Bertin may show a spectrum of uptake of ^{99m}Tc-DTPA or ^{99m}Tc-MAG 3 ranging from minimally to markedly increased (62).

Compensatory hypertrophy develops in patients with unilateral renal disease. It may occur in patients with contralateral nephrectomy, agenesis, multicystic dysplasia, hypoplasia, or atrophy. The normal kidney increases in size to compensate for loss of overall renal mass. This compensatory hypertrophy should not be confused with renal neoplasia or pathologic renal enlargement.

Occasionally, renal inflammation mimics a neoplasm. These *inflammatory renal pseudotumors* may be caused by an abscess, xanthogranulomatous pyelonephritis, or acute pyelonephritis. Clinical features include fever, abdominal

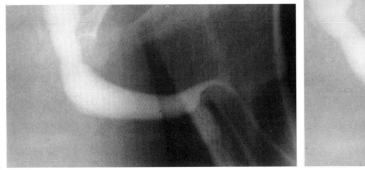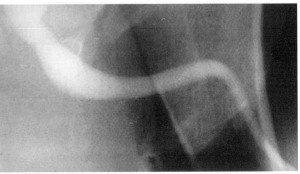

FIG. 9-29. Urinal artifact. A: Compression and angulation of the penile urethral stream of contrast media by a plastic urinal. **B:** Repeat voiding film after repositioning of the receptacle shows a normal urethra.

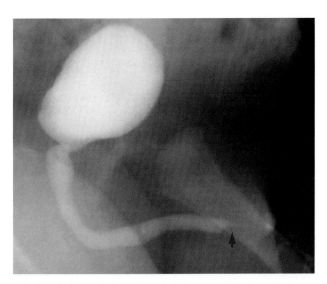

FIG. 9-30. Foreskin artifact. The foreskin has been retracted and causes extrinsic compression of the urethra *(arrow)* mimicking a distal stricture.

mass, hematuria, and pyuria. Imaging techniques show an intrarenal mass with or without displacement or distortion of collecting structures (62). US is helpful for localizing these ''masses'' by demonstrating focal change in renal echogenicity. Generalized inflammatory disease of the kidneys, such as acute pyelonephritis, may be more confusing. Intravenous urography usually shows enlargement of the kidney with poor filling of the calyces. US may simply show generalized enlargement of the kidney, loss of the corticomedullary junction, and diffuse abnormality of echogenicity. CT may be necessary to distinguish these inflammatory lesions from renal tumors, although this modality is seldom necessary for the diagnosis of ordinary pyelonephritis or glomerulonephritis. Renal cortical scanning with DMSA, contrast-enhanced CT, and color (especially power) Doppler sonography are the preferred methods for verifying the diagnosis of acute pyelonephritis (69,70).

Ureteral Pseudotumors

Filling defects in the ureter may suggest a neoplasm, but it should be remembered that ureteral neoplasms are very rare in childhood. Ureteral filling defects include vascular impressions, transverse folds, calculi, blood clots, air bubbles (after cystography or retrograde or antegrade pyelography), sloughed renal tissue from papillary necrosis, and ureteritis cystica.

Dilated ureters in conjunction with a dilated bladder may compress the rectum to form an abdominal pseudotumor (62). A barium enema may even suggest a pelvic mass. Abdominal sonography demonstrates that the pelvic mass is due to dilated ureters and a dilated bladder.

Bladder Pseudotumors

A *dilated bladder* may simulate a pelvic neoplasm. Plain films show a soft-tissue density in the pelvis with the rounded contour of the bladder. In young infants, bowel loops are often displaced by the distended bladder, particularly in the ill, premature newborn who may have functional delay in bladder emptying (62). The bladder may also become distended due to distal obstruction or in conjunction with the megacystis-microcolon-intestinal hypoperistalsis syndrome.

Cystitis occasionally results in marked edematous thickening of the bladder mucosa, which protrudes into the bladder lumen. Radiologic and even endoscopic findings may suggest an invasive neoplasm such as rhabdomyosarcoma (Fig. 9-31). Biopsy with permanent sections (frozen sections are not adequate) may be required for clarification. US has been useful for distinguishing edematous circumferential bladder wall thickening from a true mass. Bladder wall inflammation may be due to bacterial or viral cystitis, eosinophilic cystitis, cystitis cystica, cystitis in immunodeficiency states (agammaglobulinemia, chronic granulomatous disease), or cystitis associated with chemotherapy (62).

Urethral Pseudotumors

Ectopic and more commonly simple *ureteroceles* occasionally prolapse into the proximal urethra to create a filling defect mimicking a polyp (see Figs. 9-90 and 9-186). Films obtained at various phases during VCUG help distinguish these pseudotumors from true urethral masses.

Genital Pseudotumors

The *newborn uterus and vagina* are relatively large. In certain newborns, presumably because of maternal estrogen, these normal structures become markedly enlarged, resulting in a pseudotumor. The enlarged uterus and vagina produce a mass between the bladder and rectum. Hypertrophy of the vaginal mucosa and labia sometimes causes a perineal soft-tissue mass that mimics sarcoma botryoides. The uterus and vagina gradually decrease in size after the newborn period to approximately 50% of their birth size by 6 months of age (62).

Scrotal extension of healed meconium peritonitis may produce a hard, irregular mass that mimics a testicular neoplasm. This mass may contain calcifications (Fig. 9-32A) that suggest a testicular teratoma or scrotal neuroblastoma. A history of hydrocele at birth and the distribution of the calcifications help to exclude a neoplastic lesion; sonography clarifies the diagnosis (Fig. 9-32B). Calcification may also be noted in the abdomen, or there may be a history of meconium peritonitis.

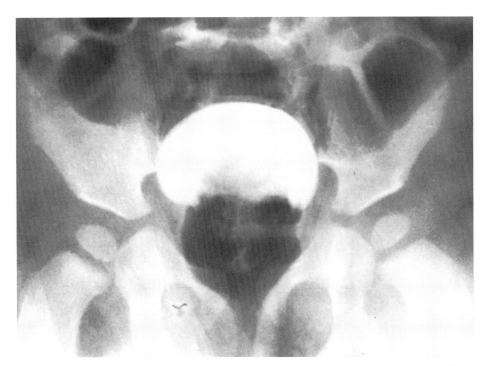

FIG. 9-31. Hemorrhagic cystitis. A 1-month-old girl with hematuria. There is marked thickening and irregularity of the bladder wall and elevation of the base of the bladder. Multiple biopsies showed only bladder mucosa with inflammatory changes. A repeat cystogram after 3 weeks of antibiotic therapy was normal. (Courtesy of Herman Grossman, M.D., Durham, NC.)

Renal Enlargement

Renal enlargement may be bilateral or unilateral. Deviations in size from normal are determined by nomograms or growth charts (see Figs. 9-11 and 9-12). Significant renal enlargement is usually taken as 2 standard deviations (SD) above normal or more. Bilateral renal enlargement (Table 9-2) is frequently due to congenital abnormalities or processes that infiltrate the kidneys. Unilateral renal enlargement (Table 9-3) is frequently due to duplication, tumor, obstruction, hypertrophy, or infection. The cause of renal enlargement is usually apparent from the history, laboratory findings, and imaging features.

Small Kidneys

Small kidneys are at least 2 SD below the mean in greatest length. The causes of bilateral small kidneys (Table 9-4) and unilateral small kidney (Table 9-5) can be categorized as congenital, inflammatory, vascular, or atrophic, plus a group of miscellaneous causes.

Cul-de-Sac Masses

Pelvic masses are common in children and may be presacral, rectovesical, uterovaginal, vesical, rectal, or perineal. The cul-de-sac is an extension of the peritoneal cavity that lies between the bladder and the rectum. It has also been called the pouch of Douglas and retrovesical space. It is only a potential space in boys. In girls, it is a small space that contains the uterus and its broad ligaments.

Cul-de-sac masses may be asymptomatic, although the proximity of the pelvic organs frequently results in bowel or bladder symptoms. Radiologic evaluation usually includes frontal and lateral radiographs of the pelvis to delineate the

TABLE 9-2. *Bilateral renal enlargement*

Congenital disorders	Tumor
Duplications[a]	Nephroblastomatosis
Cystic disease	Bilateral Wilms tumor
Polycystic disease	Metastases
Tuberous sclerosis	Infiltration
Beckwith-Wiedemann	Leukemia-lymphoma[a]
syndrome[a]	Amyloid
Tyrosinemia	Glycogen storage disease
Bartter syndrome	(von Gierke disease)
Total lipodystrophy	Sarcoidosis
Generalized	Vascular disorders
visceromegaly	Renal vein thrombosis
Infection	Acute tubular necrosis
Acute pyelonephritis[a]	Sickle cell anemia[a]
Acute	Hemolytic-uremic syndrome
glomerulonephritis[a]	Nephrotic syndrome[a]
Infectious	Obstruction[a]
mononucleosis	Extrinsic compression:
	hepatosplenomegaly

[a] More common.

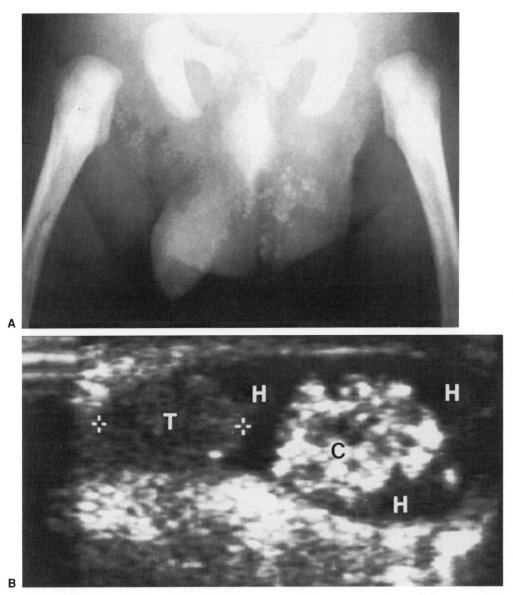

FIG. 9-32. Scrotal meconium peritonitis. A 3-day-old boy with a hard mass in the scrotum. **A:** Plain film shows multiple calcifications in the left scrotum. **B:** Longitudinal scrotal sonography shows a normal left testis *(T)*. The echogenic mass *(C)* within hydrocele fluid *(H)* is due to scrotal extension of healed meconium peritonitis.

mass, identify any calcifications, and assess the integrity of the spine and sacrum. US is used next because it is noninvasive. Excellent images of the pelvis are obtained using the urine-filled bladder as an acoustic window (Fig. 9-33A). Usually either CT (Fig. 9-33B) or MRI is required to evaluate the extent of complex inflammatory disease or malignancy. Rarely, a double study (simultaneous cystogram and rectogram) or triple study (simultaneous cystogram, rectogram, and vaginogram) is needed for further clarification.

The differential diagnosis of cul-de-sac masses includes enlarged or ectopic normal structures, inflammatory disease, benign or malignant tumors, blood secondary to trauma, ureteral dilatation, bladder diverticula, ectopic ureterocele, ectopic pregnancy, and normal pregnancy (Table 9-6). The

history, laboratory results, and imaging features usually lead to the correct diagnosis.

Urinary Tract Obstruction

Obstruction is one of the most common indications for radiologic evaluation of the urinary tract in children. The terminology used for urinary tract obstruction may be confusing (71,72). *Hydronephrosis* is defined as dilatation of the renal pelvis and calyces. *Hydroureter* indicates ureteral dilatation of any cause (71). *Hydroureteronephrosis* includes both hydronephrosis and hydroureter; it has also been termed *ureteropyelocaliectasis.*

TABLE 9-3. Unilateral renal enlargement

Congenital disorders
  Duplication[a]
  Cystic disease
    Multicystic dysplastic kidney[a]
    Multilocular cyst
    Dysplasia
    Simple cyst
    Polycystic disease
Infection
  Acute pyelonephritis[a]
  Inflammatory mass
    Abscess
    Xanthogranulomatous
      pyelonephritis
  Tuberculoma
  Echinococcosis
  Acute glomerulonephritis
    (asymmetric)
Tumor
  Mesoblastic nephroma
  Wilms tumor[a]
  Nephroblastomatosis
  Angiomyolipoma
  Sarcoma
  Carcinoma
  Metastasis
  Lymphoma-leukemia
Vascular disorders
  Renal vein
    thrombosis[a]
  Infarct
  Transplants
    Rejection
    Tubular necrosis
    Vascular
      occlusion
Trauma
  Contusion[a]
  Hematoma[a]
  Urinoma
Obstruction[a]
  UPJ obstruction[a]
  Primary
    megaureter
  Other
Hypertrophy
  Compensatory
    hypertrophy[a]
  Hemihypertrophy

[a] More common.

TABLE 9-5. Unilateral small kidney

Congenital disorders
  Hypoplasia
  Dysplasia[a]
Infection
  Chronic pyelonephritis[a]
  Tuberculosis
Vascular disorders
  Venous thrombosis[a]
  Arterial
    Emboli
    Occlusion
Atrophy
  Obstructive atrophy[a]
  Reflux and scarring[a]
Miscellaneous disorders
  Partial nephrectomy
  Radiation

[a] More common.

It is sometimes difficult to distinguish nonobstructive dilatation of the urinary tract from obstruction. Methods to confirm or exclude obstruction include VCUG, Doppler sonography, furosemide (Lasix) intravenous urography, furosemide nuclear scintigraphic renography, and the Whitaker test.

TABLE 9-4. Bilateral small kidneys

Congenital disorders
  Dysplasia
    Cystic dysplasia
    Congenital obstruction
  Hypoplasia
  Syndromes
    Prune belly syndrome
    Laurence-Moon-Biedl syndrome
    Jeune syndrome
Infection
  Chronic pyelonephritis[a]
Vascular disorders
  Renal vein thrombosis[a]
  Arterial disorders
    Emboli
    Occlusion
  Cortical necrosis
  Medullary necrosis
  Arteriolar nephrosclerosis: hypertension
Atrophy
  Obstructive atrophy[a]
  Reflux and scarring[a]
Miscellaneous disorders
  Chronic nephritis
    Glomerulonephritis
    Radiation
    Henoch-Schönlein purpura
  Hereditary nephritis: Alpert disease
  Collagen vascular disease
    Scleroderma
    Lupus erythematosus
    Periarteritis
    Medullary cystic disease

[a] More common.

TABLE 9-6. Cul-de-sac masses

Normal structures
  Fluid-filled loops of small bowel[a]
  Ectopic kidney
  Large normal uterus[a]
  Torsion of normal ovary
Inflammatory
  Abscess from ruptured appendicitis[a]
  Pelvic inflammatory disease[a]
  Peritonitis
Tumor
  Teratoma
  Sarcoma botryoides
  Rhabdomyosarcoma
  Leiomyosarcoma
  Hydrometrocolpos[a]
  Lymphoma
  Ovarian tumor[a]
  Yolk sac tumor
  Neurogenic tumor
Trauma
  Intraperitoneal blood
  Ruptured viscus
    Bladder
    Rectum
Miscellaneous
  Ovarian torsion
  Ureteral dilatation
    Hydroureters, especially obstructed ectopic ureters
    Ectopic ureterocele
  Pregnancy[a]
  Bladder diverticulum

[a] More common.

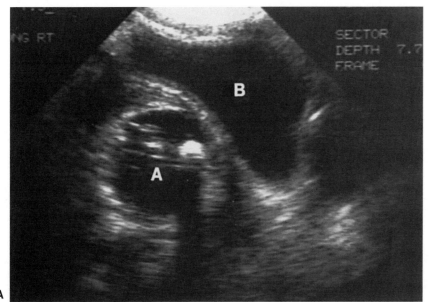

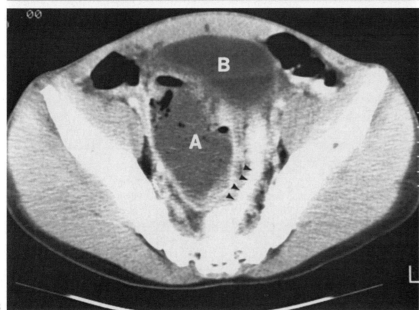

FIG. 9-33. Cul-de-sac abscesses secondary to perforated appendicitis. A: A 2-year-old boy with vomiting and abdominal distention. Longitudinal sonography shows a complex mass *(A)* in the cul-de-sac. The pelvic abscess contains an echogenic appendicolith with acoustic shadowing. Note the extrinsic compression of the bladder *(B)*. **B:** A 15-year-old boy with abdominal pain, vomiting, and a pelvic mass. CT demonstrates a cul-de-sac abscess *(A)* containing fluid and air. This mass also compresses the bladder *(B)*. Note the inflammatory thickening of the wall of the rectosigmoid colon *(arrowheads)*.

Urinary tract dilatation may have physiologic, functional, or mechanical causes. Physiologic causes of urinary tract dilatation include a full bladder and severe chronic constipation. Functional causes of dilatation of the urinary tract include neurogenic dysfunction of the bladder, increased urine flow (diabetes insipidus, Bartter syndrome, juvenile nephronophthisis), vesicoureteral reflux, inflammatory disease, and prune-belly syndrome. Vesicoureteral reflux and mechanical obstruction are the most common causes of dilatation of the calyces, pelves, and ureters in infants and children. Mechanical obstruction may be congenital or acquired. In infants and children, most causes of mechanical obstruction are congenital.

In considering the differential diagnostic possibilities, urinary tract obstruction may be divided into causes affecting the upper urinary tract and those affecting the lower urinary tract. Upper urinary tract obstruction involves the kidneys or ureters and can be unilateral or bilateral (Table 9-7). Lower urinary tract obstruction involves the bladder or urethra (Table 9-8). The specific causes of urinary tract obstruction are discussed in detail later in this chapter.

Systemic Hypertension

Systemic hypertension is much less common in children than in adults. Several large studies have now defined normal blood pressure for children from birth to age 16. Contrary to the much lower incidence in adults, secondary causes of hypertension in children are demonstrated in 42% to 70%

TABLE 9-7. *Causes of upper urinary tract obstruction*

Kidney
  Calyceal obstruction
    Congenital
      Intrinsic
      Extrinsic, vascular (Fraley syndrome)
    Tuberculosis
  Congenital ureteropelvic junction obstruction[a]
    Intrinsic: stenosis[a]
    Extrinsic: crossing vessel
  Tumor
    Wilms tumor
    Carcinoma
Ureter
  Physiologic
    Full bladder
    Chronic constipation
  Stricture
  Valve
  Retrocaval ureter
  Retroiliac ureter
  Retroperitoneal fibrosis
  Polyp
  Calculus
  Blood clot
  Inflammatory disease
    Tuberculosis
    Bilharziasis
    Appendicitis[a]
    Crohn disease[a]
    Pelvic inflammatory disease
    Osteomyelitis of an adjacent bone
  Hydrometrocolpos
  Adhesions
  Neoplasm
    Neuroblastoma
    Lymphoma
    Genitourinary neoplasm
  Primary megaureter[a]
  Ectopic ureter
  Ectopic ureterocele[a]
  Simple ureterocele

[a] More common.
Source: Modified from Friedland (71,72).

TABLE 9-8. *Causes of lower urinary tract obstruction*

Bladder
  Ureterocele
    Simple
    Ectopic[a]
  Foreign body
  Neoplasm
    Rhabdomyosarcoma
    Neurofibroma
  Neurogenic dysfunction[a]
  Calculus
  Blood clot
Posterior urethra
  Valves[a]
  Polyp
  Ureterocele, prolapsing[a]
  Rhabdomyosarcoma of prostate
  Calculus
Anterior urethra
  Diverticulum
  Valve
  Megalourethra
  Calculus
  Stricture
    Traumatic[a]
    Inflammatory
  Cowper duct cyst
  Duplication (dorsal channel only)
  Meatal stenosis[a]
  Phimosis[a]

[a] More common.
Source: Modified from Friedland (71,72).

Clinical Presentation

Systemic hypertension may be asymptomatic, found only on routine physical examination. Occasionally, however, hypertension in children is a clinical emergency. These patients have pulmonary edema, hypertensive encephalopathy, subarachnoid hemorrhage due to rupture of an aneurysm, or a hypertensive crisis. Less dramatic clinical symptoms include transient facial nerve palsy, headache, irritability, unsteadiness of gait, sweating, tachycardia, dizziness, and anxiety. The symptoms may be episodic.

Imaging Evaluation

Persistent, unexplained, nonuremic hypertension requires vigorous search for a renovascular cause. Although renovascular lesions account for less than 10% of pediatric hypertension, they are usually treatable. In the past, rapid sequence intravenous urography and radionuclide flow studies were used to search for renovascular causes of hypertension. However, both procedures have unacceptably high false-negative rates due to the high frequency of bilateral or intrarenal (and therefore obscure) renovascular lesions. Most unilateral renal causes of hypertension present with a smaller

of cases (46,73,74). The incidence of idiopathic hypertension increases with increasing age. Idiopathic (essential) hypertension may begin in childhood, particularly in black teenagers.

Hypertension in children may be primary or secondary (Table 9-9). There is a correlation between essential hypertension and positive family history, sodium intake, and obesity. Secondary hypertension in children may be due to a renal parenchymal lesion, aortic disease, renal vascular disease, or a tumor (Table 9-9). One of the most common secondary types of hypertension in children is renovascular disease due to fibromuscular dysplasia.

TABLE 9-9. *Causes of hypertension in children*

Primary causes
    Essential hypertension: familial,[a] racial[a]
    Obesity[a]
Secondary causes
    Renal parenchymal lesions
        Glomerulonephritis[a]
            Acute
            Chronic
        Chronic renal disease[a]
            Cortical necrosis
            Medullary necrosis
            Collagen vascular disease
        Atrophic pyelonephritis: reflux and scarring[a]
        Obstructive atrophy[a]
        Segmental renal hypoplasia: Ask-Upmark kidney
        Renal vein thrombosis
        Hemolytic uremic syndrome
        Hydronephrosis
    Vascular disease
        Coarctation of aorta[a]
        Postcoarctectomy syndrome
        Abdominal coarctation
        Neurofibromatosis
        Tuberous sclerosis
        Chronic granulomatous disease
        Arteritis
    Renovascular disease
        Fibromuscular dysplasia[a]
        Neurofibromatosis
        Abdominal coarctation
        Radiation
        Homocystinuria
        Vasculitis
            Idiopathic
            Autoimmune
        Hypercalcemia
            Williams syndrome
        Trauma
            Avulsion
            Occlusion
            Thrombosis
        Tuberous sclerosis
        Rubella syndrome
        Renal vein thrombosis
        Periarteritis
        Arteriovenous fistula
    Tumors
        Wilms tumor
        Reninoma
        Pheochromocytoma
        Neuroblastoma

[a] More common.

kidney on the affected side and a normal or perhaps hypertrophied kidney on the contralateral side. If sonography demonstrates a length differential of >1 cm between the two kidneys or local renal parenchymal disease in a hypertensive child, differential renal function studies should be performed with ^{99m}Tc-DTPA or ^{99m}Tc-MAG 3 to determine the functional importance of the sonographic finding. Captopril enhancement has increased the sensitivity of renal scintigraphy in the adult (75); this technique is being used increasingly in hypertensive children.

Renal angiography remains the standard for diagnosing renovascular causes of pediatric hypertension; it demonstrates the morphology and hemodynamic significance of the lesion and indicates the surgical approach. Cure or significant reduction in hypertension by angioplasty, surgical therapy, or both is possible in 87% to 95% of children with renovascular hypertension. Renal angiography and renal vein renin sampling should be performed in all children with persistent, unexplained hypertension (46).

Etiology

Renal artery stenosis, usually due to fibromuscular dysplasia, is the most common cause of renovascular hypertension in children. The stenotic lesions may be bilateral (17%) and commonly involve the middle or distal third of the main renal artery. Not infrequently (64%), segmental renal arteries (Fig. 9-34A) are involved. If segmental stenosis is identified, segmental renal vein renin should be analyzed. Rarely, stenotic lesions involve the origins of the main renal arteries in patients with neurofibromatosis (Fig. 9-35), Williams syndrome, and after transplantation (Fig. 9-36).

Other causes of hypertension demonstrable by angiography include vasculitis, renin-producing tumors, chronic pyelonephritis, trauma (Fig. 9-37), homocystinuria, hydronephrosis, coarctation of the abdominal aorta, pheochromocytoma, and aldosteronoma (46).

Intrarenal Collaterals

Collateral circulation develops because of a decrease in blood flow to part of the kidney. This ischemia causes dilatation of preexisting anastomotic connections. Whether extrarenal or intrarenal collateral pathways dominate depends on the site of the vascular occlusion. Intrarenal collaterals would be expected in children with intrarenal stenotic lesions, which are usually due to fibromuscular dysplasia.

There are several sources of intrarenal collateral circulation (Fig. 9-34B). The pericalyceal complex (Fig. 9-34) is a communication between adjacent interlobar arteries. Direct communications also exist between intrarenal vessels and extrarenal collateral networks. Flow in these intrarenal collaterals may be in either direction, depending on the site of renal ischemia (Fig. 9-34B).

Intrarenal collaterals are frequently identified in hypertension in children. They should not be confused with tumor vascularity or vascular malformations. The presence of these collaterals indicates significant renal artery stenosis regardless of the segmental or main renal vein renin levels. Although there is an excellent opportunity for cure by angioplasty or surgery, intrarenal stenotic lesions require precise demonstration in order to revascularize and preserve renal parenchyma (46).

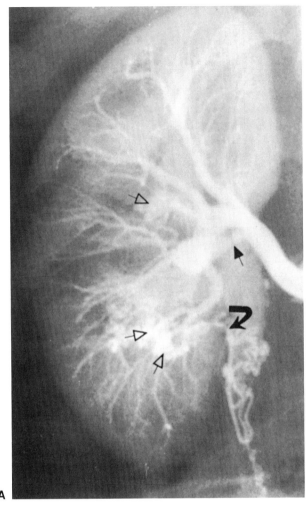

A

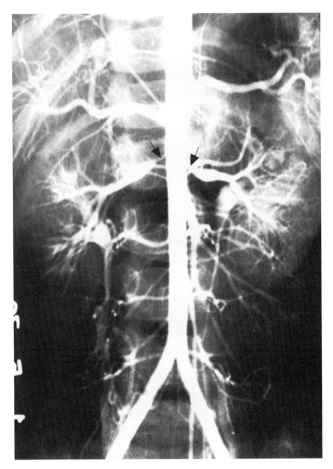

FIG. 9-35. Main renal artery stenoses. A 6-year-old girl with neurofibromatosis and hypertension. There are bilateral stenoses *(arrows)* of the origins of the renal arteries.

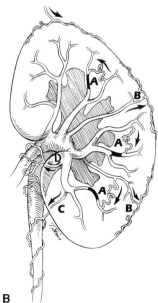

B

FIG. 9-34. Intrarenal collateral circulation. A: Segmental renal artery stenosis. A 12-year-old boy with a blood pressure of 140/100 mm Hg. Late arterial phase of a selective right renal arteriogram. There is stenosis of the ventral branch of the renal artery *(solid arrow)* and poststenotic aneurysmal dilatation. Pericalyceal collaterals *(open arrows)* between ad-

The results of renal artery angioplasty in children with fibromuscular dysplasia have been excellent; there is an 80% to 100% long-term patency rate and frequently a return to normotensive status (76). Patients with stenosis due to neurofibromatosis and Williams syndrome have less success with angioplasty, perhaps because of greater intimal proliferation and longer segments of involvement (76). Balloon angioplasty of postoperative stenotic lesions has also been successful (Fig. 9-36); there are few significant complications.

jacent interlobar arteries are evident. There is a direct communication *(curved arrow)* between interlobar arteries and the periureteric complex. **B:** Routes of intrarenal collateral circulation. *A*, pericalyceal collaterals between adjacent interlobar arteries; *B*, perforating capsular arteries connecting intrarenal parenchymal vessels to the extrarenal capsular complex; *C*, direct communication between an interlobar artery and the extrarenal periureteric complex; *D*, direct communication between an interlobar artery and the extrarenal peripelvic complex. Note that the direction of collateral flow indicated by *arrows* is schematic. This flow may be in either direction, depending on the exact site of renal ischemia. From Kirks (46).

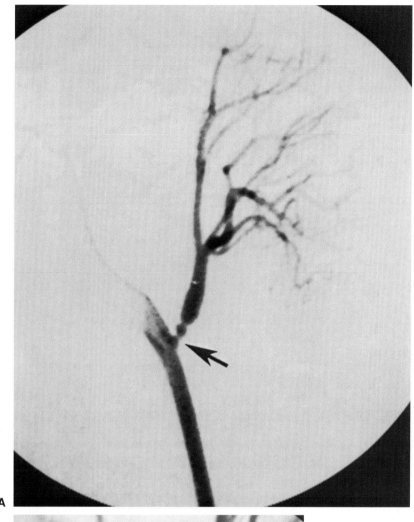

A

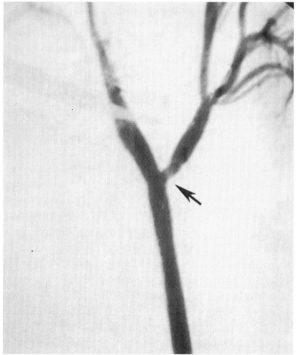

B

FIG. 9-36. Successful angioplasty of renal artery stenosis in a transplanted kidney. A: Digital subtraction angiography demonstrates stenosis of the orifice of the transplanted renal artery *(arrow)* at its origin from the left common iliac artery. **B:** Same patient after dilatation with a 6-mm angioplasty balloon catheter. Note the significant increase in the diameter of the vessel *(arrow).*

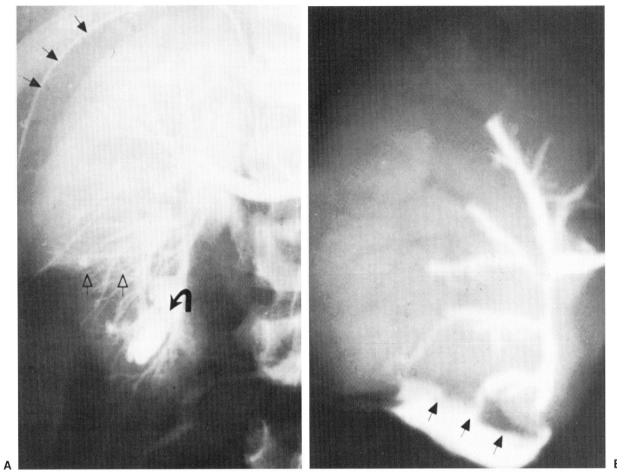

FIG. 9-37. Fractured kidney. A 14-year-old boy with hematuria and uncontrollable hypertension after a sledding accident. **A:** A selective right renal arteriogram shows a fracture across the lower pole of the kidney *(open arrows)*. There is intrarenal contrast extravasation *(curved arrow)* and displacement of the superior capsular artery *(solid arrows)* due to a perirenal hematoma. The hypertension in this patient is presumably due to both intrarenal arterial damage (Goldblatt phenomenon) and renal capsular compression (Page kidney). **B:** Injection of the nephrectomy specimen. There is contrast extravasation *(arrows)* at the lower pole fracture. From Kirks (46).

Urinary Tract Calcification

Causes of urinary tract calcification include nephrocalcinosis and urolithiasis. Nephrocalcinosis, which is less common in children than in adults, is defined as calcium deposition within the renal parenchyma. The etiology may be idiopathic, but it is usually due to hypercalciuria, hypercalcemia, or renal tissue damage (Table 9-10). Calcium deposition in nephrocalcinosis is in the tubular lumen, tubular epithelium, or interstitium.

When present on plain radiographs, calcifications in nephrocalcinosis are granular or stippled. These calcifications are usually bilateral in the medullary pyramids. Excretory function at IVU is frequently normal. Some patients with nephrocalcinosis also have urolithiasis. US is more sensitive to nephrocalcinosis than conventional radiography (Fig. 9-38) and is the best screening modality. The most common cause of pediatric nephrocalcinosis is chronic diuretic therapy in infants, for bronchopulmonary dysplasia or congenital heart disease (77).

Urolithiasis is defined as the presence of a calculus in the collecting system of the kidneys or lower in the urinary tract. Calculi formed in the kidney may pass into the distal urinary tract, growing by accretion. Urolithiasis is uncommon in children in the Western hemisphere with certain geographic exceptions and is usually idiopathic (78). Specific causes of urolithiasis in children include infection, immobilization, urinary stasis, foreign bodies, enteric abnormalities, and metabolic disorders (Table 9-11). Enteric causes of pediatric urolithiasis include oxalate urolithiasis due to interruption of the enterohepatic circulation of bile salts and uric acid lithiasis due to loss of fluid and bicarbonate (79). Sonography may demonstrate echogenic stones in the kidney (Fig. 9-39). Because sonography sometimes has difficulty identifying calcifications in ureters, intravenous urography is still performed in some patients suspected of having urolithiasis.

TABLE 9-10. *Differential diagnosis of nephrocalcinosis*

Idiopathic[a]
Hypercalciuria or hypercalcemia
  Hyperparathyroidism
  Malignancies
  Renal tubular acidosis[a]
  Cushing disease
  Steroids
  Osteoporosis
  Immobilization[a]
  Total parenteral nutrition[a]
  Hypervitaminosis D
  Hypovitaminosis D
  Sarcoidosis
  Idiopathic hypercalciuria
  Williams syndrome
  Bartter syndrome
  Diuretics[a]
  Hypophosphatasia
  Osteogenesis imperfecta
  Osteopetrosis
  Oxalosis, oxaluria
  Aminoaciduria
  Cystinuria
  Hyperuricemia
Tissue damage
  Renal cortical necrosis[a]
  Renal papillary necrosis
  Chronic glomerulonephritis
  Congenital nephritis
  Chronic pyelonephritis
  Tuberculosis
  Medullary sponge kidney[a]
  Heavy-metal poisoning
  Drugs: sulfonamide
  High altitude
  Renal infarcts
  Malignancies: Wilms tumor
  Xanthogranulomatous pyelonephritis

[a] More common.

Source: Modified from Chrispin et al. (3) and Reeder and Felson (11).

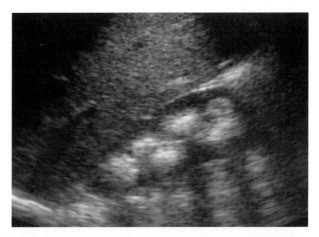

FIG. 9-38. Sonography of nephrocalcinosis. Supine, longitudinal renal sonography demonstrates echogenic pyramids in a child with medullary nephrocalcinosis. There is also some posterior acoustic shadowing.

the abdomen, and loops of air-filled bowel are seen floating in the center of the abdomen (see Fig. 9-68). A urinoma produces a retroperitoneal mass. IVU, in association with VCUG, demonstrates extravasation of contrast media into the perirenal fascia (Fig. 9-68A). Frequently, contrast material may be seen extending into the peritoneal cavity. The site of upper urinary tract perforation as well as the cause of the distal obstruction may be demonstrated by VCUG (Fig. 9-68). US is excellent for demonstrating hydronephrosis, perirenal urinoma, and ascites (13).

Spiral CT may occasionally be helpful in verifying urolithiasis.

Urine Ascites and Urinoma

Intraperitoneal urine is one of the most common causes of neonatal ascites (Table 9-12) (80). Most neonates with urine ascites are boys with urethral obstruction due to posterior urethral valves or an anterior urethral diverticulum (see Fig. 9-68). Distal obstruction is thought to cause perforation of the upper urinary tract, usually at the fornix of a calyx, which allows urine to escape into the perirenal space. If urine remains in a perinephric location, it produces a urinoma. Usually urine escapes from the perirenal space into the peritoneal cavity either through a tear or by transudation.

In patients with urine ascites, there is uniform density to

TABLE 9-11. *Differential diagnosis of urolithiasis*

Idiopathic[a]	Metabolic
Hypercalciuria	Renal tubular
Normocalciuria	syndromes
Stasis	Renal tubular
Hydronephrosis	acidosis[a]
Megacalyces	Carbonic
Medullary sponge kidney[a]	anhydrase
Calyceal diverticulum	inhibitors
Ureteric obstruction	Cystinuria
Ectopic ureterocele	Glycinuria
Neurogenic dysfunction	Enzyme disorders
Immobilization[a]	Primary hyperoxaluria
Enteric	Xanthinuria
Oxalate urolithiasis	Hypercalcemia[a] (see
(interruption of	Table 9-10)
enterohepatic circulation)[a]	Infection: Proteus
Uric acid lithiasis (loss of fluid	Uric acid lithiasis
and bicarbonate)	Idiopathic
Diarrhea	Secondary
Ileostomy	Enteric
Tissue breakdown from	Tumor lysis from
chemotherapy	chemotherapy
	Foreign body[a]

[a] More common.

Source: Modified from Kirks (79) and Walther et al. (78).

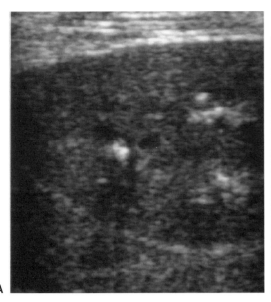
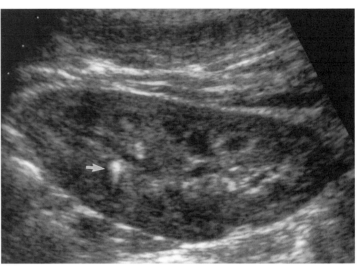

FIG. 9-39. Sonography of urolithiasis. A: The small, echogenic uric acid stone *(arrow)* causes some posterior acoustic shadowing. **B:** A 13-year-old child with cystinuria. Sonography of the left kidney shows an echogenic focus *(arrow)* with a comet tail distal shadow. The sonographic appearance is typical of a noncalcified (cystine) renal stone.

SPECIFIC ABNORMALITIES

Congenital Abnormalities

Pelvic and Ureteral Obstruction

Ureteropelvic Junction Obstruction

Ureteropelvic junction (UPJ) obstruction is the most common congenital obstruction of the urinary tract (71,72, 81,82). There is obstruction to the flow of urine from the renal pelvis to the proximal ureter. UPJ obstruction is very common in the fetus and neonate, but it can present for the first time at any age. UPJ obstruction is often bilateral but is usually asymmetric in severity.

In the past, children with UPJ obstruction usually came to attention because of a palpable flank mass, intermittent flank pain, hematuria after minor trauma, or urinary tract infection. Today, UPJ obstruction is frequently a prenatal diagnosis (83). In the older child, however, hematuria after minor trauma continues to be a fairly common presentation.

UPJ obstruction may coexist with other urinary tract abnormalities such as vesicoureteral reflux (84) and uretero-vesical junction obstruction (85). It may also occur in the lower moiety of a duplex kidney (Fig. 9-40) (86) and is the most common cause of obstruction of a horseshoe kidney (Fig. 9-41).

Etiology. There is considerable controversy regarding the etiology of UPJ obstruction. The surgeon usually finds intrinsic, probe-patent narrowing of the UPJ. Intrinsic narrowing may be caused by congenital intrinsic stricture (Fig. 9-42), abnormal orientation of the longitudinal musculature, disordered peristalsis, fibrosis due to collagen deposition,

prior ischemia, high ureteral insertion into the renal pelvis, and redundant ureteral mucosal folds. Rarely, a polyp (Fig. 9-43) is the cause of intrinsic UPJ obstruction.

Extrinsic obstruction may be caused by fibrous bands or aberrant vessels. Extrinsic compression of the ureter by a crossing blood vessel is usually due to a normal lower pole renal artery. The diagnosis of extrinsic UPJ obstruction may be difficult because symptoms (pain and hydronephrosis) tend to be intermittent.

Imaging. If UPJ obstruction is severe, plain radiographs may show a soft-tissue mass in the renal area and displacement of bowel gas. Plain radiographs are normal if the obstruction is mild. Stones may form in the dilated renal pelvis or in a calyx because of urinary stasis; these calculi may be visible on plain radiographs (Fig. 9-44).

Ultrasonography. US is usually the first imaging modality performed in patients with possible UPJ obstruction. When hydronephrosis has been diagnosed prenatally, US during the first few days of life may underestimate its severity because of the normal postnatal oliguria (Fig. 9-45) (87). In some instances, a multicystic dysplastic kidney consisting of only a few large cysts cannot be sonographically distinguished from hydronephrosis due to UPJ obstruction.

The normal central pelvicalyceal echo complex may contain a small amount of urine, particularly in the prone position (88). If this echolucent zone is as thick as the renal cortex, there is pathologic dilatation. Sonography of UPJ obstruction without coexisting abnormalities shows hydronephrosis without hydroureter (89). There are multiple hypoechoic cystic spaces, the largest being medial and representing the dilated renal pelvis. The cysts intercommunicate, and one can usually identify infundibula and calyces as well as surrounding renal parenchyma. There is no evidence of ure-

TABLE 9-12. *Causes of neonatal ascites*

Urine
    Anterior urethral diverticulum
    Anterior urethral valve
    Posterior urethral valve[a]
    Neurogenic bladder
    Extrinsic bladder mass
    Bladder rupture
    Ureterovesical junction obstruction
    Ureteropelvic junction obstruction
    Renal rupture
Edema—transudate
    Erythroblastosis fetalis[a]
    Primary liver disease[a]
    Portal vein obstruction[a]
    Hypoproteinemia[a]
    Volvulus, bowel ischemia[a]
    Intestinal lymphangiectasia
    Cardiac disease
    Mesenteric vessel occlusion
Pus—exudate
    Peritonitis[a]
    Syphilis
    Toxoplasmosis
    Volvulus, complicated[a]
    Meconium peritonitis
Gastrointestinal contents
    Meconium peritonitis
    Perforation[a]
Blood
    Trauma[a]
    Rupture[a]
        Spleen[a]
        Liver[a]
Chyle
    Chylous ascites
    Lymphangiectasia
Bile
    Obstruction: common bile duct
    Perforation
        Gallbladder
        Cystic duct
        Hepatic duct
        Common bile duct
Cyst fluid
    Ruptured ovarian cyst
    Ruptured omental cyst
    Ruptured mesenteric cyst
    Ruptured choledochal cyst
Indeterminate

Source: Modified from Griscom et al. (80).

[a] More common.

Modified form Griscom et al. (80).

teral dilatation and the bladder is normal. The hydronephrosis can be described as mild (pelvic dilatation without calyceal dilatation), moderate (pelvic and calyceal dilatation), or severe (pelvic and calyceal dilatation with parenchymal thinning; the kidney may be merely a large cystic mass). If the hydronephrosis is so massive that the dilated pelvicalyceal system extends down into the pelvis next to the bladder, UPJ obstruction can be mistaken for ureterovesical junction (UVJ) obstruction (Fig. 9-46).

Identification of a dilated ureter or a thick-walled bladder suggests lower obstruction rather than UPJ obstruction. US should also attempt to evaluate renal parenchymal thickness. The amount of parenchymal thinning is related to the severity and duration of obstruction and the amount of atrophy (3). If a cystic mass consistent with hydronephrosis is identified, a VCUG should be the next diagnostic procedure. It is

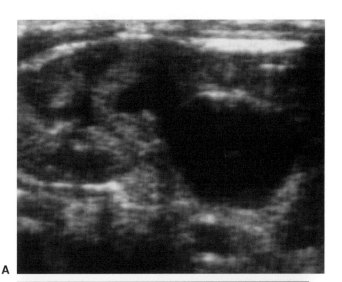

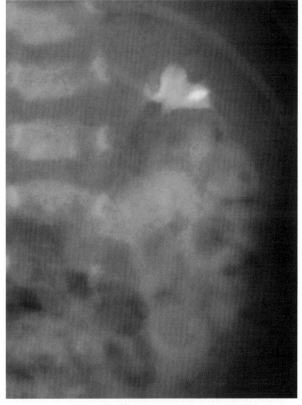

FIG. 9-40. Lower pole UPJ obstruction. A: Ultrasonography. Dilated pelvicalyceal system of the lower pole moiety of the left kidney. **B:** IVU. The upper pole moiety of the left kidney is not obstructed. There is obstructive hydronephrosis of the lower pole due to UPJ obstruction.

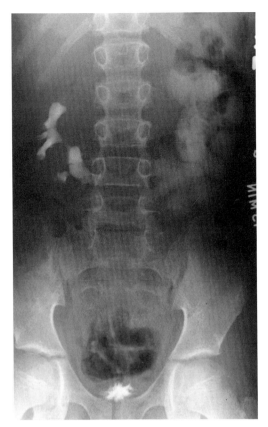

FIG. 9-41. UPJ obstruction of a horseshoe kidney. Because the two kidneys are joined by an isthmus of renal tissue, the lower poles are closer to the spine than the upper poles. There is UPJ obstruction on the left.

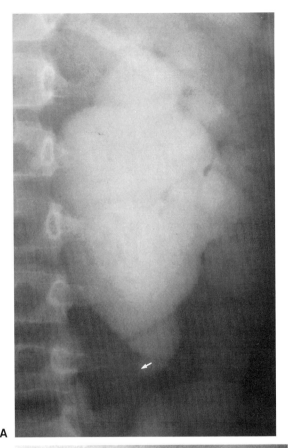

A

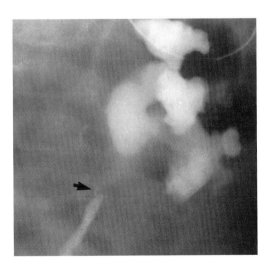

FIG. 9-42. UPJ obstruction due to intrinsic ureteral stricture. Retrograde ureteropyelogram shows marked narrowing at the ureteropelvic junction *(arrow)*.

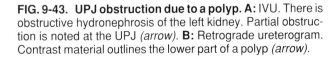

FIG. 9-43. UPJ obstruction due to a polyp. A: IVU. There is obstructive hydronephrosis of the left kidney. Partial obstruction is noted at the UPJ *(arrow)*. **B:** Retrograde ureterogram. Contrast material outlines the lower part of a polyp *(arrow)*.

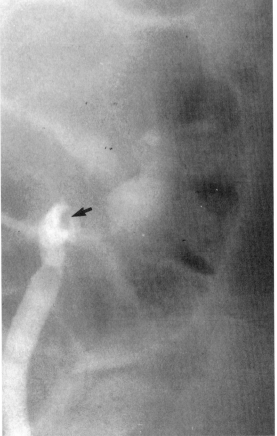

B

performed to exclude reflux, urethral obstruction, or both (27). Renal scintigraphy or intravenous urography should be performed to confirm the cause and site of obstruction as well as to determine the function of the kidneys.

Voiding cystourethrography. Because the sonographic finding of hydronephrosis can be due to UPJ obstruction alone, vesicoureteral reflux alone, or UPJ obstruction with coexisting reflux, a VCUG should always be performed (Fig. 9-47). The coexistence of UPJ obstruction and reflux is suggested on VCUG by obstruction of the refluxed contrast material at the level of the UPJ, dilution of contrast as it enters the dilated renal pelvis, and delay in drainage from the renal pelvis (Fig. 9-47). Renal pelvic dilatation due to UPJ obstruction may lead to overestimation of the severity of vesicoureteral reflux. Lack of ureteral tortuosity suggests that renal pelvic dilatation is not due to reflux alone. If reflux

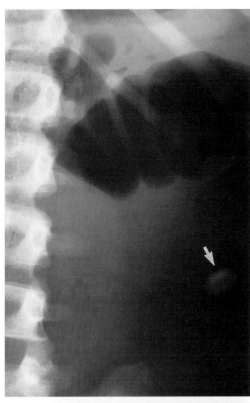

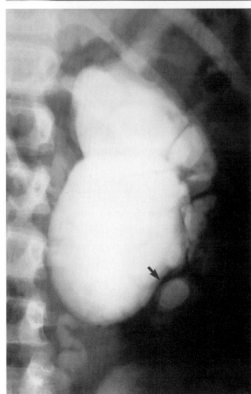

FIG. 9-44. UPJ obstruction with stone formation. A: There is a soft-tissue mass in the left flank. An opaque calculus *(arrow)* is identified. **B:** IVU. There is obstructive hydronephrosis due to intrinsic UPJ obstruction. The renal stone *(arrow)* is in a lower pole calyx.

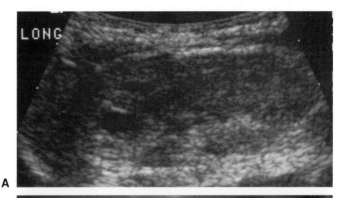

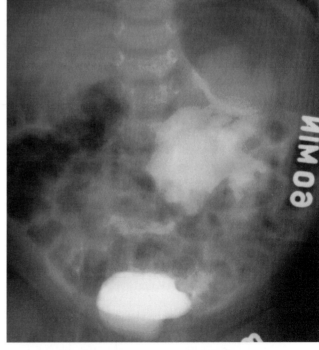

FIG. 9-45. Underestimation of hydronephrosis. A: Longitudinal sonography at 1 day of age in a child with the prenatal diagnosis of hydroephrosis. There is no evidence of hydronephrosis. **B:** IVU at 2 months of age. A delayed film (1 hour after injection) shows severe left UPJ obstruction.

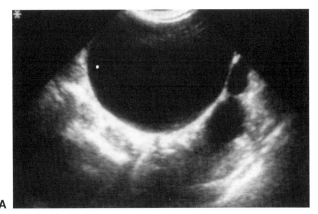

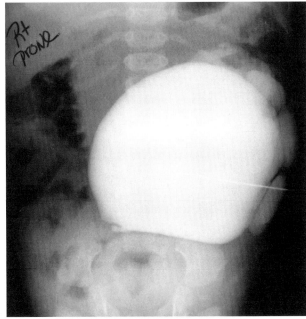

FIG. 9-46. Severe UPJ obstruction mimicking UVJ obstruction. A: Transverse ultrasonography through the bladder. The markedly dilated calyces to the left of the bladder mimic a dilated, tortuous left ureter. **B:** Antegrade pyelogram. Severe hydronephrosis due to UPJ obstruction. The ureter is normal.

coexists with UPJ obstruction, a catheter should be placed in the urinary bladder prior to IVU or renal scintigraphy. An empty bladder prevents confusion between excreted and refluxed contrast material or radiotracer (see Fig. 9-6). The coexistence of UPJ obstruction and reflux affects the order of surgical intervention; pyeloplasty may be followed by resolution of reflux so that ureteral reimplantation becomes unnecessary (84).

Scintigraphy. Renal nuclear scintigraphy (both dynamic and static) may be performed with ^{99m}Tc-MAG 3 or ^{99m}Tc-DTPA. This technique, particularly with diuretic (furosemide) provocation, is very useful to assess renal function and the severity of UPJ obstruction quantitatively (see Fig. 9-9).

Intravenous urography. Intravenous urography, with or

without furosemide, can also be useful in diagnosing UPJ obstruction; it qualitatively assesses renal function, qualitatively determines the degree of obstruction, and further defines the anatomy. IVU demonstrates delayed (or even lack of) excretion, dilution of excreted contrast by urine retained in the renal pelvis, and dilatation of the pelvicalyceal system while failing to visualize a dilated ureter. The papillary ducts (ducts of Bellini) are dilated in chronic obstruction and become visible as circular or beaded collections of contrast medium adjacent to calyces (90). Moreover, contrast retention within groups of collecting tubules that have been reoriented due to calyceal distention produce curvilinear dense bands, termed calyceal crescents, adjacent to the dilated renal pelvis (Fig. 9-48) (91). If the patient is known to have vesicoureteral reflux, the IVU must be performed with a catheter in the urinary bladder as noted above.

UPJ obstruction due to a crossing vessel may be suggested on IVU if there is visualization of the angled proximal ureter just above the obstructing vessel (Fig. 9-49) (92). UPJ obstruction due to a crossing renal vessel may also be suggested by a characteristic appearance at sonography (Fig. 9-50A), retrograde ureterography (Fig. 9-50B), antegrade pyelography, and CT. Obstruction by a crossing vessel is characteristically intermittent, so that imaging may be completely normal when the child has no pain. The sequence of hydronephrosis with pain and no hydronephrosis when pain-free should make one highly suspicious of a crossing renal vessel (92).

An extrarenal pelvis, particularly in an ectopic kidney, can mimic UPJ obstruction. Contrast may accumulate in the dilated, patulous extrarenal pelvis, even without obstruction. In this situation, as well as in other patients with possible UPJ obstruction, a furosemide challenge helps to confirm or exclude obstruction.

Whitaker test. The diagnosis of UPJ obstruction occasionally remains equivocal. A pressure-flow study (Whitaker test) may then be helpful. If a child's kidney can tolerate a flow of 10 cc/minute without the pressure gradient between the renal pelvis and bladder rising to more than 15 cm of water, the diagnosis of significant UPJ obstruction is excluded. The Whitaker test is invasive. Furosemide renography can usually exclude or confirm obstruction and does not require percutaneous renal puncture.

Natural History and Treatment. Some patients with UPJ obstruction demonstrate spontaneous regression of the obstruction, whereas most show no change for many years, having a persistently dilated central collecting system. The third and most troublesome group has progressive obstruction (Fig. 9-51) and sometimes deterioration in renal function.

Most pediatric urologists perform a dismembered pyeloplasty for patients with severe UPJ obstruction and follow those who have only mild or moderate UPJ obstruction with periodic (every 6 months to 1 year) sonography. Long-standing severe obstruction may result in persistent caliectasis and pyelocaliectasis, even after successful pyeloplasty. Neonatal kidneys are more resilient after treatment for UPJ obstruction

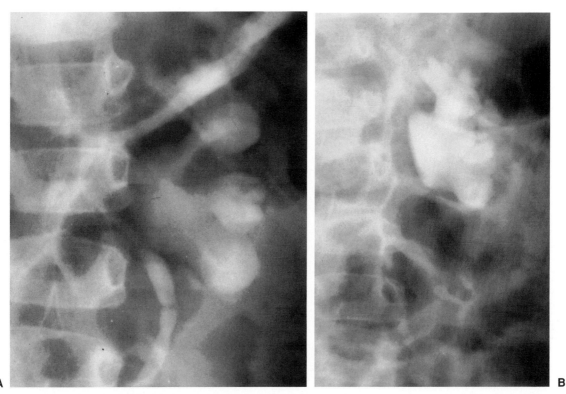

A   B

FIG. 9-47. UPJ obstruction and reflux. A: VCUG. There was some delay in passage of contrast material from the ureter up into the dilated renal pelvis. Note also the subtle dilution of contrast material in the dilated pelvicalyceal system. **B:** A drainage film shows contrast material trapped above the narrowed UPJ.

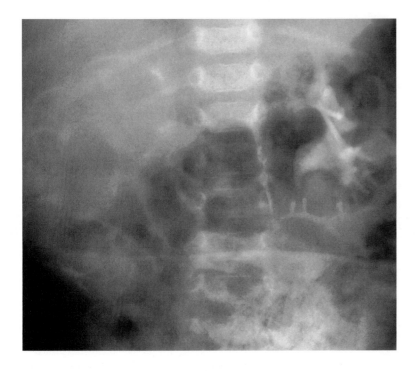

FIG. 9-48. Calyceal crescents in obstructive hydronephrosis. The calyceal crescents in the hydronephrotic right kidney are due to reorientation of distal collecting ducts surrounding dilated calyces. On delayed images, the dilated calyces will fill with contrast material and the crescents will disappear. The left kidney is normal.

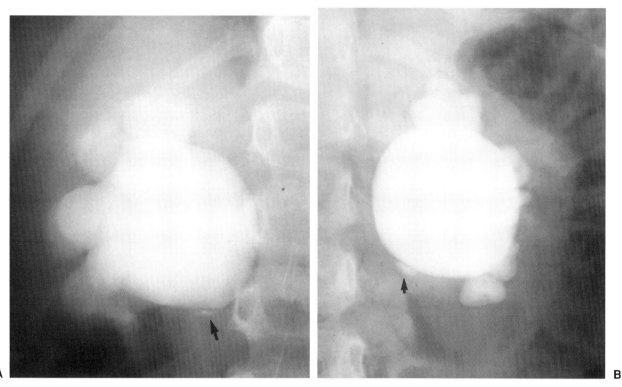

FIG. 9-49. UPJ obstruction due to a crossing renal vessel. A: 12-year-old boy. There is a linear, angled collection of contrast material *(arrow)* in the proximal ureter. **B:** 13-year-old girl. There is obstruction just below the UPJ *(arrow)* due to an extrinsic renal vessel.

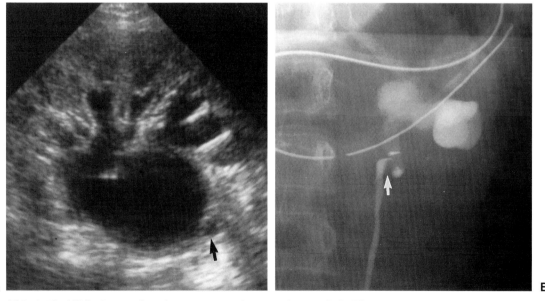

FIG. 9-50. UPJ obstruction due to a crossing renal vessel. A: There is dilatation of the left renal pelvis, calyces, and proximal ureter *(arrow)*. **B:** Retrograde ureteropyelogram. There is characteristic extrinsic compression of the ureter by a crossing renal vessel. Note that the ureter is draped over the vessel *(arrow)*.

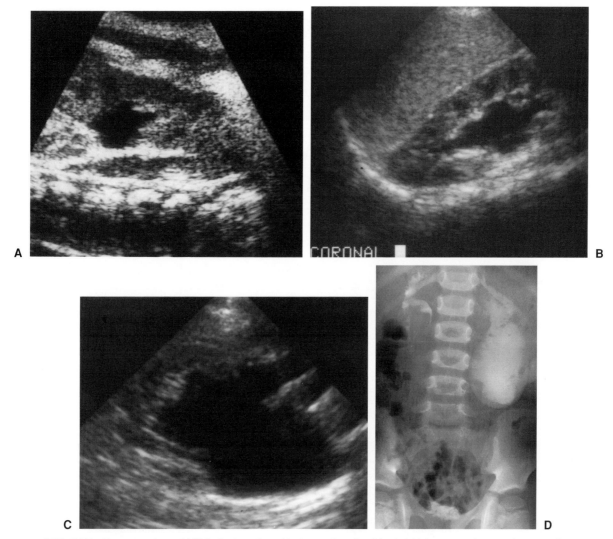

FIG. 9-51. Progression of UPJ obstruction. Hydronephrosis of the left kidney was detected prenatally. **A:** Ultrasonography at 1 week of age shows mild dilatation of the renal pelvis. **B:** At 18 months of age, there had been no significant change. **C:** Routine follow-up at 4 years of age shows marked worsening of the hydronephrosis. **D:** IVU confirms left-sided obstructive hydronephrosis due to UPJ obstruction. The child remained completely asymptomatic.

than those of older children; their renal collecting structures usually return to normal size. The indications and timing of surgery for UPJ obstruction are continually being reassessed (93–97).

Multicystic Dysplastic Kidney

Multicystic dysplastic kidney is frequently categorized and discussed with renal cystic diseases. However, this is both misleading and incorrect. The central embryonic event in the formation of a multicystic dysplastic kidney is severe obstruction, most often due to ureteropelvic atresia during the metanephric stage of renal development; the abnormality is therefore best included in a discussion of ureteral obstruction.

The site of atresia determines the type of multicystic dysplastic kidney. In the more common type of pelvoinfundibular multicystic dysplastic kidney, the proximal ureter, renal pelvis, and infundibula are all atretic (98). In the most severe form, the multiple cysts are actually dilated calyces (Fig. 9-52). Grossly, the kidney consists of grape-like, smooth-walled cysts of variable size that do not communicate (Fig. 9-53B); there is atresia of the entire pelvis and infundibular system. Cores of rudimentary renal tissue and dysplastic glomeruli with tubular atrophy are found between the cysts. Relatively well-differentiated renal tissue is present in 5% to 20% of the kidneys (27). If the proximal ureter alone is very severely stenotic, the cysts represent dilatation of both the pelvis and calyces; this "hydronephrotic" form of multicystic dysplastic kidney is uncommon (approximately 5%) (Fig. 9-52) (99).

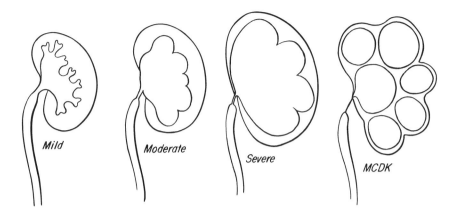

FIG. 9-52. Multicystic dysplastic kidney. Spectrum of UPJ obstruction, from mild to pelvoinfundibular atresia type of multicystic dysplastic kidney.

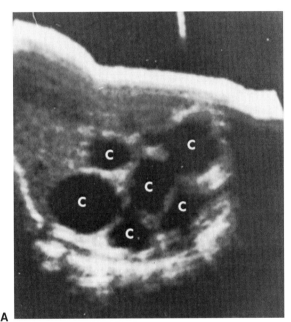

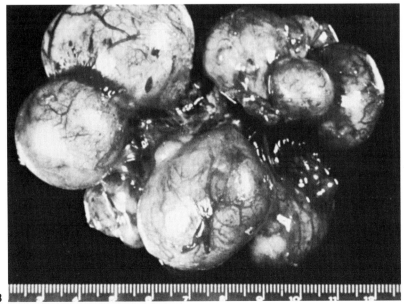

FIG. 9-53. Multicystic dysplastic kidney. A: Supine longitudinal ultrasonography of the right kidney shows many anechoic cysts *(c)* separated by septa. The largest of these cysts is not in the position of the renal pelvis. **B:** There is a grape-like appearance of the resected kidney due to the multiple cysts caused by pelvoinfundibular atresia. From Kirks et al. (27).

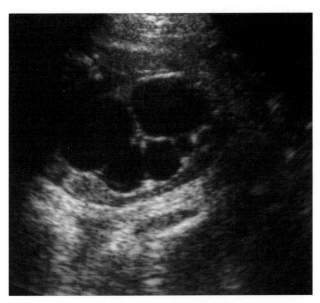

FIG. 9-54. In utero diagnosis of multicystic dysplastic kidney. Prenatal sonography at 36 weeks gestation. In the left kidney, there are many cysts of varying size without evidence of intercommunication. (Courtesy of Judy Estroff, M.D., Boston, MA.)

In the past neonates with multicystic dysplastic kidney were identified because of a large flank mass, and IVU showed nonfunction of the involved kidney. A nephrectomy was performed to confirm the diagnosis. Most cases are now diagnosed by prenatal US (Fig. 9-54); this expedites postnatal evaluation and management.

Imaging. The prenatal or postnatal sonographic visualization of many round anechoic regions of variable size in the kidney, without a definable central renal pelvis and with little or no intervening normal-appearing renal tissue, is diagnostic of multicystic dysplastic kidney (Figs. 9-53A and 9-

54) (100,101). It may be difficult or impossible to distinguish multicystic dysplastic kidney sonographically from true hydronephrosis because they form a continuum; in hydronephrosis the ''cysts'' communicate with a large central cystic structure, the dilated renal pelvis. It is critical to examine both kidneys since at least 10% to 15% of patients with multicystic dysplastic kidney have an abnormality of the contralateral kidney or vesicoureteral reflux (27).

Renal scintigraphy with MAG 3 or DTPA confirms the absence of perfusion and lack of function on static images. There is no tracer accumulation within the renal pelvis on 4-hour images. However, delayed films at 24–48 hours occasionally show a small amount of isotope puddling in the cysts, depending on the amount of functioning renal parenchyma (27). The diagnosis may also be confirmed by renal cortical scintigraphy using DMSA (Fig. 9-55). There is seldom any uptake of radiopharmaceutical on the affected side (14). IVU, although not generally used for this entity, permits assessment of the anatomy and function of the contralateral kidney. If a multicystic dysplastic kidney remains undiagnosed, the cysts may turn up in later life as rounded, calcified, cystic renal masses of small or moderate size (27).

Because multicystic dysplastic kidney is due to early atresia of the pelvis or ureteropelvic junction, it is not surprising that some degree of UPJ obstruction is frequently found in the contralateral kidney. The fetus with bilateral multicystic dysplastic kidney usually dies in the neonatal period because of pulmonary hypoplasia caused by severe oligohydramnios. A reflux study (VCUG or RNC) is often performed in patients with unilateral multicystic dysplastic kidney to determine whether treatment for contralateral reflux is necessary to protect the normal kidney (102). If vesicoureteral reflux is detected, the treatment may be either prophylactic antibiotic therapy or ureteral reimplantation. It should be noted that there is occasionally reflux into the unused ureter below a

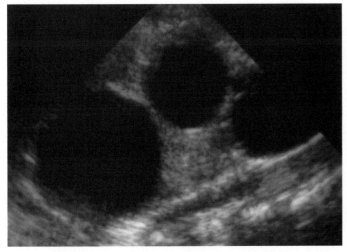

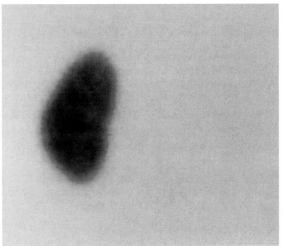

FIG. 9-55. Multicystic dysplastic kidney. A: Longitudinal ultrasonography of the right kidney. There are several cysts of varying sizes without a definable central renal pelvis and little intervening renal tissue. **B:** Posterior DMSA renal scintigraphy. There is complete absence of activity on the right.

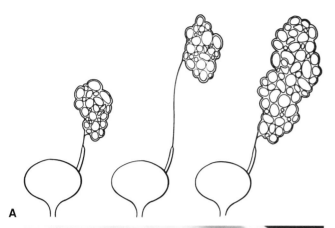

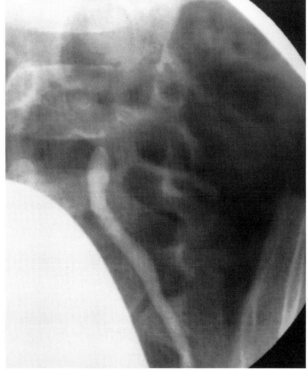

FIG. 9-56. Reflux into the ureter of multicystic dysplastic kidney. A: If reflux does not extend all the way to the flank, the MCDK may have a pelvic location *(left)*, a long atretic segment of ureter *(middle)*, or huge size with a short ureter *(right)*. **B:** Characteristic rounded upper end of the ureter at the point of atresia in a patient with a left pelvic MCDK.

multicystic dysplastic kidney (98) (Fig. 9-56). Focal multicystic dysplastic kidney may occur in the upper or lower moiety of a duplex kidney (Fig. 9-57A), in a portion of a horseshoe kidney (Fig. 9-57B), in a pelvic kidney, or in crossed renal ectopia.

Management. In the past, nephrectomy was the usual treatment. However, imaging can now establish the diagnosis without surgery. Most patients are treated nonoperatively (103–106). If there is bowel obstruction or respiratory compromise (both are rare) due to a large multicystic dysplastic kidney, nephrectomy or cyst aspiration is performed. Because of the fear of possible increased risk of malignancy

and hypertension (107,108), some pediatric urologists still recommend nephrectomy. However, recent data suggest that the incidence of malignancy is not increased in multicystic dysplastic kidneys; it is better to monitor blood pressure and to perform a nephrectomy only if hypertension develops (103).

Most multicystic dysplastic kidneys will slowly decrease in size (Fig. 9-58). Although the kidney does not actually disappear, the small amount of residual, dysplastic renal tissue is no longer discernible by imaging techniques (105). Many cases of apparent unilateral renal agenesis probably represent involution of multicystic dysplastic kidneys (109,110).

Congenital Midureteral Obstruction

Although it is less common than involvement of the upper and lower ends of the ureter, the midureter may also be obstructed by either a congenital valve or a stricture (111,112). Because of its rarity, midureteral obstruction is frequently misdiagnosed as low UPJ obstruction or the long aperistaltic segment of a primary megaureter. The distinction between a ureteral valve and a stricture of the midureter is difficult (Fig. 9-59), even with careful histologic examination (113). However, this distinction is not important for management.

The embryologic events leading to congenital midureteral obstruction are not completely understood. Hypothetical causes of midureteral valves include persistence of normal fetal ureteral folds (114) and persistence of ureteral membranes (115). Theories for the development of congenital midureteral strictures are residua of intrauterine ureteritis (116), compression by blood vessels (117), and failure of normal ureteral recanalization in fetal life (118).

Patients with congenital midureteral obstruction may present with prenatal hydronephrosis, urinary tract infection, or flank pain. The diagnosis of midureteral obstruction is made by sonography, IVU, or retrograde ureterography. Precise localization of the site of obstruction, to guide surgical planning is critical. Treatment is usually excision of the narrowed segment and end-to-end ureteroureterostomy.

Ureterovesical Junction Obstruction

Many conditions cause the ureter to dilate. Not all of them are obstructive and require surgery. Reflux and obstruction can coexist; a VCUG should always be performed to exclude reflux even when definite obstruction is present (72). Obstruction at the distal ureter or ureterovesical junction may be congenital or acquired. Congenital causes are primary megaureter, primary megaureter with reflux, primary megaureter with bladder saccule, simple ureterocele, ectopic ureterocele, and ectopic ureter (72). Acquired causes of distal ureteral obstruction are stricture formation from previous ureteral reimplantation, neurogenic bladder, complications of infection, and calculus formation (72).

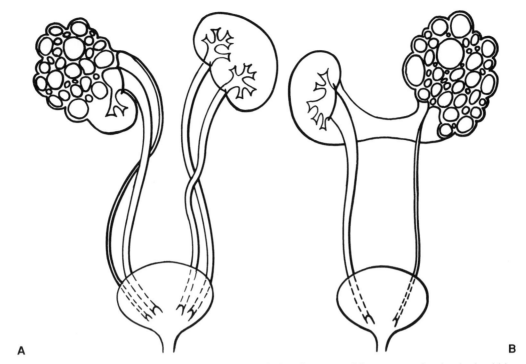

FIG. 9-57. Focal multicystic dysplastic kidney. A: Involvement of the upper pole of a duplex kidney. **B:** Involvement of half of a horseshoe kidney.

Primary Megaureter

In primary megaureter, there is dilatation above a short aperistaltic normal-caliber juxtavesical section of a normally inserted ureter (119). The normal ureter proximal to the aperistaltic segment dilates because of relative obstruction (Fig. 9-60). This phenomenon is somewhat similar to achalasia and Hirschsprung disease, in which the esophagas or bowel dilates above a segment of abnormal peristalsis. The cause of distal ureteral aperistalsis is not known; it may be due to a paucity of ganglion cells in the connective tissue (Waldeyer sheath) that surrounds the distal ureter (120).

The general term *megaureter* describes a dilated, usually tortuous ureter without implying its cause. Primary megaure-

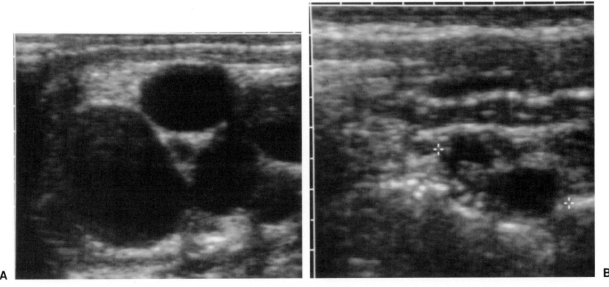

FIG. 9-58. Involution of multicystic dysplastic kidney. A: Sonography at 3 weeks of age. Enlarged kidney with multiple cysts of varying sizes. **B:** Sonography at 2 years of age. The renal length *(between cursors)* has decreased from 4.8 to 2.5 cm. Only two tiny cysts are now seen.

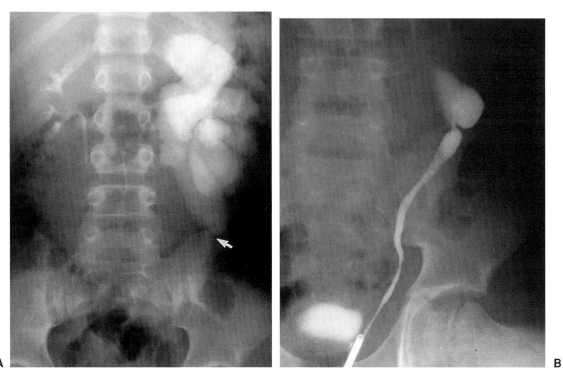

A

B

FIG. 9-59. Congenital midureteral obstruction. A: IVU. There is partial obstruction in the midportion of the left ureter *(arrow)* at the level of the iliac crest. **B:** Retrograde ureterography confirms the ureteral obstruction. It is often impossible to distinguish between a congenital midureteral stricture and an obstructing valve.

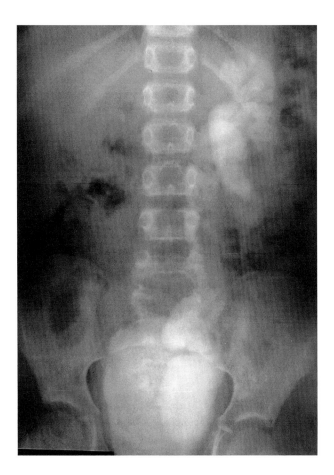

FIG. 9-60. Primary megaureter. A delayed IVU shows left hydroureteronephrosis down to a juxtavesical, aperistaltic ureteral segment.

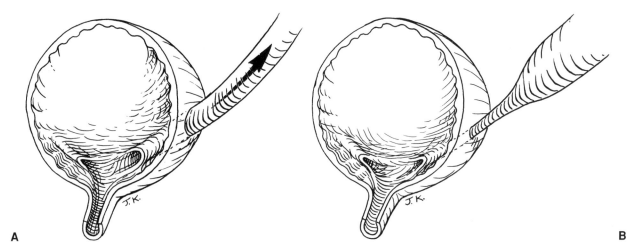

FIG. 9-61. Anatomy of distal ureter. A: Reflux. The ureter is dilated in its entirety. **B:** Primary megaureter. The dilatation begins above the aperistaltic, juxtavesical segment.

ter is usually congenital and is usually discovered early in childhood. It affects boys more than girls, involves the left side more than half of the time, and is bilateral in 20% of cases (119). Before the era of prenatal sonography, patients with primary megaureter usually presented with urinary tract infection. Today, the dilated ureter is frequently detected prenatally, and the diagnosis is made soon after birth.

Imaging. Sonography shows hydronephrosis and ureteral dilatation above the distal segment. Real-time imaging reveals active peristaltic waves passing to and fro in the dilated ureter above the narrowing (32,121). In patients suspected of having a primary megaureter, it is critical to perform a VCUG to distinguish between reflux, obstruction at the ureterovesical junction, and a combination of the two (122). The entire ureter is dilated in vesicoureteral reflux, but the juxtavesical, aperistaltic segment is of normal caliber in primary megaureter (Fig. 9-61). IVU also shows ureteral dilatation above a distal segment (Figs. 9-60 and 9-62). Although dilated, the proximal ureter may not be tortuous. The calyces are frequently not dilated, but this depends on the degree of obstruction. Fluoroscopy shows active peristaltic waves passing through the dilated ureter down to the distal segment.

Sonography and VCUG are usually followed by IVU or nuclear scintigraphy to assess the degree of UVJ obstruction and amount of renal function. Diuretic renography may be extremely helpful in confirming the presence and severity of obstruction caused by primary megaureter.

Natural History and Treatment. The severity of obstruction due to primary megaureter is usually stable. In fact, there is evidence that the ureteral and pelvicalyceal dilatation in mild cases actually decreases with age (119).

Sequential sonography (6- to 12-month intervals) is performed in unoperated patients to detect any increase in hydroureteronephrosis. Ureteral reimplantation is seldom performed in patients with mild or moderate primary megaureter (123). Severe primary megaureter usually requires both ureteral reimplantation and plication or tapering.

Many believe that reimplantation of severe primary megaureter should not be performed unless there is well-documented deterioration of renal function. The coexistence of reflux with primary megaureter increases the complexity of management decisions.

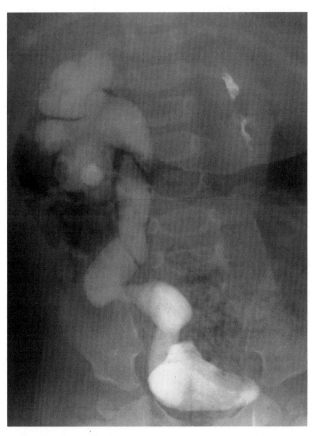

FIG. 9-62. Primary megaureter. IVU shows severe right hydroureteronephrosis but preservation of the concentrating ability of the kidney. The left kidney is normal.

Retrocaval Ureter

The midureter may be obstructed if it courses behind the inferior vena cava (IVC). Although termed *retrocaval ureter,* a more precise term is *preureteral vena cava* because the anomalous course is due to abnormal caval rather than ureteral development.

The IVC develops from complicated anastomoses and regressions of the posterior cardinal, subcardinal, and supracardinal paired venous systems. In the usual form of retrocaval ureter, an infrarenal vascular segment that normally involutes persists; the ventral position of the anomalous IVC causes the ureter to pass behind it before descending to the bladder.

Sonography shows hydroureteronephrosis (Fig. 9-63A) and an abnormal course of the dilated midureter (124). IVU shows abrupt narrowing of the ureter as it passes medially and superiorly before descending behind the IVC (Fig. 9-63B). A retrocaval ureter may also be diagnosed by renal scintigraphy (125).

Retrocaval ureter may be an incidental finding. Surgical correction is indicated only if there is significant obstruction, when the ureter is transected and reanastomosed in front of the IVC.

Urethral Obstruction

Posterior Urethral Valves

Despite an incidence of only 1 in 10,000 live births (126), posterior urethral valves (PUV) are still the most common cause of urethral obstruction in the male infant, child, and adolescent. Because the entire outflow of urine is impeded, PUVs are often devastating. At least one third of affected patients have impaired renal function (127).

Distal remnants of the Wolffian or mesonephric ducts normally form mucosal ridges or folds that migrate laterally and posteriorly to attach to the posterior urethral wall. These normal folds become the plicae colliculae and extend distally from the verumontanum to attach to the posterior urethral wall. Normal plicae and their prominent distal insertions are often seen (see Fig. 9-27). If the margins of the normal mucosal folds fuse (usually anteriorly), circumferentially obstructing PUVs are formed (128).

Young initially classified PUV into three types: type I valves are a pair of folds of tissue emanating from the distal end of the verumontanum; type II are valves occurring above the verumontanum; type III valves are a diaphragm with a central aperture (129). It is now clear that there is really only one type, formerly called type I (130). The valves are fused from above downward so that the residual lumen of the urethra is near its floor; the lateral view on VCUG shows the narrowed urinary stream to be posteroinferior rather than central (Fig. 9-64).

The bladder, as it attempts to empty, responds to urethral

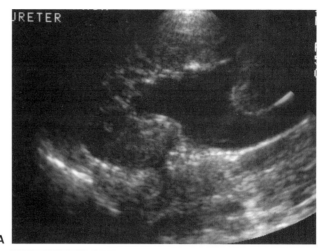

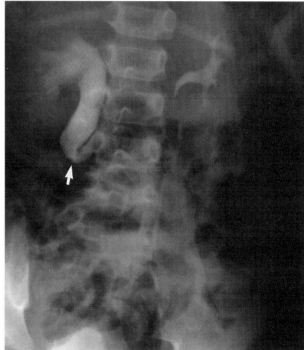

FIG. 9-63. Retrocaval ureter. A: Longitudinal renal sonography. The upper right ureter and pelvicalyceal system are dilated. **B:** IVU shows the typical "fish hook" appearance *(arrow)* of the right ureter. The ureter passes medially and superiorly and then descends behind the inferior vena cava. (Courtesy of Roy G.K. McCauley, M.D., Boston, MA.)

obstruction by hypertrophy, seen on VCUG as trabeculation. The bladder base remains smooth. Until muscle failure occurs, the bladder empties satisfactorily, but the intraluminal pressure rises and ureteral emptying is impeded both by the elevated bladder pressure and by distal ureteral obstruction due to thickening of the bladder wall. Urinary retention occurs only when the bladder finally decompensates, after a long period of high-pressure voiding. An analogy is the development of congestive heart failure in patients long after the onset of aortic valvular stenosis.

Prenatal US is currently the usual method of detecting

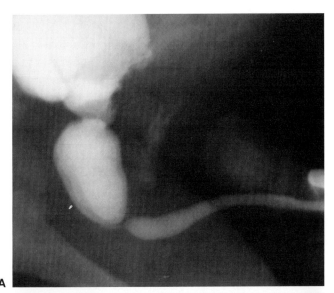

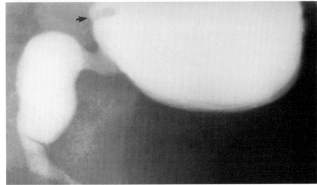

FIG. 9-64. Posterior urethral valves. A: The dilated posterior urethra produces a classic spinnaker-sail appearance. The ureteral narrowing is just distal to the verumontanum. **B:** The posterior urethra is markedly dilated and tortuous. There is hypertrophy of the interureteric ridge *(arrow)*.

PUV. Abnormalities are most evident when the valves are severely obstructing and may include oligohydramnios, bladder distention, bilateral hydroureteronephrosis, and occasionally fetal ascites (131,132). The volume of amniotic fluid is the most useful indicator of fetal renal function since much of it is fetal urine (133). In addition to PUV, other causes of bilateral fetal hydroureteronephrosis in the male fetus are bilateral ureterovesical junction obstruction, bilateral reflux, a combination of reflux and obstruction, and, rarely, prune-belly syndrome. In bilateral fetal hydroureteronephrosis, these four conditions together outnumber PUV.

Endoscopic visualization of PUV may be difficult for the inexperienced (134), and the radiologist may be the first to suggest the diagnosis. One should consider PUV in a male infant, child, or adolescent with voiding difficulties, dilatation of the upper urinary tracts, and urinary tract infection. Although postnatal sonography may be normal, there is usually bilateral hydroureteronephrosis and a thick-walled or dilated bladder. Careful examination of the posterior urethra by sonography, particularly through a perineal window, may

demonstrate dilatation of the posterior urethra (135). However, VCUG is the best diagnostic method (Fig. 9-64). Vesicoureteral reflux occurs in only 50% of patients with valves; this is unilateral in about 35% and bilateral in 15%. As in patients without PUV, reflux is unusual in black boys with valves (136).

PUVs have various effects on the kidney and bladder (Fig. 9-65). Kidneys exposed to reflux at high pressure because of urethral obstruction do not develop normally; the kidney affected by reflux functions less well than the kidney that is affected only by obstruction (Fig. 9-65A). At sonography, the more echogenic the kidney and the less well defined its corticomedullary junction, the more likely it is to be dysplastic because of the long-standing obstruction. Such dysplastic kidneys are small and echogenic with poor corticomedullary differentiation; there may be associated macrocysts (Fig. 9-66). Calyceal rupture at the fornix and decompression may allow the kidney to develop in a more normal fashion (Fig. 9-65A). Imaging may show urinary ascites or a perirenal urinoma (137).

Although reflux without extravasation damages the kidney, it protects the developing bladder (Fig. 9-65B). Conversely, if there is no reflux, the kidney develops more normally, but there is marked hypertrophy of the bladder wall and sometimes subsequent abnormal function (Fig. 9-65B).

Oligohydramnios or decreasing amounts of amniotic fluid on serial prenatal sonographic examinations is the only indication for fetal or maternal intervention when hydronephrosis is discovered; this is extremely rare, even when posterior urethral valves are diagnosed in utero. If bilateral hydroureteronephrosis is discovered in a male fetus but amniotic fluid volume remains normal, the patient should be delivered at term and the urethra evaluated by VCUG within 24 hours. Although the diagnosis of PUV must be made expeditiously, it is not a middle-of-the-night emergency because the patient has had urethral obstruction for many months. The diagnosis of PUV is urgent, not emergent.

Catheterization of the infant with PUV is sometimes difficult; the tip of the catheter can enter the posterior-superior recess of the dilated posterior urethra rather than the bladder. A coudé catheter with the curved end directed anteriorly will almost always enter the bladder. The catheter tip can also be directed into the bladder by a finger in the boy's rectum.

The bladder is frequently thickened and trabeculated by cellules or saccules (intraluminal collections of contrast material between hypertrophied muscle bundles) and diverticula (extraluminal herniation of mucosa through weaknesses in the bladder wall). Bladder capacity is often significantly decreased by the bladder wall thickening. The interureteric ridge may be hypertrophied and, in lateral projection, appears as a filling defect on the posteroinferior aspect of the bladder wall (Fig. 9-64B). Cellules and saccules only occur above the interureteric ridge, while diverticula most often occur at the ureteral hiatus. When the boy voids and the catheter is removed, in addition to the valves and the dilatation of the supravalvular posterior urethra, there may be re-

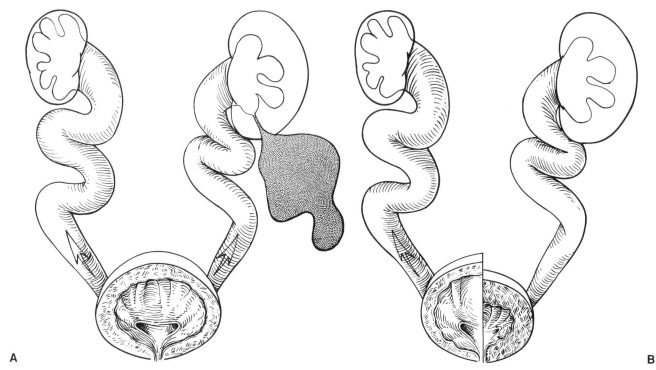

A   **B**

FIG. 9-65. Effects of posterior urethral valves. Diagrammatic representation of the relationships between extravasation, renal function, reflux, and subsequent bladder function. **A:** Reflux without extravasation *(right kidney)* damages the developing kidney. Extravasation *(left kidney)* vents the pressure and tends to protect the developing kidney. **B:** Reflux without extravasation *(right kidney)* damages the kidney but protects the developing bladder. If there is no vesicoureteral reflux *(left kidney)*, the kidney develops more normally but there is hypertrophy of the wall of the bladder, which then functions abnormally.

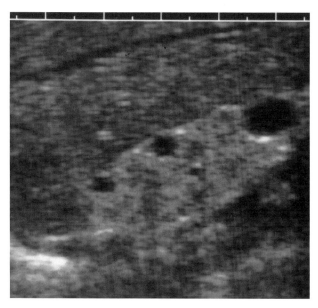

FIG. 9-66. Renal dysplasia due to posterior urethral valves. Sonography of a 2-week-old boy with posterior urethral valves and vesicoureteral reflux. The right kidney is small and markedly echogenic. There are three cortical macrocysts.

flux into prostatic ducts, ejaculatory ducts, or the prostatic utricle. Vesicoureteral reflux sometimes vents the bladder and therefore reduces urethral dilatation. The bladder neck will appear elongated as it passes through the thickened bladder wall. If there is vesicoureteral reflux, the baby should be recatheterized immediately after voiding so that drainage from the upper tracts can be assessed. This information helps predict the adequacy of drainage after fulguration of valves or vesicostomy. During voiding, the posterior urethra is dilated and the obstructing valves produce a bulging spinnaker-sail appearance (Fig. 9-64). This is best demonstrated by a steep oblique or lateral view of the urethra (138,139). The urethral catheter should be removed during voiding, not only so that the area of narrowing can be seen and a missed diagnosis avoided, but also as a basis for comparison with postoperative studies (64,140).

Even if there is no reflux, catheter drainage of the bladder is performed until the obstruction is relieved by surgical ablation of the valves. Like many congenital anomalies, valves occur with a spectrum of severity from mild to severe. Milder forms of valvular obstruction without other renal abnormalities may not be manifest until late childhood, adolescence, or even young adult life. Very mild valve formation may be extremely difficult to differentiate from normal mucosal folds.

Boys with severely obstructing valves need very close clinical follow-up; this should include urodynamic studies to assess bladder function. Some children may develop abnormalities of bladder function included in the term "valve bladder": muscle failure, detrusor hyperreflexia, and bladder hypertonia (141). This problem should be identified early so that treatment by anticholinergic medication, intermittent catheterization, and sometimes bladder augmentation can preserve renal function. Reflux in patients with PUV tends to protect the bladder (the pop-off phenomenon) and make the development of a valve bladder less likely (Fig. 9-65) (142).

Anterior Urethral Diverticulum

Anterior urethral diverticulum, although uncommon, is the second most common cause of congenital urethral obstruction in boys (143). These diverticula are termed *saccular* or *diffuse*. The saccular type is a localized protrusion from the lumen into the ventral wall of the anterior urethra (143). The diffuse type is a generalized dilatation of the entire anterior urethra; this has also been called megalourethra or urethral ectasia. The diffuse type is much less common than the saccular type and is frequently associated with prune-belly syndrome.

Congenital saccular diverticulum may produce anterior urethral obstruction by the valve-like mechanism of the distal lip of the diverticulum. As urine fills the diverticulum during voiding, the thin distal lip is elevated (Fig. 9-67). Because the distal lip forms an acute angle with the ventral urethra, further filling of the diverticulum presses this lip against the dorsal wall of the urethra (143). This action obstructs the distal end of the urethra and limits the flow of urine.

As the anterior lip of the diverticulum obstructs the urinary stream, the penis swells (Fig. 9-67). Intermittent obstruction of the urinary stream and simultaneous swelling of the penis strongly suggest an anterior urethral diverticulum. The urethrographic appearance of a saccular diverticulum is characteristic (Figs. 9-68 and 9-69). Contrast material fills an oval ventral outpouching of the anterior urethra (Fig. 9-67). The diverticulum usually involves the midportion of the penile urethra but occasionally involves the bulbous urethra. Preoperative renal sonography and IVU or renal scintigraphy must be used to assess the anatomy and function of the upper urinary tract. There may be extravasation of contrast material from a ruptured fornix into the perirenal space (Fig. 9-68A).

The cause of congenital anterior urethral diverticulum is unknown. Hypotheses include distal urethral obstruction in the fetus, dilatation of periurethral glands, an incomplete urethral groove, and faulty development of the corpus spongiosum of the penis (143).

The primary differential diagnostic considerations are anterior urethral valve and dilatation of a Cowper gland duct. An *anterior urethral valve* is rare. Most reported cases of anterior urethral valves are in fact congenital saccular di-

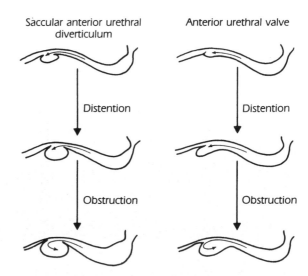

FIG. 9-67. Postulated pathophysiology of congenital saccular anterior urethral diverticulum and anterior urethral valve. From Kirks and Grossman (143).

verticula with a prominent distal lip. There may be dilatation of the anterior urethra proximal to a valve, which mimics a diverticulum (Fig. 9-67). However, the proximal urethral dilatation of an anterior urethral valve forms an obtuse angle with the ventral floor of the urethra (Fig. 9-67); the proximal lip of an anterior urethral diverticulum, however, forms an acute angle with the ventral floor of the urethra (Fig. 9-68B). A true anterior urethral valve may be treated by transurethral resection, whereas an anterior urethral diverticulum usually requires diverticulectomy and urethroplasty. *Dilated Cowper gland ducts* may fill during VCUG. A tubular channel arises from the ventral surface of the bulbous urethra, parallels the undersurface of the bulbomembranous urethra, and terminates in the urogenital diaphragm (see Figs. 9-107 and 9-108).

Vesicoureteral Reflux

Vesicoureteral reflux (VUR) remains a controversial topic. Considerable information has been gained regarding the prevalence, pathogenesis, radiologic diagnosis, and importance of VUR. Guidelines for medical and surgical management are constantly being reassessed (144).

Prevalence

VUR is usually found during radiologic evaluation of urinary tract infection (UTI) or prenatally diagnosed hydrone-

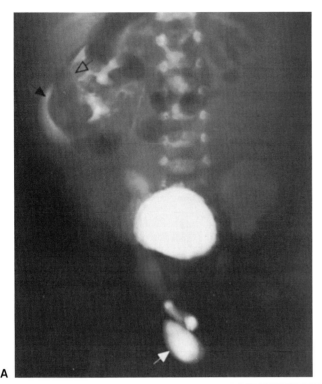

A

FIG. 9-68. **Congenital saccular anterior urethral diverticulum.** Newborn boy with abdominal distention, poor urinary stream, and a soft mass at the penoscrotal junction. **A:** Postvoiding cystourethrogram. The bowel gas is centrally located because of urine ascites. Residual contrast material is noted in an anterior urethral diverticulum *(white arrow)*. The bladder is mildly trabeculated and there is vesicoureteral reflux on the right. Contrast material has extravasated from a ruptured fornix *(open arrow)* into the perirenal space *(black arrow)*. **B:** VCUG. The lucent distal tip *(solid arrow)* and proximal lip *(open arrow)* of the anterior urethral diverticulum are shown well. There is dilatation of the proximal anterior urethra and entire posterior urethra. From Kirks and Grossman (143).

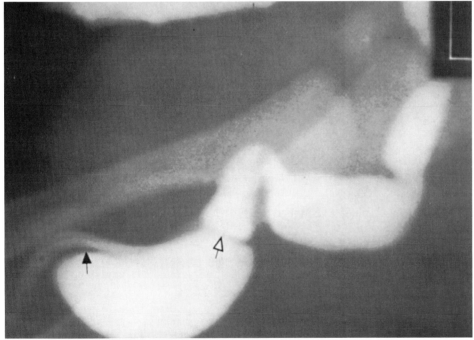

B

phrosis. The prevalence of VUR in asymptomatic children is <0.5% (144). Its presence is pathologic, although it often disappears spontaneously. VUR is present in anywhere from 29% to 50% of children with UTI (144,145). This common association with UTI decreases with age and is lower in black children (144,146). There is a high prevalence (8% to 40%) in siblings of children with VUR. Moreover, children of parents with a history of VUR have an incidence of reflux as high as 66% (145–149). These familial associations sup-

port the concept that VUR is a primary abnormality, not a secondary one.

Pathogenesis

In VUR, urine flows in a retrograde fashion from the urinary bladder into the ureter (Fig. 9-70). VUR is usually greatest during voiding and it may be demonstrated only then.

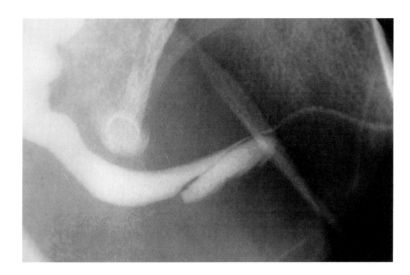

FIG. 9-69. Anterior urethral diverticulum. During voiding, the diverticulum fills with contrast material. The anterior lip of the diverticulum is elevated and obstructs the urethral lumen.

The understanding of VUR has changed dramatically over the past several years. VUR was originally considered secondary to distal obstruction. It was assumed that if there was reflux during voiding, it must be due to obstruction of normal bladder outflow, at or below the bladder neck. Later, it was argued that urinary tract infection, not obstruction, was the cause of VUR. Today, most agree that reflux is in almost all instances a primary phenomenon due to incompetence of the ureterovesical junction and is not secondary to either obstruction or infection (61,150). Radiologic studies in patients with reflux rarely show obstruction. Even when PUV cause obstruction, VUR may be unilateral or not present at all. Indirect evidence that infection does not cause reflux is based, among other things, on the disappearance of VUR despite recurrence of UTI in some children (145,150). The increased incidence of reflux in siblings and an incidence that is 20 times as high in nonblack as in black children support the concept that reflux is primary (150). Moreover, Gross and Lebowitz have shown that the vast majority (88%) of children with reflux have sterile urine and that there is no significant difference in the incidence of sterile (88% to 90%) and infected (10% to 12%) urine in nonrefluxing children compared with those with reflux (150). Therefore, reflux is thought to be a primary immaturity or maldevelopment, of the ureterovesical junction with resultant incompetence of its anti-reflux, flap-valve action. Rarely, VUR is secondary to voiding dysfunction. Moreover, it is possible that a few children with borderline anatomy have transient, mild reflux due to UTI with inflammation of the bladder wall and the intravesical ureteral segment (150).

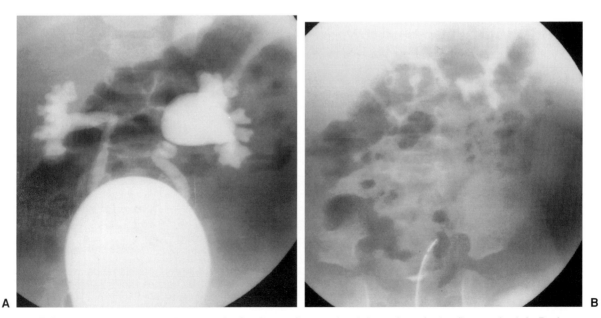

A   B

FIG. 9-70. Vesicoureteral reflux. A: Grade 3 reflux on the right and grade 4 reflux on the left. **B:** A drainage film shows no obstruction.

The normal valve mechanism of the ureterovesical junction is due to the oblique entry of the ureter into the bladder and an adequate length of the intramural ureter, especially of its submucosal segment (144). This valve mechanism is primarily passive, although there is an active component from the ureterotrigonal longitudinal muscles and from ureteral peristalsis. VUR is thought to result from a deficiency or immaturity of the longitudinal muscle of the submucosal ureter. The severity of this disturbance can be assessed cystoscopically by the degree of lateral displacement of the ureteral orifice, its shape and degree of patulousness, and the length of the submucosal tunnel (144). VUR is particularly common in the neonate and infant. With growth, the submucosal ureter elongates and the ratio between the submucosal tunnel and ureteral diameter increases, making incompetence of the valve mechanism less likely (144).

Association with Renal Scarring

Hodson noted the association of VUR with renal parenchymal scarring (51). There is radiologic evidence of renal scarring in 30% to 60% of children with VUR, and VUR is present in almost all children with severe renal scarring (151). Bisset et al. have demonstrated the direct correlation between the prevalence of scarring and the grade of VUR. In their study, 8% of girls with UTI and grade I VUR had scarring whereas 100% of girls with UTI and grade IV VUR had scars (145). Although it has been suggested that sterile

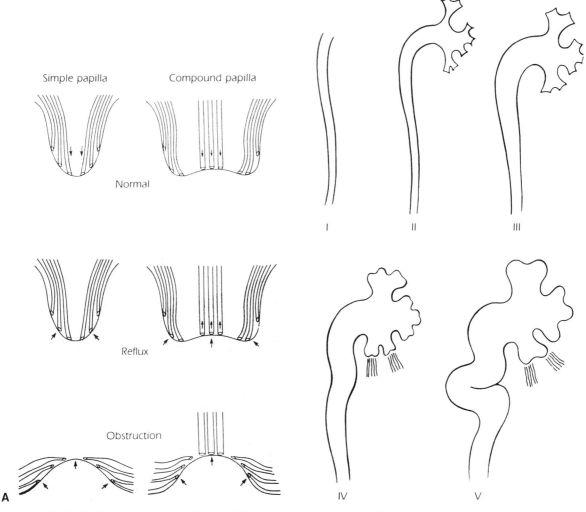

FIG. 9-71. Vesicoureteral reflux. A: Simple and compound papillae. Intrarenal reflux tends to occur in the central parts of a compound papilla. Obstruction with hydronephrosis causes reorientation of the tubules of both simple and compound papillae to produce calyceal crescents. Modified from Ransley and Risdon (153,156,157). **B:** Grading of vesicoureteral reflux. Grading is based on the level of reflux, dilatation, forniceal blunting, and papillary impressions. Intrarenal reflux rarely occurs with grade II reflux and is infrequent with grade III reflux. Modified from Levitt et al. (144).

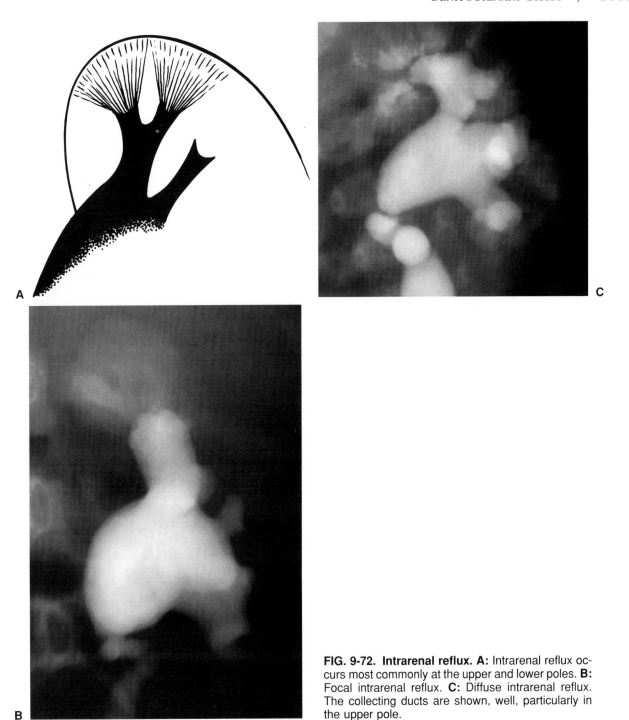

FIG. 9-72. Intrarenal reflux. A: Intrarenal reflux occurs most commonly at the upper and lower poles. **B:** Focal intrarenal reflux. **C:** Diffuse intrarenal reflux. The collecting ducts are shown, well, particularly in the upper pole.

VUR causes renal scarring, most experimental studies (152,153) and longitudinal studies (145) indicate that the appearance of renal scarring or the extension of established renal scars requires infection. A history of UTI can usually be elicited in children with VUR and renal scarring. The higher the grade of reflux (Fig. 9-71B), the more likely the development of new or progressive scarring after urinary tract infection (144,145).

Experimental work on the pathogenesis of renal scarring has emphasized the importance of intrarenal reflux (144,153–157). Intrarenal reflux is the extension of VUR into the collecting tubules of the nephrons (Figs. 9-71A and 9-72) and allows urinary microorganisms access to the renal parenchyma with subsequent infection and scarring. That sterile intrarenal reflux produces similar scars by chemical or hydrodynamic effects is less likely (51).

A simple papilla is defined as a conical papilla in a calyx not containing other papillae (153,156,157). These convex papillae are nonrefluxing, as the crescentic or slit-like openings of their collecting ducts open obliquely into the calyx

(Fig. 9-71A). A compound papilla is defined as a papilla formed from fusion of pyramids at their tips (153,156,157). These concave or flat papillae are refluxing papillae, as the collecting ducts open at right angles from the flat portion of the papilla into the calyx (Fig. 9-71A). The vast majority of compound papillae occur at the polar regions, whereas simple papillae are usually in the midzones of the kidneys (155). This polar concentration of compound papillae, with their propensity for intrarenal reflux, may explain the frequency of reflux scarring there (51).

Intrarenal reflux occurs at much lower pressures in compound papillae than in simple papillae. It is hypothesized that the obliquely oriented, slit-like duct orifices of cone-shaped simple papillae are easily closed by a rise in the intrapelvic pressure. This closure mechanism produces a check-valve effect and prevents intrarenal reflux (153,156,157). Conversely, the large, open papillary duct orifices situated on the concave surface of a compound papilla cannot be closed by a pressure rise and thus allow intrarenal reflux (155). Moreover, increasingly high pressures are required to produce intrarenal reflux over the first 12 months of life (155), which suggests that increasingly effective defenses against intrarenal reflux are developing then. The kidney is particularly susceptible to scarring from intrarenal reflux during the first year of life (155). The "big bang" theory postulates that this vulnerable period is the critical time during which UTI with VUR causes renal scarring (157). This theory states that, if there is no infection during this time, later UTI is unlikely to cause significant scarring.

Recent observations of renal scarring associated with in utero VUR refute the "big bang" theory (158). Moreover, renal scarring in the neonate after in utero VUR suggests that sterile reflux may cause renal damage in the fetus.

Importance

The relevance of VUR is both complicated and controversial. As previously discussed, VUR may lead to intrarenal reflux and subsequent renal scarring. VUR of infected urine may lead to acute pyelonephritis. VUR, with or without infection, may also interfere with the normal growth of the kidney and produce hypertension (144). Severe renal scarring may cause hypertension (Fig. 9-73) and even later renal failure. There is evidence that segmental renal hypoplasia (the Ask-Upmark kidney), a lesion commonly associated with severe hypertension, is caused by infected reflux (144,159). High-grade reflux of sterile urine may also interfere with renal growth (160). However, acute pyelonephritis occurs in children even without VUR (161). All patients with VUR should have careful follow-up for assessment of renal growth and for detection of renal scarring or hypertension. UTI in children will be discussed in detail later in this chapter.

Megacystis-Megaureter Association

The megacystis-megaureter association is the extreme in the spectrum of primary VUR; reflux is so massive that most of the bladder urine refluxes into one or both upper tracts and only a small amount is expelled via the urethra (Fig. 9-74). The refluxed urine then drains back into the urinary bladder. This constant recirculation of urine between ureter and bladder (aberrant micturition) results in a very distended urinary bladder and extreme dilatation of one or both upper collecting systems (Fig. 9-75).

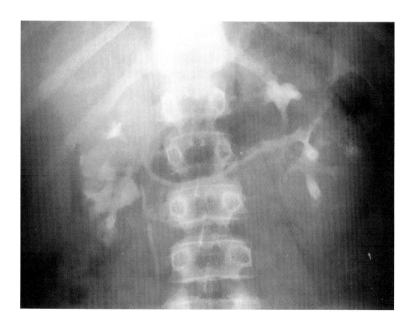

FIG. 9-73. Lower pole scarring in a duplex kidney. A 10-year-old boy with hypertension. IVU shows a small right duplex kidney with extensive loss of cortical parenchyma, particularly of the lower pole.

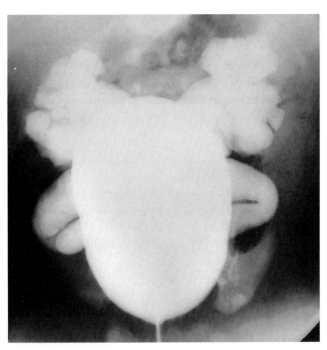

FIG. 9-74. Megacystis-megaureter association. The bladder is large and smooth-walled. There is severe bilateral vesicoureteral reflux.

Imaging Evaluation

VUR is defined as the retrograde passage of urine from the bladder into the upper urinary tract. Occasionally, the presence of VUR is suggested by IVU (by the presence of pelvic striations [162] or ureteral dilatation) or US. However, both IVU and renal sonography may be completely normal in patients with gross VUR. For this reason, cystography

should be performed to document the presence and grade of VUR in many situations. Either a radiographic VCUG or RNC can be used to diagnose VUR (163). Nuclear cystography is usually used for follow-up of patients with known VUR.

The prenatal detection of hydronephrosis, hydroureteronephrosis, or dilatation of part of a double collecting system is an indication for evaluation for reflux after delivery (131,164,165). Prenatal sonography should assess the degree of hydronephrosis, the gestational age at which it is identified, and any changes in urinary tract dilatation during the pregnancy. After delivery, these neonates should be placed on a prophylactic antibiotic and evaluated by VCUG.

Some patients with UTI, especially those with presumed pyelonephritis, are also evaluated for VUR. It is critical to diagnose UTI accurately and localize the probable site (upper or lower tract) of infection. Because a positive culture may be due to contamination by perineal or preputial bacteria, a bagged specimen is not acceptable for culture. Documentation of UTI in babies requires a specimen obtained by catheterization or suprapubic aspiration. Clean-catch specimens in older children are accurate if the interlabial area is cleaned in girls and the foreskin is retracted in uncircumcised boys. It is also important to localize the infection if possible to the lower urinary tract (cystitis, urethritis) or the upper urinary tract (pyelonephritis), to maximize the yield of imaging. This distinction grows easier with age. An older child with signs and symptoms of cystitis (frequency, urgency, dysuria, no fever or systemic illness) will usually not have reflux and will not benefit from VCUG. Conversely, children with pyelonephritis are more likely to have reflux and should be evaluated by VCUG. A third group of patients who should be evaluated are those with a sibling or a parent with VUR.

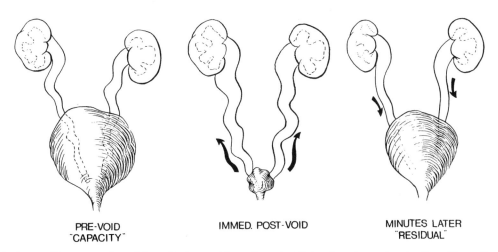

PRE-VOID "CAPACITY"   IMMED. POST-VOID   MINUTES LATER "RESIDUAL"

FIG. 9-75. Aberrant micturition. During voiding, there is bilateral vesicoureteral reflux. The refluxed urine drains back into the bladder *(right)*, giving the false impression that the bladder did not empty completely.

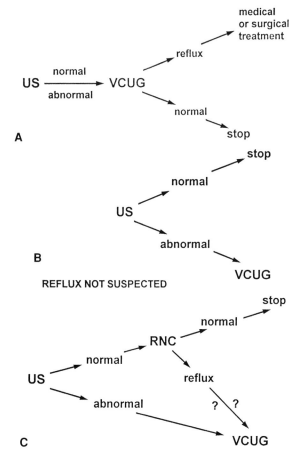

FIG. 9-76. Algorithms for imaging children with urinary tract infection. A: High-risk patient. VCUG is performed regardless of the sonographic findings. **B:** Reflux not suspected. If sonography is normal, VCUG is not performed. **C:** Reflux not suspected but confirmation required. Even if sonography is normal, radionuclide cystography (RNC) is performed for verification.

It is important to provide information to referring urologists, family practitioners, and pediatricians regarding the imaging evaluation of UTI and VUR. This information may be presented as an algorithm (Fig. 9-76), a guideline for preprocedural antibiotic therapy (Fig. 9-77), or a letter including algorithms. A sample letter to referring physicians is as follows:

Dear Doctor:

Our updated recommendations for studying the urinary tract of infants and children who have had urinary tract infection (UTI) and may have vesicoureteral reflux (VUR) are as follows: In any child suspected of having VUR, i.e., anyone thought to have had pyelonephritis because of a positive urine culture plus fever or systemic illness, or with an abnormal ultrasonogram or a strong family history of reflux, a VCUG is recommended. The younger the child, the more important it is to perform VCUG. These infants and children should usually be on antibiotic therapy until they have had their VCUG. Remember that VUR is rare in black children.

In children with only bladder or urethral signs and symptoms as well as a normal ultrasonogram, reflux is unlikely.

Therefore, neither VCUG nor radionuclide cystography (RNC) is recommended.

In anyone *not* suspected of having VUR (i.e., UTI, but without fever or systemic illness and a normal ultrasonogram) in whom you need to be certain, RNC is recommended because of its lower radiation exposure.

RNC is also recommended for (a) screening of patients with family history (sibling, parent) of VUR and (b) follow-up of previously diagnosed VUR.

If you have any questions about these recommendations, please give us a call.

These algorithms and recommendations are only guidelines. Individual patients may require other imaging approaches. Babies and young children with presumed pyelonephritis are placed on prophylactic antibiotic therapy after treatment of the acute infection, at least until their imaging studies have been performed.

Ultrasonography. US is used to assess the renal parenchyma, the collecting system, and any associated abnormalities such as ectopic ureterocele. However, normal sonography does not exclude VUR. Changing degrees of hydronephrosis during real-time scanning is highly suggestive of VUR. Although nonspecific, urothelial thickening may also be seen in patients with reflux (166,167).

Gray scale sonography is much less sensitive to acute pyelonephritis and renal scarring than cortical scintigraphy (41,168–171). In children over 3–4 years of age who have signs only of lower UTI, VCUG is not recommended if renal ultrasonography is normal. However, if sonography is abnormal, VCUG or RNC should be performed.

Voiding Cystourethrography. Babies and young children with a well-documented UTI should have cystography looking for VUR. Precise anatomic delineation requires VCUG. RNC does not suffice, although some advocate the use of RNC in girls because abnormalities on VCUG other than reflux are uncommon and because the radiation dose from RNC is significantly less (145,172). The International Reflux Study classifies VUR into five grades (Fig. 9-71B) (173). VCUG should document the presence or absence of VUR and its grade according to this classification. The site of insertion of the ureter into the bladder must be determined

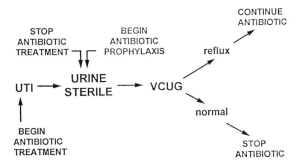

FIG. 9-77. Preprocedural prophylactic antibiotic therapy. Antibiotics are recommended for the interval between the cessation of treatment of an infection and the performance of VCUG. This will protect the child from another infection.

and the presence or absence of dilution of refluxed contrast material noted. One must carefully search for intrarenal reflux. Any delay in drainage of refluxed contrast material must be documented. Both of these features are critical in characterizing VUR and for guiding therapy. The ureter normally inserts into the bladder approximately one quarter of the distance from the base to the dome of the full bladder; an insertion lower than this is abnormal. Occasionally, the ureter inserts into a bladder diverticulum. It is unlikely that reflux will resolve without surgery if there is an ectopic ureteral insertion or if the ureter inserts into a diverticulum.

Reflux can coexist with obstruction (84). Clues on VCUG to the combination of these two abnormalities are as follows: (a) hold-up of reflux of the column of contrast medium at the site of obstruction; (b) dilution of contrast medium by urine above the site of obstruction; (c) poor drainage of refluxed contrast medium after bladder emptying.

Intrarenal reflux is defined as reflux into the ducts of Bellini (Fig. 9-72) (157). Its presence should be documented at VCUG. Although patients with intrarenal reflux are at particular risk for serious sequelae of ascending infection, its presence does not change the grade or treatment of VUR.

Radionuclide Cystography. Because of its lower radiation dose, RNC is preferred to VCUG in four situations: (a) screening children whose siblings or parents have VUR; (b) follow-up of children with previously detected VUR; (c) exclusion of VUR when it is not seriously suspected but the referring physician desires confirmation; (d) postoperative evaluation of ureteral reimplantation. Many institutions use RNC rather than VCUG in all girls (145). Because the anatomy is not as precisely defined as with VCUG, VUR is divided into only three grades by RNC (Fig. 9-78).

Cortical Scintigraphy. The most sensitive method of identifying pyelonephritis and renal scarring has been cortical scintigraphy with DMSA (41,168,169,174). Acute pyelonephritis shows photopenic areas in the kidney (see Fig. 9-132A). In addition to decreased activity, the renal scarring of chronic pyelonephritis also causes a decrease in renal volume (see Fig. 9-132B). Doppler sonography and contrast-enhanced spiral CT are also sensitive methods for diagnosing pyelonephritis (69,70).

Natural History

Most mild VUR resolves spontaneously unless there is dysfunctional voiding (175,176) or an anatomic abnormality (ureteral ectopia, a bladder diverticulum); this spontaneous resolution usually occurs by age 5–6 years of age in girls and slightly earlier in boys. The resolution of VUR with age is another suggestion that the ureterovesical junction was underdeveloped and has matured. The likelihood that primary reflux will resolve spontaneously depends on the age at detection (the younger the better) and the grade of reflux (the lower the better) (177–180).

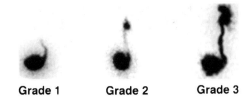

FIG. 9-78. Vesicoureteral reflux by radionuclide cystography. Three different patients, with grade 1, grade 2, and grade 3 vesicoureteral reflux.

Treatment

If there are no anatomic, age, or functional reasons why reflux should not resolve spontaneously and the family is reliable, treatment other than prophylactic antibiotics is seldom required. Patients are reevaluated with RNC after 9–12 months; the antibiotic therapy is discontinued when the reflux has resolved. Surgical reimplantation of the ureter should be considered if VUR has not resolved over a reasonable time interval, if breakthrough infections occur frequently, or if compliance with medical therapy is unreliable.

The two traditional operations for ureteral reimplantation are the Politano-Leadbetter procedure and the cross-trigonal or Cohen procedure. Sonography commonly shows thickening and impressions on the bladder base after reimplantation (181,182). Patients with high-grade VUR with marked dilatation may also require tapering or plication of the distal ureter. Some centers, primarily in Europe, treat VUR with endoscopic submucosal injection of collagen or teflon rather than surgical reimplantation. However, this technique is not widely accepted in the United States (183–185). In the future, laparoscopic ureteral reimplantation may be possible; this less invasive surgical procedure will further shorten the child's hospital stay.

Ureteropelvic Duplications

Nephrogenesis is induced when the ureteric bud (a branch of the mesonephric [Wolffian] duct) meets the metanephric blastema during the fifth week of embryonic development. If a second ureteric bud forms and meets the same blastema, there is duplication of the ureter (not duplication of the kidney). The term *duplex kidney* refers to this configuration of two ureters draining one kidney. An analogy is a duplex house, a single structure with two exits.

Duplication is by far the most common anomaly (1 in 160 patients) of the upper collecting system and ureter. It occurs in a spectrum, from a bifid renal pelvis to complete duplication in which two ureters enter the bladder through separate orifices. In the incomplete form of duplication, the bifurcation can be high (bifid renal pelvis), anywhere along the ureter (bifid mid-ureter), or near the bladder (low bifid ureter) (186). In a few cases, the duplicated ureters join at or within the wall of the bladder.

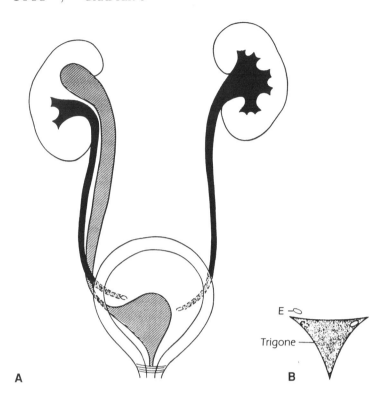

FIG. 9-79. Weigert-Meyer rule. A: Typical features of ectopic ureterocele. There is usually duplication of the upper urinary tract. Flattening of the lower pole calyces produces a "drooping lily" appearance. The ureter of the lower pole moiety is displaced laterally on the side of the ureterocele. The mass in the bladder is due to a ureterocele of the distal ureter of the upper pole moiety. The Weigert-Meyer rule states that the ectopic ureteral orifice of the upper pole moiety is medial and inferior to its normal location. **B:** Frequently, the ureteral orifice of the lower pole moiety is slightly ectopic *(E)*, being lateral and superior to its normal location. There may be vesicoureteral reflux into the ureter that drains the lower pole moiety.

Ureteropelvic duplication is thought to be due to premature division of the ureteral bud or the development of two ureteral buds from the same Wolffian duct. Incomplete duplication is twice as frequent as complete duplication; each is five times as common unilaterally as bilaterally. The two pelvicalyceal systems lie one above the other, the upper segment being smaller and having fewer calyces. The distal ends of the two ureters are contained in a common sheath. If ureteropelvic duplication is complete (each segment has

its own ureteral orifice in the bladder), the Weigert-Meyer rule applies. This rule states that the ureteral orifice of the upper pole moiety inserts into the bladder medial and inferior both to its normal location and to the orifice of the ureter draining the lower renal segment (Fig. 9-79).

Duplications are familial. Generally benign, they are frequently noted on screening ultrasound examinations (Fig. 9-80). Patients with incomplete duplication have a frequency of urinary tract disease similar to patients without duplica-

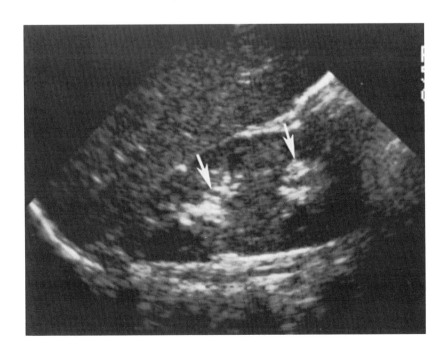

FIG. 9-80. Renal duplication. A 5-year-old girl with urinary tract infection. Supine, longitudinal sonography of right kidney demonstrates separation of the central pelvicalyceal complex into superior and inferior components *(arrows)*.

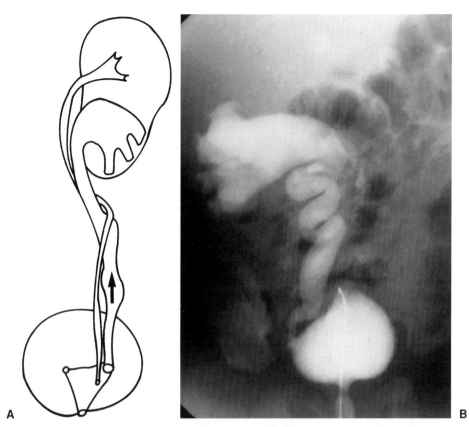

FIG. 9-81. Reflux into lower moiety of duplex kidney. A: Diagrammatic representation of left lower moiety vesicoureteral reflux. **B:** Grade 4 reflux into the lower moiety of the right kidney.

tion. Children with complete duplication have a higher incidence of urinary tract infection, VUR, parenchymal scarring, and obstruction (187,188). If there is neither reflux into the lower moiety nor obstruction of the upper moiety, a duplex kidney is considered a normal variant. A duplex kidney with ureteral duplication has two separate renal sinus echo complexes at sonography (Fig. 9-80). This appearance is considered an incidental finding and requires no further evaluation unless reflux or obstruction is suspected.

The pelvicalyceal system and ureter associated with the lower moiety of a duplex kidney are analogous to those associated with a kidney that has a single collecting system. Abnormalities such as UPJ obstruction and VUR may occur. If duplication is complete, reflux usually involves the ureter draining the lower moiety of the kidney (Fig. 9-81A). Reflux into the lower pole on VCUG has a characteristic appearance (Fig. 9-81B). A line drawn through the upper and lower calyces of a refluxing, nonduplicated system points to the contralateral shoulder. However, a similar line through a duplex kidney points to the ipsilateral shoulder (Fig. 9-81). If the upper moiety is small and nonfunctioning or if reflux into the lower moiety is massive, the diagnosis of complete duplication is easy to miss (188).

Reflux and infection may produce scarring of the lower moiety (see Fig. 9-73). The natural history of reflux into the lower pole of a duplicated collecting system without obstruction is the same as that of reflux into a single collecting system (189–191).

Ureterocele

A ureterocele is the dilated distal end of the ureter. The dilatation lies between the mucosal and muscular layers of the bladder (192). Ureteroceles are divided into the simple type and the ectopic type (Fig. 9-82).

Simple Ureterocele

A simple ureterocele consists of dilatation of only the most distal end of the ureter. The ureterocele is submucosal in the bladder and is located at the lateral margin of the trigone. It rarely measures more than 1 cm in diameter. The ureteral orifice is usually stenotic (Fig. 9-82). Simple ureteroceles sometimes occur bilaterally.

A simple ureterocele may be demonstrated by VCUG, IVU, or sonography. A radiolucent filling defect is present at VCUG. Occasionally, during a VCUG, the ureterocele everts to mimic a bladder diverticulum. At IVU, contrast material collects within the ureterocele to produce a rounded or oval density surrounded by the radiolucent halo of the ureterocele wall, causing the classic cobra-head appearance

Ureterocele

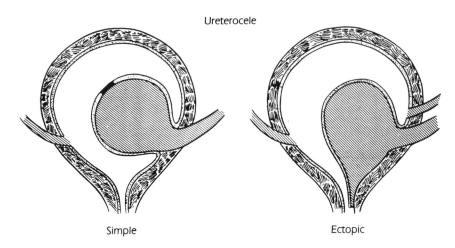

Simple   Ectopic

FIG. 9-82. Ureteroceles. Simple ureterocele and ectopic ureterocele.

(Fig. 9-83). Early during IVU, or if renal function is diminished, a simple ureterocele may appear as a round, radiolucent defect in the bladder because of inadequate accumulation of contrast material in the distal ureter. Simple ureteroceles are not necessarily associated with hydroureteronephrosis.

Ectopic Ureterocele

An ectopic ureterocele is the cyst-like protrusion into the bladder lumen of the dilated submucosal distal portion of an ectopic ureter (Fig. 9-82). It is almost invariably associated with duplication, is at the end of the ureter of the upper renal moiety, and is more inferiorly placed than a simple ureterocele. It is usually unilateral, is far more common in girls than in boys (192,193), and is rare in blacks. The contralateral kidney is duplex in about half of cases (194). The involved ureter may be dilated and tortuous depending on severity and chronicity (Fig. 9-84). The upper moiety frequently is not visualized on IVU and may be dysplastic. The ureterocele may extend through the bladder neck into the submucosal portion of the proximal urethra (see Fig. 9-186). Ureteroceles interfere with the muscular support of the orifice of the ipsilateral duplicated ureter, so that reflux into the lower moiety is common. Moreover, the ureter draining the lower moiety may be located superior and lateral to its normal trigonal position (see Fig. 9-79), which apparently also predisposes to VUR. The ureterocele may fill the base of the bladder, obstruct the entire urinary tract, and produce hydronephrosis of the opposite kidney and of the ipsilateral lower pole. In girls, a ureterocele may present as a perineal interlabial mass if it prolapses through the urethra (195).

The most common type of ectopic ureterocele is stenotic, in which the ureteral orifice is inherently tiny (Fig. 9-85). Other types are the sphincteric, in which the urethral sphincter or bladder neck obstructs the distal ureter when the child is not voiding; the sphincterostenotic, in which there are two causes of obstruction; and rare forms, including the cecoureterocele (Fig. 9-85) (1,3,192).

The sonographic appearance of an ectopic ureterocele is characteristic (Figs. 9-86 and 9-87). The upper pole of a duplex kidney is dilated and connects with a dilated, tortuous ureter (Fig. 9-86). There may also be dilatation of the lower moiety due to either VUR (Fig. 9-86B) or extrinsic UPJ obstruction of the lower pole by the crossing dilated upper pole ureter. At the level of the bladder, the hydroureter terminates in a round, thin-walled anechoic intravesical ureterocele (Fig. 9-86C, D). If hydroureteronephrosis is demon-

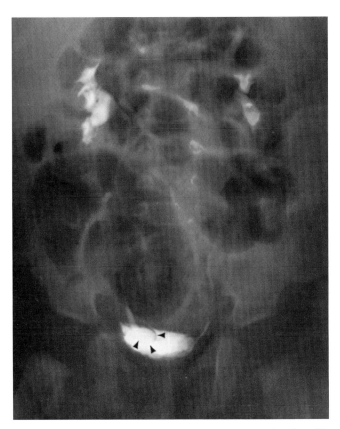

FIG. 9-83. Simple ureterocele. IVU shows a "cobra head" appearance due to contrast material within a simple ureterocele on the right *(arrowheads).*

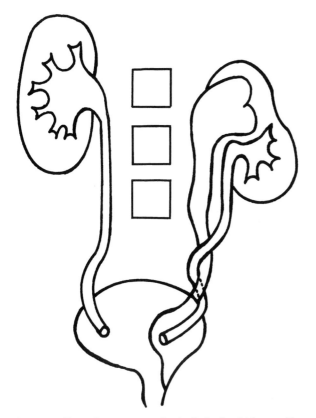

FIG. 9-84. Ectopic ureterocele. Left duplex kidney with an obstructed upper pole moiety. The orifice of the ureterocele (submucosal distal portion of the upper pole ureter) is stenotic. The normal lower pole ureter wraps around the dilated upper pole ureter. The lower pole of the kidney and its ureter are farther from the spine than normal; the lower pole collecting system has a characteristic "drooping lily" axis.

strated by renal sonography, particularly with disproportionate dilatation of the upper moiety (Fig. 9-86), the bladder should be carefully assessed for an ectopic ureterocele (Fig. 9-86C, D). A ureterocele may not be sonographically visible if the bladder is empty and the urine-filled ureterocele is mistaken for the bladder or if the bladder is very full and the ureterocele is pressed against the bladder wall (Fig. 9-88A).

A ureterocele may be seen as a rounded filling defect within the bladder on VCUG (Figs. 9-89A and 9-90A). Reflux into the ipsilateral lower pole ureter is frequently associated. However, unless done meticulously, VCUG may not demonstrate an ectopic ureterocele, as contrast medium is highly radiopaque and filling the bladder may flatten, intussuscept, or even evert the ureterocele (Fig. 9-88). When VCUG is performed for suspected ectopic ureterocele, it is important to use dilute contrast material (17%) in small amounts. Early filling should be fluoroscoped in oblique and sometimes lateral projections as well as a straight AP projection. The ureterocele may evert through a defect in the bladder musculature or intussuscept into the lumen of the upper pole ureter (Figs. 9-88B and 9-89B). Because the appearance of a ureterocele changes rapidly, fluoroscopy is critical. An everted ureterocele with reflux into the ipsilateral lower pole ureter may be mistaken for a paraureteral diverticulum with reflux into a single collecting system (Fig. 9-89B) (196). A ureterocele can also prolapse into the urethra during voiding (Fig. 9-90).

If performed, IVU will usually show a hydronephrotic upper pole moiety and, in the contrast-filled bladder, a lucent filling defect representing the ectopic ureterocele filled with

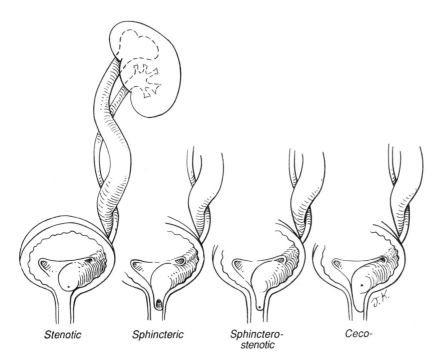

Stenotic   *Sphincteric*   *Sphinctero-stenotic*   *Ceco-*

FIG. 9-85. Types of ectopic ureteroceles. The stenotic ureterocele is obstructed because of an abnormally small orifice. Although the sphincteric ureterocele has a patulous orifice, it is obstructed by the closed urethral sphincter and bladder neck when the patient is not voiding. The sphincterostenotic type has a small orifice and is also obstructed by the closed sphincter and bladder neck. The cecoureterocele has a portion of dilated ureter distal to the stenotic orifice. Only the sphincteric type of ureterocele has vesicoureteral reflux.

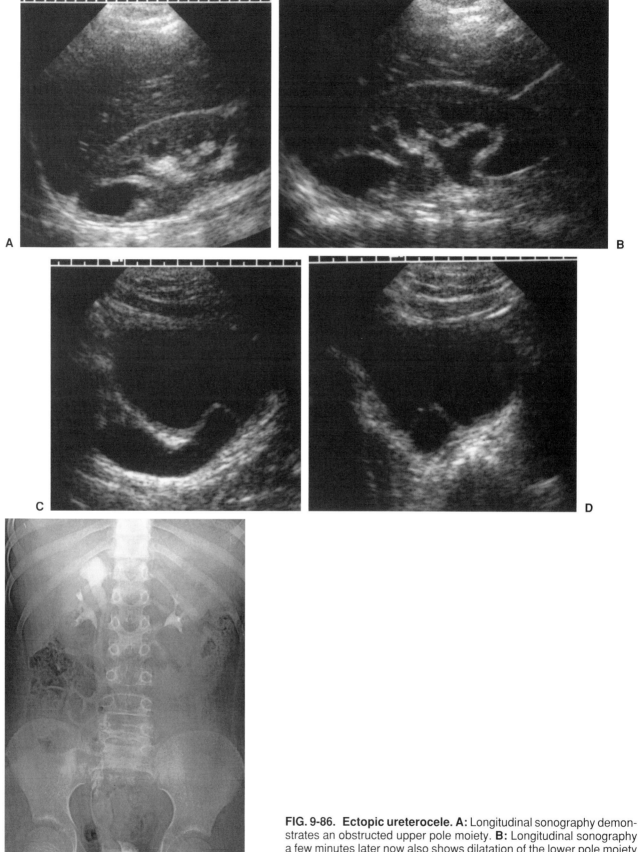

FIG. 9-86. Ectopic ureterocele. A: Longitudinal sonography demonstrates an obstructed upper pole moiety. **B:** Longitudinal sonography a few minutes later now also shows dilatation of the lower pole moiety due to vesicoureteral reflux. Longitudinal **(C)** and transverse **(D)** views demonstrate a dilated right ureter emptying into an ectopic ureterocele. **E:** IVU. There is good function of a dilated upper pole moiety. The ureterocele is filled with dilute contrast material.

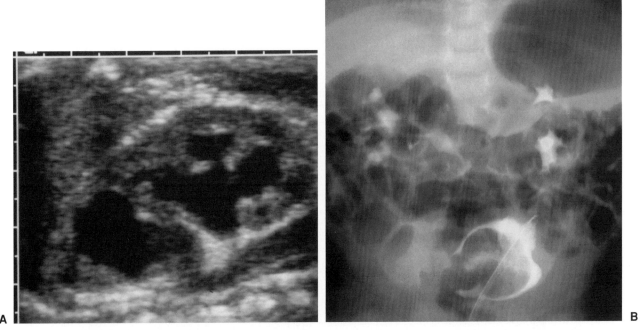

FIG. 9-87. Ectopic ureterocele. A: Longitudinal sonography of the right kidney shows both upper and lower pole hydronephrosis. **B:** IVU. There is a duplex left kidney. There is nonvisualization of the upper moiety of the duplex right kidney as well as mild dilatation of the lower pole pelvicalyceal system. Note the large ureterocele in the bladder.

nonopaque urine. The filling defect in the bladder is usually oval, the long axis of the ureterocele pointing to the affected side. Large ectopic ureteroceles are often rounded. They may almost completely fill the bladder. An IVU or renal scintigraphy is sometimes performed to evaluate the function of the upper renal moiety. If function is good, the upper pole caly-

ces, the ureter, and then the ureterocele will fill with tracer or contrast (Fig. 9-86E). If there is little or no upper moiety function, the upper pole collecting system will not be visualized and the ureter will not fill with contrast. If reflux co-exists, these studies should be performed with constant catheter drainage of the bladder, unless the child is able to empty

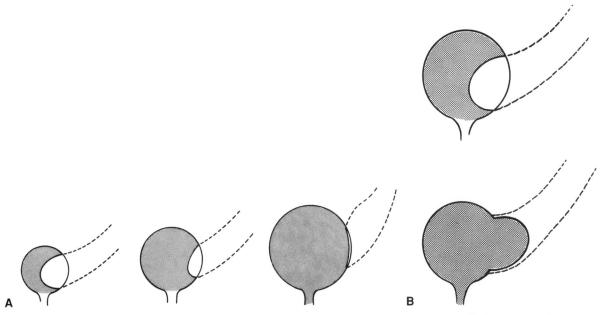

FIG. 9-88. Ectopic ureterocele. A: Effacement of ureterocele with bladder filling. **B:** Intussusception or eversion. The ureterocele may intussuscept (*above*) or evert (*below*) into or adjacent to its own ureter.

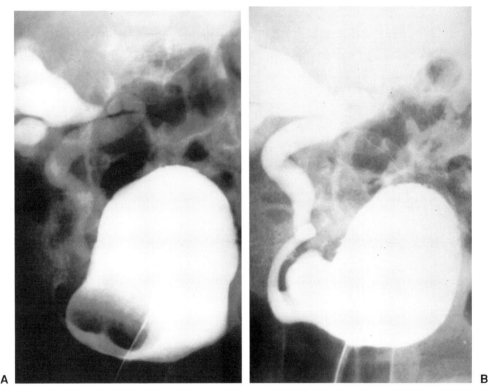

A   B

FIG. 9-89. Everting ureterocele. A: VCUG. There is a large right ureterocele with reflux into the lower pole moiety. **B:** The ureterocele has everted and mimics a refluxing ureter inserting into a bladder diverticulum.

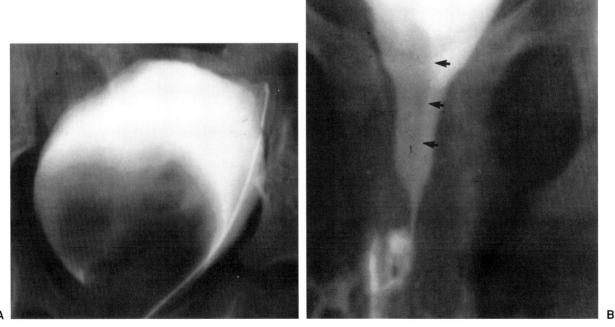

A   B

FIG. 9-90. Prolapsing ureterocele. A: A large ureterocele is visualized during bladder filling. **B:** During voiding, the ureterocele prolapses into the urethra *(arrows).*

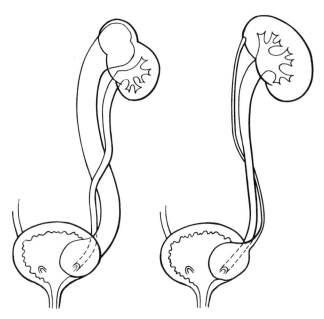

FIG. 9-91. Ureterocele disproportion. On the left is the typical proportionality in the sizes of the dilated upper pole moiety, dilated ureter, and ureterocele. On the right the ureterocele is of comparable size, but both the upper pole moiety and its draining ureter are diminutive; this is called *ureterocele disproportion.*

the bladder frequently. Rarely, lower pole UPJ obstruction is caused by the dilated, tortuous ureter of the upper pole (86).

Occasionally, a ureterocele is associated with a very tiny upper renal moiety; the ureterocele is disproportionately large compared to the amount of upper pole renal cortex (Figs. 9-91 and 9-92). This appearance, termed *ureterocele disproportion,* can be confusing on sonography (Fig. 9-92) (197). The ureterocele is frequently visible within the urinary bladder, but the ipsilateral kidney has the appearance of a normal single system (Fig. 9-92A) rather than a duplex kidney with upper pole obstruction. The diagnosis of ureterocele disproportion can be confirmed with endoscopic, retrograde injection of the ureterocele (Fig. 9-92B).

In the past, upper pole nephroureterectomy with or without lower pole reimplantation was the mainstay of the treatment of ectopic ureteroceles. Although this is still required in some patients, endoscopic incision of ureteroceles with careful follow-up is now advocated (Fig. 9-93) (198,199). The optimal result of endoscopic incision of an ectopic ureterocele is relief of upper moiety obstruction and resolution of lower pole reflux (Fig. 9-94). Other possible results include no change in lower pole reflux and the creation of upper pole reflux (Fig. 9-94). Preliminary work suggests that

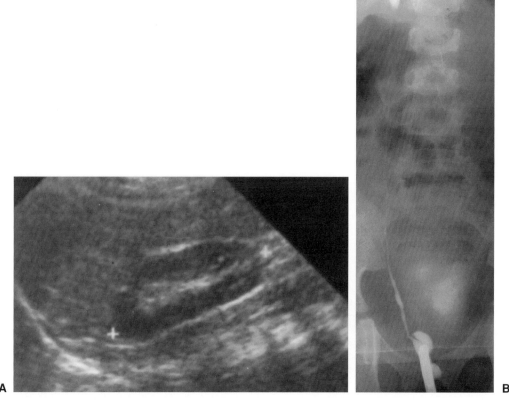

FIG. 9-92. Ureterocele disproportion. A: Longitudinal ultrasonography. There is no evidence of hydronephrosis or duplication. **B:** Ureterocele injection. Despite the negative ultrasonography, there is a diminutive upper pole moiety and draining ureter.

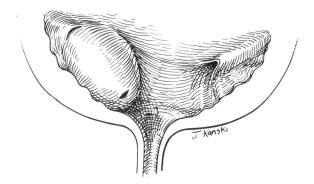

FIG. 9-93. Endoscopic incision of ureterocele. There is an endoscopic incision at the lower end of a right ectopic ureterocele. The distorted lower pole orifice is the slit at the upper end of the ureterocele. Note the undermining of the right side of the trigone by the large ureterocele.

endoscopic ureterocele incision is the only surgery required in approximately 70% of cases (199). Additional late outcome studies are required to define the utility of this procedure.

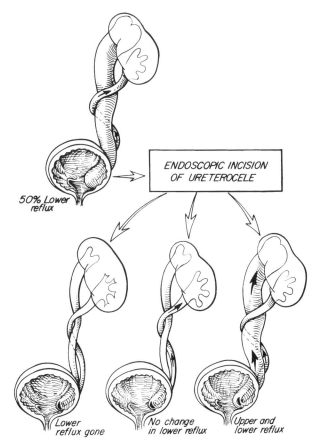

FIG. 9-94. Possible results of endoscopic incision of a ureterocele. About half of patients with an ectopic ureterocele have ipsilateral lower pole reflux. After endoscopic incision, the upper pole may be decompressed with resolution of or no change in the lower pole reflux. Alternatively, the upper pole obstruction may be relieved, but with the development of upper pole reflux and unchanged lower pole reflux.

Ectopic Ureter

The primitive ureter arises from the mesonephric (Wolffian) duct rather than directly from the bladder. The orifice migrates to lie in the bladder concomitant with a caudal migration of the remainder of the duct, which in boys contributes to the formation of the genital tract. In the process there is a reversal of position so that the mesonephric duct terminates more distally. Failure of the ureter to separate from the duct results in the ureteral orifice being carried to some point distal to its normal location. The result is ureteral ectopia, which is much more frequent in girls than in boys (Fig. 9-95).

In girls, this anomaly is usually associated with a duplex

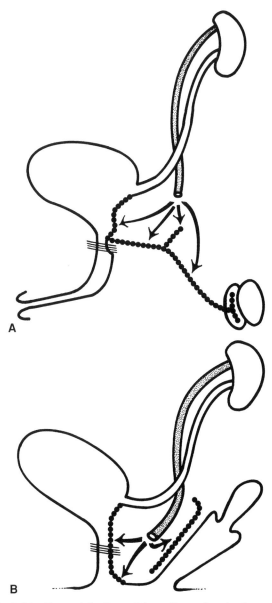

FIG. 9-95. Potential sites of insertion of ectopic ureter. The *black dots* indicate possible sites for an ectopic ureteral orifice. **A:** Boys. The opening is never below the urethral (external) sphincter. **B:** Girls. The upper pole ureteral orifice is usually below the sphincter. Modified from Johnston and Scholtmeijer (543).

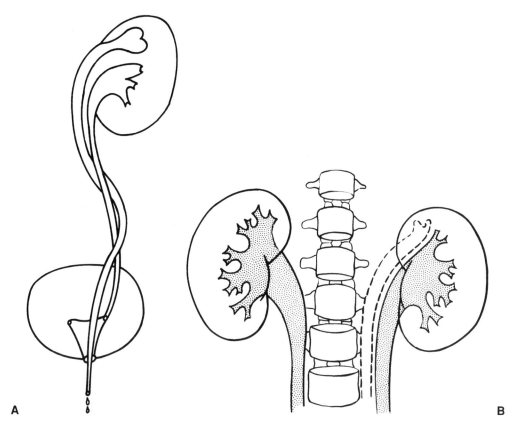

A   **B**

FIG. 9-96. Ureteral ectopia in girls with wetting. **A:** The infrasphincteric ureteral orifice is usually from the upper pole moiety of a duplex kidney. **B:** IVU. The upper pole moiety often functions too poorly to be visualized directly; a common error is to mistake the lower pole moiety for a complete collecting system. The clue is the inferolateral displacement of the visualized calyces and pelvis.

kidney, and it is the upper segment that terminates ectopically. Fewer than 10% of ectopic ureters in girls drain a nonduplicated collecting system. The ectopic orifice in the female patient most commonly empties into the urethra, vestibule, or vagina (Fig. 9-95B). Rarely, it empties into the uterus, cervix, or rectum.

Because the opening of the ectopic ureter in girls is usually distal to the urethral sphincter, a common clinical presentation is incontinence due to continuous leakage of small amounts of urine. The child is wet, both day and night, despite successful toilet training (200). Renal sonography to exclude a duplex kidney may be misleading; the upper moiety in these patients may be too small to be detected. The IVU in nearly all cases verifies ureteral duplication (by secondary signs, not by direct visualization) even with considerable upper pole dysplasia (Fig. 9-96). A duplex kidney on one side in a girl who is always wet suggests contralateral occult duplication with ureteral ectopia of the upper moiety as the cause. If the history is compelling and the IVU is not diagnostic, CT may detect a tiny, dysplastic upper pole (201).

The upper moiety of a duplex kidney can be obstructed if its ureter inserts ectopically into the urethra at the level of the sphincter (Fig. 9-97). The ureter is obstructed when the girl is not voiding, and urine may reflux into the ureter when the sphincter is relaxed during voiding. In this situation, demonstration of VUR is optimized by a cyclic VCUG (25,26).

Although far less common, ectopic insertion of a ureter of a single collecting system may also cause incontinence in girls (Fig. 9-98) (202,203). The involved kidney is usually small and dysplastic, and may not be visible on ultrasound or IVU. CT is useful in locating a small, poorly functioning dysplastic kidney (Fig. 9-98B) (204,205).

Ectopic ureters are less likely to be associated with duplex kidneys in boys. Ectopic ureteral openings may be in the posterior urethra, ejaculatory ducts, seminal vesicles, vas deferens, or rectum (Fig. 9-95A). Because none of these structures lie below the urethral sphincter, boys with ectopic ureters do not have urinary incontinence. However, hydroureteronephrosis, infection, prostatitis, or epididymitis may be present. Ureteral ectopia in a boy may not be found until early adulthood.

IVU may suggest the diagnosis by directly visualizing the termination of the ectopic ureter or, more frequently, by verifying the presence of a nonfunctioning superior renal moiety, inferred from the appearance of the lower renal segment (see Fig. 9-96). The visualized calyces are frequently fewer than normal, and there may be lateral and inferior displacement of the lower moiety of the kidney and shift of the longitudinal renal axis.

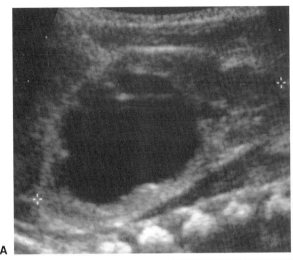

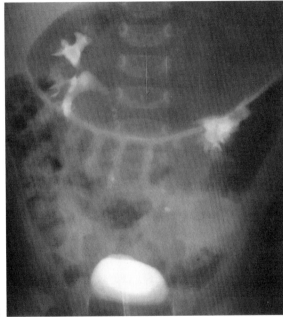

FIG. 9-97. Ectopic ureter without ureterocele. A: Longitudinal sonography shows an obstructed upper pole moiety. **B:** IVU. There is an obstructed upper pole moiety on the left. No ureterocele is identified in the bladder. There was obstruction of an ectopic, extravesical upper pole ureter.

Filling of the ectopic ureter by VCUG is possible if it terminates in the urethra or by vaginography if it terminates in the vagina. A cyclic VCUG is helpful in filling ectopic ureters that drain into the urethra (25,26). Ectopic ureters in boys, which frequently drain nonduplicated kidneys and enter the genital tract, are usually associated with minimally functional remnants of renal parenchyma. The diagnosis should be considered in a boy with a retrovesical, pararectal mass and ipsilateral nonvisualization of the kidney on ultrasound or IVU. In general, the portion of the kidney served by an ectopic ureter is itself abnormal (usually dysplastic) when it is drained into an extra-urinary structure.

Bladder Abnormalities

Bladder Diverticula

Bladder diverticula are protrusions of mucosa through a defect in the muscular wall of the urinary bladder (Fig. 9-99) (206). Most bladder diverticula are primary and are due

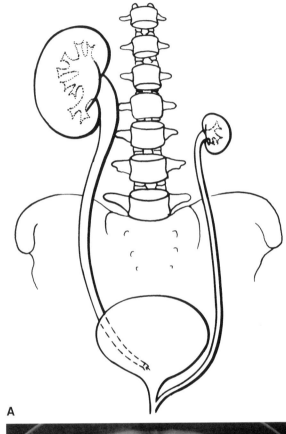

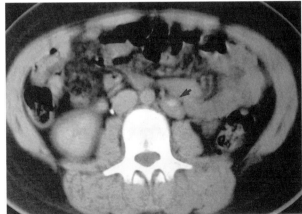

FIG. 9-98. Single-ureter ectopia in a girl with wetting. A: An ectopic ureter usually drains a small, dysplastic, malpositioned kidney without hydronephrosis. **B:** Teenage girl with continuous wetting. IVU showed no left kidney. Contrast-enhanced CT at the level of the lower pole of the right kidney demonstrates a tiny, dysplastic, poorly functioning left kidney (arrow).

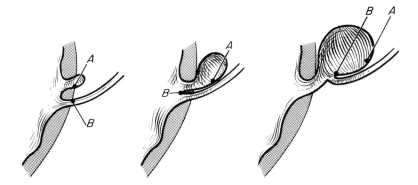

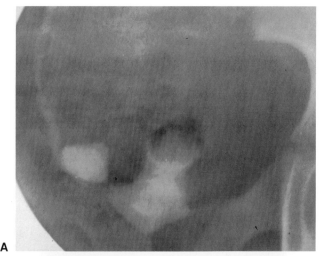

FIG. 9-99. Reflux due to bladder diverticulum. As a bladder diverticulum enlarges, the bladder mucosa is distorted and draws the ureteral orifice into the diverticulum. There is distortion of the submucosal tunnel and consequent vesicoureteral reflux. *A,* bladder diverticulum. *B,* wall of the ureter near its orifice.

to a congenital defect or point of weakness in the muscle wall (206).

Diverticula are often incidental findings but may become symptomatic. Complications of bladder diverticula reflect their location and size (206). First, the bladder may be transformed into a multichambered cavity with the potential for stagnation of urine and subsequent infection, bleeding, or stone formation. Second, they may deform the ureterovesical junction to produce VUR or ureteral obstruction (Fig. 9-99). Bladder diverticula in a periureteric location are termed Hutch diverticula (207). VUR is due to distortion of the ureteral orifice and submucosal tunnel (Fig. 9-99). Approximately half of Hutch diverticula are associated with VUR (206). It is easy to mistake an everting ureterocele with lower moiety reflux (see Fig. 9-89) for a congenital periureteral diverticulum with reflux into a single collecting system (Fig. 9-100) (196). Finally, bladder diverticula may become so large that they produce urethral obstruction (206,208–212).

Although it once was thought that many diverticula of the bladder in children were secondary to obstruction, most diverticula are in fact primary developmental anomalies (206). The most common types of obstruction causing secondary diverticula are posterior urethral valves and obstruction at the external urethral sphincter in children with neurogenic dysfunction, usually due to myelomeningocele (206). Many irregularities of the bladder wall in patients with obstruction are really protrusions of mucosa between hypertrophied muscle bundles; these are not true diverticula but cellules or saccules.

Bladder diverticula may also be iatrogenic and follow reimplantation, placement of a suprapubic cystostomy, or repair of high anorectal malformation with rectovesical fistula. Some are ureterocele remnants or ureteral stumps (206). Table 9-13 lists other conditions associated with bladder diverticula.

Small bladder diverticula are difficult to demonstrate by IVU. VCUG with fluoroscopy and oblique positioning is the only reliable method of diagnosing bladder diverticula (Fig. 9-100) (213). Most patients with small diverticula are asymptomatic.

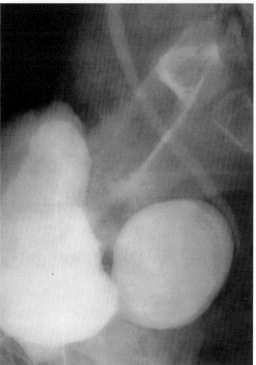

FIG. 9-100. Bladder diverticula. A: Right ureter inserts into a small bladder diverticulum. **B:** Left ureter inserts into a large bladder diverticulum.

TABLE 9-13. *Bladder diverticula in children*

Primary diverticula
  Hutch diverticula[a]
    Without vesicoureteral reflux
    With vesicoureteral reflux
  Urachal diverticulum
  Diverticula at other locations[a]
Secondary diverticula
  Obstruction
  Neurogenic dysfunction[a]
Iatrogenic diverticula
  Postreimplantation
    New ureteric hiatus
    Old ureteric hiatus
  Site of suprapubic tube
  Enlarged remnant of rectovesical fistula in anorectal malformation
  Ureterocele remnant
  Ureteral stump
Associated with other conditions
  Prune belly syndrome
  Kinky hair syndrome (Menke syndrome)
  Williams syndrome
  Ehlers-Danlos syndrome
  Cutis laxa

[a] More common.
Source: Modified from Boechat and Lebowitz (206).

Bladder Trabeculation

The Latin root *trab* means "beam" or "timber"; a "trabeculum" is a small beam or bar. Trabeculations are irregularities in a bladder wall thickened by muscular hypertrophy.

Bladder trabeculation is due to obstruction of the egress of urine. This may be due to an intrinsic urethral abnormality such as posterior urethral valves or to failure of appropriate, coordinated relaxation of the urethral sphincter (bladder sphincter dyssynergy) (214). Many newborn boys with severe posterior urethral valves and some neonates with myelomeningocele already have trabeculated bladders (215). The fetus voids in utero and has months to develop changes secondary to bladder outlet obstruction. If a patient has a trabeculated bladder without a urethral abnormality, urodynamic testing for voiding dysfunction should be performed. Because the bladder and urethra are innervated by the second, third, and fourth sacral nerves, the patient should be examined for spinal dysraphism, and plain films of the spine should be assessed for lumbosacral anomalies.

Thickening due to trabeculation is diagnosed by sonography when the bladder wall measures >3 mm when distended or 5 mm when empty. Wall thickening is inferred at cystography by elevation of the base of the bladder above the pelvic floor, an irregular mucosal contour, or the presence of many cellules or saccules. Because of its cholinergic innervation, the base of the bladder remains smooth despite trabeculation in its body.

Bladder Exstrophy-Epispadias Spectrum

Exstrophy of the bladder is caused by a failure of midline closure of the infraumbilical abdominal wall. The entire anterior wall of the bladder and the overlying skin and skeletal muscle are absent. The edges of the remaining posterior part of the bladder are joined to the skin at a mucocutaneous junction. There is also defective development of the anterior wall of the urogenital sinus and the genital tubercle (216). Exstrophy is the most common anomaly in a spectrum that includes epispadias, diphallus, urethral duplication of the epispadiac type, superior vesical fissure, and cloacal exstrophy (216). Inguinal hernia, rectal prolapse, hydrometrocolpos, anorectal malformations, and spinal dysraphism may coexist. The bladder neck is open anteriorly, as is the urethra; the urethra has not formed into a tube but remains a rectangular sheet of mucosa.

Epispadias is failure of dorsal closure of the urethra. It occurs with all degrees of severity, from an open bladder neck and urethra to involvement of only the distal urethra. The urethral sphincter is deficient and the functional problem is incontinence. Because closure of the bladder and the urethra in the embryo occurs from cranial to caudal, exstrophy of the bladder always includes epispadias, but epispadias can exist without exstrophy.

The bladder exstrophy-epispadias spectrum of abnormalities is felt to be caused by an abnormal persistence, position, or overgrowth of the cloacal membranes in the first 6 weeks of embryonic life (217,218). This causes a low midline abdominal wall defect and varying degrees of exposure of the vesicourethral mucosa. This mucosa may show histologic abnormalities such as islands of adenomucosa, foci of inflammation, and cystitis glandularis. There may also be disorganization and fibrosis of the musculature (219).

The incidence of exstrophy is 3 in 100,000 births. Epispadias without exstrophy is slightly less common (2 in 100,000 births) (216). Exstrophy has a male predominance of 3:1. Nearly all patients with epispadias are boys (216).

The normal distance between the two pubic bones as seen on AP radiographs of the pelvis varies from 5 to 9 mm during the first 2 years of life and from 4 to 8 mm at 2–13 years of age (221). With exstrophy of the bladder, there is widening of the symphysis pubis due to outward rotation of the iliac bones, outward rotation of the pubic bones, and lateral displacement of the iliac bones (Fig. 9-101) (221,222). The amount of bony separation is proportional to the severity of the malformation. Approximately 66% of all patients with true widening of the pubic symphysis have exstrophy of the bladder or one of its variants; another 25% occurs in patients with epispadias; and 10% occurs in unusual clinical entities, such as anorectal malformation, urethral duplication, diphallus, congenital hydrometrocolpos, and pseudoexstrophy (221). Widening of the pubic symphysis in patients with exstrophy is different from the local skeletal abnormality of cleidocranial dysostosis, in which the apparent widening is

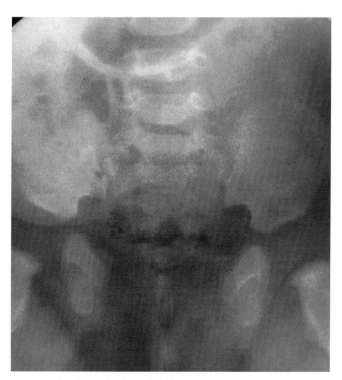

FIG. 9-101. Bladder exstrophy. A 3-month-old girl. The pubic bones are widely separated.

due to delayed mineralization of the pubic bones rather than to a true separation.

In patients with exstrophy, the rectus abdominis muscles are widely separated inferiorly, and there is frequently an umbilical hernia. The bladder is usually small and lies open and everted on the anterior abdominal wall. The ureteral orifices are visible and are slightly prolapsed. The phallus tends to be bifid (split). The lower ends of the ureters make a wide lateral sweep and pass medially and slightly upward to traverse the wall of the bladder almost perpendicularly, in contrast to the normal oblique intramural course (216). There is usually slight dilatation of the distal ureters, and the appearance has been referred to as a hurley-stick (hockey-stick) configuration (216). This appearance is usual in patients with exstrophy of the bladder and should not be interpreted as a sign of obstruction. The kidneys are normal at birth except in patients with cloacal exstrophy, who may have renal ectopia (220). An initial renal sonogram should be performed as a baseline at 1–2 weeks of age.

The diagnosis of bladder exstrophy is obvious on physical examination at birth. Plain radiographs of the pelvis show separation of the pubic bones (Fig. 9-101). The only increase in the incidence of spinal cord tethering in this spectrum is in cloacal exstrophy; in the latter group of patients, MRI or US of the spine is necessary to diagnose spinal cord abnormalities, which cannot be excluded by conventional radiographs of the lumbosacral spine (223,224).

In patients with epispadias, the bladder capacity is low,

the ureterovesical junction frequently permits reflux, and inadequate sphincteric development tends to cause incontinence. Abnormal separation of the pubic bones may occur in patients with epispadias even without exstrophy. The degree of separation is proportional to the severity of the epispadias (216). The goals of treatment are to preserve renal function, establish urinary continence, achieve a cosmetically pleasing result, and optimize sexual function and fertility.

Cystectomy with ureterosigmoidostomy was formerly the usual treatment for bladder exstrophy. However, it is now recognized that patients with ureterosigmoidostomies are at risk for adenocarcinoma at the ureterosigmoid suture line caused by bathing of mucosa with a mixture of stool and urine (225–228). Current therapy is usually a multistage procedure which includes bladder and urethral closure, bladder neck reconstruction and repair of epispadias for continence, antireflux surgery, and cosmetic as well as functional correction of abnormalities of the phallus. If the bladder is too small, it can be augmented. The initial bladder closure is now done on the first day or two of life to protect the mucosa from injury and infection and to take advantage of the malleability of the neonatal pelvis, which allows approximation of the pubic bones. Periodic renal sonography to detect hydronephrosis or renal scarring is worthwhile. Complete preoperative and postoperative imaging evaluation is important to ensure adequate reconstruction of the lower urinary tract and to verify lack of secondary damage to the upper urinary tract (1,3).

Urachal Abnormalities

Embryologically, there is a normal communication between the apex of the bladder and the umbilicus. This closes before birth. A patent urachus is the persistence of this communication. The lumen of the urachus is not occluded, and urine can pass from the dome of the bladder to the umbilicus. The neonate presents with an umbilical sinus draining urine. A patent urachus may be demonstrated by VCUG with the patient in the lateral projection or by direct injection of the tract (Fig. 9-102A). A persistent urachus frequently coexists with congenital lower urinary tract obstruction such as PUV or prune-belly syndrome. It may also occur with ventral abdominal wall defects, such as omphalocele. A urachal sinus is persistence of the ventral part of the urachus at its abdominal wall end; this sinus tract ends blindly (Fig. 9-102B). A urachal diverticulum is persistence of the urachus at its bladder end; a diverticulum of variable size arises anteriorly from the dome of the bladder. US shows a tubular or cyst-like structure communicating with a full bladder. There may be a fibrous tract or sinus extending from the diverticulum to the umbilicus or occasionally a thin persistent tubular channel. A urachal cyst is encapsulation of fluid within the urachus, closed at both bladder and abdominal wall ends (Fig. 9-102C). Children with urachal cysts may have a palpable

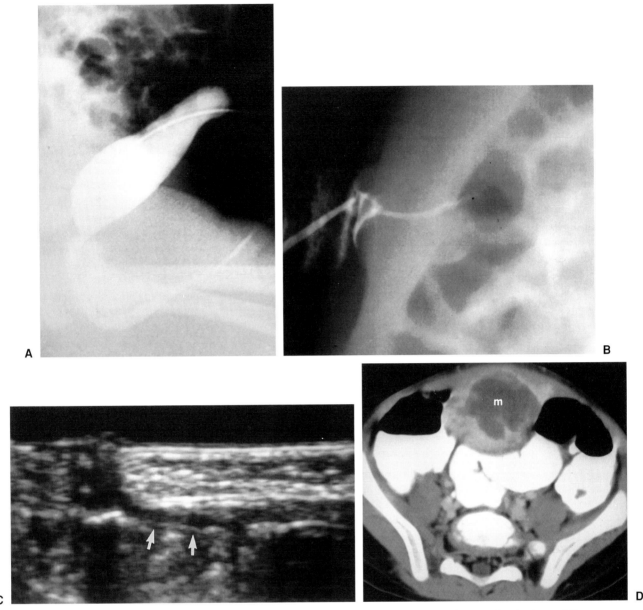

FIG. 9-102. Urachal abnormalities. A: Patent urachus. A catheter placed in the opening in the umbilicus enters the bladder. **B:** Urachal sinus. Contrast material injected into an opening in the umbilicus fills a blind-ending sinus tract. **C:** Urachal cyst. Longitudinal sonography demonstrates a rounded cyst just beneath the umbilicus. A tract *(arrows)* from this cyst extends toward the dome of the bladder. **D:** Infected urachal cyst. Contrast-enhanced CT at the level of the umbilicus shows an inflammatory mass *(m).*

midline mass or fever due to superimposed infection (Fig. 9-102D). US (Fig. 9-102C) or CT (Fig. 9-102D) shows a cystic mass located anteriorly in the midline (1,3). Stones may occur in urachal cysts.

Other Urethral Abnormalities

Hypospadias

Hypospadias is an abnormality in boys in which failure of closure of the urethral lumen leads to an abnormally proximal meatus. The urethral orifice is on the ventral (under-neath) side of the penis. There is failure of the normal proximal-to-distal fusion of the urogenital folds, probably caused by underproduction of androgens by the fetal testes. There is also incomplete formation of the spongy urethra. Normal ectodermal ingrowth still occurs in boys with hypospadias, so that there appears to be a meatus at the tip of the penis, but this is actually just a blind-ending dimple.

The malposition of the urethral opening may be minor (low on an otherwise normal glans penis), intermediate, or extreme (perineal, with associated penile hypoplasia). The position of the urethral meatus determines the type of hypo-

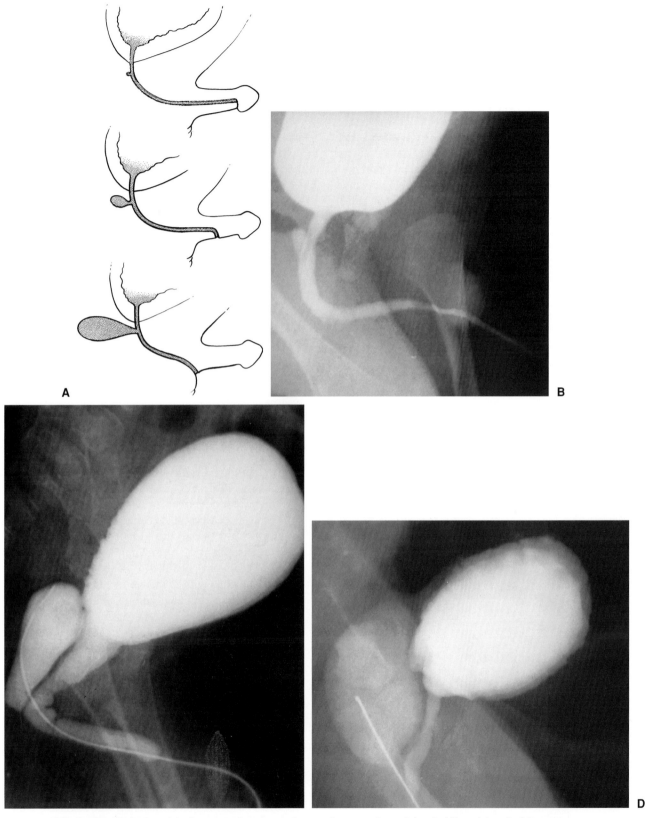

FIG. 9-103. Relationship between hypospadias and prostatic utricle. A: Minor (glanular) hypospadias and small utricle *(top)*. Moderately severe (penile) hypospadias and moderate-sized utricle *(middle)*. Severe (penoscrotal) hypospadias and very large utricle *(bottom)*. The penile hypoplasia often seen in penoscrotal hypospadias is not depicted. **B:** Mild hypospadias and small utricle. **C:** Penile hypospadias. The catheter has been inadvertently passed from the midshaft hypospadias into a fairly large utricle. **D:** Perineal hypospadias and very large utricle.

spadias: glanular, penile, penoscrotal, or perineal. The incidence of hypospadias is approximately 1 in 300 male births; the glanular and penile types account for about 80% of these. The prostatic utricle is usually enlarged. The more extreme the hypospadias, the larger the utricle (Fig. 9-103). Associated meatal stenosis is common in the less extreme forms of hypospadias.

Imaging is not necessary in most boys with hypospadias. However, in patients requiring extensive urethroplasties, VCUG demonstrates urethral anatomy and shows the size of the utricle. Following repair of hypospadias, there may be a stricture or diverticulum that requires radiologic evaluation. There is some evidence that abnormalities of kidney ascent and rotation are more common in boys with hypospadias. However, even if present, these minor renal abnormalities tend to be of no clinical significance; routine ultrasound evaluation of the kidneys is probably not necessary (229,230).

Urethral Duplication

Duplication of the urethra is rare in boys and virtually unknown in girls. In boys, there are three types of urethral

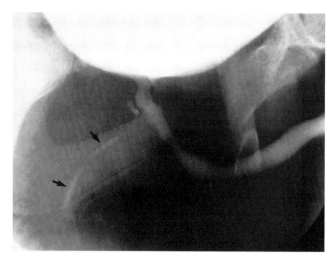

FIG. 9-105. Congenital urethroperineal fistula. This resembles duplication of the urethra of the hypospadiac type. However, the urethra is located normally. The fistula *(arrows)* extends from the posterior urethra to the perineum.

duplication: (a) a blind-ending accessory urethral channel originating independently from a single bladder; (b) a complete accessory urethral channel originating from a normal urethra, independently from a single bladder, or from the phallus; and (c) two urethras arising independently from a duplicated or septated bladder. The first two types are duplications in the sagittal plane whereas the third is a side-by-side duplication. The second type is the most common.

Almost all blind-ending urethral duplications originate in the phallus. These tracts usually arise dorsal to the functional urethral meatus, regardless of whether it is normally placed or hypospadiac. Most blind channels extend from the glanular meatus back toward the base of the penis in boys with hypospadias. This type of urethral duplication usually produces no symptoms, and the incidence is unknown (231).

Most patients with a patent urethral duplication are asymptomatic or complain only of double urinary stream, although incontinence, dysuria, obstruction, and infection are occasionally present (231). The accessory urethra may have an epispadiac, glanular, or hypospadiac meatus (Fig. 9-104). Renal sonography should be performed, as occasionally upper urinary tract anomalies, renal agenesis, or hydronephrosis is present. Retrograde urethrography and VCUG are usually required for adequate evaluation and surgical planning (231). The ventrally positioned (underneath) urethral channel, regardless of the position of its meatus, is almost always the more functional channel and therefore more easily catheterized (231). The pubic bones are abnormally separated in patients with an epispadiac meatus (231).

Patients with urethral duplication who also have duplication of the bladder or penis may have doubling of other portions of the caudal end of the body, particularly the distal parts of the genital and gastrointestinal tracts (231). These rare cases of double urethra and double bladder usually are discovered during evaluation for associated caudal anomalies.

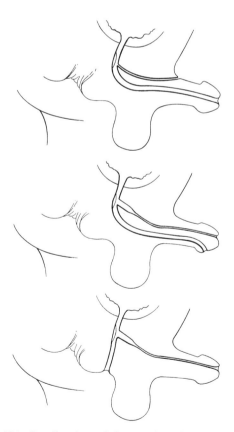

FIG. 9-104. Duplication of the urethra. There is a continuum of duplication of the urethra with the accessory urethra in an epispadiac position *(top)*, both urethras in the penis *(middle)*, and one urethra in a hypospadiac position *(bottom)*. The ventral (underneath) urethra is almost always the more functional.

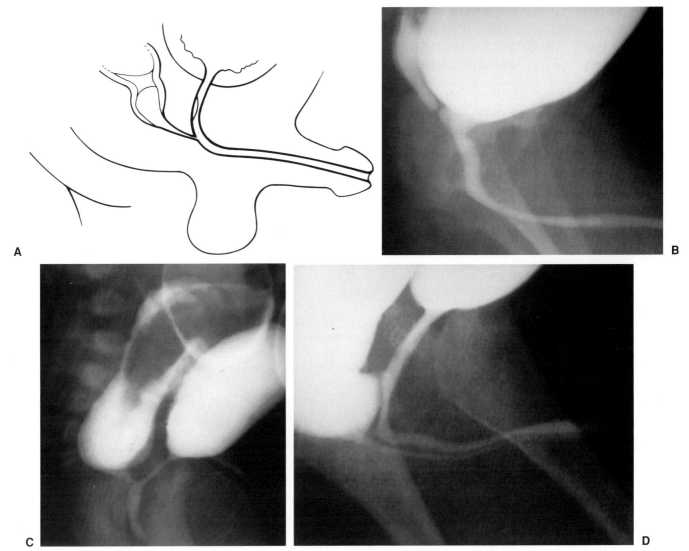

FIG. 9-106. Rectourethral fistulas in boys with imperforate anus. A: Fistulous communication to the membranous urethra. The connection between the rectum and the lower urinary tract can be located anywhere from the bladder to the urethral meatus. **B:** Fistula to the urethra just below the bladder neck. **C:** The rectum communicates with the membranous portion of the urethra, the most common situation. **D:** The rectourethral fistula parallels the urethra and joins it near the urethral meatus.

Congenital Urethroperineal Fistula

Despite some similarities, the hypospadiac form of urethral duplication and a congenital urethroperineal fistula are different entities and must be distinguished. Boys with congenital urethroperineal fistula have normal micturition through the penile urethra, and only a few drops of urine pass through the perineal opening (Fig. 9-105) (232). In boys with the hypospadiac form of urethral duplication, the main urinary stream is through the ventral (perineal) meatus (Fig. 9-104). In congenital urethroperineal fistula, the dorsal urethra is the functionally normal channel (Fig. 9-105). Ventral channel excision is curative in a congenital urethroperineal fistula; it may be disastrous in the hypospadiac form of urethral duplication which requires an extensive repair.

Imperforate Anus with Rectourethral Fistula

Infants with high imperforate anus usually have a diverting colostomy soon after birth without radiologic evaluation other than plain films of the chest and abdomen. All boys with high imperforate anus have a connection from the rectum to the lower urinary tract (Fig. 9-106). The fistula in girls with high imperforate anus usually enters the vagina. When the rectum is connected to the urinary tract by a fistula (only in boys), urine and meconium can mix in the colon in utero and the meconium may calcify (233). Urine and meconium can also mix and calcify in girls, but only in the cloacal malformation. The shape and distribution of the intracolonic calcifications on plain radiographs suggest their intraluminal position and distinguish them from meconium peritonitis (233). In difficult cases, ultrasound may show the location of the calcifications (234).

There is no need to define the fistulous connection between the bowel and the genitourinary system until just before definitive repair, usually at 1–2 years of age. Full visualization is best achieved by injecting water-soluble contrast material into the distal limb of the colostomy. It may be helpful to occlude the stoma of this distal colon segment with an inflated Foley balloon (235). A VCUG may also show the fistulous communication. In boys, the fistula between the rectum and lower urinary tract is usually at the level of the prostatic urethra; more distal and proximal communications do occasionally occur (Fig. 9-106) (236).

Following rectal pull-through and excision of the rectourethral fistula, a small fistula stump may be visualized; this small remnant is usually of no clinical significance (237). However, the stump may enlarge, especially in the setting of urethral obstruction, and may look like a diverticulum. It may cause hematuria or urinary tract infection, especially epididymitis. A rectourinary fistula occasionally recurs many years after surgery (237). Fistula stumps and recurrent fistulas may not fill on retrograde urethrography; they are best shown with the external sphincter open during the micturition phase of VCUG.

Renal agenesis and ectopia occur with increased frequency in patients with imperforate anus, and imaging of the kidneys with ultrasound is recommended (238,239).

Abnormalities of Cowper Gland Ducts

The bulbourethral glands (Cowper glands) are paired paraurethral glands located in the urogenital diaphragm near the bulbous urethra. Their secretions pass through paired Cowper ducts, which enter the ventral surface of the proximal bulbous urethra (Fig. 9-107A). The secretions have lubricating and spermatozoa-protecting functions.

A *retention cyst of a Cowper gland duct* is caused by obstruction of the duct and gland; it causes a smooth, rounded filling defect in the bulbous urethra just proximal to the expected site of Cowper duct insertion (Figs. 9-107B and 9-108A, B). Although usually asymptomatic, large retention cysts may cause urethral obstruction (240). Retention cysts are best shown on VCUG; they may be effaced by the urethral distention that occurs during retrograde urethrography (241).

Occasionally, *Cowper gland ducts* are filled during urethrography. Reflux into these ducts is caused by a patulous orifice, rupture of a retention cyst due to urethral instrumentation, spontaneous rupture of a retention cyst, or distal urethral obstruction (Figs. 9-107B and 9-108C, D). A Cowper's duct should not be confused with a urethral diverticulum, partial duplication, ectopic ureter, fistula, blood vessel, or Müllerian duct remnant.

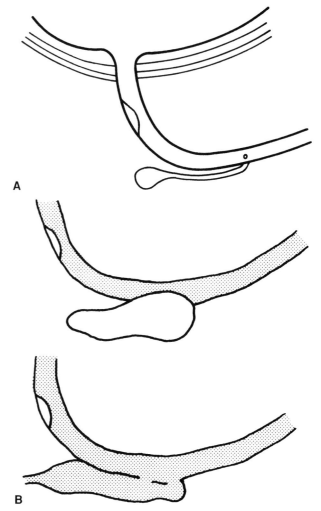

FIG. 9-107. Anatomy and abnormalities of Cowper glands. A: The paired Cowper glands are located in the external sphincter. The ducts open into the bulbous urethra. **B:** Cowper gland duct cyst *(top).* Reflux into a dilated Cowper gland duct *(bottom).*

Renal Agenesis

Renal agenesis may be unilateral or bilateral. Unilateral renal agenesis occurs in 1 in 1000 births; the fatal bilateral form occurs in 1 to 3 in 10,000 births (242). Agenesis can occur with other conditions such as vaginal or uterine duplication and the VATER association. Renal agenesis occurs when the ureteral bud (metanephric diverticulum) fails to form or degenerates. The ipsilateral hemitrigone of the bladder is usually absent. Without induction of nephron development in the metanephric mesoderm by penetration by the ureteral bud, the kidney fails to form (243).

Because amniotic fluid is largely composed of fetal urine, the diagnosis of bilateral renal agenesis should be suggested when prenatal sonography shows severe oligohydramnios and absence of definable kidneys. Bilateral renal agenesis is more common in boys. Newborns with bilateral renal

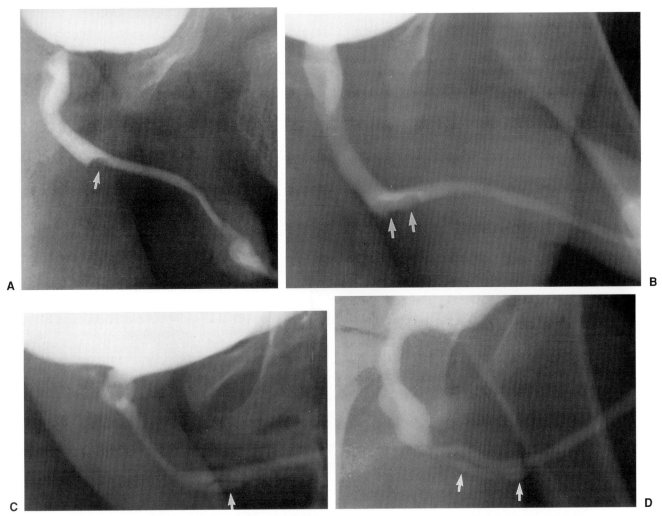

FIG. 9-108. Abnormalities of Cowper gland ducts. A, B: Retention cysts. The filling defects in the floor of the bulbous urethra may be lobular *(arrow)* or bilobed *(arrows)*. **C, D:** Reflux into Cowper gland ducts during VCUG. Reflux into a patulous or ruptured Cowper gland duct may be moderate *(arrow)* or more marked *(arrows)*.

agenesis are often premature. They are stillborn or die soon after birth. Almost all have a characteristic facial appearance, called Potter facies: large, flattened, low-set, cartilage-deficient ears; prominent epicanthal folds; hypertelorism; nasal flattening; and micrognathia. Pulmonary hypoplasia is almost always present, also apparently a result of severe oligohydramnios (by way of intrauterine chest compression), and is frequently complicated by pneumothorax and pneumomediastinum. The ureters are usually absent and the trigone is poorly defined. The renal arteries are absent. Other anomalies of the genitourinary tract and gastrointestinal tract are frequent. Radiologic investigation may be prompted by anuria. No functioning renal tissue can be identified by nuclear scintigraphy, and no renal structure can be clearly identified by US. In renal agenesis, the elongated adrenal gland can assume a cylindrical shape and simulate the appearance

of a kidney on both prenatal and newborn sonography.

The prognosis for a patient with unilateral renal agenesis depends on the status of the other kidney. A solitary kidney usually develops normally and undergoes compensatory hypertrophy. The hypertrophied kidney may be an incidental finding or may, because of its size or ectopic location, be thought an abdominal mass. Damage to a solitary kidney by infection, reflux, calculus disease, or trauma may be lethal.

Intravenous urography, nuclear scintigraphy, and US show that there is only one kidney. The anatomic splenic flexure of the colon occupies the renal fossa in patients with left renal agenesis or ectopia (Fig. 9-109) (244). The colon remains in normal position in patients with left renal dysplasia or left nephrectomy using a posterior, extraperitoneal approach. Nephrectomy performed by an anterior approach mobilizes the colon and produces findings similar to left

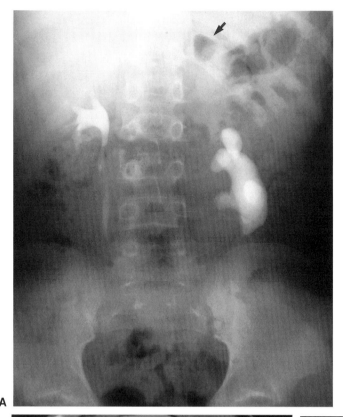

A

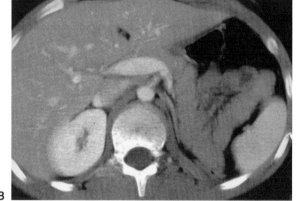

B

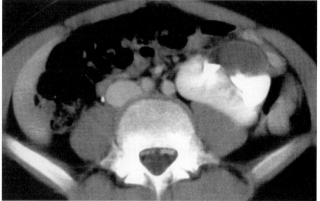

C

FIG. 9-109. Left renal ectopia. A: IVU. The air-filled colon *(arrow)* is above the lesser curvature of the stomach and fills the left renal fossa. The malrotated left kidney is low in position. **B:** CT section at the level of the right kidney. Colon fills the left renal fossa. **C:** CT section at the level of L4. The left kidney is ectopic and malrotated.

renal agenesis or ectopia. Colon that is filled with liquid or stool and located in the left renal fossa can mimic a left kidney at sonography (245). Malformations of the lower urinary tract, genitalia, and other organs are common in patients with unilateral renal agenesis.

Renal Hypoplasia

Renal hypoplasia and dysplasia are the two major developmental aberrations that result in small, malformed kidneys. *Renal hypoplasia* is the term for a congenitally small kidney that shows no pathologic evidence of dysplasia (187). *Simple hypoplasia* refers to a congenitally small kidney re-

sembling a miniaturized normal kidney. There is frequently a reduced number of reniculi, recognized radiologically by a decrease in the number of calyces (187). Hypoplastic kidneys may be ectopic or malrotated and are prone to develop recurrent infection with pyelonephritic scarring.

Segmental hypoplasia is a particular type of unilateral renal hypoplasia, which, when associated with hypertension, has been referred to as the Ask-Upmark kidney. The kidney is small and has a narrow main renal artery and a reduced number of reniculi (187). The characteristic pathologic finding is a transverse groove in the capsular surface over an area of marked parenchymal thinning and an elongated recess arising from the renal pelvis. Radiologically, one sees a small kidney with indentation of the renal outline adjacent to a dilated and elongated expansion of the renal pelvis. These appearances are difficult or impossible to distinguish from chronic pyelonephritis (187). Many observers think that the Ask-Upmark lesion is actually a form of reflux nephropathy; indeed, most such kidneys are found in association with VUR.

Oligonephronic hypoplasia is a rare form of bilateral hypoplasia with extremely small kidneys that are usually unirenicular or birenicular (187). The number of nephrons is greatly reduced, and those that are present are enlarged and hypertrophied. During the early stages of renal failure, IVU may demonstrate the underdeveloped collecting system.

Renal Dysplasia

Renal dysplasia is characterized by disorganization of renal parenchyma associated with abnormally developed and immature nephrons and ductal structures that resemble those normally found during fetal life. Anomalous metanephric differentiation is frequently associated with cyst formation (187). Dysplasia may involve the entire kidney or may affect a particular segment. Dysplastic kidneys are almost invariably found in association with congenital abnormalities of the ureter or lower urinary tract. For this reason, renal dysplasia is best regarded as an anomaly of the entire urinary tract (187). Renal dysplasia is classified into various types: hypoplastic dysplasia; multicystic dysplasia; aplasia; segmental dysplasia of the upper pole of a duplex kidney; and dysplasia associated with bilateral hydronephrosis (187). Radiologic evaluation is helpful not only for distinguishing renal hypoplasia from renal dysplasia but also for clarifying other abnormalities of the urinary tract (187).

Renal Ectopia; Anomalies of Fusion and Rotation

Renal ectopia is the abnormal position of a kidney. It may be due to failure of complete ascent of the kidney from its primitive location at the S1–2 level or to excessive cranial migration. *Renal fusion* is the union of two kidneys. Each kidney maintains its own collecting system. Fusion abnormalities presumably result from failure of separation of primitive nephrogenic cell masses or fusion of the two blastemas during abdominal ascent. Because of their common features and frequent association, renal ectopia, anomalies of fusion, and abnormalities of rotation are grouped together. These renal anomalies are common, occurring in approximately 1 in 500 children.

Renal ectopia is the term used for abnormal position of the kidney without fusion with the opposite kidney. Rarely, the kidney is too high, being located in the posterior thorax. More commonly, the ectopic kidney lies in the lumbar, iliac, or pelvic area and is malrotated. Ectopic kidneys may also be in a cul-de-sac or presacral location. There is a tendency for the calyces, infundibula, and renal pelvis to be positioned on the surface of the kidney, not incorporated into the body of the renal parenchyma (246). This anatomic configuration can make it difficult, on sonography, to identify an ectopic kidney because it may not have the normal central sinus echo complex (246). The abnormal position of the kidney and any malrotation are readily identified on IVU (Fig. 9-109A). CT demonstrates colon filling the left renal fossa if the left kidney is ectopic (Fig. 9-109B) and the abnormal position and rotation of the kidney (Fig 9-109C). The length of the ureter is appropriate for the position of the kidney, which distinguishes renal ectopia from renal ptosis.

Crossed renal ectopia is a condition in which the affected kidney is located entirely or primarily on the opposite side of the abdomen. The ectopic kidney lies below the normal contralateral kidney, and the two organs are almost always fused (Fig. 9-110A). There is usually malrotation of the lower kidney, and both pelves point toward the midline. The ureter of the upper renal component descends normally, on the ipsilateral side into the bladder. The ureter of the crossed ectopic kidney courses from the lower renal component across the midline to enter the bladder on the contralateral side (Fig. 9-110B). Crossed fused ectopia is commonly seen in anorectal malformations. There may be accompanying renal dysplasia or VUR (Fig. 9-110B).

Horseshoe kidney is the most common type of renal fusion, occurring in about 1 in 600 births. There is fusion of the lower poles of the two kidneys across the midline by an isthmus, which usually lies anterior to the aorta and inferior vena cava. The connecting tissue can be functioning renal parenchyma or fibrous tissue. The isthmus prevents complete renal ascent, and horseshoe kidneys lie lower than normal. Moreover, the connecting isthmus also prevents normal renal rotation so that the renal pelves and ureters leave the horseshoe kidney ventrally rather than ventromedially (Fig. 9-111). Lateral films show that both lower poles are located anteriorly. The anomaly may be confirmed by US, and the position and function may be clarified by nuclear scintigraphy or IVU. The hilus of the horseshoe kidney is a complex structure, usually with a multiplicity of renal vessels that arise from and divide nearer to the aorta than normal. The infundibula frequently drain to an extrarenal pelvis. Complications due to the complexity of the renal hilus include obstruction of the upper ureter, pelvis, or infundibula. There is also a slightly increased incidence of Wilms tumor, renovascular hypertension, and adenocarcinoma in patients with horseshoe kidney (3).

It may be difficult to identify a horseshoe kidney by sonography. Overlying bowel obscures the connecting isthmus. Abnormalities of the renal axis and rotation are better shown by IVU (Fig. 9-111). The isthmus of renal tissue may be well demonstrated by renal scintigraphy or CT (Fig. 9-112).

Renal malrotation is the most common and least significant renal anomaly. As the kidney ascends from its original location in the pelvis to its final position opposite the second lumbar vertebra, it undergoes a 90° rotation about its longitu-

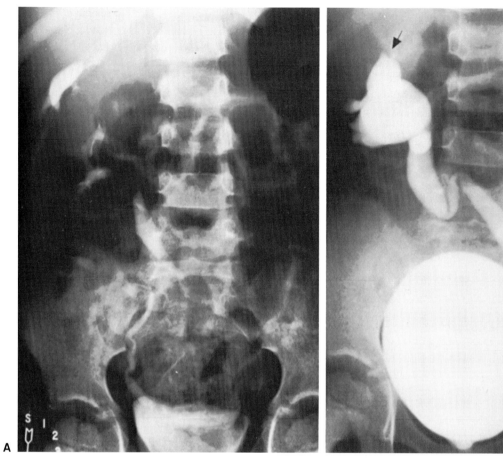

FIG. 9-110. Crossed fused renal ectopia. A 4-year-old boy with urinary tract infection. **A:** IVU. There is fusion of the ectopic lower kidney with the upper kidney. The ureter of the upper renal component descends on the ipsilateral side to enter the right side of the bladder, as expected. The ureter of the crossed lower ectopic kidney passes across the midline to enter the bladder on the left. **B:** VCUG. Vesicoureteral reflux extends up the distal left ureter to the crossed fused ectopic kidney. Note the intrarenal reflux (arrow).

dinal axis. The renal hilus becomes directed medially and slightly forward. If this rotation is deficient or absent, the renal pelvis projects anteromedially or anteriorly. If, as is less common, the rotation is excessive (more than 90°), the pelvis faces posteriorly. In reverse rotation, the kidney rotates outwardly so that the renal pelvis is directed laterally. Renal malrotation is fairly frequent and may occur as an isolated event, either unilaterally or bilaterally. There is an association of malrotation with renal ectopia and anomalies of fusion. Ureteropelvic obstruction is a common complication.

Congenital Megacalyces

Congenital megacalyces is a nonobstructive enlargement of the calyces accompanied by hypoplasia of the medullary pyramids. This entity is important because it can be confused radiologically with obstructive or refluxing hydronephrosis. The nonobstructive nature of this condition should be realized so that needless surgery is avoided. The relatively be-

nign nature of this condition should also be appreciated, so that treatment for any coexisting problem elsewhere is not withheld because the child is thought to have major renal disease (247).

The renal pyramids are well defined, the corticomedullary junction is distinct, and the cortical parenchyma is of normal thickness. The most striking pathologic finding is thinning of the renal medulla. The papillae are flat or inapparent, and the remaining medullary tissue assumes a semilunar configuration (247). The calyx is therefore flat or convex toward the renal surface. The condition is probably a congenital fault in development during early divisions of the ureteral bud as it joins with the metanephric blastema (248,249).

Congenital megacalyces is a benign, nonprogressive condition that usually has no effect on renal function. There may be mild impairment of concentrating ability or occasional stone formation and hematuria (248,249). It is usually discovered in children who are being evaluated for urinary infection, hematuria due to nephrolithiasis, or other abnormalities (247). The incorrect interpretation of the radiologic

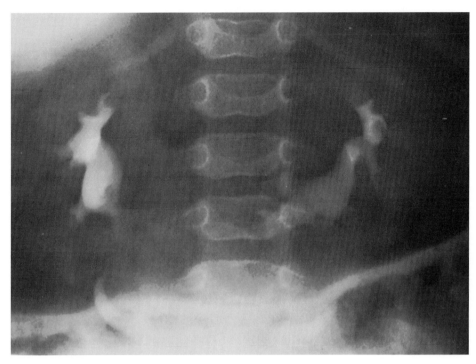

FIG. 9-111. Horseshoe kidney. The lower poles of the kidneys are medial in location, and the axes of the main renal masses are vertical. An isthmus of tissue fuses the lower poles of the two kidneys.

findings may lead to unnecessary surgery. If there is super-imposed renal disease, such as urinary tract infection, it should be treated as if the kidneys were anatomically normal.

The radiologic features of congenital megacalyces are characteristic (Fig. 9-113) (247–249). There is calyceal dilatation, which may affect all or a few of the calyces of one or both kidneys. The infundibula are short and broad and the pelves and ureters are normal. There is no radiologic evidence of obstruction of the ureters, bladder, or urethra. VUR is not a feature of this disease; if present, it is an incidental finding (247). The kidneys are larger than normal

for age, and fetal lobation is prominent. There is an increase in the number of calyces. Moreover, these calyces are polygonal in shape and faceted in appearance (Fig. 9-113) (247). The calyces have no definable fornices or papillary impressions on IVU (247) and renal sonography (250). There is a prompt nephrographic phase on IVU, but opacification of the pelvis and ureters may be delayed because the volume of contrast required to fill the calyces is large. Nephrolithiasis may be present. US shows the increased number of dilated calyces, the normal thickness of the renal cortex, and thinning or attenuation of the medulla (250).

Congenital megacalyces may coexist with primary megaureter. In that circumstance, the presence of congenital megacalyces may only become evident after surgical relief of distal ureteral obstruction (251).

Cystic Diseases of the Kidney

Cystic disease of the kidney is a complex topic. There are a number of proposed classifications (252–259) based on the postulated etiology, pathology, anatomic location of the cysts, and radiologic features. However, the etiology and pathophysiology of most renal cystic diseases is unclear. Histologic features are not specific, and clinical classifications have too much overlap (256). The classification shown in Table 9-14 is modified from previous publications (13,255–258). Unfortunately, certain entities without much clinical similarity are still lumped together. However, perhaps this classification can simplify the approach to renal

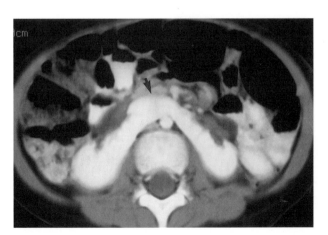

FIG. 9-112. Horseshoe kidney. Contrast-enhanced CT. An isthmus of renal tissue *(arrow)* extends across the midline in front of the aorta and vena cava.

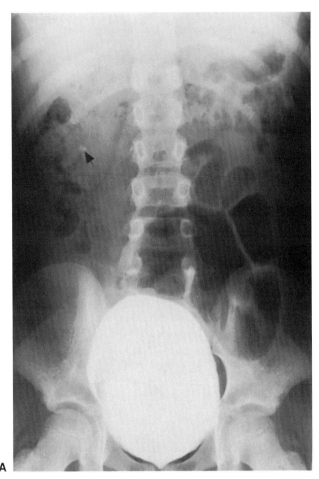

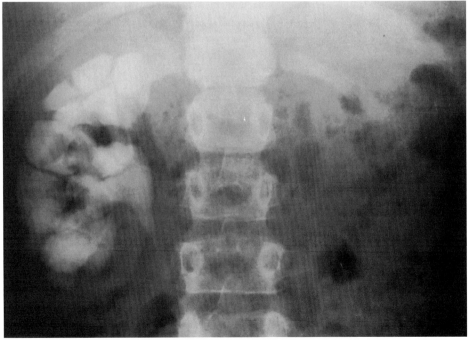

FIG. 9-113. Congenital megacalyces. An 8-year-old boy with urinary tract infection. **A:** Cystogram. There is a right renal stone *(arrow)* and the splenic flexure is located medically. **B:** IVU. The solitary right kidney has an increased number of calyces. These calyces are polygonal in shape and faceted in appearance. The pelvis and ureter are not dilated, and there is no radiologic evidence of ureteral obstruction.

TABLE 9-14. *Renal cysts in children*

Autosomal recessive polycystic kidney disease (ARPCKD)
Autosomal dominant polycystic kidney disease (ADPCKD)
Medullary cystic disease, juvenile nephronophthisis
Glomerulocystic kidney disease
Dysplasia related to obstruction (UPJ, PUV, MCDK)
Syndromic:
    Tuberous sclerosis
    Meckel-Grüber
    Zellweger
    Beckwith-Wiedemann
    von Hippel-Lindau
    Trisomy 13, 18, 21
    Ehlers-Danlos
Simple cysts

UPJ, ureteropelvic junction; PUV, posterior urethral valves; MCDK, multicystic dysplastic kidney.

cystic disease and aid in the understanding of radiologic features. Many cystic diseases have radiologic features that must be understood on an individual basis rather than forced into a system of classification.

Simple Renal Cyst

A simple cyst is the most common adult renal mass. Prior to the use of ultrasound, simple renal cysts were infrequently diagnosed in children, but now they are seen often (260,261). A simple renal cyst is unilocular and solitary and contains a single layer of flattened epithelium with a fibrous wall (261). There is no communication between the cyst cavity and the renal collecting system. Simple renal cysts of the kidneys discovered in children may be detected during evaluation of hematuria following trauma or for other symptoms

unrelated to the cyst (260,261). The pathogenesis of simple renal cysts is unknown. They may represent a focal reaction to intrarenal obstruction or ischemia or be the sequelae of calyceal diverticula (261). Cysts are also seen in end-stage renal disease.

Sonography shows that a simple renal cyst is an anechoic mass with a sharp posterior wall and increased through-transmission (Fig. 9-114). There are no central echoes even at high gain settings (260). Doppler sonography shows no evidence of blood flow within the simple renal cyst and distinguishes it from a vascular abnormality. A complex renal cyst contains other material in addition to fluid. The fluid in a simple cyst is usually serous, but it may be blood from previous trauma or pus related to superimposed infection (260). IVU shows a solitary renal mass that distorts the renal collecting system or produces a lobular external contour. Correlation with clinical presentation and urinalysis should lead one to the appropriate diagnosis or indicate the need for further evaluation. Percutaneous needle puncture is occasionally performed for confirmation. Periodic physical examination, urinalysis, and sonographic examinations are probably the best methods for follow-up (260). In the usual case, neither biopsy nor excision is warranted.

Occasionally, a single cyst is the first sign of previously undiagnosed familial cystic disease of the kidney. If there is any suggestion of a family history of renal disease, sonography of the parents and siblings is warranted. If there is no family history of renal disease, laboratory examinations are normal, and the child is normotensive, further imaging is usually not performed (262). There have been reports of children with renal cysts, hypertension, and elevated renin levels who become normotensive with cyst decompression (263). If the cyst is large (>1 or 2 cm in diameter) or the

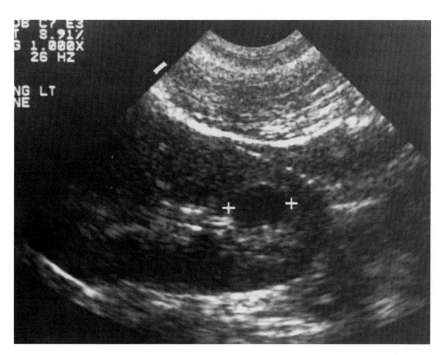

FIG. 9-114. Simple renal cyst. Longitudinal renal sonography demonstrates an anechoic mass *(cursors)* in the lower pole of the left kidney. The wall of the renal cyst is smooth and well defined.

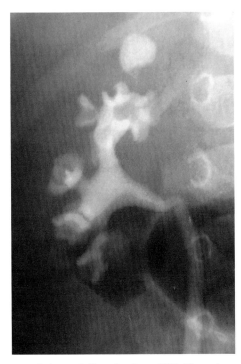

FIG. 9-115. Calyceal diverticulum. IVU. The calyceal diverticulum is attached to a fornix of an upper calyx and fills with contrast material.

patient has flank pain, percutaneous drainage and sclerosis should be considered. An IVU should be performed to exclude the possibility of a calyceal diverticulum.

Calyceal Diverticulum

A calyceal diverticulum is a round, cyst-like structure that connects to the renal collecting system, usually via a fornix, and is lined by transitional epithelium. Calyceal diverticula fill with contrast material on IVU and have a characteristic radiographic appearance (Fig. 9-115). The etiology of calyceal diverticula is unknown. Although usually asymptomatic, incidental imaging findings, large calyceal diverticula may occasionally be painful. Some simple renal cysts may actually be calyceal diverticula that no longer have a demonstrable connection to the collecting system. Calyceal diverticula are not associated with systemic diseases or syndromes.

Autosomal Recessive Polycystic Kidney Disease

Autosomal recessive polycystic kidney disease (ARPCKD), also known as childhood polycystic disease of the kidneys and liver (Potter type I), is inherited as an autosomal recessive trait; there is usually no family history of renal disease. A spectrum of abnormalities includes both microcystic and macrocystic renal disease and variable degrees of hepatic fibrosis and biliary ectasia (252,264,265). The

findings range from severe renal tubular ectasia and minimal liver involvement (infantile polycystic kidney disease) to severe fibrotic liver disease and minimal renal disease (juvenile polycystic kidney disease or renal tubular ectasia with hepatic fibrosis) (259).

Infantile ARPCKD includes perinatal, neonatal, and infantile forms. All three of these entities present within the first several months of life with palpable kidneys and variable degrees of renal failure. There is mild to moderate periportal fibrosis and bile duct proliferation. From 10% to 90% of renal tubules are involved. Numerous small cysts (1–2 mm diameter) are seen in both the cortex and the medulla, and there is hypoplasia and dilatation of the interstitial portions of the collecting tubules. The ultrasonographic appearance is virtually diagnostic; there is renal enlargement with diffusely increased echogenicity of the kidneys (Fig. 9-116) due to small cysts that obscure the normal echo complex of the central collecting system (264). There may be a hypoechoic subcapsular rim of renal tissue, which probably represents the radial orientation of fluid-filled, dilated peripheral tubules (266). Liver echogenicity in the infantile form is usually normal. IVU, although now rarely performed, shows poor renal function and bilateral nephromegaly. Linear striations, attributable to stasis of contrast medium in dilated tubules, radiate from the cortex to the center of the kidney (Fig. 9-116B). MRI demonstrates enlarged lobular kidneys with dilated tubules and absence of corticomedullary differentiation.

Occasionally, renal enlargement in ARPCKD may by asymmetric (264, 267). Sonographic follow-up has shown that absolute renal length may actually decrease as the child grows (268). Enlarged kidneys with echogenic medullary pyramids resembling nephrocalcinosis may rarely be seen (269). Liver disease in ARPCKD seldom dominates the clinical picture in the neonatal period. However, if the infant survives, increased portal echoes due to fibrosis and biliary duct proliferation as well as beaded dilatation of the hepatic ducts may develop (Fig. 9-117).

Juvenile ARPCKD (renal tubular ectasia with congenital hepatic fibrosis) usually presents after 10 years of age with hepatosplenomegaly and portal hypertension. Fewer than 10% of renal tubules are involved, but there is gross hepatic fibrosis. The kidneys are normal or large with cysts of variable size, predominantly in the medulla but also in the cortex. There is marked periportal fibrosis and bile duct proliferation. IVU may show only a faint pyramidal blush resembling renal tubular ectasia in the adult. Because both renal tubular ectasia (a normal variant in the adult) and medullary sponge kidney seldom occur in childhood, one should suspect juvenile polycystic kidney disease in a child with the radiologic features of tubular ectasia. US demonstrates kidneys that are normal in size or enlarged. There is marked echogenicity of the kidney, with loss of the normal corticomedullary junction. Increased echogenicity may also be present in the liver because of hepatic fibrosis.

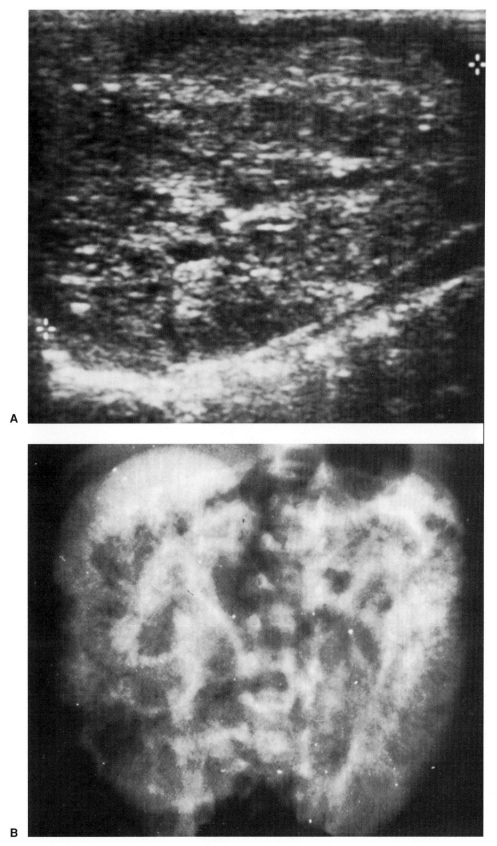

FIG. 9-116. Autosomal recessive polycystic kidney disease. A: Renal sonography. Longitudinal sonography demonstrates a markedly enlarged and echogenic kidney *(cursors)*. The other kidney was similar. **B:** IVU. There is stasis of contrast material within ectatic tubules, which radiate from the peripheral cortex toward the renal pelvis. The small white dots are artifactual.

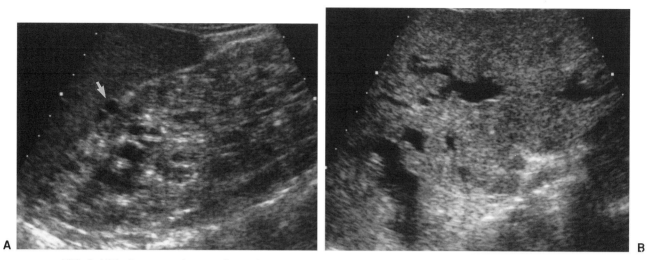

FIG. 9-117. Autosomal recessive polycystic kidney disease. A: Longitudinal renal sonography. The kidney *(arrows)* is enlarged and markedly echogenic and has tiny peripheral cysts. **B:** Transverse liver sonography. There is beaded dilatation of the hepatic ducts.

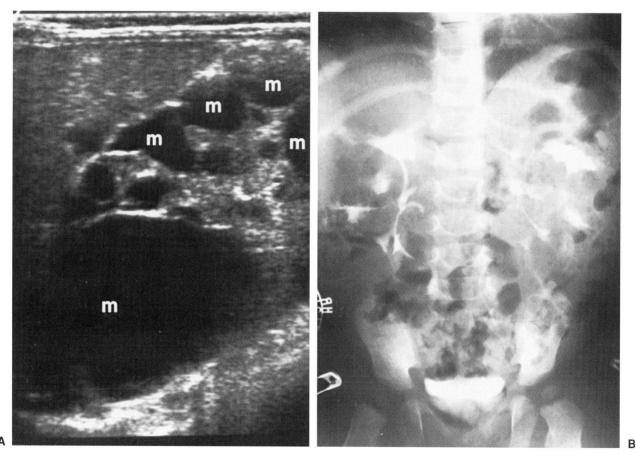

FIG. 9-118. Autosomal dominant polycystic kidney disease. A 1-year-old boy with bilateral flank masses and a paternal history of kidney disease. **A:** Longitudinal sonography of the right kidney demonstrates renal enlargement and many large anechoic masses *(m)* with good through-transmission. **B:** IVU. There is bilateral nephromegaly and gross distortion of the calyces.

Autosomal Dominant Polycystic Kidney Disease

Autosomal dominant polycystic kidney disease (ADPCKD), also known as adult polycystic disease of the kidneys and liver (Potter type III), has variable penetrance. Sporadic cases occur. The cysts are of variable size and involve both cortex and medulla. There are intervening areas of normal parenchyma. As the cysts enlarge, normal tissue is compressed and destroyed, and the collecting system becomes distorted. Hepatic cysts occur in approximately one third of adults with the disease, but there is usually no periportal fibrosis. Cysts may also be found in the pancreas, lungs, spleen, ovaries, seminal vesicles, and testes. Approximately 10% of patients have intracranial berry aneurysms.

Although it is common, ADPCKD usually is not diagnosed until early adulthood when hypertension, hematuria, or renal failure begin to appear. The process is slowly progressive; the average patient succumbs at the age of 50. However, ADPCKD can appear in the neonate as a unilateral or bilateral abdominal mass (27). Therefore, the designation ''adult polycystic disease'' is not really correct. In fact, US of the fetus may suggest the diagnosis (270). The family history is usually diagnostic. Children with ADPCKD may also present with one or only a few detectable renal cysts that slowly progress to multiple cysts.

IVU, if performed, shows enlarged kidneys with grossly distorted calyces and pelves (Fig. 9-118B). The disease is always bilateral pathologically, although it may be asymmetric radiologically. US shows enlarged kidneys with anechoic masses (Fig. 9-118A). During infancy the sonographic and IVU findings of ADPCKD may be similar to those of ARPCKD (13). As the child becomes older, the cysts coalesce and assume the typical adult appearance. CT shows

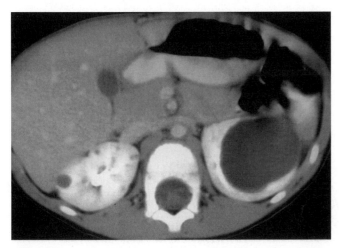

FIG. 9-119. Autosomal dominant polycystic kidney disease. Contrast-enhanced CT. There is a large cyst in the left kidney. There are many cysts of varying size in the right kidney. Note that the renal tissue between the cysts enhances normally.

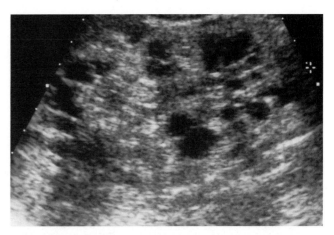

FIG. 9-120. Glomerulocystic disease. A 3-year-old girl with bilateral flank masses. The enlarged, echogenic kidneys contain many cysts. The sonographic appearance is indistinguishable from autosomal recessive and autosomal dominant polycystic kidney disease.

normal enhancing renal tissue between cysts of varying size (Fig. 9-119). Normal renal sonography in infancy does not exclude ADPCKD (271). Cysts in other organs are usually not detectable by sonography until adolescence or adulthood (272,273).

Glomerulocystic Kidney Disease

Glomerulocystic kidney disease (GCKD) is a rare disorder characterized by cystic dilatation of Bowman's space and the first portion of the proximal convoluted tubule. The etiology is unknown; most cases are sporadic. Occasionally, the disease occurs in association with the cerebrohepatorenal and orofacial-digital syndromes (274). The kidneys become enlarged and echogenic early in infancy. Small cortical cysts are sometimes identified (274,275). As the child grows, the kidney length may normalize for age (274). The renal sonographic appearance may be indistinguishable from polycystic kidney disease (Fig. 9-120). The identification of normal hypoechoic medullary pyramids suggests GCKD rather than ARPCKD (276). Liver cysts may be present in infants with GCKD (277). The diagnosis of GCKD is established definitively by renal biopsy.

Cystic Dysplasia Associated with Lower Urinary Tract Obstruction

Cystic dysplasia can coexist with severe hydroureteronephrosis caused by lower urinary tract obstruction. The most common etiology is posterior urethral valves. The cystic dysplasia is usually apparent at sonography or IVU (278). Occasionally, reflux during VCUG fills the multiple dysplastic tubules and cysts (Fig. 9-121). As previously discussed, multicystic dysplastic kidney is another example, due to ureteropelvic obstruction, of cystic dysplasia of the kidney.

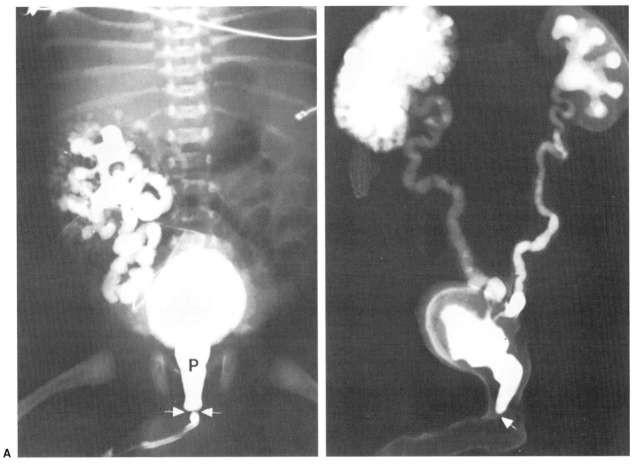

FIG. 9-121. Cystic dysplasia due to obstruction. Newborn boy with renal failure and poor urinary stream. **A:** Portable cystogram shows vesicoureteral reflux on the right and filling of many intrarenal dysplastic cysts. There is dilatation of the posterior urethra *(P)* due to partial obstruction by posterior urethral valves *(arrows)*. **B:** Postmortem injection shows obstruction by posterior urethral valves *(arrow)*, a thick-walled bladder, bilateral vesicoureteral reflux, and filling of many dysplastic cysts of the right kidney.

Juvenile Nephronophthisis and Medullary Cystic Disease

Juvenile nephronophthisis and medullary cystic disease of the kidney are related hereditary diseases characterized by polyuria, polydipsia, decreased renal concentrating ability, anemia, and eventual renal failure (279). Tubulointerstitial nephritis and medullary cysts are present (280). *Juvenile nephronophthisis* tends to become symptomatic in childhood and is inherited as an autosomal recessive trait; *medullary cystic* disease becomes symptomatic in adulthood and is inherited as an autosomal dominant trait (279). Symptoms of juvenile nephronophthisis are usually apparent by age 5 and progress to overt renal insufficiency in adolescence (280). The cysts in medullary cystic disease are clearly evident macroscopically, whereas in juvenile nephronophthisis they usually are not (281). Some patients with juvenile nephronophthisis have extrarenal manifestations including congenital hepatic fibrosis and cone-shaped epiphyses (272, 282).

US demonstrates small kidneys, diffuse increased parenchymal echogenicity (Fig. 9-122) due to microscopic cysts, a widened central echo pattern that may be due to small cysts, and well-defined cystic structures when larger medullary cysts predominate (282). Visible macrocysts are uncommon in juvenile nephronophthisis (280). IVU shows reduction in kidney size and a prolonged nephrogram (281). There is diminished excretion of contrast material. Medullary tubular ectasia is a common finding but usually is only apparent by retrograde pyelography, which sometimes also opacifies medullary cysts. Renal biopsy is necessary to confirm the diagnosis, although this may be complicated by a perirenal hematoma (281), due to loss of cortical tissue next to large vessels on the surface of the fibrotic kidney (281).

Hydrometrocolpos

Hydrocolpos is a dilatation of the vagina proximal to a congenital obstruction. If the uterus is also dilated, the condition is termed *hydrometrocolpos* (283). If the obstruction is at the level of the cervix and only the uterus dilates, it forms

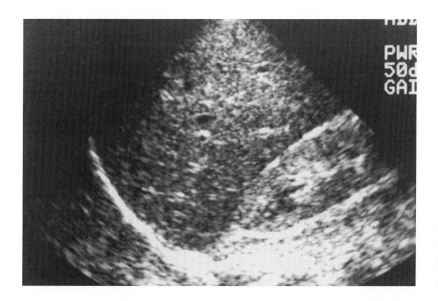

FIG. 9-122. Juvenile nephronophthisis. An 11-year-old boy with anemia, protein-uria, and mild renal failure. Longitudinal sonography shows a small right kidney, decreased in both length and volume. There is a marked increase in renal parenchymal echogenicity.

a *hydrometra*. The dilatation is due to accumulation of secre-tions (Fig. 9-123). The dilated vagina and uterus usually produce a palpable, fixed midline mass (Fig. 9-124). If large enough, the mass can cause obstruction of venous return from the lower extremities, ureteral obstruction, and hydro-nephrosis. Occasionally, there is associated plastic, adhesive peritonitis due to the retrograde passage of secretions through the fallopian tubes into the peritoneal cavity.

Imperforate Hymen

If the vaginal obstruction is due to an imperforate hymen, the condition is fairly benign. This type of vaginal obstruc-tion may be found during the neonatal period but is more commonly recognized during early adolescence when men-ses begin (Fig. 9-124). There is no increased incidence of congenital anomalies elsewhere in patients with imperforate hymen.

Vaginal or Cervical Atresia

If the obstruction is due to atresia, it is a serious congenital malformation often manifest during the neonatal period (Fig. 9-123). Almost all patients with vaginal or cervical stenosis or atresia have other congenital anomalies, usually multiple and severe (283). These anomalies include rectogenital fistu-las, bicornuate uterus, urogenital sinus, renal hypoplasia or agenesis, ectopic ureter, imperforate anus, gastrointestinal atresias, and congenital heart disease.

Imaging

Plain films may show a lower, midline abdominal mass (Fig. 9-123A). US confirms the presence of a tubular midline mass arising from the pelvis. The mass is cystic and contains scattered echoes suggesting cellular debris, mucoid material, or blood in the dilated vagina and uterus (Figs. 9-123 and 9-124) (284). US also demonstrates the anatomy of the uterus and kidneys. Cross-sectional imaging, such as MRI, may help confirm the nature of the mass (Fig. 9-124B).

Imperforate Vagina with Vaginourethral Communication

Imperforate vagina with vaginourethral communication is an unusual congenital anomaly characterized by an imper-forate vagina with otherwise normal external genitalia (285). There is communication between the patent proximal vagina and a normal female urethra. Hydrometrocolpos may be present at birth.

This anomaly is the result of defective development of the lower urogenital tract. It probably represents a rare form of persistence of the primitive urogenital sinus, coincident with the failure of distal migration of the primitive vaginal plate or failure of development or canalization of the distal vagina (285). Recognition of this anomaly is of practical importance. Failure to close the vaginourethral communica-tion at the time of definitive vaginoplasty may result in con-tinuing pooling of urine and secretion in the vagina leading to vaginitis, perineal irritation, and urinary tract infection (285). Contrast material appearing in a hydrocolpos during excretory urography or VCUG is an indirect sign of vagi-nourethral or vesicovaginal communication. The communi-cation is best shown on the voiding films of a VCUG with the patient in the lateral position. Selective injection may be necessary for precise demonstration (285).

Cryptorchidism

During prenatal development, the testicle becomes at-tached to fibers of the gubernaculum, a cord-like structure

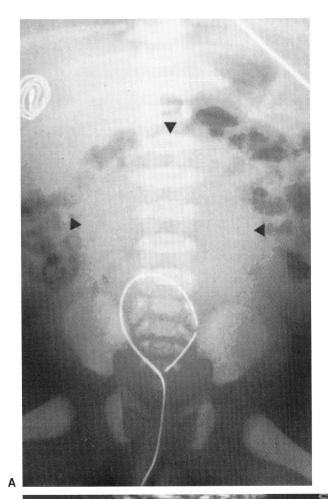

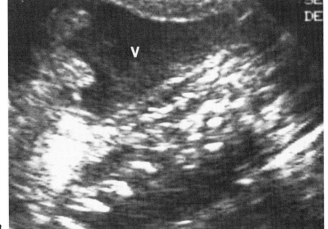

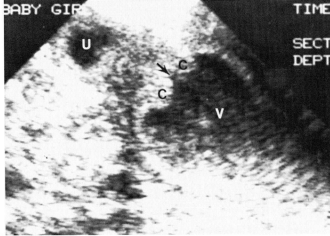

FIG. 9-123. Hydrometrocolpos due to vaginal atresia. Newborn female with a central, fixed abdominal mass. **A:** Abdominal radiograph with catheter draining bladder. There is a large, midline soft-tissue mass *(arrowheads)*. **B:** Longitudinal pelvic sonography. There is marked dilatation of the vagina *(V)*. **C:** Longitudinal sonography of the lower abdomen. There is marked dilatation of the vagina *(V)* and mild dilatation of the uterine cavity *(U)*. Note the lips of the cervix *(C)* and the cervical os *(arrow)*.

extending from the testis to the scrotum, at the site of the future inguinal canal. The contractile muscle fibers of the gubernaculum are believed to cause the testicle to migrate through the inguinal canal into the scrotum. Testicular descent into the scrotum normally occurs in the seventh month of gestation. However, approximately 4% of boys have an undescended testicle at birth. This number decreases to 1.8% at 1 month of age and 0.8% at 9 months (286). Withdrawal of maternal estrogen at birth causes a rise in testosterone

and stimulation of testicular descent (286). Spontaneous testicular descent does not occur after the age of 1 year. Cryptorchidism is bilateral in 30% of cases. Complications of cryptorchidism include infertility, increased risk of malignancy in the cryptorchid testis, an associated inguinal hernia, torsion of the undescended testis, and the psychological effects of the empty scrotum. An undescended testis is histologically normal at birth; developmental failure and atrophy are noted by the end of the first year of life, and there is a

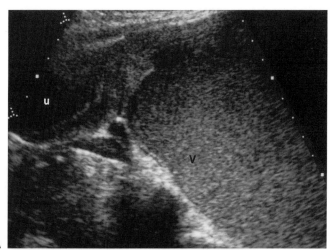

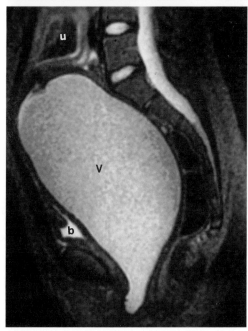

FIG. 9-124. Hydrometrocolpos due to imperforate hymen. A 12-year-old girl with a large pelvic mass. **A:** Longitudinal pelvic sonography. Echogenic material is seen within the markedly distended vagina *(v)*. There is only mild distention of the uterus *(u)*. **B:** T2-weighted MRI. The urinary bladder is nearly empty *(b)*. There is distention of the vagina *(V)* and uterine cavity *(u)*.

dramatic reduction in the number of germ cells by 2 years of age. Orchiopexy is therefore usually performed between 1 and 2 years of age. It should be stressed that cryptorchid testes may coexist with other congenital anomalies, including the prune-belly syndrome, imperforate anus, Noonan syndrome, intersex abnormalities, and various urologic abnormalities (287–292).

The undescended testicle is palpable in 80% of boys with cryptorchidism. Of testes that are cryptorchid or otherwise not palpable, 15% are at the external inguinal ring, 55% are

in the inguinal canal, 20% are intraabdominal, and 10% are absent because of agenesis or in utero torsion.

Because the majority of cryptorchid testes are located in the inguinal canal, US should be performed first (Fig. 9-125). The normal testis is scanned to confirm its size and parenchymal echogenicity. Then, on the affected side, careful scanning of the path of descent (renal hilum, iliac vessels, inguinal canal, and scrotum) is performed. An undescended testis may be located anywhere along this normal path of descent, The processus vaginalis is usually patent. An ectopic testis descends normally but is located in a subcutaneous, extrascrotal position.

Undescended, dysplastic testes are sometimes confused with lymph nodes. The bulbous end of the gubernaculum might also be mistaken for an undescended testicle (293).

MRI provides multiplanar imaging of the inguinal and retroperitoneal regions; it is more sensitive than US to intra-abdominal testes. Undescended testes, like scrotal testes, are usually hypointense on T1-weighted images and hyperintense on T2-weighted images. However, if the testis is dysplastic and atrophic, it may not be hyperintense on T2-weighted sequences (294–296).

Ambiguous Genitalia

The discovery of ambiguous genitalia prompts radiologic evaluation (297). The phenotypic sex of an individual is determined by numerous factors. An intersex state exists when there are contradictions in the morphology of the genital tract. An evaluation of intersex problems requires prompt assignment of sex before gender imprinting complicates reassignment (29). The incidence of ambiguous genitalia is somewhere between 1 in 700 births (if perineal hypospadias is included [297]) and 1 in 1500 births (29). Diagnostic studies that may be used include sex chromatin pattern, external genital anatomy, internal genital anatomy,

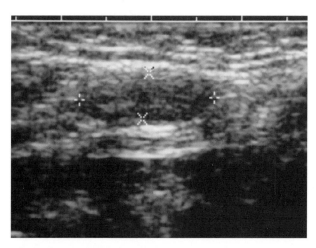

FIG. 9-125. Inguinal testis. A 5-year-old boy with empty left scrotum. Longitudinal sonogram of the left inguinal region demonstrates a left testis *(between cursors)*.

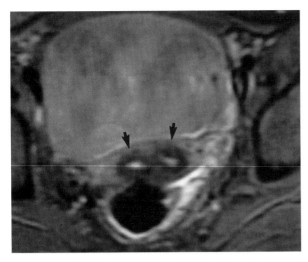

FIG. 9-126. Uterine didelphys. Axial proton density MRI. Two separate cervices *(arrows)* are identified.

urinary hormonal excretion, and gonadal biopsy (29). Not all of these evaluations are needed for the neonatal assignment of gender.

Internal genital anatomy is well characterized by sonography. US readily establishes the presence or absence of a vagina and uterus during the neonatal period. Investigation of the sex chromatin pattern and urinary hormone excretion and biopsy of the gonads should be carried out later before definitive surgery. Genitography may be used to demonstrate the anatomy of the genital passages and the presence or absence of a vaginal cavity. MRI may be used to search for undescended testes, and map uterine and vaginal anatomy (Fig. 9-126) (312).

Sexual Differentiation

The genetic sex of the embryo is determined at the time of fertilization. However, the gonads of the developing embryo do not develop gender-specific characteristics until the seventh week of gestation. At this time, the primordial germ cells migrate from the yolk sac to the undifferentiated gonads. The Y chromosome directs differentiation of the gonads into testes, causing development of the primary sex cords into seminiferous tubules. In the absence of a Y chromosome and the presence of two X chromosomes, normal ovaries develop. If there is only one X chromosome (Turner syndrome), dysgenetic or streak ovaries develop (298).

The gonads subsequently determine the differentiation of the other internal and external genitalia. The presence of testicular androgens leads to differentiation of the mesonephric (Wolffian) duct into the epididymis, vas deferens, and seminal vesicles. Müllerian-inhibiting factor, also produced by each testis, causes involution of the ipsilateral paramesonephric (Müllerian) duct. If this factor is absent, but testicular androgens are present, Müllerian structures may continue to develop in an otherwise normal male. In the

absence of both androgens and Müllerian inhibiting factor, and even in the absence of ovaries, the mesonephric ducts regress and the paramesonephric ducts develop into fallopian tubes, the uterus, and the upper vagina (299). Nontesticular androgens can virilize an otherwise normal female fetus; these androgens are most commonly produced by the fetal adrenal gland.

Types of Intersex Abnormalities

Genital ambiguity includes cryptorchidism, fused labia, incomplete scrotal fusion, small penis, clitoral hypertrophy, epispadias, and hypospadias. Imaging evaluation may require US, VCUG, genitography, and MRI.

There are many ways to classify intersex abnormalities (300). The most common classification is as follows, in order of decreasing frequency: female pseudohermaphroditism, male pseudohermaphroditism, gonadal dysgenesis, and true hermaphroditism.

Female pseudohermaphroditism is the presence of ovaries but masculinization of the lower genital tract and external genitalia. There is usually an enlarged clitoris and prominent, fused labia. Congenital adrenal hyperplasia, due to 21-hydroxylase deficiency, is by far the most common cause of female pseudohermaphroditism (Fig. 9-127). Serum sodium and chloride should be assayed and the skin chromatin pattern determined. Clitoral hypertrophy and hirsutism may also occur in older girls due to excessive androgen effect from an adrenal adenoma or carcinoma. US confirms the genetic sex by demonstrating the ovaries and uterus. Occasionally, female pseudohermaphroditism may be idiopathic.

Male pseudohermaphroditism is the presence of testes but feminized genitalia. It is due to decreased androgen production or an abnormal response by target organs (testicular feminization syndrome). Although US may not always be successful in locating undescended testes, it can exclude the presence of ovaries and uterus.

Gonadal dysgenesis includes a variety of abnormalities characterized by having at least one streak gonad. Streak gonads do not elaborate normal hormones and are at increased risk of malignancy (301–305).

True hermaphroditism is the presence of ovarian and testicular tissue in the same individual. The ovaries and testes may be separate at the sides of the pelvis or joined as an ovotestis. Internal and external genital anatomy is variable, and the presence of the uterus depends on Müllerian stimulation. US can identify the uterus if it is present and occasionally visualizes the gonads for biopsy. Final diagnosis is based on the histology of the gonads. This is a very rare and poorly understood condition.

Classification by Genitography

Shopfner described a classification for the genitographic findings in patients with ambiguous genitalia (29). One of

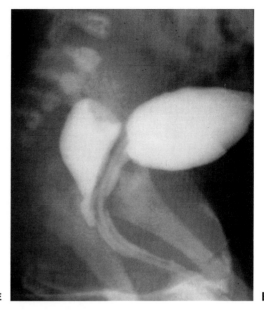

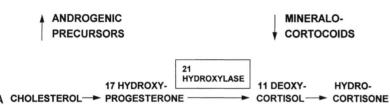

FIG. 9-127. Adrenogenital syndrome. A: Adrenogenital syndrome due to deficiency of the enzyme 21-hydroxylase. Due to block of the synthetic pathway, there is decreased mineralocorticoid production with an increase in androgenic precursors leading to virilization. **B:** VCUG. There is reflux of contrast material from the urogenital sinus into the vagina. Note the cervical impression at the apex of the vagina.

the limitations of genitography is that it demonstrates only the anatomy that communicates with the exterior. However, when the results of sonography, VCUG, genitography, and MRI are integrated, it is usually possible to assign a practical gender to an intersex patient (29). One should consider intersex anomalies as deviations from the normal female; any fetus will develop into a female in the absence of testes (29).

Type I anatomy is normal female urethral structures with clitoral hypertrophy. The urethra is female and a normal vagina is present (Fig. 9-128A). This condition is usually caused by androgenizing (masculinizing) effect on the genital tubercle (29). Type II is the anatomy of the female pseudohermaphrodite. It is due to an abnormality of induction caused by congenital adrenal cortical hyperplasia, i.e., administration of androgenizing hormones to the mother during the first months of pregnancy. It may also be a congenital condition associated with anal atresia or an idiopathic anomaly (29). US demonstrates ovaries, a uterus, and a vagina. There is a fairly long urogenital sinus with a normal, short female urethra and a normal vagina entering this sinus (Fig. 9-128B). Type III represents even more masculinization of the internal genitalia (Fig. 9-128C). The urogenital sinus is small, and there is lengthening of the urethra but without a verumontanum. A fully formed uterus is present. The gonads may be testes, ovotestes, or gonadal streaks. Type IV is even more masculinized. The vagina is extremely small and may or may not be capped by a rudimentary uterus. The urethra is definitely male with a verumontanum (Fig. 9-128D). The vagina may open into the posterior urethra rather than the perineum (29). Type V is due to additional masculinization, the fetal vagina remaining in its original position to produce

the utricle (Fig. 9-128E). The urethra lengthens and has a verumontanum. A uterus is not present. The urethral orifice may be perineal or hypospadiac. Type VI or hypospadias is in reality a variant of an intersex state as it represents incomplete masculinization of the external genitalia (29). The urethral orifice may be hypospadiac or perineal, and a verumontanum and utricle are present (Fig. 9-128F).

Imaging

Radiologic evaluation is performed urgently, not emergently, and is done for psychosocial reasons. A genitogram or VCUG shows the anatomy of the urethra, vagina, and utricle. A urogenital sinus is usually present (Fig. 9-127B). A cervical impression on the superior margin of the vagina distinguishes it from an enlarged utricle (male analog of the vagina). However, absence of a visible cervical impression by genitography does not exclude the presence of a uterus. Accurate demonstration of the junction between the vagina and the urethra is extremely helpful for surgical planning (306,307).

Ultrasound is able to identify uterus and ovaries. The kidneys and adrenal glands should also be examined. Although the adrenal glands may be large or have a cerebriform contour in congenital adrenal hyperplasia, normal-appearing adrenal glands do not exclude the diagnosis (308–310). US may identify an ovotestis in true hermaphroditism (311). Although MRI has been used to demonstrate the internal genitalia in patients with intersex states, it is probably most helpful in verifying uterine anomalies (4,312).

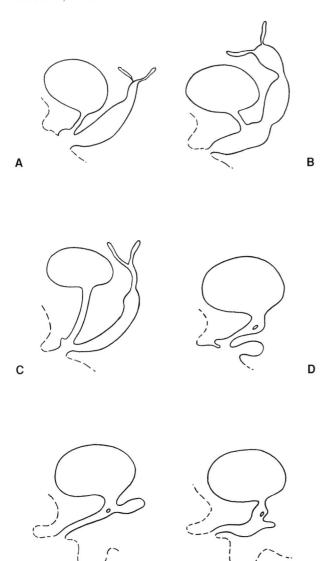

FIG. 9-128. Intersex states. Classification of genitographic findings in patients with ambiguous genitalia. **A**, type I; **B**, type II; **C**, type III; **D**, type IV; **E**, type V; **F**, type VI. Modified from Shopfner (29).

Cloacal Malformation

Cloacal malformation, which is quite different from cloacal exstrophy, is a persistence of an early embryonic state in which the urinary, genital, and gastrointestinal tracts all drain through a common perineal opening (Fig. 9-129A). This rare anomaly has an incidence of 1 in 50,000 newborns (313) and occurs only in genotypic girls. There have been reports of the prenatal diagnosis of cloacal malformation (314).

Although not completely understood, the cloacal malformation is believed to result from failure of the urorectal septum (separating the allantois from the hindgut) to join the cloacal membrane during the fourth to sixth week of embryonic life. This produces a channel called a cloaca (Latin for ''sewer'').

There are different types of cloacal malformations, depending on the way in which the three systems join. The cloacal channel may have a urethral configuration or a (wider) vaginal configuration. It may join the urinary tract at the level of the urethra so that there is a normal urinary sphincter and a well-formed proximal urethra. However, the cloacal channel may join the urinary tract at the level of the urinary bladder. In this type of cloaca, there is no mechanism for continence, the urethra and urethral sphincter being absent. The rectal communication is usually at the level of the vagina or cloaca. If there is a septated (double) vagina, as is common, the rectum usually inserts into its midline septum. In the cloacal variant, an anteriorly placed anus exits through the perineum just posterior to a urogenital sinus (315).

Plain radiographs demonstrate a pelvic mass, usually a distended vagina or uterus and not the bladder. Gas within the pelvic mass implies a rectal communication (283). Calcified meconium peritonitis may be seen because of gastrointestinal or vaginal perforation (316). Meconium can also enter the peritoneal cavity through dilated Fallopian tubes without any demonstrable vaginal or gastrointestinal perforation (283,317,318). Intraluminal colonic calcifications in the fetus or neonate occur when fetal urine and meconium are in contact with each other; this implies a cloacal malformation in a girl or an imperforate anus with a urinary-rectal fistula in a boy. Imperforate anus in a girl does not result in the mixing of fetal urine and meconium because the colonic communication is with the vagina and not the urinary tract (233). Intraluminal calcifications are also found in cases of multiple intestinal atresias as is discussed in Chapter 8.

Water-soluble contrast material should be injected into the cloaca. After demonstration of the anatomy, a catheter can be advanced into the bladder and a VCUG performed. Over half of girls with the cloacal malformation will have VUR, sometimes of high grade (315).

A diverting colostomy is performed to separate the fecal stream from the urinary tract (319). Prior to definitive surgical repair, the distal limb of the colostomy is injected to demonstrate the anatomy and clarify the site of rectal communication (Fig. 9-129).

The bony structures and spinal cord should be assessed in all patients with the cloacal malformation. There is a 40% incidence of agenesis or hypoplasia of the sacrum, a 70% incidence of pubic diastasis, and a 14% incidence of spinal dysraphism (315). Pubic diastasis occurs in patients with the more severe anomalies, including duplication of the bladder, absent vagina, and vaginal malposition (315,320). Approximately one half of patients with the cloacal malformation will also have abnormalities of the spinal cord, usually tethering (315). Normal plain radiographs of the spine do not exclude spinal cord abnormalities. Spinal sonography in the neonatal period is an excellent screening examination for diagnosing tethering of the cord. In older children, evaluation for a tethered cord requires MRI (321).

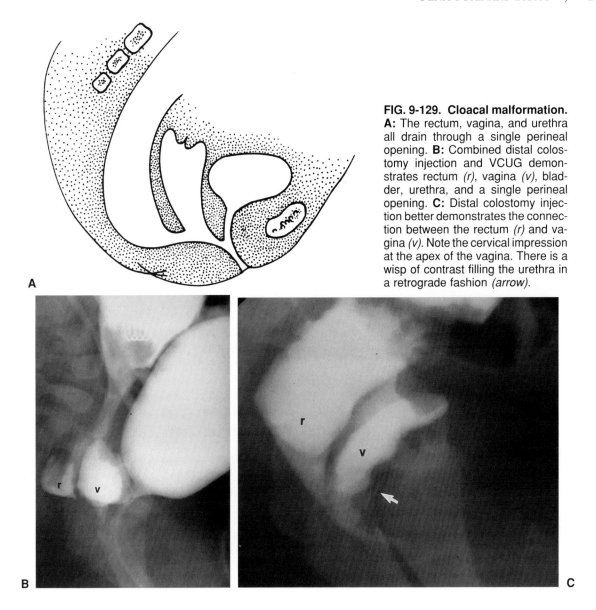

FIG. 9-129. Cloacal malformation. A: The rectum, vagina, and urethra all drain through a single perineal opening. **B:** Combined distal colostomy injection and VCUG demonstrates rectum *(r)*, vagina *(v)*, bladder, urethra, and a single perineal opening. **C:** Distal colostomy injection better demonstrates the connection between the rectum *(r)* and vagina *(v)*. Note the cervical impression at the apex of the vagina. There is a wisp of contrast filling the urethra in a retrograde fashion *(arrow)*.

Cloacal Exstrophy

Cloacal exstrophy, which is quite different from the cloacal malformation, is the most severe anomaly in the bladder exstrophy-epispadias spectrum. There is failure of fusion of the infraumbilical midline structures at the cloacal stage of embryonic development. Although the external abnormalities in the cloacal malformation may be subtle at birth, cloacal exstrophy is obvious. The usual components of cloacal exstrophy are omphalocele, imperforate anus, exstrophy of two hemibladders, lateral cecal fissure between the two hemibladders, ambiguous genitalia, and spinal dysraphism (322). The ileum may prolapse through the cecal defect and sometimes looks like an elephant's trunk. In the cloacal malformation, all affected individuals are genetic females; in cloacal exstrophy, two thirds are genetic males. Because the phallus is rudimentary, most boys undergo orchiectomy and are reared as girls (322).

Cloacal exstrophy is extremely rare, occurring in 1 in 200,000 to 1 in 400,000 live births (323–325). It is believed to result from premature disruption of the cloacal membrane prior to complete descent of the urorectal septum (323,326); prenatal sonography suggests that this is not the complete explanation (327). The occurrence of cloacal exstrophy in siblings suggests a genetic basis (328,329).

The symphysis pubis is always widely diastatic (Fig. 9-130). There is an increased incidence of spinal dysraphism (Fig. 9-130), scoliosis, kyphosis, and club feet (330). Renal ectopia is common (331).

Patients are usually repaired during the first few days of life to prevent bacterial colonization of the exposed viscera. This repair includes separation of the urinary and intestinal tracts, joining of the two hemibladders (usually with an enteric augmentation cystoplasty), colonic pull-through or colostomy, orchiectomy in genetic males, and closure of the

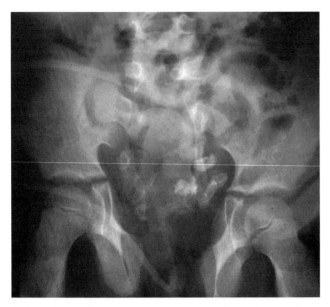

FIG. 9-130. Cloacal exstrophy and spinal dysraphism. There is wide separation of the pubic bones. Note the bony changes of sacral dysraphism. There are several calculi in a pelvic kidney.

abdominal wall defect (322). Despite the high frequency of undescended testes and malrotation (332), imaging for these abnormalties is not performed until primary surgical repair has been performed.

After surgery and stabilization, the infant should be screened for abnormalities of the spinal cord. There is a 50% to 100% incidence of occult abnormalities of the spinal cord (224,333–335). It is not clear whether sonography or MRI should be performed to evaluate for cord tethering and other anomalies.

Most genetic females with cloacal exstrophy have two widely separated vaginas and hemiuteri; obstruction of the genital tract at various levels is common (336). If possible, the better formed vagina is brought to the perineum and the other is excised. Definitive vaginal reconstruction can be deferred for several years but must be performed before puberty to allow for the egress of menstrual flow (322). Genitography, ultrasonography, and MRI of pelvic structures are helpful in the evaluation of cloacal exstrophy.

Prune-Belly Syndrome

The classic triad of the prune-belly (Eagle-Barrett) syndrome is hypoplasia of the abdominal muscles, cryptorchidism, and abnormalities of the urinary system (Fig. 9-131A). Other abnormalities may include microcephaly, scoliosis, hip dislocation, foot and leg deformities, polydactyly, syndactyly, pectus deformities, congenital heart disease, intestinal malrotation, and imperforate anus. The kidneys have a decrease in the number of functioning nephrons, varying degrees of dysplasia, and sometimes cystic changes. The ureters and bladder show patchy absence of smooth muscle, replaced by fibrous collagenous tissue. The prune-belly syndrome occurs almost exclusively in boys.

There appear to be two groups of patients with prune-belly syndrome. The first group has an obstructing lesion of the urethra that leads to death shortly after birth. The obstruction may be urethral atresia or posterior urethral valves. The bladder is hypertrophied and has a large urachal diverticulum; the kidneys are severely hydronephrotic with cystic dysplasia due to obstruction. In the second group of patients, there is a functional abnormality of bladder emptying but no urethral obstruction. The urinary bladder in these patients is usually large, a urachal diverticulum is frequently present (Fig. 9-131B), severe hydronephrosis is noted, and the urethra has an abnormal configuration. The second group survives the neonatal period and may develop chronic urinary tract problems (13).

A variety of radiologic findings have been described in the prune-belly syndrome (Fig. 9-131). These abnormalities include bulging flanks, gaseous distention of bowel, flaring of the lower ribs, flared iliac wings, decreased iliac indices, renal agenesis, hydronephrosis, ureteral atresia, trabeculated bladder tapering toward an umbilical attachment, bladder diverticula, patent urachus, VUR, tapering of the bladder base into a dilated posterior urethra, dilated prostatic utricle, urethral valves, urethral diverticulum, urethral stenosis, urethral atresia, and megalourethra (337). Calcifications in a urachal cyst and in the dome of the bladder have also been reported (337). These calcifications are probably related to urinary stasis.

Infection

Urinary Tract Infection

UTI is the most common disease of the urinary tract in children and the second most common site of infection (61,154,338), exceeded only by the upper respiratory tract. Overt UTIs occur in approximately 5% to 10% and asymptomatic bacteriuria is present in 1% to 2% of all school-aged girls (145,339). UTI frequently occurs during infancy and is especially common in the neonate. Not only is UTI exceedingly common, but it is also dangerous because of the frequency of delay in diagnosis and treatment, the high relapse rate, and the potential for damage leading to chronic renal disease.

Definition

A UTI is defined as the presence of bacteria in the urine and is documented by culture of a properly collected specimen. A bacterial count of more than 100,000 colonies/ml^3 of a single organism in urine collected by the midstream clean-catch method is considered to represent infection. Fewer than 100,000 colonies/ml^3 may be significant if urine is collected by catheterization or suprapubic aspiration (338).

infections of the kidney have been many and varied. This has led to confusion within and between medical specialties about the nature of UTI. The descriptor *acute pyelonephritis* should be used only when referring to acute tubulointerstitial inflammatory disease of the kidney caused by bacterial infection (340). Other terms such as *lobar nephronia, phlegmon, lobar nephronitis, focal acute bacterial nephritis, pre-abscess, renal cellulitis,* and *renal carbuncle* should seldom or never be used; there is little agreement on their meaning or their implications for therapy.

Etiology

UTI beyond the neonatal period is usually due to bacteria that gain access to the bladder through the urethral meatus. More than 80% of first UTIs in children are due to *Escherichia coli,* presumably from the gastrointestinal tract (61,338). These bacteria have ready access to the female bladder through the short urethra; this difference may account for the higher incidence of UTI in girls. Bacteria subsequently reach the kidney by VUR. Acute pyelonephritis can also occur by hematogenous spread of bacteria from an infection elsewhere. Although uncommon in older children, this may be the most common origin of UTI in the neonate (61,338). The usual organism in hematogenous spread is *Staphylococcus.* When urinary tract calculi are present, infection may be due to *Proteus* species (338).

Clinical Features

The younger the child with a UTI, the greater is the likelihood that symptoms will be nonspecific. These include anorexia, lethargy, vomiting, irritability, diarrhea, fever of unknown etiology, and failure to thrive (61,338). The classic symptoms of UTI—chills, fever, flank pain, dysuria, and urinary frequency—are usually not present in young children.

Barriers to Urinary Tract Infections

Urinary tract infection occurs when bacterial virulence outweighs host resistance (154,338). Imaging is usually not done to discover why a child has or had a UTI; the cause is usually humoral, cellular, or bacteriologic, and causality is often multifactorial. Factors that protect against urinary infection include the presence of antibodies (enhanced by breast-feeding in the neonatal period), male sex beyond infancy (circumcision protects during the newborn period), lower density of bacterial receptor sites on host epithelial cells, lack of perineal colonization by virulent fecal bacteria, and unimpeded urinary flow. Factors that enhance bacterial virulence include the presence of bacterial adhesins (fimbriae or pili), rapid generation time, production of specific endotoxins, and the ability to sequester important nutrients such as iron (338,341–347).

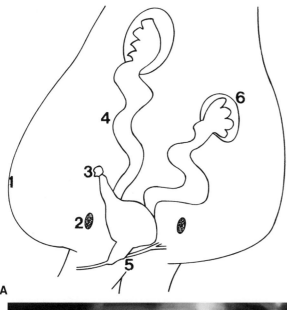
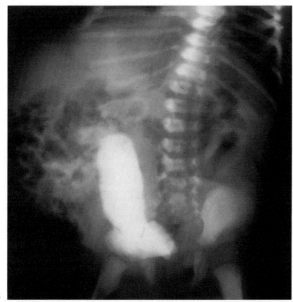

FIG. 9-131. Prune-belly syndrome. A: Common abnormalities. *1,* Deficiency of abdominal musculature; *2,* undescended testes; *3,* urachal abnormality; *4,* hydroureteronephrosis; *5,* deficiency of prostate and reflux into genital ducts; *6,* renal dysplasia. **B:** Cystogram. There is bulging of the flanks due to deficiency of the abdominal muscles. A very large urachal diverticulum protrudes superiorly from the bladder.

The presence of more than one type of organism in a culture or an organism count of between 10,000 and 100,000 bacterial colonies/ml³ in a clean-catch urine specimen is indeterminate; the culture should be repeated. A bagged urine specimen is unacceptable for diagnosing UTI (338).

Terminology

Precise terminology promotes understanding and improves treatment. Unfortunately, the terms used to describe

There are at least four anatomic or biological barriers that prevent bacterial organisms in feces from reaching the kidneys in normal children (154,338). The first barrier is the biological resistance of the perineum, related to the pH of vaginal fluids and inhibition of bacterial growth on both vaginal and distal urethral cells. The second barrier is the biological resistance of the bladder. If bacteria reach the bladder and there is neither VUR nor a significant residual volume, organisms are normally cleared during voiding. There is also racially and genetically determined inherent resistance in the bladder; other factors are urine pH, urea content, and osmolarity (154). Certain bacteria have a greater ability than others to attach to bladder mucosa and proliferate; the host may have decreased antibody production against attachment by bacteria (338). The third anatomic and functional barrier is the ureterovesical junction. This barrier prevents VUR. Components of this third barrier include the muscles of the bladder and submucosal ureter, the oblique course of the ureter through the bladder, the length of the submucosal tunnel, ureteral peristalsis, and ureteral urine flow. The final barrier is related to calyceal structure. Intrarenal reflux is more likely to occur in compound papillae than in simple papillae (see Fig. 9-71A) (153,155–157). Furthermore, during the first year of life, only a low pressure is required to produce intrarenal reflux. These factors explain the distribution of intrarenal reflux and scarring, which are discussed in greater depth in the earlier section on VUR.

Myths About Urinary Tract Infection

Some of the myths and misconceptions about UTI are as follows: all reflux is secondary to distal obstruction; infection causes all reflux; reflux always causes infection; obstruction always causes infection; stones always cause infection; clubbed and scarred kidneys are susceptible to recurrent infections; and sexual intercourse does not increase the risk of infection (61,144,154,338).

Imaging Evaluation

Physicians generally agree that boys should be studied radiologically after the first UTI and that any girl with two episodes of UTI should be evaluated (61). There are now reasons to think that first-time infection should be investigated in both boys and girls (154,338). The purpose of this evaluation is to diagnose causative structural or physiologic abnormalities, identify renal damage, provide a baseline for subsequent evaluation of renal growth, and establish the prognosis (61,144,154,338).

Most patients need no imaging during the acute phase of pyelonephritis. In a few patients, imaging to distinguish upper from lower UTI will affect treatment. This distinction is made with cortical scintigraphy using DMSA (Fig. 9-132A) (41,168–170,174), color Doppler US (70), or con-

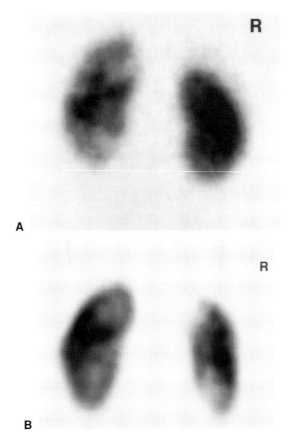

FIG. 9-132. Pyelonephritis. A: Acute pyelonephritis. Posterior DMSA scan shows a normal right kidney and several left-sided photopenic areas due to acute pyelonephritis. **B:** Chronic pyelonephritis. Posterior DMSA scan. There are photopenic areas in the poles of both kidneys, more marked on the right than the left, due to scarring. Note the decrease in size of the right kidney.

trast-enhanced spiral CT (69). Certain patients require detailed imaging evaluation. If the response to therapy for acute pyelonephritis is delayed, imaging should be performed to detect preexisting structural abnormalities and to search for complications.

The first imaging examination is usually US, to look for hydronephrosis, renal or perinephric abscess, pararenal fluid or abscess, and renal scarring (Fig. 9-133). Sometimes infected fluid collections are so echogenic that they are difficult to distinguish from the surrounding renal parenchyma. Color Doppler sonography can help to distinguish vascularized tissue from drainable pus. If sonography is normal but complications are still suspected, unenhanced CT (to look for stones) and enhanced CT (to identify defects in vascularization) may be helpful; CT is more sensitive than US to abscesses.

Acute Pyelonephritis

Acute pyelonephritis in infants and young children may merely cause fever, irritability, and vague abdominal

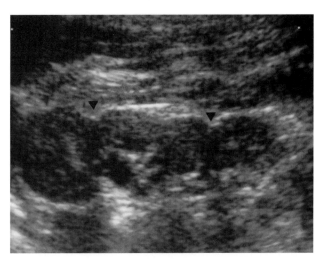

FIG. 9-133. Chronic pyelonephritis. A 12-year-old female with known recurrent urinary tract infection and vesicoureteral reflux. Longitudinal ultrasonography of the left kidney. The kidney is small and is focally scarred *(arrowheads)*.

pain. In older children, fever and flank pain may be found. The diagnosis of acute pyelonephritis is confirmed by urinalysis and urine culture. Blood cultures are occasionally positive.

Children with acute pyelonephritis are rarely evaluated before their infection is successfully treated. If radiologic evaluation is performed to rule out a renal abscess or pyonephrosis, US is the modality of choice. Findings of early acute pyelonephritis include renal enlargement and decreased echogenicity. In some patients diffusely increased echogenicity is found. There is blurring of the corticomedullary junction because of edema. Intravenous urography, is usually normal and is rarely performed; it occasionally shows unilateral or bilateral renal enlargement, decreased renal function, and calyceal distortion (62). Renal cortical scanning agents provide a functional map of renal tubular mass and high-resolution images of the renal parenchyma (14,348,349). A relatively specific pattern in acute pyelonephritis has been described by Handmaker: flare-shaped regions of decreased renal activity radiating from the pelvicalyceal structures toward the periphery of the kidney (350). These areas (sometimes they are spherical) of decreased activity are due to cortical vasoconstriction with inflammatory cells obstructing the paratubular capillaries or, more likely, metabolic alterations in transport mechanisms of radiopharmaceutical across tubular cell membranes by inflammation (348,349). Color Doppler sonography strengthens the diagnosis of acute pyelonephritis by demonstrating decreased blood flow (70). Sonographic contrast agents will further improve the rate of detection of acute pyelonephritis. Contrast-enhanced CT (especially spiral CT) can also be used effectively to diagnose acute pyelonephritis (69).

Chronic Pyelonephritis

Pathophysiology

Chronic pyelonephritis is defined anatomically as an alteration in the renal parenchyma resulting from previous bacterial infection (51). The condition may be focal. The chronic reaction begins in the medulla as a localized area of fibrosis and scar formation that enlarges and involves the entire thickness of the renal substance. The outer margin of the kidney is retracted inward, the renal papilla is pulled outward, and there is secondary distortion of the calyx (see Fig. 9-23). In addition to being focal and full thickness, the scars are frequently polar.

Radiologic Appearance

Most cases of chronic atrophic pyelonephritis affect children, and even those that are first recognized during adult life presumably originated in childhood (51). Measurements of the thickness of the renal substance by IVU are equal in the midportions of the two kidneys and at all four polar regions (see Fig. 9-13) (51).

The earliest radiologic sign of chronic atrophic pyelonephritis is loss of renal substance. Pathologic changes may be focal, areas of scarring involving various cortical and medullary portions of the kidney. Scarring is often manifest as a slight reduction in renal substance thickness at one of the renal poles; this is why it is desirable to see the entire renal outline in every child's renal sonogram and IVU. With scar maturation and contraction, there may be retraction of the adjacent pyramid. A distorted calyx may extend beyond the normal central echo complex as either a sonolucent region filled with urine or an echogenic focus of scar tissue. The polar regions are usually the most adversely affected (Fig. 9-133) (51). The affected kidney is usually reduced in length and volume (Fig. 9-132B); frequently, there is VUR.

Differential Diagnosis

Fetal lobation (see previous) is a normal lobular contour of the kidney that often persists into infancy and occasionally is seen in adults. The renal contour is scalloped at the sites of fusion of the lobes of the kidney. The junction of these lobar fusions is marked by depressions or grooves in the renal outline. Because each renal lobe has its own calyx or calyces, the residual grooves are not directly opposite the calyces as in the pyelonephritic scar, but are between calyceal groups (see Fig. 9-23). Fetal lobation does not cause calyceal distortion.

Papillary necrosis (medullary necrosis) is caused by decreased blood flow in the vasa recta (1). In the older child or adult it is frequently associated with diabetes, sickle cell disease, and analgesic abuse. Most cases of papillary necrosis in younger children are probably secondary to pyelonephritis (351). It may or may not be associated with a pyelonephritic scar. Papillary necrosis is frequently focal, so that it may be difficult to distinguish the everted calyx of atrophic pyelonephritis from loss of tissue due to papillary necrosis (see Fig. 9-23) (338).

The imaging findings of papillary necrosis vary according to the severity and extent of necrosis. Early changes on excretory urography include large papillae and dense, prolonged opacification of the pyramids. Within the pyramids, small cavities develop and communicate with the calyces. As the papillae are partially detached, contrast surrounds them on IVU or CT to produce a crescent, sinus, ''ring,'' or ''egg-in-cup'' appearance, but the latter findings are unusual in children (1). Further sloughing of the papilla results in obliteration of the tip of the pyramid and clubbing of the calyces. End-stage, generalized medullary necrosis causes clubbing of all the calyces associated with uniform cortical loss; this resembles reflux nephropathy and chronic pyelonephritis. Calcifications may develop in cortical necrosis (1).

There are many causes of a *unilateral small kidney* (see Table 9-5). Some of the more important causes including hypoplasia, dysplasia, chronic atrophic pyelonephritis, reflux nephropathy, chronic renal vein thrombosis, obstructive atrophy, and irradiation. In several of these conditions the kidney is evenly affected throughout. This is not true in chronic atrophic pyelomephritis, the most common cause of a small, scarred kidney in childhood (61).

Complications of Renal Parenchymal Infection

Focal acute pyelonephritis may expand and produce a focal mass. Renal parenchymal infection may not be diagnosed before suppurative necrosis and abscess formation. If infection extends beyond the renal capsule but is contained within Gerota's fascia, it is termed a *perirenal abscess.* If the inflammatory reaction extends beyond Gerota's fascia, it is considered a *pararenal abscess* (19).

Organisms causing renal parenchymal infections may reach the kidney by hematogenous spread (usually grampositive organisms) or by the ascending route (usually gramnegative organisms). VUR is the most common pathogenesis of renal parenchymal infection (19). Patients with renal parenchymal infections may be otherwise well, have an underlying urinary abnormality, have an abnormality of another organ system, or have an abnormality of host response to infection.

Renal Abscess

Renal abscess is renal parenchymal infection in which suppuration and necrosis results in a mass lesion.

When acute pyelonephritis becomes an abscess, sonography demonstrates a complex echogenic and hypoechoic mass. The hypoechoic regions may represent liquefaction, necrosis, or distorted and dilated calyces. US is particularly helpful in showing perinephric extension (19). IVU may show scoliosis concave to the side of involvement, decreased kidney motion with respiration, inhomogeneities and focal lobar defects on the nephrogram, loss of renal outline, and frank mass lesions (19). CT is more sensitive than gray scale US and confirms the presence of an intrarenal mass and verifies its extent. Imaging modalities other than US and CT are rarely indicated.

Perirenal Abscess

Perirenal (perinephric) abscess is the extension of a renal parenchymal infection to form an abscess beyond the renal capsule but not beyond Gerota's fascia. The usual etiology is extension of infection from the kidney to this potential anatomic space rather than hematogenous spread. US is of particular value in demonstrating this abnormality. A mass of mixed echogenicity is noted inside and just outside the kidney. Although inflammation breaks through the renal capsule, it is usually confined by Gerota's fascia. CT shows the precise anatomy adjacent to the kidney very well.

Xanthogranulomatous Pyelonephritis

Xanthogranulomatous pyelonephritis (XPN), a specific type of chronic renal infection, is rare in children. There are focal and diffuse types. The focal type of XPN is much more common in girls and pathologically shows the presence of xanthomatous foam cells (macrophages filled with lipid material) without other evidence of chronic pyelonephritis. Because foam cells and xanthomatous reaction are nonspecific and are frequently found in children with chronic infection, it is thought that the focal form of XPN is merely an unusual manifestation of chronic inflammation or abscess (352).

The diffuse type of XPN is much more common in adults than in children and in males than in females. The pathologic criteria for this diffuse type require the association of chronic pyelonephritis (interstitial fibrosis with an inflammatory infiltrate of lymphocytes, plasma cells, and, occasionally, neutrophils); dilatation and contraction of tubules with atrophy of the epithelium; concentric fibrosis about Bowman's capsule; vascular changes similar to those of benign or malignant arteriosclerosis; and xanthomatous reaction (foam cells producing yellowish nodules) (352).

The symptoms are recurrent fever, dysuria, leukocytosis, and, frequently, a palpable mass. The general condition of the child is usually poor, and anemia is common. Causative organisms include *Proteus vulgaris, Escherichia coli,* and *Staphylococcus aureus.* The frequency of stenotic endarteritis and thrombotic phlebitis of the distal renal veins in the diffuse types suggests a vascular etiology (352).

The radiologic features of the localized type of XPN are identical to those of a renal abscess. However, the diffuse type of XPN has specific radiologic features (352): unilateral involvement, calcification in the kidney, a complex ultrasonographic mass, and nonfunction at IVU (352). Angiography, rarely performed, is nonspecific and shows only splaying of intrarenal arteries and poorly marginated vascular defects. There is mild hypervascularity but no evidence of arteriovenous shunting (353).

The diagnosis of XPN is based on the histologic findings. The focal type is frequently confused with an intrarenal mass such as Wilms tumor. Treatment is surgical removal or drainage of the focal type and nephrectomy for the diffuse type. The long-term prognosis is good (353).

Pyonephrosis

The term *pyonephrosis* refers to an obstructed, infected kidney. Renal sonography demonstrates a dilated collecting system. The fluid may be abnormally echogenic, suggesting infection. There may be a urine-debris level (Fig. 9-134). However, the lack of echogenic fluid in a dilated collecting system does not exclude the condition (354,355). Because of potential damage to the kidney, percutaneous aspiration of fluid might be warranted to exclude or confirm the diagnosis. If pyonephrosis is confirmed by aspiration, a percutaneous nephrostomy catheter is placed for drainage.

Cystitis

Bacterial cystitis is frequently present in combination with pyelonephritis, although it may occur alone. The causes of cystitis include bacterial or viral infection, drug therapy (particularly cyclophosphamide [Cytoxan]), and noxious agents (ether, hydrogen peroxide).

The features of cystitis are much more apparent at sonography than at VCUG. In the well-distended bladder, a wall thickness of >3 mm is abnormal. This measurement is a nonspecific but sensitive indicator for cystitis (Fig. 9-135). Patients with moderate to severe cystitis demonstrated by cystoscopic examination may have normal VCUGs and IVUs. If radiographic abnormalities are present, they usually consist of marginal irregularities of the bladder due to spasm and mucosal edema. If there is extensive hemorrhage associated with cystitis, blood clots may create echogenic debris within the bladder. Occasionally, there is marked thickening of the wall and a mass-like indentation on the bladder lumen that mimics a malignancy (see Fig. 9-31). Cystitis may coexist with VUR.

Pelvic Inflammatory Disease

Pelvic inflammatory disease (PID) is common in the sexually active adolescent female. Usually bilateral, it is caused

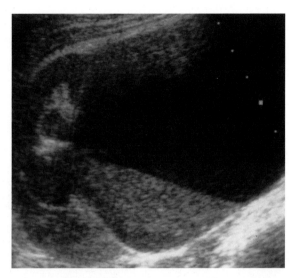

FIG. 9-134. Pyonephrosis. A 13-year-old boy with known UPJ obstruction and spiking fevers. Longitudinal sonography shows a markedly dilated renal pelvis with a fluid-debris level. An emergency percutaneous nephrostomy was performed.

by gonorrhea and other sexually transmitted diseases. Other causes of PID include complications of pregnancy, attempted abortion, and extension of an abscess into the pelvis.

Sexually transmitted PID spreads along the mucosa of the pelvic organs, initially infecting the cervix and uterus (endometritis), the fallopian tubes (acute salpingitis), and, finally, the ovaries and the peritoneum. Pyosalpinx develops when a fallopian tube becomes occluded.

There is a spectrum of sonographic findings (356). Acutely, the pelvic sonogram can be normal. Endometrial thickening or fluid in the uterus may indicate endometritis. With the development of pyosalpinx, low-level echoes are seen within a fluid-filled tubular or ovoid structure adjacent to the uterus. Transvaginal sonography is able to distinguish pyosalpinx from other adnexal masses (357). Pus may be demonstrated in the cul-de-sac; unlike serous fluid, it contains echogenic material. As PID worsens, tuboovarian abscesses develop; these appear as multiloculated, complex adnexal masses. In more extensive cases of PID, the pelvis is diffusely filled with heterogeneous echogenic material that obscures the pelvic soft-tissue planes and uterine margins (356). In children, the primary differential diagnostic consideration is appendicitis with perforation.

Tumors

Wilms Tumor

Wilms tumor (nephroblastoma) is a malignant, embryonic neoplasm containing epithelial, blastemal, and stromal elements (Fig. 9-136). It has almost the same overall incidence as neuroblastoma and accounts for approximately 8% of all childhood malignant tumors. Wilms tumor is the most com-

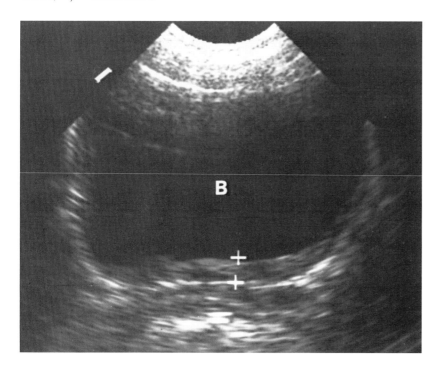

FIG. 9-135. Cystitis. A transverse sonographic section through a distended bladder *(B)* demonstrates a thick (4.5 mm) posterior bladder wall *(cursors)* in a child with cystoscopic evidence of hemorrhagic cystitis.

mon solid abdominal mass and by far the most common renal malignancy of childhood (1,3,8,358). Advances in the understanding and management of Wilms tumor have occurred, in large measure, as a result of cooperative studies such as the National Wilms Tumor Study (NWTS).

History

Max Wilms (1867–1918), the son of a lawyer, was born near Aachen, Germany in 1867. He studied at a number of German universities and obtained his doctorate at Bonn in 1890. In 1899, while working at the Institute of Pathology,

Wilms wrote a monograph on the pathology of mixed tumors of the kidney. This account by Wilms, written at the age of 32, was the first that classified this renal neoplasm as an embryonal sarcoma (358).

Clinical Features

The peak incidence of Wilms tumors is between $2\frac{1}{2}$ years and 3 years of age; 78% of all cases are detected between 1 and 5 years of age. Wilms tumor affects approximately one child in 10,000 before the age of 15 years worldwide; the annual incidence is approximately 7.8 per 1 million children.

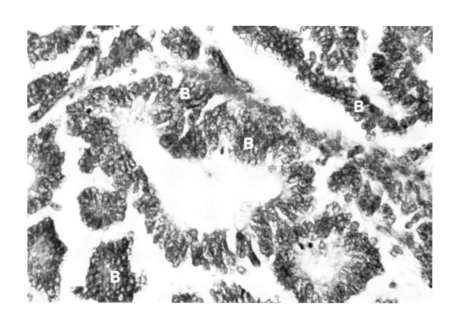

FIG. 9-136. Histology of Wilms tumor. The triphasic embryonic neoplasm consists of blastemal *(B)*, epithelial (tubular), and stromal elements.

About 500 new cases are reported each year in the United States. The tumor constitutes 6.2% of all cancers in white American children and 7.9% in black American children (359–362). The worldwide sex ratio is 1:1, although some reports have shown a slightly higher incidence in the United States in boys (8,358,359).

An asymptomatic abdominal mass is the most common clinical presentation. It may be noted by the patient, parent, or examining physician. Uncommon clinical presentations include abdominal pain, fever, anorexia, hematuria, and hypertension. Dysuria and renal failure are rare. An occasional child presents with hematuria after minor trauma.

Associations

Although most Wilms tumors are sporadic, at least 1% are familial (363). The mode of inheritance is usually autosomal dominant with variable penetrance and expressivity (364). It is important to recognize these familial cases, not only for genetic counseling but also for early diagnosis and therapy. A child with a sibling or parent with bilateral Wilms tumor has a risk of up to 30% for development of the tumor.

Extrarenal abnormalities occur in 7.6% of patients with Wilms tumor (365). These abnormalities include overgrowth disorders, sporadic aniridia, genital malformations, and other malformations.

There is an association of overgrowth disorders with neoplasia; there are specific associations with congenital hemihypertrophy and Beckwith-Wiedemann syndrome. The genetic abnormality in Beckwith-Wiedemann syndrome has been localized to chromosome 11p15.5, although the pattern of inheritance has not yet been fully elucidated (365). Isolated congenital hemihypertrophy appears to be a sporadic malformation. The mean age of diagnosis of Wilms tumor in Beckwith-Wiedemann syndrome and isolated hemihypertrophy is similar to that in the general Wilms tumor population. However, Wilms tumor occurs at an earlier age in association with aniridia and Drash syndrome (pseudohermaphroditism and renal failure) (363). Several other overgrowth disorders, including Soto syndrome (cerebral gigantism), neurofibromatosis, and Klippel-Trenaunay-Weber syndrome, have weak associations with Wilms tumor.

Aniridia is rare. Two thirds of affected individuals have autosomal dominant aniridia. These patients are not at increased risk for the development of Wilms tumor. The remaining one third have sporadic nonfamilial congenital aniridia with a chromosome 11p13 deletion. Wilms tumor develops in approximately one third of individuals with this type of aniridia, usually in the first 3 years of life. Approximately 1% of all Wilms tumor patients have aniridia (8,358). The most common association between sporadic aniridia and Wilms tumor is in the WAGR syndrome (Wilms tumor; Aniridia; Genital anomalies; mental Retardation). Wilms tumor has also been associated with trisomy 18, Bloom syndrome, Perlman syndrome, 45,X chromosomal abnormality, various chromosomal translocations, and linear sebaceous nevus syndrome (8,365,366).

Wilms tumor is bilateral in approximately 5% of patients. Bilateral tumors are frequently associated with sporadic aniridia, genitourinary anomalies, hemihypertrophy, and nephroblastomatosis.

Pathology

A Wilms tumor is usually bulky and replaces most of the involved kidney. The tumor may arise in any portion of the kidney. It may be exophytic but usually expands within the renal parenchyma to displace and distort the pelvicalyceal system (Fig. 9-137). The tumor is usually solid and has a pseudocapsule that separates it from normal renal parenchyma. The renal capsule is usually intact; rarely, the tumor breaks through this capsule and extends into the extrarenal spaces. Areas of central hemorrhage and necrosis may produce a cystic appearance. Calcification is identified on pathologic examination in up to 15% of patients (8), although it is radiographically visible much less commonly. There are frequently local metastases to regional lymph nodes. Occasionally there may be urothelial spread. Wilms tumor may invade the renal vein and inferior vena cava. Venous extension of Wilms tumor follows the "rule of 10's": 10% extend into the renal vein; 10% of that group extend into the IVC; 10% of the latter further extend into the right atrium. This type of venous extension (Figs. 9-138 and 9-139) is particularly important to document preoperatively; it often changes the surgical approach. Distal metastases most commonly involve the lungs; the liver is the next most common site (367).

Wilms tumor, an embryonal renal neoplasm, is presumed to develop from abnormal histogenesis. Renal blastema tissue (nephrogenic rests) is thought to be the precursor of Wilms tumor; this is somewhat analogous to the existence of neuroblastoma in situ in neonates. Nephrogenesis is normally complete by 36 weeks of gestation, and kidneys of normal term newborn infants contain no foci of renal blastema. Nodules of renal blastema are found in approximately 15% of kidneys involved by Wilms tumor and are particularly common if the tumor is bilateral (358,368). Nephrogenic rests are of two distinct types, perilobar and intralobar, distinguished primarily by their position in the renal lobe. "Panlobar" includes both perilobar and intralobar types. Perilobar nephrogenic rests are confined to the lobar periphery. Intralobar nephrogenic rests may be found anywhere in the renal lobe, in the wall of the pelvicalyceal system, and in the renal sinus. Nephrogenic blastemal cells arising earlier in gestation tend to be situated deeper in the lobe; intralobar nephrogenic rests have a higher association with the subsequent development of Wilms tumor (369). Nephrogenic rests are classified into four subtypes based on gross and microscopic characteristics: incipient or dormant, regressing or sclerosing, hypoplastic, and neoplastic (370).

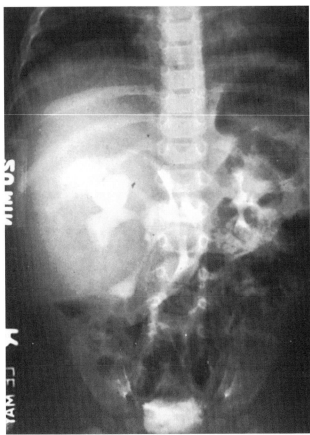

FIG. 9-137. Wilms tumor. A 1-year-old boy with right abdominal mass. **A:** Intravenous urography shows a large intrarenal mass in the right kidney that displaces and distorts the pelvicalyceal system. The left kidney is normal. **B:** A retrograde ureteral injection of the nephrectomy specimen confirms distortion of the renal pelvis and calyces by the intrarenal mass. From Kirks et al. (27).

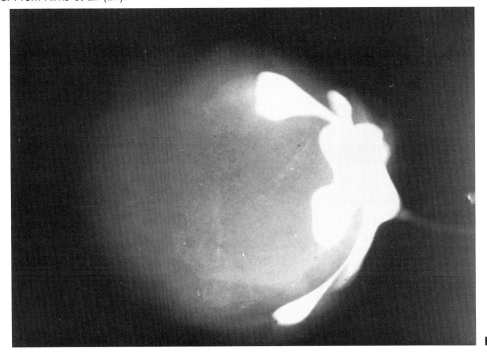

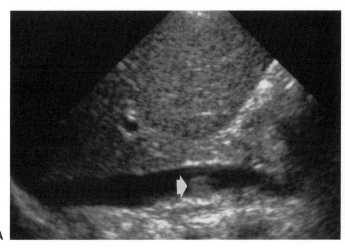

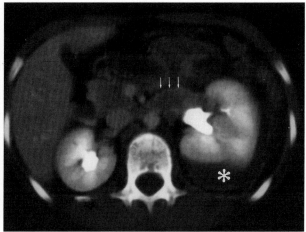

FIG. 9-138. Wilms tumor with tumor thrombus in left renal vein and inferior vena cava. A: Longitudinal sonography of IVC. There is a tumor thrombus *(arrow)* within the inferior vena cava. **B:** Contrast-enhanced CT. The Wilms tumor *(asterisk)* involves the posterior part of the left kidney and is contained within the renal capsule. The left renal vein is distended by a tumor thrombus *(arrows)*.

Histologically, Wilms tumor usually consists of fairly well-differentiated renal tissue with embryonic or abortive glomeruli and tubule formation surrounded by spindle cell stroma (see Fig. 9-136). There may be components of striated muscle, fibrous tissue, cartilage, bone, and even fat.

The most important prognostic factor in Wilms tumor is histology. Approximately 10% of all Wilms tumors have unfavorable histology with anaplasia (variability in size and shape of nuclei, large nuclei, large numbers of mitotic figures) (371).

Wilms tumor is bilateral in approximately 5% of cases and is unilateral but multicentric in 7% (372). Bilateral tumors are diagnosed at initial presentation (synchronous) in two thirds of cases and are detected anywhere from 3 weeks to 10 years later (metachronous) in the other third (368).

The patient survival rate with synchronous tumors is approximately 87%; the survival rate with metachronous tumors is only 40% (8). CT and MRI are particularly helpful for following the therapeutic response of bilateral Wilms tumor.

The two major tumor types defined by the NWTS are favorable histology (no anaplasia, nonsarcomatous) and unfavorable histology (anaplasia, sarcomatous) (372). In patients with bilateral Wilms tumor, the histology may be different on the two sides. The tumor frequently shows a mixed pattern with an abundance of differentiated epithelial tissue forming glandular acini. However, there may be a predominance of either blastemal or stromal elements.

Renal vein extension explains the high frequency (12% to 20%) of hematogenous lung metastases at diagnosis. Although many lung metastases are detected by chest radiogra-

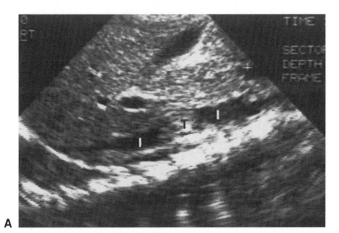

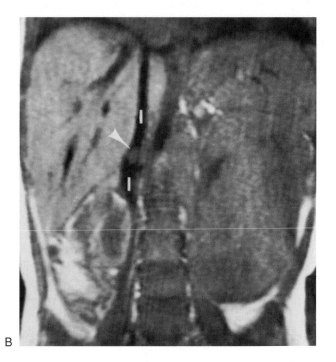

FIG. 9-139. Wilms tumor with tumor thrombus in inferior vena cava. A: Sonography of IVC. There is a tumor thrombus *(T)* in the inferior vena cava *(I)*. **B:** MRI. Coronal T1-weighted MRI demonstrates a tumor thrombus *(arrowhead)* in the infrahepatic inferior vena cava *(I)* at the insertion of the left renal vein. Note the large left Wilms tumor.

phy, CT is important to verify the presence or absence of small metastases. Pneumothorax occasionally complicates metastases from the anaplastic type of Wilms tumor. Liver metastases are present in 8% to 10% of all patients (373). There are occasionally bony metastases, which are usually osteolytic. Bone metastases are almost always from anaplastic tumors.

Staging

Staging of Wilms tumor depends on involvement as determined by imaging modalities, surgery, and pathologic examination. Anatomic staging of Wilms tumor is as follows: stage I, tumor limited to the kidney and completely resected; stage II, tumor extending beyond the kidney but completely resected; stage III, residual tumor confined to the abdomen without hematogenous spread; stage IV, hematogenous metastases to lung, liver, bone, or brain; stage V, bilateral renal involvement appearing initially or during the course of treatment of disease (3,8,374). Advances in multidrug adjuvant chemotherapy have significantly improved the prognosis, even in patients with metastatic disease or bilateral renal involvement, particularly if the histology is favorable.

Imaging

Imaging of Wilms tumor should define the size and location of the primary tumor, any local spread, and any distant metastases. Imaging is also used for surveillance of individuals at risk for primary or recurrent Wilms tumor.

There is disagreement about the optimal selection of imaging studies in the evaluation of Wilms tumor. As recently as 1993, a position paper from members of the NWTS recommended IVU and US (375). However, in most large pediatric centers in the United States, cross-sectional techniques (US, CT, MRI) are the main investigative methods; IVU is now rarely performed for tumor.

Abdominal Radiography. Abdominal radiography usually shows a soft-tissue mass that displaces bowel. Calcification is shown by conventional radiography in approximately 5% of Wilms tumors (373,376). This dystrophic calcification may be curvilinear or amorphous. It can usually be distinguished from the stippled or flaky calcifications that occur in 55% of neuroblastomas. Organized ossification is rare in Wilms tumor.

Intravenous Urography. Intravenous urography was once the mainstay for evaluating children with abdominal masses; cross-sectional imaging modalities are now almost always used. IVU shows stretching and distortion of the pelvicalyceal system (see Fig. 9-137). Wilms tumor may also compress the renal pelvis to produce obstructive hydronephrosis. In approximately 10% of patients with a Wilms tumor, there is no function of the kidney by IVU; this is usually caused by a massive tumor with extension into the renal pelvis and occlusion of the ureter or renal vein.

Ultrasonography. US is usually the first imaging modality for a child with a palpable abdominal mass. Wilms tumor is usually shown to be large, sharply marginated, and of increased echogenicity; tumor echogenicity is usually equal to or slightly greater than that of adjacent liver and less heterogeneous than that of neuroblastoma (Fig. 9-140) (377,378). Hypoechoic areas in the tumor may represent hemorrhage, necrosis, or dilated calyces (378,379). A solid renal mass demonstrated by sonography in an older infant or child is most commonly a Wilms tumor (358).

Because of the high frequency of extension of Wilms tumor into the renal vein, inferior vena cava, and even right atrium, careful evaluation for tumor thrombus using color Doppler sonography is mandatory. This requires longitudinal, transverse, and oblique imaging with duplex sonography. Venous extension is diagnosed when an intravascular echogenic focus is identified (Figs. 9-138A and 9-139A). However, because Wilms tumors are usually large and bulky, precise evaluation of the inferior vena cava may be difficult because of marked extrinsic displacement and compression by the tumor mass. This situation may prevent adequate sonographic evaluation of venous structures, particularly in uncooperative children. CT (Fig. 9-138B) or MRI (Fig. 9-139B) may be necessary.

Computed Tomography. CT confirms the presence of an intrarenal mass, determines the extent of the Wilms tumor, visualizes vascular structures, identifies nodal involvement, evaluates the presence or absence of liver metastases, and images the opposite kidney (380). CT defines the location and extent of the intrarenal tumor and its morphologic characteristics (Fig. 9-138B and 9-140B). The tumor mass usually has a rounded appearance, low attenuation, and inhomogeneous contrast enhancement. The mass is usually solid but may contain cystic areas due to hemorrhage or necrosis; it may appear to be septated because of fibrous stroma. Small calcifications, not appreciated by conventional radiography, may be apparent on CT; calcifications are identified by CT in up to 15% of cases (380). The adjacent tissue planes are well defined, and a pseudocapsule is frequently identified. The vessels are displaced, not encased as in neuroblastoma. Even if the mass crosses the midline, the tumor does not extend behind the aorta. Abdominal CT also evaluates the renal arteries and veins, inferior vena cava, adjacent lymph nodes, liver, and contralateral kidney. The contralateral kidney is better evaluated by CT than by US. Chest CT is also usually performed, as pulmonary metastases are present in as many as 20% of patients at the time of diagnosis.

CT is an excellent method for following patients after resection of Wilms tumor. The tumor bed may be difficult to assess by US, as it frequently contains loops of bowel. CT after the administration of oral and intravenous contrast media provides precise anatomic delineation of the tumor bed. It is also usually able to detect ipsilateral recurrence or contralateral development of tumor. Moreover, the lungs and liver can be evaluated for metastases.

Magnetic Resonance Imaging. Despite excellent anatomic delineation by CT, MRI is rapidly becoming the preferred imaging modality for Wilms tumor (Fig. 9-141) (381–383). The multiplanar imaging capability of MRI is useful in depicting the renal origin of the tumor, its margins,

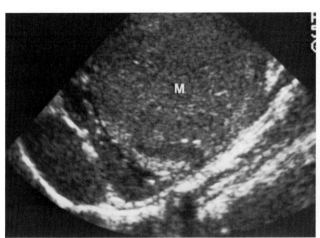
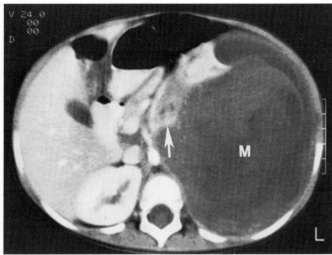

FIG. 9-140. Imaging of Wilms tumor. A 1-year-old girl with a left abdominal mass. **A:** Renal sonography. Longitudinal ultrasonography shows a large, echogenic mass *(M)* arising from the left kidney. **B:** CT. The left renal mass *(M)* distorts the remnant of functioning kidney *(arrow)*. Low attenuation areas within the tumor mass are due to necrosis. The right kidney and inferior vena cava are normal.

and local extensions. Excellent inherent contrast between vessels and adjacent soft tissues permits accurate delineation of extension into the renal veins and inferior vena cava (see Fig. 9-139). As a general rule, Wilms tumors have prolonged T1 and T2 relaxation times. However, the signal intensity may be quite variable because of hemorrhage and necrosis in the tumor. Intravenous contrast shows an inhomogeneous enhancement pattern and improves the delineation of tumor margins (383). MRI is also an excellent modality for detecting recurrent or metastatic abdominal tumor.

Angiography. Less invasive imaging modalities have made angiography unnecessary in patients with Wilms tumor. Most Wilms tumors are markedly hypervascular at angiography. Angiography may play a role in a patient with a solitary kidney or bilateral disease when a partial nephrectomy is being considered.

Differential Diagnosis

Neuroblastoma. A neuroblastoma, the other common pediatric abdominal malignancy, may look like a Wilms tumor on US. Conversely, an exophytic Wilms tumor may mimic a neuroblastoma. The appearance of neuroblastoma is described in detail in a subsequent section of this chapter. An important differential feature is that the mass effect of neuroblastoma is extrarenal. Because of their exquisite spatial resolution, CT and MRI can usually correctly diagnose neuroblastoma even when it has invaded the kidney. By CT or MRI, neuroblastoma tends to be an irregular, ill-defined, calcified mass that displaces, surrounds, and frequently encases vessels. There is frequently involvement of adjacent lymph nodes and extension across the midline as well as to the paravertebral region (384).

Nephroblastomatosis. Nephroblastomatosis is a rare group of dysontogenic lesions of the infantile kidney that should be considered intermediate between a malformation and neoplasm. It is related to and a precursor of Wilms tumor. The complex of nephroblastomatosis includes rests of renal blastema (nephrogenic rests), nodular renal blastema, and confluent nephroblastomatosis.

Normal renal development results from the merger of the ureteric (metanephric) ducts and the metanephric blastema, which lies peripherally in the subcapsular and intralobular spaces. Nephrogenesis is complete in the normal fetus at 34–36 weeks of gestation; metanephric blastema does not normally persist after this stage of development (358).

Rests of renal blastema are found in most cases of bilateral Wilms tumor but are also found in about 1% of autopsies of patients under 3 months of age. These nephrogenic rests, or ''Wilms tumor in situ,'' may be perilobar, intralobar, or panlobar. They may occur singly or in multiples, with or without Wilms tumor, and may be present in the same kidney, the opposite kidney, or both in the presence of Wilms tumor. Beckwith has proposed that nephroblastomatosis is multiple or diffuse nephrogenic rests (NRs) (370).

Intralobar NRs and perilobar NRs differ in a number of characteristics. Patients with Wilms tumors arising in association with intralobar NRs are significantly younger than those with perilobar NRs; this has implications for the duration of patient surveillance. The kidneys of children with Beckwith-Wiedemann syndrome, trisomy 18, and hemihypertrophy (Fig. 9-142) more commonly have perilobar NRs than intralobar NRs; children with sporadic aniridia and Drash syndrome usually have intralobar NRs. Both types of NRs are associated with Wilms tumor; perilobar NRs are more commonly associated with synchronous bilateral tumors, intralobar NRs with metachronous Wilms tumors.

NRs and nodular renal blastema resemble Wilms tumor

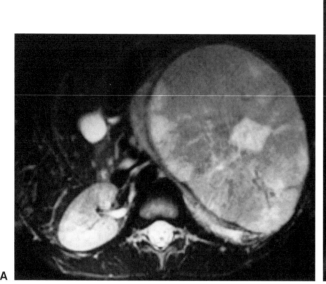
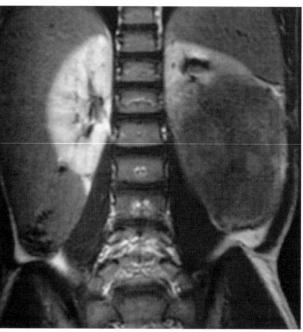

A

B

FIG. 9-141. **Magnetic resonance imaging of Wilms tumor.** A 4-year-old boy with right hemihypertrophy and left flank mass. Renal sonography at 3 months of age was normal. **A:** T2-weighted axial MRI. There is a well-circumscribed, intrarenal mass of the left kidney with central necrosis. The right kidney is normal. **B:** Contrast-enhanced coronal T1-weighted MRI. The Wilms tumor arises from the lower pole of the left kidney.

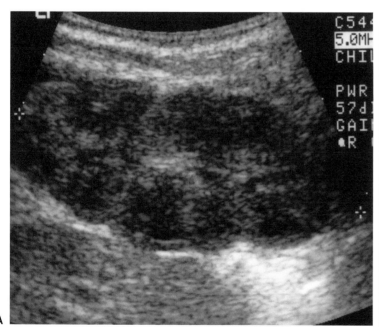
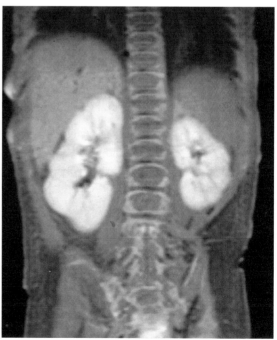

A

B

FIG. 9-142. **Hemihypertrophy with ipsilateral benign nephromegaly.** A 3-week-old girl with right hemihypertrophy and an enlarged kidney detected by prenatal sonography. **A:** Longitudinal sonography of the right kidney. The kidney is enlarged *(cursors)* and has prominent fetal lobations. **B:** Contrast-enhanced coronal T1-weighted MRI. The right kidney is enlarged but otherwise normal.

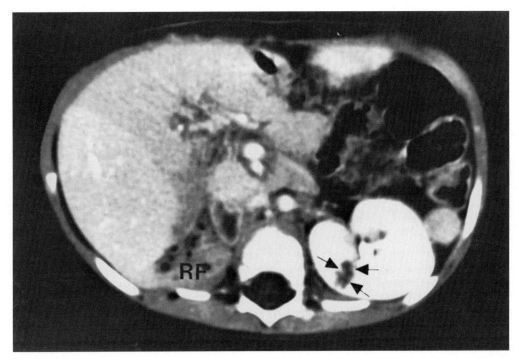

FIG. 9-143. Nephroblastomatosis: Nodular renal blastema. A 4-year-old boy evaluated 1 year after a nephrectomy for a right Wilms tumor. There is no evidence of tumor recurrence in the right renal fossa *(RF)*. An irregular, low-attenuation, subcortical mass is present in the left kidney *(arrows)*. Biopsy confirmed nodular renal blastema. From Kirks et al. (358).

microscopically but have no mitoses. NRs may be seen as hypoechoic nodules by US. Occasionally, these nodules are isoechoic or hyperechoic (385,386). Contrast-enhanced CT is more sensitive than US for identification of nephroblastomatosis (387); nodular renal blastema appears as a low-attenuation intrarenal lesion (Fig. 9-143). Nodular renal blastema may be associated with (Fig. 9-144) or progress to Wilms tumor (388).

The massive or confluent form of nephroblastomatosis is frequently confused with bilateral Wilms tumors. Although related to Wilms tumor and a precursor of it, confluent nephroblastomatosis is recognized as a separate entity. The growth and histologic location of the tumor aid in differentiation, and this distinction is also prognostically important.

Infants with confluent nephroblastomatosis are usually under 2 years old and have bilateral flank masses. The pro-

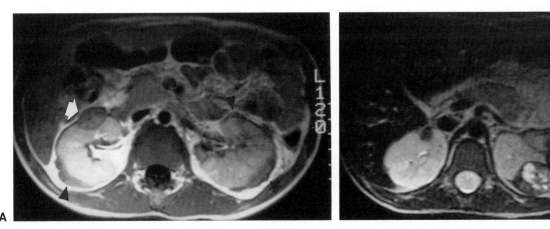

FIG. 9-144. Nephroblastomatosis and Wilms tumor. A: Contrast-enhanced axial T1-weighted MRI. There are plaque-like *(arrowheads)* and nodular *(arrow)* nephrogenic rests of homogeneous signal intensity. **B:** Axial T2-weighted MRI. In addition to nodular foci in the right kidney, there is an inhomogeneous mass arising from the posterior surface of the upper pole of the left kidney. Biopsy of the left-sided mass demonstrated Wilms tumor.

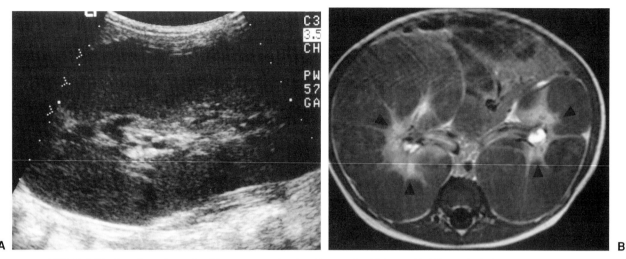

A

B

FIG. 9-145. Confluent nephroblastomatosis. An 11-month-old boy with bilateral abdominal masses. **A:** Longitudinal sonography. The right kidney is large. There is marked thickening of the renal parenchyma and loss of the corticomedullary differentiation. **B:** Contrast-enhanced axial T1-weighted MRI. There are many bilateral, lobulated, homogeneous renal masses in a perilobar distribution. The masses are hypointense when compared to the normal but compressed renal parenchyma *(arrowheads)*.

cess is diffuse and involves the entire subcapsular portion of the kidneys. The tumor is uniform, pink, fleshy, and firm. There is no definite capsule, and there is an absence of necrosis or hemorrhage. Microscopically, confluent masses of nephrogenic epithelial cells are located beneath the renal capsule; these cells form immature tubules and glomeruli. Sonography confirms mixed echogenic and hypoechoic subcortical tissue and bilaterally enlarged kidneys (Fig. 9-145A). CT demonstrates low-attenuation subcapsular tumor

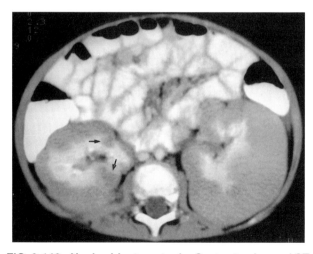

FIG. 9-146. Nephroblastomatosis. Contrast-enhanced CT. There are many bilateral, subcapsular, low-attenuation masses that compress normal renal parenchyma. This is consistent with perilobar confluent nephroblastomatosis. Moreover, there are intralobar *(arrows)* foci that presumably represent nodular renal blastema. Biopsy confirmed the diagnosis of nephroblastomatosis.

nodules and compression of adjacent normal renal parenchyma (Fig. 9-146). MRI shows hypointense renal masses in a perilobar distribution; the masses compress normal renal parenchyma (Fig. 9-145B).

Patients with confluent nephroblastomatosis are usually treated with chemotherapy. The subcapsular masses may completely resolve with this therapy. However, Wilms tumor may develop, and imaging surveillance is critical.

MRI may detect NRs as small as 4 mm in diameter (383). Preliminary results suggest that MRI can distinguish nephroblastomatosis from Wilms tumor (Fig. 9-144) (383). Foci of sclerosing and hyperplastic nephroblastomatosis are plaquelike, ovoid, or lenticular in shape as opposed to Wilms tumors, which are spherical. Moreover, in contrast to the heterogeneity of Wilms tumor, foci of nephroblastomatosis are of homogeneous signal intensity on all imaging sequences (Fig. 9-144). On contrast-enhanced MRI, NRs remain homogeneously hypointense compared to normal kidney tissue, whereas Wilms tumors enhance inhomogeneously (383).

Mesoblastic Nephroma. Mesoblastic nephroma (fetal renal hamartoma) is the most common neonatal renal neoplasm (389). It is almost always discovered during the first few months of life, although rarely it is detected in older children or even in adults.

Occasionally, pregnancy is complicated by dystocia or hydramnios (390). A solid fetal renal mass may be diagnosed by prenatal sonography. The neonate usually has a large, nontender abdominal mass with no other abnormalities; occasionally, hematuria is present. There is a 2 : 1 male predominance. The mean age at diagnosis is 3.4 months (391). Previously, it was believed that Wilms tumor had a better prognosis in neonates than in older children. In fact, the vast majority of these renal tumors occurring during the first weeks of life are benign mesoblastic nephromas (389). Mesoblastic nephroma is distinguished from Wilms tumor by its earlier presentation, more favorable outcome, and histologic features.

The pathology of mesoblastic nephroma explains the imaging findings (Fig. 9-147). The typical lesion is a solid, yellowish tan, encapsulated mass arising in the medulla; it measures 8–30 cm in diameter and replaces as much as 75% of the renal parenchyma (358,392). The cut surface has a whorled appearance that resembles a uterine fibroid (Fig. 9-147C). The tumor margins blend imperceptibly with normal kidney parenchyma. Although the neoplasm may penetrate the renal capsule and extend into the perinephric space or retroperitoneum, it is histologically benign and does not invade the renal pedicle, extend into the renal pelvis, or metastasize to distant sites. Local recurrence may result from capsular penetration or incomplete resection. Hemorrhage and necrosis are uncommon, but the neoplasm may show gross cystic changes, especially at the junction of the tumor and uninvolved kidney. These cystic changes in the tumor may resemble multilocular cystic nephroma.

Microscopically, mesoblastic nephroma consists of benign-appearing spindle cells. The histologic appearance of the lesion is so distinctive that it is considered a unique hamartomatous lesion unrelated to Wilms tumor (389). At the interface with normal kidney, sheets of spindle cells grow between intact nephrons. Foci of calcification may be present. The central portion of the tumor is primarily mesenchymal but may contain tubules and glomeruli (Fig. 9-147D). Because they are smaller than normal and dysplastic, it is uncertain whether they are nephrons that have been trapped by the tumor or have differentiated from the metanephrogenic blastema (358).

A subgroup of patients have the cellular form of mesoblastic nephroma. These tumors are highly cellular, have a very large number of mitotic cells, and sometimes recur locally and metastasize distantly (393).

Plain films of the abdomen show a large soft-tissue abdominal mass that is rarely calcified. Sonography usually shows a mixed echogenic intrarenal mass indistinguishable from Wilms tumor as seen in the older child (Fig. 9-147A). A distinctive ring sign has been described (394). Occasionally, the mass may be relatively hypoechoic, anechoic, or of mixed echogenicity with anechoic areas (390). Sonographic findings are usually similar to that of a noncalcified uterine leiomyoma—a solid mass with low-level internal echoes. Although seldom performed, contrast-enhanced CT shows a solid intrarenal mass surrounded by a variable amount of functioning renal parenchyma (395). Because these neoplasms are vascular, they may show minimal contrast enhancement. Moreover, the trapped tubules and glomeruli within the tumor may permit excretion of contrast material at IVU, CT, or nuclear scintigraphy (Fig. 9-147B) (395).

MRI shows a well-defined intrarenal mass with mixed signal intensity on T1-weighted images (Fig. 9-148); T2-weighted images show predominantly high signal intensity

(396). Imaging cannot differentiate between a typical mesoblastic nephroma and the potentially more aggressive cellular form of the tumor.

Congenital mesoblastic nephroma is an unusual, benign hamartomatous renal neoplasm that typically has no distant metastases. It is the most common solid renal neoplasm occurring during the first few months of life and differs from Wilms tumor by its earlier presentation, benign biological behavior, and more favorable outcome. The prognosis after complete surgical removal is excellent in most patients, so that adjuvant chemotherapy and irradiation not only are unwarranted but may produce unnecessary morbidity (389). In children with the cellular form of mesoblastic nephroma, the age of diagnosis determines prognosis. Patients undergoing resection prior to 3 months of age are less likely to develop local recurrence or metastatic disease than older children (393). Chemotherapy and radiation are therefore generally reserved, in the cellular form of mesoblastic nephroma, for children older than 3 months of age with either extensive local tumor, metastases, or recurrent disease (390,391,393).

Multilocular Cystic Renal Tumors. Multilocular cystic renal tumors are two histologically distinct but grossly identical lesions: multilocular cystic nephroma (multilocular renal cyst, cystadenoma) and cystic partially differentiated nephroblastoma (CPDN, well-differentiated cystic Wilms tumor) (397,398). Multilocular cystic nephroma is a cystic mass containing many septa composed entirely of differentiated tissues, without blastemal, embryonal, or other malignant elements. CPDN is also a multilocular lesion without solid or nodular components, but its septa contain blastemal or other embryonal cells. Grossly, multilocular cystic renal tumors have a solitary, well-circumscribed, multiseptated mass of noncommunicating, fluid-filled cysts surrounded by a thick, fibrous capsule. Cyst herniation into the renal pelvis has been described (399).

Multilocular cystic tumors mainly affect boys in early childhood, when a substantial fraction of these lesions contain embryonal elements (CPDN), and adult women, whose lesions commonly contain only mature cells (multilocular cystic nephroma). Children with multilocular cystic renal tumors present with a painless abdominal mass. Symptoms (pain, hematuria, urinary tract infection) are more common in adults.

Multilocular cystic nephroma and CPDN cannot be distinguished by imaging or gross pathologic appearance. Sonographically, the tumor usually consists of multiple anechoic cystic spaces with septa (Fig. 9-149A). However, lesions with small cysts have many acoustic interfaces and may resemble a solid mass.

Typical CT findings include a well-circumscribed, multiseptated mass; the attenuation value of the cyst contents is similar to water (Fig. 9-150). Even by CT, when very small cysts are present, the mass may appear solid (400). Although there is contrast enhancement of the septa, contrast material does not accumulate in the cysts.

MRI findings have been described in a few cases

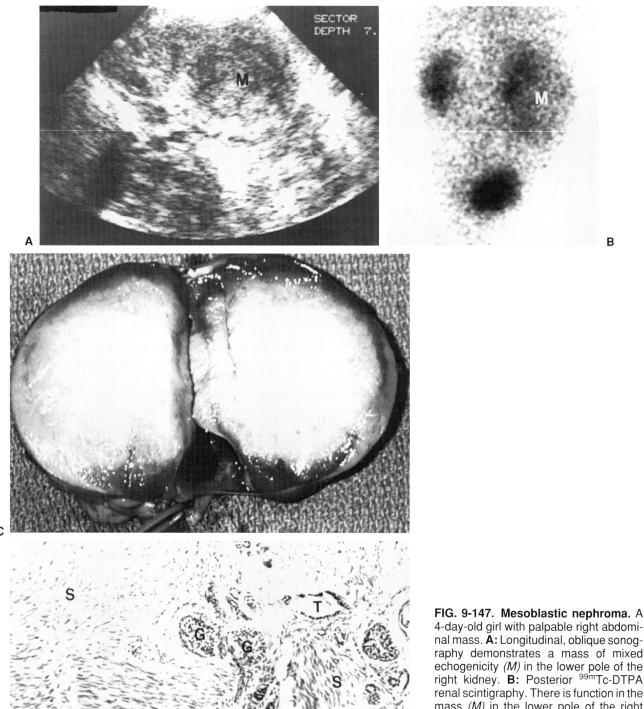

FIG. 9-147. Mesoblastic nephroma. A 4-day-old girl with palpable right abdominal mass. **A:** Longitudinal, oblique sonography demonstrates a mass of mixed echogenicity *(M)* in the lower pole of the right kidney. **B:** Posterior ^{99m}Tc-DTPA renal scintigraphy. There is function in the mass *(M)* in the lower pole of the right kidney. **C:** The cut surface of the mesoblastic nephroma has a whitish, glistening, trabeculated surface that resembles a uterine fibroid. **D:** Histologic section demonstrates glomeruli *(G)* and tubules *(T)* trapped within sheets and whorls of spindle cells *(S)* of tumor stroma. From Kirks and Kaufman (395).

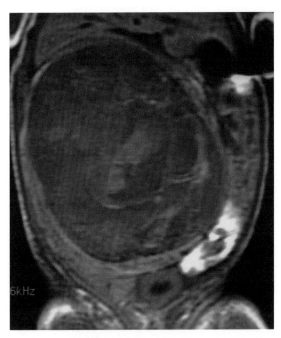

FIG. 9-148. Mesoblastic nephroma. Neonate with large abdominal mass. Coronal T1-weighted MRI. There is a well-circumscribed, inhomogeneous mass arising from the right kidney.

(397,401,402). The variable signal intensity from the cysts is felt to be due to different concentrations of protein and blood products. The septa of the cysts usually enhance after the administration of gadolinium (Fig. 9-149B) (397).

The histogenesis of multilocular cystic renal tumors is unknown. Most authorities consider the neoplasms to be benign equivalents of nephroblastoma or hamartoma (403). It

is highly doubtful that they represent congenital cystic dysplasia. It is impossible for current imaging methods to distinguish a benign multilocular cystic nephroma from a well-differentiated cystic Wilms tumor (CPDN), multilocular cystic nephroma containing foci of renal blastema, ordinary Wilms tumor, or renal cell carcinoma. The presence of thick or irregular septa seen by sonography or CT is suggestive of a multilocular nephroblastoma (well-differentiated Wilms tumor) (358). This type of multilocular nephroblastoma frequently contains blastemal elements within the cyst walls and is considered a cystic variant of Wilms tumor. The treatment of multilocular cystic nephroma with or without Wilms tumor or blastemal elements is nephrectomy. Regular postoperative surveillance is advised in patients with the CPDN variant (398).

Renal Cell Carcinoma. Renal cell carcinoma is rare during the first two decades of life. The mean age of affected children is significantly greater than that of patients with Wilms tumor (404–406). Although renal cell carcinoma is much more common in male adults, there is an almost equal sex incidence in children. Presenting symptoms include a palpable mass (60%), flank pain (50%), and hematuria (30%). US and CT show a nonspecific, solid intrarenal mass (358,404). There is a higher frequency of calcification in renal cell carcinoma (25%) (Fig. 9-151) than in Wilms tumor (5% to 15%). There may be extension of tumor or thrombus into the inferior vena cava (Fig. 9-151).

This tumor, rare in childhood, should be included in the differential diagnosis of intrarenal mass lesions, particularly in older children with hematuria or calcification in the mass. The prognosis, as in the adult, depends on the stage of disease at diagnosis (358).

Renal Lymphoma. Although rarely found early, renal in-

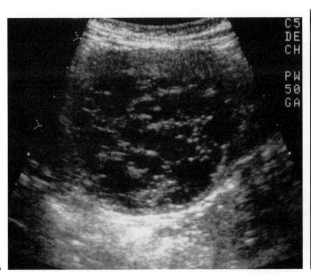

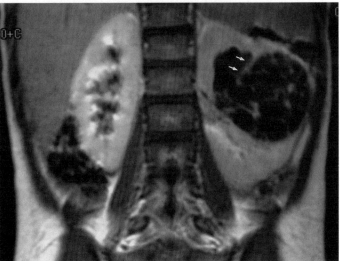

A B

FIG. 9-149. Multilocular cystic nephroma. A 4-year-old boy with gross hematuria. **A:** Longitudinal renal sonography. The left intrarenal mass is well-circumscribed and multiloculated. **B:** Contrast-enhanced coronal T1-weighted MRI. There is contrast enhancement *(arrows)* of the linear septa in the cystic mass.

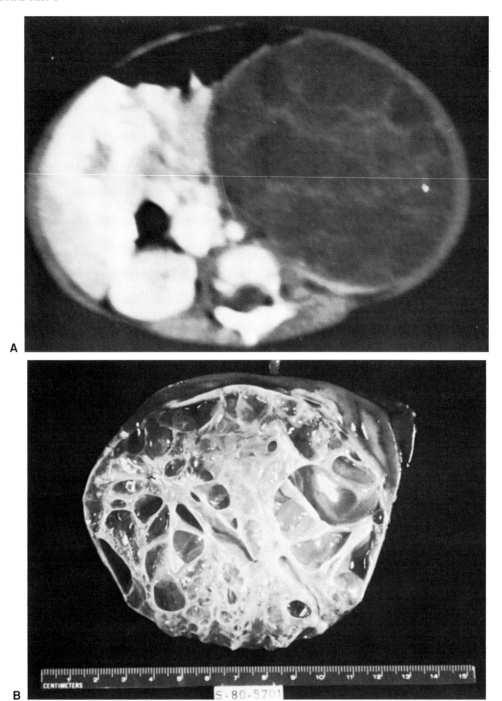

FIG. 9-150. Multilocular cystic nephroma. A 2-year-old girl with a left abdominal mass. **A:** CT with contrast enhancement. The left intrarenal mass contains areas of decreased attenuation. These low-density spaces are separated by fine, linear septa. **B:** Transverse section of the lower pole of the nephrectomy specimen. The gross pathology correlates with findings on CT. From Kirks et al. (27).

volvement is often present in the terminal phases of lymphoma, particularly non-Hodgkin lymphoma (8,407). There may be many small nodules, large confluent masses, or a diffuse infiltrative process. Lymphoma sometimes causes bilateral renal enlargement (see Table 9-2). Vascular compromise due to lymphomatous involvement can cause hypertension.

Diffuse renal lymphoma usually produces a decrease in parenchymal echogenicity (8). Bilateral nodules may be hypoechoic or anechoic, and they may distort the renal contour and disrupt the normal intrarenal architecture. CT demonstrates bilateral renal masses that enhance less than the adjacent renal parenchyma. Retroperitoneal or mesenteric adenopathy almost always coexists (408). Rarely, lymphoma presents as a focal, unilateral mass that suggests a primary renal neoplasm (409).

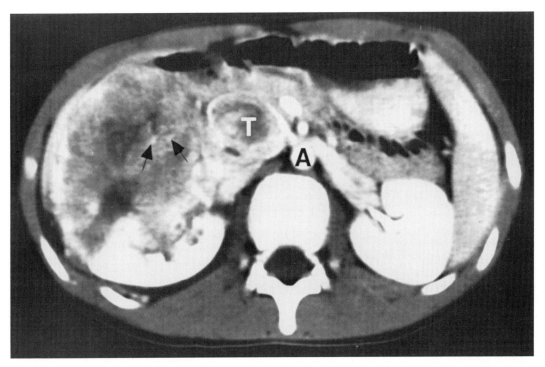

FIG. 9-151. Renal cell carcinoma. A 13-year-old girl with right abdominal pain and a palpable abdominal mass. CT with contrast enhancement shows a large inhomogeneous mass arising from the right kidney. The mass contains calcifications *(arrows)*. A pseudocapsule was not identified. Note the large tumor thrombus *(T)* within the markedly dilated inferior vena cava. The aorta *(A)* is normal. From Kirks et al. (358).

Renal Leukemia. Leukemic involvement of the kidneys, usually causing nephromegaly, may be detected at the time of initial diagnosis or during remission (8). Although most commonly diffuse, renal leukemia is occasionally focal. Leukemic infiltration can also cause decreased renal function (15,410).

Clear Cell Sarcoma of the Kidney. Clear cell sarcoma of the kidney (CCSK) is a highly malignant renal neoplasm of childhood with a propensity for bone metastases. Formerly considered to be an unfavorable type of Wilms tumor, it is now known to be a distinct pathologic entity. Although the age distribution is identical to that of Wilms tumor, CCSK has a higher rate of relapse and greater morbidity. Because no imaging permits distinction between CCSK and Wilms tumor, the diagnosis is based on histology. In patients with CCSK, bone scintigraphy is extremely useful for staging and for postoperative follow-up (5).

Rhabdoid Tumor of the Kidney. Rhabdoid tumor of the kidney (RTK) is a highly malignant neoplasm that is also considered to be distinct from Wilms tumor. RTK occurs in infants and young children and is extremely rare over the age of 5. RTK has a high relapse rate and a mortality of over 80%; it is one of the most malignant tumors of childhood. Metastatic spread to the lungs, liver, and brain is common. Bone metastases can also occur (5). Sonography, CT, and MRI show a large intrarenal soft-tissue mass that compresses the normal renal parenchyma. There is frequently a large amount of subcapsular fluid (Fig. 9-152). The renal capsule is irregularly thickened and there may be subcapsular nodules (411).

Tumor Surveillance of High-Risk Individuals

Children with sporadic aniridia, hemihypertrophy, Beckwith-Wiedemann syndrome, Drash syndrome, and nephroblastomatosis are all at increased risk for the development of Wilms tumor. Ultrasound is currently the best modality for tumor surveillance, although MRI may ultimately prove more sensitive (383). Because no longitudinal studies have been performed, recommendations for tumor surveillance by imaging are arbitrary (388,413). Most centers recommend follow-up imaging at 3- to 6-month intervals for any child with any of these conditions. The fact that most Wilms tumors not diagnosed through screening programs are very large at presentation and yet carry an excellent prognosis supports less frequent intervals between studies. Screening of high-risk children can probably be stopped between the ages of 6 and 10 years; fewer than 15% of all Wilms tumors occur after the age of 6 years and fewer than 1% after age 10. Moreover, Wilms tumor associated with the syndromes listed above are diagnosed at a younger age than other Wilms tumors. A metachronous Wilms tumor almost always develops within 2 years of the first tumor (371,414); in children

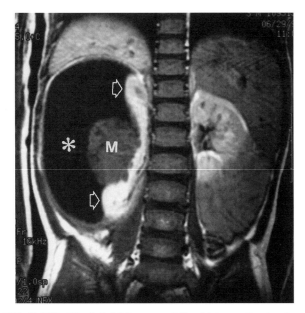

FIG. 9-152. Rhabdoid tumor of the kidney. Contrast-enhanced coronal T1-weighted MRI. There is an intermediate-intensity mass *(M)* arising from the lateral part of the compressed right kidney *(arrows)*. There is a large subcapsular fluid collection *(asterisk)*.

without any special risk factors, follow-up imaging for tumor surveillance can be discontinued after 2 years.

Treatment and Prognosis

Survival of patients with Wilms tumor has increased from approximately 10% in the 1920s to over 90% in the 1990s (5,9,415). The treatment is surgical plus adjuvant chemotherapy. The contralateral kidney is explored to exclude bilaterality. Radiation therapy may also be used after surgery.

Although staging is always performed, histology is by far the most important prognostic factor. Most pediatric oncologists consider that two years free of disease indicates cure. Surgery with supplementary chemotherapy and irradiation has led to a 2-year survival rate of well over 90% in patients with favorable histology. Mortality remains high in children with unfavorable histology. In NWTS III, patients with clear cell sarcomas responded well to chemotherapy; the 2-year survival after three-drug therapy was similar to that of Wilms tumor with favorable histology (372). In contrast, the prognosis of children with rhabdoid tumor is extremely poor. There is only a 19% 3-year survival after triple-agent chemotherapy.

Neuroblastoma

Neuroblastoma is one of the most enigmatic, biologically intriguing, diagnostically interesting, and therapeutically frustrating neoplasms of childhood (384). It is the most com-

mon extracranial solid malignant tumor in children and the third most common malignancy of childhood, surpassed in incidence only by leukemia and by primary brain tumors grouped together. Neuroblastoma accounts for at least 10% of all pediatric neoplasms. Approximately 525 new cases are diagnosed in the United States each year (416). At least 15% of cancer deaths in children are due to neuroblastoma. Neuroblastoma is the second most common abdominal malignancy in the older infant and child, occurring in the abdomen almost as frequently as Wilms tumor (8,27). Over the last 30 years, there has been modest improvement in the outcome for infants and for older children with local or regional disease. However, the prognosis has not improved significantly for older children with metastases at the time of diagnosis.

Neuroblastoma is a malignant tumor of primitive neural crest cells (neuroblasts) that may arise anywhere in the sympathetic ganglion chain or adrenal medulla. The tumor usually involves the abdomen, thorax, or lower neck. It has a tendency for direct spread, metastases to bone and liver, and tumor calcification.

Clinical Features

Neuroblastoma is slightly more common in boys than girls; the male/female ratio is 1.2:1 (8,9,12,384). The median age at diagnosis is 22 months; 6% of patients are diagnosed by the age of 1 year, 79% by 4 years, and 97% by 10 years (417).

Neuroblastoma is usually silent until it invades or compresses adjacent structures, metastasizes, or produces a paraneoplastic syndrome. The general signs and symptoms are nonspecific; they include fever, weight loss, irritability, and anemia. Abdominal neuroblastoma commonly presents as a firm, nodular abdominal mass. There may be local symptoms and signs due to ureteral obstruction or compression of the rectum, bladder, or blood vessels. Although extradural tumor extension is common with thoracic neuroblastomas, it is rare in abdominal tumors.

The proportion of patients presenting with localized, regional, or metastatic disease is age-dependent. The incidence of localized tumors, regional lymph node spread, and disseminated disease is 19%, 13%, and 68%, respectively, in older children as compared to 39%, 18%, and 53% in infants. Approximately 18% of infants have stage IV-S disseminated disease (417).

Metastatic spread, the cause of the presenting symptoms and signs in many patients with neuroblastoma, is lymphatic and hematogenous. Common sites of metastases are the skeleton, bone marrow, liver, lymph nodes, and skin. Patterns of metastatic spread vary greatly with age. Bone metastases are common in children >1 year of age, often involving the long bones and orbits and frequently causing bone pain or proptosis. However, bony metastases occur in fewer than

5% of newborns, whereas massive hepatic involvement and skin lesions are frequent in patients <1 year of age. Patients of any age may have bone marrow involvement, adenopathy, and liver metastases (384).

Despite the high frequency of increased catecholamine secretion by neuroblastomas, no more than 10% of children have hypertension (384). Approximately 90% to 95% of patients with neuroblastoma excrete an excess of catecholamine metabolites [vanillylmandelic acid (VMA), homovanillic acid, norepinephrine, and dopamine] in the urine (418). Although spot VMA tests may be positive in neuroblastoma, there are high false-positive and high false-negative rates; therefore, 24-hour urine collections are usually tested. Increased excretion of catecholamine metabolites indicates the presence of a neural crest neoplasm. An increase or decrease in the excretion of these metabolites with treatment suggests that the tumor is growing or regressing.

Two unusual but well-described paraneoplastic syndromes occur in children with neuroblastoma: myoclonic encephalopathy of infancy (MEI) and the syndrome of diarrhea with hypokalemia. MEI is often associated with neurogenic tumors of ganglion cell origin. It includes the triad of opsoclonus, myoclonus, and cerebellar ataxia (419,420). As many as 4% of patients with neuroblastoma have MEI (418,421). Although some reviews state that almost half of all children with MEI have an associated neurogenic tumor (420), the true incidence is unknown; there probably is a bias in favor of publishing cases associated with neoplasms (384,417). However, all patients with MEI should be evaluated for a neurogenic tumor.

MEI-associated neuroblastoma differs from classic neuroblastoma in three ways: equal sex incidence, greater frequency of thoracic tumors, and improved prognosis (419,421,422). Approximately half of children with neuroblastoma and MEI will have posterior mediastinal tumors. Chest radiography is therefore essential. The initial imaging of MEI should include chest radiography and then abdominal US or CT. Neck CT or MRI, chest CT or MRI, or abdominal MRI may be required in some patients. The precise pathogenesis of MEI is unknown, although an immune response to tumor that cross-reacts with cerebellar tissue has been postulated (384,419).

The second paraneoplastic syndrome, present in approximately 7% of children with neural crest tumors, consists of intractable watery diarrhea, hypokalemia, and achlorhydria. The cause is an excessive secretion of vasoactive intestinal peptides (VIPs) as well as catecholamines. Elevated VIP levels may occur in as many as 25% of patients with neuroblastoma, but many of these children do not have the syndrome (384).

Helpful laboratory studies for diagnosing neuroblastoma include a complete blood count and differential, bone marrow aspiration, liver function tests, blood coagulation studies, and urinary catecholamine metabolite assays. Bone marrow aspiration is critical for staging.

Pathology

Neuroblastoma and its more differentiated forms, ganglioneuroblastoma and ganglioneuroma, arise from primitive sympathetic neuroblasts of the embryonic neural crest. The tumor consists microscopically of small, round cells (Fig. 9-153) that may be difficult to differentiate from those of Ewing sarcoma, rhabdomyosarcoma, leukemia, and lymphoma. Neuroblastoma is the only one of these malignancies that commonly forms tumor rosettes in both blood and bone marrow.

The three pediatric neural crest tumors (neuroblastoma, ganglioneuroblastoma, ganglioneuroma) are differentiated by the degree of cellular maturation. Neuroblastoma, a frankly malignant tumor, is composed of undifferentiated sympathoblasts. The tumor contains gross or microscopic calcification and is usually well demarcated but lacks a capsule. It has nests of primitive round cells with dark-staining nuclei and scanty cytoplasm (Fig. 9-153). Tumor cells may form rosettes and contain fibrils. Ganglioneuroblastoma is also a malignant tumor; it contains undifferentiated neuroblasts but also mature ganglion cells. The tumor may be partially or totally encapsulated and frequently contains granular calcifications. Because the histologic appearance may vary in a single tumor, the pathologic distinction between ganglioneuroblastoma and neuroblastoma has been criticized as arbitrary (423). A prognostic classification for ganglioneuroblastoma based on age and histopathologic features has been developed by Shimada (424). The tumors are graded according to their degree of differentiation, amount of stroma, and mitosis-karyorrhexis index (number of cells per 5000 showing mitosis or nuclear fragmentation). Preliminary results suggest that this histologic pattern predicts outcome; tumor stage may be prognostically less important than histologic grade (423). Ganglioneuroma is a benign tumor of mature ganglion cells. It is well circumscribed, encapsulated, and usually contains gross calcification.

Many young infants who die of other causes have pathologic evidence of neuroblastoma in situ. In the normal child, these clumps of primitive neuroblastic cells tend to involute or mature. In a few others, the primitive rests apparently progress to neuroblastoma. Both primary and metastatic neuroblastoma have a tendency to change spontaneously into a less malignant tumor in the ganglioneuroma-neuroblastoma series, especially in neonates and young infants.

Approximately two thirds of neuroblastomas are located in the abdomen, and two thirds of these lesions arise from the adrenal gland. The other abdominal and pelvic tumors almost always originate in the paravertebral sympathetic chain or the presacral area, with an occasional abdominal tumor arising in the celiac axis or organ of Zuckerkandl. Fifteen percent of neuroblastomas are thoracic, usually arising from the sympathetic ganglia of the posterior mediastinum. Other sites of origin include the pelvis (5%), cervical sympathetic plexuses (5%), and cerebrum (0.2%). Primary cerebral neuroblastomas are now considered in the spectrum

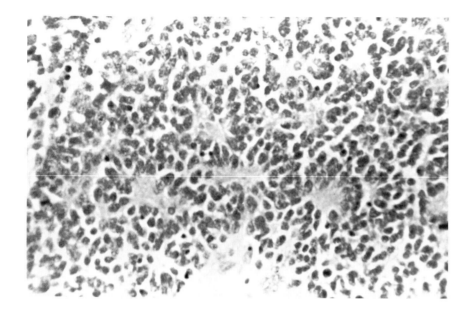

FIG. 9-153. Histology of neuroblastoma. The neoplasm consists of small, round, dark-staining cells that form tumor rosettes. From Bousvaros et al. (384).

of primitive neuroectodermal tumors (PNET). Ten to twelve percent of neuroblastomas are disseminated but have no known site of origin (417).

Staging

Three systems are currently available for staging neuroblastomas. In the past, the Evans system was universally used, and it is still used widely. Stage I is tumor confined to the structure of origin. Stage II includes tumor extension in continuity beyond the structure of origin but not across the midline. This stage includes tumors arising in midline structures, such as the organ of Zuckerkandl. Regional lymph nodes may be involved on the same side as the tumor or, in midline tumors, on one side. Stage III tumors extend in continuity across the midline, including bilateral extension of a midline tumor. Regional lymph nodes may be involved bilaterally. Stage IV is disseminated disease with metastases involving the skeleton, soft tissues, distant lymph nodes, or other distant organs. A unique group of patients is assigned to stage IV-S, in which the primary tumor would be considered stage I or II but there is metastatic disease limited to liver, skin, or bone marrow. Patients with bony metastases (positive bone scintigraphy or skeletal survey) are not in stage IV-S (384). It is apparent that the size of the tumor, its extension across the midline, and the presence of metastases are the three most important criteria in the Evans system (8). The incidence of neuroblastoma by Evans staging is stage I 13.5%, stage II 11%, stage III 8.4%, stage IV 43.9%, stage IV-S 9.1%, and unknown stage 14.1% (384).

The Pediatric Oncology Group (POG) staging is based on tumor resectability and lymph node involvement. The International Neuroblastoma Staging System (INSS) is based on tumor resectability, lymph node involvement, rela-

tionship of tumor to the midline, and sites of tumor dissemination (425–428).

Although each system has its strengths, their differences have made it difficult to compare results and determine which better indicates prognosis. Staging by current imaging techniques is more adapted to the Evans system, as tumor extension across the midline is readily detected by CT or MRI. Because CT and MRI cannot predict lymph node involvement accurately, the POG staging system and INSS require surgicopathologic correlation. Although only recently developed, the INSS has received widespread acceptance by pediatric oncologists (427,428).

Imaging

During the 1980s, CT became the imaging modality of choice for patients with neuroblastoma (384). Either CT or MRI is essential for the confirmation, localization, and staging of neuroblastoma, whether the tumor is abdominal, pelvic, thoracic, cervical, or intracranial in location. Imaging is used to identify the primary tumor mass, to document the extent of disease at presentation, and to assess response to therapy.

Because of superior spatial resolution, current INSS recommendations are for diagnostic evaluation of the abdomen by CT or MRI (427,428). In particular, it is recommended that three-dimensional measurements of the primary tumor and large metastases be obtained by either CT or MRI to determine response to therapy . It is also recommended that metaiodobenzylguanidine (MIBG) scanning be performed if available (428).

Abdominal Radiography. Plain radiography demonstrates calcification in as many as 55% of patients with abdominal neuroblastoma but in only 5% of patients with Wilms tumor. This calcification may be diffuse, mottled, finely stippled, or (less frequently) coalescent (8,9,384). Other plain film findings include displacement of bowel gas, paravertebral widening in the lower chest, bone destruction, and widened interpediculate distances indicating tumor extension into the vertebral canal. One should carefully evaluate the vertebral bodies and pedicles for spinal extension, the paravertebral soft tissues for direct extension, and the liver for enlargement due to hematogenous metastases.

Ultrasonography. Unless tumor calcifications have been shown by a radiograph, US is usually the next imaging mo-

dality for a child with a palpable abdominal mass. Neuroblastoma can usually be distinguished from Wilms tumor by its extrarenal location. The sonographic characteristics of the mass may provide additional diagnostic information. Neuroblastoma is inhomogeneous in echogenicity because of increased tumor cellularity, hemorrhage, necrosis, and dystrophic calcification. Wilms tumor has a more homogeneous echogenicity.

Sonography is inferior to CT and MRI for assessing the character and extent of neuroblastoma. It has limited ability

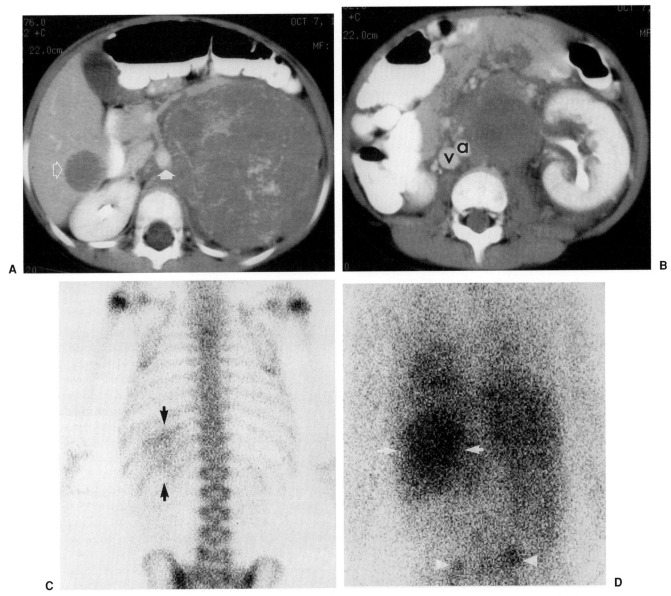

FIG. 9-154. Stage IV neuroblastoma. A 5-year-old girl with the recent onset of fever, abdominal cramps, abdominal distention, and constipation. **A:** Contrast-enhanced axial CT. There is a large, calcified left upper quadrant mass that surrounds the great vessels and displaces the aorta *(white arrow)* ventrally. There is a metastasis to the posterior segment of the right lobe of the liver *(open arrow)*. **B:** A lower CT section shows necrotic tumor extending across the midline and displacing the aorta *(a)* and inferior vena cava *(v)* to the right. **C:** Posterior ^{99m}Tc-MDP bone scintigraphy. There is uptake of tracer *(arrows)* by the large tumor. **D:** Posterior ^{123}I-MIBG scintigraphy shows tracer uptake in the abdominal tumor *(arrows)* and bony pelvic metastases *(arrowheads)*.

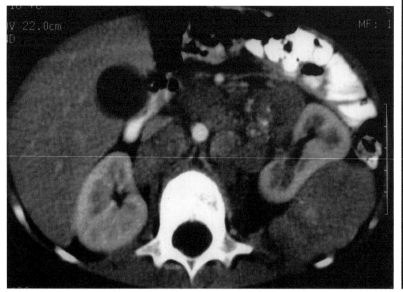
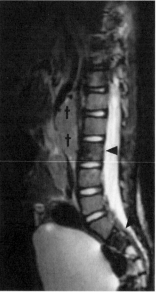

FIG. 9-155. Unresectable stage IV neuroblastoma arising from organ of Zuckerkandl. A: Contrast-enhanced axial CT. There is a large, midline, calcified mass that surrounds the aorta, inferior vena cava, and superior mesenteric artery. The kidneys are displaced laterally. This tumor is not resectable. **B:** Sagittal T2-weighted MRI. Tumor mass *(t)* surrounds and displaces the inferior vena cava anteriorly. There is hypointensity of the L3 and S2 vertebral bodies *(arrowheads)*. Bone marrow biopsy was positive for neuroblastoma.

to detect metastases in retroperitoneal and retrocrural lymph nodes and is usually unable to detect extradural extension of tumor. If conventional radiography demonstrates typical calcifications in a patient with a palpable abdominal mass, one should proceed directly to CT or MRI (384).

Computed Tomography. CT is superior to sonography for defining tumor morphology and extent. CT is able to detect prevertebral extension of tumor across the midline as well as encasement of the celiac axis or superior mesenteric artery by neuroblastoma (Figs. 9-154 to 9-156). CT can also show extension of tumor to retroperitoneal lymph nodes, to liver, around central vessels, and into the vertebral canal. CT is excellent for demonstrating retrocrural and paravertebral tumor extension to the chest, which is common in abdominal neuroblastoma.

CT detects abdominal neuroblastoma with a sensitivity approaching 100% (384). The mass is commonly suprarenal or paravertebral. The tumor is usually lobulated and lacks an identifiable capsule. Hemorrhage, necrosis, and calcification cause inhomogeneous attenuation. Calcification is identified by CT in at least 85% of patients. Intravenous contrast enhancement is helpful in showing vascular displacement and encasement, either of which is a contraindication to immediate surgical resection (Figs. 9-154A, 9-155A, and 9-156A).

In the past, CT myelography was routinely performed for all paraspinal neurogenic tumors because of their propensity to extend extradurally into the vertebral canal. MRI has now replaced this more invasive technique.

Magnetic Resonance Imaging. MRI is excellent for eval-

uating the location, extent, and spread of neuroblastoma (412,429,430). These tumors usually have prolonged T1 and T2 relaxation times, like most malignancies (Figs. 9-155B, 9-156B, and 9-157). Although focal areas of calcification may not be detected, large calcific regions are recognizable by their low signal intensity.

Advantages of MRI over CT and sonography include (a) multiplanar imaging (useful for assessing invasion of adjacent organs); (b) detection of extradural tumor extension without intrathecal contrast injection; (c) identification of bone marrow metastases (useful for staging); and (d) delineation of intraabdominal vascular displacement or encasement without dependence on intravenous contrast (Figs. 9-155B, 9-156B, and 9-157).

Changes in signal intensity are seen with therapy, although their significance is not known (412). As previously discussed, MRI has replaced CT myelography for the demonstration of extradural tumor extension (Fig. 9-158). MRI is also very sensitive to bone marrow metastases (Fig. 9-155B); unfortunately, this MRI appearance is not specific.

Nuclear Scintigraphy. Approximately 70% of patients with neuroblastoma have primary tumor uptake of ^{99m}Tc-labeled phosphate compounds (431,432). The exact mechanism of this uptake is not known. If there is uptake of skeletal tracer by an abdominal mass, neuroblastoma should be strongly considered (Fig. 9-154C). MIBG (I-131 and I-123) has been used in recent years to localize neuroblastomas. Uptake of this tracer occurs in metabolically active neural crest tumors (Fig. 9-154D). The agent can detect primary, recurrent, and metastatic disease. The current INSS recom-

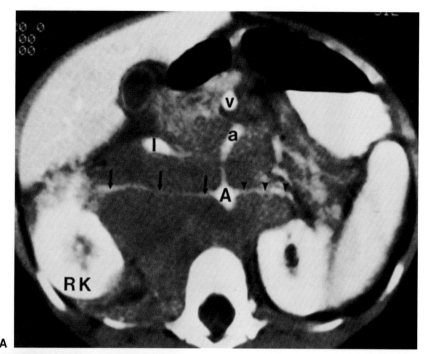

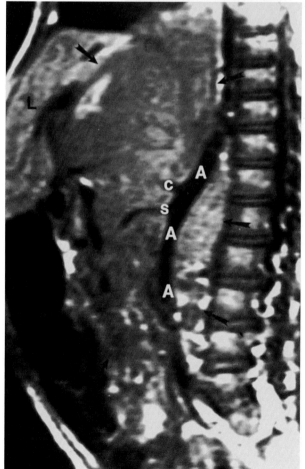

FIG. 9-156. Unresectable stage IV neuroblastoma. A 3-year-old boy with a palpable abdominal mass. **A:** Contrast-enhanced CT. The large retroperitoneal mass displaces the right kidney *(RK)* laterally and inferiorly. Neuroblastoma extends across the midline behind the aorta *(A)*. Note that the aorta, superior mesenteric artery *(a)*, superior mesenteric vein *(v)*, inferior vena cava *(l)*, right renal artery *(arrows)*, and left renal artery *(arrowheads)* are completely surrounded and encased by the tumor, which is not resectable. **B:** Sagittal proton-density MRI. The large neuroblastoma *(arrows)* surrounds and encases the aorta *(A)*, celiac axis *(c)*, and superior mesenteric artery *(s)*. *L*, liver.

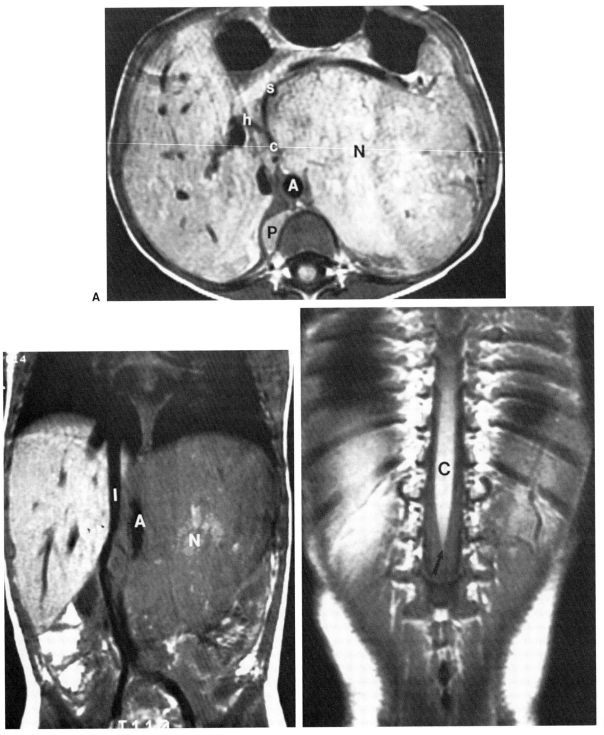

FIG. 9-157. Unresectable stage III neuroblastoma. A 1-year-old boy with a left abdominal mass. **A:** Proton density axial MRI. There is a large mass *(N)* in the left abdomen that crosses the midline. There is paravertebral *(P)* tumor extension on the right. The aorta *(A)* is displaced ventrally. The celiac axis *(c)* is encased by tumor, and there is displacement of the hepatic artery *(h)* and splenic artery *(s)*. **B:** Coronal MRI. The large neuroblastoma *(N)* contains areas of calcification and hemorrhage. The aorta *(A)* is surrounded by tumor; there is displacement of the infrahepatic portion of the inferior vena cava *(I)* to the right. **C:** Coronal MRI. There is excellent visualization of the spinal cord *(C)* and the tip of the conus medullaris *(arrow)*. There is no evidence of extradural tumor extension.

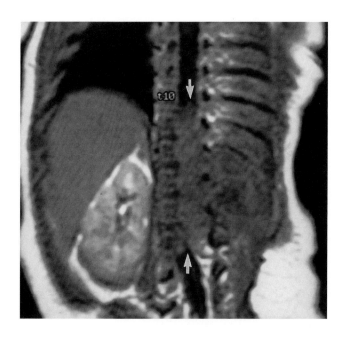

FIG. 9-158. Extradural extension of abdominal neuroblastoma. A 6-week-old boy with a left-sided back mass. Contrast-enhanced coronal T1-weighted MRI. There is a lobulated left paraspinal mass. Note the extradural extension at several levels *(between arrows).*

mendation is for MIBG scanning, if available. MIBG scintigraphy is particularly useful in distinguishing residual active tumor from fibrosis and is more sensitive than bone scintigraphy for assessing the response of tumor involving cortical bone (433,434). Problems with MIBG scintigraphy include its lack of wide availability, its generally inferior spatial resolution compared to bone scintigraphy, and the fact that not all primary tumors and metastases are MIBG-avid.

Imaging of Unique Types of Neuroblastoma

Stage IV-S tumors usually occur in infants less than 6 months of age. Sonography is ideal for demonstrating the primary tumor as well as metastatic disease in the liver (Fig. 9-159). MRI is excellent for confirming the primary neuroblastoma as well as hepatic involvement (Fig. 9-160); MR spectroscopy has considerable potential for evaluating this unique type of neuroblastoma as well as its response to therapy (384). Bone scintigraphy should be performed to exclude bony metastases.

Since approximately half of all children with neuroblastoma and *myoclonic encephalopathy of infancy* will have tumors of the posterior mediastinum, chest radiography is mandatory (419); the tumor is further evaluated with CT or MRI and nuclear scintigraphy. Sonography is the ideal screening modality for patients with possible abdominal tumors; anatomic detail is shown by CT or MRI.

Differential Diagnosis

Neonatal Adrenal Hemorrhage. Adrenal hemorrhage, a more common abnormality of the neonate than neuroblastoma, may present as an asymptomatic flank mass. The symptoms and signs, when present, include hypovolemic shock, anemia, and jaundice (27,435). The etiology of adrenal hemorrhage is not clear, but birth trauma, stress, hypoxia, and dehydration have been implicated. Surgical intervention is usually unnecessary unless there is secondary infection and an adrenal abscess forms. It may occasionally be difficult to distinguish cystic adrenal neuroblastoma (Fig. 9-161) from neonatal adrenal hemorrhage; sequential sonography or MRI is helpful.

US classically shows a suprarenal anechoic mass (Figs. 9-162 and 9-163) compressing the upper pole of the kidney. However, on the first sonographic examination, the hemorrhage may appear as an echogenic, solid lesion. The more typical anechoic appearance develops as the hematoma liquefies (Fig. 9-163B) (436,437). The mass may become echogenic again as clot and calcification develop (Figs. 9-162B and 9-163D). Sequential US shows shrinkage of the mass and eventual disappearance or calcification over several months.

The major differential diagnostic considerations in a neonate with a suprarenal mass are adrenal hemorrhage and neuroblastoma. US should almost always be able to distinguish between neuroblastoma (echogenic and vascular) and neonatal adrenal hemorrhage (anechoic and avascular). Moreover, since congenital adrenal neuroblastoma has an excellent prognosis, serial US is an acceptable way to identify the exceedingly rare case in which history, physical examination, and sonography are not diagnostic (27,436). If immediate differentiation is imperative, MRI may be used to confirm adrenal hemorrhage (438).

Other Adrenal Neoplasms. Other childhood adrenal neoplasms occasionally mimic neuroblastoma. These neoplasms, which may or may not be functional, include teratoma, dermoid, cortical adenoma, adrenal carcinoma, and

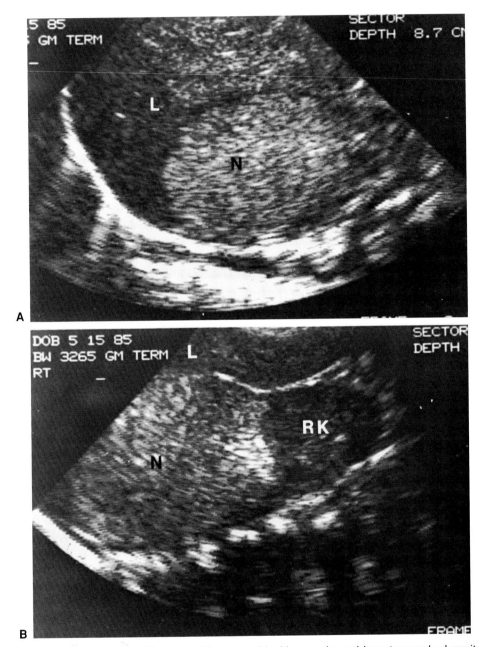

FIG. 9-159. Stage IV-S neuroblastoma. Newborn girl with anemia and hepatomegaly. Longitudinal sonography of the right upper quadrant **(A)** and right retroperitoneum **(B)** demonstrate marked heterogeneity and altered echogenicity of the liver *(L)*. There is a large echogenic mass *(N)* above the right kidney *(RK)*. From Bousvaros et al. (384).

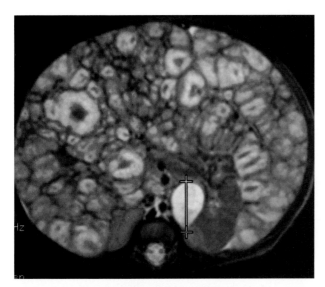

FIG. 9-160. MRI of stage IV-S neuroblastoma. A 1-month-old with rapidly increasing abdominal girth. Axial T2-weighted MRI. There is massive enlargement of the liver with many nodules of high signal intensity. The left adrenal mass *(between cursors)* also has increased signal intensity.

pheochromocytoma. Nonfunctioning adrenocortical neoplasms are frequently malignant (8,9).

Other Retroperitoneal Tumors. Wilms tumor usually distorts the pelvicalyceal system of the kidney and is thus usually distinguishable from neuroblastoma, which displaces the kidney with little distortion. Occasionally, an intrarenal malignancy grows in an exophytic manner and displaces the kidney, simulating neuroblastoma. CT or MRI usually clarifies the organ of origin and determines the presence or absence of calcification. *Hydronephrosis* of the upper pole moiety of a duplicated collecting system may become ob-

structed, as in ectopic ureterocele or ureteral ectopia, and simulate neuroblastoma. US clarifies the cystic characteristics of the mass and shows the dilated ureter draining the upper pole. The filling defect of an ectopic ureterocele in the bladder may be demonstrated by US, VCUG, or IVU. *Retroperitoneal lymph node enlargement* due to leukemia, lymphoma, or metastases may rarely simulate neuroblastoma by displacing a kidney inferiorly and laterally (8,9). *Hepatoblastoma* of the right lobe of the liver can displace the right kidney inferiorly and laterally. If calcification is present, differentiation from neuroblastoma may be very difficult. MRI, particularly in the coronal plane, helps distinguish these two neoplasms. A *splenic mass* (epidermoid, cyst, hamartoma) may depress the left kidney to mimic a left adrenal neuroblastoma (9). *Lymphatic malformations* (439) and *teratomas* may involve the retroperitoneum; CT or MRI will demonstrate the tissue content of these tumors.

Treatment and Prognosis

The preferred treatment for stage I or II tumors is complete surgical resection. If a tumor is nonresectable because of its large size or its relation to critical vessels, it may be advisable to confirm the diagnosis by surgical biopsy, treat with radiation therapy or chemotherapy, and perform second-look surgery after the expected response is documented. The surgical removal of a stage IV tumor does not improve survival but may be palliative (384).

Spontaneous regression sometimes occurs in patients with stage IV-S disease. Treatment is therefore reserved for patients with morbidity due to local disease. An occasional serious complication of stage IV-S disease is respiratory compromise secondary to massive hepatomegaly. This has been treated with low-dose radiation therapy, small doses

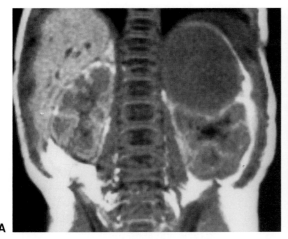
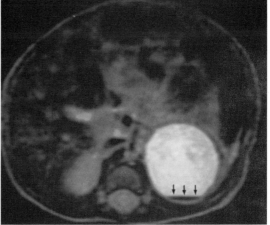

FIG. 9-161. Cystic adrenal neuroblastoma. Neonate with cystic suprarenal mass. There was no change in size on sequential sonography. **A:** Coronal T1-weighted MRI. There is a homogeneous, hypointense left suprarenal mass. **B:** Axial T2-weighted MRI. The left suprarenal mass is predominantly hyperintense and has a fluid-fluid level *(arrows)*. The dependent fluid is of low signal intensity consistent with blood products. A cystic adrenal neuroblastoma was completely resected.

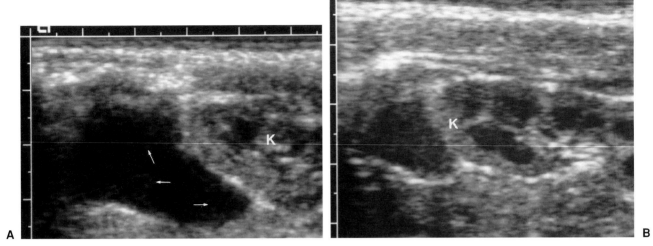

FIG. 9-162. Neonatal adrenal hemorrhage. A 2-week-old infant with Taybi-Rubinstein syndrome referred for screening ultrasound examination of the kidney. **A:** Longitudinal sonography shows an anechoic mass containing thin strands of echogenic tissue *(arrows)* above the right kidney *(K)*. **B:** Follow-up sonography at 2 months of age. The mass is smaller and more echogenic. *K,* right kidney.

of chemotherapy, and surgical decrease of intraabdominal pressure with a Silastic patch.

The most important determinants of prognosis in patients with neuroblastoma are age, stage, and location of disease at diagnosis. The younger the patient, the better the prognosis. Stages I, II, and IV-S have a much better prognosis than stage III and IV disease. Thoracic neuroblastoma has better survival than abdominal tumors.

The outcome for infants <1 year of age is substantially better than that for older patients with the same stage of disease, especially in the more advanced stages. This improved survival in young patients may be due to less widespread disease at diagnosis, a higher incidence of spontaneous regression, a lower propensity for bony metastases, and a greater response to intensive multiagent chemotherapy. The prognosis for disease-free survival of patients with stage I, II, and IV-S neuroblastoma is between 75% and 90%; those with stages III and IV disease have a survival of only 10% to 30%. Tumors arising in the abdomen and pelvis have the worst prognosis, with adrenal tumors having the highest mortality. Thoracic neuroblastomas have an overall 61% survival rate compared to 20% for abdominal tumors. Perhaps this improved survival in thoracic tumors is due to diagnosis at an earlier stage of disease.

Infants with INSS stage IV (disseminated disease) tumors treated with intensive multiagent chemotherapy have a relapse-free survival rate of 75% (440,441). Some of these patients also received irradiation. However, an even larger group of infants with disseminated disease were treated with low-dose chemotherapy or low-dose chemotherapy followed by delayed removal of the primary tumor; 60% of this group remained disease-free (417). These observations demonstrate that a significant subset of infants have a high probability of cure without intensive multidrug chemotherapy or ra-

diation and suggest that aggressive multimodality therapy should be reserved for stage IV-S infants who are not responding to initial therapy (440,441). Identification of higher risk infants with disseminated disease may now be possible by measuring tumor DNA content and N-myc copy number.

The highest risk population is children over 12 months of age with INSS stage IV. The overall survival for this risk group has remained unchanged for the last 30 years at <15%. More intensive chemotherapy has improved temporary disease control. The dose-limiting myelosuppression that occurs with this approach has prompted the search for alternative methods of tumor therapy. These include immunotherapy, bone marrow transplantation, and cytokines. ^{131}I-MIBG and ^{125}I-MIBG therapy may also offer improved survival. Chemotherapy may cause significant shrinkage of the primary tumor, make an unresectable mass resectable, and improve survival.

The relation of the tumor to the abdominal great vessels (aorta, inferior vena cava, celiac axis, superior mesentery artery) is more critical for resectability and prognosis than the relation of the tumor to the midline (384).

Pheochromocytoma

Pheochromocytoma arises from neural crest cells and is usually benign. Approximately 70% of pheochromocytomas arise from the adrenal medulla. Extraadrenal tumors may occur anywhere that chromaffin tissue is present, usually along the thoracic and abdominal sympathetic chains. Pheochromocytoma may also arise in the sympathetic ganglia located adjacent to the aorta and in the carotid body, organ of Zuckerkandl, bladder wall, and ureter (8,9). Approximately 5% of pheochromocytomas occur in children, and

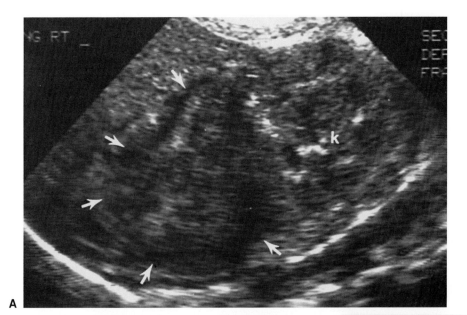

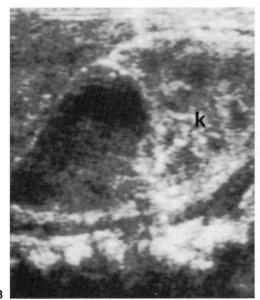

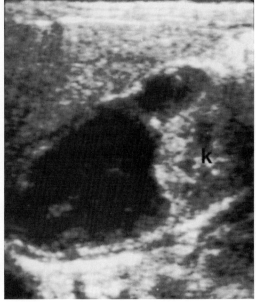

FIG. 9-163. Neonatal adrenal hemorrhage. Newborn with anemia, jaundice, and a questionable right abdominal mass. **A:** One day of age. Longitudinal sonography demonstrates an inhomogeneous mass *(arrows)* above the right kidney *(k)*. **B:** 1 week *(left)* and 2 weeks *(right)* of age. Sequential sonography demonstrates an adrenal hemorrhage above the right kidney *(k)* that becomes smaller and more hypoechoic with time. *(Continued)*

approximately 5% of those tumors are malignant. Pheochromocytomas are usually discovered during evaluation of a child with hypertension. In contrast to the adult, the hypertension of pheochromocytoma in children is usually sustained, not paroxysmal (8,9). Occasionally, there is a palpable mass. Polyuria and polydypsia mimicking diabetes insipidus, episodes of sweating, and headaches also may occur.

Bilateral disease occurs in approximately 5% of children with pheochromocytoma. These children are likely to have a positive family history. Pheochromocytomas occurring in multiple endocrine neoplasia (MEN) syndrome are more likely to be bilateral and malignant. There is also an increased incidence of pheochromocytoma in neurofibromatosis, Sturge-Weber syndrome, and von Hippel-Lindau syndrome (Fig. 9-164).

Pheochromocytomas secrete norepinephrine. Screening tests include assays of catecholamines and metabolites of epinephrine and norepinephrine. The most reliable laboratory test is the 24-hour urinary excretion of metanephrine (8,9).

[123]I- or ^{131}I-MIBG scintigraphy should be the initial imaging modality in patients suspected of having a pheochromocytoma (Fig. 9-165A). If an area of increased uptake is identified, CT or MRI should follow (Fig. 9-165B). Pheochromocytomas have long T1 and T2 relaxation times at MRI (Fig. 9-165B). If biochemical tests are positive, a blocking agent should be administered prior to injection of contrast material for IVU, CT, or angiography. The tumors are usually highly vascular, and contrast medium enters venous pools in the periphery of the tumor to produce a whorled appearance. This type of hypervascularity may be demon-

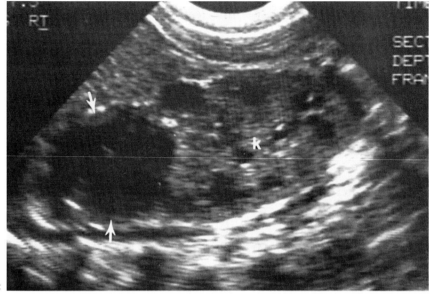

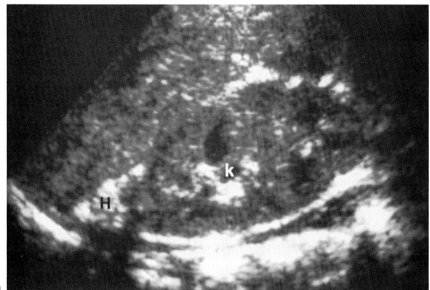

FIG. 9-163. *Continued.* **C:** 1 month of age. The adrenal hemorrhage *(arrows)* above the right kidney *(k)* is now smaller and still anechoic. **D:** 5 months of age. There is an echogenic focus *(H)* above the right kidney *(k)*. Plain films demonstrated suprarenal calcification.

strated by CT or angiography. Imaging cannot differentiate benign from malignant tumors (442).

Resection of benign pheochromocytomas is usually curative. Recurrence of hypertension suggests the presence of a second, sometimes contralateral neoplasm. Malignant pheochromocytomas frequently recur, but long survival is still possible. The 5-year survival rate following appropriate therapy is 96% for benign pheochromocytoma and 44% for malignant pheochromocytoma (8,9).

Gonadal Tumors

Testicular Neoplasms

Testicular neoplasms have an annual incidence of 2 per million population in the United States (443); 70% to 90% are of germ cell origin. In prepubertal boys, endodermal sinus tumor and teratoma are the most common testicular neoplasms (444,445). After puberty, embryonal cell carcinoma, choriocarcinoma, and teratocarcinoma occur most frequently. Stromal (nongerm cell) tumors account for 10% to 30% of testicular neoplasms and include Sertoli and Leydig cell tumors. Sertoli cell tumors generally occur in the first year of life and are usually benign. Leydig cell tumors present in boys 3–6 years old, often in association with precocious puberty, and are always benign (Fig. 9-166). Metastatic tumors, including leukemia and lymphoma, account for fewer than 10% of testicular masses. More than 60% of boys with leukemia have testicular involvement at autopsy, although it is clinically apparent in only 5% to 30% of patients (446,447). Testicular leukemia can present as unilateral or bilateral testicular enlargement. Neuroblastoma also occasionally metastasizes to the testis (448).

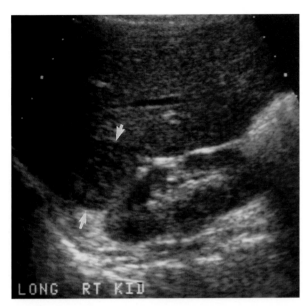

FIG. 9-164. Pheochromocytoma. An 11-year-old boy with a family history of von Hippel-Lindau syndrome and recent onset of night sweats. Longitudinal sonography. The right suprarenal mass *(arrows)* is isoechoic to the adjacent renal cortex.

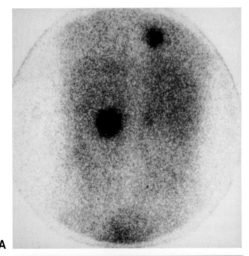

A

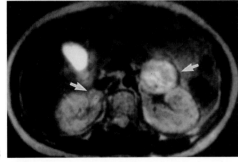

B

FIG. 9-165. Multiple pheochromocytomas. A 14-year-old girl with aggressive behavior and hypertension. **A:** Posterior ¹²³I-MIBG scintigraphy of the thorax and abdomen. There is tracer uptake in right posterior mediastinal, left adrenal, and right adrenal pheochromocytomas. **B:** Axial T2-weighted MRI. There are bilateral adrenal masses *(arrows)*, larger on the left.

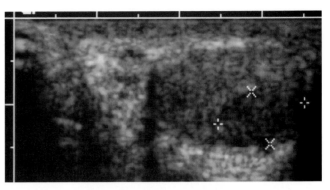

FIG. 9-166. Leydig cell tumor of the testis. An 8-year-old boy with precocious puberty and an enlarged right testis. Longitudinal sonography of right testis. There is a well-defined, hypoechoic testicular mass *(within cursors)*.

The usual testicular neoplasm presents as a firm, painless scrotal mass. The primary goal of imaging is to define the local extent of the mass and detect metastases to paraaortic lymph nodes, lung, liver, and bone. Sonography is used first. There are no sonographic features that permit differentiation between the various tumor types. Furthermore, other abnormalities such as orchitis, abscess, and infarction may have similar sonographic findings. Hydrocele coexists with 25% of testicular neoplasms (449); any boy with a hydrocele and an abnormal testis on clinical examination should therefore have ultrasound. If a solid intratesticular mass is found (Fig. 9-167), the examination should include an evaluation of the retroperitoneum up to the level of the renal hila for paraaortic and paracaval lymph nodes. When malignancy is likely, further evaluation of the abdomen with CT or MRI is performed to rule out metastases. Chest CT should also be performed to exclude or diagnose metastatic disease.

Luker and Siegel studied seven boys with testicular malignancies using US and color Doppler imaging (450). Testicular echogenicity was normal in four prepubertal patients (although their testes were large), whereas discrete intratesticular masses were seen in all three postpubertal patients. Increased blood flow was documented in six of seven neoplasms. Three of the four boys with normal gray scale echo-

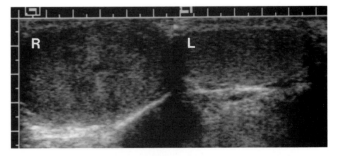

FIG. 9-167. Testicular teratocarcinoma. Teenage boy with right scrotal swelling. Longitudinal testicular sonography. The left testis *(L)* is normal. The right testis *(R)* is enlarged and its parenchyma is inhomogeneous.

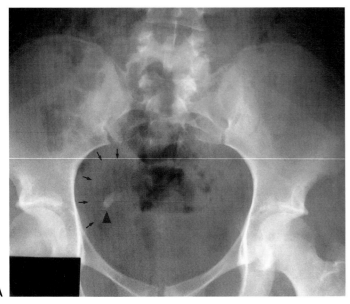
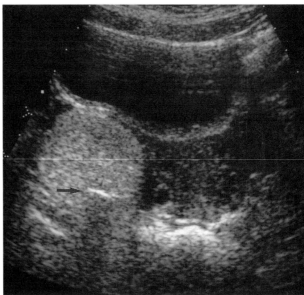

A   B

FIG. 9-168. Benign ovarian teratoma. A 17-year-old girl with a right adnexal mass. **A:** Supine radiograph of the pelvis demonstrates a tooth in the right adnexa *(arrowhead)* surrounded by lucent fat *(arrows)*. **B:** Transverse sonography of the right adnexa. The right ovarian echogenic mass contains calcification *(arrow)* with distal shadowing.

genicity had diffuse hypervascularity and one had a focal hypovascular mass on color Doppler imaging. In all cases, the vasculature was disorganized and abnormal (450,451). Although color Doppler US permitted identification of abnormal vasculature in the affected testis, it did not identify the type of tumor or distinguish between primary neoplasms and metastases.

Paratesticular Tumors

Testicular tumors arising from mesenchymal tissue are rare. Embryonal rhabdomyosarcoma may arise from either the spermatic cord or epididymis.

Ovarian Tumors

Ovarian tumors occur with an annual incidence of 2.2 per million population in the United States (443). In children, some are nonfunctioning and present as pelvic or abdominal masses. If functional, they may cause precocious puberty (granulosa-thecal cell tumor) or virilization (gonadoblastoma, arrhenoblastoma). Other types include teratoma, dysgerminoma, Brenner tumors, mesometanephric rest tumors, and adrenal rest tumors.

Ovarian Teratoma. Ovarian teratoma is the most common ovarian neoplasm in children. The ovary is second only to the sacrococcygeal region as the site of origin of teratomas (1,444). Ovarian teratomas may be malignant. Cystic ovarian teratomas are the most common variety and are usually benign. Solid teratomas, although less common, are often malignant.

Most ovarian teratomas occur in adolescent girls; how-

ever, they may occur in younger children or even infants. They are usually not discovered until they grow large enough to produce a palpable mass or twist on their pedicle, causing abdominal pain.

Plain films of the abdomen may show an abdominal or pelvic mass. Calcification or ossification is present in approximately two thirds of ovarian teratomas. Recognizable fat (Fig. 9-168A) is more frequent in older patients. US confirms the pelvic origin of the mass and delineates the characteristics of its components. Ovarian teratomas usually have a cystic component, but increased echogenicity due to calcification or fat is also present (Fig. 9-168B). If performed, CT examination shows soft tissue, calcific, and fatty components. MRI also identifies various tumor components (Fig. 9-169) and helps stage patients with malignant disease.

Neonatal Ovarian Cysts. A neonatal ovarian cyst is a fairly common abdominal mass. It may be discovered by prenatal sonography or postnatal physical examination. The cause is unknown, but perhaps these cysts develop because of follicular stimulation by maternal hormones. They are usually of germinal or Graafian epithelial origin.

Neonatal ovarian cysts may be very large. Plain films show an abdominal mass that displaces bowel gas. Frequently, the mass appears to be more abdominal than pelvic. US confirms that the mass is cystic and often shows that it is more abdominal than pelvic (Fig. 9-170). Renal sonography demonstrates normal kidneys separate from the cystic mass (27).

Treatment of neonatal ovarian cysts is controversial. Both conservative observation (452) and surgical excision (453) have been recommended. Percutaneous drainage of neonatal

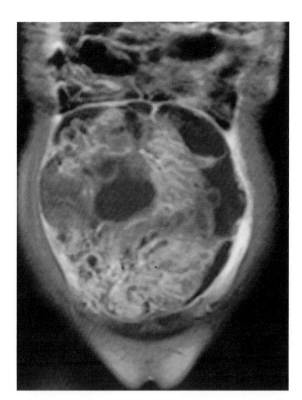

FIG. 9-169. Immature ovarian teratoma. A 9-year-old girl with increasing abdominal distention. Coronal T1-weighted MRI with gadolinium enhancement. There is a large abdominal mass that contains cystic (low intensity) and solid enhancing components.

ovarian cysts has also been successfully performed (454). Most simple ovarian cysts resolve spontaneously and should be treated conservatively. Large ovarian cysts (>6 cm in diameter) have a greater risk of torsion, so that percutaneous drainage or surgical excision may be indicated.

Ovarian Cysts in Older Girls and Adolescents. A simple ovarian cyst is the most common ovarian mass in adolescents. Functional or retention cysts occur when a normal, mature follicle fails to involute. Physiologic follicular cysts are <5 cm in diameter. In the absence of symptoms, a cyst

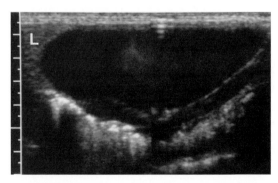

FIG. 9-170. Neonatal ovarian cyst. A 3-week-old girl with an abdominal mass identified on a prenatal sonogram. Longitudinal sonography demonstrates a huge unilocular cyst extending from the pelvis up to the liver *(L)*.

<5 cm in diameter is treated nonoperatively. Bleeding into an ovarian cyst often causes pelvic pain. Cysts may also predispose to ovarian torsion.

Paraovarian cysts arise in the broad ligament from Wolffian duct remnants. However, unlike ovarian cysts, they are not subject to hormonal control and do not change in size. Girls with a history of pelvic inflammatory disease or who have undergone pelvic surgery may develop inclusion cysts due to trapping by peritoneal adhesions of ovarian fluid from ruptured follicles (455).

Follicular cysts usually contain clear fluid and tend to be found in the lower abdomen or pelvis of older girls and adolescents. Since ovarian cysts are often hemorrhagic, a fluid/debris level or clot may be identified.

Polycystic Disease. Polycystic disease of the ovaries (Stein-Leventhal syndrome) may cause primary amenorrhea or irregular menses. This disorder is due to an abnormal feedback loop between the pituitary, hypothalamus, and ovary; it is best diagnosed by demonstrating an elevated ratio of luteinizing hormone to follicle-stimulating hormone (456,457). US can be used to document the absence of a virilizing ovarian or adrenal mass. Transvaginal sonography more accurately demonstrates the enlargement and abnormal stroma of the polycystic ovaries (458).

Ovarian Torsion. Torsion of the uterine adnexa is uncommon. It sometimes occurs in women of reproductive age, usually in association with an underlying ovarian abnormality such as a cyst or tumor. Torsion of normal adnexa occurs even less frequently, predominantly in premenarchal girls. Several predisposing factors have been postulated, including the relative mobility of the adnexa in young girls, permitting torsion of the mesosalpinx, and circumstances causing acute changes in intraabdominal pressure, such as pushing or lifting of heavy objects (459,460).

Because of its rarity and nonspecific clinical presentation, the diagnosis of ovarian torsion is usually delayed. Symptoms include lower abdominal pain, nausea, vomiting, and low-grade fever. A palpable mass is found in two thirds of patients.

The sonographic findings of adnexal torsion vary. An adnexal cyst or tumor may be present. A spectrum of ischemic changes may be seen, depending on the degree of vascular compromise. Edema and enlargement of the ovary, due to impaired venous and lymphatic drainage, are seen. Peripheral follicular distention due to transudation of fluid is seen by sonography or CT in 75% of cases and strongly suggests torsion (460,461). Free fluid in the cul-de-sac is identified in about one third of cases (460). Persistent edema and venous congestion eventually lead to arterial thrombosis and ovarian necrosis. The twisted, engorged, edematous ovary will be seen as a hypoechoic mass with good sound transmission. In the absence of peripheral follicular cysts, the differential diagnosis includes hemorrhagic ovarian cyst, ovarian teratoma, and appendiceal abscess.

Amputation of the infarcted ovary (see following discussion) may follow adnexal torsion (462). Plain films may demonstrate abdominal or pelvic calcifications (Fig. 9-

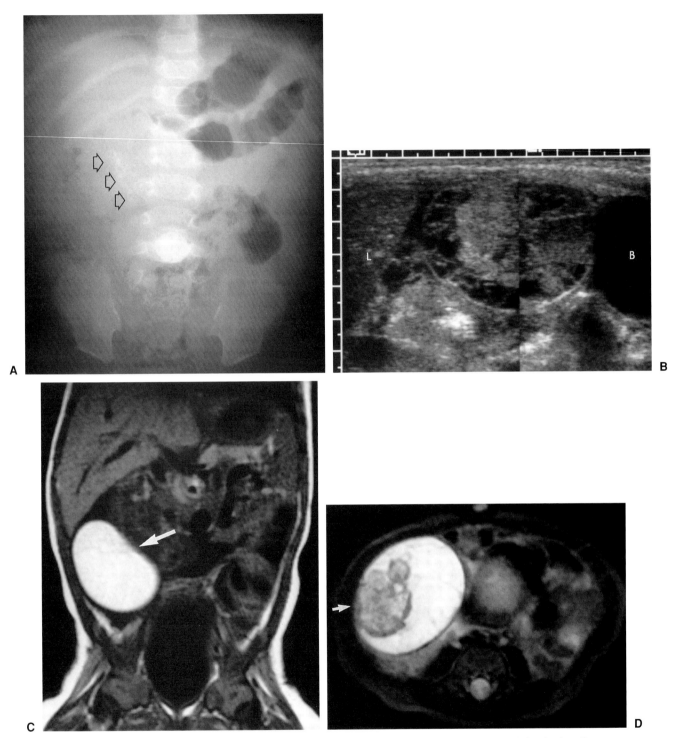

FIG. 9-171. Ovarian torsion and infarction. A 5-month-old asymptomatic girl. **A:** Abdominal radiograph shows punctate calcifications in the right midabdomen *(open arrows)*. **B:** Composite longitudinal sonogram demonstrates a well-circumscribed, complex mass extending from the bladder *(B)* to the liver *(L)*. **C:** T1-weighted coronal MRI. The mass *(arrow)* is of high intensity, which suggests that its contents are hemorrhagic. **D:** T2-weighted axial MRI. There is a low-intensity, solid portion *(arrow)* of the mass surrounded by a high-intensity cystic component.

171A), seen in different locations on serial examinations. Sonography in chronic ovarian torsion will show a complex mass (Fig. 9-171B). MRI may verify the hemorrhagic and cystic components of the twisted, infarcted ovary (Fig. 9-171C, D).

Amputated Ovary. Amputation of the ovary is a rare cause of abdominal calcification. Plain films demonstrate an area, often oval, of coarsely stippled calcification in the pelvis that may be seen in different locations at various times (463). Amputation is presumably a late effect of torsion of the adnexa and infarction. If signs and symptoms are not severe enough during the acute event to prompt evaluation, there may be amputation of the ovary and subsequent dystrophic calcification (463). The differential diagnosis of this type of calcification in the pelvis of a girl includes an enterolith in the appendix or Meckel diverticulum, ovarian teratoma, ingested foreign body, ureteral calculus, and bladder calculus. If it moves, an amputated ovary is likely (463). Calcifications in amputated ovaries tend to be ovoid, whereas calcifications and ossifications in teratomas have a somewhat irregular shape. Other, rare causes of mobile abdominal calcifications include amputated appendices epiploicae, deposits in the omentum, mummified pieces of free small bowel, enteroliths, liquid calcifications in psoas abscess, gallstones, ureteral stones, and calcifications in omental or mesenteric cysts. Opaque intraperitoneal and intraluminal gastrointestinal foreign bodies may also be mobile.

Rhabdomyosarcoma

Rhabdomyosarcoma is the most common pediatric soft-tissue sarcoma and the seventh most frequent cause of death due to malignant disease in children (8,9). It is the only common pediatric tumor that can arise from virtually any tissue or organ in the body except the brain (12,464,465). It accounts for approximately 10% of all childhood solid tumors. Its frequency is exceeded only by central nervous system tumors, lymphoma, neuroblastoma, and Wilms tumor. It is extremely malignant and has a propensity for local invasion, early recurrence, and metastases by hematogenous and lymphatic routes (466). If untreated, 90% of patients die within a year (8,9).

Boys and girls are equally affected by rhabdomyosarcoma. There is no racial predilection. The tumor occurs throughout childhood; there are peaks between 2 and 6 years of age and between 14 and 18 years of age (464). Tumors of the bladder and vagina occur primarily in infants. Rhabdomyosarcoma has been reported in newborns; its occurrence during the first year of life carries an extremely poor prognosis.

Pathology

Rhabdomyosarcoma is thought to develop from primitive rhabdomyoblasts or totipotential mesenchymal cells. It may arise even in areas where striated muscle is not normally present (8,467).

The histologic diagnosis may be extremely difficult; there are currently no universally accepted diagnostic criteria (464). In the United States, the most widely used histologic classification is that of the Intergroup Rhabdomyosarcoma Study (468). The histologic types include embryonal, alveolar, embryonal-botryoid, pleomorphic, undifferentiated, and other. The embryonal form is the most common in children and has the best prognosis. The alveolar form usually involves the extremities in older children and has the worst prognosis (9). Many authorities consider the alveolar form a variant of the embryonal type. The pleomorphic type occurs primarily on the trunk or extremities in adults and is rarely seen in children. Sarcoma botryoides is a unique form of embryonal rhabdomyosarcoma with a distinctive grape-like appearance (Fig. 9-172). This polypoid tumor originates submucosally in hollow organs and grows into the lumen. The histologic features of various types of rhabdomyosarcoma may be present in the same tumor.

The most common sites of origin of rhabdomyosarcomas in children are the pelvis and genitourinary tract (39%) and the head and neck (31%) (3,8). Head and neck rhabdomyosarcomas may arise in the orbit, nasopharynx, paranasal sinuses, oropharynx, hypopharynx, middle ear, or external auditory canal (3). Approximately 21% of rhabdomyosarcomas in children arise in the genitourinary tract (468); the tumor may involve the upper or lower urinary tract, prostate gland (Fig. 9-173), spermatic cord, testis, paratesticular tissues, penis, vagina (Fig. 9-174), uterus, pelvic floor, or perineum (3).

Imaging

Urinary Tract. Rhabdomyosarcoma may arise anywhere in the urinary tract, from the kidney to the external genitalia. The urinary bladder is the most common site of origin. Boys are affected twice as frequently as girls. The tumor usually presents during the first 3 years of life as either a solid infiltrating lesion or a polypoid mass in the bladder. The tumor usually arises from the trigone or bladder base (2,8,9).

US is an excellent modality for verification of lesions of the bladder base (469). CT and MRI are used to demonstrate the full extent of the tumor more accurately (470,471). Voiding cystourethrography or cross-sectional imaging demonstrates a polypoid (bunch of grapes) mass in the urinary bladder (Fig. 9-172) and thickening, elevation, and infiltration of the bladder wall. There may be partial obstruction of the lower ureters and hydroureteronephrosis. The tumor may prolapse into or invade the urethra. It may be difficult to decide whether the tumor arises from the bladder or prostate gland in boys, or bladder or vagina in girls.

Tumors arising from the bladder base are usually botryoid, but occasionally present as a single intravesicular mass that may be confused with a blood clot. Rarely, the main growth

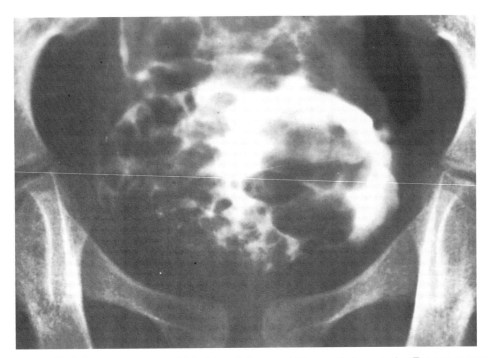

FIG. 9-172. Rhabdomyosarcoma of bladder. A 3-year-old boy with hematuria. Excretory urogram shows many rounded and oval filling defects in the bladder. The base of the bladder is elevated. Biopsy confirmed the sarcoma botryoides type of bladder rhabdomyosarcoma. (Courtesy of Herman Grossman, M.D., Durham, NC.)

of the tumor is extravesical with only slight indentation of the bladder base.

Prostate Gland. Rhabdomyosarcoma of the prostate gland usually presents with voiding difficulties and symptoms of prostatism. There is early invasion of the base of the bladder and posterior urethra and there may be partial obstruction of the rectum or lower ureters. Voiding cystourethrography, US, CT (Fig. 9-173), and MRI may demonstrate extrinsic compression and displacement of the bladder.

The mass may extend into the ischiorectal fossa (Fig. 9-173B) and occasionally invades the bladder or urethral lumen.

Vagina. Rhabdomyosarcoma is the most common primary tumor of the vagina and external genitalia in girls (8,9). It is usually of the sarcoma botryoides type. The clinical symptoms include vaginal discharge, bleeding, vaginal mass, and protrusion of polypoid tissue from the vaginal orifice. There is often a delay in diagnosis. This tumor usu-

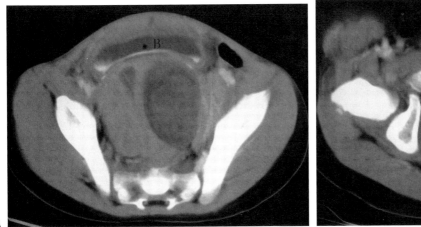
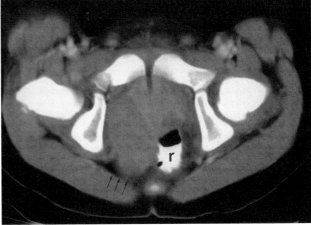

FIG. 9-173. Embryonal rhabdomyosarcoma of the prostate. A 5-year-old boy with abdominal pain and urinary retention. **A:** Contrast-enhanced CT. There is a large, inhomogeneous pelvic mass that extrinsically compresses and displaces the bladder *(B)*. **B:** The tumor extends into the right ischiorectal fossa *(arrows)* and displaces the rectum *(r)* to the left.

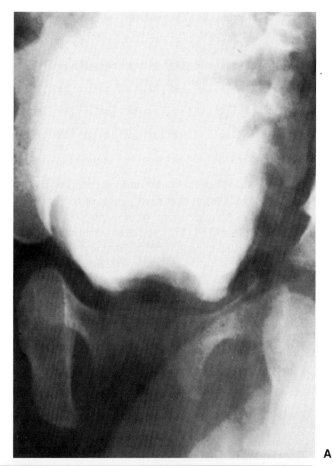

FIG. 9-174. Vaginal rhabdomyosarcoma. A 10-month-old girl with soft-tissue mass at the vaginal introitus. **A:** A cystogram shows crescentic extrinsic compression and elevation of the base of the bladder. **B:** A computed tomogram through the pelvis shows a soft-tissue mass *(M)* in the cul-de-sac between the bladder *(B)* and rectum *(R)*. It is elevating and secondarily invading *(arrows)* the base and posterior portion of the bladder. (Courtesy of Robert A: Kaufman, M.D., Memphis, TN.)

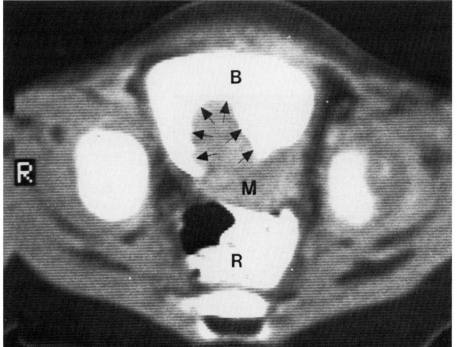

ally arises from the upper third of the anterior vaginal wall with growth into the vaginal lumen and infiltration of the vesicovaginal septum, posterior bladder wall, and urethra (Fig. 9-174A). In adolscent girls the tumor may grow toward the uterine cervix. The extent of the intravaginal mass and any involvement of the bladder or rectum are well demonstrated by CT (Fig. 9-174B) or MRI.

Trauma

Renal Trauma

Renal injury is one of the most common results of blunt abdominal trauma. During childhood, causes of renal injury include falls (25%), vigorous and reckless play (25%), and vehicular accidents (50%) (472). Contrast-enhanced CT has replaced IVU for the evaluation of renal trauma in infants and children (473–475). Hydronephrotic (Fig. 9-175) and ectopic kidneys are at increased risk of injury, which may follow even minor trauma.

A functional classification of renal injury includes minor injury, major injury, and critical injury (472). *Minor injury* is parenchymal damage (contusion, hematoma, contained laceration) without a capsular tear or extension into the pelvicalyceal system. It accounts for 50% of renal injuries due to blunt trauma during childhood (472). *Major injury* is parenchymal damage with capsular tear or extension into the pelvicalyceal system and includes complete laceration (renal fracture). Major injury accounts for 25% of renal injuries due to blunt abdominal trauma during childhood (472). *Critical injury* includes complete fragmentation or shattering of the kidney and injury to renal vessels in the form of avulsion or thrombosis; it accounts for approximately 25% of blunt renal trauma during childhood (472). Injuries in the young

child are often quite severe; this is presumably because of the lower renal position with less protection by the ribs, the relatively greater size of the kidneys, the more elastic properties of the lower ribs, and the lack of development of the perirenal capsule (472). Potential renal injuries are shown in Fig. 9-176 (476). Only the more extreme injuries are likely to result in permanent loss of renal function or to develop complications such as urinoma, sepsis, and persistent hypertension (477).

Clinical Features

Hematuria (more than 50 red blood cells per high power field in a centrifuged specimen) is almost always present in children with renal injury from blunt trauma (477). There is poor correlation between microscopic hematuria and definable renal parenchymal injury (478). Other symptoms and signs include pain or tenderness in the flank or upper abdomen over the affected kidney. Although these findings raise the suspicion of renal injury, definition of the extent of injury depends on imaging (475,478–482).

Imaging

Abdominal Radiography. Plain films of the abdomen may show a lung contusion; pleural effusion; peritoneal fluid; fractures of pelvic bones, ribs, or vertebrae; and bowel distention due to adynamic ileus. Conventional radiography seldom provides direct evidence about the state of the kidneys.

Intravenous Urography. Prior to CT, IVU was considered the basic radiologic examination in the evaluation of renal injury (472,476). With major injury, there may be extravasation of contrast material beyond the renal capsule or from the pelvicalyceal system. In critical injury there may be little or no urographic function. Because early assessment is mandatory, and severe injury or multiple organ injury may be present, CT is the imaging method of choice. An abdominal radiograph or CT Scoutview is obtained after contrast-enhanced CT to assess further the upper and lower urinary tracts.

Ultrasonography. The role of US in renal trauma is still being defined, but the approach is promising. Power Doppler and ultrasound contrast agents may prove useful in the evaluation of renovascular injuries. However, renal sonography is often difficult in patients with abdominal trauma because of abdominal tenderness and gaseous distention of the bowel.

Nuclear Scintigraphy. Radionuclide scanning, when performed with dynamic, early blood pool imaging and SPECT, provides valuable information regarding renal vascularity and parenchymal damage. Less anatomic detail is obtained with this method than with other imaging studies. Moreover, scintigraphy is organ-specific, which limits the evaluation of multiorgan injury.

Computed Tomography. CT is more accurate than IVU

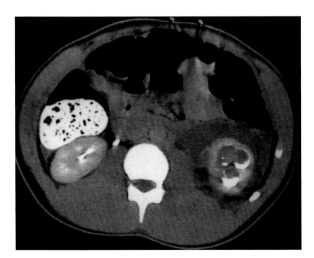

FIG. 9-175. Renal trauma in patient with hydronephrosis. Contrast-enhanced CT. The right kidney is normal. There is left pelvicaliectasis with fluid-contrast levels. The left renal hematoma primarily involves the perirenal space. The hydronephrosis is due to congenital UPJ obstruction.

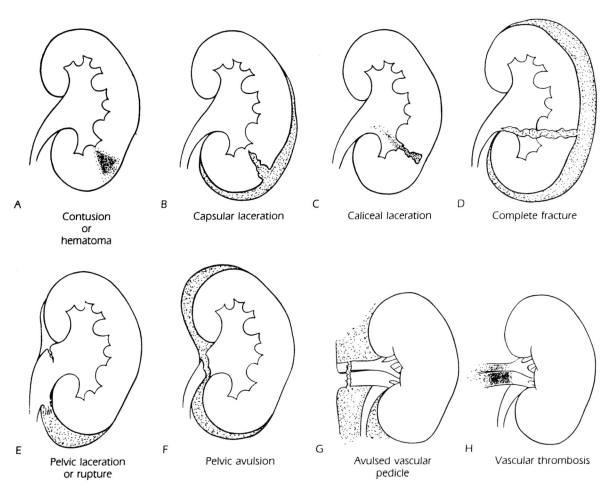

FIG. 9-176. Potential renal injuries. Modified from Macpherson and Decter (476).

A Contusion or hematoma B Capsular laceration C Caliceal laceration D Complete fracture

E Pelvic laceration or rupture F Pelvic avulsion G Avulsed vascular pedicle H Vascular thrombosis

in assessing the presence and extent of renal injury (472–475,479–481). Minor contusions or lacerations are frequently seen as areas of nonfunction in the nephrographic phase, and contrast material persists in these regions on delayed scans. The most common injury diagnosed by CT is a fracture or laceration extending to the renal capsule and associated with a perirenal hematoma or urinoma (Fig. 9-177). These lesions may be missed or underestimated by IVU. A renal fracture causes an irregular, often wedge-shaped, low-density defect that is optimally visualized after bolus contrast enhancement (475). A contused kidney has one or more areas of nonfunction in the nephrographic phase of the contrast examination. A fresh hematoma may be denser than the unenhanced renal parenchyma. Subcapsular hematomas are usually lenticular or oval and frequently deform the renal contour (480). Perirenal fluid collections are larger, are confined by Gerota's fascia, and partially surround the kidney. Shearing fractures and fragmentation of the kidney are beautifully demonstrated by CT (Fig. 9-177) (480). They may be treated nonoperatively or, rarely, with partial nephrectomy; there may be complete healing or formation of a renal scar.

If there is severe damage to the renal vascular pedicle,

the kidney may appear nearly normal on nonenhanced CT. After contrast enhancement, avascularity of the kidney is apparent (Fig. 9-178A), which is an indication for prompt surgery after (Fig. 9-178B) or without renal angiography. Rarely, a cortical rim of enhancement is seen even after complete renal artery disruption because of perfusion of the renal surface through capsular arteries (474). The time of warm ischemia that can be tolerated by the kidney is less in children (2–4 hours) than in adults (4–6 hours). Surgery should not be delayed for angiographic confirmation of renal pedicle injury beyond this critical time period (483). Although follow-up scans are not routinely performed after minor trauma, signs of repair are usually apparent on CT within 2 weeks of the insult. Resolution of perirenal and subcapsular hematomas is complete within 3 months (480).

Treatment

Both minor and major injury categories usually receive conservative (nonoperative) management. This conservatism is easier if one knows the precise extent of renal injury, which is best delineated by CT. Moreover, other organs are

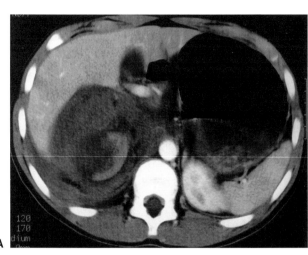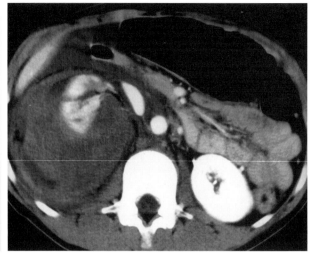

A   B

FIG. 9-177. Severe renal trauma. A teenage boy in motor vehicle accident. **A:** Contrast-enhanced CT. The upper part of the fractured right kidney is poorly perfused. Extensive hemorrhage is identified in the perirenal and pararenal spaces. **B:** Lower CT section. The lower part of the kidney is normally perfused. There is a linear renal fracture. The right renal hematoma displaces and elevates the inferior vena cava.

frequently injured (18%) when only renal injury is suspected clinically, and these other injuries are best detected by CT (480). However, avulsion of the vascular pedicle and vascular thrombosis require emergency surgical intervention.

Ureteropelvic Junction Disruption

Traumatic disruption of the ureter from the renal pelvis is a rare pediatric injury probably caused by extreme thoracolumbar hyperextension (484). Because of the greater flexibility of the child's skeleton, children can survive this type of injury, whereas adults rarely do. CT immediately after the injury may be normal, show only a nonspecific perinephric fluid collection, or show leakage of contrast material near the renal pelvis (485,486). Because early imaging by CT tends to be nondiagnostic and the injury is rare, the recognition of UPJ disruption is frequently delayed (487,488).

Bladder Trauma

Bladder injuries are uncommon in children, even in the presence of pelvic fractures. When investigating possible bladder injury, a retrograde urethrogram should be obtained before a retrograde cystogram is attempted (481).

Rupture of a distended urinary bladder may lead to urine extravasation into the peritoneal cavity or into the extraperitoneal spaces (Fig. 9-179). Bladder rupture may be associated with pelvic fractures (Fig. 9-179B) (489).

Although rupture of the bladder may be evident on CT, cystography is sometimes necessary. Children with bladder injury are usually successfully managed with continuous

catheter drainage of the bladder until healing is complete (489).

In patients with pelvic fractures, there may be no perforation of the bladder but a large pelvic hematoma that elevates, displaces, or deforms the bladder, sometimes to the shape of a pear.

Urethral Trauma

Straddle injuries and other types of perineal trauma can result in injuries to the male urethra, usually at the level of the inferior pubic ramus. These injuries are sometimes but not always associated with pelvic fractures. Urethral injuries are best evaluated with retrograde urethrography (Fig. 9-180). Traumatic disruptions of the urethra may be partial or complete. Complete disruption frequently leads to erectile dysfunction. Urethral strictures often follow healing of both minor injuries and complete urethral disruption (490).

In children, unlike adults, urethral strictures are almost never infectious in origin. They are almost always due to trauma, either from a perineal injury as noted above, from catheterization, or from endoscopy. If a stricture is strongly suspected, a RUG may be the only study needed. Strictures in boys are almost always in the proximal bulbous portion of the urethra. When a stricture is first seen on VCUG, the lumen of the urethra is often so narrow and the flow so reduced that the normal urethra beyond the stricture does not distend and the length of the stricture cannot be determined. In this situation, RUG immediately after VCUG will show the true length of the strictured segment. After repair of urethral stricture, either by dilatation, ure-

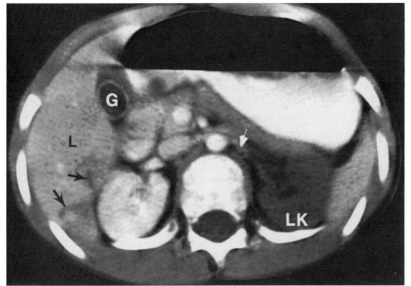

FIG. 9-178. Renal pedicle injury. An 8-year-old boy who fell 15 feet from a rooftop. He was seen approximately 1 hour later with abdominal tenderness, elevated liver enzymes, and gross hematuria. **A:** Contrast-enhanced CT. There is no perfusion of the left kidney *(LK)*. Stasis of contrast was noted in the proximal left renal artery *(white arrow)*. There are linear fractures *(black arrows)* of the posterior segment of the right lobe of the liver *(L)*, and there is free intraperitoneal blood in the space of Morison and surrounding the gallbladder *(G)*. **B:** Aortogram. The aorta *(A)* and right renal artery *(R)* are normal. There is abrupt termination *(arrow)* of the main left renal artery *(L)* due to thrombosis. At surgery, there was an intimal tear of the left renal artery and secondary thrombosis.

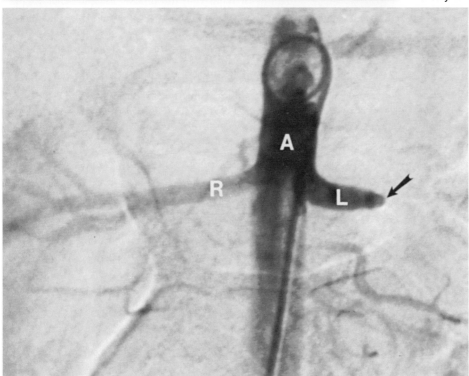

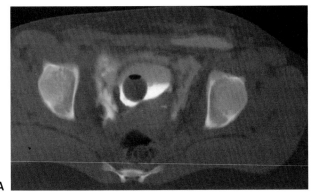

A

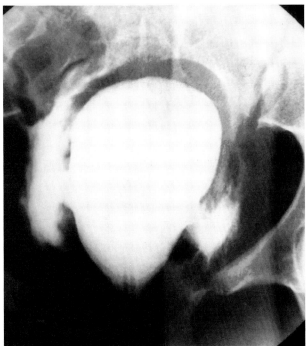

B

FIG. 9-179. Bladder rupture. A: Teenage boy struck by automobile. A Foley catheter is in the bladder. There is extraperitoneal extravasation of contrast material from the bladder. **B:** Teenage girl with pelvic fractures. The bilateral extravasation of contrast material from the bladder is extraperitoneal.

throtomy, or urethroplasty, the appropriate follow-up study is RUG.

Miscellaneous Abnormalities

Renal Vein Thrombosis

Renal vein thrombosis, a serious condition, may be acute or chronic (491). Lesions associated with renal vein thrombosis include renal tumor, extrarenal tumor, phlebitis involving the vena cava or renal veins, dehydration, lymphoma, membranous glomerulonephritis, and renal amyloidosis (492). Neonatal renal vein thrombosis is a serious complication in the dehydrated, polycythemic, or septic infant; it is frequently associated with maternal diabetes (491).

Clinical Features

Sudden and complete occlusion of the renal vein leads to hemorrhagic infarction of the kidney. Acute renal vein thrombosis may cause pain, nephromegaly, and hematuria, and be associated with thromboembolic phenomena elsewhere (492). Chronic renal vein thrombosis may have an insidious onset characterized by proteinuria, usually severe. Platelets are frequently depleted. Neonates with renal vein thrombosis may have hematuria, a flank mass, proteinuria, and transient hypertension.

Renal vein thrombosis is usually treated nonoperatively with or without anticoagulation. Occasionally, it is a cause of renal failure in the neonate. In most cases, renal function returns to normal.

Imaging

Prompt diagnosis of renal vein thrombosis is required to institute proper therapy. Although renal vein thrombosis in children may have a classic clinical presentation, the diagnosis in neonates is difficult.

US is a safe, rapid, noninvasive technique for diagnosing both acute and chronic renal vein thrombosis. The pathologic features of renal vein thrombosis include renal edema and hemorrhage during the acute stage followed by cellular infiltration and fibrosis (12,492). Early sonographic features are decreased cortical echogenicity and nephromegaly, presumably due to edema and hemorrhage. Within 10 days to 2 weeks there is increased cortical echogenicity with preservation of the corticomedullary definition and variable renal size (492). US of acute renal vein thrombosis demonstrates

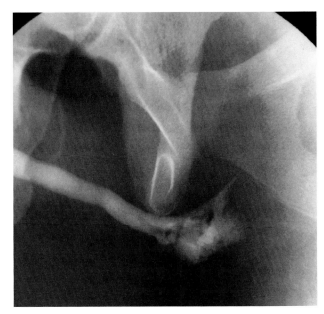

FIG. 9-180. Urethral trauma. Teenage boy with perineal injury. Retrograde urethrogram. There is partial transection of the urethra and contrast extravasation.

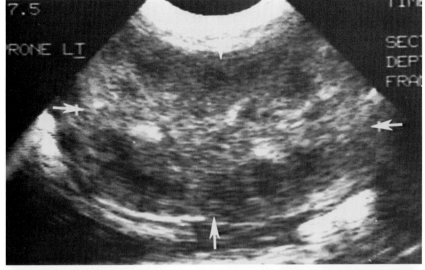

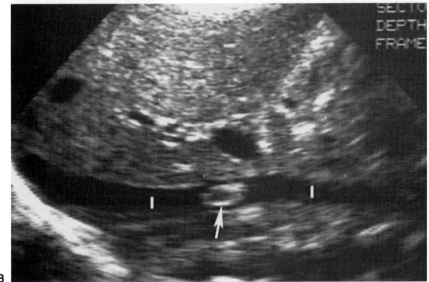

FIG. 9-181. Renal vein thrombosis. A 1-week-old infant of a diabetic mother with hematuria, proteinuria, and a questionable left upper quadrant mass. **A:** Prone longitudinal sonography demonstrates a markedly enlarged and echogenic left kidney *(arrows)*. The central echo complex is obliterated. **B:** Longitudinal sonography through the inferior vena cava *(I)* demonstrates an echogenic thrombus *(arrow)* at the level of the left renal vein.

decreased echogenicity in an enlarged kidney. Focal areas of increased and decreased echogenicity due to cellular infiltration and fibrosis follow (Fig. 9-181A). Late changes include increased parenchymal echoes, continued loss of corticomedullary definition, and a decrease in renal size due to fibrosis. Clot or tumor is occasionally seen in the renal vein or inferior vena cava (Fig. 9-181B). Color Doppler and duplex US may show a decrease or absence of venous pulsations and flow (492). Duplex and color Doppler US are extremely helpful in making the diagnosis of renal vein thrombosis; the inferior vena cava, renal arteries, and renal veins should be assessed for thrombus and abnormal blood flow. The sonographic findings evolve more quickly in the neonate (491). Renal enlargement, diffuse increased echogenicity, and loss of the normal central echo complex may develop within 7–10 days (Fig. 9-181A).

Chronic renal vein thrombosis may cause vascular calcifications (Fig. 9-182A) and diminution in kidney size. Sonog-

raphy of the inferior vena cava may show an echogenic thrombus (Fig. 9-182B).

Bladder Stones

Bladder stones (Fig. 9-183) are endemic in developing countries but are common in industrialized countries only in a few circumstances. Postpubertal patients who catheterize their bladders regularly may introduce a foreign body, which then acts as a nidus for stone formation (Fig. 9-183). Any foreign body, including a surgical staple, can serve as a stone nidus (493). Infection with the urea-splitting organism *Proteus mirabilis* and surgical reconstruction of the urinary tract using intestinal mucosa also puts patients at risk for bladder stones (494). The endoscopic, submucosal injection of Teflon paste immediately inferior to the ureterovesical junction in treatment of reflux may cause a hyperechoic focus with distal shadowing that mimics the sonographic appearance of calcification in the bladder (184,185).

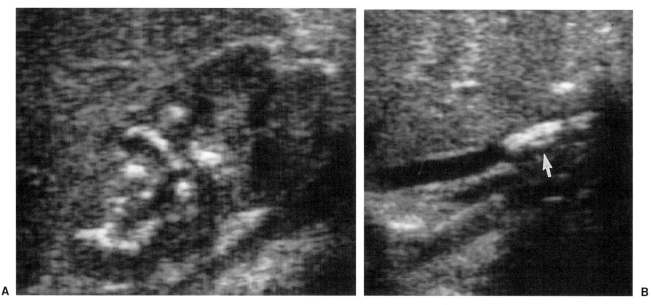

FIG. 9-182. Chronic renal vein thrombosis. A 6-month-old boy with right renal calcifications on abdominal radiograph. **A:** Longitudinal sonography. There are linear, branching echogenicities within the right kidney. **B:** Longitudinal sonography through the inferior vena cava demonstrates an echogenic thrombus *(arrow)* at the level of the right renal vein.

Renal Transplantation

The success rate of renal transplantation continues to improve because of improvements in graft preservation, surgical techniques, and immunosuppressive drug therapy. Transplantation is the treatment of choice in children with end-stage renal disease. Older children now do as well as adults after renal transplantation, although children under 4 years do less well. The difficulties to be overcome in the very young include surgical problems caused by the small size

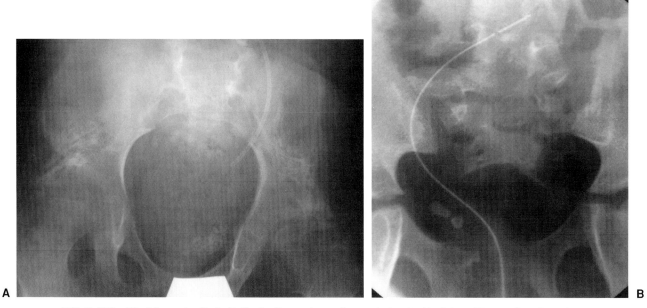

FIG. 9-183. Bladder calculi. **A:** Patient with myelomeningocele treated by intermittent self-catheterization. Many bladder stones are present. Note the spinal dysraphism, traumatic gluteal calcifications (perhaps secondary to stretching contracted poorly innervated muscles), and ventriculoperitoneal shunt catheter. **B:** A scout film for a VCUG in a patient with cloacal malformation who catheterizes her bladder every 4 hours. There are two stones in the right side of the bladder. Note also the sacral anomalies and widening of the symphysis pubis.

of the recipient and the fact that young patients do not recover from rejection as well as older patients. When considering renal transplantation, the cause of end-stage renal disease must be taken into account. Certain disorders, such as focal glomerulosclerosis and oxalosis, may recur in the allograft (495). Bladder dysfunction, as in patients treated for posterior urethral valves who have developed a ''valve bladder,'' can contribute significantly to allograft problems (496).

Most renal allografts are placed in the pelvis in an extraperitoneal position with anastomoses between the recipient internal iliac artery and donor renal artery and between the recipient external iliac vein and donor renal vein. If the child is very small, the allograft is placed in the abdomen, and the vascular anastomoses are to the recipient's distal aorta and inferior vena cava. The anastomosis of the donor ureter to the recipient's urinary bladder is termed a ureteroneocystostomy.

In about 25% of recipients, the native kidneys are removed. Indications for native kidney nephrectomy include serious chronic urinary tract infection, renovascular disease causing hypertension, congenital nephrotic syndrome with large protein losses, and young age.

Complications of Renal Transplantation

Acute Tubular Necrosis. Acute tubular necrosis (ATN) is caused by ischemic damage to the donor kidney. This is rare in kidneys from living relatives unless there is prolonged ischemia during transplantation or the recipient has hypotension during or soon after surgery. Most cadaver allografts have suffered enough ischemia to cause some degree of ATN. This damage is usually reversible, and the allograft recovers spontaneously. ATN is rarely manifest in the first 24 hours after transplantation but is evident soon thereafter.

Graft Rejection: Hyperacute, Acute, Chronic. *Hyperacute rejection* occurs immediately after transplantation, is due to the presence of circulating antibodies, and results in thrombosed arterioles and cortical necrosis. *Acute rejection* occurs from 24 hours to 4 months after transplantation with a peak incidence between the second and fifth postoperative week (38). Acute rejection is divided into vascular and interstitial forms. The vascular form is caused by endovasculitis and thrombosis. The interstitial form is characterized by interstitial edema, capillary and lymphatic infiltration with lymphocytes, and sparing of the arterioles and arteries (38). *Chronic rejection* is a slow, relentless, progressive process that develops months or years after transplantation. Biopsy of kidneys undergoing chronic rejection shows sclerosing vasculitis and interstitial fibrosis.

Fluid Collections. Hematomas, urinomas, lymphoceles, and abscesses may form in, around, or near a transplanted kidney. A hematoma may be intrarenal, subcapsular, or perirenal. Subcapsular hematomas, if large enough, can cause parenchymal compression and decreased perfusion. Urino-

mas tend to occur at or near the ureteroneocystostomy because of an anastomotic leak or ischemia of the distal ureter. Lymphoceles usually occur within a month of transplantation, but can occur later.

Complications in the Allograft Vasculature. The transplanted renal artery or vein may become thrombosed. This is particularly a problem in small children because of kinking of vessels or because of a great discrepancy in size between the donor and recipient vessels. The renal artery anastomosis is prone to stenosis and pseudoaneurysm formation. Biopsy of the transplant kidney may lead to a pseudoaneurysm or arteriovenous fistula in the renal parenchyma.

Ureteral Dilatation. Immediately after transplantation, there tends to be some degree of ureteral dilatation due to swelling at the ureteroneocystostomy; this usually resolves gradually without intervention. Obstruction of the transplanted ureter can be due to intraluminal blood clots, ischemic stricture, and compression by fluid collections. Rarely extrinsic ureteral obstruction is caused by a lymphoproliferative mass, due to immunosuppression and Epstein-Barr viral disease. Vesicoureteral reflux is a nonobstructive cause of ureteral dilatation.

Imaging of Renal Transplants

Imaging of renal transplants requires detailed knowledge of the type of allograft, date of transplantation, type of anastomoses, nature of any surgical difficulties, and current clinical concerns. The current study must always be compared to previous examinations. Evaluation without a detailed history and the earlier studies is of limited value (497).

Duplex and color Doppler US and renal scintigraphy with ^{99m}Tc-DTPA are used to evaluate transplanted kidneys. US evaluates renal size, parenchymal appearance, presence or absence of perinephric fluid collections, renal vascularity, and masses. Scintigraphy assesses both renal perfusion and function. Increase in renal size (30% volume increase over baseline), enlarged medullary pyramids, mottled or increased renal parenchymal echogenicity, decrease in prominence of central sinus echoes, and loss of corticomedullary differentiation are all signs of rejection (Fig. 9-184). Unfortunately, these sonographic findings are also nonspecific (498). The size, location, and echotexture of any intrarenal or perinephric fluid collections should always be noted. Acute hemorrhage tends to be echogenic; there are low-level echoes during the intermediate stages, and eventually an anechoic clot forms. Noninfected urinomas are anechoic. Most lymphoceles contain septations.

Renal artery and renal vein patency should be documented by both duplex and color Doppler sonography. On Doppler interrogation, renal artery stenosis causes turbulence and high-frequency shifts and eventually absence of definable flow (499).

The value of changes in the resistive index (RI) (peak systolic minus end diastolic divided by peak systolic veloc-

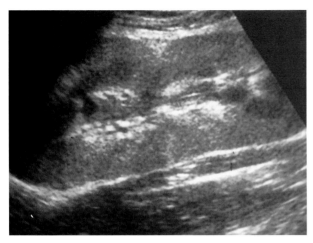

FIG. 9-184. Acute renal transplant rejection. Longitudinal sonography of a transplanted kidney. There is diffuse increase in echogenicity of the renal parenchyma and loss of corticomedullary differentiation.

ity) remains controversial. There is considerable overlap between the normal RI and the RI found in various complications. Although nonspecific (500,501), correlation of clinical information and careful assessment of RI may be useful (497,502). An increased RI may be seen in rejection, severe ATN, extrarenal compression, obstructive uropathy, renal vein obstruction, and pyelonephritis (497,503). Renal allografts undergoing the vascular form of acute rejection tend to have a very high RI (504). A normal RI does not exclude rejection, particularly of the interstitial type (505). Diastolic reversal of flow in the renal artery indicates a poor prognosis for the transplanted kidney (506).

Renal scintigraphy assesses allograft perfusion and function. Both ATN and rejection have normal or decreased perfusion, decreased DTPA uptake, and delayed tracer excretion. Sequential scintigraphy shows a return to normal with reversal of ATN but worsening with rejection. Ureteral obstruction and urine leaks can also be shown by renal scintigraphy (507).

Angiography is still performed in selected patients when the diagnosis is unclear and when interventional therapy for a pseudoaneurysm is indicated. The role of MRI in the evaluation of renal transplants has not yet been determined (35,508,509).

Urethral Polyps

A solitary fibroepithelial polyp of the posterior urethra is an occasional cause of obstruction, infection, and hematuria in boys. Urethral polyps are covered by the same uroepithelium that lines the urethra and have a stalk attached to the verumontanum. The fibrovascular core of these polyps is covered by transitional cell epithelium that may rarely contain foci of squamous metaplasia or glandular rests (510,511). Congenital posterior urethral polyps are benign;

their etiology is not known. Some believe that urethral polyps represent mesonephric duct remnants and are analogous to the cervical polyps seen in girls (510,512,513). Other hypotheses include defective formation of the urethral wall, metaplastic epithelial change secondary to estrogen stimulation during gestation, and response to infection.

Signs and symptoms of a urethral polyp include obstruction (48%), hematuria (27%), retention (25%), infection (19%), azotemia (8%), and enuresis (6%) (510). Although these features are nonspecific, they should prompt radiologic evaluation.

Bladder sonography may demonstrate a mobile, intravesical mass of mixed echogenicity if the polyp has prolapsed back into the bladder. VCUG shows a filling defect in the urethra, if it has prolapsed into the prostatic urethra during voiding, or bladder (Fig. 9-185) (510).

A look-alike for urethral polyp is a prolapsing ureterocele (see Fig. 9-90; Fig. 9-186) (514). If contrast surrounds the inferior margin of the filling defect when it is located in the urinary bladder, the lesion originates from the bladder and is probably not a urethral polyp (Fig. 9-186). However, if contrast surrounds the superior margin of the filling defect when it is located in the urethra, the lesion originates inferiorly and is probably a urethral polyp (Fig. 9-185). US may be able to distinguish between the two conditions. A ureterocele is anechoic, whereas a polyp is echogenic.

Other differential diagnostic considerations include nonopaque stone, foreign body, blood clot, rhabdomyosarcoma of the bladder base, and hypertrophy of the verumontanum (510). Most polyps of the posterior urethra are treated by endoscopic excision; they do not recur (510,515).

Nontumorous Scrotal and Testicular Abnormalities

Testicular Torsion

Approximately 40% of boys with acute scrotal pain have testicular torsion. Torsion of the testicle is an axial twisting of the spermatic cord and attached testis. Although torsion can occur at any age, it is most common in the neonatal period and in adolescence.

The normal testis is partially covered on its anterior surface by the tunica vaginalis, a serosal membrane derived from the processus vaginalis of the peritoneum. When the tunica vaginalis invests not only the testicle but the epididymis and distal spermatic cord as well (''bell-clapper'' deformity), the testis and cord may twist in this serosal space and become ischemic. The abnormality of the tunica vaginalis is frequently bilateral. In neonates with torsion, fixation of the testis to the scrotum is not necessarily abnormal, and the mechanism of torsion appears to be different. Neonatal torsions are usually extravaginal, the entire testis and tunica vaginalis rotating within the lax subcutaneous tissues of the scrotum.

After the neonatal period, testicular torsion produces acute

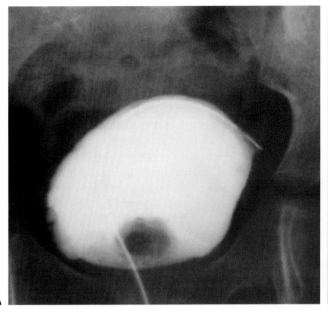
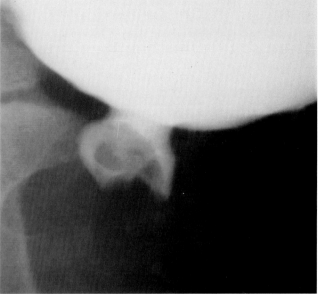

A

B

FIG. 9-185. Posterior urethral polyp. A: Cystogram. A rounded lucent filling defect is noted at the base of the bladder. **B:** VCUG. During voiding the polyp prolapses into the posterior urethra and produces a large filling defect.

scrotal pain and swelling. Prompt diagnosis and therapy are imperative; preservation of hormonal and spermatogenetic function is usually possible only in patients whose ischemia is relieved within 6–10 hours. Neonates with testicular torsion may have no pain or discomfort and often present with

a firm, painless mass in a discolored scrotum (516). Salvage of twisted neonatal testes is extremely rare.

Testicular perfusion depends on whether torsion or detorsion of the testis is present at the time of the examination. In the past, testicular scintigraphy was the best imaging mo-

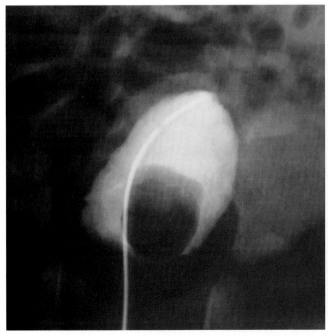
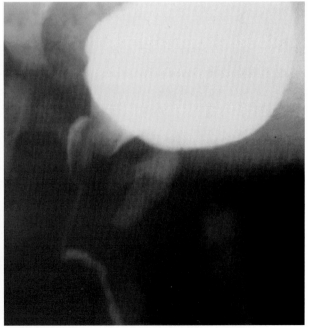

A

B

FIG. 9-186. Ureterocele mimicking urethral polyp. A: Cystogram. There is a large lobular filling defect at the base of the bladder. It was sonolucent at sonography and was connected to a dilated ureter. **B:** VCUG. The ureterocele prolapses into the urethra and causes partial obstruction. The appearance may be confused with that of a posterior urethral polyp.

dality for the diagnosis of acute testicular torsion (517,518). With torsion of less than 24 hours duration, perfusion of the affected testis is decreased and there is less radiotracer uptake than on the normal side. Within a few days of complete torsion, scrotal vessels produce a rim of increased perfusion around the avascular testis.

Recently, color Doppler sonography has become the preferred screening method for boys with acute scrotal symptoms. Morphology and perfusion of both the testis and other scrotal contents can be assessed noninvasively and, if necessary, repeatedly. Unfortunately, even state-of-the-art equipment may be unable to detect intratesticular arterial flow in normal babies and small children (519–521).

The sonographic appearance of testicular torsion depends on the time since the twist occurred. In most cases of acute torsion, edema makes the affected testis slightly larger and more hypoechoic than the normal testis (Fig. 9-187) (522). The epididymis is usually enlarged. After approximately 10 hours, the testicular parenchyma becomes heterogeneous because of hemorrhage and necrosis. A hydrocele may develop. Color Doppler sonography demonstrates absence of perfusion in acute testicular torsion. Conversely, patients with torsion of a testicular appendix, epididymitis, or epididymoorchitis will demonstrate increase in both epididymal and testicular flow. There is increased peritesticular flow in patients with chronic testicular torsion (Fig. 9-188) (523).

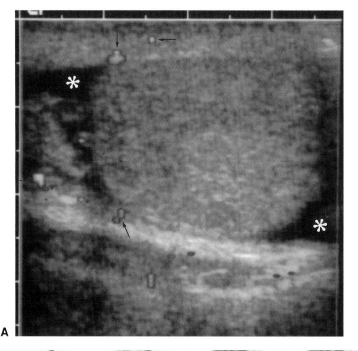

A

FIG. 9-187. Acute testicular torsion. A 16-year-old boy with 3 hours of left scrotal pain. **A:** Longitudinal sonography. The left testis is enlarged. There was no evidence of intratesticular flow with color Doppler imaging. There is an associated hydrocele *(asterisks)*. **B:** Radionuclide angiography. There is relatively symmetric scrotal perfusion, although a photopenic region can be faintly identified in the left hemiscrotum. **C:** Tissue-phase image with converging collimator. There is photopenia of the left hemiscrotum. **D:** Tissue phase image with pinhole collimator. This confirms the photopenic region corresponding to the left testicle. At surgery, a 180° torsion was found. Detorsion and bilateral orchiopexies were performed. Follow-up studies demonstrated normal left testicular morphology and perfusion.

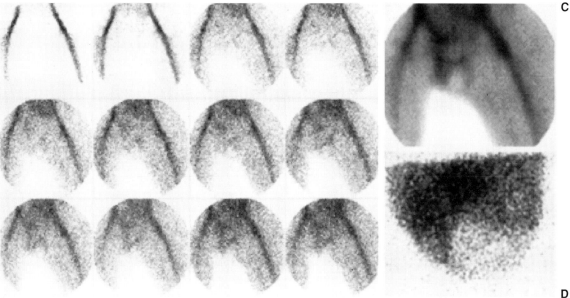

B

C

D

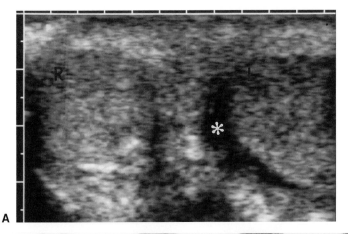

FIG. 9-188. Chronic testicular torsion. A 14-year-old boy with pain and swelling of the left hemiscrotum for 3 days. **A:** Transverse sonography of the scrotum demonstrates a mildly hypoechoic, inhomogeneous, and slightly enlarged left testis *(L)*. The right testicle *(R)* is normal. There is a small left hydrocele *(asterisk)*. **B:** Radionuclide angiography shows increased scrotal perfusion surrounding an area of absent perfusion. Static images with converging **(C)** and pinhole **(D)** collimators verify a rounded region of decreased tracer localization surrounded by a rim of increased tracer localization *(arrows)*. There was a 540° torsion of the left spermatic cord and a necrotic left testicle.

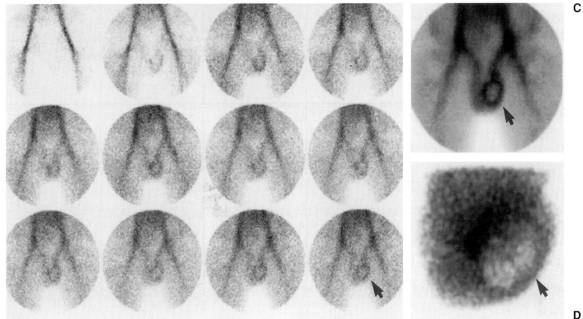

Patients with testicular torsion should be explored promptly. If surgical detorsion and fixation are performed within 6 hours of torsion, approximately 90% of testes will survive. The viability of the testis decreases rapidly after more than 6 hours, and orchiectomy is usually required. In the latter situation, the necrotic testis is removed and the contralateral testis is fixed to the scrotum to prevent future torsion. In neonates with testicular torsion and loss of viability of the testis, emergency surgery is performed to remove the necrotic testicle and to fix the normal testicle to the scrotum.

Epididymoorchitis

Epididymitis and orchitis were said in the past to be rare in the prepubertal boy in the absence of congenital genitourinary anomalies, chronic infection, or prior instrumentation. Most cases were thought to occur in adolescents and to be secondary to gonorrheal infection. However, preadolescent epididymitis and orchitis are more common than was formerly believed. They are usually not secondary to known causes (521,524–526). Orchitis is usually associated with epididymitis and presumably represents a direct extension of inflammation. Isolated orchitis is unusual and is most commonly viral or posttraumatic.

US with color Doppler imaging distinguishes painful epididymo-orchitis from other causes of scrotal pain, testicular torsion in particular. The inflamed epididymis appears swollen and hypoechoic. Testicular enlargement occurs with orchitis and there may be a focal or generalized decrease in echogenicity. A reactive hydrocele is commonly present. Scrotal scintigraphy usually demonstrates diffusely increased perfusion of the symptomatic hemiscrotum because of epididymal and testicular hyperemia (Fig. 9-189). Complications of epididymoorchitis include abscess, pyocele, and testicular ischemia. Ischemia occurs when testicular venous outflow is compressed by an inflamed, edematous epididymis. Diagnosing this decreased arterial blood flow requires comparison with the opposite testis.

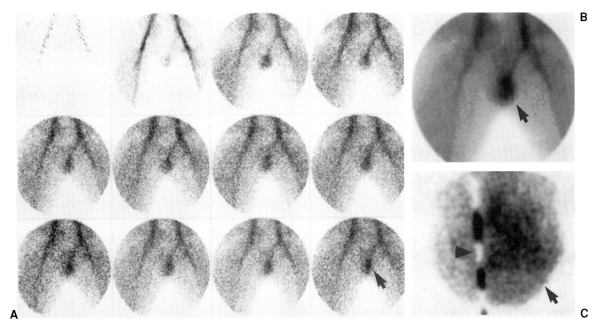

FIG. 9-189. Epididymoorchitis. Radionuclide angiography **(A)** shows increased perfusion of the left hemiscrotum *(arrow)*. Static images obtained with converging **(B)** and pinhole **(C)** collimators demonstrate diffusely increased tracer localization there *(arrows)*. A cobalt-57 marker indicates the median raphe on the pinhole image *(arrowhead)*.

Torsion of the Testicular Appendage

The testicular appendages are vestigial remnants of the mesonephric and Müllerian ducts and include the appendix testis, the appendix epididymis, and the paradidymis. The classic clinical presentation of torsion of a testicular appendage is a firm, exquisitely tender, pea-sized nodule attached to the testis or epididymis in the upper scrotum. However, the clinical features may be indistinguishable from those of testicular torsion, and marked scrotal edema as well as a reactive hydrocele may make physical examination difficult or impossible. Sonography shows a normal testis with normal blood flow. A mass of increased echogenicity with a central hypoechoic region may be found next to the testicle (527,528). Others have described epididymal enlargement with increased blood flow by color Doppler sonography, a pattern indistinguishable from that of epididymitis (Fig. 9-190) (520). Scrotal scintigraphy may also demonstrate increased blood flow and radiotracer uptake identical to that of epididymoorchitis (520).

Scrotal Trauma

US is ideal for imaging the scrotum after trauma. Testicular integrity can be assessed and any focal alterations in parenchymal echogenicity documented. Areas of increased or decreased echogenicity suggest hemorrhage or infarction. Scrotal hematoceles appear as fluid collections that may contain low-level echoes. Color Doppler sonography is used to

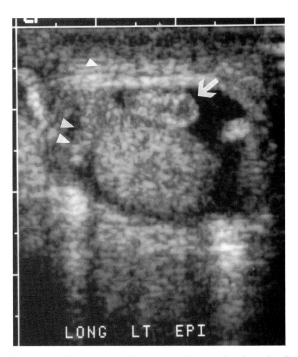

FIG. 9-190. Torsion of the appendix testis. Longitudinal sonogram of the left testis shows an enlarged appendix testis *(arrow)* near the head of the epididymis *(arrowheads)*. There is a hydrocele of moderate size. Duplex Doppler sonography demonstrated normal testicular blood flow.

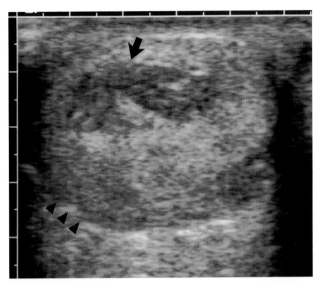

FIG. 9-191. Intratesticular hematoma. A 14-year-old boy who was kicked in the scrotum. A longitudinal sonogram of the right testicle shows a lobulated parenchymal hematoma *(arrow)*. The posterosuperior testicular margin is ill defined *(arrowheads)*, which suggests testicular fracture.

demonstrate testicular perfusion. An intratesticular hematoma is an avascular mass of abnormal echogenicity (Fig. 9-191) that causes displacement of peripheral vessels.

Hydrocele

A hydrocele is the most common scrotal mass in childhood. It may be congenital (representing incomplete closure of the processus vaginalis) or acquired as a result of testicular torsion, inflammation, trauma, or neoplasm. A completely open processus vaginalis not only permits peritoneal fluid to collect around the testis but provides a route for visceral herniation into the scrotum. Hydroceles are readily diagnosed with transillumination. US is useful in identifying an associated testicular abnormality when the physical examination is equivocal. Simple hydroceles usually do not have loculations. The presence of septations raises the possibility of an additional abnormality such as hemorrhage, infection, or tumor. In most infants, a patent processus vaginalis undergoes spontaneous closure. Surgery is required only if a simple hydrocele persists into the second year of life or if there is an associated hernia.

Spermatocele

A spermatocele usually occurs after trauma or chronic epididymitis and is due to cystic dilatation of epididymal tubules (529). This abnormality is usually located in the head of the epididymis and is easily identified as a predominantly anechoic, cystic structure. Occasionally, it may contain echogenic debris (530).

Varicocele

A varicocele is an acquired dilatation of the pampiniform plexus caused by increased pressure in the spermatic vein or its tributaries, with reversal of venous blood flow. Although usually left-sided, varicoceles are bilateral in 10% of cases. They are rare before puberty.

Varicoceles are identified by their increase in size in the erect position or with a Valsalva maneuver. In prepubertal boys US is useful to exclude a mass obstructing gonadal venous drainage. Especially in a prepubertal boy, a varicocele may lead to a smaller testicle on that side; this may cause decreased fertility (531). Although the normal right–left difference in testicular volume has not been established for prepubertal boys, postpubertal volumes should differ by no more than 1 cm³. If the testis on the side of the varicocele is smaller, venous ligation is recommended (532). Doppler examination of a varicocele demonstrates a mass of anechoic tubes with venous blood flow (Fig. 9-192). Nonoperative obliteration of varicoceles is performed by retrograde catheterization of the gonadal vein and embolization (533).

Idiopathic Scrotal Edema

Idiopathic scrotal edema is rare and consists of bilateral scrotal swelling, sometimes with eosinophilia. It is self-limited, has no known sequelae, and tends to affect young boys. Sonography demonstrates thickened, ill-defined scrotal tissues.

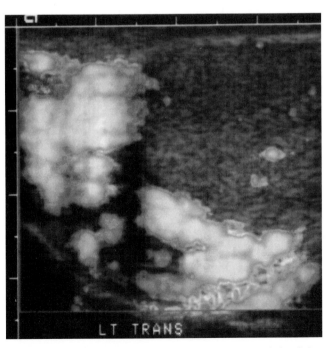

FIG. 9-192. Varicocele. Power Doppler image of the left hemiscrotum. There is dramatically increased flow in the dilated veins.

Scrotal Extension of Healed Meconium Peritonitis

Scrotal extension of healed meconium peritonitis may produce a hard, irregular mass mimicking a testicular neoplasm. A history of hydrocele at birth or of meconium peritonitis is highly suggestive. The distribution of the calcification on abdominal plain films and the appearance at scrotal sonography are helpful in excluding a neoplasm (see Fig. 9-32), although neuroblastoma has been known to metastasize to the scrotum and calcify there.

Testicular Microlithiasis

Testicular microlithiasis is an uncommon, nonprogressive entity with a characteristic sonographic appearance. There are innumerable tiny echogenic foci throughout both testes (Fig. 9-193). These hyperechoic foci represent calcified concretions within the lumina of seminiferous tubules. Microlithiasis is typically discovered incidentally during investigation of unrelated testicular symptoms. The condition may be associated with Klinefelter syndrome, male pseudohermaphroditism, cryptorchidism, varicocele, epididymitis, and testicular neoplasms (534–536).

Precocious Puberty

There is considerable variation in the age at which puberty begins in the normal child. However, the development of secondary sexual characteristics prior to 8 years of age in girls and 9 years in boys is considered precocious. Precocious pubertal development is classified as true precocious puberty or precocious pseudopuberty. *True precocious puberty* is always isosexual and includes both early development of secondary characteristics and an increase in size and activity of the gonads. In *precocious pseudopuberty,* the secondary sex characteristics may be either isosexual or heterosexual. However, there is no activation of the hypothalamic-pituitary gonadal axis, and the gonads do not mature. A form of precocious puberty that is gonadotropin-independent has recently been described. These children resemble those with true precocious puberty, but the hypothalamic-pituitary axis is not involved. The condition is usually sporadic and is much more common in girls.

In the past, precocious puberty was thought to be idiopathic in 80% to 90% of girls and 50% of boys. These numbers have changed dramatically with the development of CT and MRI; causative factors are found in more patients. In girls, cysts and tumors of the central nervous system, hydrocephalus, postencephalitic scarring, ovarian tumors, feminizing adrenocortical tumors, exogenous sources of estrogen, and the McCune-Albright syndrome must be considered. In boys, the differential diagnosis includes the same central nervous system lesions, as well as the adrenogenital syndrome, a Leydig cell tumor, and a gonadotropin-producing hepatoma.

Precocious Puberty in Girls

Early development of secondary sexual characteristics in girls is termed *precocious thelarche* if breast enlargement occurs prior to 7 years of age, *precocious pubarche* if pubic hair develops prior to 8 years of age, and *precocious menarche* if vaginal bleeding occurs prior to 8 years of age (537). There is usually a hypothalamic cause for precocious puberty in girls. However, an autonomously functioning ovarian cyst or tumor is occasionally the source of estrogen or androgen secretion. Girls with precocious puberty should undergo comprehensive evaluation, including abdominal US, serum endocrinologic studies, radiography of the hand and wrist for assessment of skeletal maturation, and sometimes CT or MRI of the head.

Sonographic evaluation of a girl with precocious sexual development should include imaging of the uterus and ovaries and accurate measurement in three dimensions (538). Any ovarian cysts are similarly measured (539). Bilateral ovarian enlargement is a reliable indicator of true isosexual precocious puberty, whereas unilateral ovarian enlargement in combination with macrocysts (>9 mm in diameter) suggests precocious pseudopuberty (540). Smaller ovarian cysts do not appear to be specific (539,540). When precocious puberty is due to hypothalamic dysfunction, treatment with gonadotropin-releasing hormone is usually started. Serial sonography is used to assess response. With therapy, uterine and ovarian volumes will usually return to normal or remain only slightly above normal (541). If a solitary ovarian tumor or a large cyst is identified, it is removed (540).

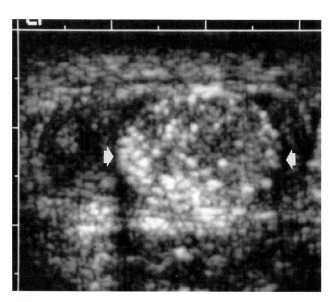

FIG. 9-193. Testicular microlithiasis. A longitudinal sonogram of the left hemiscrotum demonstrates many punctate, hyperechoic foci in the testis *(between arrows).* The right testis had a similar sonographic appearance.

Precocious Puberty in Boys

The diagnosis of male precocious puberty is based on premature testicular and penile enlargement as well as the development of pubic hair. It may be idiopathic, caused by unusually early but otherwise normal development of the hypothalamic-pituitary axis. However, more often it is secondary to a testicular or adrenal tumor, a gonadotropin-secreting tumor, or a disorder of the central nervous system involving the hypothalamus. Hypothalamic involvement may be due to pressure, scarring, or tumor invasion. Other causes of precocious puberty in boys include the adrenogenital syndrome and gonadotropin-independent precocious puberty.

The history and physical examination usually provide clues to the diagnosis. In the adrenogenital syndrome, the testes are small compared to the degree of sexual maturation. Leydig cell tumors and hepatomas will usually be detected by physical examination. A family history of sexual precocity is suggestive of gonadotropin-independent precocious puberty. Even when brain CT or MRI is normal, a boy with precocious puberty must be carefully followed for several years before an intracranial abnormality can be excluded.

Sonography should evaluate the adrenal glands, liver, retroperitoneum, and testes (542). The testes are measured in three dimensions so therapy can be monitored quantitatively.

REFERENCES

General Information

1. Aaronson IA, Cremin BJ. *Clinical paediatric uroradiology.* New York: Churchill Livingstone, 1984.
2. Silverman FN, Kuhn JP eds. *Caffey's pediatric x-ray diagnosis: an integrated imaging approach.* 9th ed. St. Louis: Mosby, 1993.
3. Chrispin AR, Gordon I, Hall C, Metreweli C. *Diagnostic imaging of the kidney and urinary tract in children.* Berlin: Springer-Verlag, 1980.
4. Cohen MD, Edwards MK. *Magnetic resonance imaging of children.* Philadelphia: BC Decker, 1990.
5. Cohen MD. *Imaging of children with cancer.* St. Louis: Mosby–Year Book, 1992.
6. Hilton SW, Edwards DK III, eds. *Practical pediatric radiology.* 2nd ed. Philadelphia: W.B. Saunders, 1994.
7. Lebowitz RL. *Postoperative pediatric uroradiology.* New York: Appleton-Century-Crofts, 1981.
8. Miller JH, ed. *Imaging in pediatric oncology.* Baltimore: Williams and Wilkins, 1985.
9. Parker BR, Castellino RA. *Pediatric oncologic radiology.* St. Louis: CV Mosby, 1977.
10. Poznanski AK. *Practical approaches to pediatric radiology.* Chicago: Year Book, 1976.
11. Reeder MM, *Reeder and Felson's gamuts in radiology: comprehensive lists of roentgen differential diagnosis.* 3rd ed. New York: Springer-Verlag, 1993.
12. Slovis TL, Sty JR, Haller JO. *Imaging of the pediatric urinary tract.* Philadelphia: WB Saunders, 1989.
13. Swischuk LE. *Imaging of the newborn and young infant.* Baltimore: Williams and Wilkins, 1989.
14. Treves ST. *Pediatric nuclear medicine.* 2nd ed. New York: Springer-Verlag, 1995.
15. Sty JR, Wells RG, Starshak RJ, Gregg DC. *Diagnostic imaging of infants and children.* Gaithersburg, MD: Aspen Publications, 1992.

Techniques

16. Shopfner CE, Hutch JA. The normal urethrogram. *Radiol Clin North Am* 1968;6:165–189.
17. Shopfner CE. Cystourethrography. *Med Radiogr Photogr* 1971;47:2–31.
18. Hass EA, Solomon DJ. Telling children about diagnostic radiology procedures. *Radiology* 1977;124:521.
19. Lebowitz RL, Fellows KE, Colodny AH. Renal parenchymal infections in children. *Radiol Clin North Am* 1977;15:37–47.
20. Leibovic SJ, Lebowitz RL. Reducing patient dose in voiding cystourethrography. *Urol Radiol* 1980;2:103–107.
21. Ben-Ami T, Boichis H, Hertz M. Fused labia. Clinical and radiologic findings *Pediatr Radiol* 1978;7:33–35.
22. Koff SA. Estimating bladder capacity in children. *Urology* 1983;21:248.
23. Berger RM, Maizels M, Moran GC, et al. Bladder capacity (ounces) equals age (years) plus 2 predicts normal bladder capacity and aids in diagnosis of abnormal voiding patterns. *J Urol* 1983;129:347–349.
24. Jequier S, Jequier J-C. Reliability of voiding cystourethrography to detect reflux. *AJR* 1989;153:807–810.
25. Wyly JB, Lebowitz RL. Refluxing urethral ectopic ureters: recognition by the cyclic voiding cystourethrogram. *AJR* 1984;142:1263–1267.
26. Paltiel HJ, Rupich RC, Kiruluta HG. Enhanced detection of vesicoureteral reflux in infants and children with use of cyclic voiding cystourethrography. *Radiology* 1992;184:753–755.
26a. Nogrady MB, Dunbar JS, Delayed concentration and prolonged excretion of urographic contrast medium in the first month of life. *AJR* 1968;104:289–295.
27. Kirks DR, Merten DF, Grossman H, Bowie JD. Diagnostic imaging of pediatric abdominal masses: an overview. *Radiol Clin North Am* 1981;19:527–545.
28. Magill HL, Clarke EA, Fitch SJ, et al. Excretory urography with Iohexol: evaluation in children. *Radiology* 1986;161:625–630.
29. Shopfner CE. Genitography in intersexual states. *Radiology* 1964;82:664–674.
30. Grant EG, White EM, eds. *Duplex sonography.* New York: Springer-Verlag, 1988.
31. LeQuesne GW. Patterns of ultrasonic abnormality in the renal parenchyma in childhood. *Ann Radiol* 1978;21:225–230.
32. Shkolnik A. B-mode ultrasound and the nonvisualizing kidney in pediatrics. *AJR* 1977;128:121–125.
33. Slovis TL, Perlmutter AD. Recent advances in pediatric urological ultrasound. *J Urol* 1980;123:613–620.
34. Teele RL. Ultrasonography of the genitourinary tract in children. *Radiol Clin North Am* 1977;15:109–128.
35. Steinberg HV, Nelson RC, Murphy FB, et al. Renal allograft rejection: evaluation by Doppler US and MR imaging. *Radiology* 1987;162:337–342.
36. Bude RO, Rubin JM, Adler RS. Power versus conventional color Doppler sonography: comparison in the depiction of normal intrarenal vasculature. *Radiology* 1994;192:777–780.
37. Fobbe F, Siegert J, Fritzsch T, et al. Color-coded duplex sonography and ultrasound contrast media—detection of renal perfusion defects in experimental animals. *Rofo Fortschr Geb Rontgenstr Neuen Bildgeb Verfahr* 1991;154:242–245.
38. Surratt JT, Siegel MJ, Middleton WD. Sonography of complications in pediatric renal allografts. *RadioGraphics* 1990;10:687–699.
39. Kleinman PK, Diamond DA, Karellas A, et al. Tailored low-dose fluoroscopic voiding cystourethrography for the reevaluation of vesicoureteral reflux in girls. *AJR* 1994;162:1151–1154.
40. Lebowitz RL. Tailored low-dose fluoroscopic voiding cystourethrography for the reevaluation of vesicoureteral reflux in girls. Commentary. *AJR* 1994;162:1155–1156.
41. Majd M, Rushton HG. Renal cortical scintigraphy in the diagnosis of acute pyelonephritis. *Semin Nucl Med* 1992;22:98–111.
42. Majd M. Nuclear medicine in pediatric nephrology and urology. In: Seibert JJ, ed. *Syllabus: Current concepts: a categorical course in pediatric radiology.* Oak Brook, IL: The Society for Pediatric Radiology, 1994, 83–90.
43. Berger PE, Munschauser RW, Kuhn JP. Computed tomography and ultrasound of renal and perirenal diseases in infants and children. Relationship to excretory urography in renal cystic disease, trauma and neoplasm. *Pediatr Radiol* 1980;9:91–99.
44. Kuhn JP, Berger PE. Computed tomography of the kidney in infancy and childhood. *Radiol Clin North Am* 1981;19:445–461.

45. Kuhns LR. Computed tomography of the retroperitoneum in children. *Radiol Clin North Am* 1981;19:495–501.
46. Kirks DR. Pediatric renal angiography. *Appl Radiol* 1978;11:83–91.
47. Whitaker RH. Diagnosis of obstruction in dilated ureters. *Ann R Coll Surg Engl* 1973;53:153–166.

Normal Genitourinary Tract

48. Currarino G. Roentgenographic estimation of kidney size in normal individuals with emphasis on children. *AJR* 1965;93:464–466.
49. Eklof O, Ringertz H. Kidney size in children. A method of assessment. *Acta Radiol* 1976;17:617–625.
50. Moskowitz PS, Carroll BA, McCoy JM. Ultrasonic renal volumetry in children: accuracy and simplicity of the method. *Radiology* 1980; 134:61–64.
51. Hodson CJ. The radiological contribution toward the diagnosis of chronic pyelonephritis. *Radiology* 1967;88:857–871.
52. Patriquin H, Lefaivre J-F, Lafortune M, et al. Fetal lobation. An anatomo-ultrasonographic correlation. *J Ultrasound Med* 1990;9: 191–197.
53. Han BK, Babcock DS. Sonographic measurements and appearance of normal kidneys in children. *AJR* 1985;145:611–616.
54. Hricak L, Slovis TL, Callen CW, et al. Neonatal kidneys: sonographic anatomic correlation. *Radiology* 1983;147:699–702.
55. Cohen HL, Shapiro MA, Mandel FS, Shapiro ML. Normal ovaries in neonates and infants: a sonographic study of 77 patients 1 day to 24 months old. *AJR* 1993;160:583–586.
56. Haber HP, Mayer EI. Ultrasound evaluation of uterine and ovarian size from birth to puberty. *Pediatr Radiol* 1994;24:11–13.
57. Cohen HL, Tice HM, Mandel FS. Ovarian volumes measured by US: bigger than we think. *Radiology* 1990;177:189–192.
58. Fonkalsrud EW. Testicular undescent and torsion. *Pediatr Clin North Am* 1987;34:1305–1317.
59. Zachmann M, Prader A, Kind HP, et al. Testicular volume during adolescence. Cross-sectional and longitudinal studies. *Helv Paediatr Acta* 1974;29:61–72.

Normal Variants and Pseudotumors

60. Hoffer FA, Hanabergh AM, Teele RL. The interrenicular junction: a mimic of renal scarring on normal pediatric sonograms. *AJR* 1985; 145:1075–1078.
61. Lebowitz RL, Colodny AH. Urinary tract infection in children. *CRC Crit Rev Clin Radiol Nucl Med* 1973;4:457–475.
62. Taybi H. Pseudoneoplastic masses (pseudotumors) in children. Part two: pseudotumors of abdomen, skeleton, and soft tissue. *Med Radiogr Photogr* 1978;54:41–71.
63. Kirks DR, Currarino G, Weinberg AG. Transverse folds in the proximal ureter: a normal variant in infants. *AJR* 1978;130:463–464.
64. Lebowitz RL, Avni FE. Misleading appearances in pediatric uroradiology. *Pediatr Radiol* 1980;10:15–31.
65. Allen RP, Condon VR. Transitory extraperitoneal hernia of the bladder in infants (bladder ears). *Radiology* 1961;77:979–982.
66. Firlit CF. Urethral abnormalities. *Urol Clin North Am* 1978;5:31–55.
67. Saxton HM, Borzyskowski M, Mundy AR, Vivian GC. Spinning top urethra: not a normal variant. *Radiology* 1988;168:147–150.
68. Currarino G, Fuqua F. Cowper's glands in the urethrogram. *AJR* 1972; 116:838–842.
69. Dacher JN, Boillot B, Eurin D, et al. Rational use of CT in acute pyelonephritis: findings and relationships with reflux. *Pediatr Radiol* 1993;23:281–285.
70. Dacher JN, Pfister C, Monroc M, et al. Power Doppler sonographic pattern of acute pyelonephritis in children: comparison with CT. *AJR* 1996;166:1451–1455.

Urinary Tract Obstruction

71. Friedland GW. Hydronephrosis in infants and children. Part I. *Curr Probl Diagn Radiol* 1978;7:1–52.
72. Friedland GW. Hydronephrosis in infants and children. Part II. *Curr Probl Diagn Radiol* 1978;7:1–34.

Systemic Hypertension

73. Clayman AS, Bookstein JJ. The role of renal arteriography in pediatric hypertension. *Radiology* 1973;108:107–110.
74. Korobkin M, Perloff DL, Palubinskas AJ. Renal arteriography in the evaluation of unexplained hypertension in children and adolescents. *J Pediatr* 1976;88:388–393.
75. Sfakianakis GN, Bourgoignie JJ, Jaffe D, et al. Single-dose captopril scintigraphy in the diagnosis of renovascular hypertension. *J Nucl Med* 1987;28:1383–1392.
76. Ball WL. Radiographic evaluation and intervention in the child with hypertension related to renal disease. In: Loggie J, ed. *Pediatric and adolescent hypertension.* Boston: Blackwell Scientific, 1992.

Urinary Tract Calcification

77. Myracle MR, McGahan JP, Goetzman BW, Adelman RD. Ultrasound diagnosis of renal calcification in infants on chronic furosemide therapy. *J Clin Ultrasound* 1986;14:281–287.
78. Walther PC, Lamm D, Kaplan GW. Pediatric urolithiases: a ten-year review. *Pediatrics* 1980;65:1068–1072.
79. Kirks DR. Lithiasis due to interruption of the enterohepatic circulation of bile salts. *AJR* 1979;133:383–388.

Urine Ascites and Urinoma

80. Griscom NT, Colodny AH, Rosenberg HK, et al. Diagnostic aspects of neonatal ascites: report of 27 cases. *AJR* 1977;128:961–969.

Congenital Abnormalities

81. Alton DJ. Pelviureteric obstruction in childhood. *Radiol Clin North Am* 1977;15:61–70.
82. Brown T, Mandell J, Lebowitz RL. Neonatal hydronephrosis in the era of sonography. *AJR* 1987;148:959–964.
83. Preston A, Lebowitz RL. What's new in pediatric uroradiology. *Urol Radiol* 1989;11:217–220.
84. Lebowitz RL, Blickman JG. The coexistence of ureteropelvic junction obstruction and reflux. *AJR* 1983;140:231–238.
85. McGrath MA, Estroff J, Lebowitz RL. The coexistence of obstruction at the ureteropelvic and ureterovesical junctions. *AJR* 1987;149: 403–406.
86. Fernbach SK, Zawin JK, Lebowitz RL. Complete duplication of the ureter with ureteropelvic junction obstruction of the lower pole of the kidney: imaging findings. *AJR* 1995;164:701–704.
87. Laing FC, Burke VD, Wing VW, et al. Postpartum evaluation of fetal hydronephrosis: optimal timing for follow-up sonography. *Radiology* 1984;152:423–424.
88. Fernbach SK. The dilated urinary tract in children. *Urol Radiol* 1992; 14:34–42.
89. Chopra A, Teele RL. Hydronephrosis in children: narrowing the differential diagnosis with ultrasound. *J Clin Ultrasound* 1980;8: 473–478.
90. Griscom NT, Kroeker MA. Visualization of individual papillary ducts (ducts of Bellini) by excretory urography in childhood hydronephrosis. *Radiology* 1973;106:385–389.
91. Dunbar JS, Nogrady MB. The calyceal crescent—a roentgenographic sign of obstructive hydronephrosis. *AJR* 1970;110:520–528.
92. Hoffer FA, Lebowitz RL. Intermittent hydronephrosis: a unique feature of ureteropelvic junction obstruction caused by a crossing renal vessel. *Radiology* 1985;156:655–658.
93. MacNeily AE, Maizels M, Kaplan WE, et al. Does early pyeloplasty really avert loss of renal function? A retrospective review. *J Urol* 1993;150:769–773.
94. Koff SA, Campbell KD. The nonoperative management of unilateral neonatal hydronephrosis: natural history of poorly functioning kidneys. *J Urol* 1994;152:593–595.
95. Ransley PG, Dhillon HK, Gordon I, et al. The postnatal management of hydronephrosis diagnosed by prenatal ultrasound. *J Urol* 1990; 144:584–587.
96. Duckett JW Jr. When to operate on neonatal hydronephrosis. *Urology* 1993;42:617–619.
97. Woodard JR. Hydronephrosis in the neonate. *Urology* 1993;42: 620–621.

98. Griscom NT, Vawter GF, Fellers FX. Pelvoinfundibular atresia. *Semin Roentgenol* 1975;10:125–131.

99. Felson B, Cussen LJ. The hydronephrotic type of unilateral congenital multicystic disease of the kidney. *Semin Roentgenol* 1975;10:113–123.

100. Avni EF, Thoua Y, Lalmand B, et al. Multicystic dysplastic kidney: evolving concepts. In utero diagnosis and post-natal follow-up by ultrasound. *Ann Radiol* 1986;29:663–668.

101. Avni EF, Thoua Y, Lalmand B, et al. Multicystic dysplastic kidney: natural history from in utero diagnosis and postnatal followup. *J Urol* 1987;138:1420–1424.

102. Flack CE, Bellinger MF. The multicystic dysplastic kidney and contralateral vesicoureteral reflux: protection of the solitary kidney. *J Urol* 1993;150:1873–1874.

103. Wacksman J, Phipps L. Report of Multicystic Kidney Registry: preliminary findings. *J Urol* 1993;150:1870–1872.

104. Rickwood AMK, Anderson PAM, Williams MPL. Multicystic renal dysplasia detected by prenatal ultrasonography. Natural history and results of conservative management. *Br J Urol* 1992;69:538–540.

105. Strife JL, Souza AS, Kirks DR, et al. Multicystic dysplastic kidney in children: US follow-up. *Radiology* 1993;186:785–788.

106. Peters CA, Mandell J. *The multicystic dysplastic kidney*, vol 8. Houston: American Urological Association, 1989;50–55.

107. Susskind MR, Kim KS, King LR. Hypertension and multicystic kidney. *Urology* 1989;34:362–366.

108. Emmert GK Jr, King LR. The risk of hypertension is underestimated in the multicystic dysplastic kidney: a personal perspective. *Urology* 1994;44:404–405.

109. Hitchcock R, Burge DM. Renal agenesis: an acquired condition? *J Pediatr Surg* 1994;29:454–455.

110. Mesrobian HGJ, Rushton HG, Bulas D. Unilateral renal agenesis may result from in utero regression of multicystic renal dysplasia. *J Urol* 1993;150:793–794.

111. Gallegos CRR, Iyer SK, Massouh H. Congenital ureteric valves. *Br J Urol* 1991;68:656.

112. Docimo SG, Lebowitz RL, Retik AB, et al. Congenital midureteral obstruction. *Urol Radiol* 1989;11:156–160.

113. Reinberg Y, Aliabadi H, Johnson P, Gonzalez R. Congenital ureteral valves in children: case report and review of the literature. *J Pediatr Surg* 1987;22:379–381.

114. Mering JH, Steel JF, Gittes RF. Congenital ureteral valves. *J Urol* 1972;107:737–739.

115. Chwalle R. The process of formation of cystic dilatations of the vesical end of the ureter and of diverticula at the ureteral ostium. *Urol Cutan Rev* 1927;31:499–504.

116. Campbell MF. The dilated ureter in children; a brief consideration of its causes, diagnosis and treatment. *Am J Surg* 1938;39:438.

117. Allen TD. Congenital ureteral strictures. *Birth Defects* 1977;13:17–18.

118. Ruano-Gil D, Coca-Payeras A, Tejedo-Mateu A. Obstruction and normal recanalization of the ureter in the human embryo. Its relation to congenital ureteric obstruction. *Eur Urol* 1975;1:287–293.

119. Meyer JS, Lebowitz RL. Primary megaureter in infants and children: a review. *Urol Radiol* 1992;14:296–305.

120. Docimo SG, Dikkes P, Horton CE. Primary obstructive megaureter: a neuroanatomic disease? *American Academy of Pediatrics Section on Urology Program*, 1988.

121. Teele RL, Share JC. *Ultrasonography of infants and children*. Philadelphia: WB Saunders, 1991.

122. Blickman JG, Lebowitz RL. The coexistence of primary megaureter and reflux. *AJR* 1984;143:1053–1057.

123. Keating MA, Escala J, Snyder HM III, et al. Changing concepts in management of primary obstructive megaureter. *J Urol* 1989;142:636–640.

124. Schaffer RM, Sunshine AG, Becker JA, et al. Retrocaval ureter: sonographic appearance. *J Ultrasound Med* 1985;4:199–201.

125. Yen T-C, Yeh S-H. Retrocaval ureter in newborn demonstrated by Tc-99m DTPA renal scintigram. *Clin Nucl Med* 1993;18:989.

126. Casale AJ. Early urethral surgery for posterior urethral valves. *Urol Clin North Am* 1990;17:361–372.

127. Parkhouse HF, Woodhouse CRJ. Long-term status of patients with posterior urethral valves. *Urol Clin North Am* 1990;17:373–378.

128. Friedland GW, Fair WR, Govan DE, Filly R. Posterior urethral valves. *Clin Radiol* 1977;28:367–380.

129. Young HH, Frontz WA, Baldwin JC. Congenital obstruction of the posterior urethra. *J Urol* 1919;3:289–354.

130. Dewan PA, Zappala SM, Ransley PG, Duffy PG. Endoscopic reappraisal of the morphology of congenital obstruction of the posterior urethra. *Br J Urol* 1992;70:439–444.

131. Patten RM, Mack LA, Wang KY, Cyr DR. The fetal genitourinary tract. *Radiol Clin North Am* 1990;28:115–130.

132. Dinneen MD, Dhillon HK, Ward HC, et al. Antenatal diagnosis of posterior urethral valves. *Br J Urol* 1993;72:364–369.

133. Reinberg Y, de Castano I, Gonzalez R. Prognosis for patients with prenatally diagnosed posterior urethral valves. *J Urol* 1992;148:125–126.

134. Cremin BJ. The "spinnaker sail" appearance of the posterior urethral valve in infants. *J Can Assoc Radiol* 1975;26:188–191.

135. Cohen HL, Susman M, Haller JO, et al. Posterior urethral valve: transperineal US for imaging and diagnosis in male infants. *Radiology* 1994;192:261–264.

136. Nancarrow PA, Lebowitz RL. Primary vesicoureteral reflux in blacks with posterior urethral valves: does it occur? *Pediatr Radiol* 1988;19:31–33.

137. Feinstein KA, Fernbach SK. Septated urinomas in the neonate. *AJR* 1987;149:997–1000.

138. Eklof O, Ringertz H. Pre- and postoperative urographic findings in posterior urethral valves. *Pediatr Radiol* 1975;4:43–46.

139. Eklof O, Olsson H. The variability of urographic findings in posterior urethral valves. *Pediatr Radiol* 1983;13:215–218.

140. Ditchfield MR, Grattan-Smith JD, de Campo JF, Hutson JM. Voiding cystourethrography in boys: does the presence of the catheter obscure the diagnosis of posterior urethral valves? *AJR* 1995;164:1233–1235.

141. Campaiola JM, Perlmutter AD, Steinhardt GF. Noncompliant bladder resulting from posterior urethral valves. *J Urol* 1985;134:708–710.

142. Kaefer M, Keating MA, Adams MC, Rink RC. Posterior urethral valves, pressure pop-offs and bladder function. *J Urol* 1995;154:708–711.

143. Kirks DR, Grossman H. Congenital saccular anterior urethral diverticulum. *Radiology* 1981;140:367–372.

144. Anonymous. Medical versus surgical treatment of primary vesicoureteral reflux. *Pediatrics* 1981;67:392–400.

145. Bissett GS III, Strife JL, Dunbar JS. Urography and voiding cystourethrography: findings in girls with urinary tract infection. *AJR* 1987;148:479–482.

146. Askari A, Belman AB. Vesicoureteral reflux in black girls. *J Urol* 1982;127:747–748.

147. Jerkins GR, Noe HN. Familial vesicoureteral reflux: a prospective study. *J Urol* 1982;128:774–778.

148. Van den Abbeele AD, Treves ST, Lebowitz RL, et al. Vesicoureteral reflux in asymptomatic siblings of patients with known reflux: radionuclide cystography. *Pediatrics* 1987;79:147–153.

149. Noe HN, Wyatt RJ, Peeden JN Jr, Rivas ML. The transmission of vesicoureteral reflux from parent to child. *J Urol* 1992;148:1869–1871.

150. Gross GW, Lebowitz RL. Infection does not cause reflux. *AJR* 1981;137:929–932.

151. Smellie JM, Normand ICS, Katz G. Children with urinary tract infection: a comparison of those with and those without vesicoureteral reflux. *Kidney Int* 1981;20:717–722.

152. Newman L, Bucy JG, McAlister WH. Experimental production of reflux in the presence and absence of infected urine. *Radiology* 1974;111:591–595.

153. Ransley PG, Risdon RA. Reflux and renal scarring. *Br J Radiol* 1978;14.

154. Friedland GW. Recurrent urinary tract infections in infants and children. *Radiol Clin North Am* 1977;15:19–35.

155. Funston MR, Cremin BJ. Intrarenal reflux—papillary morphology and pressure relationships in children's necropsy kidneys. *Br J Radiol* 1978;51:665–670.

156. Ransley PG. Opacification of the renal parenchyma in obstruction and reflux. *Pediatr Radiol* 1976;4:226–232.

157. Ransley PG, Risdon RA. The renal papilla, intrarenal reflux, and chronic pyelonephritis. In: Hodson J, Kincaid-Smith P, eds. *Reflux nephropathy*. New York: Masson, 1979, 126–133.

158. Najmaldin A, Burge DM, Atwell JD. Reflux nephropathy secondary to intrauterine vesicoureteric reflux. *J Pediatr Surg* 1990;25:387–390.

159. Arant BS Jr, Sotelo-Avila C, Bernstein J. Segmental "hypoplasia" of the kidney (Ask-Upmark). *J Pediatr* 1979;95:931–939.

160. Shimada K, Matsui T, Ogino T, et al. Renal growth and progression of reflux nephropathy in children with vesicoureteral reflux. *J Urol* 1988;140:1097–1100.

161. Ditchfield MR, de Campo JF, Cook DJ, et al. Vesicoureteral reflux: an accurate predictor of acute pyelonephritis in childhood urinary tract infection? *Radiology* 1994;190:413–415.

162. Friedland GW, Forsberg L. Striation of the renal pelvis in children. *Clin Radiol* 1972;23:58–60.

163. Strife JL, Bisset GS III, Kirks DR, et al. Nuclear cystography and renal sonography: findings in girls with urinary tract infection. *AJR* 1989;153:115–119.

164. Schwoebel MG, Sacher P, Bucher HU, et al. Prenatal diagnosis improves the prognosis of children with obstructive uropathies. *J Pediatr Surg* 1984;19:187–190.

165. Anderson N, Clautice-Engle T, Allan R, et al. Detection of obstructive uropathy in the fetus: predictive value of sonographic measurements of renal pelvic diameter at various gestational ages. *AJR* 1995;164:719–723.

166. Avni EF, Van Gansbeke D, Thoua Y, et al. US demonstration of pyelitis and ureteritis in children. *Pediatr Radiol* 1988;18:134–139.

167. Babcock DS. Sonography of wall thickening of the renal collecting system. A nonspecific finding. *J Ultrasound Med* 1987;6:29–32.

168. Rushton HG, Majd M, Chandra R, Yim D. Evaluation of ^{99m}technetium-dimercapto-succinic acid renal scans in experimental acute pyelonephritis in piglets. *J Urol* 1988;140:1169–1174.

169. Rushton HG, Majd M. Dimercaptosuccinic acid renal scintigraphy for the evaluation of pyelonephritis and scarring: a review of experimental and clinical studies. *J Urol* 1992;148:1726–1732.

170. Verboven M, Ingels M, Delree M, Piepsz A. 99m Tc-DMSA scintigraphy in acute urinary tract infection in children. *Pediatr Radiol* 1990;20:540–542.

171. Bjorgvinsson E, Majd M, Eggli KD. Diagnosis of acute pyelonephritis in children: comparison of sonography and 99m Tc-DMSA scintigraphy. *AJR* 1991;157:539–543.

172. Conway JJ, Cohn RA. Evolving role of nuclear medicine for the diagnosis and management of urinary tract infection. *J Pediatr* 1994;124:87–90.

173. Lebowitz RL, Olbing H, Parkkulainen KV, et al. International system of radiographic grading of vesicoureteric reflux. International Reflux Study in Children. *Pediatr Radiol* 1985;15:105–109.

174. Mastin ST, Drane WE, Iravani A. Tc-99m DMSA SPECT imaging in patients with acute symptoms or history of UTI. Comparison with ultrasonography. *Clin Nucl Med* 1995;20:407–412.

175. Koff SA, Murtagh DS. The uninhibited bladder in children: effect of treatment on recurrence of urinary infection and on vesicoureteral reflux resolution. *J Urol* 1983;130:1138–1141.

176. Allen TD. Vesicoureteral reflux and the unstable bladder. *J Urol* 1985;134:1180.

177. Lenaghan D, Whitaker JG, Jensen F, Stephens FD. The natural history of reflux and long-term effects of reflux on the kidney. *J Urol* 1976;115:728–730.

178. Dwoskin JY, Perlmutter AD. Vesicoureteral reflux in children: a computerized review. *J Urol* 1973;109:888–890.

179. McLorie GA, McKenna PH, Jumper BM, et al. High grade vesicoureteral reflux: analysis of observational therapy. *J Urol* 1990;144:537–540.

180. Gordon AC, Thomas DFM, Arthur RJ, et al. Prenatally diagnosed reflux: a follow-up study. *Br J Urol* 1990;65:407–412.

181. Rypens F, Avni EF, Bank WO, et al. The ureterovesical junction in children: sonographic findings after surgical or endoscopic treatment. *AJR* 1992;158:837–842.

182. Zerin JM, Smith JD, Sanvordenker JK, Bloom DA. Sonography of the bladder after ureteral reimplantation. *J Ultrasound Med* 1992;11:87–91.

183. Dewan PA, Guiney EJ. Endoscopic correction of primary vesicoureteric reflux in children. *Urology* 1992;39:162–164.

184. Gore MD, Fernbach SK, Donaldson JS, et al. Radiographic evaluation of subureteric injection of teflon to correct vesicoureteral reflux. *AJR* 1989;152:115–119.

185. Mann CI, Jequier S, Patriquin H, et al. Intramural teflon injection of the ureter for treatment of vesicoureteral reflux: sonographic appearance. *AJR* 1988;151:543–545.

186. Glassberg KI, Braren V, Duckett JW, et al. Suggested terminology for duplex systems, ectopic ureters and ureteroceles. *J Urol* 1984;132:1153–1154.

187. Risdon RA, Young LW, Chrispin AR. Renal hypoplasia and dysplasia: a radiological and pathological correlation. *Pediatr Radiol* 1975;3:213–225.

188. Share JC, Lebowitz RL. The unsuspected double collecting system on imaging studies and at cystoscopy. *AJR* 1990;155:561–564.

189. Ben-Ami T, Gayer G, Hertz M, et al. The natural history of reflux in the lower pole of duplicated collecting systems: a controlled study. *Pediatr Radiol* 1989;19:308–310.

190. Peppas DS, Skoog SJ, Canning DA, Belman AB. Nonsurgical management of primary vesicoureteral reflux in complete ureteral duplication: is it justified? *J Urol* 1991;146:1594–1595.

191. Lee PH, Diamond DA, Duffy PG, Ransley PG. Duplex reflux: a study of 105 children. *J Urol* 1991;146:657–659.

192. Friedland GW, Cunningham J. The elusive ectopic ureteroceles. *AJR* 1972;116:792–811.

193. Williams DI, ed. *Paediatric urology.* London: Butterworths, 1968, 195–212.

194. Lundin E, Riggs W. Upper urinary tract duplication associated with ectopic ureterocele in childhood and infancy. *Acta Radiol* 1968;7:13–24.

195. Nussbaum AR, Lebowitz RL. Interlabial masses in little girls: review and imaging recommendations. *AJR* 1983;141:65–71.

196. Bellah RD, Long FR, Canning DA. Ureterocele eversion with vesicoureteral reflux in duplex kidneys: findings at voiding cystourethrography. *AJR* 1995;165:409–413.

197. Share JC, Lebowitz RL. Ectopic ureterocele without ureteral and calyceal dilatation (ureterocele disproportion): findings on urography and sonography. *AJR* 1989;152:567–571.

198. Husmann DA, Ewalt DH, Glenski WJ, Bernier PA. Ureterocele associated with ureteral duplication and a nonfunctioning upper pole segment: management by partial nephroureterectomy alone. *J Urol* 1995;154:723–726.

199. Blyth B, Passerini-Glazel G, Camuffo C, et al. Endoscopic incision of ureteroceles: intravesical versus ectopic. *J Urol* 1993;149:556–559.

200. Stannard MW, Lebowitz RL. Urography in the child who wets. *AJR* 1978;130:959–962.

201. Braverman RM, Lebowitz RL. Occult ectopic ureter in girls with urinary incontinence: diagnosis by using CT. *AJR* 1991;156:365–366.

202. Weiss JP, Duckett JW, Snyder HM. Single unilateral vaginal ectopic ureter: is it really a rarity? *J Urol* 1984;132:1177–1179.

203. Gotoh T, Morita H, Tokunaka S, et al. Single ectopic ureter. *J Urol* 1983;129:271–274.

204. Gharagozloo AM, Lebowitz RL. Detection of a poorly functioning malpositioned kidney with single ectopic ureter in girls with urinary dribbling: imaging evaluation in five patients. *AJR* 1995;164:957–961.

205. Korogi Y, Takahashi M, Fujimura N, et al. Computed tomography demonstration of renal dysplasia with a vaginal ectopic ureter. *J Comput Tomogr* 1986;10:273–275.

206. Boechat MI, Lebowitz RL. Diverticula of the bladder in children. *Pediatr Radiol* 1978;7:22–28.

207. Hutch JA. Saccule formation at the ureterovesical junction in smooth walled bladders. *J Urol* 1961;86:390–399.

208. Vates TS, Fleisher MH, Siegel RL. Acute urinary retention in an infant: an unusual presentation of a paraureteral diverticulum. *Pediatr Radiol* 1993;23:371–372.

209. Bellinger MF, Gross GW, Boal DK. Bladder diverticulum associated with ureteral obstruction. *Pediatr Radiol* 1985;15:207–208.

210. Livne PM, Gonzalez ET Jr. Congenital bladder diverticula causing ureteral obstruction. *Urology* 1985;25:273–276.

211. Verghese M, Belman AB. Urinary retention secondary to congenital bladder diverticula in infants. *J Urol* 1984;132:1186–1188.

212. Taylor WN, Alton D, Toguri A, et al. Bladder diverticula causing posterior urethral obstruction in children. *J Urol* 1979;122:415.

213. Hernanz-Shulman M, Lebowitz RL. The elusiveness and importance of bladder diverticula in children. *Pediatr Radiol* 1985;15:399–402.

214. Amis ES Jr, Blaivas JG. Neurogenic bladder simplified. *Radiol Clin North Am* 1991;29:571–580.

215. Kopp C, Greenfield SP. Effects of neurogenic bladder dysfunction in utero seen in neonates with myelodysplasia. *Br J Urol* 1993;71:739–742.

216. White P, Lebowitz RL. Exstrophy of the bladder. *Radiol Clin North Am* 1977;15:93–107.

217. Marshall VF, Muecke EC. Variations in exstrophy of the bladder. *J Urol* 1962;88:766–796.

218. Mildenberger H, Kluth D, Dziuba M. Embryology of bladder exstrophy. *J Pediatr Surg* 1988;23:166–170.

219. Culp DA. The histology of the exstrophied bladder. *J Urol* 1964;91:538–548.

220. Hayden PW, Chapman WH, Stevenson JK. Exstrophy of the cloaca. *Am J Dis Child* 1973;125:879–883.

221. Muecke EC, Currarino G. Congenital widening of the pubic symphysis: associated clinical disorders and roentgen anatomy of affected bony pelves. *AJR* 1968;103:179–185.

222. Loder RT, Dayioglu MM. Association of congenital vertebral malformations with bladder and cloacal exstrophy. *J Pediatr Orthop* 1990;10:389–393.

223. Jaramillo D, Lebowitz RL, Hendren WH. The cloacal malformation: radiologic findings and imaging recommendations. *Radiology* 1990;177:441–448.

224. Warf BC, Scott RM, Barnes PD, Hendren WH III. Tethered spinal cord in patients with anorectal and urogenital malformations. *Pediatr Neurosurg* 1993;19:25–30.

225. Hammer E. Cancer du colon sigmoide dix ans apres implantation des ureteres d'une vessie exstrophiee. *J Urol Nephrol (Paris)* 1929;28:260–263.

226. Warren RB, Warner TFCS, Hafez GR. Late development of colonic adenocarcinoma 49 years after ureterosigmoidostomy for exstrophy of the bladder. *J Urol* 1980;124:550–551.

227. Gittes RF. Carcinogenesis in ureterosigmoidostomy. *Urol Clin North Am* 1986;13:201–205.

228. Kliment J, Luptak J, Lofaj M, et al. Carcinoma of the colon after ureterosigmoidostomy and trigonosigmoidostomy for exstrophy of the bladder. *Int Urol Nephrol* 1993;25:339–343.

229. Rozenman J, Hertz M, Boichis H. Radiological findings of the urinary tract in hypospadias: a report of 110 cases. *Clin Radiol* 1979;30:471–476.

230. Davenport M, MacKinnon AE. The value of ultrasound screening of the upper urinary tract in hypospadias. *Br J Urol* 1988;62:595–596.

231. Effmann EL, Lebowitz RL, Colodny AH. Duplication of the urethra. *Radiology* 1976;119:179–185.

232. Bates DG, Lebowitz RL. Congenital urethroperineal fistula. *Radiology* 1995;194:501–504.

233. Berdon WE, Baker DH, Wigger HJ, et al. Calcified intraluminal meconium in newborn males with imperforate anus. Enterolithiasis in the newborn. *AJR* 1975;125:449–455.

234. Anderson S, Savader B, Barnes J, Savader S. Enterolithiasis with imperforate anus. Report of two cases with sonographic demonstration and occurrence in a female. *Pediatr Radiol* 1988;18:130–133.

235. Gross GW, Wolfson PJ, Pena A. Augmented-pressure colostogram in imperforate anus with fistula. *Pediatr Radiol* 1991;21:560–562.

236. Currarino G, Votteler TP, Kirks DR. Anal agenesis with rectobulbar fistula. *Radiology* 1978;126:457–461.

237. Lebowitz RL, Lamego C. Rectourethral fistula on the urethrogram. *Urol Radiol* 1979;1:53–59.

238. Hall JW, Tank ES, Lapides J. Urogenital anomalies and complications associated with imperforate anus. *J Urol* 1970;103:810–814.

239. Smith ED. Urinary anomalies and complications in imperforate anus and rectum. *J Pediatr Surg* 1968;3:337–349.

240. Moskowitz PS, Newton NA, Lebowitz RL. Retention cysts of Cowper's duct. *Radiology* 1976;120:377–380.

241. Colodny AH, Lebowitz RL. Lesions of Cowper's ducts and glands in infants and children. *Urology* 1978;11:321–325.

242. Carter CO, Evans K. Birth frequency of bilateral renal agenesis. *J Med Genet* 1981;18:158.

243. Daneman A, Alton DJ. Radiographic manifestations of renal anomalies. *Radiol Clin North Am* 1991;29:351–363.

244. Mascatello V, Lebowitz RL. Malposition of the colon in left renal agenesis and ectopia. *Radiology* 1976;120:371–376.

245. Teele RL, Rosenfield AT, Freedman GS. The anatomic splenic flexure: an ultrasonic renal impostor. *AJR* 1977;128:115–120.

246. Barnewolt CE, Lebowitz RL. Absence of a renal sinus echo complex in the ectopic kidney of a child: a normal finding. *Pediatr Radiol* 1996;26:318–323.

247. Kozakewich HPW, Lebowitz RL. Congenital megacalyces. *Pediatr Radiol* 1974;2:251–258.

248. Talner LB, Gittes RF. Megacalyces. *Clin Radiol* 1972;23:55–61.

249. Talner LB, Gittes RF. Megacalyces: further observations and differentiation from obstructive renal disease. *AJR* 1974;121:473–486.

250. Garcia CJ, Taylor KJW, Weiss RM. Congenital megacalyces. Ultrasound appearance. *J Ultrasound Med* 1987;6:163–165.

251. Vargas B, Lebowitz RL. The coexistence of congenital megacalyces and primary megaureter. *AJR* 1986;147:313–316.

252. Osathanondh V, Potter EL. Pathogenesis of polycystic kidneys. *Arch Pathol* 1964;77:466–473.

253. Hayden CK Jr, Swischuk LE. Renal cystic disease. *Semin Ultrasound CT MR* 1991;12:361–373.

254. Wood BP. Renal cystic disease in infants and children. *Urol Radiol* 1992;14:284–295.

255. Elkin M, Bernstein J. Cystic diseases of the kidney—radiological and pathological considerations. *Clin Radiol* 1969;20:65–82.

256. Elkin M. Renal cystic disease—an overview. *Semin Roentgenol* 1975;10:99–102.

257. Faure C. Renal cysts and cystlike conditions in infancy and childhood. *Curr Concepts Pediatr Radiol* 1977;1:76.

258. Grossman H, Winchester PH, Chisari FV. Roentgenographic classification of renal cystic disease. *AJR* 1968;104:319–331.

259. Six R, Oliphant M, Grossman H. A spectrum of renal tubular ectasia and hepatic fibrosis. *Radiology* 1975;117:117–122.

260. Bartholomew TH, Slovis TL, Kroovand RL, Corbett DP. The sonographic evaluation and management of simple renal cysts in children. *J Urol* 1980;123:732–736.

261. Gordon RL, Pollack HM, Popky GL, Duckett JW Jr. Simple serous cysts of the kidney in children. *Radiology* 1979;131:357–361.

262. McHugh K, Stringer DA, Hebert D, Babiak CA. Simple renal cysts in children: diagnosis and follow-up with US. *Radiology* 1991;178:383–385.

263. Hoard TD, O'Brien DP III. Simple renal cyst and high renin hypertension cured by cyst decompression. *J Urol* 1976;115:326–327.

264. Boal DK, Teele RL. Sonography of infantile polycystic kidney disease. *AJR* 1980;135:575–580.

265. Premkumar A, Berdon WE, Levy J, et al. The emergence of hepatic fibrosis and portal hypertension in infants and children with autosomal recessive polycystic kidney disease. Initial and follow-up sonographic and radiographic findings. *Pediatr Radiol* 1988;18:123–129.

266. Currarino G, Stannard MW, Rutledge JC. The sonolucent cortical rim in infantile polycystic kidneys. Histologic correlation. *J Ultrasound Med* 1989;8:571–574.

267. Kogutt MS, Robichaux WH, Boineau FG, et al. Asymmetric renal size in autosomal recessive polycystic kidney disease: a unique presentation. *AJR* 1993;160:835–836.

268. Blickman JG, Bramson RT, Herrin JT. Autosomal recessive polycystic kidney disease: long-term sonographic findings in patients surviving the neonatal period. *AJR* 1995;164:1247–1250.

269. Herman TE, Siegel MJ. Pyramidal hyperechogenicity in autosomal recessive polycystic kidney disease resembling medullary nephrocalcinosis. *Pediatr Radiol* 1991;21:270–271.

270. Pretorius DH, Lee ME, Manco-Johnson ML, et al. Diagnosis of autosomal dominant polycystic kidney disease in utero and in the young infant. *J Ultrasound Med* 1987;6:249–255.

271. Worthington JL, Shackelford GD, Cole BR, et al. Sonographically detectable cysts in polycystic kidney disease in newborn and young infants. *Pediatr Radiol* 1988;18:287–293.

272. Hartman DS. Renal cystic disease in multisystem conditions. *Urol Radiol* 1992;14:13–17.

273. Alpern MB, Dorfman RE, Gross BH, et al. Seminal vesicle cysts: association with adult polycystic kidney disease. *Radiology* 1991;180:79–80.

274. Fitch SJ, Stapleton FB. Ultrasonographic features of glomerulocystic disease in infancy: similarity to infantile polycystic kidney disease. *Pediatr Radiol* 1986;16:400–402.

275. McAlister WH, Siegel MJ, Shackelford G, et al. Glomerulocystic kidney. *AJR* 1979;133:536–538.

276. Fredericks BJ, de Campo M, Chow CW, Powell HR. Glomerulocystic renal disease: ultrasound appearances. *Pediatr Radiol* 1989;19:184–186.

277. Taxy JB, Filmer RB. Glomerulocystic kidney. Report of a case. *Arch Pathol Lab Med* 1976;100:186–188.

278. Pinckney LE, Currarino G, Weinberg AG. Parenchymal reflux in renal dysplasia. *Radiology* 1981;141:681–686.

279. Chamberlin BC, Hagge WW, Stickler GB. Juvenile nephronophthisis and medullary cystic disease. *Mayo Clin Proc* 1977;52:485–491.

280. Garel LA, Habib R, Pariente D, et al. Juvenile nephronophthisis: sonographic appearance in children with severe uremia. *Radiology* 1984;151:93–95.

281. Jones DN, Risdon RA, Hayden K, et al. Juvenile nephronophthisis. Clinical, radiological and pathological correlationships. *Pediatr Radiol* 1973;1:164–171.

282. Rosenfield AT, Siegel NJ, Kappelman NB, Taylor KJ. Gray scale ultrasonography in medullary cystic disease of the kidney and congenital hepatic fibrosis with tubular ectasia: new observations. *AJR* 1977;129:297–303.

283. Reed MH, Griscom NT. Hydrometrocolpos in infancy. *AJR* 1973;118:1–13.

284. Wilson DA, Stacy TM, Smith EI. Ultrasound diagnosis of hydrocolpos and hydrometrocolpos. *Radiology* 1978;128:451–454.

285. Kirks DR, Currarino G. Imperforate vagina with vaginourethral communication. *AJR* 1977;129:623–628.

286. Berkowitz GS, Lapinski RH, Dolgin SE, et al. Prevalence and natural history of cryptorchidism. *Pediatrics* 1993;92:44–49.

287. Goulding FJ, Garrett RA. Twenty-five-year experience with prune belly syndrome. *Urology* 1978;12:329–332.

288. Marshall FF, Shermeta DW. Epididymal abnormalities associated with undescended testis. *J Urol* 1979;121:341–343.

289. Pappis CH, Argianas SA, Bousgas D, Athanasiades E. Unsuspected urological anomalies in asymptomatic cryptorchid boys. *Pediatr Radiol* 1988;18:51–53.

290. Puchner PJ, Santulli TV, Lattimer JK. Urologic problems associated with imperforate anus. *Urology* 1975;6:205–208.

291. Raghavaiah NV. Noonan's syndrome associated with cake kidney. *Urology* 1975;5:640–642.

292. Rajfer J, Walsh PC. The incidence of intersexuality in patients with hypospadias and cryptorchidism. *J Urol* 1976;116:769–770.

293. Rosenfield AT, Blair DN, McCarthy S, et al. The pars infravaginalis gubernaculi: importance in the identification of the undescended testis. *AJR* 1989;153:775–778.

294. Fritzsche PJ, Hricak H, Kogan BA, et al. Undescended testis: value of MR imaging. *Radiology* 1987;164:169–173.

295. Kier R, McCarthy S, Rosenfield AT, et al. Nonpalpable testes in young boys: evaluation with MR imaging. *Radiology* 1988;169:429–433.

296. Beomonte Zobel B, Vicentini C, Masciocchi C, et al. Magnetic resonance imaging in the localization of undescended abdominal testes. *Eur Urol* 1990;17:145–148.

297. Cremin BJ. Intersex states in young children: the importance of radiology in making a correct diagnosis. *Clin Radiol* 1974;25:63–73.

298. Blyth B, Duckett JW, Jr. Gonadal differentiation: a review of the physiological process and influencing factors based on recent experimental evidence. *J Urol* 1991;145:689–694.

299. Grimes CK, Rosenbaum DM, Kirkpatrick JA Jr. Pediatric gynecologic radiology. *Semin Roentgenol* 1982;17:284–301.

300. Izquierdo G, Glassberg KI. Gender assignment and gender identity in patients with ambiguous genitalia. *Urology* 1993;42:232–242.

301. Manuel M, Katayama PK, Jones HW Jr. The age of occurrence of gonadal tumors in intersex patients with a Y chromosome. *Am J Obstet Gynecol* 1976;124:293–300.

302. Cortes D, Thorup J, Graem N. Bilateral prepubertal carcinoma in situ of the testis and ambiguous external genitalia. *J Urol* 1989;142:1065–1069.

303. Muller J, Skakkebaek NE. Testicular carcinoma in situ in children with the androgen insensitivity (testicular feminisation) syndrome. *Br J Med* 1984;288:1419–1420.

304. Muller J, Skakkebaek NE, Ritzen M, et al. Carcinoma in situ of the testis in children with 45, X/46, XY gonadal dysgenesis. *J Pediatr* 1985;106:431–436.

305. Scully RE. Neoplasia associated with anomalous sexual development and abnormal sex chromosomes. In: Josso N, ed. *The intersex child*. Vol 8. New York: Karger, 1981, 203.

306. Horowitz M, Glassberg KI. Ambiguous genitalia: diagnosis, evaluation and treatment. *Urol Radiol* 1992;14:306–318.

307. Hendren WH, Crawford JD. Adrenogenital syndrome: the anatomy of the anomaly and its repair. Some new concepts. *J Pediatr Surg* 1969;4:49–58.

308. Bryan PJ, Caldamone AA, Morrison SC, et al. Ultrasound findings in the adreno-genital syndrome (congenital adrenal hyperplasia). *J Ultrasound Med* 1988;7:675–679.

309. Sivit CJ, Hung W, Taylor GA, et al. Sonography in neonatal congenital adrenal hyperplasia. *AJR* 1991;156:141–143.

310. Avni EF, Rypens F, Smet MH, Galetty E. Sonographic demonstration of congenital adrenal hyperplasia in the neonate: the cerebriform pattern. *Pediatr Radiol* 1993;23:88–90.

311. Eberenz W, Rosenberg HK, Moshang T, et al. True hermaphroditism: sonographic demonstration of ovotestes. *Radiology* 1991;179:429–431.

312. Gambino J, Caldwell B, Dietrich R, et al. Congenital disorders of sexual differentiation: MR findings. *AJR* 1992;158:363–367.

313. Karlin G, Brock W, Rich M, Pena A. Persistent cloaca and phallic urethra. *J Urol* 1989;142:1056–1059.

314. Cilento BG, Jr, Benacerraf BR, Mandell J. Prenatal diagnosis of cloacal malformation. *Urology* 1994;43:386–388.

315. Jaramillo D, Lebowitz RL, Hendren WH. The cloacal malformation: radiologic findings and imaging recommendations. *Radiology* 1990;177:441–448.

316. Stephenson CA, Ball TI Jr, Ricketts RR. An unusual case of meconium peritonitis associated with perforated hydrocolpos. *Pediatr Radiol* 1992;22:279–280.

317. Bear JW, Gilsanz V. Calcified meconium and persistent cloaca. *AJR* 1981;137:867–868.

318. Griscom NT. The roentgenology of neonatal abdominal masses. *AJR* 1965;93:447–463.

319. Hendren WH. Cloacal malformations: experience with 105 cases. *J Pediatr Surg* 1992;27:890–901.

320. Steidle CP, Kennedy HA, Mitchell ME, Rink RC. Symphyseal diastasis in the absence of the exstrophy-epispadias complex. *J Urol* 1988;140:349–350.

321. Carson JA, Barnes PD, Tunell WP, et al. Imperforate anus: the neurologic implication of sacral abnormalities. *J Pediatr Surg* 1984;19:838–842.

322. Lund DP, Hendren WH. Cloacal exstrophy: experience with 20 cases. *J Pediatr Surg* 1993;28:1360–1368.

323. Thomalla JV, Rudolph RA, Rink RC, Mitchell ME. Induction of cloacal exstrophy in the chick embryo using the CO2 laser. *J Urol* 1985;134:991–995.

324. Tank ES, Lindenauer SM. Principles of management of exstrophy of the cloaca. *Am J Surg* 1970;119:95–98.

325. Hurwitz RS, Manzoni GA, Ransley PG, Stephens FD. Cloacal exstrophy: a report of 34 cases. *J Urol* 1987;138:1060–1064.

326. Johnston JH, Penn IA. Exstrophy of the cloaca. *Br J Urol* 1966;38:302–307.

327. Langer JC, Brennan B, Lappalainen RE, et al. Cloacal exstrophy: prenatal diagnosis before rupture of the cloacal membrane. *J Pediatr Surg* 1992;27:1352–1355.

328. Smith NM, Chambers HM, Furness ME, Haan EA. The OEIS complex (omphalocele-exstrophy-imperforate anus-spinal defects): recurrence in sibs. *J Med Genet* 1992;29:730–732.

329. Chitrit Y, Zorn B, Filidori M, et al. Cloacal exstrophy in monozygotic twins detected through antenatal ultrasound scanning. *J Clin Ultrasound* 1993;21:339–342.

330. Greene WB, Dias LS, Lindseth RE, Torch MA. Musculoskeletal problems in association with cloacal exstrophy. *J Bone Joint Surg Am* 1991;73:551–560.

331. Herman TE, Cleveland RH, Kushner DC. Pelvic kidney in cloacal exstrophy. *Pediatr Radiol* 1986;16:306–308.

332. Meglin AJ, Balotin RJ, Jelinek JS, et al. Cloacal exstrophy: radiologic findings in 13 patients. *AJR* 1990;155:1267–1272.

333. Appignani BA, Jaramillo D, Barnes PD, Poussaint TY. Dysraphic myelodysplasias associated with urogenital and anorectal anomalies: prevalence and types seen with MR imaging. *AJR* 1994;163:1199–1203.

334. Rivosecchi M, Lucchetti MC, Zaccara A, et al. Spinal dysraphism detected by magnetic resonance imaging in patients with anorectal anomalies: incidence and clinical significance. *J Pediatr Surg* 1995;30:488–490.

335. Karrer FM, Flannery AM, Nelson MD Jr, et al. Anorectal malformations: evaluation of associated spinal dysraphic syndromes. *J Pediatr Surg* 1988;23:45–48.

336. Visnesky PM, Texter JH, Galle PC, et al. Genital outflow tract obstruction in an adolescent with cloacal exstrophy. *Obstet Gynecol* 1990;76:548–551.

337. Kirks DR, Taybi H. Prune belly syndrome. An unusual cause of neonatal abdominal calcification. *AJR* 1975;123:778–782.

Infection

338. Lebowitz RL, Mandell J. Urinary tract infection in children: putting radiology in its place. *Radiology* 1987;165:1–9.

339. Anonymous. Sequelae of covert bacteriuria in school girls. A four-year follow-up study. *Lancet* 1978;2:889–893.

340. Talner LB, Davidson AJ, Lebowitz RL, et al. Acute pyelonephritis: can we agree on terminology? *Radiology* 1994;192:297–305.

341. Lomberg H, Hanson LA, Jacobsson B, et al. Correlation of P blood group, vesicoureteral reflux, and bacterial attachment in patients with recurrent pyelonephritis. *N Engl J Med* 1983;308:1189–1192.

342. Majd M, Rushton HG, Jantausch B, Wiedermann BL. Relationship among vesicoureteral reflux, P-fimbriated Escherichia coli, and acute pyelonephritis in children with febrile urinary tract infection. *J Pediatr* 1991;119:578–585.

343. Fussell EN, Kaack MB, Cherry R, Roberts JA. Adherence of bacteria to human foreskins. *J Urol* 1988;140:997–1001.

344. Wiswell TE. Prepuce presence portends prevalence of potentially perilous periurethral pathogens. *J Urol* 1992;148:739–742.

345. Svanborg C. Resistance to urinary tract infection. *N Engl J Med* 1993; 329:802–803.

346. Kallenius G, Mollby R, Svenson SB, et al. Occurrence of P-fimbriated Escherichia coli in urinary tract infections. *Lancet* 1981;2:1369–1372.

347. Israele V, Darabi A, McCracken GH Jr. The role of bacterial virulence factors and Tamm–Horsfall protein in the pathogenesis of Escherichia coli urinary tract infection in infants. *Am J Dis Child* 1987;141:1230–1234.

348. Sty JR, Wells RG, Schroeder BA, Starshak RJ. Diagnostic imaging in pediatric renal inflammatory disease. *JAMA* 1986;256:895–899.

349. Sty JR, Wells RG, Starshak RJ, Schroeder BA. Imaging in acute renal infection in children. *AJR* 1987;148:471–477.

350. Handmaker H. Nuclear renal imaging in acute pyelonephritis. *Semin Nucl Med* 1982;12:246–253.

351. Kessler WO, Gittes RF, Hurwitz SR, Green JP. Gallium-67 scans in the diagnosis of pyelonephritis. *West J Med* 1974;121:91–93.

352. Garel L, Brunelle F, Montagne J.Ph. Les pyelonephrites xanthogranulmateuses de l'enfant. *Ann Radiol* 1979;22:207–212.

353. Fahr K, Oppermann HC, Scharer K, Greinacher I. Xanthogranulomatous pyelonephritis in childhood. Report of three cases and a review of the literature. *Pediatr Radiol* 1979;8:10–16.

354. Schneider K, Helmig FJ, Eife R, et al. Pyonephrosis in childhood—is ultrasound sufficient for diagnosis? *Pediatr Radiol* 1989;19:302–307.

355. Yoder IC, Pfister RC, Lindfors KK, Newhouse JH. Pyonephrosis: imaging and intervention. *AJR* 1983;141:735–740.

356. Swayne LC, Love MB, Karasick SR. Pelvic inflammatory disease: sonographic-pathologic correlation. *Radiology* 1984;151:751–755.

357. Tessler FN, Perrella RR, Fleischer AC, Grant EG. Endovaginal sonographic diagnosis of dilated Fallopian tubes. *AJR* 1989;153:523–525.

Renal Tumors

358. Kirks DR, Kaufman RA, Babcock DS. Renal neoplasms in infants and children. *Semin Roentgenol* 1987;22:292–302.

359. Crist WM, Kun LE. Common solid tumors of childhood. *N Engl J Med* 1991;324:461–471.

360. Breslow NE, Beckwith JB. Epidemiological features of Wilms tumor: results of the National Wilms Tumor Study. *JNCI* 1982;68:429–436.

361. Breslow N, Olshan A, Beckwith JB, Green DM. Epidemiology of Wilms tumor. *Med Pediatr Oncol* 1993;21:172–181.

362. Stiller CA, Parkin DM. International variations in the incidence of childhood renal tumours. *Br J Cancer* 1990;62:1026–1030.

363. Breslow N, Beckwith JB, Ciol M, Sharples K. Age distribution of Wilms tumor: report from the National Wilms Tumor Study. *Cancer Res* 1988;48:1653–1657.

364. Matsunaga E. Genetics of Wilms tumor. *Hum Genet* 1981;57:231–246.

365. Clericuzio CL. Clinical phenotypes and Wilms tumor. *Med Pediatr Oncol* 1993;21:182–187.

366. Miller RW, Fraumeni JF, Manning MD. Association of Wilms tumor with aniridia, hemihypertrophy, and other congenital malformations. *N Engl J Med* 1964;270:922–927.

367. Breslow NE, Churchill G, Nesmith B, et al. Clinicopathologic features and prognosis for Wilms tumor patients with metastases at diagnosis. *Cancer* 1986;58:2501–2511.

368. Malcolm AW, Jaffe N, Folkman MJ, Cassady JR. Bilateral Wilms tumor. *J Radiat Oncol Biol Phys* 1980;6:167–174.

369. Beckwith JB, Kiviat NB, Bonadio JF. Nephrogenic rests, nephroblastomatosis, and the pathogenesis of Wilms tumor. *Pediatr Pathol* 1990; 10:1–36.

370. Beckwith JB. Precursor lesions of Wilms tumor: clinical and biological implications. *Med Pediatr Oncol* 1993;21:158–168.

371. Beckwith JB, Palmer NF. Histopathology and prognosis of Wilms tumors: results from the First National Wilms Tumor Study. *Cancer* 1978;41:1937–1948.

372. D'Angio GJ, Evans AE, Breslow N, et al. Results of the Third National Wilms Tumor Study (NWTS-3). A preliminary report. *Proc Am Assoc Cancer Res* 1984;25:183.

373. Clark RE. Roentgen evaluation of Wilms tumor. *CRC Crit Rev Radiol Sci* 1972;3:543–576.

374. Farewell VT, D'Angio GJ, Breslow N, Norkool P. Retrospective validation of a new staging system for Wilms tumor. *Cancer Clin Trials* 1981;4:167–171.

375. D'Angio GJ, Rosenberg H, Sharples K, et al. Position paper: imaging methods for primary renal tumors of childhood: costs versus benefits. *Med Pediatr Oncol* 1993;21:205–212.

376. Shackelford GD, McAlister WH. Errors in the diagnosis of Wilms tumors. *CRC Crit Rev Radiol Sci* 1972;3:171–196.

377. De Campo JF. Ultrasound of Wilms tumor. *Pediatr Radiol* 1986;16:21–24.

378. Jaffe MH, White SJ, Silver TM, Heidelberger KP. Wilms tumor: ultrasonic features, pathologic correlation, and diagnostic pitfalls. *Radiology* 1981;140:147–152.

379. Cremin BJ. Wilms tumour: ultrasound and changing concepts. *Clin Radiol* 1987;38:465–474.

380. Reiman TA, Siegel MJ, Shackelford GD. Wilms tumor in children: abdominal CT and US evaluation. *Radiology* 1986;160:501–505.

381. Dietrich RB, Kangarloo H. Kidneys in infants and children: evaluation with MR. *Radiology* 1986;159:215–221.

382. Belt TG, Cohen MD, Smith JA, et al. MRI of Wilms tumor: promise as the primary imaging method. *AJR* 1986;146:955–961.

383. Gylys-Morin V, Hoffer FA, Kozakewich H, Shamberger RC. Wilms tumor and nephroblastomatosis: imaging characteristics at gadolinium-enhanced MR imaging. *Radiology* 1993;188:517–521.

384. Bousvaros A, Kirks DR, Grossman H. Imaging of neuroblastoma: an overview. *Pediatr Radiol* 1986;16:89–106.

385. Franken EA Jr, Yiu-Chiu V, Smith WL, Chiu LC. Nephroblastomatosis: clinicopathologic significance and imaging characteristics. *AJR* 1982;138:950–952.

386. Montgomery P, Kuhn JP, Berger PE, Fisher J. Multifocal nephroblastomatosis: clinical significance and imaging. *Pediatr Radiol* 1984;14:392–395.

387. Fernbach SK, Feinstein KA, Donaldson JS, Baum ES. Nephroblastomatosis: comparison of CT with US and urography. *Radiology* 1988;166:153–156.

388. White KS, Kirks DR, Bove KE. Imaging of nephroblastomatosis: an overview. *Radiology* 1992;182:1–5.

389. Berdon WE, Wigger HJ, Baker DH. Fetal renal hamartoma—a benign tumor to be distinguished from Wilms tumor. *AJR* 1973;118:18–27.

390. Hartman DS, Lesar MS, Madewell JE, et al. Mesoblastic nephroma: radiologic-pathologic correlation of 20 cases. *AJR* 1981;136:69–74.

391. Howell CG, Othersen HB, Kiviat NE, et al. Therapy and outcome in 51 children with mesoblastic nephroma: a report of the National Wilms Tumor study. *J Pediatr Surg* 1982;17:826–831.

392. Kirks DR, Rosenberg ER, Johnson DG, King LR. Integrated imaging of neonatal renal masses. *Pediatr Radiol* 1985;15:147–156.

393. Beckwith JB. Wilms tumor and other renal tumors of childhood: an update. *J Urol* 1986;136:320–324.

394. Chan HSL, Cheng MY, Mancer K, et al. Congenital mesoblastic nephroma: a clinicoradiologic study of 17 cases representing the pathologic spectrum of the disease. *J Pediatr* 1987;111:64–70.

395. Kirks DR, Kaufman RA. Function within mesoblastic nephroma: imaging-pathologic correlation. *Pediatr Radiol* 1989;19:136–139.

396. Wootton SL, Rowen SJ, Griscom NT. Pediatric case of the day. Congenital mesoblastic nephroma. *RadioGraphics* 1991;11:719–721.

397. Agrons GA, Wagner BJ, Davidson AJ, Suarez ES. Multilocular cystic renal tumor in children: radiologic-pathologic correlation. *Radio-Graphics* 1995;15:653–669.

398. Joshi VV, Beckwith JB. Multilocular cyst of the kidney (cystic

nephroma) and cystic, partially differentiated nephroblastoma. Terminology and criteria for diagnosis. *Cancer* 1989;64:466–479.

399. Madewell JE, Goldman SM, Davis CJ Jr, et al. Multilocular cystic nephroma: a radiographic-pathologic correlation of 58 patients. *Radiology* 1983;146:309–321.

400. Banner MP, Pollack HM, Chatten J, Witzleben C. Multilocular renal cysts: radiologic-pathologic correlation. *AJR* 1981;136:239–247.

401. Abara OE, Liu P, Churchill BM, Mancer K. Magnetic resonance imaging of cystic, partially differentiated nephroblastoma. *Urology* 1990; 36:424–427.

402. Dikengil A, Benson M, Sanders L, Newhouse JH. MRI of multilocular cystic nephroma. *Urol Radiol* 1988;10:95–99.

403. McAlister WH, Siegel MJ, Askin FB, et al. Multilocular renal cysts. *Urol Radiol* 1979;1:89–92.

404. Chan HS, Daneman A, Gribbin M, Martin DJ. Renal cell carcinoma in the first two decades of life. *Pediatr Radiol* 1983;13:324–328.

405. Lack EE, Cassady JR, Sallan SE. Renal cell carcinoma in childhood and adolescence: a clinical and pathological study of 17 cases. *J Urol* 1985;133:822–828.

406. Hartman DS, Davis CJ Jr, Madewell JE, Friedman AC. Primary malignant renal tumors in the second decade of life: Wilms tumor versus renal cell carcinoma. *J Urol* 1982;127:888–891.

407. Schey WL, White H, Conway JJ, Kidd JM. Lymphosarcomas in children. A roentgenologic and clinical evaluation of 60 children. *AJR* 1973;117:59–72.

408. Mukerji PK, Hilfer CL. Burkitt's lymphoma with mandible, intra-abdominal and renal involvement-initial presentation of HIV infection in a 4-year-old child. *Pediatr Radiol* 1993;23:76–77.

409. Capps GW, Das Narla L. Renal lymphoma mimicking clear cell sarcoma in a pediatric patient. *Pediatr Radiol* 1995;25:S87–S89.

410. Sty JR, Starshak RJ, Miller JH. *Pediatric nuclear medicine.* Norwalk: Appleton-Century-Crofts, 1983.

411. Sisler CL, Siegel MJ. Malignant rhabdoid tumor of the kidney: radiologic features. *Radiology* 1989;172:211–212.

412. Cohen MD, Weetman R, Provisor A, et al. Magnetic resonance imaging of neuroblastoma with a 0.15-T magnet. *AJR* 1984;143: 1241–1248.

413. DeBaun MR, Brown M, Kessler L. Screening for Wilms' tumor in children with high-risk congenital syndromes: considerations for an intervention trial. *Med Pediatr Oncol* 1996;27:415–421.

414. Shearer P, Parham DM, Fontanesi J, et al. Bilateral Wilms tumor. Review of outcome, associated abnormalities, and late effects in 36 patients treated at a single institution. *Cancer* 1993;72:1422–1426.

415. D'Angio GJ, Breslow N, Beckwith JB, et al. Treatment of Wilms tumor. Results of the Third National Wilms Tumor study. *Cancer* 1989;64:349–360.

Neuroblastoma and Other Retroperitoneal Tumors

416. Young JL Jr, Ries LG, Silverberg E, et al. Cancer incidence, survival and mortality for children younger than age 15 years. *Cancer* 1986; 58:598–602.

417. Brodeur GM, Castleberry RP. Neuroblastoma. In: Pizzo PA, Poplack DG, eds. *Principles and practice of pediatric oncology.* 3rd ed. Philadelphia: Lippincott-Raven, 1997, 761–797.

418. Graham-Pole J, Salmi T, Anton AH, et al. Tumor and urine catecholamines (CATs) in neurogenic tumors. Correlation with other prognostic factors and survival. *Cancer* 1983;51:834–839.

419. Baker ME, Kirks DR, Korobkin M, et al. The association of neuroblastoma and myoclonic encephalopathy: an imaging approach. *Pediatr Radiol* 1985;15:184–190.

420. Farrelly C, Daneman A, Chan HS, Martin DJ. Occult neuroblastoma presenting with opsomyoclonus: utility of computed tomography. *AJR* 1984;142:807–810.

421. Roberts KB. Cerebellar ataxia and "occult neuroblastoma" without opsoclonus. *Pediatrics* 1975;56:464–465.

422. Altman AJ, Baehner RL. Favorable prognosis for survival in children with coincident opso-myoclonus and neuroblastoma. *Cancer* 1976; 37:846–852.

423. Dehner LP. Classic neuroblastoma: histopathological grading as a prognostic indicator. The Shimada System and its progenitors. *Am J Pediatr Hematol Oncol* 1988;10:143–154.

424. Shimada H, Chatten J, Newton WA Jr, et al. Histopathologic prognostic factors in neuroblastic tumors: definition of subtypes of ganglio-

neuroblastoma and an age-linked classification of neuroblastomas. *J Natl Cancer Inst* 1984;73:405–416.

425. Evans AE, D'Angio GJ, Randolph J. A proposed staging for children with neuroblastoma. Children's Cancer Study Group A. *Cancer* 1971; 27:374–378.

426. Nitschke R, Smith EI, Shochat S, et al. Localized neuroblastoma treated by surgery: a Pediatric Oncology Group Study. *J Clin Oncol* 1988;6:1271–1279.

427. Brodeur GM, Seeger RC, Barrett A, et al. International criteria for diagnosis, staging and response to treatment in patients with neuroblastoma. *J Clin Oncol* 1988;6:1874–1881.

428. Brodeur GM, Pritchard J, Berthold F, et al. Revisions of the international criteria for neuroblastoma diagnosis, staging, and response to treatment. *J Clin Oncol* 1993;11:1466–1477.

429. Forman HP, Leonidas JC, Berdon WE, et al. Congenital neuroblastoma: evaluation with multimodality imaging. *Radiology* 1990;175: 365–368.

430. Kornreich L, Horev G, Kaplinsky C, et al. Neuroblastoma: evaluation with contrast enhanced MR imaging. *Pediatr Radiol* 1991;21: 566–569.

431. Podrasky AE, Stark DD, Hattner RS, et al. Radionuclide bone scanning in neuroblastoma: skeletal metastases and primary tumor localization of 99mTc MDP. *AJR* 1983;141:469–472.

432. Martin-Simmerman P, Cohen MD, Siddiqui A, et al. Calcification and uptake of Tc-99m diphosphonates in neuroblastomas: concise communication. *J Nucl Med* 1984;25:656–660.

433. Shulkin BL, Shapiro B, Hutchinson RJ. Iodine-131-metaiodobenzylguanidine and bone scintigraphy for the detection of neuroblastoma. *J Nucl Med* 1992;33:1735–1740.

434. Parisi MT, Greene MK, Dykes TM, et al. Efficacy of metaiodobenzylguanidine as a scintigraphic agent for the detection of neuroblastoma. *Invest Radiol* 1992;27:768–773.

435. Koch KJ, Cory DA. Simultaneous renal vein thrombosis and bilateral adrenal hemorrhage: MR demonstration. *J Comput Assist Tomogr* 1986;10:681–683.

436. Heij HA, Taets van Amerongen AHM, Ekkelkamp S, Vos A. Diagnosis and management of neonatal adrenal hemorrhage. *Pediatr Radiol* 1989;19:391–394.

437. Wu C-C. Sonographic spectrum of neonatal adrenal hemorrhage: report of a case simulating solid tumor. *J Clin Ultrasound* 1989;17: 45–49.

438. Willemse APP, Coopes MJ, Feldberg MAM, et al. Magnetic resonance appearance of adrenal hemorrhage in a neonate. *Pediatr Radiol* 1989;19:210–211.

439. Leonidas JC, Brill PW, Bhan I, Smith TH. Cystic retroperitoneal lymphangioma in infants and children. *Radiology* 1978;127:203–208.

440. Hachitanda Y, Hata J. Stage IVS neuroblastoma: a clinical, histological, and biological analysis of 45 cases. *Hum Pathol* 1996;27: 1135–1138.

441. Paul SR, Tarbell NJ, Korf B, et al. Stage IV neuroblastoma in infants. Long-term survival. *Cancer* 1991;67:1493–1497.

442. Velchik MG, Alavi A, Kressel HY, Engelman K. Localization of pheochromocytoma: MIGB, CT, and MRI correlation. *J Nucl Med* 1989;30:328–336.

Gonadal Tumors

443. Ries LA, Hankey BF, Miller BA, et al, eds. *Cancer statistics review 1973–1988.* Bethesda: NIH Publication No. 91-2789, 1991.

444. Castleberry RP, Cushing B, Perlman E, Hawkins EP. Germ cell tumors. In: Pizzo PA, Poplack DG, eds. *Principles and practice of pediatric oncology.* 3rd ed. Philadelphia: Lippincott-Raven, 1997, 921–945.

445. Castleberry RP, Kelly DR, Joseph DB, Cain WS. Gonadal and extragonadal germ cell tumors. In: Fernbach DJ, Vietti TJ, eds. *Clinical pediatric oncology.* 4th ed. St. Louis: Mosby–Year Book, 1991, 577–594.

446. Askin FB, Land VJ, Sullivan MP, et al. Occult testicular leukemia: testicular biopsy at three years continuous complete remission of childhood leukemia: a Southwest Oncology Group Study. *Cancer* 1981;47:470–475.

447. Crist WM, Pullen DJ, Rivera DK. Acute lymphoid leukemia. In: Fernbach DJ, Vietti TJ, eds. *Clinical pediatric oncology.* 4th ed. St. Louis: Mosby–Year Book, 1991, 305–335.

448. Casola G, Scheible W, Leopold GR. Neuroblastoma metastatic to the testis: ultrasonographic screening as an aid to clinical staging. *Radiology* 1984;151:475–476.

449. Exelby PR. Testicular cancer in children. *Cancer* 1980;45: 1803–1809.

450. Luker GD, Siegel MJ. Pediatric testicular tumors: evaluation with gray-scale and color Doppler US. *Radiology* 1994;191:561–564.

451. Middleton WD, Thorne DA, Melson GL. Color Doppler ultrasound of the normal testis. *AJR* 1989;152:293–297.

452. Zachariou Z, Roth H, Boos R, et al. Three years' experience with large ovarian cysts diagnosed in utero. *J Pediatr Surg* 1989;24:478–482.

453. Brandt ML, Luks FI, Filiatrault D, et al. Surgical indications in antenatally diagnosed ovarian cysts. *J Pediatr Surg* 1991;26:276–281.

454. Widdowson DJ, Pilling DW, Cook RCM. Neonatal ovarian cysts: therapeutic dilemma. *Arch J Dis Child* 1988;63:737–742.

455. Hoffer FA, Kozakewich H, Colodny A, Goldstein DP. Peritoneal inclusion cysts: ovarian fluid in peritoneal adhesions. *Radiology* 1988; 169:189–191.

456. Hann LE, Hall DA, McArdle CR, Siebel M. Polycystic ovarian disease: sonographic spectrum. *Radiology* 1984;150:531–534.

457. Futterweit W, Yeh H-C, Thornton JC. Lack of correlation of ultrasonographically determined ovarian size with age, ponderal index, and hormonal factors in 45 patients with polycystic ovarian disease. *Int J Fertil* 1987;32:456–459.

458. Ardaens Y, Robert Y, Lemaitre L, et al. Polycystic ovarian disease: contribution of vaginal endosonography and reassessment of ultrasonic diagnosis. *Fertil Steril* 1991;55:1062–1068.

459. Worthington-Kirsch RL, Raptopoulos V, Cohen IT. Sequential bilateral torsion of normal ovaries in a child. *J Ultrasound Med* 1986;5: 663–664.

460. Graif M, Itzchak Y. Sonographic evaluation of ovarian torsion in childhood and adolescence. *AJR* 1988;150:647–649.

461. Helvie MA, Silver TM. Ovarian torsion: sonographic evaluation. *J Clin Ultrasound* 1989;17:327–332.

462. Currarino G, Rutledge JC. Ovarian torsion and amputation resulting in partially calcified, pedunculated cystic mass. *Pediatr Radiol* 1989; 19:395–399.

463. Nixon GW, Condon VR. Amputed ovary: a cause of migratory abdominal calcification. *AJR* 1977;128:1053–1055.

Rhabdomyosarcoma

464. Agamanolis DP, Dasu S, Krill CE Jr. Tumors of skeletal muscle. *Hum Pathol* 1986;17:778–795.

465. Feldman BA. Rhabdomyosarcoma of the head and neck. *Laryngoscope* 1982;92:424–440.

466. Wexler LH, Helman LF. Rhabdomyosarcoma and the undifferentiated sarcomas. In: Pizzo PA, Poplack DG, eds. *Principles and practice of pediatric oncology*. 3rd ed. Philadelphia: Lippincott-Raven, 1997, 799–829.

467. Hornback NG, Shidnia H. Rhabdomyosarcoma in the pediatric age group. *AJR* 1976;126:542–549.

468. Maurer HM, Beltangady M, Gehan EA, et al. The Intergroup Rhabdomyosarcoma Study—I. A final report. *Cancer* 1988;61:209–220.

469. Bahnson RR, Zaontz MR, Maizels M, et al. Ultrasonography and diagnosis of pediatric genitourinary rhabdomyosarcoma. *Urology* 1989;33:64–68.

470. Tannous WN, Azouz EM, Homsy YL, et al. CT and ultrasound imaging of pelvic rhabdomyosarcoma in children. A review of 56 patients. *Pediatr Radiol* 1989;19:530–534.

471. Bartolozzi C, Selli C, Olmastroni M, et al. Rhabdomyosarcoma of the prostate: MR findings. *AJR* 1988;150:1333–1334.

Trauma

472. Young LW, Wood BP, Linke CA. Renal injury from blunt trauma in childhood. Radiological evaluation and review. *Ann Radiol* 1975;18: 359–376.

473. Herschorn S, Radomski SB, Shoskes DA, et al. Evaluation and treatment of blunt renal trauma. *J Urol* 1991;146:274–276.

474. Bretan PN Jr, McAninch JW, Federle MP, Jeffrey RB Jr. Computerized tomographic staging of renal trauma: 85 consecutive cases. *J Urol* 1986;136:561–565.

475. Yale-Loehr AJ, Kramer SS, Quinlan DM, et al. CT of severe renal trauma in children: evaluation and course of healing with conservative therapy. *AJR* 1989;152:109–113.

476. Macpherson RI, Decter A. Pediatric renal trauma. *J Can Assoc Radiol* 1971;22:10–21.

477. Abdalati H, Bulas DI, Sivit CJ, et al. Blunt renal trauma in children: healing of renal injuries and recommendations for imaging follow-up. *Pediatr Radiol* 1994;24:573–576.

478. Taylor GA, Guion CJ, Potter BM, Eichelberger MR. CT of blunt abdominal trauma in children. *AJR* 1989;153:555–559.

479. Kaufman RA, Towbin R, Babcock DS, et al. Upper abdominal trauma in children: imaging evaluation. *AJR* 1984;142:449–460.

480. Kuhn JP, Berger PE. Computed tomography in the evaluation of blunt abdominal trauma in children. *Radiol Clin North Am* 1981;19: 503–513.

481. Pollack HM, Wein AJ. Imaging of renal trauma. *Radiology* 1989;172: 297–308.

482. Moore EE, Shackford SS, Pachter HL, et al. Organ injury scaling: spleen, liver and kidney. *J Trauma* 1989;29:1664–1666.

483. Smith SD, Gardner MJ, Rowe MI. Renal artery occlusion in pediatric blunt abdominal trauma-decreasing the delay from injury to treatment. *J Trauma* 1993;35:861–864.

484. Reda EF, Lebowitz RL. Traumatic ureteropelvic disruption in the child. *Pediatr Radiol* 1986;16:164–166.

485. Seiler RK, Filmer RB, Reitelman C. Traumatic disruption of the ureteropelvic junction managed by ileal interposition. *J Urol* 1991;146: 392–395.

486. Howerton RA, Norwood SN. Proximal ureteral avulsion from blunt abdominal trauma. *Milit Med* 1991;156:311–313.

487. Onuora VC, Patil MG, al-Jasser AN. Missed urological injuries in children with polytrauma. *Injury* 1993;24:619–621.

488. Boone TB, Gilling PJ, Husmann DA. Ureteropelvic junction disruption following blunt abdominal trauma. *J Urol* 1993;150:33–36.

489. Hochberg E, Stone NN. Bladder rupture associated with pelvic fracture due to blunt trauma. *Urology* 1993;41:531–533.

490. Baskin LS, McAninch JW. Childhood urethral injuries: perspectives on outcome and treatment. *Br J Urol* 1993;72:241–246.

Miscellaneous Abnormalities

491. Rosenberg ER, Trought WS, Kirks DR, et al. Ultrasonic diagnosis of renal vein thrombosis in neonates. *AJR* 1980;134:35–38.

492. Rosenfield AT, Zeman RK, Cronan JJ, Taylor KJW. Ultrasound in experimental and clinical renal vein thrombosis. *Radiology* 1980;137: 735–741.

493. Dangman BC, Lebowitz RL. Urinary tract calculi that form on surgical staples: a characteristic radiologic appearance. *AJR* 1991;157: 115–117.

494. Lebowitz RL, Vargas B. Stones in the urinary bladder in children and young adults. *AJR* 1987;148:491–495.

495. Fine RN, Tejani A. Renal transplantation in children. *Nephron* 1987; 47:81–86.

496. Reinberg Y, Gonzalez R, Fryd D, et al. The outcome of renal transplantation in children with posterior urethral valves. *J Urol* 1988;140: 1491–1493.

497. Taylor KJW, Marks WH. Use of Doppler imaging for evaluation of dysfunction in renal allografts. *AJR* 1990;155:536–537.

498. Slovis TL, Babcock DS, Hricak J, et al. Renal transplant rejection: sonographic evaluation in children. *Radiology* 1984;153:659–665.

499. Stringer DA, O'Halpin D, Daneman A, et al. Duplex Doppler sonography for renal artery stenosis in the post-transplant pediatric patient. *Pediatr Radiol* 1989;19:187–192.

500. Genkins SM, Sanfilippo FP, Carroll BA. Duplex Doppler sonography of renal transplants: lack of sensitivity and specificity in establishing pathologic diagnosis. *AJR* 1989;152:535–539.

501. Kelcz F, Pozniak MA, Pirsch JD, Oberly TD. Pyramidal appearance and resistive index: insensitive and nonspecific sonographic indicators of renal transplant rejection. *AJR* 1990;155:531–535.

502. Rifkin MD, Needleman L, Pasto ME, et al. Evaluation of renal transplant rejection by duplex Doppler examination: value of the resistive index. *AJR* 1987;148:759–762.

503. Don S, Kopecky KK, Filo RS, et al. Duplex Doppler US of renal allografts: causes of elevated resistive index. *Radiology* 1989;171: 709–712.

504. Frauchiger B, Bock A, Eichlisberger R, et al. The value of different resistance parameters in distinguishing biopsy-proved dysfunction of renal allografts. *Nephrol Dial Transplant* 1995;10:527–532.

505. Drake DG, Day DL, Letourneau JG, et al. Doppler evaluation of renal transplants in children: a prospective analysis with histopathologic correlation. *AJR* 1990;154:785–787.

506. Kaveggia LP, Perrella RR, Grant EG, et al. Duplex Doppler sonography in renal allografts: the significance of reversed flow in diastole. *AJR* 1990;155:295–298.

507. Preston DF, Luke RG. Radionuclide evaluation of renal transplants. *J Nucl Med* 1979;20:1095–1097.

508. Helenon O, Attlan E, Legendre C, et al. Gd-DOTA-enhanced MR imaging and color Doppler US of renal allograft necrosis. *Radio-Graphics* 1992;12:21–33.

509. Hricak H, Terrier F, Marotti M, et al. Posttransplant renal rejection: comparison of quantitative scintigraphy, US and MR imaging. *Radiology* 1987;162:685–688.

510. Kearney GP, Lebowitz RL, Retik AB. Obstructing polyps of the posterior urethra in boys: embryology and management. *J Urol* 1979;122:802–804.

511. Foster RS, Garrett RA. Congenital posterior urethral polyps. *J Urol* 1986;136:670–672.

512. Selzer I, Nelson HM. Benign papilloma (polypoid tumor) of the cervix uteri in children: report of 2 cases. *Am J Obstet Gynecol* 1962;84:165–169.

513. Huffman JW. Mesonephric remnants in the cervix. *Am J Obstet Gynecol* 1948;56:23–39.

514. Diard F, Eklof O, Lebowitz R, Maurseth K. Urethral obstruction in boys caused by prolapse of simple ureterocele. *Pediatr Radiol* 1981;11:139–142.

515. Gleason PE, Kramer SA. Genitourinary polyps in children. *Urology* 1994;44:106–109.

516. Zerin JM, DiPietro MA, Grignon A, Shea D. Testicular infarction in the newborn: ultrasound findings. *Pediatr Radiol* 1990;20:329–330.

517. Kim CK, Zuckier LS, Alavi A. The role of nuclear medicine in the evaluation of the male genital tract. *Semin Roentgenol* 1993;28:31–42.

518. Mendel JB, Taylor GA, Treves S, et al. Testicular torsion in children: scintigraphic assessment. *Pediatr Radiol* 1985;15:110–115.

519. Paltiel HJ, Rupich RC, Babcock DS. Maturational changes in arterial impedance of the normal testis in boys: Doppler sonographic study. *AJR* 1994;163:1189–1193.

520. Atkinson GO Jr, Patrick LE, Ball TI Jr, et al. The normal and abnormal scrotum in children: evaluation with color Doppler sonography. *AJR* 1992;158:613–617.

521. Yazbeck S, Patriquin HB. Accuracy of Doppler sonography in the evaluation of acute conditions of the scrotum in children. *J Pediatr Surg* 1994;29:1270–1272.

522. Bird K, Rosenfield AT, Taylor KJ. Ultrasonography in testicular torsion. *Radiology* 1983;147:527–534.

523. Burks DD, Markey BJ, Burkhard TK, et al. Suspected testicular torsion and ischemia: evaluation with color Doppler sonography. *Radiology* 1990;175:815–821.

524. Bickerstaff KI, Sethia K, Murie JA. Doppler ultrasonography in the diagnosis of acute scrotal pain. *Br J Surg* 1988;75:238–239.

525. Melekos MD, Asbach HW, Markou SA. Etiology of acute scrotum in 100 boys with regard to age distribution. *J Urol* 1988;139:1023–1025.

526. Gislason T, Noronha RF, Gregory JG. Acute epididymitis in boys: a 5-year retrospective study. *J Urol* 1980;124:533–534.

527. Cohen HL, Shapiro MA, Haller JO, Glassberg K. Torsion of the testicular appendage. Sonographic diagnosis. *J Ultrasound Med* 1992;11:81–83.

528. Hesser U, Rosenborg M, Gierup J, et al. Gray-scale sonography in torsion of the testicular appendages. *Pediatr Radiol* 1993;23:529–532.

529. Wakely CPG. Cysts of the epididymis, the so-called spermatocele. *Br J Surg* 1943;31:165–171.

530. Rifkin MD, Kurtz AB, Goldberg BB. Epididymis examined by ultrasound. Correlation with pathology. *Radiology* 1984;151:187–190.

531. Sayfan J, Soffer Y, Manor H, et al. Varicocele in youth. A therapeutic dilemma. *Ann Surg* 1988;207:223–227.

532. Finkelstein MS, Rosenberg HK, Snyder HM III, Duckett JW. Ultrasound evaluation of scrotum in pediatrics. *Urology* 1986;27:1–9.

533. Reyes BL, Trerotola SO, Venbrux AC, et al. Percutaneous embolotherapy of adolescent varicocele: results and long-term follow-up. *JVIR* 1994;5:131–134.

534. Janzen DL, Mathieson JR, March JI, et al. Testicular microlithiasis: sonographic and clinical features. *AJR* 1992;158:1057–1060.

535. Backus ML, Mack LA, Middleton WD, et al. Testicular microlithiasis: imaging appearances and pathologic correlation. *Radiology* 1994;192:781–785.

536. Doherty FJ, Mullins TL, Sant GR, et al. Testicular microlithiasis. A unique sonographic appearance. *J Ultrasound Med* 1987;6:389–392.

537. Salardi S, Orsini LF, Cacciari E, et al. Pelvic ultrasonography in girls with precocious puberty, congenital adrenal hyperplasia, obesity, or hirsutism. *J Pediatr* 1988;112:880–887.

538. Shawker TH, Comite F, Rieth KG, et al. Ultrasound evaluation of female isosexual precocious puberty. *J Ultrasound Med* 1984;3:309–316.

539. King LR, Siegel MJ, Solomon AL. Usefulness of ovarian volume and cysts in female isosexual precocious puberty. *J Ultrasound Med* 1993;12:577–581.

540. Fakhry J, Khoury A, Kotval PS, Noto RA. Sonography of autonomous follicular ovarian cysts in precocious pseudopuberty. *J Ultrasound Med* 1988;7:597–603.

541. Hall DA, Crowley WF, Wierman ME, et al. Sonographic monitoring of LHRH analogue therapy in idiopathic precocious puberty in young girls. *J Clin Ultrasound* 1986;14:331–338.

542. Vanzulli A, DelMaschio A, Paesano P, et al. Testicular masses in association with adrenogenital syndrome: US findings. *Radiology* 1992;183:425–429.

543. Johnston JH, Scholtmeijer RJ. *Problems in paediatric urology.* Amsterdam: Excerpta Medica, 1972, 57–58.

APPENDIX 1
Preparation of Pediatric Patients for Radiographic Procedures

1. **Genitourinary tract.** If both genitourinary and gastrointestinal radiographic examinations are to be performed on the same day, genitourinary studies or sonography should be performed first. Explanation sheets written in layman's terms are sent to the parents before the examination.

   A. **Excretory urogram (intravenous urogram).** No solids the morning of the examination or 4 hours before the examination. Fluids should be given freely. For infants, skip the last feeding before the examination. Bring bottle to feed afterwards.

   B. **Voiding cystourethrogram (VCUG).** No preparation is necessary.

   C. **Retrograde urethrogram.** No preparation is necessary.

   D. **Vaginogram.** No preparation is necessary.

   E. **Genitogram in intersex situations.** No preparation is necessary.

2. **Gastrointestinal tract.** Genitourinary examinations, sonographic, and nuclear scintigraphic examinations should precede gastrointestinal studies if more than one examination is to be performed. Explanation sheets written in layman's terms are sent to the parents before the examination.

   A. **Barium swallow, upper gastrointestinal series, small bowel follow through.**

   Newborns—6 months: Nothing by mouth (NPO) 2–3 hours before the examination.

   6 months—3 years: Nothing by mouth (NPO) 3–4 hours before the examination.

   Over 3 years: Nothing by mouth (NPO) 6 hours before the examination.

   B. **Double-contrast UGI.** NPO 8 hours before the examination.

   C. **Barium enema (single contrast).** No preparation is necessary.

   D. **Barium enema (air contrast).** Air contrast enemas are indicated rarely in young children and almost never in infants. Because of the vigorous preparation necessary, each case should be discussed with the radiologist before the enema is scheduled. The preparation protocols outlined below should be considered to be guidelines rather than absolute prescriptions. No preparation should be given to children when severe inflammatory bowel or acute abdominal disease is suspected. Doses must be adjusted for age and size.

   Neonate: Liquid diet for 24 hours before the examination, with clear liquids for the last 12 hours.

   1–3 years: Liquid diet for 24 hours before the examination, with clear liquids for the last 12 hours. Castor oil 1–2 teaspoons (depending on age) or magnesium citrate 1.5 oz on the day before the examination. A repeat dose may be necessary.

   Over 3 years: Low residue diet for 3 days before the examination, with clear liquids for the last 24 hours. Day before exam: castor oil 2 teaspoons (young children) to 2 tablespoons (older children and young adults) *or* magnesium citrate 1.5–7 oz, depending on age and size or 1–2 Bisacodyl tablets (5 mg) in children old enough to swallow tablets. Fleet enema the morning of examination.

3. **Ultrasonography.** Sedation is seldom needed for any type of sonographic examination.

   A. **Abdomen.** NPO 4 hours before the examination; for infants, NPO 1–2 hours.

   B. **Pelvis.** Older patients should drink 24–32 oz of fluids 2 hours before the examination and should not urinate until after the examination.

4. **Computed tomography.** NPO 4 hours before the examination except for oral contrast (see Appendix 7). Sedation may be required (see Appendix 6).

5. **Magnetic resonance imaging.** NPO 4 hours before the examination. Sedation may be required (see Appendix 6).

1171

APPENDIX 2
Pediatric Radiographic Projections

I. General information

  A. If views are not specified on the requisition, follow this list.

  B. In trauma, manipulation of the part to be examined should be minimized.

  C. Shield gonads in all cases, except when the shield covers the specific part to be examined.

  D. In any questionable case, check with the radiologist.

II. Routine projections

  A. Skull and face. Examinations below marked with a superscript *a* may be more appropriately performed by CT; check with radiologist.

    1. Routine skull: Anteroposterior (AP), Towne, lateral (of affected side if convenient).

    2. Mastoids[a]: Towne; both laterals with 25–30° caudal angulation; Stenvers, or Arcelin if patient is over 2 years and cooperative.

    3. Petrous bones[a]: Submentovertex; AP to show petrous base through orbits; Stenvers, or Arcelin if patient is over 2 years and cooperative.

    4. Sinuses: Caldwell, Waters, lateral (all upright if possible).

    5. Facial bones: Waters (upright when possible), Caldwell, lateral; if zygoma is affected, Towne of facial area.

    6. Nasal bones: Waters; lateral on detail film.

    7. Mandible: AP; lateral oblique of each side; Towne and Panorex optional.

    8. Temporomandibular joints: Towne; laterals of each side (30° caudal angulation) with mouth open and closed.

    9. Orbits[a]: PA, Waters (upright when possible), lateral.

    10. Optic foramina[a]: PA oblique of each foramen.

  B. Neck and upper airway.

    1. Adenoids: Lateral of nasopharynx and neck during inspiration through nose with mouth closed.

    2. Lateral airway: Lateral on inspiration, AP on inspiration; (croup and epiglottitis: these patients should remain sitting upright).

  C. Spine: Oblique and flexion-extension views only if requested.

    1. Cervical: AP and lateral; AP open mouth if over 5 years.

    2. Thoracic: AP and lateral; use breathing lateral over age 6.

    3. Lumbar: AP and lateral.

    4. Sacrum and coccyx: Angled AP (straight AP for young children) and lateral.

    5. Scoliosis films: Erect 6-foot PA only; lateral for kyphosis; include entire spine from external auditory meatus to anterior superior iliac crest; bending films only if requested.

  D. Extremities. In trauma, comparison views are obtained when needed but only after consultation with radiologist.

Comparison views are frequently obtained when joint disease is suspected.

    1. Finger, hand, foot, ankle: AP or PA, oblique, and lateral. If examination of the foot is for congenital or positional abnormalities, obtain both AP and lateral films with weight-bearing or forced dorsiflexion. Spread fingers apart with different degrees of flexion at the metacarpophalangeal joints on lateral view of hand.

    2. Humerus, elbow, forearm, wrist, femur, knee, tibia-fibula: AP and lateral.

    3. Scapula: AP and lateral.

    4. Shoulder: AP in neutral rotation, transthoracic lateral in major trauma, Y-view or axillary view for dislocation; external and internal rotation AP views optional.

    5. Clavicle: AP and AP with 15° cranial angulation.

    6. Pelvis: AP; obliques as requested.

    7. Hips: AP neutral and AP frog-leg lateral. Gonad shielding on all films except:

      a) First exam on girls <1 year old: shield only frog-leg lateral

      b) Patients with diagnosis of metastases, osteomyelitis, pelvic trauma, or females with reconstruction of acetabulum.

    8. Calcaneus: Lateral, Harris (tangential).

    9. Bone age.

      a) Below 1 year: Left hemiskeleton (AP shoulder to finger tips, AP mid-thigh to toe tips).

      b) Above 1 year: PA left hand and wrist.

    10. Skeletal survey or metastatic series: Lateral skull to include cervical spine, AP long bones including hands and feet, lateral thoracic and lumbar spine, AP abdomen to include pelvis and lumbar spine (bone technique), AP chest (bone technique).

    11. Skeletal survey for child abuse: AP and lateral skull; AP humeri, radii-ulnae, femurs, tibiae-fibulae; AP feet; PA hands; AP and lateral lumbar spine; AP abdomen; AP pelvis (bone technique); AP and lateral chest (bone technique); additional views if needed after radiologist reviews films.

    12. Long bones: AP both upper extremities (shoulder to wrist), AP both lower extremities (hips to ankles).

    13. Bow-legs: AP erect of lower extremities; lateral views (recumbent).

  E. Chest.

    1. Routine chest:

      a) Newborn and infant: use supine position until baby sits with minimal support (about 1 year); AP recumbent, lateral cross–table.

      b) All other age groups: PA upright, lateral upright.

    2. Chest for foreign body: PA or AP during inspiration

and expiration, lateral during inspiration; check with radiologist for possible fluoroscopy or decubitus films.

3. **Chest and abdomen for swallowed foreign body:** AP chest and abdomen, lateral upper airway to include entire nasopharynx.

4. **Ribs:** AP and oblique of involved side.

5. **Sternum:** RAO and lateral.

F. **Abdomen.**

1. **Abdomen, single view:** AP supine, diaphragm to pubic bones.

2. **Abdomen, two views:** AP supine; upright or left lateral decubitus or cross–table lateral.

3. **Abdomen, three views:** AP supine, PA prone, AP erect or left lateral decubitus.

APPENDIX 3

Typical Radiographic Exposures and Doses

SID = focal spot to image receptor distance (cm)
PID = patient exit plane to image receptor distance (cm)
Grd Rat = grid ratio
Pat Thick = patient thickness (cm)
Free A Expos = free in air exposure without scatter (mR)
M/F = male/female; no gonadal shielding used

Patient age or thickness	SID (cm)	PID (cm)	Grd Rat	kVp	mAs	Pat thick (cm)	Free A expos. (mR) ±10%	Doses (mrad) Skin ±15%	Doses (mrad) Midline ±30%	Doses (mrad) M/F gonads[a] ±30%
PA CHEST (400 speed system)										
Adult	183	5	8	130	1.0	24	7.0	7.3	2.2	0.000/0.035
10–15 yr	183	5	—	85	2.4	19	7.5	7.5	2.3	NA
6–10 yr	183	5	—	80	2.3	17	6.2	6.1	2.2	NA
3–6 yr	183	2	—	75	2.1	14	4.9	4.8	2.1	0.000/0.034
1–3 yr	183	2	—	70	2.1	13	4.2	4.0	1.8	0.000/0.008
3–12 mo	107	1	—	65	0.8	12	4.8	4.6	2.2	NA
Newborn	107	1	—	60	0.8	10	3.9	3.6	2.1	0.012/0.047
LATERAL CHEST (400 speed system)										
Adult	183	5	8	130	3.0	34	23	24	3.6	0.000/0.060
10–15 yr	183	5	—	100	2.4	28	11	11	2.0	NA
6–10 yr	183	5	—	95	2.3	26	9.6	9.8	2.0	NA
3–6 yr	183	2	—	90	2.1	19	7.3	7.4	2.4	0.000/0.073
1–3 yr	183	2	—	85	2.1	16	6.3	6.3	2.5	0.000/0.082
3–12 mo	107	1	—	70	0.8	13	5.7	5.5	2.5	NA
Newborn	107	1	—	64	0.8	10	4.5	4.3	2.5	0.027/0.023
3 FOOT SPINE PA (1100 speed system)										
25–30 cm	183	4	10	85	30	27	103	103	17	1.9/31
20–25 cm	183	4	10	80	24	23	70	69	15	NA
17–20 cm	183	4	10	75	20	18	49	48	15	NA
13–17 cm	183	4	10	70	16	15	33	32	12	4.3/12
3 FOOT SPINE LAT (1100 speed system)										
35–40 cm	183	4	10	95	60	32	272	277	35	2.0/30
30–35 cm	183	4	10	90	48	29	189	191	29	NA
27–30 cm	183	4	10	85	40	25	135	135	26	NA
23–27 cm	183	4	10	80	32	22	93	92	22	15/26
AP ABDOMEN (400 speed system)										
Adult	107	8	8	85	5.0	21	63	63	15	1.6/18
10–15 yr	107	8	8	80	5.0	18	52	51	15	NA
6–10 yr	107	8	8	75	3.8	16	33	32	11	NA
3–6 yr	107	8	8	75	3.0	14	25	24	10	3.1/8.9
1–3 yr	107	8	8	70	3.0	13	21	20	8.6	2.2/7.4
3–12 mo	107	8	8	65	2.2	12	15	14	6.4	NA
Newborn	107	8	8	65	1.5	10	8.6	8.2	4.5	1.2/4.8
AP PELVIS & HIPS (400 speed system)										
Adult	107	8	8	85	4.0	22	51	51	11	14/5.1
10–15 yr	107	8	8	80	4.0	19	43	43	11	NA
6–10 yr	107	8	8	80	2.0	17	20	20	6.4	NA
3–6 yr	107	8	8	70	1.9	15	14	13	4.7	14/5.2
1–3 yr	107	8	8	70	1.5	14	12	12	4.5	12/4.4
3–12 mo	107	8	8	70	1.5	13	11	11	4.5	NA
Newborn	107	8	8	65	1.3	11	7.6	7.2	3.6	7.6/4.3

SID = focal spot to image receptor distance (cm)
PID = patient exit plane to image receptor distance (cm)
Grd Rat = grid ratio
Pat Thick = patient thickness (cm)
Free A Expos = free in air exposure without scatter (mR)
M/F = male/female; no gonadal shielding used

Patient age or thickness	SID (cm)	PID (cm)	Grd Rat	kVp	mAs	Pat thick (cm)	Free A expos. (mR) ±10%	Doses (mrad)		
								Skin ±15%	Midline ±30%	M/F gonads[a] ±30%
AP LUMBAR SPINE (400 speed system)										
Adult	107	8	8	85	6.0	21	75	75	18	0.30/9.0
10–15 yr	107	8	8	80	5.2	18	54	53	16	NA
6–10 yr	107	8	8	80	3.8	16	38	38	13	NA
3–6 yr	107	8	8	75	3.0	14	25	24	9.9	2.8/6.3
1–3 yr	107	8	8	70	2.2	13	16	15	6.5	1.7/5.1
3–12 mo	107	8	8	70	2.0	12	14	13	6.2	NA
Newborn	107	8	8	70	1.5	10	10	10	5.5	1.1/4.3
LUMBAR SPINE LAT (400 speed system)										
Adult	107	8	8	95	12.0	28	222	226	33	0.29/15
10–15 yr	107	8	8	90	10.0	24	150	152	29	NA
6–10 yr	107	8	8	85	7.6	22	98	98	21	NA
3–6 yr	107	8	8	85	6.0	18	70	70	21	9.1/16
1–3 yr	107	8	8	80	3.2	16	32	32	11	6.4/14
3–12 mo	107	8	8	75	3.0	13	24	23	10	NA
Newborn	107	8	8	75	1.5	10	11	11	6.3	3.3/4.7
AP or LAT ELBOW (100 speed system)										
Adult	107	1	—	76	1.8	9	14	14	8.8	0.000/0.000
10–15 yr	107	1	—	74	1.3	8	9.2	8.9	6.2	NA
6–10 yr	107	1	—	72	1.1	7	7.2	6.9	5.2	NA
3–6 yr	107	1	—	68	0.9	6	5.2	5.0	4.1	0.000/0.000
1–3 yr	107	1	—	66	0.9	4	4.7	4.5	3.9	0.000/0.000
3–12 mo	107	1	—	64	0.9	3	4.3	4.1	3.7	NA
Newborn	107	1	—	62	0.9	2	3.9	3.7	3.4	0.000/0.000
AP HAND (100 speed system)										
Adult	107	1	—	68	1.0	4.5	5.6	5.4	3.6	0.000/0.000
10–15 yr	107	1	—	68	0.8	3.5	4.4	4.2	3.0	NA
6–10 yr	107	1	—	66	0.7	2.5	3.5	3.3	2.6	NA
3–6 yr	107	1	—	64	0.7	2.5	3.3	3.1	2.6	0.000/0.000
1–3 yr	107	1	—	62	0.7	2.0	3.1	2.9	2.6	0.000/0.000
3–12 mo	107	1	—	60	0.7	1.5	2.8	2.6	2.5	NA
Newborn	107	1	—	58	0.6	1.0	2.2	2.0	1.9	0.000/0.000
AP or LAT KNEE (100 speed system)										
Adult	107	1	—	75	2.5	12	20	19	9.5	NA
10–15 yr	107	1	—	75	2.1	11	16	16	8.4	NA
6–10 yr	107	1	—	72	1.5	9	10	10	6.1	NA
3–6 yr	107	1	—	72	0.7	7	4.6	4.4	3.3	NA
1–3 yr	107	1	—	70	0.7	6	4.3	4.0	3.2	NA
3–12 mo	107	1	—	66	0.7	4	3.6	3.4	3.0	NA
Newborn	107	1	—	62	0.7	3	3.1	2.9	2.7	NA
AP FOOT (100 speed system)										
Adult	107	1	—	72	1.4	8	9.4	9.0	6.2	NA
10–15 yr	107	1	—	72	0.8	7	5.3	5.1	3.8	NA
6–10 yr	107	1	—	70	0.8	6	4.8	4.6	3.8	NA
3–6 yr	107	1	—	68	0.8	5	4.5	4.3	3.7	NA
1–3 yr	107	1	—	66	0.8	4	4.2	4.0	3.5	NA
3–12 mo	107	1	—	64	0.6	3	2.9	2.8	2.5	NA
Newborn	107	1	—	62	0.6	2	2.6	2.4	2.3	NA
AP SKULL (400 speed system)										
Adult	107	8	8	75	11.0	20	105	102	24	0.000/0.000
10–15 yr	107	8	8	75	9.0	18	83	81	23	NA
6–10 yr	107	8	8	75	7.4	16	65	63	21	NA
3–6 yr	107	8	8	75	5.6	15	48	47	17	0.000/0.000
1–3 yr	107	8	8	70	3.7	14	27	26	10	0.000/0.000
3–12 mo	107	8	8	70	2.9	13	21	20	8.6	NA
Newborn	107	8	8	70	2.3	12	16	15	7.1	0.000/0.000

SID = focal spot to image receptor distance (cm)
PID = patient exit plane to image receptor distance (cm)
Grd Rat = grid ratio
Pat Thick = patient thickness (cm)
Free A Expos = free in air exposure without scatter (mR)
M/F = male/female; no gonadal shielding used

Patient age or thickness	SID (cm)	PID (cm)	Grd Rat	kVp	mAs	Pat thick (cm)	Free A expos. (mR) ±10%	Doses (mrad)		
								Skin ±15%	Midline ±30%	M/F gonads[a] ±30%
AXIAL (Towne) SKULL (400 speed system)										
Adult	107	8	8	85	11.0	22	141	141	31	0.000/0.000
10–15 yr	107	8	8	85	9.0	21	111	111	26	NA
6–10 yr	107	8	8	85	7.4	18	86	86	26	NA
3–6 yr	107	8	8	85	5.6	17	63	63	21	0.000/0.000
1–3 yr	107	8	8	80	3.7	16	37	37	13	0.000/0.000
3–12 mo	107	8	8	80	2.9	15	28	28	11	NA
Newborn	107	8	8	80	2.3	14	22	22	9.2	0.000/0.000
LATERAL SKULL (400 speed system)										
Adult	107	8	8	70	11.0	18	87	84	22	0.000/0.000
10–15 yr	107	8	8	70	9.0	16	69	66	21	NA
6–10 yr	107	8	8	70	7.4	15	55	53	19	NA
3–6 yr	107	8	8	70	5.6	14	41	39	15	0.000/0.000
1–3 yr	107	8	8	65	3.7	12	22	20	9.4	0.000/0.000
3–12 mo	107	8	8	65	2.9	11	17	16	8.1	NA
Newborn	107	8	8	65	2.3	10	13	12	6.9	0.000/0.000
PA SINUSES (400 speed system)										
Adult	115	4	8	85	6.9	22	84	84	19	0.000/0.000
10–15 yr	115	4	8	85	6.6	21	78	78	19	NA
6–10 yr	115	4	8	80	6.2	18	61	60	19	NA
3–6 yr	115	4	8	80	5.9	17	57	56	19	0.000/0.000
1–3 yr	115	4	8	75	5.5	16	46	45	15	0.000/0.000
3–12 mo	115	4	8	70	3.7	15	26	25	9.0	NA
WATERS PROJECTION SINUSES (400 speed system)										
Adult	115	4	8	90	6.9	22	93	94	22	0.000/0.000
10–15 yr	115	4	8	90	6.6	21	86	87	22	NA
6–10 yr	115	4	8	85	6.2	18	69	69	22	NA
3–6 yr	115	4	8	85	5.9	17	64	64	22	0.000/0.000
1–3 yr	115	4	8	80	5.5	16	52	51	18	0.000/0.000
3–12 mo	115	4	8	75	3.7	15	30	29	11	NA
LATERAL SINUSES (400 speed system)										
Adult	115	4	8	70	8.0	18	52	50	14	0.000/0.000
10–15 yr	115	4	8	70	7.6	16	48	46	15	NA
6–10 yr	115	4	8	70	7.2	15	44	42	15	NA
3–6 yr	115	4	8	70	6.8	14	41	39	16	0.000/0.000
1–3 yr	115	4	8	60	6.4	12	27	25	11	0.000/0.000
3–12 mo	115	4	8	60	4.3	11	18	17	8.3	NA

Modified from Godderidge [Chapter 1, reference 2], with permission.

[a] The gonadal doses are calculated from the free in air exposure without scatter and conversion factors yielded from experimental data based on phantoms of varying sizes. No experimental data are available for some age ranges; therefore, some gonadal doses are not available.

NA, not available.

Following is a listing of the equipment used to collect the data that resulted in the dose calculations in the above table.

I. Generator: three-phase, midfrequency, 80 kilowatts
II. Table
   A. Tabletop to image receptor distance (PID) = 8 cm
   B. Tabletop equivalence: 0.75 mm aluminum (Al) @ 100 kVp
   C. Automatic exposure control pickup attenuation = 0.3 mm Al @ 100 kVp
   D. Grid ratio = 8:1; 103 lines/in.; focused 34–44 in.
III. X-ray tube assembly
   A. 2.7 mm equivalent total filtration

    B. Standard source to image receptor distances (SID)
       1. Routine table bucky exams = 107 cm
       2. Routine tabletop exams = 107 cm
       3. Vertical wall bucky or cassette holders = 183 cm
       4. Sinus exams = 115 cm
    C. Half value layer at 80 kVp = 2.97 mm Al
    D. Radiation output = 13.5 mR/mAs @ 70 kVp @ 61 cm from focus
 IV. Wall bucky
    A. Grid mounted on front rails to allow easy removal
    B. Wall bucky front to image receptor distance = 5 cm
    C. Wall bucky front equivalence: 0.4 mm Al @ 100 kVp
    D. Automatic exposure control pickup equivalence: 0.3 mm Al @ 100 kVp
    E. Removable grids
       1. Grid Number 1: Used for upright abdomens
          Grid Ratio 8:1; 103 lines/in.; 34–44 in. focus
       2. Grid Number 2: Used for chest exams
          Grid Ratio 8:1; 103 lines/in.; 48–72 in. focus
  V. Wall cassette holder for 36″ films (scoliosis exams)
    A. Grid plane to image receptor distance = 4 cm
    B. Grid ratio = 10:1; 103 lines/in.; 60–72 in. focus
 VI. Upright cassette holder mounted on tabletop (upright chests of 1- to 5-year-old children)
    A. Holder has no front or grid
    B. Patient exit plane to image receptor distance = 2 cm
VII. Image receptor and processing
    A. Nominal 400 speed image receptor (routine work)
       Cassette front equivalence: 1.7 mm Al @ 100 kVp
    B. Nominal 100 speed image receptor (extremities)
       Cassette front equivalence: 1.7 mm Al @ 100 kVp
    C. Nominal 1100 speed image receptor (36 in. film exams)
    D. Processing parameters
       Film manufacturer's chemistry and processing parameters are used.

APPENDIX 4
Radiographic Technique Guidelines

Examination	SID[a] (in.)	Grid	mAs-kVp, by age[b]				
			6 Months	2 Years	6 Years	12 Years	15 Years
AP supine chest	42	No	0.8–65	*	*	*	*
Lateral supine chest	42	No	0.8–75	*	*	*	*
Upright PA chest	72	No	*	2.1–72	2.4–80	2.6–80	1–120**
Upright lateral chest	72	No	*	2.1–90	2.4–95	2.6–100	1–120**
AP abdomen	42	Yes	2.8–70	4–70	4–75	6.5–80	6.5–85
AP pelvis	42	Yes	2–70	2.6–75	3.6–80	5–80	6.5–85
AP lumbar spine	42	Yes	2.8–70	4–70	4–75	6.5–80	6.5–85
Lateral lumbar spine	42	Yes	4–75	4.2–75	10–85	16–85	25–90
AP thoracic spine	42	Yes	2–70	2.6–75	3–75	5–80	6.5–85
Lateral thoracic spine	42	Yes	2–80	3.2–85	5–85	60 kVp*** 20 mA 6000 ms	65 kVp*** 20 mA 6000 ms
AP cervical spine	42	Yes	2.5–68	2.5–72	2.5–75	3–80	3.5–84
Lateral cervical spine	72	No	2.5–76	2.5–80	3–80	4–85	5–85
Skull, AP or PA	42	Yes	4.8–70	6–70	7–75	12–75	15–75
Skull, lateral	42	Yes	4.8–65	6–65	7–70	12–70	15–70
Lateral airway	72	No	2.8–70	4–70	5–75	6.5–80	6.5–85
AP ankle	42	No	0.8–60	0.8–64	0.8–68	0.7–80	0.8–80
AP elbow	42	No	0.5–64	0.5–66	0.5–70	0.7–74	0.7–76
PA hand	42	No	0.5–56	0.5–58	0.6–58	0.6–60	0.6–62
AP femur	42	No	0.5–64	0.5–70	0.6–75	0.8–78	0.9–80
AP knee	42	No	0.5–64	0.5–68	0.6–72	0.8–75	0.9–75
AP upper GI	42	Yes	1.2–100	1.6–100	2.5–100	3.2–100	3.2–100
AP BE	42	Yes	1.2–100	1.6–100	2.5–100	3.2–100	5–100

[a] Studies are done at 42 in. because of custom-made tubes with 0.3 + 0.6 mm focal spot to assure adequate film coverage.

[b] Generator: 150 kVp, 300 mA, three-phase. Bucky grid: 8:1. Film/screen: Kodak Pediatric Insight with carbon front cassette (360 relative speed). Detail Pediatric Insight (240 relative speed) used on all extremities. mAs, milliampere-second; kVp, kilovolt peak; mA, milliampere; ms, millisecond; AP, anteroposterior; BE, barium enema; GI, gastrointestinal tract; PA, posteroanterior; SID, source image distance.

* Children under 1 year usually are radiographed supine; over 1 year, upright.

** Done with grid technique at age 15 and older.

*** Done with breathing technique.

APPENDIX 5

Commonly Used Pediatric Contrast Media

Generic name	% in Solution	Trade name	Iodine (mg/ml)	Osmolality (mOsm/l)	Mfr.[a]	Use[b]
Diatrizoate meglumine	18	Dilute Cystografin	85	386	B	VCUG
Iothalamate meglumine	17.2	Cysto-Conray II	81	400	M	VCUG, GI, Antegrade Pyelogram
Diatrizoate Sodium 8% Meglumine 52%	60	Renografin 60	292.5	1420	B	EU, CT
Diatrizoate meglumine	60	Reno-M 60	282	1500	B	EU, CT
Diatrizoate sodium	50	Hypaque 50%	300	1550	N	EU, CT
Diatrizoate meglumine	60	Hypaque 60%	282	1415	N	EU, CT
Diatrizoate Sodium 10% Meglumine 66%	76	Renografin 76	370	1940	B	AG
Diatrizoate Sodium 10% Meglumine 66%	76	Hypaque 76	370	2016	N	AG
Diatrizoate Sodium 25% Meglumine 50%	75	Hypaque M, 75%	385	2108	N	AG
Iothalamate sodium	66.8	Conray 400	400	2300	M	AG
Ioversol	74	Optiray 350	350	792	M	AG
	68	Optiray 320	320	702	M	AG, EU, CT
	51	Optiray 240	240	502	M	AG, DSA
	34	Optiray 160	160	355	M	DSA, GI, Bronch
Iopamidol	76	Isovue 370	370	796	B	AG
	61	Isovue 300	300	616	B	EU, CT, AG
	41	Isovue 200	200	413	B	DSA, CT
	41	Isovue M 200	200	413	B	M
	26	Isovue 128	128	290	B	DSA, GI, Bronch
Ioxaglate Sodium 19.6% Meglumine 39.3%	59	Hexabrix	320	600	M	AG, EU, CT
Iohexol	75.5	Omnipaque	350	862	N	AG
	64.7	Omnipaque	300	709	N	EU, CT, AG
	51.8	Omnipaque	240	504	N	M, DSA, CT
	38.8	Omnipaque	180	411	N	M, DSA, CT, GI, Bronch

[a] B, Bracco Diagnostics, Inc., Princeton, NJ (previously Squibb); M, Mallinckrodt, Inc., St. Louis, MO; N, NYCOMED, Inc., New York, NY (previously Winthrop Pharmaceuticals).

[b] VCUG, voiding cystourethrography; EU, excretory urogram (intravenous urogram); CT, computed tomography; AG, conventional angiography; DSA, digital subtraction angiography; M, myelography; GI, gastrointestinal tract; Bronch, bronchogram.

Modified from Fischer HW. Catalog of intravascular contrast media. *Radiology* 1986;159:561–563.

APPENDIX 6

Sedation Formulary

Age	Medication	Recommended dosage	Route of administration	Additional instructions	Precautions/ contraindications
<12 mo	Chloral hydrate[a]	50–100 mg/kg	PO, Rectal	May repeat every 30 minutes to *maximum of 100 mg/kg*	Alternative sedation should be considered in patients who have impaired liver function, since proper metabolic degradation of chloral hydrate may not occur and sedation may be prolonged. Use caution with *any* sedation including chloral hydrate for patients with upper respiratory obstruction and patients with cyanotic or decompensated cardiac disease.
>12 mo	Pentobarbital (Nembutal)	2–3 mg/kg	IV	If necessary to give additional IV sedation, a repeat bolus of 2–3 mg/kg may be given after 30–60 seconds. *Maximum of 6 mg/kg*	Patients on barbiturate therapy for seizures may be refractory to the indicated doses of pentobarbital.
>12 mo	Fentanyl citrate[b]	1 μg/kg	IV	May be used in conjunction with pentobarbital but only when additional minimal sedation and pain control is desired. Titrate 1 μg/kg every 5 minutes to a *maximum of 3 μg/kg*	In children with impaired respiratory function, unstable or cyanotic cardiac disease, or evidence of increased intracranial pressure, alternative methods of sedation should be used. Impaired respiratory function specifically includes former premature infants at less than 60 weeks estimated gestational age with or without a history of apnea.
>12 mo	Midazolam (Versed)[c]	0.05 mg/kg	IV	Administer via slow IV push over 2–3 minutes to avoid respiratory depression. Titrate as needed to a *maximum dose of 0.15 mg/kg. Maximum total dose of 5 mg.*	The combination of midazolam with any narcotic causes greater respiratory depresssion and cardiac depression than either drug used alone. This technique is designed for conscious sedation. The nurse monitoring the patient should be in contact with him or her and may need to prompt the patient to breathe deeply.

[a] In children older than 12 months who have low body weight due to failure to thrive or malnutrition, oral chloral hydrate may also be effective.

[b] Fentanyl citrate is used to relieve pain and may be combined with midazolam or pentobarbital for interventional procedures.

[c] Midazolam is mainly used in interventional cases.

mo, month; mg, milligram; kg, kilogram; μ, microgram; PO, per oral; IV, intravenous.

APPENDIX 7

Oral Contrast Dosage for Computed Tomography

A. *Preparation of Contrast Solution*

Use either a dilute (1–2%) barium solution or a water-soluble, iodine-based contrast agent. 10 cm^3 of 37% Gastrografin can be mixed into 8 oz (240 ml) of any liquid *except* milk or apple juice. (This dilutes 37% Gastrografin to 1.5%)

B. *Oral Contrast Regimen*

Age	Amount given 60 min before study (oz)	Amount given 15 min before study (oz)
<1 month	2–3	1–1.5
1 month–1 year	4–8	2–4
1–5 years	8–12	4–6
6–12 years	12–16	6–8
13–15 years	16–20	8–10
>15 years	20	11

For children who have difficulty tolerating large amounts of contrast, the time from administration of oral contrast to the CT examination can be increased to 4 hours or overnight, particularly if the patient is an outpatient to be scanned the following day. Note that 1 ounce (oz) is 30 ml.

APPENDIX 8
Computed Tomography Protocols

The following guidelines are designed for general screening. Many examinations must be tailored to the particular clinical indications.

Brain

1. Patient supine with head placed in foam head holder on the table.
2. Tilt chin down 15° or adjust gantry angle to achieve scan plane parallel to a line drawn between the orbital roof and the external auditory meatus.
3. Field-of-view (FOV) 20–25 cm.
4. 7–10 mm contiguous axial sections from skull base to vertex.
5. 5-mm contiguous axial sections in neonates.
6. 5-mm contiguous axial sections through posterior fossa if indicated.
7. If intravenous (IV) contrast is necessary, then administer 2 ml/kg of 300–320 mg/ml nonionic contrast medium (maximum dose of 100 ml). Begin scan immediately after completion of injection.
8. Use "standard" algorithm for image reconstruction.

Sinus, orbits, facial bones

A. Direct coronal scan (contraindicated in presence of cervical spine, neck, or airway abnormality)
   1. Position patient supine or prone in the coronal head holder with a 15° angle sponge under the shoulders and encourage the patient to achieve a maximal but comfortable degree of extension.
   2. From the lateral scout view, angle gantry to achieve a scan plane perpendicular to the hard palate.
   3. 3- to 5-mm contiguous sections from the posterior wall of the sphenoid sinus to nasal bones.
   4. FOV depends on patient size (usually 20 cm).
   5. Use "bone" algorithm for image reconstruction.
B. Axial scan
   1. Position the patient supine in foam head holder on the table with a 15° angle sponge under the shoulders.
   2. From the lateral scout view, angle gantry to achieve a scan plane parallel to the hard palate.
   3. 3- to 5-mm contiguous sections from the hard palate through the frontal sinus.
   4. FOV depends on patient size (usually 20 cm).
   5. Use "bone" algorithm for image reconstruction.

Temporal bone

A. Direct coronal scan (contraindicated in presence of cervical spine, neck, or airway abnormality)
   1. Position patient supine or prone in the coronal head holder with a 15° angle sponge under the shoulders and encourage the patient to achieve a maximal but comfortable degree of extension.

2. From the lateral scout view, angle gantry to achieve a scan plane perpendicular to the hard palate.
   3. 1- to 3-mm contiguous sections through the petromastoid portions of the temporal bones.
   4. FOV depends on patient's size (usually 20 cm).
   5. Use "bone" algorithm for image reconstruction.
B. Axial scan
   1. Position the patient supine in foam head holder on the table with a 15° angle sponge under the shoulders.
   2. From the lateral scout view, angle gantry to achieve a scan plane parallel to the hard palate.
   3. 1- to 3-mm contiguous sections through the petromastoid portion of the temporal bone.
   4. FOV depends on patient's size (usually 20 cm).
   5. Use "bone" algorithm for image reconstruction.

For choanal atresia

1. Position the patient supine with the chin tilted upward about 15° and the head in a foam head holder on the table.
2. From the lateral scout view, angle gantry to achieve a scan plane parallel to the nasal passage.
3. 1- to 3-mm contiguous sections through the nasopharynx.
4. Use FOV of 15 cm.
5. Use "standard" and "bone" algorithms for image reconstruction.

Neck

1. Position the patient's head flat on the table with patient's arms at his or her side for IV accessibility.
2. From the lateral scout view, 5 mm contiguous axial sections from the medial ends of the clavicles to the skull base.
3. Administer 2 ml/kg of 300–320 mg/ml nonionic contrast medium (maximum dose 100 ml). For incremetal CT systems, initiate scan when 50% of the contrast has been injected. For helical CT systems, initiate scan immediately after the contrast has been administered.
4. For incremental CT systems, use minimum interscan delay ("dynamic" mode) and scan during quiet respiration. For helical CT systems, scan with a pitch of 1 and a section thickness of 5 mm.
5. Use "standard" algorithm for image reconstruction.

Cervical spine

1. Position the patient flat on the table. Do not use sponges if patient is in a cervical collar. Remove all high-density external objects when possible. Patient's arms are at his or her side with head rotated as little as possible.
2. For screening, use 3- to 5-mm axial sections over the region of interest. Use 1-mm sections for sagittal or coronal reformatting and 3-D reconstructions.
3. Use a FOV of 15 cm.

4. Use both "bone" algorithm and "standard" algorithm for image reconstruction.

Thoracic spine

1. Position the patient as parallel to the long axis of the table as possible. Use a bolster under the knees to help relax the patient's back. The arms are raised over the head. Remove all high-density external objects if possible.
2. For screening, use 3- to 5-mm axial sections over the region of interest. Use 1-mm sections for sagittal or coronal reformatting and 3-D reconstructions.
3. Use a FOV of 15 cm.
4. Use both "bone" algorithm and "standard" algorithm for image reconstruction.

Lumbar spine

1. Position the patient as parallel to the long axis of the table as possible. Use a bolster under the knees to help relax the patient's back and flatten the lumbar spine. The arms are raised over the head. Remove all high density external objects if possible.
2. From the lateral scout view, use 3- to 5-mm axial sections over the region of interest. It is sometimes better to angle the section plane to be parallel to the disk spaces.
3. Use a FOV of 15 cm.
4. Use both "bone" algorithm and "standard" algorithm for image reconstruction.

Chest

A. For conventional (incremental) CT systems.
   1. Patient supine on CT table with arms raised above head.
   2. From the anterposterior (AP) scout view, 10-mm contiguous transaxial sections from thoracic inlet to just below the diaphragm to include all of each lung base. 5-mm contiguous sections used in neonates. If necessary, rescan with 1- to 5-mm sections for higher spatial resolution for evaluation of the parenchyma or for clarification of suspicious findings on the initial scan.
   3. For evaluation of mediastinum and hila, IV contrast should be used. 2 ml/kg of 300–320 mg/ml of nonionic contrast with rapid hand injection technique. Start scan after 75% of the contrast has been administered.
   4. Suspended inspiration for acquisition of each section in the cooperative older child or adolescent. Scan during quiet respiration in the young or sedated child.
   5. Use "standard" algorithm for reconstruction of mediastinum and hila. Use a high-contrast algorithm such as "bone" or "lung" algorithm for reconstruction of lung parenchyma.
B. For helical CT systems.
   1. Patient supine on CT table with arms raised above head.
   2. From AP scout view, scan from the thoracic inlet to the lung bases with the following parameters:

Age	Pitch	Section thickness
Newborn–2 years	1.5	5 mm
>2 years	1.5	8 mm

You may choose to reconstruct with smaller interval than the section thickness, but with overlap no more than 50% of the original section thickness.
   3. For evaluation of mediastinum and hila, IV contrast should be used. 1.5 ml/kg of 300–320 mg/ml of nonionic contrast with a rapid hand injection technique. Start scan 10–15 seconds after the end of the injection.
   4. Breath-hold technique in the cooperative adolescent after practice trials. Scan through quiet respiration in the young or sedated child.

Abdomen

A. For conventional (incremental) CT systems.
   1. Oral contrast preparation as indicated in Appendix 7 (oral contrast not necessary in trauma cases).
   2. Patient supine on CT table with arms raised above head.
   3. From the AP scout view of the abdomen and pelvis, scan from the domes of the diaphragms to the pubic symphysis with 10-mm contiguous sections. Thinner collimation used to evaluate suspicious areas further for improved spatial resolution and to decrease partial volume artifact. Use 5-mm contiguous sections in neonates.
   4. IV contrast should be used. 2 ml/kg of 300–320 mg/ml of nonionic contrast with a rapid hand injection technique. Start scan after 75% of the contrast has been administered. If pathology is suspected in the pelvis, one third of the total dose of contrast can be given as a rapid bolus as the scan plane reaches the level of the iliac crest.
   5. Scan during quiet respiration with minimum interscan delay through the abdomen.
   6. Use "standard" algorithm for reconstruction.
B. For helical CT systems.
   1. Oral contrast preparation as indicated in Appendix 7 (oral contrast not necessary in trauma cases).
   2. Patient supine on CT table with arms raised above the head.
   3. From the AP scout view of the abdomen and pelvis, scan from the domes of the diaphragms to the pubic symphysis with the following parameters:

Age	Pitch	Section thickness
Newborn–2 years	1.5	5 mm
>2 years	1.5	10 mm

You may choose to reconstruct with smaller interval than section thickness, but with overlap no more than 50% of the original section thickness.
   4. IV contrast should be used (1.5 ml/kg of 300–320 mg/ml of nonionic contrast). Start scan 20–30 seconds after the end of the injection.
   5. Scan during quiet respiration with minimum interscan delay through the abdomen and pelvis. If the entire volume cannot be scanned in one sequence, use consecutive sequences from the domes of the diaphragms to iliac crests, then without delay, from the iliac crest to the pubic symphysis.
   6. Use "standard" algorithm for reconstruction.

APPENDIX 9
MR Neuroimaging Protocols

These protocols are based on experience with the General Electric Signa 1.5T unit (General Electric, Milwaukee, WI) at the 4.8 hardware/software configuration. Choices of sequences and coils are limited by the available hardware and software. The protocols are designed for general use. Each examination may be further tailored to fit the particular clinical indication.

Brain

Use standard head coil; may use extremity coil for small infants.

Basic imaging sequences:

Sequence	TR	TE	TI	α	Nex	ϕ	FOV	Thick	Skip
CSE T1 Sag	600	20	—	—	2	128	24	5	1.0 or 2.5
FSE PD Ax	2000	17	—	—	1	192	24	5	2.5
FSE T2 Ax	3200	85	—	—	1	192	24	5	2.5

Other sequences, if appropriate:

Sequence	TR	TE	TI	α	Nex	ϕ	FOV	Thick	Skip
FSE T2 Cor[a]	3200	85	—	—	1	192	24	5	2.5
CSE T1 Cor/Sag/Ax (Gd)[b]	600	20	—	—	2	128–192	24	5	1.0–2.5
SPGR Ax (T1-GE)[c]	24	5	—	50	2	128	20	5	1
MPGR Ax (PD-GE)[d]	500	20	—	20	2	128	20	5	1
MPGR Ax (T2*-GE)[e]	500	40	—	15	2	128	20	5	1
CSE T1 Ax (Hi Res)[f]	600	20	—	—	2	192	24	3	1

Spine

Use surface coil

Basic imaging sequences:

Sequence	TR	TE	TI	α	Nex	ϕ	FOV	Thick	Skip
CSE T1 Sag[g]	400	17	—	—	1	128	32	5	1
FSE PD/T2 Sag	2500	16, 96	—	—	2	192	24	4	1
CSE T1 Ax	600	15	—	—	2	192	12–18	5	1

Other sequences, if appropriate:

Sequence	TR	TE	TI	α	Nex	ϕ	FOV	Thick	Skip
CSE T1 Sag (Gd)[h]	400	15	—	—	2	192	24	4	1
CSE T1 Cor (Gd)[h]	400	15	—	—	2	192	24	4	1
CSE T1 Ax (Gd)[h]	600	15	—	—	2	192	12–18	5	1
FMPIR Sag[i]	4000	51	150	—	1	256	24	4	1
MPGR Ax (T2*-GE)[j]	500	20	—	20	4	128	16	5	1

For the infant spine (<1 year), the following sequences are often appropriate:

Sequence	TR	TE	TI	α	NEX	ϕ	FOV	Thick	Skip
CSE T1 Sag[g]	400	17	—	—	1	128	24	4	1
FSE PD/T2 Sag	2500	16, 96	—	—	2	192	21	4	1
CSE T1 Ax	600	15	—	—	2	192	12–16	5	1
CSE T1 (Gd)[h]	400	15	—	—	2	192	21	3	0
CSE T1 Sag/Cor (±Gd)[h]	400	15	—	—	2	192	21	3	0
CSE T1 Ax (±Gd)[h]	600	15	—	—	2	192	12–16	5	1

[a] For the evaluation of a seizure disorder; angled perpendicular to the hippocampus.

[b] For the evaluation of intracranial masses or infection.

[c] For the evaluation of vascular flow.

[d] For the evaluation of CSF flow.

[e] For the detection of mineralization and hemorrhage.

[f] For the use with and without fat suppression and gadolinium for the evaluation of the orbits, the sellar region, and the internal auditory canals and cerebellopontine angles.

[g] Localizer sequence to guide the remaining sequences.

[h] May be used for the evaluation of spinal masses; for the evaluation of metastatic seeding, the entire neural axis is imaged from the cranial vertex to the sacral tip.

[i] May be used for the detection of spinal cord pathology not detected by gadolinium-enhanced CSE T1 images; also used for the detection of bone marrow abnormalities.

[j] For the "myelogram effect."

TR, repetition time in milliseconds; TE, echo time in milliseconds; TI, inversion time in milliseconds; α, flip angle in degrees; Nex, number of excitations or signal averages; ϕ, number of phase-encoding steps; FOV, field of view in centimeters; Thick, thickness of section in millimeters; Skip, distance between consecutive sections in millimeters; CSE, conventional spin-echo; FSE, fast spin-echo; SPGR, spoiled gradient-recalled; MPGR, multiplanar gradient-recalled; FMPIR, fast multiplanar inversion recovery; Sag, sagittal; Cor, coronal; Ax, axial; ±, with or without; Gd, gadolinium; T1-GE, gradient-recalled echo sequence with T1-type contrast; PD-GE, gradient-recalled echo sequence with proton density–type contrast; T2*-GE, gradient-recalled echo sequence with T2*-type contrast.

APPENDIX 10
MR Body Imaging Protocols

These protocols are based on experience with the General Electric Signa 1.5T unit (General Electric, Milwaukee, WI) at the 4.8 hardware/software configuration. Choices of sequences and coils are limited by the available hardware and software. The protocols are designed for general use. Each examination may be further tailored to fit the particular clinical indication.

Abdomen, Pelvis

Coil selection:

<18 months	head coil
18 months–6 years	flat surface coil (e.g. 5 × 11 in.)
older patients	body coil

Superior and inferior presaturation on all CSE and FSE sequences.
Gradient moment nulling (flow compensation) on all gradient-recalled echo sequences.
Respiratory-ordered phase encoding (respiratory compensation) on all sequences.

For general imaging:

Sequence	TR	TE	TI	α	Nex	ϕ	FOV	Thick	Skip
FMPIR Sag[a]	4000	51	150	—	2	128–192	24–40	5	1
CSE T1 Cor	600	min	—	—	2	192	24–36	5	1
FSE T2 Ax fat sat	4000	96	—	—	2	256	20–32	5–8	1–2
GRASS Ax[b]	33	14	—	30	2	192	20–32	6	0
CSE T1 Cor (Gd)[c]	600	min	—	—	2–4	192	24–36	5–8	1–2
FMPIR Cor[c]	4000	51	150	—	2	128–192	24–40	5–8	1–2

For vascular malformations and hemangiomas:

Sequence	TR	TE	TI	α	Nex	ϕ	FOV	Thick	Skip
GRASS Ax	33	14	—	30	2	192	24–40	10	0
CSE T1 Cor	600	min	—	—	2	192	24–36	5–8	1–2
FSE T2 Ax fat sat	4000	96	—	—	2	256	20–32	5–8	1–2
CSE T1 Cor/Ax (Gd)[d]	600	min	—	—	2–4	192	24–36	5–8	1–2
MRA 2D TOF[e]	45	min	—	60	2	192	24–36	2.9	0

Heart, Vascular Rings

Coil selection:

| Infants, small toddlers | head coil |
| older children | body coil |

Electrocardiographic gating for all CSE sequences.

Sequence	TR	TE	TI	α	Nex	ϕ	FOV	Thick	Skip
FGRE Sag/Cor/Ax[f]	min	min	—	30	1	128	28–30	5–10	0
CSE T1 Sag	RR	20	—	—	2	192	20–32	5	1
CSE T1 Ax[f]	RR	20	—	—	2	192	20–32	8	2
CSE T1 Ax[g]	RR	20	—	—	2	192	20–32	3–5	0–1
CSE T1 Cor[g]	RR	20	—	—	2	192	20–32	3–5	0–1
CSE T1 Obl[h]	RR	20	—	—	2	192	20–32	3–5	1
Cine GRASS	25	min	—	20	2	128	32–40	6–10	0
Cine 2D-PC[i]	25	min	—	20	4	128	32–40	6–10	0

Musculoskeletal (must have radiographs before MR examination)

For hips:

	Patient position	Coil
one hip	supine	shoulder coil
both hips	prone	flat surface coil (<5 years old)
	supine	body coil (>5 years old)

Sequence	TR	TE	TI	α	Nex	ϕ	FOV	Thick	Skip
MPGR Ax	250	13	—	20	2	192	see *j*	5	0
CSE T1 Cor	200	11	—	—	2	192	see *j*	4	0[k]
MPGR Cor	200	min	—	20	4	192	see *j*	4	0
FSE T2 Cor	3200	96	—	—	2–4	256–512	see *j*	3	1
FSE T2 Sag[l]	3200	96	—	—	2–4	256–512	see *j*	3	1

For knees:

Use extremity surface coil; if knee is in cast, use head coil or flexible surface coil.

Sequence	TR	TE	TI	α	Nex	ϕ	FOV	Thick	Skip
MPGR Ax	300	13	—	20	2	192	20	4	0
CSE T1 Cor	300	min	—	—	2	192	16	4	0[m]
CSE PD/T2 Sag	2000	min, 80	—	—	2	192	16	3	1
FSE T2 Sag or Cor (fat sat)[n]	3600	85	—	—	2	192	16	3	1

For screening of congenital and developmental abnormalities, and cartilaginous abnormalities of the extremities:

Sequence	TR	TE	TI	α	Nex	ϕ	FOV	Thick	Skip
MPGR Ax	300	13	—	20	2	192	16	5	0
CSE T1 Cor	300	13	—	—	2	192	16	4	0[o]
MPGR Cor	300	13	—	20	2	192	16	4	0[o]
CSE PD/T2 Sag (fat sat)	2000	min, 80	—	—	1	192	16	3	1

For evaluation of tumor or osteomyelitis or other bone marrow abnormality:

Sequence	TR	TE	TI	α	Nex	φ	FOV	Thick	Skip
CSE T1 Cor[p]	600	16	—	—	1	192	36–40	5	1.5
CSE T1 Sag	600	min	—	—	1	128	16–24	5	1
FMPIR Cor or Sag	4000	51	150	—	2	256	18–24	5	1
FSE PD Ax (fat sat)	4000	36	—	—	2	256	18	6	2
CSE T1 Sag[q]	600	min	—	—	1	192	16–24	5	1
GRASS Ax[r]	34	13	—	45	2	128	16	5	0

[a] Use as localizer to start an examination.

[b] As needed for identification of vessels.

[c] Optional; especially useful in evaluation of paraspinal, adrenal, and renal masses.

[d] Consider giving Gd before T2 sequence to allow time for Gd to diffuse into a large venous malformation.

[e] Optional.

[f] Use as a localizer to start an examination.

[g] Thin sections to evaluate for small pulmonary arteries and aorto-pulmonary collaterals as seen in cases of tetralogy of Fallot and pulmonary atresia.

[h] For the evaluation of the aortic arch, usually for coarctation.

[i] 16–24 phases in one cardiac cycle; velocity-encoding value of 150 to 250 cm/sec typically used.

[j] 24–32 cm for evaluation of both hips; 18 cm for one hip.

[k] Interleaved.

[l] Sagittal plane is optional; useful to evaluate degree of anterior coverage.

[m] Interleaved sections.

[n] Optional; useful for detection of marrow abnormalities.

[o] Interleaved sections.

[p] Done in body coil to evaluate the entire bone for skip lesions.

[q] Can be done with or without fat suppression; pre- and post-Gd administration.

[r] To evaluate for patency of vessels, usually during a preoperative evaluation.

TR, repetition time in milliseconds; TE, echo time in milliseconds; TI, inversion time in milliseconds; α, flip angle in degrees; ϕ, number of phase-encoding steps; Nex, number of signal averages; FOV, field-of-view in centimeters; Thick, thickness of each section in millimeters; Skip, distance between consecutive sections in millimeters; CSE, conventional spin-echo; FSE, fast spin-echo; SPGR, spoiled gradient-recalled; MPGR, multiplanar gradient-recalled; GRASS, gradient-recalled acquisition in the steady-state; FMPIR, fast multiplanar inversion recovery; FGRE, fast gradient-recalled echo; 2D-PC, two-dimensional phase contrast; cm/sec, centimeter per second; Sag, sagittal; Cor, coronal; Ax, axial; Obl, oblique; Gd, gadolinium; min, minimum time allowed for TE and TR; RR, duration of one cardiac cycle; MRA, magnetic resonance angiography.

Subject Index

A *t* following a page number indicates tabular material and an *f* following a page number indicates an figure.

1195